ABNORMAL LABORATORY FINDINGS (continued)

Osteolysis
  Osteomyelitis
  Osteoporosis
Granulomatous disease
Acidosis
Spurious
  Hyperalbuminemia

Decreased
Eclampsia
Renal secondary
  hyperparathyroidism
Hypoalbuminemia
Hypomagnesemia
Hypoparathyroidism
Pancreatitis
Rhabdomyolysis
Dietary
  Hypovitaminosis D
  Excess dietary phosphorus
C-cell thyroid tumors
Malabsorption
Hypercalcitoninism
  Iatrogenic
Parathyroidectomy
Phosphate enemas
Intravenous phosphate
  administration
Alkalosis
Ethylene glycol
Spurious
  EDTA contamination
  Oxalate contamination

Chloride
  Increased
Dehydration
Metabolic acidosis
Bromide therapy

  Decreased
Gastric vomiting
Metabolic alkalosis

Cholesterol
  Increased
Cholestasis
Endocrine disease
  Hypothyroidism
  Hyperadrenocorticoidism
  Diabetes mellitus
Postprandial
Dietary
Nephrotic syndrome
Primary hyperlipidemia
  Idiopathic hypercholesterolemia
  Primary hyperchylomicronemia
    (cats)
  Lipoproteinlipase deficiency (cats)

  Decreased
Protein-losing enteropathy
Portosystemic shunt
Malassimilation
  Malabsorption
  Maldigestion
  Lymphangiectasia
  Starvation
Liver failure
Hypoadrenocorticism

Cholinesterase
  Decreased
Organophosphates
Carbamates

Cobalamin (B$_{12}$)
  Decreased
Bacterial overgrowth

Creatinine
  Increased
Azotemia
  Prerenal
  Renal
  Postrenal

  Decreased
Decrease muscle mass

Creatine kinase (CK)
  Increased
Muscle inflammation
  Immune mediated
  Eosinophilic myositis
  Masticatory muscle myositis
  Endocarditis
  Infectious
    Toxoplasmosis
    Neosporum caninum
Nutritional
  Hypokalemia (polymyopathy)
  Taurine deficiency
Trauma
  Exertional myositis
  Surgical
  Intramuscular injections
  Hypothermia
  Pyrexia
  Prolonged recumbency
  Post-infarct ischemia
    Cardiomyopathy
    Disseminated intravascular
      coagulation

Fibrinogen
  Increased
Inflammation
Pregnancy

  Decreased
Liver failure
Coagulopathies
Primary hypofibrinogenemia

Folate
  Increased
Bacterial overgrowth

Fructosamine
  Increased
Diabetes mellitus

  Decreased
Spurious
Hypoproteinemia
Anemia (false)

Gamma glutamyltransferase (GGT)
  Increased
Cholestasis
  Intrahepatic
  Extrahepatic
Drugs (canine)
  Glucocorticoids
  Anticonvulsants
    Primadone
    Phenobarbital

  Decreased
Spurious
Hemolysis

Globulin
  Increased
Dehydration (albumin and total
  protein)

Inflammation
Gammopathy
  Monoclonal
    Plasma cell myeloma
    Ehrlichia
    Dirofilariasis
  Polyclonal
    Chronic inflammatory disease
    Feline infectious peritonitis
    Dental disease
    Dermatitis
    Inflammatory bowel disease
    Parasitic diseases
    Immune-mediated diseases
    Neoplasia

  Decreased
Neonatal
Immunodeficiency
  Congenital
  Acquired
Blood loss
Protein-losing enteropathy

Glucose
  Increased
Endocrine
  Acromegaly
  Diabetes mellitus
  Hyperadrenocorticism
Pancreatitis
Stress (cats)
Drugs
  Intravenous glucose administration
  Glucocorticoids
  Xylazine
  Progestagens (Ovaban and others)

  Decreased
Liver failure
Endocrine
  Hypoadrenocorticism
  Hypopituitarism
Starvation
Neoplasia
Hyperinsulinism
  Iatrogenic
  Insulinoma
Idiopathic
  Puppies
  Toy breed dogs
Septicemia
Polycythemia
Leukemia
Glycogen storage disease
Artifact
  Delayed serum separation

Iron
  Increased
Hemolysis

  Decreased
Chronic blood loss
Dietary deficiency

Lactate dehydrogenase (LDH)
  Increased
Organ/tissue damage
Hemolysis
  In vivo
  In vitro
Hepatocytes
Muscle
Kidney
Spurious
  Failure to separate serum from
    RBCs

Lipase
  Increased
Pancreatic disease
  Pancreatitis
  Necrosis
  Neoplasia
Enteritis
Renal disease
Glucocorticoids

Magnesium
  Decreased
Dietary
Diabetic Ketacidosis
Potential causes:
  gastrointestinal
    malabsorption
    chronic diarrhea
  renal
    glomerular disease
    tubular disease
  drugs
    diuretics
    Amphotericin B
  others

Phosphorus
  Increased
Reduced GFR
  Renal
    Acute
    Chronic
  Postrenal
Hemolysis
Hyperthyroidism
Neonates
Intoxication
  Hypervitaminosis D
  Jasmine ingestion
Dietary excess
Iatrogenic
  Phosphate enemas
  Intravenous phosphate
    administration
Osteolysis
Hypoparathyroidism
Spurious
  Delayed serum separation

  Decreased
Hyperparathyroidism
  Primary
  Nutritional secondary
Neoplasia
  PTH-like hormone
  C-cell thyroid tumors
Insulin therapy
Diabetic ketoacidosis
Dietary deficiency
Eclampsia
Hyperadrenocorticism

Potassium
  Increased
Renal failure
  Distal RTA
  Oliguric/anuric
Postrenal
  Obstruction
  Ruptured bladder
Spurious
  Breed idiosyncracy (Akitas)
  Leukemias
  Thrombocytosis
  Collection in potassium
    heparin
  Collection in potassium EDTA
Hypoadrenocorticism

58 Jaundice 210
Jan Rothuizen

59 Bleeding Disorders: Epistaxis
and Hemoptysis 213
Orla Mahony

60 Petechiae and Ecchymoses 218
Mary Beth Callan

61 Hyponatremia and Hypokalemia 222
Yonatan Peres

62 Hyperkalemia and Hypernatremia 227
Michael Schaer

63 Abnormalities of Magnesium, Calcium,
and Chloride 232
Lisa K. Kurosky

Section II
Dietary Considerations of Systemic Problems

64 Nutrition of Healthy Dogs and Cats in
Various Stages of Adult Life. 236
James G. Morris
Quinton R. Rogers

65 Neonatal and Pediatric Nutrition 241
Johnny D. Hoskins

66 Developmental Orthopedic Disease
of Dogs 245
Daniel C. Richardson
Steven C. Zicker

67 Adverse Reactions to Foods: Allergies
Versus Intolerance 251
Philip Roudebush
W. Grant Guilford

68 Nutritional Management of Gastrointestinal,
Hepatic, and Endocrine Diseases 258
Kathryn E. Michel

69 Dietary Modifications in Cardiac Disease 262
Stephen J. Ettinger

70 Dietary Considerations for
Urinary Diseases 269
Cathy A. Brown
Scott A. Brown
Joseph W. Bartges
Delmar R. Finco
Jeanne A. Barsanti

71 Enteral and Parenteral Nutritional Support 275
Stanley L. Marks

72 Hyperlipidemias 283
John E. Bauer

Section III
Therapeutic Considerations in Medicine

73 Principles of Drug Therapy 294
Dawn Merton Boothe

74 Antimicrobial Drugs 301
Mark G. Papich

75 Glucocorticoid Therapy 307
John M. MacDonald

76 Over-the-Counter Pharmaceuticals. 318
Etienne Côté

77 Adverse Drug Reactions 320
Jill Maddison

78 Fluid Therapy, Electrolytes,
and Acid-Base Control 325
Rebecca Kirby
Elke Rudloff

79 Blood Banking and Transfusion Medicine. 348
Ann E. Hohenhaus

80 Toxicology. 357
Steven S. Nicholson

81 Common Plant Toxicities 363
    Lynn Hovda

82 Acupuncture in Small Animal Practice 366
    Luc A.A. Janssens

83 Complementary/Alternative Cancer
    Therapy—Fact or Fiction? 374
    Gregory K. Ogilvie
    Narda G. Robinson

SECTION IV

INFECTIOUS DISEASE

84 Frequently Asked Questions
    About Zoonoses 382
    Michael G. Groves
    Kathleen S. Harrington
    Joseph Taboada

85 Bacterial Diseases 390
    Craig E. Greene

86 The Rickettsioses 400
    Edward B. Breitschwerdt

87 Protozoal and Miscellaneous Infections 408
    Michael R. Lappin

88 Canine Viral Diseases 418
    Johnny D. Hoskins

89 FeLV and Non-Neoplastic
    FeLV-related Disease 424
    Julie K. Levy

90 FIV and FIV-related Diseases 433
    Margaret C. Barr
    Tom R. Phillips

91 FIP-related Disease 438
    Rosalind Gaskell
    Susan Dawson

92 Other Feline Viral Diseases 444
    Alice M. Wolf

93 Systemic Mycoses 453
    Joseph Taboada

SECTION V

CANCER

94 Tumor Biology 478
    Cheryl London

95 Principles of Chemotherapy 484
    Antony S. Moore
    Angela E. Frimberger

96 Practical Radiation Therapy 489
    Alain Théon

97 Paraneoplastic Syndromes 498
    Gregory K. Ogilvie

98 Hematopoietic Tumors 507
    David M. Vail

99 Tumors of the Skin 523
    Susan A. Kraegel
    Bruce R. Madewell

100 Soft Tissue Sarcomas
    and Hemangiosarcomas 529
    Rodney L. Page
    Donald E. Thrall

101 Bone and Joint Tumors 535
    Rodney C. Straw

102 Tumors of the Urogenital System and
    Mammary Glands 541
    Deborah W. Knapp
    David J. Waters
    Bradley R. Schmidt

TEXTBOOK
OF
VETERINARY
INTERNAL
MEDICINE
DISEASES OF THE DOG AND CAT

TEXTBOOK
OF
VETERINARY
INTERNAL
MEDICINE

DISEASES OF THE DOG AND CAT

Fifth Edition   **VOLUME 2**

STEPHEN J. ETTINGER, D.V.M.
California Animal Hospital, Los Angeles, California

EDWARD C. FELDMAN, D.V.M.
University of California, Davis, California

W.B. SAUNDERS COMPANY
A Division of Harcourt Brace & Company
Philadelphia   London   Toronto   Montreal   Sydney   Tokyo

W.B. SAUNDERS COMPANY
A Division of Harcourt Brace & Company

The Curtis Center
Independence Square West
Philadelphia, Pennsylvania 19106

Library of Congress Cataloging-in-Publication Data

Textbook of veterinary internal medicine: diseases of the dog and cat / [edited by]
Stephen J. Ettinger, Edward C. Feldman.—5th ed.

p.   cm.

ISBN 0–7216–7256–6 (2 vol. set)

1. Dogs—Diseases.   2. Cats—Diseases.   3. Veterinary internal medicine.
I. Ettinger, Stephen J.   II. Feldman, Edward C.

SF991.T48 2000   636.7′0896—dc21   98–34212

Volume 1 ISBN 0–7216–7257–4
Volume 2 ISBN 0–7216–7258–2
Set ISBN 0–7216–7256–6

TEXTBOOK OF VETERINARY INTERNAL MEDICINE:
Diseases of the Dog and Cat

Printed in the United States of America.

Last digit is the print number: 9   8   7   6   5   4   3   2   1

CONTENTS

VOLUME 1

SECTION I
CLINICAL MANIFESTATIONS OF DISEASE

General

1 Clinical Genetics 2
Urs Giger

2 Hyperthermia and Hypothermia 6
James B. Miller

3 Weakness and Syncope 10
Stephen J. Ettinger

4 Acute Vision Loss 17
Susan A. McLaughlin
Holly L. Hamilton

5 Pain: Identification 20
Spencer A. Johnston

6 Pain: Management 23
Elizabeth M. Hardie

Skin and Subcutaneous

7 The Skin as a Sensor of Internal
Medical Disorders 26
Stephen D. White

8 Alopecia 29
Gail A. Kunkle

9 Pruritus 31
Peter J. Ihrke

10 Cutaneous and Subcutaneous Lumps,
Bumps, and Masses 36
D.N. Carlotti

11 Erosions and Ulcerations 39
Ian S. Mason

12 Pustules and Papules 43
Edmund J. Rosser, Jr.

13 Scaling and Crusting Dermatoses 47
Anthony A. Stannard
Andrea G. Cannon
Thierry Olivry

14 Diagnostic Cytology of Skin Lesions 51
George P. Reppas
Paul J. Canfield

15 Changes in Pigmentation 55
Zeineb Alhaidari

16 External Parasites: Identification
and Control 58
Karen L. Campbell

17 Subcutaneous Space Accumulations 62
David Feldman

18 Red Eye 66
Joan Dziezyc

Physique

19 Obesity 70
Karen J. Wolfsheimer

20 Cachexia 72
Deborah S. Greco

21 Failure to Grow 74
Sherri L. Ihle

22 Swollen Joints and Lameness 77
Michael L. Magne

Urogenital

23 Vaginal and Preputial Discharge 80
Hans-Klaus Dreier

24 Polyuria and Polydipsia 85
Susan Meric Taylor

25 Incontinence, Enuresis, Dysuria,
and Nocturia 89
George E. Lees

26 Urinary Obstruction and Functional
Urine Retention 93
India F. Lane

27 Discolored Urine 96
Joseph W. Bartges

28 Proteinuria 100
Donald R. Krawiec

Gastrointestinal-Abdominal

29 Anorexia 102
William E. Monroe

30 Polyphagia 104
Ellen N. Behrend

31 Ptyalism 107
Linda J. DeBowes

32 Gagging 111
Mark J. Kopit

33 Dysphagia and Regurgitation 114
Christine C. Jenkins

34 Vomiting 117
David C. Twedt

35 Diarrhea 121
Todd R. Tams

36 Melena and Hematochezia 126
W. Grant Guilford

37 Constipation, Tenesmus, Dyschezia, and
Fecal Incontinence 129
Brent Jones

38 Flatulence and Borborygmus 135
W. Grant Guilford

39 Abdominal Distention, Ascites,
and Peritonitis 137
Stephen A. Kruth

Neurologic

40 Shivering and Trembling 139
David Lipsitz
Anne E. Chauvet

41 Ataxia, Paresis, and Paralysis 142
Joane Parent

42 Altered States of Consciousness: Coma
and Stupor 144
Linda Shell

43 Seizures 148
Andrée D. Quesnel

44 Sleep Disorders 152
Joan C. Hendricks

45 Behavioral Disorders 156
Ilana R. Reisner
Katherine A. Houpt

Cardiothoracic

46 Coughing 158
Stephen J. Ettinger

47 Dyspnea and Tachypnea 166
Grant H. Turnwald

48 Abnormal Heart Sounds and
Heart Murmurs 170
Wendy A. Ware

49 Pulse Alterations 174
John-Karl Goodwin

50 Hypertension 179
Meryl P. Littman

51 Hypotension 183
Douglass K. Macintire

52 Pleural Effusion 186
Kenneth J. Drobatz

53 Cardiopulmonary Arrest and Resuscitation 189
Mary Anna Labato

54 Sneezing and Nasal Discharge 194
Brendan C. McKiernan

Hematologic-Chemical

55 Anemia 198
Kenita S. Rogers

56 Polycythemia 203
Andreas H. Hasler
Urs Giger

57 Cyanosis 206
Rebecca L. Stepien

SECTION VI

THE NERVOUS SYSTEM

103 Neurologic Manifestations of
Systemic Disease.......................... 548
Michael Podell

104 Diseases of the Brain 552
William R. Fenner

105 Multifocal Neurologic Disease................ 603
Rodney S. Bagley

106 Diseases of the Spinal Cord 608
Richard A. LeCouteur
Jacqueline L. Grandy

107 Neuro-Ophthalmology—Pupils
That Teach.................................. 657
B. Keith Collins

108 Peripheral Nerve Disorders 662
Karen Dyer Inzana

109 Disorders of the Skeletal Muscles.............. 684
Stéphane Blot

SECTION VII

THE CARDIOVASCULAR SYSTEM

110 Pathophysiology of Heart Failure and
Clinical Evaluation of Cardiac Function 692
Helio Autran de Morais

111 Therapy of Heart Failure 713
Mark D. Kittleson

112 Congenital Heart Disease..................... 737
D. David Sisson
William P. Thomas
John D. Bonagura

113 Acquired Valvular Heart Disease............... 787
Clarence Kvart
Jens Häggström

114 Electrocardiography........................... 800
Stephen J. Ettinger
Gérard Le Bobinnec
Etienne Côté

115 Echocardiography 834
John D. Bonagura
Virginia Luis Fuentes

116 Primary Myocardial Disease in the Dog 874
D. David Sisson
William P. Thomas
Bruce W. Keene

117 Feline Cardiomyopathies 896
Philip R. Fox

118 Pericardial Disorders......................... 923
Matthew W. Miller
D. David Sisson

119 Dirofilariasis in Dogs and Cats................. 937
Ray Dillon

120 Peripheral Vascular Disease................... 964
Philip R. Fox
Jean-Paul Petrie
Peter F. Suter

INDEX i

VOLUME 2

SECTION VIII
EYES, EARS, NOSE, AND THROAT

121 Ocular Manifestations of
Systemic Diseases 984
Cecil P. Moore

122 Diseases of the Ear 986
Rod A. W. Rosychuk
Patricia Luttgen

123 Diseases of the Nose and Nasal Sinuses 1003
Autumn P. Davidson
Kyle Mathews
Philip Koblik
Alain Théon

124 Diseases of the Throat 1025
Anjop J. Venker–van Haagen

SECTION IX
THE RESPIRATORY SYSTEM

125 Clinical Evaluation of the Patient With
Respiratory Disease 1034
Brendan Corcoran

126 Diseases of the Trachea 1040
Stephen J. Ettinger
Brett Kantrowitz
Kyle Brayley

127 Diseases of the Bronchus 1055
Lynelle Johnson

128 Pulmonary Parenchymal Diseases 1061
Eleanor C. Hawkins

129 Mediastinal Disease 1091
David S. Biller

130 Pleural and Extrapleural Diseases 1098
Theresa W. Fossum

SECTION X
THE GASTROINTESTINAL SYSTEM

131 Oral and Salivary Gland Disorders 1114
Mark M. Smith

132 Dentistry—Genetic, Environmental, and
Other Considerations 1122
John E. Saidla

133 Dentistry: Periodontal Aspects 1127
Linda J. DeBowes

134 Dentistry: Endodontic and Restorative
Treatment Planning 1135
Edward R. Eisner

135 Diseases of the Esophagus 1142
Robert J. Washabau

136 Diseases of the Stomach 1154
Jean A. Hall

137 Diseases of the Small Intestine 1182
Edward J. Hall
Kenneth W. Simpson

138 Diseases of the Large Intestine 1238
Albert E. Jergens
Michael D. Willard

139 Rectoanal Disease 1257
Robert C. DeNovo, Jr.
Ronald M. Bright

Section XI

Diseases of the Liver and Pancreas

140 History, Physical Examination, and Signs of Liver Disease............................ 1272
Jan Rothuizen
Hein P. Meyer

141 Laboratory Diagnosis of Hepatobiliary Disease........................ 1277
Cynthia R. Leveille-Webster

142 Indications and Techniques for Liver Biopsy............................. 1294
Deborah G. Day

143 Chronic Hepatic Disorders..................... 1298
Susan E. Johnson

144 Acute Hepatic Disorders and Systemic Disorders That Involve the Liver.............. 1326
Susan E. Bunch

145 Diseases of the Gallbladder and Extrahepatic Biliary System 1340
Michael D. Willard
Theresa W. Fossum

146 Exocrine Pancreatic Disease and Pancreatitis ... 1345
David A. Williams

Section XII

The Endocrine System

147 Acromegaly................................. 1370
Ad Rijnberk

148 Diabetes Insipidus 1374
Ad Rijnberk

149 Disorders of the Parathyroid Glands........... 1379
Edward C. Feldman

150 Hyperthyroidism............................. 1400
Mark E. Peterson

151 Hypothyroidism 1419
J. Catharine R. Scott-Moncrieff
Lynn Guptill-Yoran

152 Insulin-Secreting Islet Cell Neoplasia.......... 1429
Richard W. Nelson

153 Diabetes Mellitus............................ 1438
Richard W. Nelson

154 Hyperadrenocorticism........................ 1460
Edward C. Feldman

155 Hypoadrenocorticism 1488
Claudia E. Reusch

156 Gastrointestinal Endocrine Disease 1500
Carole A. Zerbe
Robert J. Washabau

Section XIII

The Reproductive System

157 Estrous Cycle and Breeding Management of the Healthy Bitch 1510
Auke C. Schaefers-Okkens

158 Ovarian and Estrous Cycle Abnormalities...... 1520
Autumn P. Davidson
Edward C. Feldman

159 Abnormalities in Pregnancy, Parturition, and the Periparturient Period.................. 1527
Catharina Linde-Forsberg
Annelie Eneroth

160 Early Spay and Neuter 1539
Margaret V. Root Kustritz
Patricia N. Olson

161 Contraception and Pregnancy Termination 1542
J. Verstegen

162 Cystic Endometrial Hyperplasia, Pyometra, and Infertility 1549
Edward C. Feldman

163 Vaginal Disorders............................ 1566
Beverly J. Purswell

164 Semen Evaluation, Artificial Insemination,
and Infertility in the Male Dog 1571
Gary C. W. England

165 Inherited and Congenital Disorders of the
Male and Female Reproductive Systems 1581
Mushtaq A. Memon
W. Duane Mickelsen

166 Feline Reproduction 1585
J. Verstegen

S E C T I O N   X I V

THE URINARY SYSTEM

167 Clinical Approach and Laboratory
Evaluation of Renal Disease 1600
Stephen P. DiBartola

168 Acute Renal Failure 1615
Larry D. Cowgill
Denise A. Elliott

169 Chronic Renal Failure 1634
David J. Polzin
Carl A. Osborne
Frédéric Jacob
Sheri Ross

170 Glomerular Disease 1662
Gregory F. Grauer
Stephen P. DiBartola

171 Bacterial Infections of the Urinary Tract 1678
Gerald V. Ling

172 Prostatic Diseases 1687
Margaret V. Root Kustritz
Jeffrey S. Klausner

173 Familial Renal Disease in Dogs and Cats 1698
Stephen P. DiBartola

174 Disorders of Renal Tubules 1704
Joseph W. Bartges

175 Feline Lower Urinary Tract Diseases 1710
Carl A. Osborne
John M. Kruger
Jody P. Lulich
David J. Polzin
Chalermpol Lekcharoensuk

176 Canine Lower Urinary Tract Disorders 1747
Jody P. Lulich
Carl A. Osborne
Joseph W. Bartges
Chalermpol Lekcharoensuk

S E C T I O N   X V

HEMATOLOGY AND IMMUNOLOGY

177 Regenerative Anemias Caused by Blood
Loss or Hemolysis 1784
Urs Giger

178 Non-regenerative Anemia 1804
Susan M. Cotter

179 Platelets and von Willebrand's Disease 1817
Rafael Ruiz de Gopegui
Bernard F. Feldman

180 Coagulopathies and Thrombosis 1829
Marjory Brooks

181 Leukocyte Changes in Disease 1842
Gary J. Kociba

182 Non-Neoplastic Disorders of the Spleen 1857
C. Guillermo Couto
Rance M. Gamblin

S E C T I O N   X V I
JOINT AND SKELETAL DISORDERS

183 Joint Diseases of Dogs and Cats 1862
Niels C. Pedersen
Joe P. Morgan
Philip B. Vasseur

184 Skeletal Diseases 1887
Kenneth A. Johnson
A. D. J. Watson

A P P E N D I C E S

Appendix 1 Client Information Series 1918

Neurologic

    Disc Disease. 1919
    Richard A. LeCouteur
    Seizures 1920
    Michael Podell

Cancer

    Chemotherapy 1921
    Susan A. Kraegel
    Hemangiosarcoma in the Dog . . . 1922
    Mona P. Rosenberg
    Lymphoma 1923
    Susan A. Kraegel
    Mast Cell Tumors in Dogs 1924
    Mona P. Rosenberg
    Osteosarcoma 1925
    Susan A. Kraegel
    Solar-Induced Squamous Cell
    Carcinoma in Cats. 1926
    Mark M. Smith
    Vaccine-Induced Sarcoma
    in Cats 1927
    Susan A. Kraegel
    Canine Mammary Tumors. 1928
    Deborah W. Knapp

Endocrine

    o,p'-DDD Treatment of Pituitary
    Cushing's. 1929
    Edward C. Feldman
    Diabetes Mellitus in Dogs
    and Cats. 1930
    Edward C. Feldman
    Hyperthyroidism in Cats 1931
    Edward C. Feldman
    Canine Hypothyroidism 1932
    J. Catharine R. Scott-Moncrieff

Reproduction

    Birth Control Alternatives 1933
    Autumn P. Davidson
    Breeding Management of
    the Bitch 1934
    Autumn P. Davidson
    Whelping in the Bitch 1935
    Margaret V. Root Kustritz
    and Autumn P. Davidson
    Dystocia in the Bitch 1936
    Autumn P. Davidson
    Pyometra. 1937
    Autumn P. Davidson

Gastrointestinal Tract/Liver

    Colitis 1938
    Albert E. Jergens
    Chronic Hepatitis in the Dog 1939
    Richard E. Goldstein
    Dental Disease in Dogs
    and Cats. 1940
    M. J. Lommer and F. J. M. Verstraete
    Flatulence 1941
    W. Grant Guilford
    Gastrointestinal Food Allergies . . 1942
    Michael D. Willard
    Gastric Dilatation–Volvulus 1943
    W. Grant Guilford
    Hepatic Lipidosis in Cats. 1944
    Richard E. Goldstein
    Managing PEG Tubes
    and Feeding Tubes 1945
    Theresa M. Ortega and
    Marcella F. Harb-Hauser
    Megaesophagus 1946
    Michael D. Willard
    Non-Neoplastic Infiltrative Bowel
    Diseases 1947
    Albert E. Jergens
    Pancreatitis 1948
    David A. Williams

Cardiothoracic

Canine and Feline
Cardiomyopathy 1949
Stephen J. Ettinger
Collapsing Trachea 1950
Stephen J. Ettinger
Congential Heart Disease 1951
Stephen J. Ettinger
Canine Valvular Insufficiency
and Congestive Heart Failure 1952
Stephen J. Ettinger
Canine Heartworm Disease 1953
Clarke Atkins
Feline Bronchitis ("Feline
Asthma") 1954
Carol Norris
Pneumonia 1955
Alfred M. Legendre

Infections

Feline Immunodeficiency
Virus 1956
Alfred M. Legendre
Feline Leukemia Virus Vaccinations
in Cats 1957
Alfred M. Legendre
Parvovirus in Dogs 1958
Alfred M. Legendre
Canine Distemper 1959
Alfred M. Legendre

Immune-Mediated Hematologic

Immune-Mediated Hemolytic
Anemia and Immune-Mediated
Thrombocytopenia 1960
Carol Norris
Immune-Mediated Arthritis 1961
David Feldman
von Willebrand's Disease 1962
*Rafael Ruiz de Gopegui and
Bernard F. Feldman*

Kidney & Urinary Tract

Chronic Renal Failure 1963
David J. Polzin
Chronic and/or Recurrent Urinary
Tract Infections 1964
Gerald V. Ling
Ethylene Glycol Toxicity
(Radiator Fluid) 1965
Denise A. Elliott
Urinary Stones: Cause;
Treatment; Prevention 1966
Carl A. Osborne
Does Your Cat Have Lower
Urinary Tract Disease? 1967
Carl A. Osborne

Drugs

"Steroid" Therapy 1968
Edward C. Feldman
Antibiotics 1969
Etienne Côté

Skin/Ears

Canine Demodicosis 1970
Terese C. DeManuelle
Fleas and Flea Allergy
Dermatitis 1971
Terese C. DeManuelle
Food Hypersensitivity 1972
Terese C. DeManuelle
Canine Atopic Dermatitis 1973
Sandra Merchant
Otitis Externa 1974
Sandra Merchant

Appendix 2 Congenital Defects of the Cat 1975
Johnny D. Hoskins

Appendix 3 Congenital Defects of the Dog 1983
Johnny D. Hoskins

INDEX i

Abnormal Laboratory Findings

Conditions Associated With Hematologic Change

Urinalysis Abnormalities . . . . Found on the inside covers
Robert M. DuFort

SECTION VIII

EYES, EARS, NOSE, AND THROAT

CHAPTER 121

OCULAR MANIFESTATIONS OF SYSTEMIC DISEASES

Cecil P. Moore

The value of ocular examination in providing clues to the recognition of systemic disorders is well recognized. Depending on the specific disease process, virtually any component of the eye may be involved. Ocular manifestations of systemic diseases are discussed using a problem-based approach, whereby the presenting finding is noted (i.e., the clinical ocular condition) and the systemic disease that may be associated with the particular ocular finding is considered.

EXOPHTHALMOS

Exophthalmos, the forward displacement of the eye resulting from a space-occupying orbital lesion, is the most common orbital manifestation of systemic disease. Orbital involvement may occur either unilaterally or bilaterally. Lymphosarcoma is the most frequent systemic cause of exophthalmos. Retrobulbar hemorrhage resulting from systemic clotting disorders may also cause exophthalmos, as can immune-mediated disorders. In dogs, autoimmune muscle diseases result in inflammatory infiltrates of either masticatory muscles or extraocular muscles, but usually not both. Myositis of the temporalis and masseter muscles occurs with highest incidence in German shepherd dogs, whereas extraocular muscle myositis occurs most often in golden retrievers. Immune-mediated pathogeneses are suspected for these myopathies.

BLEPHARITIS

Acute swelling of the eyelids, or blepharedema, may occur as an allergic reaction to vaccines, ingested allergens, or insect stings. Swelling results from an acute IgE-mast cell–mediated hypersensitivity reaction triggering local release of vasoactive amines. Inflammatory skin diseases that may also cause blepharitis include staphylococci, dermatophyte infections, and demodicosis. Granulomatous blepharitis may occur with systemic mycoses or as a sterile granulomatous disease and may result in focal or multifocal thickening of the eyelids. Fistulas associated with eyelid granulomas suggest foreign body or filamentous bacterial or fungal infection. Culture of exudates and histopathology of eyelid granulomas are essential for definitive diagnosis.

Autoimmune blepharitis may be associated with lupus erythematosus or pemphigus and can result in alopecia, crusting, or ulceration of the eyelids. Although discoid lupus erythematosus most commonly involves the planum nasale, lesions may also affect the eyelids. In pemphigus foliaceus, lesions often involve the face and head, including the periocular area. Diagnosis of these autoimmune diseases depends on typical histologic changes or appropriate immunohistochemical procedures.

CONJUNCTIVAL CHANGES

Conjunctival color changes may accompany systemic conditions, including anemia (blanched, pale), icterus (yellow, amber), and cyanosis (blue, purple). Intense conjunctival hyperemia most typifies severe conjunctival inflammation, although it may also reflect vascular changes with toxemias and heat stress.

Besides conjunctival hyperemia, conjunctivitis is characterized by chemosis and marked ocular discharge. Viral agents are the most notable causes of conjunctivitis as an ocular manifestation of systemic disease in dogs and cats. Mucosal epithelial viral replication occurs with canine distemper virus and feline herpesvirus and, in each instance, may result in intense conjunctivitis. *Chlamydia psittaci* is an important cause of infectious conjunctivitis in cats.

NICTITANS PROTRUSION

Protrusion of the nictitating membrane results from infiltration of the nictitans by orbital neoplasia (e.g., lymphosarcoma). In the absence of a mass lesion, relaxation and protrusion of the nictitans occur with sympathetic denervation in Horner's syndrome, in which upper eyelid droop (ptosis), constricted pupil (miosis), and enophthalmos are accompanying clinical findings.

KERATITIS

Keratoconjunctivitis sicca (KCS) is a common ocular disease in dogs. Although the majority of cases are believed to be caused by local immune-mediated events, certain systemic conditions may induce or predispose to canine KCS, including viral disease (canine distemper), drug toxicity (sulfonamides), or metabolic disease (hypothyroidism).

The significance of corneal edema (diffuse bluing) as a manifestation of systemic disease is that it may indicate severe intraocular inflammation (uveitis). Many systemic infectious diseases may cause uveitis (see later). In dogs, intense diffuse corneal edema may occur as an immunologic reaction to canine adenovirus.[1]

Deep corneal vascularization, referred to as interstitial or stromal keratitis, indicates subacute or chronic intraocular inflammation (see Uveitis later). This pattern of vascularization is characterized by small, straight vessels that occur circumferentially around the limbus and, therefore, are sometimes referred to as "circumciliary."

Corneal stromal deposition of lipids, primarily cholesterol, can occur in hypercholesteremic states.[2] Dense white material accompanied by fibrovascular infiltration is commonly present in the perilimbal cornea. Diagnostic evaluation for primary and secondary hypercholesterolemias is indicated with this problem.

CATARACTS

Systemic causes of cataracts include nutritional or metabolic abnormalities. Neonates supplemented with artificial milk replacers may develop cataracts. Diabetes mellitus is a common cause of acquired cataracts in dogs, but not cats. Laboratory tests to screen for diabetes mellitus are indicated in dogs with cataracts before proceeding with cataract surgery. Inflammatory cataracts commonly occur secondary to anterior uveitis in dogs and cats and should prompt inquiry into the cause of the uveitis.

UVEITIS

Because uveal tissues harbor the majority of intraocular blood vessels, the uvea is an extremely important site for ocular manifestations of systemic disease. Infectious, neoplastic, and metabolic diseases may affect uveal tissues, causing vasculitis, inflammatory cell infiltrates, leakage of proteins or lipids into the eye, or proliferative disease.[3–9] Failure to detect uveitis or failure to distinguish it from other causes of ocular disease may result in progression of potentially life-threatening systemic illnesses.

Findings indicative of acute uveitis include episcleral vascular injection, corneal edema, miosis, aqueous flare, and iris congestion. Keratic precipitates are accumulations of inflammatory cells on the corneal endothelium characteristic of granulomatous uveitis. Signs of uveitis are caused by release of multiple inflammatory mediators and disruption of the blood-aqueous barrier. Hyphema or hypopyon indicates a severe breakdown of the blood-uvea barrier. Intraocular pressure is generally low in cases of uveitis unless a secondary glaucoma has developed. Chronic uveitis is characterized by iris-lens adhesions (posterior synechiae), which may account for disparity in pupil sizes and result in lens capsule pigment.

When there is a clinical diagnosis of uveitis, an attempt should be made to identify the cause. The potential causes of uveitis are numerous (Table 121–1), however, and this is not always possible. A thorough history and general physical examination are indicated in all animals with uveitis. A complete blood count, serum biochemical profile, urinalysis, and thoracic radiographs are recommended as a minimal database. Serologic tests for infectious agents are usually indicated. Ocular centesis with cytology and/or culture of anterior chamber, vitreous, or subretinal exudates may be necessary for definitive diagnosis. Skin biopsy may be needed to diagnose uveal-dermal depigmentation syndrome (Vogt-Koyanagi-Harada–like syndrome).[10] The selection of specific diagnostic tests is dictated by physical examination findings and knowledge of diseases endemic to a given region.

Dogs and cats with primary or secondary hyperlipidemias may have a milky-appearing aqueous humor, referred to as lipemic aqueous. Similarly, lipid-laden retinal vessels, termed lipemia retinalis, may also be noted. The degree of turbidity may increase dramatically following ingestion of a fatty meal; conversely, fasting may result in clearing. Lipemic aqueous or lipemia retinalis typically results from hypertriglyceridemia, with breed-predisposed hyperlipidemia and diabetes mellitus being relatively common causes.

CHORIORETINITIS

Similar to uveitis, retinal and/or choroidal lesions may occur with many systemic diseases, including infectious,[11] neoplastic,[8] vascular,[12] or parasitic[13] disorders (Table 121–2). Therefore, funduscopic examination is an extremely important part of the complete ophthalmic evaluation. The appearance of funduscopic lesions varies with the tissue involved (vascular, neuronal, or both), whether the condition is active or inactive, and whether the lesion involves tapetal or nontapetal regions.

Retinal edema; pre-, intra-, or subretinal exudates; perivascular infiltrates; or retinal hemorrhages are indicative of acute inflammatory or vascular (hypertensive) disease. Subretinal exudation may cause retinal detachment when the neurosensory retina separates from the retinal pigment layer. By contrast, chronic inflammation may result in tapetal hyperreflectivity, hyperpigmented foci, vascular attenuation, or optic nerve changes (e.g., pallor). The optic nerve may lose definition, becoming pale or dark with atrophy. Atrophic retinas may be predisposed to detachment.

OPTIC NEURITIS

Either unilateral or bilateral, optic neuritis may be associated with systemic disease and may cause blindness in affected eyes. When optic neuritis extends to the globe, the papilla appears swollen, elevated, and hyperemic. Retrobulbar optic neuritis is more difficult to diagnose, because the optic papilla may appear normal. If optic neuritis is treated promptly and if the cause is reversible, vision may be preserved. Uncontrolled optic neuritis results in optic nerve atrophy. Causes of optic neuritis are included in Table 121–2.

TABLE 121–1. SYSTEMIC CAUSES OF UVEITIS

CANINE	FELINE
Mycoses (blastomycosis, histoplasmosis, cryptococcosis, coccidioidomycosis)	Feline infectious peritonitis
Spirochetes (leptospirosis, Lyme disease?)	Toxoplasmosis
Brucellosis	Feline leukemia virus
Leishmaniasis	Feline immunodeficiency virus
Tick-borne diseases (ehrlichiosis, Rocky Mountain spotted fever)	Mycoses (see Canine)
Parasites (dirofilariasis)	Neoplasia (lymphosarcoma)
Neoplasia (metastatic intraocular tumor, lymphosarcoma)	
Immune-mediated (adenovirus reaction, Vogt-Koyanagi-Harada–like syndrome, thrombocytopenia)	

TABLE 121–2. SYSTEMIC CAUSES OF CHORIORETINAL AND OPTIC NERVE DISEASE

CHORIORETINITIS	OPTIC NEURITIS
Viral (canine distemper [ICD], feline infectious peritonitis [FIP])	Viral (ICD, FIP, feline leukemia virus)
Canine ehrlichiosis	Granulomatous meningoencephalitis
Rocky Mountain spotted fever	Neoplasia (lymphosarcoma, metastatic disease)
Mycoses (blastomycosis, histoplasmosis, cryptococcosis, coccidioidomycosis)	Mycoses (see Chorioretinitis)
Prototheosis	Toxoplasmosis
Toxoplasmosis	
Leishmaniasis	
Parasites (larval migrans, ophthalmomyiasis)	
Immune-mediated (Vogt-Koyanagi-Harada–like syndrome, systemic lupus erythematosus, thrombocytopenia)	
Vascular disease (hypertension)	
Neoplasia (lymphosarcoma, metastatic disease, multiple myeloma)	
Nutritional retinopathy (vitamin E deficiency)	
Drug-induced toxicity	

REFERENCES

1. Carmichael LE: The pathogenesis of ocular lesions of infectious canine hepatitis. Pathol Vet 2:344, 1965.
2. Crispin SM, Barnett KC: Arcus lipoides cornea secondary to hypothyroidism in the Alsatian. J Small Anim Pract 19:127, 1978.
3. Buyukmihci NC: Ocular lesions of blastomycosis in the dog. JAVMA 180:426, 1982.
4. Swanson JF: Uveitis associated with *Ehrlichia canis* infection. Proc Am Coll Vet Ophthalmol, 1982, pp 204–214.
5. Angel JA, et al: Ocular lesions associated with coccidioidomycosis in dogs: 35 cases (1980–1985). JAVMA 190:1319, 1987.
6. Davidson MG, et al: Ocular manifestations of Rocky Mountain spotted fever in dogs. JAVMA 194:777, 1989.
7. Davidson MB, et al: Feline anterior uveitis: A study of 53 cases. J Am Anim Hosp Assoc 27:77, 1991.
8. Krohne SDB, et al: Ocular involvement in canine lymphosarcoma: A retrospective study of 94 cases. Proc Am Coll Vet Ophthalmol, 1987, pp 68–84.
9. Olin DD, et al: Lipid-laden aqueous humor associated with anterior uveitis and concurrent hyperlipemia in two dogs. JAVMA 168:861, 1976.
10. Morgan RV: Vogt-Koyanagi-Harada syndrome in humans and dogs. Comp Contin Educ Small Anim Pract 11:1211, 1989.
11. Fischer C: Retinal and retinochoroidal lesions in early neuropathic canine distemper. JAVMA 158:740, 1971.
12. Morgan RV: Systemic hypertension in four cats: Ocular and medical findings. J Am Anim Hosp Assoc 22:615, 1986.
13. Gwin RM, et al: Ophthalmomyiasis interna posterior in two cats and a dog. J Am Anim Hosp Assoc 20:481, 1984.

CHAPTER 122

DISEASES OF THE EAR

Rod A. W. Rosychuk and Patricia Luttgen

GENERAL CONCEPTS

Several concepts are important when evaluating an animal suspected or known to have ear disease:

1. Signalment (age, breed, sex) may suggest more likely differential diagnoses (e.g., otitis externa in dogs and cats younger than 6 months of age is often due to *Otodectes* infestations).

2. Questions regarding history should emphasize when the problem started, its progression, seasonality, any association with pain and/or pruritus, therapies, and any response to therapy.

3. Many diseases of the external ear (i.e., pinna, vertical and horizontal canals) are extensions of more generalized skin disease, such as atopy. A thorough dermatologic history and physical examination should be performed on all pets with ear disease.

4. Because the middle and inner ear are closely associated with the facial, sympathetic, parasympathetic, and vestibu-
locochlear nerves, evidence of Horner's syndrome, facial palsy, or keratoconjunctivitis sicca may suggest middle ear disease. Severe otitis media may be associated with pain on opening the mouth.

5. Inner ear disease is suggested by head tilt, spontaneous nystagmus, or ataxia.

6. The ear examination must include an evaluation of both the concave and convex (inner and outer) aspects of the pinna and palpation of the auricular cartilages of the canals for pain, thickening, and/or calcification. A thorough otoscopic examination of the ear canals and tympanic membrane is mandatory.

CLINICAL MANIFESTATIONS, DIAGNOSIS, AND THERAPY FOR SPECIFIC DISEASES OF THE PINNA

A complete list of differential diagnoses is presented in Table 122–1.

TABLE 122–1. DIFFERENTIAL DIAGNOSIS OF DISEASES OF THE PINNA

NONPRURITIC ALOPECIA

Canine

Pinnal alopecia syndrome of short-coated breeds
Periodic alopecia of miniature poodles
Color dilution alopecia
Idiopathic follicular dysplasia
Estrogen-responsive dermatosis
Alopecia areata
Demodicosis
Dermatophytosis
Hypothyroidism (especially in giant breeds)
Congenital alopecias
Ectodermal defects

Feline

Idiopathic pinnal alopecia
Demodicosis
Dermatophytosis
Alopecia areata
Iatrogenic hypothyroidism (after radioiodine or surgical thyroidectomy)
Iatrogenic hyperadrenocorticism

EAR MARGIN DERMATOSIS

Canine

Sarcoptic mange
Fly strike dermatitis
Zinc-responsive dermatosis
Proliferative thrombovascular necrosis
Vasculitis
Ear margin seborrhea
Idiopathic hyperkeratosis of Boston terriers
Idiopathic lymphocytic/plasmacytic dermatitis
Ear fissures
Frostbite
Hypothyroidism

Feline

Actinic dermatitis
Squamous cell carcinoma
Notoedric mange
Frostbite

INFLAMMATION/ULCERATION/NECROSIS OF THE EAR APEX

Canine

Vasculitis
Proliferative thrombovascular necrosis
Superficial necrolytic dermatitis
Systemic lupus erythematosus
Discoid lupus erythematosus
Dermatomyositis
Pemphigus complex
Fly strike dermatitis
Drug eruption
Frostbite
Cold agglutinin disease

Feline

Relapsing polychondritis
Iatrogenic hyperadrenocorticism
Frostbite
Actinic dermatitis
Squamous cell carcinoma

DIFFUSE ERYTHEMA

Canine

Atopy
Food sensitivity
Contact/irritant dermatitis
Idiopathic erythema/edema
Actinic dermatitis
Drug eruption
Demodicosis
Dermatophytosis
Juvenile cellulitis
Mycosis fungoides (cutaneous lymphosarcoma)
Pheochromocytoma (flushing)
Carcinoid syndrome (flushing)
Mast cell tumors (flushing)

Feline

Actinic dermatitis
Atopy
Food sensitivity
Mastocytosis (flushing)

CRUSTING/INFLAMMATION

Canine

Demodicosis
Dermatophytosis
Zinc responsive dermatosis
Sarcoptic mange
Lichenoid psoriasiform dermatosis of the springer
    spaniel
Pemphigus complex
Systemic lupus erythematosus
Drug eruption
Sebaceous adenitis
Dermatomyositis
Superficial necrolytic dermatitis

Feline

Pemphigus complex
Dermatophytosis
Drug eruption

PUSTULES/VESICLES/BULLA (DOG AND CAT)

Pemphigus complex
Bullous pemphigoid
Drug eruption
Contact/irritant dermatitis

PAPULES/NODULES

Canine

Neoplasia
Eosinophilic folliculitis/furunculosis
Eosinophilic granuloma
Sterile nodular histiocytic granuloma
Bacterial pyoderma

Feline

Neoplasia
Mosquito bite hypersensitivity
Eosinophilic (collagenolytic) granuloma
Xanthoma

ENT

Nonpruritic Alopecia

Canine Pinnal Alopecia. A progressive, symmetric alopecia of the pinna is seen primarily in dachshunds, but it also occurs in Boston terriers, Chihuahuas, whippets, Manchester terriers, and Italian greyhounds. The cause is unknown, but a vasculopathy, follicular dysplasia, or both may be involved. The alopecia seldom develops before 1 year of age and is slowly progressive. Chronically affected skin may become hyperpigmented and dry, leather-like, and scaly. The remainder of the coat is normal. Diagnosis is based on the process of elimination and on the results of skin biopsy. Histopathologic examination reveals small hair follicles. There is an anecdotal suggestion that pentoxifylline, melatonin, or mibolerone may produce significant hair re-growth.

Periodic Pinnal Alopecia of Miniature Poodles and Siamese Cats. These two popular breeds are known to undergo a sudden loss of hair over one or both ears. Over several months there is progression to complete bilateral pinnal alopecia, and hair re-growth may be noted within several months. The etiology of this disease is not known, but telogen effluvium, drug eruptions, and alopecia areata have been mentioned.

Ear Margin Dermatoses

Sarcoptic and Notoedric Mange. *Sarcoptes scabiei* produces an intensely pruritic dermatitis primarily directed at the head, convex (outer) aspect of the pinna, lateral elbows, stifles, and ventrum of the dog. Although the head and ears may be most prominently affected, widespread pruritus is common. Pinnal lesions consist of patchy alopecia, erythema, scaling, and crusting. The ear margin is often significantly affected, becoming alopecic, inflamed, thickened, and, as the disease progresses, crusty. Rubbing the apex of the pinnal margins should elicit a hind limb scratch, a non-specific reaction. Diagnosis is made by skin scrapings, response to trial therapy, or, when available, serologic testing. Therapy involves oral ivermectin or milbemycin oxime administered once weekly until lesions and pruritus have completely resolved (usually 4–6 weeks). Good responses have also been noted with every-other-day dosing of milbemycin oxime continued for 3 weeks. Alternatively, ivermectin can be given subcutaneously every 10 to 14 days until pruritus and lesions have resolved (Table 122–2). To hasten resolution and reduce the potential for contagion, topical therapy with 2 per cent lime sulfur dips administered once weekly, or amitraz (Mitaban), 0.025 per cent administered once weekly, may be considered. Systemic glucocorticoids may be used to reduce pruritus during the initial stages of therapy.

Notoedres cati primarily affects cats but may be found on foxes, dogs, and rabbits. Lesions are pruritic and begin on the margins of the ears and spread to the rest of the ear, face, and neck. The distal extremities and perineum may also be affected. There is alopecia, thickening, and marked crusting. Large numbers of mites are found on skin scrapings. Ivermectin is an effective therapy.

Fly Strike Dermatitis. Fly strike dermatitis is most commonly caused by the bites of *Stomoxys calcitrans* (stable flies) and, less commonly, *Simulium* species (black flies) and tabanids (deer flies, horse flies). Lesions consist of small erythematous papules or ulcers with hemorrhagic crusts. Pruritus and pain are variable. The lesions are found on the convex side of the apex of the ear in erect-eared dogs or over the dorsalmost part of the convex aspect of the pinna in floppy-eared dogs. Diagnosis is based on history (flies often seen in the environment; horses nearby) and physical examination. Resolution can be facilitated be restricting outdoor exposure and/or using commercial or homemade fly protectants or repellants at least twice daily. A homemade formulation can be made by mixing petroleum jelly with a small amount of diethyltoluamide (DEET), a pyrethrin, or a pyrethroid. Use of a topical glucocorticoid/antibiotic or of oral prednisone/prednisolone at anti-inflammatory dosages may hasten the resolution of the inflammation.

Canine Ear Margin Seborrhea. Oily/waxy or scaly accumulations are restricted to the margins of the ears. The debris is variably adherent and yellow to brown. Partial alopecia in affected areas is common. Pruritus is varible. Clinically and histologically, the lesions are variably inflammatory. Non-inflammatory ear margin seborrhea is characterized histologically by marked hyperkeratosis (variable parakeratosis), variable acanthosis, and variably present mild perivascular mononuclear infiltrates (lymphocytes, macrophages). Inflammatory ear margin seborrhea commonly shows an interface accumulation of lymphocytes and plasma cells. Pigmentary incontinence may be present.

Therapy for non-inflammatory ear margin seborrhea is directed at loosening and removing debris. Ceruminolytics (e.g., propylene glycol 50:50 with water) can be applied daily, followed in several hours by antiseborrheic shampoos (sulfur-salicylic acid, benzoyl peroxide, or coal tar), which are allowed to remain on the ear for 5 to 10 minutes and then thoroughly rinsed off. Once accumulations are controlled, the frequency of applications is reduced to a maintenance regimen. Retinoids (especially etretinate or acitretin) may be of some benefit. For inflammatory ear margin seborrhea, therapeutic alternatives include topical glucocorticoids, oral glucocorticoids, pentoxifylline, or tetracycline/niacinamide (see Table 122–2).

Actinic Dermatitis and Squamous Cell Carcinoma. Actinic dermatitis represents sun-induced damage to non-pigmented (white), usually sparsely haired skin. Cats are more commonly affected than dogs. Affected cats are generally older (mean age, 12 years).[1] Non-pigmented areas of the margins and apex of the ears are involved initially. Affected areas are erythematous, with variable degrees of alopecia and scaling. More advanced cases may ulcerate and crust. Pruritus and/or pain is variable. Pinnal margins may curl and take on a scalloped appearance. This is a pre-cancerous condition that may lead to carcinoma in situ or squamous cell carcinoma. Diagnosis is based on history, physical examination, and results of skin biopsy.

Therapy for pre-cancerous actinic dermatitis includes sun restriction, especially between the times of 10 A.M. and 4 P.M., topical sunscreens (SPF of 15 or greater; with waterproof base) applied at least twice daily, topical glucocorticoids (1 to 2.5 per cent hydrocortisone every 12 to 24 hours), and possibly a short course of oral prednisone at anti-inflammatory dosages.

Although etretinate may benefit both cats and dogs with actinic dermatitis[2] (see Table 122–2), this drug has recently been discontinued. Its replacement, acetretin, may be of benefit but has not been thoroughly evaluated in the dog and cat. With etretinate, initial response should be seen within 4 to 6 weeks. Every-other-day administration may be tried for maintenance. Squamous cell carcinomas appear to be poorly responsive to retinoid therapy. However, etretinate (and therefore, possibly acetretin) may be used as adjunctive therapy along with more specific treatment for established

TABLE 122–2. DRUGS USED IN TREATMENT OF EAR DISEASES

GENERIC	TRADE	DOSAGE	ROUTE	FREQUENCY	DESCRIPTION
Prednisone/prednisolone	Many and generic	0.25–0.5 mg/lb (0.5–1 mg/kg)	Orally	q24h	Canine anti-inflammatory/antipruritic
		0.5–1 mg/lb (1.0–2.0 mg/kg)	Orally	q24h	Feline anti-inflammatory/antipruritic
		0.5–1.0 mg/lb (1.0– 2.0 mg/kg)	Orally	q12h	Canine immunosuppressive
		1.0–2.0 mg/lb (2.0–4.0 mg/kg)	Orally	q12h	Feline immunosuppressive
Dexamethasone	Many and generic	0.05 mg/lb (0.1 mg/kg)	Orally	q12 h or q24h	Idiopathic pinnal erythema
Etretinate	Tegison	0.5 mg/lb (1.0 mg/kg) or 10 mg/cat total dose	Orally	q24h	Canine acquired pattern alopecia, Canine ear margin seborrhea, Canine and feline actinic dermatitis, lichenoid-psoriasiform dermatitis
Ivermectin	Ivomec	0.15 mg/lb (0.3 mg/kg)	Orally	Once weekly	Sarcoptic mange, notoedric mange, canine and feline ear mites
		0.15 mg/lb (0.3 mg/kg)	SQ	q10–14 days	
Lime sulfur	Lym Dyp	2%	Dip	Once weekly	Sarcoptic mange, notoedric mange
Amitraz	Mitaban	.025%	Dip	Once weekly	Sarcoptic mange, notoedric mange
Dapsone	Dapsone USP	0.5 mg/lb (1.0 mg/kg)	Orally	q8h	Idiopathic vasculitis; potentially toxic; see elsewhere for specifics
Sulfasalazine	Azulfidine	10–20 mg/lb (20–40 mg/kg)	Orally	q8h	Idiopathic vasculitis; potentially toxic; see elsewhere for specifics
Fluocinolone 0.01%, DMSO 60%	Synotic	2–12 drops; varies with size of ear	Topically	q12h initially, q48–72h maintenance	Potent anti-inflammatory; moderate to severe allergic otitis; Cocker hyperplastic/proliferative otitis
Hydrocortisone 1.0%	HB101, Burrows H	2–12 drops; varies with size of ear	Topically	q12h initially, q24–48h maintenance	Mild anti-inflammatory/astringent; mild to moderate allergic otitis; swimmer's otitis; ceruminous (seborrheic) otitis
Hydrocortisone 0.5%, sulfur 2%, acetic acid 2.5%	Clear X Ear Treatment	2–12 drops; varies with size of ear	Topically	q12–24h initially, q24–48h maintenance	Mild anti-inflammatory/astringent/germicidal; allergic otitis; swimmer's otitis; ceruminous (seborrheic) otitis
Lactic acid 2.5%, salicylic acid 0.1%, DSS, propylene glycol, malic acid, benzoic acid	Epi-Otic	Fill ear	Topically	q24 or 48h or as necessary	Ceruminolytic/drying agent; mild antibacterial, antifungal activity
Propylene glycol, malic acid, benzoic acid, salicyclic acid	Oti-Cleans	Fill ear	Topically	q24–48h or as necessary	Ceruminolytic/drying agent; mild antibacterial/antifungal activity
Dioctyl sodium sulfo-succinate 6.5%, urea (carbamide) peroxide 6%	Clear X Ear Cleansing Solution	1–2 mL/ear	Topically	As necessary	May be irritating in awake animals
Chlorhexidine 2%	Nolvasan	Dilute 1:40 in water	Topically	As necessary	Ear flushing
Chlorhexidine 1.5%		Dilute 2% in propylene glycol		q12h	Refractory *Pseudomonas* otitis; may be irritating
Povidone-iodine 10%	Betadine Solution	Dilute 1:10 to 1:50 in water	Topically	As necessary	Ear flushing
Polyhydroxidine iodine 0.5%	Xenodyne	Dilute 1:1 to 1:5 in water	Topically	As necessary (Ef); once weekly (Em); q12h (RPo)	Ear flushing (Ef), ear mites (Em), refractory *Pseudomonas* otitis (RPo)
Acetic acid 5%	White vinegar	Dilute 1:1 to 1:3 in water	Topically	As necessary; q12–24h for *Pseudomonas*	Ear flushing; *Pseudomonas* otitis; may be irritating in more concentrated solutions

Table continued on following page

ENT

TABLE 122–2. DRUGS USED IN TREATMENT OF EAR DISEASES *Continued*

GENERIC	TRADE	DOSAGE	ROUTE	FREQUENCY	DESCRIPTION
Neomycin 0.25%, triamcinolone 0.1%, thiabendazole 4%	Tresaderm	2–12 drops; varies with size of ear	Topically	q12h	Bacterial, yeast, or allergic otitis; first-line therapy; ear mite therapy
Neomycin 0.25%, triamcinolone 0.1%, nystatin 100,000 U/mL	Panalog	2–12 drops; varies with size of ear	Topically	q12h	Bacterial, yeast, allergic otitis; first-line otic product
Chloramphenicol 0.42%, prednisone 0.17%, tetracaine 2%, squalene	Liquachlor	2–12 drops; varies with size of ear	Topically	q12h	Bacterial, allergic otitis; first-line otic product
Neomycin 1.75%, polymyxin B 5000 IU/mL, penicillin G procaine 10,000 IU/mL	Forte Topical	2–12 drops; varies with size of ear	Topically	q12h	First-line otic product
Gentamicin 0.3%, betamethasone valerate 0.1%	Gentocin Otic Solution	2–12 drops; varies with size of ear	Topically	q12h	Second-line otic product; *Pseudomonas* otitis
Gentamicin 0.3%, betamethasone 0.1%, clotrimazole 1.0%	Otomax	2–12 drops; varies with size of ear	Topically	q12h	Second-line otic product; refractory *Malassezia* otitis
Polymyxin B 10,000 IU/mL, hydrocortisone 0.5%	Otobiotic	2–12 drops; varies with size of ear	Topically	q12h	Second-line otic product; *Pseudomonas* otitis
Carbaryl 0.5%, neomycin 0.5%, tetracaine	Mitox Liquid	2–12 drops; varies with size of ear	Topically		Ear mite therapy
Pyrethrins .05%, squalene 25%	Cerumite	2–12 drops; varies with size of ear	Topically	q24h	Ear mite therapy
Isopropyl alcohol 90%, boric acid 2%	Panodry	Fill ear	Topically	As necessary	Ear drying (astringent); swimmer's otitis
Acetic acid 2%, aluminum acetate	Otic Domeboro	Fill ear	Topically	q12–48h	Ear drying (astringent); swimmer's otitis
Silver sulfadiazine 1%	Silvadene	Dilute 1:1 with water	Topically	q12h for 14 days	Resistant *Pseudomonas* otitis; refractory *Malassezia* otitis; should be used in a clean ear
Tris-EDTA, +/− gentamicin .03%		1 liter distilled water, 1.2 g EDTA, 6.05 g tris hydroxymethyl aminomethane, 1 mL glacial acetic acid; 2–12 drops	Topically	q12h for 14 days	Resistant *Pseudomonas* otitis; may use alone or mix with gentamicin to achieve a 0.3% gentamicin-tris-EDTA solution
Silver nitrate 5%		Use sparingly	Topically	As necessary	Cauterization for ulcerative otitis externa
Miconazole 1%	Conofite	2–12 drops; varies with size of ear	Topically	q12–24h	May use with or without a topical glucocorticoid (e.g., fluocinolone and 60% DMSO); can add 7.5 mL of dexamethasone phosphate (4 mg/mL) to 10 mL of 1% miconazole
Enrofloxacin	Baytril	1.25–2.5 mg/lb (2.5–5.0 mg/kg)	Orally	q12h	*Pseudomonas* otitis externa, otitis media
Ketoconazole	Nizoral	2.5–5.0 mg/lb (5.0–10.0 mg/kg)	Orally	q12h for 2–4 weeks; q48h for long-term maintenance	Refractory *Malassezia* otitis externa; *Malassezia* otitis media
Itraconazole	Sporanox	5 mg/lb (10 mg/kg)	Orally	q24h	Refractory *Malassezia* otitis externa
Cephalexin	Keflex or generic	5–10 mg/lb (10–20 mg/kg)	Orally	q8h	Bacterial otitis externa, otitis media
		10–15 mg/lb (20–30 mg/kg)	Orally	q12h	
Chloramphenicol	Many and generic	25 mg/lb (50 mg/kg)	Orally	q6–8h	Otitis media (dogs)

squamous cell carcinoma or for palliation in cats with inoperable squamous cell carcinoma. Isotretinoin (Accutane) has generally not been effective for treating actinic dermatitis or squamous cell carcinoma in cats or dogs.[2, 3]

Surgical excision (partial pinnectomy) is an effective therapy for progressive solar lesions and squamous cell carcinoma. Hyperthermia or cryosurgery can be used to successfully treat small, focal solar lesions or early squamous cell carcinoma.[1] However, therapy directed at the pinna may cause necrosis and sloughing. There is a higher incidence of local recurrence associated with cryosurgery than surgery. Photochemotherapy and strontium plesiotherapy (form of superficial radiotherapy) have also been used with success.[4]

Frostbite. Frostbite most commonly affects the apex of the ears of cats and some erect-eared dogs. It appears to be more common in weak or debilitated animals and those not accustomed to extended exposure to cold temperatures. After thawing, affected tissues become erythematous, scaly, alopecic, and variably painful. Subsequently, the ear tips may curl, necrose, and slough. Frozen tissue should be rapidly thawed with warm water. Erythematous, scaly skin can be lightly covered with a bland ointment such as petrolatum. In severe cases, amputation of the affected tissue should be performed, but only after enough time has elapsed to accurately identify non-viable tissue. Hairless, scarred tissue may be more susceptible to repeated freezing. Amputation of this tissue may allow for better coverage of the ear margin with hair.

INFLAMMATION/ULCERATION/NECROSIS OF THE EAR APEX

Vasculitis. Lesions of vasculitis often affect the apex of the ears, with variable patchy involvement of the concave surface of the pinna. Other areas of the body that may be affected are the lips, tail, oral mucosa, nails/nail folds, pads, and lower extremities. Lesions are erythematous, crusty, eroded, and occasionally ulcerated. With chronicity, they may become hyperpigmented and scar. A diagnosis of vasculitis is confirmed by skin biopsy.

Potential causes of vasculitis include systemic infections (e.g., rickettsial), deep staphylococcal pyoderma, systemic lupus erythematosus, discoid lupus erythematosus, dermatomyositis, familial vasculitis of German shepherd dogs, polyarteritis nodosa, systemic neoplasia, and drug reactions. Many cases are idiopathic, probably immune-mediated diseases involving immune complex deposition of unknown origin.

Therapy involves resolving underlying disease when possible. Idiopathic, suspected immune-mediated vasculitis is treated with immunosuppressive dosages of glucocorticoids, with or without other immunosuppressive drugs such as azathioprine. Alternative therapies include sulfasalazine (± glucocorticoids), pentoxifylline (± glucocorticoids) or dapsone (see Table 122-2).

Proliferative Thrombovascular Necrosis. This disease has been recognized in the dachshund, Chihuahua, terrier crosses, Labrador retriever, and Rhodesian ridgeback. Initial lesions are noted along the apex margins and spread down the concave surface of the ear. The more central area of the lesion may be ulcerated. The periphery of the lesion is often hyperpigmented. Scaling and crusting are variable. Affected areas may undergo complete necrosis. The diagnosis is confirmed by skin biopsy. Some treatment success may be achieved with pentoxifylline. Refractory cases may be managed with surgical removal.

Ear Fissures. Ear fissures often originate from the trauma of severe head shaking or scratching. Therapy is directed at relieving the underlying disease (e.g., oral glucocorticoid for atopic otitis). Some success has been achieved with the frequent use of a tissue glue applied two or three times daily. Immobilization of the ear flap may be beneficial. Medical failure usually warrants surgical amputation of the affected portion of the pinna.

Relapsing Polychondritis. A polychondritis affecting the ear margin apex has been described in cats.[5] It is suspected to be an immune-mediated disease. The distal margins of the ears are curled, erythematous, and thickened. Differential diagnoses for the curling of the ear tips include iatrogenic hyperadrenocorticism, frostbite, squamous cell carcinoma, and the normal floppy ear of the Scottish fold.[5] Diagnosis is based on pinna biopsy, and treatment consists of immunosuppressive dosages of glucocorticoids.

DIFFUSE ERYTHEMA

Atopy and Food Sensitivities. See Otitis Externa.

CELLULITIS

Juvenile Cellulitis. Juvenile cellulitis (juvenile sterile granulomatous dermatitis and lymphadenitis) is an uncommon acute dermatitis of dogs 3 weeks to 6 months of age. Breed predilections may include the golden retriever, dachshund, yellow Labrador retriever, and Lhasa apso.[6, 7] One or more individuals in a litter may be affected. Characteristic features include a marked submandibular and prescapular lymphadenopathy, and severe edema, exudation, pustules, and inflammatory nodules affecting the concave aspect of the pinna, muzzle, and periocular region. The highly exudative, purulent dermatitis of the pinna is unique for a dog this age. Diagnosis is based on history, physical examination, and results of skin biopsy of early lesions. Histopathology shows a severe pyogranulomatous to suppurative dermatitis. Treatment consists of immunosuppressive dosages of oral glucocorticoids for 1 to 2 weeks, which are then tapered over 3 to 4 weeks. Systemic antibiotics are given for suspected secondary pyoderma.

PUSTULES/VESICLES/BULLAE

When pustules, vesicles, or bullous lesions are noted on the pinna, they are most commonly seen over the more hairless concave surface. The most common causes are autoimmune diseases of the pemphigus complex and bullous pemphigoid. Bacterial infections, drug eruptions, and contact hypersensitivities may produce similar lesions. Cytologic examination of exudate taken from unbroken lesions may provide diagnostic information. The presence of large numbers of round, basophilic acantholytic keratinocytes, along with variable numbers of neutrophils and occasionally eosinophils, is strongly suggestive of the pemphigus complex.

PAPULES/NODULES

Neoplasia. Auricular tumors are found more commonly in cats than in dogs. In cats, these tumors also have a greater tendency to be malignant. Malignant aural tumors are usually locally invasive but can metastasize to regional lymph nodes, lungs, and viscera. The most common pinnal tumors in dogs are histiocytomas and papillomas; in cats, squamous cell carcinomas are noted (see earlier).[1, 8]

AURAL HEMATOMA

Aural hematomas occur in both dogs and cats and are thought to be products of head shaking. The hematoma appears to arise within the cartilage of the ear but is most evident on the concave surface of the pinna. Affected pets almost always have underlying ear disease (e.g., otitis externa due to atopy, food sensitivity, foreign body). There has been no substantiation of earlier suggestions that autoimmunity may be an underlying cause.[9–11] Aural hematomas may resolve naturally, but do so slowly, leaving residual scarring and contraction of skin and cartilage. These deformities often predispose to secondary bacterial and *Malassezia* infections.

Therapeutic options include needle aspiration (rarely successful), drainage with a self-retaining disposable teat cannula or Penrose drain, and surgical incision with postoperative maintenance of surgical apposition (e.g., mattress sutures).[12] Regardless of the therapy selected, it is important to cure or control the underlying irritative disease.[13]

DISEASES OF THE EXTERNAL EAR CANAL (OTITIS EXTERNA)

NORMAL ANATOMY AND PHYSIOLOGY

The ear canal extends from the entrance of the vertical canal to the tympanic membrane. The skin lining the canals consists of stratified squamous epithelium, sebaceous glands, and ceruminous glands (modified apocrine glands). Sebaceous glands are found superficially in the dermis, whereas the ceruminous glands have a deeper distribution. A combination of ceruminous and sebaceous secretions along with desquamated epithelium make up normal ear wax. The epidermis and dermis tend to become thinner with progression to the tympanic membrane. Numbers of hair follicles and the amount of glandular tissue also gradually decrease throughout the length of the canals to the tympanic membrane. The springer spaniel, cocker spaniel, and black Labrador retriever breeds have been shown to have relatively increased amounts of ceruminous gland tissue, which may play a role in their predisposition to otitis externa.[14] Self-cleaning of the canals is at least in part a product of lateral epithelial migration, beginning with movement of epithelial cells from the tympanum.[15]

PATHOPHYSIOLOGY

Otitis externa is generally defined as inflammation of the ear canals and may involve the more proximal portion of the pinna. The clinical signs associated with otitis externa include variable degrees of head shaking, pruritus, pain, odor, and exudation. Otitis externa is estimated to affect 5 to 20 per cent of dogs and 2 to 6 per cent of cats.[16, 17]

Primary Factors

Primary factors of otitis externa are those that are capable of initiating inflammation in otherwise normal ears.

Hypersensitivities

Atopy, Food Sensitivity, and Flea Bite Hypersensitivity. Otitis externa occurs in 50 to 80 per cent of atopic dogs and in a similar percentage of food-sensitive dogs.[18, 19] Flea bite hypersensitivities uncommonly produce otitis externa. Dogs with allergic otitis externa usually have aural pruritus (scratching, rubbing) and head shaking. "Flares" of atopic otitis may antedate the development of more obvious generalized pruritus by 1 to 2 years. Whereas 3 to 5 per cent of atopic dogs will have only ear disease, as many as 24 per cent of food-sensitive dogs have otitis externa as the only manifestation.[19] The otitis externa associated with atopy and food sensitivities is generally bilateral.

One of the earliest physical changes associated with the ear is edema in the region of the pars flaccida. This is seen as a "bleb" of edematous tissue hanging down from the dorsal wall of the horizontal canal, adjacent to the tympanum. Often more obvious is diffuse inflammation primarily noted in the more proximal portion of the concave pinna and in the proximal portion of the vertical canal. The horizontal canals tend to be relatively less affected. With chronicity, affected skin becomes thickened, cobblestone in appearance, variably hyperpigmented, and waxy/oily. Thickening may eventually result in almost complete occlusion of the entrance to the canals. In some instances, especially in erect-eared dogs, the distal two thirds of the pinna may be more significantly affected. Pets with severe chronic disease may traumatize the convex surface of the ear. Secondary *Malassezia* and bacterial infections are common.

The diagnosis of an allergic otitis externa is based on history, physical examination, results of pinnal biopsy, response to a restrictive diet, and intradermal skin testing or serologic testing for atopy.

Contact Hypersensitivities and Irritant Reactions. The neomycin or propylene glycol in topical otic products is most commonly incriminated in animals with contact hypersensitivities, causing an acute exacerbation of severe otitis while the pet is being treated. Cytologic examination of exudates often reveals inflammatory cells where they were not present in earlier cytologic examinations. Contact hypersensitivities may be difficult to differentiate from irritant otitic reactions. Irritant reactions involving alcohol, glycerin, povidone-iodine, and 2.5 per cent acetic acid have been reported.[20] Otitis-related breaks in the epithelial barrier of the ear may allow for irritation by these drugs, whereas they may not affect normal skin.

Drug Reactions. Reactions to systemically administered drugs commonly affect the ears. There is often an acute exacerbation of diffuse pinnal erythema with variable degrees of swelling and exudation, erosion, and full-thickness epidermal necrosis.

Foreign Bodies. Grass awns, foxtails, dirt, and impacted debris may all cause significant irritation within ears. Impacted debris may stretch the tympanum into the middle ear to produce a "false" middle ear. Grass awns and foxtails may migrate through the tympanum to cause otitis media.

Ectoparasites. *Otodectes cynotis* causes approximately 50 per cent of the cases of otitis in cats and 5 to 10 per cent in dogs.[18] Infestations are generally encountered in dogs and cats younger than 1 year of age. Variable hypersensitivities to the mite bite causes the inflammation associated with infestations. Some dogs and cats carry mites but remain asymptomatic. Severe inflammation may result in decreased mite numbers in affected ears.[18] Mites may also inhabit other areas of the skin (e.g., head, neck). Diagnosis is made by direct otoscopic or cytologic examination.

Demodicosis commonly causes otitis externa in dogs with generalized demodicosis, but these mites can be restricted to the ears, especially in cats. In the cat, *Demodex* infection may only cause a ceruminous otitis with large amounts of brown waxy debris. Diagnosis is often possible using mineral oil preparations of debris taken by swabs. Less commonly, hair plucking, scraping, and even skin biopsy may be necessary to confirm a diagnosis. Other ectoparasites can also cause otitis externa.

Keratinization/Sebaceous Gland Disorders (Ceruminous or Seborrheic Otitis).

Hypothyroidism, hyperestrogenism, sebaceous adenitis, and idiopathic seborrheas (e.g., in the cocker spaniel) may be associated with low-grade inflammation within the ears, possibly as a result of the accumulation of abnormal fatty acids. Affected individuals almost always have significant, more generalized cutaneous involvement.

Idiopathic Inflammatory/Hyperplastic Otitis in the Cocker Spaniel.

This disease, which must be differentiated from allergic and idiopathic seborrhea, affects only the ears. A local hypersensitivity to perhaps some component of cerumen has been hypothesized as the cause.

Other Primary Factors.

Autoimmune diseases including the pemphigus complex and systemic and discoid lupus erythematosus may cause inflammation and crusting that is usually more restricted to the more distal aspects of the medial surface of the pinna. Zinc-responsive dermatoses have a similar distribution of inflammation and scaling/crusting. These animals almost always have skin lesions involving other areas of the body that facilitate diagnosis.

Predisposing Factors

Predisposing factors are those that make the ear more susceptible to inflammation initiated by primary factors but by themselves do not cause otitis.

Temperature and Humidity.

Increases in ambient temperature, humidity, rainfall, and swimming have all been shown to have a direct correlation with the incidence of otitis externa. Increased temperature and humidity within the ear likely predisposes to otitis through alteration of the normal barrier function of the epidermis.

Anatomic Predispositions.

Numerous anatomic predispositions to otitis externa have also been noted. Pendulous ears are prone to developing otitis externa, perhaps due to poor aeration, increased humidity, and increased temperature. Recent studies have shown no difference in ear temperature in pendulous- and erect-eared dogs.[21] Hair in ears is generally not a problem unless otitis is present and hair becomes a trap for debris. Hair plucking in such cases may be beneficial. Routine hair plucking for dogs with normal ears is generally not necessary nor recommended. Congenitally stenotic ear canals are noted in certain breeds (e.g., stenotic horizontal canals in some chow chows and English Bulldogs; stenosis of the entrance to the vertical canal and at the vertical/horizontal canal junction in Shar Peis). In these ears, a relatively minor degree of inflammation results in more rapid occlusion of the canals with debris. Increased ceruminous (apocrine) gland tissue has been noted in breeds that are prone to otitis externa (cocker spaniels, springer spaniels, Labrador retrievers),[14] but the true significance of this finding is unknown.

Obstructive Ear Disease.

Neoplasia, polyps, and proliferative changes predispose to otitis by altering the normal "flushing" mechanisms of the ear and by producing a micro-environment that is prone to the development of secondary infections.

Perpetuating Factors

Perpetuating factors are those that are responsible for continuing the inflammatory response, even though the original primary factors may no longer be present or active.

Bacterial Colonization/Infection.

Bacteria are found in small numbers in normal ears. In dogs, these include *Staphylococcus epidermidis*, *Staphylococcus intermedius*, *Micrococcus* species, and occasional coliforms.[22] Bacteria that proliferate in association with otitis externa are usually opportunists but contribute significantly to pathologic changes. Infection is usually suggested by the concurrent presence of inflammatory cells and intracellular bacteria on cytologic examination. The presence of large numbers of bacteria without an inflammatory response suggests colonization. Increased numbers of bacteria may break down ceruminous components to potentially irritating products like fatty acids. For this reason, emphasis is placed on normalizing bacterial numbers in all cases of otitis externa.

The most common bacterial isolates associated with otitis externa are *Staphylococcus intermedius* (30 to 50 per cent of cases), *Pseudomonas aeruginosa*, *Proteus* species, *Streptococcus* species, *Escherichia coli*, and *Corynebacterium* species.[22, 23] Acute otitis externa is usually associated with *Staphylococcus intermedius*. As the otitis externa becomes more chronic, or if there is a history of chronic topical antibiotic therapy, the incidence of gram-negative infections increases, with that from *Pseudomonas aeruginosa* predominating.[22] The most common bacteria associated with feline otitis externa are *Staphylococcus intermedius*, *Streptococcus* species, and *Pasteurella multocida*. *Pseudomonas aeruginosa*, *Proteus* species and *E. coli* are less commonly encountered.[16]

Malassezia pachydermatis.

Malassezia pachydermatis has been identified in 20 to 49 per cent of normal dog ears and up to 23 per cent of normal cat ears.[24] *Malassezia* is considered an opportunist that proliferates in otherwise inflamed ears. Increased numbers of *Malassezia* have been observed in 50 to 80 per cent of dogs with otitis externa and have been shown to cause inflammation perhaps due to byproducts of lipid/*Malassezia* interaction (e.g., formation of peroxides) and type I reactions to *Malassezia* or its byproducts.[18, 22–27]

Proliferative Changes.

Proliferative changes within the ear canals are generally the result of chronic inflammation and irritation. Epidermal hyperkeratosis, acanthosis, dermal fibrosis, edema, and apocrine gland hyperplasia and dilation produce skin thickening that is thrown into folds. Reactive fibrous, pyogranulomatous nodules, and polyps may also develop.[28] These changes produce a microenvironment that may readily harbor bacteria, yeast, and potentially irritating components of cerumen.

Otitis Media.

Otitis media perpetuates otitis externa through its reservoir effect by harboring bacteria, yeast, and potentially irritating debris.

Contact Hypersensitivities/Irritant Dermatitis.

Both of these problems function as primary factors but may also perpetuate otitis externa once infectious components or underlying allergies are under control.

Treatment Errors, Undertreatment, and Overtreatment.

Overtreated ears often remain inflamed in spite of resolution of infections. Maceration (keeping the ear too moist) and irritation likely contribute most significantly.

ENT

Overtreated ears often accumulate large quantities of opalescent debris, as seen on otoscopic examination. Cytologic examination usually shows only large numbers of epithelial cells.

DIAGNOSTIC PRINCIPLES

Physical Examination. The most productive pathway to an appropriate diagnosis and therapy for otitis externa begins with a history, plus dermatologic, physical, and otoscopic examinations. Otoscopic examination should include notation of the following: parasites, the degree of inflammation within the canals, the size of the canals, the amount and nature of exudate, proliferative changes, and the appearance of the tympanic membrane.

Cytologic Examination. When excessive amounts of waxy debris or inflammatory exudate are encountered within the canals, a cytologic examination should be performed and repeated at each follow-up visit. Oil immersion microscopy (100×) should be used to identify and quantitate bacteria, yeast, inflammatory cells, and debris. Smears should be heat-fixed and stained with modified Wright's stain (e.g., Diff-Quick). Gram's stain is generally not necessary because the stain characteristics of the organisms can often be predicted by their morphologic appearance (i.e., rods, gram-negative; cocci, gram-positive).

Smears from normal ears generally reveal only an occasional bacterium or *Malassezia* organism per oil immersion field. Higher normal carriage rates are expected in warmer, more humid environments. The use of a scale (e.g., 1+ to 4+) to quantitate and record increased numbers of bacteria, yeasts, and inflammatory cells will facilitate the comparison of results from visit to visit. Cytologic examinations are often of most benefit in follow-up visits. If bacteria persist despite topical antibiotic therapy, consideration should be given to lack of owner compliance regarding therapy or the presence of a resistant strain of bacteria. Persistence of a significant amount of gross inflammation within the ear in spite of resolution of bacterial and yeast infections may suggest an underlying allergic or ceruminous otitis.

Culture and Sensitivity Testing. Culture and sensitivity testing are recommended only if resistant strains of bacteria are suspected. Resistance is suggested if there has been a history of chronic topical therapy or if bacteria persist in spite of appropriate therapy. If bacteria or yeasts are not seen on cytologic examination, it is unlikely that they will be recovered by culture or are significant to the pathogenesis of the disease.

This may not be true for the cytologic examination of debris taken from the middle ear. Culture results may be positive when cytologic examinations are negative.[23] Culture and sensitivity testing is recommended in all cases in which otitis media is suspected. Cultures should be taken from both the canal and middle ear.

Radiology, Computed Tomography, and Magnetic Resonance Imaging. Otitis media is an important perpetuating factor of otitis externa. In all cases of chronic or recurrent otitis externa in which the tympanic membrane is abnormal, or cannot be seen because of canal swelling or proliferation, the tympanic bulla should be radiographed. The lack of radiographic changes, however, does not always preclude the presence of middle ear disease (see Otitis Media). Radiographs can also provide prognostic information in cases of chronic proliferative otitis externa. The presence of aural cartilage calcification is usually associated with a poor prognosis for medical management.

GENERAL PRINCIPLES OF MANAGEMENT

The general goals of therapy for otitis externa are to control or remove primary factors, reduce inflammation, resolve bacterial or yeast infections, and clean and dry the ears. These endpoints are generally achieved through the appropriate use of topical and, at times, systemic therapies.

Ear Cleaning. Establishing a clean, dry ear is extremely important in the management of otitis externa. Accumulated oils, waxes, and debris may directly irritate the ear or may contain microscopic foreign material that is irritating. Debris also produces a microenvironment that is conducive to the proliferation of bacteria and yeast, and it may prevent medication from contacting the lining of the ear and may inactivate constituents of the medication (e.g., polymixin B). Debris may also significantly impair hearing.

Aggressive ear cleaning should not be attempted in severely swollen or proliferative ears. These ears are better treated first with systemic and/or topical glucocorticoids (in anti-inflammatory dosages) and antibiotics. Once the canals have "opened up," more effective ear cleaning can be achieved.

Ear cleaning is generally accomplished through the use of a topical ceruminolytic and/or a flushing system. Ceruminolytics are generally surfactants and detergents that emulsify, soften, and break up waxy debris and exudate. Examples, in decreasing order of potency, include dioctyl sodium or calcium sulfosuccinate, carbamide peroxide (acts as a humectant by releasing urea and also releases oxygen to create a foaming action), squalene, triethanolamine polypeptide elite condensate and hexamethyltetracosane, propylene glycol, glycerin, and mineral oil. Other ingredients often included with ceruminolytics include alpha-hydroxy acids (e.g., lactic, salicylic, benzoic, and malic acids), which have significant pH-reducing, keratolytic, and mild antibacterial and antifungal effects, alcohol, chlorbutanol, and isopropyl myrisate.

Ceruminolytics are usually placed in the ear 5 to 15 minutes before a flushing procedure to facilitate breakup of debris. The ceruminolytics may be flushed out with water, saline, or a germicidal solution such as chlorhexidine, povidone-iodine, polyhydroxidine iodine (Xenodyne), or acetic acid (see Table 122–2 for dilutions). Milder ceruminolytic products (often marketed as combination cleanser/dryers; e.g., Epi-Otic, Oti-Cleans) may be used by owners for at-home flushing. Ceruminolytics and flushing solutions have the potential to be ototoxic and should not be used in the presence of a perforated tympanum. Exceptions include squalene, diluted acetic acid, water, and saline (see Ototoxicity).

For most acute cases of otitis with significant ceruminous and purulent debris accumulation, sufficient cleansing may be achieved at home by the owners. Water-miscible products tend to be less messy for routine use. Milder combination cleanser/dryers are often preferred. The ear is filled with solution and massaged. The dog or cat then shakes out the solution. This procedure may be repeated daily or every other day. Flushing with an ear bulb syringe is best done by the veterinarian, technician, or responsible owner who has been thoroughly instructed regarding technique. This technique often fails to retrieve debris adjacent to the tympanic membrane.

Thorough ear cleansing is usually most effective with the animal under general anesthesia. Large particulate material, foreign bodies, and hair can usually be removed with alligator forceps through a surgical otoscope head. Ear curettes (generally size 0, 1, or 2) may be effective but must be used with great care in the region of the tympanum. Debris is most effectively and safely removed by flushing and suction. Flushing should be performed under direct visualization through a surgical otoscope head with an open-ended tomcat catheter attached to a 12-mL syringe. Suction can be obtained with the same unit. Alternatively, a 6- to 8-inch length of 3.5, 5, or 8 French feeding tube attached to a syringe may be used. More effective suction can be achieved through a regulated suction bottle attached to an "in-house" vacuum system or homemade vacuum system. The suction hose is attached to a 14- or 16-gauge, 5.5-inch Teflon catheter (Abbott Hospital, Inc., North Chicago, IL).

Flushing solutions include dilute chlorhexidine, povidone-iodine (see Table 122–2), or water/saline. Water or saline is preferred if the integrity of the tympanum is not known.

Topical Therapy. Eighty to 85 per cent of acute otitis externa cases can be managed with topical therapy alone.[16] In many of these cases, the primary factor initiating the otitis may not be defined.

Most topical medications indicated for the treatment of otitis externa contain a glucocorticoid in combination with an antifungal and/or an antibiotic. These combination products work well because otitis externa, regardless of underlying cause, tends to involve similar pathologic changes: edema, hyperemia, and thickening of the stratum corneum (hyperkeratosis) in more acute cases and epidermal hyperplasia, inflammatory cell infiltrates, ceruminous gland dilatation, and dermal fibrosis in more chronic cases. Colonization and infection with bacteria and yeast are common.

Topical glucocorticoids are vasoconstrictive, are antiproliferative, and may decrease ceruminous and sebaceous secretions. The anti-inflammatory potency of glucocorticoids is profoundly affected by the vehicles in which they are formulated. Although there are no data comparing the anti-inflammatory potency of glucocorticoids in veterinary otic preparations, empirically, products containing hydrocortisone and prednisone are considered mild; triamcinolone acetonide and isoflupredone, moderate; and dexamethasone and betamethasone, potent. Perhaps the most potent is a combination of fluocinolone and dimethysulfoxide (DMSO). DMSO may significantly potentiate the anti-inflammatory effects of glucocorticoids.

Significant systemic absorption of otic glucocorticoids occurs. Suppression of the hypothalamic-pituitary axis and abnormalities in liver enzyme activities consistent with steroid hepatopathy have been noted in 7 and 21 days, respectively, after the use of triamcinolone acetate (Panalog) and dexamethasone (Tresaderm).[29, 30] Although several weeks of topical therapy with more potent topical glucocorticoids may not be deleterious, the long-term, frequent use of potent topical products can cause iatrogenic hyperadrenocorticism.

The topical antibiotics used most commonly in the treatment of otitis externa include the aminoglycosides neomycin (e.g., Tresaderm, Panalog) and gentamicin (e.g., Otomax). Chloramphenicol (Liquachlor) and polymyxin B (Cortisporin, Surolan) are used less commonly.

Neomycin- and chloramphenicol-containing products ("first-line" therapies) work well for acute otitis that involves *Staphylococcus intermedius*. Gentamicin- and polymixin B–containing products have an enhanced gram-negative spectrum, especially against *Pseudomonas*, and as such are used when more resistant bacteria are suspected (i.e., bacteria persist in spite of appropriate first-line therapy; the ears have been frequently treated with first-line products in the past; rods predominate on cytologic examination). Product examples are listed in Table 122–2. Antibiotics for more

resistant bacterial infections are discussed further under Therapy for Specific Diseases.

Topical antifungal, and more specifically anti-*Malassezia*, ingredients commonly found in otic products include (in decreasing order of in vitro efficacy) ketoconazole, clotrimazole, miconazole, and nystatin.[26] Thiabendazole, although not effective in vitro, appears to have good effects in vivo. Ketoconazole has only recently been explored as a topical alternative medication in the dog.[31] The glucocorticoid component of most otic preparations may also inhibit *Malassezia* proliferation by normalizing the otic microenvironment and perhaps by a direct deleterious effect on the organism.[32]

Products containing predominantly glucocorticoids (e.g., hydrocortisone in BurOtic HC, fluocinolone in Synotic) are generally used for maintenance therapy in allergic ears and swimmer's ear.

Overall product choice in the management of otitis externa is dictated by the severity of inflammation and the presence and type of secondary infections. The common otic products noted earlier (e.g., Tresaderm, Panalog, Otomax) are generally used twice daily to initiate therapy. Resolution of the otitis externa can be determined only by otoscopic and cytologic examination, and therefore re-checks should be scheduled every 10 to 14 days until the problem is resolved or controlled. The majority of cases will reach this endpoint within 2 to 4 weeks.

Systemic Therapy. In otitis complicated by bacterial infection/colonization, oral antibiotics appear to be beneficial when there is moderate to severe thickening of the canals/proximal pinna (preventing adequate penetration of topical therapies) and when there is significant periaural skin dermatitis, ulcerative changes in the ear, or large numbers of inflammatory cells seen cytologically (indicating true infection or deeper skin involvement). Systemic antibiotics are indicated in all cases that involve a concurrent otitis media. Higher dosages of systemic antibiotics may be necessary to optimize responses.

Oral glucocorticoids at anti-inflammatory dosages are beneficial in the management of severe acute and chronic otitis externa, especially when allergies are the cause. They are the most effective means of reducing inflammatory and proliferative changes within the ear.

THERAPY FOR SPECIFIC DISEASES OF THE EAR CANAL

Ear Mites. Topical therapies with efficacy in treating ear mites include pyrethrin- or rotenone-containing products (generally do not kill mite eggs and as such are recommended for use throughout the 3-week life cycle of the mite); a thiabendazole-containing product (Tresaderm; believed to kill all stages of the mite, including the egg; use twice daily for 2 weeks); gentamicin, clotrimazole, betamethasone (Otomax; twice daily for 2 weeks); an iodine complex solution (Xenodyne; once daily for 4 weeks); and topical ivermectin (300–500 μg/kg once weekly for 4 to 5 weeks).[33] Because mites may inhabit other areas of the body, it is recommended that topical otic therapy be combined with a total body miticide treatment (e.g., fipronil). All dogs and cats in contact should be treated in a similar fashion.

Ivermectin, given orally once weekly for 4 weeks or subcutaneously every 10 to 14 days for two or three treatments has been effective against *Otodectes* infestations in both dogs and cats (see Table 122–2 for dosages). In milder cases, it may be used alone; in more severe cases, it is usually used in conjunction with topical treatments (e.g., Tresaderm). All animals in contact with each other are treated similarly.

Allergic Otitis Externa. Emphasis is first placed on resolving secondary bacterial and/or yeast infections with a combination antibiotic/antifungal/glucocorticoid preparation. For severely inflamed ears, consideration can be given to the use of a potent topical glucocorticoid such as fluocinolone and DMSO. Antibacterial coverage may be obtained with this product by mixing 3 to 8 mL of enrofloxacin (22.7 mg/mL) in 8 mL of fluocinolone/DMSO. If inflammation is severe or extensive and tissue proliferation is present, oral glucocorticoid therapy is often indicated at anti-inflammatory dosages for 1 to 2 weeks or longer (see Table 122–2).

Once inflammation/proliferation has been controlled, longer-term maintenance therapy can be achieved by using a mild, 0.5 to 1 per cent hydrocortisone product applied every 2 to 3 days. More severely inflamed ears may have to be treated with a potent steroid (fluocinolone/DMSO) every 2 to 3 days. When bacterial and/or yeast infections tend to be recurrent despite this therapy, consideration should be given to the use of long-term maintenance therapy with a combination product such as gentamicin/clotrimazole/betamethasone applied twice weekly. Recurrent yeast infections may be controlled with a maintenance topical miconazole solution. Debris accumulation should be minimized through the routine use of a combination cleansing/drying solution (e.g., Epi-Otic) two or three times a week.

Swimmer's Ear. In many instances, swimmers prone to otitis have underlying low-grade primary inflammatory disease (e.g., atopy). The goal of therapy, therefore, is to keep the ear clean and dry while providing some anti-inflammatory/antimicrobial activity. Drying agents for this purpose primarily contain alcohol or astringents (e.g., aluminium acetate, Domeboro Solution). Cleansing/drying products (e.g., Epi-Otic, Oti-Cleans) also have mild antibacterial and antifungal properties. Because low-grade allergies may play an underlying role in swimmer's ear, the use of a glucocorticoid-containing drying agent (hydrocortisone, aluminum acetate—BurOtic HC) is often preferred.

The aforementioned products are generally used on the day of swimming and for 2 to 5 days thereafter. For dogs that swim frequently, their routine use (either daily or every other day) may prove beneficial as maintenance therapy.

Idiopathic Inflammatory/Hyperplastic Otitis in the Cocker Spaniel. Proliferative otitis is best treated with a combination of oral glucocorticoids at anti-inflammatory dosages, a potent topical glucocorticoid/antibiotic/antifungal preparation (e.g., Otomax), and possibly oral antibiotics. Maintenance therapy often includes these more potent topical combination products on a twice-per-week basis and regular flushing with a cleanser/dryer preparation (e.g., Epi-Otic) once or twice weekly. Frequently, this regimen must be combined with the long-term use of low oral dose of glucocorticoids. Calcification of the auricular cartilages is associated with a poor response to medical therapy.

Resistant Bacterial Otitis with Emphasis on *Pseudomonas*. *Pseudomonas* infections are most commonly encountered in chronic otitis externa or after prolonged or intermittent topical antibiotic therapy. Refractory *Pseudomonas* infections may be attributed to acquired resistance, a failure to recognize and control underlying inflammatory disease (e.g., food sensitivity, atopy), otitis media, or reactions to topical medications that may be perpetuating the otitis (e.g., propylene glycol).

Suspected *Pseudomonas* infections are first empirically treated with polymixin B or gentamicin. When resistance is encountered, therapy is based on culture and sensitivity testing. Alternatives include enrofloxacin (injectable enrofoxacin 22.7 mg/mL diluted 1 part to 3 parts in saline or propylene glycol), Epi-Otic, Oti-Cleans, or fluocinolone and DMSO (instilled into a clean ear twice daily), amikacin (injectable diluted to 50 mg/mL; 4 to 6 drops twice daily), tobramycin (e.g., Tobrex ophthalmic), or ticarcillin or ticarcillin/clavulanic acid[34] (dilute to 25–100 mg/mL; frozen aliquots are good for 2 to 3 days); see Table 122–2 for specifics.

When *Pseudomonas* species are resistant to all routinely tested antibiotics, therapies to consider include silver sulfadiazine (0.1 per cent; must be used in a clean ear), polyhydroxidine-iodine complex (Xenodyne), and tris-EDTA[35, 36] (increases *Pseudomonas* sensitivity to several antibiotics, including gentamicin; often used as a pre-treatment 10 minutes before placing antibiotic in ear; can also be used as a single agent for topical maintenance therapy two to three times per week to keep *Pseudomonas* from recurring[36]). See Table 122–2 for formulations.

A topical or systemic glucocorticoid can be used, if necessary, for anti-inflammatory effects. Systemic antibiotics are commonly employed. Preference is often given to the use of enrofloxacin, 10 to 20 mg/kg given once daily. Aggressive parenteral ticarcillin therapy has also been reported to be effective.[34]

White vinegar (5 per cent) diluted 1:1 to 1:3 with water is the ear flush of choice for *Pseudomonas*-infected ears. Acetic acid solutions have specific efficacy in treating *Pseudomonas*.[18] Ulcerative lesions may be cauterized with 5 per cent silver nitrate.

Refractory or Recurrent *Malassezia* Infections. *Malassezia* infections are commonly resolved with products containing clotrimazole, miconazole, thiabendazole, or nystatin (listed in decreasing order of in vitro efficacy[26]). When *Malassezia* is refractory or recurrent, efforts must be directed toward recognizing and controlling underlying inflammatory primary factors (e.g., atopy, food sensitivity[8]). Perhaps the best overall therapy for refractory *Malassezia* is a 2- to 4-week course of oral ketoconazole (2.5–5 mg/1b or 5–10 mg/kg twice daily) or itraconazole (2.5 mg/1b or 5 mg/kg twice daily) or fluconazole (2.5 mg/1b or 5 mg/kg once daily or 30–50 mg/cat once daily for 7 to 10 days). Topical alternatives include 1 per cent miconazole (an anti-inflammatory effect can be produced by adding 7.5 mL injectable dexamethasone phosphate [4 mg/mL] to 30 mL 1 per cent miconazole or silver sulfadiazine [0.1 per cent]); used two to three times per week for the long-term management of recurrent *Malassezia* otitis.

Neoplasia. Chronic otitis externa is thought to be a predisposing factor in the development of tumors of the ear canals.[8, 37] Cocker spaniels appear to be a breed at increased risk for both benign and malignant tumors.[8]

The most common benign tumors in both dogs and cats are inflammatory polyps, papillomas, ceruminous gland adenomas, and basal cell tumors.[8, 37] Cats are prone to the development of ceruminous gland cysts, which are blue or black and contain black fluid. The most common malignant tumors in the dog are ceruminous gland adenocarcinomas, carcinomas of undetermined origin, and squamous cell carcinomas; and in cats, they are ceruminous gland adenocarcinomas, squamous cell carcinomas, and carcinomas of undetermined origin.[8, 37] In cats, ceruminous gland adenocarcinomas are variably reported as being most common, with squamous cell carcinomas reported as having an equal incidence in one study.[37]

Benign tumors in general tend to be nodular, pedunculated, and rarely ulcerated. Malignant tumors ar more likely to be broad based, ulcerated, and hemorrhagic. Twenty-five per cent of malignant tumors have evidence of bulla involvement.[8] Neurologic signs are seen in 10 per cent of dogs with malignant tumors and 25 per cent of cats with benign or malignant tumors.[8] In general, ear canal tumors tend to be locally invasive. Metastases are uncommon, with approximately 10 per cent of dogs and cats having metastases to the local lymph nodes or lungs.[8]

Malignant ear tumors in dogs tend to be less aggressive than in cats. In the dog, negative prognostic factors are bulla involvement and conservative surgical management.[8] In the cat, negative prognostic factors are neurologic signs, the presence of squamous cell carcinoma or carcinoma of undetermined origin, histopathologic evidence of lymphatic or vascular invasion, or conservative surgery.[8] Benign tumors may be treated with conservative surgeries. Malignant tumors are best treated with aggressive excision, including ear canal ablation and lateral bulla osteotomy. In general, the prognosis for malignant tumors in dogs after aggressive surgery is good (median survival of 58 months in one study[37]); in cats, the prognosis for ceruminous gland adenocarcinomas is fair (median survival, 12–49 months) but is guarded to poor for squamous cell carcinoma or carcinomas of undetermined origin (median survival, 4–6 months).[8, 37]

ROLE OF SURGERY IN THE MANAGEMENT OF OTITIS EXTERNA

Lateral ear resections are primarily indicated as adjunctive therapies to improve drainage, improve aeration, decrease canal temperature and humidity, and facilitate medication administration in animals with chronic otitis externa. They may also allow access to neoplasms of the canals for purposes of surgical resection or biopsy. They are of most value when disease is restricted to the vertical canal or when performed early in the course of the ear disease, before irreversible changes have occurred within the ear canals, tympanic membrane, or bulla. When intended to cure chronic or recurrent otitis externa, they have a high failure rate (47 to 80 per cent[38, 39]). This is attributed to the presence of intractable horizontal canal disease, otitis media, or persistent disease in the remaining vertical canal and proximal pinna (as is commonly seen with allergies).

Vertical ear canal resection is most commonly performed in dogs with tumors, traumatic injuries, or severe proliferative disease localized to the vertical canal. The procedure may also be used to alter the microclimate of the ear. Vertical ear canal resection is prone to the same shortcomings as the lateral ear resection.

Intractable disease associated with severe proliferation of the horizontal canal and calcification of the auricular cartilages is usually not amenable to successful medical management. Ablation of the entire ear canal combined with bulla osteotomy and curettage has proved extremely beneficial in such cases. In one study, 95 per cent of dogs with otitis externa and otitis were cured with this surgery.[40] Several studies suggest that hearing does not deteriorate postoperatively, although many of these dogs may be functionally deaf before surgery and hearing may only be by osseous conduction.[41, 42]

DISEASES OF THE MIDDLE AND INNER EAR

NORMAL ANATOMY AND PHYSIOLOGY

The middle ear consists of the tympanic membrane, the osseous bulla (tympanic cavity), and the auditory ossicles (malleus, incus, stapes). The osseous bulla is an air-filled space lined with a modified respiratory mucosa that includes small numbers of ciliated and secretory cells.[43] The auditory canal connects the middle ear to the caudal nasal pharynx with a mucociliary system capable of clearing material. The canine middle ear has a normal bacterial flora that includes *Corynebacterium*, *Klebsiella pneumoniae*, *Staphylococcus aureus*, *E. coli*, *Streptococcus*, and *Branhamella* species.[44]

The facial, sympathetic, and parasympathetic nerves pass through or near the middle ear. The facial nerve traverses the facial canal in the petrosal bone. In its course through the canal, a portion of the nerve is separated from the cavity of the tympanic bulla by only a small amount of loose connective tissue. Postganglionic sympathetic neurons pass through the middle ear, closely associated with the ventral surface of the petrosal bone. Parasympathetic preganglionic neurons also pass through the bulla.

The inner ear is made up of two parts, one within the other. The bony labyrinth is a series of channels in the petrous portion of the temporal bone. Inside these channels is a series of membranous structures (membranous labyrinth) that generally duplicate the shape of the bony channels. The membranous labyrinth is made up of the cochlea, vestibule (saccule and utricle), and three semicircular canals. The cochlea of the inner ear is concerned with hearing. The axons from the neurons that innervate this structure form the auditory portion of the vestibulocochlear or eighth cranial nerve and terminate in the cochlear nuclei of the medulla oblongata. From here, axons carry auditory pulses to the inferior colliculi (the centers for auditory reflexes) and the auditory cortex. The saccule, utricle, and semicircular canals provide proprioceptive function. Changes in the position of the head are mediated through the vestibular apparatus to control the tone of muscles used in maintaining posture and equilibrium. The innervation of the vestibular apparatus is by means of the vestibular branch of the eighth cranial nerve. The vestibular nerves terminate in the vestibular nuclei and cerebellum. Pathways from the vestibular nuclei project to other brain stem centers, the cerebellum, the cerebral cortex, and the spinal cord.[45] Connections between the vestibular nuclei and the motor nuclei of cranial nerves III, IV, and VI account for the nystagmus associated with disorders of the vestibular system.

OTITIS MEDIA

Otitis media generally develops as an extension of otitis externa through a perforated tympanum. Pharyngeal infection may, in rare instances, extend to the middle ear through the auditory tube. Cats may develop otitis media through this route as a sequela to upper respiratory tract disease. Both secretory and purulent (infected) otitis media have been experimentally created in dogs by obstructing the pharyngeal opening of the auditory canal.[44] Involvement of the middle ear through hematogenous spread is rarely encountered.

Organisms cultured most frequently from affected middle ears, in decreasing order of frequency, include *Pseudomonas* species, *Staphylococcus intermedius*, *Malassezia*, beta-he-

ENT

molytic *Streptococcus*, *Corynebacterium* species, *Enterococcus* species, *Proteus* species, *E. coli*, and anaerobes.[23] Infections are commonly associated with perforating foreign bodies (e.g., grass awns), or they occur as a sequela to chronic, usually proliferative or severe otitis externa. The reported incidence of tympanic membrane perforations associated with chronic otitis externa varies from 0.03 to 50 per cent.[46] This wide range may reflect the difficulty in accurately assessing the integrity of the tympanum with conventional techniques. The tympanum may also re-form after perforation. In one study, the tympanic membrane was intact in 71 per cent of 38 ears with otitis media.[23, 43] There is a direct correlation between the incidence of otitis media and the presence of calcification of the auricular cartilages. Cocker spaniels and German shepherd dogs also appear to be predisposed to the development of otitis media.

Other causes of otitis media include fungal infections (*Aspergillus*, *Candida*), foreign bodies, neoplasia, inflammatory polyps, trauma, and primary bone tumors.[16] Aural cholesteatoma is a form of epidermoid cyst that is believed to form from a pocket in the tympanic membrane.[47] The keratin-filled cyst, which may fill much of the bulla, is found in conjunction with otitis media. The canals of ears with cholesteatoma are generally stenosed, owing to inflammation/proliferative tissue and are usually calcified. Radiographic changes may reveal thinning, a change in shape, and disruption of the bony bulla. Diagnosis is confirmed on histologic examination. Therapy for cholesteatoma is generally restricted to bulla osteotomy and ear ablation,[44] although some palliation has been achieved with retinoid therapy.

Animals with otitis media generally have signs of otitis externa (e.g., head shaking, rubbing or scratching at ears, discharge, odor). Signs more suggestive of the presence of otitis media include otic pain, swelling or stenosis of the ear canal, purulent otitis externa, or facial nerve palsy (drooping of the ear or lip, inability to move these structures, drooling of saliva, decreased or absent palpebral reflex, or exposure keratitis) and/or Horner's syndrome (ptosis, miosis, enophthalmos, protrusion of the third eyelid). Signs of abnormal peripheral vestibular function (head tilt, nystagmus, ataxia) suggest the presence of otitis interna.

Para-aural abscesses have also been associated with otitis media.

The diagnosis of otitis media is first suspected on a thorough physical examination. The temporomandibular joints should be palpated and manipulated for masses or pain. Pain on opening the mouth has been associated with middle ear neoplasia in the cat. The pharyngeal region should be examined for pathologic changes in the region of the auditory canals.

A thorough otoscopic examination should be performed. The finding of a perforated tympanum strongly supports the presence of otitis media. One must be aware that, especially when large amounts of debris are wedged into the deep horizontal canal, the tympanum may stretch into the bulla space, creating an apparently longer horizontal canal (also referred to as a "false" middle ear). This may give a false sense of perforation. The false middle ear phenomenon can only be ascertained by thorough cleaning, direct visualization, and/or gentle tapping (e.g., with catheter tip) to suggest apparent tympanum-like tissue covering bony structures on the medial wall of the tympanic cavity. Direct contact with bone often gives a different "feel." With medical therapy, the tympanum rapidly returns to a more normal position (e.g., often within one to two weeks), which would be faster than expected for complete regrowth of a severely perforated tympanum. The integrity of the tympanum can sometimes be assessed by placing a small, fixed amount of water or saline (e.g., 1 mL) in the horizontal canal at the level of the suspected perforation. Because the bulla in most medium-sized dogs will accept 2 to 5 mL, loss or inability to draw back this saline would suggest the presence of a perforation. This "test" is invalidated if the bulla is full of debris.

The lack of visible perforation does not preclude a diagnosis of otitis media. In one study, the tympanic membrane was intact in 70 per cent of dogs with otitis media.[23] The tympanum may re-form after perforation. Any significant discoloraton or bulging of the tympanum suggests the possibility of otitis media.

Radiographic studies of the bulla are indicated whenever otitis media is suspected, but the tympanum or a tympanic rupture cannot be visualized. Recommended views are dorsoventral, lateral, lateral obliques, and a rostroventral-caudodorsal open-mouth oblique (open-mouth bulla view). Increased tissue opacity within the bulla may signify acute or chronic otitis media, neoplasia, or hemorrhage. Sclerosis and thickening of the bulla wall are considered to be normal changes in aged animals (primarily cats), chronic otitis media, and nasopharyngeal polyps. Lysis of the tympanic bulla and/or petrous temporal bone is seen with malignant neoplasia, chronic otitis media, and osteomyelitis.[48] Thinning of the bulla wall is generally seen with slowly growing, compressive lesions such as cholesteatoma or benign neoplasia. Unfortunately, the absence of radiographic changes does not preclude a diagnosis of otitis media. In one study, 25 per cent of 19 clinical cases failed to show radiographic changes when otitis media was confirmed by surgical exploration.[49] These may represent more acute cases. Computed tomography and magnetic resonance imaging provide more definitive, non-invasive diagnostic data.[48]

When otitis media is suspected based on clinical signs or imaging studies, but the tympanum is visualized and intact, myringotomy may be performed to harvest samples for cytologic examination and culture and sensitivity testing. Myringotomy may also relieve pain and pressure and allow for lavage and instillation of medication. Myringotomy is performed with the dog or cat anesthetized and after thorough flushing/lavage of the canals. The caudoventral aspect of the pars tensa is perforated with a 20-gauge spinal needle (under direct visualization through an otoscope). Suction can be applied through the needle, or the needle may be replaced with an open-ended tomcat catheter. Flushing with 0.5 to 1 mL of sterile saline may be necessary if samples are not readily retrievable. Alternatively, a sterile culture swab (Calgiswab, Spectrum Laboratories, Inc, Dallas, TX) may be passed into the middle ear. Surgical exploration may be the most accurate and cost-effective means of diagnosing otitis media in questionable cases.

If medical management is to be attempted, debris should initially be retrieved from the canals and middle ear for cytologic examination and culture and sensitivity testing. In one study comparing cultures from the middle ear versus those from ear canals, differences in isolates and in the sensitivity patterns of isolates were seen in 90 per cent of ears.[23] Culture was also reported to be more accurate than cytology in defining infections within the middle ear.[23]

The external ear canals and middle ear should be thoroughly flushed with sterile saline while the animal is under general anesthesia. Over the course of therapy, several general anesthesias may be necessary for purposes of cleaning.

Pending culture and sensitivity testing, therapies are based on cytologic findings. With a perforated tympanum, every effort should be made to use topical medications that are least likely to be ototoxic. Topical therapies that do not appear to be ototoxic include (1) enrofloxacin and ticarcillin; (2) glucocorticoids in saline (e.g., dexamethasone phosphate), fluocinolone, DMSO; and (3) flushing agents—dilute acetic acid (1:1–1:3), saline, and Constant Cleans Dermal Wound Cleanser (Sherwood Medical, St. Louis, MO). If necessary, topical therapies with ototoxic potential may be necessary (see Ototoxicity).

Systemic antibiotic therapy with enrofloxacin, cephalexin, clavulanic acid/amoxicillin, or trimethoprim-sulfamethoxazole (see Table 122–2) is recommended for at least 4 to 6 weeks. Oral glucocorticoids (e.g., prednisone) may also be considered to reduce canal swelling and facilitate flushing. This is especially effective when allergy is an underlying factor. At-home flushing should be continued daily or every other day initially. Aggressive attempts must also be made to concurrently resolve otitis externa. Topical and systemic therapy should be continued until all evidence of infection has resolved.

Dogs that undergo rupture of the tympanum intentionally by myringotomy or iatrogenically during removal of a foreign body from the ear canal typically sustain a puncture wound that heals within 2 weeks.[50] Acutely destroyed tympanic membranes (involving the entire pars tensa) were completely healed between days 21 and 35 in otherwise healthy dogs.[50] When medical therapy fails to resolve the otitis media, consideration should be given to ventral bulla osteotomy or ear ablation and lateral bulla osteotomy. If the tympanum fails to heal, the structure of the ear encourages the re-accumulation of debris. In such cases, regular flushing, possibly combined with a lateral ear resection to facilitate drainage, may offer control. Otherwise, a surgical resolution of the problem should be considered (ear ablation and bulla osteotomy).

NEOPLASIA OF THE MIDDLE EAR

Neoplasms originating from the middle ears of dogs and cats are rare.[51, 52]

INFLAMMATORY POLYPS OF THE MIDDLE EAR IN CATS

Inflammatory polyps composed of an admixture of macrophages, neutrophils, and plasma cells and lymphocytes are known to originate from the lining of the tympanic cavity, auditory canal, and nasopharynx of the cat.[53] They may occur as a result of ascending infection from the nasopharynx or from prolonged infection of the middle ear. The finding of lesions in 6-month-old sibling kittens with no evidence of underlying inflammation suggests a congenital predisposition.[53]

Affected cats tend to be younger (1 to 5 years of age), but cats of all ages are susceptible. Clinical signs usually include respiratory stridor, dyspnea, dysphagia, and evidence of external or middle/inner ear disease. Diagnosis is based on careful oropharyngeal evaluation and otoscopic and radiographic examination of the middle and nasal cavity. Treatment is surgical excision.[54, 55]

OTITIS INTERNA

Otitis interna most commonly arises as a progression from infection or neoplastic disease related to otitis media. In some instances, the inflammation may be an extension of inflammatory/neoplastic disease from the middle ear.[52]

The clinical signs of otitis interna include asymmetric ataxia (animal falls or drifts to side of lesion), head tilt usually toward the side of the lesion, circling to the side of the lesion, horizontal or rotatory nystagmus with the quick phase away from the side of the lesion, and positional or vestibular strabismus with the eyeball ipsilateral to the lesion deviated ventrally. Facial nerve paralysis or Horner's syndrome may be present. Signs of paresis or proprioceptive deficits associated with a head tilt usually indicate central vestibular disease. Bilateral vestibular disease does not produce a head tilt. The animal will walk in a crouched fashion.

The diagnosis and treatment of otitis interna is generally established on the basis of neurologic examination and an evaluation for otitis media. Aggressive medical or surgical management is indicated to prevent the spread of infectious disease into the brain stem.

PROGNOSIS FOR OTITIS MEDIA/INTERNA

The prognosis for the medical management of infectious otitis media/interna is poor if the ear canals remain stenotic, if the middle ear cannot be thoroughly cleaned and kept clean, if there is osteomyelitis or significant bony proliferation/lysis, or if resistant organisms are encountered. In chronic otitis media/interna, neurologic deficits are often permanent, especially in the cat.[52] However, many dogs and cats learn to compensate for vestibular disorders. Facial paralysis and keratoconjunctivitis sicca, when encountered, are usually permanent.

OTOTOXICITY

Ototoxic drugs affect the cochlea, the vestibule, and the semicircular canals, with subsequent effects on hearing, vestibular function, or both. Toxic drugs (Table 122–3) reach the inner ear either by means of local application or hematogenously. The development of topical ototoxicity generally

TABLE 122–3. OTOTOXIC DRUGS*

AMINOGLYCOSIDE ANTIBIOTICS	ANTISEPTICS
Amikacin A†	Chlorhexidine
Kanamycin A†	Ethanol
Streptomycin V†	Iodine (iodophor)
Neomycin A + V†	Benzalkonium chloride
Gentamicin A + V†	Benzethonium chloride
Tobramycin A + V†	Cetrimide
OTHER ANTIBIOTICS	**MISCELLANEOUS**
Erythromycin	Propylene glycol
Poymyxin B, E	Cisplatin
Minocycline	Trialkyl tin compounds
Vancomycin	(trimethyl tin chloride
Chloramphenicol	and triethyl tin bromide)
LOOP DIURETICS	Quinine
	Lead
Furosemide	Mercury
Bumetanide	Arsenic
Ethacrynic acid	Salicylates
	Detergents

*Ototoxicity only critically evaluated for gentamicin, neomycin, streptomycin, and chlorhexidine in cats and hygromycin C, furosemide, bumetanide, and cisplatin in dogs. All other reports involved laboratory animal experiments or reports of human toxicities.

†Predominant functional impairment: V = vestibular; A = auditory.

requires a perforated tympanum and deposition of the material within the middle ear. Absorption into the inner ear is through the round or oval window. With otitis media, the round window may become more permeable to macromolecules.[52] Ototoxicity after systemic drug therapies (primarily aminoglycosides) usual follows high dosages, prolonged therapy (over 14 days), or concurrent renal failure (affecting drug excretion). There may be selective damage to the cochlea or vestibular apparatus or both. Damage may occur to the hair cells, the stria vascularis, the organ of Corti, the neuroepithelium of the vestibular appartus, or associated neurons.

The true prevalence of ototoxicity associated with topical use of these drugs is open to question:

1. Much of this information is anecdotal.
2. Studies were performed in chinchillas and guinea pigs, known for their increased sensitivity to ototoxicity when compared with other species.
3. Studies used topical concentrations of drugs that far exceed the concentrations found in proprietary medications.
4. Studies used administration protocols that do not mimic clinical situations.
5. Studies looked only at normal animals, whereas the presence of inflammatory middle/inner ear disease may enhance toxicity.[56–58]
6. Reactions may be idiosyncratic.

Toxicity from aminoglycosides (commonly used in humans[59]) after topical otic therapy in dogs with a ruptured tympanum appears to be rare in clinical practice. However, it is wise to use aminoglycosides only if indicated by cytologic findings or results of culture and sensitivity testing.

IDIOPATHIC VESTIBULAR/FACIAL NERVE DISEASES

Idiopathic Facial Paralysis. It is imperative that an infectious otitis media/interna be ruled out before the institution of therapy. Prognosis is generally good without therapy.

Congenital Vestibular Syndromes. Congenital vestibular syndromes have been reported in purebred dogs and cats. Deafness may also be noted. There is no therapy.

DEAFNESS

Causes of Deafness. The two major categories of deafness are conduction deafness and sensorineural deafness. Conduction deafness occurs when there is a failure of proper transmission of sound vibration to the inner ear and auditory nervous system. Abnormalities of, or diseases affecting, the external ear canal, tympanic membrane, auditory ossicles, and/or middle ear can cause conduction deafness. Examples include occlusion of the external ear canal with waxy debris, destruction of the tympanic membrane, and severe otitis externa/media.

In comparison, sensorineural deafness results from abnormalities of the inner ear structures, cochlear (auditory) nerve, and/or central auditory pathways in the brain stem, thalamus, and cerebrum. Causes of sensorineural deafness include inherited deafness, neural damage from ototoxic substances, and age-related or senile deafness.

Signalment. Inherited deafness has been reported to occur in numerous breeds of dogs (Table 122–4) and cats. It is a sensorineural deafness due to degeneration of inner ear structures and neurons of the spiral ganglion, with clinical signs apparent from a few weeks to a few months of age. Dogs with predominantly white, merle, or piebald coat coloring seem predisposed to inherited deafness. The mode of inheritance of deafness in dogs is predominantly autosomal dominant; however, recessive inheritance has been described in the bull terrier.[60] Many of these dogs also have associated ocular abnormalities. In Dalmatians, inherited deafness is presumed to be associated with white coat color arising from a gene for coat color spotting.[61] Inherited deafness in cats has not been documented by breed but is clearly associated with a dominant gene for white coat color.[61] In addition, blue eye color in white cats has a strongly positive correlation for deafness.[62]

History. There should be documentation of the animal's age at the onset of deafness (inherited vs. acquired deafness), head shaking, ear scratching, pinna and canal irritation or discharge that might indicate the presence of excessive wax accumulation, otitis or foreign bodies, previous head trauma or illnesses such as viral or rickettsial infection, and previously administered medications (ototoxicity). The owners should specifically be asked about signs suggestive of vestibular or other neurologic dysfunction.

Clinical Evaluation of Hearing Loss. Degree of hearing loss varies greatly, depending on the nature and severity of the underlying cause and the extent of involvement (unilateral or bilateral). Behavioral changes or abnormalities suggestive of hearing loss are usually recognized by the owners of animals with complete or nearly complete bilateral hearing loss.

Behavioral Evaluation. An animal suspected of being deaf should be challenged with sounds of varying intensity and frequency from different directions and observed for a response. Sometimes behavioral responses are difficult to interpret. Care should be taken to avoid making sounds that could alert the animal through "feel" (e.g., slamming a door) or visual cueing (e.g., clapping hands in front of the animal). To avoid visual cueing, other animals and people should not be present during the evaluation. Some animals

TABLE 122–4. CANINE BREEDS WITH REPORTED INHERITED DEAFNESS

Akita	Great Dane
American Staffordshire terrier	Great Pyrenees
Australian blue heeler	Greyhound
Australian shepherd	Ibizan hound
Beagle	Kuvasz
Border collie	Maltese
Boston terrier	Miniature poodle
Boxer	Mongrel
Bull terrier	Norwegian dunkerhound
Catahoula leopard dog	Old English sheepdog
Cocker spaniel	Papillon
Collie	Pointer
Dalmatian	Rhodesian ridgeback
Dappled dachshund	Rottweiler
Doberman pinscher	Saint Bernard
Dogo Argentino	Scottish terrier
English bulldog	Sealyham terrier
English setter	Shetland sheepdog
Foxhound	Shropshire terrier
Fox terrier	Walker American foxhound
German shepherd	West Highland white terrier

Strain GM: Congenital deafness in dogs and cats. Compend Contin Ed Small Anim Pract 13:245–250, 1991.

will acclimatize to repetitive sound, or just not react, and appear to be deaf when they are not. Frightened or uncooperative animals may be impossible to evaluate.

Physical Examination. Abnormalities of the external ear canals and tympanic membranes, along with the presence or absence of excessive ear wax accumulation, foreign bodies, and/or infection or irritation, should be noted. Compliance of the tympanic membrane can be visually observed with an appropriately equipped otoscope. If evidence of additional neurologic dysfunction is found, additional diagnostic tests such as cerebrospinal fluid analysis, blood and cerebrospinal fluid titers, and computed tomography or magnetic resonance imaging of the head may need to be performed.

Electrodiagnostic Evaluation of Hearing Loss. Impedance audiometry and auditory-evoked response testing provide a quantitative way to determine the type (conduction vs. sensorineural) and degree (partial vs. complete) of deafness present and the symmetry (unilateral vs. bilateral) of dysfunction. Both tests require specialized equipment, thereby requiring referral to neurologic specialty centers in most cases.

Impedance Audiometry: Tympanometry and Acoustic Reflex Testing. Tympanometry determines the status of middle ear function by evaluating the integrity and compliance of the tympanic membrane, the mobility of the bony ossicles, and the function of the middle ear muscles and their attachments, as well as the size of the external ear canal.[62] Tympanometric abnormalities would indicate conduction deafness, whereas normal results in a hearing-impaired animal would support a diagnosis of sensorineural deafness.

When a loud noise is presented to the ear, the muscles of the middle ear reflexively contract to dampen the effect of the loudness on the inner ear. This is known as the stapedial or acoustic reflex. The auditory nerve is the afferent arm of the reflex arc, and the trigeminal (tensor tympani muscle) and facial (stapedius muscle) nerves are the efferent arm. The acoustic reflex can be measured during tympanometry. Ipsilateral and contralateral response muscle reflexes are recorded. If the reflex is present, it is a strong indicator that the auditory system is intact.

Auditory Evoked Responses. Early latency (1–10 ms) auditory evoked responses to externally applied auditory stimuli have proved extremely valuable in the assessment of hearing function in animals. Early latency responses are believed to arise mainly from brain stem generators, thus the term *brain stem auditory-evoked response* (BAER). In normal animals, BAER consists of five to seven reproducible waves that represent various levels of the auditory nervous system beginning with the auditory nerve (wave I). Most animals do not require drug restraint for testing. However, BAER is little affected by level of consciousness so sedation or general anesthesia can be used without significantly altering the response recorded. Middle (10–15 ms) and late (50–250 ms) latency responses to auditory stimulation have been studied in animals, but they are of little clinical usefulness and are altered significantly by sedation or general anesthesia. Puppies and kittens are not born with a mature auditory system. BAER latencies and amplitudes have been shown to approach adult values as early as 2 weeks of age but more frequently mature between 6 and 8 weeks of age.[62] This must be kept in mind when evaluating puppies and kittens for inherited deafness to avoid labeling an immature BAER as abnormal. Breeders often want to test early to eliminate deaf puppies from the litter as soon as possible. However, it is advisable to wait until at least 6 weeks of age to perform

screening BAER tests for inherited deafness to avoid erroneous conclusions.

In normal animals, BAER wave amplitudes and latencies vary depending on the intensity level of auditory stimulation and the rate of stimulus presentation. Increasing stimulus intensity produces a corresponding decrease in latency and increase in amplitude of waveforms recorded. An increase in stimulus rate causes a decrease in wave amplitude and increase in latency. Most BAER clinical tests are performed leaving stimulation rate constant and increasing intensity in regular increments over a set range of decibels (e.g., 75 to 105 dB). Auditory responses are recorded simultaneously from the right and left sides of the brain from electrodes placed on the head in a standardized montage. Several hundred stimulus responses are averaged together to produce the recognizable waveforms of the BAER. In a normal animal, there are many cross-over connections between left and right sides of the brain stem so that stimuli presented to one ear will be "heard" by both sides of the brain, resulting in nearly identical left- and right-side BAER responses.

In animals, the main clinical use of BAER has been in the evaluation of deafness, particularly inherited and senile deafness. However, it should be remembered that the auditory pathways traverse the brain stem extensively from side to side and back to front. Consequently, BAER provides a fairly good evaluation of brain stem integrity in general and can be used in cases of head trauma, inflammatory disease, and other conditions when an animal is comatose and cranial nerve reflexes cannot be evaluated.

Conduction deafness in effect reduces the intensity of air-conducted sound stimuli by failing to present the stimuli to the inner ear properly. At low-intensity stimulation, BAER may not be recognized, but increasing the intensity of the stimulus will often "drive out" a response. When recorded, wave I will often have a prolonged latency and perhaps a reduced amplitude. Bone-conducted BAER bypasses these impediments by stimulating the cochlea directly. A normal bone-conducted BAER in the presence of an abnormal air-conducted BAER confirms the presence of conduction deafness.

Sensorineural deafness can cause abnormalities in any part of the BAER, depending on the anatomic site of the lesion. Most sensorineural deafness (e.g., inherited, ototoxicity, otitis interna) is due to disease of the cochlea and/or peripheral nerve. As a result, no BAER waveforms are generated. If the injury is further back in the auditory system, initial waves may be present, but waves generated beyond the point of the lesion will not appear. By knowing the location of generators of individual waveforms, a lesion can be localized. BAER can also be used to evaluate a return of function that may occur secondary to withdrawal of ototoxic drugs.

Senile or age-related deafness can be entirely sensorineural or a combination of sensorineural and conduction if chronic otitis or otosclerosis is also a component of the dysfunction. Evaluation of senile deafness has become increasingly important with the availability of hearing aids for pet animals. Most animals with senile deafness have some remaining sensorineural function. The BAER is then used to determine if enough hearing remains to warrant the expense and effort of training an animal to accept a hearing aid and which ear has the best remaining function and therefore should be fitted with the aid. Few animals learn to tolerate the presence of the hearing aid in their ear canal. Before spending a great deal of money on BAER testing and a hearing aid, owners of pets with age-related hearing loss can place foam ear plugs in the external ear canals of their pet as a "trial run." The foam ear plugs will cost only a few dollars at most, a less risky expenditure than the several hundred dollars required for testing and purchasing a hearing aid.

REFERENCES

1. Kirpensteijn J: Aural neoplasms. Semin Vet Med Surg (Small Anim) 8:17, 1993.
2. Marks SL, et al: Clinical evaluation of etretinate for the treatment of canine solar-induced squamous cell carcinoma and preneoplastic lesions. J Am Acad Dermatol 27:11, 1992.
3. Evans AG, et al: A trial of 13-cis-retinoic acid for treatment of squamous cell carcinoma and preneoplastic lesions on the head of cats. Am J Vet Res 46:2553, 1985.
4. Peaston AE: Photodynamic therapy for nasal and aural squamous cell carcinoma in cats. JAVMA 202:1261, 1993.
5. Bunge MM, et al: Relapsing polychondritis in a cat. J Am Anim Hosp Assoc 28:203, 1992.
6. Gross TL, et al: Veterinary Dermatopathology. St. Louis, Mosby–Year Book, 1992.
7. White SD, et al: Juvenile cellulitis in dogs: 15 cases (1979–1988). JAVMA 195:1609, 1989.
8. Vail DM, Withrow SJ: Tumors of the skin and subcutaneous Tissues. In Withrow SJ, MacEwen GE (eds): Small Animal Clinical Oncology, Philadelphia, WB Saunders, 1996, p 167.
9. Kuwahara J: Canine and feline aural hematoma: Clinical, experimental and clinicopathologic observations. Am J Vet Res 47:2300, 1986.
10. Kuwahara J: Canine and feline aural hematoma: Results of treatment with corticosteroids. J Am Anim Hosp Assoc 22:641, 1986.
11. Joyce JA, Day MJ: Immunopathogenesis of canine aural hematoma. J Small Anim Pract 38:152, 1997.
12. Fossum TW: Surgery of the ear. In Fossum TW, et al (eds): Small Animal Surgery. St. Louis, Mosby–Year Book, 1997, p 171.
13. Joyce JA: Treatment of canine aural haematoma using an indwelling drain and corticosteroids. J Small Anim Pract 35:341, 1994.
14. Stout-Graham M, et al: Morphologic measurements of the external horizontal ear canal of dogs. Am J Vet Res 51:990, 1990.
15. Logas DB: Diseases of the ear canal. In Rosychuk RAW, Merchant SR (eds): Ear, Nose and Throat. Vet Clin North Am Small Anim Pract 24:905, 1994
16. Macy DW: Diseases of the ear. In Ettinger SJ (ed): Textbook of Veterinary Internal Medicine. Philadelphia, WB Saunders, 1989, pp 246–262.
17. August J: Otitis externa, a disease of multifactorial etiology. Vet Clin North Am Small Anim Pract 18:731, 1988.
18. Griffin CE: Otitis externa and otitis media. In Griffin CE, et al (eds): Current Veterinary Dermatology. St. Louis, Mosby–Year Book, 1998, pp 245–262.
19. Rosser EJ: Diagnosis of food allergy in dogs. JAVMA 203:259, 1993.
20. Mansfield PD: Preventive ear care for dogs and cats. Vet Clin North Am 18:845, 1988.
21. Huang HP, Shih HM: Use of infrared thermometry and effect of otitis externa on external ear canal temperature in dogs. JAVMA 213:76, 1998.
22. Kowalski JJ: The microbial environment of the ear canal in health and disease. Vet Clin North Am Small Anim Pract 18:743, 1988.
23. Cole LK, et al: Microflora and antimicrobial susceptibility patterns of isolated pathogens from the horizontal ear canal and middle ear in dogs with otitis media. JAVMA 212:534, 1998.
24. Merchant SR: Pathogenesis of otitis externa. In Ear Care: Veterinary Learning Systems for Schering-Plough Animal Health, Trenton, NJ, 1992, p 8.
25. Mansfield PD, et al: Infectivity of Malassezia pachydermatis in the external ear canal of dogs. J Am Anim Hosp Assoc 26:93, 1990.
26. Kiss G, et al: New combination for the therapy of canine otitis externa: I. Microbiology of otitis externa. J Small Anim Pract 38:51, 1997.
27. Morris DO, et al: Type I hypersensitivity reactions to Malassezia pachydermatis extracts in atopic dogs. Am J Vet Res 59:836, 1998.
28. Eger LE, Lindsay P: Effects of otitis on hearing in dogs characterised by brainstem auditory evoked response testing. J Small Anim Pract 38:380, 1997.
29. Moriello KA, et al: Adrenocortical suppression associated with topical otic administration of glucocorticoids in dogs. JAVMA 193:329, 1988.
30. Meyer DJ, et al: Effect of otic medications containing glucocorticoids on liver function. JAVMA 196:743, 1990.
31. Kiss G, et al: New combination for the therapy of canine otitis externa: II. Efficacy in vitro and in vivo. J Small Anim Pract 38:57, 1997.
32. Mason KV, Steward LJ: Malassezia and canine dermatitis. In Ihrke PJ, et al (eds): Advances in Veterinary Dermatology, vol 2. New York, Oxford, 1993.
33. Gram D: Treatment of ear mites (Otodectes cynotis) in cats: Comparison of subcutaneous and topical ivermectin. In: Proceedings of 7th Annual Symposium of AVD/ACVD. Scottsdale, AZ, 1991, p 26.
34. Nuttall TJ: Use of ticarcillin in the management of canine otitis externa complicated by Pseudomonas aeruginosa. J Small Anim Pract 39:165, 1998.
35. Farco AM, et al: Potentiating effect of EDTA-tris on the activity of antibiotics against resistant bacteria associated with otitis, dermatitis and cystitis. J Small Anim Pract 38:243, 1997.
36. Foster AP, DeBoer DJ: The role of Pseudomonas in canine ear disease. Compend Small Anim 20:909, 1998.
37. London CA et al: Evaluation of dogs and cats with tumors of the ear canal: 145 cases (1978–1992). JAVMA 208:1413, 1996.
38. Lane JG: Surgery of the externa and middle ear. Vet Rep 3:4, 1990.
39. Bellah JR: How and when to perform lateral and vertical ear canal resections. Vet Med 92:535, 1997.
40. Beckman SC, et al: Total ear canal ablation combining bulla osteotomy and curettage in dogs with chronic otitis externa and media. JAVMA 196:84, 1990.
41. Krahwinkel DJ: Effect of total ablation of the externa acoustic meatus and bulla osteotomy on auditory function in dogs. JAVMA 202:949, 1993.
42. Bellah JR: When should you recommend total ear canal ablation and lateral bulla osteotomy? Vet Med 92:544, 1997.
43. Little CJL, et al: Inflammatory middle ear disease of the dog: The pathology of otitis media. Vet Rec 128:293, 1991.
44. Tojo M, et al: Experimental induction of secretory and purulent otitis media by the surgical obstruction of the eustachian tube in dogs. J Small Anim Pract 26:81, 1985.
45. Oliver JE, et al: Handbook of Veterinary Neurology. Philadelphia, WB Saunders, 1997.
46. Little CJL, Lane JG: An evaluation of tympanometry, otoscopy and palpation for assessment of the canine tympanic membrane. Vet Rec 124:5, 1989.
47. Little CJL, et al: Inflammatory middle ear disease of the dog: The clinical and pathological features of cholesteatoma, a complication of otitis media. Vet Rec 1228:319, 1991.
48. Hoskinson J: Imaging techniques in the diagnosis of middle ear disease. Semin Vet Med Surg (Small Anim) 8:10, 1993.
49. Remidios AM, et al: A comparison of radiographic versus surgical diagnosis of otitis media. J Am Anim Hosp Assoc 27:183, 1991.
50. Steiss JE, et al: Healing of experimentally perforated tympanic membranes demonstrated by electrodiagnostic testing and histopathology. J Am Anim Hosp Assoc 28:308, 1992.
51. Little CJL, et al: Neoplasia involving the middle ear cavity of dogs. Vet Rec 124:54, 1989.
52. Trevor PB, Martin RA: Tympanic bulla osteotomy for treatment of middle-ear disease in cats: 19 cases (1984–1991). JAVMA 202:123, 1993.
53. Rogers KS: Tumors of the ear canal. Vet Clin North Am Small Anim Pract 18:859, 1988.
54. Kapatkin AS, et al: Results of surgery and long-term follow-up in 31 cats with nasopharyngeal polyps. J Am Anim Hosp Assoc 26:387, 1990.
55. Faulkner JE, Budsburg SC: Results of ventral bulla osteotomy for treatment of middle ear polyps in cats. J Am Anim Hosp Assoc 26:496, 1990.
56. Merchant SR, et al: Ototoxicity assessment of a chlorhexidine otic preparation in dogs. Prog Vet Neurol 4:72, 1993.
57. Strain GM, et al: Ototoxicity assessment of a gentamicin sulfate otic preparation in dogs. Am J Vet Res 56:532, 1995.
58. Mansfield PD: Ototoxicity in dogs and cats. Compend Contin Ed Small Anim Pract 12:331, 1990.
59. Mawson SR, Ludman H: Mawson's Diseases of the Ear. London, Edward Arnold, 1988, p 618.
60. Strain GM: Congenital deafness in dogs and cats. Compend Contin Ed Small Anim Pract 13:245, 1991.
61. Holliday TA, et al: Unilateral and bilateral brainstem auditory-evoked response abnormalities in 900 Dalmation dogs. J Vet Intern Med 6:166, 1992.
62. Sims MH: Electrodiagnostic evaluation of auditory function. Vet Clin North Am Small Anim Pract 18:913, 1988.

CHAPTER 123

DISEASES OF THE NOSE AND NASAL SINUSES

Autumn P. Davidson, Kyle G. Mathews, Philip D. Koblik, and
Alain Théon

ANATOMY OF THE NOSE AND NASAL SINUSES

The nasal cavity is divided into two non-communicating, symmetric sides along the sagittal midline by a cartilaginous septum rostrally and a bony septum caudally. During inhalation, air flowing past a nostril (external naris) enters the nasal vestibule, largely filled with the alar fold (rostral aspect of the ventral nasal concha) (Figs. 123–1 through 123–3). Inhaled air is then directed into three longitudinally oriented chambers, the ventral, middle, and dorsal nasal meatuses. Next to the septum the vertically oriented, slit-like, common nasal meatus connects the other three meatuses. Air entering the dorsal nasal meatus moves over the surface of the olfactory neuroepithelium located on the ethmoidal concha near the cribriform plate. The cribriform plate is the fenestrated portion of the ethmoid bone that separates the nasal cavity from the cranial vault and is crossed by olfactory nerve fibers. Inhaled air passes through the meatuses and is warmed, humidified, and filtered as it passes over the well-vascularized, ciliated, pseudocolumnar mucosa lining the delicate, scroll-like conchae that separate these chambers. The conchae are cartilaginous rostrally and ossified caudally. They consist of the rostrally located ventral (maxilloturbinates) conchae, the smaller dorsal (dorsal nasoturbinates) conchae, and the caudally located ethmoidal conchae (ethmoturbinates). After passage through the meatuses and over the conchae, inspired air exits the nasal cavity through the paired nasal conchae located between the caudal aspect of the hard palate and the vomer. Air then enters the nasopharynx dorsal to the soft palate.

Each side of the nasal cavity is largely surrounded and protected by bone, including but not limited to the frontal bone, maxilla, and nasal bones dorsally, the maxilla laterally, and the incisive bones, maxilla, vomer, and palatine bones ventrally. The mobile rhinarium rostral to the nasal and incisive bones is supported by cartilage. Caudally, the frontal sinuses are situated primarily between the outer (dorsal) and inner (ventral) tables of the frontal bones. There are three separate non-communicating frontal sinuses on each side in the dog and a single chamber on each side of the midline in the cat (Figs. 123–3 and 123–4). The frontal sinuses may be small or completely absent in some brachycephalic dogs. Each frontal sinus is hollow, lined with a ciliated mucous membrane, and drains by means of separate ostia (nasofrontal ducts). In the dog, a large maxillary recess is present in the nasal surface of the maxilla dorsal to the tooth roots of the upper fourth premolar. This recess is small in the cat. Cats have a sphenoidal sinus, which extends caudally from the nasal cavity into the sphenoid bone ventral to the brain. Dogs do not have a sphenoidal sinus.

DIAGNOSTIC APPROACH TO NASAL DISORDERS

Abnormal nasal discharge, sneezing, paroxysmal reverse sneezing, stertor, halitosis, muzzle pain, discoloration of the

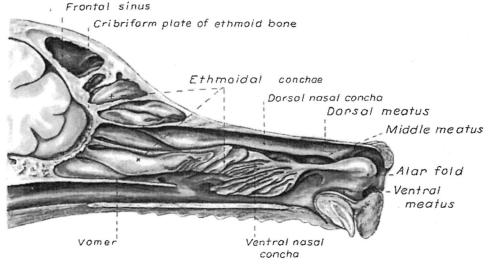

Figure 123–1. Sagittal section, canine nasal cavity. (From Evans HE [ed]: Miller's Anatomy of the Dog, 3rd ed. Philadelphia, WB Saunders, 1993, p 468.)

Frontal sinus
Cribriform plate of ethmoid bone
Ethmoidal conchae
Dorsal nasal concha
Dorsal meatus
Middle meatus
Alar fold
Ventral meatus
Vomer
Ventral nasal concha

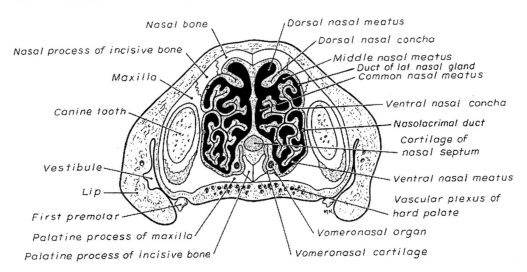

Figure 123–2. Transverse section, canine nasal cavity. (From Evans HE [ed]: Miller's Anatomy of the Dog, 3rd ed. Philadelphia, WB Saunders, 1993, p 468.)

nares, and distortion of the nasal surfaces are common signs of nasal passage or sinus disease. The veterinarian should consider the animal's signalment, history, environment, and physical examination findings when formulating a differential diagnosis and diagnostic plan (see Chapter 54). Diagnostic approaches to nasal disease include assisted physical examination using rhinoscopy, as well as radiologic, cytologic, histopathologic, microbiologic, and serologic evaluations. Because most procedures require general anesthesia, prior performance of a complete blood cell count, serum chemistry profile, and urinalysis are indicated as a database and to evaluate for the presence of concurrent or contributing disorders. Coagulation profiles, cross-matching, and blood transfusions should all be considered, depending on the severity of the disease, history of epistaxis, and the invasiveness of the examination procedure. Because hemorrhage secondary to internal nasal examination will confound the results of radiographs, computed tomography (CT) or magnetic resonance imaging (MRI) of the nasal cavity, imaging studies should be performed first.

DIAGNOSTIC IMAGING OF THE NASAL CAVITY

Diagnostic imaging of the nasal cavity and paranasal sinuses is an important component evaluating dogs and cats with signs of nasal disease. The objective of the imaging study is to permit evaluation of the extent and character of

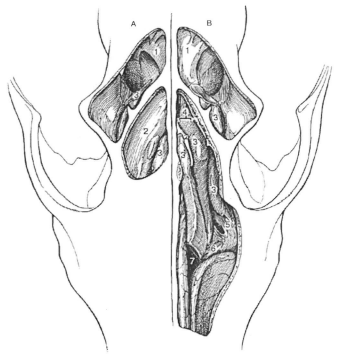

Figure 123–3. Canine frontal sinuses, dorsal view with portions of the frontal bone removed. A, Lateral sinus (1), rostral sinus (2), and ethmoidal conchae (3). B, The floor of the rostral sinus has been removed to expose the more ventrally located medial sinus (4). Relative locations of the nasofrontal ducts' openings from the lateral (5), medial (6), and rostral (7) frontal sinuses (Modified from Slatter D [ed]: Textbook of Small Animal Surgery, 2nd ed. Philadelphia, WB Saunders, 1993, p 697.)

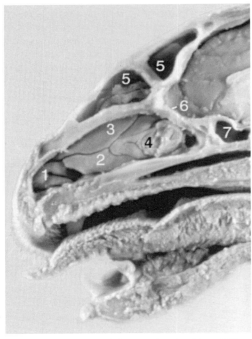

Figure 123–4. Sagittal section, feline nasal cavity. Ventral (1), middle (2), dorsal (3), and ethmoidal (4) conchae; frontal sinus (5), cribriform plate (6), and sphenoidal sinus (7).

involvement of the calvarial bones and teeth, nasal turbinates and air passages, and paranasal sinus cavities, as well as to determine if the lesion has extended into the brain cavity or retrobulbar space. Survey radiography, CT, and MRI can all be used to image the nasal cavity and paranasal sinuses. Each modality has its relative merits. Survey radiography is universally available and relatively inexpensive but requires general anesthesia and close attention to positioning and exposure factors and provides a limited view of regional anatomy. CT is available at most academic veterinary hospitals, in many large referral practices, and through access to cooperative human hospitals. CT is generally more expensive than survey radiography, although in many academic institutions not significantly so. Although CT studies performed on traditional scanners require general anesthesia, studies performed on new spiral CT systems may be acquired in a matter of a few minutes, enabling them to be performed on sedated animals. CT produces images that represent thin, cross-sectional slices of the skull, avoiding the problem of superimposition inherent to survey radiography. CT, relative to survey radiography, also provides better tissue contrast, permitting improved visualization of fine bony structures. At present, access to MRI is limited and the studies tend to be expensive. The principal advantages of MRI compared with CT are that, with MRI, cross-sectional slices of the skull can be produced in any imaging plane and a variety of pulse sequences can be used to improve discrimination of solid mass lesions from accumulations of fluid. However, little useful MRI signal is generated by dense connective tissue, limiting the use of this modality to evaluate bone involvement.

SURVEY RADIOGRAPHY

Several technical factors determine the diagnostic quality of radiographic studies of the nasal cavity and paranasal sinuses in dogs and cats. All studies must be performed with the animal under general anesthesia to ensure proper skull positioning, to avoid motion artifacts, and to allow proper radiation safety practices. Close attention must be paid to radiographic positioning and exposure for comparison of structures in the right versus left side of the skull and to ensure that the full extent of the nasal cavity and the sinuses have been included on the various views. On all views it is important to prop the mouth open and to keep the endotracheal tube and tongue out of the way by binding them to the mandible. The proper exposure should be one that uses a relatively low kVp (65–70 kVp) and appropriate mAs for the film-screen system being used. In a properly exposed view, one should be able to easily visualize soft tissues along the outside of the nasal cavity (lips and nasal planum) as well as the ethmoidal turbinates in the caudal part of the nasal cavity. Overexposure will tend to diminish visualization of subtle lesions in the nasal cavity; underexposure will tend to lead to false impression of fluid or swelling of the nasal mucosa. Finally, because of the delicate and intricate nature of the turbinates, a high-detail film-screen combination or non-screen mammography film should be used.

Comprehensive descriptions of the various nasal cavity and paranasal sinus radiographic projections in the dog and cat are available.[1, 2] These projections include the intraoral dorsoventral view, open mouth ventrodorsal view, lateral view, oblique view, and frontal view. The dorsoventral or ventrodorsal views provide the most information regarding the nasal cavity. In one report, the intraoral dorsoventral or open mouth ventrodorsal views satisfactorily showed relevant radiographic lesions in more than 80 per cent of cases described.[3] The open mouth ventrodorsal view, if performed properly, will display the entire nasal cavity, including the frontal sinuses, although some distortion of these structures is inevitable because the x-ray beam is not perpendicular to the x-ray film (Fig. 123–5). The intraoral dorsoventral view avoids this minor distortion problem but fails to display the caudal nasal cavity in most dogs. Lateral and oblique views are useful to help visualize the upper dental arcades, facial bones, and frontal sinuses. The tangential frontal view provides an unobstructed view of the frontal sinuses in most dogs. Coulson provides a similar description of radiographic techniques in the cat.[2]

Virtually every report describing the radiographic features of nasal disease has stressed the importance of evaluating the integrity of the nasal turbinates (conchae). Loss of the so-called normal trabecular pattern is regarded as a sign of aggressive nasal disease such as neoplasia or destructive rhinitis. However, not all normal turbinates are created equal. The nasal and maxillary turbinates in the mid to rostral portion of the nasal cavity consist of nasal epithelium covering fine bony conchae and create predominantly soft tissue radiographic shadows. The striated pattern created by these turbinates and the interposed air passages will be obliterated by the presence of fluid in the nasal cavity. The ethmoidal turbinates in the caudal nasal cavity have much coarser bony conchae and create definite bone dense radiographic shadows that cannot be obliterated by the presence of fluid alone.[4] However, whereas there is a general symmetry of structures in the two halves of the nasal cavity, there will not be a perfect correspondence in shape or position of individual turbinates. This lack of perfect symmetry is particularly apparent in dogs with short noses and in cats.

There have been numerous reports describing the radiographic features of nasal disease in the dog. Most authors have chosen to divide these diseases into three basic categories. Although the exact descriptions vary from author to author, these three categories represent (1) non-destructive nasal disease, which includes viral, bacterial, and immune-mediated rhinitis as well as simple nasal hemorrhage or edema; (2) destructive rhinitis, usually associated with fungal infection but also occasionally seen with chronic rhinitis due to a nasal foreign body; and (3) nasal tumors, usually of epithelial origin but also including squamous cell carcinomas and a variety of sarcomas. The common or typical radiographic findings for these three general groups of nasal lesions are as follows:

Non-destructive Nasal Disease (Fig. 123–6)[1–3, 8]

- Patchy increase in opacity throughout most of the nasal cavity; usually bilateral involvement
- Loss of turbinate pattern (obliteration of air spaces) in the mid to rostral portion of the nasal cavity
- Frontal sinuses usually unaffected
- No evidence of bony destruction involving caudal turbinates, vomer bone, or surrounding facial bones
- No evidence of external soft tissue swelling or mass

Destructive Rhinitis (Fig. 123–7)[1–3, 5, 8]

- Areas of decreased opacity (turbinate destruction) within the nasal cavity; lesions can be unilateral or bilateral (if bilateral extent of involvement is usually asymmetric)
- Poorly circumscribed mass lesions possible in the caudal nasal cavity and frontal sinuses (aspergillomas)

ENT

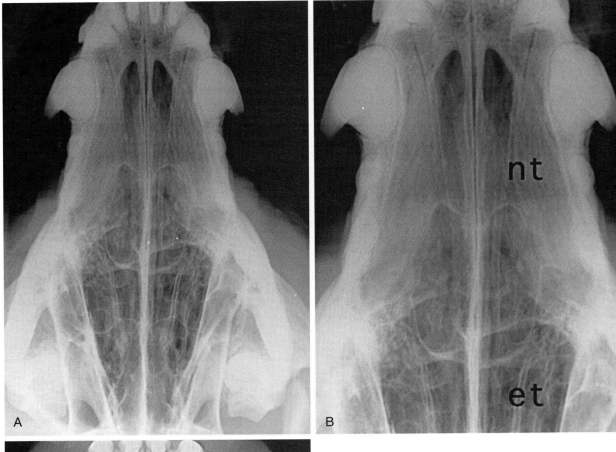

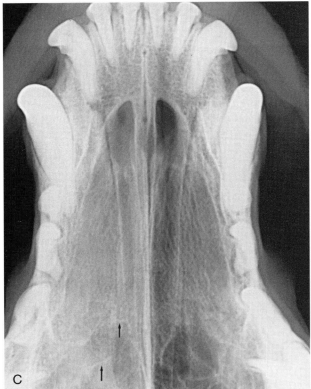

Figure 123–5. Open-mouth ventrodorsal radiograph of a normal dog *(A, B)*. This projection allows visualization of the entire nasal cavity. On the close-up view *(B)*, note the difference of appearance of the nasal turbinates (nt) and ethmoidal turbinates (et). Shadows representing the nasal turbinates are created solely by soft tissue dense structures (cartilage and nasal epithelium) and intervening air passages. Shadows representing the ethmoidal turbinates are a mixture of bone and soft tissue dense structures. The presence of fluid in the nasal cavity (C) tends to obliterate visualization of the nasal turbinates; however, the bony shadows associated with the ethmoidal turbinates (arrows) remain visible.

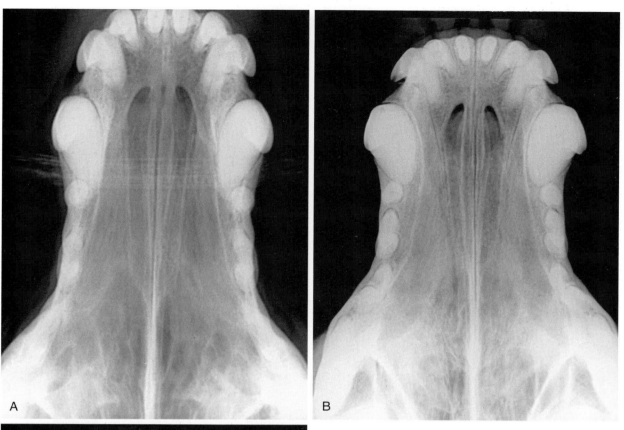

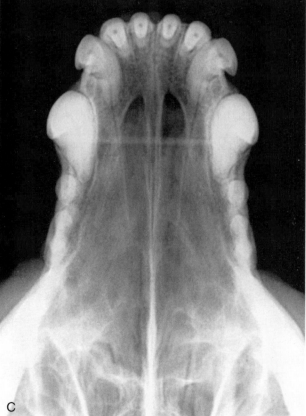

ENT

Figure 123–6. *A* to *C*, Open-mouth ventrodorsal radiographs of three different dogs with non-destructive nasal disease. Nasal biopsy specimens from all three dogs were interpreted as lymphocytic/plasmacytic rhinitis. Excessive fluid and edema of the nasal epithelium has resulted in focal areas of increased opacity and loss of nasal turbinate detail bilaterally within the nasal cavity.

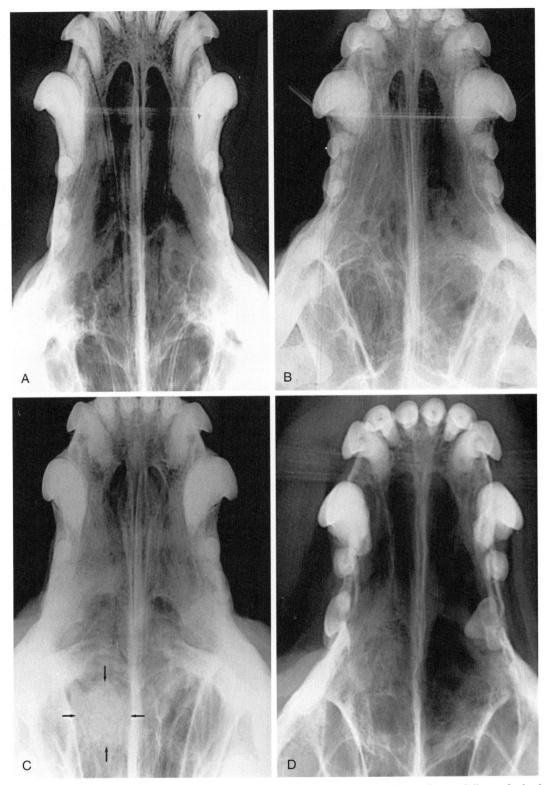

Figure 123–7. *A* to *D*, Open-mouth ventrodorsal radiographs of four different dogs with destructive nasal disease. In the dog in *A* there is a classic radiographic presentation of nasal aspergillosis. There is marked bilateral destruction of nasal turbinates creating widespread areas of increased lucency. Similar, but less obvious, turbinate destruction is evident in the left side of the nasal cavity in the dog in *B*. In addition, this dog had fluid within the left frontal sinus causing an increased opacity in the caudal aspect of the nasal cavity. The dog in *C* had mild turbinate lysis in the mid-nasal cavity. A well-defined granuloma (arrows) was present in the right frontal sinus. The radiographic lesions in this dog could easily be confused with nasal neoplasia. The dog in *D* had been treated with radiation therapy for a nasal tumor. The resultant turbinate atrophy appears similar to fungal rhinitis.

- Frontal sinus involvement common in chronic or severe cases
- Facial bone lysis and production (osteomyelitis) possible in severe cases

Neoplasia (Fig. 123–8)[1–3, 6–8]

- Soft tissue mass with associated turbinate, vomer bone, hard palate, and facial bone destruction
- Punctate to geographic areas of decreased opacity associated with destruction of the hard palate and/or overlying facial bones
- Usually unilateral; vomer bone distortion or destruction if bilateral
- Frontal sinus involvement common
- External soft tissue swelling or mass; occurs in approximately half of the cases

These guidelines are by no means perfect. Early tumors, particularly if associated with copious nasal discharge, can be difficult to detect. Bony lysis of the hard palate or overlying facial bones can create areas of increased lucency that can mimic destructive rhinitis. Fungal granulomas create mass lesions and can be associated with osteomyelitis of adjacent bony structures. Surprisingly, there has only been one published paper evaluating the accuracy of nasal radiography in an extended population of subjects. Harvey and associates applied guidelines similar to those listed previously to review radiographic studies on 40 dogs with chronic nasal disease.[8] Fifteen of 18 dogs with confirmed nasal tumors were correctly diagnosed; the other 3 dogs were misdiagnosed as having fungal rhinitis. Nine of 15 dogs with fungal rhinitis were correctly diagnosed; 2 other dogs were incorrectly diagnosed as having nasal tumors, and 4 other dogs were undiagnosed. Only 1 of 7 dogs with diseases other than a tumor or fungal rhinitis were correctly diagnosed.

COMPUTED TOMOGRAPHY

CT offers several advantages relative to survey radiography, the most important being its ability to produce cross-sectional tomographic slices that avoid the problem of superimposing of structures inherent in "flat film" radiography. Because CT generates digital images, it is possible to adjust the contrast scale so that optimum optical density of the entire nasal cavity/paranasal sinus region can be displayed. Manipulation of the contrast scale also allows better discrimination of soft tissue structures from those that are only faintly mineralized, which improves visualization of even the fine turbinate structures in the rostral part of the nasal cavity.

Nasal CT is most easily performed with the animal in ventral recumbency with the head secured in such a way that the hard palate is parallel to the table. It is important to attempt to keep the sagittal plane of the head perpendicular to the plane of the gantry. It is also important to avoid using endotracheal tubes with metal fittings or radiopaque markers because these can cause significant image artifacts. The resulting set of transverse images is usually sufficient to evaluate the entire nasal cavity and frontal sinus region. Comprehensive descriptions of the CT anatomy of the nasal cavity and paranasal sinuses are available for the dog[9–11] and cat.[12] It is also possible to place an animal in either dorsal or lateral recumbency with the neck flexed so that dorsal plane images can be obtained. This imaging plane has been shown to provide better visualization of the cribriform plate in dogs.[13]

Other technical considerations include slice thickness and size of the field-of-view. Choice of slice thickness is a compromise between the superior image quality of thinner slices and the practical time limitations for acquiring, processing, and reviewing studies that contain large numbers of slices. Most CT scanners offer a limited selection of slice thickness, typically 1.5 mm, 3 or 5 mm, and 10 mm. One approach is to determine the total distance to be imaged for each patient and choose a slice thickness that will cover that distance in 20 to 40 slices. With spiral CT scanners, image data are acquired for an entire volume. Thickness of slices is chosen after the study is acquired and can be altered to suit different portions of the anatomy. Field of view affects the size of the image for display and the in-slice resolution of each image. Most CT scanners have a few standard choices for field-of-view size (i.e., large body, medium body, head, and infant). The best choice is the option that provides the small field-of-view and offers a standard reconstruction algorithm (usually the "infant" setting). Most scanners also allow the images to be "targeted," providing an even smaller field-of-view. If this option is available, one should acquire an untargeted slice through the thickest portion of the anatomy that is going to be scanned. One then defines the center for the field-of-view and the magnification factor that results in an image that nearly fills the display screen. If the scanner software allows a choice of image matrix size, the largest matrix available should be chosen.

There are a few pitfalls in interpreting CT nasal studies. One should be aware that there is a zone in the rostral nasal cavity in the area of the first and second premolar teeth where the turbinates become numerous and are delicate and the air passages between turbinates are quite convoluted. The net result is that the air passages become indistinct and blend with adjacent turbinates. This appearance mimics the presence of fluid within the air passages. Farther caudally in the area of the fourth premolar, the mucosal lining of the ventral nasal concha and endoturbinate III becomes quite thick and can be mistaken for a mass (Fig. 123–9).

The initial reports describing the use of CT to evaluate the nasal cavity compared the information gained by performing CT versus radiography in dogs with nasal tumors.[14, 15] Not surprisingly, CT proved to be superior in defining the extent of involvement of the lesions. CT was more accurate at determining whether the lesions were unilateral versus bilateral; whether the lesions involved the paranasal sinuses; whether lesions had caused bony lysis of the hard palate, surrounding facial bones, sphenoid bone, or cribriform plate; and whether lesions had extended into the cranial cavity, retrobulbar space, or oral cavity. By giving a more accurate representation of the extent of involvement, CT was deemed to be more valuable in staging tumors, predicting treatment-related complications, and planning either surgery or radiation therapy (Fig. 123–10).

The criteria used to diagnose nasal tumors, fungal rhinitis, and non-destructive nasal disease of CT are identical to those used on survey radiography. Burk reviewed CT studies performed on 100 dogs with nasal disease representing 69 with nasal tumors, 27 with non-fungal rhinitis, and 4 with nasal aspergillosis, looking for features that best distinguished neoplastic from non-neoplastic lesions.[16] He found that regions of patchy increased attenuation within a surrounding soft tissue lesion, ethmoid, maxillary, or nasal bone destruction, and extension into the retrobulbar space were all good predictors of neoplasia. However, no single finding or combination of findings was "absolutely definitive" for neoplasia.

ENT

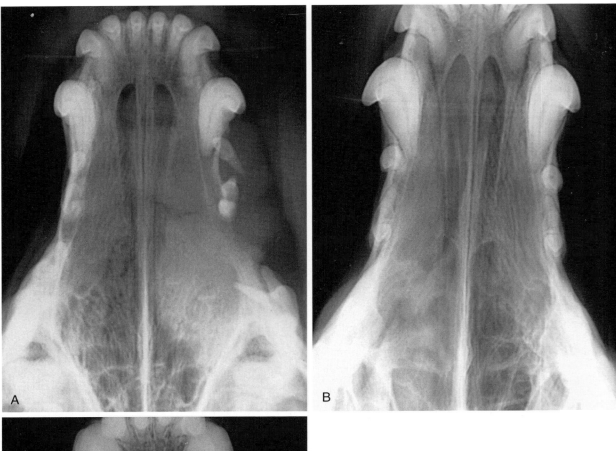

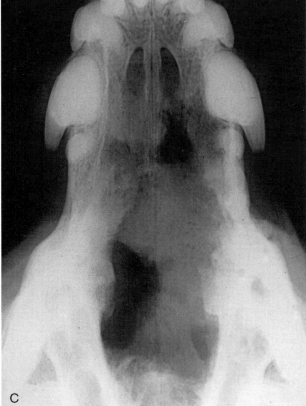

Figure 123–8. *A* to *C,* Open-mouth ventrodorsal radiographs of three different dogs with nasal tumors. In the dog in *A* there is a classic radiographic presentation of a nasal tumor with a well-defined mass in the mid left nasal cavity. Marked bone destruction involves turbinate structures and adjacent facial bones. The nasal tumor in dog *B* is much less advanced. As is typical with nasal adenocarcinomas, this tumor is centered in the region of the maxillary recess (right side). The mass is less well defined, and there is less bone destruction compared with the dog in *A*. Early nasal tumors can be easily confused with rhinitis. The dog in *C* has a very advanced nasal tumor involving both sides of the nasal cavity. Focal areas of hard palate destruction create regions of increased lucency superimposed over portions of the nasal cavity and create the potential for an incorrect diagnosis of fungal rhinitis.

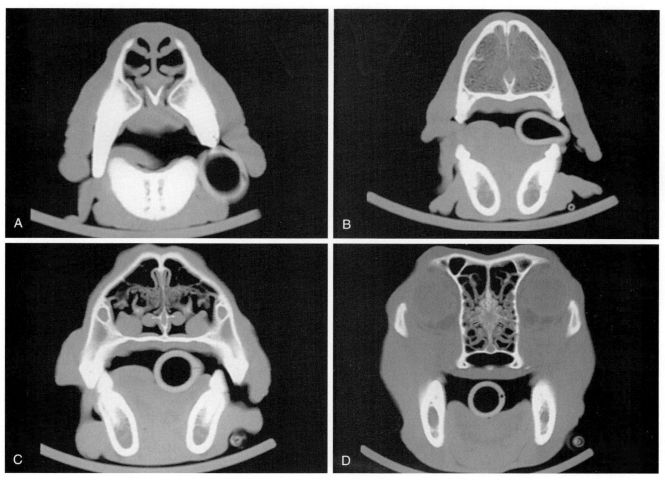

Figure 123–9. Four transverse CT slices of the nasal cavity in a normal dog. Slices are arranged in a rostral *(A)* to caudal *(D)* progression. Slice *A* is at the level of the upper canine teeth. At this level there are relatively few turbinates and the air passages are prominent. Slice *B* is at the level of the rostral premolars. At this level the nasal turbinates are numerous and quite fine with a complex labyrinth of intervening air passages. The normal "turbinate pattern" can be difficult to appreciate in this region, particularly if thick slices were acquired. This appearance can mimic the changes seen with non-destructive rhinitis. Slice *C* is at the level of the molar teeth. There is a more heterogeneous appearance of the turbinates in this region. The ventral nasal concha and endoturbinate III create prominent soft tissue structures and must not be mistaken for mass lesions. Slice *D* is at the level of the cribriform plate (arrows). The ethmoidal turbinates form a complex scroll composed of both bone dense and soft tissue dense structures. These turbinates extend into the rostral aspect of the frontal sinuses.

ENT

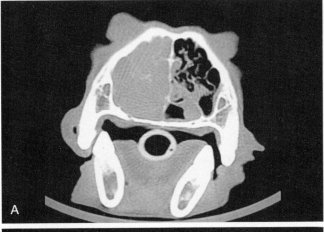

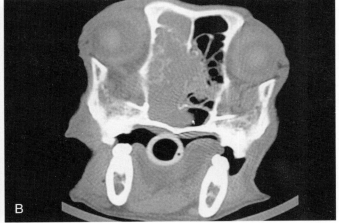

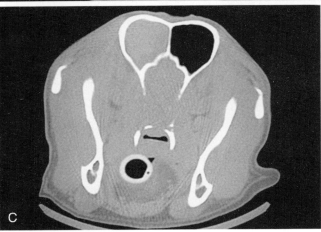

Figure 123–10. Three transverse CT slices from a dog with a nasal tumor. Slices are arranged in a rostral *(A)* to caudal *(C)* progression. A large mass is present throughout the right nasal cavity. Destruction of turbinates in the ventral aspect of the nasal cavity is evident. In slice *B,* the mass can be seen extending into the nasal choanae and there is destruction of the right half of the cribriform plate. In slice *C* the mass also extends into the basilar portion of the skull with marked destruction of the basisphenoid and pterygoid bones bilaterally. This pattern of bone lysis without any obvious productive response is often seen with nasal adenocarcinomas. Uniform soft tissue opacity is present within the right frontal sinus. It is difficult to differentiate fluid from a soft tissue mass with CT, although use of intranasal or intravenous contrast material may help outline a mass lesion if it is surrounded by fluid.

CT has provided a new appreciation for the aggressive nature of fungal rhinitis (Figs. 123–11 through 123–13). Whereas mild cases of nasal aspergillosis result in relatively little structural change within the nasal cavity other than the regional lysis of nasal turbinates, chronic cases often demonstrate dramatic turbinate destruction, gross epithelial thickening, formation of dense fungal colonies and granulomas, and penetration into adjacent bone, causing hyperostosis and, in some instances, gross bony destruction. Dogs with nasal aspergillosis frequently have copious, thick nasal exudate, which can obscure the presence of granulomas. Administration of intranasal iodinated contrast medium can help define mass lesions in the presence of surrounding fluid.[17]

The CT appearance of non-destructive nasal disease is as expected. Air passages are obliterated by the presence of fluid and/or epithelial edema. With appropriate windowing, one can confirm the integrity of the underlying turbinates (Fig. 123–14). CT can provide an accurate picture of the morphologic changes occurring within the nasal cavity and paranasal sinuses and by doing so allows a more accurate diagnosis to be rendered. There is, however, little information to estimate how much more accurate CT is compared with traditional radiography. The only published report comparing the two modalities in a group of dogs in which the diagnosis was not known before imaging involved only 11 animals and did not examine test performance in any rigorous fashion.[18]

MAGNETIC RESONANCE IMAGING

There are several theoretical advantages of MRI compared with CT. With CT, images of the head can only be acquired in the transverse or dorsal plane. Re-formatted sagittal or oblique slices can be re-constructed through computer manipulation of the original image data; however, these images lack sufficient resolution to be of much use in evaluating fine bony detail. MR images of the head can be acquired directly in any imaging plane, without any loss of resolution. Compared with CT, MRI also provides superior soft tissue contrast. With MRI, signal intensity associated with soft tissue structures is dependent on the local ultrastructural and biochemical environment of hydrogen protons. For example, on CT it can be difficult to differentiate mass from fluid, especially in the caudal nasal cavity and frontal sinuses. With MRI, this is an easy task. A variety of different MRI pulse sequences can be used to further amplify signal intensity differences among normal tissues and between pathologic versus normal tissues, making it much easier to detect subtle lesions such as brain edema. This attribute is particularly helpful in evaluating animals suspected of having a nasal tumor invading the cranial cavity or retrobulbar space. The only two published reports discussing the use of MRI to evaluate animals with nasal disease both dealt exclusively with this particular scenario and consisted of five dogs with nasal tumors that had invaded the brain and a cat with a nasal tumor that had invaded the retrobulbar space.[19, 20] In one of these reports, both CT and MRI studies were available and the authors concluded that the MRI studies were superior in demonstrating the anatomic features of the primary tumor masses as well as secondary features of brain pathology (edema) in response to the tumor invasion (Fig. 123–15).[19]

There are also some disadvantages of MRI compared with CT. Bone produces no useful MRI signal, making it difficult

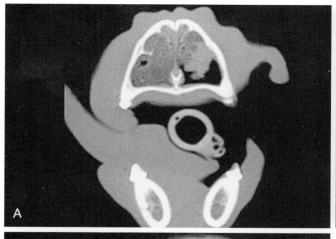

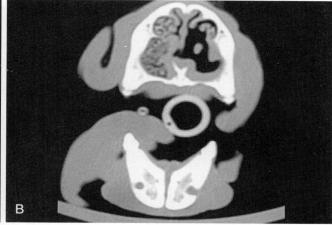

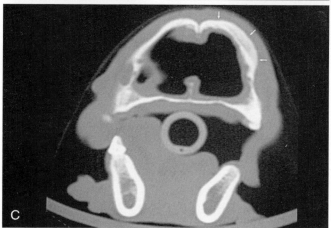

Figure 123–11. Transverse CT slices from three different dogs with nasal aspergillosis. These images show a progression of turbinate destruction from mild *(A)* to severe *(C)*. Note the hyperostosis involving the left maxillary bone in *C*, which is a common manifestation of chronic fungal rhinitis.

ENT

to differentiate bone from adjacent soft tissues with most of the typical clinical pulse sequences. Furthermore, many MR imagers available for clinical veterinary use may not be capable of producing contiguous slice studies, or slices as thin as can be obtained with most CT scanners. In-plane resolution also is an issue with MRI because the field of view with MRI must encompass the entire volume of the part being scanned. MRI studies that consist of multiple pulse sequences and multiple imaging planes take considerably longer to obtain than a CT study.

APPROACHES TO EXAMINATION OF THE NASAL CAVITY

With the increasing use of non-invasive diagnostic techniques (e.g., computed tomography, rhinoscopy) and treatment methods (e.g., radiation therapy, topical antifungal therapy), the need for and use of aggressive surgery of the canine and feline nasal cavity is becoming less frequent. Some exceptions to that statement include the repair of oronasal communications (primary or secondary cleft palate and oronasal fistulae (see 4th edition, Chapter 80), palliative debulking of some nasal tumors, removal of large fungal granulomas, and foreign body retrieval. Approaches to the nasal cavity for collection of cytologic and biopsy specimens and for microbiologic testing vary from minimally invasive (e.g., rostrally through the nares) to invasive (e.g., dorsal rhinotomy). The least invasive option to achieve the desired goal should be chosen.

ROSTRAL ACCESS TO THE NASAL CAVITY

Numerous techniques have been described to obtain tissue specimens for definitive histopathologic diagnosis of nasal diseases through the nares. General anesthesia is usually required, with a cuffed endotracheal tube placed to prevent aspiration of blood and lavage fluids. The external surface of the nasal cavity should be visually and digitally examined for evidence of swelling, asymmetry, and ulceration. This includes a thorough oral examination with visualization of the nasopharynx with either a flexible fiberoptic scope or an angled, warmed dental mirror. Placement of pre-counted gauze sponges in the pharynx, for further protection of the airways, is then performed. Larger laparotomy sponges should be used if possible, because these are less easily swallowed by dogs that may respond to manipulation of the nasal tissues. The clinician can then measure the distance from the nares to the area of interest on radiographs or other imaging studies. This distance serves as a guide for the attainment of nasal biopsy specimens. In addition, before any instrument is inserted in the nasal cavity, the distance from the nares to the medial canthus of the eye is noted and should not be exceeded or penetration of the cribriform plate may result. Rhinoscopy can then be performed while the animal is in sternal recumbency. Limited examination of the rostral nasal cavity may be performed with an otoscope. A rigid arthroscope with a 1.9- to 2.7-mm outside diameter and a 5- to 25-degree angle of view (Richard Wolf Medical Instruments Corporation, Rosemont, IL) is commonly used. A flexible bronchoscope with a 3.5- to 4.8-mm outside

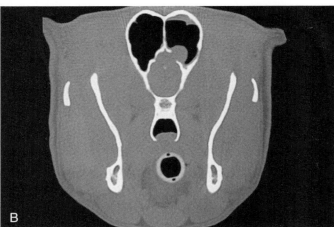

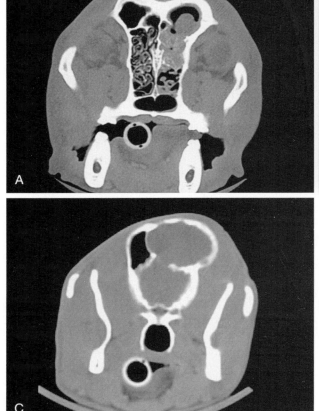

Figure 123–12. *A* to *C,* Transverse CT slices from three different dogs with nasal aspergillosis. All three dogs had granuloma lesions involving the caudal nasal cavity and frontal sinuses. Areas of osteomyelitis are often encountered with these lesions. The granuloma seen in *B* has caused a focal area of lysis of the internal table of the frontal bone whereas the granuloma seen in *C* presents as an expansile mass with both production and destruction of the surrounding frontal bone. Hence, these granulomas share many CT features with neoplastic lesions.

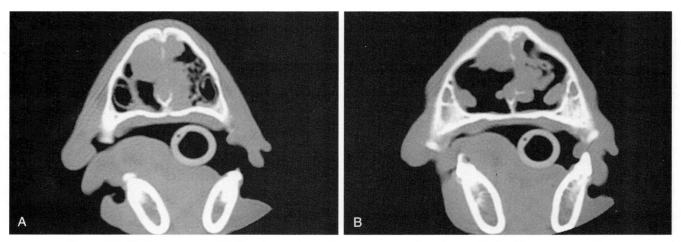

Figure 123–13. Two transverse CT slices from a dog with a nasal tumor and nasal aspergillosis. Slices are arranged in a rostral *(A)* to caudal *(B)* progression. Turbinate destruction is evident. In addition, there is a soft tissue mass with destruction of the nasal septum. Based on the CT study, this case was originally diagnosed as fungal rhinitis; however, nasal biopsy results indicated a nasal squamous cell carcinoma and nasal aspergillosis.

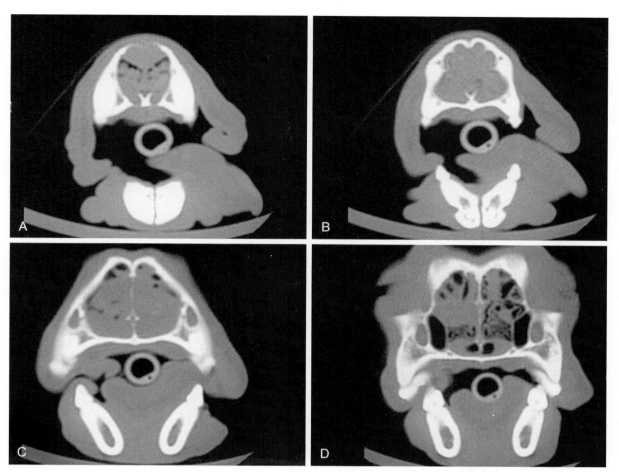

Figure 123–14. Four transverse CT slices from a dog with non-destructive rhinitis. Slices are arranged in a rostral *(A)* to caudal *(D)* progression. There is excessive fluid within both sides of the nasal cavity obscuring turbinate detail. With appropriate adjustment of the window level and width it is usually possible to demonstrate that the turbinates are intact. Note there is also no evidence of a "mass effect."

diameter (Olympus Corporation, Lake Success, NY) has the added benefit of allowing visualization of the nasopharynx by retroflexing the scope around the soft palate. Light resistance is usually felt while inserting the scope through the nares. The scope can then be directed ventrally into the ventral nasal meatus toward the nasopharynx or dorsally into the dorsonasal meatus toward the olfactory epithelium, openings (ostia) of the frontal sinuses, and the cribriform plate. The advantages of direct visualization of the nasal cavity are that a more thorough understanding of the nature of the disease process can be obtained and a biopsy instrument can be placed specifically at the area of interest. Small foreign bodies, such as grass awns, which enter through the nares, are unlikely to be dislodged using simple flushing techniques but may be retrieved using rhinoscopy. Larger foreign bodies, such as sharp bones that have penetrated the soft or hard palate, will often have to be removed by means of rhinotomy. Many scopes are equipped with biopsy ports or sleeves that simplify tissue sampling. In addition, a biopsy instrument, such as a uterine or gastric biopsy forceps, may be inserted alongside the scope if room permits. Disadvantages of rhinoscopy are the need for expensive equipment and poor visualization if excessive nasal discharge exists or hemorrhage occurs. Some degree of hemorrhage is inevitable. The nasal mucosa is richly endowed with blood vessels that allow for efficient heat exchange; in addition, the neovascularization of mucosa that occurs with inflammatory

conditions and neoplasia results in a propensity for hemorrhage after biopsy or even light trauma by a rhinoscope. Generally, hemorrhage from nasal biopsy specimens obtained through the nares, although frustrating to the rhinoscopist, is self-limiting. Concurrent lavage of the nasal cavity with physiologic saline can improve visualization. Ice packs may be applied to the bridge of the nose and digital pressure placed on the rostral cartilaginous portion of the nasal cavity to reduce hemorrhage. Lavage of the nasal cavity with chilled saline or instillation of epinephrine (1:100,000) may also be of benefit. Because of this propensity for hemorrhage, thorough examination of the entire nasal cavity should be performed before biopsy. Biopsy specimens should be placed in formalin for future histopathologic examination, in appropriate media for bacterial and fungal cultures, and rolled onto glass slides for immediate cytologic examination. After cessation of hemorrhage and before recovery from anesthesia, pharyngeal gauze sponges must be re-counted to be sure they have been removed and the pharynx suctioned as needed.

Indirect methods of obtaining tissue specimens through the nares have also been described. As with rhinoscopic examination, pre-biopsy imaging studies are recommended, biopsy instruments should never be inserted beyond the level of the medial canthus, and protection of the airways under general anesthesia is recommended. The simplest of these techniques involves flushing the nasal cavity with saline in

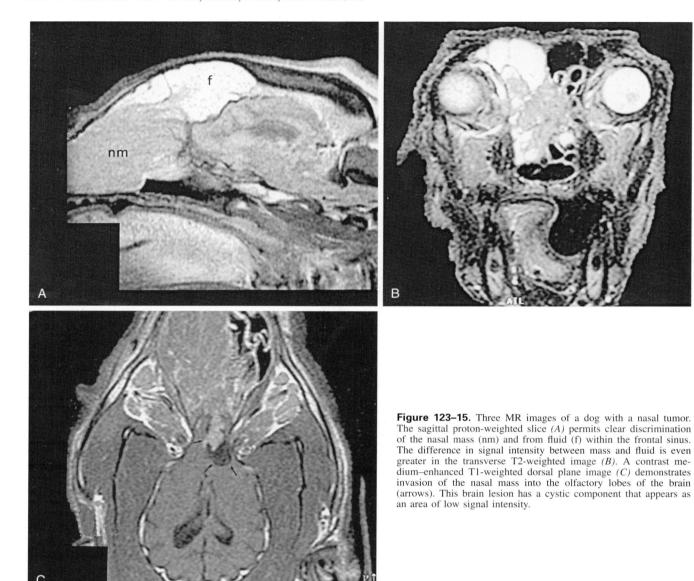

Figure 123–15. Three MR images of a dog with a nasal tumor. The sagittal proton-weighted slice *(A)* permits clear discrimination of the nasal mass (nm) and from fluid (f) within the frontal sinus. The difference in signal intensity between mass and fluid is even greater in the transverse T2-weighted image *(B)*. A contrast medium–enhanced T1-weighted dorsal plane image *(C)* demonstrates invasion of the nasal mass into the olfactory lobes of the brain (arrows). This brain lesion has a cystic component that appears as an area of low signal intensity.

an attempt to dislodge inflammatory or neoplastic cells. A catheter can be placed in the nares or retroflexed 180 degrees around the soft palate. Gauze sponges are used to catch tissues that are flushed out through the nares or into the pharynx.[21] More aggressive blind techniques include flushing the nasal cavity while reaming the area of interest with a stiff plastic tube, sampling with a biopsy needle (Tru-Cut Disposable Biopsy Needle; Travenol Laboratories, Inc, Morton Grove, IL) or plastic catheter, or applying suction to a Foley urethral catheter.[22–24] These techniques do not allow characterization of the disease process that is possible with direct visualization, and in some cases result in non-diagnostic or misleading tissue samples. However, they do not require specialized equipment, are easy to perform, and often result in a definitive diagnosis. If the cytologic diagnosis is inconsistent with the signalment, history, or imaging studies, the veterinarian should repeat the procedure or consider one that allows direct visualization of the area of interest. Catheters have also been placed through the nares and into the dorsonasal meatus to administer antifungal medications in dogs.[17, 25]

CAUDAL ACCESS TO THE NASAL CAVITY

In some animals, the nasopharynx is the primary area of interest, as determined by results of imaging studies and nasopharyngeal examination. Tissue samples may be obtained from this area by means of a flexible scope, surgical splitting of the soft and/or hard palate (see Ventral Access to the Nasal Cavity), or retroflexion of a catheter dorsal to the soft palate followed by lavage and/or suction.

DORSAL ACCESS TO THE NASAL CAVITY AND FRONTAL SINUSES

Neoplastic and infectious disease processes will occasionally result in lysis of bone dorsal to the nasal cavity (frontal, nasal, or maxillary bones) with subsequent extension to the overlying soft tissues. These areas may be sampled directly with a biopsy needle or by incisional biopsy. Sedation with provisions for appropriate analgesia is often all that is needed; however, general anesthesia may be required to fully evaluate the extent of the disease process (e.g., CT studies), and biopsy can be performed during the same anesthetic episode. Subtle lytic defects that are detected, or suspected, on evaluation of imaging studies may be amenable to ultrasound-guided biopsy. Limited dorsal rhinotomy or sinusotomy can be performed by incision of the skin, subcutaneous tissues, and periosteum directly over the site of the lesion. A small window in the overlying bone can be made with an oscillating bone saw, Steinmann pin, Michelle's trephine, or osteotome and enlarged with rongeurs. Bone that is involved in the disease process may be submitted for histopathologic examination. Representative samples of affected nasal turbinates and masses should then be collected by curettage. If a small window was made into one of the frontal sinuses, the sinus may be examined by inserting a sterile rigid arthroscope through the opening. Trephination or osteotomy of each lateral frontal sinus can begin at a point halfway between the dorsal midline and the zygomatic process of the frontal bone. Penetration of the frontal bones caudal to these processes increases the risk of penetration through the floor of the frontal sinus or directly into the brain case. In the cat, the sinuses are much less extensive and so there is less room for error when making this approach. Each sinus drains rostrally and ventrally into the nasal cavity through separate ostia. It has been shown that surgical damage to the ostia will result in granulation tissue and new bone formation that can block sinus drainage and result in fluid accumulation.[26] Techniques that involve curettage of this area during biopsy, or placement of catheters through sinus ostia for the treatment of fungal rhinitis, could theoretically result in similar obstruction. Inflammatory, infectious, and neoplastic diseases can also result in ostia obstruction and subsequent fluid accumulation within the sinuses. Resection of the midline intersinus septum to improve drainage in cases of unilateral sinusitis may be of little value because mucociliary flow is directed away from this septum.[27] Medications that are administered into the lateral frontal sinuses in dogs may not be distributed to the other sinuses. Intranasal administration of infusate with canine cadavers placed in dorsal recumbency resulted in better distribution than did techniques that mimicked antifungal administration through sinusotomy.[28] After sinusotomy "vent" tubes are typically placed to limit formation of subcutaneous emphysema.

In cats, trephination of the frontal sinuses has been performed to allow instillation of medications for the treatment of chronic secondary bacterial rhinitis/sinusitis. Trephination of the frontal sinuses in cats should be performed with an intramedullary pin, trephine, nitrogen-powered drill, or a 16- to 18-gauge bone marrow biopsy needle. In kittens, the hole is made just off of the midline, halfway between the medial canthus of the eye and the zygomatic process of the frontal bone; in mature cats, the hole should be slightly more caudal, rostral to a line drawn between the zygomatic processes on either side. The trephine holes may be connected with an osteotomy and a bone flap created if obliteration of the sinuses is planned. Chronic sinusitis is unlikely to resolve unless the frontal sinuses are obliterated surgically.[29] Feline frontal sinus obliteration requires a more aggressive sinusotomy followed by removal of the mucous membrane, plugging the sinus ostia with fascia, and packing the sinuses with autogenous fat.[30–32] Reduction of nasal discharge after packing of the frontal sinuses with gentamicin-impregnated bone cement has also been reported.[33]

The classic dorsal rhinotomy involves exposure and elevation of a large bone flap. Typically, a dorsal midline skin incision is made and the frontal and nasal bones exposed by periosteal elevation over the area of interest. Either a unilateral or a bilateral rhinotomy and sinusotomy may be performed. Excessive lateral dissection may predispose to postoperative subcutaneous emphysema formation. A three-sided bone flap is left attached to the soft tissues at its rostralmost aspect. The flap is then separated from its deep attachments with an osteotome and rocked forward. Biopsy, foreign body retrieval, or palliative reduction of nasal tumors can then be performed. Hemorrhage with this procedure may require blood transfusion, so cross-matching should have been performed preoperatively. In addition, temporary ligation of the common carotid arteries may decrease blood loss.

Because of well-developed collateral circulation originating from the vertebral arteries in dogs, this procedure can be performed with no notable adverse effects. This is not true for the cat, in which bilateral carotid ligation may result in death.[34–37] Given the presence of collateral circulation in the dog, the actual benefit of carotid ligation for reducing blood loss during nasal surgery has been brought into question. Hemorrhage usually subsides after curettage of the nasal turbinates but occasionally will persist and require continuous direct pressure by packing the nasal cavity with petrolatum-impregnated gauze. The gauze is placed so that it can be retrieved through the nares 24 to 48 hours postoperatively. Closure of the dorsal rhinotomy may include replacement of the bone flap, which is typically stabilized with orthopedic cerclage wire placed through pre-drilled holes in the dorsolateral aspect of the flap, with similar holes in the parent bone. If the flap is to be included in a radiation field for treatment of nasal neoplasia, some have advised elimination of the cerclage because electron ejection from the metal may result in an extremely high radiation dose around the wires with subsequent bone necrosis. Others have reported that failure to replace the bone flap results in little if any cosmetic defect.[38, 39] Discarding the bone flap is recommended if neoplastic invasion of the flap exists, or if there are concerns regarding necrosis of the flap (e.g., if it will be included in a radiation field). One of the most common complications that occurs after dorsal rhinotomy is the development of subcutaneous emphysema. Strategies to decrease the likelihood of this complication have included the placement of "vent" tubes in the osteotomy site that act as a low-resistance pathway along which air can escape nasal passages. Flexible urinary catheters or sterile tubing from a fluid administration set is typically cut into two sections 5 to 8 cm in length. The tubes are then placed in the dorsolateral aspects of the osteotomy and are sutured to the skin using a finger-trap pattern. An Elizabethan collar should be placed because many animals will attempt to dislodge the tubing. An alternative is to create a rhinostomy at the dorsal aspect of the surgical site that is allowed to heal by second intention. Persistent serous discharge and or recurrent bacterial rhinitis may occur in dogs after extensive surgical damage to the nasal mucosa, as seen with some rhinotomy procedures. Although the cause for this is unclear, owners need to be warned of this possible sequela to radical turbinectomy.

VENTRAL ACCESS TO THE NASAL CAVITY

Given the potential problems associated with dorsal rhinotomy (such as subcutaneous emphysema), the need to reposition an animal (twice) if carotid artery ligation is to be performed, and the relative dissatisfaction of owners with

ENT

the appearance of their pets in the immediate postoperative period, ventral rhinotomy has been investigated.[40] After aseptic preparation of the oral cavity, and the ventral cervical region if carotid artery ligation is to be performed, a ventral midline incision is made through the mucoperiosteum of the hard palate centered over the region of interest. Additional lateral exposure is achieved with a periosteal elevator, being careful not to damage the major palatine arteries caudolaterally. A rectangular window is created in the hard palate with a burr (compressed nitrogen, electric, or battery powered). The midline incision may be extended caudally to include the soft palate, if preoperative imaging studies have shown that the tissue or mass to be accessed is dorsal to the junction of the hard and soft palates. Closure of the palatal mucoperiosteum is accomplished with a single layer of simple interrupted absorbable sutures. Closure of soft palate incisions is accomplished with two to three layers of absorbable sutures. Animals are placed on a soft diet for several weeks postoperatively. Dehiscence is rarely a problem after ventral rhinotomy, subcutaneous emphysema has not been reported, and cosmesis is improved in the immediate postoperative period. Access to caudal nasopharyngeal tumors, fungal granulomas, and foreign bodies can be gained by incision of the soft palate alone. Acquired nasopharyngeal stenosis has been described in cats as a possible sequela to chronic rhinitis. Soft palate splitting with surgical excision of the membrane is apparently curative.[41]

CATEGORIES OF DISEASE IN THE NOSE AND NASAL SINUSES

INFLAMMATORY RHINITIS

Inflammatory nasopharyngeal polyps in young cats may originate from the middle ear or the eustachian tube and subsequently protrude into the nasopharynx. Purulent nasal discharge, dyspnea, and stridorous respiration may follow. Once the polyp is visualized dorsal to the soft palate, radiographs or CT studies of the tympanic bullae are recommended to look for evidence of otitis media. The polyp can then be avulsed by grasping the base and applying gentle traction. Visualization is improved by retracting the soft palate rostrally with a spay hook. Recurrence is unlikely if ipsilateral ventral bulla osteotomy is performed simultaneously.[42]

Rostral polypoid rhinitis in the dog occurs rarely in conjunction with *Rhinosporidium seeberi* infection. Diagnosis is based on cytologic and histopathologic findings. Aggressive surgical removal of the affected tissue is indicated in most cases, although spontaneous remissions have been reported. Medical therapy with dapsone can inhibit growth of the organism, but the drug can be associated with severe hematologic side effects.[43]

Lymphocytic plasmacytic rhinitis has been described as an immune-mediated cause of chronic nasal disease in the dog. The diagnosis is based on the finding of severe diffuse lymphoplasmacytic infiltrate in nasal biopsy specimens and the exclusion of other causes of nasal disease. Immunosuppressive corticosteroid administration for at least 2 weeks is indicated; thus, the exclusion of other infectious causes of nasal disease is a prerequisite to therapy.[44]

INFECTIOUS RHINITIS

Bacterial and Viral Rhinitis

Primary bacterial rhinitis is uncommon in both the dog and cat. In the dog, bacterial rhinitis occurs most commonly as a sequela to the presence of a foreign body or as a consequence of gross anatomic changes (primarily loss of turbinates) resulting from prior mycotic disease, trauma, or irradiation. Feline bacterial rhinitis most commonly occurs in conjunction with viral upper respiratory tract infections (feline herpesvirus-1 and calicivirus). *Chlamydia psittaci* causes primary upper respiratory tract disease in a small number of cats. Opportunistic infection involving normal respiratory flora occurs most commonly. Bacterial culture of nasal discharge is usually not warranted. Administration of a broad-spectrum antibiotic and appropriate nursing care (intermittent nasal decongestants, nutritional support, and cleansing of the nares) are indicated.

At least 90 per cent of feline upper respiratory tract disease is caused by the feline herpesvirus-1 and feline calicivirus.[45] Confirming the diagnosis of viral rhinitis is best accomplished by virus isolation from tonsillar/oropharyngeal swabs. Cytology and serology are generally unrewarding diagnostically. Chronically affected cats should be evaluated for feline leukemia virus and feline immunodeficiency virus.

Parasitic Rhinitis

Parasitic rhinitis is rare in the dog and cat and is most commonly associated with the nasal mite *Pneumonyssoides caninum* and the nasal nematode *Capillaria aerophila*. The visualization of the mites during rhinoscopy and the identification of the nematode from histopathologic sampling and/or fecal examination permit diagnosis. Therapy with ivermectin (0.2 mg/kg SC or PO, given twice over a 3-week period) is reported to be successful.

Mycotic Rhinitis

Canine nasal aspergillosis is characterized by colonization and invasion of the nasal passages and frontal sinuses, most commonly by *Aspergillus fumigatus*, a ubiquitous, saprophytic species of filamentous fungus. Destruction and necrosis of the nasal mucosa and underlying turbinate bones result, often accompanied by frontal sinus osteomyelitis. *Aspergillus* is regarded as an opportunistic pathogen, suggesting that some pre-existing immunologic defect allowed its establishment.[46] Alternatively, an in-vitro inhibition of B- and T-lymphocyte transformation by *A. fumigatus* products is described, suggesting that immunosuppression may result from infection.[47] The clinical signs, diagnosis, and management of nasal aspergillosis are well reviewed.[48]

Therapeutic recommendations for nasal aspergillosis have included surgery as well as systemic and topical antimycotic medications. Rhinotomy and turbinectomy with perioperative thiabendazole administration resulted in improvement in less than or equal to 50 per cent of cases. Oral ketoconazole administration was efficacious in 47 per cent of cases, oral fluconazole in 60 per cent, and oral itraconazole in 60 to 70 per cent. Enilconazole applied topically through frontal sinus tubes, twice daily for 7 to 10 days, was efficacious in 80 to 90 per cent of cases but is not readily available in the United States.[48] Invasive surgical exposure of the nasal passages and frontal sinuses, topical 10 per cent povidone iodine application, with delayed closure 6 to 8 weeks postoperatively was recommended for refractory cases but had poor client acceptance.[49]

Clotrimazole is a synthetic imidazole derivative. At concentrations achieved during systemic use, imidazoles impair the biosynthesis of ergosterol, the major component of fungal cell membranes, resulting in interference with certain membrane-bound enzyme systems and fungistatic inhibition of growth.[50] Clotrimazole is fungicidal at higher concentrations (1.5×10^{-4}M). Electron microscopic observations indicate clotrimazole causes alteration in the cell membrane with consequent changes in permeability and leakage of cellular constituents in a manner similar to the effect of polyene antifungal antibiotics.[51]

Clotrimazole is available as human topical preparations for cutaneous, oral, or vaginal applications. Orally, clotrimazole is poorly absorbed and the small amount absorbed undergoes hepatic metabolism and biliary excretion. Gastrointestinal irritation and cutaneous pruritus are reported side effects in humans.

Clotrimazole solution has been used successfully for the topical treatment of nasal aspergillosis in the dog.[52] Ideally, diagnostics (radiology, rhinoscopy, biopsies, and cultures) are performed during the same period of anesthesia as the therapy. Rhinoscopic evidence of fungal plaques and turbinate destruction lends strong clinical support for the diagnosis of nasal aspergillosis. Mycologic, histologic, and serologic studies provide confirmation of aspergillosis. Dogs should receive inhalation anesthesia with a cuffed endotracheal tube in place. A 24-French Foley catheter is placed per os so that the tip of the catheter lies dorsal to the soft palate. A mouth gag is placed, and an assistant pulls the tongue rostrally to improve visualization during catheter placement. The catheter is advanced until the balloon is dorsal to the junction of the hard and soft palates. The balloon of the Foley catheter is then inflated to occlude the nasopharynx. The balloon can be palpated through the soft palate to confirm its position just caudal to the hard palate. Moistened laparotomy sponges are counted and then placed in the pharynx so that the catheter cannot migrate caudally, and to absorb any infusate that might escape around the balloon. During sponge placement, the index finger of the opposite hand is used to maintain balloon position. The mouth gag is removed. One 10-French polypropylene infusion catheter is then advanced through each nostril. Beginning dorsomedially, each catheter is advanced into the dorsal nasal meatus to the level of the medial canthus of the ipsilateral palpebral fissure. A Foley catheter (12 French) is then inserted into each nostril and the balloons inflated so that they lie just caudal to, and occlude, the nostrils. Occasionally, a nylon suture is placed across each nostril to prevent cranial migration of the nasal balloons. The three Foley catheters (one nasopharyngeal, two nasal) are placed, and their balloons are inflated, to slow the leakage of clotrimazole from the nasal cavity and frontal sinuses. The dogs are then re-positioned in dorsal recumbency, and an additional laparotomy sponge is placed just caudal to the upper incisors between the endotracheal tube and the incisive papilla to control leakage of clotrimazole through the incisive duct.

One gram of clotrimazole in 100 mL of polyethylene glycol 200 (1 per cent solution) is then evenly divided between two 60-mL syringes (50 mL/syringe). The clotrimazole is slowly infused over 1 hour (50 mL/infusion catheter). The polypropylene catheters are maintained in a horizontal position, parallel to the table, throughout infusion. When fluid is noted within the lumen of a Foley catheter it is clamped shut. Each animal should be positioned so that its nose protrudes beyond the edge of the treatment table, allowing clotrimazole to escape around the nasal catheters and drip into a receptacle.

While the dog's body is maintained in dorsal recumbency, its head is rotated and maintained in the following positions to ensure drug contact with all nasal surfaces: dorsal recumbency (15 minutes), left lateral recumbency (15 minutes), right lateral recumbency (15 minutes), dorsal recumbency (15 minutes). The dog should then be placed in sternal recumbency, the catheters and sponges removed and counted, the medication allowed to drain rostrally, the pharynx and proximal esophagus suctioned, and the anesthesia discontinued.

Some dogs with advanced disease may require multiple 1-hour clotrimazole infusions. Most will experience resolution of their nasal discharge after one treatment. Ideally, a CT scan should be performed before the infusion to best evaluate the integrity of the cribriform plate, because infusion of clotrimazole into the central nervous system causes severe meningitis. In addition, severity of disease on CT correlates with the likely need for multiple infusions. A favorable response to clotrimazole therapy is reflected by resolution of the signs of nasal aspergillosis and can be confirmed rhinoscopically and histologically. Nasal discharge, depigmentation, facial pain, and sneezing diminish markedly from 1 to 2 weeks after therapy. Persistence of symptoms 2 to 4 weeks after therapy indicates the need for additional infusions.

Nasal cryptococcosis occurs most frequently in the cat. Canine cryptococcosis commonly involves the central nervous system. Diagnosis is based on recovery of *Cryptococcus neoformans* in cytologic specimens or by a positive latex antigen test. Surgical removal of isolated lesions is possible, but most cases require systemic antifungal therapy, of which itraconazole is most efficacious. Fluconazole is indicated in cases in which central nervous system involvement has occurred.

NEOPLASIA OF THE NASAL PLANE, NASAL CAVITY, AND PARANASAL SINUSES

Exact nasal cavity tumor location is sometimes difficult to determine because these tumors can be extensive and involve surrounding tissues (external nose, orbit, and oral cavity). Intranasal tumors are more common in dogs than in cats. They are the most common cause of unilateral epistaxis, facial deformity, and epiphora in aged dogs and cats. Tumors of the nasal plane and nasal vestibule are rare in the dog and more common in the cat.

The most common tumor type of the nasal plane is squamous cell carcinoma (SCC). Other tumors in this site are lymphoma, fibrosarcoma, hemangioma, melanoma, mast cell tumor, and fibroma. SCCs are usually seen in adult or aged animals. They may arise de novo or from skin damaged by sun exposure. Generally, SCCs are locally invasive but late to metastasize.

In dogs, SCC is an erosive and deeply infiltrative tumor. Epistaxis, sneezing, swelling, and ulceration of the nasal plane are common presenting signs.[53] The tumor appears to be more common in males than in females.[53, 54] At the time of presentation, dogs typically have advanced, invasive lesions.[53] In cats, excessive sunlight exposure and lack of skin pigmentation are two major risk factors associated with development of SCC. The risk for white cats is 13.4 times greater than for non-white cats.[55] Sunlight-induced SCC is often preceded by a protracted course of disease (months to years) that progresses through the following clinical stages: waxy, dark epithelial crusting and erythema corresponding histologically to actinic keratosis; superficial erosions and ulcers corresponding to carcinoma in situ or early SCC; and finally deeply invasive and erosive lesions.[56] These tumors usually develop in multiple sites, including the eyelids and pinnae if lacking pigment.

Advanced SCC of the nasal plane tends to invade underlying cartilage. Lesions of the columella invade the upper lip and premaxilla. Lesions arising on the lateral alae or the nasolabial junction tend to infiltrate deeply into the nasal vestibule, and lateral spread occurs into the lip and external nose. For advanced lesions it is sometimes impossible to determine if a tumor originates from the vestibule or extends into it. Lesions involving the vestibule are quite deceptive because they are always more extensive than predicted from physical findings. SCC of the nasal plane may be locally invasive but only rarely metastasizes. Distant metastases may be seen in dogs with advanced disease.[57] In a study of 90 cats with SCC of the nasal plane, 6 had metastasis to mandibular lymph nodes and 1 had pulmonary metastases.[58]

Tumors should be sampled with a deep wedge to determine degree of invasion and histologic type. These biopsies require a brief general anesthetic because of the sensitivity of the nasal plane. Regional lymph nodes (buccal and mandibular) should be palpated. If lymphadenopathy is present, the nodes should be evaluated with cytology or histology. Thoracic radiographs are recommended for advanced cases.

In dogs with SCC of the nasal plane, the probability of cure with any conventional form of treatment is low. The fact that most dogs with carcinomas of the nasal plane are presented with advanced disease deeply infiltrating bone or cartilage and extending into the nasal vestibule may explain the poor response to treatment. For invasive superficial SCC, amputation of the nasal plane can be performed.[59] Functional and cosmetic results are usually marginal. Treatment is indicated for SCC confined to the nasal plane with no extension to the lip or surrounding skin. Careful evaluation of the surgical margins is required to ensure that the resection is complete. If the surgical resection is incomplete, adjuvant post-operative radiation therapy may be recommended. Intratumoral administration of a slow-release formulation of antineoplastic drugs including cisplatin, carboplatin, 5-fluorouracil, and bleomycin has not been found effective. Tumors appear responsive but recur promptly (2–3 months) after treatment. For advanced lesions, surgical resection and/or radiation therapy are not effective.[54, 59]

Cats with actinic keratosis, carcinoma in situ, and early SCC lesions can be managed effectively by limited surgical resection or conservative treatments including cryosurgery, phototherapy, or irradiation. Brachytherapy radiation using a strontium-90 radioactive applicator is the treatment of choice for lesions 2 to 3 mm thick. The treatment field includes the gross lesion and a 2-mm biologic margin, and the radiation surface dose ranges from 200 to 250 Gy depending on the thickness of the area to be treated. For treatment areas larger than the active surface of the applicator, a multiple abutting field technique is used with overlapping areas restricted to tumor tissues. The 1-year local control rate with a single application is 90 per cent, and the cosmetic results are excellent.[60] Similar efficacy may be obtained with photodynamic therapy, but equipment cost and photosensitizer-related toxicity may limit its application. In one study, local control rate for non-invasive lesions (<1.5 cm in diameter) was 90 per cent at 1-year. Treatment complications included skin photosensitization and drug-related cardiovascular reactions.[61] Cryotherapy is the least effective treatment and is associated with substantial local reactions, including temporary obstruction of the nares and delayed wound healing. In a series of 90 cats treated with liquid nitrogen, the 1-year

local control rate with a single treatment was 70 per cent.[62] For invasive SCC, amputation of the nasal plane can be performed in cats with acceptable functional and cosmetic results.[59] When available, external-beam radiation therapy is often preferred as primary treatment because of the good functional and cosmetic results. In addition, it allows treatment of a large field including the overt tumor and the precancerous non-invasive lesions that often are located within the surrounding sun-damaged skin. Radiation therapy is indicated for treatment of extensive superficial or invasive tumors. In cats with invasive lesions treated with orthovoltage irradiation, the 1-year local control rate was 85 per cent for lesions less than 2 cm in diameter and 67 per cent for lesions 2 to 4 cm in diameter. Tumor response is rapid and often complete by the end of the course of radiation therapy. During the last portion of the treatment and the first 2 weeks after treatment, epilation is common and the mucosa of the vestibule and the skin included in the treatment field develop radiation reactions. Severity of these reactions may be aggravated by self-trauma and superimposed infection. Mild reactions including erythema and dry desquamation do not require any medication. Severe reactions include moist desquamation in which the epidermis is shed, exposing the dermis. Moist desquamation is characterized by oozing of serous exudate and superficial crust formation and is associated with pruritus. Management of moist desquamation of the skin focuses on preventing trauma with an Elizabethan collar and preventing infection. Areas of moist desquamation should be kept clean and crusts may be removed by soaking with a 1:1 solution of 3 per cent hydrogen peroxide and normal saline (full-strength 3 per cent hydrogen peroxide is harmful to granulation tissue and must be avoided). Patient comfort may be improved with systemic administration of corticosteroids. Acute radiation reactions usually resolve within 2 to 3 weeks of treatment. After treatment, the new epidermis is thin, fragile, and pink, although it thickens over time. Hair regrowth may be incomplete or abnormal with distorted whiskers and whitening. Radiation complications including stenosis of the nares, chronic rhinitis, and ulceration of the nasal and lip margins may develop several months after treatment. In one study, cats infected with feline immunodeficiency virus had an increased incidence of severe chronic radiation complications compared with cats free of this virus.[58]

Intratumoral administration of a slow-release formulation of carboplatin has been found safe and effective for treatment of superficial invasive SCC. Treatment includes a series of four injections with carboplatin (1.5 mg/cm^3 of tissue including the gross tumor and a margin of normal tissue) incorporated in a drug carrier given at 1-week intervals (Fig. 123–16). The 1-year local control rate was 100 per cent for lesions 2 to 4 cm in diameter.[63] Because of the specific and dose-related toxicity of cisplatin and 5-fluorouracil in cats, their use should be avoided for large invasive tumors because cumulative dosage may result in severe systemic toxicosis. For advanced lesions, deeply infiltrating maxillary bone, or cartilage, the goals of treatment are essentially palliation. Radiation therapy (median survival, 9 months) and intratumoral chemotherapy with carboplatin (median survival, 5 months) improves the quality and duration of survival.

In dogs, SCC of the nasal plane is associated with a poor, long-term prognosis. In cats, prognosis depends on tumor size and location. Early (Tis to T1) SCC of the nasal plane is curable, but later development of new sites of neoplasia on other areas of the plane or the facial skin damaged by the sun is common. Small and minimally invasive tumors

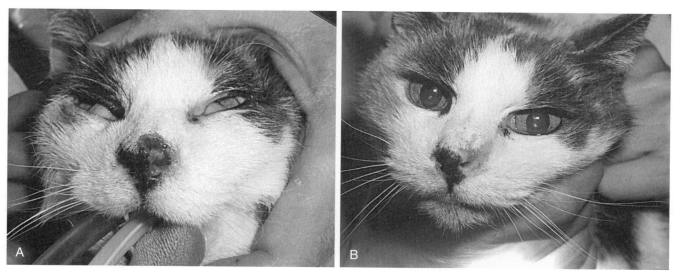

Figure 123–16. Cat with a squamous cell carcinoma of the nasal plane *(A)*. This cat received four intratumoral administrations of carboplatin in a water/sesame seed/oil emulsion. The tumor is in complete remission 12 months after treatment *(B)* with no evidence of local or systemic toxicity.

ENT

have a good prognosis, whereas advanced tumors have invariably a poor prognosis. It is expected that development of an optimum radiation protocol using daily fractionation and high total doses may improve efficacy. Tumors affecting the columella and floor of the nasal vestibule have a poor prognosis. Decreased control rates may be explained in this site by the occult extension of the tumor into the floor of the nasal vestibule, nasal septum, lip, and premaxilla. Tumor proliferative fraction, as estimated by use of a proliferating cell nuclear antigen immunohistochemistry method, is another factor that has been found to have a prognostic value for cats treated with orthovoltage irradiation. A high proliferation index was associated with a poorer prognosis.[58]

Tumors of the sinonasal cavities account for 1 to 2 per cent of all canine and feline neoplasms.[64] Nasal tumors are more common in middle-aged and old animals. Most tumors in dogs and cats are malignant. The malignant nature of intranasal tumors is reflected more by their progressive local invasiveness than by distant metastasis, which usually occurs late in the course of the disease.

In dogs, no sex or breed predisposition has been found. The median age of affected dogs is between 8 and 10 years. Eighty per cent of canine intranasal tumors are malignant and, approximately two thirds of them are of epithelial origin.[65] The three most common intranasal carcinomas are adenocarcinoma, SCC, and undifferentiated carcinoma. Nonepithelial sinonasal tumors are reported less frequently and include chondrosarcomas, fibrosarcomas, undifferentiated sarcomas, osteosarcomas, lymphomas, and transmissible venereal tumors. The metastatic rate is generally low at the time of initial diagnosis but may rise to 40 per cent by the end of the animal's life. Lymph nodes and lungs are the most common metastatic sites.[66] Benign adenoma/papilloma, fibroma, chondroma, or osteoma is rarely identified.

Approximately 90 per cent of all feline intranasal nasal tumors are malignant.[65] Carcinomas are more commonly diagnosed. Lymphoma, fibrosarcoma, and chondrosarcoma are less frequently seen.[67] When compared with dogs, cats (usually feline leukemia virus negative) have a higher risk for lymphoma.

Neoplasia of the sinonasal cavities is characterized by insidious onset and protracted clinical course. The period between the development of clinical signs and diagnosis is 3 months on average. Clinical signs include nasal discharge, sneezing, epistaxis, facial and/or oral deformity, epiphora due to obstruction of the nasolacrimal duct, stertor, exophthalmos due to a retrobulbar mass effect, and central neurologic signs usually due to expansion of the tumor through the cribriform plate. In a report of 104 dogs with sinonasal neoplasia, the most common clinical signs included epistaxis, nasal discharge, seizures, sneezing, and dyspnea.[66] The nasal discharge is usually unilateral initially. As the disease progresses and the integrity of the nasal septum is lost, the discharge becomes bilateral and serosanguineous. Although these clinical signs overlap with those of other causes of intranasal disease, a strong suspicion of intranasal neoplasia can be made in older animals with an intermittent and progressive history of nasal discharge/epistaxis. The presence of facial deformity and, to a lesser degree, epiphora increases the risk that the nasal disease is neoplasia. A definitive diagnosis of intranasal neoplasia requires a tissue biopsy, even though diagnostic imaging and historical information can be highly suggestive.

The complex anatomy of the nasal cavity and paranasal sinuses and their proximity to the orbit and cranial vault make precise evaluation of tumor extent difficult. CT is the most accurate imaging technique for staging of sinonasal tumors. Although the risk for nasal neoplasia to metastasize is low, fine-needle aspiration or biopsy of clinically enlarged regional nodes and thoracic radiographs should be obtained to rule out this possibility. If any signs of central nervous system disease exist, a CT or MRI study should be performed and a sample of cerebrospinal fluid evaluated to help in determining tumor invasiveness.

Dogs and cats with intranasal tumors are too often presented at a late stage with, in most cases, extensive bony involvement. The life expectancy of an untreated animal depends largely on the owner's tolerance of the signs. The usual period between diagnosis and euthanasia or natural death in a dog with an untreated nasal tumor is 3 to 5 months; it may be longer in cats. Treatment of animals with nasal tumors is directed primarily at control of local disease. Radiation therapy is the mainstay of treatment for intranasal tumors. It is the only form of treatment that improves the quality and duration of survival. Cytoreductive surgery alone does not increase survival time or the disease-free interval in dogs or cats with intranasal tumors. The poor response to surgery is attributed to the local invasiveness of most nasal tumors. The high rate of acute and chronic postoperative morbidity, particularly in cats, without significant prolongation of life should preclude the use of surgical curettage unless other adjuvant treatments such as irradiation are available.[68] Chemotherapy, immunotherapy, and cryosurgery have not been shown to improve survival when used in the treatment of intranasal tumors.

Radiation therapy has the advantage of treating the entire nasal cavity and paranasal sinuses, including any bone extension, which surgery cannot remove. The poor overall treatment efficacy indicates that optimum irradiation techniques and treatment protocols have not been identified. Access to modern equipment and computerized treatment planning may allow precise delivery of high doses of radiation to the tumor volume while sparing normal surrounding tissues (eye, brain, oral mucosa). The current recommendation for irradiation technique is to use high-energy (megavoltage) radiation generated by a medical linear accelerator or a cobalt unit with CT-based treatment planning (Fig. 123–17). Median survival time was 13 months for dogs[69, 70] and 11.5 months for cats[71] with non-lymphoproliferative nasal tumors treated with megavoltage irradiation. The use of lower radiation energy (orthovoltage) is not recommended because of the poor penetration of radiation in tissues and the substantial risk of bone radionecrosis and severe skin reaction. The median survival time for dogs treated with orthovoltage irradiation (3 mm Cu HVL) was 4 months.[72]

Irradiation of intranasal tumors results in some damage to the normal tissue included in the treatment field. The incidence of radiation effects on normal tissues increases with the magnitude of the dose per fraction, the total dose, and the volume of tissue included in the field of irradiation irradiated and with a decrease of overall treatment time. Radiation effects on normal tissues appear to be less severe in cats than in dogs. With treatment protocols using large doses per fraction (3–5 Gy) and short overall time (3–4 weeks) the risk of radiation damage to normal tissue, particularly in the eyes included in the radiation field, is high.[69, 73] It is important to inform the owner about the potential side effects of treatment. During the last portion of the treatment and the first 2 weeks after treatment, radiation-induced mucosal inflammation in the nasal cavity, referred to as rhinitis, is manifested by nasal stuffiness, increased mucous production, and bloody nasal discharge. These clinical signs are always overshadowed by the reactions of the adjacent tissues, including the skin, oral mucosa, eyelid, and eye. Oral mucositis, rhinitis, and conjunctivitis occur earlier than skin reactions, and healing usually proceeds more rapidly. Oral mucositis is manifested by increased salivation, accumulation of tenacious mucus, tenderness of the mouth, and halitosis. Highly palatable food is recommended during a course of radiation therapy, because radiation effects to the oral and nasal cavity may reduce smell and taste sensation. Mild to moderate mucositis may be treated with irrigation with a solution of 1:2 hydrogen peroxide 3 per cent in normal saline placed in an atomizer and used as a spray. Commercial mouthwashes containing alcohol or glycerin oils prolong mucositis and should be avoided. Management of severe oral mucositis include topical chlorhexidine (0.2 per cent solution without alcohol) and systemic corticosteroid and antibiotic therapy. Severe reactions may result in

anorexia and secondary debilitation. Salivary substitutes (Salivart) may be used to keep the mucosa moist, mobile, and free of debris.

With the use of megavoltage radiation (linear accelerator and cobalt units) skin reactions are usually mild. Epilation is common. In areas where the skin may be irradiated tangentially, including the dorsum of the nose, nasal plane, and lips, the radiation dose may be excessive and result in punctate areas of moist desquamation. Skin care includes gentle cleansing with one-half strength hydrogen peroxide. Topical antiseptics including sulfadiazine (Silvadene) may be used to reduce the severity of the reaction and prevent superimposed infection.

When the eye and adnexal tissues are included in the treatment field, ocular reactions are the most painful side effects of radiation therapy. During a course of treatment, patients develop moderate symptoms of conjunctivitis and eyelid irritation. Conjunctivitis is often self-limiting, and treatment of inflammatory changes includes topical administration of corticoid suspension (Pred Forte, 1 per cent) or ointments. Unless all of the lacrimal tissue has received the full radiation dose, these clinical signs generally resolve completely within 2 to 3 weeks after treatment. If most of the eye is in the field, irradiation of lacrimal glands induces a decrease in the quantity and quality of the tears. The loss of the lubricating and cleansing effect of the tears can lead to corneal irritation and abrasion. This condition can progress to a painful keratitis, keratoconjunctivitis sicca, or corneal ulceration and may be aggravated by secondary infection. Acute conjunctivitis and keratoconjunctivitis can be managed with artificial tear supplementation (Tears Naturale, Bion Tears), topical administration of corticosteroid, and specific antibiotics. Tear film production must be monitored closely to avoid corneal ulceration. Corneal ulceration is manifested clinically by blepharitis, blepharospasm, and ocular discharge. Permanent damage to the lacrimal gland may result in chronic keratoconjunctivitis sicca and require long-term medical management, including viscous artificial tears preparations (Celluvisc, AquaSite) and cyclosporine ophthalmic ointment (Optimmune, 2 per cent). Radiation of the globe is relatively well tolerated. The most sensitive structure is the lens, and cataract formation occurs with radiation doses below therapeutic range. Cataracts usually take years to mature. Other ocular complications include nasolacrimal duct obstruction, retinopathy, and optic nerve injury. Blindness secondary to radiation retinopathy or optic nerve injury is recognized in people but is rarely diagnosed in dogs and cats; pets may not survive long enough to develop radiation-induced blindness. In dogs and cats with tumors involving the root of the nasal cavity and the frontal sinuses, a portion of the brain may be included in the treatment field. In these animals, a transient central nervous system syndrome, including disorientation and lethargy, may develop during or shortly after treatment.[69] Therapy is symptomatic with systemic anti-inflammatory corticosteroids. With tumor extension into the cribriform plate, cerebrospinal fluid leakage may occur as tumor size decreases after irradiation, resulting in ataxia and disorientation. With megavoltage radiation and computerized treatment planning, the risk of permanent damage to the brain, including brain necrosis, is low. Efforts to alleviate radiation damage to the brain, eye, and eyelid focus on improved treatment planning and use of low dose fractions. Because of the direct association between size of dose per fraction and probability of complications, any increase in total radiation dose to improve efficacy will

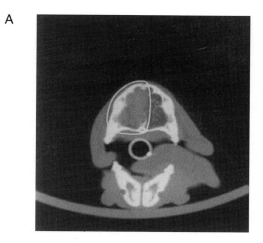
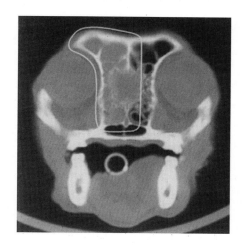
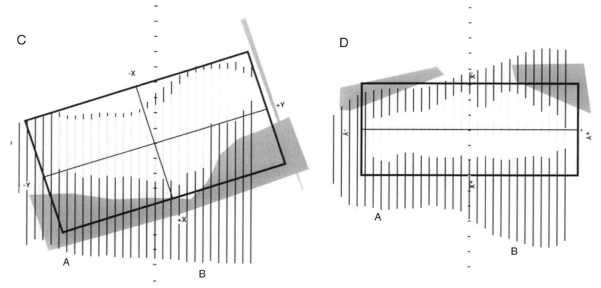

Figure 123–17. Dog with an intranasal tumor, showing the tumor volume and head contour as wire-frame surfaces reconstructed from serial CT slices from the vantage point of the radiation beam (beam's-eye view). A three-field technique (two parallel opposed lateral fields and one dorsal field) was used. Projection of CT slices *A* and *B* are shown on panels *C* and *D*. The central area on panels *C* and *D* shows a beam's-eye view display of the target volume defined on CT slices (panel *C* for dorsal radiation portal and panel *D* for lateral radiation portal). The remainder of the rectangular radiation beam is blocked by a lead alloy to protect adjacent normal structures. Beam's-eye view display provides a valuable tool for selecting portal size and shape that give the best coverage of the target volume with minimal radiation dose to surrounding normal tissues.

be achieved by using a larger number of dose fractions (≤ 3 Gy) rather than by an increase in the size of dose per fraction.

In humans, treatment of nasal and sinus tumors includes surgery or radiation therapy for small tumors without bone invasion and a combination of surgery and radiation for large tumors with bone invasion.[74] The benefit of cytoreductive surgery before irradiation has been shown in dogs and cats when orthovoltage radiation is used or when treatment is given with a few large dose fractions.[72, 75–77] The efficacy of surgery in combination with an optimal radiation treatment protocol using megavoltage radiation has not been determined.

Overall, the prognosis for non-lymphoproliferative nasal tumors is poor and most animals die or are euthanized as a result of local disease progression. A poorer prognosis has been associated with SCC and undifferentiated carcinoma, compared with nasal adenocarcinoma or sarcoma.[72] In one study, dogs with nasal chondrosarcoma had a better prognosis than dogs with adenocarcinoma.[69] It was suggested that the longer survival for dogs with chondrosarcoma may reflect a slower regrowth rate after irradiation rather than a true difference in response to radiation. Intranasal lymphoma (stage I) is the only tumor type currently curable with radiation therapy.[78] The World Health Organization tumor staging scheme has not been found to have a prognostic value. A modified staging scheme based on radiograph findings found that bilateral neoplasia extending into the frontal sinuses, with erosion of any bone of the nasal passages, was associated with a poorer prognosis.[69] The use of CT scanning will improve staging of intranasal tumors and may allow analysis of the prognostic value of tumor extent.

REFERENCES

1. Morgan JP: Radiographic study of the nasal cavity and paranasal sinuses of the dog. Small Animal Veterinary Medicine Series Update Series #9. Princeton, NJ, Veterinary Publications, 1978.
2. Coulson A: Radiology as an aid to diagnosis of nasal disorders in the cat. Vet Annual 28:150, 1988.
3. Gibbs C, et al: Radiological features of intra-nasal lesions in the dog: A review of 100 cases. J Small Anim Pract 20:515, 1979.
4. Schmidt M, Voorhout G: Radiography of the canine nasal cavity: Significance of the presence or absence of the trabecular pattern. Vet Radiol Ultrasound 33:83, 1992.
5. Sullivan M, et al: The radiological features of aspergillosis of the nasal cavity and frontal sinuses in the dog. J Small Anim Pract 27:167, 1986.
6. Morgan JP, et al: Tumors in the nasal cavity of the dog: A radiographic study. Vet Radiol 13:18, 1972.
7. Sullivan M, et al: The radiological features of sixty cases of intra-nasal neoplasia in the dog. J Small Anim Pract 28:575, 1987.
8. Harvey CE, et al: Chronic nasal disease in the dog: Its radiographic diagnosis. Vet Radiol 20:91, 1979.
9. Burk RL: Computed tomographic anatomy of the canine nasal passages. Vet Radiol Ultrasound 33:170, 1992.
10. Feeney DA, Fletcher TF, Hardy RM: Atlas of Correlative Imaging Anatomy of the Normal Dog—Ultrasound and Computed Tomography. Philadelphia, WB Saunders, 1991.
11. Assheur J, Sager M: MRI and CT Atlas of the Dog. Oxford, Blackwell Scientific Publications, 1997.
12. Losonsky JM, et al: Computed tomography of the normal feline nasal cavity and paranasal sinuses. Vet Radiol Ultrasound 38:251, 1997.
13. Koblik PD, Berry CR: Dorsal plane computed tomographic imaging of the ethmoid region to evaluate chronic nasal disease in the dog. Vet Radiol 31:92, 1990.
14. Thrall DE, et al: A comparison of radiographic and computed tomographic findings in 31 dogs with malignant nasal cavity tumors. Vet Radiol 30:59, 1989.
15. Park RD, et al: Comparison of computed tomography and radiography for detecting changes induced by malignant nasal neoplasia in dogs. JAVMA 201:1720, 1992.
16. Burk RL: Computed tomographic imaging of nasal disease in 100 dogs. Vet Radiol Ultrasound 33:177, 1992.
17. Mathews KG, et al: Computed tomographic assessment of non-invasive infusion in dogs with fungal rhinitis. Vet Surg 25:309, 1996.
18. Codner EC, et al: Comparison of computed tomography with radiography as a noninvasive diagnostic technique for chronic nasal disease in dogs. JAVMA 202:1106, 1993.
19. Moore MP, et al: MR, CT and clinical features from four dogs with nasal tumors involving the rostral cerebrum. Vet Radiol 32:19, 1991.
20. Voges AK, Ackerman N: MR evaluation of intra- and extracranial extension of nasal adenocarcinoma in a dog and cat. Vet Radiol Ultrasound 36:196, 1995.
21. MacEwen EG, Withrow SJ, Patnaik AK: Nasal tumors in the dog: Retrospective evaluation of diagnosis, prognosis, and treatment. JAVMA 170:45, 1977.
22. Withrow SJ: Diagnostic and therapeutic nasal flush in small animals. J Am Anim Hosp Assoc 13:704, 1977.
23. Withrow SJ, Susaneck SJ, Macy DW, et al: Aspiration and punch biopsy techniques for nasal tumors. J Am Anim Hosp Assoc 21:551, 1985.
24. Love S, Barr A, Lucke VM, et al: A catheter technique for biopsy of dogs with chronic nasal disease. J Small Anim Pract 28:417, 1987.
25. Mathews KG, Davidson AP, Koblick PD, et al: Comparison of topical administration of clotrimazole through surgically versus non-surgically placed catheters for treatment of nasal aspergillosis in dogs: 60 cases (1990–1996). JAVMA (in press).
26. Walsh TE: Experimental surgery of the ostium and nasofrontal duct in postoperative healing. Laryngoscope 53(2):75, 1943.
27. Dolezal RF, Baker SR: Mucociliary flow in the canine frontal sinus. Ann Otol Rhinol Laryngol 92(1 Pt 1):78, 1983.
28. Richardson EF, Mathews KG: Patterns of distribution of topical agents administered in the frontal sinuses and nasal cavity of dogs: A comparison between current treatment protocols for treatment of nasal aspergillosis and a new noninvasive technique. Vet Surg 24:476, 1995.
29. Winstanley EW: Trephining frontal sinuses in the treatment of rhinitis and sinusitis in the cat. Vet Rec 95:289, 1974.
30. Bright RM, Thacker HL, Brunner RD: Fate of autogenous fat implants in the frontal sinuses of cats. Am J Vet Res 44:22, 1983.
31. Tomlinson MJ, Schenck NL: Autogenous fat implantation as a treatment for chronic frontal sinusitis in a cat. JAVMA 167:927, 1975.
32. Anderson GI: The treatment of chronic sinusitis in six cats by ethmoid conchal curettage and autogenous fat graft sinus ablation. Vet Surg 16:131, 1987.
33. Norsworthy GD: Surgical treatment of chronic nasal discharge in 17 cats. Vet Med 88:526, 1993.
34. Gillian LA: Extra- and intra-cranial blood supply to the brains of dogs and cats. Am J Anat 146:237, 1976.
35. King AS: Arterial supply to the central nervous system. In Physiological and Clinical Anatomy of the Domestic Mammals, vol I, p 1. Oxford, Oxford University Press, 1987.
36. Holmberg DL: Sequelae of ventral rhinotomy in dogs and cats with inflammatory and neoplastic nasal pathology: A retrospective study. Can Vet J 37:483, 1996.
37. Holmberg DL, Pettifer GR: The effect of carotid artery occlusion on lingual arterial blood pressure in dogs. Can Vet J 38:629, 1997.
38. Thrall DE, Harvey CE: Radiotherapy of malignant nasal tumors in 21 dogs. JAVMA 183:663, 1983.
39. Birchard SJ: A simplified method for rhinotomy and temporary rhinostomy in dogs and cats. J Am Anim Hosp Assoc 24:69, 1988.
40. Holmberg DL, Fries D, Cockshutt J, et al: Ventral rhinotomy in the dog and cat. Vet Surg 18:446, 1989.
41. Mitten RW: Nasopharyngeal stenosis in four cats. J Small Anim Pract 29:341, 1988.
42. Kapatkin AS, Matthiesen DT, Noone KE, et al: Results of surgery and long-term follow-up in 31 cats with nasopharyngeal polyps. J Am Anim Hosp Assoc 26:387, 1990.
43. Wilson RB: Canine rhinosporidiosis. Compend Contin Ed Small Anim Pract 11:48, 1989.
44. Burgener DC, Slocombe RF, Zerbe CA: Lymphoplasmacytic rhinitis in 5 dogs. J Am Anim Hosp Assoc 23:565, 1987.
45. Ford RB: Viral upper respiratory infection in cats. Compend Contin Ed Small Anim Pract 13:20, 1991.
46. Washburn RG, Kennedy DWW, Begley MG, et al: Chronic fungal sinusitis in apparently normal hosts. Medicine (Baltimore) 67:231, 1988.
47. Sharp NJ, Harvey CE, Sullivan M: Canine nasal aspergillosis and penicilliosis. Compend Contin Ed Vet 13:41, 1991.
48. Sharp NJ: Nasal aspergillosis. In Kirk RW (ed): Current Veterinary Therapy X. Philadelphia, WB Saunders, 1989, p 1106.
49. Pavletic MM, Clark GN: Open nasal cavity and frontal sinus treatment of chronic canine aspergillosis. Vet Surg 20:43, 1991.
50. Bodey GP: Azole antifungal agents. Clin Infect Dis 14(Suppl 1):S161, 1992.
51. Iwata K, Yamaguchi H, Hiratani T: Mode of action of clotrimazole. Sabouraudia 11:158, 1973.
52. Davidson AP, Komtebedde J, Pappagianis D, et al: Treatment of nasal aspergillosis with topical clotrimazole. In Proceedings of the 10th Annual Veterinary Medical Forum, Denver, CO, ACVIM, 1992, p 807.
53. Rogers KS, Hellman RG, Walker MA: Squamous cell carcinoma of the canine nasal planum: Eight cases (1988–1994). J Am Anim Hosp Assoc 31:373, 1995.
54. Thrall DE, Adams WM: Radiotherapy of squamous cell carcinomas of the canine nasal plane. Vet Radiol 23:193, 1982.
55. Dorn CR, Taylor ON, Schneider R: Sunlight exposure and risk of developing cutaneous and oral squamous cell carcinoma in white cats. J Natl Cancer Inst 46:1073, 1971.
56. Evans AG, Madewell BR, Stannard AA: A trial of 13-cis-retinoic acid for treatment of squamous cell carcinoma and preneoplastic lesions of the head in cats. Am J Vet Res 46:2553, 1985.
57. Théon AP, Madewell BR, Moore AS, et al: Localized thermo-cisplatin therapy: A pilot study in spontaneous canine and feline tumours. Int J Hyperthermia 7:881, 1991.
58. Théon AP, Madewell BR, Shearn V, Moulton JE: Prognostic factors associated with radiotherapy of squamous cell carcinoma of the nasal plane in cats. JAVMA 206:991, 1995.
59. Withrow SJ, Straw RC: Resection of the nasal planum in nine cats and five dogs. J Am Anim Hosp Assoc 26:219, 1990.
60. VanVechten MK, Théon AP: Strontium-90 plesiotherapy for treatment of early squamous cell carcinomas of the nasal planum in 30 cats. Vet Radiol Ultrasound, in press.
61. Magne M, Rodriguez CO, Autry SA, et al: Photodynamic therapy of facial squamous cell carcinoma in cats using a new photosensitizer. Lasers Surg Med 20:202, 1997.
62. Clarke RE: Cryosurgical treatment of feline cutaneous squamous cell carcinoma. Aust Vet Pract 21:148, 1991.
63. Théon AP, VanVechten MK, Madewell BR: Intratumoral administration of carboplatin for treatment of squamous cell carcinomas of the nasal plane in cats. Am J Vet Res 57:205, 1996.
64. Moulton JE: tumors of the respiratory system. In Tumors in the Domestic Animals, 3rd ed. Berkeley, University of California Press, 1990, pp 308–318.
65. Madewell BR, Priester WA, Gillette EL, et al: Neoplasms of the nasal passages and paranasal sinuses in domestic animals as reported by 13 veterinary colleges. Am J Vet Res 37:851, 1976.
66. Patnaik AK: Canine sinonasal neoplasms: Clinicopathological study of 285 cases. J Am Anim Hosp Assoc 25:103, 1989.
67. Cox NR, Brawner WR, Powers RD et al: Tumors of the nose and paranasal sinuses in cats: 32 cases with comparison to a national database (1977–1987). J Am Anim Hosp Assoc 27:339, 1991.
68. Laing EJ, Binnington AG: Surgical therapy of canine nasal tumors: A retrospective study (1982–1986). Can Vet J 29:809, 1988.
69. Théon AP, Madewell BR, Harb MF, Dungworth DL: Megavoltage irradiation of neoplasms of the nasal and paranasal cavities in 77 dogs. JAVMA 202:1469, 1993.
70. McEntee MC, Page RL, Heidner GL, et al: A retrospective study of 27 dogs with intranasal neoplasms treated with cobalt radiation. Vet Radiol 32:135, 1991.
71. Théon AP, Peaston AE, Madewell BR, Dungworth DL: Irradiation of nonlymphoproliferative neoplasms of the nasal cavity and paranasal sinuses in 16 cats. JAVMA 204:78, 1994.
72. Adams WM, Withrow SJ, Walshaw R, et al: Radiotherapy of malignant nasal tumors in 67 dogs. JAVMA 191:311, 1987.
73. Roberts SM, Lavach JD, Severin GA, et al: Ophthalmic complications following megavoltage irradiation of the nasal and paranasal cavities in dogs. JAVMA 100:43, 1987.

74. Parsons JT, Stringer SP, Mancuso AA, et al: Nasal vestibule, nasal cavity, and paranasal sinuses. In Millon RR, Cassisi NJ (eds): Management of Head and Neck Cancer: A Multidisciplinary Approach, 2nd ed. Philadelphia, JB Lippincott, 1994.
75. Thrall DE, Harvey CE: Radiotherapy of malignant nasal tumors in 21 dogs. JAVMA 183:663, 1983.
76. Morris JS, Dunn KJ, Dobson JM, et al: Effects of radiotherapy alone and surgery

and radiotherapy on survival of dogs with nasal tumors. J Small Anim Pract 35:567, 1994.
77. Evans SM, Goldschmidt M, McKee LJ, Harvey CE: Prognostic factors and survival after radiotherapy for intranasal neoplasms in dogs: 70 cases (1974–1985). JAVMA 194:1460, 1989.
78. Straw RC, Withrow SJ, Gillette EL, et al: Use of radiotherapy for the treatment of intranasal tumors in cats: six cases (1980–1985). JAVMA 15:835, 1986.

CHAPTER 124

DISEASES OF THE THROAT

Anjop J. Venker–van Haagen

ENT

FUNCTIONAL CONSIDERATIONS

THE SWALLOWING PROCESS

Swallowing (deglutition) is the sum of activities involved in the mechanism to transport material from the oral cavity into the stomach. The most obvious function of swallowing is the transport of food and fluids during eating and drinking. However, swallowing also occurs frequently, independent of the intake of food and fluid, during periods of consciousness and during arousal from sleep, its function being to clear saliva and debris from the nasal pharynx and from the respiratory tract. This protects the respiratory tract from aspiration of saliva and debris.[1–3]

Much of the knowledge about the swallowing process in dogs and cats has been derived from experimental work in dogs and other animals, using videofluorography and electromyography.[4, 5] Deglutition is usually described as having three stages: the oral preparatory phase, the pharyngeal phase, and the esophageal phase. In the oral phase, small portions of food are taken into the oropharyngeal cavity and a bolus is formed. This action is immediately followed by contractions of the pharyngeal muscles that lift the food bolus up and pass it through the relaxed cricopharyngeal sphincter into the esophagus. This is the pharyngeal phase, and during this phase there is coordination of the respiratory cycle so that respiration is inhibited. The respiratory tract is protected by closure of the pharyngeal isthmus and the laryngeal inlet. Closure of the oropharyngeal cavity during this action promotes the one-way propulsion of the bolus.[1, 3, 4] During the esophageal phase, the food is propelled through the cervical and thoracic parts of the esophagus. There may be more than one bolus passing through the esophagus at the same time.

Neurophysiologic control of the swallowing process involves regulatory mechanisms that include the afferent signals, the efferent innervation of the musculature, and the control systems in the brain stem and the cortex. Swallowing can be evoked without influence of the cortex. The cerebral cortex controls voluntary aspects of feeding, such as food preparation in the oral phase.[1, 6] The sensory nerves involved

are the trigeminal, glossopharyngeal, cranial laryngeal, and the pharyngeal branches of the vagus. The muscles involved in the oral phase of the swallowing process are the mandibular and facial, innervated by the trigeminal and facial nerves, respectively. The movement of the tongue is determined by the intrinsic and extrinsic (hyoid) muscles of the tongue. The intrinsic muscles are innervated by the hypoglossal nerve and the extrinsic by the first two cervical nerves. In the pharyngeal phase, the muscles of the soft palate, the pharyngeal muscles, and the base of the tongue act together with the hyoid muscles. This involves the trigeminal nerve, the pharyngeal plexus, and the hypoglossal and cervical nerves, respectively. The esophagus is innervated by the pharyngeal plexus and the vagus nerves.[7] In dogs, the pharyngeal plexus innervates the soft palate and the hyopharyngeal, thyropharyngeal, and cricopharyngeal muscles. Each of these muscles has a double but strictly ipsilateral innervation from the glossopharyngeal nerve and the pharyngeal branch of the vagus nerve.[4]

Swallowing occurs as a result of sequential activity in the pharyngeal muscles, which moves material in a caudal direction. Pharyngeal swallowing depends on a central pattern generator located in the brain stem, an interneuronal network that programs the sequential motor pattern and timing during swallowing (Figs. 124–1 and 124–2).[8] However, regulation is markedly disturbed by peripheral transection of pharyngeal plexus components,[5] and stimulation of peripheral pathways influenced the contraction timing during swallowing in dogs.[8]

Laryngeal action during swallowing has not been clearly characterized by electromyographic studies, but some aspects can be described. During the pharyngeal phase of swallowing, respiration is inhibited and hence there is no abduction of the vocal folds. Closing of the vocal folds by muscular action may occur during deglutition,[7] but leakage of food through the laryngeal inlet into the trachea occurs when swallowing is disturbed by transection of the pharyngeal branch of the vagus nerve, leaving the cranial laryngeal nerves and the recurrent laryngeal nerves intact.[4] Further studies of the regulation of swallowing and the combined action of the pharyngeal and laryngeal muscles are needed.

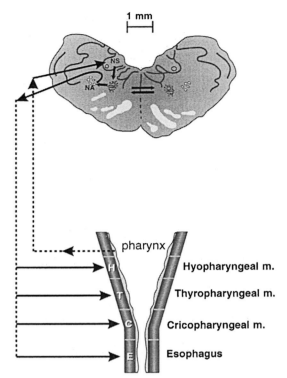

Figure 124–1. Diagram showing the functional relationship between the pharynx and the brain stem (transverse section) in pharyngeal swallowing. Afferent fibers in the glossopharyngeal, pharyngeal branch of the vagus, and cranial laryngeal nerves activate the solitary nucleus (NS). When the pathways synapsing with the interneurons of the central pattern generator are excited, sequential activation of the motorneurons in the nucleus ambiguus (NA) generates pharyngeal swallowing.

REGULATION AND CONDITIONING OF THE INSPIRATORY AND EXPIRATORY AIRFLOW

The laryngeal action during the respiratory cycle has been studied in dogs and cats. Abduction of the glottis during inspiration and adduction during expiration can be observed by laryngoscopy. Recordings of electrical activity via wire electrodes placed in intrinsic laryngeal abductor and adductor muscles revealed increased activity in the abductor, the dorsal cricoarytenoid muscle, at the end of expiration and particularly at the beginning of inspiration, whereas increased activity in the adductors, the muscles of the vocal folds, started at the end of inspiration, increased during expiration, and continued until the beginning of the following inspiration.

The synchronization of laryngeal and pharyngeal activity was shown in electromyographic recordings from the muscles of the soft palate and the pharynx, in which electrical activity was synchronous with respiration during quiet breathing under sedation.[4] The activity was most pronounced during inspiration but continued partly into the expiratory phase. These findings indicate that under quiet circumstances, the motor units contributing to the pharyngeal plexus are also activated by the respiratory center in the brain stem.

DISEASES OF THE PHARYNX

HISTORY AND CLINICAL SIGNS

Diseases of the pharynx are usually associated with abnormal deglutition. However, dyspnea may be the sole sign of disease when the nasopharynx is obstructed. Snoring, an inspiratory stridor, occurs when passage of air is still possible. Complete obstruction of the nasopharynx results in clinical signs of nasal obstruction but without nasal discharge.

The history in cases of dysphagia can be confusing, because a variety of signs such as coughing, vomiting, regurgitation, and nasal discharge may accompany the "swallowing disorder." The diagnosis of dysphagia by use of a standardized questionnaire was compared with the results of videofluorographic findings.[9] The questionnaire was found to be helpful in detecting pharyngeal dysphagia but cannot replace videofluorography.

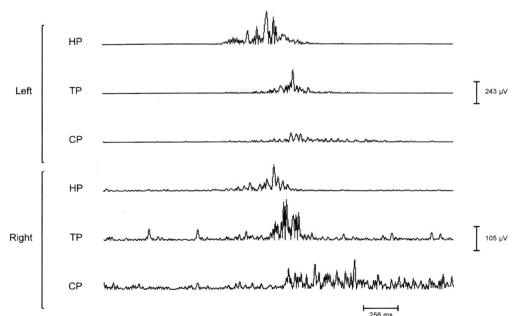

Figure 124–2. Digital high-pass filtered and rectified EMG recordings of swallowing activity in the left and right hyopharyngeal (HP), left and right thyropharyngeal (TP), and left and right cricopharyngeal (CP) muscles during stimulation of the right cranial laryngeal nerve in a dog under anesthesia. The central pattern generator located in the brain stem programs the bilateral sequential motor activity after unilateral afferent stimulation. (From Venker–van Haagen AJ, et al: Effect of stimulating peripheral and central neural pathways on pharyngeal muscle contraction timing during swallowing in dogs. Brain Res Bull 45:131, 1998. With permission from Elsevier Science.)

Clinical signs in acute pharyngeal disease may be dominated by pain. The animal usually refuses to eat or drink. The neck is extended, there is often drooling of saliva, and there are weak swallowing movements independent of intake.

In chronic pharyngitis, the predominant signs are gagging, regurgitation, and often sudden episodes of pica. When the last occurs, it is usually the dominant finding in the history, because it involves eating such things as houseplants, carpets, and wallpaper.

PHYSICAL EXAMINATION

Dogs and cats with pharyngeal disease require a thorough physical examination. Pharyngeal disease is a component of many systemic diseases, but at the same time it can be complicated by such things as abscesses following foreign body trauma, by pneumonia associated with dysphagia, or by metastasis in the case of pharyngeal tumors. The results of this general examination will, together with the history, lead to decisions and plans for further examination.

SPECIAL DIAGNOSTIC PROCEDURES

Inspection of the pharynx usually follows the general examination. Since a thorough inspection of the pharyngeal cavities cannot be performed without anesthesia, plans should be made for electromyography and radiography while the animal is sedated. It may be helpful to have the radiographs at hand during inspection of the pharynx.

Inspection of the pharyngeal cavities includes inspection of the oral cavity. Thorough inspection of the teeth, tongue, and frenulum precedes inspection of the palatine tonsils and their fossae, the base of the tongue, and the soft palate. The soft palate should be inspected for edema, abnormal color, vascular abnormalities, and, especially in the cat, lymphoid nodules. Soft palate length is important, because congenital hypoplasia is a common cause of swallowing abnormalities. The overlong soft palate, most often seen in brachycephalic breeds, may cause airway obstruction and regurgitation. The soft palate can be palpated to evaluate the lumen of the middle and caudal parts of the nasopharynx. The inspection of the nasopharynx can be facilitated by use of a Mathieu retractor and a dentist's mirror or a flexible endoscope, which can be turned through 180 degrees. During inspection of the entrance to the esophagus, the airway should be kept open by an endotracheal tube, since the inspection is facilitated by depressing the larynx with the blade of the laryngoscope.

Plain radiographs are most useful for finding radiopaque foreign bodies such as stones, needles, and bones. Radiographs provide no useful information about pharyngitis, tonsillitis, or congenital hypoplasia of the soft palate. Radiographic examination of the pharynx in brachycephalic dogs can be misleading, because a thick soft palate can resemble an overlong soft palate in a laterolateral projection. Abnormal radiographic findings in the pharyngeal area always should be confirmed by pharyngeal inspection before diagnostic conclusions are made.

Computed tomography is extremely helpful in diagnosis of lesions in the rostral part of the nasopharynx and at the base of the skull. In our experience, the most useful information is the location and extent of neoplasms, particularly with regard to the surgical risks and the prognosis.[10]

Contrast videofluorography is almost indispensable in diagnostic studies of dysphagia. Recordings are made while the animal eats food (ground meat) mixed with barium. The procedure needs the cooperation of the patient and is extremely time consuming, even in a routine set-up. Most dogs are cooperative, but fasting for more than 1 day may be necessary before some will eat in unfamiliar surroundings. These studies are virtually impossible in cats. All phases in the swallowing process can be studied repeatedly once the video recording has been made. The diagnosis is based on a detailed description of the process of formation of the bolus, the relaxation of the cricopharyngeal muscle, and the passage of the bolus through the cervical and thoracic parts of the esophagus and into the stomach. Leakage of fluid or food into the larynx and the trachea is a definite indication of dysfunction and can be recognized with certainty on the video recordings.

Electromyography of the pharyngeal muscles is useful when no abnormalities are found during inspection. In clinical electromyography, bipolar needle electrodes are preferred. The procedure is described in detail elsewhere.[4] In previously denervated pharyngeal muscles, the finding of fibrillation potentials was dominant.[4] In dogs with histologic evidence of muscular dystrophy in the pharyngeal muscles, there were fibrillation potentials, positive sharp waves, and complex repetitive discharges.[11] In our experience, the cervical esophagus can be included in these studies when a specially designed holder for the needle electrode is used.[11]

DYSPHAGIA

Dysphagia or abnormal deglutition can occur as a symptom in systemic diseases or as an isolated disorder. It can be caused by malfunction as a result of anatomic abnormalities, inflammation, neoplasia, or neurologic, neuromuscular, or muscular diseases. Pain in the pharyngeal area can block the regulatory mechanisms for swallowing.

Neurogenic dysphagia can be caused by interruption of the peripheral innervation or by abnormalities within the brain. In pharyngeal-esophageal dysphagia caused by peripheral nerve interruptions, both sensory and motor innervation are affected. Spontaneous unilateral denervation may be caused by a process near the tympanic bulla. Tumors near the pontine angle in the brain stem usually affect more cranial nerves (V, VII, VIII, XII), and dysphagia is not the primary sign. Other brain tumors may cause dysphagia, but this disorder is usually associated with a wide variety of complex dysfunctions.

Neuromuscular dysphagia is represented by myasthenia gravis. The German shepherd seems to be affected more than other breeds.[12] Dysphagia in these cases is usually associated with a megaesophagus, easily recognized on plain radiographs.

Myogenic dysphagia is a rare sign in polymyopathies of various causes but was the main sign in muscular dystrophy described in 24 Bouviers.[11] Eleven of these dogs were male, and their ages ranged from 6 months to 9 years. This study in Bouviers is interesting because comparable dystrophies could affect other breeds in the same way. The clinical signs differed from those of a described degenerative myopathy in Bouviers,[13] in that there was no generalized weakness, exercise intolerance, or abnormalities in the limbs.

CONGENITAL MALFORMATION

Congenital malformation of pharyngeal structures may be due to hypoplasia, usually involving an incomplete closure

ENT

between the nasopharynx and the oropharynx, or hyperplasia such as a thick and overlong soft palate. Hypoplasia usually results in an opening between the oropharynx and the naso- pharynx. Depending on the size of the defect, clinical signs may be negligible or considerable, including swallowing problems and misdirection of milk and, later, food in the pup or kitten. When the cleft does not continue as an orona- sal fistula, clinical signs are often mild, and in many cases the diagnosis is not made until the animal is over 1 year of age. Surgical repair has the best prognosis when the cleft only involves the soft palate and there is still a substantial muscular layer.[14] In some cases, no soft palate has developed. Having the animal eat and drink from an elevation in such a way that the head is held with the nose pointing almost upward diminishes the leakage of food and water into the nasal cavity.

Hyperplasia of the soft palate is associated with brachy- cephaly and a relatively narrow pharynx. It is believed that the genetic defect responsible for shortening the nose does not affect the soft tissue, so that there is too much tongue and soft palate in a narrow pharyngeal cavity. Clinical signs associated with an overlong soft palate consist of snoring, regurgitation, and dyspnea, usually increasing in severity during the second and third years of the dog's life. Not all brachycephalic dogs have similar pharyngeal disproportions. In some dogs, the pharyngeal mucosa and soft palate are very thick and the musculature is insufficient, resulting in snoring during closed-mouth breathing. When at a later age these dogs develop dyspnea, little can be done. This is in contrast to the overlong soft palate, which can be reduced in length so that it no longer covers the laryngeal inlet.[14] When hypoplasia of the larynx or other brachycephalic anomalies are present, success in diminishing the dyspnea is much dependent on the narrowest of the abnormal upper airway passages.

PHARYNGITIS

Acute pharyngitis is a typical symptom of viral infections. It is characterized by pain, fever, and extreme discomfort. The dog or cat does not attempt to eat, often salivates, and makes inefficient swallowing movements. The neck is held extended, and palpation of the pharyngeal area evokes reac- tions indicating discomfort or pain. General examination of the animal and laboratory findings will guide further steps in diagnosis and treatment. Symptomatic treatment of acute pharyngitis consists of parenteral broad-spectrum antibiotics. In addition to analgesics, intravenous administration of fluids or parenteral/enteral nutrition may become lifesaving "pro- cedures." Periods of extreme pain may persist for 3 to 5 days, followed by a week of convalescence in which recov- ery also depends on the severity of the viral infection. In this period, liquid food may be given in small portions several times a day, until the animal begins to exibit interest in more normal foods. Pharyngeal pain during swallowing of food continues for 2 weeks.

Chronic pharyngitis is characterized by retching indepen- dent of the intake of food, normal swallowing, and sudden periods of pica. In most cases in dogs and cats, the cause is obscure. Inspection reveals that the pharyngeal mucosa is thickened and sometimes irregularly reddened. All symptom- atic treatment is directed at diminishing the irritation of the pharyngeal mucosa. Moistening the food and feeding it in smaller portions may be helpful. In periods of gagging and retching, nonsteroidal anti-inflammatory drugs (NSAIDs)

may diminish the mucosal inflammation, and bouts of pica can be subdued by phenobarbital in a moderate dose (1 mg/ lb [2 mg/kg] body weight twice daily), starting when the first signs appear (licking, restlessness).

TONSILLITIS

In small animal practice, tonsillitis usually refers to in- flammation of the palatine tonsils. The clinical signs are not always clear, since tonsillitis is seldom a separate disease but rather one component of pharyngitis. After prolonged periods of inflammation, both tonsils may be indurated and enlarged. They can hinder the passage of food in the narrow oral pharynx. Pain during swallowing may persist even though the pharyngitis has long since subsided. Only in such cases should the tonsils be removed. In cats, the tonsils are enlarged in inflammatory diseases affecting the pharynx and in feline leukemia and lymphoma. Biopsy of the tonsils will lead to the diagnosis.

PHARYNGEAL MUCOCELE

The pharyngeal mucocele is a rather common anomaly in dogs and a rare finding in cats.[15,16] It consists of a large cyst containing mucus, and it is located in the wall of the phar- ynx. The clinical signs are related to its location and consist of dyspnea and, to a lesser extent, dysphagia. Such cysts are not usually connected to salivary glands or ducts. They probably originate from the mucus-producing glands in the pharyngeal wall or occasionally from those in the soft palate. Therapy consists of removal of the thick mucus and excision of the bulging and obstructing tissue.

NASOPHARYNGEAL POLYPS

Nasopharyngeal polyps occur in the middle area of the nasopharynx in cats. They occur at various ages, even in kittens. The polyps consist of inflammatory tissue originating in the middle ear. The stalk of the polyp emerges from the eustachian tube. In the uncomplicated stage, the clinical signs are dominated by dyspnea as a result of bilateral obstruction of the nasal airway but, surprisingly, no nasal discharge. The polyp may depress the rostral part of the soft palate, causing a bulge that is sometimes visible during inspection of the oropharynx. Radiography reveals a rounded density in the nasopharynx, just caudal to the hard palate. For visualization and removal of the polyp, the cat should be anesthetized, its mouth opened widely, and the soft palate pulled rostrally until the polyp is visible. A curved mosquito forceps is introduced into the nasopharynx between the polyp and the roof of the nasopharynx in order to clamp the stalk of the polyp. The stalk is then twisted around, and the polyp is removed with a sharp tug. Bleeding is stopped by applying pressure on the area of the eustachian tube.

PHARYNGEAL TRAUMA AND FOREIGN BODIES

Pharyngeal injuries most often result from foreign bodies such as needles, fish hooks, and bones in both cats and dogs and wooden sticks or grass awns (foxtails) in dogs.[17] The animal's initial response to penetration of a fish hook or needle is to try to remove it by movements of the tongue, by gagging and chewing, and, in cats, by use of the front paws. These efforts are accompanied by excessive salivation. At this stage, the foreign body is usually still visible and can be removed without difficulty when the animal is anesthetized.

Trauma in the pharyngeal area caused by bite wounds may include fracture of the hyoid bone, large hematomas, and lacerations causing subcutaneous emphysema. A tracheostomy, suturing of the pharyngeal mucosa, and placement of drains are the principal steps in treatment. Removal of the fractured parts of the hyoid bone is possible, but the surgery should be postponed for several weeks after the initial trauma because it may prove to be unnecessary because of absence of clinical signs.

NEOPLASMS

In dogs and cats, most tumors of the pharyngeal area are malignant. The most common tumors are squamous cell carcinomas in dogs and lymphomas in cats. The tonsillar carcinoma in the dog is remarkable because of its misleading presentation as a painful process rather than an obvious mass in the oropharyngeal area.[10] The major clinical sign is a slowly progressive difficulty in swallowing, first manifested by frequent interruptions of eating and by swallowing movements without taking up more food. The ipsilateral superficial retropharyngeal lymph node can be seen beside the larynx. Chemotherapy has not been successful. The pain caused by this tumor gradually becomes severe, and it provides adequate motivation for euthanasia.

In cats, lymphomas arising in the tonsils or other sites in the pharyngeal cavity lead to difficulty in swallowing. The tumors are found during inspection of the pharyngeal cavity, and biopsy specimens should be obtained for histologic examination. If chemotherapy is not available or is refused by the owner, corticosteroids may be used to temporarily diminish the signs.

Melanomas occur in the oropharyngeal area in dogs and cats. They are generally malignant and often metastasize before causing signs that come to the attention of the owner.

REVERSE SNEEZING

Reverse sneezing is a familiar sign in dogs. It consists of short periods (1 to 2 minutes) of severe inspiratory dyspnea characterized by extension of the neck, bulging of the eyes, and abduction of the elbows. Swallowing causes the attack to stop. The sound can be mimicked by a person who closes the lumen of the caudal nasopharynx by pressing the base of the tongue upward and then tries to inhale through the nose. The incomplete closure of the nasopharynx results in the snoring sounds. This closure is normal during swallowing and is inhibited at the end of the swallowing process, which explains the effect of swallowing in releasing the apparently fixed position of the pharynx and tongue to stop an attack of reverse sneezing. The owner should be instructed to induce the dog's swallowing reflex by massaging the pharyngeal area or briefly closing the nares.

GLOSSOPHARYNGEAL NEURALGIA

This uncommon but dramatic phenomenon is characterized by attacks of severe pharyngeal pain, causing the dog to scream and salivate. Cramping of the neck muscles may also be observed. The attacks last for several seconds but

may occur many times daily. The therapy prescribed in humans is carbamazepine alone or in combination with phenytoin.[18] In our experience in dogs, this was never successful. We have never observed spontaneous recovery.

DISEASES OF THE LARYNX

HISTORY AND CLINICAL SIGNS

The history and clinical signs in laryngeal disease reflect dysfunction of the larynx in its regulation of the airflow or vocalization, its insufficiency in protecting the airway, or the resulting irritation of the "cough receptors." In dysfunction of regulation of the airflow, it is the inability of abduction that causes the predominant signs of dyspnea and stridor on exertion. A dramatic change in vocal ability in dogs and cats is usually a sign of laryngeal tumor rather than laryngeal paralysis. Irritation of the laryngeal mucosa, as in laryngitis, results in coughing. Without accompanying bronchitis, the cough is loud and dry and persistent.

PHYSICAL EXAMINATION

The procedure for examining the dog or cat with laryngeal disease depends largely upon the degree to which the respiration is impaired.[19] If the animal appears severely dyspneic or is in rapidly increasing distress, emergency laryngotracheal intubation should precede clinical examination. Laryngoscopy can be completed after the animal is stabilized.

When dyspnea is not the predominant sign, clinical examination begins with listening to the animal's stridor or cough. Palpation of the larynx can reveal information about the degree of inflammation of the laryngeal mucosa. If the inflammation is severe, a harsh, dry cough is produced immediately when the larynx is touched. The tone of the stridor will change when soft pressure is applied to the larynx. Palpation can also reveal a change in location of the larynx or a deformation.

DIAGNOSTIC PROCEDURES

A lateral radiograph can be helpful in detecting ossification and neoplasia. Since even moderate respiratory distress can influence the configuration of air pockets in and around the laryngeal structures, care must be taken in the interpretation of these radiographs.

Laryngoscopy, the direct inspection of the larynx via the oropharyngeal cavity, is most informative. When the appropriate anesthesia is used, the respiratory movements of the arytenoid cartilages and the vocal folds can be assessed. Laryngeal inspection should take place as soon as the animal stops resisting opening of its mouth. The use of lidocaine spray is indispensable in cats. The larynx of the cat should be examined with a minimum of touching of the laryngeal mucosa, which is prone to develop edema. Electromyography of the intrinsic laryngeal muscles is indicated when the clinical signs and the insufficient glottic movements revealed by laryngoscopy both indicate laryngeal paralysis. The procedure is described in detail elsewhere.[19]

LARYNGEAL PARALYSIS

Laryngeal paralysis is a complete or partial loss of function of the larynx caused by neurologic, muscular, neuromus-

ENT

cular, or ankylotic (cricoarytenoid articulation) disease. The severity of the clinical signs (dyspnea and laryngeal stridor) is predominantly related to the degree of abductor dysfunction. Owners usually seek veterinary care as a result of their dog's exercise intolerance and extremely noisy respiratory sounds. Diagnosis is subjectively made under an extremely light plain of anesthesia and documenting non-retracted vocal folds during breathing.

Most commonly, laryngeal paralysis is a slowly progressive disease with or without other signs of polyneuropathy. The neurogenic origin of the disease was demonstrated in several studies by histologic examination of the affected muscles and nerves.[20, 21] The hereditary transmission of progressive neurogenic laryngeal paralysis was demonstrated in Bouviers and in crossbred Huskies.[22]

The study in the family of Bouviers and crossbred Bouviers included histologic examination of the recurrent laryngeal nerves and the nucleus ambiguus.[10] There were characteristic changes of both degeneration and regeneration of nerve endings in the intrinsic laryngeal muscles, and there was axon degeneration of the intramuscular branches of the nerves. Wallerian degeneration in the left and right recurrent laryngeal nerves was also observed. In the brain stem, there was a distinctly smaller number of motor neurons in the left and right nucleus ambiguus than were found in Bouviers without laryngeal paralysis, as well as degeneration of motor neurons and proliferation of oligodendroglia. The disease was progressive, as evidenced by the increase in number of affected intrinsic laryngeal muscles detected by electromyographic recordings during the first 3 months of life and by the increase in degeneration of recurrent laryngeal nerves of dogs presumed to be affected to a similar degree, when examined at ages between 10 and 24 weeks. The disease is inherited as an autosomal dominant trait.[10]

Laryngeal paralysis caused by a muscular disease is rare but has been demonstrated in bull terriers and dogs of various other breeds. Laryngeal paralysis is never the sole disorder in these cases, but rather one aspect of a polymyositis or general muscular disease. Similarly, a neuromuscular disease such as myasthenia gravis may involve the intrinsic laryngeal muscles in some cases.

Except for muscular and neuromuscular laryngeal paralysis, which should be treated according to the nature of the disease, the only way to restore the obstructed laryngeal passage is by surgical intervention. Lateral fixation of one arytenoid and vocal fold is the least traumatic method that usually leads to satisfactory results, especially when the larynx has a normal cartilaginous structure.[19, 23] The surgery is performed mostly in dogs but has been reported to be applicable in the rare case of laryngeal paralysis in a cat.

CONGENITAL MALFORMATION

Hypoplasia of the laryngeal structures, causing laryngeal collapse, is a common finding in brachycephalic breeds. Strong cartilaginous structures normally support the laryngeal opening and the function of the intrinsic laryngeal muscles. In brachycephalic breeds, the cartilages of the larynx are soft and underdeveloped in shape, which results in a narrow air passage and dysfunction of the abductors. The dogs are dyspneic, and a laryngeal stridor indicates the insufficiency of the laryngeal opening. There is no satisfactory treatment as yet.

In dogs and cats, congenital malformations are found occasionally and usually cause laryngeal dysfunction, indicated by stridorous breathing and dyspnea at an early age. When laryngeal function is limited, the prognosis is poor.

LARYNGITIS

Acute laryngitis is more common in dogs than in cats and is often caused by infectious tracheobronchitis, commonly called kennel cough. Laryngotracheitis caused by viral or bacterial infection is characterized initially by a persistent, rough, dry cough and no further signs of illness. Bronchitis or bronchopneumonia may complicate the infection. Acute laryngitis is therefore treated with house rest and cough syrups to limit irritation of the laryngeal mucosa. There is no indication for antibiotic treatment, but daily measurement of the dog's temperature gives the owner and veterinarian warning of the development of complications. In cats, viral tracheobronchitis also causes acute inflammation of the larynx, but the symptoms are dominated by fever and distress, salivation, conjunctivitis, and sometimes dyspnea caused by edema of the laryngeal mucosa. Antibiotic treatment and fluid therapy are indicated, and if there is severe salivation for more than a day, the serum potassium concentration should be assessed.

Acute laryngeal edema can be caused by insect poison or other allergens. Corticosteroids are indicated, and when necessary, a tracheostomy should be performed without hesitation. The cause of the edema is not always found. The tracheostomy cannula can be removed after laryngeal inspection in 3 to 5 days if the airway is patent.

Chronic laryngitis is rather common in dogs. Continuous barking, panting, and straining on the leash during training cause and maintain the irritation. The cartilage of the chronically irritated larynx may ossify, this being recognized by palpation and on radiographs. Severe chronic laryngitis may influence the function of the larynx and induce changes in the glottis such as fibrosis of the vocal folds. The dysfunction and laryngeal irritation are then permanent and result in recurrent coughing and a hoarse voice. Slight relief may only be obtained with intermittent corticosteroid treatment. Chronic irritation of the larynx may cause laryngeal spasm. This occurs in dogs under constant stress during training sessions. The laryngeal spasm causes severe dyspnea, a heavy stridor, and cyanosis. The spasm usually occurs during special exercises in the training program. It becomes a permanent hazard for the dog and can be avoided only by stopping the training.

TRAUMA

Laryngeal trauma is often life-threatening because the passage of the air through the larynx is obstructed. Trauma caused by the bite of a dog, which is a combined blunt and sharp trauma, can result in damage to the cartilage and considerable narrowing of the laryngeal passage. When the larynx is partially lacerated, emphysema develops in the cervical area. Surgical examination of the larynx and suturing of the laceration are necessary. In most cases of severe trauma, a tracheostomy is indicated. The initial swelling and hemorrhage prevent an accurate diagnosis, but when a tracheal cannula is introduced, time is obtained for partial recovery. Radiographs do not elucidate details of the traumatic wounds, and the prognosis is more easily determined when the primary wounds are healed. Although spontaneous recovery may seem remarkable, it is not rare.

Stenosis of the glottis can occur after laryngeal surgery. Any surgical intervention involving the vocal folds and arytenoids can cause stenosis, but if the mucosa remains intact, permanent stenosis is avoided. In cats, the risk of stenosis is even greater than it is in dogs. One of the most feared complications is webbing, the forming of scar tissue in the laryngeal lumen.[19] Bilateral interruption of the mucosa, as in removal of the vocal folds, is hazardous. The contraction of the scar tissue immobilizes the larynx, and mobility is seldom restored after removal of the web.

In cats, almost every intervention in the larynx causes edema, and thus corticosteroids are indicated when the first signs of laryngeal obstruction are observed. Prophylactic administration of corticosteroids may be indicated in special circumstances.

NEOPLASMS

Primary laryngeal tumors occur occasionally in dogs and cats. In dogs, leiomyomas, rhabdomyosarcomas, and squamous cell carcinomas, as well as other types of tumors, have been reported.[24–29] In cats, lymphosarcoma and squamous cell carcinoma are the most frequent tumors. Squamous cell carcinomas and lymphosarcomas invade the laryngeal structures rapidly and are inoperable by the time they are diagnosed. Rhabdomyosarcoma may originate from one of the vocal muscles, and this tumor can be removed via a ventral midline approach to the laryngeal lumen.[19] Complete removal of the larynx is the theoretic solution for other tumors, but not many veterinary surgeons will take this hurdle.

REFERENCES

1. Miller AJ: Neurophysiological basis of swallowing. Dysphagia 1:91, 1986.
2. Kennedy JG III, Kent RD: Physiological substrates of normal deglutition. Dysphagia 3:24, 1988.
3. Dodds WJ: The physiology of swallowing. Dysphagia 3:171, 1989.
4. Venker–van Haagen AJ, et al: Contributions of the glossopharyngeal nerve and the pharyngeal branch of the vagus nerve to the swallowing process in dogs. Am J Vet Res 47:1300, 1986.
5. Venker–van Haagen AJ, et al: Continuous electromyographic recordings of pharyngeal muscle activity in normal and previously denervated muscles in dogs. Am J Vet Res 50:1725, 1989.
6. Buchholz MD: Neurologic causes of dysphagia. Dysphagia 1:152, 1987.
7. Dyce KM, et al: Textbook of Veterinary Anatomy. Philadelphia, WB Saunders, 1987.
8. Venker–van Haagen AJ, et al: Effect of stimulating peripheral and central neural pathways on pharyngeal muscle contraction timing during swallowing in dogs. Brain Res Bull 45:131, 1998.
9. Peeters ME, et al: Evaluation of a standardised questionnaire for detection of dysphagia in 69 dogs. Vet Rec 27:211, 1993.
10. Venker–van Haagen AJ: Diseases of the throat. In Ettinger SJ, Feldman EC: Textbook of Veterinary Internal Medicine, 4th ed. Philadelphia, WB Saunders, 1995, pp 567–575.
11. Peeters ME, et al: Dysphagia in Bouviers associated with muscular dystrophy; evaluation of 24 cases. Vet Quart 13:65, 1991.
12. Pedroia V: Disorders of the skeletal muscles. In Ettinger SJ (ed): Textbook of veterinary Internal Medicine, 3rd ed. Philadelphia, WB Saunders, 1989, pp 733–744.
13. Braund KG, Steinberg MS: Degenerative myopathy of Bouviers des Flandres. Proc 7th ACUIM Forum, San Diego, May 1989, p 995.
14. Nelson AW: Upper respiratory system. In Slatter D (ed): Textbook of Small Animal Surgery, 2nd ed. Philadelphia, WB Saunders, 1993, pp 733–804.
15. Weber J, et al: Pharyngeal mucoceles in dogs. Vet Surg 15:5, 1986.
16. Feinman JM: Pharyngeal mucocele and respiratory distress in a cat. JAVMA 179:1179, 1990.
17. White RAS, Lane JG: Pharyngeal stick penetration injuries in the dog. J Small Anim Pract 29:13, 1988.
18. Ballenger JJ: Headache and neuralgia of the face. In Ballenger JJ, Snow JB (eds): Otorhinolaryngology: Head and Neck Surgery, 15th ed. Philadelphia, Williams & Wilkins, 1996, pp 158–162.
19. Venker–van Haagen AJ: Diseases of the larynx. Vet Clin North Am Small Anim Pract 22:1155, 1992.
20. Gaber CE, et al: Laryngeal paralysis in dogs: A review of 23 cases. JAVMA 186:377, 1985.
21. Braund KG, et al: Laryngeal paralysis in immature and mature dogs as one sign of a more diffuse polyneuropathy. JAVMA 194:1735, 1989.
22. O'Brien JA, Hendricks JC: Inherited laryngeal paralysis. Analysis in the Husky cross. Vet Quart 8:301, 1986.
23. White RAS: Unilateral arytenoid lateralisation: An assessment of technique and long term results in 62 dogs with laryngeal paralysis. J Small Anim Pract 30:543, 1989.
24. Bright RM, et al: Laryngeal neoplasia in two dogs. JAVMA 184:738, 1984.
25. Calderwood Mays MB: Laryngeal oncocytoma in two dogs. JAVMA 185:677, 1984.
26. Crowe DT, et al: Total laryngectomy for laryngeal mast cell tumor in a dog. JAAHA 22:809, 1986.
27. Flanders JA, et al: Laryngeal chondrosarcoma in a dog. JAVMA 190:68, 1987.
28. Ndikuwera J, et al: Malignant melanoma of the larynx in a dog. J Small Anim Pract 30:107, 1989.
29. Saik JE, et al: Canine and feline laryngeal neoplasia: A 10-year survey. JAAHA 22:359, 1986.

ENT

SECTION IX

THE RESPIRATORY SYSTEM

CHAPTER 125

CLINICAL EVALUATION OF THE PATIENT WITH RESPIRATORY DISEASE

Brendan Corcoran

Respiratory diseases, common clinical problems in small animal practice, can prove difficult to diagnose. The most common respiratory infections (cat flu and kennel cough) are readily diagnosed on the basis of history and clinical signs. Difficulty arises with chronic airway and lung diseases and with pleural and mediastinal diseases, where without biopsy material, a definitive diagnosis is not possible. In this chapter the clinical investigative approach to the respiratory case is outlined, starting with the clinical history and physical examination. The remainder of the chapter outlines the operation of the various ancillary diagnostic tests available and the utility of these tests in aiding diagnosis.

HISTORY

As with all other body systems, obtaining a thorough clinical history is important, particularly in the case of chronic respiratory disease, where the historical information may cover several years. Diseases of other body systems can have profound effects on the respiratory system, and this has to be considered in the history. The close interrelationship between the cardiovascular and respiratory systems should also be borne in mind. Typically, respiratory cases present with clinical signs such as sneezing, nasal discharge, cough, dyspnea, and exercise intolerance. Other less typical presentations include vomiting, regurgitation, dysphagia, ataxia, collapsing and syncope, dysphonia, obesity, abdominal distention, pyrexia, lethargy, inappetence, and cachexia. Prior malignancy surgery, trauma, or toxin exposure is significant. Consideration has to be given to the owner's accuracy in describing events and their timing. Many owners have trouble quantifying respiratory difficulty and describing abnormal respiratory sounds.

Signalment. Age and breed predisposition are well-recognized features of respiratory diseases. Contagious infectious diseases are seen mainly in young, unvaccinated animals, whereas neoplasia, chronic bronchitis, and laryngeal paralysis are seen in middle-aged to old animals. Examples of breed predispositions include brachycephalic airway syndrome and tracheal collapse in toy breeds. Laryngeal paralysis is common in aged Labrador retrievers, and nasal neoplasia and nasal aspergillosis are noted mainly in dolichocephalic breeds. Asthma in cats is reported to be more prevalent in the Siamese than in other breeds,[1] and a suspected primary immunodeficiency resulting in bronchopneumonia has recently been reported in the Irish wolfhound.[2]

Environment. Environmental factors that predispose to respiratory disease should be identified. With appropriate environmental exposure, unvaccinated cats are susceptible to upper respiratory tract viral infections (feline herpesvirus, feline calicivirus, *Chlamydia psittaci*) and dogs to kennel cough (*Bordetella bronchiseptica*, parainfluenza, canine adenovirus, and distemper virus). Animals that are allowed to roam have a greater risk of trauma, and strangulation can occur when excitable dogs are left tied and unattended. Dogs that readily scavenge or travel through heavy undergrowth are more likely to inhale foreign bodies. Exposure to environmental pollutants is an important factor. The possible role of passive smoke in the development of respiratory disease in animals is a consideration but is unproved. More likely is the association between inhalation of human dander and house dust mite feces and feline asthma.[1] Allergen load might be a function of the home microenvironment, and there is suspicion that centrally heated, air-conditioned, double-glazed, fully carpeted homes may be a contributing factor in asthma in humans and cats. Consumption of toxins causing respiratory disease is well documented, with paraquat and coumarin-based rodenticides being the best examples.[3]

The geographic distribution of certain diseases is also well recognized. Pulmonary mycoses are commonly seen in the midwestern and southwestern areas of the United States, whereas bronchopulmonary aspergillosis is a particular problem in western Australia. Infection with the nasal mite (*Pneumonyssoides caninum*) is well documented in Scandinavia but is rare in other parts of Europe. *Dirofilaria immitis* infection is important in many regions of North America, the Mediterranean basin, and Australia, whereas *Angiostrongylus vasorum* is common in southwest Britain and France.

Hunting behavior should be recorded in cats, as this is the method of transmission of the lungworm *Aelurostrongylus abstrusus*. Infection with *Crenosoma vulpis* or *Capillaria* spp. also requires consumption of a paratenic host. *Oslerus osleri* is transmitted from dam to newborn offspring and is typically associated with kenneled dogs (racing greyhounds, hunt packs).

Primary Complaint. The duration and progression of the primary complaint should be noted. The frequency of the presenting sign should be recorded, as well as whether it is continuous or intermittent. If multiple signs are contemporaneous, determine whether there is a direct association between them. Attempt to quantify the severity of the clinical signs, and identify any association with specific events such as exercise, excitement, or resting. The nature of any coughing can be useful in diagnosis but should be interpreted with caution. A soft, ineffectual cough is often seen with lung parenchymal disease, whereas a harsh, hacking cough is seen with large airway disease. A goose-honk or seal-bark sound is a common finding with tracheal collapse. Assessment of dyspnea from the history can be difficult if the pet is relatively normal during the consultation, and persistent questioning of the owner is often necessary to determine the course of events.

Response to Therapy. The response to any previous therapy should be noted but not relied on to make a diagnosis. A rapid and marked response to glucocorticosteroids alone suggests a hypersensitivity disorder. Significant response to antibacterial agents implies only that bacterial pathogens are involved and does not identify the disease entity or the etiology.

GENERAL PHYSICAL EXAMINATION

Respiratory disease can be acutely life-threatening. The clinician should quickly check for the presence of respiratory embarrassment and institute emergency medical procedures as appropriate. The demeanor and overall activity of the animal and the general physical appearance should be noted. Body temperature is recorded, bearing in mind the effect of external factors such as stress, excitement, and panting. Body condition can be confirmed by palpation, the skin and adnexa examined (color, temperature, body surface masses), the peripheral lymph nodes palpated, and hydration assessed. Abdominal examination should be thorough, with attention paid to identifying enlarged organs, masses, and free fluid. The head and neck should be assessed for changes attributable to mediastinal disease (Horner's syndrome, subcutaneous edema of the head and neck).

A detailed examination of the cardiovascular system is required in any case presenting with respiratory signs. This is outlined in Chapter 110. The oral cavity can be inspected for dental, gingival, and tongue disease and for oral foreign bodies, and the gag reflex should be assessed. The thorax should be percussed to assess resonance. A high-pitched sound is found with lung hyperinflation or pneumothorax and a dull note with lung consolidation and pleural effusion. The presence of a pleural fluid line can often be appreciated with percussion, and asymmetric changes in percussion suggest that there is a unilateral thoracic problem. Percussion can also elicit coughing and give information on the likely site of disease.

The external nares should be checked for discharges, conformity, and patency, and the frontal bones palpated for evidence of deformity, pain, and softening. The larynx and cervical trachea can be palpated for abnormality and the presence of a cough confirmed on tracheal pinching. The presence of dyspnea and tachypnea should be noted, taking into account external factors such as excitement, stress, hyperthermia, and physiologic panting. The assessment of dyspnea is easiest if breathing is relatively slow and purposeful. Open-mouth breathing, orthopnea (positional dyspnea), and an abdominal component to respiration (expiratory effort) are abnormal findings.

Auscultate the respiratory system from the nares to the periphery (Table 125–1). During slow breathing, rhonchus sounds (stridor and stertor if the upper airways are affected) are abnormal findings. The presence of wheezes and crackles is abnormal irrespective of the respiratory rate. When all sounds are present together, complicated harmonics make identification of specific sounds difficult. Expiratory dyspnea is best appreciated close to the end-expiratory point and is

TABLE 125–1. CLASSIFICATION OF RESPIRATORY SOUNDS

DESCRIPTION	DEFINITION
Breath sounds	The normal airway and lung sounds audible during quiet tidal breathing; they are barely perceptible in normal cats
Stertor	Noise generated from the nasal passages
Stridor	High-pitched inspiratory sound generated from turbulent airflow in the extrathoracic airways (typically the larynx)
Rhonchus	Low-pitched, continuous inspiratory or expiratory sound associated with rapid airflow through the larger airways
Wheeze	High-pitched, continuous inspiratory or expiratory sound associated with narrowing of smaller airways
Crackle (coarse or fine)	High-pitched, discontinuous inspiratory sound associated with reopening of airways that closed during expiration
Rales, vesicular or bronchovesicular	These terms are less widely used in human and veterinary respiratory medicine, as they are difficult to define

Modified from the American Thoracic Society Classification.

often appreciated with tracheal collapse, masses compressing larger bronchi, and lung hyperinflation in feline asthma. In dogs with long-standing expiratory dyspnea, hypertrophy of the abdominal musculature can be detected.

DIAGNOSTIC TECHNIQUES IN RESPIRATORY MEDICINE

The applicability of the various diagnostic tests available for the investigation of respiratory diseases must be considered, and the tests chosen must be expected to give valuable diagnostic data. The potential hazard of any test must be taken into account, particularly with life-threatening respiratory disease. The specificity and sensitivity of the tests available should also be understood, and caution in interpreting the results of diagnostic tests is necessary.

HEMATOLOGY, BIOCHEMISTRY, AND SEROLOGY

Hematology and biochemical profiles are invaluable in determining an animal's overall health status and in identifying nonrespiratory diseases that impinge on the respiratory system (e.g., anemia, endocrinopathies). Polycythemia can be seen as a response to chronic hypoxia in respiratory disease. Leukocytosis with neutrophilia and a left shift is often found with acute bacterial bronchopneumonia, and a circulating eosinophilia can be associated with pulmonary infiltration with eosinophilia (PIE) and feline asthma.[1, 4] A circulating basophilia is highly supportive of a diagnosis of PIE or *Dirofilaria immitis* infection.[1] Pleural effusion can be associated with hypoalbuminemia, and noncardiogenic pulmonary edema can be associated with systemic illnesses. If biochemical abnormalities are detected, further dynamic tests are usually necessary. Coagulation profiles are carried out if unexplained hemorrhage is present.

Serology profiles, with or without agent isolation, can be used to identify respiratory-specific viral infections and infections that result in respiratory disease because of compromised immune function (feline leukemia virus, feline immunodeficiency virus). Serology is also beneficial in the diagnosis of pulmonary mycotic diseases. Serology tests have been proposed as potentially useful diagnostic tests for the identification of culprit allergens in feline asthma by assessing allergen-specific IgE levels,[5] but further work is required in this area.

DIAGNOSTIC IMAGING

Radiography

Radiography is still the most important diagnostic technique in respiratory medicine. It is applicable to the investigation of the upper respiratory tract, the thoracic cage, and the lower airways and lungs. Furthermore, it allows assessment of the mediastinum and cardiovascular system, diseases of which impinge on respiratory function.

The major limitation of radiography is its lack of diagnostic specificity and sensitivity. Attention to radiographic quality can improve its sensitivity, as can using standardized radiographic technique, attaining appropriate clinical proficiency in radiograph interpretation, and consulting colleagues with postgraduate specializations in radiology. Adequate exposure charts have to be derived and updated for individual radiographic equipment setups.

Quality is also a function of the equipment available (unit output, exposure times, screens, grids, and so forth), the use of proper positioning and restraining devices, and the use of appropriate exposure and development procedures. Movement blur can be so severe as to make accurate identification of subtle intrathoracic structures impossible.[6, 7] The presence of air in the respiratory system adds excellent contrast for respiratory radiography, and this fact should be used to improve radiographic quality. Sedation allows proper restraint and positioning and has safety implications for staff. Positioning aids are used to prevent the limbs from overlying structures of interest; prevent rotation of the head, neck, and thorax; and raise the sternum in the lateral position. If general anesthesia is used, lung inflation immediately before taking a thoracic radiograph is required to reverse the positional atelectasis of the dependent lung lobes.[7]

The standard respiratory radiography views include the lateral head view, intraoral dorsoventral and ventrodorsal views (occlusal), frontal sinus view, right lateral larynx and cervical trachea, and right lateral and ventrodorsal thorax. In addition, a left lateral thoracic view may give valuable information.[8] The views should be as close as possible to the end-inspiratory point to maximize air contrast. In the case of suspected tracheal collapse, an end-expiratory view is preferable so as to demonstrate intrathoracic tracheal narrowing. Standing lateral views may be informative in cases of pleural effusion or pneumothorax, but potential radiation hazard must also be considered. When there is severe pathology, a poorer-quality radiograph may be acceptable, particularly if attempting to get better-quality films would be hazardous to the animal. The animal's conformity, including the shape of the thoracic cage (breed variability) and degree of obesity, should also be noted in the interpretation.

The assessment of any radiograph should follow a set procedure, and the clinician should not have preconceived ideas as to the likely radiographic abnormality. With difficult chronic respiratory cases, where dramatic radiographic changes are not noted, clinicians are often tempted to find radiographic changes to explain the clinical presentation, even when such conclusions would not hold up to scrutiny. There should be no other distractions in the immediate viewing area during film reading, and sufficient time should be set aside for proper assessment. The author's approach is to first assess quality: positioning, the level of contrast (exposure factors, body conformity, body fat, and stage of respiration), and the presence of artifacts. Attempting to assess the radiographic appearance of structures implies that the observer has a good working knowledge of respiratory radiographic anatomy.

The nasal passages should be checked for symmetry, and the integrity of the nasal septum assessed.[6] The adjacent bony structures should be examined for changes (typically neoplastic). The nasal chambers have a fine trabecular bony (turbinate) pattern, which is destroyed or obscured with infection and neoplasia. The frontal sinuses should also be checked, as they communicate with the nasal passages. The position and width of the soft palate can be assessed, and the structure of the hyoid apparatus appreciated. Apart from neoplasia (chondrosarcoma), pyogranulomatous lesions, and extraluminal masses, few other abnormalities can be appreciated radiographically in the larynx.

The integrity of the thoracic cage should be assessed, paying attention to the bony structures of the thorax, the adjacent appendicular skeleton, and the diaphragm. The presence of pleural abnormalities (pleural line, pleural effusion) should be noted. The cranial mediastinum is then checked for changes. The position and dimensions of the trachea are noted, and assessment of the cardiovascular system is made. Evidence of intrathoracic lymphadenopathy (sternal and hilar) should be noted. The airways and lungs can then be inspected.

In the normal lung, the major radiographic feature is blood vessels with their attendant airways. Although the lung parenchyma adds a degree of density to the lung field, this is minimal if the lungs are properly inflated. The bronchial walls are not normally seen, except in the central areas or if they are calcified (age-related changes). The presence of readily visible, thickened bronchi suggests pathologic changes. Affected bronchi are best appreciated end-on as ringlike structures (doughnuts) but can also be appreciated as parallel linear markings (tramlines). Alterations in the interstitial pattern can often be difficult to identify. This particular pattern is markedly affected by radiographic quality (stage of respiration, obesity, exposure factors). It is best described as a linear density (similar to vascular markings) giving a hazy appearance to the lung field. When severe, interstitial changes become difficult to distinguish from a true alveolar pattern. The presence of air bronchograms indicates that there is uniform consolidation of lung tissue adjacent to the bronchi and is the best indicator of a true alveolar pattern. Alveolar patterns are also described as fluffy, cotton wool–like coalescing densities and can be localized or diffuse. With sufficient lung consolidation, an alveolar pattern becomes difficult to distinguish from other soft tissue densities such as neoplastic masses. Lastly, a mixed pattern may be present, consisting of increased bronchial, interstitial, and alveolar densities. In many situations the radiographic changes are so equivocal as to make a tentative diagnosis difficult, and further diagnostic tests are required.

Ultrasonography

Ultrasonography is used in respiratory medicine mainly to assist in the identification of pleural effusions and intrathoracic masses, to image structures in the mediastinum, and to allow more accurate needle biopsy sampling.[8] More importantly, ultrasonography (echocardiography) is required to exclude a cardiac explanation for the clinical presentation.

Scintigraphy

Pulmonary scintigraphy, and expertise in its interpretation, is available in only a limited number of specialist centers worldwide. Its major use is in the diagnosis of pulmonary thromboembolism, using technetium 99m–labeled aerosols, enabling identification of underperfused lung areas. Scintigraphy has also been used to demonstrate poor mucociliary clearance in dogs with primary ciliary dyskinesia and chronic bronchitis.[9]

ENDOSCOPY (RHINOSCOPY AND BRONCHOSCOPY)

Endoscopy is a valuable diagnostic technique in respiratory medicine and has been standard procedure in referral practice for many years. Endoscopy allows direct visualization of the respiratory tract to assess for abnormality, as well as accurate collection of samples and retrieval of foreign material. Endoscopy is a requirement in all chronic airway and lung disease cases but can be of little value if the animal is in clinical remission.[10]

A wide variety of endoscopes are available. Rigid endoscopes are particularly useful for examination of the rostral nasal chamber. Fiberoptic bronchoscopes and flexible videoendoscopes are the most versatile, allowing inspection of the caudal nasal chamber (retroflex technique) and inspection of all the lobar bronchi with ease.[11] Human bronchoscopes, which are widely used in small animal veterinary practice, have a working length of approximately 50 cm and a diameter of 5 to 6 mm, making examination of the more distal airways in large dogs difficult and introduction into toy breeds and cats hazardous. Longer and wider human gastroscopes can be used for small animal bronchoscopy but are of use only in large dogs. A wide range of low-cost veterinary-dedicated endoscopes of suitable length are available, but the technical specification and quality of the image are usually not as good as with human scopes. A light source, cleaning brushes, biopsy catheters, and storage system are also required. A suction unit is a useful item, and an automated washing system improves care and cleaning. Increased

ease of use, better image quality, and storage of images can be obtained using video attachments.

All airway endoscopy should be carried out under general anesthesia with the animal intubated, except for inspection of the larynx and cervical trachea. Anesthesia should be under the control of a competent person, as the hazards of airway occlusion by the scope can be considerable.

Rhinoscopy invariably results in significant bleeding, and visualization of structures in the rostral nasal chamber can be difficult. The caudal part of the nasal chamber is best visualized by retroflex positioning of the tip of a flexible bronchoscope. Rhinoscopy allows identification of foreign bodies, polyps, tumors and other masses, and fungal plaques.

Bronchoscopy can be carried out in either sternal or lateral recumbency, depending on the operator's preference. In lateral recumbency, periodic lung inflation will reverse atelectasis. The procedure should be carried out in a managed and methodical manner but with a degree of urgency, considering that the scope is occluding the airway, and the airway is reacting to the scope (mucus secretion). A relatively rapid (within the first 30 seconds of scoping) initial assessment of the amount of mucoid material in the tracheobronchial tree should be made. Normal tracheobronchial mucosa has a light salmon-pink color (paler in cats), and blood vessels should be visible beneath the ciliated pseudostratified columnar epithelium (Fig. 125–1). The amount, color, and viscosity of secretions are noted. The presence of a roughened bronchial mucosa with nodular changes is abnormal. Each lung lobe bronchus should be inspected in turn, bearing in mind any localized lesion noted on radiography. A bronchoscopic airway anatomic nomenclature system exists for the dog,[12] but beyond the entrance to the lobar bronchi, it is easy to become disoriented, and identification of further bronchial divisions can be difficult. The presence of mucus plugging, foreign bodies (right side mainly), and dynamic collapse of the airways (extraluminal compression) should be noted (Table 125–2). With the endotracheal tube removed, the dynamic movement of the trachea and main stem bronchi is assessed. Inspection of the larynx is best achieved using a laryngoscope. The larynx is assessed for anatomy, inflammatory diseases, masses, and function (under light anesthesia).

Once the examination is complete, an immediate record of the findings should be made. For inexperienced operators, bias can be a major problem in interpretation of endoscopic findings.

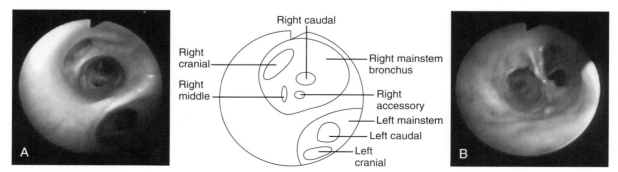

Figure 125–1. Contrasting bronchoscopic images of the dog airway (normal and abnormal). *A,* Normal bronchoscopic image (with line drawing) of the division of the carina, demonstrating the position of the right and left main stem bronchi; the right cranial, middle, accessory, and caudal bronchi; and the left cranial and caudal lobe bronchi. The mucosa has a light salmon-pink color, and blood vessels are visible beneath the mucosa. *B,* Bronchoscopic image of a dog with severe chronic bronchitis and bronchiectasis, illustrating severe changes. There is overall dilatation of the main stem bronchi, with loss of mucosal surface detail and accumulation of mucopurulent material. The divisions between the airways appear paper thin and have a distorted anatomy.

TABLE 125-2. TYPICAL BRONCHOSCOPIC FINDINGS

CONDITION	COMMON BRONCHOSCOPIC FINDINGS
Tracheal collapse	Redundancy of the dorsal membrane, varying degrees of dorsoventral flattening of the trachea
Oslerus osleri infection	Greyish, yellow, or brown nodules at the carina, localized acute mucosal inflammatory reaction
Airway foreign body	Foreign body visible in bronchus (typically right side), localized mucopurulent reaction
Chronic bronchitis	Nodular roughening of the airway mucosa, blanching of mucosa, excess mucus, loss of vascular detail
Bronchopneumonia	Accumulations of mucopurulent material in the large airways, material exiting from specific lobar bronchi, relatively normal bronchial mucosa
Pulmonary neoplasia	Compression of bronchi, blood-tinged mucoid material, airway wall mucosal distortion
Pulmonary fibrosis	Normal bronchial mucosa, dynamic collapse of main stem or lobar bronchi

RESPIRATORY SAMPLING TECHNIQUES

Respiratory sampling techniques are invaluable in the diagnosis of nasal, airway, and lung diseases and are used to assess the cytology profiles and for culture and sensitivity testing.[13] A wide variety of sampling brushes, catheters, and biopsy forceps are available for sampling. For bronchial washes, three aliquots (2 mL for cats and up to 20 mL for dogs) of warmed normal saline are usually sufficient. In normal dogs and cats, up to 95 per cent of cells in bronchoalveolar lavage are undifferentiated macrophages, with low numbers of neutrophils, eosinophils, and lymphocytes.[12] In bronchial washes, ciliated epithelial cells are commonly seen, either singly or as rafts of cells. Epithelial cells are the dominant cell type in nasal washes from normal dogs. Although the presence of eosinophils in bronchial samples of dogs and cats with respiratory disease is considered significant, relatively high numbers of eosinophils may also be present in up to 25 per cent of apparently healthy cats.[14] The distal airways of the dog and cat are sterile. In respiratory cases in which organisms can be grown, gram-negative organisms such as *Escherichia coli*, *Pasteurella* spp., *Pseudomonas* spp., *Proteus* spp., and *Klebsiella* spp. predominate.[15] In cats, *Pasteurella* spp. are the most common isolates.

Nasal Sampling (Nasal Flushing and Nasal Biopsy)

Samples from the nasal passages and caudal nasal chamber are obtained by using a combination of catheter flushing and needle and biting biopsy forceps.[16] Biopsy sampling of the nasal passages results in significant bleeding, and care should be taken to avoid puncturing the cribriform plate. Samples should include the nasal mucosa and some of the underlying bone to check for osteomyelitis.

Tracheobronchial Sampling (Brushes, Washes, and Biopsy Sampling)

Samples for the trachea and bronchi can be obtained by blind sampling using transtracheal or translaryngeal (entry point at the cricothyroid ligament) techniques or via an endotracheal tube. Material can be sampled more accurately with endoscope guidance, and this gives better results than blind sampling. For transtracheal sampling, the animal is sedated, and an area over the midcervical trachea is aseptically prepared and infiltrated with local anesthetic. With the animal held in the sternal position with the neck partially dorsiflexed, a small skin incision is made and a large-bore (14-gauge) needle is passed between the cartilage rings. A suitable catheter is passed through the needle and positioned roughly at the level of the carina. Warmed normal saline (up to 20 mL) is instilled and immediately aspirated. In some instances, little material is retrieved, and the procedure can be repeated.

Bronchial biopsy requires the use of an endoscope for accuracy and is used primarily for the diagnosis of chronic bronchitis or for the sampling of masses within the airway lumen.[9]

Bronchoalveolar Lavage

Sampling from the distal airways and the alveoli requires endoscope-guided catheter placement. Select the airway of interest, and advance the scope until the airway is occluded. Instill the sampling solution, and collect after 10 seconds. Typically, 40 to 60 per cent of the instillate is recovered in successful bronchoalveolar lavage. The procedure can be repeated at the operator's discretion at different sites.

TRANSTHORACIC NEEDLE BIOPSY

This technique is invaluable in the diagnosis of pulmonary neoplasia, and in modified form it is used to sample pleural effusions (thoracocentesis). It is less valuable in the diagnosis of other diffuse lung diseases.[17] Samples can be collected using large-bore biopsy or fine-needle aspiration techniques. The site for sampling is carefully selected using radiography, and the accuracy of sampling can be improved by using ultrasound guidance (recommended for mediastinal sampling). The chest wall is aseptically prepared and instilled with local anesthetic. Care should be taken not to cause pneumothorax, but this is a rare complication with fine-needle aspiration.[17] Material collected is smeared onto glass slides, air-dried, and processed. A full report from a qualified diagnostic cytopathologist should be obtained. Collected pleural fluid should be assessed for color, turbidity, specific gravity, cell count, protein determination, cell type, cholesterol-triglyceride ratio, and culture and sensitivity testing.

OPEN-CHEST LUNG BIOPSY

Open-chest lung biopsy is a diagnostic test of last resort because of the invasiveness, degree of morbidity, and danger of mortality associated with the technique. The adoption of video-assisted thoracoscopic lung biopsy techniques in veterinary medicine may overcome some of these problems. Biopsy material is often collected during exploratory thoracotomy and can allow confirmation of pulmonary metastases and the definitive diagnosis of pulmonary interstitial fibrosis.

BLOOD GAS ANALYSIS

Blood gas analysis is an invaluable tool in the assessment of an animal's gas exchange capacity and acid-base balance.

Formula for the calculation of Alveolar (A) to arterial (a)

gradient

$$A\text{-}a = (150 - (Pa_{CO_2}/0.8) - Pa_{O_2}$$

Normal	Hypoventilation	V/Q Mis-match
$Pa_{O_2}=95$; $Pa_{CO_2}=40$	$Pa_{O_2}=60$; $Pa_{CO_2}=60$	$Pa_{O_2}=60$; $Pa_{CO_2}=40$
(predicted A-a <10mmHg)	(predicted A-a <15mmHg)	(predicted A-a > 15-20mmHg)

A-a $= (150 - (40/0.8))$ $- 95$ $= 5$ mmHg	A-a $= (150 - (60/0.8))$ $- 60$ $= 15$ mmHg	A-a $= (150 - (40/0.8))$ $- 60$ $= 40$ mmHg

Figure 125–2. Examples of the use of the alveolar (A) to arterial (a) oxygen gradient (A-a) to distinguish hypoventilation from ventilation-perfusion mismatch.

It is a more sensitive indicator of changes in lung function and lung pathology than any other diagnostic test but is relatively insensitive in the early stages of disease and in mild respiratory conditions.[18] The main aim of blood gas analysis is to assess arterial oxygen (Pa_{O_2}) and carbon dioxide (Pa_{CO_2}) tensions and determine the degree of hypoxia or hypercapnia. Normal arterial oxygen tension is 90 to 100 mmHg. At Pa_{O_2} of 80 to 90 mmHg, oxygen saturation approaches 100 per cent, but at values less than 60 mmHg, significant hypoxia exists. When Pa_{O_2} drops below 40 to 50 mmHg, cyanosis develops. Hypercapnia is present at Pa_{CO_2} values greater than 60 mmHg, resulting in respiratory acidosis. The major respiratory abnormalities affecting arterial gas tensions include hypoventilation, ventilation-perfusion mismatch (V_A/Q), and diffusion abnormalities (uncommon cause).

Hypoventilation typically occurs with upper airway obstruction and pleural effusions and results in hypoxemia and hypercapnia, and less commonly, with drug-induced central depression, neuropathies affecting diaphragmatic and intercostal muscle control and neuromuscular diseases.[18] With V_A/Q mismatch, hypoxia with normocapnia or hypocapnia is usually present, and the hypoxia can be reversed by increasing the oxygen fraction of inspired air. V_A/Q typically is associated with significant lower airway and lung parenchymal disease. With diseases causing diffusion impairment, by the time clinical signs are apparent, concurrent V_A/Q mismatch is usually also present. Blood gas analysis also allows differentiation of alveolar hypoventilation from V_A/Q mismatch by calculation of the alveolar-arterial oxygen gradient ($(A\text{-}a)P_{O_2}$) (Fig. 125–2).

Respiratory acidosis, the second most common acid-base

disturbance, is associated with hypercapnia and, consequently, is seen mainly with alveolar hypoventilation.[18] Reversal of respiratory acidosis is best achieved by treating the underlying cause (e.g., upper airway obstruction). Oxygen supplementation is beneficial, particularly if there is acute hypercapnia associated with life-threatening hypoxia, but it is less beneficial in chronic hypercapnia, where there is blunted hypoxic ventilatory drive. Maintenance of normal plasma chloride levels is important with chronic hypercapnia, as it is required for the renal excretion of excess HCO_3^-.

PULMONARY FUNCTION TESTING

Pulmonary function testing is widely used for the assessment of respiratory function in chronic respiratory disease in humans, but widespread adoption of these techniques in veterinary medicine has not occurred. In general, abnormalities of pulmonary function (mechanics) are best appreciated in animals with severe respiratory impairment.[19]

REFERENCES

1. Corcoran BM, et al: Feline asthma syndrome: A retrospective study of the clinical presentation in 29 cats. J Small Anim Pract 36:481, 1995.
2. Leisewitz AL, et al: Suspected primary immunodeficiency syndrome in three related Irish wolfhounds. J Small Anim Pract 38:209, 1997.
3. Darke PGG, et al: Acute respiratory distress in the dog associated with paraquat poisoning. Vet Rec 100:275, 1977.
4. Corcoran BM, et al: Pulmonary infiltration with eosinophils in 14 dogs. J Small Anim Pract 32:494, 1991.
5. Halliwell REW: Efficacy of hyposensitization in feline allergic disease based upon results of in vitro testing for allergen-specific immunoglobulin E. J Am Anim Hosp Assoc 33:282, 1997.
6. Kealy JK: The thorax. In Kealy JK (ed): Diagnostic Radiology of the Dog and Cat, 2nd ed. Philadelphia, WB Saunders, 1987, p 171.
7. Suter PF: Normal radiographic anatomy and radiographic examination. In Suter PF, Lord PF (eds): Thoracic Radiogrpahy. Weittseil, Switzerland, PF Suter, 1984, p 1.
8. Stowater JL, Lamb CR: Ultrasonography of noncardiac thoracic diseases in small animals. JAVMA 195:514, 1989.
9. Padrid PA, et al: Canine chronic bronchitis; a pathological evaluation of 18 cases. J Vet Intern Med 4:172, 1990.
10. Venker–van Haagen AJ, et al: Bronchoscopy in small animal clinics: An analysis of the results of 228 bronchoscopies. J Am Anim Hosp Assoc 21:521, 1985.
11. McKiernan B: Bronchoscopy in the small animal patient. In Kirk RW, Bonagura JD (eds): Current Veterinary Therapy X. Philadelphia, WB Saunders, 1989, p 219.
12. Rebar AH, et al: Bronchopulmonary lavage cytology in the dog: Normal findings. Vet Pathol 17:294, 1980.
13. Hawkins EC, et al: Bronchoalveolar lavage in the evaluation of pulmonary disease in the dog and cat. J Vet Intern Med 4:267, 1990.
14. Padrid PA, et al: Cytologic, microbiologic, and biochemical analysis of bronchoalveolar lavage fluid obtained from 24 healthy cats. Am J Vet Res 52:1300, 1991.
15. Angus JC, et al: Microbiological study of transtracheal aspirates from dogs with suspected lower respiratory tract disease: 264 cases (1989–1995). JAVMA 210:55, 1997.
16. Withrow SJ, et al: Aspiration and punch biopsy techniques for nasal tumours. J Am Anim Hosp Assoc 21:551, 1985.
17. Teske E, et al: Transthoracic needle aspiration biopsy of lung in dogs with pulmonic diseases. J Am Anim Hosp Assoc 27:289, 1991.
18. DiBartola SP, De Morais HSA: Respiratory acid-base disorders. In DiBartola SP (ed): Fluid Therapy in Small Animal Practice. Philadelphia, WB Saunders, 1992, p 258.
19. Dye JA, et al: Pulmonary function in cats with bronchopulmonary disease and acute response to IV bronchodilator challenge. J Vet Intern Med 6:140, 1992.

RES

CHAPTER 126

DISEASES OF THE TRACHEA

Stephen J. Ettinger, Brett Kantrowitz, and Kyle Brayley

ANATOMY AND PATHOPHYSIOLOGY

The normal trachea is a semirigid, flexible tubular passageway connecting the larynx to the bronchi. It is made up of 35 to 45 C-shaped cartilages, each alternating with an elastic annular ligament. The cartilage-free, dorsal part of the trachea is composed of mucosa, connective tissue, and tracheal muscle (the dorsal tracheal membrane). The trachea bifurcates into the main stem bronchi at the level of the fourth or fifth thoracic vertebra.

The cranial and caudal thyroid arteries are the major blood supply to most of the trachea. The recurrent laryngeal and vagus nerves supply parasympathetic innervation to the tracheal mucosa and its smooth muscle, which stimulates muscular and glandular secretion. The inhibitory sympathetic fibers arise from the middle cervical ganglion and sympathetic trunk.

The tracheal mucosal layer is composed of a pseudostratified, ciliated columnar epithelium with goblet cells; mucus-secreting tubular glands are found in the submucosa. The ciliated cells of the epithelium act as part of the mucociliary transport system to propel mucus and inspired debris toward the pharynx.

As is true of other tissue in the body, the trachea has a limited number of ways to respond to an insult. Changes seen during examination of the trachea are usually not pathognomonic for a given disease state. The immediate response of the tracheal mucosa to irritation of any cause is increased mucus secretion. With continued insult, epithelial cells desquamate, and goblet cell hyperplasia occurs. Squamous metaplasia takes place if continued insults occur with insufficient time for healing between episodes. Superficial defects in the tracheal mucosa can begin to heal as early as two hours after cessation of an injury. Large areas of damaged epithelium devoid of functional cilia can impair the mucociliary transport system, predisposing to infection and delayed healing.

The primary pathophysiologic response to stenotic disease is increased airway resistance that cannot be overcome through mouth breathing and decreased pulmonary compliance. With impaired airflow, hypoventilation and respiratory acidosis occur. Chronic obstruction can result in secondary pulmonary hypertension and right heart failure (cor pulmonale).

HISTORY AND PHYSICAL EXAMINATION

The most commonly recognized clinical signs of tracheal disease are coughing, stertorous noisy inspiratory sounds, stridulous or wheezing expiratory sounds, pulmonary edema, and occasionally cyanosis. See Chapter 46 for the clinical differentiation of coughing and its most commonly encountered causes.

A thorough physical examination is the first diagnostic step to take after the history in evaluating animals with suspected tracheal disease. The physical examination should cover all aspects of the animal, with particular attention to the entire upper and lower respiratory tracts as well as the cardiovascular system. The entire neck should be palpated for evidence of surrounding disease such as subcutaneous emphysema, lymphadenopathy, abscess, cyst, neoplasia, thyroid gland enlargement, or any other mass that may involve the trachea. In most animals, except for the heavy or obese, the trachea can be palpated from the larynx to the thoracic inlet. The trachea is relatively noncollapsible, and obvious borders or angles usually cannot be felt. Often, a cough can be elicited with light tracheal palpation at the thoracic inlet when laryngeal or tracheal irritation and inflammation are present.

Auscultation of the lung sounds, as well as respiratory sounds directly over the trachea, larynx, and nose, should be compared to help localize the site of the lesion. Sounds are usually most intense near their site of origin. Examination of the oral and pharyngeal cavities is best done with the aid of anesthesia (propofol, thiopental) or light sedation.

DIAGNOSTIC TESTS

RADIOGRAPHY

Two views of the trachea should be obtained for routine radiographic examination: lateral and ventrodorsal or dorsoventral. Radiographs to evaluate the cervical trachea should be obtained separately from those of the thoracic trachea. The lateral radiographic examination must be performed with careful positioning of the animal to avoid artifactual deviations of the trachea, especially in the caudal cervical and cranial mediastinal regions. Excessive flexion of the occipitoatlantal articulation may cause deviations of the trachea, which may artifactually suggest extratracheal masses (Fig. 126–1). Dorsal deviation of the intrathoracic trachea can be due to ventroflexion of the neck. Other causes include cardiac enlargement, pleural effusions, and cranial mediastinal masses. Ventral deviation of the thoracic trachea can be seen with a dilated esophagus or with diseases of the dorsal cranial mediastinum. Ventrodorsal views are used to evaluate the course of the trachea. Ventrodorsal oblique views are occasionally needed when the thoracic tracheal lumen is superimposed over the vertebral column and sternum, preventing sufficient radiographic detail. These views are usually not necessary, however, because the trachea normally courses to the right of the cranial mediastinum and reaches the midline only at the tracheal bifurcation (carina).

Tracheal radiographs should be surveyed for luminal filling defects, continuity of the mucosal lining, diameter, and placement within the cervical and thoracic regions. Normal aging may result in dystrophic mineralization of tracheal rings, which is not pathologic. The normal tracheal diameter

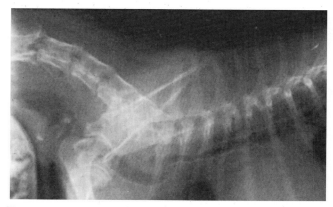

Figure 126–1. The kinking of the trachea that may occur with excessive flexion of the neck in small animals and in those with tracheal malacia. These undesirable causes of narrowing of the trachea must be avoided while radiographing the dog and, more importantly, while it is recovering from an anesthetic.

generally decreases slightly from cranial to caudal. The normal diameter of the trachea at the third rib should be approximately three times the width of the third rib at the level of the trachea.[1] Another method of determining tracheal diameter uses the ratio of the inner diameter of the trachea at the thoracic inlet to the distance between the ventral edge of the first thoracic vertebra and dorsal edge of the manubrium. The normal ratio is 0.16 or greater.[1] The tracheal lumen is similar to the caudal laryngeal lumen. One recent study determined that accurate measurement of the degree of tracheal stenosis is not possible with currently available methodology.[2]

Motion studies (fluoroscopy) of the diseased trachea are highly desirable for evaluating pathodynamics. Image intensification equipment is necessary to safely obtain adequate radiographic detail. These studies are extremely valuable for the study of the collapsed trachea and other coughing syndromes. Animals should be placed in lateral recumbency and the entire trachea visualized. A cough usually can be induced by digital pressure applied at the thoracic inlet. Videotape recordings add to the usefulness of dynamic studies. Playback observations in slow motion can result in the detection of functional features missed during the initial examination.

Fluoroscopic equipment may not be available to the general practitioner. Motion dynamics of the trachea can often be inferred from static images obtained at different phases of respiration. Lateral inspiratory and expiratory projections are used to evaluate changes in the tracheal lumen. A forced expiration can be obtained by inducing a cough with tracheal palpation. Mild physiologic changes in tracheal diameter during respiration is normal. The cervical trachea may narrow slightly with inspiration, whereas the intrathoracic trachea and carina narrow slightly during expiration.

Contrast studies of the trachea and bronchi (bronchography) have been advocated in the past for further evaluation of the trachea and airways. This procedure has generally been replaced by bronchoscopy, a more effective and safer technique for evaluation of the lumen and lining of the major airways.

TRACHEOSCOPY AND BRONCHSCOPY

Endoscopic examination is a useful tool for evaluating pathologic states of the trachea. It may be performed with a rigid or flexible scope to help localize the site and extent of a lesion. Endoscopy directly visualizes the tracheal mucosa and identifies inflammation, ulceration, and edema. It is used to visualize and to obtain biopsy specimens of tumors and masses; for brush cytology, fluid aspiration, and cultures; for removal of foreign bodies; for demonstration of collapsed, hypoplastic, stenotic, disrupted, or compressed areas; and for evaluation of disease progression or response to therapy.

Small animal respiratory endoscopy requires general anesthesia. The use of atropine sulfate generally is not recommended because of its detrimental effects of thickening and decreasing respiratory epithelial secretions. There are several options for sedation for tracheoscopy. Short-acting barbiturates (propofol) permit the rapid and gentle sedation of an animal for intubation and can be given on a continuous basis if the procedure is to be relatively short. Maintenance for a longer period is best handled using isoflurane gaseous anesthesia, because the animal may be quickly awoken after the procedure with few side effects and short duration of sedation. On occasion, ketamine-diazepam–type sedation proves useful for longer procedures, but the problems associated with waking up are enhanced, especially in difficult to manage pets such as those with severe lung disease, obese animals, and brachycephalic breeds. Another option is oxymorphone (Numorphan), although its respiratory depressive effects may necessitate manual (bagged) breathing for the animal.

TRACHEOBRONCHIAL CULTURE AND CYTOLOGY

Examining cytologic specimens can often be an efficient and practical means of helping to support a diagnosis while ruling out others. There are multiple ways to obtain diagnostically significant samples from the trachea for culture and cytology. In all cases, culture specimens should be obtained before cytology specimens. If tracheal endoscopy is being performed and the equipment has a biopsy port, specimens may be obtained through this instrument with sterile endoscopic brushes. A protected sterile culture swab or cytology brush can also be introduced directly through the mouth and larynx and into the trachea for specimen retrieval. Bronchoalveolar lavage is the preferred method of obtaining cytologic and culture samples from the lower respiratory tract and occasionally from the upper portions of the tract. The endoscope is cleaned externally and the channels flushed with sterile saline. It is then repositioned at the sampling site and gently wedged into position. Multiple aliquots of sterile saline are passed through the channel and immediately suctioned back into the syringe. Samples may be obtained in this manner from one or more positions using bronchoalveolar lavage. Another method[1] that works well in smaller animals is to place a sterile endotracheal tube, flush a small amount of sterile saline through the tube and into the trachea, hold the animal upside down, and collect draining fluid in a sterile vial as it runs out of the endotracheal tube. Although this method is not as precise as other methods, it is practical and easy to perform with equipment found in most small animal hospital settings. An alternative technique that does not usually require general anesthesia is transtracheal aspiration. This usually requires either local anesthesia or mild sedation while a long sterile needle is used to puncture the midcervical trachea or cricothyroid membrane. A catheter designed to pass through the needle is threaded into the tracheal lumen and is used for aspiration.

Numerous bacterial culture studies have been made from

RES

transtracheal and bronchoscopic aspirations. These samples have principally but not exclusively been taken from lower tracheal and respiratory tract. In a study evaluating 264 cases of lower respiratory tract specimens, 203 bacterial species were isolated in 116 of 264 dogs. Most (57 percent) contained a single species of bacteria. Those cultured most commonly were *Escherichia coli* (45.7 percent), *Pasteurella* (22.4 percent), obligate anaerobes (21.6 per cent), beta-hemolytic streptococcus (12.1 per cent), *Bordetella bronchiseptica* (12.1 per cent), nonhemolytic *Streptococcus/Enterococcus* spp. (12.1 per cent), coagulase-positive *Staphylococcus* (9.5 per cent), and *Pseudomonas* (7.8 per cent). Of these cultures, the most active antimicrobial agents for aerobic microorganisms inhibiting over 90 per cent of the isolates were amikacin, ceftizoxime sodium, enrofloxacin, and gentamicin sulfate.[3] *Mycoplasma* recovery in normal dogs and those with pulmonary disease was about 25 per cent. Only young dogs under 1 year of age and those with *Bordetella* or streptococci isolations had a significant association between their disease and *Mycoplasma* recovery during tracheobronchial lavage.[4] *Bordetella bronchiseptica* infection was reported in a series of cats mostly younger than 8 weeks old with dry nonproductive coughing. Transtracheal washings were positively cultured for *B. bronchiseptica*.[5]

Bronchoalveolar lavage cytology from 33 normal dogs identified alveolar macrophages (79.4 per cent), lymphocytes (13.5 per cent), eosinophils (3.6 per cent), mast cells (2.1 per cent), epithelial cells (0.8 per cent), and neutrophils (0.6 per cent).[6] These numbers vary from earlier reports of limited numbers of macrophages and lymphocytes.[7] Deviations from these numbers, although not usually diagnostic, provide valuable information on the type of response and the type of disease process present. Neutrophilic inflammation most often results from bacterial infection, which can be secondary to a number of other problems, including, but not limited to, collapsed trachea, chronic bronchitis, neoplasia, allergic disease, and viral, mycotic, or parasitic infections. Such cytologic findings could include an increased number of neutrophils, degenerative changes within the neutrophils, and phagocytized bacteria.[8] Eosinophilic inflammation is usually considered significant, although it has been noted in clinically normal dogs and cats.[8, 9] Eosinophils and mast cells imply an allergic or parasitic tracheobronchitis.[10] A concurrent, nonseptic neutrophilic or chronic inflammatory response is frequently present. Major differential diagnoses include allergic bronchitis, pulmonary parasites, heartworm disease, and hypersensitivity responses secondary to bacterial, protozoal, fungal, or neoplastic diseases. Chronic inflammation is indicated by a mixed inflammatory cell population with a predominant number of activated macrophages.[8] This type of response is nonspecific and has a long list of differentials. All slides should be carefully examined for organisms or atypical cells. Tight coils of inspissated mucus can be washed out in association with small airway disease.[10] Hemorrhagic inflammation consists of chronic or chronic-active inflammatory cells with erythrophagocytosis and increased numbers of red blood cells.[8] Many diseases of the respiratory tract can cause hemorrhage, but systemic clotting disorders should also be considered. Large numbers of reactive lymphocytes and plasma cells are nonspecific indicators of immune stimulation.[8] Primary ciliary dyskinesia may be suggested when associated with chronic bronchopneumonial ultrastructural abnormalities and a lack of sperm motility on testicular aspiration.[11] Neoplastic cells may be identified. Differentiation of criteria of malignancy in epithelial cells is often difficult, especially when accompanied by marked

inflammation. Histologic examination may be necessary. Organisms may be found cytologically to give a definitive diagnosis. However, their absence does not eliminate infectious disease as a diagnosis.

CLINICOPATHOLOGIC STUDIES

Tracheal diseases only rarely have definitive, demonstrable clinicopathologic findings. Hematologic and biochemical analysis of the blood, as well as serology and a urinalysis, should be used as a reflection of the animal's overall health as well as to indicate systemic or allergic disease. Blood gas analysis is helpful to demonstrate severity of the disease and acid-base status.

SPECIFIC TRACHEAL DISEASES

NONINFECTIOUS TRACHEITIS

Etiology. Tracheitis refers to an inflammation of the epithelial lining of the trachea. This inflammatory response may be infectious or noninfectious, primary or secondary. The noninfectious causes of chronic tracheitis are probably more common and are discussed as a group. Noninfectious tracheitis is usually a secondary problem related to prolonged barking, collapsing trachea, chronic cardiac disease, or disease of the oropharynx. Tracheitis is unusual in cats and most commonly is associated with infectious feline respiratory diseases. Allergic lower airway disease may also promote secondary tracheitis.

Clinical Signs and Diagnosis. Because tracheitis may be primary (inhalation of smoke or other noxious gases) or secondary, the history varies with the etiology. Most animals with tracheitis are asymptomatic except for a cough, which is characterized as resonant, harsh, paroxysmal, and often terminated by nonproductive or slightly productive gagging. The physical examination is often normal, and no fever is present. Palpation of the trachea near the thoracic inlet elicits the typical tracheal cough. Examination of the oral cavity and oropharynx is unlikely to reveal abnormalities unless the tracheitis is secondary to an oropharyngeal disease process. The tonsils may be enlarged and extend further out of the crypts than normal. Auscultation of the heart is usually normal. If a cardiac murmur or arrhythmia exists, cardiac disease must be eliminated as the cause for coughing (see Chapter 46) or as the cause of chronic tracheitis. If chronic cardiac coughing causes secondary tracheitis, snapping of the second heart sound as a result of increased pulmonary resistance may be present over the pulmonic valve region. Findings on auscultation of the lungs are normal unless tracheitis is secondary to pulmonary disease (see Chapter 128), in which case coarse bronchial lung sounds may be heard.

Tracheitis as a primary disease often has no specific radiographic features. In acute tracheitis, edema of the mucosal lining may result in a reduction of the lumen diameter. Care must be taken not to confuse this for a fixed, hypoplastic trachea. The radiographic features that occur when tracheitis is secondary to other diseases are included in the discussions of those conditions. Hematology and blood chemistries are usually within reference ranges unless affected by the primary disease, or unless systemic disease states concurrently exist.

Therapy. Therapy should be directed at the primary underlying disease process, and these treatments are discussed in their appropriate sections. The cough associated with secondary tracheitis may act as a continued source of irritation, perpetuating the tracheitis, and a vicious circle ensues. Treatment of the underlying disease process may not always be adequate to relieve the cough because of this cycle of cough-induced tracheitis, perpetuating the cough as well as the tracheitis. Therefore, treatment aimed specifically at the tracheitis is often beneficial, if not mandatory.

Tracheal coughing is often treated with antitussive and bronchodilating preparations (Table 126–1). Many of these preparations also contain expectorants. Occasionally, short-term therapy with corticosteroids may be warranted. It is important to emphasize that this provides symptomatic relief only, and it may exacerbate the primary condition. With chronic coughing, nebulization four to six times daily may help to liquefy mucoid material collecting in the trachea. When nebulization is not possible, the dog or cat can be placed in a bathroom filled with steam from a hot shower. This procedure should last 15 to 20 minutes, three times daily. Following either method, gentle coupage of the chest wall helps to loosen secretions and stimulate expectoration.

INFECTIOUS TRACHEOBRONCHITIS

Etiology. Infectious canine tracheobronchitis, also known as canine respiratory disease complex and kennel cough, is not a single disease but a clinical disease syndrome. Involved in this multietiology syndrome are infectious agents such as viruses, bacteria, mycoplasmas, fungi, and parasites. The most commonly incriminated agents are canine parainfluenza virus, canine adenovirus, canine herpesvirus, reovirus, *Bordetella bronchiseptica,* mycoplasmas, and occasionally canine distemper virus.[12] Most cases of infectious canine tracheobronchitis involve a primary viral infection. *B. bronchiseptica* infection in cats is unusual but has been described.[5, 13] The role of *B. bronchiseptica* in infectious tracheobronchitis in dogs has recently been reviewed.[47]

Clinical Signs and Diagnosis. Infectious canine tracheobronchitis is highly contagious and most commonly occurs where groups of dogs of different ages and susceptibility are congregated. There is almost always a history of exposure to other animals, as in a kennel, hospital, or dog show. Aerosol or direct contact is considered the main source of exposure. Clinical signs usually develop three to five days after initial exposure. The clinical signs are generally mild and self-limited. A dry, hacking, paroxysmal cough is the most consistent sign. A purulent nasal discharge may be noted. Generally, the animal is healthy in other respects.

Diagnosis is made most often on the basis of circumstantial evidence. History of exposure with a dry hacking cough is usually sufficient. Thoracic auscultation, thoracic radiographs, and hemograms are usually unremarkable. Tracheal cytology may reveal increased numbers of neutrophils and bacteria. Bacterial or mycoplasmal isolation, as well as virus isolation and serologic evaluation, can be performed but are usually unnecessary. *B. bronchiseptica* commonly associated with this condition may require three months for full clearance to occur.

Therapy. Uncomplicated cases of tracheobronchitis probably do not require antimicrobials. Even though antibiotics have not been shown to reach significant concentrations in tracheobronchial secretions or to shorten the course of infection, prophylactic therapy has been recommended by some.[14] Antibiotic treatment is indicated if there is deeper respiratory involvement or if the animal is showing signs of systemic illness. Drugs chosen should be based on results of bacterial culture and sensitivity testing. In the absence of culture results, choices of oral antibiotics used by the authors include chloramphenicol, fluoroquinolones, or cephalosporins. Macrolide antibiotics are effective in young dogs against *B. bronchiseptica* (clarithromycin and azithromycin), and tetracyclines in adult dogs may be the preferred antimicrobial agent.[47] More potent injectable agents such as amikacin, gentamicin, and ceftizoxime should be chosen only after culture results indicate their effectiveness.

Glucocorticoids, administered at anti-inflammatory doses, can be effective in suppressing the cough of uncomplicated infectious tracheobronchitis. However, glucocorticoids do not appear to shorten the clinical course of the disease.[14] They may worsen the illness in immunocompromised individuals. If glucocorticoids are used, a bactericidal antibiotic should be chosen over a bacteriostatic one for concurrent use.

Antitussives, either alone or in combination with bronchodilators, are recommended. Narcotic cough suppressants seem to be the most effective. These agents can compromise ventilation and should not be used in the presence of concurrent bacterial pneumonia. Methylxanthine bronchodilators may also be of benefit in suppressing the cough through their ability to prevent bronchospasm. Animals with tracheobronchial disease also benefit from nebulization, which can help to loosen excessive accumulations of bronchial and

TABLE 126–1. DRUGS USED FOR TRACHEAL DISEASES

GENERIC NAME AND PREPARATION	TRADE NAME	DOSAGE
Aminophylline	—	5 mg/lb q6–12h PO as needed
Theophylline	Elixophyllin, Theolixir; Theo-Dur	5 mg/lb q6–16h PO as needed
Theophylline with glyceryl guaiacolate	Quibron	1 capsule q8–12h for larger dogs; ¼–1 tbsp elixir q8–12h for smaller dogs
Aminophylline with ¼ or ½ gr phenobarbital	—	½–1 tablet q6–12h PO
Ephedrine sulfate	—	1 mg/lb q8h PO
Terbutaline	Brethine; Bricanyl	1.25–5 mg q8–12h PO
Prednisone with trimeprazine	Temaril-P	1 tablet per 20 lb q12h PO
Dextromethorphan	Benylin DM; Pertussin	0.5–1 mg/lb q6–8h PO
Dextromethorphan with guaifenesin	Robitussin-DM	Dosage similar to that for adults and children
Codeine	—	0.5–1 mg/lb q6–8h PO
Hydrocodone bitartrate with homatropine	Hycodan; Tussigon	½–1 tablet (or tsp) q6–24h PO
Butorphanol tartrate	Torbutrol	0.25 mg/lb q6–12h PO

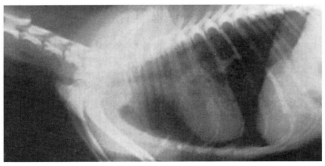

Figure 126–2. Lateral thoracic radiograph of an immature male terrier showing multiple nodules in the lumen of the caudal trachea due to *Oslerus osleri*. Note the hyperexpansion of the thoracic cavity, which is probably due to increased resistance within the trachea during expiration.

tracheal secretions. Nebulization with sterile saline is as acceptable as mucolytic agents.

LUNGWORM

Etiology. *Oslerus osleri* (formerly *Filaroides osleri*) is a worldwide parasitic disease seen most often in dogs younger than 2 years of age. It can occur in individual situations but is more commonly a kennel-related problem (especially in greyhounds).[1] Although most often described in young dogs, it does persist in older animals, often without significant pathophysiologic effects.

Although described as a lungworm, this parasite most commonly affects the region proximal to the tracheal carina. Occasionally, it affects the lumen and lining of the larger bronchi, but only rarely does it extend deeper into the pulmonary system.

Reports of direct transmission through larvae in the stool and saliva suggest that this metastrongyle may not require an intermediate host to complete its life cycle. First-stage larvae are directly transmitted through salivary and airway secretions. These molt in the small bowel, followed by migration of the larvae to the lungs and bronchi. Experimental and natural direct transmission has been demonstrated.[1] Transmission to pups has also been reported to occur through parental food regurgitation and licking and cleaning of pups by a nursing bitch.[15]

Clinical Signs and Diagnosis. Dogs usually present with chronic, mild to severe inspiratory wheezing sounds, dyspnea, coughing, and/or debilitation. Panting usually is not prominent except in advanced cases. The severity of the clinical signs may be overplayed in the literature. Most dogs experience definite but mild, often nonprogressive respiratory signs. Exercise intolerance occasionally occurs, and coughing is typically characterized as a harsh tracheobronchial sound associated with attempts at terminal retching. A small amount of white to blood-tinged mucus in common, but at times larger amounts of exudate are brought up.

Tracheal sensitivity occurs, but physical palpation is normal. Heart sounds are normal but may be less apparent when obvious respiratory embarrassment with wheezing, ronchi, or pulmonary edema is present.

The radiographic examination is helpful if the disease process is extensive and the nodules are large. The tracheal lining may be diffusely thickened, interrupted with indistinct solid masses, or show ill-defined, 2- to 10-mm semicircular lesions protruding into the lumen (Fig. 126–2). Endoscopically, cream-colored nodules, 1 to 5 mm high and wide, are usually diagnostic. The larvae are often seen peeking into the luminal edge of the growth. Brushings and biopsies of the nodules provide a definitive diagnosis (Fig. 126–3).

Larvae are occasionally detected in the feces. Although some flotation methods dehydrate the larvae, zinc sulfate flotation techniques are diagnostic, as is the Baermann technique. Eggs, when seen, are 50 by 80 μm, thin shelled, colorless, and larvated. The larvae are 230 μm long with a distinct kinked tail. Both larvae and eggs may be visualized in the sputum and in washings from the trachea of an affected dog.

Therapy. Many drugs have been reported to be effective

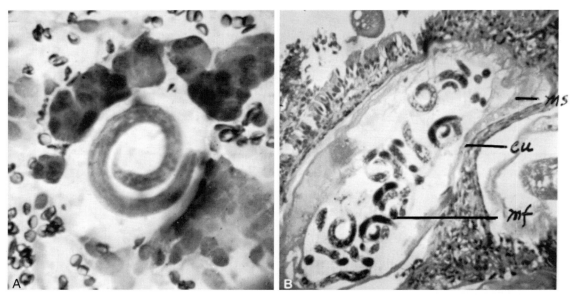

Figure 126–3. *A,* Photomicrograph of a biopsy taken from the trachea just proximal to the carina of the animal in Figure 126–2. The tracheal lining is surrounded by a larval representative of *Oslerus osleri.* Note the kinked tail characteristic of this worm larva. *B,* Parasitic tracheitis exhibiting prominent infestation by adult filarial worms. The worms contain microfilaria (mf), which are within the cuticle (cu) and are surrounded by mucosal tissue (ms) from the host's pulmonary system.

in treating lungworms, such as thiacetarsamide sodium, diethylcarbamazine, levamisole, fenbendazole, and albendazole.[1] We have treated several dogs with oral ivermectin at 1000 µg/lb once weekly for two months. The nodules were reduced in size but did not resolve entirely. All these dogs became asymptomatic and continued to thrive. Thiabendazole continues to receive favorable press; the most recent report used it at 16 mg/lb twice daily for five days and then at 32 mg/lb twice daily for 21 days. Along with thiabendazole, prednisone at 0.25 mg/lb was given twice daily every other day.[16]

Surgical removal is not recommended, owing to the large number of nodules. Removal of a large obstructing nodule may potentially be therapeutic in rare situations.

TRACHEAL HYPOPLASIA

Etiology. The hypoplastic trachea syndrome, first described in 1972, is a congenital defect resulting from inadequate growth of the tracheal rings.[1] The condition varies from mild to severe. This disease is recognized primarily in young, brachycephalic animals. The first complete report involved a series of dogs, most of which were English bulldogs.[1] In another report, the highest incidence was in English bulldogs (55 per cent), with Boston terriers also being commonly affected (15 per cent of the cases).[17] Other congenital abnormalities, including elongated soft palate, stenotic nares, cardiac defects, and megaesophagus, may be associated.

Clinical Signs and Diagnosis. Because tracheal hypoplasia is a congenital disease, it can be diagnosed early in life. In one study, the median age at diagnosis was 5 months (range, 2 days to 12 years).[17] Common clinical signs include dyspnea, stridor, and coughing. Occasionally, dogs present with a moist, productive cough, moist rales on auscultation, and a fever associated with bronchopneumonia.

Physical examination may be normal (except for a palpably small trachea) or may reveal a sensitive trachea that, when palpated, evokes coughing. Excitement is likely to exacerbate the coughing episode, which is usually more severe and serious during the day. Heart sounds are normal unless an associated congenital cardiac malformation is present. Clinical pathology reveals a leukocytosis with a left shift if there is a concurrent bronchopneumonia. The radiographic features are most important and usually provide a definitive diagnosis (Fig. 126–4). Dorsoventral and lateral radiographs of the thorax and lateral views of the cervical region should be obtained to assess the tracheal diameter and the presence or absence of pulmonary changes. Methods for measuring and determining normal trachea diameter were reviewed earlier in the chapter.

The diagnosis of hypoplastic trachea is generally made when the lumen diameter is less than two times the width of the third rib where they cross. The tracheal lumen also appears smaller than the caudal laryngeal lumen in these animals. Care must be taken in young animals in which the adult proportions of the tracheal lumen have not yet been obtained. Tracheal edema associated with tracheitis may mimic a hypoplastic trachea in the radiograph. For this reason, it is best to get radiographs when the animal is asymptomatic.

Prognosis and Therapy. The prognosis for dogs with a hypoplastic trachea depends on the degree of hypoplasia as well as the presence or absence of concurrent congenital defects. Many animals with slight to moderate hypoplastic

tracheas can live normal, satisfactory lives with only an occasional need for bronchodilator therapy and antibiotics. Young dogs with this diagnosis often outgrow the condition. One report suggests that tracheal hypoplasia may be clinically insignificant in the absence of concurrent cardiac or other obstructive upper respiratory disease. Further, it supports the idea that the degree of hypoplasia does not correlate with the presence or absence of clinical signs.[17]

Clinical experience has shown that many dogs present with this condition in various states of severity as puppies and young dogs. With effective empiric therapy, a significant number of these dogs develop and grow into healthy mature dogs. Because the initial impression is one of a very advanced condition, the veterinarian may wish to advise the client on the potential for the dog to overcome this problem. This is particularly true if there are no associated congenital defects present. Owners who are experienced with these breeds are familiar with the problem and are often quite capable of dealing with the extensive nursing care required. One should be firm, but not too insistent, on recommending therapy for these animals. Many who have suggested euthanasia have come to regret their haste after seeing some of these dogs as mature adults. The prognosis remains guarded, and it is prudent to identify the possibilities to a new pet owner who presents a pet with this condition. Similarly, the veterinarian must carefully evaluate the pet for associated congenital defects (cardiac or other upper airway).

It is important to prevent bronchopneumonia from developing by keeping the affected animal in a draft-free environment and preventing excessive exposure to moisture and cold. Prevention of excessive weight gain also helps the animal by limiting the strain placed on the respiratory system by obesity. When recurrent upper respiratory tract infections do occur, the use of antibiotics is in order, preferably as determined by culture and sensitivity testing.

It is advisable to discourage the breeding of animals affected with this congenital defect, even though at this time there is no absolute evidence indicating a hereditary basis. There are no known surgical corrective procedures.

SEGMENTAL TRACHEAL STENOSIS

Etiology. Segmental tracheal stenosis is an unusual condition affecting small animals. It may occur as a congenital lesion or it may result from trauma to the trachea. The congenital absence of tracheal rings causing a focal stenotic area has been described.[18] Multiple cases of young animals with segmental tracheal strictures of unknown cause have been recorded.[1]

Segmental tracheal stenosis can also occur secondary to a tracheotomy procedure, with necrosis and thickening of the tracheal wall from excessive endotracheal cuff pressures, as a complication of thoracic surgery, following bite wounds to the cervical area, and following massive chest trauma.

Clinical Signs and Diagnosis. This syndrome produces stridulous respiratory distress and subsequent cyanosis. Secondary upper airway tract infections may result and develop into overwhelming pulmonary disease.

Radiographic studies usually establish the diagnosis. Survey tracheal radiographs often show the stenotic region as an abrupt, segmental reduction in lumen diameter.

Inspiratory and expiratory projections or fluoroscopic examination demonstrates little dynamic change in the stenosis during the respiratory cycle. Bronchoscopy can also be used in larger animals to identify the stenotic lesion and its extent.

RES

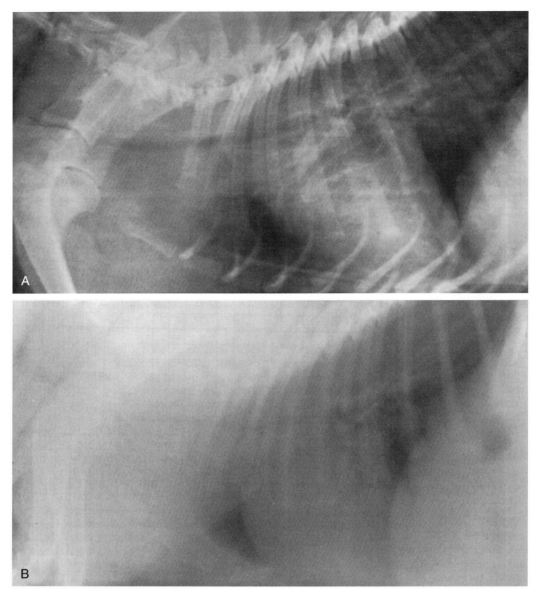

Figure 126–4. *A,* Lateral cervical and thoracic radiographs of a 1-year-old female bulldog. The radiograph of the thorax clearly demonstrates a markedly hypoplastic trachea, in addition to pulmonary changes suggesting bronchitis. The ratio of the tracheal diameter to the height of the thoracic inlet was 0.07. The normal ratio is 0.16 or greater. The indistinct outline of the trachea is due to the accumulation of large amounts of mucus in the trachea. *B,* Hypoplasia of the trachea in a 4-month-old female boxer that presented with a productive gagging cough and moderate respiratory distress. Lateral thoracic radiographs show a severely hypoplastic trachea. The ratio of the tracheal diameter to the height of the thoracic inlet was 0.05.

Therapy. The management of segmental tracheal stenosis is similar regardless of cause. The mainstay of treatment is surgical resection of the stenotic region. Several types of procedures have been used, and they are well reviewed.[1, 18, 19] In one report of a 5-month-old German shepherd, 4.5 cm of trachea (nine cartilaginous rings) was resected without excessive tension or complications.[19] Another report described the use of balloon dilatation with good success for tracheal stenosis in a cat.[20]

COLLAPSED TRACHEA

There are two types of collapsed trachea—the dorsoventral and lateral forms. The lateral form is unusual; it has been reported without obvious cause but has also developed after central chondrotomy had been performed to treat the dorsoventral form of tracheal collapse. Lateral collapse rarely occurs spontaneously, although rare cases have been described in dogs of varying sizes.[21] Dorsoventral flattening (narrowing of the trachea) is a commonly described lesion that is often associated with a pendulous, redundant dorsal tracheal membrane that prolapses into the tracheal lumen.

The collapsed trachea may involve the cervical region only, but more commonly both the cervical and thoracic areas of the trachea are involved, and the collapse frequently extends into the bronchi. Extension of the tracheal collapse to the bronchi is sometimes described as collapsing of the trachea at the carina. Extension into the cartilage of the lower airways is referred to as bronchomalacia. Regardless of the focal or diffuse nature of the problem, increasing respiratory work leads to dynamic collapse of the dorsal tracheal membrane into the tracheal lumen. This further irritates and inflames the mucous membranes, disrupts the mucociliary apparatus, and increases the risk for associated small airway problems and signs.[22] This condition has been described in cats in association with an intraluminal obstructing lesion[22] and by others but is unusual.[23]

Etiology. The etiology of collapsed trachea is unknown. The condition is an acquired disease that usually occurs in middle-aged to aged dogs, although it has been described in young dogs as a congenital lesion.[1] The clinical syndrome and findings in congenital cases are essentially similar to those described in acquired disease. In dogs with acquired collapsed tracheas, there is no loss of potential tracheal ring size, but the rings lose their ability to remain firm and subsequently collapse. They become hypocellular, and the matrix varies from normal. Glycoprotein and glycosaminoglycan are deficient or totally lacking in dogs with collapsed tracheas.[1] The essential lesion is a deficiency in the organic matrix of the tracheal cartilage. This has led some to associate the condition with tracheal and bronchomalacia. There may be a failure of chondrogenesis or simple degeneration of hyaline cartilage, decreasing its turgidity. This may, in time, lead to stretching of the dorsal membrane and finally collapse of the trachea. Biomechanical and biochemical parameters were similar when comparing cervical with thoracic tracheal rings of young and middle-aged healthy dogs.[24] Tracheal cartilage of the normal adult dogs had a significantly higher proteoglycan content and a lower water content than did that of the immature dogs.

Chronic coughing caused by long-term airway and/or pulmonary parenchymal disease, chronic cardiac disease with tracheal and bronchial compression, tracheal trauma, denervation of the dorsal tracheal membrane, congenital defects, obesity, increased mediastinal fat, and thoracic and extrathoracic masses have all been suggested as being related to collapse of the trachea. It is suggested that these are likely to be associated problems rather than primary inciting causes of the disease.

Clinical Signs and Diagnosis. Tracheal collapse produces a respiratory distress syndrome. The disease is usually paroxysmal in nature, often with a long history of chronic coughing. The cough may be described as chronic, harsh, or dry; if the owner is asked specifically, however, the cough is often described as a "goose honk" sound occurring initially during the day and occasionally into the evening hours. With rare exception, the disease is recognized in toy and miniature breeds, most often Chihuahuas, Pomeranians, toy poodles, Shih Tzus, Lhasa apsos, and Yorkshire terriers. It is often associated with chronic mitral valvular heart disease and must frequently be differentiated from heart failure due to this condition. Often, animals in a compensated cardiac state are presented with a cough due to a collapsed trachea. The pressure of the enlarged left atrium on the left main stem bronchus may aggravate or precipitate the tracheal cough, even in the absence of heart failure. The characteristic cough is elicited by excitement, tracheal pressure (such as that caused by pulling on a leash), and drinking water or eating food. Often, the owner indicates that the pet begins to cough when it is picked up or held, when excessive pressure is placed on the thoracic inlet.

Physical examination usually reveals a normal dog, which may be obese or thin. Depending on the state of anxiety and the respiratory distress of the moment, the dog's color varies from normal to cyanotic. Most are afebrile, but an elevated temperature develops with extreme respiratory distress and agitation. Hyperthermia may result if the distress is not relieved. Perhaps the most significant finding during the physical examination is the elicitation of a "goose honk" cough when the trachea is palpated in the region of the thoracic inlet. In thin animals, dorsoventral compression of the trachea and an angle at the lateral edges of the trachea can be palpated. This is not observed in obese dogs. The cardiac sounds vary from normal to that associated with simultaneous mitral valvular insufficiency. In the normal dog, the second heart sound is less pronounced than the snapping second heart sound that is often auscultated in dogs with collapsed tracheas. The lung sounds vary from normal vesicular sounds to rattling, stridulous sounds associated with sibilant rales and wheezing. Stridor implies inspiratory sounds associated with upper airway obstruction, including laryngeal paresis or paralysis, everted laryngeal saccules, and cervical tracheal collapse. Varying degrees of inspiratory or expiratory dyspnea (respiratory distress), inspiratory noises, and an expiratory grunt (abdominal press) with an abdominal effort are recognized in all cases. A significant feature of the physical examination is the frequent association of hepatomegaly. Hepatomegaly occurs in a large percentage of animals with this syndrome. It is considered to be associated with fat deposition in the liver. The relationship of this sign to the clinical syndrome is unclear; however, it is postulated to further stress respiratory movement and pulmonary compliance.

In most uncomplicated cases, there are usually no electrocardiographic abnormalities other than P-pulmonale resulting from right-sided heart strain. Examination of the oral cavity is usually normal. Culture of the tracheal lining may produce a common bacterium, but most have no growth. Tracheoscopy reveals a decreased dorsoventral diameter of the trachea with a pendulous dorsal tracheal membrane. Dynamic changes such as intrathoracic collapse are noted, as are other structural abnormalities, such as specific single or multiple flattening or collapse of tracheal rings. In most cases, the tracheal mucous membranes are hyperemic but usually show no exudate. On occasion, a copious, frothy catarrhal exudate may be present. In a study of 20 surgically managed cases, 30 per cent of the dogs were observed to have concurrent laryngeal paresis or paralysis.[1] The high figure does not correlate with our experience with large numbers of dogs that cough intermittently with this disease for many years. It may represent an important specific subset of animals, however, and should be looked for when a diagnosis of tracheal collapse is made. Further, laryngeal paresis results in stridulous inspiratory effort, in marked contrast to this expiratory wheeze, cough, and grunting syndrome. Upon completion of the visual examination, bronchoalveolar lavage, brush cytology, and/or biopsy samples are taken. The risks of bronchoscopy and tracheoscopy are relevant. Extreme caution is required; brachycephalic dogs with diminished laryngeal motility or everted saccules are additionally at risk, as may be obese animals and those with severe tracheobronchial malacia, concurrent pulmonary disease, small airway collapse, accumulated bronchial secretions, and hypoventilation. Post-bronchoscopy recovery requires careful patient attention, minimized stress, occasionally long-term intubation, and sometimes intratracheal administration of 1 per cent lidocaine spray.[25]

Radiographic examination of animals with collapsed tracheas uses both still and motion studies. The trachea should be examined on dorsoventral and lateral radiographs. Separate lateral radiographs of the cervical and cranial thoracic regions should be obtained to assess the contour of the entire trachea. Lateral radiographs made during both the maximal

RES

inspiratory and expiratory phases of the respiratory cycle are needed to demonstrate a dynamic collapsing trachea (Fig. 126–5). Collapse of the cervical tracheal segment is usually best demonstrated during the inspiratory phase. Conversely, the study made on expiration usually shows a collapse of the thoracic segment (and occasionally main stem bronchi) and an unchanged or slightly dilated cervical segment. Care should be taken not to overflex or overextend the occipitoatlantal articulation when obtaining the lateral views, because this may produce pressure on the trachea that can cause narrowing of the lumen (Fig. 126–6) or an abnormal tracheal course in the caudal cervical or thoracic region. There can be a subtle loss of radiographic detail at the dorsal luminal margin, which is produced by inversion of the dorsal tracheal membrane. The ventral margin of the tracheal lumen remains well demarcated and is unaffected by the collapsing process. The collapsed region usually involves approximately one third of the tracheal length, and the extremities of the collapse blend into normal lumen size over a distance of 2 to 3 cm. The course of the trachea is usually normal in uncomplicated cases. A redundant dorsal tracheal membrane that invaginates into the tracheal lumen can be seen as a soft tissue opacity along the dorsal aspect of the caudal cervical tracheal lumen (see Fig. 126–6A). This condition is seen in both small and large breed dogs and can be distinguished from a superimposed esophagus or other structure by the sharp soft tissue–gas interface along the ventral margin. Dorsoventral or ventrodorsal views of the thorax do not usually demonstrate changes in the trachea. Concomitant lung disease may be seen.

Motion studies of normal respiratory function and cough, using fluoroscopy, can be made in order to assess the severity of the lesion. Some cases may show collapse only during the forced expiration of coughing. Slow-motion studies of videotape recordings are often helpful in delineating the magnitude of the collapse, especially when produced by coughing.

The differential diagnosis of collapsed trachea requires consideration of such common conditions as tonsillitis, laryngeal paralysis or collapse, stenosis of the nares or trachea, eversion of the lateral saccules, elongation of the soft palate, bronchitis, primary tracheitis, foreign body tracheitis, and decompensated chronic mitral valvular disease. The list of causes of coughing that could be confused with collapsed trachea is extensive (see Chapter 46).

Therapy. The therapeutic approach to an animal with a collapsing trachea covers both the acute and the chronic state. Although both conditions are treated with the same common drugs, the need to deal quickly and aggressively with the acute state differs conceptually. Clients are often very anxious, and the pet may be equally so, thus demanding immediate attention to the pet and assurances to the owner.

In the acute state, the clinician is concerned with calming the animal as quickly as possible. This may require the use of oral antitussive agents such as butorphanol or dihydrocodeinone. In the event that these products are not rapid or potent enough, injectable butorphanol may be considered. Other agents that are effective in more advanced conditions include dilute acetylpromazine, diazepam intravenously, or morphine by injection. Separating the extremely anxious pet from the client may be very useful and allows the clinician to appropriately sedate the dog and reduce the external stimuli. Not infrequently, simply removing the pet from view of the owner calms the dog. In the event of cyanosis, oxygen in a humidified environment such as an oxygen-enriched cage or by nasal catheterization is suggested. The latter is made more difficult by the extreme anxiety of the animal. In such situations, any physical manipulation or stress may aggravate the problem, making the cure worse than the disease. The use of short-term corticosteroids has a place in such situations because there likely is tracheal edema. Injectable steroids initially, followed by oral dosages, tapered slowly, are quite helpful during acute treatment. In some cases, pets are sent home with the owner, who is instructed on the administration of dilute acetylpromazine in the event of an acute exacerbation of the problem.

Throughout treatment, bronchodilators remain effective in treating this condition. The theoretic benefits are attributable to reduction in spasm of the smaller airways, reducing intrathoracic pressures and thus decreasing the tendency of the larger airways to collapse. Additionally, there is improved mucociliary clearance and reduced diaphragmatic fatigue. In some cases, the alcoholic content of the theophylline elixir seems to benefit the animal as much as the actual medication. Caution is required concerning the side effects of methylxanthine drugs, which include vomiting and excitability. Similar

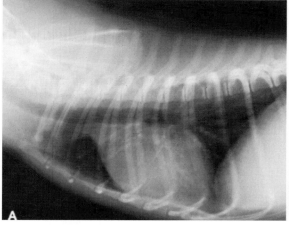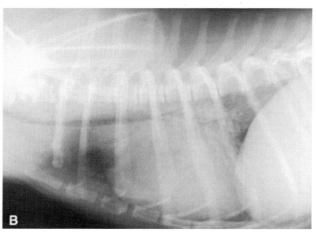

Figure 126–5. Lateral thoracic radiographs of an 8-year-old Yorkshire terrier during (*A*) peak inspiration and (*B*) peak expiration. Note the dramatic change in tracheal diameter that can occur during the respiratory cycle in animals with collapsing trachea and how important it is to obtain inspiratory as well as expiratory views. In severe cases such as this, the expiratory collapse is not limited to the thoracic segment of the trachea but extends into the cervical region as well.

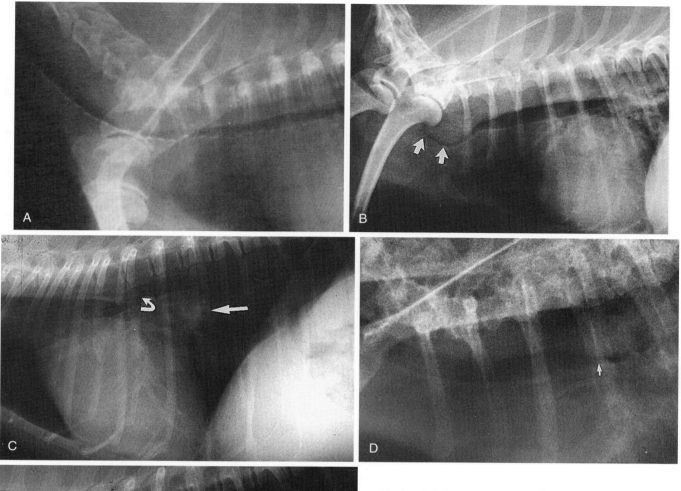

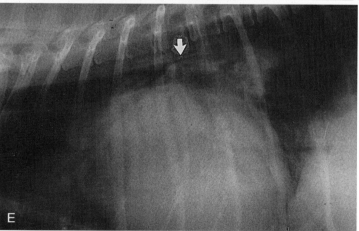

Figure 126–6. *A,* Lateral radiograph of a 13-year-old Chihuahua with a pliable, collapsible trachea showing caudal cervical tracheal collapse due to overextension of the neck. *B,* Lateral thoracic radiograph from a 14-year-old neutered male Pomeranian. Notice the reduced size of the cervical trachea *(arrows)* as compared with the thoracic trachea on inspiration. *C and D,* Eleven-year-old spayed female poodle with severe chronic coughing. There is marked left atrial enlargement *(arrow)* with bronchial dilatation *(curved arrow)* on inspiration *(C)*. On expiration *(D)* there is narrowing and reduction in size of the two main stem bronchi *(arrow)*. Such pathology usually precludes surgical correction of the disease. *E,* Lateral radiograph from a 7-year-old spayed female Pomeranian with severe coughing. Note the normal tracheal size until the carina, at which point the main stem bronchi show compression and constriction *(arrow)*. This dog required long-term aggressive medical therapy.

results may be obtained by having the owner place a small dab of an alcoholic liquid in the buccal region during acute episodes of coughing at night when at home.

Treating the animal long term on an outpatient basis uses the same principles as set out earlier, except on a more relaxed level. Usually, medications can be administered on an as-required basis and often may not be required throughout every day. The backbone of such therapy remains the bronchodilator agents (usually the methylxanthine derivatives such as aminophylline, theophylline elixir, or another bronchodilator; see Table 126–1). Beta agonists (terbutaline

and albuterol) can be used effectively in place of the methylxanthine agents. Antitussive agents butorphanol and dihydrocodeinone (hydrocodone) are quite effective in controlling symptoms. Side effects, including oversedation, anorexia, and constipation, may develop. Occasionally, longer-term low-dose steroids are given, often in combination with a sedative-antihistamine. Some combination products work well here (see Table 126–1). Often the clinician will need to change therapies from time to time to find a newer effective agent.

For an unknown reason, some animals that do not respond

to the preceding therapies are often helped with oral digoxin. The neuroendocrine effect of digitalis may play a role in the effectiveness of this product, although the treatment of the cor pulmonale is considered to be another possible role.

Weight reduction in the obese animal is essential. This is accomplished principally with high-fiber, low-fat diets, because exercise modification is unlikely. Weight loss alone can be curative in terms of dealing with the symptoms of this disease. Likewise, removal of the neck collar and using only a harness when the dog is taken outside can be most effective in reducing the clinical signs. Identification and treatment of hepatomegaly may be a complicating process in association with signs of a collapsing trachea.

The majority of cases can be successfully treated symptomatically. Bronchodilator preparations containing expectorants and sedatives usually suffice to control this disease (see Table 126–1). Nebulization or vaporization may provide additional relief. Hospitalization with sedation for a period of several days, associated with corticosteroid therapy and nebulization, helps to reduce the degree of associated tracheitis. It is important to recognize that other disease states, specifically chronic lung disease, hepatomegaly, or chronic mitral valvular fibrosis, may be present. Antibiotics are not indicated in treating this disease unless a concomitant bacterial infection is suspected. Removing the dog from respiratory irritants such as noxious gases, smoke, and dust is common sense.

Several authors have reported on the surgical correction of this condition.[1, 26–28] There is no overwhelming evidence to link central chondrotomy with effective control of this disease. In one survey evaluating 100 dogs with tracheal collapse, 71 per cent had long-term resolution of clinical signs with conservative care. Four per cent required upper airway surgery, and 11 per cent were sent for tracheal reconstruction when no other medical conditions were recognized. Only half of this latter group had an asymptomatic recovery. These authors suggest, and we concur, that surgery should be reserved only for those dogs that fail to respond to conservative care.[29]

Surgical methods that have been described include plication of the dorsal tracheal membrane, tracheal ring prostheses, and intraluminal Silastic devices. These surgical efforts may not resolve the coexisting problem of main stem bronchial collapse and usually do not effectively resolve even isolated thoracic inlet disease. Polypropylene C-shaped stent placement has been described with good results.[27, 28, 30] These authors suggest that surgery involving the thoracic portion of the trachea has been unrewarding because of high morbidity and that dogs with main stem bronchial collapse are not good surgical candidates. In a group of dogs that did have surgery, 17 of 90 (19 per cent) required a follow-up tracheostomy, and a high percentage of these developed complications due to occlusion with mucus or skinfolds. The authors believe that extraluminal placement of polypropylene C-shaped stents was an effective method of controlling the clinical signs of collapsing trachea in a large number of dogs. Weight, severity of tracheal collapse, duration of clinical signs, and need for a tracheostomy did not affect the long-term outcome. Dogs over 6 years of age had more postoperative complications and a poorer long-term outcome than did younger dogs.

Twenty-five dogs were treated surgically for tracheal collapse using extraluminal polypropylene ring prostheses plus a left arytenoid lateralization. The authors reported a lower complication rate of 4 per cent and a 75 per cent success rate. They believed that complications were reduced as a result of the tie-back procedure.[31]

Surgical correction of a 4-year-old poodle with a lateral collapsing trachea using ring prosthesis provided definitive relief of the symptoms. The authors evaluated the dog postoperatively and found little change anatomically. Because there was so much improvement, the authors attributed it to increased airway rigidity, which alleviated the effects of dynamic collapse and resulted in improvement of airflow.[21] Surgical management using polypropylene spiral ring prostheses was reported in two large breed dogs with extrathoracic tracheal collapse.[32]

OBSTRUCTIVE TRACHEAL MASSES

Etiology. Obstructive tracheal masses have varied etiologies. Lesions may be intraluminal, as in the case of primary tracheal neoplasia, or extraluminally compressive. Various forms of tracheal tumors have been described in dogs and cats. These include squamous cell carcinoma, histiocytic lymphosarcoma, lymphoblastic lymphosarcoma, osteosarcoma, adenocarcinoma, osteoma, chondroma, osteochondroma, chondrosarcoma, plasmacytoma,[46] and leiomyoma.[1, 33, 34] In both dogs and cats, primary tumors of the trachea are unusual. Other types of intraluminal masses include nodular amyloidosis, eosinophilic granulomas, abscesses, chronic granulomas,[1, 35] and inflammatory polyps.[36] A single second-stage instar larval stage of *Cuterebra* sp. was identified in a 7-year-old cat's trachea.[37]

Tracheal foreign bodies can also cause intraluminal obstruction.[38, 39] Foreign bodies are not common, but when they do occur, they are usually small enough to pass beyond the tracheal bifurcation, causing the subsequent development of inhalation pneumonia. When foreign bodies are relatively large, they are likely to come to rest at the carina.

Conditions that are extrinsic to the trachea may also cause obstruction by external compression. These include thyroid and parathyroid tumors; enlargement of the mandibular, retropharyngeal, or prescapular lymph nodes owing to infection, neoplasia, or granuloma, such as histoplasmosis or coccidioidomycosis; peritracheal abscesses and cysts; cranial mediastinal masses such as thymomas; esophageal tumors; and esophageal granulomas secondary to *Spirocerca lupi.*[40, 41]

Clinical Signs and Diagnosis. Obstructive diseases are associated with a dramatic increase in airway resistance at the point of obstruction. This impedes airflow, causing hypoventilation and respiratory acidosis.[42] Clinical signs depend on the degree of obstruction present. Up to half of the airway diameter may be compromised without obvious clinical signs.[43] Even in these cases, however, close inspection of the animal reveals an obstructive breathing pattern, which consists of a slow inspiratory phase followed by a more rapid expiratory phase.[43] Most animals present with stridor and loud rhonchi (rattling in the throat). Chronic coughing also may occur. Respiratory distress and dyspnea are usually obvious.

Overzealous examination and performance of laboratory studies may disturb the animal, thereby worsening the condition. Every effort should be made to keep the animal calm, and initial diagnostic tests should be done with as little stress as possible.

The work-up for an animal with suspected tracheal obstructive disease usually begins with radiography. Lateral views should be obtained if the animal can tolerate recumbency without struggling. Ventrodorsal radiographs often put the animal in a stressful position, so dorsoventral views should be obtained instead. Tracheal masses may decrease luminal size in a nonlinear manner, resulting in a mass protruding into the lumen. These masses are outlined by the tracheal air, which provides a good natural negative contrast medium (Fig. 126–7). Disruption of the mucosal continuity is seen at the base of the mass. This is in contradistinction to the silhouette produced by masses that are extraluminal, in which the line produced by the luminal air-mucosa interface is seen to pass uninterrupted through the mass. Non-radiopaque foreign bodies can be rendered invisible to radiographic examination if they travel distal enough in the bronchi, resulting in atelectasis of the obstructed lobe with transudation of serous fluid distal to and around the foreign body. Extraluminal masses causing tracheal obstruction are generally recognized radiographically as linear decreases in the lumen diameter over a length determined by the size of the mass (Fig. 126–8). In the mediastinal region, a mass must be quite large to result in tracheal compression. The trachea is easier to displace than to compress in this location. High-level airway obstruction is most likely to be associated with hypoinflated, small lung fields. Intrathoracic tracheal obstruction may present as a hyperinflated lung due to air

trapping as a result of narrowing of the airway during expiration. This creates a ball valve effect, trapping air distal to the obstructing lesion. In a cat with an inflammatory polyp partially obstructing the trachea, thoracic radiography suggested increased airway resistance during expiration (hyperinflated lungs and a caudally displaced flattened diaphragm).[36] Contrast esophageal studies are sometimes needed to differentiate the etiology of the tracheal narrowing or displacement in the cranial mediastinal region, particularly in brachycephalic breeds, in which cranial mediastinal masses are often difficult to delineate. Concomitant narrowing of the trachea and esophagus in the cranial mediastinum is highly suggestive of an extraluminal mass.

Bronchoscopy can also be used to visualize tracheal masses and foreign bodies (especially radiolucent foreign bodies). Bronchoscopy can also help in reaching a definitive diagnosis by allowing the retrieval of cytologic specimens of masses or even obtaining biopsies.

Therapy. In addition to its diagnostic value, bronchoscopy can be used as part of the treatment. Some foreign bodies can be removed endoscopically, and some tracheal masses may be removed by means of a suction biopsy device attached to the bronchoscope.[34]

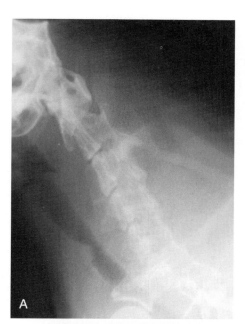

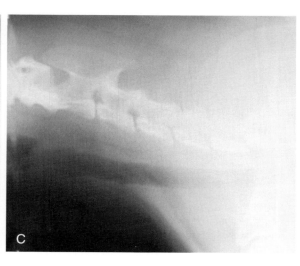

Figure 126–7. *A* and *B,* Lateral cervical radiograph of an 8-year-old cat with inspiratory dyspnea and open-mouth breathing. A tracheal mass can be seen arising from the ventral tracheal wall and growing into the lumen at the level of C4-C5. The air in the trachea provides a natural negative contrast agent. *C,* Cervical radiographs three months after surgical resection of the mass. The mass is no longer seen. Histopathologic diagnosis was tracheal adenocarcinoma.

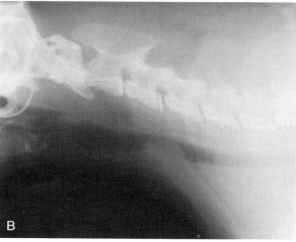

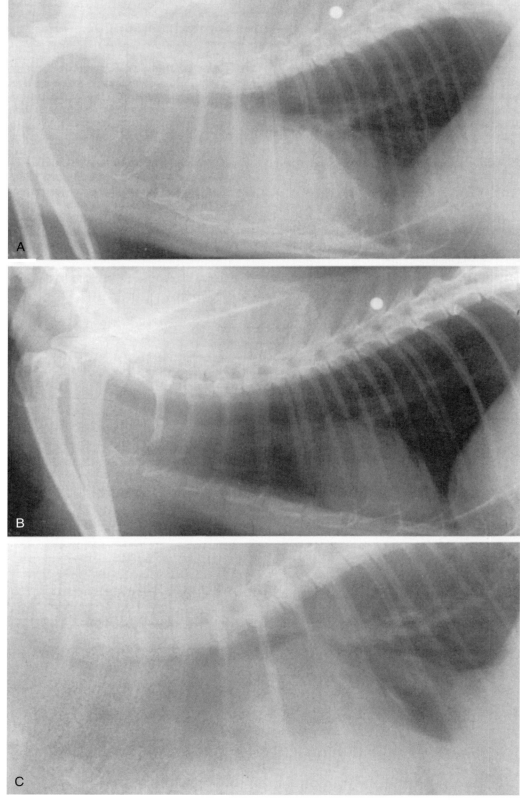

Figure 126–8. *A,* Lateral thoracic radiograph of a 5-year-old domestic shorthair cat, presented for dyspnea and emesis, shows elevation and compression of the trachea at the thoracic inlet, along with pleural fluid. The cranial lung lobes are displaced caudally. These signs were secondary to lymphosarcoma of the cranial mediastinum. *B,* The same cat, five weeks after chemotherapy. Notice the re-expansion of the previously compressed trachea. *C,* Lateral thoracic radiograph of an 8-year-old female Burmese cat with pleural fluid secondary to cardiomyopathy. Note that the tracheal elevation is not accompanied by tracheal compression, as in the previous case of a mediastinal mass.

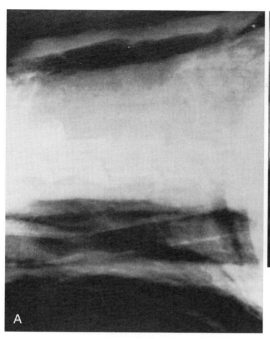
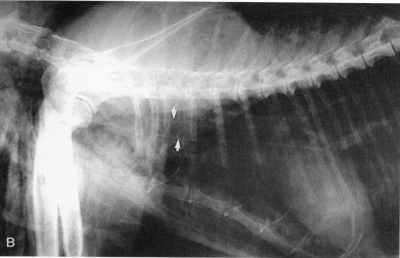

Figure 126–9. *A,* Lateral cervical radiograph of a 10-year-old male cocker spaniel with tracheal narrowing and rupture at the level of C3 resulting from a dog fight. There is extensive cervical and subcutaneous emphysema. Note that the outer tracheal wall is visible throughout its length, owing to the free extraluminal air providing contrast. *B,* Pneumomediastinum in a cat associated with subcutaneous air collection. Note the prominent tracheal stripes both dorsally and ventrally *(arrows)* as a result of the trachea being outlined by air both inside and outside of the trachea lumen.

RES

For foreign bodies that cannot be retrieved through the bronchoscope and for large or firm tracheal masses, the mainstay of therapy is surgical removal or resection. Surgical procedures of the trachea have been well described. Some foreign bodies may be removed in smaller animals by holding them upside down (head down) while under general anesthesia and gently but firmly tapping the thorax. Occasionally the foreign body is actually coughed out, and sometimes it is moved into a more proximal position for easier bronchoscopic retrieval.

The prognosis for animals with tracheal obstruction depends on the specific primary disease as well as the present degree of respiratory embarrassment, because any type of stressful diagnostic measure may push the animal into a state of decompensation. With tracheal tumors, the prognosis varies not only with the amount of trachea involved but also with the specific biologic behavior of the tumor type.

TRACHEAL TRAUMA

Etiology. With the exception of lacerations of the tracheal wall resulting in secondary subcutaneous emphysema, traumatic injury to the trachea is an unusual condition in small animals. Some relatively common causes of this condition include bite wounds to the neck incurred during a dog or cat fight, transtracheal wash procedures, and inadvertent laceration of the trachea during jugular venous puncture. An uncommon sequela to trauma is a tracheoesophageal fistula.

Clinical Signs and Diagnosis. A ventrolateral tear of the annular ligament may produce secondary subcutaneous emphysema over the entire body.[44] This latter condition develops frequently in dogs or cats involved in fights during which a tooth punctures or lacerates the tracheal wall. Air escapes from the tracheal opening and enters the subcutaneous tissue of the neck (Fig. 126–9). The subcutaneous em-

physema may involve only the peritracheal region or be more extensive and involve the entire subcutaneous area of the body. Such tears may also be responsible for the development of pneumomediastinum in both the dog and the cat (Fig. 126–10). Subcutaneous emphysema is generally recognized by the crackling sensation of the animal's skin. The tissue beneath the skin appears swollen. The presence of such a lesion should immediately indicate the possibility of a tracheal tear.

Fractures of the trachea produce radiographic signs of peritracheal, intermuscular, and subcutaneous emphysema. Pneumomediastinum may also be present with a cervical or intrathoracic lesion. Fractures or lacerations of the trachea

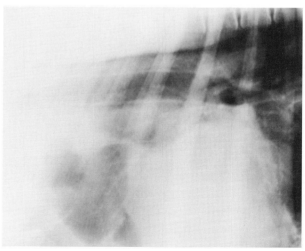

Figure 126–10. Lateral thoracic radiograph of a 10-year-old Great Dane with pneumomediastinum. Note how the free air in the mediastinum provides a negative contrast and allows detection of the dorsal tracheal wall.

or tracheobronchial tree should always be considered in cases of persistent, increasing subcutaneous emphysema, even when no cutaneous lacerations can be located. Bronchoscopy visualizes the point and extent of tracheal mucosal interruption. Occasionally, traumatic injury of the intrathoracic trachea results in a circumferential rupture, leaving the mucosal or serosal lining intact. This prevents air from dissecting into the mediastinum. Radiographs reveal the separation of the tracheal rings (Fig. 126–11). A focal widening of the tracheal lumen at the separation during inspiration and narrowing during expiration are often identified. Surgery is indicated to avoid complications of tracheal stricture.

Therapy. If the subcutaneous air collection is regressing and there are no signs of pulmonary distress, the usual recommendation is cage rest, allowing the emphysema to regress by slow absorption. If the condition is becoming further aggravated by continued air leakage, the severity of subcutaneous emphysema may be reduced by aspiration through a large-bore needle and wrapping the body with elastic bandages, being careful not to mechanically restrict respiration. In most cases, this procedure is not necessary. Perhaps of greater importance is the effort to detect other pathologic conditions such as pneumothorax or hemothorax. If another such condition is present, the clinician should consider thoracocentesis.

Surgical repair with good results were reported in three cats with intrathoracic tracheal avulsion associated with dyspnea, exercise intolerance, and exertional cyanosis.[45]

REFERENCES*

1. As reported in Ettinger SJ, Ticer JW: Diseases of the trachea. In Ettinger SJ (ed): Textbook of Veterinary Internal Medicine, 3rd ed. Philadelphia, WB Saunders, 1989, pp 795–815.
2. Huber ML, et al: Assessment of current techniques for determining tracheal luminal stenosis in dogs. Am J Vet Res 58:1051, 1997.
3. Angus J, et al: Microbiological study of transtracheal aspirates from dogs with suspected lower respiratory tract disease: 264 cases (1989–1995). JAVMA 210:1, 1997.
4. Randolph JF, et al: Prevalence of mycoplasmal and ureaplasmal recovery from tracheobronchial lavages and prevalence of mycoplasmal recovery from pharyngeal swab specimens in dogs with or without pulmonary disease. Am J Vet Res 54:3, 1993.
5. Welsh R: Bordetella bronchiseptica infections in cats. J Am Anim Hosp Assoc 32:2, 1996.
6. Vail D, et al: Differential cell analysis and phenotypic subtyping of lymphocytes and bronchoalveolar lavage fluid from clinically normal dogs. Am J Vet Res 56:3, 1995.
7. Hoffman WE, Wellman ML: Tracheobronchial cytology. In Kirk RW (ed): Current Veterinary Therapy IX. Philadelphia, WB Saunders, 1986, pp 243–247.
8. Hawkins EC: Tracheal wash and bronchoalveolar lavage in management of respiratory disease. In Kirk RW (ed): Current Veterinary Therapy XI. Philadelphia, WB Saunders, 1992, pp 795–800.
9. Padrid P: Canine and feline bronchial disease. Proc 10th ACVIM Forum, San Diego, 1992, pp 292–294.
10. Rebar AH, et al: Cytologic evaluation of the respiratory tract. Vet Clin North Am Small Anim Pract 22:5, 1992.
11. Kipperman BS, et al: Primary ciliary dyskinesia in a Gordon setter. J Am Anim Hosp Assoc 28:4, 1992.
12. Dhein CR: Canine respiratory disease complex. In Barlough JE (ed): Manual of Small Animal Infectious Disease. New York, Churchill Livingstone, 1988, pp 109–118.
13. Bemis DA: Bordetella and Mycoplasma respiratory infections in dogs and cats. Vet Clin North Am Small Anim Pract 22:5, 1992.
14. Ford RB, Vaden SL: Canine infectious tracheobronchitis. In Green CE (ed): Infectious Diseases of the Dog and Cat. Philadelphia, WB Saunders, 1990, pp 259–265.
15. Barr SC, et al: Oslerus (Filaroides) osleri in a dog. Aust Vet J 63:334, 1986.
16. Levitan DM, et al: Treatment of Oslerus osleri infestation in dog: Case report and literature review. J Am Anim Hosp Assoc 32:435, 1996.
17. Coyne BC, Fingland RB: Hypoplastic trachea in the dog: 103 cases (1974–1990). Proc Ann Mgt Am Coll Vet Surg, 1991.
18. White RAS, Kellagher REB: Tracheal resection and anastomosis for congenital stenosis in a dog. J Small Anim Pract 27:61, 1998.
19. Bradley RL, et al: Tracheal resection and anastomosis for traumatic tracheal collapse in a dog. Comp Small Anim Med 9:234, 1987.
20. Berg J, et al: Treatment of posttraumatic carinal stenosis by balloon dilation during thoracotomy in a cat. JAVMA 198:1025, 1991.
21. Johnson LR, et al: Surgical management of atypical lateral tracheal collapse in a dog. JAVMA 203:12, 1993.
22. Johnson L: Tracheal collapse and bronchomalacia. Proc 14th ACVIM Forum, 1996.
23. Hendricks JC, O'Brien JA: Tracheal collapse in two cats. JAVMA 187:418, 1985.
24. Hamaide A, et al: Effects of age and location on the biomechanical and biochemical properties of canine tracheal ring cartilage in dogs. Am J Vet Res 59:18, 1998.
25. Johnson L, McKiernan B: Diagnosis and medical management of tracheal collapse. Semin Vet Med Surg (Small Anim) 10:2, 1995.
26. Nelson AW: Lower respiratory system. In Slatter DH (ed): Textbook of Small Animal Surgery. Philadelphia, WB Saunders, 1985, pp 990–1023.
27. Fingland RB: Clinical and pathologic effects of spiral and total ring prosthesis applied to the cervical and thoracic portions of the trachea of dogs. Am J Vet Res 50:2168, 1989.
28. Fingland RB: Surgical management of cervical and thoracic tracheal collapse in dogs using extra luminal spiral prosthesis. J Am Anim Hosp Assoc 23:163, 1987.
29. White RAS, Williams JM: Tracheal collapse in the dog—is there really a role for surgery? A survey of 100 cases. J Small Anim Pract 35:4, 1994.
30. Buback JL, et al: Surgical treatment of tracheal collapse in dogs: 90 cases (1983–1993). JAVMA 208:3, 1996.
31. White RN: Unilateral arytenoid lateralization and extra luminal polypropylene ring prostheses for correction of tracheal collapse in the dog. J Small Anim Pract 36:4, 1995.

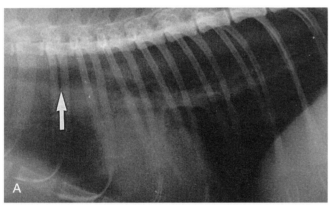

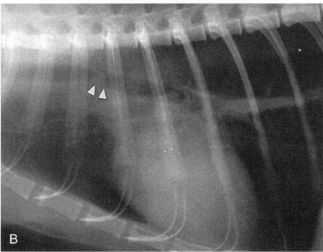

Figure 126–11. Lateral thoracic radiographs of a cat following thoracic trauma. *A,* Note the focal increased size of the trachea *(large arrow)* at the level of the fourth rib, suggesting trauma to the tracheal wall. *B,* In the lateral view taken one week later, there is marked diminution in the size of the trachea *(arrowheads)* at the fourth intercostal space due to tracheal stenosis.

*An extensive list of 64 early references (prior to 1987) may be found by consulting reference 1. Most of the references listed here are subsequent to that date and involve newly identified material relevant to the trachea.

32. Spodnick GJ, Nwadike BS: Surgical management of extrathroacic tracheal collapse in two large-breed dogs. JAVMA 211:1545, 1997.
33. Schena CJ, et al: Extra skeletal osteosarcoma in two dogs. JAVMA 194:1452, 1989.
34. Neer TM, Zeman D: Tracheal adenocarcinoma in a cat and review of literature. J Am Anim Hosp Assoc 23:327, 1987.
35. Brovida C, Massimo C: Tracheal obstruction due to eosinophilic granuloma in a dog: Surgical treatment and clinicopathologic observations. J Am Anim Hosp Assoc 28:8, 1992.
36. Sheaffer K, Dillon AR: Obstructive tracheal mass due to an inflammatory polyp in a cat. J Am Anim Hosp Assoc 32:431, 1996.
37. Fitzgerald SD, et al: A fatal case of intrathoracic cuterebriasis in a cat. J Am Anim Hosp Assoc 32:353, 1996.
38. Lotti U, Niebauer GW: Tracheobronchial foreign bodies of plant origin in 153 hunting dogs. Comp Contin Educ 14:900, 1992.
39. Dimski DS: Tracheal obstruction caused by tree needles in a cat. JAVMA 199:477, 1991.
40. Squires RA, et al: Invasive thymoma complicated by pneumothorax and hemothorax in a dog. J Small Anim Pract 27:89, 1986.
41. Tucker A: Pathophysiology of surgically correctable diseases of the respiratory system. In Slatter DH (ed): Textbook of Small Animal Surgery. Philadelphia, WB Saunders, 1985, pp 919–937.
42. Harari J, et al: Clinical and pathologic features of thyroid tumors in 26 dogs. JAVMA 188:1160, 1986.
43. Aron DN, Crow DT: Upper airway obstruction: General principles and selected conditions in the dog and cat. Vet Clin North Am 15:891, 1985.
44. Bauer MS, Currie J: Generalized subcutaneous emphysema in a dog. Can Vet J 29:836, 1988.
45. White RN, Milner HR: Intrathoracic tracheal avulsion in three cats. J Small Anim Pract 36:8, 1995.
46. Chaffin K, et al: Extramedullary plasmacytoma in the trachea of a dog. JAVMA 212:1579, 1998.
47. Keil DJ, Fenwick B: Role of Bordetella bronchiseptica in infectious tracheobronchitis in dogs. JAVMA 212:200, 1998.

CHAPTER 127

DISEASES OF THE BRONCHUS

Lynelle Johnson

RES

The bronchial tree is responsible for conduction of oxygen toward the alveoli for gas exchange and removal of respiratory secretions. The airways are covered by ciliated, columnar epithelial cells and submucosal mucous glands, which play an important role in the defense of the respiratory system. Mucus contains antimicrobial substances such as immunoglobulin, lactoferrin, and proteases that inhibit bacterial colonization. Cilia propel mucus and debris up the mucociliary escalator for removal from the respiratory tract. Diseases of the conducting airways result in clinical signs of cough and airway obstruction.

CANINE BRONCHITIS

Acute and chronic forms of bronchitis are common in dogs. Definitive causes of acute bronchitis include infection with Bordetella, Mycoplasma, and lungworm, or inflammation from heartworm disease. Chronic bronchitis is defined by the presence of a cough for two months of each year that lacks a specific etiology.[1] Neutrophilic infiltration of the bronchial mucosa results in release of proteases, elastases, and oxidizing products, with resultant mucosal injury. Histology is characterized by hypertrophy and hyperplasia of mucous glands and goblet cells, smooth muscle hypertrophy, fibrosis of the lamina propria, and epithelial erosion with squamous metaplasia.

Presentation. Chronic bronchitis is classically considered a disease of small breed dogs,[1] but large breed dogs are often affected.[2] The primary clinical complaint is an unrelenting cough, which may be dry or productive depending on the stage of disease. Obesity is common in dogs with chronic bronchitis. Lung sounds may be normal at rest, but post-tussive crackles and wheezes can generally be ausculted. Tracheal sensitivity is usually present owing to nonspecific airway inflammation. Severely affected dogs have a prolonged expiratory phase with increased expiratory effort and may have a history of cyanosis or collapse. Cardiac auscultation could reveal concurrent mitral valve insufficiency in small breed dogs. Thus congestive heart failure is an important differential diagnosis in these dogs. Typically, dogs with respiratory disease have a normal to slow heart rate with an exaggerated sinus arrhythmia rather than a tachycardia, as seen with heart failure.

Diagnostic Evaluation. The diagnosis of chronic bronchitis is one of exclusion. A peribronchial infiltrate is considered classic for chronic bronchitis, but normal chest radiographs do not rule out the diagnosis. Right-sided cardiomegaly may be seen in dogs with long-standing airway disease that develop pulmonary hypertension and/or cor pulmonale.

Arterial blood gas analysis can be used to assess pulmonary gas exchange and to follow response to treatment. Hypoxemia and abnormal distribution of ventilation on radioaerosol lung scans have been reported in dogs with chronic bronchitis.[2]

The majority of dogs with bronchitis have hyperemic airways and increased airway mucus when examined with bronchoscopy. Fibrous nodules can be seen protruding into the airway in dogs with long-standing disease (Fig. 127–1). Healthy dogs have 6 to 9 per cent neutrophils, 6 to 9 per cent eosinophils, and 65 to 70 per cent macrophages in bronchoalveolar lavage (BAL) fluid. Nondegenerate neutrophils are increased in bronchitis,[2] although some animals

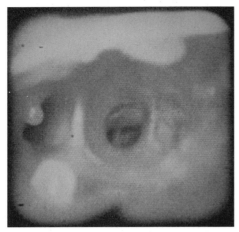

Figure 127–1. Bronchoscopic photograph of a dog with bronchitis. Fibrous nodules are seen protruding into the lumen. Increased mucus is evident at the top of the photograph. Generalized hyperemia is present throughout the airways. (Courtesy of Dr. Brendan McKiernan, University of Illinois.)

have predominantly eosinophils in BAL or tracheal wash samples. Increased mucus and squamous metaplasia may also be seen. True bacterial infection is not common in dogs with chronic bronchitis.[2] Heavy growth of a single bacterial species or an atypical resistance pattern would support the diagnosis of bronchial infection.

Treatment

Anti-inflammatories. Coexisting diseases and infectious conditions must be adequately managed before initiation of anti-inflammatory treatment. Anti-inflammatory doses of short-acting steroids are generally safe and effective in dogs with uncomplicated bronchitis. Severity of clinical signs, chronicity of infection, systemic health, and disease recurrence determine the therapeutic regimen for the individual. Decreasing the dosage of glucocorticoid as soon as possible and achieving alternate-day dosing allow normalization of the pituitary-adrenal axis. Many dogs require constant or intermittent therapy for life.

Bronchodilators. Bronchodilators may reduce signs in dogs with bronchitis or reduce the dosage of glucocorticoid required. The bronchodilators used most commonly are methylxanthine derivatives and beta-2 agonists. Methylxanthine derivatives are believed to act through antagonism of adenosine, because therapeutic levels do not inhibit phosphodiesterase or accumulate cyclic AMP. Theo-Dur tablets and Slo-bid gyrocaps achieve plasma levels in dogs that approximate the human therapeutic range of 10 to 20 μg/mL. Generic theophylline products have not been shown to be equally bioavailable in veterinary patients.

Adverse effects of methylxanthines include gastrointestinal upset, tachycardia, and hyperexcitability. Theophylline metabolism is influenced by many factors, including dietary fiber, smoke in the environment, congestive heart failure, and use of other drugs. Enrofloxacin inhibits metabolism of theophylline, and concurrent use of the two drugs results in toxic plasma theophylline levels.[3] At least a 30 per cent reduction in theophylline dose is recommended when enrofloxacin is required to treat coincident infection. If toxicity is suspected, plasma theophylline levels can be determined through a human laboratory.

Beta-2 adrenergic agonists include terbutaline and albuterol. Albuterol was efficacious in reducing cough in almost one half of dogs with chronic bronchitis.[2] In some dogs, bronchodilator therapy also reduced the severity of the pulmonary infiltrate. Side effects include excitability or tremors during initial therapy. Animals that develop toxicity to methylxanthines or beta agonists will usually tolerate therapy with adjustment of the dosage.

Antitussives. Suppression of the cough reflex before resolution of inflammation traps mucus in the lower airway, perpetuates airway inflammation, and worsens clinical signs. When inflammation has resolved, use of a narcotic cough suppressant (butorphanol or hydrocodone) is warranted to prevent repeated airway injury and cough syncope. These agents must be given at an interval that suppresses coughing but avoids excessive sedation. Long-term therapy may be required in many dogs.

Antibiotics. When infection has been documented, antibiotic treatment is warranted. Pending culture and sensitivity results, an agent with broad-spectrum efficacy against *Mycoplasma*, *Bordetella*, *Pasteurella*, *Staphylococcus*, *Streptococcus*, and various gram-negative species is recommended. Lipophilic drugs such as chloramphenicol, doxycycline, or enrofloxacin have excellent penetration of airway tissue and are relatively free of side effects (see also Bacterial Pneumonia in Chapter 128).

Nebulization. Dogs also benefit from intermittent airway humidification, which hydrates airway secretions and improves mucociliary clearance. Steam inhalation via a vaporizer is of limited benefit, because large water droplets are retained by the upper airway. A pneumatic or ultrasonic nebulizer creates smaller water particles that hydrate secretions in lower airways.[4]

Humidified, oxygenated air can be provided to hospitalized dogs by attaching the nebulizer to an enclosed cage or by constructing an oxygen or mist tent for the animal. A hand-held nebulizer can also be attached to the oxygen line of an anesthetic machine and a face mask used to deliver moisture-laden air. Fresh sterile saline should be added to the cup of the nebulizer for each treatment. A common complication of nebulization therapy is infection, and the face mask should be cold-sterilized after each use. For animals with bacterial infection, the nebulizer is replaced daily. For stable bronchitic animals, the unit can be cleaned and replaced weekly. For therapy at home, a jet nebulizer can be obtained from a hospital pharmacy and attached to a compressed air source.

Nebulization should be performed two to four times daily for 10 to 30 minutes. Animals are closely monitored for bronchospasm, overhydration, or respiratory distress. Administration of a bronchodilator immediately before therapy may benefit some dogs. Chest coupage follows nebulization. Coupage is performed by cupping the hands and gently pounding on the chest, moving from caudal to cranial and ventral to dorsal, to loosen secretions. Elevating the dog's hind legs helps achieve postural drainage.

Ancillary Treatment. Obesity worsens both clinical signs and gas exchange in dogs with chronic bronchitis, and improvements in exercise tolerance and arterial oxygenation can be seen with weight loss alone. Stresses in the environment, such as cigarette smoke, pollutants, heat, or humidity, are to be avoided.

Prognosis. Bronchitis is a chronic disease that can be controlled but never cured. The majority of animals have persistent cough and clinical signs throughout life. The goals of therapy are to control inflammation and to prevent worsening airway disease. Uncontrolled bronchitis can lead to bronchiectasis with recurrent parenchymal infections, and some dogs may be at risk for pulmonary hypertension owing to chronic hypoxia and/or vascular remodeling.

BRONCHIECTASIS

Bronchiectasis is characterized by irreversible dilatation of mid-sized bronchi with accumulation of secretions. It can be focal or diffuse and occurs with primary ciliary dyskinesia, as a sequela to chronic pulmonary disease, as a result of pulmonary injury due to smoke inhalation or airway obstruction, or as a complication of radiation-induced pneumonitis.[5] Products of inflammation destroy the muscular and elastic support structure of the airways. Surrounding lung tissue exerts a contractile force that pulls the bronchi into a dilated state. Damage to the epithelial surface causes ciliostasis, delayed clearance of bacteria and mucus, and recurrent infection.

Presentation. Bronchiectasis is most common in middle-aged to older dogs or in young dogs with ciliary dyskinesia.[6] American cocker spaniels have a high incidence of disease. A moist, productive cough is the most common complaint; recurrent bouts of pneumonia are typical. Initially, a response to antibiotic therapy is seen, but signs recur.[7] Physical examination is remarkable for moist crackles and expiratory wheezing. Purulent nasal discharge is seen with primary ciliary dyskinesia or pneumonia.

Diagnostic Evaluation. Neutrophilia, monocytosis, and hyperglobulinemia can occur owing to chronic inflammation. Chronic antigenic stimulation may lead to reactive amyloidosis with proteinuria. Arterial blood gas analysis reveals hypoxemia and an increased alveolar-arterial oxygen gradient.

Thoracic radiographs are insensitive for the diagnosis of bronchiectasis. The classic radiographic finding would be central or diffuse bronchial dilatation with thickening of bronchial walls. Mixed bronchial, interstitial, and alveolar patterns are seen, and dilated airways are more visible when a severe pneumonic infiltrate is present (Fig. 127–2).

In veterinary medicine, the most reliable method for diagnosis of bronchiectasis is bronchoscopy. Visual inspection reveals loss of the circular shape of the airway lumen owing to saccular or cylindric dilatation, mucosal hyperemia and irregularity, and trapped secretions. BAL specimens typically show suppurative inflammation with increased neutrophils and monocytes. Bacterial cultures for both aerobes and anaerobes are indicated, because purulent secretions can favor the growth of anaerobic species. In human medicine, *Pseudomonas* species are found most commonly, and mixed opportunistic flora are often present.[5] In dogs, some cases may appear to be sterile.[7]

Treatment. Severely affected animals require hospitalization for intravenous fluids, broad-spectrum antibiotics, and nebulization. Intravenous ampicillin and gentamycin are reasonable first-line antibiotics. Long-term use of antibiotics is based on culture and sensitivity results, and antibiotics that penetrate pulmonary tissue well, such as doxycycline, clindamycin, or chloramphenicol, are most efficacious. Animals with negative cultures are best treated with broad-spectrum therapy for aerobes and anaerobes, such as combined enrofloxacin and clindamycin. Antibiotics should be continued for 6 to 12 weeks, and certain cases require lifelong therapy.

Nebulization and coupage facilitate removal of viscid pulmonary secretions. Bronchodilators may be beneficial, although animals typically have irreversible airflow limitation. Cough suppressants are absolutely contraindicated, because retention of infectious and inflammatory secretions perpetuates disease. Animals with focal bronchiectasis or bronchial foreign bodies can benefit from lung lobectomy.

Prognosis. Chronic recurrent infection is likely in dogs with bronchiectasis, and resistance to antibiotic treatment may occur. Some dogs may develop amyloidosis, sepsis, or cor pulmonale.

Prevention. Appropriate therapy of infectious or inflammatory lung disease limits the occurrence of bronchiectasis. Prompt recognition with removal of bronchial foreign bodies prevents initiation of disease.

FELINE BRONCHIAL DISEASE (FELINE ASTHMA)

Airway inflammation induces reversible airflow obstruction through smooth muscle constriction, bronchial wall edema, and hypertrophy of mucous glands, resulting in signs ranging from intermittent coughing to severe respiratory distress. Hyperresponsive airways and reversible airflow obstruction have been documented in some cats.[8, 9]

Presentation. The most frequent complaints in cats with bronchial disease are coughing and abnormal respiration, described as wheezing or difficulty breathing.[9] A subset of cats presents with cyanosis and open-mouth breathing. Inciting stimuli such as upper respiratory tract infection, aerosolized irritants, bacterial infection, and allergens can sometimes be identified.

Bronchial disease is an obstructive disorder of small airways, and a prolonged expiratory phase can be seen.[9, 10] Air trapped distal to obstructed airways leads to decreased thoracic compressibility and a barrel-shaped appearance to the chest. Bronchitic cats may appear normal at rest and exhibit normal pulmonary auscultation. Most cats display increased tracheal sensitivity, and post-tussive crackles are often ausculted.

Diagnostic Evaluation. Peripheral eosinophilia was reported in 30 per cent of cats with bronchial disease in a recent review.[9] In heartworm-endemic regions, heartworm antibody and antigen tests should be considered for cats with

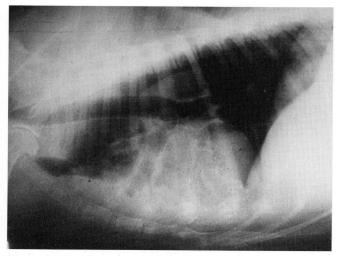

Figure 127–2. Lateral thoracic radiograph of a dog with bronchiectasis. Dilated airways can be seen extending into the cranial lung lobe. The cranioventral alveolar infiltrate and lung consolidation improve visualization of airway dilatation.

RES

TABLE 127–1. BACTERIA RETRIEVED FROM THE AIRWAYS OF HEALTHY DOGS AND CATS

Pasteurella spp.	*Enterobacter*
Mycoplasma spp.	*Pseudomonas* spp.
Streptococcus spp.	*Escherichia coli*
Staphylococcus spp.	*Klebsiella* spp.
Acinetobacter	*Bordetella bronchiseptica*
Moraxella	

Data from references 9, 12, 14.

cough or dyspnea.[11] Airway parasites may incite eosinophilic inflammation with subsequent bronchoconstriction, and fecal examinations should be performed routinely in cats with airway disease.

Interstitial, bronchial, and alveolar patterns may be observed in cats with bronchial disease, but normal chest radiographs do not rule out the diagnosis. Cats with or without obvious pulmonary infiltrates may show signs compatible with bronchoconstriction, such as air trapping, flattening of the diaphragm, or hyperinflation of the lungs. Mucus obstruction of large airways can result in alveolar infiltrates, lobar atelectasis, or consolidating lesions.

A transoral tracheal wash or bronchoscopy is performed to obtain airway specimens. Bronchoscopy may reveal mild hyperemia, increased mucus, or mucus plugs occluding large airways. In a recent study of feline bronchial disease, numbers and percentages of inflammatory cells (eosinophils and neutrophils) increased with the severity of disease.[9] However, healthy cats may exhibit 25 per cent or more eosinophils on airway cytology.[12]

Bacterial culture and antibiotic sensitivity testing should be performed in all cats, because infection has been documented in 24 to 42 per cent of cases.[9, 13] Airway infection may contribute to bronchial inflammation and hyperresponsiveness. Dye et al. found no correlation between cytologic evidence of inflammation and the presence or absence of positive bacterial cultures in diseased cats.[9] Healthy cats often have positive airway cultures, making it difficult to diagnose true bacterial infection (Table 127–1). The role of *Mycoplasma* infection in respiratory disease remains controversial. It has been isolated from tracheobronchial lavage samples in 21 to 44 per cent of cats with respiratory disease,[13, 15] but not from BAL samples from healthy cats.[12, 15]

Pulmonary function testing has shown higher airway resistance in cats with bronchial disease. Some cats also exhibit hyperresponsiveness to aerosolized methacholine.[9] Tidal breathing flow volume loops have been evaluated in unsedated cats with bronchial disease. Significant findings included increased expiratory-inspiratory time ratio, decreased peak expiratory flow rate, and decreased expiratory volume.[10]

Treatment. A cat with cyanosis and open-mouth breathing should be placed in an oxygen cage and stabilized before diagnostic testing. Parenteral administration of a beta-2 agonist may alleviate clinical signs (Table 127–2). If respiratory rate and effort do not diminish in 30 to 60 minutes, a short-acting corticosteroid is administered, although this will affect future test results.

Anti-inflammatories. Corticosteroids reduce inflammation through inhibition of phospholipase A$_2$, the enzyme that initiates conversion of arachidonic acid into inflammatory prostaglandins and leukotrienes. Corticosteroids also decrease migration of inflammatory cells into the airway, thus decreasing the concentration of granulocytic products.

The duration and dose of corticosteroid therapy depend on the severity of pulmonary infiltrates and the chronicity of respiratory disease in the cat. Initially, prednisolone is given at 1 mg/kg twice a day for one week; the dosage is decreased to 0.5 mg/kg twice a day for the second week if a good therapeutic response is seen. Cats are relatively resistant to the side effects of corticosteroids, but an attempt should be made to achieve the lowest dose of drug that controls signs. Cats that cannot be orally medicated are treated with intramuscular injection of a long-acting corticosteroid. Methylprednisolone acetate (10 to 20 mg) can be administered every two to eight weeks as needed.

Alternative drugs may help control airway inflammation in some cats. Experimentally, cyproheptadine, a serotonin receptor blocker, attenuated smooth muscle constriction in response to antigen challenge in cats.[16] Currently, serotonin levels have not been measured in naturally occurring feline bronchial disease, but some cats appear to benefit clinically from serotonin antagonists. Cyclosporine, an inhibitor of T-lymphocyte activation, attenuates bronchoconstriction in asthmatic humans and in animal models of airway hyperreactivity.[17] In cats, blood samples must be collected weekly until trough levels of 500 to 1000 ng/mL are achieved. The variable pharmacokinetics and potential toxicity of cyclosporine suggest that it should be considered only in refractory cases.

Bronchodilators. Bronchodilators can be helpful in emergency situations, in chronic management, and in control of exacerbations of disease in cats with bronchial disease. Bronchodilators may reduce the dose of steroids required to control signs.

Administration of a beta agonist results in direct bronchodilatation by relaxation of airway smooth muscle. Intravenous terbutaline has been shown to reduce airway resistance acutely in bronchitic cats,[8] and pharmacokinetic studies have established the safety of the drug.[18]

Sustained-release theophylline prevents nocturnal signs of asthma in humans and may prevent acute bronchoconstriction in predisposed felines. Current dosing recommendations apply only to Theo-Dur tablets or Slo-bid gyrocaps. One evening dose of 20 to 25 mg/kg results in peak plasma theophylline levels that are within the reported therapeutic range for human patients (10 to 20 μg/mL).[19]

Antibiotics. Antibiotic therapy is based on culture and sensitivity results. If *Mycoplasma* is suspected, a clinical trial of doxycycline can be prescribed pending culture results.

Prognosis. Feline bronchial disease is a chronic disorder, and affected cats exhibit chronic persistent signs or recurrent episodes of clinical disease. Continual medical management should be anticipated for approximately one half of cats diagnosed with bronchial disease.

Prevention. Situations that might provoke bronchoconstriction should be avoided. Cigarette smoke, dusty litters, aerosol sprays, and exposure to upper respiratory viruses may trigger clinical signs in certain cats. Beta blockers, including selective beta-1 agents, are avoided if bronchial disease is suspected. Atropine should not be used chronically in bronchial disease because it thickens bronchial secretions and encourages mucus plugging of airways.

PRIMARY CILIARY DYSKINESIA

Clearance of respiratory secretions is dependent on an intact mucociliary elevator. Cilia have a specific ultrastructure composed of two central microtubules surrounded by nine pairs of outer microtubules. Primary ciliary dyskinesia (PCD) is an inherited defect in microtubule formation affecting cilia of the respiratory tract, urogenital tract, and auditory canal.[6] Clinical defects include rhinitis, bronchiectasis, loss of hearing, hydrocephalus, dilatation of renal tubules, and infertility. Kartagener's syndrome is a specific form of PCD characterized by the triad of situs inversus (right-to-left transposition of thoracic and abdominal organs), chronic rhinitis and sinusitis, and bronchiectasis. Situs inversus may occur in approximately half of dogs with PCD.[6]

Presentation. PCD can be detected within the first few weeks of life, although some animals have mild clinical signs that are not recognized until later in life. Affected breeds include the English springer spaniel, English Pointer, Old English sheepdog, Shar Pei, and bichon frise; cats are rarely affected.[6] Clinical complaints include chronic mucopurulent nasal discharge, productive cough, exercise intolerance, and dyspnea. Signs are nonresponsive to antibiotic treatment or are recurrent in nature. Physical examination is remarkable for nasal discharge, tracheal sensitivity, inspiratory crackles, and expiratory wheezes during disease episodes.

Diagnostic Evaluation. Standard diagnostic tests reflect the severity of underlying respiratory infection or inflammation. Radiographic findings include situs inversus, bronchitis, bronchiectasis, and consolidating pneumonia in chronic cases. Airway samples should be cultured for aerobes, anaerobes, and *Mycoplasma*, and growth of one or more microorganisms is common. Different organisms may be found during recurrent episodes of clinical disease, indicating that repeat airway cultures may be needed. Tracheal mucosal transport time, measured with nuclear scintigraphy, suggests defective mucociliary transport; however, *Mycoplasma* infection and cigarette smoke can also delay transport.

Definitive diagnosis of PCD requires electron microscopic evaluation of ciliary ultrastructure in biopsies of nasal or respiratory epithelium, or in seminal samples. Normal animals may show structural abnormalities in 2 to 5 per cent of cilia; therefore, both the extent and the quality of ultrastructural abnormalities must be determined. Typical findings in PCD include shortening or loss of dynein arms, atypical microtubular orientation, and duplication or deletion of central or outer microtubule doublets.[6]

Treatment. The primary goals of therapy are to control infection and to facilitate clearance of respiratory secretions. Broad-spectrum antibiotics are employed as described for bronchiectasis. Nebulization and coupage therapy are generally helpful. Cough suppression is absolutely contraindicated, because it enhances trapping of secretions and potentiates airway inflammation.

Prognosis. Control of respiratory infection is essential to prevent debilitating sequelae such as cor pulmonale and reactive amyloidosis in dogs with PCD. Some dogs achieve good quality of life despite the ciliary defect.

Prevention. PCD is thought to be inherited as an autosomal recessive trait, and clinically normal animals can produce offspring with PCD. Diagnosis of PCD in an individual suggests that close relatives should not be included in a breeding program.

BRONCHIAL COMPRESSION

The larger airways are compressed by external mass lesions or by an enlarged left atrium, causing a nonproductive cough and/or wheeze. Hilar lymphadenopathy caused by fungal or granulomatous disease and neoplasia compresses the airway from the dorsal aspect (Fig. 127–3A). Left atrial enlargement causes dynamic collapse of the left main stem bronchus (Fig. 127–3B) and can be a significant cause of cough in the absence of heart failure.

Presentation. Bronchial compression occurs more often in dogs than in cats. Occlusion of the airway causes chronic cough but may also result in respiratory difficulty and hypoxemia. Fixed obstruction by hilar lymphadenopathy leads to

RES

TABLE 127–2. DRUGS COMMONLY USED IN CANINE AND FELINE BRONCHOPULMONARY DISEASE

DRUG	DOSAGE	SIDE EFFECTS
Bronchodilator		
METHYLXANTHINES		
Theophylline (Theo-Dur tablets)	Dog: 20 mg/kg BID Cat: 20 mg/kg PO SID (P.M.)	Multiple drug interactions, gastrointestinal upset, tachycardia
Theophylline (Slo-bid gyrocaps)	Dog: 25 mg/kg BID Cat: 25 mg/kg PO SID (P.M.)	
BETA AGONISTS		
Terbutaline	Dog/cat: 0.01 mg/kg SQ, IV Dog: 1.25–5 mg/dog PO BID Cat: 0.625 mg PO BID	Tachycardia, hypotension
Albuterol	Dog: 50 μg/kg PO BID	
Epinephrine	Dog/cat: 20 μg/kg IV, IM, SQ, IT	Arrhythmias, hypertension, vasoconstriction
Anti-Inflammatory		
Prednisolone	Dog/cat: 0.5–1 mg/kg BID and tapered	Immune suppression
Cyproheptadine	Cat: 1–2 mg/cat PO BID	Increased appetite
Cyclosporine	Cat: 10 mg/kg initially (see text)	
Antitussive		
Hydrocodone	Dog: 0.2 mg/kg PO BID–QID	Sedation
Butorphanol	Dog: 0.5–1.2 mg/kg PO BID–QID	Sedation
Antibiotic		
Doxycycline	Dog/cat: 3–5 mg/kg PO BID	Vomiting, diarrhea
Chloramphenicol	Dog/cat: 50 mg/kg PO TID	Red blood cell aplasia, induction of liver enzymes
Clindamycin	Dog/cat: 5–11 mg/kg PO BID	Diarrhea, colitis
Enrofloxacin	Dog/cat: 2.5–11 mg/kg PO BID	Cartilage deformity in young

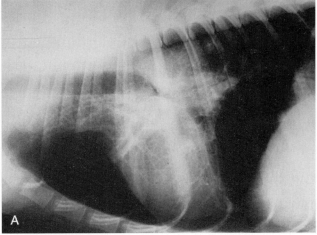

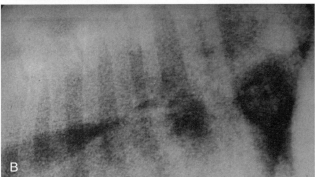

Figure 127–3. *A,* Lateral thoracic radiograph of a dog with inactive histoplasmosis. Hilar lymphadenopathy compresses the trachea from the dorsal aspect. *B,* Fluoroscopy from a dog with left atrial enlargement. During the expiratory phase of respiration, collapse of the main stem bronchi can be seen.

loud bronchial sounds or wheezing during both inspiration and expiration. Animals with dynamic collapse of the airway can have an end-expiratory snap as the intrathoracic airways close during forced expiration. Complete obstruction of a main stem bronchus may result in syncope.

Diagnostic Evaluation. Hilar mass lesions are seen on static thoracic radiographs, but diagnosis of collapse of the main stem bronchi may require fluoroscopy. Bronchoscopy characterizes the degree of bronchial compression and airway collapse and detects concurrent airway disease or bronchitis. Dogs with left atrial enlargement may require echocardiography to determine appropriate therapy.

Treatment. Hilar lymphadenopathy due to active infectious or inflammatory lung disease usually resolves substantially with treatment of the primary disease. If the lesion persists, surgical debulking may be required. Dynamic collapse of the left main stem bronchus may be partially alleviated by therapy directed at reducing left atrial volume; however, many cases appear to have persistent airway collapse despite these efforts. If airway disease is present, therapy for bronchitis is implemented. Narcotic cough suppressants are used to alleviate clinical signs when infectious and inflammatory conditions have been ruled out.

BRONCHIAL FOREIGN BODIES

Bronchial aspiration of plant material, sticks, toys, or stones occurs when the laryngeal reflex is unable to prevent access of foreign objects into the trachea. Hunting dogs commonly aspirate during physical exertion. Animals with laryngeal paralysis may be more likely to aspirate owing to a combination of poor laryngeal sensation and deficient laryngeal reflexes. Failure to intubate animals for dental procedures may lead to aspiration of teeth or dental tartar.

Presentation. Bronchial foreign bodies result in acute onset of an unrelenting cough. A large study of bronchial foreign bodies in dogs indicated that evidence of pneumonia could be detected in most cases within two weeks of aspiration.[20] Animals with bronchial foreign bodies are at risk for pleural empyema, lung abscessation, bronchoesophageal fistula, and development of bronchiectasis distal to the obstruction. A bronchial foreign body should be suspected in an animal with a recurrent, antibiotic-responsive lung infection, particularly when anaerobic infection (*Actinomyces* or *Nocardia*) is diagnosed.

Diagnostic Evaluation. Chest radiographs may outline a radiodense foreign object, but in many cases, nonspecific findings of alveolar infiltrates, distal atelectasis, or consolidation of a lung segment are seen. Definitive diagnosis can require bronchoscopic evaluation of the airways, and all segments should be examined if a foreign body is suspected. Foreign objects with rough edges are grasped with biopsy or rat-tooth forceps and removed. Stones and pebbles are a challenge to remove bronchoscopically, especially when wedged in a bronchus, and surgical intervention may be required. With plant aspiration, the foreign body is usually obscured by a heavy purulent exudate that has partially digested the organic material. Gentle lavage and suction with saline are required to identify the object, but the material may be too friable to remove endoscopically. Airway samples are cultured for both aerobes and anaerobes.

Treatment. Foreign bodies should be removed immediately with bronchoscopy or surgery. Lung lobectomy may be required for smooth-shaped foreign bodies or when lung abscessation, bronchiectasis, or fistulation has occurred. Broad-spectrum antibiotic therapy is based on culture and sensitivity results (see Bacterial Pneumonia in Chapter 128).

Prognosis. Airways are closely reexamined following foreign body removal, because bronchiectasis may develop distal to the obstruction and lead to persistent pulmonary dysfunction.

BRONCHOESOPHAGEAL FISTULA

A bronchoesophageal fistula may be congenital or acquired as a result of trauma, a penetrating esophageal foreign body, or a bronchial foreign body. Affected animals commonly develop chronic cough and recurrent pneumonia related to aspiration of esophageal contents. Respiratory signs may be relatively mild, causing a marked delay in the diagnosis of a congenital lesion.[21] In some cases, difficulty eating may be the predominant sign. The diagnosis is suspected in young animals with recurrent aspiration pneumonia or when megaesophagus or focal pulmonary densities are found in association with chronic respiratory disease. The diagnosis is confirmed with a contrast esophagram. Surgical resection of the fistula is required, and lung lobectomy is sometimes necessary owing to adhesion formation or abscessation.

BRONCHIAL MINERALIZATION

Bronchial mineralization can occur secondary to any chronic inflammatory or infectious condition. Mineralization of airways has also been reported with hyperadrenocorticism. Bronchial mineralization most likely reduces lung compliance, but its effects on gas exchange are not fully understood.

BRONCHIAL NEOPLASIA

Diagnosis and treatment of pulmonary neoplasia are described in Chapter 128.

REFERENCES

1. Wheeldon EB, et al: Chronic bronchitis in the dog. Vet Rec 94:466, 1974.
2. Padrid PA, et al: Canine chronic bronchitis: A pathophysiologic evaluation of 18 cases. J Vet Intern Med 4:172, 1990.
3. Intorre L, et al: Enrofloxacin-theophylline interaction: Influence of enrofloxacin on theophylline steady-state pharmacokinetics in the beagle dog. J Vet Pharmacol Ther 19:352, 1995.
4. Nobel JJ: Ultrasonic nebulizers. Pediatr Emerg Care 10:251, 1994.
5. Nicotra MB, et al: Clinical, pathophysiologic, and microbiologic characterization of bronchiectasis in an aging cohort. Chest 108:955, 1995.
6. Edwards DF, et al: Primary ciliary dyskinesia in the dog. In Spaulding GL (ed): Problems in Veterinary Medicine. Philadelphia, JB Lippincott, 1992, p 291.
7. Brownlie SE: A retrospective study of diagnosis in 109 cases of canine lower respiratory disease. J Small Anim Pract 31:371, 1990.
8. McKiernan BC, Johnson LR: Clinical pulmonary function testing in dogs and cats. Vet Clin North Am Small Anim Pract 22:1087, 1992.
9. Dye JA, et al: Bronchopulmonary disease in the cat: Historical, physical, radiographic, clinicopathologic and pulmonary functional evaluation of 24 affected and 15 healthy cats. J Vet Intern Med 10:385, 1996.
10. McKiernan BC, et al: Tidal breathing flow volume loops in healthy and bronchitic cats. J Vet Intern Med 7:388, 1993.
11. Atkins CE, et al: Prevalence of heartworm infection in cats with signs of cardiorespiratory abnormalities. JAVMA 212:517, 1998.
12. Padrid PA, et al: Cytologic, microbiologic, and biochemical analysis of bronchoalveolar lavage fluid obtained from 24 healthy cats. Am J Vet Res 52:1300, 1991.
13. Moise SN, et al: Clinical, radiographic, and bronchial cytologic features of cats with bronchial disease: 65 cases (1980–1986). JAVMA 194:1467, 1989.
14. McKiernan BC, et al: Bacterial isolates from the lower trachea of clinically healthy dogs. J Am Anim Hosp Assoc 20:139, 1984.
15. Randolph JF, et al: Prevalence of mycoplasmal and ureaplasmal recovery from tracheobronchial lavages and of Mycoplasma recovery from pharyngeal swabs in cats with and without pulmonary disease. Am J Vet Res 54:897, 1993.
16. Padrid PA, et al: Cyproheptadine-induced attenuation of type-1 immediate-hypersensitivity reactions of airway smooth muscle from immune-sensitized cats. Am J Vet Res 56:109, 1995.
17. Padrid PA, et al: Cyclosporine treatment in vivo inhibits airway reactivity and remodeling after chronic antigen challenge in cats. Am J Respir Crit Care Med 154:1812, 1996.
18. McKiernan BC, et al: Terbutaline pharmacokinetics in cats (abstract). Proceedings of the 9th Annual ACVIM Forum, New Orleans, LA, 1991.
19. Dye JA, et al: Sustained-release theophylline pharmacokinetics in the cat. J Vet Pharmacol Ther 12:133, 1989.
20. Lotti U, Niebauer GW: Tracheobronchial foreign bodies of plant origin in 153 hunting dogs. Comp Contin Educ 14:900, 1992.
21. Basher AW, et al: Surgical treatment of a congenital bronchoesophageal fistula in a dog. JAVMA 199:479, 1991.

RES

CHAPTER 128

PULMONARY PARENCHYMAL DISEASES

Eleanor C. Hawkins

SUPPORT OF THE COMPROMISED PATIENT

OXYGEN SUPPLEMENTATION

Hypoxemia can result from hypoventilation or ventilation-perfusion (V:Q) abnormalities. Causes of hypoventilation include upper airway obstruction, diseases affecting pulmonary or thoracic wall compliance (pleural effusion, pneumothorax, extreme abdominal distention), and decreased function of respiratory muscles (lower motor neuron paralysis, coma, certain drugs). Most pulmonary parenchymal diseases cause V:Q mismatching.

Degree of hypoxemia is readily assessed by measuring the partial pressure of oxygen in arterial blood (P_aO_2). Arterial blood gas measurement is also useful for the calculation of the alveolar-arterial oxygen gradient, which can assist in distinguishing between hypoxemia due to hypoventilation and hypoxemia due to V:Q abnormalities. Pulse oximetry is used to estimate arterial hemoglobin oxygen saturation.

Therapeutic intervention is recommended when the P_aO_2 falls below 60 mmHg or the P_aCO_2 rises above 60 to 75 mmHg.[1] More severe hypoxemia can result in tissue hypoxia, cardiac arrhythmias, mental depression, and eventually loss of consciousness. P_aCO_2 greater than 60 mmHg can be associated with significant hypoxemia and eventually respiratory depression and narcosis.[1]

In the absence of blood gas analysis, the presence of cyanosis, "muddy" mucous membranes, deterioration in mental status, or cardiac arrhythmias in conjunction with increased respiratory effort is a clear indication for treatment of hypoxemia. Any animal with increased respiratory effort may benefit substantially from treatment. Although other factors are involved, such as the red cell mass, cyanosis is generally observed at oxygen tensions less than 50 mmHg.

Some causes of hypoventilation are treated directly (e.g., bypassing or relieving upper airway obstruction, thoracocentesis for pneumothorax or pleural effusion). Otherwise, hypoventilation is corrected with ventilation therapy. Increasing the inspired concentration of oxygen may improve oxygenation but will not correct the hypercapnia and resultant alkalosis.

Hypoxemia resulting from V:Q abnormalities generally responds readily to increased alveolar oxygen concentration, which is achieved by increasing the concentration of inspired oxygen. An exception is with complete shunts, in which blood flows directly from artery to vein without passing ventilated alveoli. Some pulmonary parenchymal diseases are severe enough that blood oxygen tensions cannot be adequately maintained without prolonged administration of 100 per cent oxygen, which is toxic, or are associated with collapse of alveoli and decreased compliance. In these situations, positive-pressure ventilatory support, as well as oxygen supplementation, is necessary.

The fractional concentration of inspired oxygen can be increased over that in room air (about 21 per cent) by supplementation, although potential side effects must be addressed. Pulmonary toxicity occurs when an oxygen concentration of 50 per cent is given for longer than 24 hours, or 100 per cent for longer than 12 hours. Animals that cannot be maintained on lower concentrations of oxygen must be provided with positive-pressure ventilatory support. Airway drying can occur if oxygen administration is necessary for more than a few hours, necessitating humidification.

Oxygen supplementation can be provided through masks, transtracheal catheters, nasal catheters, oxygen cages, and tracheal tubes. Masks are used for the emergency stabilization of animals requiring oxygen support. They should fit snugly over the muzzle to minimize dead space, and ophthalmic ointment should be applied to protect against corneal drying. Fractional concentrations of 50 to 60 per cent oxygen can be achieved with a properly fitting mask and flow rates of 8 to 12 L/minute.[2] Long-term supplementation requires other methods.

Oxygen can also be administered for short periods through an intravenous catheter positioned transtracheally. The catheter is placed using the same technique as for tracheal washings. These systems cannot be maintained for prolonged periods and may result in tracheitis. Fractional concentrations of 30 to 40 per cent can be achieved with flow rates of only 1 to 2 L/minute.[2] This method has been suggested for oxygen delivery during cardiopulmonary resuscitation when intubation and positive-pressure ventilation cannot be accomplished.[3] High flow rates of 15 L/minute are suggested.[3]

Nasal catheters can be used for oxygen supplementation for longer periods of time and allow free movement of the animal's head (Fig. 128–1). They are easy to place, require no expensive supplies, and are well tolerated by animals. The technique has been described for use in dogs.[4] One milliliter of lidocaine is dripped into the nostril with the nose slightly elevated. A polyurethane or rubber catheter is lubricated with lidocaine jelly and placed in the ventral meatus by aiming the tip dorsomedially. It is inserted to the level of the carnassial tooth. The external end of the catheter is sutured to the muzzle within 1 cm of its exit from the nostril. Additional sutures can be used to tack the tube to the skin between the eyes and on the top of the head. An intravenous administration set is used to connect the catheter to the oxygen source. Fractional concentrations of oxygen of 40 per cent or more can be achieved with flow rates of 50 to 100 mL/kg body weight using the described method.[4] Potential complications include epistaxis and gastric distention.

Oxygen cages can be used to provide increased oxygen concentrations with minimal stress to the animal. The animal is in a completely isolated environment, and careful attention must be paid to temperature, humidity, and concentrations

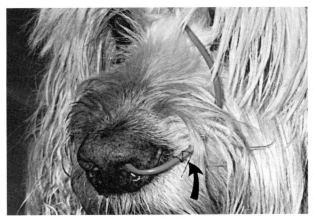

Figure 128–1. Nasal catheter is a simple means of delivering oxygen to small animal patients. The catheters are well tolerated by the animals, although an Elizabethan collar is suggested to prevent pawing. Sutures are placed as close to the naris as possible (*arrow*). Additional sutures can be used to hold the tube in position between the eyes and over the top of the head.

of oxygen and carbon dioxide within the cage. If these parameters are not controlled, considerable stress can be placed on these fragile patients. Oxygen cages can usually provide fractional concentrations of 35 to 50 per cent oxygen.

Tracheal tubes can be used to bypass upper airway obstructions and can be cuffed to allow for positive-pressure ventilation. These tubes can be placed orally for short-term management, in which case the animal must be unconscious or chemically restrained, or transtracheally (tracheostomy tube). Placement and care of tracheostomy tubes are described in many surgery textbooks and emergency manuals. Careful monitoring and frequent nursing care are required. Fractional concentrations of up to 100 per cent can be delivered.

Animals that are sedated, unconscious, or otherwise limited in mobility are at increased risk for the development of atelectasis of the dependent lung lobes and pneumonia. Recumbent animals should be turned every two hours. Coupage of conscious animals with limited mobility may encourage coughing and mobilization of airway secretions (see Bacterial Pneumonia, later in this chapter).

AIRWAY HUMIDIFICATION

Normal airway clearance mechanisms are dependent on the maintenance of adequate airway hydration. Drying of airways results in increased viscosity of secretions and decreased ciliary function, interfering with the clearance of secretions from the lungs. Additional effects of airway drying include inflammation and degeneration of the mucosa, vascular shunting, decreased compliance, atelectasis, and increased risk of infection.[2]

Maintaining airway hydration should be a consideration in all animals with lower respiratory disease. Special attention is necessary when the nasal cavity is bypassed or when oxygen supplementation is required, because canister gas does not contain water vapor.

The most important method of maintaining airway hydration is maintaining the systemic hydration of the animal. Strict attention to fluid balance is essential. The importance of systemic hydration cannot be overemphasized and should deter the clinician from arbitrarily treating a coughing animal with diuretics.

The addition of water to inspired gases is indicated in animals receiving oxygen supplementation for more than a few hours. The simplest system incorporates a canister of water into the oxygen line so that the gas is bubbled through the water. Complete water saturation of inspired air cannot be achieved because once the air becomes heated to body temperature within the airways, it can carry additional moisture. Such a system is adequate for use with intranasal catheters but is not sufficient for oxygen delivered through tracheal tubes. To provide greater saturation, humidifiers using the same principle are available that also heat the gas to body temperature. They should be placed in close proximity to the animal to minimize cooling and condensation within the tubing of the system.

Nebulizers can be used to administer saline droplets to the airways. When oxygen therapy is being used, nebulization is recommended for 10 to 30 minutes every 4 to 8 hours.[5] If nebulization is not available, sterile saline can be injected through the tube at a rate of 1 to 5 mL every 1 to 2 hours to moisten the mucosa and secretions.[5]

Disposable filters can be incorporated into the ventilation system that retain the heat and moisture from expired air to be returned with the inspired gases. These filters can interfere with the flow of air as they become plugged with secretions and can provide a site for bacterial growth. They must be changed at least every 24 hours to minimize these problems.[2]

VENTILATION

Ventilatory support can be provided on an emergency basis with an anesthetic machine or Ambu bag. Prolonged maintenance of an animal requires a ventilator and the ability to closely monitor the animal for the appearance of deleterious side effects of positive-pressure ventilation such as decreased venous return, resulting in decreased cardiac output and hypotension; ischemia of abdominal organs; pulmonary damage; pneumothorax; and impaired airway clearance.[6] Small disruptions to the system can result in death. Four types of ventilatory support are intermittent positive-pressure ventilation (IPPV), positive end expiratory pressure (PEEP), continuous positive airway pressure (CPAP), and high-frequency ventilation (HFV). Reviews of ventilatory techniques in veterinary patients have been published.[6,7]

INFECTIOUS DISEASES

VIRAL DISEASES

Canine Distemper

Canine distemper virus can infect epithelial tissues throughout the body. Pulmonary involvement is usually identified with severe disease, and bacterial pneumonia is a common complication. See Chapter 88.

Other Canine Viral Pneumonias

Viral agents other than canine distemper virus have been associated with respiratory diseases in the dog. Two of the more common of these viruses are canine adenovirus 2 and canine parainfluenza virus, which are associated with canine infectious tracheobronchitis (see Chapter 126). Mild interstitial pneumonia can be caused by viruses, but clinically apparent disease generally occurs as a result of concurrent or secondary bacterial infection (see Bacterial Pneumonia, later in this chapter). Adenovirus has been incriminated as the sole pathogen in young kennel-origin dogs with pneumonia.[8] There is no specific treatment for these viruses.

Feline Calicivirus Infection

Feline calicivirus is a major cause of feline upper respiratory infections, but the virus can infect other tissues in the body and can result in an interstitial pneumonia in cats.[9] The clinical usefulness of virus isolation tests is limited owing to the lack of specific therapy once the agent is identified. Treatment is supportive.

Feline Infectious Peritonitis

A common clinical presentation of feline infectious peritonitis (FIP) is pleural effusion. *However,* FIP can involve the pulmonary parenchyma, resulting in peribronchiolar pyogranulomatous inflammation.

Feline Retroviral Infections

Neither feline leukemia virus (FeLV) nor feline immunodeficiency virus (FIV) appears to directly cause overt lower respiratory tract disease. See Chapters 89–92.

RICKETTSIAL DISEASES

The two major rickettsial agents in dogs, *Rickettsia rickettsii* and *Ehrlichia canis,* generally result in vague, systemic signs of disease. Pulmonary signs occur more commonly with Rocky Mountain spotted fever than with ehrlichiosis.[10] See Chapter 86.

BACTERIAL DISEASES

Bacterial Pneumonia

Bacterial pneumonia is a common cause of respiratory disease in dogs but is an unusual finding in cats. Primary bacterial infection in dogs can occur as a result of *Bordetella bronchiseptica* and possibly *Streptococcus zooepidemicus.* A wide variety of other bacteria can result in pneumonia, presumably as opportunistic invaders. The more common isolates include *Escherichia coli, Pasteurella, Streptococcus, Staphylococcus, Pseudomonas,* and *Klebsiella.*[11–13]

The possibility of an underlying problem should not be overlooked in animals with bacterial pneumonia. In fact, bacterial infection can complicate nearly any other pulmonary disease process. Possible primary etiologies include aspiration (see Aspiration Pneumonia, later in this chapter), foreign body, viral infection, bronchial disease, neoplasia, contusion, lung parasites, and mycotic infection. Immune compromise secondary to viral infection, endocrinopathies, congenital abnormalities, and drug therapy and the presence of indwelling intravenous, urinary, and arterial catheters can also predispose animals to bacterial infection. Pneumonia resulting from infection with *Mycobacterium* is discussed separately.

Presentation. Animals with bacterial pneumonia often present with signs typical of lower respiratory disease. Localizing signs such as cough, exercise intolerance, respiratory distress, and nasal discharge are common, although cough is less often a complaint in feline patients. Subtle, nonspecific signs such as depression, anorexia, and weight loss may be the only complaints.

Physical findings also are typical of lower respiratory disease. Tachypnea or increased respiratory effort may be noted. Mucous membranes may be cyanotic with severe disease or following exertion. Lung sounds are usually increased, with crackles auscultable over all or part of the lung fields. The dependent (usually cranioventral) regions are often most severely affected. Bilateral mucopurulent nasal discharge may be present. Fever is an inconsistent sign. Animals with mild or localized disease may not have obvious signs, and radiographs may be necessary to support clinical intuition.

Diagnostic Evaluation. Thoracic radiographs may show only an interstitial pattern early in the disease. An alveolar pattern develops as the disease progresses. Distribution of lesions may be helpful in identifying underlying problems. Focal lesions may be associated with foreign bodies. Involvement of primarily the dependent lung lobes is supportive of concurrent airway disease or aspiration. The presence of a marked bronchial pattern suggests primary airway disease. Hematogenously borne infections (e.g., secondary to intravenous catheters) may have a caudodorsal distribution. Radiographs are carefully examined for patterns characteristic of other diseases, such as hilar lymphadenopathy, pulmonary artery enlargement, or mass lesions. Alveolar densities can mask these lesions, so repeated evaluation is indicated following resolution of pneumonia.

The complete blood count (CBC) may reveal a neutrophilic leukocytosis and left shift with a monocytosis. It is common to find only a stress response or a normal leukogram.

Tracheal wash fluid analysis is valuable for the diagnosis and treatment of bacterial infections. Fluid should be obtained before the administration of antibiotics in order to confirm the diagnosis and obtain antibiotic susceptibility information. Cytologic evaluation classically reveals septic inflammation with a predominance of degenerate neutrophils; however, signs of sepsis are not always present, and bacterial infection should remain a differential diagnosis in animals with nonseptic neutrophilic inflammation. Nonseptic neutrophilic inflammation is particularly likely to be present if antibiotics have been administered in the past few days. In a study of 42 dogs with bacterial pneumonia, only 48 per cent had septic inflammation on tracheal wash fluid analysis.[11] In another report, bacteria were visible in tracheal wash fluid from approximately one third of dogs with bacterial pneumonia.[12]

The specimen should always be cultured for identification of bacteria and sensitivity testing. Significantly more dogs with pneumonia respond to treatment based on sensitivity testing than on empiric treatment.[11, 13] *Mycoplasma* cultures should be considered, especially for evaluation of pneumonia in young dogs and in cats.[13–15] Cultures for anaerobic organisms should also be performed, particularly if abscessation is suspected.

More invasive diagnostic techniques, such as bronchoscopy or lung aspiration, may be necessary if the tracheal wash specimen is nondiagnostic. This situation may occur with localized disease. Bronchoalveolar lavage consistently demonstrated neutrophilic inflammation, and protected catheter brush specimens were consistently positive, in 16 dogs with bacterial pneumonia that underwent bronchoscopy.[16]

If an underlying cause is not obvious during the evaluation and treatment of the pneumonia, further diagnostic tests may be indicated. Considerations include FIV and FeLV tests, tests for endocrinopathies, barium swallow for decreased esophageal motility, and biopsies or motility tests for ciliary dyskinesia (see Chapter 127).

Treatment. Antibiotics are the primary treatment for bacterial infections. Antibiotics should be selected based on the results of susceptibility testing from tracheal wash or other pulmonary specimens.[11,13] Reasonable initial antibiotic choices pending results of sensitivity testing include cephalexin, trimethoprim-sulfadiazine, chloramphenicol, or amoxicillin-clavulanate (Table 128–1). If the infection is life-threatening, as with concurrent sepsis, intravenous treatment with broad-spectrum antibiotics is indicated. Possibilities include imipenem or the combination of ampicillin-sulbactam or ampicillin with either enrofloxacin or amikacin.

Aerosol administration of antibiotics, through nebulization, has been suggested for the treatment of refractory *Pseudomonas* infections.[17] This route of therapy should be used in addition to, not in place of, systemic therapy in cases of bronchopneumonia.[17]

General therapeutic measures should always be applied in addition to antibiotic therapy. Adequate oxygenation should be maintained with supplementation as needed. Airway hydration is maintained with systemic hydration, avoidance of diuretics, and, in some cases, nebulization.

Mobilization of airway secretions may be facilitated by mild activity in sufficiently stable animals. *Coupage* may also be helpful in mechanically jarring secretions and stimulating cough. The palm of the hand is used to strike the rib cage in a clapping motion over the area of the lungs. The force approaches that used in enthusiastic applause but should not be uncomfortable to the animal. The technique is performed for 5 to 10 minutes, several times daily. When teaching the technique to owners, the exact location of the lung fields should be demonstrated, because a large portion of the rib cage protects the abdominal organs. Animals that are recumbent should not be allowed to remain on one side for longer than two hours so that the same areas of lung are not always dependent.

The use of bronchodilators is controversial. Theophylline may interfere with the inflammatory response, which is undesirable in the face of infection. Bronchodilators may also contribute to V:Q mismatching. Bronchodilators are indicated for the treatment of bronchoconstriction. Bronchoconstriction is more likely to be contributing to signs in cats than in dogs and can occur immediately following aspiration in either species.

Corticosteroids and cough suppressants are avoided. Their interference with normal defense mechanisms is undesirable.

Once a plan of therapy has been established, the animal should be monitored for 48 to 72 hours. If no improvement in signs is observed during that time, therapy should be reevaluated. If improvement is observed, treatment should continue a minimum of one week beyond the total resolution of signs (including active radiographic changes). Usually a course of three to six weeks is required. Radiographs should be reevaluated approximately one week after discontinuation of therapy to detect early evidence of recurrence, to note any persistent changes suggesting an underlying disease process, and to detect complications such as consolidation or abscessation.

Prognosis. Bacterial pneumonias are generally responsive to appropriate antibiotic therapy and supportive care. The severity and chronicity of the infection, the presence of

TABLE 128–1. DRUG INDEX

GENERIC NAME (TRADE NAME)	DOSAGE	ROUTE	FREQUENCY	DESCRIPTION/ COMMENTS
Acepromazine	Dog, cat: 0.02 mg/lb	IV, SQ	q8–24h	Tranquilizer; dose modified to effect
Amikacin (Amiglyde)	Dog, cat: 2.5–4 mg/lb	IV, IM, SQ	q8h	Antibiotic
Amoxicillin/ clavulanate (Clavamox)	Dog, cat: 10 mg/lb	PO	q8h	Antibiotic
Ampicillin	Dog, cat: 10 mg/lb	PO, IV, SQ	q8h	Antibiotic
Ampicillin/ sulbactam (Unisyn)	Dog, cat: 10 mg/lb of ampicillin	IV, IM	q8h	Antibiotic
Cephalexin (Keflex)	Dog, cat: 10–15 mg/lb	PO	q8h	Antibiotic
Cephalothin (Keflin)	Dog, cat: 10–15 mg/lb	IV, SQ	q8h	Antibiotic
Chloramphenicol	Dog: 23 mg/lb Cat: 50 mg/cat	PO, IV, SQ PO, IV, SQ	q8h q12h	Antibiotic
Cyclophosphamide (Cytoxan)	Dog, cat: 50 mg/M^2	PO	q48h	Cytotoxic agent
Diethylcarbamazine	Dog: 35 mg/lb	PO	q12h for 3 days	For *Crenosoma* infection
Doxycycline	Dog, cat: 2.5–5 mg/lb	PO, IV	q12h	Antibiotic
Enrofloxacin (Baytril)	Dog, cat: 1.23–2.5 mg/lb	PO, IV	q12h	Antibiotic
Fenbendazole (Panacur)	Dog, cat: 11–23 mg/lb	PO	q12h for 10–14 days	For some lungworm infections
Furosemide (Lasix)	Dog, cat: 0.5–1 mg/lb	IV, SQ	q8–12h	Diuretic
Heparin	Dog, cat: 90–135 U/lb	SQ	q8h	Anticoagulant; dose adjusted based on PTT
	Dog, cat: 30 U/lb	SQ	q8–12h	Prevention of PTE
Imipenem/ cilastatin (Primaxin)	Dog, cat: 1.5–3 mg/lb	IV	q6–8h	Antibiotic
Morphine sulfate	Dog: 0.05 mg/lb	IV	To effect	Narcotic analgesic
Praziquantel (Droncit)	Dog, cat: 11 mg/lb	PO	q8h for 3 days	For *Paragonimus* infection
Prednisolone sodium succinate (Solu-Delta-Cortef)	Dog, cat: 10 mg/lb	IV	Once	Rapid-acting corticosteroid; shock dose
Prednisone	Dog, cat: 0.25–0.5 mg/lb	PO	q12h	Corticosteroid; initial anti-inflammatory dose; should be rapidly tapered to lowest effective dose
	Dog, cat: 0.5–1 mg/lb	PO	q12h	Initial immune-suppressive dose
Tetracycline	Dog, cat: 10 mg/lb	PO	q8h	Antibiotic
Trimethoprim/ sulfadiazine (Tribrissen)	Dog, cat: 7–15 mg/lb	PO, IM	q12h	Antibiotic
Warfarin (Coumadin)	Dog: 0.05–0.1 mg/lb Cat: 0.5 mg/cat	PO PO	q24h q24h	Anticoagulant; dose adjusted based on PT

IM = intramuscular; IV = intravenous; PO = oral; SQ = subcutaneous; PT = prothrombin time; PTE = pulmonary thromboembolism; PTT = partial thromboplastin time.

underlying disease, and the development of complications can affect the long-term prognosis.

Pulmonary Abscessation

Pulmonary abscesses, though rare, are a complication of bacterial pneumonia, foreign bodies, trauma (including aspiration), parasitic or fungal infections, and neoplasia. They are identified radiographically as nodular or cavitary lesions. The walls may be thick or thin and are often ill defined. If air is present within the cavity, a fluid line may be apparent on horizontal beam radiographs.

The diagnosis is suspected from radiographic appearance, especially during or following an episode of an associated disease. Surgery is indicated if the diagnosis must be confirmed through excision and histologic evaluation or if the lesion does not resolve after several months of aggressive antibiotic therapy. Anaerobic organisms can be involved and should be considered in the submission of specimens for culture and in the selection of antibiotics.

Mycobacterial Infections

Mycobacterial infections involving the lungs can mimic neoplasia, severe bacterial pneumonia, mycotic infection, or hypersensitivity or immune-mediated disease. Thoracic radiographs often show hilar lymphadenopathy. Interstitial patterns, granulomas, lung lobe consolidation, mineralization of pulmonary lesions, and pleural or pericardial effusions may be apparent.[18] Pulmonary hypertrophic osteopathy can occur.[18] The diagnosis depends on the identification of organisms. Although organisms may be found in tracheal wash fluid, examination of pleural fluid, lung aspirates, bronchoalveolar lavage, or lung biopsies may be required.

PROTOZOAL DISEASES

Toxoplasmosis

Pulmonary involvement with toxoplasmosis is common, particularly in cats with acute disease. Pulmonary signs were present in 9 of 12 cats with acute toxoplasmosis and in 4 of 17 cats with chronic toxoplasmosis.[19] Dyspnea was reported in 8 of 13 dogs with histologically confirmed toxoplasmosis, including 3 of 3 dogs without other identifiable primary disease.[20] Radiographs of the thorax classically reveal fluffy interstitial and alveolar densities throughout the lung fields. Nodular patterns, diffuse interstitial patterns, consolidation, and effusions can occur. Tracheal wash fluid analysis can show nonspecific inflammation, and careful examination of the fluid for tachyzoites is warranted and could provide a definitive diagnosis. Organisms can be retrieved by bronchoalveolar lavage from cats with acute toxoplasmosis, but careful inspection of concentrated slide preparations is required.[21] Pleural or peritoneal effusions are also potential sources for organism retrieval.[20] Lung biopsy for the identification of organisms is rarely feasible in an animal with acute, severe pulmonary disease. See Chapter 87.

Pneumocystosis

Pneumocystis carinii is a protozoal organism that causes pulmonary disease in immunocompromised patients. Increased awareness of this disease has occurred as a result of human immunodeficiency virus infections and immune-suppressive therapies. Latent or subclinical infections can occur in several species, including dogs and cats.[22] Clinical disease can occur in dogs, but apparently not in cats.[23,24] Clinical infections in the dog are generally limited to the lung, although systemic spread is possible. The organisms adhere to the epithelial cells lining the alveoli without invading into deeper tissues. Signs appear when the organisms multiply to a sufficient extent to interfere with alveolar ventilation.[25] Signs also can occur as a result of a severe inflammatory response. This response may be successful in eliminating the infection.[25]

Presentation. Dogs with clinical pneumocystosis present with signs reflective of chronic pneumonia, including weight loss, exercise intolerance, respiratory distress, and sometimes a nonproductive cough.[26, 27] The majority of reported cases have involved young dogs, particularly miniature dachshunds.[22, 26, 27] Careful questioning for evidence of immune-suppressive disease or therapy is indicated. Increased breath sounds may be ausculted. Pyrexia is not a feature.[26]

Diagnostic Evaluation. Radiographs typically show a diffuse alveolar pattern. Depending on the inflammatory reaction, interstitial or localized disease may be present. A CBC generally shows a neutrophilic leukocytosis, often with a left shift.[25, 27] Eosinophilia or monocytosis can be seen.

The diagnosis is made through the identification of organisms. Tracheal wash analysis has resulted in organisms in dogs,[27] but other specimens may be necessary. Bronchoalveolar lavage fluid analysis is valuable in the diagnosis of the disease in people and has been successful in a dog.[22, 28] Lung aspirates or lung biopsies can be examined. The identification of organisms can be enhanced with the application of Gomori's methenamine silver (cysts) or Giemsa stain (cysts and trophozoites), as the organisms are not obvious with routine hematoxylin-eosin stain. Immunohistochemistry and polymerase chain reaction (PCR) of pulmonary specimens are used to detect *Pneumocystis* in people, and they have been applied successfully in dogs.[22, 29]

Treatment. Three dogs have been successfully treated with potentiated sulfonamides at a dosage of either 15 mg/kg every 8 hours or 30 mg/kg every 12 hours, both for three weeks.[27] Two of these dogs were also administered cimetidine and levamisole as potential immune stimulants. Pentamidine isethionate can be administered at a dosage of 2 mg/lb (4 mg/kg) intramuscularly every 24 hours for two weeks.[25] Toxic effects include vasodilatation and hypotension, hyperglycemia, hypocalcemia, hypokalemia, renal and liver dysfunction, swelling at the injection site, and systemic anaphylaxis.[25] General therapy should include elimination of immune-suppressive factors whenever possible.

Prognosis. Few cases have been described in the dog. The prognosis has been considered poor unless the immune suppression can be reversed. However, the recent publication of successful treatment in three out of four dogs allows for a more hopeful prognosis.[27]

Zoonosis. Experimental transmission of pneumocystosis between species is difficult.[25] To the author's knowledge, no link has been found between disease in people and disease in cats or dogs.

FUNGAL DISEASES

The historic, physical, clinical, pathologic, and radiographic signs of mycotic infections involving the lungs are often the same as those signs produced by neoplasia, hypersensitivity or immune-mediated disease, or other infections. Animals showing slowly progressive lower respiratory signs in conjunction with weight loss, lymphadenopathy, fever, or chorioretinitis should be considered potential candidates for mycotic disease. A definitive diagnosis is essential, because treatment is prolonged, costly, and potentially toxic. The reader is referred to Chapter 93 for a complete discussion of fungal infections. The following discussion is limited to aspects that are unique to the respiratory system.

Histoplasmosis

Exposure to *Histoplasma capsulatum* occurs primarily through inhalation of organisms. Following exposure, most animals develop a localized, asymptomatic infection of the lungs, resolved by cell-mediated immunity. Depending on the amount of organisms inhaled and the immune status of the animal, fungal pneumonia and/or systemic dissemination may occur, and clinical signs may develop. Reactivation of a previous infection can also occur.

Presentation. Lung involvement with histoplasmosis is common, and the signs are typical of chronic lower respiratory tract disease. Lung involvement can also be present in animals presented for nonlocalizing signs such as weight loss, anorexia, fever, and depression.[30] Although unusual, pleural effusion has been reported.[31] Signs of involvement of other organs may occur concurrently with respiratory signs or as the primary presenting complaint.

Diagnostic Evaluation. Thoracic radiographs classically exhibit a diffuse interstitial pattern, which is often miliary. Alveolar patterns or areas of consolidation may occur with severe inflammation. Hilar lymphadenopathy may be present in dogs and can be sufficiently severe to cause signs from bronchial compression. Hilar lymphadenopathy is not a common finding in cats.[30] Calcification of pulmonary lesions can occur.

Tracheal wash fluid cytology may have neutrophilic, macrophagic, eosinophilic, or mixed inflammation. Hemorrhage may be evident. Macrophages should be critically examined for organisms.

Cytologic identification of organisms is the preferred method of diagnosis. Organisms frequently cannot be identified in tracheal wash fluid, and collection of other specimens may be required. Pulmonary tissue can be sampled more deeply through transthoracic needle aspiration, bronchoalveolar lavage, or biopsy. Fungal culture of specimens also increases the likelihood of organism identification.

Blastomycosis

The route of exposure to *Blastomyces dermatitidis* is probably through inhalation, with the lungs as the primary site of infection.[32] Dissemination may occur to a variety of organs. Animals may be exposed to the organism without developing clinical signs, but once clinical signs develop, the animals are generally considered to have progressive disease.[32]

Presentation. There is usually chronic progression of signs. Lower respiratory signs were present in 43 per cent of 47 dogs.[33] Disease in cats is rare. Respiratory involvement was identified in 70 per cent of cats with blastomycosis; however, the number of these cats presenting with respiratory signs was not provided.[34]

Diagnostic Evaluation. In a review of 47 dogs with blastomycosis, radiographic changes of the thorax were noted in 85 per cent of cases.[33] A diffuse, miliary interstitial pattern, as is seen with histoplasmosis, is typical (Fig. 128–2). An alveolar or bronchial pattern can also occur (Fig. 128–3). Hilar lymphadenopathy occurs, but probably less frequently than with other mycotic diseases. Pleural effusion may be apparent.

Tracheal wash fluid analysis can be unremarkable or reveal neutrophilic, macrophagic, eosinophilic, or mixed inflammation, with or without hemorrhage. Careful examination of slides should be performed to identify organisms. Of seven dogs with blastomycosis, three had organisms identified by tracheal wash fluid analysis.[35]

As is the case with histoplasmosis, cytologic identification of organisms is the preferred method of diagnosis. In addition to tracheal wash fluid, cytologic evaluation can be performed on lung aspirates or biopsies or bronchoalveolar lavage fluid (Fig. 128–4). Cytologic analysis of bronchoalveolar lavage fluid in seven dogs revealed a range of responses, including acute neutrophilic inflammation, mixed inflammation, eosinophilic inflammation, hemorrhage, lymphocytic reactivity, and normal cytologic characteristics. Organisms were seen in lavage fluid from five of the seven dogs.[35] Culture of specimens for fungus increases the likelihood of organism identification. Pleural fluid should be examined when present.

Coccidioidomycosis

Infection with *Coccidioides immitis* can occur through the respiratory tract, as with the other systemic mycoses. Localized, asymptomatic pulmonary infections occur but are rarely diagnosed. Severe pulmonary infection and systemic dissemination are responsible for clinically recognized infection.

Presentation. Animals with pulmonary disease present with slowly progressive lower respiratory signs. Coccidioidomycosis is an extremely rare disease in cats.

Diagnostic Evaluation. Thoracic radiographs are abnormal in the majority of cases, with changes similar to those seen with the other mycoses.[36] A diffuse interstitial pattern occurs, and bronchial or alveolar components are possible. Hilar lymphadenopathy was present in 74 per cent

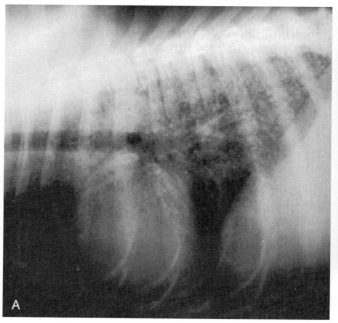

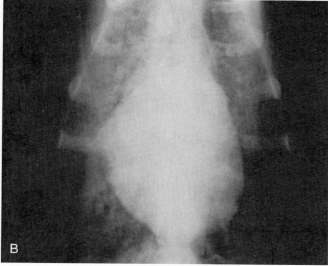

Figure 128–2. Radiographs demonstrating the typical diffuse, miliary interstitial pattern of pulmonary mycotic disease.

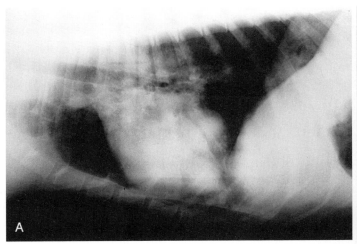
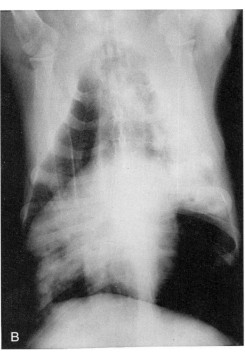

Figure 128–3. Radiographs demonstrating alveolar infiltrates and areas of consolidation in the lungs of a dog with blastomycosis. Notice the marked variation in appearance compared with the radiographs in Figure 128–2 from a different dog with blastomycosis.

of reviewed cases, and pleural effusion or thickening was noted in 47 per cent.[36]

Tracheal wash fluid may be unremarkable or reveal inflammation. Slides should be carefully examined for organisms. Cytologic identification of organisms provides a definitive diagnosis. If tracheal wash preparations are nondiagnostic, other specimens should be examined from organs suspected of being infected. Specimens can include lung aspirates or biopsies, bronchoalveolar lavage fluid, and pleural fluid.

Cryptococcosis

Cryptococcus neoformans generally affects the nasal cavity, nasal sinuses, eyes, skin, or brain of cats and the central nervous system or eyes of dogs. Pulmonary lesions have been reported in 50 per cent of feline cases, although clinical signs relative to the lower respiratory tract are rare, and an

antemortem diagnosis of pulmonary involvement is uncommon.[37] Thoracic radiographs are normal in most cases, in spite of pulmonary involvement discovered on necropsy, but can show a bronchoalveolar pattern, consolidation, or nodules.[37] Organisms were retrieved by tracheal wash and bronchoalveolar lavage in a cat with cryptococcosis that had normal radiographs.[38] The reader is referred to Chapter 87.

Aspergillosis

Aspergillosis is a disease that predominantly involves the nasal cavity and sinuses of dogs. Systemic disease, occasionally with pulmonary involvement, occurs rarely in dogs and cats. A species of *Aspergillus* other than *A. fumigatus,* that associated with most nasal infections, is usually involved. Disease is generally associated with immune compromise, and the diagnosis is often made postmortem. Disseminated aspergillosis is discussed further in Chapter 93.

PARASITIC DISEASES

Lungworms can result in a variety of clinical signs in dogs and cats as a result of both the parasites themselves and the inflammatory reaction they induce, though frequently the infections are asymptomatic. The inflammatory response is typically eosinophilic, but nonspecific mixed or chronic inflammatory changes can predominate. Secondary bacterial infections may occasionally obscure the diagnosis. A definitive diagnosis is based on the identification of organisms. The diagnosis is hampered by intermittent shedding of characteristic eggs or larvae.

The prognosis for most lungworm infections is good, because severe disease is rarely present. However, the clinical effectiveness of specific antiparasitic therapy is not well established.

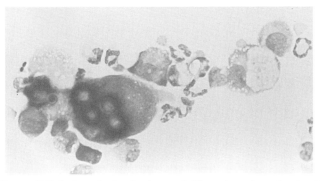

Figure 128–4. Bronchoalveolar lavage fluid cytology from the dog in Figure 128–2 demonstrates macrophages and mature nondegenerate neutrophils. A single extracellular budding yeast form of *Blastomyces dermatitidis* and a giant cell with four phagocytized yeast forms are present. The fungal forms are 10 to 20 μm in size, are deeply basophilic, and have a thick cell wall.

Paragonimus kellicotti

Paragonimus kellicotti, lung flukes, cause pulmonary disease in dogs and cats in the states surrounding the Great

Lakes and in the midwestern and southern United States. Adult flukes reside in cysts within the parenchyma of the lung. Eggs are passed into the airways, coughed up, swallowed, and passed in the feces. Aquatic snails and crayfish are required intermediate hosts. Crayfish or paratenic hosts are ingested, and the flukes migrate to the lungs through the diaphragm. The adult worms, as well as eggs trapped in alveoli and airways, result in pulmonary pathology.

Presentation. Animals may not exhibit signs as a result of *Paragonimus* infection. When they occur, clinical signs result from an inflammatory reaction to the parasite, from cyst rupture and pneumothorax, or from secondary bacterial infection. The major sign of the inflammatory disease is coughing. Occasionally hemoptysis occurs. In cats, wheezing can occur and may be confused with feline bronchitis. Acute respiratory distress occurs when cyst rupture results in pneumothorax. Crackles and wheezes may be ausculted with inflammatory disease; decreased lung sounds occur with pneumothorax.

Diagnostic Evaluation. Thoracic radiographs demonstrate air-filled cysts or tissue density masses averaging 1 cm in diameter.[39] The masses most commonly involve the caudal lung lobes and may be well defined or not, depending on the inflammatory reaction.[39] Pneumothorax may be present. Diffuse inflammatory signs may be apparent, resulting in bronchial, interstitial, or patchy alveolar patterns.[40]

A CBC and tracheal wash fluid analysis may reveal eosinophilic inflammation. Macrophagic, neutrophilic, or mixed inflammation can occur. The disease is definitively diagnosed by the identification of eggs. They may be found in tracheal wash fluid or in feces. The eggs are single-operculated, ovoid eggs 80 to 115 μm in length (Fig. 128–5).[40] Concentration techniques should be performed on fecal specimens to increase the likelihood of identifying the eggs. Sedimentation is the preferred technique and can be performed without expensive equipment.[40, 41] Eggs may be shed intermittently, and multiple fecal examinations may be necessary for their detection.

Treatment. Currently recommended treatments are praziquantel (11 mg/lb, or 25 mg/kg, every 8 hours orally for 3 days) or fenbendazole (11 to 23 mg/lb, or 25 to 50 mg/kg, every 12 hours for 10 to 14 days).[42–44] Response to treatment is monitored by thoracic radiography and periodic fecal examinations. Radiographic lesions can take many weeks to resolve, and some abnormal density may persist. Experimentally infected dogs and cats treated with praziquantel ceased

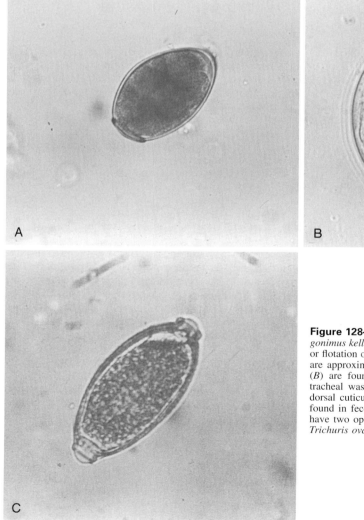

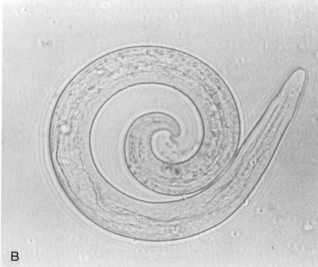

Figure 128–5. Diagnostic specimens of common lung parasites. *Paragonimus kellicotti* ova (*A*) are found in feces examined by sedimentation or flotation or in tracheal wash fluid. They have a single operculum and are approximately 90 μm in length. *Aelurostrongylus abstrusus* larvae (*B*) are found in feces examined by the Baermann technique or in tracheal wash fluid. They are characterized by ventral and prominent dorsal cuticular spines on their tails. *Capillaria aerophila* ova (*C*) are found in feces examined by flotation and in tracheal wash fluid. They have two opercula but are smaller (<70 μm) and less pigmented than *Trichuris* ova. (Courtesy of Dr. K. Kazacos.)

shedding ova in their feces two and seven days after treatment, respectively.[42] Treatment may need to be repeated in some cases.

Aelurostrongylus abstrusus

Aelurostongylus abstrusus is a small (less than 1 cm) lungworm of cats. Adult worms reside primarily within the bronchioles. First-stage larvae are coughed out of the airways, swallowed, and passed in the feces. A mollusk (snail or slug) intermediate host is required, and transport hosts such as small mammals or birds play a role in infecting cats. An inflammatory response to the parasites can result in clinical signs.

Infection with *Aelurostrongylus* is relatively common in cats, although many infections are not associated with clinical signs. Of 128 cats euthanized at a humane shelter in Alabama, 20 were infected with *Aelurostrongylus*.[45] Less than half of the cats had organisms present on histologic examination of the lungs, indicating that routine necropsy evaluation is insensitive in the detection of infection and likely results in underestimation of the incidence of infection. Infection was found in the majority of cats (90 percent) by Baermann examination of feces.

Presentation. *Aelurostrongylus* infections may be asymptomatic. Clinical signs can range from mild coughing to severe wheezing and respiratory distress. Wheezes or crackles may be auscultated. The clinical presentation mimics feline bronchitis. Secondary bacterial infections can occur.

Diagnostic Evaluation. Thoracic radiographs can show small, poorly defined, nodular densities throughout the lung fields, similar to metastatic neoplasia or mycotic disease. The caudal lung fields are most heavily involved.[39, 40] Inflammatory reactions can also result in bronchial, interstitial, and alveolar patterns. These patterns can be confused with feline bronchitis.

Tracheal wash fluid analysis may reveal eosinophilic inflammation, which can be reflected in the CBC. A macrophagic, neutrophilic, or mixed inflammatory response can also occur. The disease is definitively diagnosed by the identification of first-stage larvae in tracheal wash fluid or feces. Larvae are characterized by dorsal and ventral cuticular spines on their tails (see Fig. 128–5).[40] Multiple fecal specimens should be examined following concentration of larvae using the Baermann technique, which can be performed with very little equipment.[40, 41]

Treatment. Infection with *Aelurostrongylus* is usually self-limited, and asymptomatic infections do not necessarily warrant treatment.[40] Experimental infections were nearly resolved within six months.[46] The presence of inflammation may be an indication for treatment, because the inflammatory cells themselves can induce permanent airway changes.

Specific antiparasitic therapy can be attempted with fenbendazole (11 to 23 mg/lb, or 25 to 50 mg/kg, every 24 hours for 10 to 14 days). Ivermectin also has been used successfully (180 μg/lb, or 400 μg/kg, subcutaneously).[44, 47] Nonspecific treatment with corticosteroids and bronchodilators may be helpful in decreasing the severity of clinical signs. This response to therapy can mislead the clinician into believing a tentative diagnosis of "idiopathic" feline bronchitis. The potential for side effects and for interference with antiparasitic treatment should be considered when administering these drugs. It is preferable to treat the underlying disease directly.

Capillaria aerophila

Capillaria aerophila is a 2- to 4-cm lungworm that resides in the trachea and bronchi of dogs and cats. Eggs are coughed up, swallowed, and passed in the feces. Infection is probably direct or through earthworm intermediate hosts.[44, 48]

Presentation. The majority of cases are asymptomatic. Occasionally a chronic cough is reported.

Diagnostic Evaluation. Thoracic radiographs in symptomatic animals may reveal a bronchial or interstitial pattern. Tracheal wash fluid typically shows eosinophilic inflammation, although macrophagic, neutrophilic, or mixed inflammation is also possible. The diagnosis is made by the identification of eggs in tracheal wash fluid or in fecal specimens examined by flotation.

The eggs are double-operculated like *Trichuris* ova but are smaller (60 by 35 μm), are less pigmented, and have asymmetric terminal plugs (see Fig. 128–5).[40] Intermittent shedding of ova may occur.[48]

Treatment. Fenbendazole is recommended for treatment (11 to 23 mg/lb, or 25 to 50 mg/kg, every 12 hours for 14 days).[44] Levamisole can be used in dogs. An effective dosage for ivermectin has not been established.

Oslerus osleri

Oslerus osleri is a lungworm that resides at the carina and in the major bronchi of dogs, forming inflammatory nodules. The reader is referred to Chapter 126.

Filaroides hirthi

Filaroides hirthi is a small lungworm (less than 2 mm) that resides in the terminal bronchioles and alveoli of dogs.[40] Larvae are coughed up, swallowed, and passed in the feces. No development of larvae outside of the dog is required, and autoinfection can worsen the worm burden within the animal. The worms often induce a granulomatous inflammatory reaction. The parasite can be endemic in research colonies of dogs and interfere with interpretation of pathologic findings following experiments.

The majority of cases do not demonstrate clinical signs. Respiratory tract signs, including nonproductive cough, tachypnea, and respiratory distress, have been reported in small numbers of cases.[49, 50] Immune compromise may facilitate superinfection, resulting in severe clinical signs and even death.[50]

Thoracic radiographs may reveal a diffuse, miliary interstitial pattern or focal nodules.[44, 49] A definitive diagnosis may be difficult. Tracheal wash specimens should be evaluated for larvae or larvated eggs. Fecal specimens are best examined using zinc sulfate flotation, although the Baermann technique can be used.[40, 44] Larvae demonstrate the kinked tails characteristic of *Filaroides* spp.

Albendazole (23 mg/lb, or 50 mg/kg, every 12 hours for 5 days, repeated in 21 days) and fenbendazole (23 mg/lb, or 50 mg/kg, for 14 days) have been used to treat infections.[44, 49, 50] Signs may suddenly worsen during treatment, perhaps due to a reaction to worm death.[49] Ivermectin had an efficacy of 74 per cent when given at a relatively high dosage to infected beagles (1 mg/kg subcutaneously, repeated in one week).[51] Efficacy for eliminating first-stage larvae was 95 per cent.[51]

Crenosoma vulpis

Crenosoma vulpis is a worm that resides in the trachea, bronchi, and bronchioles of dogs. Larvae are coughed up, swallowed, and passed in the feces. Mollusks serve as intermediate hosts.[44, 52] Spines on the worms cause mucosal abrasions and can result in occlusion of smaller airways.[46] Infection is uncommon.

Dogs present with signs of tracheobronchitis. Bronchopneumonia, sneezing, and nasal discharge can occur.[46] Radiographs may reveal bronchial, alveolar, interstitial, or mixed patterns.[52] The diagnosis is made by identification of larvae in tracheal wash fluid or in fecal specimens examined by the Baermann technique. Larvae have straight tails, unlike those of *Filaroides* spp.[46]

Drugs that have been used for treatment are diethylcarbamazine (35 mg/lb, or 80 mg/kg, every 12 hours for 3 days), levamisole (3.5 mg/lb, or 8 mg/kg, orally once), and fenbendazole (23 mg/lb, or 50 mg/kg, orally every 24 hours for 3 days).[52, 53]

Angiostrongylus vasorum

Angiostrongylus is rarely diagnosed in the United States. The 2.5-cm worm resides in the pulmonary artery and right ventricle of dogs.[46, 54] The larvae are coughed up, swallowed, and passed in the feces. Mollusks serve as intermediate hosts. Pulmonary artery obstruction, endarteritis, and thrombosis occur, as well as parenchymal damage due to larval migration.[46, 54] Hemorrhages due to anticoagulant factors have been reported.[46, 54] Dogs may present with lower respiratory signs, including cough or hemoptysis, congestive heart failure, and/or subcutaneous hemorrhages. Radiographs can show pulmonary and cardiac changes similar to those of heartworm disease.[54] Larvae may be found in feces (ideally, using the Baermann technique) or tracheal washings and are identified by a small cephalic button and wavy tail.[46, 54] Levamisole (3.5 mg/lb, or 7.5 mg/kg, orally for 2 days followed by 4.5 mg/lb, or 10 mg/kg, orally for 2 days) is recommended for treatment.[54] Aspirin or corticosteroid has been suggested as concurrent therapy.[54] Mebendazole, fenbendazole, and ivermectin have also been used.[46, 54]

Intestinal Parasite Migration

Toxocara canis undergoes migration through the lungs of dogs following infection. There are generally no clinical signs at this stage, but in heavy infections, pulmonary signs may result from damage and the inflammatory reaction to the migrating larvae.[46] Coughing and tachypnea are usually noted in puppies younger than 6 weeks of age. Fecal examination may reveal characteristic ova, but larvae begin migrating before the shedding of eggs. A peripheral eosinophilia may be present.

Signs are usually mild and resolve without treatment. Glucocorticoids can be administered in low dosages to control severe signs but are rarely necessary. Routine anthelmintic therapy is not effective against the larvae but should be initiated to prevent further propagation.

Other intestinal parasites with lung migration as part of their life-cycle include *Ancylostoma caninum* and *Strongyloides stercoralis*. Transient signs, such as coughing, might be noted.[46] No specific treatment for pulmonary involvement is recommended.

HYPERSENSITIVITY AND IMMUNE-MEDIATED DISEASES

The immune system, systemic and local, plays a major role in the pathogenesis, clinical signs, progression, and recovery of virtually all pulmonary diseases. In some instances the immune response dominates the clinical disease. The resultant inflammation may be an excessive reaction to an antigenic stimulus (hypersensitivity reaction), the result of immune complex deposition, or of undetermined cause. In some cases an antigenic source is discovered, and treatment can be directed toward eliminating the cause. In most instances no offending agent can be found, and immune-suppressant therapy is necessary to control the response.

EOSINOPHILIC DISEASES

Eosinophilic pulmonary diseases can be characterized as primarily bronchial or parenchymal. Bronchial eosinophilic diseases include canine and feline allergic bronchitis (see Chapter 127).

Eosinophilic diseases predominantly involving the pulmonary parenchyma are also known as pulmonary infiltrates with eosinophils, or PIE. This terminology reflects a spectrum of diseases that can result in minimal to severe clinical signs and can be self-limited, chronic, or fatal.[55] Differential diagnoses for eosinophilic lung diseases include hypersensitivity reactions to pulmonary parasites, heartworms, drugs, or inhaled allergens. Occasionally, bacteria, fungi, or neoplasias can cause a hypersensitivity response.

The term eosinophilic pulmonary granulomatosis (EPG) has been used to describe a severe form of PIE.[55, 56] Thoracic radiographs show pulmonary nodules of varying sizes, some as large as 20 cm.[56] Mixed patterns can be present concurrently. Hilar lymphadenopathy is common. Histologically the lesions are primarily eosinophils, with smaller numbers of lymphocytes, plasma cells, and macrophages.[56] Surrounding the granulomas is a zone of epithelial proliferation and infiltrates of eosinophils and neutrophils. Thickening of interalveolar septae occurs owing to fibrosis and mononuclear infiltrates. Unlike lymphomatoid granulomatosis, there is no consistent vascular orientation. As with other forms of PIE, underlying antigenic sources, particularly heartworms, should be considered. Heartworm disease was present in 11 of 17 reported cases.[55, 56]

Presentation. Signs of PIE are extremely variable, depending on the severity of disease. Coughing is often the primary complaint.[57] Other signs of pulmonary disease can occur, as well as weight loss, depression, and anorexia. The owner should be questioned about exposure to drugs and inhaled allergens. Animals are usually normothermic. Auscultation often reveals increased breath sounds or crackles. Wheezes and decreased sounds can occur.

Diagnostic Evaluation. The CBC classically reflects the eosinophilic response; however, peripheral eosinophilia may be absent in spite of marked pulmonary involvement. Basophilia can also be present.

Radiographs can show a mild interstitial pattern, patchy alveolar densities, and even large masses that are indistinguishable from neoplasia or fungal granulomas. A bronchial component also may be present. Hilar lymphadenopathy may be severe. Dilated, tortuous pulmonary arteries may be present as a result of pulmonary hypertension and should increase the index of suspicion for heartworm disease.

Cytologic evaluation is necessary for a clinical diagnosis. Tracheal wash fluid can be obtained readily and may be adequate, particularly if there is bronchial involvement or alveolar flooding. Deeper specimens may be required with localized or interstitial disease and are obtained through bronchoalveolar lavage, thoracic aspirates, or lung biopsy.

Eosinophilic inflammation predominates, although other types of inflammatory cells are also present. Specimens should be critically evaluated for any source of antigen, including parasites, bacteria, fungi, and neoplasias.

Further evaluation for an antigenic source should be pursued with examination of multiple fecal specimens for lungworms and testing for heartworms. Animals in endemic areas also should be tested for mycotic diseases.

Lymphomatoid granulomatosis has similar presenting and radiographic signs as EPG and frequently has a component of eosinophilic inflammation. It should be considered as a differential diagnosis for dogs with suspected EPG in which the diagnosis has not been confirmed by tissue biopsy.

Treatment. When possible, an etiology should be identified and removed. If the animal is on medications, the drugs should be discontinued. Exposure to inhaled allergens should be eliminated. Infectious agents should be treated appropriately.

If no allergen can be found, immune suppression is required. Corticosteroids are frequently successful in controlling the inflammatory process, except in cases of EPG. An initial dosage of prednisone 0.5 mg/lb (1 mg/kg) every 12 hours is suggested. The animal should be reevaluated after five to seven days. Radiographs should be evaluated at that time to assess response and also to identify any change that might suggest deterioration due to an undiagnosed infectious disease.

If the process is not controlled, the initial steroid dosage can be doubled. If signs have resolved, the steroid dosage is gradually tapered to alternate-day therapy at a dosage of 0.25 mg/lb (0.5 mg/kg). Discontinuation of the drug can be attempted after three months of therapy, but long-term treatment is often required.

Cases with mass lesions consistent with EPG may exhibit clinical behavior similar to lymphomatoid granulomatosis (discussed later), and cytotoxic drugs are often required.[56]

Prognosis. If a primary allergen is identified, the prognosis is dependent on the ability to eliminate the antigen. If no source is identified, the prognosis for control is good, although many animals require long-term steroid therapy to manage the clinical signs.[57] EPG is a severe form of PIE with a guarded prognosis.[56]

VASCULITIDES

There are numerous interstitial lung diseases in humans in which the underlying etiology is unknown. Some of these diseases are inflammatory processes associated with the vasculature. Examples include Wegener's granulomatosis, lymphomatoid granulomatosis, Goodpasture's syndrome, and systemic lupus erythematosis (SLE). Wegener's granulomatosis and lymphomatoid granulomatosis are characterized by necrotizing vasculitis and granulomatous inflammation.[58] Goodpasture's syndrome is a result of anti–basement membrane antibodies that attack the glomerular basement membranes and the basement membranes of pulmonary alveoli and capillaries.[59] SLE is a multisystemic autoimmune disease, and lung vasculature is occasionally involved.[59]

Reported cases of similar diseases in dogs have included lymphomatoid granulomatosis, granulomatosis associated with a positive LE cell test, and pneumonitis as a component of SLE.[60–63] Other cases of inflammatory pneumonitis have been diagnosed in dogs and cats in which no etiology was found and resolution was achieved with immune-suppressant therapy (Figs. 128–6 and 128–7). These diseases have not been well characterized pathologically.

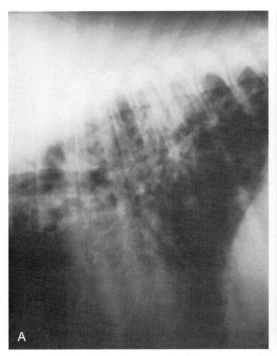
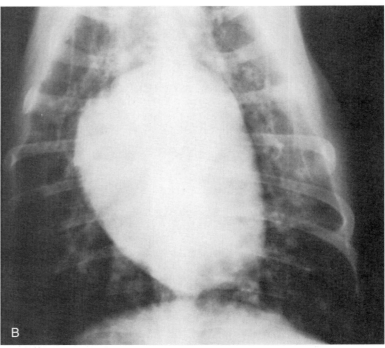

Figure 128–6. A 4-year-old dog was presented for chronic coughing and weight loss. Radiographs show a diffuse interstitial pattern with fluffy nodular densities. A tracheal wash was nondiagnostic. Granulomatous inflammation was present on bronchoalveolar lavage fluid analysis. There was no evidence of neoplasia, and no etiologic agents were seen or cultured. Fungal and toxoplasma titers and heartworm tests were negative. A thrombocytopenia was present also and was assumed to be immune mediated. Neoplastic or infectious pulmonary disease could not be completely eliminated from the differential diagnoses, but further diagnostic measures were declined, and a presumptive diagnosis of immune-mediated disease was made. An immune-suppressive dosage of prednisone was prescribed.

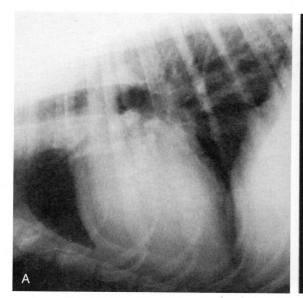
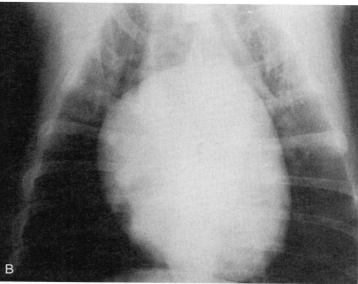

Figure 128–7. Radiographs from the dog in Figure 128–6 show marked resolution of disease after one week of corticosteroids. The thrombocytopenia also had resolved.

Inciting causes for these syndromes are rarely identified. Some infectious agents that can cause similar signs include FIP virus, rickettsia, atypical bacteria, protozoa, fungi, parasites (including *Dirofilaria*), and bacteria secondary to foreign bodies. Another differential diagnosis is pulmonary neoplasia, either of mononuclear cell origin or inciting an inflammatory response. Lymphomatoid granulomatosis is considered an early or low-grade form of lymphoma.

PULMONARY NEOPLASIA

The lungs can be affected by primary pulmonary neoplasia, metastatic neoplasia, lymphoma, and neoplasia involving adjacent tissues. Lymphomatoid granulomatosis is considered by some to be a neoplastic process. Malignant histiocytosis involving the lungs has been reported in Bernese Mountain Dogs.

PRIMARY PULMONARY NEOPLASIA

Neoplasia arising primarily from the lungs is uncommon in the dog and cat, especially when compared with the incidence in people or the incidence of metastatic pulmonary neoplasia. The great majority of primary pulmonary tumors in dogs and cats are carcinomas. Adenocarcinomas are most frequently found, accounting for 70 to 80 percent of pulmonary carcinomas,[64] followed by squamous cell and anaplastic carcinomas.[65–67] Fibrosarcomas, osteosarcomas, chondrosarcomas, hemangiosarcomas, and benign adenomas occur infrequently. Fibrosarcoma has been reported in association with infection with *Spirocerca lupi*.[68] A common primary lung tumor in people, small cell carcinoma or oat cell tumor, is rare in dogs and cats.

Metastatic disease resulting from primary lung tumors is common owing to the malignant nature of most of these tumors. Neoplastic cells frequently metastasize to other areas of the lung through blood vessels, lymphatics, or airways. The pulmonary metastatic lesions may be smaller than the original tumor, or multiple uniform nodules can occur. Uniform nodules may represent multicentric disease rather than metastases. Another common site of metastasis is the bronchial lymph nodes. The pleura is less often involved. Extrathoracic metastatic lesions can involve the long bones, intraabdominal organs, heart, brain, esophagus, mediastinal lymph nodes, and eyes.[65–67, 69–71] Involvement of multiple digits has been seen in several cats.

Clinical signs can result from the primary pulmonary tumors and intrathoracic metastases, from extrathoracic metastases, and from paraneoplastic conditions. Primary tumors and intrathoracic metastases can cause respiratory signs from compression or obstruction of airways, regional V:Q abnormalities, or pleural effusion. Inflammatory reactions to the tumors, secondary infections, intrapulmonary hemorrhage, cavitary lesions, pneumothorax, and hemothorax also can contribute to signs.

Nonrespiratory signs from the primary tumor, such as weight loss, anorexia, and depression, can occur with or without concurrent respiratory signs. Occasionally, pulmonary tumors compress the major veins within the thorax, resulting in ascites, jugular distention, or edema of the head and neck. Esophageal compression can lead to dysphagia or regurgitation. Extrathoracic metastatic disease results in signs associated with the systems involved. Animals may present for those signs alone without historic evidence of respiratory disease.

A number of paraneoplastic syndromes have been associated with primary pulmonary tumors in people, but few have been reported in small animals.[72] Hypertrophic pulmonary osteopathy (HPO) is the most frequently reported syndrome in dogs, with less frequent occurrence in cats.[66, 72, 73]

Presentation. Dogs and cats that present with primary pulmonary tumors are usually middle-aged or older animals. The mean age at presentation is 9 to 12 years, with animals as young as 2 years reported.[65–67, 74] There is no sex or breed predisposition.

Client complaints can reflect respiratory signs, signs of metastases or HPO, or nonlocalizing signs, all of which are usually chronic. Respiratory system involvement is suggested by cough, exercise intolerance, respiratory distress, and, rarely, hemoptysis. The cough is generally nonproductive. Lameness or signs of dissemination to other organs

RES

occur from metastases or HPO. Nonlocalizing signs include weight loss, anorexia, and depression. Dysphagia, vomiting, and rarely ascites or edema of the head and neck also can occur.

Physical examination can reflect signs of respiratory disease, other organ involvement, or general debilitation. The lungs should be carefully ausculted for localized areas of increased or absent lung sounds, which can occur over regions of consolidation. Crackles or wheezes may be present as a result of infiltration, inflammation, or airway obstruction. Pleural effusion or pneumothorax may result in a generalized decrease in lung sounds. Lameness may be noted owing to bone metastases or HPO, and the involved limb may be swollen and painful. The animal may exhibit poor condition and weight loss.

Abnormalities may be discovered on physical examination that are unrelated to the pulmonary neoplasia, and the tumor may be an incidental finding. Occasionally animals are presented for primary tumors elsewhere in the body.

Diagnostic Evaluation. Thoracic radiographs are the most valuable diagnostic aid in the evaluation of animals with pulmonary neoplasia. They can provide preliminary or supportive evidence of neoplasia. They also can localize abnormal tissue within the lung, which is useful for the selection of collection techniques for retrieving lung specimens for cytologic or histologic analysis. Lung patterns due to neoplasia are quite varied and include single circumscribed mass lesions, lobar consolidation, multiple circumscribed masses, and diffuse involvement (Fig. 128–8). Because metastasis has frequently occurred at the time of diagnosis, diffuse involvement is common and can be demonstrated as reticular or nodular interstitial, alveolar, or peribronchial opacities. These patterns can occur alone or in combination. Cavitation of mass lesions, hilar lymphadenopathy, and calcification of lesions can be seen.[67]

Radiographs of the lungs have important limitations that must be considered. Radiographs are insensitive to masses less than approximately 1 cm in diameter (improving the sensitivity of thoracic radiographs is discussed in the section on metastatic pulmonary neoplasia). More important to the owner and the animal, a definitive diagnosis of neoplasia cannot be made based on radiographs alone. The signalment, history, physical findings, and radiographs may strongly suggest a neoplastic process, but the definitive diagnosis is obtained through cytologic or histologic evaluation of tissue. Conditions that can mimic pulmonary neoplasia to a surprising degree include infections (especially parasitic, fungal, and atypical bacterial), foreign body reactions, mineral oil aspiration, hypersensitivity and immune-mediated diseases, and lung lobe torsions. Lung tumors that result in diffuse radiographic patterns can be indistinguishable from bacterial infection, hemorrhage, and edema in addition to the previously mentioned diseases. All these conditions offer a significantly better prognosis than primary neoplasia and should be aggressively pursued whenever possible.

Pleural effusion or pneumothorax may be present radiographically in animals with pulmonary neoplasia.[65, 67] Neoplasia of the chest is a common cause of pleural effusion in small animals. Pneumothorax is much less common. Animals should be reevaluated radiographically following the removal of fluid or air from the pleural space to allow the lungs to expand fully for accurate radiographic evaluation.

Radiographs of the bones should be evaluated in animals presenting with lameness, limb pain, or swelling for evidence of HPO or bone metastases. Signs involving other organ systems also should be pursued.

A definitive diagnosis of pulmonary neoplasia requires the cytologic or histologic evaluation of specimens. Pleural fluid, tracheal washings, bronchial brushings, and bronchoalveolar lavage fluid can be evaluated cytologically. These specimens can be collected relatively noninvasively, but collected cells often do not allow a definitive diagnosis to be made. Interpretation of such specimens must be carefully performed. Inflammatory processes can result in cytologic criteria of malignancy, especially in cells such as the pleural mesothelium or respiratory epithelium. Furthermore, the presence of non-neoplastic abnormalities, such as bacterial infection, nonseptic inflammation, or hypersensitivity responses, does not totally eliminate the possibility of underlying neoplasia.

Transthoracic or transbronchial biopsies can be obtained from lesions near the thoracic wall or involving the major airways, respectively. Transthoracic needle biopsies are best

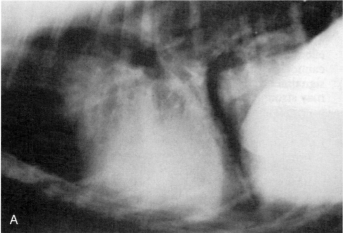

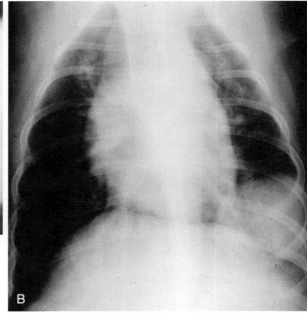

Figure 128–8. Radiographs showing a well-circumscribed mass in the left caudal lung lobe. A lobectomy was performed. The histologic diagnosis was pulmonary adenocarcinoma.

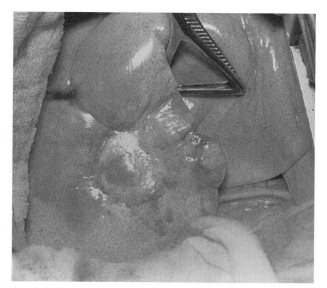

Figure 128–9. Papillary adenocarcinoma involving the left cranial lung lobe of a dog.

performed with fluoroscopic or ultrasonographic guidance. Peripheral lesions can be biopsied using two radiographic views to provide anatomic guidance. Transbronchial biopsies can be guided by visualization of lesions during bronchoscopy or fluoroscopy. A relatively small specimen is obtained and must be representative of the primary disease for an accurate diagnosis to be made. Potential complications include hemothorax, pneumothorax, and abscess rupture.

Thoracotomy is the most invasive method of obtaining lung tissue but has major advantages. Excellent specimens can be provided to the pathologist for analysis. Other lung lobes and regional lymph nodes can be examined and biopsied, and the treatment of choice, lobectomy, can be performed (Fig. 128–9).

In situations in which aggressive diagnostic evaluation is not desirable, further information can be obtained noninvasively by the repeated evaluation of thoracic radiographs over time. Radiographs taken every four to six weeks, depending on the rate of progression of clinical signs, can be evaluated to determine the course of the disease. If no change is seen radiographically after several months, the lesions may be non-neoplastic or extremely slow growing. If changes typical of malignant neoplasia occur rapidly, the clinical diagnosis of primary pulmonary neoplasia is more likely correct. This approach is not recommended for potentially resectable lesions, because the tumor may become nonresectable during the delay.

Computed tomography and thoracoscopy are being used more frequently in the evaluation of intrathoracic disease in dogs and cats. Their use is currently limited to specialized practices.

Treatment. Excision of tumor with wide surgical margins is the treatment of choice for primary pulmonary neoplasia. Lobectomy is usually required. If the disease is determined to be nonresectable at surgery, signs may be temporarily palliated with the excision of areas of major involvement. This improvement may be a result of relief of compression on adjacent tissues, elimination of sites of necrosis and inflammation, or improvement of V:Q relationships. Tumors that cannot be excised can be treated with systemic chemotherapeutic drugs, based on the tumor type, although promising results have not been published.

Prognosis. Benign neoplasia carries an excellent prognosis but is uncommon. The long-term prognosis for most primary pulmonary tumors is guarded and depends on whether metastasis has occurred. Therefore, early diagnosis and treatment are important.

A report of 15 dogs treated by lobectomy based on single lung lobe involvement without identifiable metastases or extrathoracic disease on preoperative evaluation demonstrated a mean survival of 10 months (range 7 to 19 months) in the 9 dogs that had died and a mean survival of 20 months (range 8 to 46 months) in the 6 dogs that were alive and asymptomatic at the time of publication.[75] Although the statistical significance was not present, dogs with adenocarcinoma had longer mean survival times than dogs with squamous cell carcinoma, and dogs without lymph node metastasis had longer survival times than those with lymph node involvement. A multicenter study of 76 dogs with primary lung tumors that underwent surgical excision found that remission was induced in 55 dogs based on the elimination of macroscopic evidence of tumor.[76] The dogs that went into remission had a median survival of 330 days, with 10 dogs alive at the conclusion of the study. Those dogs that did not go into remission had a median survival of 28 days. The absence of enlarged regional lymph nodes before or at the time of surgery was a good prognostic sign. A study in cats had similar findings, with a favorable prognosis associated with a lack of metastasis or lymph node involvement. Of 21 cats, 7 were still alive and asymptomatic 119 to 634 days after surgery.[77]

METASTATIC PULMONARY NEOPLASIA

The lungs are the most common site of distant metastasis. The lungs contain the first capillary system through which most circulating neoplastic cells pass.[72] Any malignant tumor can result in metastatic disease. Pulmonary metastases from thyroid carcinoma, mammary carcinoma, osteosarcoma, hemangiosarcoma, transitional cell carcinoma, oral and digital melanoma, and squamous cell carcinoma are common. Metastatic disease is often the limiting factor in the treatment of primary malignancies.

Detection of metastases is routinely attempted through the evaluation of thoracic radiographs because of the high incidence of metastases to the lung and the ability to detect metastases in the lung because of contrast with air. Unfortunately, the discovery of metastases on thoracic radiographs represents a late finding in the course of disease.

Presentation. Animals with pulmonary metastatic disease can be presented for signs caused by the primary tumor or for signs caused by the pulmonary involvement. The presenting signs related to pulmonary disease are similar to those described for primary pulmonary neoplasia.

Diagnostic Evaluation. A presumptive diagnosis of pulmonary metastatic disease is made on the basis of a histopathologically diagnosed primary malignant tumor and suggestive thoracic radiographs. Radiographic patterns associated with metastasis are the same as those described for metastasized primary pulmonary neoplasia (Figs. 128–10 and 128–11).

Clinical evidence may be sufficiently convincing to discontinue the diagnostic evaluation at this point, but the clinician should be aware that erroneous conclusions are occasionally reached owing to a lack of specificity of radiographic findings. A diagnosis of pulmonary metastases may be incorrectly made as a result of two primary tumors in

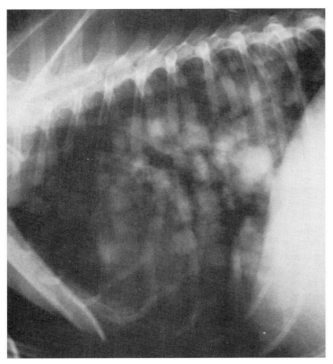

Figure 128–10. A reticular interstitial pattern with multiple nodules throughout the lung fields is suggestive of metastatic neoplasia. Fungal infection, immune-mediated disease, or other inflammatory processes must be included in the differential diagnoses and are supported by the ill-defined borders of many of the nodules. This animal had had a malignant melanoma removed from a distal limb previously, and the tumor had metastasized to the lung.

the same animal or because of misinterpretation of benign radiographic lesions. Fifteen of 29 dogs with primary pulmonary neoplasia were found to have coincidental tumors at other sites in the body.[66] In another report, two cats with mammary tumors had pulmonary masses; one was an abscess, and one was a primary lung tumor.[78] In these cases,

the pulmonary lesions were not the result of metastasis from the extrapulmonary tumors.

Benign radiographic lesions that can be misinterpreted as metastatic disease can occur as a result of atypical bacterial infections, immune-mediated or hypersensitivity diseases, parasitic infections, fungal infections, and other non-neoplastic diseases. Nonprogressive, non-neoplastic, diffuse nodular patterns, with or without mineralization, have been reported in 10 per cent of older dogs.[79] A definitive diagnosis of metastatic neoplasia is obtained through the cytologic or histologic evaluation of specimens as described for primary pulmonary tumors. Reevaluation of the animal radiographically at one- to two-month intervals can be useful in these cases.

The relative insensitivity of thoracic radiographs is well established and must be considered when radiographs are used for the detection of metastases, whether for general screening purposes or when a primary malignancy has been diagnosed. Under the best circumstances, thoracic radiographs can detect only lesions greater than 3 to 5 mm in diameter.[80] One study showed that conventional radiographs failed to detect 25 per cent of canine pulmonary metastases that were found at necropsy.[81] Three of eight dogs with pulmonary metastases from transitional cell carcinoma of the bladder were not diagnosed radiographically because the unstructured interstitial densities were interpreted as compatible with age.[82] Sensitivity can be improved by performing both right and left lateral recumbent views and by having multiple readers interpret the radiographs.[83] Improved sensitivity from two lateral views can be attributed to increased contrast in the well-aerated, nondependent lung lobes and magnification of the lung farthest from the film (Fig. 128–12).[83, 84] Radiographs should be exposed during full inspiration. If pleural effusion is present, the fluid should be removed and radiographs taken again with the lungs fully expanded.

Treatment. Surgical excision of metastatic lesions could potentially contribute to cure of disease and may palliate clinical signs. Unfortunately, metastatic disease is rarely identified before the development of diffuse, nonresectable pulmonary lesions. Chemotherapeutic agents are recom-

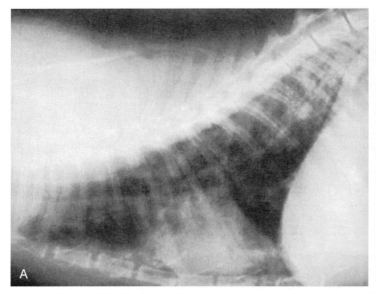

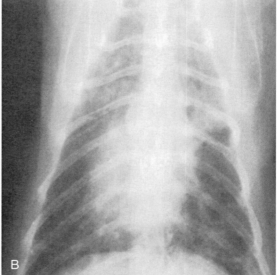

Figure 128–11. A cat with metastatic mammary gland carcinoma. The metastases are represented by a marked, diffuse interstitial pattern. A bronchial component also is visible.

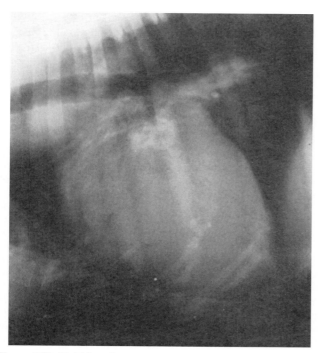

Figure 128–12. This radiograph is from the same dog as Figure 128–18 but was exposed with the animal in left lateral recumbency rather than right. The absence of air contrast in the poorly ventilated dependent lobes obscures the presence of the infiltrated lobe. Because of this effect, both lateral views should be taken to improve the sensitivity of radiographs used to screen for neoplastic disease.

mended based on the sensitivity of the primary tumor. The advanced stage at which metastases are detected may account for a generally poor long-term response.[72] Other potential treatment modalities include immunotherapy and anti-metastatic drugs.

Prognosis. The long-term prognosis for animals with pulmonary metastatic disease is grave. Therefore, the clinician should be extremely careful in making the diagnosis.

LYMPHOMA

Lymphoma can involve the pulmonary parenchyma in the multicentric form of the disease in dogs and cats (see also Chapter 98). Primary pulmonary lymphoma, which can occur in people, has not been reported.

Lung involvement is present in approximately 66 percent of dogs with multicentric lymphoma based histologic findings and bronchoalveolar lavage, although supportive radiographic changes are present in only about 33 percent of cases.[85]

Thoracic radiographs reveal an irregular reticular pattern, often with ill-defined nodular densities. Hilar, mediastinal, or sternal lymphadenopathy may be apparent (Fig. 128–13). Rarely, a single mass lesion or a peribronchial pattern occurs. Radiographic changes are similar to changes caused by inflammatory pulmonary diseases.

Neoplastic cells within the lungs may be identifiable in bronchoalveolar lavage fluid, lung aspirates, or histologic specimens, but the disease is generally diagnosed through other more accessible systems, such as the peripheral lymph nodes.

LYMPHOMATOID GRANULOMATOSIS

Lymphomatoid granulomatosis has been considered an immune-mediated vasculitis. More recent immunologic evidence in humans and dogs, in conjunction with clinical experience, supports the classification of this disease as a low-grade lymphoma.[86, 87] The disease is characterized by infiltrates of pleomorphic lymphoreticular cells, plasmacytoid cells, eosinophils, lymphocytes, and plasma cells sur-

RES

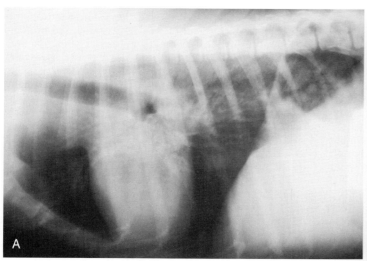

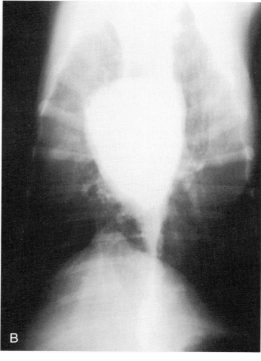

Figure 128–13. *A* and *B,* These radiographs demonstrate an increased interstitial pattern and hilar lymphadenopathy compatible with pulmonary involvement with multicentric malignant lymphoma. Inflammatory diseases or other neoplasia could result in a similar pattern.

rounding and invading the walls of small blood vessels.[60, 61] Thrombosis and necrosis of adjacent lung may be present.[60, 61] Morphologic criteria of malignancy are seen, and intrathoracic lymph nodes also may be infiltrated.[60, 61]

Presentation. Lymphomatoid granulomatosis has been described only in the dog. There is no obvious age or breed predisposition. Reported cases have ranged in age from 18 months to 14 years.[60, 61] Dogs present with any combination of respiratory signs, particularly cough and respiratory distress. Signs are usually slowly progressive. Increased breath sounds, crackles, or wheezes may be ausculted. Fever, anorexia, and weight loss may occur.

Diagnostic Evaluation. Thoracic radiographs reveal an interstitial pattern with multiple ill-defined nodules of varying size.[60, 61] Lobar consolidation can occur in one or several lobes.[60, 61] Hilar lymphadenopathy is frequently present.[60, 61] A peripheral basophilia, with or without eosinophilia, has been reported in some cases.[60] Heartworm tests and fungal serology should be performed.

Cytologic evaluation of tracheal wash fluid, bronchoalveolar lavage fluid, or lung aspirates reveals eosinophilic and neutrophilic inflammation with reactive macrophages.[60] Lymphocytes and plasma cells may also be present. Slides should be carefully examined for infectious agents. Special stains for fungal organisms or *Mycobacterium* should be considered. Histopathologic evaluation of a biopsy is required for a definitive diagnosis.

Treatment. Treatment consists of immune suppression and should be withheld pending the elimination of infectious differential diagnoses. Combination chemotherapy is recommended, as described from lymphoma (see Chapter 98). Response to prednisone alone is often poor.[60]

Prognosis. Prognosis is difficult to address because of the lack of clinical reports. Of five reported cases treated with prednisone and clyclophosphamide, three were still in complete remission 19, 27, and 32 months from the time of treatment.[60] One dog was euthanized for continued respiratory distress after six months. The other dog did not respond to treatment and developed multicentric malignant lymphoma six weeks later.

MALIGNANT HISTIOCYTOSIS

Malignant histiocytosis is a malignant proliferative disorder of morphologically atypical histiocytes and their precursors. It has been reported primarily in Bernese Mountain Dogs but has also been diagnosed in golden retrievers, rottweilers, and other dogs.[88, 89] It is believed to be inherited with a polygenic mode of inheritance in Bernese Mountain Dogs.[89] Infiltration frequently involves the lungs and lymph nodes, with infiltration also noted in liver, spleen, and other organs.[88, 89]

The majority of dogs are middle to older aged.[88–90] In a report of 15 dogs, 8 were presented with cough or respiratory distress.[90] Anorexia, weight loss, lethargy, and anemia are common complaints.[90] Radiographic abnormalities of the thorax include single or multiple mass lesions, hilar lymphadenopathy, mediastinal masses, and pleural effusion.[90]

Histopathologic examination of tissues is necessary for a diagnosis. The tumor may be difficult to distinguish from anaplastic carcinoma on light microscopic examination alone, and staining with specific markers may be necessary.[88] A review of pathologic specimens found some "hybrid" neoplasms with characteristics of both malignant histiocytosis and malignant fibrous histiocytoma.[89]

No treatment has been reported for this disease. Surgical therapy alone is unlikely to be curative owing to the presence of metastasis at the time of diagnosis. Chemotherapy with doxorubicin, cyclophosphamide, and vincristine has been useful in the treatment of a few cases.[91] The prognosis is poor.

PULMONARY THROMBOEMBOLIC DISEASE

Pulmonary thromboembolism (PTE) is a relatively common disease but is often unrecognized.[92] Lack of clinician awareness and the inability to readily make a definitive diagnosis interfere with the antemortem identification of these animals. Even with necropsy, identification requires examination of relatively fresh tissues and careful evaluation. It is essential that clinicians maintain a high index of suspicion for this disease in animals presented with tachypnea, dyspnea, or conditions associated with PTE if it is to be diagnosed and treated effectively.

Pulmonary thromboembolic disease is the result of the obstruction of pulmonary arteries and arterioles. The lungs can usually cope with small amounts of emboli and may serve a beneficial function in preventing emboli from reaching the systemic circulation and causing ischemic damage to less tolerant organs such as the kidneys, brain, or heart. Emboli can consist of bacteria, foreign bodies (e.g., intravenous catheters), air, fat, or parasites. The majority of emboli are fragments of thrombi (clots). Thrombi can develop within vessels of the lungs themselves or elsewhere in the body as a result of stasis of blood, damage to the endothelial lining of blood vessels, and systemic hypercoagulability. Blood clots are normally eliminated shortly after they form by the fibrinolytic system. In disease states, the balance between formation and dissolution is disturbed.

Multiple factors associated with PTE result in pulmonary failure. The principal result of interference in pulmonary blood flow is abnormal V:Q relationships within the lung. Ventilated regions are not perfused, resulting in regions of high V:Q or alveolar dead space. In addition, platelet degranulation can lead to vasoconstriction and bronchoconstriction, further compromising pulmonary function and contributing to pulmonary hypertension and increased workload of the right heart. Other effects of PTE that can contribute to pulmonary dysfunction include decreased surfactant production, development of pulmonary edema due to overcirculation of unaffected regions of lung, pulmonary infarction (ischemic necrosis), and development of mild pleural effusion.[93, 94] These effects of PTE result in tachypnea or dyspnea as a result of hypoxia or as a reflex initiated by receptors in the pulmonary artery.[95]

The most commonly recognized cause of PTE in small animal medicine is dirofilariasis. Other diseases that have been associated with the condition in dogs include cardiac disease, nephrotic syndrome, immune-mediated hemolytic anemia, neoplasia, sepsis, pancreatitis, hyperadrenocorticism, and disseminated intravascular coagulation.[92, 96–98] Cardiac diseases associated with PTE, in addition to heartworm disease, include cardiomyopathy, chronic valvular insufficiency, and bacterial endocarditis.[92, 93] Other conditions that can potentially result in PTE include surgery, severe trauma, hyperlipidemia, and hyperviscosity syndromes. There is little reference to feline PTE in the literature, although it is known to occur.

Presentation. Animals classically experience a peracute

onset of extremely severe respiratory distress and tachypnea that are poorly responsive to routine supportive measures. Less severely affected animals may demonstrate tachypnea only. Tachycardia is often present.[92] A loud or split second heart sound may occur as a result of pulmonary hypertension. Occasionally, cough, hemoptysis, or crackles may be present. Signs may be present related to a predisposing disease process.

Diagnostic Evaluation. Thoracic radiographs can be surprisingly normal. An animal with profound respiratory distress and minimal radiographic changes should immediately be suspected of having PTE. The predominant lung patterns reported in 21 dogs with confirmed PTE were hyperlucent zones due to regional loss of blood flow, and alveolar pulmonary infiltrates secondary to edema or hemorrhage (Fig. 128–14).[98] The alveolar infiltrates were described as having indistinct margins, as resulting in lobar consolidation, or as being triangular in shape with the base toward the heart.[98] Other potential abnormalities include interstitial pattern, mild pleural effusion, heart enlargement, and main pulmonary artery enlargement.[92, 98] Unique features associated with dirofilariasis are discussed in Chapter 119.

Arterial blood gas analysis is particularly useful in identifying pulmonary dysfunction. Typical abnormalities are hypoxemia and hypocapnia. Hypercapnia can occur with extremely severe compromise. In people, normal arterial oxygen tension does not rule out PTE.[99] Calculation of the alveolar-arterial oxygen gradient, $P_{(A-a)}O_2$, provides a more sensitive indicator of the disease and is abnormal in 95 per cent of human patients.[99] The gradient is widened in cases of PTE owing to V:Q abnormalities.

Routine blood testing is not helpful in the diagnosis of PTE. It may be useful in identifying predisposing diseases.

A definitive diagnosis of PTE is obtained with contrast radiography. The study should be performed early in the course of disease, before the partial dissolution of clots. Ideally, contrast material is injected through a catheter placed in the pulmonary artery; however, nonselective angiography can be used and is a more practical technique. A positive angiogram reveals filling defects or sudden interruptions in blood flow. Tortuous pulmonary arteries, decreased pulmonary perfusion, and delayed venous return to the left atrium are not specific for PTE.[97]

Ventilation and perfusion scanning with radioisotopes can also be performed to confirm a diagnosis of PTE. These procedures are associated with fewer complications than angiography, but the facilities for such testing in animals are limited. Perfusion studies are performed by injecting radionucleotide-labeled albumin into a peripheral vein. The particles are trapped in the pulmonary capillaries, and imaging demonstrates pulmonary blood flow (Fig. 128–15). If the perfusion scan is abnormal, ventilation scans are performed to determine whether hypoventilation could explain the decreased perfusion. It is normal for the lungs to shunt blood away from regions of the lung that have decreased ventilation (e.g., due to pneumonia or edema) in order to match ventilation and perfusion. PTE typically results in abnormal perfusion in areas with normal ventilation. Ventilation scans are not always available, even at referral hospitals. In such situations, a presumption of normal ventilation is based on an absence of abnormal radiographic densities in the region of abnormal perfusion. Unfortunately, several other factors can also result in abnormal perfusion scans, and all available clinical information must be considered in making the diagnosis; however, a normal scan can be used to rule out PTE.

Treatment. Animals with acute, severe PTE are treated for cardiovascular shock, administered oxygen, and given

RES

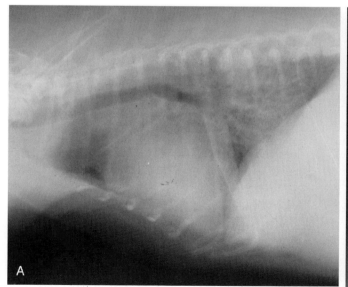

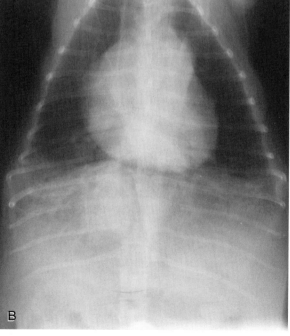

Figure 128–14. Dog with pulmonary thromboembolism. Air bronchograms in the caudal lung lobes (*A* and *B*) and lobar sign visible on the lateral view (*A*) are probably the result of edema and hemorrhage. Right heart enlargement is present. The pulmonary artery to the right caudal lung lobe was dilated, but this change cannot be appreciated in these reproductions. This dog had several radiographic signs supporting a diagnosis of pulmonary thromboembolism; however, thoracic radiographs can be completely normal or demonstrate a wide variety of patterns.

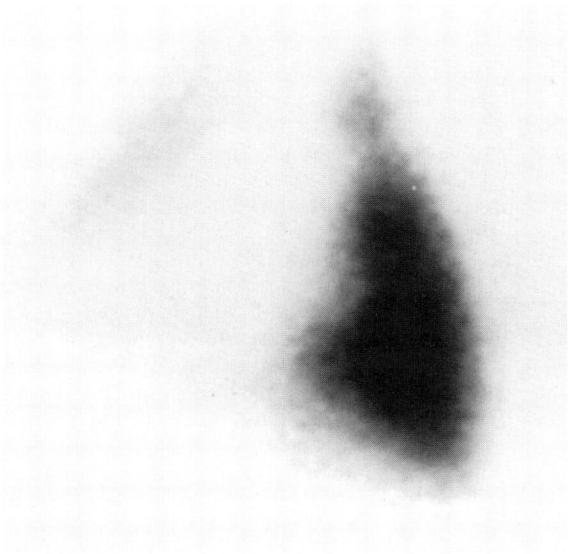

Figure 128–15. Perfusion scan of the lungs of a dog with pulmonary thromboembolism. The left lung has normal uptake of radionucleotide, represented by the dark shadow. The right lung has almost no uptake, indicating nearly complete arterial obstruction. Thoracic radiographs of this dog were unremarkable.

high doses of rapid-acting corticosteroids (e.g., prednisolone sodium succinate 10 mg/lb, or 22 mg/kg, intravenously). Dogs or cats with PTE secondary to adulticide treatment for dirofilariasis may not require further treatment. Even if clinical improvement with oxygen therapy is not obvious, administration should be continued to inhibit pulmonary vasoconstriction.

Anticoagulant therapy with heparin, and possibly warfarin, is administered to prevent further clot formation. These drugs have no effect on the existing emboli. Hemorrhage is a potential complication, and treatment is reserved for animals in which there is a high degree of suspicion for PTE. Therapeutic recommendations are based largely on limited clinical experience and human trials.

Several protocols have been suggested for heparin use in animals.[93][97][100] One protocol is an initial dosage of 90 to 135 U/lb (200 to 300 U/kg) subcutaneously every 8 hours.[100] Regardless of the administration regimen used initially, the dosage must be modified on an individual basis to maintain the partial thromboplastin time (PTT) at 1.5 to 2.5 times normal, or the activated clotting time (ACT) at 1.2 to 1.4 times normal. Clotting times are measured before initiating heparin for baseline values, and two hours after administration of a subcutaneous dose for determination of maximal effect.[95][100] Fresh or fresh frozen plasma should be administered to animals with possible antithrombin III deficiencies, such as those with nephrotic syndrome.

Excessive anticoagulation with heparin can result in hemorrhage. If clotting times are greatly prolonged or hemorrhage occurs, heparin is discontinued. Protamine sulfate can be administered to antagonize heparin if discontinuation alone is not effective. When heparin therapy is no longer needed, gradual discontinuation over several days may be advisable to prevent rebound hypercoagulable effects.

Treatment with heparin can be continued at home with subcutaneous injections. Animals that require prolonged treatment, usually because of a persistent predisposing problem that cannot be resolved, can be maintained with oral warfarin. Fatal hemorrhage is a potential side effect of treatment, and these animals must be monitored frequently. Again, treatment is based largely on information from humans and limited clinical experience in animals.

Warfarin is administered initially at a dosage of 0.05 to 0.1 mg/lb (0.1 to 0.2 mg/kg) orally every 24 hours (0.5 mg, total, for most cats), while continuing administration of heparin.[100][101] The dosage is modified after four to five days of administration to maintain a prothrombin time (PT) that is 1.5 to 2 times longer than baseline. A safer value than PT for monitoring the effect of warfarin is the international normalization ratio (INR).[101] The INR is derived from the PT, taking into account the variable strength of reagents used to run the PT. The INR or the formula for its calculation is available from the commercial laboratory performing the PT or from the company that produces the in-office kit being used. The goal of warfarin therapy is an INR of 2.0 to 3.0. Once this effect is achieved, heparin is discontinued. Some dogs and cats will maintain prolonged clotting times when administration is decreased to every 48 hours after the initial four to five days of treatment.[100] Clotting times are measured every five days initially, with the interval gradually prolonged to every four to six weeks.

Hemorrhage secondary to warfarin toxicity is treated with transfusions of fresh or fresh frozen plasma. Vitamin K_1 is administered if necessary but will prevent further anticoagulation with warfarin for up to three weeks.[100] Several commonly used drugs can interact with warfarin. The reader is advised to review the pharmacology of warfarin before using it.

Thrombolytic drugs, such as tissue plasminogen activator, have great potential for the treatment of PTE because existing clots can be dissolved. Thrombolytic drugs have not gained widespread acceptance in veterinary medicine owing to expense and lack of selectivity.

Prognosis. The prognosis is variable, depending on the severity of disease and the ability to correct predisposing problems. In most cases, the prognosis is guarded to poor.

Prevention. No studies are available in dogs or cats to determine the success of prophylactic treatment for PTE in animals at risk. The serious nature of the disease and experience in people provide some rationale for preventive therapy in high-risk animals. If prophylaxis is desired, heparin can be administered at low dosages (30 U/lb, or 70 U/kg, subcutaneously every 8 to 12 hours).[97] Such dosages are not expected to prolong ACT or PTT and in people have not resulted in excessive hemorrhage during surgery.[97] Treatment is discontinued once the predisposing factor has been controlled.

PULMONARY HYPERTENSION

Pulmonary hypertension is defined as increased pulmonary arterial pressure (in people, mean pulmonary artery pressure >25 mmHg), and it is almost always a secondary problem.[102] Causes can be classified as precapillary and postcapillary.[103] Precapillary causes include lung disease, PTE, congenital heart disease, pulmonary vasculitis, high-altitude disease, and pulmonary arteriovenous fistula.[103][104] Alveolar hypoxia, as a result of lung disease or high altitude, causes local vasoconstriction. Congenital heart diseases causing left-to-right shunts (e.g., patent ductus arteriosus and septal defects) result in increased pulmonary blood flow. A common precapillary cause of pulmonary hypertension in veterinary patients is heartworm disease. Postcapillary causes result in increased left atrial or pulmonary venous pressures and include left ventricular failure, mitral insufficiency or stenosis, left atrial masses (thrombus or neoplasia), and pulmonary venous obstruction.[103, 104] Although acutely pulmonary hypertension may be reversible, by the time of diagnosis, irreversible arterial changes secondary to the elevated pressures may have occurred.

The right heart is secondarily affected by the pressure overload, and dilatation and hypertrophy can develop. Decreased cardiac index can result in clinical signs. Cor pulmonale refers to the cardiac changes that occur in response to pulmonary hypertension from respiratory causes. With progression, overt right heart failure can develop.

Presentation. In veterinary patients, pulmonary hypertension is generally recognized during the evaluation of animals with chronic lung disease or right heart failure. Exercise intolerance, respiratory distress, or cough may be present. Pronounced or split second heart sounds may be auscultable, providing a valuable clue.

Diagnostic Evaluation. Thoracic radiographs can be normal. Right heart enlargement, enlarged pulmonary arteries, or evidence of primary pulmonary disease may be observed. Echocardiography may be a more sensitive indicator of right heart involvement, particularly in cats. Echocardiography with flow measurements can be used to estimate pulmonary pressure in some cases. Arterial blood gas measurements are useful for identifying hypoxemia. If pulmonary hypertension is suspected based on clinical evidence, a complete cardiac and respiratory evaluation is indicated to identify the primary disease. A definitive diagnosis of pulmonary hypertension requires cardiac catheterization. Risks and the need for specialized equipment generally necessitate referral for this procedure.

Treatment. Treatment is aimed at eliminating the primary cause whenever possible. For irreversible respiratory causes of pulmonary hypertension (e.g., chronic obstructive disease), oxygen therapy has been found to decrease hypertension and prolong survival in people.[103] In animals, chronic administration of oxygen is rarely feasible, but in the acute setting (such as PTE), oxygen supplementation is a crucial component of treatment.

Use of vasodilator drugs is controversial. The effect on the pulmonary vasculature in individual dogs is unpredictable, and the side effects of systemic hypotension and tachycardia can contribute to right heart dysfunction. Therefore, test doses of drug must be given while monitoring pulmonary and systemic blood pressures by cardiac catheterization before treatment is prescribed.[102, 104] Hydralazine and nifedipine have been proposed.[102, 104]

Theophyllines are recommended for animals with hypertension secondary to chronic pulmonary disease. Potential benefits in small animals include pulmonary vasodilatation, bronchodilatation, improvement of diaphragmatic contractility, and decreased respiratory muscle fatigue.[102]

Prognosis. Prognosis is dependent on the reversibility of the underlying disease and the extent of irreversible damage to the pulmonary arteries. Monitoring of animals with repeated radiographs, echocardiograms, and arterial blood gas analysis may provide some indication of progression for individual animals.

PULMONARY EDEMA

Pulmonary edema is the accumulation of excess fluid within the lungs. Fluid balance within the lung is a dynamic process with many determinants. As in other parts of the body, homeostasis is dependent on vascular and interstitial hydrostatic and oncotic pressure and vascular permeability. Blood flow, lymphatic drainage, and surfactant also contribute. There are some differences in fluid homeostasis in the lungs compared with systemic capillary beds.[105] The hydrostatic pressure in pulmonary capillaries is relatively low. Lymphatic flow in the lungs can be relatively high, possibly owing to the continual pumping action of the lungs with respiration. With chronic elevations in capillary pressures, the lymphatics can greatly expand and further increase their ability to remove excess fluid. Surfactant decreases alveolar surface tension, decreasing the tendency of fluid to be drawn into the alveoli. Because of these mechanisms, capillary hydrostatic pressures must acutely reach 23 mmHg before edema develops.[105] Pressures in excess of 40 mmHg can occur with chronic disease without the formation of edema.[105] Normal pulmonary wedge pressures in the dog (an estimate of capillary hydrostatic pressure) average approximately 5 mmHg.[106] Pulmonary edema occurs secondary to a disease process that upsets the balance of fluid accumulation and removal. It is not a primary disease.

Excess fluid within the lungs initially accumulates perivascularly and peribronchially in the interstitium. With increasing volumes, alveoli become flooded. This edema results in pulmonary dysfunction through several mechanisms. Obviously, the filling of alveoli with fluid prevents ventilation of affected regions of lung. In addition, dilution of surfactant contributes to decreased lung compliance. Increased airway resistance occurs because of edema involving the airway walls, pressure from the fluid in peribronchial tissues, and, possibly, bronchoconstriction. Other factors may also be involved. The result of these changes is V:Q mismatching, and hypoxemia occurs. With severe edema, shunting develops, and the hypoxemia becomes refractory to oxygen supplementation.

Causes of pulmonary edema can be grouped based on the major mechanism resulting in edema formation: decreased plasma oncotic pressure, vascular overload, lymphatic obstruction, increased vascular permeability, and miscellaneous or unknown mechanisms. Decreased plasma oncotic pressure occurs with low concentrations of serum albumin. Hypoalbuminemia alone is unlikely to cause pulmonary edema; however, it can be a contributing factor in conjunction with other predisposing problems. Albumin concentrations associated with edema formation are usually less than 1 g/dL. Subcutaneous edema often occurs prior to pulmonary edema. Transudative pleural effusion may also be present. In the hospital setting, excessive fluid administration resulting in vascular overload in conjunction with hypoalbuminemia is a cause of pulmonary edema. Causes of hypoalbuminemia are identified in Chapter 141. Vasculitis can cause hypoalbuminemia in conjunction with increased permeability.

Vascular overload can result from overcirculation (increased blood flow) or increased hydrostatic pressure. Cardiac disease and excessive fluid administration are the most common causes of vascular overload. Left heart failure, often due to mitral insufficiency or pump failure, is the most common cause of pulmonary edema. Left-to-right shunts and obstruction of the left atrium or pulmonary veins due to masses are less common.

Lymphatic obstruction is an uncommon cause of pulmonary edema in dogs and cats. It is usually the result of neoplasia.

Edema due to increased vascular permeability is seen in conjunction with a wide variety of pulmonary and systemic

RES

disorders. The edema, by definition, is noncardiogenic and therefore is associated with normal pulmonary wedge pressures. Because the fluid results from vascular leakage, it is relatively proteinaceous and does not readily resolve with diuretic therapy.

Acute respiratory distress syndrome (ARDS) is a form of noncardiogenic pulmonary edema. Clinically, it is identified by the severity and rapid progression of signs, although specific histologic changes occur. The wide variation in causes and severity of ARDS in people has led Murray et al. to recommend a system to be used in describing patients with this syndrome.[107] Although not all parts of their classification scheme are practical in veterinary medicine, the principles should be applied whenever possible. The description consists of chronicity, severity, and underlying cause of ARDS. Chronicity is categorized as acute or chronic. Both acute and chronic ARDS are associated with hypoxia and decreased compliance. Acute ARDS is characterized by a sudden onset of signs, with alveolar infiltrates apparent radiographically. Histologic changes include endothelial and epithelial injury, development of hyaline membranes, and the presence of edema and hemorrhage. Chronic ARDS can develop in as little as three days. Radiographic infiltrates become more organized, epithelial hypertrophy occurs, and fibrosis begins. Complete recovery from chronic change may be slow and incomplete. Severity of ARDS is determined by degree of lung involvement radiographically, blood gas analysis, and results of other pulmonary function tests.

ARDS can occur secondary to pulmonary or systemic disease. Strictly speaking, almost any inflammatory disease of the lung has a component of edema. Clinically, the signs and management of such diseases relate primarily to the inflammatory component rather than to the edema. Pulmonary diseases in which edema can result in significant signs include inhalation trauma (such as smoke inhalation, gastric acid aspiration, near drowning, and oxygen toxicity) and direct trauma (pulmonary contusions).[108] Systemic diseases that have been associated with ARDS include sepsis and endotoxemia, including parvovirus infection; pancreatitis; severe uremia; major trauma; drugs or toxins, such as cis-platinum in cats, snake venom, and paraquat; electrocution; and disseminated intravascular coagulation.[107–110] The most common causes of ARDS in a recent retrospective study were microbial pneumonia, sepsis, and aspiration pneumonia.[111]

Several other diseases have been associated with noncardiogenic pulmonary edema, although the mechanisms are not well understood. These include PTE; upper airway obstruction; neurogenic edema, often secondary to seizures or head trauma; and liver disease, unrelated to hypoalbuminemia.[106] Surprisingly, upper airway obstruction need only be transient.[112] Vasculitis, of infectious or noninfectious origin, is another cause.

Presentation. Animals with pulmonary edema show acute or subacute signs typical of lower respiratory tract disease. Depending on the severity of edema, signs can range from tachypnea alone to marked respiratory distress with blood-tinged froth visible from the mouth or nares. Dogs may present with cough, crackles, and/or wheezing that is most pronounced in the central or caudodorsal regions rather than cranioventrally, as is typical of bacterial pneumonia. Because pulmonary edema is a secondary phenomenon, historic and physical signs reflecting the underlying disease are often present. Careful questioning of the owner related to the differential diagnoses described earlier is indicated.

Cardiac auscultation and assessment of pulses are critical in the early identification of cardiogenic pulmonary edema.

Diagnostic Evaluation. As for all respiratory patients, the stress of obtaining diagnostic information must be weighed against its immediate value. Severely compromised animals are treated based only on presenting signs. Cardiac disease is usually suspected based on presenting information and can be investigated further by electrocardiogram with minimal stress. Animals with suspected hypoalbuminemia can be screened with plasma protein measurement by refractometer. Following stabilization, thoracic radiography and complete systemic evaluation are performed.

Thoracic radiographs may be normal early in the development of edema. Interstitial densities appear, followed by an alveolar pattern demonstrating alveolar flooding. In dogs with cardiogenic edema, the lesions are usually most prominent in the perihilar regions. Cats with heart failure may have patchy areas of edema. Edema secondary to increased vascular permeability is often most pronounced in the caudodorsal regions (Fig. 128–16).[112] Radiographs are carefully evaluated for signs of heart disease, venous congestion, PTE, lymphadenopathy, and pleural effusion.

Echocardiography is extremely valuable for evaluating the heart. Heart failure is a common cause of edema in veterinary patients, and determining the underlying heart disease is helpful in both treatment and prognosis. Echocardiography is useful in ruling out subtle cardiac disease.

CBC, serum biochemical analysis, and urinalysis are helpful in evaluating the systemic status of the animal. Arterial blood gas analysis is useful for determining the severity of disease and response to therapeutic intervention. Acid-base measurements also assist in patient management.

Pulmonary specimens are usually not specific or helpful, unless primary pulmonary disease is suspected. Mild neutrophilic inflammation and slight hemorrhage are commonly seen.

Treatment. Oxygen supplementation, cage rest, and possibly sedation and bronchodilators are used initially to stabilize animals with pulmonary edema. Further treatment depends on the underlying mechanism that is responsible. Oxygen should initially be provided by the least stressful method possible. If an adequate response is not seen, intubation and positive-pressure ventilation may be required. Cage rest is extremely valuable for decreasing overall oxygen requirement and cardiac workload. Sedation can be helpful for the same reasons and can also decrease anxiety. Morphine sulfate is administered to dogs as intravenous boluses of 0.05 mg/lb (0.1 mg/kg), to effect. Adverse effects of morphine are less predictable in cats, and its use is not suggested. Acepromazine can be administered at 0.02 mg/lb (0.05 mg/kg) intravenously or subcutaneously, to effect. Methylxanthines are mild diuretics and may decrease ventilatory muscle fatigue, in addition to their bronchodilating effect.

Diuretics are indicated for treatment of some forms of edema, but in hypovolemic animals, they can cause further deterioration of cardiac output. Cautious administration of fluid may actually be necessary. Maintenance of vascular volume or cardiac output may be facilitated by the concurrent administration of plasma or hetastarch to animals with hypoalbuminemia or positive inotropes to animals in heart failure.

Animals with edema due to decreased oncotic pressure are treated with plasma infusions. Edema fluid will be mobilized at less than normal plasma protein concentrations. Diuretics are useful if adequate plasma volume can be main-

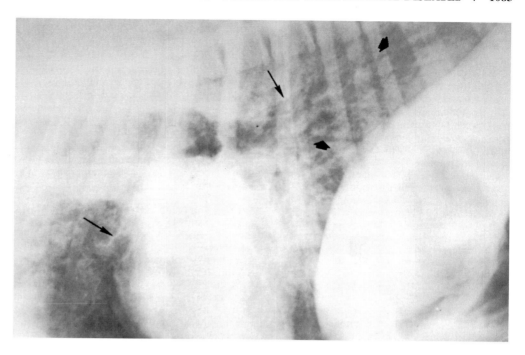

Figure 128–16. Lateral radiograph of a 4-month-old Great Dane with severe noncardiogenic pulmonary edema caused by smoke inhalation. The lung field appears mottled, and blotchy or grainy confluent densities are present. Air bronchograms (*wide arrows*) are seen, supporting a radiographic diagnosis of a disseminated alveolar pulmonary pattern. A number of ill-defined lines are seen in the dense lung field (*small arrows*). They represent an increased density of the bronchial walls and are due to edema of the bronchial walls and peribronchial tissue. The cardiac silhouette is partially obscured by the increased pulmonary density; nonetheless, one can assume that no significant cardiomegaly is present. The involvement of all lung lobes and the normal-appearing peripheries of the cranial and middle lobes are compatible with a diagnosis of lung edema rather than pneumonia. (Courtesy of S. J. Ettinger.)

tained. Aggressive management of the underlying disease is necessary, and attention must be paid to the nutritional requirements of the animal.

Edema due to volume overload from excessive fluid administration often resolves upon discontinuation of fluids. Furosemide (0.5 to 1 mg/lb, or 1 to 2 mg/kg, intravenously or subcutaneously) is administered to treat marked edema. The healthy body can adapt to large volume excesses. Consideration should be given to the possibility of subtle cardiac or renal disease in these animals. Pulmonary edema due to heart failure is discussed in Chapter 110.

Edema due to increased vascular permeability is difficult to treat. Some mild cases respond to cage rest and oxygen supplementation alone. Unfortunately, most animals with ARDS do not respond adequately. Positive-pressure ventilation, usually with PEEP, is needed. Diuretics can be administered to normovolemic animals, but they are minimally effective in most ARDS patients. The use of corticosteroids is controversial. No clear benefit is obtained from their use, except in the treatment of shock. Positive inotropes (dobutamine) may be necessary to maintain adequate cardiac output, particularly with positive-pressure ventilation. Their use in conjunction with vasodilators has been suggested, but detrimental effects such as increased shunting have also been reported.[108, 113] Other novel approaches to treatment under investigation include inhaled nitric oxide, antibodies against tumor necrosis factor, surfactant replacement, free radical scavengers, and a variety of anti-inflammatory agents.[108, 114] Management of the underlying disease is essential.

Prognosis. The prognosis of animals with edema is dependent on the severity of edema, the underlying mechanism of the edema, and the reversibility of the primary disorder. Prognoses range from excellent to grave.

CYSTIC-BULLOUS DISEASE

Grossly visible circumscribed regions of air and fluid, cavitary lesions, can occur within the lung parenchyma as a result of cysts, bullae, blebs, and pneumatoceles. Similar lesions result from parasitic cysts and abscesses (see *Paragonimus kellicotti* and Pulmonary Abscessation).

Cysts are fluid-filled or air-filled lesions surrounded by a thin wall of respiratory epithelium.[115] They may be congenital or acquired. Bullae are gross air accumulations formed by the loss of alveolar walls. They are often multiple and can occur as a progression of emphysema (bullous emphysema) or secondary to trauma.[115] Emphysema refers to the enlargement of peripheral airspaces with destruction of bronchiolar and alveolar walls due to chronic obstructive pulmonary disease, as may be seen with chronic bronchitis. In addition to airway obstruction from bronchial disease, the loss of radial traction from the alveoli can contribute to airway collapse. Alveoli are able to fill with air, but expiration is impeded by airway closure. Preexisting collagen defects may predispose some animals to the formation of these cavities.[116] In dogs with chronic bronchitis, the changes are usually confined to the edges of lung lobes. Bullae that occur at the pleural surface are called blebs.[115]

Pneumatoceles result from the entry of air into necrotic lesions. They may occur as a result of abscesses, granulomas, or neoplasias.[115] The term has been used to describe a variety of other cavitary lesions.

Respiratory signs reflect the primary disease process (such as pulmonary contusions or chronic bronchitis), V:Q abnormalities, interference with function of adjacent normal structures, and pneumothorax due to dissection of air or rupture of cysts. Secondary infections can occur.

Presentation. Animals generally present with signs of either primary pulmonary disease or pneumothorax. In the latter instance, acute respiratory distress can occur. Occasionally, lesions are incidental findings with no related signs. Eliciting a history of prior trauma or pulmonary disease can be helpful in determining the cause.

Diagnostic Evaluation. Most cavitary lesions are identified initially by thoracic radiography. Animals with known associated disease processes, such as traumatic contusions, severe bronchopneumonia, aspiration pneumonia, and granulomas, should be radiographed periodically for early detection of cystic change or other complications. Animals pre-

RES

sented with pneumothorax and respiratory compromise are stabilized by thoracocentesis before further diagnostic evaluation. Thoracocentesis is indicated before radiographic evaluation of the lungs because full lung expansion is necessary for an accurate interpretation of radiographic signs.

Initially, cavitary lesions may be totally obscured by overlying opacities. As silhouetting opacities resolve, the margins of the lesions can often be identified. Horizontal beam projections can be useful in enhancing the appearance of a fluid line. Bullous emphysema is rarely apparent radiographically. It is usually observed at exploratory thoracotomy or on postmortem examination of animals with chronic pulmonary disease.

Cytologic evaluation of lung specimens may provide evidence of the cause of the cavitary lesion. For example, septic inflammation or *Paragonimus* ova might be found. Transthoracic lung aspiration is contraindicated for sampling cavitary lesions because of the risk of pneumothorax.

A definitive diagnosis of cavitary lesions is obtained with thoracotomy, excision, and histopathologic examination. This aggressive approach is not always necessary or indicated, however.

Treatment. The treatment and monitoring of various primary processes are discussed elsewhere. Acute pneumothorax is managed medically as discussed in Chapter 130. Cavitary lesions may resolve with supportive care and treatment of primary disease, but total resolution may require many weeks. Surgical exploration and removal of cavitary lesions may be necessary in the presence of continued pneumothorax, unresolving localized infection, or enlargement of the lesion. A review of dogs with spontaneous pneumothorax found that recurrence was common without surgery.[117] Dry-gauze pleurodesis is suggested following removal of bleb lesions.[115] Bullous emphysema is difficult to correct surgically. Pleurodesis can be considered.[116]

Incidental or nonprogressive cavitary lesions can be approached conservatively or surgically. If observation is elected, the owner should be warned of the potential for pneumothorax. Surgical intervention may eliminate those risks but carries risks of its own.

Prognosis. Animals whose cavitary lesions result in overt clinical signs have variable prognoses, depending on the primary disease process and the extent of involvement. Resolution of the primary disease decreases the likelihood of further cavitary lesions. Localized lesions can be successfully removed surgically, if indicated. Multiple diffuse lesions may not be surgically resectable and may be associated with conditions in which recurrence is probable, such as bullae due to chronic airway disease. Prognosis in such cases is guarded, although in one report, three of six cases of recurrent pneumothorax due to bullous emphysema survived at least two years after surgery.[116]

TRAUMATIC LUNG DISEASE

Injury to the lung can occur as a result of external or internal trauma. External trauma refers to injury sustained to the lung from outside of the body, such as being hit by a car, being kicked, or falling. Also included in this category are penetrating wounds, such as from gunshots, stabbings, or bites. The subject of management of the trauma patient is too broad for this chapter, but the isolated component of pulmonary contusions is addressed. Internal trauma refers to lung injury sustained from inhalation or aspiration of damaging material. Aspiration pneumonia, near drowning, and smoke inhalation are discussed.

PULMONARY CONTUSIONS

Pulmonary contusions refer to hemorrhage and edema within the lung and occur as a result of traumatic injury. Respiratory signs develop from V:Q abnormalities as alveoli become filled with fluid or collapse. Cardiovascular shock, pain, pneumothorax, hemothorax, rib fractures, diaphragmatic hernias, and traumatic myocarditis can add to the clinical signs.

Presentation. The animal is presented with historic or physical examination findings confirming a traumatic incident. The animal may be eupneic or in severe respiratory distress, depending on the degree of injury. The lungs should be carefully auscultated. Recent hemorrhage and edema result in crackles, and consolidated lobes cause absence or enhancement of sounds. The abnormal sounds are often localized. Diffusely decreased lung sounds are suggestive of pleural involvement.

Ribs should be carefully palpated for penetrating fractures. The skin overlying the thorax should be examined thoroughly, visually and by palpation, for penetrating wounds or subcutaneous emphysema that may be obscured by the coat. Penetrating wounds, particularly from bites, should be examined critically to determine the full extent of involvement.[118] Surgical exploration may be required.[118]

The animal should be carefully monitored, even though apparently stable. Deterioration may occur for up to 24 hours after the traumatic incident.

Diagnostic Evaluation. Pulmonary contusions are evidenced radiographically by localized areas of an interstitial pattern, alveolar pattern, or consolidation. Radiographic signs may be delayed for up to 24 hours following trauma. Other trauma-induced changes may be apparent. Bite wounds are often contaminated with unpredictable organisms.[118] Material should be submitted for bacterial culture.

Treatment. The critical patient is stabilized following principles of shock-trauma management. Animals showing clinical signs of hypoxemia are provided oxygen supplementation. Short-acting corticosteroids may be indicated during stabilization.

Once the animal is stabilized, little therapy is generally required beyond cage rest. Antibiotics are recommended only for animals with penetrating wounds, not for routine prophylaxis. Careful monitoring for the early detection of infection is preferred.

Prognosis. Pulmonary contusions are a common component of external trauma. Improvement is usually seen within 24 to 48 hours of injury. Complications occasionally develop, and reevaluation of animals radiographically following trauma is indicated for the early detection of bacterial pneumonia, abscess, atelectasis, traumatic cysts, lung lobe torsions, or other related injuries.

ASPIRATION PNEUMONIA

Aspiration pneumonia occurs when foreign material is inspired into the lungs. Aspiration may occur from the loss of normal protective mechanisms or iatrogenically. Normal protective mechanisms can be circumvented with megaesophagus or other esophageal disorders, cleft palate, bronchoesophageal fistula, therapeutic laryngoplasty, peripheral neuropathies, myopathies, or abnormal consciousness due to neurologic disease, severe metabolic disease, sedation, or severe debilitation. Pharyngeal abnormalities associated with brachycephalic airway syndrome may predispose some affected dogs to aspiration. Iatrogenic aspiration can occur by administering food, medication, or diagnostic compounds (such as barium) through stomach tubes, pharyngostomy tubes, or nasogastric tubes that have been incorrectly positioned in the trachea. The oral administration of mineral oil to cats to treat hairballs can result in aspiration owing to a lack of stimulation of protective reflexes by the flavorless, nonirritating oil.

Aspiration can result in respiratory signs from many mechanisms, including chemical damage by gastric acid, resulting in necrosis, hemorrhage, edema, bronchoconstriction, and severe inflammation; obstruction of airways with particulates, bronchoconstriction, and inflammation; and bacterial infection due to inhalation of contaminated material or subsequently due to damaged pulmonary clearance mechanisms.[119, 120] ARDS is a life-threatening complication. Obstruction of large airways with inhaled material is uncommon. The severity of signs is dependent on the characteristics of the aspirated material and the respiratory and systemic status of the animal prior to aspiration.

Presentation. Animals may present with acute respiratory signs following vomiting or regurgitation, loss of consciousness, or forced oral administration of mineral oil, food, or drugs. Hospitalized animals can experience aspiration during management of a predisposing problem. Those at risk for aspiration should be closely monitored for early signs.

Most cases demonstrate acute, severe respiratory distress, with signs apparent within hours of aspiration. There may be a sudden onset of coughing before the development of respiratory distress. Cardiovascular shock can occur. Other cases have a more chronic history of recurrent bacterial pneumonia.

Physical examination reveals crackles and sometimes wheezes, especially in the dependent (usually cranioventral) lung fields. A fever may be present. A thorough oral examination should be performed to identify vomitus or foreign material, cleft palate, or an abnormal gag reflex. The thoracic inlet should be observed to detect ballooning of the esophagus during expiration, characteristic of megaesophagus. A complete neurologic examination should also be performed.

Diagnostic Evaluation. The clinical diagnosis of aspiration pneumonia is based on radiographic evidence in conjunction with suggestive historic or physical findings. Thoracic radiographs characteristically show a bronchoalveolar pattern involving primarily the dependent lung lobes (Fig. 128–17). Consolidation may be present. The typical cranioventral distribution may not be present if aspiration occurred with the animal in other than a sternal position. Further, bacterial pneumonia is most often of bronchial origin and results in a similar distribution of lesions without the overt aspiration of gross material into the lungs. Mineral oil aspiration in cats can cause a diffuse, nodular, interstitial pattern that can mimic neoplastic, fungal, and parasitic disease.

Radiographic changes may be inapparent initially, then gradually progress for up to 24 hours following aspiration. Radiographs should be critically examined for megaesophagus.

Tracheal wash fluid analysis is indicated to verify the presence of infection and obtain antimicrobial susceptibility information. Acidic gastric contents may be sterile, although the marked inflammatory response mimics infection. Mixed infections are common, making selection of effective antibiotics difficult. Cytologic analysis shows acute or chronic inflammation, depending on the duration of injury. Hemorrhage can be present. Food particles or fat may be present in the fluid or within macrophages.

Bronchoscopy can be performed to remove large pieces of foreign material. Examination of airways and specimen collection can also be performed. Because general anesthesia is required and these animals are usually unstable, scoping is indicated primarily if large airway obstruction is suspected.

Hematocrit, protein concentration, electrolyte status, and blood gas measurements are useful for emergency management. Once the animal is stabilized, further diagnostic evaluation can be performed to identify underlying diseases. The search for such a problem should be aggressive, because aspiration is a secondary problem and is likely to recur without elimination of the underlying cause. Potential diagnostic tests include contrast radiography (barium swallow), thorough oral and pharyngeal examination, and tests of neuromuscular function.

Treatment. The severely distressed animal needs immediate oxygen supplementation. Positive-pressure ventilation may also be necessary to overcome decreased lung compliance. Intravenous fluid therapy is indicated. High volumes are often required initially to treat shock. Fluid administra-

RES

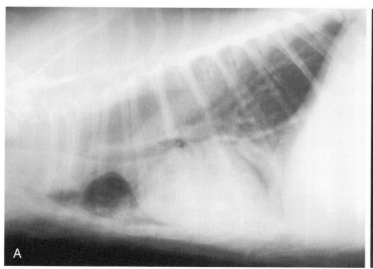
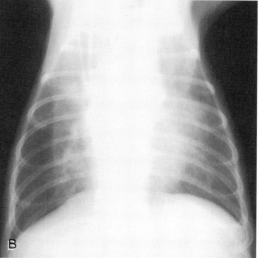

Figure 128–17. *A* and *B,* Megaesophagus and aspiration pneumonia are apparent in these radiographs. The pneumonia is characterized by a lobar alveolar pattern in the dependent lung lobes.

tion is continued to maintain systemic hydration, which is essential to promote airway clearance. Overhydration may contribute to the formation of pulmonary edema. Nothing is administered orally until the animal is stabilized and the underlying abnormality has been addressed.

If material is still present in the upper airways based on radiographs or auscultation, airway suctioning or bronchoscopy and foreign body removal should be performed. These procedures may require sedation, and ventilatory support should be available. Routine suctioning is not useful unless it is performed immediately following aspiration. Low-pressure, intermittent suction should be used to minimize collapse of lung lobes. Suctioning should be followed by several "sighs" of positive-pressure ventilation using an anesthesia or Ambu bag. Therapeutic lavage is not recommended.[119, 120]

Bronchodilators can be beneficial in the immediate management of aspiration to overcome acute bronchoconstriction (see Chapter 127). Continued use is controversial (see Bacterial Pneumonia).

The use of corticosteroids for treatment of acute aspiration is also controversial. Although these drugs decrease inflammation and stabilize membranes, they can also inhibit helpful protective responses of the lung. In acute cases in which the animal is deteriorating, administration of short-acting corticosteroids is justified. They should not be continued beyond 24 to 48 hours.

In people, antibiotics may not be used initially in the treatment for aspiration of gastric contents because the material is sterile, secondary infections are common, and the secondary infections will likely be from resistant organisms if antibiotics are used initially.[119] However, unlike people, dogs often aspirate esophageal contents that have not been affected by gastric acid, and dogs and cats commonly have dental disease. This author recommends the routine use of first-line, broad-spectrum antibiotics. Amoxicillin-clavulanate or ampicillin-sulbactam is a good initial choice, because both are effective against anaerobes. Second-line antibiotics such as fluoroquinolones, aminoglycosides, and imipenem are reserved for animals with documented life-threatening, refractory, or resistant infections. Tracheal wash is recommended before the initiation of antibiotics.

Careful monitoring is essential, because a population of resistant bacteria can develop in spite of antibiotic therapy. Repeated cytologic and microbiologic analysis of tracheal wash fluid is indicated in animals that later develop signs of bacterial infection or undergo clinical deterioration.

Animals with minimal signs due to aspiration of barium or mineral oil often require no specific therapy. They should be monitored for the development of further signs or sequelae.

The reader is referred to the section on bacterial pneumonia for further discussion of antibiotic therapy, supportive care, and monitoring.

Prognosis. Prognosis is dependent on the amount and character of the material aspirated, the condition of the animal before aspiration, and the inciting cause of aspiration. The prognosis can be excellent, as with mild aspiration of barium or mineral oil, or grave. Long-term complications can occur, and radiographs should be evaluated following recovery to identify such problems. Possible sequelae include abscesses, granulomas, and consolidated lobes.

Prevention. Guidelines for the prevention of aspiration generally pertain to the management of animals with full stomachs before the induction of anesthesia and are dis-

cussed in surgery and anesthesia texts. The management of megaesophagus is discussed in Chapter 135.

NEAR DROWNING

Near drowning occurs as a result of submersion in water. Carbon dioxide concentrations in the bloodstream rise, stimulating breathing efforts. Aspiration occurs in most cases and results in severe pulmonary damage. In 10 per cent of cases, laryngospasm prevents the aspiration of water.[121] Dry drowning results, and pulmonary disease is absent.

Pulmonary damage occurs through a variety of mechanisms. Surprisingly, large volumes of water are not usually aspirated.[122] Fresh water reaching the alveoli dilutes the surfactant, resulting in alveolar collapse and decreased compliance. Salt water is hypertonic, causing interstitial fluid to diffuse into the alveoli (secondary drowning), contributing to alveolar filling. The result of both situations is severe V:Q abnormalities or shunt.[121, 122]

Aspiration pneumonia can occur from the inhalation of vomitus and debris or chemicals the water. Bacteria may be present in the water, potentially causing complicating infection. ARDS can occur secondary to near drowning. In people, it is recommended that all victims be observed in the hospital for 24 hours for early recognition of ARDS.[123] Cerebral edema, herniation, and ultimately death can occur as a result of profound hypoxemia, complicated by metabolic acidosis.[121]

Presentation. History provides the diagnosis of near drowning, because animals are always presented following a rescue. Physical examination generally reveals loss of consciousness and either severe respiratory distress or respiratory arrest. Cardiovascular shock and hypothermia are common, and pulses may be difficult to palpate. Auscultation of the lungs reveals severe crackles and possibly wheezes. Propeller injury from boats can be a complication. Neurologic status is closely monitored for signs of cerebral edema.

Diagnostic Evaluation. Stabilization is the first priority. Following stabilization, thoracic radiographs are useful to determine the extent of involvement. Radiographic changes may lag 24 to 48 hours behind clinical signs.[121]

A mixed bronchial, alveolar, and interstitial pattern is commonly seen. The presence of radiopaque material filling airways—sand bronchograms—is a potentially fatal complication. Radiographic evaluation should be continued during and following recovery for the detection of bacterial pneumonia, consolidation, or abscessation. Recovering cases should show rapid resolution of alveolar densities.[121] Overall radiographic improvement is expected within 10 days.[121]

Tracheal wash evaluation is indicated if secondary bacterial infection is suspected. Bacterial culture and sensitivity testing are performed in addition to cytologic analysis. Systemic status is monitored routinely.

Treatment. Ventilation should be initiated as soon as possible. Mouth-to-muzzle resuscitation can be initiated on site, following the clearing of any debris or obstruction from the oral cavity. Pressing the larynx upward and compressing the cervical esophagus decrease the amount of air entering the stomach during resuscitation.[124] Oxygen supplementation is provided when available. The Heimlich maneuver or postural drainage is not recommended unless airway obstruction is evident, because aspiration of gastric contents can result.[125]

In the hospital, positive-pressure ventilation is often required in addition to supplemental oxygen therapy. Shock is aggressively treated. Animals with abnormal consciousness following metabolic stabilization or other suggestive signs are treated for cerebral edema (see Chapter 104). Routine administration of corticosteroids or prophylactic antibiotics is not recommended.[125] Animals that have been resuscitated before arrival at the hospital and are stable should be observed for 24 hours because of the potential for the development of ARDS.

Prognosis. Prognosis is dependent on the animal's condition on presentation. Poor prognostic indicators are coma, blood pH less than 7, and the need for resuscitation or mechanical ventilation.[121] Once metabolic stabilization has been achieved, the neurologic status should be closely monitored. As long as the neurologic status shows continued improvement, time should be allowed for functional recovery to occur.

Prevention. Client education is necessary for prevention. In one survey, half the dogs in immersion accidents were 4 months old or younger.[121] Cold water and rapid currents are particularly exhausting, even for an experienced swimmer. Pools, ditches, and some rivers provide no avenues for exit. Boating accidents occur when dogs leap from boats, often unobserved, for no apparent reason. Given these predisposing situations, the settings for owner education are obvious.

SMOKE INHALATION

Pulmonary damage due to the inhalation of chemicals can occur during exposure to pollutants, poorly ventilated housing, exhaust from gasoline or diesel engines, improperly functioning heaters, and a variety of other sources.[126] The most commonly identified source of inhalation damage is smoke inhalation as a result of fire.

Smoke inhalation results in respiratory signs through several mechanisms.[126] Carbon monoxide inhalation results in the formation of carboxyhemoglobin with the displacement of oxygen from hemoglobin. Tissue hypoxia results. Inhalation of high concentrations of carbon dioxide can cause severe acidosis. Heat from the fire can injure the upper airways to the level of the larynx, and the resultant inflammation and edema can cause upper airway obstruction. Thermal injury can occur to deeper airways through the inhalation of heated particles. These particles can cause injury themselves and can carry chemicals that are caustic to the epithelial cells of the lungs. Chemicals released from the combustion of plastic and other materials can be directly toxic to lung tissue. Pulmonary macrophage function and the mucociliary apparatus are adversely affected by smoke inhalation, predisposing the lungs to secondary bronchopneumonia.[127] Concurrent burns to the skin can worsen the pulmonary status, perhaps owing to the release of depressant factors, inhibition of immune mechanisms, development of disseminated intravascular coagulation, or increase in pulmonary vascular permeability.[127] Burn patients are highly susceptible to septicemia.

Presentation. Animals presented with smoke inhalation are generally brought from the scene of a fire. The presence of burns around the face, signed vibrissae, oral inflammation, and soot-stained nasal discharge or saliva are supportive of inhalation exposure. The absence of these signs does not eliminate the possibility that significant exposure occurred.

Mucous membranes may be bright red, due to carboxyhemoglobin, or cyanotic. Cyanosis may not be apparent if high concentrations of carboxyhemoglobin are present, even with extremely low blood oxygen content.[127] Furthermore, carbon monoxide intoxication may be significant in the absence of the characteristic reddening of mucous membranes.[126] Therefore, animals with suspected carbon monoxide exposure should be treated as such, pending confirmatory laboratory results.

Stridor may be audible owing to laryngeal edema. Wheezes may be auscultated as a result of airway edema and bronchoconstriction. Crackles may also be heard.

Animals that appear stable on initial presentation must be closely monitored for at least 24 hours. Laryngeal edema can develop over 12 to 24 hours.[127, 128] ARDS and secondary infections may occur days later.[129]

Diagnostic Evaluation. Thoracic radiographs are particularly valuable in following the progression and resolution of injury.[129] Common pulmonary patterns, in order of frequency, are diffuse bronchial patterns, diffuse patchy consolidation, hyperinflation, and massive consolidation, especially of dorsal lung fields (see Fig. 128–16).[129] As with other traumatic disease, radiographic signs may lag behind clinical signs.[129]

Blood gas analyses must be evaluated with caution. The P_aO_2 is a reflection of dissolved oxygen and in most instances provides an indication of whole blood oxygen content; however, with carbon monoxide poisoning, the P_aO_2 may be normal in spite of decreased oxygen content, because the carbon monoxide interferes with the oxygen saturation of hemoglobin. The P_aO_2 can be used as an indication of pulmonary function in these animals.

Carboxyhemoglobin concentrations in venous blood can be measured by human hospitals. Specimens must be transported on ice. Treatment should not pend results, but recovery can be monitored by such evaluation.

The animal's cardiac and neurologic status should be carefully monitored with electrocardiograms and serial neurologic examinations. Routine monitoring of systemic status is also recommended.

Deterioration in respiratory status following initial stabilization can be a result of ARDS or bacterial infection. Animals may require further evaluation with radiographs, blood gas analysis, tracheal wash analysis, or bronchoscopy. Cytologic evaluation and culture and sensitivity testing of collected specimens can provide useful information.

Treatment. A patent airway is essential, and animals with laryngeal obstruction may require tracheostomies. In compromised patients, oxygen supplementation should begin as soon as an airway is established. Supplementation can be initiated at the scene of the fire by face mask when rescue personnel are in attendance. Carbon monoxide is eliminated by the lungs, and removal is greatly facilitated by the administration of 100 per cent oxygen. The half-life of carboxyhemoglobin is 4 hours in room air and 30 minutes in 100 per cent oxygen.[127] Oxygen therapy should be continued until carboxyhemoglobin concentrations are less than 10 per cent.[126]

Pulmonary injury should be managed using general principles of therapy, including oxygenation, airway humidification, and physiotherapy. Positive-pressure ventilation may be necessary in animals with depressed respiratory effort or severe edema. Bronchodilators may be useful acutely. Antibiotic therapy generally should be withheld until signs of infection occur.[127, 128] Careful monitoring for evidence of infection is essential. Corticosteroids may be necessary for acute stabilization, but continued use should be avoided owing to potential interference with already damaged protective mechanisms.

Cardiovascular abnormalities often respond to correction of hypoxemia and fluid and electrolyte derangements. Intra-

RES

venous fluid therapy is necessary to maintain cardiac output, but overhydration should be avoided. Deterioration in neurologic signs may suggest cerebral edema. Skin burns require meticulous management.

Treatment of pulmonary sequelae, such as bronchitis, bronchopneumonia, abscesses, and consolidation, are discussed in other sections. The animal should be monitored, including evaluation of thoracic radiographs, following apparent recovery to detect persisting disease.

Prognosis. Animals presented with minimal signs of smoke inhalation on physical and radiographic examination have a good prognosis, assuming marked deterioration does not occur within the first 24 to 48 hours.[129] The prognosis is progressively more guarded with increasingly severe respiratory signs, neurologic signs, and cutaneous burns. Bronchopneumonia is more likely to develop when factors besides inhalation injury are involved, such as use of a tracheostomy tube or cutaneous burns.[127]

MISCELLANEOUS CONDITIONS

PULMONARY MINERALIZATION

Mineralized thoracic densities in the airways, pleura, parenchyma, or lymph nodes may be incidental radiographic findings. Chondrodystrophoid dogs may demonstrate airway mineralization at an early age. Mineralization of the airways or the pleura can occur in aged dogs of any breed, although the increased pleural opacity is usually the result of fibrosis.[79] No correlation with disease has been made. Diffuse nodular mineralization of unknown etiology involving the pulmonary parenchyma can be a nonprogressive lesion and can be misinterpreted as metastatic neoplasia.[79] Mineral densities in the local lymph nodes can result from the prior aspiration of barium.

Mineralization can also occur in areas of inflammation or necrosis, such as in the center of masses resulting from fungal infections, tuberculosis, parasites, or neoplasia. The mineralized densities often persist following resolution of active disease.

Systemic diseases resulting in soft tissue mineralization, such as renal secondary hyperparathyroidism and hyperadrenocorticism, can result in mineral deposition in the lungs and other organs. The presenting signs generally reflect the primary disease.

OBESITY (PICKWICKIAN SYNDROME)

Obesity can affect the lungs in a variety of ways. Intrathoracic and intra-abdominal fat may interfere with expansion of the thoracic cavity and lungs during inspiration, causing decreased thoracic wall compliance. Obesity may reflect relatively low levels of exercise and conditioning. Work of breathing, oxygen consumption, and cardiac output during activity are increased in people with excess body mass.[130] Ultimately, V:Q abnormalities resulting in hypoxemia occur owing to decreased ventilation of peripheral lung regions.

Pickwickian syndrome refers to a specific condition in humans characterized by obesity, somnolence, hypoventilation, and erythrocytosis.[131] A central neurologic abnormality may be involved.[131] It has been defined by extreme obesity, elevated P_aCO_2, and an absence of pulmonary disease.[131] The term should not be used indiscriminately to describe all obese patients with respiratory disease. As more is learned

about breathing disorders, terms such as obesity-hypoventilation syndromes (obese patients with concurrent decreased ventilatory response to hypoxia) and sleep apnea syndromes appear to more accurately describe such patients.

The specific contribution of obesity to clinical pulmonary disease in small animal medicine is not well characterized. The clinician should be careful not to use obesity as an excuse to avoid pursuing specific disease entities; however, the beneficial effects of weight reduction in animals with chronic bronchial or pulmonary disease can be dramatic.

LOBAR CONSOLIDATION

Consolidation refers to the filling of alveoli and airways with cells or fluid and can occur with inflammatory, neoplastic, or hemorrhagic disease. V:Q abnormalities occur as blood flow persists through unventilated regions of lung. An entire lung lobe becomes involved when localized lesions coalesce, when processes spread through channels of collateral ventilation throughout the lung lobe, and when there is complete bronchial obstruction.[80] Lobar consolidations are recognized radiographically as soft tissue densities with visible lung lobe borders (Fig. 128–18).

Consolidation can be a result of any severe inflammatory disease process. Primary pulmonary neoplasia results in a consolidated pattern in a small percentage of cases, and pulmonary hemorrhage (contusion) and lung lobe torsions can also cause lobar consolidation. If treatment of the primary disease does not result in resolution of the consolidation, surgical excision may be necessary.

ATELECTASIS

Atelectasis refers to the collapse (or incomplete expansion) of lung due to the loss of air from the alveoli. Atelectasis commonly results from pneumothorax and pleural effusion. Reexpansion almost always follows removal of the air or fluid from the pleural space. Atelectasis occasionally occurs as a complication of pulmonary disease due to total airway obstruction and the absorption of alveolar gases into the blood. The obstruction may be a result of foreign bodies but is more often caused by mucus, inflammation, airway collapse, or airway compression. Atelectasis can also be caused by the loss of surfactant. Decreased surfactant is a common problem in premature infants but can occur in acquired diseases such as ARDS and near drowning. Inhalation anesthesia, prolonged recumbency, or decreased ciliary clearance can potentiate the tendency for atelectasis to occur.

The primary differential diagnosis for atelectasis is pulmonary consolidation resulting from the replacement of alveolar air with fluid or cells. Atelectatic lobes may have concave margins and result in rearrangement of the unaffected lung lobes, evident by changes in location of the interlobar fissures and shifting of the mediastinum.[80] The lobes are not always completely shrunken, because edema and inflammatory infiltration can be present within the parenchyma.[80]

Treatment is directed at the inciting cause. Prolonged atelectasis can potentially result in abscessation or fibrosis, and surgical intervention may be necessary if signs are persistent following correction of the underlying problem.

Atelectasis of the cranial or right middle lung lobes of cats with bronchitis does not seem to contribute significantly to clinical signs, and lobectomy is not recommended.

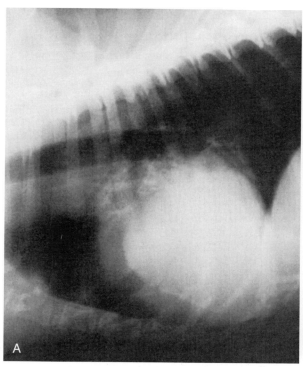
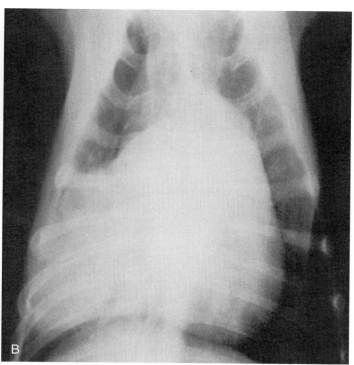

Figure 128–18. A 12-year-old dog was presented for coughing and shortness of breath of a two-week duration. Radiographs show consolidation of the right middle lung lobe. The bronchus was compressed and could not be entered bronchoscopically. Bronchoalveolar lavage fluid revealed mild, chronic inflammation. A lobectomy was performed, and torsion of the lobe was found. On microscopic examination, infarction and fibrosis were identified. There was no evidence of an active inflammatory process or neoplasia.

RES

REFERENCES

1. Haskins SC: Management of pulmonary disease in the critical patient. *In* Zaslow IM (ed): Veterinary Trauma and Critical Care. Philadelphia, Lea & Febiger, 1984, p 339.
2. Court MH, et al: Inhalation therapy. Vet Clin North Am Small Anim Pract 15:1041, 1985.
3. Branditz FK, et al: Continuous transtracheal oxygen delivery during cardiopulmonary resuscitation: An alternative method of ventilation in a canine model. Chest 95:441, 1989.
4. Fitzpatrick RK, Crowe DT: Nasal oxygen administration in dogs and cats: Experimental and clinical investigations. J Am Anim Hosp Assoc 22:293, 1986.
5. Haskins SC: Physical therapeutics for respiratory disease. Semin Vet Med Surg Small Anim 1:276, 1986.
6. Pascoe PJ: Short-term ventilatory support. *In* Kirk RW (ed): Current Veterinary Therapy IX. Philadelphia, WB Saunders, 1986, p 269.
7. Moon PF, Concannon KT: Mechanical ventilation. *In* Kirk RW, Bonagura JD (eds): Current Veterinary Therapy XI. Philadelphia, WB Saunders, 1992, p 98.
8. Ducatelle R, et al: Immunoperoxidase study of adenovirus pneumonia in dogs. Vet Q 7:290, 1985.
9. Hoover EA, Kahn DE: Experimentally induced feline calicivirus infections: Clinical signs and lesions. JAVMA 166:463, 1975.
10. Greene CE: Rocky Mountain spotted fever. JAVMA 191:666, 1987.
11. Thayer GW, Robinson SK: Bacterial bronchopneumonia in the dog: A review of 42 cases. J Am Anim Hosp Assoc 20:731, 1984.
12. Hirsch DC: Bacteriology of the lower respiratory tract. *In* Kirk RW (ed): Current Veterinary Therapy IX. Philadelphia, WB Saunders, 1986, p 247.
13. Jameson PH, et al: Comparison of clinical signs, diagnostic findings, organisms isolated, and clinical outcome in dogs with bacterial pneumonia: 93 cases (1986–1991). JAVMA 206:206, 1995.
14. Randolph JF, et al: Prevalence of mycoplasmal and ureaplasmal recovery from tracheobronchial lavages and prevalence of mycoplasmal recovery from pharyngeal swab specimens in dogs with or without pulmonary disease. Am J Vet Res 54:387, 1993.
15. Randolph JF, et al: Prevalence of mycoplasmal and ureaplasmal recovery from tracheobronchial lavages and prevalence of mycoplasma recovery from pharyngeal swab specimens in cats with or without pulmonary disease. Am J Vet Res 54:897, 1993.
16. King RR, et al: Reliability of a protected catheter brush in the diagnosis of pneumonia in dogs (abstract). Proceedings of the 7th Veterinary Respiratory Symposium of the Comparative Respiratory Society, Chicago, 1988.

17. Boothe DM, McKiernan BC: Respiratory therapeutics. Vet Clin North Am Small Anim Pract 22:1231, 1992.
18. Clercx C, et al: Tuberculosis in dogs: A case report and review of the literature. J Am Anim Hosp Assoc 28:207, 1992.
19. Petrak M, Carpenter JD: Feline toxoplasmosis. JAVMA 146:728, 1965.
20. Dubey JP, et al: Fatal toxoplasmosis in dogs. J Am Anim Hosp Assoc 25:659, 1989.
21. Hawkins EC, et al: Cytologic identification of *Toxoplasma gondii* in bronchoalveolar lavage fluid of experimentally infected cats. JAVMA 210:648, 1997.
22. Sukura A, et al: *Pneumocystis carinii* pneumonia in dog: A diagnostic challenge. J Vet Diagn Invest 8:124, 1996.
23. Hagler DN, et al: Feline leukemia virus and *Pneumocystis carinii* infection. J Parasitol 73:1284, 1987.
24. Shiota T, et al: *Pneumocystis carinii* infection in corticosteroid-treated cats. J Parasitol 76:441, 1990.
25. Greene CE, Chandler FW: Pneumoncystosis. *In* Greene CE (ed): Infectious Diseases of the Dog and Cat. Philadelphia, WB Saunders, 1990, p 854.
26. Farrow BRH, et al: Pneumocystis pneumonia in the dog. J Comp Pathol 82:447, 1972.
27. Lobetti RG, et al: *Pneumocystis carinii* in the miniature dachshund: Case report and literature review. J Small Anim Pract 37:280, 1996.
28. Mann JM, et al: Nonbronchoscopic lung lavage for diagnosis of opportunistic infection in AIDS. Chest 91:319, 1987.
29. Furuta T, et al: Spontaneous *Pneumocystis carinii* infection in the dog with naturally acquired generalised demodecosis. Vet Rec 134:423, 1994.
30. Wolf AM: Feline histoplasmosis: A literature review and retrospective study of 20 new cases. J Am Anim Hosp Assoc 20:995, 1984.
31. Kowalewich N, et al: Identification of *Histoplasma capsulatum* organisms in the pleural and peritoneal effusions of a dog. JAVMA 202:423, 1993.
32. Legendre AM: Blastomycosis. *In* Greene CE (ed): Infectious Diseases of the Dog and Cat. Philadelphia, WB Saunders, 1990, p 669.
33. Legendre AL, et al: Canine blastomycosis: A review of 47 clinical cases. JAVMA 178:1163, 1981.
34. Miller PE, et al: Feline blastomycosis: A report of three cases and literature review (1961–1988). J Am Anim Hosp Assoc 26:417, 1990.
35. Hawkins EC, DeNicola DB: Cytologic analysis of tracheal wash specimens and bronchoalveolar lavage fluid in the diagnosis of mycotic infections in dogs. JAVMA 197:79, 1990.
36. Millman TM, et al: Coccidioidomycosis in the dog: Its radiographic diagnosis. J Am Vet Radiol Soc 20:50, 1979.
37. Barsanti JA: Cryptococcosis. *In* Greene CE (ed): Clinical Microbiology and Infectious Diseases of the Dog and Cat. Philadelphia, WB Saunders, 1984, p 700.

38. Hamilton TA, et al: Bronchoalveolar lavage and tracheal wash to determine lung involvement in a cat with cryptococcosis. JAVMA 198:655, 1991.
39. Kneller SK: Thoracic radiography. *In* Kirk RW (ed): Current Veterinary Therapy IX. Philadelphia, WB Saunders, 1986, p 250.
40. Barsanti JA, Prestwood AK: Parasitic diseases of the respiratory tract. *In* Kirk RW (ed): Current Veterinary Therapy VIII. Philadelphia, WB Saunders, 1983, p 241.
41. Hawkins EC: Disorders of the pulmonary parenchyma. *In* Nelson RW, Couto CG (eds): Small Animal Internal Medicine, 2nd ed. St. Louis, CV Mosby, 1998, p 297.
42. Bowman DD, et al: Evaluation of praziquantel for treatment of experimentally induced paragonimiasis in dogs and cats. Am J Vet Res 52:68, 1991.
43. Dubey JP, et al: Fenbendazole for treatment of *Paragonimus kellicotti* infection in dogs. JAVMA 174:835, 1979.
44. Reinemeyer CR: Parasite of the respiratory system. *In* Bonagura JD, Kirk RW (eds): Current Veterinary Therapy XII. Philadelphia, WB Saunders, 1995, p 895.
45. Willard MD, et al: Diagnosis of *Aelurostrongylus abstrusus* and *Dirofilaria immitis* infections in cats from a humane shelter. JAVMA 192:913, 1988.
46. Urquhart GM, et al: Veterinary Parasitology. Essex, England, Longman Scientific and Technical, 1987.
47. Kirkpatrick CE, Megella C: Use of ivermectin in treatment of *Aelurostrongylus abstrusus* and *Toxocara cati* infections in a cat. JAVMA 190:1309, 1987.
48. Greenlee PG, Noone KE: Pulmonary capillariasis in a dog. J Am Anim Hosp Assoc 20:983, 1984.
49. Rubash JM: *Filaroides hirthi* infection in a dog. JAVMA 189:213, 1986.
50. Pinckney RD, et al: *Filaroides hirthi* infection in two related dogs. JAVMA 193:1287, 1988.
51. Bauer C, Bahnemann R: Control of *Filaroides hirthi* infections in beagle dogs by ivermectin. Vet Parasitol 65:269, 1996.
52. Stockdale PHG, Smart ME: Treatment of crenosomiasis in dogs. Res Vet Sci 18:178, 1975.
53. Peterson EN, et al: Use of fenbendazole for treatment of *Crenosoma vulpis* infection in a dog. JAVMA 202:1483, 1993.
54. Bolt G, et al: Canine angiostrongylus: A review. Vet Res 135:447, 1994.
55. Neer TM, et al: Eosinophilic pulmonary granulomatosis in two dogs and literature review. J Am Anim Hosp Assoc 22:593, 1986.
56. Calvert CA, et al: Pulmonary and disseminated eosinophilic granulomatosis in dogs. J Am Anim Hosp Assoc 24:311, 1988.
57. Corcoran BM, et al: Pulmonary infiltration with eosinophils in 14 dogs. J Small Anim Pract 32:494, 1992.
58. Stokes LT, Turner-Warwick M: Lungs and connective tissue disorders. *In* Murray JF, Nadel JA (eds): Textbook of Respiratory Medicine. Philadelphia, WB Saunders, 1988, p 1462.
59. Tizard I: Veterinary Immunology: An Introduction. Philadelphia, WB Saunders, 1987, p 337.
60. Postorino NC, et al: A syndrome resembling lymphomatoid granulomatosis in the dog. J Vet Intern Med 3:15, 1989.
61. Berry CR, et al: Pulmonary lymphomatoid granulomatosis in seven dogs (1976–1987). J Vet Intern Med 4:157, 1990.
62. Berkwitt L, et al: Pulmonary granulomatosis associated with immune phenomena in a dog. J Am Anim Hosp Assoc 14:111, 1978.
63. Drazner FH: Systemic lupus erythematosus in the dog. Comp Contin Educ Pract Vet 2:243, 1980.
64. Moulton JE, et al: Classification of lung carcinomas in the dog and cat. Vet Pathol 18:513, 1981.
65. Barr FJ, et al: The radiological features of primary lung tumours in the dog: A review of 36 cases. J Small Anim Pract 27:493, 1986.
66. Brodey RS, Craig PH: Primary pulmonary neoplasms in the dog: A review of 29 cases. JAVMA 147:1628, 1965.
67. Koblik PD: Radiographic appearance of primary lung tumors in cats: A review of 41 cases. Vet Radiol 27:66, 1986.
68. Stephens LC, et al: Primary pulmonary fibrosarcoma associated with *Spirocerca lupi* infection in a dog with hypertrophic pulmonary osteoarthropathy. JAVMA 182:496, 1983.
69. Moore JA, Taylor HW: Primary pulmonary adenocarcinoma in a dog. JAVMA 192:219, 1988.
70. Hamilton HB, et al: Pulmonary squamous cell carcinoma with intraocular metastasis. JAVMA 185:307, 1984.
71. Gionfriddo JR, et al: Ocular manifestations of a metastatic pulmonary adenocarcinoma in a cat. JAVMA 197:372, 1990.
72. Madewell BR, Theilen GH: Tumors of the respiratory tract. *In* Theilen GH, Madewell BR (eds): Veterinary Cancer Medicine. Philadelphia, Lea & Febiger, 1987, p 535.
73. Gram WD, et al: Feline hypertrophic osteopathy associated with pulmonary carcinoma. J Am Anim Hosp Assoc 26:425, 1990.
74. Hahn KA, McEntee MF: Primary lung tumors in cats: 86 cases (1979–1994). JAVMA 211:1257, 1997.
75. Mehlhaff CJ, et al: Surgical treatment of primary pulmonary neoplasia in 15 dogs. J Am Anim Hosp Assoc 20:799, 1984.
76. Ogilvie GK, et al: Prognostic factors for tumor remission and survival in dogs after surgery for primary lung tumor: 76 cases (1975–1985). JAVMA 195:109, 1989.
77. Hahn KA, et al: Prognostic factors for tumor remission and survival in cats after surgery for primary lung tumors: 21 cases (1979–1994) (abstract). J Vet Intern Med 11:125, 1997.
78. Nafe LA, et al: Mammary tumors and unassociated pulmonary masses in two cats. JAVMA 175:1194, 1979.
79. Reif JS, Rhodes WH: The lungs of aged dogs: A radiographic-morphologic correlation. J Am Vet Radiol Soc 7:5, 1966.
80. Suter PF: Lower airway and pulmonary parenchymal disease. *In* Thoracic Radiography. Wettswil, Switzerland, Peter F. Suter, 1984, p 517.
81. Reif JS, et al: Canine pulmonary disease and the urban environment I: The validity of radiographic examination for estimating the prevalence of pulmonary disease. Arch Environ Health 20:676, 1970.
82. Walter PA, et al: Radiographic appearance of pulmonary metastases from transitional cell carcinoma of the bladder and urethra of the dog. JAVMA 185:411, 1984.
83. Lang J, et al: Sensitivity of radiographic detection of lung metastases in the dog. Vet Radiol 27:74, 1986.
84. Biller DS, Meyer CW: Case examples demonstrating the clinical utility of obtaining both right and left lateral thoracic radiographs in small animals. J Am Anim Hosp Assoc 23:381, 1987.
85. Hawkins EC, et al: Cytologic analysis of bronchoalveolar lavage fluid from 47 dogs with multicentric malignant lymphoma. JAVMA 203:1418, 1993.
86. Smith KC, et al: Canine lymphomatoid granulomatosis: An immunophenotypic analysis of three cases. J Comp Pathol 115:129, 1996.
87. Luce JA: Lymphoma, lymphoproliferative disease, and other primary malignant tumors. *In* Murray JF, Nadel JA (eds): Textbook of Respiratory Medicine, 2nd ed. 2 Philadelphia, WB Saunders, 1994, p 1597.
88. Padgett GA, et al: Inheritance of histiocytosis in Bernese Mountain Dogs. J Small Anim Pract 36:93, 1995.
89. Kerlin RL, Hendrick M: Malignant fibrous histiocytoma and malignant histiocytosis in the dog: Convergent or divergent phenotypic differentiation? Vet Pathol 33:713, 1996.
90. Schmidt ML, et al: Clinical and radiographic manifestations of canine malignant histiocytosis. Vet Q 14:117, 1993.
91. Withrow SJ: Tumors of the respiratory system. *In* Withrow SJ, MacEwen EG (eds): Clinical Veterinary Oncology. Philadelphia, JB Lippincott, 1989, p 215.
92. LaRue MJ, Murtaugh RJ: Pulmonary thromboembolism in dogs: 47 cases (1986–1987). JAVMA 197:1368, 1990.
93. Wall RE: Respiratory complications in the critically ill animal. Problems Vet Med 4:365, 1992.
94. Dennis JS: The pathophysiologic sequelae of pulmonary thromboembolism. Comp Contin Educ Pract Vet 13:1811, 1991.
95. Center D, McFadden R: Pulmonary defense mechanisms. *In* Sodeman WA, Sodeman TM (eds): Sodeman's Pathologic Physiology Mechanisms of Disease. Philadelphia, WB Saunders, 1985, p 460.
96. Klein MK, et al: Pulmonary thromboembolism associated with immune-mediated hemolytic anemia in dogs: Ten cases (1982–1987). JAVMA 195:246, 1989.
97. Baty CJ, Hardie EM: Pulmonary thromboembolism: Diagnosis and treatment. *In* Kirk RW, Bonagura JD (eds): Current Veterinary Therapy XI. Philadelphia, WB Saunders, 1992, p 137.
98. Fluckiger MA, Gomez JA: Radiographic findings in dogs with spontaneous pulmonary thromboembolism or embolism. Vet Radiol 25:124, 1984.
99. Cvitanic O, Marino PL: Improved use of arterial blood gas analysis in suspected pulmonary embolism. Chest 95:48, 1989.
100. Meric SM: Drugs used for disorders of coagulation. Vet Clin North Am Small Anim Pract 18:1217, 1988.
101. Harpster NK, Baty CJ: Warfarin therapy of the cat at risk of thromboembolism. *In* Bonagura JD, Kirk RW (eds): Current Veterinary Therapy XII. Philadelphia, WB Saunders, 1995, p 868.
102. Johnson LR, Hamlin RL: Recognition and treatment of pulmonary hypertension. *In* Bonagura JD, Kirk RW (eds): Current Veterinary Therapy XII. Philadelphia, WB Saunders, 1995, p 887.
103. Rubin LJ: Approach to the diagnosis and treatment of pulmonary hypertension. Chest 96:659, 1989.
104. Perry LA, et al: Pulmonary hypertension. Comp Contin Educ Pract Vet 13:226, 1991.
105. Guyton AC: Textbook of Medical Physiology, 7th ed. Philadelphia, WB Saunders, 1986, p 287.
106. Harpster N: Pulmonary edema. *In* Kirk RW (ed): Current Veterinary Therapy X. Philadelphia, WB Saunders, 1989, p 385.
107. Murray JF, et al: An expanded definition of the adult respiratory distress syndrome. Am Rev Respir Dis 138:720, 1988.
108. Frevert CW, Warner AE: Respiratory distress resulting from acute lung injury in the veterinary patient. J Vet Intern Med 6:154, 1992.
109. Moon ML, et al: Uremic pneumonitis-like syndrome in ten dogs. J Am Anim Hosp Assoc 22:687, 1986.
110. Turk J, et al: Coliform septicemia and pulmonary disease associated with canine parvoviral enteritis: 88 cases (1987–1988). JAVMA 196:771, 1990.
111. Parent C, et al: Clinical and clinicopathologic findings in dogs with acute respiratory distress syndrome: 19 cases. JAVMA 208:1419, 1996.
112. Drobatz KJ, et al: Noncardiogenic pulmonary edema in dogs and cats: 26 cases (1987–1993). JAVMA 206:1732, 1995.
113. Molly WD, et al: Treatment of canine permeability pulmonary edema: Short-term effects of dobutamine, furosemide, and hydralazine. Lab Invest 72:1365, 1985.
114. Rossaint R, et al: Inhaled nitric oxide for the adult respiratory distress syndrome. N Engl J Med 328:399, 1993.
115. Anderson GI: Pulmonary cavitary lesions in the dog: A review of seven cases. J Am Anim Hosp Assoc 23:89, 1987.
116. Kramek BA, et al: Bullous emphysema and recurrent pneumothorax in the dog. JAVMA 186:971, 1985.

117. Holtsinger RH, et al: Spontaneous pneumothorax in the dog: A retrospective analysis of 21 cases. J Am Anim Hosp Assoc 29:195, 1993.
118. McKiernan BC, et al: Thoracic bite wounds and associated internal injury in 11 dogs and 1 cat. JAVMA 184:959, 1984.
119. Khawaja IT, et al: Aspiration pneumonia: A threat when deglutition is compromised. Postgrad Med 92:165, 1992.
120. Broe PJ, et al: Aspiration pneumonia. Surg Clin North Am 60:1551, 1980.
121. Farrow CS: Near-drowning. In Kirk RW (ed): Current Veterinary Therapy VIII. Philadelphia, WB Saunders, 1983, p 167.
122. Ornato JP: Special resuscitation situations: Near drowning, traumatic injury, electric shock, and hypothermia. Circulation 74 (Suppl 4):23, 1986.
123. Denison D: Disorders associated with diving. In Murray JF, Nadel JA (eds): Textbook of Respiratory Medicine. Philadelphia, WB Saunders, 1988, p 1664.
124. Amis TC, Haskins SC: Respiratory failure. Semin Vet Med Surg 1:261, 1986.
125. Modell JH: Near drowning. Circulation 74 (Suppl 4):27, 1986.
126. Carson TL: Toxic gases. In Kirk RW (ed): Current Veterinary Therapy IX. Philadelphia, WB Saunders, 1986, p 203.
127. Tams TR: Pneumonia. In Kirk RW (ed): Current Veterinary Therapy X. Philadelphia, WB Saunders, 1989, p 376.
128. Shepphard D: Chemical agents. In Murray JF, Nadel JA (eds): Textbook of Respiratory Medicine. Philadelphia, WB Saunders, 1988, p 1631.
129. Farrow CS: Inhalation injury. In Kirk RW (ed): Current Veterinary Therapy VIII. Philadelphia, WB Saunders, 1983, p 173.
130. Cherniack RM, et al: Obesity. Am Rev Respir Dis 134:827, 1986.
131. West JB: Disorders of ventilation. In Braunwald E, et al (eds): Harrison's Principles of Internal Medicine, 11th ed. New York, McGraw-Hill, 1987, p 1129.

CHAPTER 129

MEDIASTINAL DISEASE

David S. Biller

RES

The mediastinum is the anatomic space that divides the thorax into right and left pleural cavities. It contains a number of vital structures, including the heart, trachea, esophagus, thymus, vagus nerves, and great vessels. Mediastinal abnormalities are most often detected when disease processes affect structures that are either within or adjacent to the mediastinum. However, mediastinal disease can also be associated with systemic disorders such as coagulopathies.

Survey radiography is usually the first step in the recognition of mediastinal lesions. Other diagnostic modalities are often required to arrive at a definitive diagnosis. These include other imaging techniques (e.g., contrast radiography, computed tomography), clinical pathology (e.g., coagulogram, fungal serology, cytology), thoracotomy, and histologic evaluation of biopsy specimens.

ANATOMY

The mediastinum is a potential space centrally located between the right and left pleural cavities and lined on each side by parietal pleura (mediastinal pleura). It is bordered dorsally by the spine, ventrally by the sternum, caudally by the diaphragm, and cranially by the thoracic inlet. Anatomic regions of the mediastinum are often subdivided to facilitate radiographic description of mediastinal disease. For these purposes, the mediastinum can be divided by frontal and transverse planes into five regions: craniodorsal, cranioventral, middle, caudodorsal, and caudoventral (Table 129–1). The mediastinum is typically incomplete, and the pleura that covers it is not fenestrated.[1] For this reason, most unilateral pleural cavity diseases in dogs and cats that cause effusion or pneumothorax ultimately become bilateral. The mediastinum is not a closed compartment; it communicates cranially with the fascial planes (periesophageal, peritracheal, perivascular) of the neck and caudally with the retroperitoneal space through the aortic hiatus. These communications create pathways for the spread of disease between the neck, thorax, and peritoneal and retroperitoneal areas.

HISTORY AND CLINICAL SIGNS

Events that should prompt the clinician to consider mediastinal disease include recent trauma to the head, neck, or thorax; recent foreign body ingestion; or previous invasive diagnostic or therapeutic procedures involving the trachea, esophagus, or cervical region. Physical examination findings of mediastinal disease may include dysphagia, regurgitation, dyspnea (especially if associated with thoracic pain), cough, vocalization changes, Horner's syndrome, and poor compressibility of the cranial thorax. Edema of the head, neck, and forelimbs secondary to venous and lymphatic obstruction (vena cava syndrome) may be present in animals with large cranial mediastinal masses. Extrathoracic signs of illness (peripheral lymphadenopathy, weight loss, polyuria) may be detected when mediastinal disease is a component of systemic or multicentric disease, such as lymphoma or systemic fungal infection.

DIAGNOSTIC EVALUATION OF THE MEDIASTINUM

The mediastinum is not easily accessible for clinical examination because of its location within the thorax. Therefore, noninvasive evaluation is usually dependent on utilization of appropriate imaging techniques such as radiography, ultrasonography, and endoscopy. Invasive techniques for evaluation of the mediastinum include fine-needle aspiration, percutaneous biopsy, and surgical biopsy.

TABLE 129–1. MEDIASTINAL ANATOMY

REGION	ORGANS	BOUNDARIES
Craniodorsal	Cranial vena cava Aortic arch Mediastinal lymph nodes Trachea Esophagus Thoracic duct Arteries, veins, and nerves	Between the thoracic inlet and carina and from the ventral edge of the spine to just ventral to the trachea
Cranioventral	Thymus Sternal lymph nodes	From just ventral to the trachea to the sternum; from the thoracic inlet to the heart
Middle	Esophagus Trachea Main stem bronchi Thoracic duct Heart Pulmonary arteries and veins Hilar lymph nodes Azygous vein Aorta Arteries, veins, and nerves	From ventral edge of the spine to the sternum; from the cranial edge to the caudal edge of the heart
Caudodorsal	Esophagus Thoracic duct Azygous vein Aorta Arteries, veins, and nerves	Dorsal to the caudal vena cava to the ventral edge of the spine; from the caudal edge of the heart to the diaphragm
Caudoventral	Caudal vena cava	Ventral to the caudal vena cava to the sternum; from the caudal edge of the heart to the diaphragm

SURVEY RADIOGRAPHY

The normal mediastinum appears radiographically as an unclear anatomic area that is often difficult to evaluate because of the lack of contrasting tissue densities. All mediastinal structures, with the exception of the air-filled trachea, demonstrate soft tissue opacity. This results in border effacement, which causes the structures within the mediastinum to appear confluent, preventing their visualization as distinct organs or vessels. The cranioventral region is often more radiopaque than other areas of the mediastinum owing to its greater thickness. On dorsoventral (DV) and ventrodorsal (VD) radiographs, the craniodorsal and caudodorsal regions of the mediastinum appear as midline structures that are normally no more than one and a half times the width of the spine. The craniodorsal region may appear wider in obese animals owing to accumulation of fat, but its boundaries normally remain smooth and straight. The craniodorsal and cranioventral regions of the mediastinum are usually incompletely evaluated on DV or VD radiographs because of their superimposition on the sternum and spine. In young dogs, the thymus may be visualized as a triangular, sail-shaped soft tissue dense structure in the cranioventral region of the mediastinum.

Survey radiography is the imaging modality of choice for localizing mediastinal disease and establishing differential diagnoses. It is used to assess the size, shape, opacity, and position of the mediastinum, as well as the visibility of structures within the mediastinum. Positional radiographs, which permit free fluid to move away from the mediastinum, often improve visualization of the mediastinum in animals with pleural effusion. Mediastinal disease can be manifested radiographically as an abnormal position of the mediastinum (mediastinal shift), pneumomediastinum, or increased size and/or opacity of the mediastinum.

Abnormal positioning of the mediastinum is usually indicative of disease originating in the lungs, bronchi, thoracic wall, or pleura. It may result from the presence of an intrathoracic mass or from uneven inflation of the right and left lungs associated with a unilateral increase or decrease in lung volume. A mediastinal shift is identified radiographically by a difference in size between the right and left hemithoraces as assessed on a VD or DV view. In addition, lateral displacement of major mediastinal structures (such as the cardiac silhouette or trachea) may be apparent.

Pneumomediastinum is characterized radiographically by visualization of mediastinal structures that are not normally seen (such as the esophagus, aorta, azygous vein, cranial vena cava, and serosal surface of the trachea) because the presence of air within the mediastinum provides excellent contrast to adjacent soft tissue structures (Fig. 129–1). Pneumomediastinum is usually not recognized on VD or DV radiographs. Pneumothorax, pulmonary overinflation, and deep-chested conformation in thin dogs can cause a radiographic appearance that may be mistaken for pneumomediastinum. In addition, a gas-distended esophagus may drape over the trachea and rarely the great vessels, creating a false impression of pneumomediastinum.

Increased mediastinal size is usually manifested radiographically as diffuse or focal widening of the mediastinum as assessed on a VD or DV view. Diffuse widening can be caused by mediastinal inflammation, hemorrhage, or edema or by the accumulation of fluid within the mediastinum associated with effusive pleural cavity disease. Positional radiography and ultrasonography are helpful in differentiating mediastinal fluid accumulation from other causes of diffuse mediastinal widening. Focal mediastinal widening is

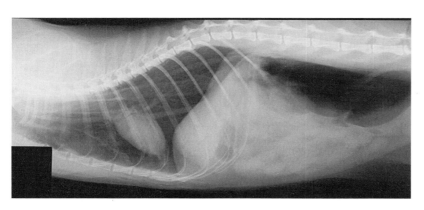

Figure 129–1. Lateral whole body radiograph of a 5-year-old female spayed cat presented after being in a fight with a dog. Numerous mediastinal structures, including cranial vena cava, aorta, serosal surface of the trachea, and esophagus, are well visualized owing to the presence of mediastinal gas (pneumomediastinum). There is a large accumulation of retroperitoneal gas, causing displacement of the kidneys and bowel ventrally.

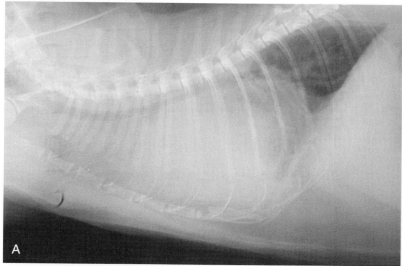

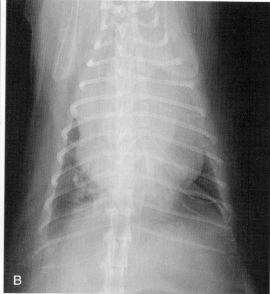

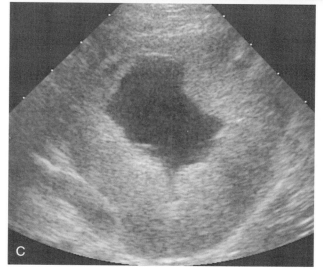

RES

Figure 129–2. Lateral *(A)* and ventrodorsal *(B)* radiographs and an axial ultrasonogram *(C)* of the thorax of a 7-year-old domestic longhair cat presented with tachypnea and cough. Radiographs demonstrate a slightly narrowed trachea that is displaced dorsally and to the right. The carina and lung fields are caudally displaced. The border of the cardiac silhouette is effaced by the cranial mediastinal mass. All these changes are consistent with a large cranial mediastinal mass. The ultrasonogram demonstrates that the mass is thick walled and cystic. This mass was removed surgically and was diagnosed as a thymoma histologically.

usually the result of a mass lesion associated with a neoplastic or inflammatory process. Pathologic mediastinal widening must be differentiated from diffuse widening associated with accumulation of fat in obese animals, which is a common radiographic finding in older dogs, especially in brachycephalic breeds.

Contrast radiographic procedures are often helpful in the further evaluation of structures within the mediastinum that cannot be adequately visualized on survey radiographs, such as the esophagus and great vessels. In the case of a suspected esophageal perforation, the contrast medium of choice should be a water-soluble iodinated product.

ULTRASONOGRAPHY

Thoracic ultrasonography provides poor visualization of the normal mediastinum because air in adjacent lung lobes prevents transmission of sound waves. However, sonographic evaluation may provide useful information in animals with pleural effusion or cranial mediastinal disease.[2] Ultrasonography allows visualization of most cranial mediastinal masses. Very large masses can be imaged from almost anywhere on the craniolateral thoracic wall. Placing the transducer in a parasternal position or using the heart as an

acoustic window may be necessary for adequate evaluation of smaller masses, such as enlarged sternal lymph nodes. In addition to identifying a mediastinal mass, ultrasonography helps to define its internal architecture as solid, cystic, cavitated, or fluid filled (Fig. 129–2). It also allows localization of vascular structures relative to the mass. Although ultrasonography alone usually does not allow indentification of the tissue of origin, it can be used to direct needle placement for fine-needle or tissue core biopsy.[2, 3] Transesophageal ultrasonography provides excellent visualization of the heart base, major cranial mediastinal vessels, descending aorta, and occasionally part of the azygous vein.[4]

OTHER IMAGING MODALITIES

Computed tomography (CT) provides the most detailed anatomic analysis of mediastinal structures.[5] It is valuable in defining the margins and size of mass lesions and can be used to guide placement of a needle or percutaneous biopsy instrument (Fig. 129–3). Disadvantages of CT include an inability to distinguish mediastinal masses from adjacent collapsed lung lobes, limited availability in veterinary practice, and the need for anesthesia. Thyroid scintigraphy using

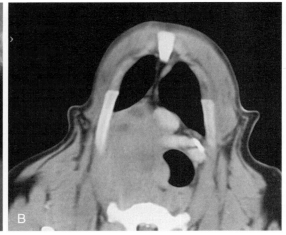

Figure 129–3. Lateral radiograph *(A)* and axial computed tomograph *(B)* of the cranial thorax of a 9-year-old male golden retriever presented with lameness of the right front leg and right-sided Horner's syndrome. The lateral radiograph demonstrates a lobulated craniodorsal mediastinal mass. The computed tomograph demonstrates a fluid opaque mass originating in the right craniodorsal mediastinum and causing displacement of the craniodorsal mediastinal structures to the left. Histology of the mass from necropsy indicated an undifferentiated sarcoma of the mediastinum.

technetium 99m or iodine 131 can be used to identify ectopic or metastatic thyroid tissue within the mediastinum.[6]

DISEASES OF THE MEDIASTINUM

PNEUMOMEDIASTINUM

Pneumomediastinum (the presence of gas within the mediastinum) can develop spontaneously (usually in animals with preexisting respiratory disease), or it can result from damage to the esophagus, trachea, or lungs associated with cervical trauma, mechanical ventilation, transtracheal aspiration, tracheostomy, or central venous catheter placement.[7] In addition, because of the normal communications between the mediastinum, retroperitoneum, and fascial planes of the neck, air may enter the mediastinum from subcutaneous tissues or the retroperitoneum (see Fig. 129–1). The most common cause of pneumomediastinum is bronchial or alveolar rupture (secondary to either pulmonary pathology or mechanical ventilation), with subsequent dissection of air along perivascular or peribronchial spaces to the pulmonary hilus. A sudden increase in intrathoracic pressure associated with coughing or severe dyspnea may induce spontaneous pneumomediastinum.

Pneumomediastinum does not occur secondary to pneumothorax. However, pneumothorax is often present in animals with pneumomediastinum and is caused either by rupture of the mediastinal pleura or by airway or alveolar rupture associated with underlying pulmonary disease. Subcutaneous emphysema and pneumoretroperitoneum may also occur secondary to pneumomediastinum. Clinical signs in animals with pneumomediastinum are usually limited to the presence of associated subcutaneous emphysema. Dyspnea is typically absent unless concurrent pneumothorax is present. Animals with esophageal rupture often present with pain, fever, and dysphagia. Acute development of severe pneumomediastinum may cause signs of circulatory collapse secondary to decreased venous return resulting from compression of the vena cava and azygous vein.

The air trapped in a pneumomediastinum is usually benign. Therefore, pneumomediastinum itself does not require therapy and will spontaneously resolve within two weeks if there is not an ongoing source of mediastinal air. Similarly, concurrent subcutaneous emphysema does not require needle aspiration unless the volume is large enough to cause the animal discomfort. Other therapy should be aimed at resolution of underlying disease.

MEDIASTINITIS

Mediastinal inflammation is manifested radiographically as either focal or diffuse mediastinal widening. It may result from esophageal or tracheal perforation, from deep cervical soft tissue infections that extend along fascial planes into the cranial mediastinum,[8] or from extension of infection from the pericardium, pulmonary parenchyma, or pleural space. In addition, chronic granulomatous mediastinitis may be caused by fungal *(Histoplasma, Blastomyces, Cryptococcus, Coccidioides)* or bacterial *(Actinomyces, Nocardia, Corynebacterium)* organisms.[9, 10] Abscessation of the mediastinum may result from progression of chronic infectious or neoplastic mediastinal disorders.[11] Both mediastinal abscesses and granulomas typically appear on radiographs as mediastinal masses and thus may be mistaken for neoplasia. Clinical signs that have been associated with mediastinitis include tachypnea (probably related to thoracic pain), dyspnea, fever, cough, head or neck edema, regurgitation, and voice changes secondary to recurrent involvement of laryngeal nerves. Pneumomediastinum often accompanies mediastinitis that is caused by esophageal or tracheal perforation.

Therapeutic measures for mediastinitis include efforts to resolve the underlying cause (e.g., surgical repair of esophageal perforation) combined with appropriate antimicrobial therapy and supportive care. Thoracostomy tube drainage is often necessary in animals with acute infectious mediastinitis. Mediastinal abscesses and granulomas often require surgical resection and/or drainage.[12]

MEDIASTINAL EDEMA

Mediastinal edema results from the same pathophysiologic mechanisms that produce edema in other areas of the body.

Potential causes include hypoproteinemia, lymphatic or venous obstruction, vasculitis, and heart failure. Clinical signs from mediastinal edema are minimal and are often overlooked because of accompanying pleural effusion.

MEDIASTINAL HEMORRHAGE

Hemorrhage into the mediastinum usually results from either trauma[13] or coagulopathy but has also been associated with neoplastic erosion of mediastinal vessels and with rapid thymic involution.[14] The latter is characterized by spontaneous mediastinal hemorrhage in young dogs.[15, 16] Most of the clinical signs associated with mediastinal hemorrhage are related to the effects of acute blood loss (e.g., pale mucous membranes, weak pulses). Dyspnea may occur if mediastinal hemorrhage progresses to hemothorax. Treatment of hemomediastinum should be aimed at the underlying cause of the hemorrhage.

MEDIASTINAL CYSTS

Benign cysts of pleural, branchial, lymphatic, bronchogenic, or thymic origin occur rarely in the mediastinum.[17, 18] Clinical signs are usually absent. Radiographically, a cyst can mimic a solid mass lesion. Ultrasonographically, a cyst can be differentiated from a solid mass, but solid neoplasias, abscesses, or granulomas may have cystic components. Fine-needle aspiration with or without ultrasound guidance may be helpful in differentiating cysts from other mediastinal lesions.

MEDIASTINAL MASS LESIONS

Mediastinal masses are common in dogs and cats and are usually caused by primary or metastatic neoplasia associated with structures within the mediastinum. Other potential causes of mediastinal masses include abscesses, granulomas, hematomas, cysts, esophageal foreign bodies, infectious lymphadenopathy, diaphragmatic hernias, gastroesophageal intussusception, and vascular lesions involving the great vessels.

Radiographically, mediastinal masses appear as thoracic opacities on or near the midline that frequently cause displacement of adjacent mediastinal or thoracic structures, such as the heart, esophagus, and trachea (see Fig. 129–2). The carina, which is normally located at the fifth or sixth intercostal space in the dog and at the sixth intercostal space in the cat, is displaced caudally by cranial mediastinal masses. Esophageal masses usually cause ventral displacement of the trachea; however, most other mediastinal masses displace the trachea dorsally and to the right. Other radiographic changes associated with mediastinal masses include increased opacity in the cranial thorax; widening of the mediastinum; tracheal compression; and loss of distinct, smooth, straight mediastinal borders. Masses that are in contact with a mediastinal structure may not have clearly defined borders. Mediastinal masses are frequently classified by location as cranioventral, craniodorsal, perihilar, caudoventral, or caudodorsal (Table 129–2).

Pleural effusion may imitate a mediastinal mass because of the associated tracheal elevation, which is caused by the dorsal displacement of the lungs.[19] Repeat radiographs obtained after removal of the pleural fluid are often helpful in distinguishing pleural effusion from a mediastinal mass.

TABLE 129–2. LESIONS ASSOCIATED WITH FOCAL MEDIASTINAL ENLARGEMENT

REGION	DISEASES
Cranioventral	Lymphadenopathy; abscess; thymic mass; ectopic thyroid; hematoma; granuloma; obesity; vascular mass (aorta, cranial vena cava); hematoma, esophageal mass, foreign body, or dilatation; tracheal mass
Craniodorsal	Esophageal mass, foreign body, or dilatation; heart base mass; neurogenic tumor; paraspinal or spinal mass; hematoma; lymphadenopathy; aortic stenosis, patent ductus arteriosus; mediastinal abscess; mediastinal hematoma; tracheal mass
Perihilar	Lymphadenopathy; left atrial enlargement; esophageal mass, foreign body, or dilatation; main pulmonary artery mass (post-stenotic dilatation); heart base or right atrial mass; spinal or paraspinal mass
Caudodorsal	Esophageal mass, foreign body, or dilatation; hiatal hernia; diaphragmatic hernia or mass; *Spirocerca lupi;* spinal or paraspinal mass; aortic aneurysm; gastroesophageal intussusception
Caudoventral	Diaphragmatic hernia (peritoneopericardial hernia); mediastinal abscess, granuloma, or hematoma

Other lesions that may be confused with a mediastinal mass include the normal thymus in young animals, mediastinal fat in obese animals, lung masses (especially those involving the accessory lobe or the cranial tips of left and right cranial lung lobes), very large right and left caudal pulmonary arteries, and perihilar edema. The presence of an air bronchogram within a suspected mediastinal mass indicates that it is actually a pulmonary lesion.

MEDIASTINAL NEOPLASIA

Mediastinal tumors can originate from structures within the mediastinum (e.g., lymph nodes, thymus, great vessels, trachea, esophagus, paravertebral tissue), from ectopic thyroid or parathyroid tissue, or from extension of neoplastic lesions in adjacent tissues (e.g., lung, mesothelium, thyroid). In addition, mediastinal neoplasms may be metastatic lesions or components of a multicentric neoplastic process, such as lymphoma, malignant histiocytosis,[20] or mastocytosis.[21] Clinical signs associated with mediastinal tumors are usually caused by compression or invasion of structures such as the great vessels, thoracic duct, esophagus, and trachea. Signs include coughing, dyspnea, dysphagia, regurgitation, and edema of the head, neck, and forelimbs (cranial vena caval syndrome). Signs caused by peripheral nerve entrapment are less common and could include laryngeal paralysis, vocalization changes, or Horner's syndrome. Signs associated with multicentric neoplasia may reflect other sites of neoplastic involvement or may be related to paraneoplastic syndromes.

Mediastinal lymphoma originates from either lymph node or thymic tissue in the cranial mediastinum. In cats, mediastinal lymphoma usually occurs in young cats infected with feline leukemia virus. It is often associated with pleural effusion, which may initially obscure radiographic visualization of the cranial mediastinal mass. The diagnosis of mediastinal lymphoma in a cat can often be confirmed by cytologic identification of neoplastic lymphocytes in either a sample of pleural fluid or a sample obtained via fine-needle aspiration of the mediastinal mass. In dogs, mediastinal lymphoma is often associated with hypercalcemia, and the presence of a mediastinal mass is a poor prognostic indicator in hypercalcemic dogs with lymphoma.[22] Less common lymphatic-based tumors that can cause mediastinal masses in dogs and cats include lymphangiosarcoma and lymphangioma.[23–25]

Chemodectomas, which are usually aortic body tumors or carotid body tumors, are most often identified as heart base masses in older brachycephalic dogs.[26] Affected animals may be presented for dysphagia, dyspnea, heart failure, or cervical swelling. Because these tumors often invade and surround the roots of the great vessels at the heart base, surgical resection is difficult.

MEDIASTINAL LYMPHADENOPATHY

Lymph node pathology is the most common cause of mediastinal mass lesions in dogs and cats. There are three sets of lymph nodes within the mediastinum: (1) cranial mediastinal lymph nodes, which lie along the major vascular structures and just ventral to the trachea; (2) sternal lymph nodes, which are just dorsal to the sternum, medial to the second costal cartilage, and cranioventral to the internal thoracic vessels; and (3) tracheobronchial (hilar) lymph nodes, which are found at the bifurcation of the trachea and proximal bronchi. None of these lymph nodes are normally visible on survey thoracic radiographs.

Enlarged sternal or tracheobronchial lymph nodes are most easily visualized on a lateral radiograph, whereas cranial mediastinal lymphadenopathy is better appreciated on a VD or DV view. Radiographic findings associated with enlargement of the tracheobronchial lymph nodes include separation of the main stem bronchi, elevation of the trachea cranial to the carina (Fig. 129–4), and ventral deviation of the main caudal lobe bronchi caudal to the carina. Left atrial enlargement is the main differential diagnosis for this radiographic appearance.

Mediastinal lymphadenopathy in small animals is usually the result of either neoplastic infiltration or infection with bacterial, fungal, or mycobacterial organisms. Lymphoma, in addition to causing a cranial mediastinal mass in some dogs (see earlier), is often associated with sternal and/or tracheobronchial lymphadenopathy.[27] Lymphomatoid granulomatosis is a rare neoplastic/inflammatory disease of unknown etiology that causes hilar lymphadenopathy, pulmonary masses, and pleural effusion in young dogs.[28] It is often associated with peripheral eosinophilia, basophilia, and leukocytosis. Evidence of eosinophilic inflammation may also be present in cytologic samples of pleural fluid or tissue aspirates.

Mediastinal lymphadenopathy (especially of the tracheobronchial nodes) is often detected in animals with blastomycosis, coccidioidomycosis, histoplasmosis, and cryptococcosis and may be the primary radiographic finding in these animals. Systemic atypical mycobacteriosis, although rare, has also been associated with mediastinal lymphadenopathy in dogs.[29] Bacterial infections that may be associated with mediastinal lymphadenopathy include pyothorax and mediastinitis. In addition, because lymphatic drainage to the sternal lymph node includes the abdomen, inflammatory or neoplastic abdominal disorders (e.g., pancreatitis, carcinomatosis) may result in sternal lymphadenopathy.[7]

DISORDERS OF THE THYMUS

The thymus extends from the thoracic inlet caudally to the fifth rib in the dog and the sixth rib in the cat. Dorsally it lies next to the phrenic nerves and cranial vena cava. Laterally it is bounded by the cranial lung lobes. Thymic

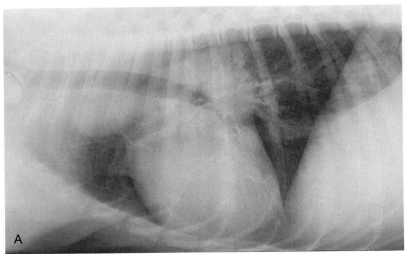

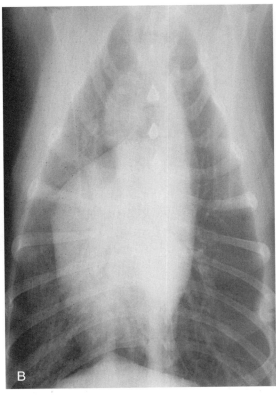

Figure 129–4. Lateral *(A)* and ventrodorsal *(B)* thoracic radiographs of a 1-year-old golden retriever presented with anorexia, weight loss, and fever of unknown origin. The radiographs demonstrate mass lesions (lymphadenopathy) in the craniodorsal and hilar regions. On the lateral radiograph the main stem bronchi are being displaced ventrally. There is mild main stem bronchial compression of both right and left sides on the ventrodorsal radiograph. Final diagnosis was lymphoma.

involution in small animals occurs concurrently with the onset of sexual maturity and the loss of deciduous teeth.[30] Spontaneous thymic hemorrhage may occur in association with thymic involution and is usually fatal.[15, 16] Dogs younger than 2 years of age (especially German shepherds and cocker spaniels) are most often affected. Thymic branchial cysts, which arise from remnants of branchial pouch epithelium, are generally identified as multiple small cysts in the cranial mediastinum. They are usually encountered in older dogs and appear radiographically as a mediastinal mass.

THYMOMA

Thymomas are rare canine and feline tumors that arise from the epithelial cells of the thymus.[31, 32] They appear radiographically as large, poorly defined soft tissue masses in the cranial mediastinum (see Fig. 129–2). Expansion and invasion into adjacent tissues are common, but in some cases the masses are well encapsulated and fairly noninvasive. Metastasis has been reported in dogs but not in cats.[33] Pleural effusion is a variable finding and may hinder visualization of the thymic mass. Sonographically, thymomas can appear as either solid or cystic masses (see Fig. 129–2). Cytologic examination of fine-needle aspirates reveals a variable number of mature lymphocytes, which makes cytologic differentiation of thymoma from mediastinal lymphoma difficult. Mast cells are also frequently identified in cytologic samples from thymomas. Surgical or ultrasound-guided percutaneous biopsy is required for a definitive diagnosis. Paraneoplastic syndromes are commonly associated with thymoma in both dogs and cats. The most well described is myasthenia gravis, which is often associated with megaesophagus in dogs with thymoma.[31] Myasthenia is less common in cats with thymoma, in which it typically causes signs of weakness such as neck ventroflexion. Other paraneoplastic disorders that have been associated with thymoma include polymyositis and hypercalcemia. Surgical resection is the treatment of choice for thymoma, but recurrence is common.

REFERENCES

1. Dyce K, Sack WO, Wensing CJG: Textbook of Veterinary Anatomy. Philadelphia, WB Saunders, 1996, pp 406–407.
2. Konde LJ, Spaulding K: Sonographic evaluation of the cranial mediastinum in small animals. Vet Radiol 32:178, 1991.
3. Burk RL, Ackerman N: Small Animal Radiology and Ultrasonography. Philadelphia, WB Saunders, 1996, pp 91–92.
4. St.-Vincent RS, Pharr JW: Transesophageal ultrasonography of the normal canine mediastinum. Vet Radiol Ultrasound 39:197, 1998.
5. Burk RL: Computed tomography of thoracic diseases in dogs. JAVMA 199:617, 1991.
6. Adams WH, et al: Treatment of differentiated thyroid carcinoma in 7 dogs utilizing 131 I. Vet Radiol Ultrasound 36:417, 1995.
7. Thrall DE: The mediastinum. In Thrall DE (ed): Textbook of Veterinary Diagnostic Radiology. Philadelphia, WB Saunders, 1994, pp 289–290.
8. Myer W: Radiographic review: The mediastinum. J Am Vet Radiol Soc 21:198, 1978.
9. Schmidt M, Wolvekamp P: Radiographic findings in ten dogs with thoracic actinomycosis. Vet Radiol 32:301, 1991.
10. Meadows RL, et al: Chylothorax associated with cryptococcal mediastinal granuloma in a cat. Vet Clin Pathol 22:109, 1993.
11. Salisbury SK, et al: Peritracheal abscesses associated with tracheal collapse and bilateral laryngeal paralysis in a dog. JAVMA 196:1273, 1990.
12. Barrett RJ, et al: Use of ultrasonography and secondary wound closure to facilitate diagnosis and treatment of a cranial mediastinal abscess in a dog. JAVMA 203:1293, 1993.
13. Mason GD, et al: Fatal mediastinal hemorrhage in a dog. Vet Radiol 31:214, 1990.
14. Klopfer U, et al: Spontaneous fatal hemorrhage in the involuting thymus in dogs. J Am Anim Hosp Assoc 21:261, 1985.
15. Coolman BR, et al: Severe idiopathic thymic hemorrhage in two littermate dogs. JAVMA 205:1152, 1994.
16. Glaus TM, et al: Acute thymic hemorrhage and hemothorax in a dog. J Am Anim Hosp Assoc 29:489, 1993.
17. Malik C, et al: Benign cranial mediastinal lesions in three cats. Aust Vet J 75:183, 1997.
18. Ellison GW, et al: Idiopathic mediastinal cyst in a cat. Vet Radiol Ultrasound 35:347, 1994.
19. Snyder PS, et al: The utility of thoracic radiographic measurement for the detection of cardiomegaly in cats with pleural effusion. Vet Radiol 31:89, 1990.
20. Schmidt ML, et al: Clinical and radiographic manifestations of canine malignant histiocytosis. Vet Q 15:117, 1993.
21. Pollack MJ, et al: Disseminated malignant mastocytoma in a dog. J Am Anim Hosp Assoc 27:435, 1991.
22. Rosenberg MP, et al: Prognostic factors in dogs with lymphoma and hypercalcemia (abstract). Proceedings of the 9th Annual Conference of the Veterinary Cancer Society, Raleigh, NC, 1989.
23. Stobie D, Carpenter JL: Lymphangiosarcoma of the mediastinum, mesentery, and omentum in a cat. J Am Anim Hosp Assoc 29:78, 1993.
24. Remedios A, et al: Mediastinal cystic lymphangioma in a dog. J Am Anim Hosp Assoc 26:161, 1990.
25. Myers NC, et al: Chylothorax and chylous ascites in a dog with mediastinal lymphosarcoma. J Am Anim Hosp Assoc 32:263, 1996.
26. Obradovich JE, et al: Carotid body tumors in the canine: 11 cases (abstract). Proceedings of the 8th Annual Conference of the Veterinary Cancer Society, Estes Park, CO, 1988.
27. Starrak GS, et al: Correlation between thoracic radiographic changes and remission/survival duration in 270 dogs with lymphosarcoma. Vet Radiol Ultrasound 38:411, 1997.
28. Berry CR, et al: Pulmonary lymphomatoid granulomatosis in seven dogs (1976–1987). J Vet Intern Med 4:157, 1990.
29. Grooters AM, et al: Systemic Mycobacterium smegmatis infection in a basset hound. JAVMA 206:200, 1995.
30. Davenport DJ: The lymphoid system. In Hoskins JD (ed): Veterinary Pediatrics. Philadelphia, WB Saunders, 1990, pp 405–414.
31. Klebanow ER: Thymoma and acquired mysasthenia gravis in the dog: A case report and review of 133 additional cases. J Am Anim Hosp Assoc 28:63, 1992.
32. Atwater SW, et al: Thymoma in dogs: 23 cases (1980–1991). JAVMA 205:1007, 1994.
33. Sorde A, et al: Psychomotor epilepsy associated with metastatic thymoma in a dog. J Small Anim Pract 35:377, 1994.

RES

CHAPTER 130

PLEURAL AND EXTRAPLEURAL DISEASES

Theresa W. Fossum

DISORDERS OF THE DIAPHRAGM

DIAPHRAGMATIC HERNIAS

Diaphragmatic hernia (DH) is a term that refers to disorders of the diaphragm that allow abdominal contents to enter the thoracic cavity, either within the pleural space (pleuroperitoneal hernias) or within the pericardial sac (peritoneopericardial diaphragmatic hernias). DHs are common in dogs and cats and may be the result of trauma or may be congenital. Clinically recognized congenital DHs are usually pericardial in nature because pleuroperitoneal hernias usually result in death upon, or shortly after, birth.[1] The incidence of congenital DH in humans has been estimated to range from 0.08 per 1000 to 0.45 per 1000 births.[2] Similar epidemiologic studies have not been reported for diaphragmatic herniation in domestic animals.

Congenital DHs in children are associated with pulmonary hypoplasia, and controversy exists as to whether the primary pathology is the diaphragmatic defect with secondary pulmonary hypoplasia, or whether pulmonary hypoplasia leads to intrathoracic herniation of the diaphragm.[3] True DHs, also known as eventration, are defined as subtotal diaphragmatic tears in which the serosa on the diaphragmatic surface of the diaphragm remains intact, precluding direct communication between the pleural and pericardial sacs. A cat with a true DH in which only falciform fat was herniated into the thoracic cavity has been reported.[4] A thoracic mass was noted in the caudal thorax of abdominal films during evaluation of the aforementioned cat for recurrent, intermittent diarrhea. Whether the DH was congenital or traumatic was not determined. Hernias involving the esophageal hiatus are typically congenital in nature and are known as hiatal hernias (see Chapter 136).

Traumatic DHs are more commonly recognized in small animal veterinary patients than are congenital hernias and are frequently associated with motor vehicle accidents.[5, 6] The abrupt increase in intra-abdominal pressure that accompanies forceful blows to the abdominal wall causes the lungs to rapidly deflate (if the glottis is open), resulting in a large pleuroperitoneal pressure gradient. This pressure gradient causes the diaphragm to tear at its weakest points, generally in the muscular portions. The location and size of the tear(s) depend on the position of the animal at the time of impact and location of the viscera. Traumatic DHs are often associated with significant respiratory embarrassment; however, chronic DHs are commonly diagnosed in asymptomatic animals.

Traumatic Diaphragmatic Hernias

Signalment and History. Young male dogs between the ages of 1 and 2 years are most commonly diagnosed

with traumatic DH because of their propensity to roam and sustain vehicular trauma or other forceful blows to the abdomen or chest (e.g., being kicked by horses or cattle). The duration of DH may range from a few hours to years. In one study, 20 per cent of animals with traumatic DH were not diagnosed until at least 4 weeks after the injury had occurred (chronic DH).[7] Affected animals may be presented in shock following the injury and often have associated injuries, such as fractures. With chronic DH, clinical signs are most often referable to either the respiratory or gastrointestinal systems and may include dyspnea, exercise intolerance, anorexia, depression, vomiting, diarrhea, weight loss, and/or pain following ingestion of food.

Physical Examination Findings. Animals with traumatic DH are frequently presented in shock; thus clinical signs may include pale or cyanotic mucous membranes, tachypnea, tachycardia, and/or oliguria. Cardiac arrhythmias are common and are associated with significant morbidity. Other clinical signs are dependent upon which organs herniate and may be attributed to the gastrointestinal, respiratory, or cardiovascular systems. The liver is the most common herniated organ and is often associated with hydrothorax as a result of entrapment and venous occlusion. Extrahepatic biliary obstruction may also occur.[8] Concomitant gastric dilatation volvulus and DH have been reported and should be suspected in cats presenting with abdominal enlargement and dyspnea.

Diagnosis. Definitive diagnosis of pleuroperitoneal DH is typically made either on thoracic radiographs or by ultrasonography of the diaphragm and cranial abdomen.[9] Ultrasound examination of the diaphragmatic silhouette is most helpful in animals in which hepatic herniation is present or when large volumes of pleural effusion mask identification of abdominal contents in the thoracic cavity. If significant pleural effusion is present, thoracentesis is often necessary for diagnostic radiographs. Radiographic signs of DH include loss of the diaphragmatic line, loss of the cardiac silhouette, dorsal or lateral displacement of lung fields, presence of gas or a barium-filled stomach or intestines in the thoracic cavity, and pleural effusion (Figs. 130–1 and 130–2). Positive-contrast celiography, using a water-soluble contrast agent, may occasionally be needed for the diagnosis. However, caution should be used when interpreting positive-contrast celiograms because omental and fibrous adhesions may seal the defect, resulting in false-negative films.

Management. Although DHs are a surgical disorder, immediate surgical intervention is not warranted in many animals. Many animals have associated thoracic trauma (i.e., pulmonary contusion and/or hemorrhage) and are best stabilized prior to being anesthetized for definitive repair of the diaphragmatic defect. An exception to this may be animals with herniation of the stomach. These animals must be

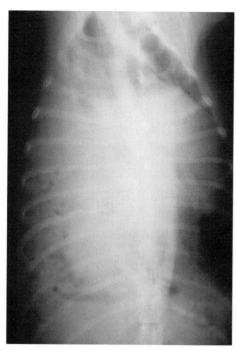

Figure 130–1. Ventrodorsal thoracic radiograph of a dog with a traumatic diaphragmatic hernia. Notice the gas-filled loops of small intestine in the right hemithorax.

carefully evaluated for gastric distention and operated on as soon as they can safely be anesthetized because acute gastric distention within the thorax may cause rapid, fatal respiratory impairment. Initially, if the animal is dyspneic, oxygen should be provided by face mask, nasal insufflation, or an oxygen cage. Positioning the animal in sternal recumbency with the forelimbs elevated may help ventilation. If moderate or severe pleural effusion is present, thoracentesis should be performed. Fluid therapy and antibiotics should be given if the animal is in shock (see Chapter 78). Readers are referred to a surgery textbook for details of surgical correction of DH.

Peritoneopericardial Diaphragmatic Hernias

Peritoneopericardial diaphragmatic hernias (PPDHs) occur when there is a congenital communication between the abdomen and the pericardial sac. As with traumatic DHs, they may be associated with severe respiratory embarrassment or affected animals may be asymptomatic. Although PPDH may arise in human beings as a result of trauma (the diaphragm forms one wall of the pericardial sac in human beings), they are always congenital in dogs and cats because there is no direct communication between the pericardial and peritoneal cavities after birth. The most widely accepted theory regarding the embryogenesis of this defect is that the hernia arises because of faulty development or prenatal injury of the septum transversum. This could be a result of a teratogen, genetic defect, or prenatal injury. The embryotoxic herbicide nitrofen, when given to rats during a critical period in gestation, induces a high incidence of right- and left-sided DH.[3] PPDH has been reported to be the most common congenital heart defect diagnosed in cats 2 years of age or older.[10]

Cardiac abnormalities and sternal deformities often occur concomitantly with PPDH.[11] The combination of congenital cranial abdominal wall, caudal sternal, diaphragmatic, and pericardial defects has been reported in dogs, often associated with ventricular septal defects or other intracardiac defects (Fig. 130–3). Pulmonary vascular abnormalities have been noted in children with congenital DH, and persistent pulmonary hypertension is thought to contribute to the morbidity/mortality of this disease in affected children.[12] Polycystic kidneys have been reported in association with PPDH in cats. For information regarding the signalment, history, physical examination findings, diagnosis, and management of PPDH, please see Chapter 114.

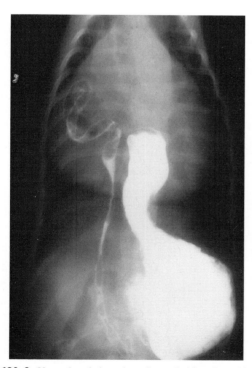

Figure 130–2. Ventrodorsal thoracic radiograph of a dog with a peritoneopericardial diaphragmatic hernia after administration of barium. Notice that the pylorus and proximal small intestine are located in the thoracic cavity.

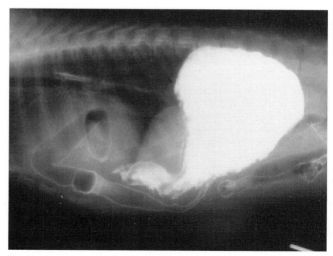

Figure 130–3. Lateral thoracic radiograph of a dog with a peritoneopericardial diaphragmatic hernia. This dog also had a cranial abdominal wall hernia and a ventricular septal defect. (From Fossum TW: Small Animal Surgery. St. Louis, CV Mosby, 1997, p 685.)

RES

DIAPHRAGMATIC DISPLACEMENT/DYSFUNCTION

Caudal diaphragmatic displacement may be associated with pleural cavity disease (e.g., pneumothorax, pleural effusion) or obstructive airway disease that causes air trapping and pulmonary hyperinflation. Typically, the displacement is bilateral and may be difficult to recognize if pleural effusion masks identification of the diaphragmatic silhouette. Unilateral caudal displacement is uncommon but may occur with unilateral pleural effusion, particularly chylothorax or pyothorax.

Cranial displacement of the diaphragm may also occur. Enlargement (e.g., late-term pregnancy) or gas distention of abdominal contents, such as occurs with gastric dilatation–volvulus, may cause marked cranial diaphragmatic displacement and contribute to respiratory difficulties in affected animals. Removal of a lung lobe or pulmonary atelectasis or consolidation may result in unilateral cranial advancement of the diaphragm.

Paralysis of the diaphragm may occur unilaterally or bilaterally. The diaphragm is innervated by the phrenic nerves, which arise from C4 to C7. These nerves traverse the mediastinum and pericardium to supply the diaphragm; thus infiltrative masses, surgical transection (during pericardiectomy or mass removal), as well as neuropathies, may cause unilateral diaphragmatic paralysis. Unilateral diaphragmatic paralysis seldom causes clinically evident abnormalities in respiration; however, bilateral paralysis may be associated with significant ventilatory abnormalities. Bilateral paralysis is most frequently associated with cervical spinal trauma or fracture. Radiographically, cranial displacement of the diaphragm may be noted; however, unilateral cranial displacement is more apparent on thoracic films than is bilateral displacement. Lack of movement of the diaphragm during fluoroscopic evaluation may lead to increased suspicion of this condition.

DISORDERS OF THE CHEST WALL

CHEST WALL TRAUMA

Thoracic wall injury may be due to either blunt (i.e., motor vehicular accidents, being kicked by a horse) or penetrating trauma. The most common causes of penetrating injuries of the thorax in dogs are bite wounds and gunshot injuries. Both blunt and penetrating trauma may cause extensive soft tissue damage of the thoracic wall. Although soft tissue damage is rarely the cause of major morbidity or mortality, in some animals it may be the only external evidence of severe thoracic trauma. Occasionally, pain associated with muscular tears may lead to altered respiration because the animal is unwilling to breathe deeply. Unless associated with pulmonary parenchymal damage, alterations in ventilation that lead to hypoxemia seldom occur with chest wall trauma.

Subcutaneous emphysema may occur with both blunt and penetrating trauma but is usually of little significance. This occurs when air is forced into subcutaneous tissues and dissects along muscular and fascial planes. The air may reach the subcutaneous tissues through a disruption of the pleura and intercostal muscles, by direct communication with an external wound, or as an extension of mediastinal emphysema. Treatment of subcutaneous air should be directed at its cause. Similarly, isolated rib fractures are seldom associated with major morbidity. Occasionally rib fractures produce sharp fragments that may injure a major vessel or lacerate the lung. Rib fractures may interfere with ventilation if the animal splints the thorax in an attempt to reduce pain by decreasing motion of the fragments.

Flail chest occurs when several ribs on both sides of the point of impact are fractured such that the intervening rib segments lose their continuity with the remainder of the thorax. Paradoxic movement of the chest wall occurs during respiration as a result of intrapleural pressure changes; the fractured segment moves inward during inspiration and outward during expiration. Respiratory abnormalities in patients with flail chest include decreased vital capacity, reduced functional residual capacity, hypoxemia, decreased compliance, increased airway resistance, and increased work of breathing. These abnormal respiratory parameters were once thought to be due primarily to the movement of the flail segment; however, it is now believed that the underlying lung damage and hypoventilation from chest pain are more important factors in the development of respiratory insufficiency.

PECTUS EXCAVATUM

Pectus excavatum (PE) is a deformity of the sternum and costocartilages that results in a dorsal to ventral narrowing of the thorax.[13] Pectus carinatum is a protrusion of the sternum that occurs much less frequently than PE. Synonyms for PE include funnel chest, chondrosternal depression, chonechondrosternon, koilosternia, and trichterbust.

The cause or causes of PE in animals are unknown (Fig. 130–4). Theories proposed include shortening of the central tendon of the diaphragm, intrauterine pressure abnormalities, and congenital deficiency of the musculature in the cranial portion of the diaphragm. Abnormal respiratory gradients appear to play a role in the development of this disease in some animals, as brachycephalic dogs are most commonly affected, many of which have concurrent hypoplastic tracheas. PE may be associated with "swimmer's syndrome," which is a poorly characterized disease of neonatal dogs in which the limbs tend to splay laterally, impairing ambulation. Abnormalities of the joints of the limbs and the long bones may also occur. Although the etiology of PE is uncertain, multiple animals in some litters have been affected; thus

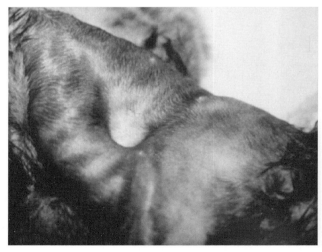

Figure 130–4. A cat with pectus excavatum. Notice the palpable depression of the caudal sternum. (From Fossum TW, et al: Pectus excavatum in 8 dogs and 6 cats. J Am Anim Hosp Assoc 25:595, 1989.)

breeding should not be undertaken and affected animals should be neutered.

Patients with PE may have abnormalities of both respiratory and cardiovascular function. Circulatory disorders in animals with PE may occur as a result of abnormal cardiac positioning resulting in kinking of the large veins and disturbance of venous return, compression of the heart predisposing to arrhythmias (particularly the auricles), restriction of ventricular capacity, and decreased respiratory reserve. Cardiac murmurs are common in patients with PE and appear to be associated with the cardiac malpositioning. These murmurs often disappear following surgical correction of the defect or a change in the patient's position. Systolic murmurs in some patients appear to be related to kinking of the pulmonary artery or to exaggeration of the artery's normal vibrations resulting from its proximity to the chest wall. Animals with PE and innocent systolic murmurs must be differentiated from those that have underlying cardiac defects, such as pulmonic stenosis or atrial septal defects.

Signalment and History. PE is a congenital abnormality in dogs and cats. In symptomatic animals, clinical signs are usually present at birth or shortly thereafter. PE may occur in any breed, but brachycephalic dogs appear to be predisposed. A sex predisposition has not been identified. Many animals with PE are asymptomatic; however, the defect is usually palpable and this may prompt owners to seek veterinary care, despite lack of obvious clinical signs. Symptomatic animals may present for evaluation of exercise intolerance, weight loss, hyperpnea, recurrent pulmonary infections, cyanosis, vomiting, persistent and productive coughing, inappetence, and/or mild episodes of upper respiratory disease. A correlation between severity of clinical signs and severity of anatomic or physiologic abnormalities has not been observed.

Physical Examination Findings. The sternal deformity is usually palpable. Other physical examination findings may include cardiac murmurs and harsh lung sounds. Dyspnea is variable, but rapid, shallow respirations may be noted.

Diagnosis. Thoracic radiographs show abnormal elevation of the sternum in the caudal thorax. Objective assessment of the deformity may be determined by measuring the frontosagittal and vertebral indices on thoracic radiographs.[14] Frontosagittal index is calculated by taking the ratio of the width of the chest at the tenth thoracic vertebra, measured on a dorsoventral or ventrodorsal radiograph, and the distance between the center of the ventral surface of the tenth thoracic vertebra and the nearest point on the sternum. Vertebral index is calculated as the ratio of the distance between the center of the dorsal surface of the selected vertebral body to the nearest point on the sternum and the dorsoventral diameter of the center of the same vertebral body. It has been proposed that the severity of PE be characterized as mild, moderate, or severe based on frontosagittal index and vertebral index. Such determination may aid in the objective assessment of improvement of thoracic diameters following surgery.

Thoracic radiographs should be evaluated for the evidence of concurrent abnormalities (i.e., tracheal hypoplasia, cardiac abnormalities, pneumonia). Most animals with PE have abnormally positioned hearts (Fig. 130–5), which may cause the heart to appear enlarged radiographically; thus, true cardiac enlargement cannot always be distinguished from apparent enlargement due to abnormal heart position.

Management. Animals with merely a flat chest may contour to a normal or near-normal configuration without

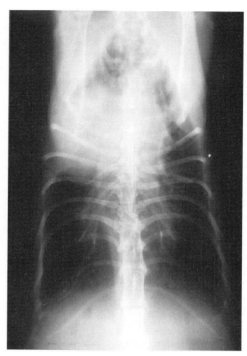

Figure 130–5. Thoracic radiograph showing malpositioning of the heart in a puppy with pectus excavatum. (From Fossum TW, et al: Pectus excavatum in 8 dogs and 6 cats. J Am Anim Hosp Assoc 25:595, 1989.)

RES

surgical intervention. However, owners should be encouraged to regularly perform medial-to-lateral compression of the chest on these young animals. Animals with severe elevation of the sternum will not benefit from this technique or from splintage that simply provides medial-to-lateral compression and does not correct the malpositioned sternum. Other medical management includes treatment of respiratory tract infections and, if the animal is severely dyspneic, oxygen therapy.

THORACIC WALL AND STERNAL NEOPLASIA

Primary tumors of the rib are uncommon in the dog; however, these tumors are usually malignant, have a high metastatic rate, and generally develop in young dogs, with a mean reported age in one study of 4.5 years.[15] Osteosarcomas are the most common neoplasm of the canine rib, followed by chondrosarcoma; the costochondral junction is the usual site of origin of these tumors. Most rib tumors cause a localized swelling of the thoracic wall; however, pleural effusion without evidence of a thoracic mass has been reported in two dogs with primary rib tumors and metastatic pulmonary lesions.[15] Other clinical signs of rib tumors are weight loss and dyspnea.

A tentative diagnosis of the cell type can usually be made by fine-needle aspiration of the mass; however, definitive diagnosis usually requires histologic examination of a biopsy specimen. Although pleural effusion is common in dogs with rib tumors, identification of neoplastic cells in the fluid is very uncommon. Owing to the high rate of pulmonary metastasis, the prognosis for dogs with rib tumors is poor. In one study of 15 dogs with primary rib tumors, greater than 90 per cent of the dogs died or were euthanized within 4 months of the diagnosis.[15]

Although also rare, both metastatic and primary tumors of

the sternum have been reported in dogs.[16] In humans, metastatic tumors involving the sternum are more frequently recognized than primary tumors. The distant primary site is most commonly in the thyroid, kidney, breast, testicle, lung, stomach, or rectum. Primary neoplasms of the bony chest comprise 7 to 8 per cent of all bone tumors in humans, and although primary rib tumors are frequently benign, tumors of the sternum are typically malignant. Similar generalizations are difficult to make in the dog, owing to the infrequency with which sternal tumors have been reported. However, chondrosarcomas and osteosarcomas involving the sternebrae have been reported in dogs.[17]

When a diagnosis of sternal neoplasia is made, the diseased bone as well as normal surrounding tissue should be removed. Unlike most bones in the body, the sternebrae can be removed with little compromise of function.[18] Successful treatment of sternal osteomyelitis following resection of large portions of the sternebrae has been reported in dogs and human beings, and the procedure would likely benefit dogs with primary sternal neoplasia.

PLEURAL EFFUSION

One of the more common diagnostic problems encountered by practitioners is pleural effusion. Although the cause of the pleural effusion may be readily apparent, such as when it is associated with cardiac disease, oftentimes the underlying disease is obscure and difficult to ascertain. Analysis of pleural fluid and categorization according to specific physical, biochemical, and cytologic parameters facilitate the formation of a rational therapeutic plan in animals with pleural effusion.

ANATOMY OF THE PLEURAL SPACE

The pleural space is lined by the visceral and parietal pleura. The visceral pleura covers the surface of the lungs, whereas the parietal pleura covers the diaphragm, costal surface, and mediastinum. The pleura consists of mesothelial cells and a thin layer of connective tissue through which blood vessels and lymphatics pass. Normally, the small amount of pleural fluid that is present within the pleural space is removed by parietal pleural lymphatics and lymphatics on the diaphragmatic and mediastinal surfaces.[19] Cells, large proteins, and particulate matter are transported to the blood stream via lymphatics in the parietal pleura. There is some experimental evidence that suggests that stomas exist between the mesothelial cells of the parietal pleura and the endothelial cells of the pleura lymphatics.[20] Movement through these stomas may be facilitated by muscle movement during respiration. Obstruction of these stomas by fibrinous material may decrease the absorption of exudative pleural effusions and increase the likelihood of formation of fibrosing pleuritis. In normal animals, a small amount of fluid (probably <2 mL) exists in the pleural space and serves to lubricate the surfaces of the lungs during respiration. This fluid differs from blood in that it is composed primarily of mesothelial cells and monocytes. The protein content of the pleural fluid is similar to other interstitial compartments; however, differences in electrolyte composition between pleural fluid and blood suggest that active transport or selective diffusion may modify an ultrafiltrate of plasma in the normal animal.[21]

ETIOLOGY

Pleural effusions develop when disease alters the forces that control the formation and absorption of pleural fluid.[21] Changes in hydrostatic and oncotic pressures and vascular or lymphatic permeability may increase pleural fluid production and/or decrease its resorption, resulting in pleural effusion.

Some of the more common causes of pleural effusion result in increased vascular permeability by inducing a vasculitis, or by obstructing, or increasing, the permeability of lymphatics. Increased vascular permeability may be caused by vascular engorgement or chemical mediators such as histamine that are released during an inflammatory process. As permeability increases, increased amounts of protein and fluid leak into the pleural space. This fluid must be removed from the pleural space by lymphatics, and failure to do so will result in a clinical effusion with a relatively high protein content. Effusions with a high protein content (generally >3.0 g/dL) imply that there is either increased vascular permeability or decreased lymphatic removal, or both, and should suggest to clinicians that the cause of these effusions is inflammation, neoplasia, or diseases of the lymphatic system.[21] Effusions with low protein content, on the other hand, are generally caused by cardiac, hepatic, or renal disease and are known as transudates. Hepatic hydrothorax is defined as a large pleural effusion occurring in a patient with cirrhosis of the liver in the absence of primary pulmonary or cardiac disease.[22] Abdominal effusion may or may not be present in affected patients. These effusions often recur and may be associated with peritoneopleural communications in the diaphragm or occur via transdiaphragmatic lymphatic drainage of the cranial abdomen.

A well-recognized cause of vasculitis-induced pleural effusion in cats is feline infectious peritonitis (FIP). Immune-mediated diseases, such as systemic lupus erythematosus and rheumatoid arthritis, may also manifest primarily as pleural effusion secondary to vasculitis.[23] Uremia and pancreatitis may cause vasculitis and pleural effusion. Other inflammatory or infectious causes of pleural effusion include bacterial, viral, fungal, or parasitic pneumonia. Neoplasia (e.g., lymphosarcoma, metastatic mammary neoplasia, mesothelioma) when associated with parietal pleural deposits may obstruct lymphatic drainage or lead to an increase in capillary permeability; visceral pleural deposits may reduce capillary absorption. Elevated cardiac pressure may increase lymphatic permeability and decrease lymphatic drainage, thereby resulting in pleural effusion.

Increased systemic venous hydrostatic pressure is a potential cause of pleural effusion. The most common cause of increased venous hydrostatic pressure is congestive heart failure secondary to cardiomyopathy. With high venous pressures, lymphatic drainage of the pleural space may be impeded resulting in either a transudative effusion or chylothorax. Other causes of increased systemic venous hydrostatic pressure include pericardial effusion and cardiac tamponade, heartworm disease, diaphragmatic hernia, lung lobe torsion, and neoplasia.

Increased negative pressure of the pleural space may be seen in animals with fibrosing pleuritis. In these animals, because the lungs cannot reexpand as pleural fluid is absorbed or removed, the pressures in the pleural space may become increasingly negative.[21] These negative pressures promote rapid reaccumulation of fluid in the pleural space. A second potential cause of increased negative pleural pressure resulting in effusion is severe upper airway obstruction.

Decreased oncotic pressure may also manifest as pleural

effusion. Reduced osmotic pressures result in increased filtration of fluid from the capillaries of the parietal pleura and decreased reabsorption from the capillaries of the visceral pleura. Causes of decreased oncotic pressure include hypoalbuminemia secondary to liver disease (decreased production), protein-losing enteropathy or nephropathy (increased loss), and neoplasia. Serum albumin levels of less than 1.5 g/dL may be associated with pleural effusion.

CLINICAL SIGNS

Clinical signs associated with pleural effusion vary depending on the underlying etiology, rapidity of fluid accumulation, and volume of fluid. Most animals do not exhibit clinical signs until there is significant impairment of ventilation; hence, pleural effusion may first be noted by veterinarians on careful physical examination, prior to the presence of obvious clinical signs. Both short- and long-term effects of pleural effusion on lung function may be noted.

The most common clinical sign noted in dogs or cats with pleural effusion is dyspnea. The dyspnea is usually marked by a forceful inspiration, with delayed expiration. The latter may make the animal appear to be holding its breath. Other clinical signs include tachypnea, cyanosis, open mouth breathing, muffled heart and lung sounds, and coughing. Coughing may be a result of irritation caused by the effusion, or may be related to the underlying disease process (such as cardiomyopathy or thoracic neoplasia). Coughing may be the first clinical sign observed with chronic forms of pleural effusion, such as chylothorax. Thus, animals with coughing that do not respond to standard treatment of nonspecific respiratory problems should be evaluated for pleural effusion. Additional findings in patients with pleural effusion may include fever, depression, anorexia, weight loss, pale mucous membranes, arrhythmias, murmurs, ascites, and pericardial effusion.

Removal of even small amounts of pleural effusion may greatly improve the animal's ability to ventilate. Large amounts of pleural effusion may interfere with normal movement of the diaphragm and chest wall. Inversion of the diaphragm, as occurs with massive pleural effusion, may cause it to move paradoxically with respiration. Thus, removal of small amounts of pleural effusion, if associated with the diaphragm returning toward normal contour, may cause significant relief of dyspnea. Animals that remain dyspneic following removal of pleural fluid should be suspected of having underlying pulmonary parenchymal or pleural disease, such as fibrosing pleuritis.

Fibrosing pleuritis has been associated with chylothorax, pyothorax, FIP, and hemothorax.[24] Although the etiology of the fibrosis is unknown, it apparently can occur subsequent to any prolonged exudative or blood-stained effusion. Exudates are characterized by a high rate of fibrin formation and degradation. Increased fibrin formation probably occurs because chronic inflammatory exudates, such as chylothorax and pyothorax, induce changes in mesothelial cell morphology, resulting in increased permeability, mesothelial cell desquamation, and triggering of both pathways of the coagulation cascade. These desquamated mesothelial cells have also been shown to produce type III collagen in cell culture, promoting fibrosis. Additionally, the chronic presence of pleural fluid might lead to an impairment in the mechanism of fibrin degradation. Decreased fibrinolysis may occur for several reasons: (1) direct injury to mesothelial cells may reduce inherent fibrinolytic activity of the cells, and/or (2)

the increased fluid volume may dilute local plasminogen activator. Plasminogen activator converts the precursor plasminogen to its active form, plasmin. Fibrinolytic activity in mammals is due primarily to this serine protease. Whatever the cause of the fibrosis in these animals with exudative effusions, the pleura is thickened by diffuse fibrous tissue that restricts normal pulmonary expansion. There is decreased vital capacity and static compliance, necessitating greater negative intrapleural pressures for any given change in lung volume, when compared with normal animals.

Diagnosis of fibrosing pleuritis is difficult. The atelectatic lobes may be confused with metastatic or primary pulmonary neoplasia, lung lobe torsion, or hilar lymphadenopathy (Figs. 130–6 and 130–7). Radiographic evidence of pulmonary parenchyma that fails to reexpand after removal of pleural fluid should be considered possible evidence of atelectasis with associated fibrosis. Fibrosing pleuritis should also be considered in animals with persistent dyspnea in the face of minimal pleural fluid.

DIAGNOSIS

Diagnostic Approach

Physical examination of animals with pleural effusion should include thorough evaluation of the cardiac and respiratory systems. Thoracic percussion may reveal hyporesonance with moderate or severe amounts of pleural fluid. With the animal standing or in sternal recumbency, a line of normal resonance may be percussed dorsal to an area of decreased resonance (fluid line). Chest compression should be performed in all cats with suspected pleural effusion. A noticeable decrease in the ability to compress the anterior chest is present in many cats with cranial mediastinal masses and pleural effusion. Thoracic auscultation may reveal muffled heart and lung sounds, particularly ventrally. Cardiovascular abnormalities such as murmurs or arrhythmias may be present in some animals. Increased bronchovesicular sounds may be heard in some animals, particularly in the dorsal lung fields. Jugular pulses may be present in animals with right-sided heart failure (e.g., pericardial effusion).

Thoracentesis. Thoracentesis should be performed *prior* to taking radiographs in dyspneic animals in which pleural effusion is suspected. Removal of even small amounts of pleural effusion may significantly improve the ventilatory

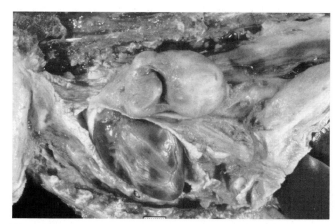

Figure 130–6. Necropsy specimen of a dog with fibrosing pleuritis and chronic chylothorax. Notice the small, consolidated lung lobes and the thickened pleura. (From: Fossum TW: Small Animal Surgery. St. Louis, CV Mosby, 1997, p 681.)

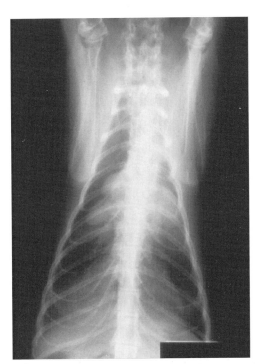

Figure 130–7. Thoracic radiograph of a cat with fibrosing pleuritis secondary to chronic chylothorax. Note the rounded appearance of the lung lobes. They are collapsed and covered by a thickened layer of pleura. The lung lobes in this cat could be mistaken for neoplastic masses. (From Fossum TW: Small Animal Surgery. St. Louis, CV Mosby, 1997, p 693.)

capabilities of the animal, allowing safer manipulation of the patient for radiographic procedures.

Needle thoracentesis is best performed with a small-gauge (No. 19 to No. 23) butterfly needle attached to a three-way stopcock and syringe, or an over-the-needle catheter attached to an extension tubing, three-way stopcock, and syringe. The appropriate site for thoracentesis is selected based on physical examination findings or, if available, radiographic findings. Usually, aspiration of either side of the thorax will adequately drain the contralateral hemithorax because the mediastinum in dogs and cats is fenestrated. However, with some diseases, particularly chylothorax and pyothorax, unilateral effusions may occur as a result of thickening of the mediastinum associated with chronic inflammation (Fig. 130–8). Thoracentesis is commonly performed at the sixth, seventh, or eighth intercostal space, just below the level of the costochondral junction.

The selected site should be clipped and, if needed, a local anesthetic block performed (this is seldom necessary). Most dyspneic animals will allow thoracentesis to be performed with minimal restraint; general anesthetics should be avoided. The animal should be allowed to remain in sternal recumbency and oxygen provided by face mask if the animal will tolerate it. The site is aseptically prepared and the needle introduced into the middle of the selected intercostal space. Care should be taken to avoid the large vessels associated with the rib margins. The needle is advanced into the pleural space until the pleura is punctured. Aspirating fluid while the needle is being advanced will allow prompt recognition of the appropriate depth of needle placement. Once the pleura has been punctured, the needle should be positioned against the body wall (rather than directed straight into the chest) to help prevent inadvertent damage to the lung as it expands. Facing the bevel of needle toward the lung (vs. the

body wall) will assist in fluid collection. Fluid should be gently aspirated, and 5-mL samples placed in an EDTA tube and clot tube for analysis of cell counts and biochemical parameters, respectively. Additionally, six to eight direct smears should be made for cytologic evaluation and appropriate samples submitted for aerobic and anaerobic cultures. If cell counts are low, cytocentrifuge preparations should be made for cytologic evaluation.

Radiography and Ultrasonography. If the animal is not overtly dyspneic, thoracic radiographs should be taken to confirm the diagnosis of pleural fluid. Taking dorsoventral (rather than ventrodorsal views) and "standing lateral" radiographic views, minimizing handling, and supplementing oxygen by face mask during the radiographic procedures may help prevent further compromise of respiration. If the animal is not dyspneic and only small amounts of fluid are suspected, ventrodorsal and expiratory views may help delineate the effusion.[25]

Radiographic signs associated with pleural effusion include blurring of the cardiac silhouette, interlobar fissure lines, rounding of lung margins at the costophrenic angles, widening of the mediastinum, separation of the lung borders from the thoracic wall, and scalloping of the lung margins at the sternal border (Fig. 130–9). The latter may be the earliest radiographic sign of pleural effusion.

Radiographically, fluid may be classified as free or encapsulated.[25] Free fluid moves easily to both sides of the pleural space because its distribution is affected by gravity. Encapsulated fluid is confined by fibrinous adhesions, and its distribution is not affected by gravity. Encapsulated fluids are commonly associated with chylothorax and pyothorax.[25] Ultrasonography should be performed prior to fluid removal because the fluid acts as an "acoustic window," enhancing visualization of thoracic structures. Ultrasonography is used to evaluate cardiac function, valvular lesions and function, congenital cardiac abnormalities, the presence of pericardial

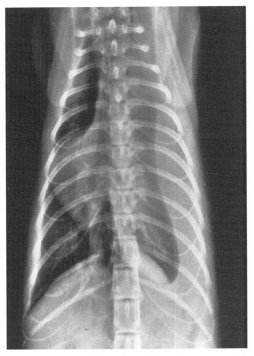

Figure 130–8. Ventrodorsal thoracic radiograph of a cat with unilateral pleural effusion associated with chronic chylothorax. (From Fossum TW: Small Animal Surgery. St. Louis, CV Mosby, 1997, p 677.)

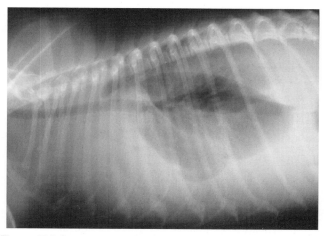

Figure 130–9. Lateral thoracic radiograph of a dog with severe pleural effusion. Notice the loss of the cardiac silhouette and separation of the lung at the vertebral diaphragmatic borders.

result of irritation to the pleura. In response, the pleura proliferates and exfoliates cells into the fluid, modifying it from a transudate to a modified transudate.

Modified transudates may arise from chronic transudates as noted above, or they may be associated with increased vascular hydrostatic pressure as seen with cardiac disease and neoplasia, or lymphatic leakage of high-protein lymph. Modified transudates can also be produced in the acute stages of an inflammatory process that will ultimately become an exudative effusion. Color and transparency vary, depending on the cause of the effusion (see Table 130–1).

Exudates are usually the result of an inflammatory process, although they may also be associated with neoplasia or chylothorax. They are characterized by high protein and nucleated cell counts and range in color from white to amber or red.

Because many modified transudates and exudates have physical characteristics that overlap, and chronicity may alter the physical characteristics of the effusion, additional methods of classifying effusions have been investigated.[27] Unfortunately, there have been too few high-quality prospective clinical studies of pleural effusion to validate or determine the usefulness of these parameters in veterinary medicine. The analyses most commonly employed in veterinary medicine include determination of triglyceride, cholesterol, pH, lactic dehydrogenase (LDH), and glucose concentrations.[27–29] LDH has been shown to be greater than 200 U/L in exudative fluids.[27] In humans, increased levels of LDH in pleural fluid are found with disorders associated with cell damage or inflammation (i.e., emphysema, chronic obstructive pulmonary disease, pneumothorax, pulmonary embolism, empyema, and pulmonary fibrosis). In contrast, lung cancer not associated with hepatic metastasis does not cause elevations in LDH.[30] Glucose and pH levels may help to differentiate septic and nonseptic effusions. Although septic effusions are often exudates, some may originate as modified transudates. Additionally, septic exudates typically are comprised primarily of degenerative neutrophils; however, some bacterial organisms may be present in low numbers or produce only weak toxins such that they do not cause degenerative changes. Studies have shown that glucose and pH tend to parallel each other in effusions and that pleural effusion acidosis results from the production of CO_2 and lactate by cells in the pleura or effusion. Lactate and CO_2 are the end products of glucose metabolism and accumulate in the effusion, resulting in it becoming acidotic. Studies of pleural effusion in cats have demonstrated that a glucose less than 10 mg/dL and a pH less than 6.9 are supportive of a septic effusion.[27] Additionally, evaluating the pH of an effusion

effusion, and mediastinal masses. With color Doppler imaging, a color signal has been noted to develop within pleural effusions during respiratory and cardiac cycles, and such a color Doppler signal ("fluid color sign") may be useful for detection of minimal or loculated pleural effusions that could be aspirated.[26]

The presence of pleural fluid will often prevent satisfactory radiographic evaluation of the structures of the thoracic cavity. Since adequate visualization of the entire thorax is necessary in order to rule out anterior mediastinal masses such as lymphosarcoma or thymoma, radiographs should be repeated following removal of most of the pleural fluid.

Pleural Fluid Evaluation

Examination of pleural fluid is based on biochemical, cytologic, and physical characteristics. Physical characteristics (i.e., color, transparency, total protein, total nucleated cell count [TNCC]) are used to classify fluids as either transudates, modified transudates, or exudates.

Transudates and Exudates. Pure transudative fluids are clear and colorless with a low total protein and low cellularity (Table 130–1). Transudates may occur with plasma protein greater than 1.5 g/dL, but a concurrent increase in vascular hydrostatic pressure or vascular permeability is necessary. Chronic transudates are altered by increased cell numbers and slightly increased protein as a

TABLE 130–1. CHARACTERISTICS OF FLUID TYPES

	TRANSUDATE	MODIFIED TRANSUDATE	EXUDATE	PYOTHORAX	CHYLOTHORAX	FIP
Protein content (g/dL)	<2.5	2.5–4	>3	>3.5	Variable	>5
TNCC* (cells/μL)	<1500	1000–7000	>7000	>7000	<10,000	<10,000
Color	Clear	Yellow, whitish-pink, red	White, amber, red	Amber to red or white	Usually white or pink	Straw to gold colored
Transparency	Colorless	Hazy to turbid	Opaque (usually) Turbid (rarely)	Turbid or opaque	Opaque	Hazy
Biochemical parameters			LDH >200 U/L	Glucose <10 mg/dL pH <6.9	Triglyceride > serum triglyceride	
Predominant cell types	Mesothelial cells, macrophages	Mesothelial cells, macrophages, eosinophils, lymphocytes	Neutrophils (most common) Lymphocytes, macrophages, mesothelial cells, neoplastic cells	Degenerative neutrophils	Lymphocytes or neutrophils	Nondegenerative neutrophils

*TNCC = total nucleated cell count.

may be helpful in differentiating between a malignant and nonmalignant effusion; malignant effusions typically have a pH greater than 7.2.[27]

Cytologic evaluation, including determination of the cell populations that comprise the TNCC, the predominant cell type, and cellular characteristics, is helpful in classifying an effusion and determining underlying causes. Cells commonly found in pleural effusions include neutrophils, macrophages, mesothelial cells, lymphocytes, eosinophils, mast cells, and neoplastic cells. With transudates, because of the low TNCC, cytologic evaluation is best accomplished by concentrating the cells by cytospin preparations or pelleting the cells with low-speed centrifugation, prior to making glass slide smears. The nucleated cell population of transudates consists of predominantly mesothelial cells and macrophages, with lesser numbers of lymphocytes and neutrophils.

Nucleated cell types seen with modified transudates depend on the cause and include mesothelial cells, macrophages, neutrophils, and lymphocytes. Less commonly seen are mast cells, eosinophils, and neoplastic cells. If the sample is turbid, glass slide smears of adequate cellularity for cytologic evaluation can be made directly from the fluid. If the fluid is hazy, concentration of the cells as previously described for pure transudates is best prior to cytologic evaluation.

Owing to the high TNCC found in exudates, direct smears are of adequate cellularity for cytologic evaluation. As with other effusive processes, the nucleated cell population of exudates varies depending on the cause. Since most exudates are due to inflammatory processes, neutrophils are often the predominant cell type. The presence of degenerative neutrophils denotes a septic process and should prompt the observer to look for free or intracellular bacteria. Even if bacteria are not seen cytologically, aerobic and anaerobic culture of the fluid is indicated. If nondegenerative neutrophils predominate, a nonseptic process or low-grade sepsis should be suspected. Microbial culture is recommended in these animals if a cause is not determined.

Determination of degenerative characteristics of neutrophils is useful in identifying a septic or nonseptic process. The presence of degenerative neutrophils in well-preserved areas of the smear indicates the presence of a bacterial toxin (Fig. 130–10). Nondegenerative neutrophils are similar in appearance to neutrophils in peripheral circulation.

Other nucleated cell types found in exudates include lymphocytes, macrophages, mesothelial cells, and neoplastic cells. A predominance of small lymphocytes indicates a

chylous effusion; however, chronic chylous effusions will result in a mixed population of cells with increasing numbers of neutrophils and macrophages. Macrophages can be present in any long-standing effusion. If a pyogranulomatous inflammation (an equally mixed population of neutrophils and macrophages) is present, a fungal or foreign body reaction should be considered. Mesothelial cells are found in all effusions and may be either quiescent or reactive. Highly reactive mesothelial cells may be very bizarre in appearance and exhibit characteristics of malignancy. *Differentiating reactive mesothelial cells from neoplastic carcinoma cells is difficult and should be done with extreme caution in the presence of inflammation.*[31] Neoplastic cells that can exfoliate into pleural effusions include lymphoblasts, carcinoma cells, mast cells, and malignant melanoma cells. Immunocytochemistry is used to diagnose, classify, and prognosticate pleural effusions in human beings.[32] Tumor markers and recombinant DNA technology are also being studied in humans.

PYOTHORAX

Pyothorax is an accumulation of pus in the pleural space. The fluid is classified as an exudate, and cytologically the nucleated cells consist primarily of degenerative neutrophils, but nondegenerative neutrophils can predominate, depending on the causative agent (see above). Effusions associated with fungi and higher bacterial agents such as *Actinomyces* and *Nocardia* may contain nondegenerative neutrophils and macrophages[33] if the organisms produce only sufficiently large enough quantities of (or strong enough) toxins to cause degenerative changes in those cells found in close proximity to the organisms.

Macrophages and reactive mesothelial cells are present in purulent effusions in variable numbers depending on the cause and the chronicity of the fluid. Macrophages are often seen engulfing debris and neutrophils (leukophagocytosis) in chronic effusions. Effusions associated with fungal or foreign body inflammation contain large numbers of macrophages. Mesothelial cells are present in all fluids with varying degrees of reactivity. As mentioned earlier, reactive mesothelial cells can exhibit criteria of malignancy and should not be confused with neoplastic cells. Occasionally, fungal elements may be noted in the pleural effusion of animals with fungal disease involving the pulmonary parenchyma.

The route by which the pleura becomes infected in animals with pyothorax is usually not evident. Possible routes of infection include hematogenous spread, migrating foreign objects such as plant awns, penetrating wounds (particularly bite wounds), extension from diskospondylitis, extension from pneumonia (e.g. aspiration pneumonia), pulmonary neoplasia and abscessation, pulmonary or thoracic wall trauma, and postoperative infection. Although diseases that result in immunosuppression (e.g., FeLV and FIV) should be excluded in animals with pyothorax, there is no evidence that development of this disease requires debilitation or an increased susceptibility to infection.

Although the cause of the effusion in animals with pyothorax is often not discernible, attempts should be made to find and correct, if possible, underlying diseases. Management of these animals needs to be aggressive. Following the diagnosis, a chest tube should be placed. If available, continuous-suction devices are ideal; however, most animals can be managed with intermittent aspiration. Lavage should be per-

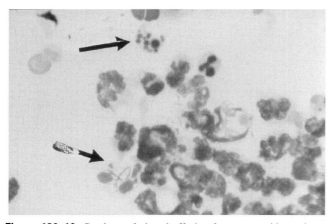

Figure 130–10. Cytology of pleural effusion from a cat with pyothorax. Karyorrhexis is present in some cells (arrows).

formed two to four times daily. Isotonic fluid, such as saline or lactated Ringer's solution (warmed to room temperature), should be used at a dosage of 10 mL/lb (20 mL/kg) body weight. The fluid is allowed to remain in the thoracic cavity for 1 hour and is then removed.

The addition of antibiotics to the lavage fluid offers no advantage over the use of appropriate systemic antibiotics. If they are used, the systemic dose should be decreased in order to minimize toxicity. The use of proteolytic enzymes is controversial and is no longer recommended by most authors. However, the addition of heparin (1500 units/100 mL of lavage) appears to be beneficial. Lavage may be required for 5 to 7 days. Systemic antibiotic therapy should be based on results of microbial culture and sensitivity testing. Appropriate antibiotics should be continued for a minimum of 4 to 6 weeks.

Surgical intervention is indicated if no improvement occurs in the first 3 to 4 days of therapy. The thorax may be approached via an intercostal thoracotomy if an abnormality can be localized to one hemithorax, or median sternotomy if localization is not possible. The thoracic cavity should be explored for abscesses, foreign bodies, or other abnormalities, and affected tissues removed. Prior to closure, the thoracic cavity should be lavaged with warmed sterile saline solution. If the pyothorax is chronic or localized, or the patient remains dyspneic in the absence of significant volumes of pleural fluid, surgical intervention and decortication may be warranted. Long-standing empyema may resorb, leaving a pleural "peel," which is a thick sheet of fibroblasts and inflammatory cells attached to the visceral pleura. This pleural peel may inhibit normal expansion of lung tissue. Decortication is recommended in human beings if lung entrapment is suspected. Decortication should be performed in animals once the empyema is mature, but before it adheres to the pleura and becomes vascularized (3 to 4 weeks is recommended).

FELINE INFECTIOUS PERITONITIS

Feline infectious peritonitis (FIP) is caused by a strain of feline coronavirus, termed FIP virus, that has a predilection for mononuclear cells of the spleen, liver, and lymph nodes. The effusive form of FIP causes a fairly characteristic fluid that accumulates in the abdomen and/or thorax. The effusion is straw to gold colored and hazy owing to fibrin flecks. The high protein and fibrin content causes the fluid to be thick and viscous. Occasionally the fluid will clot when exposed to air. The TNCC is typically low to moderate in comparison with other exudates, although some fluids may be highly cellular ($>$25,000 cells/μL). Cytologically, the fluid contains predominantly nondegenerative neutrophils with lesser numbers of macrophages, mesothelial cells, lymphocytes, and plasma cells. In chronic cases, macrophages and mesothelial cell populations increase. The nucleated cells are mixed with a stippled, eosinophilic precipitous background as a result of the high protein content.

The characteristically high protein content of the effusion in animals with FIP is an important distinguishing feature. However, other diseases can produce effusions with high protein contents; therefore, electrophoretic evaluation of the fluid protein fractions may be of value.[34] The protein content of FIP fluid is similar to that of the patient's serum, with a substantial portion of the protein content being immunoglobulin. Occasionally, local production of immunoglobulin in the fluid may result in a higher immunoglobulin level than

that seen in the serum. One study showed that effusions with a gamma globulin greater than 32 per cent had a high positive predictive value that the fluid was due to FIP, whereas fluids with less than 32 per cent globulin content were not likely to be due to FIP. Effusions with a greater than 48 per cent albumin content, and an albumin to globulin ratio greater than 0.81, were also not likely to be due to FIP virus.[34]

CHYLOTHORAX

Chyle is the term used to denote lymphatic fluid arising from the intestine and therefore containing a high quantity of fat. Chylothorax is a collection of chyle in the pleural space. In most animals, abnormal flow or pressures within the thoracic duct (TD) are thought to lead to exudation of chyle from intact, but dilated, thoracic lymphatic vessels (known as thoracic lymphangiectasia; Fig. 130–11). These dilated lymphatic vessels may form in response to increased lymphatic flow (due to increased hepatic lymph formation), decreased lymphatic drainage into the venous system as a result of high venous pressures, or both factors acting simultaneously to increase lymph flows and decrease drainage. Any disease or process that increases systemic venous pressures (i.e., right heart failure, mediastinal neoplasia, cranial vena cava thrombi, or granulomas) may cause chylothorax. Trauma is an uncommonly recognized cause of chylothorax in dogs and cats because the TD heals rapidly following injury and within 1 to 2 weeks the effusion resolves without treatment.

Possible causes of chylothorax include anterior mediastinal masses (mediastinal lymphosarcoma, thymoma), heart disease (cardiomyopathy, pericardial effusion, heartworm infection, foreign objects, tetralogy of Fallot, tricuspid dysplasia, or cor triatriatum dexter), fungal granulomas, venous thrombi, and congenital abnormalities of the TD. It may occur in association with diffuse lymphatic abnormalities including intestinal lymphangiectasia and generalized lymphangiectasia with subcutaneous chyle leakage. In a majority of animals, despite extensive diagnostic work-ups, the underlying etiology is undetermined (idiopathic chylothorax). Because the treatment of this disease varies considerably depending on underlying etiology, it is imperative that

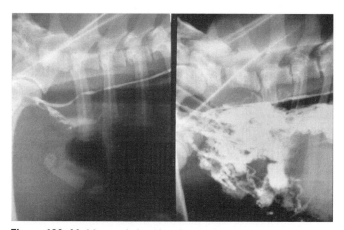

Figure 130–11. Mesenteric lymphangiogram from a normal dog (left) and a dog with idiopathic chylothorax (right). Notice the entrance of the thoracic duct into the venous system in the normal dog and the marked lymphangiectasia in the dog with chylothorax. Chylothorax is thought to occur as a result of leakage from these dilated, tortuous cranial mediastinal lymphatics.

RES

clinicians identify concurrent disease processes prior to instituting definitive therapy.

Any breed dog or cat may be affected; however, a breed predisposition has been suspected in the Afghan hound for a number of years. It has been suggested that the Shiba Inu breed may also be predisposed to this disease. Among cats, Oriental breeds (i.e., Siamese and Himalayan) appear to have an increased prevalence. Chylothorax may affect animals of any age; however, in one study older cats were more likely to develop chylothorax than were young cats.[35] This finding was believed to indicate an association between chylothorax and neoplasia. While Afghan hounds appear to develop this disease when middle aged, affected Shiba Inus have been less than 1 year old. A sex predisposition has not been identified.

Fluid recovered by thoracentesis should be placed in an EDTA tube for cytologic examination. Placing the fluid in an EDTA tube rather than a "clot-tube" will allow cell counts to be performed. Although chylous effusions are routinely classified as exudates, the physical characteristics of the fluid may be consistent with a modified transudate. The color varies depending on dietary fat content and the presence of concurrent hemorrhage. The protein content is variable and often inaccurate as a result of interference of the refractive index by the high lipid content of the fluid. Chronic chylous effusions may contain low numbers of small lymphocytes owing to the inability of the body to compensate for continued lymphocyte loss. Nondegenerative neutrophils may predominate with prolonged loss of lymphocytes or if multiple therapeutic thoracenteses have induced inflammation. Degenerative neutrophils and sepsis are uncommon findings as a result of the bacteriostatic effect of fatty acids but can occur iatrogenically owing to repeated aspirations. To help determine if a pleural effusion is truly chylous, several tests can be performed, including comparison of fluid and serum triglyceride levels; Sudan III stain for lipid droplets; and the ether clearance test. The most diagnostic test is comparison of serum and fluid triglyceride levels. If the effusion is truly chylous, it will contain a higher concentration of triglycerides than simultaneously collected serum.

Any cause of respiratory distress or coughing should be considered a differential diagnosis. Once pleural effusion has been identified, differentials include diseases causing exudative pleural effusion, such as pyothorax. Although chylous effusions have a characteristic appearance, the physical characteristics of chylous effusions and other exudative effusions may be similar. Additionally, the appearance and cell populations of chylous effusions can be altered by diet and chronicity.

Pseudochylous effusion is a term that has been misused in the veterinary literature to describe effusions that look like chyle, but in which a ruptured TD is not found. Given the known causes of chylothorax in dogs and cats, this term should be reserved for effusions in which the pleural fluid cholesterol is greater than the serum cholesterol concentration and the pleural fluid triglyceride is less than or equal to the serum triglyceride. Pseudochylous effusions are extremely rare in veterinary patients but may be associated with tuberculosis.

If an underlying disease is diagnosed, it should be treated and the chylous effusion managed by intermittent thoracentesis. If the underlying disease is effectively treated, the effusion often resolves; however, complete resolution may take several months. Surgical intervention should be considered only in animals with idiopathic chylothorax, or those that do not respond to medical management. Chest tubes should be placed only in those animals with suspected chylothorax secondary to trauma (very rare), with rapid fluid accumulation, or following surgery. Electrolytes should be monitored because hyponatremia and hyperkalemia have also been documented in dogs with chylothorax undergoing multiple thoracentesis. A low-fat diet may decrease the amount of fat in the effusion, which may improve the animal's ability to resorb fluid from the thoracic cavity.

Commercial low-fat diets are preferable to homemade diets; however, if commercial diets are refused, homemade diets are a reasonable alternative. Medium-chain triglycerides (once thought to be absorbed directly into the portal system, bypassing the TD) are transported via the TD of dogs. Thus, they may be less useful than previously believed. It is unlikely that dietary therapy will cure this disease, but it may help in the management of animals with chronic chylothorax. Clients should be informed that with the idiopathic form of this disease there is no effective treatment that will stop the effusion in all animals. However, the condition may spontaneously resolve in some animals after several weeks or months.

Benzopyrone drugs have been used for the treatment of lymphedema in humans for years. Whether these drugs might be effective in decreasing pleural effusion in animals with chylothorax is unknown; however, preliminary findings suggest that greater than 25 per cent of animals treated with rutin (25 mg/lb, PO, tid) had complete resolution of their effusion 2 months after initiation of therapy. Whether the effusion resolved spontaneously in these animals, or was associated with the drug therapy, requires further study.

Surgical intervention may be warranted in animals that do not have underlying disease and in which medical management has become impractical or is ineffective. Surgical options in animals that do not have severe fibrosing pleuritis include mesenteric lymphangiography and TD ligation, passive pleuroperitoneal shunting, active pleuroperitoneal or pleurovenous shunting, and pleurodesis. The mechanism by which TD ligation is purported to work is that following TD ligation abdominal lymphaticovenous anastomoses form for the transport of chyle to the venous system. Chyle bypasses the TD, and the effusion resolves. Unfortunately, TD ligation results in complete resolution of pleural effusion in only about 50 per cent of animals operated upon.[36, 37] The advantage of TD ligation is that, if it is successful, it results in complete resolution of pleural fluid (as compared with palliative procedures such as passive or active pleuroperitoneal shunting). Disadvantages include a long operative time (problematic in debilitated animals), a high incidence of continued or recurrent chylous or nonchylous (from pulmonary lymphatics) effusion, and that mesenteric lymphangiography may be difficult to perform (particularly in cats). Without mesenteric lymphangiography, complete ligation of the TD cannot be ensured; however, this technique may not be uniformly successful in verifying complete ligation of the TD. Some small branches of the TD system may be present and yet not fill with dye during lymphangiography. Readers are referred to a surgery textbook for a detailed explanation and description of these techniques.

NEOPLASTIC PLEURAL EFFUSION

Pleural effusion may be associated with either primary thoracic neoplasia, such as pleural mesothelioma, or metastatic pulmonary tumors. The clinical signs in these patients are often secondary to the presence of fluid that reaccumulates rapidly following thoracentesis, rather than from growth of the tumor itself in the pleura, lungs, or on the chest wall. There have been few reports of the treatment of pleural effusion of malignant origin in the veterinary literature.[38] Malignant effusions are apparently much more common in human beings, accounting for between 25 and 53 per cent of pleural effusion seen in general hospitals.[39] In fact, the most common causes of exudative effusions in human beings are malignancies. The tumors most commonly associated with pleural effusion in human beings are those arising from the lungs, breasts, and ovaries, and the lymphomas.[39]

Treatment of malignant pleural effusion should be directed at controlling the primary tumor. When there is no effective systemic treatment and clinical signs related to the effusion predominate, treatment of the effusion may be indicated in order to prolong the animal's life. Intracavitary instillation of chemotherapeutic agents or radioactive isotopes has been effective in the treatment of malignant pleural effusions in humans; the latter was reported in a dog.[38] Although the mechanism of action of most intracavitary agents in human beings is unknown, their effectiveness appears to be due to their ability to cause pleurodesis, rather than their antineoplastic effects. Pleurodesis has been reported in the dog for the treatment of pleural effusion; however, its effectiveness is unproven. Such details as proper agent, dose, and instillation method have been adapted primarily from clinical trials in human beings or from experimental studies in other species, and need to be more closely examined in the dog.

Mesotheliomas are rare tumors in dogs that arise from mesodermal cells of the pleural, pericardial, and peritoneal surfaces. In human beings, there is a documented association between mesothelioma and exposure to asbestos, and in one study three of five dogs with mesotheliomas had asbestos particles in their lungs at necropsy; asbestos particles were not found in the lungs of control dogs in the same study.[40] These tumors are highly effusive, and clinical signs are usually related to the presence of large amounts of serosanguineous fluid that inhibits normal respiration. Diagnosis of mesothelioma is generally made by open biopsy; examination of pleural fluid is rarely helpful because reactive mesothelial cells and neoplastic mesothelial cells are difficult to differentiate cytologically.

Metastasis of mesotheliomas to intrathoracic organs is common in dogs, and therapy is generally restricted to controlling pleural effusion. In human beings, intracavitary administration of chemotherapeutic agents and pleurectomy have resulted in significant clinical improvement in some patients. However, median survival in human patients treated with intrapleural therapy was only 8 months in one study.[41] The prognosis in dogs for long-term survival is similarly poor.[42]

PNEUMOTHORAX

Traumatic pneumothorax is the most frequent type of pneumothorax in dogs. It is usually closed (there is no free communication between the pleural space and the external environment) and most often occurs as a result of blunt trauma (i.e., vehicular accidents, being kicked by a horse), but has been reported after venipuncture in a kitten.[43] Rupture of the lung or bronchial tree typically occurs when the thorax is forcefully compressed against a closed glottis. Alternately, pulmonary parenchyma may be torn owing to

shearing forces on the lung. Pulmonary trauma occasionally results in subpleural bleb formation, similar to those seen with spontaneous pneumothorax (see below). Open pneumothorax occurs less commonly but is also frequently due to trauma (i.e., gun shot, bite or stab wounds, lacerations secondary to rib fractures). Some penetrating injuries are called "sucking chest wounds" because large defects in the chest wall allow an influx of air into the pleural space when the animal inspires. These large, open chest wounds may allow enough air to enter the pleural space that lung collapse and marked reduction in ventilation occur. There is a rapid equilibration of atmospheric and intrapleural pressure through the defect, interfering with normal mechanical function of the thoracic bellows that normally provides the necessary pressure gradient for air exchange. Pneumomediastinum may be associated with pneumothorax; tracheal, bronchial, or esophageal defects; or may be due to subcutaneous air migration along fascial planes at the thoracic inlet.

Spontaneous pneumothorax occurs in previously healthy animals without antecedent trauma and may be primary (i.e., an absence of underlying pulmonary disease) or secondary (underlying disease such as pulmonary abscesses, neoplasia, chronic granulomatous infections, pulmonary parasites such as *Paragonimus*, or pneumonia are present).[44, 45] Based on the histologic appearance of the pulmonary lesion, both cysts and bullae have been reported in dogs. Primary spontaneous pneumothorax in dogs may be due to rupture of subpleural blebs; the remaining lung tissue may appear normal. These blebs are most commonly located in the apices of the lungs (Fig. 130–12). Secondary spontaneous pneumothorax is more common in dogs than the primary form. In these animals, the subpleural blebs are associated with diffuse emphysema or other pulmonary lesions. It has been shown that volume strain from expansive pressure within the lung increases disproportionately at the apex as height increases. A majority of affected people are cigarette smokers, suggesting that the underlying pulmonary disease could be a result of interference of the normal function of alpha$_1$-antitrypsin in inhibiting elastase. It is believed that alpha$_1$-antitrypsin is inactivated in people who smoke, allowing increased elastase-induced destruction of pulmonary parenchyma.

Traumatic pneumothorax is most common in young dogs because they are more likely to be hit by cars or receive other trauma that may result in pulmonary damage. For similar reasons, males may be more commonly affected than

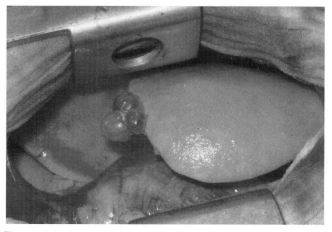

Figure 130–12. A dog with spontaneous pneumothorax. Notice the large pleural bleb at the periphery of the lung margin.

females. Although traumatic pneumothorax occurs in cats, it is less common than in dogs. Spontaneous pneumothorax usually occurs in large and "deep-chested" dogs; however, it may occur in small dogs. Dogs of any age may develop spontaneous pneumothorax; however, the majority of affected dogs are middle aged. Male and female dogs appear to be equally affected.

Pneumothorax secondary to trauma usually results in acute dyspnea. The history of trauma is often vague or unknown, complicating the differentiation of traumatic from spontaneous pneumothorax. Although the history of dogs with spontaneous pneumothorax varies depending on underlying etiology, most animals present with an acute history of dyspnea. Occasionally a chronic cough or fever may be noted. Recurrence of dyspnea in an animal previously treated for pneumothorax suggests spontaneous rather than traumatic pneumothorax.

Most animals with pneumothorax have bilateral disease and present with an acute onset of severe dyspnea. Other evidence of trauma (i.e., rib fractures, limb fractures, traumatic myocarditis, pulmonary contusions) may be evident in animals sustaining trauma. Most animals with pneumothorax exhibit a restrictive respiratory pattern (i.e., rapid, shallow respirations). If hypoventilation causes hypoxemia, they may appear cyanotic, and the heart and lung sounds are often muffled dorsally. Dogs are able to tolerate massive pneumothorax by increasing their chest expansion. Respiration becomes ineffectual in animals with tension pneumothorax as the chest becomes barrel shaped and fixed in maximal extension. This condition is life-threatening. Occasionally, subcutaneous emphysema will be noted in animals with pneumomediastinum and pneumothorax. The air may migrate from the mediastinal space to the thoracic inlet and be noticeable under the skin over the neck and trunk.

Thoracic radiographs should be delayed until after thoracentesis in dyspneic animals. Pneumothorax usually occurs bilaterally in animals because air easily diffuses across the thin mediastinum. Pneumothorax results in an increased width of air-filled space in the pleural cavity. The most sensitive view is a horizontal beam, laterally recumbent thoracic radiograph. On a recumbent lateral thoracic radiograph, the lungs collapse and retract from the chest wall and the heart usually appears to be elevated from the sternum. This apparent elevation of the heart is not noticeable on a standing lateral radiograph. Partially collapsed or atelectic lung lobes appear radiopaque when compared with the air-filled pleural space. As the lungs collapse, the vascular pattern will not extend to the chest wall; this may be particularly noticeable in the caudal thorax on a ventrodorsal view. Radiographs should be carefully evaluated for underlying pulmonary disease (i.e., abscess, neoplasia) or associated trauma (i.e., rib fractures, pulmonary contusion). Pulmonary blebs found in some animals with spontaneous pneumothorax are seldom visible radiographically. This is probably because the large blebs have ruptured, causing the pneumothorax. In such cases, surgical identification of bullae is necessary. Air-filled bullae may be incidental findings on thoracic radiographs of some animals. Pneumomediastinum is characterized by the ability to visualize thoracic structures (i.e., aorta, thoracic trachea, vena cava, esophagus) that are not usually apparent on thoracic radiographs.

Thoracic radiographs usually adequately identify the presence of free pleural air; however, if the diagnosis is uncertain, diagnostic thoracocentesis should allow retrieval of air. Because the management of animals with primary and spontaneous pneumothorax differs, once the animal has been stabilized, efforts should be directed at differentiating between the causes of pneumothorax.

Medical management of an animal with pneumothorax consists of initially relieving dyspnea by thoracentesis. If the pleural air accumulates quickly or cannot be effectively managed with needle thoracentesis, a chest tube should be placed. Tube thoracostomy is typically required in animals with spontaneous pneumothorax. Intermittent or continuous pleural drainage may be used, depending on the speed with which air accumulates. Continuous drainage may cause quicker resolution of pneumothorax in animals with large, traumatic defects. Providing an enriched oxygen environment may be beneficial, particularly in animals with concurrent pulmonary trauma (e.g., pulmonary contusion/hemorrhage). Providing analgesics to animals with fractured ribs or severe soft tissue damage may improve ventilation. *Surgical intervention is seldom required in animals with traumatic pneumothorax.* Thoracentesis should be performed as necessary to prevent dyspnea while the pulmonary lesion heals, usually within 3 to 5 days. Recurrence is uncommon. Conversely, animals with spontaneous pneumothorax commonly have recurrence of the pneumothorax if they are not operated upon.

An open chest wound should be covered immediately with any readily available material. Once the animal is admitted to the hospital, a sterile occlusive dressing should be applied as rapidly as possible and intrapleural air evacuated by thoracentesis or tube thoracostomy. Surgical therapy of animals with traumatic pneumothorax is seldom necessary (see above). However, nonsurgical management of spontaneous pneumothorax usually results in a less than satisfactory outcome. Mechanical pleurodesis of the lungs may decrease the recurrence of pneumothorax in animals operated upon for spontaneous pneumothorax. Mechanical pleurodesis damages the pleura such that healing results in adherence of the visceral and parietal pleura. Postoperative pneumothorax or pleural effusion must then be prevented, as they will result in separation of the parietal and visceral pleura, precluding adhesion formation.

REFERENCES

1. Valentine BA, Cooper BJ, Dietze AE, et al: Canine congenital diaphragmatic hernia. J Vet Intern Med 2:109, 1988.
2. Langham MR, Kays MR, Ledbetter DJ, et al: Congenital diaphragmatic hernia. Clin Perinatol 23:671, 1996.
3. Wilcox DT, Irish MS, Holm BA, et al: Pulmonary parenchymal abnormalities in congenital diaphragmatic hernia. Clin Perinatol 23:771, 1996.
4. Voges AK, Bertrand S, Hill RC, et al: True diaphragmatic hernia in a cat. Vet Radiol Ultrasound 38:116, 1997.
5. Downs MC, Bjorling DE: Traumatic diaphragmatic hernias: A review of 1674 cases. Vet Surg 16:87, 1987.
6. Wilson GP, III, Hayes HM, Jr: Diaphragmatic hernia in the dog and cat: A 25 year overview. Semin Vet Med Surg Small Anim 1:318, 1986.
7. Boudrieau RJ, Muir WW: Pathophysiology of traumatic diaphragmatic hernia in dogs. Compend Contin Educ Pract Vet 9:379, 1987.
8. Cornell KK, Jakovljevic S, Waters DJ, et al: Extrahepatic biliary obstruction secondary to diaphragmatic hernia in two cats. J Am Anim Hosp Assoc 29:502, 1993.
9. Edwards MA: Presurgical considerations in the treatment of diaphragmatic hernia. Mod Vet Pract September/October:493, 1987.
10. Neiger R: Peritoneopericardial diaphragmatic hernia in cats. Compend Contin Educ Pract Vet 18:461, 1996.
11. Bellah JR, Whitton DL, Ellison GW, et al: Surgical correction of concomitant cranioventral abdominal wall, caudal sternal, diaphragmatic, and pericardial defects in young dogs. JAVMA 195:1722, 1989.
12. O'Toole SJ, Irish MJ, Holm BA, et al: Pulmonary vascular abnormalities in congenital diaphragmatic hernia. Clin Perinatol 23:781, 1996.
13. Boudrieau RJ, Fossum TW, Hartsfield SM, et al: Pectus excavatum in dogs and cats. Compend Contin Educ Pract Vet 12:341, 1990.
14. Fossum TW, Boudrieau RJ, Hobson HP: Pectus excavatum in eight dogs and six cats. J Am Anim Hosp Assoc 25:595, 1989.

15. Feeney DA, Johnston GR, Grindem CB, et al: Malignant neoplasia of canine ribs: Clinical, radiographic, and pathologic findings. JAVMA 180:927, 1982.

16. Russell RG, Walker M: Metastatic and invasive tumors of bone in dogs and cats. Vet Clin North Am Small Anim Pract 13:163, 1983.

17. Atwell RB, Seiler R: Primary osteosarcoma of the sternum of a dog. Aust Vet J 54:585, 1978.

18. Fossum TW, Hodges CC, Miller MW, et al: Partial sternectomy for sternal osteomyelitis in the dog. J Am Anim Hosp Assoc 25:435, 1989.

19. Miserocchi G: Physiology and pathophysiology of pleural fluid turnover. Eur Respir J 10:219, 1997.

20. Wang N-S: The preformed stomas connecting the pleural cavity and the lymphatics in the parietal pleura. Am Rev Respir Dis 111:12, 1975.

21. Black LF: Pleural effusion. In Staub NC, Taylor AE (eds): Edema. New York, Raven Press, 1984, p 695.

22. Hahn K, Hahn PY, Gadallah SF, et al: Hepatic hydrothorax: Possible etiology of recurring pleural effusion. Am Fam Physician 56:523, 1997.

23. Sahn SA: Immunologic diseases of the pleura. Clin Chest Med 6:83, 1985.

24. Fossum TW, Evering WN, Miller MW, et al: Severe bilateral fibrosing pleuritis associated with chronic chylothorax in 5 cats and 2 dogs. JAVMA 201:317, 1992.

25. Myer W: Radiography review: Pleural effusion. J Am Vet Radiol Soc 19:75, 1978.

26. Yang P-C: Applications of colour Doppler ultrasound in the diagnosis of chest diseases. Respirology 2:238, 1997.

27. Stewart A, Padrid P, Lobingier R: Diagnostic utility of differential cell counts and measurement of LDH, total protein, glucose and pH in the analysis of feline pleural fluid (abstract). Proceedings of the 8th ACVIM Forum, 1990, p 1121.

28. Fossum TW, Jacobs RM, Birchard SJ: Evaluation of cholesterol and triglyceride concentrations in differentiating chylous and nonchylous pleural effusions in dogs and cats. JAVMA 188:49, 1986.

29. Tyler RD, Cowell RL: Evaluation of pleural and peritoneal effusions. Vet Clin North Am Small Anim Pract 19:743, 1989.

30. Drent M, Cobben NAM, Henderson RF, et al: Usefulness of lactate dehydrogenase and its isoenzymes as indicators of lung damage or inflammation. Eur Respir J 9:1736, 1996.

31. Clinkenbeard KD: Diagnostic cytology: Carcinomas in pleural effusions. Comp Cont Educ Pract Vet 14:187, 1992.

32. Bedrossian CWM: Special stains, the old and the new: The impact of immunocyto-chemistry in effusion cytology. Diagn Cytopathol 18:141, 1998.

33. Meyer DJ, Franks PT: Effusion: Classification and cytologic examination. Compend Contin Educ Pract Vet 9:123, 1987.

34. Shelly SM, Scarlett-Kranz J, Blue JT: Protein electrophoresis on effusions from cats as a diagnostic test for feline infectious peritonitis. J Am Anim Hosp Assoc 24:495, 1988.

35. Fossum TW: Feline chylothorax. Proceedings of the 12th Kal Kan Symposium, 1991, p 97.

36. Fossum TW, Birchard SJ, Jacobs RM: Chylothorax in 34 dogs. JAVMA 188:1315, 1986.

37. Kerpsack SJ, McLoughlin MA, Birchard SJ, et al: Evaluation of mesenteric lymphangiography and thoracic duct ligation in cats with chylothorax: 19 cases (1987–1992) (abstract). JAVMA 205:711, 1994.

38. Shapiro W, Turrel J: Management of pleural effusion secondary to metastatic adenocarcinoma in a dog. JAVMA 192:530, 1988.

39. Malden LT, Tattersall MHN: Malignant effusions. Q J Med 58:221, 1986.

40. Becklake MR: Asbestos-related diseases of the lung and other organs: Their epidemiology and implications for clinical practice. Am Rev Respir Dis 114:187, 1976.

41. Markman M, Cleary S, Pfeifle C, et al: Cisplastin administered by the intracavitary route as treatment for malignant mesothelioma. Cancer 58:18, 1986.

42. Morrison WB, Trigo FJ: Clinical characterization of pleural mesothelioma in seven dogs. Compend Contin Educ Pract Vet 6:342, 1984.

43. Godfrey DR: Bronchial rupture and fatal tension pneumothorax following routine venipuncture in a kitten. J Am Anim Hosp Assoc 33:260, 1997.

44. Forrester SD, Fossum TW, Miller MW: Pneumothorax in a dog with a pulmonary abscess and suspected infective endocarditis. JAVMA 200:351, 1992.

45. Holtsinger RH, Ellison GW: Spontaneous pneumothorax. Compend Contin Educ Pract Vet 17:197, 1995.

RES

SECTION X

THE GASTROINTESTINAL SYSTEM

CHAPTER 131

ORAL AND SALIVARY GLAND DISORDERS

Mark M. Smith

ORAL NEOPLASIA

Neoplasia of the oral and pharyngeal cavities is relatively common in the dog and cat, being the fifth and seventh most common diseases, respectively.[1] Benign and malignant neoplastic disease may be of dental or nondental origin.[2] The annual incidence of oral and pharyngeal neoplasia in dogs is 20 per 100,000, with malignant melanoma and squamous cell carcinoma (SCC) diagnosed most commonly.[1] The annual incidence rate is lower in cats (11 per 100,000), with the predominant neoplastic types being SCC and fibrosarcoma.[1, 3]

Predisposing factors in the development of oral neoplasia include age, sex, breed, size, and pigmentation of oral mucosa. Geriatric animals are predisposed in general; however, fibrosarcoma has been reported to occur more frequently in young, large breeds.[2] Papillary SCC, virus-induced papillomatosis, and undifferentiated malignancies may also be included in the differential diagnosis for young dogs with oral masses.[4, 5] Male dogs have been reported to be at risk for malignant melanoma and fibrosarcoma. Breeds with an increased risk for oral neoplasia irrespective of type include the German shepherd and short-haired Pointer, Weimaraner, golden retriever, Boxer, and cocker spaniel.[6] Large breed dogs have a higher incidence of fibrosarcoma and nontonsillar SCC, whereas small breeds have a higher incidence of malignant melanoma and tonsillar SCC.[6] Finally, dogs with heavily pigmented oral mucosa are predisposed to malignant melanoma.

BENIGN NEOPLASMS

Papilloma, fibroma, lipoma, chondroma, osteoma, hemangioma, hemangiopericytoma, histiocytoma, and epulis are reported in the oropharyngeal region in the dog.[6] Papilloma and epulis are common benign oral neoplastic conditions in the dog.

Canine oral papillomatosis (COP) consists of multiple lesions of viral etiology. Grossly, COP appears on the mucosa as pale, smooth elevations that develop a rough surface early in the disease process (Fig. 131–1).[7] Older lesions of three to four weeks' duration usually have deep and closely packed fronds. Lesions observed during regression appear shriveled and dark grey. Complete regression requires one to two weeks, with no apparent scarring.

Epulides originate from the periodontal stroma and are often located in the gingiva near incisor teeth (Fig. 131–2). The epulides are separated into three types based on histologic origin: fibromatous or fibrous epulis, ossifying epulis, and squamous or acanthomatous epulis.[6] The fibromatous and ossifying epulides are pedunculated, nonulcerating, non-

invasive masses. Acanthomatous epulis, although benign, has characteristics of malignancy, including local invasiveness and bone destruction.[6] However, acanthomatous epulis does not metastasize.

Periodontal epulides may be considered odontogenic neoplasms because they are closely associated with or may contain dental structures. The more common odontogenic neoplasms are ameloblastoma and odontoma. Ameloblastomas arise from vestigial layers of the dental laminae of the mandible, generally in the incisor region. These neoplasms emanate from enamel organ tissue but do not produce dental hard products. They are expansile, slow-growing neoplasms.[6] Odontomas are of odontogenic origin and resemble the embryologic pattern of tooth development. Enamel, dentin, cementum, and sometimes small teeth may compose the mass. Odontomas may form on or near the crown or root of a normal tooth and may resemble displaced or extra teeth. Lesions with characteristics resembling normal teeth are considered compound, whereas complex odontomas have a more disorganized arrangement.[6]

MALIGNANT NEOPLASMS

Malignant melanomas grow rapidly and are characterized by early gingiva and bone invasion. Metastasis to regional lymph nodes occurs early in the disease process, with the

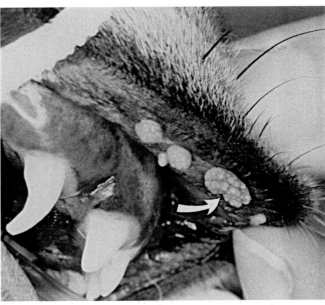

Figure 131–1. Papillomatosis *(arrow)* of the labial mucosa in a young dog.

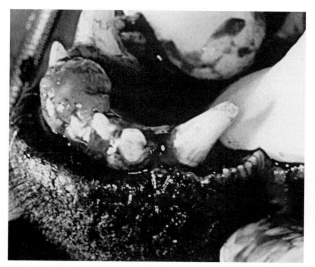

Figure 131–2. Intraoperative view of acanthomatous epulis of the mandibular incisor area in a dog.

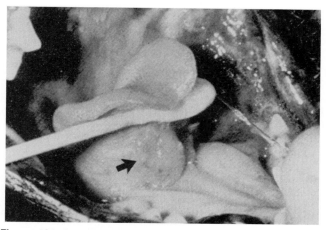

Figure 131–4. Sublingual squamous cell carcinoma *(arrow)* in a cat. (From Norris AM, et al: Oropharyngeal neoplasms. *In* Harvey CE (ed): Veterinary Dentistry. Philadelphia, WB Saunders, 1985.)

lung the most common site for visceral metastasis.[6, 8] Malignant melanomas are dome-shaped or sessile, with varying amounts of pigmentation ranging from black and brown through mottled, or they may be nonpigmented (Fig. 131–3). A minority (25 per cent) of oral melanocytic neoplasms may be benign, but all suspected melanomas should be considered malignant pending histologic evaluation. Melanomas of the mucocutaneous junction are invariably malignant.

Squamous cell carcinoma may project from the gingival mucosa but more commonly is an ulcerated, erosive lesion. It frequently involves the gingiva mesial to the canine teeth in dogs and ventral to the tongue in cats (Fig. 131–4). Other common oral sites include buccal and labial mucosa, hard palate, and tongue.[3, 6, 9–12] SCC destroys mucosa and submucosa and is locally invasive in muscle and bone. Bone involvement is particularly common in dogs, with a 77 per cent occurrence rate. Metastasis to local and regional lymph nodes is common, whereas visceral metastasis to the lung is rare and occurs late in the disease process.

Fibrosarcoma occurs in similar oral locations as SCC, with a greater frequency along the lateral maxillary arcade between the canine and fourth premolar teeth.[6] The neoplasm is firm and smooth with nodules that may become ulcerated (Fig. 131–5). Fibrosarcomas are invasive, and recurrence following local excision is common. Regional lymphatic and visceral metastasis is unusual. Low-grade fibrosarcomas appear to be clinically benign and rarely present with ulceration. However, these tumors are biologically malignant and require a high index of suspicion by both the clinician and the pathologist.[13]

CLINICAL SIGNS, DIAGNOSIS, AND STAGING

Clinical signs associated with oral neoplasms depend on size and location. Food prehension may be abnormal and cause ulceration secondary to trauma in animals with larger neoplasms. Inability to swallow or associated pain may result

GI

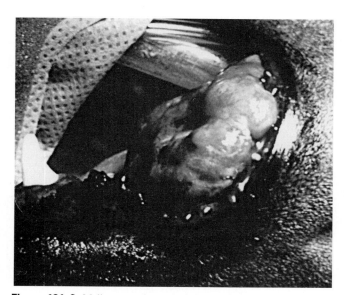

Figure 131–3. Malignant melanoma of the mandibular buccal mucosa in a dog.

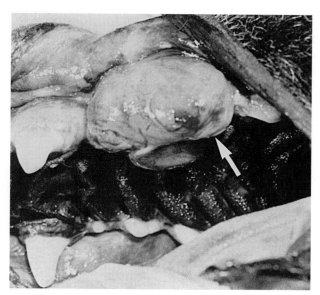

Figure 131–5. Fibrosarcoma *(arrow)* of the maxillary premolar area in a dog.

in the appearance of saliva drooling from the lip commissures at inappropriate times. The saliva is blood-tinged when concomitant with ulcerated lesions. Clinical signs associated with dental disease may be related to abnormal mastication. Painful dental structures or partial obstruction of functional dental areas leads to disuse. Subsequent periodontal disease is related to excessive plaque and calculus accumulation in these areas. Severe destructive periodontal disease, halitosis, and tooth loss are potential sequelae.

Diagnosis of oral neoplastic conditions is based on histopathologic examination (Fig. 131–6). The differential diagnosis includes malignant and benign neoplasms. Recent advances in the development and application of immunohistochemistry techniques in veterinary medicine may provide methods in the future for the early detection of malignant neoplasms.[14–16] Although severe destructive periodontitis is not associated with a mass lesion, it is often associated with bone lysis and may appear similar to SCC.

Staging of the neoplastic disease should be considered an active investigative process to be performed in concert with the diagnostic evaluation (Table 131–1).[17] The final result of this process is potentially valuable prognostic information. A complete blood count (CBC), chemistry profile, and urinalysis should be reviewed to determine organ abnormalities related to metastatic disease or concurrent disease that would alter the type or preclude the use of general anesthesia. Thoracic radiographs (right and left lateral, ventrodorsal views) are taken to evaluate visceral metastasis to the lung. The size of the neoplasm is estimated in the awake animal and may be more accurately assessed after administration of

general anesthesia. Skull radiographs taken during anesthesia provide information concerning the presence of bone invasion. Regional lymph nodes should also be evaluated. Enlargement indicates either metastasis or reactivity related to oral inflammation. Regardless of size, regional lymph nodes should be evaluated by fine-needle aspiration (false-negative results are possible) and by incisional or excisional biopsy. Minor surgery to remove a regional lymph node provides worthwhile prognostic information that may influence the owner's decision to pursue definitive treatment.[18] The most accessible regional lymph nodes are the submandibular and parotid; the medial retropharyngeal receives afferent lymphatics from these lymph nodes. Lymph node should be differentiated from salivary tissue, the latter having a tan color with distinct lobulations. A negative lymph node biopsy does not preclude the possibility of regional metastasis, which may occur along perineural or vascular routes, or metastasis to other less accessible lymph nodes such as the retropharyngeal. Unfortunately, oral malignant neoplasms are often detected late in the disease process because their location may not be readily observed by the owner or veterinarian. Consequently, oral neoplasms have usually progressed to at least stage II disease at the time of diagnosis. Higher T-stage tumors with bone involvement are associated with a poorer prognosis.[8]

TREATMENT

Animals with no radiographic signs of visceral metastasis to the lung should be considered for aggressive therapy.

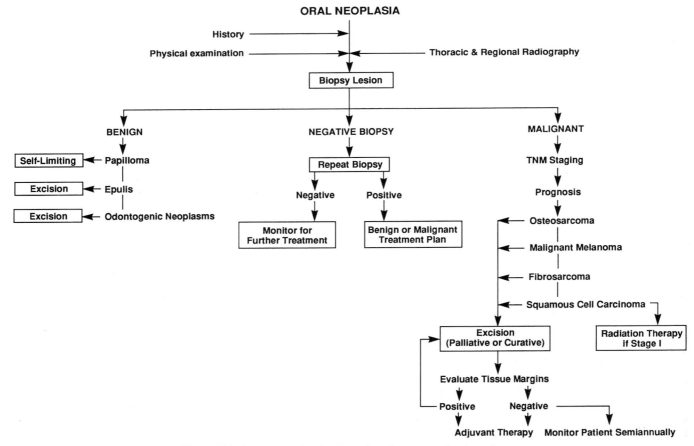

Figure 131–6. Algorithm for the diagnosis and treatment of oral neoplasms.

TABLE 131–1. CLINICAL STAGING SYSTEM FOR TUMORS OF THE ORAL CAVITY

T: *Primary tumor*
  T_0 No evidence of tumor
  T_1 Tumor < 2 cm maximum diameter
    T_{1a} Without bone invasion
    T_{1b} With bone invasion
  T_2 Tumor 2 to 4 cm maximum diameter
    T_{2a} Without bone invasion
    T_{2b} With bone invasion
  T_3 Tumor > 4 cm maximum diameter
    T_{3a} Without bone invasion
    T_{3b} With bone invasion

N: *Regional lymph nodes (RLN)*
  N_0 No evidence of RLN involvement
  N_1 Movable ipsilateral nodes
    N_{1a} Nodes histologically negative
    N_{1b} Nodes histologically positive
  N_2 Movable contralateral or bilateral nodes
    N_{2a} Nodes histologically negative
    N_{2b} Nodes histologically positive
  N_3 Fixed nodes

M: *Distant metastasis*
  M_0 No evidence of distant metastasis
  M_1 Distant metastasis present

STAGE GROUPINGS

Stage	T	N	M
I	T_1	N_0, N_{1a}, or N_{2a}	M_0
II	T_2	N_0, N_{1a}, or N_{2a}	M_0
III*	T_3	N_0, N_{1a}, or N_{2a}	M_0
IV	Any T		
	Any T	Any N_{2b} or N_3	M_0
	Any T	Any N	M_1

*Any bone involvement.
From World Health Organization: *Report of the Second Consultation on the Biological Behavior and Therapy of Tumors of Domestic Animals.* WHO, Geneva, 1978.

The concept of complete local excision of all visible tumor followed by, or concurrent with, chemotherapy or radiation therapy for treatment of presumed micrometastasis has achieved marked acceptance in human oncologic therapy and is being applied in veterinary medicine.[17, 19–21] Surgery is integral to this multimodality treatment plan, especially for large, aggressive neoplasms.[22–25] Resective surgery plus radiation and/or chemotherapy is usually well tolerated by dogs and cats, leaving conservative management for only the more debilitated and/or geriatric animals.[26]

The goal of surgery for oral neoplasms in small animals is generally curative resection or palliation.[27] The ideal surgical procedure is one that offers the greatest possibility of cure, restores or maintains function, and has an acceptable cosmetic result. Benign neoplasms that do not involve bone are surgically excised. Malignant neoplasms are also excised; however, an attempt to acquire tumor-free margins is critical.[28–30] A 2-cm margin of tumor-free tissue is recommended, often necessitating ostectomy as a component of the operative procedure.[31] Neoplasms with radiographic evidence of local bone metastasis require resective procedures including maxillectomy and mandibulectomy. Hemimaxillectomy and hemimandibulectomy are procedures that maximize the removal of the entire bony component of the neoplastic process. Segmental bone resective procedures resulting in partial maxillectomy or mandibulectomy, without the opportunity for frozen section analysis of tissue margins, risk incomplete resection owing to intrabony perineural and microvascular metastatic routes.[32, 33] This is of particular importance for mandibular lesions, in which case hemimandibulectomy may

be preferred to partial or segmental mandibulectomy, because cosmesis and function are acceptable despite a greater degree of resection.[26] Extended dissection from the primary site may improve the incidence of free margins related to surgical resection of direct metastatic pathways, especially for neoplasms of the floor of the mouth. The cranial cervical area may be approached in conjunction with reconstructive surgery. Direct observation of regional lymph nodes allows assessment of gross transcapsular spread of the tumor, which may warrant wider margins for adhered lymph nodes.[34]

Epulides are treated by aggressive surgical resection. Based on common locations for this neoplasm compared with malignant neoplasms, the operative procedure would be either rostral mandibulectomy or rostral maxillectomy.[35, 36]

Odontogenic tumors are treated by local excisional surgery requiring partial or segmental ostectomy.[37–39]

Radiation therapy may be particularly indicated for stage I SCC or following resective surgery for SCC with non-free margins. This form of treatment is most effective if used in combination with surgical excision of stage II through IV SCC or possibly for affected regional lymph nodes.[9] Recent studies report encouraging results of radiation therapy for the treatment of canine SCC, fibrosarcoma, and malignant melanoma.[8, 40] This modality should be considered for treatment of oral malignancies with or without surgery. However, as with surgery, larger, more caudally located tumors have a poorer prognosis. Severe, acute radiation reactions may occur approximately 16 per cent of the time; the most common chronic reaction is bone necrosis and fistula formation.[8] Although the latter reaction may be difficult to treat successfully, a relatively low percentage of chronic reactions to radiation therapy may be considered expected sequelae of effective treatment.[8]

Acanthomatous epulides are sensitive to radiation therapy; however, malignant neoplastic disease development at the irradiated site in approximately 18 per cent of dogs makes surgical excision a more appropriate therapeutic option if morbidity is minimized.[41, 42] However, the type of radiation administered (orthovoltage vs. megavoltage) may have an influence on the potential carcinogenic effect of radiation.[43] Epulides of smaller size located in the rostral portion of the oral cavity have a more favorable prognosis following radiation therapy compared with larger, more caudal lesions.[43] Acute and chronic radiation reactions may occur, as in the treatment for oral malignant neoplasms.

Chemotherapy may provide short-term palliation for oral neoplasia not amenable to surgery or for recurrence following surgical excision. Cisplatin has been used in dogs for oral SCC, and doxorubicin and cyclophosphamide have been used for oral fibrosarcoma and SCC in cats.[2] Results of clinical research with radiosensitizing agents (e.g., etanidazole) may show improvement in median survival times for small animals with oral neoplasms.[44–46] Intratumoral administration of carboplatin has been shown to be efficacious in treating SCC of the nasal plane in cats[47] and may have application for the treatment of oral SCC.

PROGNOSIS

Malignant oral neoplasms have a guarded to poor prognosis regardless of size or location in the oral cavity. Prognosis may be affected by the size of the lesion, the age of the animal, and the species. Dogs younger than 6 years old with SCC mesial to the second premolar have an improved prognosis compared with older dogs with neoplasms in other

GI

locations. Cats with oral SCC have a shorter tumor-free interval compared with dogs, regardless of the type of treatment.[48, 49] The most positive prognosis for oral SCC in dogs is attained with both surgery and radiation therapy. Treatment of oral SCC in cats is strictly palliative, with no improved survival interval.[2, 48] Oral malignant melanoma may be resected locally with tumor-free margins; however, regional or distant metastasis usually occurs. Tumor-free margins for oral fibrosarcoma are more difficult to achieve, making local recurrence likely. One-year survival rates of 71 per cent have been reported for dogs with mandibular osteosarcoma receiving surgery only; another study indicated less favorable results with surgery only, reporting a median survival time of 5.5 months.[50, 51]

Benign oral neoplasms, epulides, and odontogenic neoplasms have an excellent prognosis following complete surgical excision.[36–39]

SELECTED ACQUIRED DISEASES OF THE LIPS, CHEEKS, AND PALATE

Feline eosinophilic granuloma complex (FEGC) includes eosinophilic ulcer, plaque, and linear granuloma. Oral lesions are usually linear granuloma or eosinophilic ulcer; the latter has a predisposition for the maxillary lips (80 per cent).[52] Intraoral lesions appear as one or more discrete, firm, raised nodules (Fig. 131–7). Clinical signs include dysphagia and/or ptyalism. Although the etiology for this disease is unknown, bacterial and viral infections and immune-mediated and hypersensitivity diseases have been associated with FEGC.[52, 53] Biopsy of the lesion, with the aforementioned diseases in mind, should be performed to confirm the diagnosis and differentiate it from neoplastic disease. Ancillary tests should include a CBC, which usually shows an absolute eosinophilia. Concurrent or potentially causative hypersensi-

tivity diseases should be considered during the diagnostic phase of treatment. The mainstay of FEGC treatment is corticosteroid therapy. Intralesional triamcinolone (3 mg weekly), oral prednisolone (0.5 to 1 mg/lb twice a day), and subcutaneous methylprednisolone acetate (20 mg every 2 weeks) administered until FEGC resolution are efficacious treatments.[52] Progestational compounds (progesterone or medroxyprogesterone) are often used to treat FEGC. These compounds are not approved for use in cats and have potential side effects that make their use undesirable, including adrenocortical suppression, polydipsia, polyuria, polyphagia, obesity, personality change, reproduction abnormalities, mammary hypertrophy, neoplasia, and diabetes mellitus. Cats with untreated chronic lesions, responsive previous lesions, or lesions refractory to corticosteroid therapy have a 50 per cent recurrence within five months.[52] Failure of treatment is usually related to inadequate dosage or premature cessation of therapy. Animals not responding to either corticosteroids or progestational compounds have a poor prognosis and are candidates for more aggressive therapy such as irradiation, cryosurgery, laser therapy, or immunotherapy.[53–55]

Stomatitis is inflammation of the oral mucosa. Oral inflammatory lesions in dogs and cats have multiple causes, necessitating a consistent and logical diagnostic approach. A complete history and thorough physical examination are essential. Dogs and cats with no evidence of debilitating systemic disease should receive a short-acting intravenous anesthetic to allow an unimpeded visual and tactile oral examination. Oral ulcerations occur in at least four different immune-mediated diseases, including systemic lupus erythematosus, bullous (pemphigus) disease, idiopathic vasculitis, and toxic epidermal necrosis. The many infectious diseases that are manifested by lesions in the oral cavity include feline leukemia virus, feline immunodeficiency virus, feline syncytium-forming virus, feline calicivirus, feline herpesvirus, and feline infectious peritonitis (see Section IV).[56] Canine distemper and feline panleukopenia virus may cause stomatitis, although other organs are more severely affected. Candidiasis *(Candida albicans)* may cause severe stomatitis in dogs and cats.[52, 57] Many cats with stomatitis have immune-suppressive disease or systemic debilitation or have received chronic immune-suppressive therapy. Although the oral manifestation may appear as a white pseudomembrane covering the tongue, lesions are usually irregular ulcerated areas within zones of inflamed mucosa. Further description of the disease, diagnosis, and treatment is presented in Chapter 93.

Feline oral inflammatory disease ranges from simple gingivitis to varying degrees of stomatitis in which inflammation extends beyond the mucogingival junction into the oral mucosa.[58] Cats with chronic gingivitis or stomatitis may have ulceration and extension of granulation tissue involving the palatoglossal folds and fauces. Clinical signs include halitosis, ptyalism, dysphagia, inappetence, and weight loss. Extensive disease is marked by root resorption and possibly bony sequestrae in edentulous areas. See Chapters 132 to 134 for an extensive review of dental-related oral disease.

Stomatitis may be described as idiopathic despite a thorough diagnostic evaluation. Immune-mediated ulcerative gingivitis or stomatitis afflicts Maltese terriers, but the etiology is verified in only 20 per cent of animals.[52] It is appropriate to assume that there may be an immune-mediated component to idiopathic stomatitis following negative diagnostic testing. A prudent treatment plan includes regular teeth cleaning, oral preventive medicine at home, and inter-

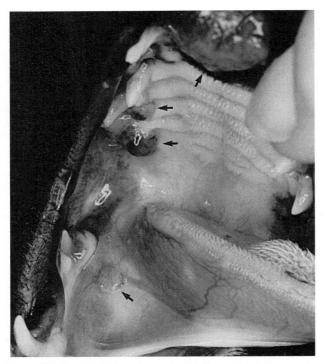

Figure 131–7. Oral lesions *(arrows)* of feline eosinophilic granuloma complex. (Courtesy of Dr. M. Leib.)

mittent or chronic provocative corticosteroid therapy. Antimicrobial therapy (e.g., metronidazole, amoxicillin, clavulanic acid/amoxicillin) emphasizing anaerobic pathogens may be administered on an intermittent, chronic basis.

SELECTED ACQUIRED DISEASES OF THE SALIVARY GLANDS

Neoplasia involving the salivary glands is uncommon. There is evidence that spaniel breeds and poodles are predisposed to neoplasia of the salivary glands. In a report of 28 primary salivary tumors in dogs, the parotid gland was involved twice as often as the other major salivary glands; the mean age of the 28 dogs studied was 10 years. A more recent study indicates that the mandibular gland is most commonly affected.[59] Multiple tumor types affecting the salivary glands have been described, including mucoepidermoid tumors, SCC, malignant mixed tumors, adenoid cystic carcinoma, acinic cell carcinoma, adenocarcinoma, undifferentiated carcinoma, and sarcoma. Although primary SCC of the sublingual salivary gland occurs, it should be considered only after an invasive carcinoma involving the oral mucosa or accessory oral salivary glands has been ruled out. Prevalence of salivary gland neoplasms in cats is almost twice that in dogs. The most common neoplasms affecting salivary glands in dogs and cats are carcinoma and adenocarcinoma. Adenocarcinoma, regardless of the gland affected, is locally infiltrative, with frequent metastasis to the lung and regional lymph nodes. Salivary neoplasms should be staged according to the TNM system to permit the appropriate prognostication and treatment plan. Thoracic radiographs and incisional biopsy of the neoplasm and nearest regional lymph provide necessary information.

Total surgical excision of malignant salivary neoplasms is difficult because of their invasive characteristics and the intricate neurologic and vascular anatomy of the salivary gland region. Therefore, local treatment should include radiotherapy, with or without surgical intervention, to debulk the neoplasm.

Mucocele is the most common clinically recognized disease of the salivary glands in dogs. A mucocele is an accumulation of saliva in the subcutaneous tissue and the consequent tissue reaction to saliva. The mucocele has a nonepithelial, nonsecretory lining consisting primarily of fibroblasts and capillaries. The incidence of salivary mucocele reportedly is fewer than 20 in 4000 dogs. Although the condition has been reported in dogs as young as 6 months of age, salivary mucocele occurs most often in dogs between 2 and 4 years of age. Salivary mucocele occurs more frequently in German shepherds and miniature poodles.

Trauma has been proposed as the cause of salivary mucocele because of the activity of young dogs and the documented damage to the salivary gland–duct complex and the formation of mucocele. The inability to induce salivary mucocele traumatically in healthy dogs suggests the possibility of a developmental predisposition in affected dogs.

The sublingual gland is the most common salivary gland associated with salivary mucocele. Sialography has shown that the origin of the mucocele is most often in the rostral portion (that portion of the sublingual gland superimposed on the mandible) of the sublingual gland–duct complex. Regardless of the location of origin, mucocele usually forms near the intermandibular area (cervical mucocele). Other locations associated with the formation of mucocele because of a sublingual gland–duct defect include under the tongue, which involves the floor of the mouth (sublingual mucocele), and the pharynx (pharyngeal mucocele).

The clinical signs associated with salivary mucocele depend on its location. A cervical mucocele is initially an acute, painful swelling resulting from an inflammatory response. Cessation of the inflammatory response results in a marked decrease in swelling. A decreased inflammatory response allows for the more common presenting history of a slowly enlarging or intermittently large, fluid-filled, nonpainful swelling (Fig. 131–8). Blood-tinged saliva secondary to trauma caused by eating, poor prehension of food, or reluctance to eat are clinical signs that can be associated with sublingual mucocele. The most common clinical signs associated with mucocele of the pharyngeal wall are respiratory distress and difficulty in swallowing secondary to partial obstruction of the pharynx.

Zygomatic salivary mucoceles are infrequently reported in dogs. A visible periorbital mass is usually the presenting clinical sign of zygomatic mucocele. Ophthalmic signs secondary to the mucocele depend on its location and the size (i.e., exophthalmos or enophthalmos).

Diagnosis of salivary mucocele is based on clinical signs, history, and results of paracentesis (Fig. 131–9). Mucocele paracentesis reveals a stringy, sometimes blood-tinged fluid with low cell numbers. Mucin and amylase analyses of the fluid are not reliable diagnostic procedures. A chronic cervical mucocele may contain palpable firm nodules that are remnants of sloughed inflammatory tissue previously lining the mucocele. Sialoliths are concretions of calcium phosphate or calcium carbonate and may occur with chronic mucocele.

Physical examination and history usually denote the origin of the mucocele. Cervical mucoceles that appear on the midline usually shift to the originating side when the animal is placed in exact dorsal recumbency. Sialography can be used to determine the affected side if careful observation and palpation are unsuccessful. The most common indication for sialography is to determine the location of a salivary gland–duct defect in animals with salivary mucocele. Sialography is also a diagnostic aid when considering traumatic injury to one of the salivary glands, salivary neoplasia, a mass or fistulous tract of unknown origin in the head or neck region, or a foreign body in the head or neck. The disadvantages of sialography include the need for general anesthesia and the difficulty associated with locating the duct openings.

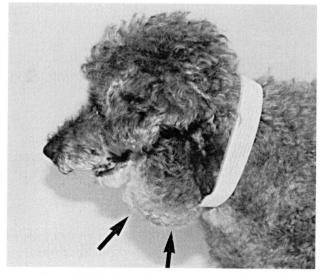
Figure 131–8. Cervical mucocele (arrows) in a poodle.

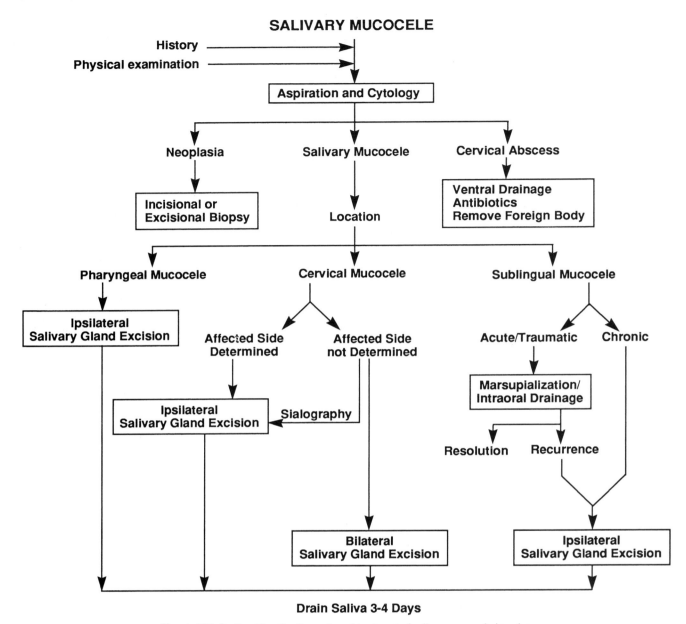

Figure 131–9. Algorithm for diagnosis and treatment of salivary mucocele in a dog.

Various approaches have been used to treat cervical mucoceles. Mucocele drainage, removal of the mucocele only, and chemical cauterization of the mucocele have been reported. The basis for these therapies was the belief that a mucocele was a true cyst with a secretory lining. The fact that a mucocele is not a cyst but is a reactive, encapsulating structure has prompted surgical removal of the affected gland-duct complex. The intimate anatomic association of the sublingual and mandibular glands and their ducts requires resection of both structures. Surgical removal of both the sublingual and mandibular salivary glands, combined with drainage of the mucocele, has been advocated for treating cervical mucoceles.

Pharyngeal and sublingual mucoceles are treated by removing the mandibular and sublingual salivary glands, based on the common etiology of a sublingual gland–duct defect. Another technique for treating these mucoceles involves marsupialization. However, resective surgery is preferred for pharyngeal mucoceles, because life-threatening upper airway compromise and morbidity from swallowing dysfunction (e.g., aspiration pneumonia) are potential complications of conservative management or recurrence.

The zygomatic salivary gland can be affected by neoplasia, inflammation, or mucocele. The clinical signs for zygomatic mucocele and neoplasia are similar. Additional signs, such as osteolytic changes of the zygomatic arch and enlargement of the submandibular lymph node, may accompany neoplasia originating in the zygomatic gland. Surgical removal of the zygomatic gland is indicated either for neoplasia or for mucocele of zygomatic origin.

REFERENCES

1. Dorn RC, Priester W: Epidemiology. *In* Theilen GK, Madewell BR (eds): Veterinary Cancer Medicine. Philadelphia, Lea & Febiger, 1987, p 27.

2. Klausner JS, Hardy RM: Alimentary tract, liver, and pancreas. *In* Slatter DK (ed): Textbook of Small Animal Surgery. Philadelphia, WB Saunders, 1993, pp 2088–2105.
3. Stebbins KE, et al: Feline oral neoplasia: A ten year survey. Vet Pathol 26:2, 1989.
4. Ogilvie GK, et al: Papillary squamous cell carcinoma in three young dogs. JAVMA 192:933, 1988.
5. Patnaik AK, et al: A clinicopathologic and ultrastructural study of undifferentiated malignant tumors of the oral cavity in dogs. Vet Pathol 23:170, 1986.
6. Theilen GH, Madewell BR: Tumors of the digestive tract. *In* Theilen GK, Madewell BR (eds): Veterinary Cancer Medicine. Philadelphia, Lea & Febiger, 1987, pp 499–534.
7. Madewell BR, Theilen GH: Tumors of the skin and subcutaneous tissue. *In* Theilen GK, Madewell BR (eds): Veterinary Cancer Medicine. Philadelphia, Lea & Febiger, 1987, pp 233–325.
8. Theon AP, et al: Analysis of prognostic factors and patterns of failure in dogs with malignant oral tumors treated with megavoltage irradiation. JAVMA 210:778, 1997.
9. Evans SM, Shofer F: Canine oral nontonsillar squamous cell carcinoma. Vet Radiol 29:3, 1988.
10. Bradley RL, et al: Oral neoplasia in 15 dogs and four cats. Semin Vet Med Surg (Small Anim) 1:1, 1986.
11. Beck ER, et al: Canine tongue tumors: A retrospective review of 57 cases. J Am Anim Hosp Assoc 22:4, 1986.
12. Carpenter LG, et al: Squamous cell carcinoma of the tongue in dogs. J Am Anim Hosp Assoc 29:17, 1990.
13. Ciekot PA, et al: Histologically low-grade, yet biologically high-grade, fibrosarcomas of the mandible and maxilla in dogs: 25 cases (1982–1991). JAVMA 204:610, 1994.
14. Stromberg PC, et al: Evaluation of oncofetal protein-related mRNA transport activity as a potential early cancer marker in dogs with malignant neoplasms. Am J Vet Res 56:1559, 1995.
15. Oliver JL, et al: Isolation and characterization of the canine melanoma antigen recognized by the murine monoclonal antibody IBF9 and its distribution in cultured canine melanoma cell lines. Am J Vet Res 58:46, 1997.
16. Gamblin RM, et al: Overexpression of P53 tumor suppressor protein in spontaneously arising neoplasms of dogs. Am J Vet Res 58:857, 1997.
17. Owen LN (ed): World Health Organization TNM Classification of Tumors in Domestic Animals, 1st ed. Geneva, World Health Organization, 1980.
18. Smith, MM: Surgical approach for lymph node staging of oral and maxillofacial neoplasms. J Am Anim Hosp Assoc 31:514, 1995.
19. Forastiere AA: Review: Management of advanced stage squamous cell carcinoma of the head and neck. Am J Med Sci 291:405, 1986.
20. Lo TCM, et al: Radiotherapy for cancer of the head and neck. Otolaryngol Clin North Am 18:521, 1985.
21. Hammer AS, Couto CG: Adjuvant chemotherapy for sarcomas and carcinomas. Vet Clin North Am Small Anim Pract 20:1015, 1990.
22. Page RL, Thrall DE: Clinical indications and applications of radiotherapy and hyperthermia in veterinary oncology. Vet Clin North Am Small Anim Pract 20:1075, 1990.
23. Bradney IW, et al: Rostral mandibulectomy combined with intermandibular bone graft in treatment of oral neoplasia. J Am Anim Hosp Assoc 23:6, 1987.
24. Salisbury SK, Lantz GC: Long-term results of partial mandibulectomy for treatment of oral tumors in 30 dogs. J Am Anim Hosp Assoc 24:3, 1987.
25. White RAS: Mandibulectomy and maxillectomy in the dog: Long term survival in 100 cases. J Small Anim Pract 32:2, 1991.
26. Fox LE, et al: Owner satisfaction with partial mandibulectomy or maxillectomy for treatment of oral tumors in 27 dogs. J Am Anim Hosp Assoc 33:25, 1997.
27. White RAS: Mandibulectomy and maxillectomy in the dog: Results of 75 cases. Vet Surg 16:1, 1987.
28. Harvey HJ: Surgery. *In* Theilen GH, Madewell BR (eds): Veterinary Cancer Medicine. Philadelphia, Lea & Febiger, 1987, pp 121–127.
29. Zarbo RJ, Crissman JD: The surgical pathology of head and neck cancer. Semin Oncol 15:10, 1988.
30. Chen TY, et al: The clinical significance of pathological findings in surgically resected margins of the primary tumor in head and neck carcinoma. Int J Radiat Oncol Biol Phys 13:833, 1987.
31. Carpenter LG, et al: Squamous cell carcinoma of the tongue in 10 dogs. J Am Anim Hosp Assoc 29:17, 1993.
32. Batsakis JG: Surgical margins in squamous cell carcinomas. Ann Otol Rhinol Laryngol 97:213, 1987.
33. Kotwall C, et al: Metastatic patterns in squamous cell carcinoma of the head and neck. Am J Surg 154:439, 1987.
34. Close LG, et al: Microvascular invasion and survival in cancer of the oral cavity and oropharynx. Arch Otolaryngol Head Neck Surg 115:1304, 1989.
35. Carter RL, et al: Radical neck dissections for squamous carcinomas: Pathological findings and their clinical implications with particular reference to transcapsular spread. Int J Radiat Oncol Biol Phys 13:825, 1987.
36. White RAS, Gorman NT: Wide local excision of acanthomatous epulides in the dog. Vet Surg 18:1, 1989.
37. Bjorling DE, et al: Surgical treatment of epulides in dogs: 25 cases (1974–1984). JAVMA 190:10, 1987.
38. Frankel M: Surgical removal of an odontoma in a dog. J Vet Dent 5:4, 1988.
39. Walsh KM, et al: Epithelial odontogenic tumours in domestic animals. J Comp Pathol 97:5, 1987.
40. Blackwood L, Dobson JM: Radiotherapy of oral malignant melanomas in dogs. JAVMA 209:98, 1996.
41. Valentine BA, et al: Compound odontoma in a dog. JAVMA 186:2, 1985.
42. Thrall DE: Orthovoltage radiotherapy of acanthomatous epulides in 39 dogs. JAVMA 184:826, 1984.
43. Theon AP, et al: Analysis of prognostic factors and patterns of failure in dogs with periodontal tumors treated with megavoltage irradiation. JAVMA 210:785, 1997.
44. White RAS, et al: Sarcoma development following irradiation of acanthomatous epulis in two dogs. Vet Rec 118:24, 1986.
45. Evans SM, et al: Technique, pharmacokinetics, toxicity, and efficacy of intratumoral etanidazole and radiotherapy for treatment of spontaneous feline oral squamous cell carcinoma. Int J Radiat Oncol Biol Phys 20:703, 1991.
46. Ogilvie GK, et al: Efficacy of mitoxantrone against various neoplasms in dogs. JAVMA 198:9, 1991.
47. Theon AP, et al: Intratumoral administration of carboplatin for treatment of squamous cell carcinomas of the nasal plane in cats. Am J Vet Res 57:205, 1996.
48. Postorino, NC, et al: Oral squamous cell carcinoma in the cat. J Am Anim Hosp Assoc 29:438, 1993.
49. Sarosy G, et al: The systemic administration of intravenous melphalan. J Clin Oncol 6:1768, 1988.
50. Straw RC, et al: Canine mandibular osteosarcoma: 52 cases (1980–1992). J Am Anim Hosp Assoc 32:438, 1996.
51. Hammer AS, et al: Prognostic factors in dogs with osteosarcomas of the flat or irregular bones. J Am Anim Hosp Assoc 31:321, 1995.
52. Harvey CE: Oral medicine. *In* Harvey CE (ed): Veterinary Dentistry. Philadelphia, WB Saunders, 1989, pp 34–58.
53. Tscharner C, et al: The eosinophilic granuloma complex. J Small Anim Pract 30:4, 1989.
54. MacEwen EG, Hess PW: Evaluation of effect of immunomodulation on the feline eosinophilic granuloma complex. J Am Anim Hosp Assoc 23:5, 1987.
55. Manning TO, et al: Three cases of feline eosinophilic granuloma complex (eosinophilic ulcer) and observations on laser therapy. Semin Vet Med Surg (Small Anim) 11:3, 1987.
56. Pederson NC: Inflammatory oral cavity diseases of the cat. Vet Clin North Am Small Anim Pract 22:1323, 1992.
57. McKeever PJ, Klausner JS: Plant awn, candidal, nocardial, and necrotizing ulcerative stomatitis in the dog. J Am Anim Hosp Assoc 22:1, 1986.
58. Williams CA, Aller MS: Gingivitis/stomatitis in cats. Vet Clin North Am Small Anim Pract 22:1361, 1992.
59. Spangler WL, Culbertson MR: Salivary gland disease in dogs and cats: 245 cases (1985–1988). JAVMA 198:465, 1991.

GI

CHAPTER 132

DENTISTRY: Genetic, Environmental, and Other Considerations

John E. Saidla

Hereditary dental abnormalities, particularly in dogs and occasionally in cats, are a source of controversy as to cause and where to affix blame. Variations in the number of teeth, placement, head and face dysmorphism, maxillofacial defects, and numerous other variations from normal are implicated as either genetic or developmental (environmental) in origin. This chapter addresses the major variations, their causes, and whether an examiner can be reasonably sure of the cause. A thorough oral examination, including radiographs, should be performed on all animals with dental or skeletal abnormalities of the head. The relative position of both mandibular premolar one teeth should be noted, as they serve as landmarks for determining proper occlusion (Fig. 132–1).

DENTAL FORMULAS AND NOMENCLATURE

The dog has 28 deciduous teeth: (I3/3, C1/1, PM3/3) × 2 = 28. Adult dogs have 42 permanent teeth: (I3/3, C1/1, PM4/4, M2/3) × 2 = 42. Maxillary premolar four and mandibular molar one are designated the carnassial teeth. There are no deciduous first premolar teeth. Williams and Evans were unable to determine for certain whether the first premolar is a member of the deciduous or permanent dentition; however, they prefer to regard it as a member of the latter.[1] Because premolar one has no deciduous precursor from which to grow, it can be assumed that it forms from a rostral extension of the dental lamina in the cranial premolar area, similar to the way in which molar teeth develop from the caudal premolar dental lamina.

The cat has 26 deciduous teeth: (I3/3, C1/1, PM3/2) × 2 = 26. Adult cats have 30 permanent teeth: (I3/3, C1/1, PM3/2, M1/1) × 2 = 30. Maxillary premolar four and mandibular molar one are also designated the carnassial teeth in the cat. Because cats have fewer teeth than dogs, the maxillary premolar teeth are designated the second, third, and fourth premolars, followed by molar one; the mandibular premolars are designated the third and fourth premolars, followed by molar one.

VARIATIONS IN NUMBERS OF TEETH

Prehistoric dog skeletal remains indicate that as early as 20,000 years ago, when it is presumed that selective breeding was not practiced, some dogs did not have a full complement of teeth. The mandibular fourth premolar was missing from *Canis ferus* Bourg; radiographs indicated that no traces of alveolar formation were present in the diastema between the third premolar and the first molar.[2] In another prehistoric canid, *Canis spelaeus* Goldf, the third premolar was missing from the mandible, and no alveolar traces were found.[2] This indicates that a genetic predisposition for missing teeth was or may have been present in the "original foundation" dogs. These data from prehistoric skeletons have been used to shift blame from certain modern breeding stock dogs for being the ancestral source of missing teeth. However, the current dog with missing teeth must have inherited the defect from somewhere, and one of these ancestral dogs is a possible choice.

Bodingbauer[2] described oligodontia and anodontia in terms of embryonic jaw development and either hypo- or hyperdevelopment of tooth germs from the dental lamina. He suggested that infection from the distemper virus may contribute to abnormal budding of the dental germinal tissue, as well as delay or prevent eruption. This theory was more plausible during the era when distemper was globally pandemic. Arnall[3] radiographically examined 140 live animals between the ages of 6 months and 5 years and found 53 per cent with anodontia of one or more teeth. Of the 50 dogs at the age and stage of development calculated to show the full complement of permanent teeth, radiographic evidence indicated that 44 per cent had anodontia. The total number of teeth absent in the 50 dogs was 49, with the maximum number in one dog being six. The most common missing tooth was mandibular molar three, followed by mandibular premolar one and two. The teeth not found missing in this study were the maxillary fourth premolar and mandibular first molar, the carnassial teeth. This same study also found that supernumerary teeth were generally duplicates of the normal adjacent tooth and were less common than the absence of teeth. The frequency of supernumerary teeth was between 10 and 12 per cent, and they were found only in permanent dentition. The maxillary first premolar was the most commonly duplicated tooth, and it was frequently bilateral.

RETENTION OF DECIDUOUS TEETH

In most breeds, normal eruption of deciduous or primary teeth begins at about 1 month of age for the central incisors. The middle incisors erupt at around 1 1/2 months of age, the lateral incisors erupt at 2 months of age, and the canine teeth erupt by 3 months of age. The resorption of the tip of the roots of deciduous teeth begins almost immediately as the developing permanent teeth start to form.[4]

Retention of deciduous teeth is caused by failure of the

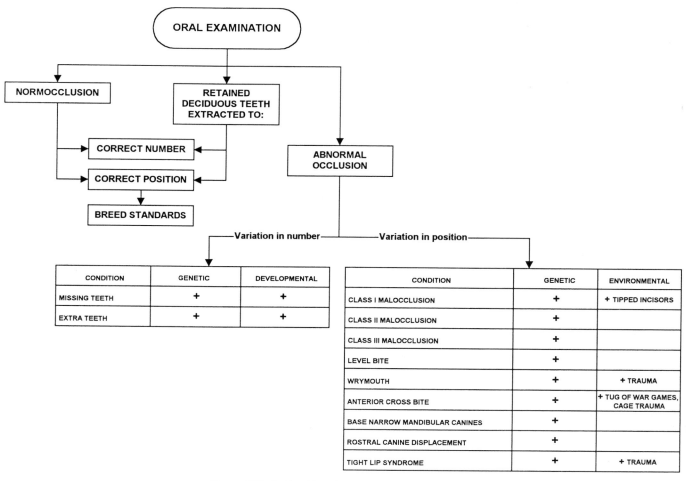

Figure 132–1. Algorithm of occlusion assessment in dogs.

deciduous roots to be reabsorbed during permanent tooth development. In normal root resorption, odontoclasts are activated in part by the pressure of the adjacent developing crown and root. The position of the permanent tooth to the deciduous tooth is approximately dorsal in the maxilla and ventral in the mandible for all teeth except the canine teeth. Special attention must be given to retained deciduous teeth, as they may cause permanent teeth to erupt out of their normal position. Retention of the upper deciduous canine tooth causes the permanent canine tooth to erupt mesially to the deciduous tooth, resulting in misalignment between the canine and incisors of the opposing jaw. Retention of the lower deciduous canine tooth causes eruption of the permanent canine tooth lingually to the deciduous tooth. This usually causes the displaced canine tooth to either grow into the hard palate or grow laterally at a more acute angle. Because these permanent teeth do not develop directly under the deciduous teeth, odontoclasts are not stimulated as much to reabsorb the root and prepare for the extrusion of the permanent crown. Any abnormally retained deciduous tooth should be extracted as soon as possible. The best rule is never to allow two teeth to occupy the same space at the same time.

EFFECT OF DECIDUOUS TEETH ON MAXILLA AND MANDIBLE DEVELOPMENT

The rates of growth of the maxillae and mandibles are different. Eruption of deciduous canine teeth may have a significant impact on the growth of either the maxilla or the mandible. If, for example, the mandibular canine teeth are distal to but touching the maxillary canine teeth, a dental interlock created by the canine teeth may keep the mandible from reaching its maximal length. Most puppies are born with a somewhat shorter mandible than maxilla. The mandible grows in a downward and forward direction and at a faster rate than the maxilla.[4] To bypass the dental interlock, the anterior deciduous teeth (incisors and canines) should be removed at an early age (8 to 12 weeks) in either the maxilla or mandible, whichever is shorter. This may allow the shorter jaw to grow unimpeded to its normal potential. This is called interceptive orthodontics and has been reported to be effective in 30 to 50 per cent of cases.[5]

GENETIC INFLUENCES ON HEAD AND MAXILLOFACIAL DEVELOPMENT

Malocclusion problems do not begin when a litter of puppies is born and they have bad "bites." Instead, the problems begin when two dogs that have numerical variations, misalignment of teeth, imperfect occlusion, or the genes to produce bad bites are bred. The German shepherd breed is considered a classic representative of the ancestral or wild type of dog, and all other breeds are variations from its "standard" form.[6] In dogs carrying the achondroplastic gene, their extremity deformities are attributed to a simple, single-factor dominant expression, but the genetics of the short achondroplastic head modification, such as that found in the bulldog and other similar breeds, is much more complex.[6] Certain factors in the complex influence distinct parts of the head in either a dominant or a recessive fashion. These modifications of different bones and structural units of the head are inherited more or less independently, and as a consequence, frequent dysharmonies occur among the parts,[6] often disturbing the functional efficiency. Structural regulatory processes are ineffective in correcting or adjusting for many of these defects. Structural asymmetry in the growth of the mandible and maxilla produces varying degrees of dental malocclusion and is a widely prevalent condition in both dogs and people and less so in cats.

OCCLUSION AND MALOCCLUSION

The shape of the head, the proportions of the facial bones, and the shape and length of the jaws determine occlusion or malocclusion for a particular breed or individual animal. Skulls differ more in size and shape among domestic dogs than in any other mammalian species. In fact, the skull of the dog varies more in size and shape than any other part of the skeleton.[6] In 1941, Stockard demonstrated that discrepancies in the pattern between the maxilla and the mandible in dogs are inherited and developed as separate and independent characters.[6]

Malocclusion in purebred dogs and cats results from selective breeding that produces a puppy or kitten with a bad bite; additionally, it results from the expression of achondroplastic genes, especially in certain breeds of dogs and cats. Dogs have been selectively bred by humans for centuries to satisfy a variety of needs, creating over 300 different breeds of various sizes and shapes (morphologic characteristics) worldwide. Various breeds over time may be selected for different types of heads that lengthen the muzzle, square the face, shorten the face, and even widen the face and muzzle.

Achondroplasia is caused by an autosomal dominant gene with partial penetrance, which means that the trait will be expressed more dramatically in some individuals than in others.[7] Many breeds of dogs carry the gene for achondroplasia; animals affected with the condition have deficient growth of cartilage. The results include extremely short extremities and an underdeveloped midface. The dachshund is the classic example, but the trait is predominant in many other breeds, especially the terriers and bulldogs.[8] The occasional puppy with a pronounced malocclusion may best be explained not on the basis of inherited jaw size or shape but by the extent to which achondroplasia was expressed in that animal. Many different breeds have undergone extensive inbreeding involving the achondroplasia trait in the past. Breeds without achondroplasia genes and canids that have not been bred by humans have little or no malocclusion.

Nongenetic influences resulting in malocclusion include individual congenital accidents (faulty patterns in germinal epithelial placement or failure of a permanent tooth bud to develop), developmental problems such as retained deciduous teeth, and injuries and mischievous chewing habits or tug-of-war games, especially in adolescents. Determining the exact cause of any malocclusion is usually difficult or impossible. In purebred animals it is best to consider the cause to be genetic until proved otherwise and to refrain from using affected animals for breeding.

GENETIC CONCERNS

The basic tenet underlying veterinary dentistry is that it is unethical to correct malocclusions in breeding animals. This is because the variable pattern of inheritance of malocclusion makes it risky to include animals with malocclusion in the genetic pool. Malocclusion in purebred dogs is thought to be by polygenic inheritance, whereas malocclusion in humans is inherited as a recessive trait with incomplete penetrance. This means that not all individuals who are homozygous for the recessive trait of malocclusion will exhibit the malocclusion phenotypically. Thus only some affected animals will exhibit malocclusion. There is often no identifiable affected individual in the family line preceding or following individuals with malocclusion.

CLASSIFICATION OF OCCLUSION AND MALOCCLUSION

In order to simplify the discussion of states of occlusion and malocclusion, it is best to identify the mandible as either brachygnathic (shorter than the maxilla, Class 2 malocclusion) or prognathic (longer than the maxilla, Class 3 malocclusion). It should also be remembered that the lengths of the mandible and maxilla are inherited independently.

Normal Occlusal Patterns. The normal occlusal pattern is classified as an incisor scissors bite in approximately 53 per cent of all dog breeds. A scissors bite occurs when the mandibular incisors are behind and resting on the cingulum of the maxillary incisors. The mandibular canine teeth interlock rostral with the maxillary canines and equidistant between the canines and the lateral incisors. When the dog's mouth is viewed from the side, the premolars show a perfect sawtooth pattern of interdigitation. The reference tooth for determining occlusion or malocclusion in the dog is the mandibular first premolar: it should be one half an interdental space rostral to the maxillary first premolar tooth, and the rest of the maxillary and mandibular premolars should interdigitate with each opposing tooth (Fig. 132–2). The mesial two thirds of the mandibular first molar should form a shearing surface with the maxillary fourth premolar forming the carnassial teeth. The distal one third of the mandibular first molar is in contact with the mesiopalatal occlusal

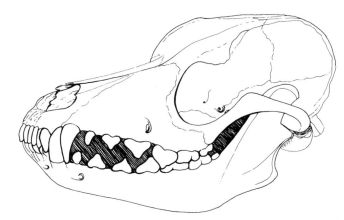

Figure 132–2. Normal occlusion; classified when the maxillary incisors are rostral to the mandibular incisors, the mandibular canine teeth are an equal distance between the maxillary canine teeth and the lateral incisors, and the mandibular premolar one is half an interdental space rostral to the maxillary premolar one and the premolars are in an interdigitating pattern.

surface of the maxillary first molar. The distal palatal surface of the maxillary first molar and the occlusal surface of the maxillary second molar occlude with the occlusal surfaces of the mandibular first and second molars.

Any deviation from normal occlusion is classified as some degree of malocclusion. Several breed standards allow variations of the normal scissors bite, such as the level or even bite and the reverse scissors bite. The reverse scissors bite differs in that the mandibular incisors are rostral to the maxillary incisors, with the maxillary incisors contacting the lingual surface of the mandibular incisors.

Class 1 Malocclusion. Class 1 malocclusion shares the same skeletal relationship as normal occlusion. The most subtle of the Class 1 changes is seen as a shift or change in the relationship of the maxillary and mandibular premolar interdigitation. This occurs when the maxillary premolars are shifted slightly rostral or distal from the normal position while the canine and incisor relationship is still normal. The mandibular canine teeth may also be shifted forward and contact the maxillary lateral incisor.

Class 1 malocclusion may also evidence an altered line of occlusion (Fig. 132–3). The line of occlusion is the relative position of each tooth to the rest of the teeth in the same jaw. If a line were drawn from the maxillary second molar around to the other maxillary second molar or around the mandible, the tips or occlusal surfaces should be in a relatively continuous line. Tipped or drifted incisors, canines, or premolar teeth; missing teeth; and rotated teeth alter or break this line of occlusion.

Class 2 Malocclusion. Class 2 malocclusion is also called mandibular brachygnathism and overbite. The mandible is shorter than the maxilla, and the mandibular incisors are distal and not touching the maxillary incisors. This malocclusion is unacceptable in any breed of dog or cat for showing.

Class 3 Malocclusion. Class 3 malocclusion may be called mandibular prognathism, underbite, prognathism, or undershot jaw and is considered normal in approximately 20 per cent of dogs (brachycephalic breeds) and in several breeds of cats. The mandible is always longer than the

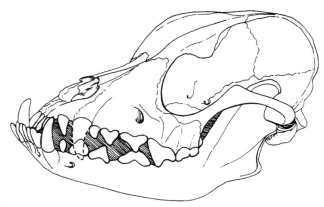

Figure 132–4. Class 3 malocclusion. The mandible is always longer than the maxilla and symmetric in length. This is an accepted malocclusion in several breeds of dogs and cats. Owing to the shortening of the maxilla, the premolars are usually rotated lingually at 90 degrees to provide space for each tooth.

maxilla, and this arrangement is considered abnormal when it occurs in breeds that are supposed to have normal scissors bites. The acceptable Class 3 bite variations must be symmetric, meaning that the teeth on each side of the jaw must be an equal distance from each other and that the number, position, and size of the teeth are the same on both sides of the dental arcade. The Boxer breed requirement faults an unserviceable bite or teeth that show when the mouth is closed.[9] Persian cats are faulted if any tooth is showing when the mouth is closed (Fig. 132–4).

Owing to severe or pronounced shortening of the maxilla, the first three premolars and particularly the fourth may be rotated and set transversely across the maxilla at right angles to the normal position. The molars, instead of being arranged almost in a straight line, follow an angular course with the apex, which projects out laterally, resulting in varying degrees of molar malocclusion.[6]

Level Bite. A level bite occurs when the incisal surfaces of the maxillary incisors rest on the incisal surfaces of the mandibular incisors, resulting in opening of the mouth. This type of bite has an open freeway space in the premolar area owing to the position of the incisors. The premolar crowns do not touch. Level or even bites may be accepted as normal in some breeds as long as the malocclusion is mildly expressed. Level bite represents a mild expression or form of Class 3 malocclusion (Fig. 132–5).

Wry Mouth. An asymmetric malocclusion called wry mouth or wry bite is not acceptable in any breed. This occurs when one hemisection or side of the skull is larger or longer than the other. This size discrepancy results in a deviation of the oral structures, causing the right mandible and maxilla to be longer or shorter than those on the left side. Open bites occur when any of the incisors do not touch and an open space can be seen when looking at the teeth (Fig. 132–6).

Anterior Crossbite. Anterior crossbite occurs with wry bites when the left maxillary incisors are rostral to the left mandibular incisors and the right maxillary incisors are distal to the right mandibular incisors, or vice versa. This condition can also occur when incisors on the right or left side are tipped forward or backward while the other side is in a normal scissors position. This condition is fairly common in many breeds and is one reason for incisors to be out of the normal line of occlusion. Possible causes are tug-of-war

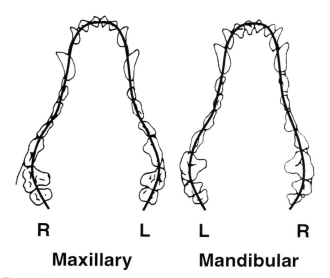

R   L   L   R
Maxillary   **Mandibular**

Figure 132–3. Normal line of occlusion. This imaginary line is used to identify teeth that are not in this continual line. The teeth may be on either side of the line (lingual or buccal), missing, or rotated. A mouth with an altered or broken line of occlusion is representative of a Class 1 malocclusion.

GI

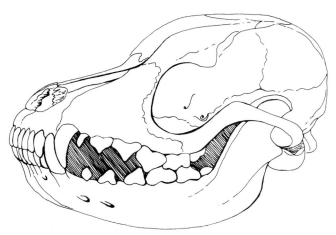

Figure 132–5. Level bite. This is thought to be a variation of a Class 3 malocclusion. Either the mandible is slightly longer than normal or the maxilla is shorter, resulting in the tips of the crowns of the mandibular incisors resting on the crown tips of the maxillary incisors. This usually results in functional loss of the shearing action of the carnassial teeth.

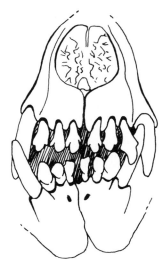

Figure 132–6. Wry mouth. This malocclusion results from one hemimandible and/or maxilla growing longer than the other side, resulting in obvious asymmetry of the mouth and possibly the head. Normal incisor function is usually lost.

games, injuries, asymmetric growth in any one of the four quadrants of the head, and genetics.

Base Narrow Mandibular Canine Teeth. This condition occurs when the mandible is too narrow. The mandibular canine teeth may enter the hard palate inside of the maxillary canine teeth, resulting in deep depressions or penetrations in the hard palate and, in severe cases, penetration of the nasal passages by the teeth. Crowded incisors are a result of breeding for smaller, narrower, "more refined" heads. As a result, the dental arches are smaller, with not enough room for all the incisors to line up side by side in the normal line of occlusion. This condition is also considered a genetic problem.

Rostral Displacement of Maxillary Canine Teeth in Shetland Sheepdogs. Sheltie puppies 6 to 10 months of age can present with the maxillary canine teeth growing forward, pushing the lips outward and forward. This condition has been observed by the author only in Shelties. The teeth truly erupt rostrally instead of following the normal downward arc made by normally erupting maxillary canine teeth. These cases can be corrected orthodontically, but the animal should be neutered at the same time.

Tight Lip Syndrome. This syndrome is caused by the lower lip curling up over the mandible, resulting in lingual displacement of the incisor and canine teeth and interference with the normal growth of the mandible. It has recently been reported in Shar Pei puppies.[10] The lips and tongue form part of the equilibrium forces of the oral cavity. These additional forces pushing on teeth in one direction without opposing counterforces result in an increased incidence of anterior crossbite and mandibular brachygnathism in the Shar Pei. In this breed it is genetic in origin. In animals with lip lesions that heal in contraction, resulting in tightening of the lip margins, similar dental changes may result, especially in young animals.

REFERENCES

1. Evans HE: The digestive apparatus and abdomen. *In* Evans HE (ed): Millers' Anatomy of the Dog. Philadelphia, WB Saunders, 1993, p 392.
2. Bodingbauer J: Oligodontia and polydontia in prehistoric dogs. Vet Rec 75:668, 1963.
3. Arnall L: Some aspects of dental development in the dog. III: Some common variations in the dentitions. J Small Anim Pract 2:195, 1961.
4. Harvey CE: Oral, dental, pharyngeal and salivary gland disorders. *In* Ettinger SJ (ed): Textbook of Veterinary Internal Medicine, 3rd ed. Philadelphia, WB Saunders, 1989, pp 1203–1253.
5. Eisner ER: Malocclusions in cats and dogs. Vet Med 83:1006, 1988.
6. Stockard CR: The Genetic and Endocrine Basis for Differences in Form and Behavior No. 19. The American Anatomical Memoirs. Philadelphia, Wistar Institute of Anatomy and Biology, 1941, pp 150–153.
7. Mulligan TE: Malocclusions—genetic or acquired? Proceedings of the American Veterinary Dental Association, San Francisco, 1990, pp 35–42.
8. Emily P: The genetics of occlusion: Malocclusion in dogs and cats. Vet Forum June:22, 1990, pp 22–23.
9. AKC: Official Standard for the Boxer. New York, American Kennel Club, 1992.
10. McCoy DE: Surgical management of the tight lip syndrome in the Shar Pei dog. J Vet Dent 14:95, 1997.

CHAPTER 133

DENTISTRY: Periodontal Aspects

Linda J. DeBowes

Periodontal disease is the most common disease affecting dogs and cats.[1] Periodontal disease is a general term referring to any disease or inflammation of the structures surrounding the teeth. It is a nonspecific term referring to conditions ranging from mild gingival disease to severe, painful, periodontitis that may result in tooth loss. Gingivitis or inflammation limited to the gingival tissue is reported to be present in at least 70 per cent of cats and dogs by the time they are 2 years of age.[2] Periodontitis, inflammation of the structures supporting the tooth, does not develop in all dogs and cats after the establishment of gingivitis. By 5 years of age most dogs have some degree of periodontitis.[3] The incidence of periodontal disease increases with increased age in dogs and cats and decreases with increased size in dogs.[3] Small and toy breeds are especially prone to gingivitis and periodontitis.

Factors that predispose dogs and cats to the development of periodontal disease include malocclusions, crowding of the teeth, specific plaque bacteria, developmental teeth defects, and host immunity.[3, 4] Diabetes mellitus, nephritis, hepatitis, and retroviral infection may also affect periodontal disease.

ANATOMY AND PHYSIOLOGY OF THE HEALTHY PERIODONTIUM

The gingiva, periodontal ligament, alveolar bone, and cementum are the tissues partly covering and supporting the teeth (Fig. 133–1). Collectively, these tissues are referred to as the periodontium. These are the tissues involved in periodontal disease.

The gingival epithelium attaches to the tooth surface at or slightly below the cemento-enamel junction (CEJ) and is referred to as the junctional epithelium. The gingival sulcus is the area coronal to the junctional epithelium between the tooth and free gingival tissue. The gingival sulcus may be absent in healthy gingiva. The "normal" depth of the gingival sulcus in health is considered to be less than 3 mm in dogs and less than 0.5 mm in cats. The junctional epithelium is attached to the tooth enamel via hemidesmosomes.[5] The junctional epithelium acts as a barrier providing protection for the underlying tissues. Leukocytes, mainly neutrophils, migrate through the junctional epithelium into the gingival sulcus and are part of the host's normal defense barrier. Gingival sulcus fluid contains complement, antibodies, and other defense mechanisms similar to those of blood for preventing and controlling infection. Gingival fibroblasts are important for producing and maintaining collagen and other components of the gingival extracellular matrix. They also play a role in protecting the connective tissues from degradation by producing tissue inhibitors of matrix metalloproteinases (TIMPs).

The alveolar bone that surrounds the root forms the alveolus. The alveolus has dense cortical bone to which the fibers forming the periodontal ligament attach, anchoring the tooth in the alveolus. Alveolar bone formation and resorption are tightly balanced and regulated in healthy tissues to maintain the alveolar crestal bone slightly apical to the CEJ.

Cementum is a specialized calcified tissue that covers the root surfaces. Cementum is a nonvascular, noninnervated tissue that serves to attach the periodontal ligament fibers to the tooth root.

The periodontal ligament is a highly vascularized and cellular connective tissue that is attached to both the cementum and alveolar bone and therefore anchors the tooth. The periodontal ligament is also important in distributing the forces of mastication and chewing into the surrounding alveolar bone.[5]

BASIC TERMINOLOGY

Calculus (tartar): hard, mineralized plaque
Dental stain: stained or discolored pellicle (clinically insignificant)
Gingivitis: inflammation of the gingiva
Pellicle: salivary glycoproteins that adhere to the tooth surface
Periodontal: around or near the tooth
Periodontal pocket: distance from free gingival margin to the attached junctional epithelium in patients with periodontitis
Periodontitis: inflammation extending beyond the gingiva affecting other tissues of the periodontium
Periodontium (supporting structures of the teeth): gingiva, periodontal ligament, cementum, alveolar bone
Plaque: a sticky yellow- to tan-colored material that contains bacteria, extracellular polysaccharides, cellular debris, leukocytes, macrophages, lipids, carbohydrates, and salivary glycans[4]

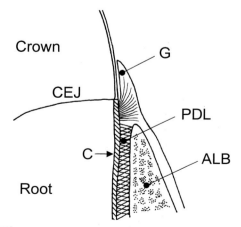

Figure 133–1. Structures of the periodontium. CEJ = cemento-enamel junction; G = gingiva; C = cementum; PDL = periodontal ligament; ALB = alveolar bone.

PATHOBIOLOGY OF PERIODONTAL DISEASE

The initial step in bacterial attachment to the tooth surface is the formation on the tooth surface of a material, the pellicle, to which bacteria can adhere. The pellicle is composed of salivary glycoproteins and coats cleaned and polished tooth surfaces as soon as oral fluids make contact with them.[6, 7] Gram-positive bacteria express adhesins that bind to the salivary glycoproteins.[7] These adhesins are important for bacterial colonization and growth of supragingival plaque. Gram-negative bacteria bind to the gram-positive bacteria within days of initial plaque formation. If left on the tooth surface, the tightly adherent bacterial plaque becomes visible at the gingival margin within days. Plaque is the yellowish-whitish soft material that can be easily rubbed from the tooth surface. Marginal gingivitis occurs as the host develops an acute inflammatory response against the supragingival plaque. Gingivitis does not progress in all patients to the more destructive periodontitis.[3, 8] In individuals susceptible to periodontitis, plaque accumulation continues subgingivally and the elicited immuno-inflammatory response causes further tissue destruction.

Periodontitis is present when destruction of the cementum, periodontal ligament, and alveolar bone results from the plaque-induced inflammation. Initially, the junctional epithelium's attachment to the tooth is compromised and the coronally situated cells become "unattached," effectively converting to pocket epithelial cells. Unless accompanied by gingival recession, this change leads to the formation of periodontal "pockets." Substances released from the bacteria, such as lipopolysaccharide (LPS), activate the release of the proinflammatory cytokines interleukin-1β (IL-1β), tumor necrosis factor-α (TNF-α), and interferon-β (IFN-β).[7] These induce and enhance the production of matrix metalloproteinases (MMPs) and prostaglandin E_2 (PGE$_2$). LPS also activates the release of proinflammatory cytokines IL-8 and IL-1α from the junctional and pocket epithelium. These cytokines attract and activate more neutrophils. Microbial products (toxins, LPS, enzymes) stimulate the release of degradative enzymes from the local and recruited cell populations.[9] They also stimulate an immune response that results in release of proinflammatory cytokines from mononuclear cell infiltrates. Indigenous cells of the periodontal tissues such as fibroblasts, keratinocytes, endothelial cells, and possibly osteoblasts are capable of expressing a degradative phenotype in response to cytokines and other proinflammatory mediators.[9]

Attachment loss associated with periodontitis results from degradation of the periodontal ligament and alveolar bone. The MMPs degrade the constituents of unmineralized connective tissues (e.g., collagen). The bone destruction is mediated through the release of PGE$_2$.[7] As the pocket epithelium is exposed, more of the subgingival bacteria and bacterial substances gain access to the gingival connective tissues and microcirculation, leading to continued production of degradative products and tissue destruction.

Proinflammatory cytokines enhance the recruitment of inflammatory cells. Endothelial cells of the gingival microcirculation express intercellular adhesion molecule–1 (ICAM-1).[7] These endothelial cells may be activated by LPS or cytokines (IL-1β, TNF-α) to express the E-selectin receptor. Early in the inflammatory process, neutrophils, followed later by macrophages and lymphocytes, bind to the E-selectin receptor and then the ICAM-1 and subsequently migrate into the extravascular compartment, forming an inflammatory infiltrate. Periodontal pocket formation is associated with an inflammatory infiltrate of neutrophils, lymphocytes, and monocyte-macrophages. Bacterial antigens and proinflammatory cytokines activate the infiltrating T and B lymphocytes. Activated lymphocytes and monocytes secrete a number of cytokines (TNF-α, IFN-γ), MMPs, and PGE$_2$, which are involved in the destructive inflammatory process. Fibroblasts exposed to LPS and cytokines secrete high levels of MMP and low levels of TIMP throughout the inflamed tissue. Alveolar bone destruction is mediated by PGE$_2$ and, to a lesser extent, by IL-1β, IL-6, and TNF-α.[7]

Mediators that suppress the immuno-inflammatory response are also secreted by the cells involved in the generation of the proinflammatory response. Interleukin-4, IL-10, and transforming growth factor–β (TGF-β) are especially important in down-regulation of proinflammatory cytokine production. There is an imbalance favoring tissue destruction when periodontitis becomes active.

PERIODONTAL DISEASE AND SYSTEMIC DISEASE

The gram-negative bacteria associated with periodontal disease release endotoxin (LPS) into the gingival crevicular fluid (GCF).[10] Phagocytic, endothelial, and epithelial cells are stimulated by LPS to release cytokines and other inflammatory mediators. Concentrations of inflammatory cytokines (e.g., IL-1, TNF-α, IL-6) in the GCF may reach levels sufficient to produce systemic effects.[11]

Numerous studies have identified periodontal disease as a risk factor for systemic disorders in humans.[7, 8, 12–17] Periodontal disease in humans is a risk factor for various cardiac diseases, thromboembolism formation, stroke, and preterm low-birth-weight babies. The association between maternal infection and preterm low-birth-weight babies has been demonstrated and is thought to result from the presence of systemic and placental bacterial toxins and inflammatory mediators.[18]

In the veterinary literature, numerous anecdotal reports suggest that periodontal disease has a systemic effect in dogs and cats.[19] One study demonstrated a positive correlation between severity of periodontal disease and histologic changes in various organs and tissues from dogs; the results of this study suggest that periodontal disease may be associated with systemic effects in dogs.[19] In this study, an association between severity of periodontal disease and the presence of histologic changes was identified in the myocardium and in renal and hepatic tissues.

The bacteria, LPS, cytokines, and other inflammatory mediators may all enter the general circulation, resulting in systemic effects. Production and secretion of potentially toxic cytokines and inflammatory molecules continue as long as bacterial plaque remains.

COMPLICATIONS ASSOCIATED WITH PERIODONTAL DISEASE

Severe periodontitis can result in several local problems and complications. Common manifestations of periodontitis include halitosis, gingival recession, tooth mobility, and tooth loss. The maxillary canine teeth, especially in smaller breeds with narrow noses (e.g., dachshund, poodle), frequently have deep periodontal pockets on their palatal aspect. There is a thin layer of bone between the nasal cavity and the canine tooth root. Destruction of the bone occurs with severe periodontitis, resulting initially in an "inapparent" oronasal fistula. An inapparent oronasal fistula may not cause clinical signs. On the other hand, sneezing may be present and in chronic cases with increased inflammation and infection a nasal discharge may be seen. The character of the nasal discharge may vary from serous to purulent, and in some cases frank hemorrhage occurs. Maxillary canine teeth that are severely compromised periodontally become loose and may eventually exfoliate or in some cases be dislodged into the nasal cavity while the pet is chewing on a hard object.

Apparent oronasal fistulas occur when the canine tooth spontaneously exfoliates or is extracted because of severe periodontitis. Sneezing and nasal discharge are common presenting signs associated with apparent oronasal fistulas. A single-flap procedure is usually successful in closing oronasal fistulas.[20] Large or recurrent fistulas may require a double-flap procedure for successful closure. When the surgery results in creation of tension on the soft tissues, the procedure often fails.

The buccal mucosa in contact with dental plaque on the teeth may become severely inflamed and ulcerated. The ulceration is usually mild and does not cause any significant clinical signs. Severe ulceration may result in significant oral pain, causing difficulty in eating, anorexia, pain on opening the mouth, and ptyalism. When ulceration of the oral tissues occurs in locations where the tissues are not in contact with bacterial plaque, causes other than association with periodontal disease should be considered. Immune-mediated, infectious, and neoplastic conditions should be in the differential diagnosis for ulcerated, inflamed oral tissues. A biopsy specimen of the affected area should be obtained and examined histologically if the etiology is questionable.

Other infrequently encountered problems include severe hemorrhage, osteomyelitis, and infection. Patients with coagulopathies may have severe hemorrhage associated with gingivitis, periodontitis, or dental procedures (e.g., tooth extraction). Osteomyelitis of the alveolar bone may occur as an extension of severe periodontitis. The author has seen a few cases of osteomyelitis in dogs presented with sequestered bone and severe bone remodeling around periodontally affected teeth. Another unusual presentation has been severe osteomyelitis with necrotic bone surrounding the periodontally involved teeth. Extensive surgical removal of all affected bone has been necessary to resolve the problem. Periodontal pockets may accumulate significant bacteria with formation of a periodontal abscess. Abscesses resulting from

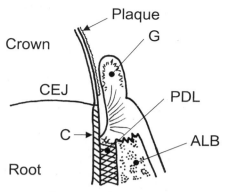

Figure 133–3. Periodontitis.

periodontitis usually drain at the gingival margin or form a fistula and drain at or coronal to the mucogingival junction.

CLINICAL SIGNS OF PERIODONTAL DISEASE

GINGIVITIS

Gingivitis is the earliest stage of periodontal disease (Table 133–1). It occurs when supragingival plaque elicits an inflammatory response in the marginal gingiva. Clinical signs of early disease include gingival erythema and rounding of the gingival margin (edema formation) (Fig. 133–2). As the inflammatory response continues, the entire gingiva (free and attached) may become involved. Gingival bleeding occurs more readily as inflammation progresses, and bleeding may occur with toothbrushing, mastication, or chewing on objects. Halitosis is also a feature of established gingivitis. Because the inflammation is limited to the soft tissues of the gingiva, there are no radiographic abnormalities.

PERIODONTITIS

Periodontitis is present when tissue inflammation and destruction extend beyond the gingiva to affect the other tissues of the periodontium (e.g., periodontal ligament, cementum, alveolar bone) (Fig. 133–3; see Table 133–1). Clinical signs of periodontitis include gingival recession, alveolar bone loss, furcation exposure (Figs. 133–4 and 133–5), and tooth

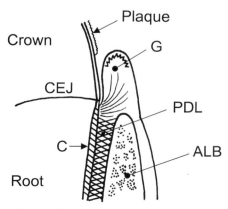

Figure 133–2. Early "marginal" gingivitis.

TABLE 133–1. STAGES OF PERIODONTAL DISEASE

OBSERVATION	STAGE			
	I	*II*	*III*	*IV*
Gingival				
Inflammation	+*	+−++	++−++	++−+++
Edges	Rounded	Rounded	Rounded	Rounded
Recession	No	No	No	+/−
Pocket formation	Absent	Absent	Early	Yes
Radiographic evidence of alveolar bone loss	None	None	Rounding of alveolar crestal bone	Bone loss present
Mobility	No	No	No	+/−

Adapted from Wiggs RB, Lobprise HB: Veterinary Dentistry: Principles and Practice. Philadelphia, Lippincott-Raven, 1997.
* + = mild; + + = moderate; + + + = severe.

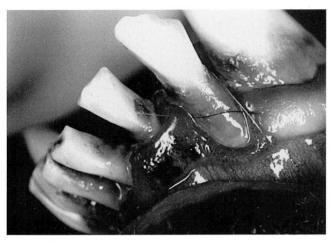

Figure 133–4. Severe periodontitis resulting in alveolar bone loss and gingival recession.

TABLE 133–2. INDICES USED TO EVALUATE AND RECORD THE EXTENT OF PERIODONTAL DISEASE

Gingival index (1–3)
1. Gingiva inflamed (rounding of the margins, red margins), no bleeding on probing
2. Gingiva inflamed, mild to moderate bleeding on probing
3. Spontaneous bleeding from gingiva or bleeding on slight touch or "excessive" or severe bleeding on probing

Furcation index (1–3)
1. Minimal bone loss in furcation
2. Approximately 50 per cent bone loss in furcation
3. Complete ("through and through") bone loss in furcation

Mobility index (1–3)
1. Less than 0.5 mm
2. 0.5–1 mm
3. Greater than 1 mm

mobility. Behavioral changes and changes in eating may be caused by periodontal pain and discomfort. Severe halitosis is often present. Bleeding of the gingiva may occur spontaneously or with mild abrasion. Findings on dental examination may include the presence of gingivitis, gingival recession, alveolar bone loss, periodontal pockets, furcation exposure, and loose teeth (Table 133–2).

In areas of quiescent periodontitis, severe inflammation is absent. Areas of active periodontitis show evidence of attachment loss as well as severe inflammation.[3]

Full-mouth radiography in dogs and cats is recommended for complete evaluation of all dental patients and especially for the older patients with more severe disease.[21, 22] The radiographic changes associated with periodontitis include resorption of the alveolar crest, widening of the periodontal space, loss of lamina dura, and alveolar bone destruction (Fig. 133–6A and B).[23] Resorption of the crestal portion of the alveolar bone (process) is the initial radiographic evidence of periodontitis.[23] Intraoral dental radiographs are valuable for determining the type (horizontal, vertical) and extent of alveolar bone loss. This information is important in determining the prognosis as well as the appropriate treatment plan. Dental radiographs are also important for determining the presence and type of combined periodontic and endodontic lesions.[23]

INDICATIONS FOR PROFESSIONAL DENTAL CLEANING

Professional dental cleaning involves the removal of supragingival and subgingival plaque and calculus to resolve or slow the progress of periodontal disease. Removal of subgingival plaque and calculus is crucial in the treatment of periodontal disease. If not removed, subgingival plaque continues to stimulate an inflammatory response and tissue destruction may progress. Gingivitis that does not resolve with daily mechanical plaque removal (e.g., toothbrushing) performed by the owner at home should be managed with professional dental cleaning. Toothbrushing may be effective in removing supragingival plaque and subgingival plaque up to about 1 mm below the free gingival margin.[4] Failure to resolve gingivitis with appropriate daily toothbrushing suggests the presence of remaining subgingival plaque, which needs to be removed. Periodontal inflammation limited to gingivitis is completely reversible if all dental plaque is removed followed by plaque removal at home on a daily basis. Calculus (supragingival and subgingival) on the tooth surface should be removed by professional dental cleaning. The use of a handscaler to remove supragingival calculus in an awake patient is discouraged.[4] This method is more likely to cause trauma to the soft tissues and, more important, does not permit removing subgingival plaque and calculus or polishing the teeth. Esthetically, the teeth may look better, but nothing has been done to prevent progression of disease if subgingival plaque and calculus remain.

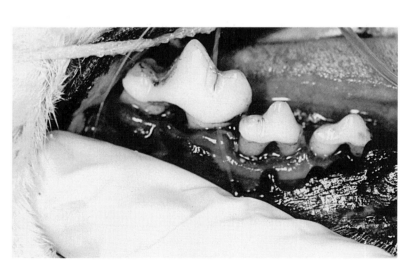

Figure 133–5. Severe periodontitis resulting in alveolar bone loss and furcation exposure.

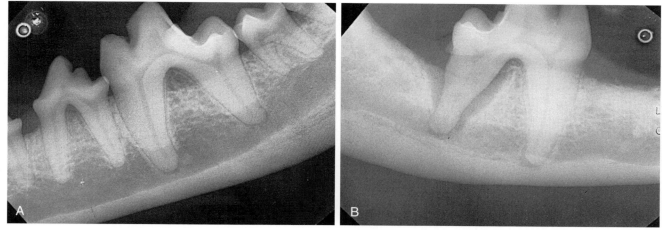

Figure 133–6. Radiographs of mandibular teeth with periodontitis. *A,* Resorption of alveolar crest bone. *B,* Severe alveolar bone loss, loss of lamina dura, and destruction of PDL.

Periodontal root débridement (root planing) is indicated for treatment of periodontal pockets. Periodontal pockets larger than 5 mm are best treated in conjunction with periodontal surgery to allow maximal visualization and root débridement.[24]

PLAQUE AND CALCULUS REMOVAL

General anesthesia is required to perform a complete dental examination, scale and polish the teeth, perform root débridement, and perform other procedures that may be required. A secured endotracheal tube should be in place to protect the lower airways during the dental procedures.

Aerosolization of oral bacteria occurs during the dental procedure when power instruments with water as a coolant are used. This contaminates the dental operatory and exposes the people in the immediate vicinity to oral bacteria. A 0.12 per cent chlorhexidine (CHX) rinse applied to the teeth before the scaling procedure may decrease the magnitude of aerosolized bacteria.[4] Personnel in the area should wear protective face shields or face masks and protective eyewear. The dental operatory is not a sterile room; therefore, other surgical procedures requiring sterility should not be performed in the same suite as dental procedures.

Scaling of the teeth may be done with hand instruments alone.[20] However, using a power-driven scaler is just as effective and decreases the procedure time.[25] This prevents operator fatigue and decreases the anesthetic time for patients. Power-driven scalers that may be used are either ultrasonic or sonic scalers. A rotary scaler bur on a high-speed handpiece is generally not recommended, and if it is used the operator should be highly experienced.[4, 20] Ultrasonic and sonic scalers are preferred over the rotary scaler because they cause less damage to the tooth surface. The vibrations of the power scalers loosen the calculus from the tooth surface. Ultrasonic scalers vibrate at a higher frequency than sonic scalers, which means that they are usually quicker in dislodging calculus from the tooth surface. Ultrasonic scalers generate a significant amount of heat at the instrument tip. Therefore, if used improperly, they have the potential to heat the tooth excessively, causing pulpitis or pulpal necrosis resulting in tooth death. As a general guideline, to prevent thermal damage, the scaler tip should not be used on one tooth for longer than 5 to 15 seconds at a time.[4]

Ultrasonic scaler tips should not be placed subgingivally unless specifically designed for that purpose. Several new tips have been designed to be used in sonic and ultrasonic powered scaling units for treatment of periodontal pockets.[20, 25] Tips designed for subgingival scaling are narrower and have internal water channels to keep them cool. Sonic scalers vibrate at a lower frequency than the ultrasonic scalers. As a result, minimal heat is generated and there is little potential for excessive heating of the tooth and pulp damage. Periodontal tips for sonic scalers may be used subgingivally. Rotary scaler burs rotate at high speed and have the greatest potential of the power-driven scalers to damage the tooth surface. When ultrasonic and sonic scalers are used, the operator should use the side of the instrument rather than the point of the tip.[4, 20] The vibrations of the scaler tip do not effectively dislodge calculus if the point is used, and more damage to the tooth surface is caused by the "jackhammer" motion against the tooth.

Hand instruments used for scaling teeth are scalers and curettes. Scalers have sharp points on their tips and should be used exclusively for supragingival calculus removal. Curettes are used for subgingival scaling and root planing. Curettes are designed with a rounded tip and smooth back to decrease soft tissue trauma when placed subgingivally. The hand instruments must be sharpened as frequently as necessary to maintain a sharp cutting edge.[20] The time for sharpening is one reason why using hand instruments alone takes more time than using power-driven scalers.[25]

The basic techniques used to scale teeth with hand instruments include (1) holding the instrument with a modified pen grasp, (2) using a finger from the working hand to establish a "finger rest" and provide a fulcrum point, (3) placing the working surface of the instrument at a 70- to 80-degree angle to the tooth surface, and (4) positioning the working end of the instrument so that it is used in an apical-to-coronal motion to prevent soft tissue injury and subgingival lodging of calculus.

POLISHING

Polishing the teeth after scaling is recommended. The power-driven scalers and hand instruments leave scratches in the enamel surface that increase the tooth surface area, making it more plaque retentive. Polishing the teeth smooths

GI

the tooth surface and thereby helps to decrease plaque accumulation after the dental procedure. A low-speed handpiece, prophy angle, rubber polishing cups, and polishing paste are used for the polishing procedure.[4, 20] Significant heat is generated when polishing the teeth. Increased speed (revolutions per minute), pressure of the polishing cup against the tooth, and length of polishing time all contribute to excessive heat production that may injure or kill a tooth. Light pressure should be used when placing the polishing cup against the tooth surface. The polishing cup is just a carrier for the polishing paste and does not itself provide any polishing benefit. Plenty of polishing paste should be used to ensure adequate polishing. The power to the low-speed handpiece should be adjusted and maintained between 2000 and 4000 revolutions per minute. To be safe, each tooth should be polished no longer than 5 to 8 seconds at a time. When all the tooth surfaces have been polished, the oral cavity and gingival sulcus should be rinsed to remove any debris (e.g., calculus, blood clots, polishing paste) that could cause pharyngeal obstruction, be inhaled after extubation, or cause subgingival irritation (e.g., polishing paste). A final rinse with 0.12 per cent CHX may be beneficial in providing a residual antimicrobial effect.[4]

ROOT DÉBRIDEMENT (ROOT PLANING)

Root débridement (root planing) is a procedure intended to remove subgingival plaque and calculus as well as remove bacterial toxins from the root surface. Power-driven scalers with specially designed tips may be used.[25] Curettes are hand instruments designed for working below the gum line and for treatment of deep periodontal pockets. They have a long shank and short working tip to allow access to the apical portion of deep pockets and to narrow pockets while minimizing soft tissue damage.[20] The curette is placed apically, near the epithelial attachment, and used with multiple short pulling strokes to clean and smooth the root surface. Excessive instrumentation resulting in cementum removal and dentin exposure must be avoided. It is now known that endotoxin adheres weakly to the root surface rather than being deeply embedded in the root surface.[25] "Sonic and ultrasonic (power-driven) instruments can be used to accomplish definite root *detoxification* and maximal wound healing without over instrumentation of root and without extensive cementum removal."[25]

Periodontal pockets larger than 5 mm cannot be adequately treated without periodontal surgery (e.g., gingival flaps) to provide adequate exposure and access for complete root débridement.

PERIODONTAL SURGERY

Deep periodontal pockets (e.g., >5 mm) usually cannot be adequately treated with conservative nonsurgical approaches.[24] Periodontal surgery is indicated to provide better access and root débridement. Client compliance with recommended oral hygiene care and recall visits is of paramount importance in the success or failure of any periodontal surgical procedure.[24] The expense of periodontal surgery and poor owner or pet compliance are the major problems. Periodontal surgery is aimed at reducing the depths of periodontal pockets, eliminating periodontal pockets, and allowing areas with attachment loss to be better maintained with home oral hygiene care.[24]

In the first year after periodontal surgery, increased oral care by the owner as well as the veterinarian is required. Maintaining excellent oral hygiene enhances healing and the ultimate success of the procedure. The diet and chewing habits of the pet must be modified for 2 to 4 weeks after surgery to allow optimal healing. Recall visits for teeth cleaning have been recommended at 6 weeks, 6 months, and 9 months after periodontal surgery.[24] If the recommended home care and follow-up during the first year are complied with, yearly teeth cleaning with home oral hygiene is usually sufficient to maintain periodontal health.[24]

ANTIMICROBIAL THERAPY

CONTROLLED LOCAL DELIVERY

Local delivery of antimicrobials for treatment of periodontitis has several benefits over systemic antibiotic administration.[26] The antimicrobial is delivered directly to the site of infection, and higher concentrations of antimicrobial are reached at the site with minimal systemic uptake.

Local delivery of antimicrobials in periodontal pockets more than 5 mm deep decreases inflammation and supports soft tissue healing.[26] Actisite is a local delivery product approved by the Food and Drug Administration and used in human dentistry. Actisite is a flexible fiber polymer saturated with tetracycline hydrochloride that allows slow, constant delivery of the tetracycline to the subgingival site for 14 days. A second visit is required to remove the fiber, and this feature makes Actisite a less desirable product for veterinary dentistry. A liquid biodegradable local drug delivery system containing doxycycline has been developed for use in dogs (Heska Periodontal Disease Therapeutic) and humans (Atridox).[26] For placement and adequate retention of the gel, the pocket should be at least 5 mm deep. The liquid gel is placed in the periodontal pocket and hardens within a few minutes, allowing it to be packed below the gingival margin. Unlike the Actisite antimicrobial local delivery system used in treating humans with periodontitis, the Heska Periodontal Disease Therapeutic is completely resorbable and a second visit for removal is not required. This local delivery system has been experimentally evaluated in beagles with severely infected periodontal pockets.[27] It was concluded from this study that the subgingival doxycycline delivery system led to a substantial improvement in periodontal health. A controlled-release biodegradable CHX chip has been developed for use in human dentistry.[28] The chip releases therapeutic levels of CHX within the periodontal pocket for 7 to 10 days after placement. When used as an adjunct to traditional periodontal pocket therapy, the CHX chip enhanced the improvement in periodontal health.[28] Because the Perio Chip is biodegradable and contains a proven antimicrobial (CHX), it may be beneficial in treating severe periodontitis in dogs.

SYSTEMIC ANTIBIOTICS

Systemic antibiotics may be useful in the treatment of dogs and cats with severe ulcerative stomatitis or periodontitis. They may enhance healing in patients with severe periodontitis when administered in the period after periodontal surgery. Recommended antibiotics include amoxicillin–clavulanic acid (Clavamox), clindamycin (Antirobe), and metronidazole.

PERIPROCEDURAL ANTIBIOTICS

Bacteremias of dental origin occur in patients with periodontal disease during mastication, flossing, and dental procedures.[29] The potential exists for the development of infection at a distant site as a result of the bacteremia. The risk of such an infection and which individuals are susceptible have not been determined. Veterinary dentists have different opinions about which patients should receive preoperative antibiotics.[4, 29] Patients considered at risk in human dentistry include those with cardiovascular disease, prosthetic joints, and an immune response altered by medications (e.g., chemotherapeutics) or disease (e.g., diabetes mellitus).[30]

Factors to consider when determining whether treatment with antibiotics is necessary or would be beneficial before periodontal procedures include (1) the patient's risk of developing a distant-site infection resulting from the procedure-induced bacteremia and (2) the possibility of development of resistant infection and bacteremia with bacteria not sensitive to current antibiotic therapy.

Preoperative antibiotics should be administered to patients at risk for developing a distant-site infection from the procedure-induced bacteremia. Antibiotics are usually administered 1 hour before initiation of the procedure to provide therapeutic blood levels during the procedure and 1 hour after completion. Long procedures may require administration of a second dose of antibiotics 4 to 6 hours after the initial administration.

HOME CARE

The purpose of oral hygiene on a regular basis for dogs and cats is to prevent accumulations of plaque and subsequent development or progression of periodontal disease. Plaque removal is accomplished by mechanical removal and/or by antimicrobial therapy. Mechanical removal is the primary method utilized in home care programs and may include one or all of the following: manual brushing of teeth, dietary means of plaque removal, and providing toys or chewing devices. Antimicrobials may be used to decrease plaque accumulation; this may be especially helpful after dental procedures that require temporary cessation of mechanical plaque removal.

MECHANICAL PLAQUE REMOVAL

Mechanical removal of dental plaque may be accomplished with a number of different toothbrushing devices designed for veterinary use or selected devices used for dental hygiene in people. Veterinary brushes or manual plaque-removing devices include toothbrushes of various sizes and designs, gauze pads, and other materials. Ideally, the frequency of toothbrushing should be once daily. The extent of existing disease, the temperament of the pet, and the owner's schedule determine the ultimate home care plan to be recommended.

Brushing the teeth to remove plaque accumulation is the mainstay of periodontal disease prevention. Owners should work with and train their young puppies and kittens to accept handling of the head, face, and oral cavity as well as the toothbrushing. Older dogs and cats can also be taught to accept oral hygiene care, but it may take longer than in a young patient. Patients with gingival inflammation or more advanced dental disease that causes pain are understandably resistant to oral hygiene methods. When preexisting disease that causes facial, oral, or dental pain is present, it should be managed first and tissues should be allowed to become less inflamed and painful before toothbrushing is started.

DENTIFRICES

Using a veterinary dentifrice rather than a human product is recommended. Depending on the ingredients in the dentifrice, veterinary products may have specific antiplaque properties or just be flavored to improve patients' compliance. The reasons given for not using human dentifrices are the potential for irritation of the gastric mucosa when the paste is swallowed and topical irritation and burning caused by the paste. Owners may be aware of sodium bicarbonate or sodium bicarbonate dentifrices for humans; these are not recommended for veterinary patients. Patients with a low tolerance for or contraindications to increased sodium consumption may be especially at risk for complications if sodium bicarbonate is used for toothbrushing. Ingredients in veterinary dentifrices include "active" ingredients such as CHX, enzymes with antimicrobial properties, and flavors to enhance palatability and compliance.

TOOTHBRUSHING METHODS AND TRAINING

When an appropriate mechanical device (i.e., toothbrush) and dentifrice have been selected for the patient, the owner may commence with the training phase.

Pets show more resistance to handling and toothbrushing when their mouth is opened. For this reason, the goal with most dogs and cats is to prevent plaque accumulation on the buccal and labial surfaces of the teeth. This can be accomplished while gently holding the mouth closed in most dogs and cats. Fortunately, plaque accumulation is often minimal on the palatal and lingual surfaces of the teeth. Patients with "heavy" plaque and calculus on the palatal or lingual tooth surfaces may be trained to allow toothbrushing of these surfaces.

Steps to follow in training a dog or cat to accept oral examination and toothbrushing:

1. Acceptance of head and face handling. Gradually work on petting, scratching, and stroking the face and muzzle area until the pet accepts it.

2. Acceptance of handling the lips. While gently holding the muzzle to keep the mouth closed, gradually work on lifting the lips to be able to visualize and touch the teeth. Do not proceed beyond this stage until the pet accepts it with no adverse behavior (Fig. 133–7A).

3. Acceptance of finger and/or brushing device placement on the teeth. Initially, this may be one tooth (e.g., canine) for 5 seconds; gradually, over a period of hours, days, or weeks, work up to longer periods of time as well as more teeth. Acceptance occurs at varying rates, depending on the pet's temperament and the comfort level of the person working with the pet.

Owners must be made aware of the importance of brushing harder to reach teeth such as the fourth premolars and molars (Fig. 133–7B).

ADVANCED ORAL HYGIENE CARE

Pets that become comfortable with and accept regular toothbrushing may also allow toothbrushing on the palatal

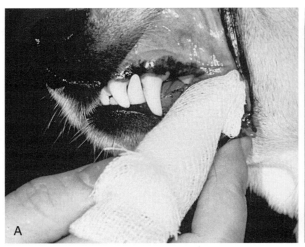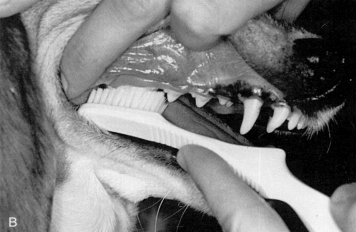

Figure 133–7. Home oral hygiene—toothbrushing. *A*, Dog accepting handling of the lips. *B*, Brushing buccal surface of premolars or molars.

and lingual surfaces. An aid for the owner in accomplishing this is to place a syringe case wrapped with surgical tape or other soft material behind the canines to hold the mouth slightly open while toothbrushing is performed. The size of the syringe case or other soft object should be appropriate for the size of the patient; too large an object may be uncomfortable for the pet and result in resistance.

DIETARY METHODS FOR DECREASING PLAQUE ACCUMULATION

Complete maintenance diets are available for dogs (Hill's Science Diet Canine t/d) and cats (Hill's Science Diet Feline t/d; Friskies Dental Diet) to decrease plaque accumulation. These diets are specially formulated kibbles that mechanically remove dental plaque when the dog or cat bites into the kibble. The diet is not effective in plaque removal if the pet swallows the kibble without chewing it.

Ideally, these diets are used as part of an oral home hygiene care program that includes toothbrushing. In situations in which toothbrushing is not possible, is unlikely, or is sporadic, the "dental" diet provides some oral health benefit for the patients. The dental diets should be used to prevent plaque accumulation and not to treat preexisting calculus accumulation. The patient's teeth should be professionally scaled and polished to treat existing calculus accumulation and periodontal disease.

REFERENCES

1. University of Minnesota Center for Companion Animal Health: Preliminary data, National Companion Animal Study. J Vet Dent 13:56, 1996.
2. Wiggs RB, Lobprise HB: Veterinary Dentistry: Principles and Practice. Philadelphia, Lippincott-Raven, 1997.
3. Harvey CE: Periodontal disease in dogs: Etiopathogenesis, prevalence, and significance. Vet Clin North Am Small Anim Pract 28:1111, 1998.
4. DuPont GA: Prevention of periodontal disease. Vet Clin North Am Small Anim Pract 28:1129, 1998.
5. Lindhe J: The anatomy of the periodontium. *In* Textbook of Clinical Periodontology. Copenhagen, Munksgaard, 1989, pp 19–69.
6. Hefferren JJ, Schiff TG, Smith MR: Assessment methods and clinical outcomes: Chemical and microbial composition, formation, and maturation dynamics of pellicle, plaque, and calculus. J Vet Dent 11:75, 1994.
7. Page RC: The pathobiology of periodontal diseases may affect systemic diseases: Inversion of a paradigm. Ann Periodontol 3:108, 1998.
8. Williams RC: Periodontal disease: The emergence of a new paradigm. Compend Contin Educ Dent (special issue suppl) 19(1):4–10, 1998.
9. Birkedal-Hansen H: Host-mediated extracellular matrix destruction by metalloproteinases. *In* Genco R, et al (eds): Molecular Pathogenesis of Periodontal Disease. Washington, DC, American Society for Microbiology, 1994, pp 191–202.
10. Fine DH, Mendieta C, Barnett ML, et al: Endotoxin levels in periodontally healthy and diseased sites: Correlation with levels of gram-negative bacteria. J Periodontol 63:897, 1992.
11. DeBowes LJ: The effects of dental disease on systemic disease. Vet Clin North Am Small Anim Pract 28:1057, 1998.
12. Beck J, Garcia R, Heiss G, et al: Periodontal disease and cardiovascular disease. J Periodontol 67:1123, 1996.
13. Loesche WJ: Periodontal disease as a risk factor for heart disease. Compend Contin Educ Dent 15:976, 1994.
14. Mattila KJ, Nieminen MS, Valtonen V, et al: Association between dental health and acute myocardial infarction. Br Med J 298:779, 1989.
15. Cohen DW, Rose LF: The periodontal-medical risk relationship. Compend Contin Educ Dent 19(1):11–24, 1998.
16. Offenbacher S, Beck JD: Peridontitis: A potential risk factor for spontaneous preterm birth. Compend Contin Educ Dent (special issue suppl) 19(1):32–39, 1998.
17. Genco R, Glurich I, Haraszthy V: Overview of risk factors for periodontal disease and implications for diabetes and cardiovascular disease. Compend Contin Educ Dent (special issue suppl) 19(1):40–45, 1998.
18. Offenbacher S, Katz V, Fertik G, et al: Periodontal infection as a possible risk factor for preterm low birth weight. J Periodontol 67:1103, 1996.
19. DeBowes LJ, Mosier D, Logan E, et al: Association of periodontal disease and histologic lesions in multiple organs from 45 dogs. J Vet Dent 13:57, 1996.
20. Holmstrom SE, Frost P, Eisner ER: Veterinary Dental Techniques for the Small Animal Practitioner. Philadelphia, WB Saunders, 1998.
21. Verstraete FJM, Kass PH, Perpak CH: Diagnostic value of full-mouth radiography in cats. Am J Vet Res 59:692, 1998.
22. Verstraete FJM, Kass PH, Perpak CH: Diagnostic value of full-mouth radiography in dogs. Am J Vet Res 59:686, 1998.
23. Gorrel C: Radiographic evaluation. Vet Clin North Am Small Anim Pract 28:1147, 1998.
24. Grove TK: Treatment of periodontal disease. Vet Clin North Am Small Anim Pract, 28:1147, 1998.
25. Drisko CH: Root instrumentation, power-driven versus manual scalers, which one? Dent Clin North Am 42:229, 1998.
26. Killoy WJ, Polson AM: Controlled local delivery of antimicrobials in the treatment of periodontitis. Dent Clin North Am 42:263, 1998.
27. Polson AM, Southard GL, Dunn RL, et al: Periodontal pocket treatment in beagle dogs using subgingival doxycycline from a biodegradable system. I. Initial clinical responses. J Periodontol 67:1176, 1996.
28. Jeffcoat MK, Bray KS, Ciancio SG, et al: Adjunctive use of a subgingival controlled-release chlorhexidine chip reduces probing depth and improves attachment level compared with scaling and root planing alone. J Periodontol 69:989, 1998.
29. DeBowes LJ: Management of dental disease in the special patient. *In* Veterinary Dentistry: Managing the Dental Patient. Proceedings, Symposium, January 1997, Orlando. Pfizer Animal Health. VLS, 1997.
30. Lockhart PB, Schmidtke MA: Antibiotic considerations in medically compromised patients. Dent Clin North Am 38:381, 1994.

CHAPTER 134

DENTISTRY: Endodontic and Restorative Treatment Planning

Edward R. Eisner

The goal of endodontic therapy is to salvage the tooth.[1-4] When possible the vitality of the tooth should be preserved with a direct pulp cap, indirect pulp cap, or pulpotomy procedure. When resultant vitality is not possible, the goal is to salvage the tooth by pulpectomy. The tooth should be treated in a manner that removes as little tooth structure and is as least invasive as possible in an effort to return the tooth to former form and function. Root canal therapy involves removing the source of infection (pulpectomy); and if a small amount of residual infection remains periapically, the body's defense mechanisms will successfully eliminate it.

Damaged teeth can be restored using in-office techniques or by using assistance from an outside dental laboratory in fabricating the restoration. The purpose of restorative dentistry is to restore the form and function of damaged teeth. Restorative materials should be easily delivered and compatible with the adjacent tissues. The materials used for surface restoration should be strong enough to withstand the traumatic and chemical forces to which they will be subjected and should display minimal expansion and contraction with temperature variations.[5, 6] The best material for the procedure depends on the desired look, the extent of trauma the tooth will be subjected to, the ability and experience of the clinician, and the economic wishes of the client. Carnivore dentition is designed for puncturing, grasping, shearing, and tearing functions, with only the two maxillary and three mandibular molars of the dog, and no teeth in the cat, designed for maceration of food. The purpose of restorative dentistry in household dogs and cats is usually focused on restoring the surface of the tooth and protecting either the inner structure of the tooth or the inner therapeutic materials. Full or partial crown restoration is appropriate for aesthetic purposes and for full oral functional restoration in field dogs, protection dogs, and service dogs.

INDICATIONS FOR PERFORMING ENDODONTICS

Endodontic treatment is indicated to preserve a tooth when injury or a carious infection exposes either the pulp chamber or the root canal.[7] It is also indicated when a pulp injury is present that results in hemorrhage or necrosis either in a closed pulp canal or when a pulp or periapical abscess of the tooth is present. Additionally, endodontic treatment should be performed when a clinician exposes the pulp during a restorative or endodontic procedure, when periodontal disease extends to the apex, resulting in an ascending pulpal infection, or when a tooth root is affected by interrupted and incomplete development.[8]

RATIONALE FOR ENDODONTIC TREATMENT

Optimum health for a dog or cat requires the proper functioning of every system in the body. The mouth is the beginning of the alimentary system. If there is pain or infection in one or more teeth, the animal may be irritable and can potentially endanger people and other animals. If the dog or cat is not eating well, its health will be compromised. Moreover, a pet with an infected mouth poses a potential public health problem because pathogenic bacteria can be transmitted to family members. A pet may also be shunned or banished from contact with family members because it has halitosis secondary to infection.[9-11]

Most dogs do not exhibit pain in a fractured tooth once pulp death occurs,[12-14] until periapical pathology occurs. Endodontic pain occurs as a result of fluid pressure changes experienced through exposed and open dentinal tubules. Once the pulp is necrotic in a fractured tooth the exposed dentinal tubules become sealed by a smear layer of tooth debris, plaque, or dirt and the patient is thus more comfortable. If the fractured tooth is alive and recently traumatized, many dogs will flinch if the tooth is percussed with a probe or other instrument. Some animals shear or macerate food only on the side of the mouth opposite the traumatized tooth or drool and produce increased calculus on the injured side. Hunting dogs may refuse their training dummies, utility dogs may refuse their dumbbells, and apprehension dogs may either hesitate to bite or bite and release repetitively because of dental pain.[15]

When the pulp is exposed, secondary to a coronal fracture or by a carious erosion,[13-15] eventually pathogenic bacteria will descend into the pulp canal to cause an abscess either within the canal itself or periapically by extension of the infection. Infection that has escaped through the apical end of the root canal can cause osteomyelitis and bone loss. Periapical infection can spread, contributing to pathologic fractures of the jaw, or result in weakened necrotic bone with eventual oronasal fistula from any of the maxillary teeth.

The advantages of endodontic therapy are (1) it is an efficient procedure to perform; (2) it is less invasive and less traumatic than surgical extraction of a large canine or carnassial tooth; (3) it is more aesthetically pleasing to the owner than surgical extraction; and (4) the cost of root canal therapy is not much more than that of surgical extraction. Another advantage of small animal endodontics is that a well-performed procedure is highly successful because the patient has a relatively short life span compared with that of humans.

The goal of endodontic therapy in cases of coronal fracture is to perform therapy within 48 hours of the trauma to increase the likelihood of preserving vitality in the injured tooth. In cases of older injuries, the goal is to eliminate the source of the infection from within the pulp canal of a tooth by removing the pulp itself from the canal. If a tooth is dead or fractured with exposed pulp, the therapy of choice is endodontic treatment rather than extraction. If a clinic is unable to provide the indicated treatment, the client should be informed where such service is available and referred to a clinic where appropriate treatment can be performed, if the service is desired.

ENDODONTIC SIGNS AND TREATMENT PLANNING

Endodontic disease should be included in the differential diagnosis of (1) an ophthalmic problem if the animal is rubbing its eye, (2) a respiratory disease when a unilateral nasal discharge is present, (3) allergies if sneezing is reported, (4) digestive or systemic disease if there is reluctance to eat or food is dropped from the mouth, (5) uremia if halitosis is evident, or (6) renal and pancreatic disease because of reported polydipsia and polyuria.

A fractured or discolored dead tooth should be endodontically treated or extracted. A dead tooth, by definition, has a necrotic pulp, and a necrotic pulp tends to putrefy and abscess. Any maxillary tooth may abscess into the nasal passages, creating a chronic sinusitis or rhinitis. A caudal tooth abscess may lead to a suborbital or retrobulbar abscess. An abscessed mandibular tooth may cause progressive lytic bone pathology that will weaken the jaw and can result in pathologic fracture. Unlike a worn tooth that has a dark-brown–stained central dentinal color, a tooth with pulp exposed for months or years will often have a black-stained central dentinal color. The defect may not be penetrable by an explorer instrument because of dirt ground tightly into the perforating defect, but if the surface color is black, almost certain infection lies beneath. During endodontic treatment, when anatomic anomalies are encountered and as new information is discovered that affects the strength and soundness of the tooth structure during treatment, it is necessary to update and adjust the plan. The variable signs of discomfort may be a unilateral swelling of the muzzle, suborbital tissue, or ventral mandible that coincides with the anatomic location of the apex of the infected tooth root. Further development of a periapical abscess may lead to a fistula on either the external surface of the mouth or the mucosal surface. When a tooth has endodontic pathology it should be treated appropriately with endodontic therapy. If this is not possible, it should be extracted. Extraction is indicated to avoid more expensive endodontic therapy, to remove infection, or to relieve pain if endodontic therapy is declined. Extraction is preferable to waiting for a bone-damaging abscess to occur. Teeth should also be extracted in cases of combined periodontal/endodontic involvement when the extent of periodontal involvement is such that the infection cannot be adequately controlled or the tooth stabilized in its socket.[16] If an extraction undesirably alters the anatomy of the face, or weakens the jaw, a synthetic, freeze-dried, or autogenous osseous implant can be placed to strengthen the bone or a prosthetic tooth can be implanted.

ENDODONTIC TREATMENT PLANNING FOR NON-FRACTURED TEETH

ENDODONTICALLY HEALTHY TEETH

A vital, clean, healthy tooth will be varying shades of white and will be translucent when backlit by a penlight in a dark room. It will be no more sensitive to percussion than its adjacent teeth. The adjacent attached gingiva and mucogingival line will be void of any swelling or parulis (abscess of the gingiva). If a tooth is stained intrinsically, the discoloration cannot be polished away. If this tooth is translucent, it is a vital tooth and no endodontic treatment is indicated.

SENSITIVITY

An endodontically affected tooth may be sensitive to percussion and may have a medical history that includes signs of dental discomfort: the animal (1) rubs its face on inanimate objects or paws at its face; (2) refuses hard treats or breaks them with the teeth of only the opposite side of its mouth; (3) eats dry food more slowly or eats only canned or softened food; (4) has hyperptyalism; (5) is irritable when petted on the head or touched near or on certain teeth; and (6) has aimless incessant circling behavior.

RADIOGRAPHY

Affected teeth may show signs of endodontic pathology radiographically, such as radiographic evidence of periapical lysis, internal tooth resorption, or root end resorption. These teeth should receive endodontic treatment, as should a tooth that radiographically has a larger pulp canal than the contralateral tooth, indicating pulp death has occurred when the animal was younger.

DISCOLORED OPAQUE TEETH

Non-fractured teeth that are discolored and opaque may be pink, purple, tan, or gray. They are dead or dying teeth and should receive endodontic therapy. If a tooth has been traumatized within the last 24 hours but not broken and has a light pink hue, it has pulpitis. Acute pulpitis occasionally may respond to a 3-week decreasing dose of corticosteroids administered orally at an anti-inflammatory dose. If no response is seen, endodontic treatment should be performed.

AGE OF PATIENT

If the patient is younger than 2 years old and the tooth is translucent and lacking radiographic signs of pathology, anti-inflammatory medication should be prescribed and the tooth should then be re-checked and radiographed at 3- to 6-month intervals until either the tooth is dead or radiographic signs of endodontic disease are seen. If the pulp dies or abscesses, either extraction or apexification and periodic radiographs should be performed, followed by standard root canal therapy. The young, developing tooth has a wide-open apex, which gradually closes as the tooth matures. In most dogs and cats, the apex is closed by 12 months but has been reported open as long as 3 years.[17] As the tooth matures, the pulp canal gradually becomes narrow and the deposition of secondary dentin thickens the dentinal wall, strengthening the tooth. Any time a tooth is operated on, it may die. If it dies before development is complete, the patient may have a thin-walled tooth that is more prone to fracture. It is best in young dogs and cats to treat a tooth conservatively in the hopes that even if it is slowly dying it will continue to develop as long as possible. If the tooth subsequently dies, as determined by appearance, transillumination, and radiographs, root canal therapy (pulpectomy, which by definition kills the tooth) should be performed to prevent abscess.

If the animal is 2 years old or older, almost all of its dental development has occurred. If the tooth is assessed to be dying or dead, standard root canal therapy is indicated. An algorithm of treatment planning for fractured teeth is presented in Figure 134–1. A fractured tooth that has pulp exposed is considered to be infected and should receive endodontic treatment to prevent dental death or the development of an abscess that invades surrounding bone. A black spot at the center of wear or at the depth of a fracture defect in a broken or worn tooth is evidence of prior pulp exposure and infection whether or not a clinician can insert an explorer into that exposure.

ENDODONTIC TREATMENT PLANNING FOR THE FRACTURED TOOTH

Black has developed a dental caries classification system[5] that classifies defects according to location (Table 134–1).[18] Black's system has also been used when referring to defects in the tooth surface for fractures and abrasions.[19] The Basrani classification system for dental fractures[20] takes into account the extent of tooth damage (Table 134–2) and is used in this chapter. The two systems complement each other in aiding the clinician in treatment planning.[19] Other factors that determine the best therapy for a broken tooth are the age of the animal as relates to the development of its teeth, the vitality of the tooth, and the length of time since pulp insult (Table 134–3).

CROWN FRACTURE—CHIP

If the tooth has an enamel chip injury only (Class A1; see Table 134–2) and the tooth is vital as determined by physical examination, radiograph, and transillumination, the best ap-

TABLE 134–1. BLACK'S CLASSIFICATION OF CAVITIES

Class I: Pits and fissures located in the occlusal surface of the premolars and molars
Class II: Cavities in the proximal surfaces of the premolars and molars
Class III: Cavities in the proximal surfaces of the incisors and canines that do not involve the removal and restoration of the incisal angle
Class IV: Cavities in the proximal surfaces of the incisors and canines that require the removal and restoration of the incisal angle
Class V: Cavities that are not pit defects in the gingival third of the labial, buccal, or lingual surfaces of the teeth
Class VI: Defects on the incisal edges of the anterior teeth or the cusp tips of the canines or posterior teeth

Adapted from Black GV: Technical procedures: Restorations in the teeth. *In:* Black's Operative Dentistry, vol 2. Chicago, Medico-Dental Publishing, 1955, pp 11–15.

TABLE 134–2. BASRANI'S CLASSIFICATION OF FRACTURES

Class A1: Crown; enamel chips only
Class A2a: Crown; enamel perforation and into the dentin, but with no pulp exposure
Class A2b: Crown; enamel and dentin perforation, and pulp exposed
Class B: Root fractures
Class C: Crown and root both included in the fracture line

Adapted from Basrani E: Fractured Teeth. Philadelphia, Lea & Febiger, 1985.

proach is to either perform odontoplasty to smooth the defect, and reduce the chance of future enamel stripping, or to restore the defect with enamel bonding. A dental radiograph is used for re-evaluation of the treatment at the next appointment. If the client elects no treatment, the clinician should recommend that a radiograph be taken at the next dental appointment to review the status of the tooth.

CROWN FRACTURE—ENAMEL AND DENTIN WITHOUT PULP EXPOSURE

If the tooth crown has deeper trauma, involving the enamel and dentin without pulp exposure, and if there is more than 0.5 mm of dentin remaining between the defect and the pulp, vitality may be protected by an indirect pulp cap procedure followed by surface restoration. If there is less than 0.5 mm of dentin between the defect and the pulp, a pink hue will be seen at the site of the near exposure. A direct pulp cap and surface restoration may be performed to insulate and protect the pulp from further traumatic, thermal, or chemical insult. In both treatments, the health of the tooth should be evaluated visually and radiographically in 6 months. If the client declines treatment, the clinician should recommend that a radiograph be taken at the time of the animal's next routine teeth cleaning.

Direct Pulp Capping

Direct pulp capping is a similar procedure to vital pulpotomy (described later) but is performed after purposeful or accidental iatrogenic pulpal exposure.[9–11, 21] The pulp may be intentionally exposed in a disarming procedure in which the length of all four canines is coronally reduced to the level of the adjacent incisors. This procedure may also be performed on one or two maloccluded mandibular canines after coronal reduction to relieve traumatic penetration of the upper gingiva or palate. This procedure is performed aseptically. The pulp does not need disinfecting because the teeth are invaded in a sterile manner.[21–25]

TABLE 134–3. CLASSIFICATION OF ENDODONTIC LESIONS AS THEY RELATE TO CONCOMITANT PERIODONTIC DISEASE

Class 0:   Primarily an endodontic lesion
Class I: Endoperio lesion: primarily endodontic with secondary periodontic involvement
Class II: Perioendo lesion: primarily periodontal with secondary endodontic involvement
Class III: True combined endodontic and periodontic lesion

GI

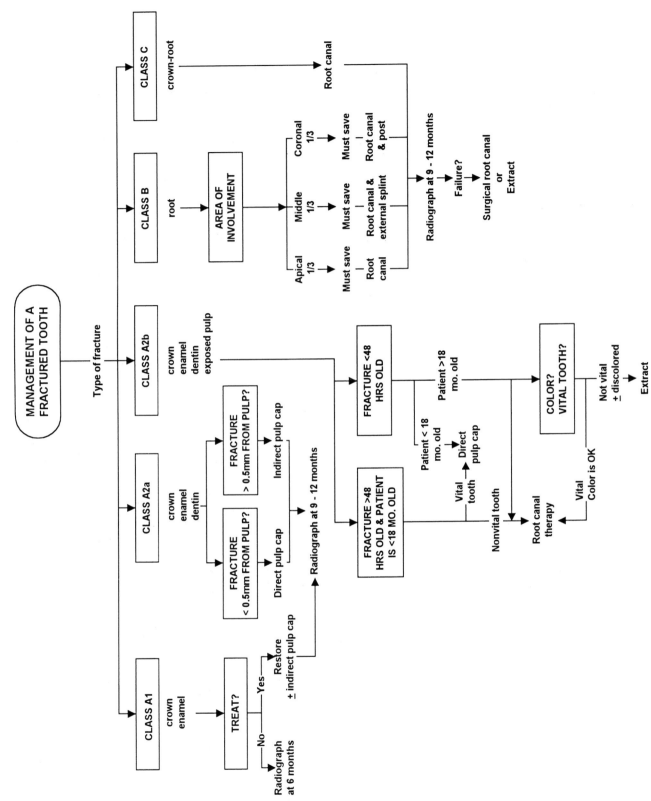

Figure 134–1. Protocol for management of a fractured tooth.

Indirect Pulp Capping

Indirect pulp capping is a restorative procedure performed when the preparation of a carious lesion does not penetrate the pulp but is periously close (0.5 mm) to it.[9-11, 21] A therapeutic and insulating base layer of 2.0 to 4.0 mm of calcium hydroxide powder covered by a thin layer of quick-setting calcium hydroxide paste is installed to protect the pulp, and the tooth defect is filled with a surface restorative. The procedure has been described in detail.[22, 23]

CROWN FRACTURE—WITH PULP EXPOSURE

If the tooth crown is fractured, pulp exposure is evidenced by a bleeding or black area at the depth of the lesion. Therapeutic decisions are based on whether the injury is more than 48 hours old; if the animal is more than 18 months old; if most of the crown is still intact; and the importance of the tooth relative to the risk of failure. If there is a chance that the tooth will be vital, it is best to try to preserve its vitality.

Recent Injury—Immature Patient

If the injury is less than 48 hours old and the animal is younger than 18 months old, the tooth is still considered a developing tooth and as such the apical constriction and the dentinal wall are both still maturing. If the tooth is not yet mature, it is best to perform a vital pulpotomy. If the pulp proceeds to die, it will often do so slowly enough that the tooth will have succeeded in becoming further developed. In the event that root canal therapy is later necessary, the tooth will have developed a thicker, stronger dentinal wall and the apex will have closed, thus improving the chances for successful root canal therapy and the salvage of a stronger, more functional tooth.

Vital Pulpotomy

Vital pulpotomy is the treatment of choice for recent fractures to preserve the dental pulp in a healthy state. Removing the exposed, contaminated pulp and gently disinfecting the remaining pulp and access site constitutes vital pulpotomy. Physiologic saline is recommended for irrigation in vital pulpotomy therapy. Calcium hydroxide is applied to the pulp to stimulate the formation of a protective dentinal bridge. If the defect is on an occlusal surface, a strong base interface is recommended to support the surface restoration of metal or composite material. The procedure has been described in detail.[18, 19, 21, 25, 26]

Recent Injury in a Mature Patient

A determination of risk should be made. A vital pulpotomy is indicated if the injury is less than 48 hours old; the animal is older than 18 months old; it is one of the principal teeth, such as a canine or carnassial tooth; the crown is mostly intact; and it is a field or service dog for which the oral grasp is important. The client's wishes are important because they may be governed by vanity or economics. A pulpotomy performed on a tooth injured for more than 48 hours has a greater risk of failure than does root canal therapy. The incidence of complications is greatly reduced if a vital pulpotomy is performed within 48 hours of the fracture of a mature tooth. The time period may be extended to 2 or 3 weeks after the fracture of an incompletely developed adult tooth.[21, 22] In the case of service dogs, field dogs, competition obedience, or agility dogs, it may be worth the risk of a long-term failure of a vital pulpotomy, in the hope that the tooth will remain vital. In such cases, if necessary, remedial root canal therapy can be performed at a later time.

Older Injury in an Immature Patient

If the injury is more than 48 hours old, if the patient is younger than 18 months old, and if the tooth appears vital, a vital pulpotomy is the treatment of choice. Signs of vitality include fresh pulpal bleeding and a normally colored crown that is translucent and shows no radiographic signs of pulpal or periapical disease. If the tooth appears nonvital and the dentinal wall is determined radiographically to be thin, the tooth should be extracted, unless it is important to the client to attempt to salvage the tooth. In the case of a partially developed tooth that is functionally or aesthetically important, apexification therapy may justify the attendant multiple procedures and expense. The treatment encourages further apexigenesis and apexification and should be monitored by radiographs every 3 to 6 months. Further treatment may be necessary if periapical pathology is noted. It may take from 6 to 24 months for apexification to be complete; and at the completion of apexification therapy, standard root canal therapy is performed on the tooth to prevent an eventual abscess. If the apexification therapy is unsuccessful in stimulating further apexigenesis or apexification, the tooth should be extracted.

Apexification

Apexification is performed on an immature adult tooth that has a nonvital pulp and an open apex. It stimulates apical closure so that standard root canal therapy can be successfully performed. This procedure may need to be repeated to be successful. Apexification involves removing the pulp from the entire pulp canal. Once the canal is cleaned, it is irrigated, dried, and filled with calcium hydroxide paste. The paste is either purchased commercially or made by combining 9 parts calcium hydroxide powder and 1 part barium sulfate powder and adding physiologic saline solution to make a paste of creamy consistency. The pH of the paste is basic, and its presence at the apex stimulates apical closure, which is verified by follow-up radiographs every 3 months after the procedure is performed. When the closure is complete, the contents of the pulp canal are removed, standard root canal therapy is performed, and the surface defect is restored.[21, 22, 25-28]

Standard Root Canal Therapy

Standard root canal therapy is also known as either a pulpectomy or normograde root canal therapy. The essence of a standard root canal procedure is to achieve access to the pulp through the crown, remove all the pulp in the tooth, and débride and shape the root canal to remove any overhangs. The root canal is disinfected, dried, and obturated (filled) with a disinfectant root canal sealer such as zinc oxide and eugenol cement. It is filled with an inert material (e.g., gutta-percha points) to seal the apex and the walls of the canal. An intermediate restorative material (e.g., zinc phosphate cement) is placed as a hard base to support a surface restorative. Finally, the access sites are restored with a quick-setting, hard restorative material.[14, 22, 24]

GI

ROOT FRACTURE

If the crown of the tooth is intact but a root fracture exists (Class B tooth fracture) (see Table 134–2), usually the treatment of choice will be extraction. If the fracture is a nondisplaced fracture in the coronal one third of the root, and is in the "must save" category, standard root canal therapy is indicated and an endodontic post should be inserted spanning the fracture site. If the root fracture involves the middle one third of the root, the tooth is nonvital, and salvage therapy is requested, then standard root canal therapy should be performed and the tooth stabilized with external splinting. If the fracture involves the apical one third of the root and salvage therapy is requested, standard root canal therapy should be performed. Follow-up radiographs should be taken no longer than 1 year after any endodontically treated root fracture; and if the procedure has failed, surgical root canal therapy or extraction should be performed. A guarded prognosis should be given for any standard root canal procedure of a Class B tooth fracture.

Apicoectomy

Apicoectomy (retrograde or surgical root canal therapy) is indicated after the failure of standard root canal therapy. Apicoectomy is also the therapeutic remedy indicated when anatomic or mechanical problems encountered during standard root canal treatment prevent the completion of an adequate seal of the apical one third of the root canal. Apicoectomy is performed on adult teeth in dogs and cats after standard root canal therapy by approaching the apex of the root surgically through the alveolus.[22, 27–33] This procedure is required infrequently in small animals but has a high success rate in treating difficult cases when greater access and visibility are required.[31–34]

FRACTURES INVOLVING BOTH THE CROWN AND ROOT

A Class C fracture involves both the crown and the root, and if it involves one of the anterior teeth, the others all being in place, standard root canal therapy to salvage the retained root may prevent drift of the adjacent teeth. The procedure will provide better abutment support if an endodontic post insertion and crown build-up is performed and a pontic built directly or fabricated by an outside laboratory to fit on top of the post. The pontic should be supported by pins or external devices anchored in or to the adjacent teeth. If the client declines endodontic therapy, the tooth should be extracted to prevent development of an abscess of the root.

RESTORATIVE DENTISTRY

The purpose of restorative dentistry is to restore the form and function of damaged teeth. The best material depends on the desired look and how much trauma the tooth will be subjected to in the future. Surface defects, whether iatrogenic (e.g., from drilling into a tooth) or due to a fracture, should be filled to protect the interior of the tooth from infection and to protect the deterioration of deeper filling materials that have been used in treating the tooth. The cause of fractured and nonvital teeth is usually occlusal trauma, which occurs when the mandibular teeth strike the maxillary teeth, when the animal chews on objects harder than its teeth, or

when an object is caught between the upper and lower teeth. This trauma can occur, for example, when a dog plays Frisbee or chews on bones or hard plastic or when external forces are directed against the teeth. In most cases the pet will subject its teeth to further trauma after the tooth has been treated.

Surface defects can also occur secondary to infection. Caries can penetrate the enamel, undermine the enamel as it penetrates deeper, and eventually penetrate into the pulp, resulting in endodontic disease. Surface defects can also be present as odontoclastic resorptive lesions, as found most commonly in domestic cats and captive cats in zoologic gardens. Surface defects can be seen, as well, in varying depths and severity as congenital, developmental, and hereditary enamel hypoplastic defects.

A restoration will protect the integrity of the dental crown and return it to its former form and function. The restoration must be confluent with the margin of the defect and be as smooth as possible, thereby delaying the formation of plaque and calculus on its surface and preventing moisture leakage at its margins. Unless one is very familiar with dental materials, most predictable results will be obtained by using only one manufacturer's products throughout a procedure, rather than, for example, one manufacturer's primer, another's adhesive, and yet another's restorative resin.

DENTAL RESTORATIVE MATERIALS

Five types of restorative materials are commonly used in veterinary dentistry: (1) amalgam (silver alloys), (2) direct composites (plastics), (3) indirect composites (plastic onlays or fabricated crowns), (4) Class II glass ionomers, and (5) full-coverage metal or porcelain-fused-to-metal crowns.

Amalgam

Of all restoratives, amalgam withstands the greatest compressive force but is the least cosmetic. It is most often used to fill defects on the occlusal surface of molars in dogs and sometimes of canine cusps of service dogs. Amalgam is most consistently successful and easiest to work with when purchased in prepared capsules containing a protective membrane between the amalgam alloy and mercury. These capsules are safer for chairside assistants and the clinician because there is less contact with the mercury by the fingers. Amalgam is held in place mechanically and requires a greater undercut preparation than composites or glass ionomers. Making a greater undercut structurally weakens smaller teeth. Although amalgam is considered self-sealing, the process is corrosive. When the seal is complete, the margin of the restoration is seen as a black corrosive line. The use of amalgam presents a potential health hazard to both dental health care workers and to patients.

High-copper amalgam is commonly used today. Specific techniques in the use of amalgam and available products have been published.[19, 22, 23, 27, 31–41] The keys to success will be the depth of the restoration, the cleanliness of the canal, the compactness of the filling, and the lack of microleakage of the restoration.[7]

All amalgam contracts when mixed and expands slightly after the restoration has completely hardened. This shifting under a static load, known as "static creep" is acceptable. Amalgam also undergoes "dynamic creep," which is a shifting of the material secondary to masticatory forces. A product that experiences less than 3.0 per cent creep is acceptable in dental practice. Additionally, corrosion leads to a delayed excessive expansion caused by remaining microscopic hydrogen.

Composite

Composites are second only to amalgam in hardness, and they are more aesthetic. Composites are most often installed on the rostral teeth and premolars. Direct composites are those installed as a one-visit, single-stage procedure by the clinician. They must be applied in a dry environment. Indirect composite restorations require two stages. The first visit is to prepare the site and make impressions and models for the dental laboratory, and the second stage is to cement the product in place.

Composite is the most commonly used class of restorative material in veterinary dentistry. It is wise to use a third- or fourth-generation composite. As with other dental restoratives, composites are manufactured for use in people. Dogs have a bite three times more powerful than people do and abuse their teeth more than people do. Four generations of composite are currently available and used in veterinary dentistry. Many articles have described restorative techniques with dental composites.[19, 20, 23, 35, 36, 39–41]

The fourth-generation composites are stronger than their predecessors, adhering to the tooth better and resisting abrasive and compressive forces nearly as well as amalgam. These composites, which are light cured, provide chemical bonding with the dentin as well as with the enamel. They also provide macromechanical bonding when the clinician undercuts a defect's margins. Two newer composites are Z-100 (3M, St. Paul, MN), and Herculite XRV (Kerr Corp., Romulus, MI). The newer bonding agents have critical expiration dates, but some bond to all surfaces, including metal. One such bonding agent is All-Bond (Bisco, Itasco, IL). It can be installed beneath full-coverage metal crowns and orthodontic appliances.

Glass Ionomers

Glass ionomers are not as strong as amalgam and plastics but bond very well with dentin. They deliver fluoride to the dentinal wall and do not shrink. One advantage is that glass ionomers do not require an absolutely moisture-free installation site. In cases in which the restoration will be subjected to abrasive forces, ionomers can be used as an adherent base beneath a surface composite that can better withstand these forces. Glass ionomers are best suited to fill defects in nonocclusal surfaces, and they are well suited to fill the access sites in the cusps of the domestic feline canine tooth because of the limited chewing habits of domestic cats. They are most often used for the restoration of feline and canine cervical line lesions, which sustain minimal compressive forces and are particularly useful for small teeth because they require minimal surface preparation. Glass ionomers are also more compatible with the tooth than are composites and amalgam in that they are less susceptible to expansion and contraction. In addition, glass ionomers contain fluoride. Over a period of several months, they deliver the fluoride into the dentin, strengthening it.[24] A number of good products are on the market including Ketac-Fil Aplicap, Chelonfil (ESPE America, Norristown, PA), Vitrebond and Vitremer (3M, St. Paul, MN), Fuji Type II (G. C. International, Dallas, TX), and Restore FL-1 (Veterinary Prescription Co, Harbor City, CA.).

Full-Coverage Fabricated Crowns

Full-coverage metal crowns are used to protect the surface of the endodontically treated tooth from further injury and to provide renewed height, shape, and function of severely deformed, fractured teeth. Preparing the tooth to receive the crown can weaken the tooth. Porcelain-fused-to-metal crowns are more cosmetically pleasing than metal crowns. Crowns can also be fabricated of a very tough reinforced composite (In-ceram, Vident, Brea, CA) that can be installed similarly to metal crowns, in a two-stage procedure. With any type of full-coverage crown, careful evaluation of tooth size, stage of tooth development, and oral habits of the animal is imperative to achieve successful results.[19, 23, 35, 42–44] In many patients it is unwise to install full-coverage crowns, whether metal, porcelain-fused-to-metal, or In-ceram.[19, 36, 44, 45]

The value of fabricating full-coverage crowns in dogs is controversial. In many cases, the disadvantages of crowning a dog's tooth outweigh the advantages.[44] Metal crowns covering a carnivore's tooth do strengthen the surface of the tooth and protect any restoration beneath them, but they do not strengthen the whole tooth appreciably. In fact, the reduction of the tooth structure, which is usually needed to prepare for the crown, weakens the remaining tooth, putting it at greater risk when subjected to the severe leverage, shear, compression, and tensile forces of "bite work" during protection training. Particularly poor candidates are young dogs with immature adult teeth. In dogs younger than 18 months old, the dentinal walls are not fully developed; and reducing this dental structure will severely jeopardize the success of the case. If a mature tooth has been extensively damaged, a post-and-core technique is required. After the standard root canal procedure, a straight-walled chamber two-thirds the length of the root canal is drilled in the canal to receive a post. But this may further weaken the tooth because the canal is widened in the process, reducing the thickness of the dentinal wall.[19, 36, 44] One technique involves placing parapulpar pins, as an antirotational device may also create stress-related weakness in the finished product.[19, 36] Fabricating crowns and correctly installing them requires an expertise shared by few veterinarians. Improved strength and success has been achieved in cases in which minimal preparation has been performed, utilizing the enamel layer for cementation.[44]

Full-coverage metal crowns should be reserved for special cases. Unless the animal's owner requests the tooth appear identical to the original, the success rate will be higher if the cusps of broken teeth are not be restored to their original height. The ideal dog to receive a full-coverage crown is not the service dog that will further abuse its teeth but the pet that fractured its tooth in an isolated accident. Full-coverage crowns will protect the surface of the tooth's crown from further trauma, however, and can restore the full height, width, and cosmetic attributes of the original tooth. A number of texts and articles have described the technical aspects of crown preparation and fabrication.[19, 23, 35, 36, 39, 40, 44, 46, 47]

REFERENCES

1. Ross DL: Veterinary dentistry. In Ettinger SJ (ed): Textbook of Veterinary Internal Medicine. Philadelphia, WB Saunders, 1975, pp 1047–1067.
2. Harvey CE, O'Brien JA, Rossman LE, Stoller NH: Oral, dental, pharyngeal, and salivary gland disorders. In Ettinger SH (ed): Textbook of Veterinary Internal Medicine, 2nd ed. Philadelphia, WB Saunders, 1983, pp 1126–1190.
3. Harvey CE: Oral, dental, pharyngeal, and salivary gland disorders. In Ettinger SJ (ed): Textbook of Veterinary Internal Medicine, 3rd ed. Philadelphia, WB Saunders, 1989, pp 1203–1254.

GI

4. West-Hyde L, Floyd M: Dentistry. *In* Ettinger SJ (ed): Textbook of Veterinary Internal Medicine, 4th ed. Philadelphia, WB Saunders, 1995, pp 1097–1123.
5. Eisner ER: Selecting equipment, instruments, and materials for endodontic procedures. Vet Med 87(May):435–449, 1992.
6. Wiggs RB, Lobprise HB: Basic materials and supplies. *In* Veterinary Dentistry: Principles and Practice. Philadelphia, Lippincott-Raven, 1997, pp 29–54.
7. Ross DL: The oral cavity. *In* Kirk RW (ed): Current Veterinary Therapy VI. Philadelphia, WB Saunders, 1977, pp 921–923.
8. Emily P, Penman S: Endodontics. *In* Handbook of Small Animal Dentistry. New York, Pergamon Press, 1990, pp 65–84.
9. Eisner ER: Symposium on endodontics in small animal practice: Expanding your option for treating injured teeth. *In* Symposium on Endodontics in Dogs and Cats. Vet Med 87(5):416–458, 1992.
10. Eisner ER: Endodontics in small animal practice: An alternative to extraction. *In* Symposium on Endodontics in Dogs and Cats. Vet Med 7(5):418–434, 1992.
11. Eisner ER: Endodontics: An alternative to extraction. Vet Forum October 60–61, 1994.
12. Mulligan TW: Endodontics. *In* Kirk RW (ed): Current Veterinary Therapy X. Philadelphia, WB Saunders, 1989, pp 454–459.
13. Ross DL, Meyers JW: Endodontic therapy for canine teeth in the dog. JAVMA 157:1713–1718, 1992.
14. Wiggs RB, Lobprise HB: Basic endodontic therapy. *In* Veterinary Dentistry: Principles and Practice. Philadelphia, Lippincott-Raven, 1997, pp 280–324.
15. Eisner ER: Standard root canal therapy: The preoperative examination and root canal access. Vet Med 88:1:42–52, 1993.
16. Schloss AJ, Manfra Marretta S: Prognostic factors affecting teeth in the line of mandibular fractures. J Vet Dent 7(4):7–9, 1990.
17. Harvey CE, Hodges C, Venner M: Development of canine teeth in dogs: A radiographic study (abstract). J Vet Dent 4:2, 1987.
18. Black GV: Technical procedures; restorations in the teeth. *In* Black's Operative Dentistry, Vol 2. Chicago, Medico-Dental Publishing, 1955, pp 11–15.
19. Holmstrom SE, Frost P, Eisner ER: Restorative dentistry. *In* Veterinary Dental Techniques, 2nd ed. Philadelphia, WB Saunders 1998, pp 319–394.
20. Basrani E: Fractured Teeth. Philadelphia, Lea & Febiger, 1985.
21. Eisner ER: Three endodontic procedures: Pulp capping, pulpotomy and apexification. Vet Med 87(5):450–458, 1992.
22. Holmstrom SE, Frost P, Eisner ER: Endodontics. *In* Veterinary Dental Techniques, 2nd ed. Philadelphia, WB Saunders, 1998, pp 255–318.
23. Harvey CE, Emily PP: Restorative dentistry. *In* Small Animal Dentistry. St. Louis, CV Mosby, 1993, pp 213–265.
24. Eisner ER: Standard root canal therapy: Preparing and filling the root canal. Vet Med 88(3):252–262, 1993.
25. Camp JH: Pediatric endodontic treatment. *In* Cohen S, Burns RC (eds): Pathways to the Pulp, 6th ed. St. Louis, CV Mosby, 1994, pp 633–671.
26. Grossman LI, Oliet S, Del Rio CE: Pulpotomy and apexification. *In* Endodontic Practice, 11th ed. Philadelphia, Lea & Febiger, 1988, pp 102–115.
27. Harvey CE, Emily PP: Endodontics. *In* Small Animal Dentistry. St. Louis, Mosby, 1993, pp 156–212.
28. Wiggs RB, Lobprise HB: Advanced endodontic therapies. *In* Veterinary Dentistry—Principles and Practice. Philadelphia, Lippincott-Raven, 1997, pp 325–350.
29. Grossman LI, Oliet S, Del Rio CE: Endodontic surgery. *In* Endodontic Practice, 11th ed. Philadelphia, Lea & Febiger, 1988, pp 289–312.
30. Carr GB: Surgical endodontics. *In* Cohen S, Burns RC (eds): Pathways to the Pulp, 6th ed. St. Louis, CV Mosby, 1994, pp 531–567.
31. Eisner ER: Surgical root canal therapy: A dental care service well within your grasp. Vet Med 90:646, 1995.
32. Eisner ER: Performing surgical root canal therapy in dogs and cats. Vet Med 90:648–661, 1995.
33. Eisner ER: Standard and surgical root canal therapy performed as a one-stage procedure in a dog. Vet Med 90:680–686, 1995.
34. Eisner ER: 353 sequential canine and feline endodontic cases: A retrospective study in an urban veterinary practice. JAAHA 28(6):533–538, 1992.
35. Wiggs RB, Lobprise HB: Operative and restorative dentistry. *In* Veterinary Dentistry—Principles and Practice. Philadelphia, Lippincott-Raven, 1997, pp 351–394.
36. Eisner ER: Restoring a tooth to form and function after endodontic treatment. Vet Med 90:662–679, 1995.
37. Oakes AB: Amalgam in veterinary dentistry. Compend Contin Ed Vet Small Anim 6:1531–1538, 1994.
38. American Dental Association: Amalgam and mercury. *In* Dentist's Desk Reference, 2nd ed. Materials, Instruments and Equipment. Chicago, ADA, 1983, pp 53–68.
39. Shipp AD, Fahrenkrug P: Dental materials. *In* Practitioners' Guide to Veterinary Dentistry. Beverly Hills, CA, Dr. Shipp's Laboratories, 1992, pp 175–192.
40. Emily P, Tholen M: Veterinary restorative dentistry. *In* Bojrab MJ, Tholen M (eds): Small Animal Medicine and Surgery. Philadelphia, Lea & Febiger, 1990, pp 194–231.
41. Craig RG, O'Brien WJ, Powers JM: Glossary. *In* Dental Materials, Properties and Manipulation, 4th ed. St. Louis, CV Mosby, 1987, pp 314–322.
42. Lindfelder KF, Lemons JE: Dental amalgam. *In* Clinical Restorative Materials and Techniques. Philadelphia, Lea & Febiger, 1988, pp 1–48.
43. Wiggs RB, Lobprise HB: Crowns and prosthodontics. *In* Veterinary Dentistry—Principles and Practice. Philadelphia, Lippincott-Raven, 1997, pp 395–434.
44. Van Foreest A, Roeters J: Evaluation of the clinical performance and effectiveness of adhesively-bonded metal crowns on damaged canine teeth of working dogs over a two- to 52-month period. J Vet Dent 15:13–19; 1998. Amended and augmented version of article originally published in the Veterinary Quarterly 19(23)28, 1997.
45. Mulligan TW: Custom crown restorations and crown lengthening procedures. *In* Proceedings of the 7th Annual Veterinary Dental Forum. Auburn, AL, Auburn University, 1993, pp 93–96.
46. Freeman SP, Duchan BS, Danbury Hospital: Tooth preparation for full-coverage restorations using the enamel milling technique. Compend Contin Ed Dent 12(6):370–376, 1991.
47. Grove TK: Functional and esthetic crowns for dogs and cats. Vet Med Rep 2:409–420, 1990.

CHAPTER 135

DISEASES OF THE ESOPHAGUS

Robert J. Washabau

ANATOMY

The transport of ingested liquids and solids from the oral cavity to the stomach is the major function of the esophagus. Anatomic structures that permit this function are the striated muscle of the upper esophageal sphincter (cricopharyngeus), the striated and smooth muscle of the esophageal body, and the smooth muscle of the lower esophageal sphincter. An important species difference between the dog and cat is in the musculature of the esophageal body. The full length of the canine esophageal body is composed of striated muscle, whereas the distal one third to one half of the feline esophageal body is composed of smooth muscle. The striated muscle of the upper esophageal sphincter and esophageal body is innervated by somatic branches (glossopharyngeal, pharyngeal, and recurrent laryngeal) of the vagus nerve arising from the brain-stem nucleus ambiguus. The smooth muscle of the esophageal body and lower esophageal sphincter is innervated by autonomic branches (esophageal) of the vagus nerve arising from the dorsal motor nucleus of the vagus.[1]

PHYSIOLOGY

The physiology of the canine and feline esophagus has been reviewed in detail.[2–6] During fasting, the elevated pressures of the upper and lower esophageal sphincters prevent movement of food and chyme into the esophageal body from the oral cavity and stomach, respectively. When an animal swallows, the upper esophageal sphincter relaxes to permit the movement of liquids and solids into the proximal esophageal body. Swallowing also initiates a wave of peristaltic contractions (primary peristalsis) in the esophagus that transports food into the distal esophageal body. Primary peristaltic contractions are reinforced by a secondary wave of contraction (secondary peristalsis) physiologically mediated by intraluminal distention. The lower esophageal sphincter relaxes in advance of the propagated pressure wave to permit food to empty into the stomach. Once the bolus of food has passed into the stomach, the lower esophageal sphincter resumes its high resting pressure.

DIAGNOSIS OF ESOPHAGEAL DISEASE

HISTORY

A careful history is useful in differentiating clinical signs of esophageal disease from oropharyngeal disease (see Chapter 131) and in planning diagnostic tests needed in the evaluation of the patient. Signs consistent with esophageal disease include regurgitation, odynophagia (painful swallowing), dysphagia (difficulty in swallowing), multiple swallowing attempts, and excessive salivation.

Regurgitation is the most important clinical sign of esophageal disease and should be differentiated from vomiting, gagging, and dysphagia. Regurgitation differs from vomiting in that it is characterized by the passive retrograde evacuation of undigested food from the esophagus. Vomiting is characterized by coordinated activities of the gastrointestinal, musculoskeletal, and nervous systems culminating in the active evacuation of digested or partially digested food from the gastrointestinal tract.[7] Vomiting usually signifies disease below the lower esophageal sphincter. The severity of clinical signs with esophageal disease is somewhat dependent on the pathogenesis of the disease. Animals with vascular ring anomaly may have severe regurgitation, but the appetite is usually excellent because of secondary malnutrition. Animals with inflammatory esophageal disease (e.g., esophagitis) may have anorexia, dysphagia, odynophagia, and salivation, without much evidence of regurgitation. The latter group clearly presents a diagnostic challenge because of the differing clinical signs. Finally, signs referrable to aspiration pneumonia (e.g., coughing and dyspnea) may be the major presenting complaint in some animals. A good history will usually elicit the other signs of esophageal disease in those patients.

PHYSICAL EXAMINATION

The physical examination findings are often minimal in animals with primary esophageal disease. Severe regurgita-

tion and malnutrition may result in mild to moderate cachexia. Fever and pulmonary crackles or wheezes occur in association with aspiration pneumonia. An occasional foreign body or esophageal dilation may be palpated during the physical examination. The physical examination is important from the standpoint of excluding other gastrointestinal or systemic disease.

DIAGNOSTIC TESTS

An approach to the diagnosis of regurgitation associated with esophageal disease is depicted in Figure 135–1. Initial laboratory testing should include routine hematology, serum biochemistry, urinalysis, and fecal parasitologic examination. This database will be useful in excluding systemic or metabolic disease as a cause of secondary esophageal signs. In the absence of systemic or metabolic disease, hypoproteinemia (associated with malnutrition) and leukocytosis (associated with esophageal inflammation or aspiration pneumonia) are the only laboratory abnormalities that are occasionally encountered.

Survey radiography, contrast radiography, and esophageal endoscopy are the diagnostic methods currently available in private veterinary practice.[6, 8] Survey radiography of the neck and thorax should be performed in all animals suspected of having esophageal disease. Definitive diagnosis or evidence in support of a diagnosis may be obtained with survey radiographs in many cases, including esophageal foreign body, megaesophagus, neoplasia, hiatal hernia, and gastroesophageal intussusception (see Fig. 135–1). Thoracic radiographs will also identify some of the complications of esophageal disease, including aspiration pneumonia, pleural effusion, mediastinitis, and pneumothorax.

Contrast radiography can be performed to identify esophageal lesions or to confirm a tentative diagnosis (see Fig. 135–1). Disorders not readily diagnosed by survey radiography (e.g., radiolucent foreign body, esophagobronchial fistula, esophagitis, diverticula, and stricture) may be more readily diagnosed by contrast radiography. Dynamic contrast studies (e.g., videofluoroscopy) should be used instead of static barium radiographs whenever possible. In addition to structural information, dynamic studies will provide some information about esophageal motility. Contrast studies may be performed using barium paste (80 to 100 per cent weight/volume), barium suspension (30 per cent weight/volume), barium-coated meals, or iodinated contrast agents. Specific contrast agents used depend on the esophageal disease suspected.

Esophageal endoscopy has become a very useful tool in the diagnosis and treatment of esophageal disease. Often performed after survey radiographic assessment, endoscopy is particularly useful in diagnosing esophageal stricture, esophagitis, intraluminal mass, foreign body, and diverticula.[6, 8, 9] In many instances, endoscopy is performed instead of contrast radiography. Endoscopy may also be used therapeutically to remove foreign bodies, to dilate esophageal strictures, or to place gastrostomy feeding tubes.

Ultrasonography has proved useful in the diagnosis of peri-esophageal masses or other mediastinal disease. Esophageal manometry is useful for diagnosing cricopharyngeal achalasia, generalized esophageal motility disorders, and lower esophageal sphincter incompetence,[5, 8, 10, 11] but the technique is currently only performed at major referral centers and university teaching hospitals. Nuclear scintigraphy and esophageal pH monitoring have also been used to diag-

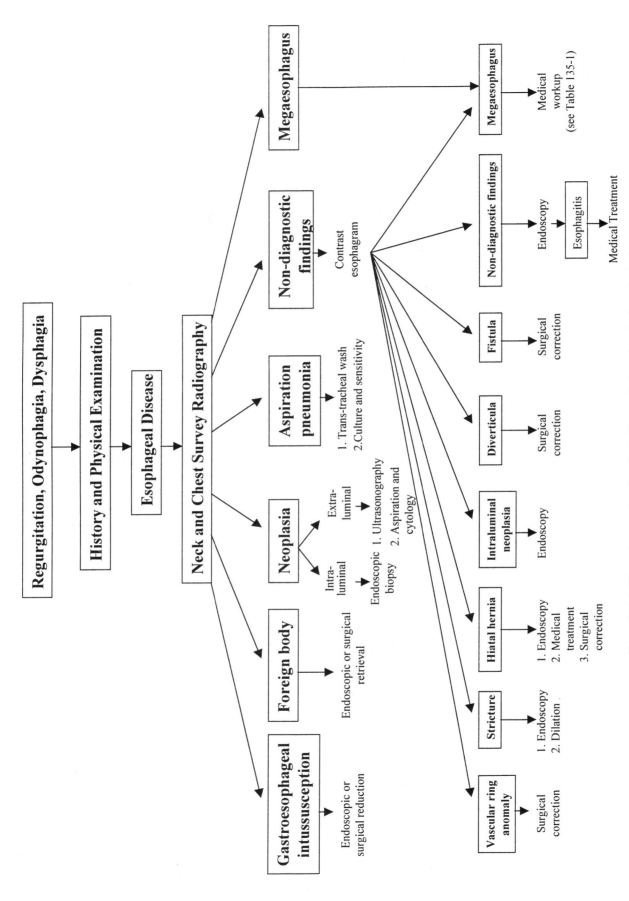

Figure 135–1. Diagnostic approach to the animal with regurgitation, odynophagia, or dysphagia.

nose esophageal motility disorders and gastroesophageal reflux, respectively.[6]

CRICOPHARYNGEAL ACHALASIA

Cricopharyngeal achalasia is a neuromuscular disorder of young dogs characterized by hypertension of the cricopharyngeal sphincter and inadequate relaxation of the sphincter with swallowing. Dysfunction of the inhibitory neuron mediating sphincteric relaxation has been postulated, but the etiology, pathogenesis, and breed predisposition are unknown.

Clinical Signs. Affected animals have progressive dysphagia and regurgitation soon after weaning. They typically make repeated, unproductive swallowing attempts that culminate in regurgitation of undigested food. Coughing and pulmonary crackles may develop as a consequence of food being aspirated into the airways. Physical examination is usually non-remarkable.

Diagnosis. Because of the inability to evaluate the rapid and complex series of events that occur during swallowing, survey and static barium contrast radiographs are not useful in diagnosing the disorder. Diagnosis of cricopharyngeal achalasia requires the use of videofluoroscopy and esophageal manometry. The videofluoroscopic finding of multiple, unproductive attempts at swallowing barium liquid or paste is consistent with a diagnosis of cricopharyngeal achalasia. Definitive diagnosis, however, requires the manometric demonstration of elevated basal pressures and inadequate relaxation with swallowing.[5, 12] If manometry is unavailable and the diagnosis is still questionable, electromyography of the oropharyngeal musculature should be performed to exclude the possibility of an oropharyngeal disorder.

Treatment. It is difficult to generalize based on the small number of cases that have been reported, but the disorder is probably best treated with cricopharyngeal myotomy. Most animals experience immediate relief after surgery,[13] and the prognosis after surgery is generally good to excellent. Effective medical management has not been described for this disorder. The prognosis is guarded to poor without surgery. Untreated animals will suffer from malnutrition and recurrent bouts of aspiration pneumonia.

VASCULAR RING ANOMALIES

Vascular ring anomalies are congenital malformations of the major arteries of the heart that, because of altered anatomic relationships, entrap the esophagus and trachea. Persistent right aortic arch, persistent right or left subclavian arteries, persistent right dorsal aorta, double aortic arch, left aortic arch and right ligamentum arteriosum, and aberrant intercostal arteries have been described in both dogs and cats.[14, 15] Persistent right aortic arch is the most common vascular ring anomaly found in dogs and cats. Circular compression of the esophagus by the right fourth aortic arch results in physical obstruction of the esophagus and/or trachea. The anomaly is considered to be a familial disease with evidence of a hereditary basis in German shepherds.[16] Aberrant subclavian arteries are the second most common vascular ring anomaly. The latter anomalies result in significant esophageal compression from the left subclavian artery and brachycephalic artery.

Clinical Signs. Affected puppies and kittens present at a young age with the major complaints of regurgitation and failure to thrive. Animals usually do well until weaning. Aspiration pneumonia develops in some animals as a result of constant regurgitation, but signs of tracheal compression are uncommon. Physical examination most often reveals a thin, stunted animal that is apparently malnourished but normal in other respects. Occasionally, a dilated esophagus can be observed or palpated in the cervical region.

Diagnosis. Laboratory findings are usually normal. As with other esophageal disorders, regenerative neutrophilia can be associated with aspiration pneumonia and hypoproteinemia can be associated with malnutrition. The diagnosis of a vascular ring anomaly is based on a compatible history and the barium contrast radiographic finding of esophageal body dilation cranial to the base of the heart; a proximal diverticulum occasionally forms with long-standing untreated vascular ring anomalies. The caudal esophagus usually appears normal, but there might be a mild dilation with reduced motility. Angiography is occasionally performed to clarify complex or atypical vascular ring anomalies or to determine the best surgical approach. Endoscopy can be performed to differentiate intraluminal stricture from extraluminal compression. With vascular ring anomaly, pulsations of the major arteries can be observed in the region of esophageal narrowing. Furthermore, vascular ring anomalies occur at the base of the heart, whereas intraluminal strictures can occur in any segment of the esophageal body. The most important differential diagnosis for vascular ring anomaly is intraluminal stricture. Strictures resulting from ingestion of foreign bodies or chemical irritants, or from malignancy, are more common in adult animals.

Treatment. Persistent right ductus arteriosus, aberrant right subclavian artery, and double aortic arch are best approached by right intercostal thoracotomy. Persistent right aortic arch is best managed surgically using a left intercostal approach. Surgical ligation and division of the ligamentum arteriosum is recommended in cases of persistent right aortic arch. At surgery, areas of peri-esophageal fibrosis should be reduced, and the strictured site should be dilated with a balloon dilation catheter or bougienage tube.[6] Other techniques to resect, reduce, or replace the redundant esophagus have not proven beneficial.

Many animals will have persistent esophageal hypomotility and clinical signs after corrective surgery. These animals may benefit from forced elevated feedings. Unfortunately, there are no drugs to improve striated muscle contraction in the canine esophagus. Cisapride may be of some benefit in cats with esophageal motility disorders, but only those confined to the smooth muscle of the distal esophageal body.[17]

The best outcomes are obtained with early diagnosis and early surgical intervention. In undiagnosed cases, progressive esophageal dilation causes irreversible myenteric nerve degeneration and esophageal hypomotility. Surgery in the latter group of animals often fails to improve clinical signs. Clients should be informed that, although surgical correction is the preferred treatment, clinical signs may persist after surgery.

ESOPHAGEAL DIVERTICULA

Esophageal diverticula are circumscribed sacculations in the wall of the esophagus that interfere with the normal esophageal motility patterns. Both congenital and acquired forms have been described.[18] Congenital diverticula have been attributed to abnormalities in embryologic development that permit herniation of the mucosa through a defect in the muscularis. Acquired diverticula are subdivided into either traction or pulsion forms, depending on the pathogenesis. Traction diverticula tend to develop in the cranial and mid-esophageal body and result from peri-esophageal inflammation and fibrosis. Adhesions to adjacent tissue (e.g., lung, bronchus, lymph node) distort the esophageal lumen and create sacculations. Abscess development from grass awn migration is a common cause of traction diverticula in the western United States. Pulsion diverticula develop in association with increases in intraluminal esophageal pressure, with abnormal regional esophageal motility, or when normal peristalsis is obstructed by a stenotic lesion.[6, 8] Pulsion diverticula may develop as a consequence of vascular ring anomalies in the cranial esophagus or from foreign bodies that become lodged in the distal esophagus, in which case they are referred to as epiphrenic diverticula.

Clinical Signs. The clinical features of esophageal diverticula are typical of many other esophageal disorders and include regurgitation, odynophagia, and retching. Signs usually result from impaction of food and/or fluid in the sacculated segment. On rare occasions, weakening of the muscularis results in perforation of the diverticulum, leakage of food and fluid into the mediastinum, and signs of sepsis.

Diagnosis. Survey radiographs may reveal an air-filled or tissue-density mass adjacent to or involving the esophagus. Contrast radiographs are necessary, however, because it may be impossible to differentiate an esophageal diverticulum from a peri-esophageal, mediastinal, or pulmonary mass. An epiphrenic diverticulum could also easily be confused with a hiatal hernia or gastroesophageal intussusception on survey radiographs. Contrast radiographs will demonstrate a focal dilated segment of esophageal lumen that fills partially or completely with contrast media. Videofluoroscopy might also demonstrate an underlying esophageal motility disorder associated with the diverticulum. Endoscopy will confirm the diagnosis, although it may be necessary to suction food and fluid to visualize the diverticulum. The differential diagnoses for cranial and mid-esophageal diverticula should include esophageal or peri-esophageal abscess, necrotic tumor, and pulmonary mass. Hiatal hernia and gastroesophageal intussusception are the major differential diagnoses for epiphrenic diverticula. The normal redundancy of the canine esophagus frequently seen in the brachycephalic breeds should not be confused with the sacculation of an esophageal diverticulum.

Treatment. Small diverticula may be managed by feeding liquid or semiliquid diets to minimize impaction of solid food in the diverticulum. Surgical excision and reconstruction of the esophageal wall are required for larger diverticula. Even small pulsion diverticula should probably be treated surgically because food impaction might cause them to enlarge.

Most cases warrant a guarded prognosis because segmental esophageal hypomotility may persist after surgery. Animals are also at some risk for esophageal stricture after corrective surgery. In cases of traction diverticula, the prognosis will also be somewhat dependent on the pathogenesis and resolution of the peri-esophageal inflammation.

ESOPHAGEAL FOREIGN BODIES

Esophageal foreign bodies are a frequent clinical problem in dogs and, to a lesser extent, cats. The most common esophageal foreign bodies found in dogs are bones or bone fragments, whereas play objects are more commonly found in cats. Many foreign bodies are regurgitated or transported into the distal gastrointestinal tract, but others remain lodged in the esophageal body. Those that are too large to pass through the esophagus cause mechanical obstruction. The severity of esophageal damage is dependent on foreign body size, angularity or sharp points, and the duration of obstruction.[19]

Clinical Signs. In many cases there is a history of foreign body ingestion. Some cases go unnoticed, however, particularly those associated with garbage ingestion. The onset of clinical signs will depend on the severity of esophageal obstruction. Animals with complete esophageal obstruction often have acute signs, whereas animals with incomplete obstruction may have signs of days to weeks' duration. Relevant clinical features include regurgitation, excessive salivation, foul breath odor, odynophagia, anorexia, dysphagia, retching, and respiratory distress.

Diagnosis. Bone foreign bodies can occasionally be palpated if they become lodged in the cervical esophagus, but definitive diagnosis usually requires radiographic studies. Radiodense foreign bodies can be detected with survey radiography, but confirmation of radiolucent foreign bodies requires administration of contrast agents. Iodine contrast agents should be used instead of barium to avoid barium pleuritis if esophageal perforation is suspected. Foreign bodies may subsequently be confirmed (and removed) during endoscopy. A tentative diagnosis of esophageal foreign body may be made in animals that present with esophageal signs after a history of foreign-body ingestion. Without a compatible history, the most important differential diagnoses would include esophageal stricture, neoplasia, hiatal hernia, and gastroesophageal intussusception. Each of these conditions can be differentiated with radiography and/or endoscopy.

Treatment. Esophageal foreign bodies should be removed promptly. Prolonged retention increases the likelihood of esophageal mucosal damage, ulceration, and perforation. Rigid or flexible fiberoptic endoscopic retrieval should be the initial approach to treating an esophageal foreign body. A rigid endoscope is most useful in retrieving large foreign bodies, particularly bones.[19] Large grasping forceps are passed through the rigid endoscope to retrieve the foreign body; and, in many cases, the foreign body can be pulled into the endoscope for safe removal. Large foreign bodies that cannot be safely removed through the mouth can occasionally be pushed into the stomach and removed by gastrotomy. Smaller foreign bodies are best managed with a flexible fiberoptic endoscope and various types of retrieval forceps (e.g., basket, tripod, or snare). Flexible endoscopes are particularly useful in retrieving fishhooks.[20]

Affected animals should be fasted for 24 to 48 hours after foreign body removal. Longer periods of fasting may be required if the esophagus is necrotic or ulcerative. In the latter circumstance, animals may instead be fed through a gastrostomy tube placed at the time of endoscopy. Specific therapy for esophagitis should include oral sucralfate suspensions (0.5–1.0 g PO tid). Suspensions of sucralfate are more therapeutic than intact tablets.[21] Anti-inflammatory doses of glucocorticoids should also be considered in those animals at risk for esophageal stricture. The risk of esophageal stricture is greatest in animals with 180-degree or greater transmucosal ulceration. Finally, broad-spectrum antibiotics should be considered in animals with severe ulceration and/or small perforations.

Surgery is indicated if endoscopy fails or if there is evidence of esophageal perforation. Gastrotomy is preferred to esophagotomy for distal esophageal foreign bodies because of the poorer healing properties of the esophagus and the potential for stricture formation. However, esophagotomy would certainly be indicated in those cases in which the foreign body could not be removed through gastrotomy. Surgery is also indicated to repair esophageal perforation.

The prognosis for most esophageal foreign bodies is generally good, especially if they are removed immediately. A worse prognosis is associated with foreign bodies that are large, have sharp points, or are retained for a prolonged period of time. Immediate complications include complete obstruction or laceration, whereas late complications include perforation, fistulation, and diverticula or stricture formation.

ESOPHAGEAL FISTULA

An esophageal fistula is an abnormal communication between the esophagus and adjacent structures. Most esophageal fistulas involve the lungs or airway structures (e.g., esophagopulmonary, esophagobronchial, or esophagotracheal fistulas). Occasionally, esophageal fistulas expand into the pleural space or cervical tissues. Both congenital and acquired fistulas have been described. Congenital fistulas are rare and result from incomplete separation of the tracheobronchial tree from the digestive tract, from which it is formed embryologically. An increased incidence of congenital esophageal fistulas (and esophageal diverticula) has been reported in the Cairn terrier.[6] Affected animals often have concurrent esophageal foreign bodies, presumably because of abnormalities in esophageal motility associated with the fistula.

Acquired esophageal fistulas typically result from foreign body ingestion, esophageal perforation, and extension of inflammation into adjacent tissues. Bones and grass awns are most commonly incriminated. A traction diverticulum often also develops because of the inflammatory reaction between the esophagus and bronchus. Secondary complications that may occur with esophagobronchial fistula are localized pneumonias, pulmonary abscess, and pleuritis. The severity of the secondary complications usually depends on the duration and size of the fistula.

Clinical Signs. Animals with congenital esophageal fistula usually develop clinical signs shortly after weaning, whereas animals with acquired fistula develop signs much later in life. Clinical features in nearly all cases are related to the respiratory system and include coughing and dyspnea. Other features that may develop include regurgitation, lethargy, anorexia, fever, and weight loss. Regurgitation is usually reported in relation to an esophageal foreign body.

Diagnosis. The radiographic manifestations of esophagobronchial fistula consist of localized alveolar, bronchial, and/or interstitial lung patterns. The right caudal, right intermediate, and left caudal lung lobes are most often involved. The esophagus appears radiographically normal unless a radiopaque esophageal foreign body is observed. Definitive diagnosis of esophageal fistulas requires contrast radiography or endoscopy. An esophagogram should be performed with a thin mixture of barium sulfate (30 per cent weight/volume) to elucidate the fistula. Use of iodinated contrast agents should be avoided because these agents are hyperosmolar and chemically irritating to the lung. Endoscopy may also be useful in documenting an esophageal fistula, although small fistulas are occasionally missed. Lobar pneumonia is the most important differential diagnosis for esophagobronchial fistula. Aspiration, bacterial, and foreign-body pneumonias can all mimic esophagobronchial fistula.

Treatment. Surgical excision and repair provide the most successful outcomes in animals with esophagobronchial fistula. The fistula is surgically excised, and the defect in the esophagus is closed. Resection of the affected lung lobe is also generally warranted. A postoperative course of antibiotics should be prescribed in all cases. The prognosis is guarded if secondary complications, such as pneumonia, pulmonary abscesses, or large quantities of pleural fluid, are present. In the absence of such complications, the prognosis is generally good.

ESOPHAGEAL NEOPLASIA

Esophageal cancer accounts for less than 0.5 per cent of all cancers in the dog and cat.[22] Tumors of the esophagus may be of primary esophageal, peri-esophageal, or metastatic origin. The most common primary esophageal tumors in the dog are osteosarcomas and fibrosarcomas, particularly in areas of *Spirocerca lupi* endemicity. Spirocercal esophageal granulomas may undergo metaplastic or neoplastic transformation to fibrosarcomas and osteogenic sarcomas.[23] Squamous cell carcinoma is the most common primary esophageal tumor in the cat. Less commonly reported primary esophageal tumors of the dog and cat include leiomyo(sarco)ma, scirrhous carcinoma, and adenocarcinoma. Metastatic lesions appear to be the most common esophageal tumors in dogs and cats and include thyroid, pulmonary, and gastric carcinomas. Tumors of the peri-esophageal structures (lymph node, thyroid, thymus, and heart base) cause local esophageal invasion and/or direct mechanical obstruction.

Clinical Signs. The primary features of esophageal neoplasia are regurgitation, dysphagia, odynophagia, and weight loss. Clinical signs develop gradually and reflect progressive esophageal obstruction or abnormal esophageal motility. Animals with metastatic disease have general debilitation and manifestations of other organ system involvement, such as dyspnea or cough. Physical examination may reveal little more than cachexia, although some peri-esophageal and esophageal tumors may be palpable if they involve the cervical esophagus.

Diagnosis. Peri-esophageal tumors are often readily diagnosed by survey radiography or thoracic ultrasonography. Diagnosis of intraluminal or metastatic lesions often requires barium contrast radiography or endoscopy and superficial biopsy.[9] The major differential diagnoses for intraluminal esophageal neoplasia are benign fibrosing stricture and foreign bodies. Radiography and endoscopy will usually differentiate these disorders.

Treatment. Therapy for malignant esophageal tumors is usually not successful because the disease is well advanced in most cases. Chemotherapy, radiation therapy, and surgical resection are the only treatment options available for malignant esophageal neoplasia. These modalities generally have a poor outcome. Surgical resections are further complicated by inadequate surgical exposure, lengthy resections, tension on the anastomosis, and poor healing properties of the thoracic esophagus.[24] Lymphosarcoma may be treated in some cases with chemotherapy or immunotherapy. Benign esophageal neoplasms (e.g., leiomyoma), generally have a favorable prognosis after surgical resection. Except for the rare, benign lesion or lymphosarcoma, the overall prognosis for esophageal tumors is very poor for cure or palliation.

ESOPHAGITIS

Esophagitis is an acute or chronic inflammatory disorder of the esophageal mucosa that occasionally involves the

GI

underlying submucosa and muscularis. It most often results from chemical injury from swallowed substances, esophageal foreign bodies, or gastroesophageal reflux. The esophageal mucosa has several important barrier mechanisms to withstand caustic substances, including stratified squamous epithelium with tight intracellular junctions, mucous gel, and surface bicarbonate ions. Disruption of these barrier mechanisms results in inflammation, erosion, and/or ulceration of the underlying structures. Signs and symptoms are related to the type of chemical injury, the severity of inflammation, and the involvement of structures underlying the esophageal mucosa (e.g., muscularis). Esophagitis may occur at any age; however, young animals with congenital esophageal hiatal hernia may be at increased risk for reflux esophagitis. Anesthesia, poor patient preparation, and poor patient positioning during anesthesia place other animals at risk for gastroesophageal reflux and esophagitis.[25]

Clinical Signs. Signs characteristic of esophagitis include regurgitation, salivation, odynophagia, extension of the head and neck during swallowing, and avoidance of food. Coughing may be observed in some animals with concurrent aspiration pneumonia. The physical examination is often non-remarkable in affected animals, although fever and drooling may occur. Pulmonary wheezes and coughing occur with aspiration pneumonia.

Diagnosis. Leukocytosis and neutrophilia may be found in animals with severe ulcerative esophagitis or aspiration pneumonia. Results of routine hematology, serum biochemistry, and urinalysis are otherwise non-remarkable. The esophagus often appears normal on survey thoracic radiographs. Aspiration pneumonia may be evident in the dependent portions of the lung. Barium contrast radiographic findings include irregular mucosal surface, segmental narrowing, esophageal dilation, and/or diffuse esophageal hypomotility. Stricture formation may also be apparent in severely affected animals. Endoscopy and biopsy are the most reliable means of diagnosing this disorder. In severe cases of esophagitis, the mucosa will appear hyperemic and edematous with areas of ulceration and active bleeding. Milder cases of esophagitis may appear endoscopically normal. Mucosal biopsy will be necessary to confirm the diagnosis in the latter cases. Esophagitis will have several important differential diagnoses, including esophageal foreign body, esophageal stricture, hiatal hernia, megaesophagus, esophageal diverticulum, and vascular ring anomaly. Each of these disorders can be differentiated by survey or contrast radiography or by endoscopy.

Treatment. Animals with mild esophagitis may be managed on an outpatient basis. Oral food intake should be withheld for 2 to 3 days in cases of mild esophagitis. Animals with more severe esophagitis (e.g., complete anorexia, dehydration, aspiration pneumonia) may require hospitalization. Food and water should be withheld in such cases, and animals should be maintained either by gastrostomy tube feedings or total parenteral nutrition.

Oral sucralfate suspensions (0.5–1.0 g PO tid) are the most important and specific therapy for esophagitis.[21, 26] Sucralfate suspensions are more therapeutic than intact sucralfate tablets because the liquid suspension will bind more readily to an erosive or ulcerative site. Gastric acid secretory inhibitors (e.g., cimetidine, 2.5–5.0 mg/lb PO or IV tid–qid; ranitidine, 0.5–1.0 mg/lb PO or IV bid–tid; omeprazole, 0.35 mg/lb PO sid) might be useful in suspected cases of gastroesophageal reflux esophagitis. Broad-spectrum antibiotics should be used in animals with aspiration pneumonia or severe ulcerative esophagitis.

Animals with mild esophagitis generally have a favorable prognosis. Ulcerative esophagitis, on the other hand, warrants a more guarded prognosis. The most important complication of esophagitis is esophageal stricture. Animals affected with esophageal stricture develop progressive regurgitation, weight loss, and malnutrition. Esophagitis and stricture also place animals at risk for aspiration pneumonia.

ESOPHAGEAL STRICTURE

Esophageal stricture is an abnormal narrowing of the esophageal lumen. The most important causes of stricture are chemical injury from swallowed substances, esophageal foreign bodies, esophageal surgery, and intraluminal or extraluminal mass lesions (neoplasia or abscesses). Anesthesia, poor patient preparation, and poor patient positioning during anesthesia place some animals at risk for gastroesophageal reflux, esophagitis, and subsequent stricture formation.[25] Fibrosis and mass compression are the most important mechanisms involved in the pathogenesis of stricture formation.

Clinical Signs. Clinical features are related to severity and extent of the stricture. Progressive regurgitation and dysphagia are the most important. At the outset, the animal's appetite is unaffected. Regurgitation occurs shortly after feeding, and the animal may attempt to re-ingest the regurgitated meal. An important sign is that liquid meals are often better tolerated than solid meals. With progressive esophageal narrowing and inflammation, affected animals develop complete anorexia, weight loss, and malnutrition. Some animals also develop aspiration pneumonia. The physical examination is remarkable for salivation, cachexia, and malnutrition. Pulmonary signs (wheezes and cough) may also be detected in animals affected with aspiration pneumonia.

Diagnosis. As with other esophageal disorders, the diagnosis is based on clinical history and radiographic and endoscopic findings. Intraluminal or extraluminal mass lesions may be evident on survey radiographs in animals with compressive esophageal stricture. Survey radiographs are usually non-remarkable in animals with fibrosing esophageal stricture. Segmental or diffuse narrowing observed with barium contrast radiography is usually diagnostic of the disorder (Fig. 135–2). There may also be some esophageal dilation proximal to the stricture site. Ultrasonography has not proved useful in diagnosing fibrosing stricture, but it may be useful in diagnosing compressive stricture. Some mediastinal and other peri-esophageal lesions have been successfully aspirated with ultrasound guidance. Endoscopy should be performed in all animals to confirm the site and severity of stricture and to exclude the possibility of intraluminal malignancy. Fibrosing esophageal stricture must be differentiated from vascular ring anomaly, esophagitis, intraluminal esophageal masses, and extraluminal peri-esophageal masses. These disorders can usually be differentiated with survey and contrast radiography, endoscopy, and/or thoracic ultrasonography.

Treatment. Oral feedings should be withheld in cases of severe stricture. In such cases, a temporary gastrostomy tube may be placed at the time of esophageal dilation as a means of providing continuous nutritional support. Liquid meals should be used when re-instituting oral feedings. Animals may be discharged from the hospital after adequate rehydration, dilation of the affected esophageal segment, nutritional intervention, and appropriate therapy for aspiration pneumonia. Esophageal strictures are best managed with mechanical dilation. Dilation may be achieved with balloon dilation catheters or bougienage tubes.[27–29] Balloon dilations are prob-

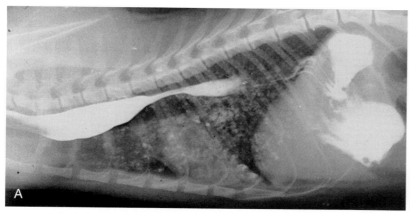
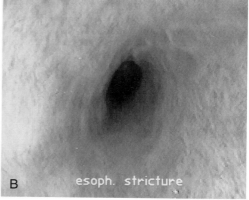

Figure 135–2. Radiographic *(A)* and endoscopic *(B)* appearance of an esophageal stricture in an 8-year-old domestic shorthair cat.

ably safer and more effective in applying radial forces to expand the stricture site. A greater risk of perforation is associated with the use of bougienage tubes due to shearing forces applied by the instrument. Re-dilation at 1- to 2-week intervals may be necessary with either approach until the stricture is resolved.

Medical therapies aimed at treating the inflammatory component of this lesion are best used as adjunctive therapy to mechanical dilation. Animals with concurrent esophagitis should be treated with oral sucralfate suspensions (0.5–1.0 g PO tid) and gastric acid secretory inhibitors (cimetidine, 2.5–5.0 mg/lb PO or IV tid–qid; ranitidine, 0.5–1.0 mg/lb PO or IV bid–tid; or omeprazole, 0.35 mg/lb PO sid). Anti-inflammatory doses of corticosteroids (e.g., prednisone 0.25–0.5 mg/lb PO or IM bid) have also been advocated to prevent fibrosis and re-stricture during the healing phase after esophageal dilation.

Surgical resection of esophageal strictures has been reported, but surgical failures and stricture recurrences are common. Therefore, surgical resection cannot be recommended at the present time. Surgical correction by jejunal interposition[30] or by creation of a traction diverticulum[31] has been attempted, but only in a small number of cases.

Strictures associated with foreign body ingestion or esophagitis have a guarded-to-fair prognosis. Multiple dilations are often required to achieve an adequate esophageal lumen. Esophageal perforation is a potentially life-threatening complication of esophageal stricture dilation. Perforations usually occur at the time of esophageal dilation, although they have been observed several days to weeks afterward. Malignant strictures have a poor prognosis. Surgical resection is often the only possible recourse.

IDIOPATHIC MEGAESOPHAGUS

Idiopathic megaesophagus is the most common cause of regurgitation in the dog. Aside from dysautonomia, megaesophagus is a rare finding in the domestic cat. The disorder is characterized by moderate to severe esophageal dilation and ineffective esophageal peristalsis. Several forms of the syndrome have been described: congenital idiopathic, acquired idiopathic, and acquired secondary megaesophagus.

Congenital idiopathic megaesophagus is a generalized dilation and hypomotility of the esophagus causing regurgitation and failure to thrive in puppies shortly after weaning. An increased breed incidence has been reported in the Irish setter, Great Dane, German shepherd, Labrador retriever, Chinese Shar Pei, and Newfoundland breeds, but heritability has been demonstrated only in the miniature schnauzer and fox terrier breeds. The pathogenesis of the congenital form is incompletely understood, although studies point to a defect in the vagal afferent innervation to the esophagus.[11, 32, 33] Congenital idiopathic megaesophagus has also been reported in several cats,[34, 35] although megaesophagus may have been secondary to pyloric dysfunction in one group of cats.[35]

Acquired secondary megaesophagus may develop in association with a number of other conditions (Table 135–1). Myasthenia gravis accounts for at least 25 per cent of the secondary cases.[36, 37] In some cases of myasthenia gravis, regurgitation and weight loss may be the only presenting signs of the disease, whereas in most other cases of acquired secondary megaesophagus regurgitation is but one of many clinical signs.

Most cases of adult-onset megaesophagus have no known etiology and are referred to as acquired idiopathic megaesophagus. The syndrome occurs spontaneously in adult dogs between 7 and 15 years of age without sex or breed predilection. The disorder has been compared (erroneously) with esophageal achalasia in humans. Achalasia is a failure of relaxation of the lower esophageal sphincter and ineffective peristalsis of the esophageal body. A similar disorder has never been rigorously documented in the dog. Several important differences between idiopathic megaesophagus in the dog and achalasia in humans have been observed.[38] More recent studies have instead suggested a defect in the afferent neural response to esophageal distention.[39, 40] The responses of the upper and lower esophageal sphincters to swallowing appear to be intact, but esophageal distention does not initiate peristaltic contractions in affected animals. The exact site of this abnormality in the afferent neural response has not yet been determined.

Clinical Signs. Regurgitation is the most frequent sign associated with megaesophagus. The frequency of regurgitation may vary from as little as one episode every few days to many episodes per day. Regurgitation associated with megaesophagus occurs several minutes to several hours after feeding, whereas the regurgitation associated with oropharyngeal or cricopharyngeal disorders usually occurs immediately after feeding. As in many other esophageal disorders, affected animals suffer from malnutrition and aspiration pneumonia. Physical examination often reveals excessive salivation, mild to moderate cachexia, coughing, and pulmonary crackles or wheezes.

GI

TABLE 135–1. MEDICAL INVESTIGATION AND TREATMENT OF MEGAESOPHAGUS

CAUSE	WORK-UP	TREATMENT
Congenital Megaesophagus		
Myasthenia gravis	Edrophonium response ± electrophysiology	Pyridostigmine (0.5–1.5 mg/lb PO bid)
Neuropathy	Esophageal manometry ± electrophysiology	Elevated, small frequent feedings
Hiatal hernia	Survey and contrast chest radiography	Diaphragmatic crural apposition, esophagopexy and gastropexy
Glycogen or lipid storage disease	Muscle or liver biopsy, white blood cell or fibroblast enzyme assays, urine metabolic screening	Enzyme replacement therapy?; supportive care
Acquired Idiopathic Megaesophagus		
Neuropathy	Esophageal manometry ± electrophysiology	Elevated, small frequent feedings
Acquired Secondary Megaesophagus		
Myasthenia gravis	Nicotinic acetylcholine receptor antibody, edrophonium response, ± electrophysiology	Pyridostigmine (0.5–1.5 mg/lb PO bid) ± prednisone (0.5–1.0 mg/lb PO or SQ bid)
Polymyositis/polymyopathy	Serum creatine phosphokinase, muscle biopsy ± electrophysiology	Prednisone (0.5–1.0 mg/lb PO or SQ bid)
Systemic lupus erythematosus	Anti-nuclear antibody	Prednisone (0.5–1.0 mg/lb PO or SQ bid)
Hypoadrenocorticism	Adrenocorticotropic hormone stimulation	Prednisone (0.05 mg/lb PO bid), fludrocortisone (0.005 mg/lb PO bid)
Hiatal hernia	Contrast radiography and esophageal endoscopy	Sucralfate (0.5–1.0 g PO tid), cimetidine (2.5–5.0 mg/lb PO tid), omeprazole (0.35 mg/lb PO sid); corrective surgery
Gastric dilation/volvulus	Survey ± contrast radiography	Reduce volvulus, gastropexy
Lead toxicity	Hematology, blood lead concentrations	Chelation with calcium EDTA
Organophosphate toxicity	Whole blood cholinesterase activity	Atropine (0.1 mg/lb SQ once), pralidoxime chloride (5–7.5 mg/lb IM or SQ bid–tid) for acute exposure; supportive care
Esophagitis	Esophageal endoscopy	Sucralfate (0.5–1.0 g PO tid), cimetidine (2.5–5 mg/lb PO tid), omeprazole (0.35 mg/lb PO sid)
Hypothyroidism?	Thyroid function tests	Levothyroxine (10 μg/lb PO bid)
Dermatomyositis	Skin and muscle biopsy	Prednisone (0.5–1.0 mg/lb PO bid)
Distemper	Cerebrospinal fluid analysis	Supportive care
Thymoma	Chest radiography, thymic aspirate and/or resection	Surgical resection
Dysautonomia (cats)	Clinical diagnosis	Supportive care

Diagnosis. Routine hematology, serum biochemistry, and urinalysis should be performed in all cases to investigate possible secondary causes of megaesophagus (e.g., hypoadrenocorticism, lead poisoning). Thereafter, survey radiographs will diagnose most cases of megaesophagus. A contrast study should always be performed to confirm the diagnosis, evaluate motility, and exclude foreign bodies or obstruction as the cause of the megaesophagus. Endoscopy may be performed and is often useful in identifying concurrent esophagitis. One risk factor analysis suggests that esophagitis increases the risk for the development of megaesophagus.[40] It is not yet clear whether esophagitis is a cause or consequence of megaesophagus.[40]

If acquired secondary megaesophagus is suspected, additional diagnostic tests should be considered, for example, serology for nicotinic acetylcholine receptor antibody, thyroid function testing, adrenocorticotropic hormone stimulation, serology for antinuclear antibody, serum creatine phosphokinase activity, electromyography and nerve conduction velocity, and muscle biopsy. The additional work-up depends on the individual case presentation (see Table 135–1). Although hypothyroidism has been cited repeatedly as a potential cause or complicating factor in the development of canine megaesophagus, it was not identified as a risk factor in a case-control study, suggesting that hypothyroidism should be considered only on a case-by-case basis.[40]

Treatment. Animals with secondary acquired megaesophagus should be appropriately diagnosed and treated (see Table 135–1). For example, dogs affected with myasthenia gravis should be treated with pyridostigmine (0.5–1.5 mg/lb PO bid) and/or corticosteroids (prednisone, 0.5–1.0 mg/lb PO or SQ bid), dogs affected with hypothyroidism should be treated with levothyroxine (10 μg/lb PO bid), and dogs affected with polymyositis should be treated with prednisone (0.5–1.0 mg/lb PO bid). If secondary disease can be excluded, therapy for congenital or acquired idiopathic megaesophagus should be directed at nutritional management and treatment of aspiration pneumonia.

Affected animals should be fed a high-calorie diet, in small frequent feedings, from an elevated or upright position to take advantage of gravity drainage through a non-peristaltic esophagus. Dietary consistency should be formulated to produce the fewest clinical signs. Some animals handle liquid diets quite well, whereas others do better with solids. Animals that cannot maintain adequate nutritional balance with oral intake should be fed by temporary or permanent tube gastrostomy. Gastrostomy tubes can be placed surgically or percutaneously with endoscopic guidance.

Pulmonary infections should be identified by culture and sensitivity and an appropriate antibiotic selected for the offending organism(s). This may be accomplished by transtracheal wash or by bronchoalveolar lavage at the time of endoscopy.

Medical therapies have been advocated for stimulating esophageal peristalsis (e.g., metoclopramide or cisapride) or diminishing lower esophageal sphincter tone (e.g., anticholinergics or calcium channel antagonists) in affected animals. Metoclopramide and cisapride are smooth muscle prokinetic agents that will not likely have much of an effect on the striated muscle of the canine esophageal body.[17, 41, 42]

Esophageal 5-HT$_4$ receptors are present in many animal species, but they are apparently absent in canine esophageal striated muscle.[43] Because of its known prokinetic effects on lower esophageal sphincter tone, cisapride may, in fact, decrease esophageal transit rate in the dog, as suggested by a preliminary study.[44] Thus, cisapride should not be recommended for the treatment of canine idiopathic megaesophagus unless there is a concurrent gastric emptying disorder.[41, 42] Metoclopramide is also without effect on canine striated esophageal musculature.[42, 45] Calcium channel antagonists have potent hypotensive effects on vascular smooth muscle but very little effect on canine lower esophageal sphincter smooth muscle.[46] Anti-cholinergic usage would likely be associated with too many side effects to be clinically useful. Unfortunately, there do not appear to be any clinically useful drugs for improving esophageal peristalsis in canine acquired idiopathic megaesophagus at this time.

Historically, cardiomyotomy (Heller's myotomy) was recommended as a therapeutic measure in the belief that megaesophagus was an achalasic disorder. Because the lower esophageal sphincter is normotensive and relaxes appropriately with swallowing in affected dogs,[39] cardiomyotomy cannot be recommended for the treatment of the disorder. Indeed, many animals treated with myotomy have had poorer outcomes than untreated animals.

Animals with congenital idiopathic megaesophagus have a fair prognosis. With adequate attention to caloric needs and episodes of aspiration pneumonia, many animals will develop improved esophageal motility over several months. The pet owner must be committed to potentially months of physical therapy.

The morbidity and mortality of acquired idiopathic megaesophagus remain unacceptably high. Many animals eventually succumb to the effects of chronic malnutrition and repeated episodes of aspiration pneumonia. A poor prognosis must be given in such cases.

Animals with acquired secondary megaesophagus have a more favorable prognosis if the underlying disease can be promptly identified and successfully managed. Refractory cases result from chronic esophageal distention, myenteric nerve degeneration, and muscle atrophy.

DYSAUTONOMIA

Dysautonomia, formerly known as the Key-Gaskell syndrome, is a generalized autonomic neuropathy that was originally reported in cats in the United Kingdom but that has now been documented in dogs and cats throughout Western Europe and the United States. The clinical signs reflect a generalized autonomic dysfunction, but megaesophagus, esophageal hypomotility, and regurgitation are fairly consistent findings.[47] Pathologically, degenerative lesions are found in autonomic ganglia, intermediate gray columns of the spinal cord, and some sympathetic axons. Despite an intensive search for genetic, toxic, nutritional, and infectious etiologic agents, no definitive etiology has ever been established.

Clinical Signs. The most frequently reported features are depression, anorexia, constipation, and regurgitation or vomiting. Fecal and urinary incontinence have been reported less commonly. Physical examination findings consistent with dysautonomia include dry mucous membranes, pupillary dilation, prolapsed nictitating membranes, reduced or absent pupillary light reflex, bradycardia, and areflexic anus. Paresis and conscious proprioceptive deficits have been reported in a small number of animals.[47]

Diagnosis. A clinical diagnosis is made in most cases based on the historical and physical examination findings. Additional findings consistent with the diagnosis would include (1) esophageal dilation and hypomotility on survey and barium contrast radiographs; (2) delayed gastric emptying on barium contrast radiographs; (3) reduced tear production in Schirmer tear tests; (4) atropine-insensitive bradycardia; and (5) bladder and colonic distention on survey radiographs. There are few differential diagnoses to consider in a cat presenting with the myriad manifestations of the syndrome. Early in the course of the illness, however, other differential diagnoses to consider are colonic or intestinal obstruction, other causes of megaesophagus, and feline lower urinary tract disease.

Treatment. Supportive care (e.g., artificial tears, elevated feedings, expressing the urinary bladder, antibiotics) is still the basis of therapy in this disorder, although some cats are reported to show improvement with parasympathomimetic drugs (e.g., bethanechol or metoclopramide). Gastrostomy tube feedings or total parenteral nutrition may sustain some animals until they regain neurologic function.

In general, dysautonomia carries a guarded to poor prognosis for long-term survival in both the dog and the cat. Twenty to 40 per cent of affected cats are likely to recover, although it may take 2 to 12 months. Complete recovery is uncommon, and many cats are left with residual impairment (e.g., intermittent regurgitation, dilated pupils, and fecal or urinary incontinence).

GASTROESOPHAGEAL REFLUX

GI

Gastroesophageal reflux is a disorder of the lower esophageal sphincter permitting reflux of gastrointestinal fluids or ingesta into the esophagus. Varying degrees of esophagitis result from prolonged contact of gastric acid, pepsin, trypsin, bile salts, and duodenal bicarbonate with the esophageal mucosa. The frequency of reflux and composition of the refluxed material determines the severity of the esophagitis. Gastric acid alone produces a mild esophagitis, whereas combinations of acid and pepsin or trypsin, bicarbonate, and bile salts produce a severe esophagitis.[48] The risk of reflux esophagitis is also greater with multiple episodes than with a single long episode of acid exposure.[49] Gastroesophageal reflux has been poorly documented in dogs and cats, but it is undoubtedly more common than previously thought. Chronic vomiting, disorders of gastric emptying, hiatal hernia, and anesthesia-induced decreases in lower esophageal sphincter pressure are the major causes of gastroesophageal reflux in dogs and cats.

Clinical Signs. The features of gastroesophageal reflux are similar to those of esophagitis. In severe cases, animals may develop regurgitation, salivation, odynophagia, extension of the head and neck during swallowing, and total avoidance of food. In milder cases, however, affected animals may have only an occasional episode of regurgitation in the early morning hours. The latter cases result from transient relaxations of the lower esophageal sphincter during sleep.[10] The physical examination is usually non-remarkable, but fever and excessive salivation may be detected in animals with severe ulcerative esophagitis.

Diagnosis. The diagnosis of gastroesophageal reflux may be little more than clinical suspicion. Survey radiographs do not usually aid in the diagnosis. Videofluoroscopy may demonstrate intermittent gastroesophageal reflux, but this finding may also be observed in normal animals without esophagitis.[50] Endoscopy is the current best means for documenting mucosal inflammation consistent with reflux esophagitis. Definitive diagnosis would require determinations of lower esophageal sphincter pressure and 24-hour intraluminal pH measurment; however, these techniques are available only in major referral centers. Hiatal hernia and esophageal stricture are the most important differential diagnoses for gastroesophageal reflux.

Treatment. Because dietary fat delays gastric emptying and reduces lower esophageal sphincter pressure, animals should be fed fat-restricted diets. Pet owners should also avoid late night feedings because this would tend to reduce lower esophageal sphincter pressure during sleep. In addition to nutritional considerations, rational medical therapy for this disorder includes diffusion barriers (e.g., sucralfate), gastric acid secretory inhibitors (e.g., cimetidine, ranitidine, or omeprazole), and prokinetic agents (e.g., cisapride or metoclopramide). Diffusion barriers are perhaps the most important medical therapy in gastroesophageal reflux. Sucralfate (0.5–1.0 g PO tid), for example, protects against mucosal damage from gastroesophageal reflux and promotes healing of existing esophagitis.[21, 26] Refractory cases of gastroesophageal reflux should also be medicated with acid secretory inhibitors and/or prokinetic agents. The H_2 histamine receptor antagonists cimetidine (2.5–5.0 mg/lb PO or IV tid–qid) and ranitidine (0.5–1.0 mg/lb PO or IV bid–tid) inhibit gastric acid secretion and reduce the amount of acid reflux. Omeprazole (0.35 mg/lb PO sid), an H^+, K^+-ATPase inhibitor, could also be used to inhibit gastric acid secretion. Cisapride (0.05–0.25 mg/lb PO bid–tid) and metoclopramide (0.1–0.2 mg/lb PO tid–qid) are useful in treating gastroesophageal reflux because they promote gastric emptying and increase lower esophageal sphincter pressure. The prognosis for most animals with gastroesophageal reflux is good with medical management.

HIATAL HERNIA

Two types of hiatal hernia have been recognized in the dog and cat: (1) sliding hiatal hernia, in which the abdominal segment of the esophagus and parts of the stomach are displaced craniad through the esophageal hiatus, and (2) paraesophageal hiatal hernia, in which the abdominal segment of the esophagus and lower esophageal sphincter remain in a fixed position but a portion of the stomach herniates into the mediastinum alongside the thoracic esophagus. Sliding hiatal hernia is the most common form and may occur as a congenital or acquired lesion in the dog and cat.

Congenital sliding hiatal hernias have been reported in the Chinese Shar Pei and chow. The hernia results from incomplete fusion of the diaphragm during early embryonic development. Affected animals develop clinical signs shortly after weaning.[51]

Acquired hiatal hernia may occur in any breed of dog or cat. The pathogenesis of acquired hiatal hernia is incompletely understood but may result from increased intra-abdominal pressure with chronic vomiting disorders or from increases in the negative intrathoracic pressure in animals with intermittent airway obstruction (e.g., laryngeal paralysis).

Clinical Signs. Regurgitation, vomiting, and hypersalivation are the most important clinical signs in congenital hiatal hernia. Regurgitation and hypersalivation result from the chemical effects of gastric juice (e.g., H^+ and pepsins) on esophageal mucosa, whereas vomiting may result from the obstructive effects of the hernia.[51] Dyspnea and coughing may also occur with severe obstruction and/or aspiration pneumonia. The physical examination findings are usually non-remarkable but may include dehydration, pulmonary crackles or wheezes, and decreased body weight. Clinical findings are usually similar, but less severe, in animals with acquired hiatal hernia; these animals may have inspiratory stridor associated with laryngeal paralysis.

Diagnosis. The survey radiographic finding of a caudodorsal gas-filled intrathoracic soft tissue opacity is consistent with the diagnosis of hiatal hernia[51] (Fig. 135–3A). Affected animals may also have esophageal dilation and dependent alveolar consolidation consistent with aspiration pneumonia. Barium contrast studies will confirm the diagnosis (see Fig. 135–3B) and further delineate esophageal dilation and hypomotility. Videofluoroscopy should always be performed if a hiatal hernia is suspected but not proved by survey radiographs. Endoscopic findings consistent with the diagnosis include cranial displacement of the lower esophageal sphincter and a large esophageal hiatus. Because young animals

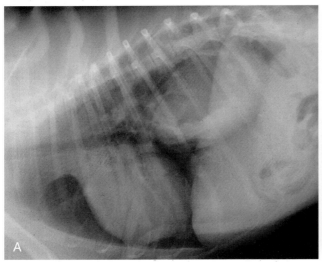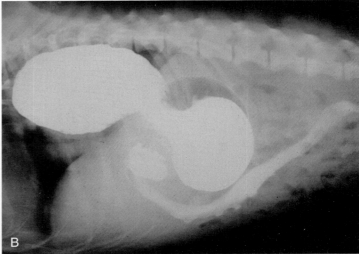

Figure 135–3. Survey (*A*) and contrast (*B*) radiographic appearance of congenital hiatal hernia in a 6-month-old Chinese Shar Pei puppy.

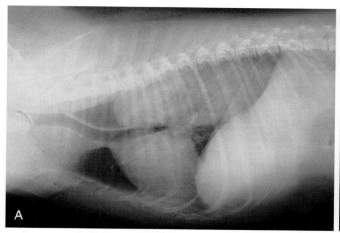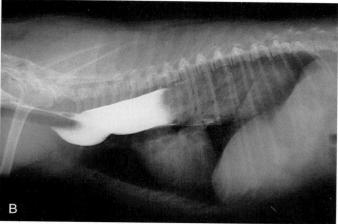

Figure 135–4. Survey *(A)* and contrast *(B)* radiographic appearance of gastroesophageal intussusception in a 12-month-old mixed breed dog.

with congenital hiatal hernia have varying degrees of esophageal dilation, a misdiagnosis of congenital idiopathic megaesophagus could be made if herniation at the hiatus is not readily apparent. Therefore, the finding of esophageal dilation in a young Shar Pei or other breed should raise a high index of suspicion of an underlying hiatal hernia.[51] Gastroesophageal reflux, gastroesophageal intussusception, epiphrenic diverticulum, and diaphragmatic hernia are the other major differential diagnoses for hiatal hernia.

Treatment. A sliding hiatal hernia is not always associated with clinical signs, particularly in the acquired form of the disease. When animals develop clinical signs, medical therapy should be attempted first. Medical therapy is similar to that for gastroesophageal reflux and should be directed at reducing gastric acid secretion (e.g., H_2 receptor antagonism), restoring the health of the esophageal mucosa (e.g., sucralfate), and increasing the tone of the lower esophageal sphincter (e.g., cisapride or metoclopramide). Many acquired sliding hiatal hernias will respond to conservative medical therapy, although laryngeal surgery (e.g., partial laryngectomy or lateralization of the vocal folds) should be considered if laryngeal paralysis has contributed to the pathogenesis of the hernia. Congenital hiatal hernias usually require surgical correction. Diaphragmatic crural apposition, esophagopexy, and gastropexy are usually sufficient to restore normal hiatus anatomy.[52, 53] Fundoplication procedures are generally not necessary.

The prognosis for surgical correction is generally favorable. Animals have few signs and symptoms after restoration of the normal anatomy.

GASTROESOPHAGEAL INTUSSUSCEPTION

Gastroesophageal intussusception is a rare condition of young dogs (most younger than 3 months of age) resulting from invagination of the stomach into the esophagus, with or without other abdominal organs (e.g., spleen, duodenum, pancreas, and omentum).[54] The disorder is more common in males than in females, with a higher incidence reported in the German shepherd. Many affected animals have pre-existing esophageal disease, most importantly idiopathic megaesophagus. The role of idiopathic megaesophagus in the pathogenesis of gastroesophageal intussusception is not clear, but it may be that the greatly enlarged capacity of a dilated esophagus permits and accommodates the invagination of the stomach. Gastroesophageal intussusception is a true gastrointestinal emergency that culminates in the death of the animal if untreated.

Clinical Signs. The initial features are vomiting or regurgitation, dyspnea, hematemesis, and abdominal discomfort. If diagnosis and therapy are delayed, these clinical signs are rapidly followed by marked deterioration in condition, shock, respiratory and cardiac arrest, and death.

Diagnosis. Survey radiographs will reveal proximal esophageal dilation, consolidation or mass effect between the cardiac silhouette and the diaphragm, and gastric rugal folds within the intrathoracic esophagus (Fig. 135–4A). Contrast radiographic studies usually reveal that the column of barium traverses the proximal esophageal body but does not enter the distal esophagus or stomach (see Fig. 135–4B). Endoscopy will confirm an intra-esophageal mass that completely obstructs the lumen of the esophagus. The major differential diagnoses are hiatal hernia, epiphrenic diverticulum, and diaphragmatic hernia. It is sometimes difficult to distinguish these entities from gastroesophageal intussusception. Because the defining characteristic of a gastroesophageal intussusception is the invagination of the stomach into the esophagus, gastric rugal folds are often readily identified within the lumen of the esophagus on survey or contrast radiographs.

Treatment. The recommended therapy is a brief period of stabilization followed by definitive endoscopic or surgical reduction. After reduction of the intussusception, a gastropexy should be performed to prevent recurrence. If disease of the esophageal hiatus is involved in the pathogenesis of the intussusception, then restorative surgery (e.g., diaphragmatic crural apposition) should also be performed. The prognosis is poor unless the disorder is quickly recognized and treated. Mortality rates have been reported in excess of 95 per cent.[54]

REFERENCES

1. Venker-van Haagen AJ, et al: Contributions of the glossopharyngeal nerve and the branch of the pharyngeal branch of the vagus nerve to the swallowing process in dogs. Am J Vet Res 47: 1300, 1986.
2. Mayrand S, et al: In vivo measurement of feline esophageal tone. Am J Physiol 267(Gastrointest Liver Physiol 30):G914, 1994.

GI

3. Blank EL, et al: Cholinergic control of smooth muscle peristalsis in the cat esophagus. Am J Physiol 257(Gastrointest Liver Physiol 20):G517, 1989.
4. Washabau RJ, et al: GABA receptors in the dorsal motor nucleus of the vagus influence feline lower esophageal sphincter and gastric function. Brain Res Bull 38:587, 1995.
5. Lang IM, et al: Videoradiographic, manometric, and electromyographic analysis of canine upper esophageal sphincter. Am J Physiol 260(Gastrointest Liver Physiol 23):G911, 1991.
6. Twedt DC: Diseases of the esophagus. In Ettinger SJ, Feldman EC (eds): Textbook of Veterinary Internal Medicine, 4th ed. Philadelphia, WB Saunders, 1994, pp 1124–1142.
7. Lang IM, et al: Pharyngeal, esophageal, and proximal gastric responses associated with vomiting in dogs. Am J Physiol 265(Gastrointest Liver Physiol 28):G963, 1993.
8. Washabau RJ: Oropharyngeal and oesophageal diseases. In Gorman N (ed): Canine Medicine and Therapeutics, 4th ed. Oxford, Blackwell Science, 1998, pp 437–455.
9. Gualtieri M: Upper gastrointestinal tract videoendoscopy. Compend Contin Ed 7: Videotape Issue #2, 1995.
10. Patrikios J, et al: Relationship of transient lower esophageal sphincter relaxation to postprandial gastroesophageal reflux and belching in dogs. Gastroenterology 90:545, 1986.
11. Tan BJK, Diamant N: Assessment of the neural defect in a dog with idiopathic megaesophagus. Dig Dis Sci 32:76, 1987.
12. Rosin ER: Quantitation of the pharyngoesophageal sphincter in the dog. Am J Vet Res 47:660, 1986.
13. Goring RL, Kagan KG: Cricopharyngeal achalasia in the dog: Radiographic evaluation and surgical management. Compend Contin Ed 4:438, 1982.
14. Patterson DF: Epidemiologic and genetic studies of congenital heart disease in the dog. Circ Res 23:171, 1968.
15. Wheaton LG: Persistent right aortic arch associated with other vascular anomalies in two cats. JAVMA 114:848, 1984.
16. Buchanan J: Causes and prevalence of cardiovascular disease. In Kirk RW, Bonagura JD (eds): Current Veterinary Therapy XI. Philadelphia, WB Saunders, 1992, pp 647–655.
17. Washabau RJ, Hall JA: Clinical pharmacology of cisapride. JAVMA 207:1285, 1995.
18. Pearson H, et al: Oesophageal diverticulum formation in the dog. J Small Anim Pract 19:341, 1978.
19. Houlton JEF, et al: Thoracic oesophageal foreign body in the dog: A review of ninety cases. J Small Anim Pract 26:521, 1985.
20. Michels GM, et al: Endoscopic and surgical retrieval of fish hooks from the stomach and esophagus in dogs and cats: 75 cases. JAVMA 207:1194, 1995.
21. Katz PO, et al: Acid-induced esophagitis in cats is prevented by sucralfate but not synthetic prostaglandin E. Dig Dis Sci 33:217, 1988.
22. Ridgway RL, Suter PF: Clinical and radiographic signs in primary and metastatic esophageal neoplasms of the dog. JAVMA 174:700, 1979.
23. Harrus S, et al: Spirocerca lupi infection in the dog: Aberrant migration. J Am Anim Hosp Assoc 32:125, 1996.
24. Withrow SJ, MacEwen EG: Esophageal cancer. In Withrow SJ, MacEwen DG (eds): Clinical Veterinary Oncology. Philadelphia, JB Lippincott, 1989, pp 190–192.
25. Pearson H, et al: Reflux oesophagitis and stricture formation after anesthesia. J Small Anim Pract 19:507, 1978.
26. Clark S, et al: Comparison of potential cytoprotective action of sucralfate and cimetidine—studies with experimental feline esophagitis. Am J Med 83:56, 1987.
27. Burk RL, et al: Balloon catheter dilation of intramural esophageal strictures in the dog and cat. Semin Vet Med Surg 2:241, 1987.
28. Harai BH, et al: Endoscopically guided balloon dilation of benign esophageal strictures. J Vet Intern Med 9:332, 1995.
29. Melendez LD, et al: Conservative therapy using balloon dilation for intramural, inflammatory esophageal strictures in dogs and cats: A retrospective study of 23 cases. Eur J Comp Gastroenterol 3:31, 1998.
30. Gregory CR, et al: Free jejunal segment for treatment of cervical esophageal stricture in a dog. JAVMA 193:230, 1988.
31. Johnson KA, et al: Correction of cervical esophageal stricture in a dog by creation of a traction diverticulum. JAVMA 201:1045, 1992.
32. Holland CT, et al: Oesophageal compliance in naturally occurring canine mega-oesophagus. Aust Vet J 70:414, 1993.
33. Holland CT, et al: Vagal afferent dysfunction in naturally occurring canine esophageal motility disorder. Dig Dis Sci 39:2090, 1994.
34. Hoenig M, et al: Megaesophagus in two cats. JAVMA 196:763, 1990.
35. Pearson H, et al: Pyloric and oesophageal dysfunction in the cat. J Small Anim Pract 15:487, 1974.
36. Shelton GD, et al: Acquired myasthenia gravis: Selective involvement of esophageal, pharyngeal, and facial muscles. J Vet Intern Med 4:281, 1990.
37. Shelton GD, et al: Risk factors for acquired myasthenia gravis in dogs. JAVMA 211:1428, 1997.
38. Diamant N, et al: Manometric characteristics of idiopathic megaesophagus in the dog: An unsuitable model for achalasia in man. Gastroenterology 65:216, 1973.
39. Washabau RJ, Gaynor A: Pathogenesis of canine megaesophagus: Neuropathy. Proc Am Coll Vet Intern Med Forum 14:583, 1996.
40. Gaynor A, et al: Risk factors for acquired megaesophagus in dogs. JAVMA 211:1406, 1997.
41. Washabau RJ, Hall JA: Gastrointestinal prokinetic therapy: Serotonergic drugs. Compend Contin Ed 19:473, 1997.
42. Washabau RJ, Hall JA: Diagnosis and management of gastrointestinal motility disorders in dogs and cats. Compend Contin Ed 19:721, 1997.
43. Cohen ML, et al: 5-HT$_4$ receptors in rat but not rabbit, guinea pig, or dog esophageal muscle. Gen Pharmacol 38:584, 1994.
44. Mears EA, et al: The effect of metoclopramide and cisapride on esophageal motility in normal beagles (abstract). J Vet Intern Med 10:156, 1996.
45. Hall JA, Washabau RJ: Gastrointestinal prokinetic drugs: Dopaminergic antagonist drugs. Compend Contin Ed 19:214, 1997.
46. Washabau RJ: Effects of calcium channel antagonism and guanylate cyclase activation on canine lower esophageal sphincter (abstract). J Vet Intern Med 7:130, 1993.
47. Sharp NJH: Feline dysautonomia. Semin Vet Med Surg 5:67, 1990.
48. Evander A, et al: Composition of the refluxed material determines the degree of reflux esophagitis in the dog. Gastroenterology 93:280, 1987.
49. Cassidy KT, et al: Continuous versus intermittent acid exposure in the production of esophagitis in a feline model. Dig Dis Sci 37:1206, 1992.
50. Watrous B, Suter PF: Normal swallowing in the dog. Vet Radiol 20:99, 1979.
51. Callan MB, et al: Congenital esophageal hiatal hernia in the Chinese Shar-pei dog. J Vet Intern Med 7:210, 1993.
52. Prymak C, et al: Hiatal hernia repair by restoration and stabilization of normal anatomy. Vet Surg 18:386, 1989.
53. Lorinson D, Bright R: Long-term outcome of medical and surgical treatment of hiatal hernias in dogs and cats: 27 cases (1978–1996). JAVMA 213:381, 1998.
54. Leib MS, Blass CE: Gastroesophageal intussusception in the dog. J Am Anim Hosp Assoc 20:783, 1984.

CHAPTER 136

DISEASES OF THE STOMACH

Jean A. Hall

ANATOMY

GROSS ANATOMY

The stomach is the largest dilatation of the alimentary canal, interposed between the esophagus and the small intestine.[1-4] It is a C-shaped musculoglandular organ in the cranial abdomen, just caudal to the liver. The stomach lies in a transverse position, more to the left of midline than to the right. Its greater curvature faces mainly to the left and its lesser curvature mainly to the right. The greater omentum attaches to the greater curvature except on the left, where its line of attachment runs obliquely across the dorsal wall of the stomach. The lesser curvature does not form an even concavity; rather, it forms an angle called the incisura angularis, an important endoscopic landmark. Lying within this angle is the papillary process of the liver. The caudal edge of the lesser omentum attaches to the lesser curvature.

The stomach consists of five anatomic regions: cardia, fundus, body, antrum, and pylorus (Fig. 136–1). The cardia is the portion of the stomach that connects with the short intra-abdominal esophagus. The fundus of the stomach is the large outpouching located to the left and dorsal to the cardia. The body of the stomach is the large middle portion of the organ. Both the body and the fundus store food and water and can dilate to accommodate food material while maintaining a constant intragastric pressure; this capacity for adaptation is known as receptive relaxation. The distal third of the stomach unites the gastric body to the duodenum. It consists of the antrum and the heavy double sphincter, the pylorus, which forms the narrowest part of the cavity of the stomach, the pyloric canal.

The position of the stomach is fixed at the cardia (where it passes through the diaphragm) and the pylorus (where the gastrohepatic and hepatoduodenal ligaments attach to the liver). Otherwise, the stomach's position changes depending on its fullness. When the stomach is empty it is located completely cranial to the thoracic outlet and nestled within the caudal concavity of the liver, being completely separated from the abdominal wall. The antrum lies to the right of the midline in an empty canine stomach. In cats, the pyloric region lies on the midline, and the lesser curvature forms a more acute angle.[5] The dilated stomach extends beyond the liver chiefly to the left and ventrally. It lies in contact with the ventral abdominal wall and protrudes beyond the costal arches, displacing the intestinal mass caudally.

The capacity of the stomach varies from 0.5 to 8 L, with puppies having a greater range in relative size than adult dogs. Gastric capacity can also be approximated as 100 to 250 mL per kilogram of body weight.

The microscopic anatomy of the stomach is reviewed elsewhere.[2]

BLOOD SUPPLY

Blood is supplied principally via the celiac artery. The celiac artery branches into the left gastric artery (supplying the lesser curvature) and the hepatic and splenic arteries. The hepatic artery branches into the right gastric and gastroduodenal arteries. At the beginning of the pyloric antrum, the larger left gastric artery anastomoses with the right gastric artery. The gastroduodenal artery gives rise to the right gastroepiploic artery. The splenic artery gives rise to the left gastroepiploic artery, which anastomoses on the greater curvature with the right gastroepiploic artery. In addition, two or more long branches of the splenic artery leave its terminal portion and supply part of the fundus of the stomach. The veins from the stomach are satellites of the arteries supplying the organ. The left gastric and left gastroepiploic veins are tributaries of the gastrosplenic vein. The right gastric and right gastroepiploic veins are tributaries of the gastroduodenal vein. Blood from the stomach enters the liver through the portal vein. All lymphatics from the

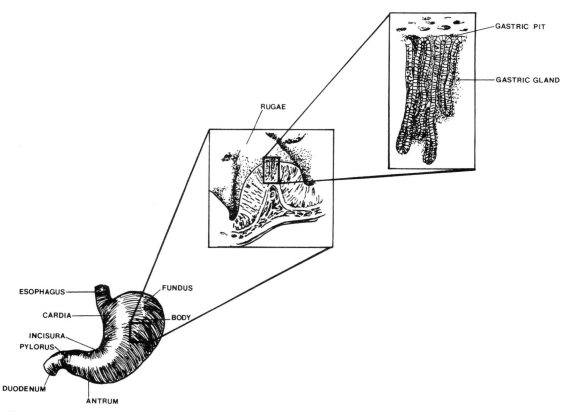

Figure 136–1. Gross and microscopic anatomy of the normal canine and feline stomach. (From Willard MD: Diseases of the stomach. *In* Ettinger SJ, Feldman EC [eds]: Textbook of Veterinary Internal Medicine, 4th ed. Philadelphia, WB Saunders, 1995, p 1144. This figure was adapted from Twedt DC, Magne ML: Diseases of the stomach. *In* Ettinger SJ [ed]: Textbook of Veterinary Internal Medicine, 3rd ed. Philadelphia, WB Saunders, 1989, p 1290.)

stomach eventually drain into the right or left hepatic lymph nodes. The left hepatic lymph node receives drainage from the splenic and gastric nodes; the right hepatic node receives drainage from the stomach via the duodenal node.

NERVE SUPPLY

Innervation of the stomach is principally autonomic. Extrinsic autonomic innervation consists of sympathetic fibers from the celiac plexus and parasympathetic fibers from the dorsal and ventral vagal trunks. Sympathetic and parasympathetic neurons interconnect with the enteric nervous system.

The stomach (and the rest of the alimentary tract) also has its own intrinsic nervous system, called the enteric nervous system. This nervous system is extensive; there are as many neurons in the intrinsic enteric nervous system as there are in the spinal cord. The myenteric plexus innervates the muscular layers, and the submucosal plexus regulates absorption and secretion. Numerous neurotransmitters have been identified in the gastrointestinal tract, including acetylcholine, norepinephrine, dopamine, 5-hydroxytryptamine, histamine, adenosine and adenine nucleotides, nitric oxide, and others.[6, 7]

PHYSIOLOGY

The stomach serves three general functions. First, it serves as a reservoir to store ingesta without the development of excessive intragastric pressure; second, it secretes hydrochloric acid and digestive enzymes to mix with the gastric contents; and third, it empties gastric contents into the duodenum at a controlled rate for final digestion and absorption.

GASTRIC FILLING

The stomach has two distinct motor regions: the proximal stomach and the distal stomach.[4, 8, 9] The two motor regions do not directly correlate with the anatomic divisions. The proximal stomach includes the cardia, fundus, and the adoral third of the gastric body. This region stores food and has a major role in gastric emptying of liquids. The distal stomach includes the aboral two thirds of the gastric body and the pylorus. The distal stomach is involved in the mechanical breakdown of food, known as trituration, and in gastric emptying of solids.

Immediately after food is swallowed, the lower esophageal sphincter and the proximal stomach relax to receive the bolus. This short-lasting relaxation of smooth muscle is called receptive relaxation. When the stomach is distended by the swallowed bolus, a further and prolonged relaxation of the proximal stomach occurs. This process is called adaptive relaxation or accommodation. Receptive relaxation and adaptive relaxation enable the proximal stomach to receive large quantities of food without an appreciable rise in intragastric pressure.[8, 10] Noncholinergic nonadrenergic vagal nerve fibers, whose neurotransmitters are most likely vasoactive intestinal polypeptide (VIP) and nitric oxide (NO), mediate relaxation.[11] The proximal stomach thus serves as the gastric reservoir. In general, a dog's stomach has a capacity of 45 to 115 mL/lb body weight, with puppies usually having a greater capacity than adults.[2]

GASTRIC ACID SECRETION

Hydrochloric acid is secreted from parietal cells by an H^+, K^+-adenosine triphosphatase (ATPase) active transport process.[12]

Parietal cells have the largest mitochondrial content of any mammalian cell; mitochondria are needed to secrete hydrogen ions against a large concentration gradient. Three local stimuli, gastrin, acetylcholine, and histamine, stimulate acid secretion by parietal cells via endocrine, neurocrine, and paracrine mechanisms, respectively (Fig. 136–2).

Gastrin is a peptide released from G cells in the antrum in the presence of food, especially aromatic amino acids.[13] Likewise, distention of the gastric antrum is a potent stimulus for gastrin release.[14] Gastrin controls acid secretion directly and by stimulating the release of histamine.[15] Ultimately, gastrin is metabolized by the kidneys. Release of gastrin from G cells is inhibited by somatostatin released from D cells. Somatostatin release is, in turn, stimulated by acidic pH in the antrum, such that an inhibitory feedback pathway, which is pH dependent, regulates gastrin release.[12] If acid secretion is blocked by antisecretory drugs in the continuing presence of food, serum gastrin concentration increases.

The transmitter acetylcholine is released from the vagus nerve and parasympathetic ganglion cells and controls acid secretion directly and by stimulating the release of histamine. Vagal fibers innervate G cells, enterochromaffin-like cells, and parietal cells. Thus, acetylcholine release has multiple actions, directly on the parietal cell but also on other cells of the acid regulatory pathway.[12]

Histamine plays a central role in the regulation of acid secretion and acts in a paracrine fashion to stimulate acid secretion directly.[15] Histamine is thought to be the most significant stimulant of acid secretion. Using H_2 receptor blockers, gastrin-stimulated acid secretion is completely inhibited, as is most of the action of acetylcholine. This indicates that stimulation of histamine release is part of the effect of gastrin and acetylcholine on acid secretion.[12] Histamine used for stimulation of parietal cells is stored in acidic granules of enterochromaffin-like cells. These paracrine cells are responsible for the release of the secretory pool of histamine. The enterochromaffin-like cells have receptors for gastrin, acetylcholine, and epinephrine. The actions of gas-

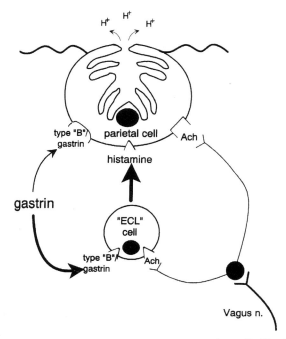

Figure 136–2. Histamine is released from enterochromaffin-like (ECL) cells and plays a central role in the stimulation of gastric acid secretion by gastrin and by acetylcholine (Ach). (From Lloyd KCK, Debas HT: Peripheral regulation of gastric acid secretion. *In* Johnson LR [ed]: Physiology of the Gastrointestinal Tract, 3rd ed. New York, Raven, 1994, p 1199.)

trin and acetylcholine on these cells are mediated by changes in intracellular calcium concentration, whereas the action of epinephrine is mediated by changes in the cyclic adenosine monophosphate (AMP) concentration. In addition, these cells have somatostatin receptors that inhibit gastrin-mediated histamine release.[16] If the gastrin stimulus is sustained for days, enterochromaffin-like cells respond with hypertrophy. They respond with hyperplasia if gastric stimulation is sustained for weeks to months.[17]

Acetylcholine, histamine, and gastrin stimulate acid secretion by activating specific receptors on the basolateral membrane of parietal cells. Acetylcholine and gastrin bind to receptors that are coupled by a guanosine triphosphatase binding protein to phospholipase C. Once activated, phospholipase C catalyzes the conversion of membrane-bound phospholipids to diacylglycerol and inositol trisphosphate. Inositol trisphosphate then causes the release of free cytosolic calcium from intracellular calcium stores. Histamine binds to histamine H_2 receptors, which are bound by a stimulatory guanosine triphosphatase binding protein to adenylate cyclase. Once activated, adenylate cyclase catalyzes the conversion of cytosolic adenosine triphosphate (ATP) to cyclic AMP, which initiates a phosphorylation cascade of cytoplasmic enzymes. Increasing cytoplasmic calcium and cyclic AMP concentrations leads to activation of the proton pump and secretion of hydrogen ions into the gastric lumen.[15]

Conversely, numerous peptides and chemicals are thought to have direct inhibitory effects on the parietal cell or have indirect effects by releasing somatostatin or prostaglandins or by modulating neural tone to the stomach.[15] For example, somatostatin, secretin, and prostaglandins E and I (PGE and PGI) may reduce gastric acid output indirectly by inhibiting gastrin release or directly by inhibiting parietal cell secretion. Interleukins may influence acid secretion indirectly through prostaglandins. Prostaglandins inhibit gastric acid secretion by decreasing production of cyclic AMP. The mechanism of action of nitric oxide is unknown, but it may mediate acid inhibition induced by interleukins. Histamine type 3 receptors, located on enterochromaffin-like cells, are pharmacologically distinct from histamine type 2 receptors and are thought to be involved in the down-regulation of histamine release.[18, 19]

Ultimately, gastric acid secretion is controlled by cephalic, gastric, and intestinal input.[15] The thought, sight, smell, taste, and swallowing of food initiate the cephalic phase of acid secretion via the aforementioned mechanisms. The gastric phase of secretion is the most important because gastric events are the most potent stimulators of acid secretion (e.g., gastric stretch receptors in the antrum). The acid-stimulating effect of circulating amino acids is gastrin independent. Thus, amino acids and amines stimulate gastrin release from canine antral G cells via different mechanisms.[20]

The status of basal acid secretion by the parietal cells in the absence of food varies among species. For example, in the dog, acid secretion does not occur in the absence of food.[12]

BICARBONATE SECRETION

Bicarbonate ion secreted by the stomach maintains a pH gradient from the surface of the gastric epithelium, through the mucus gel layer, to the gastric lumen.[21] The bicarbonate secretion alkalinizes the viscoelastic mucous gel adherent to the intact gastric mucosa and provides a first line of defense against luminal acid. Metabolism-dependent secretion of bicarbonate is a property of gastric surface epithelial cells.[21] Bicarbonate is secreted in response to increasing intragastric acidity. Bicarbonate diffuses into capillaries below the basement membrane of parietal cells. The same capillaries extend into the area under mucosal surface cells, where bicarbonate diffuses down its concentration gradient into the surface

mucosal cells. From here, the bicarbonate is secreted into the mucus layer on the surface of the mucosa. The mucosal capillaries have large pores that facilitate the diffusion of bicarbonate.[4]

Secretion of bicarbonate is thought to be controlled neurally, by prostaglandins, and by some hormones, including cholecystokinin (CCK), glucagon, and neurotensin. Bicarbonate secretion is inhibited by stress-induced sympathetic activation. Salicylates and nonsteroidal anti-inflammatory drugs (NSAIDs) that inhibit prostaglandin synthesis and bicarbonate secretion can lead to injury of the gastric mucosa.[15]

MUCUS SECRETION

The gastric mucosa is covered by a viscoelastic, lubricant layer of mucus.[22] Although mucus is a heterogeneous substance, the chief determinants of the physical and functional properties of mucous secretions are high-molecular-weight glycoproteins called mucins. Mucins are made in and secreted from goblet cells located on the mucosal surface as well as in the invaginated epithelium lining the crypts. The number of secretagogues capable of stimulating gastric mucin secretion is large, including acetylcholine, PGE_2, secretin, and beta-adrenergic agonists.[22] Suggested functional properties of mucus include lubrication of epithelial surfaces; presenting a diffusion barrier to nutrients, drugs, ions, toxins, and macromolecules; binding of bacteria, viruses, and parasites; detoxification by heavy metal binding; protection of mucosa against proteases; interaction with the immune surveillance system; and interaction of membrane mucins with actin microfilaments.[22]

DIGESTIVE ENZYME SECRETION

Pepsinogens are inactive zymogens that must be converted to active proteolytic enzymes (pepsin) under acid conditions by cleavage of an amino-terminal peptide.[23] Once formed, pepsin can catalyze its own formation from pepsinogen. Secretion of pepsinogen is highly regulated and significant amounts of enzyme are released only upon stimulation of the gastric chief cells, as occurs during feeding. Agents acting through cyclic AMP that serve as stimuli for pepsinogen secretion include secretin, vasoactive intestinal peptide, epinephrine, and prostaglandins.[23] Agents acting primarily by elevating intracellular calcium, in turn stimulating pepsinogen secretion, are acetylcholine, CCK, and gastrin.[23] Pepsinogen is released from the gastric chief cells by exocytosis.[23] Pepsin degrades proteins into polypeptides. When chyme enters the duodenum, the proteolytic activity of pepsin ceases because the enzyme is irreversibly inactivated at neutral pH. The proteolytic activity of pepsin is not essential for digestion. However, peptides generated by pepsin serve as signals for the release of gastrin and CCK, which are important regulators of digestion.[4]

GASTRIC MUCOSAL BARRIER

The normal stomach is able to resist the harmful effects of hydrochloric acid, pepsin, and intraluminal abrasive particles through several mechanisms, collectively termed the gastric mucosal barrier. The barrier consists of a layer of mucus, the cell membranes of the gastric epithelial cells, and the subepithelial vasculature.[4] The most important defense mechanisms include (1) gastric mucus secretion, (2) bicarbonate secretion, (3) barrier to back diffusion of hydrogen ions into the mucosa, (4) mucosal microcirculation allowing clearance of back-diffused hydrogen ions, (5) rapid epithelial cell turnover, (6) protective prostaglandins (especially of the E type), and (7) the mucosal immune system.[24]

Under physiologic conditions the secretion of mucus and bicarbonate from surface epithelial cells forms an unstirred layer that neutralizes hydrogen ions as they back-diffuse through the mucus.[25] Mucus also lubricates and protects the mucosa. Intracellular bicarbonate in gastric epithelial cells also protects the epithelial cells against back-diffusing acid.[4]

The mucosal barrier depends on the maintenance of normal mucosal blood flow. Exposure of gastric epithelium to acid results in reactive hyperemia.[26] The hyperemic response reflects a vascular defense mechanism.[25] The increased blood flow supplies plasma bicarbonate and removes injurious products such as back-diffused acid and inflammatory mediators.[4]

Epithelial cell turnover is rapid in the stomach. The surface mucous cells are replaced by migration of cells from the wall of the pits to the surface, a process that is completed in 3 days. Mucous neck cells, parietal cells, and chief cells turn over more slowly. Surface epithelial cells adjacent to or just beneath lost mucosal cells migrate to cover the basement membrane in areas of minor injury. This process is called epithelial restitution; it is dependent on a high concentration of bicarbonate beneath the damaged cells.[4]

The gastric mucosa can synthesize several prostaglidins such as PGE_2, $PGF_{2\alpha}$, and prostacyclin. The proposed mechanisms by which prostaglandins mediate cytoprotective actions include prevention of gastric mucosal barrier disruption, stimulation of mucus secretion, stimulation of nonparietal cell secretion, enhancement of bicarbonate secretion, stimulation of cellular transport processes, stimulation of macromolecular synthesis, stabilization of tissue lysosomes, stimulation of surface-active phospholipids, and enhancement of gastric mucosal blood flow.[25, 27–29]

Prostaglandins also modulate the activity of many immunocytes, including macrophages and mast cells.[24] The mucosa of the intestine is in a state of controlled inflammation, continuously defending against breaches of the epithelium. Even in the absence of overt inflammation, the mucosa contains a substantial number of immunocytes, including neutrophils, eosinophils, mast cells, and macrophages. Prostaglandins and nitric oxide, along with several cytokines (e.g., interleukin-10) appear to play crucial roles in regulating the immune response, which is especially important when the mucosa is inflamed.[24]

GASTRIC MOTILITY AND EMPTYING

The proximal stomach plays a major role in controlling gastric emptying of liquids via tonic contractions that regulate intragastric pressure. The rate of gastric emptying of liquids depends on the pressure gradient between the stomach and duodenum and the resistance to flow provided by the pylorus.[8–10, 30] As long as pyloric resistance to flow and intraduodenal pressure remain constant, gastric emptying of liquid increases in direct proportion to an increase in intragastric pressure. To a lesser extent, peristaltic waves in the distal stomach also affect gastric emptying of liquids because they alter intragastric pressure. Because the volume of liquid determines intragastric pressure, the primary determinant of emptying rate for liquids is volume present in the stomach.[10, 31] There are probably other mechanisms in addition to fundic tone that control the emptying rate of liquids; for example, the ratio of antral contractions to duodenal contractions may play a role.[32]

Contractions in the distal stomach are phasic rather than tonic and are called peristaltic waves. Gastric chyme is propelled toward the duodenum as a peristaltic wave passes over the middle of the antrum. Intraluminal pressure may increase to 100 cm H_2O for a duration of 1 to 4 seconds.[10, 33, 34] Chyme is not forced into the duodenum; instead, liquids with small, suspended particles are gently flushed through the pyloric orifice. Solids are retained in the stomach until they have become almost liquefied (<2 mm in diameter).[10, 33–35]

Gastric motility depends on the highly coordinated electrical activity of gastric smooth muscle cells. These cells demonstrate spontaneous fluctuations in membrane potential, which give rise to slow waves.[10, 36] Slow waves can be recorded from all smooth muscle cells in the distal stomach, but their intrinsic frequencies differ. The highest frequencies are recorded on the greater curvature of the gastric body. This region acts as the dominant gastric pacemaker and is analogous to the sinoatrial node of the heart.[37] Slow waves spread distally through longitudinal muscle fibers, from the gastric pacemaker to the pylorus. In fasted dogs, slow waves occur at a frequency of four to five per minute. The propagation velocity increases as the slow waves approach the pylorus. Two or three slow-wave fronts are present simultaneously on the stomach. Slow waves do not spread to the proximal stomach because smooth muscle cells in this region do not have membrane properties capable of supporting them. Regardless of whether gastric contractions occur, slow waves are always present in the distal stomach. In contrast to cardiac electrical activity, slow waves are not always associated with contractile activity. If contractions are present, their maximum frequency can never exceed the slow-wave frequency because contractions can occur only during a specific phase of the slow-wave cycle. Action potentials are the electrical events associated with contractions. Thus, electrical activity of the stomach consists of omnipresent, autonomous, slow waves upon which action potentials that coincide with contractions are superimposed.[8]

Even if a peristaltic wave is initiated, it may not be propagated over the full length of the distal stomach. The degree of muscle tension, the level of stimulation by excitatory nerves, and the amounts of hormones and paracrine and neurocrine substances present determine whether a contraction follows the slow-wave cycle as it passes over a particular gastric location.[8, 10]

Selective emptying is possible because of coordinated contractions in the terminal antrum and pylorus.[38] Initially, the terminal antral contraction causes the pylorus to close, thus trapping antral contents between the pyloric sphincter and the approaching peristaltic wave. The peristaltic wave causes the antral wall to contract, forming a central orifice. As the pylorus and antrum continue to contract, viscous and solid ingesta are forced back through this central orifice. The jetlike retropulsion of solid chyme results in the mechanical breakdown of solids and thorough mixing of gastric contents with gastric secretions. Once the solids have been broken into particles smaller than 2 mm in diameter, they can pass with liquids into the duodenum.

Gastric emptying of solids is determined primarily by antral motility and resistance to flow across the pylorus.[10] These, in turn, are determined by contractions of the distal stomach and gastroduodenal junction. Feeding initially stimulates antral motility. Ultimately, caloric density determines the gastric emptying rate for solids,[39, 40] because the rate of gastric emptying is controlled by receptors in the small intestine.[41] These receptors are sensitive to the concentration of acid in and osmolarity of gastric chyme and to fatty acids and tryptophan. Carbohydrates and amino acids, except for L-tryptophan, retard gastric emptying by stimulating osmoreceptors. Fats, which slow emptying by acting on fatty acid receptors, have the most potent suppressive effects on antral motility. After stimulation, these receptors delay gastric emptying.

Hormones and neural reflexes are involved in the enterogastric reflexes.[10] Acid in the duodenum stimulates secretin release, which inhibits motility in the stomach. Fats and proteins in the duodenum stimulate CCK release, which inhibits fundic motility and delays gastric emptying in dogs. Gastrin delays gastric emptying by reducing motility in the fundus, although contractions elsewhere are stimulated. In cats, gastrin and CCK release is associated with an increase in the frequency of mixing contractions in the antrum.[42] Marked distention of the stomach results in a series of protective reflexes, for example, gastroesophageal sphincter relaxation, relaxation of the body of the stomach, and contraction of the pylorus. These reflexes prevent dumping of ingesta into the duodenum and protect against gastric rupture.[4]

In the fasting state, a unique motor pattern occurs that is specialized for expelling undigested debris from the stomach. It is called the migrating myoelectric complex (MMC) or the interdigestive myoelectric complex (IDMC).[43, 44] In long-term 24-hour studies, the time from feeding to the appearance of the fasting motility pattern ranged from 6 to 16 hours in normal dogs.[45] The digestive pattern ends with a series of strong peristaltic contractions involving most of the stomach. This series is followed by a phase of motor quiescence, which lasts approximately 60 to 110 minutes. Gastric contractions then reappear, gradually increase in frequency, and culminate in a 10- to 25-minute phase of intense peristaltic contractions. Quiescence returns and the cycle repeats. Phase I is the period of quiescence, phase II is the period of increasing but irregular contractile activity, and phase III is the period of intense regular contractions. During phase III, a contraction occurs with almost every slow-wave cycle (four or five contractions per minute). The MMC passes from the stomach and small intestine to the colon in approximately 2 hours. At about the time a phase III front reaches the terminal ileum, another phase III front starts in the stomach.

Indigestible solids (e.g., plant fiber) that cannot be broken down into particles smaller than 2 mm in diameter remain in the stomach during the fed state. These particles, along with saliva, basal mucous secretions, and cellular debris, are expelled by the MMC. In the fasting state, the pylorus remains open as a contraction approaches (in the fed state, the pylorus closes as a contraction approaches). The MMC completely empties the stomach. Thus, phase III of the MMC is also called the interdigestive "housekeeper." The MMC has yet to be clearly demonstrated in cats, but a similar motility pattern is likely to occur.[4]

CLINICAL EVALUATION

The history, physical examination, clinical pathology findings, and imaging studies used to evaluate the stomach (radiology, ultrasonography, and nuclear scintigraphy) are reviewed elsewhere.[2]

ENDOSCOPY

Endoscopy allows direct inspection of the stomach and provides a noninvasive method for obtaining biopsy specimens, brush cytology, fluid aspirates, and culture samples,[46] especially in vomiting animals[47–49] and when lesions are unclear radiographically.[50] Most animals with inflammatory gastritis and many with gastric neoplasia can be diagnosed endoscopically.[2] One can remove foreign bodies and place percutaneous endoscopic gastrostomy (PEG) tubes.

Disadvantages of endoscopy include the need for potentially expensive equipment, the requirement of general anesthesia, and the inability to obtain full-thickness biopsies. Also, it is imperative that the endoscopist be able to enter, view, and obtain biopsy specimens from the duodenum, as inflammatory lesions in the duodenum, not the stomach, are more commonly the cause of vomiting.[2] Narcotic preanesthetics should not be used as they hinder passage of the scope through the pyloric sphincter and into the proximal duodenum.[2]

Animals should be fasted for at least 18 to 24 hours before induction of anesthesia because animals with gastric disease often have delayed gastric emptying. The mucosal surface should be evaluated for changes in color or consistency. Submucosal hemorrhage or small mucosal ulcerations can be observed with gastritis. Occasionally, ulcers and erosions can be difficult to find.[2] The stomach must be moderately distended so that lesions are not obscured by rugal folds. Ulcers are most often found in the antrum, lesser curvature (just inside the angularis incisura), and pylorus. A thorough examination helps to avoid missing lesions in these areas.

The terms proposed to describe abnormalities of the mucosal surface are erythema (redness), friability (ease of damage or tearing), granularity (surface texture), ulcer (focal, deep crateriform), and erosion (irregular surface irritations). The mucosa may also appear normal. Multiple biopsy specimens (cardia, midway along the greater curvature, angularis incisura, pylorus) should always be obtained from a vomiting animal, even if the mucosa appears normal.[51] There may be significant histopathologic lesions in an otherwise normal-appearing stomach and duodenum. When a lesion is observed, biopsies of the center, margin, and normal surrounding areas of the lesion are obtained. If the lesion is hard and infiltrated, it is necessary to obtain deeper pinch biopsy specimens of the submucosal areas, although this can be frustrating to accomplish.

If a foreign object is to be removed from the stomach by endoscopy, it is important to radiograph the patient immediately before anesthetizing it, as objects in the stomach for several weeks have been known to pass into the duodenum before the procedure, making endoscopic retrieval impossible. The endoscopist also needs to have appropriate grasping forceps and retrieval baskets available to remove a variety of objects.

EXPLORATORY SURGERY

Exploratory surgery is indicated as a diagnostic procedure if endoscopy in unavailable or insufficient, when an extramural lesion is suspected of causing gastric outflow obstruction, or if corrective surgery is necessary.[2] Therapeutically, surgery may be necessary to remove foreign objects, focal masses, or perforated ulcers. The stomach and duodenum should be palpated for infiltrative lesions, and multiple full-thickness biopsy specimens should always be obtained. All abdominal organs should be examined and biopsies obtained if indicated, particularly of the liver and mesenteric lymph nodes. Concerns about surgically obtained biopsies include increased anesthetic time, longer hospitalization, biopsy site and wound healing complications, risk of sepsis, and the effects of low serum proteins on tissue repair.

Fine-needle aspirates may be obtained at the time of surgery of regions of the intestinal wall, tumors, and lymph nodes from which biopsy specimens were not obtained. The diagnosis of infiltrative neoplasia, infection, and inflammation can be made or supported by the cytologic evaluation of specimens obtained by aspiration or impression of cut surfaces of resected tissues. A 12-mL syringe and 22- to 25-gauge needle are used for this technique. Cytology results may influence therapeutic plans before the histopathology results are available.[46]

OTHER METHODS OF EVALUATING THE STOMACH

Cytologic evaluation of gastric fluid is occasionally performed in the cat when searching for *Ollulanus tricuspis*.[52]

Gastric secretory testing can be performed to detect animals with relative hyper- and hypochlorhydria.[2, 53, 54]

ACUTE GASTRITIS

Acute gastritis is probably the most common cause of acute vomiting in dogs and cats.[2] Strictly defined, acute gastritis means inflammation and mucosal damage that has occurred in response to an insult to the gastric mucosa. Most affected animals become anorexic, and their vomitus usually consists of food and often bile. Many of these animals are not seriously ill, although a few may have life-threatening disease. Consequences of vomiting depend on the frequency, the volumes of food and/or fluid lost, and the underlying cause.[2] Rarely does acute gastritis warrant biopsy and histologic confirmation. The diagnosis is usually made when signs of gastric disease are acute in onset and self-limiting.[3]

CAUSES

Acute gastritis has a variety of causes,[55] although in most cases the etiology is never determined. Three general etiologic categories for acute gastritis in dogs and cats are diet-related factors, infectious agents, and toxins. Dietary indiscretion is probably the most common cause. Ingestion of rancid or spoiled foodstuffs results in "garbage can" intoxication. Fermentation products, bacterial enterotoxins, and mycotoxins can cause severe vomiting and diarrhea. Ingestion of foreign materials may irritate the mucosa and/or cause pyloric outflow obstruction. Dietary causes may also include intended foods. For example, some animals do not tolerate increased osmolality or a high fat content, whereas others have allergic or intolerance reactions to specific dietary proteins.[2]

Infectious agents causing acute gastritis include viruses such as canine distemper virus, canine hepatitis virus, parvovirus, coronavirus, and feline panleukopenia virus. In these instances, gastric lesions are part of a more extensive disease condition.[3] *Helicobacter* infection is more likely to produce a chronic gastritis. Parasites generally do not produce gastric lesions or clinical signs. *Physaloptera* spp. is the most common gastric parasite in dogs, although ascarids and tapeworms may occasionally cause gastritis and vomiting. *O. tricuspis* has been associated with gastric lesions in cats.[56, 57]

Many plants, if eaten, can cause acute gastritis, the most common probably being grass.[3] Ingestion of grass is probably a normal instinctive behavior. For reasons unknown, however, animals with gastric disease often ingest and vomit grass. Many common household plants can also cause acute gastritis.[58]

Certain drugs, such as NSAIDs,[59–62] aspirin,[63] and chemicals, can cause gastritis in dogs and cats. Chemical irritants include heavy metals (e.g., lead), cleaning agents, fertilizers, and herbicides. Antibiotics (e.g., cephalosporins and doxycycline) may also produce gastritis.[2]

A wide variety of systemic disorders or dysfunctions of other parts of the gastrointestinal tract can lead to secondary gastritis.[55] These include gastric hyperacidity (e.g., with mastocytoma[64]), reduced gastric mucosal blood flow (e.g., with shock), gastroduodenal reflux (e.g., with reduced antral motility secondary to anticholinergic administration), and compromise of the mucus-bicarbonate mucosal layer (e.g., in renal[65, 66] or hepatic disease[67, 68]).

PATHOPHYSIOLOGY

Acute gastritis results from inability of the gastric mucosal barrier to protect itself. The ability of the mucosa to withstand damage is the result of a complex mucosal defense system, which includes epithelial secretions, rapid epithelial turnover, mucosal microcirculation, and the mucosal immune system.[24] Inflammation leads to recruitment of phagocytes into the mucosa and, in turn, to mucosal injury. Neutrophil infiltration is a hallmark of inflammation. Although migration of neutrophils from the vasculature into the mucosa protects against entry of foreign material into the systemic circulation, neutrophils can also produce considerable damage to host tissue. Neutrophils amplify the inflammatory response by releasing chemotaxins such as leukotriene B_4 and reactive oxygen metabolites. Prostaglandins play an important modulatory role by down-regulating neutrophil functions that contribute to inflammation and injury.[24]

Nitric oxide also has important immunomodulatory activities. When the gastric epithelium is exposed to an irritant, one of the most rapid and important responses is an increase in mucosal blood flow. The purpose of this hyperemic response is to remove, dilute, and buffer any back-diffusing acid or toxins. This response is mediated by sensory afferent neurons just beneath the epithelium, which are activated by the back-diffusing acid. These neurons release the vasodilator calcitonin gene–related peptide, which then dilates submucosal arterioles through a nitric oxide–dependent pathway.[24]

The degree of mucosal injury depends on whether the damaging factors outweigh the protective factors.[2] Inflammation may result in either erosive or nonerosive lesions with neutrophilic infiltrates. The underlying disorder is usually self-limiting.

DIAGNOSIS

The diagnosis of acute gastritis is usually based on history and physical examination.[2] An acute onset of vomiting with a history that reveals one of the aforementioned causes is adequate for a presumptive diagnosis. Physical findings are usually unremarkable. The animal may or may not be dehydrated. Extensive laboratory testing is usually unnecessary; however, if the animal is critically ill or if the presence of other disease is suspected (e.g., renal or hepatic failure, gastric foreign body), then a complete blood count (CBC), serum chemistry panel, and abdominal radiographs are indicated. Most patients with acute gastritis have minimal changes in laboratory parameters, although a stress leukogram, hyperalbuminemia (related to dehydration), and electrolyte or acid-base abnormalities may be noted. Abdominal radiographs are usually unremarkable unless a foreign object or evidence of heavy metal (e.g., lead) ingestion is present. Canine parvoviral enteritis initially mimics acute gastritis in many dogs; anorexia and vomiting may precede fever and diarrhea by 1 to 4 days. Therefore, it is important to test a young dog with apparent gastritis for fecal parvovirus antigen early in the course of disease.[2]

THERAPY

Most animals with acute gastritis respond to symptomatic therapy within 24 to 48 hours after the onset of signs and recover completely in less than 5 days.[2] Animals that have severe clinical signs or dehydration or that fail to respond to symptomatic therapy may need additional diagnostic tests and therapeutic support. Basic therapeutic principles for gastric disease include removing the underlying cause, providing proper conditions for mucosal repair, correcting secondary complications of gastritis (vomiting, abdominal pain, infection), and correcting fluid, electrolyte, and acid-base abnormalities.[3]

Dietary Intervention

Dietary restriction should be the rule until the animal has stopped vomiting for at least 24 hours. Ingestion of food or liquid results in gastric distention and stimulates further vomiting. Both the cephalic and gastric phases of gastric acid secretion are stimulated by food.[15] This permits back diffusion of hydrogen ions and further mucosal damage. Food may also serve as an exogenous source of bacteria that could potentially invade the damaged gastric mucosa.[55]

After the period of food restriction, offer ice cubes or small amounts of water and gradually proceed to moist food. Diets high in fat and protein should be avoided; diets consisting predominantly of nonrefined carbohydrates are recommended. Dietary management is based on the knowledge that liquids are emptied from the stomach more rapidly than solids, carbohydrates are emptied more rapidly than proteins, and proteins are emptied more rapidly than lipids.[69] A low-fat, low-protein diet of liquid or semiliquid consistency should thus be fed at frequent intervals to facilitate gastric emptying and thereby avoid gastric distention. An acceptable homemade diet is a mixture of low-fat cottage cheese (one part) plus boiled rice (two parts). This can be flavored with chicken bouillon if necessary. Offer small amounts and gradually increase the amount over 2 to 4 days until the patient is able to eat and retain enough to supply daily caloric requirements. If a favorable response is obtained with dietary management, the regular diet is gradually reintroduced over several days. However, if vomiting prolongs fasting (e.g., 4 to 7 days) or if the animal is already nutritionally depleted, special nutritional support should be considered (see Chapter 71).[2]

Fluid Therapy

Animals that are only slightly dehydrated with minimal ongoing losses can usually be given oral fluids (ice cubes or iced water) in small amounts at frequent intervals. Animals that continue to vomit or those that are severely dehydrated should receive parenteral fluids. The subcutaneous route is reasonable if the patient is not in immediate need of volume replacement. If, however, the animal does not adequately absorb these fluids or if peripheral perfusion is not maintained, then the fluids should be administered intravenously. The quantity of fluids administered should be enough to supply daily maintenance needs, which are approximately 30 mL/lb body weight per day[70, 71] (although indirect calorimetry studies suggest that [15 × body weight in pounds] + 70 = daily basal water requirements in milliliters for dogs and cats),[72] correct existing dehydration deficits, and replace fluid losses that may occur with continued vomiting. The choice of fluids depends on the electrolyte and acid-base status of the animal. Vomiting in acute gastritis usually results in losses of sodium, chloride, and potassium, as well as metabolic acidosis. An isotonic balanced electrolyte solution such as Ringer's lactate solution is usually given.[3] It is rarely necessary to administer bicarbonate. Fluids should

be supplemented with potassium chloride if the vomiting is profuse, if anorexia is prolonged, and/or if the patient is hypokalemic. The serum potassium concentration should be measured before supplementation.[2] Generally, 20 mEq of potassium chloride can safely be added to each liter of fluids to prevent hypokalemia. The acidosis is usually due to lactate accumulation and resolves when peripheral perfusion is restored. Infrequently, in conditions with profuse vomiting or gastric outflow obstruction, severe hypochloremia, hypokalemia, and metabolic alkalosis may occur. Under these conditions, normal (0.9 per cent) saline is the fluid of choice. This chloride-rich therapy corrects the deficit and allows renal excretion of bicarbonate.[3]

Small animals (especially neonates) are prone to hypoglycemia, especially if they are anorexic or septicemic. Blood glucose should be monitored. If necessary, sufficient glucose is added to the intravenous fluids to create a 2.5 to 5 per cent solution.[2]

Antiemetic Therapy

Antiemetic drugs are given to control refractory vomiting associated with persistent dehydration. They are not routinely used. Although they inhibit vomiting, they do little for primary treatment of the gastritis. Centrally acting antiemetic drugs, including the phenothiazine derivatives and metoclopramide, are generally more effective than peripherally acting drugs.[73–75]

The most commonly used phenothiazine derivatives include chlorpromazine and prochlorperazine. At low doses they block the chemoreceptor trigger zone (via dopamine antagonism) and at higher doses they depress the emetic center.[3] The antiemetic dose for chlorpromazine (0.1 to 0.2 mg/lb) and for prochlorperazine (0.05 to 0.2 mg/lb), both intramuscular, three or four times per day, is generally less than that required for sedation. Prochlorperazine tends to have less sedative action than chlorpromazine.[2] Phenothiazines should not be used in dehydrated or hypotensive animals because of their alpha-adrenergic blocking action, which causes arteriolar vasodilation. Fluid therapy to correct dehydration should thus be administered before use of these agents. Phenothiazines also lower the seizure threshold in epileptic animals.[74]

Metoclopramide is probably more effective as a centrally acting antiemetic than as a gastric prokinetic agent.[76] As a dopamine antagonist, metoclopramide inhibits vomiting associated with activation of central dopaminergic D_2 receptors in the chemoreceptor trigger zone. The drug is administered parenterally at 0.1 to 0.25 mg/lb body weight every 8 hours. Constant intravenous administration of 0.5 to 1.0 mg/lb body weight in 24 hours seems to be more effective than intermittent bolus therapy. Metoclopramide should not be used when stimulation of gastrointestinal motility could be harmful, for example, in the presence of a mechanical obstruction or perforation. Metoclopramide should also be avoided in epileptic animals or those receiving other drugs that are likely to cause extrapyramidal reactions, because the frequency and severity of seizures or extrapyramidal reactions may be increased. Atropine and opioid analgesic agents may antagonize the action of metoclopramide. Additive sedative effects can occur when metoclopramide is given with narcotics or tranquilizers. Because chronic therapy with phenothiazines can produce side effects similar to those seen with metoclopramide, concomitant use of metoclopramide and phenothiazine drugs should be avoided.

GI

Miscellaneous Therapy

Anticholinergic (parasympatholytic) drugs have been used as antiemetics. Aminopentamide is a parasympatholytic drug that is reasonably effective in stopping mild to moderate vomiting but is of questionable efficacy in animals with severe vomiting.[2] It seems to work by decreasing gastrointestinal motility but might also have some central activity. Anticholinergics, including atropine, methscopolamine, and propantheline (Pro-Banthine), have the undesirable effect of reducing gastric emptying, which results in gastric distention and further acid secretion. Thus, they are poorly effective as antiemetics and tend to produce intestinal stasis, which may cause persistent vomiting.[3, 73]

Selective 5-hydroxytryptamine type 3 (5-HT$_3$) receptor antagonists may be effective antiemetics.[77] These drugs, which include ondansetron, granisetron, and tropisetron, are used in human beings for vomiting associated with *cis*-platinum chemotherapy.[78-81] *Cis*-platinum–induced emesis is mediated by 5-HT$_3$ serotoninergic receptors, either in the chemoreceptor trigger zone (in cats) or in vagal afferent neurons (in dogs).[80, 81] Cisapride also antagonizes these 5-HT$_3$ receptors and inhibits vomiting associated with *cis*-platinum chemotherapy, but this occurs at much higher doses than recommended for its gastric prokinetic effects.[78, 79] Thus, cisapride is not recommended as an antiemetic agent in chemotherapy patients if ondansetron (0.05 mg/lb intravenously 15 minutes before and 4 hours after chemotherapy in dogs) is available.[82]

Therapies of little value in acute gastritis include antibiotics, NSAIDs, corticosteroids, antacids, oral protectorants, and absorbents. There is little or no indication for antibiotic therapy in the majority of patients with acute gastritis.[2] However, if there is blood in the vomited material, which would suggest transmural disease, parenteral antibiotics should be considered. Histamine type 2 receptor antagonists are also used in patients with evidence of transmural damage, although they are probably of little value in the absence of erosions or ulcers.[83]

HEMORRHAGIC GASTROENTERITIS

Canine hemorrhagic gastroenteritis (HGE) is predominantly an intestinal disease rather than a gastric disorder; however, vomiting is typically part of the presenting complaint.[2, 84] This syndrome is unique among other causes of hemorrhagic diarrhea in the dog. HGE is characterized by peracute loss of gastrointestinal mucosal integrity with rapid movement of blood, fluid, and electrolytes into the gut lumen. The signs usually begin with acute vomiting, anorexia, and depression, which are then followed by bloody diarrhea. Dehydration and hypovolemic shock occur quickly over a period of 8 to 12 hours. Bacteria and/or toxins may cross the damaged gastric mucosal barrier and result in septic or endotoxic shock. The cause is unknown, although an immune-mediated reaction directed against the enteric mucosa has been proposed. Samples from some dogs yield pure cultures of *Clostridium perfringens* but the significance of this association is unknown. Toxigenic *Escherichia coli* has also been proposed but not confirmed as a cause of enterotoxemia. The classic signalment is a middle-aged, small-breed dog (especially miniature schnauzers, miniature poodles, Yorkshire terriers, and dachshunds) with no history of garbage, chemical, or foreign body ingestion. Hemoconcentration, with a packed cell volume (PCV) generally greater than 60 per cent, is noted. The stool is negative for parasites, enzyme-linked immunosorbent assay (ELISA) is negative for canine parvovirus, and fecal cytology reveals many red blood cells, occasional white blood cells, and possibly *C. perfringens* spores. Abdominal radiographs show fluid- and gas-filled small and large intestines. Affected dogs should be hospitalized and treated aggressively with intravenous fluids. Parenteral antibiotics are given because of the potential for septicemia. A broad-spectrum antibiotic combination with activity against *C. perfringens*, such as ampicillin plus a fluroquinolone, is recommended empirically. Fast-acting glucocorticoids are given to dogs in shock. Occasionally, disseminated intravascular coagulation (DIC) may develop. The course of the disease is generally short (lasting from 24 to 72 hours), as most patients recover with supportive therapy.

CHRONIC GASTRITIS

The definition of chronic gastritis implies that there are chronic inflammatory changes within the mucosa of the stomach coexisting with clinical signs of gastric disease.[3] In most cases of chronic gastritis, the cause is never determined. There are usually no significant abnormalities in the CBC, chemistry profile, urinalysis, or abdominal radiographs. A stress leukogram or, in cases of eosinophilic gastritis, an eosinophilia may be noted. The gastric mucosa in dogs with chronic gastritis may appear grossly normal; a precise diagnosis requires multiple gastric mucosal biopsies of all areas of the stomach.[2]

Classification of chronic gastropathies is, therefore, based on the predominant cellular infiltrate present, with lymphocytic-plasmacytic gastritis being most common.[2] Factors considered by pathologists when classifying idiopathic gastritis include the type of cellular infiltrate, the area of the mucosa affected (e.g., superficial or deep, focal or generalized), the severity of the inflammation, the mucosal thickness, and the topography (e.g., body or antrum). Idiopathic gastritis is subdivided into the following categories: nonspecific (lymphocytic-plasmacytic) gastritis, eosinophilic gastritis, and granulomatous gastritis. Nonspecific gastritis can be further subdivided into superficial gastritis, diffuse gastritis, atrophic gastritis, and hypertrophic gastritis.[85] The clinical significance of this classification scheme with regard to therapy and prognosis remains unknown.[85]

Occasionally, the primary cause of gastritis can be identified. For example, *Physaloptera* and *Ollulanus* parasites and *Helicobacter* may be associated with chronic gastritis. Chronic gastritis can also be described in terms of associated conditions, such as bilious vomiting syndrome, breed-related gastritis, systemic diseases (e.g., hepatic, renal, and endocrine diseases), and drug therapies (corticosteroids and NSAIDs).[2, 85]

CHRONIC NONSPECIFIC GASTRITIS[85]

In chronic superficial gastritis, the superficial interstitial tissue (between the gastric pits) is infiltrated by plasma cells and lymphocytes. Lymphocytic-plasmacytic infiltrates in cats are often associated with similar intestinal inflammatory infiltrates.[2] This is probably due to chronic antigenic stimulation. Superficial gastritis may resolve without progressing to diffuse gastritis, which indicates that it is probably a transient reaction to a noxious agent in the stomach.[86] In chronic diffuse gastritis, the histologic changes are similar to those of superficial gastritis but are more extensive, with plasma cells and lymphocytes infiltrating the full thickness of the mucosa, although the mucosal thickness is normal.

The gastric mucosa of dogs with atrophic gastritis is discolored and thin, and submucosal blood vessels can be observed through the mucosa. The decrease in mucosal thickness results from loss of glands and their cells. Inflammatory changes are more severe, with lymphocytes and plasma cells extending into the submucosa. These changes are reversible if the underlying cause is removed.[86] Experimentally, atrophic gastritis has been induced in the dog by repeated intradermal injections of homologous gastric juice stimulating both humoral and cell-mediated immunity.[87] End-stage atrophy results in gastric hyposecretion, which is associated with small intestinal bacterial overgrowth.[2]

Hypertrophic gastritis is characterized by diffuse or focal mucosal proliferation. Focal hypertrophy of the antral mucosa is more common (discussed under gastric outlet obstruction). Microscopically, hypertrophy and hyperplasia of the mucosa are seen, often accompanied by variable amounts of inflammatory cells (lymphocytes, plasma cells, lesser numbers of eosinophils and neutrophils) and fibrous tissue. Hypertrophic gastritis is most common in basenjis[88] and other small-breed dogs such as the Lhasa apso, shih tzu, Maltese, and miniature poodle.[89–91] Hereditary and immune-mediated factors may be involved. Hypertrophic gastritis may also result from chronic mucosal inflammation or possibly from the trophic action of histamine or gastrin on the gastric mucosa. Thus, mucosal hypertrophy can be secondary, for example, to gastrinomas, mast cell neoplasia, pancreatic polypeptide– and insulin-secreting tumors, gastric parasites, and *Campylobacter*-like organisms.[56, 85, 92–94]

Therapy for moderate to severe lymphocytic-plasmacytic infiltrates usually begins with corticosteroids (e.g., prednisone or prednisolone at 1.0 to 1.5 mg/lb body weight per day for 1 to 2 weeks before the dose is gradually reduced over a period of 2 to 3 months) on the premise that inflammation is immune mediated. Metronidazole (7 to 10 mg/lb body weight, given twice daily) may also be effective, either combined with prednisolone or used alone. If the animal responds well, the dose(s) may be slowly decreased, but no more frequently than every 1 to 2 weeks lest clinical signs recur and be less responsive to therapy. Animals with simple gastritis usually respond rapidly to corticosteroids. In contrast, animals with atrophic or hyperplastic gastritis do not respond as readily to corticosteroids. Severe cases may require concurrent cytotoxic therapy with azathioprine.[2]

The same dietary recommendations made for acute gastritis apply for animals with chronic gastritis. The ideal diet is hypoallergenic, predominantly carbohydrate, and low in fat (to avoid delayed gastric emptying). A selected (novel) protein diet should be used in case a dietary sensitivity initiated or is perpetuating the disease. Fluid, electrolyte, and acid-base derangements are less common with chronic gastritis than with acute gastritis, and fluid therapy is less important. For most animals, unless there is clinical, endoscopic, or histologic evidence of concomitant gastric erosions or ulcers, acid inhibitors, antiemetics, prokinetics, or antibiotics are not necessary or are of uncertain benefit.[2, 85]

EOSINOPHILIC GASTRITIS

Eosinophilic gastritis, which is less common than lymphocytic-plasmacytic gastritis,[2] is characterized by infiltration of the gastric mucosa with eosinophils and granulation tissue. The eosinophilic infiltration may extend throughout all layers of the stomach or, less frequently, may present as discrete granulomatous nodules.[85] The wall of the stomach can become quite thickened, resembling neoplasia. There may be an associated lymphadenitis and vasculitis.[95] In dogs, other parts of the gastrointestinal tract may be affected as well, a condition referred to as eosinophilic gastroenteritis. In cats, eosinophilic gastritis may present as one component of the hypereosinophilic syndrome, which is usually characterized by circulating hypereosinophilia and eosinophilic infiltration of organs (e.g., bone marrow, small intestine, spleen, and liver).[96] Not all cats with eosinophilic gastritis, however, have hypereosinophilic syndrome.

The cause of eosinophilic infiltration of the stomach is unknown, but it is thought to be immunologically mediated, possibly caused by an allergic hypersensitivity to dietary antigens or parasites.[85] Mechanical irritation should also be considered.[97] Laboratory tests to detect heartworms and fecal examinations for intestinal parasites should be performed to rule out parasitism as the cause of eosinophilia. Biopsy specimens taken by endoscopy or surgery are needed to demonstrate the lesions. A strict hypoallergenic diet (also called an elimination diet) should be fed as some animals respond well (no treats). If dietary therapy is not successful, prednisolone should be administered as for lymphocytic-plasmacytic gastritis. Many cats with hypereosinophilic syndrome respond poorly to therapy.[96] Higher doses of corticosteroids are often required (starting at 1 to 1.5 mg/lb every 12 hours). Azathioprine is sometimes necessary in dogs and cats with intractable eosinophilic gastritis. Surgical resection in association with a hypoallergenic diet is usually successful in dogs with eosinophilic granulomatous masses. Most animals can be controlled, rather than cured, with dietary and low-dose corticosteroid therapy.[85]

GRANULOMATOUS GASTRITIS

Granulomas are the predominant histologic finding in granulomatous gastritis. A localized granulomatous mass or diffuse inflammation may be present. Granulomatous inflammation may occur in association with eosinophilic gastritis, parasites (*Gnathostoma* nematodes), fungal diseases (phycomycosis, histoplasmosis, and cryptococcosis), feline infectious peritonitis (FIP), viral infection, foreign material, and neoplasia.[98–100] If the underlying cause can be determined, specific treatment should be instituted. If no underlying cause is found, treatment as for chronic nonspecific gastritis should be implemented.[85]

HELICOBACTER GASTRITIS

Gastric spiral bacteria, formerly assigned to the genus *Campylobacter* and now to *Helicobacter*, are spiral-shaped, gram-negative bacteria that have been isolated from the stomach of humans, nonhuman primates, cats, dogs, ferrets, and cheetahs.[101] There are at least 13 species in the new genus *Helicobacter*, the majority being proven or suspected gastrointestinal or hepatic pathogens.[102] Human research has focused on the association of *Helicobacter pylori* and chronic gastritis, peptic ulcer, and gastric neoplasia.[103] Although spiral organisms found in animals are usually a different species than *H. pylori*, which is implicated in human disease (*H. heilmannii* and *H. felis* are the two species most commonly found in dogs and cats), the role of *Helicobacter* infection in gastrointestinal disease of small animals

GI

is being investigated.[101, 104, 105] The isolation of *H. pylori, H. heilmannii,* and *H. felis* from domestic cats and human beings raises the possibility that *Helicobacter* may be a zoonotic pathogen.[101, 106, 107]

It is thought that *Helicobacter* organisms are normal inhabitants of the stomach.[101, 104, 105, 108] In a study of animal shelter cats, 97 per cent of adults were infected with *Helicobacter.*[109] In another study, 82 per cent of 122 dogs and 76 per cent of 127 cats were found to be infected.[110] Although the clinical significance of *Helicobacter* infection is unknown, most infected animals have associated mild histologic changes in the stomach.[105] Experimentally, one can infect gnotobiotic beagles with *H. pylori*[111] or *H. felis*[105] and cause gastric mucosal inflammatory infiltrates. In a case-control study of 56 dogs and 33 cats with gastrointestinal disease, gastric spiral organisms were detected in 86 and 90 per cent of clinically normal dogs and cats, respectively, and in 61 and 64 per cent of clinically abnormal dogs and cats, respectively.[112] Although evidence suggests that the usual consequence of *Helicobacter* infection is a subclinical gastritis,[112, 113] clinical signs of *Helicobacter* infection in dogs and cats reportedly include chronic vomiting and diarrhea, inappetence, pica, fever, and polyphagia. Bloody diarrhea has been described in a group of Persian cats with lymphocytic-plasmacytic gastroenterocolitis associated with a spiral-shaped organism.[114]

The pathogenicity of *Helicobacter* results in part from its ability to produce urease.[101, 115–117] Urease breaks down urea in gastric juice into ammonia and bicarbonate ions. The associated buffering effect may help *Helicobacter* colonize in an acid environment or extend the life of the organisms long enough for them to penetrate deeper within the mucus surface into a more favorable alkaline environment. Ammonia also causes histologic damage and vacuolation of epithelial cells.[118] In addition, *Helicobacter* may produce cytotoxins[119] and/or stimulate cytokines that attract the inflammatory cells responsible for inflammation and ulcerogenesis.[120] Production of the cytokine interleukin-8 contributes to the hypergastrinemia associated with *Helicobacter* infection.[121] *Helicobacter* infection is also associated with changes in the biochemical properties of mucus.[120] Pathogenicity of *Helicobacter* may correlate with motility, as some nonmotile strains cannot colonize the gastric epithelium. Typically, inflammatory changes secondary to *Helicobacter* occur deep in the gastric mucosa. Lymphoplasmacytic infiltrate and lymphoid nodules are observed on histopathologic examination of animals with chronic infection.[101]

Diagnostic tests in veterinary medicine require endoscopic or surgical biopsy.[101] Histopathologic examination relies on microscopic visualization of *Helicobacter*-like organisms. Visualization of organisms can be enhanced by the use of Warthin-Starry silver stains. Multiple biopsies, particularly of the fundus and corpus,[108] are recommended in order to maximize chances of detecting *Helicobacter.* The urease test is a rapid test used in conjunction with histopathologic examination. A color change occurs as urease breaks down ammonia, which changes the pH. Polymerase chain reaction (PCR) analysis, serologic tests, and urea breath testing are being developed to detect and monitor *Helicobacter* infection.[122, 123]

Combination therapies utilizing multiple drugs have been necessary in humans to eradicate *Helicobacter.* Acid-inhibiting drugs (e.g., H_2 receptor blockers and proton-pump inhibitors) are used along with bismuth-based compounds (e.g., bismuth subsalicylate or colloidal bismuth subcitrate). Bismuth accumulates beneath the *Helicobacter* cell wall and causes cell lysis. In human medicine, the traditional bismuth-based triple-therapy regimens consisting of bismuth, metronidazole, and either amoxicillin or tetracycline are associated with more than 90 per cent cure rates in some studies.[124] Bismuth, tetracycline, amoxicillin, ampicillin, and furazolidone have predominantly luminal activity against *Helicobacter,* whereas metronidazole has systemic effects.[125] Newer omeprazole-based triple-therapy regimens (omeprazole, amoxicillin, and tinidazole; omeprazole, amoxicillin, and clarithromycin) have 93 to 95 per cent success rates at eradicating *Helicobacter* in human beings.[126, 127]

In veterinary medicine, a combination of metronidazole (10 mg/lb), amoxicillin (10 mg/lb), and bismuth subsalicylate (8 mg/lb; Pepto-Bismol original formula) three times a day for 3 to 4 weeks is effective in eliminating infection in ferrets.[128] A combination of metronidazole, amoxicillin, and famotidine produced marked improvement of clinical signs of *Helicobacter* infection in over 90 per cent of treated dogs and cats.[125] Another suggested protocol is amoxicillin (5 mg/lb every 12 hours), metronidazole (15 mg/lb every 24 hours), and sucralfate (0.25 to 0.5 g every 8 hours) for 3 weeks. Omeprazole (0.3 mg/lb every 24 hours) can be used in place of sucralfate.[129] Triple therapy with amoxicillin (5 mg/lb every 8 hours), metronidazole (7 mg/lb every 8 hours), and bismuth subsalicylate (0.1 mL/lb every 4 to 6 hours) for 21 days has also been suggested.[101] It is likely that most of the *Helicobacter* infections in dogs and cats are asymptomatic. Treatment would therefore be most warranted for animals with obvious clinical signs and histopathologic evidence of infection.[101] Controlled studies are needed to determine the benefits of antimicrobial therapy in dogs and cats.

PARASITIC GASTRITIS

The nematode *Physaloptera* is reported to cause chronic gastritis and intermittent vomiting in otherwise healthy dogs.[130, 131] A number of *Physaloptera* species are known to exist throughout the world, but the prevalence of infection is considered to be low. Adult parasites attach to the mucosa and cause localized gastritis in both dogs and cats.[132] The intermediate hosts are beetles, crickets, and cockroaches. *Physaloptera* eggs are not easily observed after fecal concentrating techniques, and instead adult parasites are usually discovered during endoscopy, particularly with a video endoscope, which magnifies the image. Adults are 1 to 4 cm long white parasites usually found in the fundus or antrum. Immature worms are 2 to 3 mm long and are easily overlooked. Physically removing the parasite via the endoscope often resolves the vomiting. A single dose of pyrantel (2.5 mg/lb) is effective in dogs, and two doses (2.5 mg/lb) given 3 weeks apart appear to be effective in cats.[85, 131, 132]

Ollulanus tricuspis infection in cats (rarely dogs) may produce hypertrophic gastritis, gastric erosions, and/or chronic fibrosing gastritis.[56, 57, 93, 133, 134] This nematode also has a worldwide distribution. Clinical signs associated with infection can range from none to anorexia and chronic vomiting. *O. tricuspis* is usually not detected by routine parasitologic, endoscopic, and necropsy examinations.[85] These parasites are quite small (adults 1 mm long), and neither adult nor larval forms pass in the feces. Infection is often missed on histopathologic examination of gastric biopsy specimens.[135] Diagnosis is usually made by microscopic examination of the vomitus for the nematode. Transmission is due to uninfected cats eating vomitus from an infected cat. Infection is more a problem when cats are in close contact with one another, as in a cattery. Oral fenbendazole at 5 mg/lb daily for 2 days is successful in eliminating the parasite from kittens.[134]

Roundworms occasionally cause vomiting if they migrate into the stomach. Their mobility in the stomach probably causes nausea. Finding the parasite in the vomitus warrants treatment with an appropriate anthelmintic.[2]

Infection of cats with *Gnathostoma* nematodes, although worldwide in distribution, is rarely reported in the United States but is reasonably common in cats from Southeast Asia and Australia.[136] The organism produces a granulomatous mass in the stomach wall, and clinical signs vary from none to severe vomiting and even death caused by gastric perforation. Eggs may be found in the feces. Therapy usually involves surgical removal of the mass and the associated parasite, although disophenol is reported to be effective.[136]

Spirocerca lupi occasionally infects the stomach of dogs and cats.[137] Treatment is surgical removal of the nodule. Pseudomyiasis can also occur in animals that ingest garbage containing fly larvae. Identification of the larvae makes it possible to diagnose this problem, and removing the garbage source prevents recurrence.[2]

REFLUX GASTRITIS

The bilious vomiting syndrome (also called reflux gastritis) is a condition in which an otherwise normal dog tends to vomit small amounts of bile in the morning.[2] The etiology is unknown but is associated with gastroduodenal reflux of bile and bile acids into the stomach during the night. Vomiting usually occurs when the stomach is empty, especially after an overnight fast.

The condition is diagnosed by eliminating other causes of chronic vomiting and by symptomatic response to therapy. Physical examination, CBC, chemistry profile, diagnostic imaging, endoscopy and gastric biopsies are usually normal. A presumptive diagnosis is made on the basis of the history. Feed the dog a late night meal. If vomiting persists, administer a prokinetic drug late at night. The apparent dyspepsia can sometimes be controlled with H_2 receptor antagonist therapy.[2]

CHRONIC GASTRITIS ASSOCIATED WITH HEPATIC, RENAL, AND ENDOCRINE DISEASES

Chronic gastritis, erosions, and ulceration develop in animals with hepatic or renal insufficiency. Endocrine diseases associated with chronic gastritis in humans include hypothyroidism, hyperthyroidism, diabetes mellitus, and hypoadrenocorticism. Chronic gastritis occurs in dogs with hypoadrenocorticism.[85]

MISCELLANEOUS CAUSES OF GASTRIC INFLAMMATION

Basenji dogs have been reported to have a gastritis similar to that in human Ménétrier's disease, with gastric rugal hypertrophy, lymphocytic gastritis, and gastric mucosal atrophy.[88] This gastritis is associated with the immunoproliferative enteritis reported in this breed. No special therapy for the gastritis seems indicated, as the principal problem is the intestinal lesion.

Drentse patrijshond dogs have a predisposition for hyper-

trophic gastritis plus stomatocytosis, hemolytic anemia, and hepatic disease with icterus. This hereditary syndrome is called familial stomatocytosis–hypertrophic gastritis. Inflammatory cell infiltrates are commonly seen in the stomach, and hypoproteinemia may occur, similar to that in Ménétrier's protein-losing gastropathy.[138, 139]

Prolonged administration of some drugs can cause chronic gastritis. Corticosteroids and NSAIDs are reported most commonly. Food allergy is also a probable cause of acute and perhaps chronic gastritis.[85]

GASTRIC ULCERATION AND EROSION

Gastric erosions are superficial mucosal defects that do not penetrate the lamina muscularis mucosae. Gastric ulcers penetrate deeper into the muscularis mucosae layer. Gastric ulcers are less commonly observed than erosions and seem more common in dogs than in cats.[2, 140, 141]

CAUSES

Gastric ulceration or erosion may result from any of the agents that cause acute or chronic gastritis. Major causes include drugs (NSAIDs, corticosteroids), primary gastric diseases (chronic gastritis, gastric dilatation-volvulus, chemical toxins, neoplasia, pyloric outlet obstruction, mechanical irritants), stress factors (hypotension, severe illness, environmental stress), neurologic disease, metabolic disorders (renal disease, liver disease, hypoadrenocorticism), gastric hyperacidity conditions (systemic mastocytosis, gastrinoma), and miscellaneous disorders (acute pancreatitis, DIC). The most common causes of gastric ulceration in dogs and cats include drugs, neoplasia, liver disease, and shock.[85] Drugs, especially NSAIDs, and neoplasia are more commonly ulcerative, whereas other causes more commonly result in erosions.[141]

PATHOPHYSIOLOGY

The mechanisms of gastric ulcer or erosion formation and their description and location vary depending on the etiology. In all conditions the pathophysiologic factors are many. If mucosal damage exceeds the reparative process, erosions can progress to ulcers. It is not known why a single or only a few ulcers form instead of multiple mucosal lesions.[140]

Nonsteroidal Drugs[62, 142, 143]

The mechanism by which NSAIDs cause gastric ulcer or erosion formation is probably multifactorial but inhibition of prostaglandin synthesis seems important.[2] Different NSAIDs have different abilities to inhibit cyclooxygenase (the source of prostaglandins) and 5-lipoxygenase (the source of leukotrienes), which may explain the various ulcerogenic potentials of these drugs.[144] Oral administration, especially of aspirin, seems to cause gastric ulcer or erosion formation more commonly, although parenteral or suppository administration of many NSAIDs also produces gastric ulcers or erosions.[145, 146] Buffered aspirin and enteric-coated products are sometimes helpful in reducing the gastric side effects.[63, 147, 148] Risk factors for NSAID-induced gastric ulcers or erosions include higher doses, longer administration times, increased gastric acidity, and coadministration of another NSAID or a corticosteroid.[2] Dogs seem especially prone to

GI

NSAID-induced lesions, probably because these drugs often have a longer serum half-life in dogs than in people, resulting in accumulation of high concentrations of the drug. There is also marked individual variation regarding sensitivity to NSAIDs. Some dogs develop life-threatening upper gastrointestinal hemorrhage after receiving relatively small doses of aspirin.[2, 147] Absence of clinical signs, however, does not imply lack of lesions. Indomethacin, naproxen,[149, 150] piroxicam,[148, 151] flunixin meglumine,[60, 61] and ibuprofen[152–155] are particularly toxic for dogs. This correlates with their being potent inhibitors of prostaglandin synthesis and having relatively long half-lives. Naproxen also undergoes enterohepatic cycling, which allows the intestines to be exposed several times.[2] Newer NSAIDs may offer anti-inflammatory activity with less gastrointestinal toxicity.[156, 157]

Corticosteroids

Prednisone at commonly administered doses usually does not cause gastric ulcer or erosion formation, although coadministration of corticosteroids with NSAIDs appears to increase the risk in dogs significantly.[2] Administration of large dexamethasone doses (e.g., 1 mg/lb every 12 hours) has been associated with gastric ulcer or erosion formation, but such doses are seldom used except in neurosurgery patients.[2]

Stress Factors

Hypovolemic shock has been associated with gastric ulcer or erosion formation, particularly in trauma patients.[158] Septic shock results in increased gastric acid secretion in the dog.[159, 160] Neurologic disorders have also been associated with gastric ulcer or erosion formation, although it is difficult to determine whether the lesions are due to the neurologic disease or to the therapy, which includes surgery and large doses of dexamethasone.[161, 162]

Mast Cell Tumors

These tumors contain histamine, which stimulates gastric acid secretion. If a mast cell tumor degranulates (either spontaneously or because of tumor manipulation or cell death), increased circulating levels of histamine can produce gastric hyperacidity and lead to gastric ulcer or erosion formation.[163] Prophylactic therapy should be considered when a mast cell tumor is diagnosed.[2]

Gastrinomas

These are APUDomas (amine precursor uptake and decarboxylation tumors), usually found in the pancreas, which continually secrete gastrin.[3] They are more common in dogs but have also been reported in cats.[164, 165] Hypergastrinemia leads to gastric hypersecretion of acid. This results in gastric and duodenal ulceration, chronic vomiting, esophagitis (because of vomiting large volumes of acid), and diarrhea (because of loss of proximal intestinal villi caused by the large volumes of acid entering the proximal duodenum).[2]

The diagnosis is suspected in patients with recurrent gastric ulcers or erosions that do not respond to conventional therapy. Serum gastrin concentrations are usually increased; occasionally one must perform provocative testing using secretin or calcium.[3, 166] Normal dogs have a decreased gastrin response to these drugs; gastrinoma patients may have an increase. Treatment requires resection of the pancreatic tumor. Because of frequent metastasis, the prognosis is poor.

Patients may be palliated for months or years with aggressive H_2 antagonist or omeprazole therapy.[3] Other neuroendocrine tumors may also secrete gastrin in addition to other hormones.[94]

Inflammatory Bowel Disease, Hepatic and Renal Disease

Lymphocytic-plasmacytic or eosinophilic gastroenteritis may be associated with gastric or proximal duodenal ulceration.[167] How often this occurs is unknown. Canine gastric ulcer or erosion formation has also been associated with severe hepatic disease.[143] Increased gastric acidity has been speculated to be the cause of this association. Gastric bleeding may cause sudden decompensation in a patient with previously controlled chronic hepatic disease. Therefore, in patients with known hepatic disease that suddenly deteriorate, empirical therapy for gastric ulcers or erosions is indicated before ulceration is documented.[2] Gastric ulcer or erosion formation is not commonly noted in dogs and cats with renal disease, even though gastrin concentrations may be elevated with renal failure.[2]

Miscellaneous

Foreign objects rarely cause gastric ulcer or erosion formation, even when they have sharp edges and points. However, in patients with lesions any foreign object may prevent an ulcer from healing.[2] Neoplasia can cause ulcers in the stomach by disrupting the mucosal integrity.[168] Gastric adenocarcinoma and lymphosarcoma are most commonly associated with ulcers.[2] Cats have gastric ulcer or erosion formation less frequently than dogs, perhaps because owners less commonly administer NSAIDs to their cats.[2] Causes of feline lesions include abdominal mast cell tumor, gastric lymphosarcoma, inflammatory bowel disease,[167] granulomatous disease,[169] and O. tricuspis (small erosions) and Aonchotheca putorii (ulcer) infestations.[170]

CLINICAL SIGNS

Acute or chronic vomiting with or without hematemesis is the most common clinical sign associated with gastric ulcer or erosion formation.[143] Not all animals with gastric ulcers vomit, however, and not all animals that vomit blood have gastric ulcers.[171] Other clinical signs observed include anorexia, abdominal pain, melena, anemia, edema (from hypoproteinemia related to alimentary hemorrhage), and/or septicemia (from perforation). Other signs may be related to the underlying cause (e.g., liver disease, neurologic disease). Perforation of the stomach or duodenum may result in the sudden onset of severe weakness, severe abdominal pain, fever, shock, abdominal distention, and death caused by peritonitis.[140] Rarely, animals with perforated gastric ulcer have only mild signs of abdominal discomfort.[2]

DIAGNOSIS

The diagnosis of gastric ulcers or erosions requires either direct visualization with endoscopy or indirect documentation with a barium contrast study.[140] Response to medical therapy is also a rational way to diagnose gastric ulcers or erosions. If the history strongly suggests ulceration caused by NSAIDs, stress, and/or mast cell tumor, it may be reasonable to treat the patient and resort to endoscopy only if the dog does not respond as expected.[2]

Radiographic contrast studies using barium sulfate and multiple positions are usually needed to identify lesions. Ulcers vary in size from several millimeters to 4 cm in diameter. Barium may adhere to a mucosal defect or penetrate into the crater. A barium contrast study is relatively insensitive, however, and small ulcers or larger defects filled with blood or debris may not be seen.[140] Barium sulfate produces a better study than iodine contrast agents. If a perforation with peritonitis is likely, there is rarely a need for contrast radiographs.[2] Ultrasonographic features of gastric ulcer include thickening of the gastric wall, possible loss of the five-layer structure, the presence of a wall defect or crater, fluid accumulation in the stomach, and diminished gastric motility.[172]

Endoscopy is the most sensitive method for diagnosing gastric ulcers or erosions.[50] Ulcers can be observed along the greater curvature, incisura angularis, antrum, or duodenum (Fig. 136–3). Ulcers may be difficult to find, however. They may be covered by rugal folds in a poorly distended stomach, hidden in a poorly distensible pylorus, or covered by mucus, or the illumination of the endoscope may be diminished by large amounts of digested blood whose dark color absorbs light.[2] If erosions are present instead of ulcers, there may be a small spot of fresh or digested blood on the mucosa. If one wipes the blood away with biopsy forceps, there is renewed bleeding from an erosion.[2]

Biopsy samples should be collected from the edge of the ulcer to rule out neoplasia. Multiple biopsies of the same location should be taken because superficial inflammation often accompanies neoplasia. Nonlesioned areas should also have biopsies taken to identify diffuse gastritis.[140] No biopsy of the center of the ulcer bed should be obtained as it is often very friable and can be easily perforated by the biopsy forceps.

Perforation may be difficult to detect endoscopically because small lesions may seal over with omentum and fibrin. Perforation is suspected if the stomach remains distended after the stomach is deflated or if abdominal radiographs reveal free gas in the abdomen after the procedure.[140] If

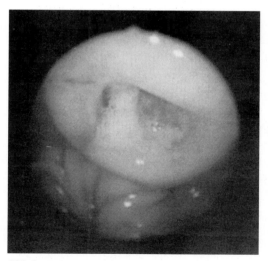

Figure 136–3. Endoscopic appearance of a gastric ulcer involving the incisura angularis in a 9-year-old cocker spaniel. Note the focal, crateriform appearance of the ulcer and the central necrotic fibrinopurulent debris. (From Jergens AE: Gastrointestinal disease and its management. Vet Clin North Am Small Anim Pract 27:1385, 1997.)

perforation is known to exist, endoscopy is contraindicated because pressurization of the stomach with air during the examination increases contamination of the abdominal cavity with gastric contents.[85]

Increased sucrose permeability has been shown to be useful in predicting the presence of endoscopically relevant gastric damage in people and in dogs experimentally treated with aspirin.[173] Healing was monitored by sequential measurements of sucrose permeability. Sucrose permeability decreased more rapidly than the gastric ulcers did, suggesting that this technique may be more sensitive to generalized mucosal damage than is the presence of discrete, endoscopically visible ulceration.

TREATMENT

Surgery should be performed if perforation is suspected or if severe bleeding is discovered. Serial evaluations of the hematocrit and cardiovascular assessment are necessary to determine whether blood loss is sufficient to warrant surgery.[2] Surgery is also indicated if the patient has not responded to *appropriate* medical therapy that has been administered for at least 5 to 7 days.[2] Lesions are resected during exploratory laparotomy. Sometimes it is difficult to locate mucosal lesions when examining the serosal surface. A thickened gastric wall may be detected, resulting from inflammatory infiltrates around the lesion. Intraoperative endoscopy is helpful in detecting lesions, so that if multiple ulcers are present they can all be located. If one does not have an endoscope and is performing surgery to look for ulcers, the stomach should be opened and thoroughly evaluated, especially in the antral and pyloric regions.[2]

Medical Therapy

The goals of medical therapy are to (1) remove the cause if possible, (2) maintain mucosal perfusion, (3) decrease gastric acidity, and (4) protect the ulcer.[2] Fluid therapy is important in dehydrated patients with gastric ulcers or erosions to maintain mucosal perfusion. Patients who are vomiting should be given antiemetics, as recommended for treatment of vomiting in acute gastritis. In addition, food should be withheld at least initially, to avoid stimulation of gastric acid and pepsin secretion.[2] Subsequent dietary management is similar to that recommended for acute gastritis. Drugs commonly used to accomplish these goals include receptor antagonists that block the interaction of secretagogues with their receptors (e.g., H_2 receptor antagonists), drugs that act on cellular metabolism to inhibit hydrogen ion secretion (e.g., prostaglandins), and proton pump inhibitors (e.g., omeprazole) that inhibit the H^+,K^+-ATPase in the apical parietal cell membrane.[85] Sucralfate is important for protecting ulcerated tissue. Antiulcer therapy should be continued for 4 to 6 weeks.

Histamine H₂ Receptor Antagonists

These drugs inhibit acid secretion by binding to the histamine H_2 receptor sites on the parietal cell, thereby preventing interaction of the receptor with histamine. Subsequently, more agonist (e.g., gastrin, histamine) is necessary to induce the same amount of acid secretion.[174] Cimetidine was the first H_2 receptor antagonist used in dogs. Inhibition of histamine-stimulated acid secretion peaks at 75 per cent within 1.5 hours, and 50 per cent inhibition of acid secretion lasts about

GI

2 hours after an oral dose.[85, 175] Drug effects are gone after 5 hours. Thus, cimetidine must be administered three to four times daily at a dose of 2.5 to 5 mg/lb to suppress gastric acid secretion in dogs.[2] Even so, there is only mild to moderate inhibition of acid secretion over a 24-hour period. The fact that it works clinically for ulcer therapy suggests that even partial suppression of gastric acid secretion is beneficial for the healing of most gastroduodenal ulcers.[176] Cimetidine is also a potent inhibitor of selected hepatic cytochrome P-450 enzymes.[176]

Ranitidine is more potent and lasts longer than cimetidine. Inhibition of acid secretion peaks at 90 per cent within 1.5 hours, and 50 per cent inhibition of acid secretion lasts about 4 hours after an oral dose.[85, 175] Ranitidine is usually effective clinically when administered at 1 mg/lb twice a day.[2] Ranitidine can be infused at a rate of 7.3 μg/lb per minute in dogs, which reduces acid secretion 70 to 80 per cent.[177, 178] In addition, ranitidine has prokinetic effects.[179] Ranitidine has minimal effects on hepatic metabolic enzymes. It can cause vomiting if rapidly administered intravenously.[2]

Famotidine may be more potent than either ranitidine or cimetidine.[174] It is administered twice (or once) daily at 0.25 to 0.5 mg/lb. It tends to be less bioavailable after oral administration than the other H$_2$ receptor antagonists and has a few drug interactions.[180]

Nizatidine is a new H$_2$ receptor antagonist, which, like ranitidine, has prokinetic activity.[181] It may be preferable in patients with gastric ulcers coexisting with a motility disorder. The dose is 1 to 2.5 mg/lb once daily.

Side effects of the H$_2$ receptor antagonists are rare.[2, 182] They include bradycardia,[183] thrombocytopenia,[184] hypersensitivity-like reactions such as drug eruption[185] or acute interstitial nephritis or polymyositis, hyperpyrexia,[186] diarrhea, granulocytopenia, and central nervous system aberrations.[187]

Prostaglandin E Analogs

These drugs inhibit adenylate cyclase, reducing cyclic AMP production and thereby reducing the protein kinase activity essential to hydrogen ion generation. In addition, these drugs increase gastric mucosal blood flow. Misoprostol is an analogue of prostaglandin E$_1$ that is administered in doses of 0.5 to 2.3 μg/lb two to three times per day. It is the drug of choice for NSAID-induced ulceration and is more effective than sucralfate or H$_2$ receptor antagonists in preventing NSAID-induced ulceration.[188–191] Some patients develop diarrhea, which is usually self-limiting.[192]

Omeprazole

Omeprazole is a substituted benzimidazole, which blocks hydrogen ion secretion in the parietal cell by inhibiting H$^+$,K$^+$-ATPase located on the apical membrane.[193] It works as a noncompetitive antagonist.[174] As a weak base, it accumulates in the acid compartment of the parietal cell, necessitating only once-daily administration. It is administered orally at doses of 0.33 to 1 mg/lb once daily.[2] Omeprazole is indicated for disease states that are not responsive to H$_2$ receptor antagonist therapy, such as nonresectable gastrinoma and systemic mast cell disease.[2] It also inhibits hepatic P-450 enzymes, and, therefore, the potential for drug interactions exists.[176] Lansoprazole, another proton pump inhibitor, does not differ significantly from omeprazole in potency or duration of action.[194]

Sucralfate

Sucralfate (Carafate) is a nonabsorbable aluminum salt of sucrose octasulfate.[195] The substance tightly adheres to the ulcerated tissue, protecting it from acid and pepsin. Sucralfate may also bind pepsin and bile acids, and it may change the gastric mucus so that it better impedes gastric acid.[196] Finally, it may stimulate prostaglandin synthesis in ulcerated areas.[197] Because absorption is minimal, it has almost no systemic effects. Long-term use may lead to constipation because of its aluminum content.[2] Sucralfate is most effective in an acidic environment but works adequately in a near-neutral pH, as might occur after H$_2$ receptor antagonist therapy.[198] It human beings, it is also used as one component of triple therapy for eradicating *H. pylori* infection.[199]

Sucralfate must be given orally, so it may be difficult to utilize this therapy in a vomiting patient. If given with other oral medication, sucralfate may adsorb and prevent, decrease, and/or delay their absorption.[2] Fluoroquinolones in particular may be adsorbed by sucralfate.[200] Absorption of H$_2$ receptor antagonists may be decreased 10 to 30 per cent by sucralfate.[174] Therefore, when treating ulcers with both types of drugs, one should administer the H$_2$ receptor antagonist first and then the sucralfate 30 to 60 minutes later.[176] There is no evidence to support an added benefit of combination therapy with sucralfate and an H$_2$ receptor antagonist, however, compared with use of either drug alone.[141, 176]

The recommended dose is 0.5 to 1 g given two to four times per day. In patients with severe blood loss, an initial loading dose of 3 to 6 g, followed by the lower dose, seems to be more effective.[2] Sucralfate is not as effective as misoprostol in preventing NSAID-induced ulcers or erosions.[144]

Miscellaneous Drugs

Oral antacids (e.g., aluminum hydroxide, magnesium hydroxide) are safe and effective at neutralizing acid, inactivating pepsin, and binding bile acids but they must be administered at least six times per day in doses sufficient to titrate gastric acid.[201] Thus, they are impractical for treatment of gastric ulcers or erosions in dogs and cats. Aluminum hydroxide has been suggested to exert some of its protective effects by generating prostaglandins and providing sulfhydryls.[202, 203] Cisapride may be helpful if the ulcer patient has a concurrent gastric motility disorder resulting in delayed gastric emptying.[82, 204] Antibiotics are usually not necessary in the treatment of gastric ulcers unless there is evidence of a microbial cause (e.g., *Helicobacter*) or gastric perforation is suspected.

GASTRIC OUTLET OBSTRUCTION

Gastric outlet obstruction refers to inability of food and/or water to exit properly from the stomach because of mechanical blockage at or near the pylorus.[2] There are four main causes of this problem: (1) foreign objects and/or intraluminal masses, (2) mucosal or muscular proliferative and/or infiltrative disease, (3) compression of the outflow tract by masses and/or organs outside the stomach, and (4) malpositioning of the stomach. Diagnosis of outflow obstruction may be made radiographically (i.e., failure of barium to leave the stomach, finding a mass or object in the pyloric antrum), endoscopically, ultrasonographically, or surgically. Clinical pathology sometimes reveals a hypochloremic, hypokalemic metabolic alkalosis as a significant complication of gastric outlet obstruction.[2, 91]

SIMPLE FOREIGN OBJECTS

Vomiting caused by foreign body ingestion is common in dogs (especially puppies) and less so in cats. Many gastric foreign bodies are removed by vomiting, are dissolved by gastric acid, or pass uneventfully through the gastrointestinal tract. Approximately 50 per cent of the objects retained in the stomach cause vomiting.[140] Unless an object obstructs the outflow or irritates the mucosa, it can remain in the animals's stomach for months without clinical signs. Thus, not all vomiting animals in which a gastric foreign body is discovered are vomiting because of the foreign body.

Diagnosis is based on history (seeing the animal eat something or have an acute onset of vomiting after some toy or object disappears), physical examination (palpation of the object), radiography (survey abdominal radiographs may demonstrate radiopaque objects, whereas a barium contrast study may be needed to demonstrate a filling defect if the object cannot be visualized), and/or endoscopy. Occasionally, a foreign body that obstructs the pylorus and causes severe clinical signs may be dislodged by vomiting yet remain in the stomach. Cyclic signs may develop as the foreign body reobstructs the pylorus. Chronic pyloric obstruction can cause delayed gastric emptying with postprandial gastric distention and discomfort, vomiting of food more than 8 hours after a meal, and weight loss.[140]

Foreign objects may be removed surgically or endoscopically to avoid the morbidity and risks associated with surgery. Useful endoscopic retrieval forceps include rat-tooth, snare, and basket forceps. It is helpful to insufflate the stomach with air to dilate the gastroesophageal sphincter. Alternatively, some foreign objects may be allowed to pass through the alimentary tract and out the anus (e.g., even glass, needles, and fishhooks), or the animal may be given an emetic and made to vomit the object. There are risks, however, that the object may cause obstruction or perforation of the small intestine if allowed to pass or esophageal laceration if vomiting is induced. Common sense and good communication with the client are essential. It is often preferable to remove objects by surgery or endoscopy to avoid potential complications.

Hair balls form in cats of all ages. Hair should empty from the stomach during the fasting state by a motility pattern similar to the MMC.[8] Gastric retention of hair, with subsequent formation of hair balls, may reflect abnormal gastric motility. Hair balls are often recurring problems, and preventive measures (petroleum-based lubricants and frequent grooming) are important to avoid repeated problems.[140]

LINEAR FOREIGN OBJECTS

Linear foreign objects may have one end lodged in the pylorus. Rapid diagnosis is preferred because of the potential for duodenal perforation as the intestine pleats itself around the end trailing off down the intestines.[205] If the foreign object is fixed at the base of the tongue and has been present for less than 2 to 3 days and if the patient does not have evidence of peritonitis, it is reasonable to cut the object at its point of attachment to see if it will pass through the gastrointestinal tract uneventfully.[206] However, the patient must be monitored for signs of abdominal pain or depression

(indications for surgery). One may also attempt to remove the foreign object endoscopically if present for less than 2 to 3 days, especially if it is a thick mass of cloth or cotton. It is possible to rupture a previously intact intestine, however, if one applies traction to a linear foreign object that has already compromised the intestine. One should not hesitate to proceed to surgery if the risk of perforation seems significant.[2]

ANTRAL PYLORIC HYPERTROPHY

Stenosis of the pyloric canal is one of the more common causes of gastric outlet obstruction.[69] The narrowing can be caused by hypertrophy of the circular muscle of the pylorus, by hyperplasia of the antropyloric mucosa, or by a combination of both muscular and mucosal thickening. Hypertrophy of the pyloric muscle exclusively is the least common form of the disease and is usually seen as a congenital disorder in boxers and Boston terriers.[85, 207] This disorder is referred to as congenital pyloric stenosis, benign muscular hypertrophy, congenital hypertrophic stenosis, or congenital pyloric muscle hypertrophy. Most adult dogs with antral pyloric hypertrophy are affected by either hypertrophy of the mucosa exclusively or a combination of muscular and mucosal hypertrophy. The hypertrophic mucosa may be focal (a polyp or single mucosal fold), multifocal (multiple polyps or folds), or generalized (involving the entire pyloric antrum). Synonyms for the adult syndrome include acquired antral pyloric hypertrophy, chronic hypertrophic pyloric gastropathy, acquired pyloric stenosis, chronic antral mucosal hypertrophy, pyloric or gastric mucosal hypertrophy, chronic hypertrophic gastritis, and multiple polyps of the gastric mucosa. For simplicity, it has been suggested that the disorder be referred to as congenital and adult forms of antral pyloric hypertrophy in recognition of the two ages of dogs affected, the involvement of the antrum in addition to the pylorus, the hypertrophic nature of the lesions, and the probability of a nonspecific etiology.[85]

Adult forms of antral pyloric hypertrophy affect older, predominantly male dogs of the smaller breeds (e.g., Lhasa apso, Pekingese, Maltese, Shih Tzu) (Fig. 136–4).[2, 85, 89–91, 208, 209] Histopathologic changes include hypertrophy of the mucosal or muscular layers of the pylorus, or both, with or

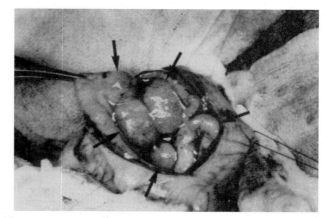

Figure 136–4. Intraoperative photograph showing large rugal folds that are pushing out through the pyloric incision in a dog with antral pyloric hypertrophy. These folds were obstructing gastric outflow. (From Willard MD: Disorders of the stomach. *In* Nelson RW, Couto CG [eds]: Essentials of Small Animal Internal Medicine, 2nd ed. St. Louis, Mosby–Year Book, 1998, p 426.)

GI

without inflammation. Gastric antral mucosal hypertrophy has also been reported in the cat.[210] The cause of the hypertrophy is unknown, although a neuroendocrine (hypergastrinemia) or stress-related cause is postulated, because many of the cases are observed in highly excitable and nervous small breeds.[211] Mild congenital pyloric stenosis or dysfunction could lead to gastric distention that in turn would stimulate gastrin secretion. Gastrin's trophic effects on pyloric musculature would eventually exacerbate the disease by encouraging pyloric muscular hypertrophy.[85] Neural dysfunction may be the underlying cause of abnormal antral motility. Antral mucosal hypertrophy may result from mucosal irritation because of chronic retention of indigestible material.

Vomiting with or without weight loss is the most common clinical sign. Dogs often have been vomiting intermittently for several months to years, and the frequency of vomiting increases as the obstruction worsens. The vomiting often occurs many hours after eating, usually contains food, and may be projectile.[85] Regurgitation caused by concurrent esophagitis is also seen.[212]

Positive-contrast radiographic studies are useful in documenting gastric outflow obstruction (delayed gastric emptying, pyloric filling defects, or a narrow and blunted pyloric canal). Ultrasonography can help identify a thick hypoechoic layer of pyloric muscle and a thickened gastric wall.[213] The diagnosis is suggested by the endoscopic appearance of an enlarged mucosal fold(s) surrounding the pyloric orifice and by exclusion of other causes, such as neoplasia, by mucosal biopsies.[214] Endoscopic biopsies are usually of sufficient quality to detect mucosal changes characteristic of the disease, but the changes are subtle.[214, 215]

Surgery is the treatment of choice for these benign lesions. Redundant tissue is resected in combination with a pyloroplasty or a pyloric antral resection (e.g., Billroth I procedure).[89, 216, 217] Biopsy of the pyloric antrum is necessary at surgery for a definitive diagnosis. Some clinicians prefer pyloromyotomy because it has fewer potential complications.[91] The prognosis is excellent if there are no postoperative problems.[2, 218, 219]

Congenital antral pyloric hypertrophy is less common than acquired antral pyloric hypertrophy. The cause is unknown. Most affected dogs are male, young to middle-aged, brachycephalic, or small breeds. The congenital form may also be seen in cats.[220] Vomiting is usually first observed in animals with congenital pyloric stenosis shortly after weaning or at an early age. The animal is usually hungry but thin and often reingests the vomitus. Chronic intermittent vomiting usually becomes more severe with time. The radiographic features of pyloric stenosis include gastric distention, delayed emptying time, and failure of contrast material to fill the pyloric canal. Stenosis may result in a "beak sign" when barium appears as a beaklike projection entering the pyloric canal. The canal may also appear elongated and narrow, with a string of contrast material passing through. In some cases, only barium mixed with food demonstrates an obstruction, whereas liquids pass through the pylorus uneventfully. Once gastric outlet obstruction has been documented, pyloric hypertrophy is diagnosed by finding muscular thickening (with perhaps redundant mucosal folds). Biopsy of the affected tissue is recommended, followed by pyloroplasty to relieve the pyloric obstruction. Pyloromyotomy is easier to perform than pyloroplasty but does not seem as reliable in enlarging the pylorus.[91, 221]

GASTRIC PHYCOMYCOSIS

Gastric phycomycosis is a systemic fungal disease caused by the ubiquitous fungus *Pythium*.[99, 100, 222, 223] It is reported most commonly in young, male, medium- to large-breed dogs from states bordering the Gulf of Mexico. Dogs are presented for chronic debilitation and vomiting because of pyloric mechanical obstruction. Diarrhea may be present, as the small intestine and colon may also be affected. An abdominal mass is often palpable on physical examination, and positive-contrast radiographic studies reveal a thickened gastric wall. Grossly, the gastric mucosa usually appears ulcerated and necrotic, often with a sharp demarcation between affected and unaffected tissue. The organism causes an intense fibrotic reaction, mimicking scirrhous carcinoma. Definitive diagnosis is made by identifying the organism with special stains in histologic sections or by fungal culture. The organism is found only in the firm, fibrotic tissues, which do not lend themselves to biopsy with a flexible endoscope. An adequate biopsy is best obtained surgically by performing an incisional biopsy.[2] Surgery is the most effective therapy for localized disease; systemic antifungal therapy has not proved effective in treating disseminated disease.

MISCELLANEOUS CAUSES

Cryptococcosis resulting in a granulomatous gastritis mimicking carcinoma has been reported in a Doberman pinscher as a cause of gastric outlet obstruction.[98] Granulomatous gastritis and severe eosinophilic gastritis can also cause pyloric obstruction. Duodenal-gastric intussusception is uncommon but has been reported in the dog.[224]

Infiltrative pyloric or duodenal neoplasia may cause mechanical obstruction of the gastric outlet. Primary gastric neoplasms include benign antral polyps and leiomyomas. Adenocarcinomas and lymphosarcomas are the most common malignant gastric tumors. Extrinsic pyloric masses, such as hepatic or pancreatic neoplasms, may cause gastric outflow obstruction via extramural compression of the pylorus. Hepatic or pancreatic abscesses and intra-abdominal neoplasia may also result in pyloric obstruction via external compression.

Iatrogenic gastric outflow obstruction in two dogs appeared to be caused by prior gastric surgery. This may be prevented by minimizing tissue inversion into the gastric lumen when surgery is performed near the pyloric outflow tract. It is important to preserve the continuity of the outflow tract when large lesions near the pylorus are resected surgically.[218]

GASTRIC DILATATION-VOLVULUS

Gastric dilatation-volvulus (GDV) is an acute life-threatening condition characterized by malposition of the stomach, rapid accumulation of air in the stomach, increased intragastric pressure, and shock. Although some progress has been made in determining risk factors, understanding the pathophysiology, and developing new treatments, the cause is still unknown.[225] The overall mortality rate for GDV is 33 per cent in dogs brought into veterinary teaching hospitals[226] and would probably be much higher if all practices were included. Early diagnosis and treatment have improved survival rate significantly, although mortality remains high at 15 per cent even with current treatments.[227–229]

Risk factors for GDV include being purebred and a large- or giant-breed dog (especially breeds with a deep and narrow thorax such as the Great Dane, Weimaraner, Saint Bernard,

Gordon setter, and Irish setter), being middle-aged to older (mean age approximately 7 years), and having a first-degree relative that had GDV.[226, 230–232] Controlled epidemiologic studies showed that eating fewer meals per day[230] and eating rapidly increased susceptibility to GDV, and dogs characterized by their owners as happy or easygoing were at lower risk than nervous or fearful dogs.[233] Epidemiologic studies have not supported a causal relationship between feeding soy-based or cereal-based dry dog food and GDV. Scientific studies do not overwhelmingly support the role of other possible contributing causes, including hypergastrinemia, exercise after ingestion of large meals of highly processed foods or water, dietary factors, and inflammatory bowel disease.[225, 226, 230, 234–237]

Delayed gastric emptying of solid particles fed with a meal has been documented in dogs with GDV after surgical treatment and recovery,[238, 239] whereas the liquid phase of gastric emptying was not similarly affected.[240, 241] Using radiopaque particles mixed with food, gastric emptying was assessed in healthy dogs not subjected to surgery, in healthy dogs 9 to 35 days after circumcostal gastropexy, and in dogs 1 to 54 months after surgical treatment and recovery from GDV. Circumcostal gastropexy surgery did not alter the 90 per cent gastric emptying time for radiopaque particles in healthy dogs. However, the 90 per cent gastric emptying time was significantly increased after circumcostal gastropexy in dogs with GDV compared with healthy dogs after the same surgical procedure and recovery period. These results suggest that dogs with GDV have delayed gastric emptying of solid particles, although it is still unclear whether delayed gastric emptying of markers in affected dogs after surgical treatment and recovery is the result or the cause of GDV. Other studies indicate that delayed gastric emptying in the GDV syndrome is associated with increased gastric slow-wave propagation velocity in the fed state.[242] Atypical fasting state phase III activity suggests that gastric emptying may be impaired in the fasting state as well.[242] These results imply that electrophysiologic abnormalities in gastric smooth muscle cells may be associated with delayed gastric emptying. Because delayed gastric emptying predisposes to chronic gastric distention, which could stretch the gastrohepatic ligament and permit increased stomach mobility, it has been hypothesized that a primary disorder of gastric motility might precede and predispose the dog to GDV.[243] Hepatogastric ligaments in GDV-affected dogs were significantly longer than those of control dogs.[243] Others have also speculated that gastric dysrhythmias may predispose to GDV.[244, 245]

Two dogs were reported to develop GDV 2 and 17 months, respectively, after splenectomy for treatment of splenic torsion. Splenic displacement and torsion may stretch the gastric ligaments, allowing increased mobility of the stomach. After splenectomy, an anatomic void may be created in the cranioventral part of the abdomen, contributing to the mobility of the stomach.[246]

Acute gastric dilatation with torsion has also been reported in cats. Two of five cats reported in one case series had concomitant diaphragmatic hernia. Clinical signs and therapeutic management are similar in cats and dogs.[247]

PATHOPHYSIOLOGY

Gastric dilatation refers to distention of the stomach, caused most often by swallowed air, fluid, and/or food. Gastric dilatation implies an innocuous condition that can easily be corrected by passing a stomach tube to relieve the distention. GDV is different, however, from simple engorgement caused by overeating (a syndrome that occurs most commonly in young animals) or gastric distention caused by aerophagia. In GDV, the air-filled stomach becomes tympanic because of the large volume of air present.[248] Dogs experiencing gastric dilatation almost invariably have gastric volvulus.[249] A fundamental abnormality associated with GDV is laxity of the hepatoduodenal and hepatogastric ligaments, leading to a high degree of mobility of the stomach within the abdomen.[249] This allows the stomach to twist about on its longitudinal axis at the esophageal cardia and the pylorus. In normal dogs, the pylorus is tightly fixed to the cranial right quadrant of the abdomen by the hepatoduodenal ligament, lesser omentum, and common bile duct. Even though the pylorus in normal dogs can be forced to the left and placed in a volvulus position, it immediately returns to its normal position when released. The stomach of a dog that has experienced GDV, however, can easily be placed in the volvulus position and remains in an abnormal position when released. Thus, both gastric dilatation and a predisposition for gastric volvulus must be present to produce the GDV syndrome.

Generally, the stomach rotates in a clockwise direction when viewed from the surgeon's perspective (with the dog on its back and the clinician standing at the dog's side, facing cranially; Fig. 136–5). The rotation may be 90 to 360 degrees but is usually 220 to 270 degrees.[250] When the stomach twists, the pylorus and duodenum move ventrally, passing under the stomach and to the left of midline, finally coming to rest dorsally above the cardia on the dog's left side. Because the spleen is attached to the greater curvature of the stomach via the gastrosplenic ligament, twisting of the stomach usually displaces the spleen to the right ventral

GI

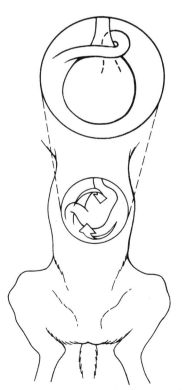

Figure 136–5. Direction of gastric rotation in most dogs with GDV. (From Fossum TW: Surgery of the stomach. *In* Fossum TW [ed]: Small Animal Surgery. St. Louis, Mosby–Year Book, 1997, p 278.)

side of the abdomen and causes congestion and splenomegaly.

Gastric torsion-volvulus results in occlusion of the cardia and obstruction of the pylorus. This prevents belching of air or vomiting of ingesta and prohibits pyloric emptying into the duodenum. It is postulated that after volvulus develops, swallowed air can pass the twisted gastroesophageal junction but cannot escape the stomach. Gastric dilatation results in increased gastric wall tension, decreased blood flow, local ischemic injury, and gastric wall necrosis. The most commonly infarcted area is along the greater curvature in the area served by the short gastric vessels.[251] GDV also causes splenic engorgement and compression of major abdominal vessels returning blood to the heart.[252] Occlusion of the portal vein and posterior vena cava reduces venous return to the heart, which in turn dramatically decreases cardiac output and mean arterial pressure, leading to hypovolemic shock. Inadequate tissue perfusion affects multiple organs, including the heart (myocardial ischemia), kidney (acute renal failure), pancreas (myocardial depressant factor, tumor necrosis factor-α),[253, 254] liver (depressed reticuloendothelial cell function prevents removal of endotoxin),[255] and small intestine (local acidosis, subepithelial hemorrhage and edema, followed by hemorrhagic enteritis). In addition, occlusion of the portal vein and caudal vena cava causes marked passive chronic congestion of the abdominal viscera. The organs suffer from ischemia as well as accumulation of endotoxin (from the gastrointestinal tract), which in turn activates many inflammatory mediators. Endotoxemia and damage to endothelium lead to activation of the coagulation cascade, and DIC may result. The enlarged stomach also encroaches on the thoracic diaphragm, which decreases tidal volume of the lungs and further impairs ventilation-perfusion matching. Ultimately, shock reaches a point of irreversibility (probably caused by endotoxemia), whereupon death ensues regardless of therapy.[249]

DIAGNOSIS

A dog with GDV may present with a history of an acute progressively distending abdomen, nonproductive retching, hypersalivation, restlessness, depression, weakness, and abdominal pain.[2] Physical examination usually reveals abdominal distention with tympany, although it may be difficult to detect gastric distention in heavily muscled large-breed or obese dogs. There is also evidence of poor perfusion and/or shock, such as weak peripheral pulses, tachycardia, prolonged capillary refill time, pale mucous membranes, or dyspnea. Often, GDV is diagnosed in the examination room on the basis of signalment, history, and physical examination, and therapy is begun immediately. If unsure, radiographic evaluation may be necessary, although caution should be exercised because positioning these dogs for radiography may further impair cardiopulmonary function. Affected animals should be decompressed before radiographs are taken. Right lateral and dorsoventral radiographic views are preferred.[256] On a right lateral view of a dog with GDV the pylorus lies dorsal and cranial to the body of the stomach and is separated from the rest of the stomach by a soft tissue fold (antral wall folding back) (Fig. 136–6). On the dorsoventral view, the pylorus appears as a gas-filled structure to the left of midline. Free abdominal air suggests gastric rupture.

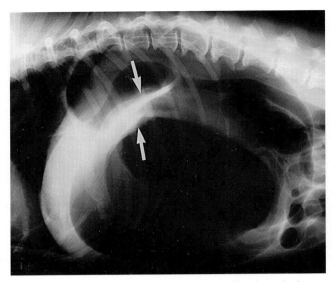

Figure 136–6. Gastric distention in the gastric dilatation-volvulus syndrome. A right lateral abdominal radiograph showing a greatly dilated stomach with a "shelf" (arrows) of tissue, demonstrating that the stomach is malpositioned (i.e., twisted). (From Willard MD: Diagnostic tests of the gastrointestinal system. *In* Nelson RW, Couto CG [eds]: Essentials of Small Animal Internal Medicine. St. Louis, Mosby–Year Book, 1992, p 289.)

MANAGEMENT OF GASTRIC DILATATION-VOLVULUS

Shock

One or more large-bore intravenous catheters are placed in either a jugular or both cephalic veins. Either high-volume isotonic fluids (40 mL/lb per hour) or low-volume hypertonic saline (7% NaCl solution in 6% dextran, 2 ml/lb over 5 to 15 minutes)[257] or hetastarch (2.5 to 4.5 ml/lb over 10 to 15 minutes) is administered.[258] The animal should be monitored closely and the isotonic fluid administration rate decreased if clinical improvement occurs. If clinical signs of shock persist, fluid administration should continue at a high rate until a response is noted. The PCV and total protein should be monitored regularly during fluid therapy for shock. Whole blood or plasma should be administered if the PCV falls below 20 per cent or total protein falls below 3.5 g/dL, respectively.[249] Although it is controversial, corticosteroids (dexamethasone sodium phosphate, 2 mg/lb or prednisone sodium succinate, 10 mg/lb, intravenously) are usually administered for endotoxemia and to stabilize lysosomal membranes.[259] Bactericidal antibiotics are usually administered intravenously (e.g., cefazolin or ampicillin plus enrofloxacin). Flunixin meglumine is recommended (0.25 to 0.5 mg/lb intravenously once) to decrease prostaglandin synthesis and attenuate the effects of endotoxemia, although it may cause severe gastrointestinal ulceration.[260] Sodium bicarbonate is administered if indicated on the basis of the blood gas analysis.[261] Sequestration of hydrogen ions in the gastric lumen can offset the lactic acidosis, causing the blood pH to be normal. Therefore, bicarbonate therapy should not be routinely administered.

Gastric Decompression

Gastric decompression should be performed at the same time shock therapy is begun.[262] Gastric decompression immediately improves cardiac output and arterial blood pressure by relieving caudal vena caval and portal venous occlusion. An orogastric tube is premeasured from the point of the nose to the last rib and a tape mark made on the tube so that when it is passed it is not advanced too far. Placing the animal in different positions (sitting, on a tilt table, or with front legs elevated on a table) may help to advance the tube by shifting the weight of the abdominal viscera. The tube is advanced with firm pressure and a twisting motion. If an orogastric tube does not pass, intragastric pressure should be reduced by gastrocentesis. Gastrocentesis is performed in an aseptically prepared area caudal to the costal arch on the right flank with several 16- to 18-gauge hypodermic needles. The region should be "pinged" using a stethoscope to determine where the spleen is located. Relief of intragastric pressure by gastrocentesis usually allows passage of an orogastric tube. Once positioned, the tube is used to remove as much gastric liquid and gas as possible. Gastric lavage using warm water may help to remove ingesta. One should note whether there is evidence of blood in the gastric contents.[2]

If necessary for intubation, the animal may be lightly sedated with oxymorphone (maximum of 0.1 to 0.2 mg/lb, intravenously to effect).[263] If the stomach tube still cannot be passed after gastrocentesis, temporary decompression may be achieved by performing a temporary gastrostomy. However, in this procedure there is a high risk for peritoneal contamination and the opening must be closed before the permanent gastropexy is performed.

Surgery

Several studies have shown no association between the time from admission to a clinic to the time of surgery and outcome.[227, 228] The presence of gastric necrosis at surgery is, however, associated with a much higher risk of dying.[227–229] If no blood is present in the gastric contents, it may be advantageous to stabilize the patient's condition for a few hours or even overnight before performing corrective surgery and gastropexy.[2] If the stomach is twisted, it continues to have impaired mucosal perfusion even when deflated[264]; therefore, surgery should be delayed only as long as necessary to give the patient the best anesthetic risk possible. The benefits of delaying surgery are that surgery can be performed at a more opportune time, the dog can be safely transported to a referral center, and a full preoperative diagnostic evaluation can be perfomed.[262] A pharyngostomy tube may be used to maintain gastric decompression. The disadvantages of delaying surgery include failure to detect necrosis or leakage of gastric contents, more time for cardiac arrhythmias to develop, and continued damage to the gastric mucosa. An electrocardiogram should be monitored to detect cardiac arrhythmias.

If the patient has blood in the gastric contents, surgery should be performed as soon as the patient is capable of withstanding anesthesia because of the danger of gastric perforation related to devitalization of the gastric wall. The stomach is repositioned and, if necessary, devitalized tissue is resected, or a partial gastric invagination technique may be performed.[265] If there is splenic necrosis or significant infarction, a partial or complete splenectomy is performed. A permanent gastropexy is performed to prevent recurrence of GDV. Many surgical procedures have been developed to attach the stomach permanently to the body wall and prevent recurrence of GDV.[266, 267] These include tube gastropexy,[268, 269] circumcostal gastropexy,[270–274] muscular flap gastropexy,[275] belt-loop gastropexy,[276] and incisional gastropexy.[277, 278] Randomized controlled trials comparing different types of gastropexy have not been conducted. The choice

of a particular technique depends on individual preference. Probably the most critical factors in success rate are the surgeon's familiarity with a technique and ability to perform it proficiently and in a timely manner.[225] Failure rates are in the range of 3 to 8 per cent. Right-sided percutaneous gastrostomy is not recommended as a means of prophylactic gastropexy.[279] Corrective pyloric surgery is not recommended.[266, 280] Intermittent gastric dilatation may occur after gastropexy.[278, 281]

Ischemia-Reperfusion Injury

Restoration of tissue perfusion and oxygenation can initiate deleterious biochemical reactions that contribute to further tissue damage. This phenomenon is called reperfusion injury.[282, 283] During ischemia, conditions develop that predispose to the production of oxygen free radicals upon reperfusion. First, ATP undergoes degradation, resulting in accumulation of hypoxanthine. Second, intracellular calcium increases and activates calpain, a protease that converts xanthine dehydrogenase to xanthine oxidase. Xanthine oxidase catalyzes the conversion of hypoxanthine to superoxide radicals in the presence of oxygen. Superoxide radicals are converted to hydrogen peroxide by superoxide dismutase. Superoxide radicals and hydrogen peroxide react, forming hydroxyl radicals.

During reperfusion an overabundance of free radicals is generated, which overwhelms the normal antioxidant defense mechanisms (superoxide dismutase, catalase, glutathione peroxidase, alpha-tocopherol, ascorbate, beta-carotene). The hydroxyl radical is a potent oxidizing agent, which initiates cell membrane lipoperoxidation. This results in increased cell membrane permeability, increased microvascular permeability, tissue edema, inflammatory cell influx, hemorrhage, and mucosal necrosis. Neutrophils play a major role in the pathophysiology of reperfusion injury. Neutrophil activation and degranulation lead to synthesis and release of numerous enzymes (proteases) and oxygen free radicals. Inhibition of neutrophil adhesion or neutrophil depletion has been shown to reduce or prevent gastrointestinal tract injury. Intestinal mucosal injury can be attenuated by both protease inhibitors and scavengers of oxygen free radicals.

Lipid peroxidation activity in the duodenum, jejunum, colon, liver, and pancreas was significantly less during reperfusion in dogs with experimentally induced GDV treated with a lipid peroxidation inhibitor.[284, 285] Free radical scavengers such as deferoxamine and allopurinol may also protect abdominal organs against reperfusion injury. These results suggest that drugs that prevent lipid peroxidation may be useful for reducing the mortality associated with GDV. Results of use of these drugs in clinical trials have, however, not been published.

Cardiac Arrhythmias

Arrhythmias are a common sequela of GDV and usually begin 12 to 36 hours postoperatively.[286, 287] Electrocardiographic monitoring of all GDV patients should be performed throughout hospitalization. Ventricular tachyarrhythmias (premature ventricular contractions, paroxysmal ventricular tachycardia, and multifocal ventricular tachycardia) are most frequently described.[286–288] They are generally self-limiting in 2 to 4 days.[249] The mechanisms that initiate and maintain these arrhythmias are varied and include acid-base abnormalities, electrolyte abnormalities, autonomic imbalances, myocardial depressant factors, and myocardial ischemia.[286] They

GI

should be treated if they are severe enough to decrease cardiac output, the origin is multifocal, ventricular rate exceeds 160 beats per minute, pulses are weak or shock is present, and subsequent premature beats are inscribed on the wave of the previous complex (R on T phenomena).[249, 250] See treatment of arrhythmias (Chapter 114). Contributing factors should be corrected. Hypokalemia, acidosis, and hypoxia promote arrhythmias and make them resistant to antiarrhythmic therapy.[2] The presence of cardiac arrhythmias may not be associated with an unfavorable outcome.[227, 228] In contrast, others have reported mortality rates as high as 38 per cent in dogs with preoperative cardiac arrhythmias.[229]

Postoperative Care

Electrolyte, fluid, and acid-base status should be monitored postoperatively. Fluid therapy is based on clinical findings. Shock that persists into the postoperative period must be treated vigorously with crystalloid fluids. Whole blood and plasma must be administered to maintain the PCV and total protein above critical levels. Intravenous fluid therapy is continued until hydration can be maintained by oral fluid intake. Hypokalemia is common and requires potassium supplementation. Sepsis and DIC are also potential complications.[289] Gastritis secondary to mucosal ischemia is also common and may result in gastric hemorrhage or vomiting. Antiemetics and H$_2$ receptor blockers (e.g., cimetidine, ranitidine, or famotidine) may be beneficial in controlling vomiting and decreasing gastric acidity. Ranitidine may also promote gastric emptying.[290] Metoclopramide may be useful as an antiemetic agent but would be unlikely to promote increased gastric emptying.[291] Cisapride is recommended as a prokinetic agent to speed gastric emptying in dogs with GDV.[82, 204]

Prognosis for GDV is guarded. Several studies have been conducted to examine survival and recurrence data after acute GDV. Dogs depressed or comatose upon admission were 3 and 36 times, respectively, more likely to die than alert dogs, and those with gastric necrosis were 11 times more likely to die.[227] The recurrence rate ranges from 54.5 to 75.8 per cent for those that do not have gastropexies and from 4.3 to 6.6 per cent for those that do.[227, 278, 292, 293]

In dogs at high risk for GDV, it may be prudent to consider gastropexy as an elective surgery to prevent GDV. Circumcostal gastropexy has not been shown to delay gastric emptying or to alter gastric myoelectric activity.[238, 294]

Chronic Gastric Volvulus

Chronic gastric volvulus[241, 295, 296] is less common and more difficult to recognize than acute GDV.[2] Malpositioning of the stomach may be constant or intermittent. Clinically, vomiting with or without abdominal distention and/or pain may be observed. These signs may be intermittent and mild so that the diagnosis of GDV is not considered initially. Multiple radiographs are needed over a period of days or weeks to confirm the diagnosis.[2]

GASTRIC MOTILITY DISORDERS

There are three general types of gastric motility disorders: accelerated gastric emptying, retrograde transit (e.g., enterogastric and gastroesophageal reflux), and delayed gastric emptying (mechanical and functional obstruction).

ACCELERATED GASTRIC EMPTYING

Gastric motility disorders associated with accelerated transit are usually iatrogenic in origin; for example, postprandial dumping syndrome may occur after gastroenterostomy.[30, 34, 297–299] Prokinetic drug therapy may also result in accelerated gastric emptying.

RETROGRADE TRANSIT

Gastric motility disorders associated with retrograde transit include vomiting, gastroesophageal reflux, duodenogastric reflux, and bilious vomiting syndrome. Vomiting is a common gastroenterologic sign and it represents the extreme form of retrograde transit.[300] Gastroesophageal reflux is a less extreme form of retrograde transit, and delayed gastric emptying may contribute to the signs of gastroesophageal reflux. Abnormalities in liquid and/or solid food emptying and in antral contractility have been observed in patients with gastroesophageal reflux.[30]

Duodenogastric reflux can be a normal physiologic event,[301–303] an epiphenomenon associated with an undetermined gastric motility disorder (abnormal pyloric function), or it may be secondary to chronic gastritis. Bilious vomiting syndrome in dogs is an idiopathic disorder associated with duodenogastric reflux of bile.[2, 85] Affected dogs tend to vomit small amounts of bile in the morning on an empty stomach after an overnight fast. The definitive diagnosis of these disorders is often based on symptomatic response to therapy.

DELAYED GASTRIC EMPTYING: MECHANICAL OBSTRUCTION

Anatomic lesions of the pylorus and adjacent duodenal segment (e.g., pyloric stenosis or chronic hypertrophic pyloric gastropathy,[89–91, 211] infiltrative pyloric or duodenal neoplasia,[304] chronic hypertrophic gastritis,[210] eosinophilic gastritis, gastric phycomycosis,[99, 100] hepatic or pancreatic abscesses, intra-abdominal neoplasia, gastric foreign bodies, antral polyps[305]) impede gastric emptying by mechanical obstruction. In general, diagnosis of mechanical obstruction is usually straightforward and involves survey and contrast radiography, ultrasonography,[213] and/or gastroscopy.[214] Surgical removal of the foreign object or the affected area is the preferred therapy. Gastrointestinal prokinetic agents are contraindicated in treating patients with mechanical obstruction.

DELAYED GASTRIC EMPTYING: FUNCTIONAL OBSTRUCTION

Functional disorders of gastric emptying (referred to as delayed gastric emptying or gastroparesis) result from one or more abnormalities in gastric motility (e.g., abnormalities in myenteric neuronal or gastric smooth muscle function) or from abnormalities in antropyloroduodenal coordination. Delayed gastric emptying is now recognized as an important cause of upper gastrointestinal tract signs (e.g., anorexia and vomiting). Gastric emptying disorders are usually diagnosed after mechanical obstruction has been ruled out.

Delayed gastric emptying has been reported in animals recovering from GDV,[238, 242] infectious and inflammatory gastric diseases,[69, 130, 306] experimental gastric ulcer,[307, 308] and radiation gastritis.[309] Pyloric dysfunction has been reported in Siamese cats with delayed gastric emptying and no visible lesions.[212] Delayed gastric emptying has also been associated with several secondary conditions, including electrolyte disturbances (e.g., hypokalemia), metabolic disorders (e.g., hypoadrenocorticism,[310–312] diabetes mellitus, hypergastrinemia,[313] and uremia), concurrent drug usage (e.g., anticholinergics, beta-adrenergic agonists, and opiates[7, 314–318]), acute stress (e.g., sympathetic stimulation or spinal cord injury), and acute abdominal inflammation.[69] More commonly, an underlying condition is not identified, and the condition is referred to as idiopathic delayed gastric emptying.

TREATMENT

Dietary management and gastric prokinetic agents are used to treat patients with delayed gastric emptying disorders.[319] Surgical procedures are often unsuccessful. Dietary management is based on the knowledge that liquids are emptied from the stomach more rapidly than solids, carbohydrates are emptied more rapidly than proteins, and proteins are emptied more rapidly than lipids. A low-fat, low-protein diet of liquid or semiliquid consistency should be fed at frequent intervals to facilitate gastric emptying. Diets should be selected for low acidity and low osmolality and should be fed at warm temperatures (72 to 100°F).

Gastric prokinetic agents should be considered for patients that fail to respond to dietary management alone. Cisapride is the drug of choice for treating delayed gastric emptying, followed by erythromycin and ranitidine or nizatidine.

Effective gastroprokinetic agents stimulate contractions in the gastropyloroduodenal area and accelerate gastric emptying. Stimulation of contractions alone is not enough to accelerate gastric emptying, as demonstrated by bethanechol chloride.[320] Bethanechol stimulates gastric contractions yet has no significant effect on the rate of gastric emptying. Thus, an effective gastroprokinetic agent must also stimulate other parameters that influence gastric emptying, such as the percentage of contractions that propagate in the stomach, the percentage of contractions that propagate from the antrum or pylorus to the duodenum, or the percentage of contractions that propagate in the duodenum.[321] Gastroprokinetic agents may affect only a few specific parameters of gastropyloroduodenal contractions. Thus, whether a particular agent works in a specific patient with delayed gastric emptying depends on the underlying disturbance in that patient and the specific parameters of gastropyloroduodenal contractions that the particular agent can influence.[321]

Cisapride is the first-choice gastric prokinetic agent.[82, 204, 321] Cisapride is representative of a group of serotonergic or 5-HT drugs that bind 5-HT$_4$ receptors on enteric postganglionic cholinergic neurons and stimulate contraction of intestinal smooth muscle. The recommended dosage of cisapride for dogs and cats has been 0.05 to 0.25 mg/lb two to three times daily by mouth. This dosage range was derived from studies of the effect of cisapride on normal gastric emptying in dogs. Higher dosages of cisapride (0.25 to 0.5 mg/lb two to three times daily by mouth) may be necessary to enhance gastric emptying in dogs with delayed gastric emptying.

Cisapride accelerates gastric emptying in dogs by stimulating pyloric and duodenal motor activity, by enhancing antropyloroduodenal coordination, and by increasing the mean propagation distance of duodenal contractions. In this regard, cisapride appears to be superior to metoclopramide

and domperidone in stimulating gastric emptying. Cisapride enhances cholinergic neurotransmission and motility in the canine antrum without activating 5-HT receptors; the neuronal receptor mediating this response has not been characterized.[322]

Cisapride lacks the antidopaminergic properties typical of metoclopramide and domperidone. Thus, cisapride does not induce the hyperprolactinemia that is typical of metoclopramide and domperidone, and cisapride has only weak antiemetic effects against apomorphine-induced vomiting in dogs. Concurrent administration of anticholinergic compounds (e.g., atropine, aminopentamide, isopropamide) would be expected to compromise some of the beneficial effects of cisapride. Concurrent administration of cimetidine, on the other hand, could lead to increased plasma cisapride concentrations, because cimetidine inhibits cytochrome P-450 enzyme systems. The facilitation of gastric emptying by cisapride could affect the rate of absorption of other drugs. Animals receiving drugs with a narrow therapeutic ratio (e.g., digoxin, anticonvulsants) should be monitored closely.

Metoclopramide may be used as a gastric prokinetic and antiemetic agent.[76, 321] The antiemetic effect is mediated through antagonism of dopaminergic D$_2$ receptors, and the prokinetic effect is mediated through agonism of serotoninergic 5-HT$_4$ receptors. The prokinetic dose of metoclopramide for use in the dog and cat is 0.1 to 0.25 mg/lb every 8 hours administered either orally or parenterally. Continuous intravenous infusions may also be administered at doses of 0.005 to 0.01 mg/lb every 1 hour or 0.5 to 1.0 mg/lb over 24 hours.

In normal dogs, gastric emptying time is not significantly shortened by metoclopramide.[321] Whereas cisapride stimulates most parameters of gastropyloroduodenal contractions that accelerate gastric emptying, metoclopramide enhances mainly the antropyloroduodenal coordination.[321] Metoclopramide may be more effective as a prokinetic agent for gastric emptying of liquids rather than solids. In one study, using a double radioisotopic technique to assess simultaneous gastric emptying of solids and liquids, metoclopramide was shown to decrease the gastric emptying time of the liquid phase 1 hour postprandially but to have no effect on the gastric emptying time of the solid phase.[323] In another study, metoclopramide was shown to speed gastric emptying of liquids but to slow the emptying of digestible solids.[324] The central antiemetic effect of metoclopramide is probably superior to its peripheral prokinetic effect.

Metoclopramide inhibits vomiting associated with activation of central dopaminergic D$_2$ receptors in the chemoreceptor trigger zone. Metoclopramide may also act peripherally to diminish the severity of vomiting through its effects on motility, by preventing gastric stasis and the retrograde peristalsis that precedes vomiting. Thus, metoclopramide is indicated for the treatment of nausea and vomiting associated with delayed gastric emptying.

If cisapride fails to improve gastric emptying, erythromycin is the second drug of choice.[325, 326] Erythromycin at low antimicrobially ineffective doses accelerates gastric emptying by inducing antral contractions that are similar, but not identical, to those associated with phase III of the MMC. Phase III contractions, which usually occur only during the fasting state, empty the stomach of indigestible solids. Erythromycin accelerates gastric emptying of solids during the fed state, so that food is inadequately triturated (i.e., food particles > 0.5 mm) and emptied into the small intestine. Previous studies have shown that the stomach empties only 6 per cent of solids as particles larger than 0.5 mm.

Because of the small surface area/mass ratio associated with large chunks of food, the small intestine may inadequately digest and absorb these nutrients. Thus, erythromycin should be used as a gastric prokinetic agent with the understanding that it is inducing an interdigestive motor pattern and not restoring a normal fed pattern of gastric motility and that food is not expelled as normally digestible particles of small size. If large particles of food in the small bowel cause intestinal distress, use of this prokinetic drug may not lead to an improvement and could actually increase symptoms despite more rapid gastric emptying.

The recommended antimicrobial dosage of erythromycin for dogs and cats is 5 to 10 mg/lb every 8 hours orally. However, the prokinetic dosage of erythromycin for dogs and cats is probably much lower, 0.25 to 0.5 mg/lb three times daily. No serious drug interactions have been reported in veterinary species.

Ranitidine and nizatidine are competitive, reversible, histaminergic H_2 receptor antagonists that were developed to inhibit gastric acid secretion. They also stimulate gastrointestinal motility by inhibiting acetylcholinesterase activity, thereby increasing the amount of acetylcholine available to bind smooth muscle muscarinic cholinergic receptors.[179, 181, 290] Prokinetic effects would be expected at the clinically recommended dosages of ranitidine used for antisecretory activity (0.5 to 1 mg/lb twice daily). Nizatidine also stimulates gastric contractions and accelerates gastric emptying comparably to cisapride at gastric antisecretory doses (1 to 2.5 mg/lb once daily).

GASTRIC NEOPLASIA

The incidence of benign and malignant gastric neoplasia in the dog and cat is low, accounting for less than 1 per cent of all malignancies.[327] Adenocarcinoma accounts for 60 to 70 per cent of cancers of the canine stomach.[327] Lymphoma is the most common gastric tumor in the cat, and most cats with gastric lymphoma are feline leukemia virus negative.[327] Gastric neoplasia impairs gastric function by causing pyloric outflow obstruction (mass effect), by preventing normal peristalsis, and by disrupting mucosal integrity (ulceration and inflammation). Chronic vomiting, anorexia, and weight loss are common clinical signs. Other signs in dogs include hematemesis, abdominal pain, melena, and anemia caused by ulceration. Lesions are often far advanced at the time of diagnosis.[2, 327, 328]

BENIGN GASTRIC TUMORS

Polyps

Polyps are one of the more common benign gastric tumors of dogs and cats.[2] They may be adenomatous or hyperplastic. Unless they produce gastric outflow obstruction, most are found incidentally during gastroscopy for other problems. Biopsies of polyps should be obtained as they cannot be distinguished from malignant tumors accurately without histopathologic examination. Because of the concern that adenomatous polyps in human beings are preneoplastic, although this has not been proved in the dog, it seems appropriate to remove them surgically in animals.[2]

Gastric Leiomyomas

These tumors are usually discrete solitary lesions found near the gastroesophageal junction.[327, 329] The average age of dogs with gastric leiomyomas is 15 years.[327] They usually do not cause clinical signs. Rarely, they may cause vomiting or result in megaesophagus if they obstruct the lower esophageal sphincter. Tumor-associated hypoglycemia has been reported with gastric leiomyomas.[330, 331] Surgical resection should be curative.[2, 331]

MALIGNANT GASTRIC TUMORS

Adenocarcinoma

Carcinomas are usually primary tumors found in older animals, more often near the lesser curvature and in the antrum and pyloric areas.[2, 168, 328] The average age of animals with carcinomas is 8 years, with a 2.5:1 male-to-female ratio.[327] These lesions are often scirrhous (firm and white serosally) because of their marked fibrous connective tissue content. They can be diffusely infiltrative, expansile with a central crater and ulceration, or polypoid.[327] Adenocarcinomas frequently spread to regional lymph nodes (70 to 80 per cent at necropsy), followed by the liver and lung.[327] Gastric adenocarcinoma is rare in the cat.[332]

Lymphosarcoma

Gastric lymphosarcoma is the most common feline gastric malignant neoplasia and the second most common malignant tumor in dogs (also more common in male dogs).[333] Gastric lymphosarcoma may be limited to the stomach or be one part of a disseminated neoplastic condition. Dogs with gastric lymphosarcoma often have involvement of the liver.[333] If limited to the stomach, the tumor may be diffuse or form a solitary mass. Mucosal erosions are often present.[2]

Others

Other reported canine malignancies include leiomyosarcoma,[334] extramedullary plasmacytoma,[335, 336] and fibrosarcoma. Metastatic tumors are uncommon. These include adenocarcinomas of mammary glands, liver, pancreas, and intestines; lymphosarcoma; hemangiosarcoma; and mast cell tumors.[337] Gastric leiomyosarcoma has been associated with persistent hypoglycemia and low serum insulin levels.[331, 338]

DIAGNOSIS

Routine clinical pathology tests and survey radiographs (abdominal and thoracic) are generally not diagnostic. Thoracic radiographs should be taken in a patient with suspected gastric neoplasia, however, because 30 per cent of dogs with gastric adenocarcinoma have visible pulmonary metastases at the time of diagnosis.[339] A microcytic, hypochromic anemia is common, and occult blood may be present in the feces. Liver enzymes may be elevated because of hepatic metastasis or bile duct obstruction. Smooth muscle tumors may be associated with persistent hypoglycemia.[331] Positive or double-contrast gastric radiography may reveal a mass lesion extending into the lumen. Delayed gastric emptying or adherence of contrast material to an ulcerated tumor may also be detected.[327] Ultrasonography is a useful tool for the detection and diagnosis of gastric epithelial neoplasia and mesenteric lymphadenopathy.[340, 341] The most common ultrasonographic finding is transmural thickening of the gastric wall associated with altered wall layering, called pseudolayering.

Diagnosis of gastric neoplasia requires cytologic or histopathologic examination of biopsy specimens from abnormal tissue.[2] Endoscopic biopsy is usually adequate but may fail to diagnose tumors in some animals.[86] This happens when the lesions are submucosal only or if gastric tumors have superficial necrosis, inflammation, and ulceration. Multiple, deep mucosal biopsy specimens should be obtained. Ultrasonography can be used to obtain diagnostic samples.[340] Open surgical biopsy is the most definitive diagnostic method.[327] The diagnosis of gastric lymphosarcoma may be missed if superficial lymphocytic infiltrates, which mimic inflammatory bowel disease, overlie lymphosarcomatous infiltrates in the deeper mucosa. Lymphocytic gastritis may also be diagnosed in a patient with a well-differentiated lymphocytic gastric lymphosarcoma.[2]

THERAPY

Except for lymphoma, surgery is the most common form of treatment for gastric neoplasia.[327] Advanced-stage disease in a difficult-to-operate area (lesser curvature, antrum, and pylorus) and metastasis may make neoplasms inoperable. (All abdominal lymph nodes should be examined for metastasis.) If the cancer is localized to the stomach, a curative resection may be attempted (wide partial gastrectomy or antrectomy followed by a gastroduodenostomy).[327] This surgery, called a Billroth I, can also be performed for obstructive lesions that cannot be completely removed at surgery in order to provide an outlet for the stomach.[216] Partial gastrectomy and gastrojejunostomy (Billroth II) can be performed palliatively to allow passage of food into the intestine, although this procedure is associated with significant postoperative morbidity (ulceration and leakage at the site of the gastrojejunostomy), and the patient eventually dies from the malignant disease. No effective chemotherapy is known for adenocarcinoma.[327]

Leiomyomas in the area of the cardia can easily be "shelled out" via midline laparotomy, gastrotomy, and submucosal removal or via intercostal thoracotomy. Lymphoma may be excised if localized but generally does not respond well to chemotherapy.[327] Radiation therapy is rarely utilized because of the poor radiation tolerance of surrounding normal tissue (liver and intestine).[327]

The prognosis for most malignant gastric cancer is poor because of the advanced nature at the time of diagnosis, surgical complications of gastric resection, and frequent metastasis.[3] Even with surgery, most patients die within 6 months as a result of recurrence or metastasis.[216, 327] For adenocarcinoma patients, palliation via bypass can be achieved for 1 to 6 months, although the short-term morbidity with radical resection can be high.[342–344] Cats with solitary lymphosarcoma might have a better prognosis than those with diffuse lymphosarcoma of the alimentary tract.[339] The median survival for dogs with gastric leiomyosarcoma that survived gastric resection was 1 year.[334] Benign tumors can be cured with complete surgical excision.

REFERENCES

1. Miller ME, Christensen GC, Evans HE. The digestive system and abdomen. *In* Miller ME, Christensen GC, Evans HE (eds): Anatomy of the Dog. Philadelphia, WB Saunders, 1964, pp 645–712.
2. Willard MD: Diseases of the stomach. *In* Ettinger SJ, Feldman EC (eds): Textbook of Veterinary Internal Medicine, 4th ed. Philadelphia, WB Saunders, 1995, pp 1143–1168.
3. Twedt DC, Magne ML: Diseases of the stomach. *In* Ettinger SJ (ed): Textbook of Veterinary Internal Medicine, 3rd ed. Philadelphia, WB Saunders, 1989, pp 1289–1322.
4. Guilford WG, Strombeck DR: Gastric structure and function. *In* Guilford WG, Center SA, Strombeck DR, et al (eds): Strombeck's Small Animal Gastroenterology, 3rd ed. Philadelphia, WB Saunders, 1996, pp 239–255.
5. Moon M, Myer W: Gastrointestinal contrast radiology in small animals. Semin Vet Med Surg 1:121–143, 1986.
6. Burks TF. Neurotransmission and neurotransmitters. *In* Johnson LR (ed): Physiology of the Gastrointestinal Tract, 3rd ed. New York, Raven, 1994, pp 211–242.
7. Dockray GJ: Physiology of enteric neuropeptides. *In* Johnson LR (ed): Physiology of the Gastrointestinal Tract, 3rd ed. New York, Raven, 1994, pp 169–209.
8. Hall JA, Burrows CF, Twedt DC: Gastric motility in dogs. Part I. Normal gastric function. Compend Contin Educ Pract Vet 10:1282–1293, 1988.
9. Kelly KA: Gastric emptying of liquids and solids: Roles of proximal and distal stomach. Am J Physiol 239:G71–G76, 1980.
10. Meyer JH: Motility of the stomach and gastroduodenal junction. *In* Johnson LR (ed): Physiology of the Gastrointestinal Tract, 2nd ed. New York, Raven, 1987, pp 613–629.
11. Barbier AJ, Lefebvre RA: Involvement of the ʟ-arginine:nitric oxide pathway in nonadrenergic noncholinergic relaxation of the cat gastric fundus. J Pharmacol Exp Ther 266: 172–178, 1993.
12. Sachs G: The gastric H,K ATPase. Regulation and structure/function of the acid pump of the stomach. *In* Johnson LR (ed): Physiology of the Gastrointestinal Tract, 3rd ed. New York, Raven, 1994, pp 1119–1138.
13. Walsh JH: Peptides as regulators of gastric acid secretion. Annu Rev Physiol 50:41–63, 1988.
14. Kovacs TO, Walsh JH, Maxwell V, et al: Gastrin is a major mediator of the gastric phase of acid secretion in dogs: Proof by monoclonal antibody neutralization. Gastroenterology 97:1406–1413, 1989.
15. Lloyd KCK, Debas HT: Peripheral regulation of gastric acid secretion. *In* Johnson LR (ed): Physiology of the Gastrointestinal Tract, 3rd ed. New York, Raven, 1994, pp 1185–1226.
16. Prinz C, Kajimura M, Scott DR, et al: Histamine secretion from rat enterochromaffinlike cells. Gastroenterology 105:449–461, 1993.
17. Hakanson R, Chen D, Sundler F: The ECL cells. *In* Johnson LR (ed): Physiology of the Gastrointestinal Tract, 3rd ed. New York, Raven, 1994, pp 1171–1184.
18. Bado A, Moizo L, Laigneau JP, et al: Pharmacological characterization of histamine H₃ receptors in isolated rabbit gastric glands. Am J Physiol 262:G56–G61, 1992.
19. Bado A, Hervatin F, Lewin MJ: Pharmacological evidence for histamine H₃ receptor in the control of gastric acid secretion in cats. Am J Physiol 260:G631–G635, 1991.
20. DelValle J, Yamada T: Amino acids and amines stimulate gastrin release from canine antral G-cells via different pathways. J Clin Invest 85:139–143, 1990.
21. Flemstrom G: Gastric and duodenal mucosal secretion of bicarbonate. *In* Johnson LR (ed): Physiology of the Gastrointestinal Tract, 3rd ed. New York, Raven, 1994, pp 1285–1309.
22. Forstner JF, Forstner GG: Gastrointestinal mucus. *In* Johnson LR (ed): Physiology of the Gastrointestinal Tract, 3rd ed. New York, Raven, 1994, pp 1255–1283.
23. Hersey SJ: Gastric secretion of pepsins. *In* Johnson LR (ed): Physiology of the Gastrointestinal Tract, 3rd ed. New York, Raven, 1994, pp 1227–1238.
24. Wallace JL: Cooperative modulation of gastrointestinal mucosal defense by prostaglandins and nitric oxide. Clin Invest Med 19:346–351, 1996.
25. Tepperman BL, Jacobson ED: Circulatory factors in gastric mucosal defense and repair. *In* Johnson LR (ed): Physiology of the Gastrointestinal Tract, 3rd ed. New York, Raven, 1994, pp 1331–1351.
26. Bruggeman TM, Wood JG, Davenport HW: Local control of blood flow in the dog's stomach: Vasodilatation caused by acid back-diffusion following topical application of salicylic acid. Gastroenterology 77:736–744, 1979.
27. Miller TA: Protective effects of prostaglandins against gastric mucosal damage: Current knowledge and proposed mechanisms. Am J Physiol 245:G601–G603, 1983.
28. Cryer B, Kimmey MB: Gastrointestinal side effects of nonsteroidal anti-inflammatory drugs. Am J Med 105:20S–30S, 1998.
29. Cryer B, Feldman M: Cyclooxygenase-1 and cyclooxygenase-2 selectivity of widely used nonsteroidal anti-inflammatory drugs. Am J Med 104:413–421, 1998.
30. Minami H, McCallum RW: The physiology and pathophysiology of gastric emptying in humans. Gastroenterology 86:1592–1610, 1984.
31. Leib MS, Wingfield WE, Twedt DC, et al: Gastric emptying of liquids in the dog: Serial test meal and modified emptying-time techniques. Am J Vet Res 46:1876–1880, 1985.
32. Miller J, Kauffman G, Elashoff J, et al: Search for resistances controlling canine gastric emptying of liquid meals. Am J Physiol 241:G403–G415, 1981.
33. Hinder RA, Kelly KA: Canine gastric emptying of solids and liquids. Am J Physiol 233:E335–E340, 1977.
34. Meyer JH, Thomson JB, Cohen MB, et al: Sieving of solid food by the canine stomach and sieving after gastric surgery. Gastroenterology 76:804–813, 1979.
35. Meyer JH, Dressman J, Fink A, et al: Effect of size and density on canine gastric emptying of nondigestible solids. Gastroenterology 89:805–813, 1985.
36. el-Sharkawy TY, Morgan KG, Szurszewski JH: Intracellular electrical activity of canine and human gastric smooth muscle. J Physiol (Lond) 279:291–307, 1978.
37. Kelly KA, Code CF: Canine gastric pacemaker. Am J Physiol 220:112–118, 1971.

GI

38. Heddle R, Miedema BW, Kelly KA: Integration of canine proximal gastric, antral, pyloric, and proximal duodenal motility during fasting and after a liquid meal. Dig Dis Sci 38:856–869, 1993.
39. Hunt JN, Stubbs DF: The volume and energy content of meals as determinants of gastric emptying. J Physiol (Lond) 245:209–225, 1975.
40. McHugh PR, Moran TH: Calories and gastric emptying: A regulatory capacity with implications for feeding. Am J Physiol 236:R254–R260, 1979.
41. Azpiroz F, Malagelada JR: Intestinal control of gastric tone. Am J Physiol 249:G501–G509, 1985.
42. Roche M, Descroix-Vagne M, Benouali S, et al: Effect of some gastrointestinal hormones on motor and electrical activity of the digestive tract in the conscious cat. Br J Nutr 69:371–384, 1993.
43. Code CF, Marlett JA: The interdigestive myoelectric complex of the stomach and small bowel of dogs. J Physiol (Lond) 246:289–309, 1975.
44. Bueno L, Rayner V, Ruckebusch Y: Initiation of the migrating myoelectric complex in dogs. J Physiol (Lond) 316:309–318, 1981.
45. Itoh Z, Aizawa I, Takeuchi S, et al: Diurnal changes in gastric motor activity in conscious dogs. Am J Dig Dis 22:117–124, 1977.
46. Hitt ME: Biopsy of the gastrointestinal tract. In Bonagura JD (ed): Kirk's Current Veterinary Therapy XII. Small Animal Practice. Philadelphia, WB Saunders, 1995, pp 675–678.
47. Tams TR: Gastroscopy. In Tams TR (ed): Small Animal Endoscopy. St. Louis, Mosby–Year Book, 1990, pp 89–166.
48. Guilford WG: Upper gastrointestinal endoscopy. Vet Clin North Am Small Anim Pract 20:1209–1227, 1990.
49. Leib MS: Endoscopic examination of the dog and cat. In Jensen SL, Gregersen H, Moody FG, et al (eds): Essentials of Experimental Surgery: Gastroenterology. Amsterdam, Harwood Academic Publishers, 1996, pp 1–10, 17.
50. Shaw PC, van Romunde LK, Griffioen G, et al: Detection of gastric erosions: Comparison of biphasic radiography with fiberoptic endoscopy. Radiology 178:63–66, 1991.
51. van der Gaag I: The histological appearance of peroral gastric biopsies in clinically healthy and vomiting dogs. Can J Vet Res 52:67–74, 1988.
52. Hasslinger MA: Ollulanus tricuspis, the stomach worm of the cat. Feline Pract 14:22, 1984.
53. Happe RP, De Bruijne JJ: Pentagastrin stimulated gastric secretion in the dog (orogastric aspiration technique). Res Vet Sci 33:232–239, 1982.
54. Youngberg CA, Wlodyga J, Schmaltz S, et al: Radiotelemetric determination of gastrointestinal pH in four healthy beagles. Am J Vet Res 46:1516–1521, 1985.
55. Guilford WG, Strombeck DR: Acute gastritis. In Guilford WG, Center SA, Strombeck DR, et al (eds): Strombeck's Small Animal Gastroenterology, 3rd ed. Philadelphia, WB Saunders, 1996, pp 261–274.
56. van der Linde-Sipman JS, Boersema JH, Berrocal A: [3 cases of hypertrophic gastritis associated with Ollulanus tricuspis infection in cats.] Tijdschr Diergeneeskd 117:727–729, 1992.
57. Hargis AM, Prieur DJ, Blanchard JL: Prevalence, lesions, and differential diagnosis of Ollulanus tricuspis infection in cats. Vet Pathol 20:71–79, 1983.
58. Garland T, Bailey EM: Toxic ornamental and garden plants. In Bonagura JD, Kirk RW (eds): Kirk's Current Veterinary Therapy XII. Small Animal Practice. Philadelphia, WB Saunders, 1995, pp 217–222.
59. Rubin SI, Papich MG: Nonsteroidal anti-inflammatory drugs. In Kirk RW (ed): Current Veterinary Therapy X. Small Animal Practice. Philadelphia, WB Saunders, 1989, pp 47–54.
60. Dow SW, Rosychuk RA, McChesney AE, et al: Effects of flunixin and flunixin plus prednisone on the gastrointestinal tract of dogs. Am J Vet Res 51:1131–1138, 1990.
61. Vonderhaar MA, Salisbury SK: Gastroduodenal ulceration associated with flunixin meglumine administration in three dogs [published erratum appears in J Am Vet Med Assoc 203:869, 1993]. JAVMA 203:92–95, 1993.
62. Wallace MS, Zawie DA, Garvey MS: Gastric ulceration in the dog secondary to the use of nonsteroidal antiinflammatory drugs. J Am Anim Hosp Assoc 26:467–472, 1990.
63. Lipowitz AJ, Boulay JP, Klausner JS: Serum salicylate concentrations and endoscopic evaluation of the gastric mucosa in dogs after oral administration of aspirin-containing products. Am J Vet Res 47:1586–1589, 1986.
64. Fox LE, Rosenthal RC, Twedt DC, et al: Plasma histamine and gastrin concentrations in 17 dogs with mast cell tumors. J Vet Intern Med 4:242–246, 1990.
65. Quintero E, Kaunitz J, Nishizaki Y, et al: Uremia increases gastric mucosal permeability and acid back-diffusion injury in the rat. Gastroenterology 103:1762–1768, 1992.
66. Quintero E, Ohning G, Guth PH: Uremia in the rat affects gastric cell growth and differentiation. Dig Dis Sci 39:1464–1468, 1994.
67. Kirk AP, Dooley JS, Hunt RH: Peptic ulceration in patients with chronic liver disease. Dig Dis Sci 25:756–760, 1980.
68. Twedt DC: Cirrhosis: A consequence of chronic liver disease. Vet Clin North Am Small Anim Pract 15:151–176, 1985.
69. Hall JA, Twedt DC, Burrows CF: Gastric motility in dogs. Part II. Disorders of gastric motility. Compend Contin Educ Pract Vet 12:1373–1391, 1990.
70. Greco DS: The distribution of body water and general approach to the patient. Vet Clin North Am Small Anim Pract 28:473–482, 1998.
71. Rudloff E, Kirby R: Fluid therapy. Crystalloids and colloids. Vet Clin North Am Small Anim Pract 28:297–328, 1998.
72. Walton RS, Wingfield WE, Ogilvie GK, et al: Energy expenditure in 104 postoperative and traumatically injured dogs with indirect calorimetry. J Vet Emerg Crit Care 6:71–75, 1996.
73. Hall JA: Clinical approach to chronic vomiting. In August JR (ed): Consultations in Feline Internal Medicine 3. Philadelphia, WB Saunders, 1997, pp 61–67.
74. Leib MS: Acute vomiting: A diagnostic approach and symptomatic management. In Kirk RW, Bonagura JD (eds): Current Veterinary Therapy XI. Small Animal Practice, 11th ed. Philadelphia, WB Saunders, 1992, pp 583–587.
75. Strombeck DR, Guilford WG: Vomiting: Pathophysiology and pharmacologic control. In Guilford WG, Center SA, Strombeck DR, et al (eds): Strombeck's Small Animal Gastroenterology, 3rd ed. Philadelphia, WB Saunders, 1996, pp 256–260.
76. Hall JA, Washabau RJ: Gastrointestinal prokinetic therapy: Dopaminergic antagonist drugs. Compend Contin Educ Prac Vet 19:214–221, 1997.
77. Marty M, Pouillart P, Scholl S, et al: Comparison of the 5-hydroxytryptamine3 (serotonin) antagonist ondansetron (GR 38032F) with high-dose metoclopramide in the control of cisplatin-induced emesis. N Engl J Med 322:816–821, 1990.
78. Gullikson GW, Loeffler RF, Virina MA: Relationship of serotonin-3 receptor antagonist activity to gastric emptying and motor-stimulating actions of prokinetic drugs in dogs. J Pharmacol Exp Ther 258:103–110, 1991.
79. Gullikson GW, Virina MA, Loeffler RF, et al: SC-49518 enhances gastric emptying of solid and liquid meals and stimulates gastrointestinal motility in dogs by a 5-hydroxytryptamine4 receptor mechanism. J Pharmacol Exp Ther 264:240–248, 1993.
80. Fukui H, Yamamoto M, Sato S: Vagal afferent fibers and peripheral 5-HT3 receptors mediate cisplatin-induced emesis in dogs. Jpn J Pharmacol 59:221–226, 1992.
81. Fukui H, Yamamoto M, Sasaki S, et al: Involvement of 5-HT3 receptors and vagal afferents in copper sulfate– and cisplatin-induced emesis in monkeys. Eur J Pharmacol 249:13–18, 1993.
82. Washabau RJ, Hall JA: Gastrointestinal prokinetic therapy: Serotonergic drugs. Compend Contin Educ Pract Vet 19:473–480, 1997.
83. Nyren O, Adami HO, Bates S, et al: Absence of therapeutic benefit from antacids or cimetidine in non-ulcer dyspepsia. N Engl J Med 314:339–343, 1986.
84. Spielman BL, Garvey MS: Hemorrhagic gastroenteritis in dogs. J Am Anim Hosp Assoc 29:341–344, 1993.
85. Guilford WG, Strombeck DR: Chronic gastric diseases. In Guilford WG, Center SA, Strombeck DR, et al (eds): Strombeck's Small Animal Gastroenterology, 3rd ed. Philadelphia, WB Saunders, 1996, pp 275–302.
86. van der Gaag I, Happe RP: Follow-up studies by peroral gastric biopsies and necropsy in vomiting dogs. Can J Vet Res 53:468–472, 1989.
87. Krohn KJ, Finlayson ND: Interrelations of humoral and cellular immune responses in experimental canine gastritis. Clin Exp Immunol 14:237–245, 1973.
88. MacLachlan NJ, Breitschwerdt EB, Chambers JM, et al: Gastroenteritis of basenji dogs. Vet Pathol 25:36–41, 1988.
89. Matthiesen DT, Walter MC: Surgical treatment of chronic hypertrophic pyloric gastropathy in 45 dogs. J Am Anim Hosp Assoc 22:241–247, 1986.
90. Sikes RI, Birchard S, Patnaik A, et al: Chronic hypertrophic pyloric gastropathy: A review of 16 cases. J Am Anim Hosp Assoc 22:99–104, 1986.
91. Bellenger CR, Maddison JE, MacPherson GC, et al: Chronic hypertrophic pyloric gastropathy in 14 dogs. Aust Vet J 67:317–320, 1990.
92. Leblanc B, Fox JG, Le Net JL, et al: Hyperplastic gastritis with intraepithelial Campylobacter-like organisms in a beagle dog. Vet Pathol 30:391–394, 1993.
93. Hargis AM, Prieur DJ, Blanchard JL, et al: Chronic fibrosing gastritis associated with Ollulanus tricuspis in a cat. Vet Pathol 19:320–323, 1982.
94. Zerbe CA, Boosinger TR, Grabau JH, et al: Pancreatic polypeptide and insulin-secreting tumor in a dog with duodenal ulcers and hypertrophic gastritis. J Vet Intern Med 3:178–182, 1989.
95. Hayden DW, Fleischman RW: Scirrhous eosinophilic gastritis in dogs with gastric arteritis. Vet Pathol 14:441–448, 1977.
96. Neer TM: Hypereosinophilic syndrome in cats. Compend Contin Educ Pract Vet 13:549–555, 1991.
97. Narama I, Kuroda J, Nagatani M, et al: Superficial eosinophilic gastritis in laboratory beagle dogs attributable probably to diet. Nippon Juigaku Zasshi 52:581–589, 1990.
98. van der Gaag I, van Niel MH, Belshaw BE, et al: Gastric granulomatous cryptococcosis mimicking gastric carcinoma in a dog. Vet Q 13:185–190, 1991.
99. Ader PL: Phycomycosis in fifteen dogs and two cats. JAVMA 174:1216–1223, 1979.
100. Miller RI: Gastrointestinal phycomycosis in 63 dogs. JAVMA 186:473–478, 1985.
101. Jenkins CC, Bassett JR: Helicobacter infection. Compend Contin Educ Pract Vet 19:267–279, 1997.
102. Fox JG: The expanding genus of Helicobacter: Pathogenic and zoonotic potential. Semin Gastroint Dis 8:124–141, 1997.
103. Bodger K, Crabtree JE: Helicobacter pylori and gastric inflammation. Br Med Bull 54:139–150, 1998.
104. Lee A, Hazell SL, O'Rourke J, et al: Isolation of a spiral-shaped bacterium from the cat stomach. Infect Immun 56:2843–2850, 1988.
105. Lee A, Krakowka S, Fox JG, et al: Role of Helicobacter felis in chronic canine gastritis. Vet Pathol 29:487–494, 1992.
106. Handt LK, Fox JG, Dewhirst FE, et al: Helicobacter pylori isolated from the domestic cat: Public health implications [published erratum appears in Infect Immun 63:1146, 1995]. Infect Immun 62:2367–2374, 1994.
107. Lavelle JP, Landas S, Mitros FA, et al: Acute gastritis associated with spiral organisms from cats. Dig Dis Sci 39:744–750, 1994.
108. Happonen I, Saari S, Castren L, et al: Occurrence and topographical mapping of gastric Helicobacter-like organisms and their association with histological changes in apparently healthy dogs and cats. Zentralbl Veterinarmed [A] 43:305–315, 1996.

109. Otto G, Hazell SH, Fox JG, et al: Animal and public health implications of gastric colonization of cats by *Helicobacter*-like organisms. J Clin Microbiol 32:1043–1049, 1994.

110. Hermanns W, Kregel K, Breuer W, et al: *Helicobacter*-like organisms: Histopathological examination of gastric biopsies from dogs and cats. J Comp Pathol 112:307–318, 1995.

111. Radin MJ, Eaton KA, Krakowka S, et al: *Helicobacter pylori* gastric infection in gnotobiotic beagle dogs. Infect Immun 58:2606–2612, 1990.

112. Yamasaki K, Suematsu H, Takahashi T: Comparison of gastric lesions in dogs and cats with and without gastric spiral organisms. JAVMA 212:529–533, 1998.

113. Geyer C, Colbatzky F, Lechner J, et al: Occurrence of spiral-shaped bacteria in gastric biopsies of dogs and cats. Vet Rec 133:18–19, 1993.

114. Feinstein RE, Olsson E: Chronic gastroenterocolitis in nine cats. J Vet Diagn Invest 4:293–298, 1992.

115. Marshall BJ, Barrett LJ, Prakash C, et al: Urea protects *Helicobacter (Campylobacter) pylori* from the bactericidal effect of acid. Gastroenterology 99:697–702, 1990.

116. Moran AP: Pathogenic properties of *Helicobacter pylori*. Scand J Gastroenterol Suppl 215:22–31, 1996.

117. Shimoyama T, Crabtree JE: Bacterial factors and immune pathogenesis in *Helicobacter pylori* infection. Gut 43(Suppl 1):S2–S5, 1998.

118. Morgan DR, Fox JG, Leunk RD: Comparison of isolates of *Helicobacter pylori* and *Helicobacter mustelae*. J Clin Microbiol 29:395–397, 1991.

119. Leunk RD: Production of a cytotoxin by *Helicobacter pylori*. Rev Infect Dis 13 (Suppl 8):S686–S689, 1991.

120. Crabtree JE: Immune and inflammatory responses to *Helicobacter pylori* infection. Scand J Gastroenterol Suppl 215:3–10, 1996.

121. Beales I, Blaser MJ, Srinivasan S, et al: Effect of *Helicobacter pylori* products and recombinant cytokines on gastrin release from cultured canine G cells. Gastroenterology 113:465–471, 1997.

122. Megraud F: Diagnosis of *Helicobacter pylori* infection. Scand J Gastroenterol Suppl 214:44–46, 1996.

123. Megraud F: Advantages and disadvantages of current diagnostic tests for the detection of *Helicobacter pylori*. Scand J Gastroenterol Suppl 215:57–62, 1996.

124. Thijs JC, van Zwet AA, Moolenaar W, et al: Triple therapy vs. amoxicillin plus omeprazole for treatment of *Helicobacter pylori* infection: A multicenter, prospective, randomized, controlled study of efficacy and side effects. Am J Gastroenterol 91:93–97, 1996.

125. DeNovo RC, Magne ML: Current concepts in the management of *Helicobacter*-associated gastritis. Proceedings 13th Annual ACVIM Veterinary Forum, Lake Buena Vista, FL, 1995, pp 57–61.

126. Axon AT, Moayyedi P: Eradication of *Helicobacter pylori*: Omeprazole in combination with antibiotics. Scand J Gastroenterol Suppl 215:82–89, 1996.

127. Thijs JC, van Zwet AA, Thijs WJ, et al: One-week triple therapy with omeprazole, amoxicillin and tinidazole for *Helicobacter pylori* infection: The significance of imidazole resistance. Aliment Pharmacol Ther 11:305–309, 1997.

128. Fox JG: *Helicobacter*-associated gastric disease in ferrets, dogs, and cats. *In* Bonagura JD (ed): Kirk's Current Veterinary Therapy XII. Small Animal Practice. Philadelphia, WB Saunders, 1995, pp 720–723.

129. Marks SL: Bacterial gastroenteritis in dogs and cats: More common than you think. Proceedings 15th Annual ACVIM Veterinary Forum, May 22–25, Lake Buena Vista, FL, 1997, pp 237–239.

130. Burrows CF: Infection with the stomach worm *Physaloptera* as a cause of chronic vomiting in the dog. J Am Anim Hosp Assoc 19:947–950, 1983.

131. Clark JA: *Physaloptera* stomach worms associated with chronic vomition in a dog in western Canada. Can Vet J 31:840, 1990.

132. Santen DR, Chastain CB, Schmidt DA: Efficacy of pyrantel pamoate against *Physaloptera* in a cat. J Am Anim Hosp Assoc 29:53, 1993.

133. Reindel JF, Trapp AL, Armstrong PJ, et al: Recurrent plasmacytic stomatitis-pharyngitis in a cat with esophagitis, fibrosing gastritis, and gastric nematodiasis. JAVMA 190:65–67, 1987.

134. Wilson RB, Presnell JC: Chronic gastritis due to *Ollanus tricuspis* infection in a cat. J Am Anim Hosp Assoc 26:137–139, 1990.

135. Guy PA: *Ollulanus tricuspis* in domestic cats—Prevalence and methods of post-mortem diagnosis. N Z Vet J 32:81–84, 1984.

136. Kirkpatrick CE, Lok JB, Goldschmidt MH, et al: Gastric gnathostomiasis in a cat. JAVMA 190:1437–1439, 1987.

137. Mense MG, Gardiner CH, Moeller RB, et al: Chronic emesis caused by a nematode-induced gastric nodule in a cat. JAVMA 201:597–598, 1992.

138. Renooij W, Schmitz MG, van Gaal PJ, et al: Gastric mucosal phospholipids in dogs with familial stomatocytosis-hypertrophic gastritis. Eur J Clin Invest 26:1156–1159, 1996.

139. Slappendel RJ, van der Gaag I, van Nes JJ, et al: Familial stomatocytosis–hypertrophic gastritis (FSHG), a newly recognised disease in the dog (Drentse patrijshond). Vet Q 13:30–40, 1991.

140. Leib MS: Diseases of the stomach. *In* Leib MS, Monroe WE (eds): Practical Small Animal Internal Medicine. Philadelphia, WB Saunders, 1997, pp 653–684.

141. Jergens AE: Gastrointestinal disease and its management. Vet Clin North Am Small Anim Pract 27:1373–1402, 1997.

142. Jones RD, Baynes RE, Nimitz CT: Nonsteroidal anti-inflammatory drug toxicosis in dogs and cats: 240 cases (1989–1990). JAVMA 201:475–477, 1992.

143. Stanton ME, Bright RM: Gastroduodenal ulceration in dogs. Retrospective study of 43 cases and literature review. J Vet Intern Med 3:238–244, 1989.

144. Cryer B, Feldman M: Effects of nonsteroidal anti-inflammatory drugs on endogenous gastrointestinal prostaglandins and therapeutic strategies for prevention and treatment of nonsteroidal anti-inflammatory drug–induced damage. Arch Intern Med 152:1145–1155, 1992.

145. Wallace JL: Prostaglandins, NSAIDs, and cytoprotection. Gastroenterol Clin North Am 21:631–641, 1992.

146. Wallace JL: Non-steroidal anti-inflammatory drug gastropathy and cytoprotection: Pathogenesis and mechanisms re-examined. Scand J Gastroenterol Suppl 192:3–8, 1992.

147. Shaw N, Burrows CF, King RR: Massive gastric hemorrhage induced by buffered aspirin in a greyhound. J Am Anim Hosp Assoc 33:215–219, 1997.

148. Aabakken L, Olaussen B, Mowinckel P, et al: Gastroduodenal lesions associated with two different piroxicam formulations. An endoscopic comparison. Scand J Gastroenterol 27:1049–1054, 1992.

149. Gilmour MA, Walshaw R: Naproxen-induced toxicosis in a dog. JAVMA 191:1431–1432, 1987.

150. Gfeller RW, Sandors AD: Naproxen-associated duodenal ulcer complicated by perforation and bacteria- and barium sulfate–induced peritonitis in a dog. JAVMA 198:644–646, 1991.

151. Thomas NW: Piroxicam associated gastric ulceration in a dog. Compend Contin Educ Pract Vet 9:1004–1006, 1030, 1987.

152. Smith KJ, Taylor DH: Another case of gastric perforation associated with administration of ibuprofen in a dog. JAVMA 202:706, 1993.

153. Scherkl R, Frey HH: Pharmacokinetics of ibuprofen in the dog. J Vet Pharmacol Ther 10:261–265, 1987.

154. Godshalk CP, Roush JK, Fingland RB, et al: Gastric perforation associated with administration of ibuprofen in a dog. JAVMA 201:1734–1736, 1992.

155. Spyridakis LK, Bacia JJ, Barsanti JA, et al: Ibuprofen toxicosis in a dog. JAVMA 189:918–919, 1986.

156. Argentieri DC, Ritchie DM, Ferro MP, et al: Tepoxalin: A dual cyclooxygenase/5-lipoxygenase inhibitor of arachidonic acid metabolism with potent anti-inflammatory activity and a favorable gastrointestinal profile. J Pharmacol Exp Ther 271:1399–1408, 1994.

157. Kirchner T, Aparicio B, Argentieri DC, et al: Effects of tepoxalin, a dual inhibitor of cyclooxygenase/5-lipoxygenase, on events associated with NSAID-induced gastrointestinal inflammation. Prostaglandins Leukot Essent Fatty Acids 56:417–423, 1997.

158. Willard MD, Toal RL, Cawley A: Gastric complications associated with correction of chronic diaphragmatic hernia in two dogs. JAVMA 184:1151–1153, 1984.

159. Arvidsson S, Falt K, Haglund U: Feline *E. coli* bacteremia—Effects of misoprostol/scavengers or methylprednisolone on hemodynamic reactions and gastrointestinal mucosal injury. Acta Chir Scand 156:215–221, 1990.

160. Arvidsson S, Falt K, Haglund U: Secretory state and acute gastric mucosal injury in sepsis. Scand J Gastroenterol 22:763–768, 1987.

161. Moore RW, Withrow SJ: Gastrointestinal hemorrhage and pancreatitis associated with intervertebral disk diseases in the dog. JAVMA 180:1443–1447, 1982.

162. Davies M: Pancreatitis, gastrointestinal ulceration and haemorrhage and necrotising cystitis following the surgical treatment of degenerative disc disease in a dachshund. Vet Rec 116:398–399, 1985.

163. Pollack MJ, Flanders JA, Johnson RC: Disseminated malignant mastocytoma in a dog. J Am Anim Hosp Assoc 27:435–440, 1991.

164. English RV, Breitschwerdt EB, Grindem CB, et al: Zollinger-Ellison syndrome and myelofibrosis in a dog. JAVMA 192:1430–1434, 1988.

165. Eng J, Du BH, Johnson GF, et al: Cat gastrinoma and the sequence of cat gastrins. Regul Pept 37:9–13, 1992.

166. Yanda RJ, Ostroff JW, Ashbaugh CD, et al: Zollinger-Ellison syndrome in a patient with normal screening gastrin level. Dig Dis Sci 34:1929–1932, 1989.

167. Jergens AE, et al: Idiopathic inflammatory bowel disease associated with gastroduodenal ulceration-erosion: A report of nine cases in the dog and cat. J Am Anim Hosp Assoc 28:21, 1992.

168. Fonda D, Gualtieri M, Scanziani E: Gastric carcinoma in the dog: A clinicopathological study of 11 cases. J Small Anim Pract 30:353–360, 1989.

169. Sheikh-Omar AR, Abdullah AS: Perforated gastric ulcer associated with disseminated staphylococcal granuloma (botryomycosis) in a cat. Vet Rec 117:131, 1985.

170. Curtsinger DK, Carpenter JL, Turner JL: Gastritis caused by *Aonchotheca putorii* in a domestic cat. JAVMA 203:1153–1154, 1993.

171. Otto CM, Dodds WJ, Greene CE: Factor XII and partial prekallikrein deficiencies in a dog with recurrent gastrointestinal hemorrhage. JAVMA 198:129–131, 1991.

172. Penninck D, Matz M, Tidwell A: Ultrasonography of gastric ulceration in the dog. Vet Radiol Ultrasound 38:308–312, 1997.

173. Meddings JB, Kirk D, Olson ME: Noninvasive detection of nonsteroidal anti-inflammatory drug–induced gastropathy in dogs. Am J Vet Res 56:977–981, 1995.

174. Shamburek RD, Schubert ML: Control of gastric acid secretion. Histamine H_2-receptor antagonists and H^+K^+-ATPase inhibitors. Gastroenterol Clin North Am 21:527–550, 1992.

175. Daly MJ, Humphray JM, Stables R: Inhibition of gastric acid secretion in the dog by the H_2-receptor antagonists, ranitidine, cimetidine, and metiamide. Gut 21:408–412, 1980.

176. Papich MG: Antiulcer therapy. Vet Clin North Am Small Anim Pract 23:497–512, 1993.

177. Frislid K, Guldvog I, Berstad A: Kinetics of the inhibition of food-stimulated secretion by ranitidine in dogs. Eur Surg Res 17:360–365, 1985.

GI

178. Ballesteros MA, Hogan DL, Koss MA, et al: Bolus or intravenous infusion of ranitidine: Effects on gastric pH and acid secretion. A comparison of relative efficacy and cost. Ann Intern Med 112:334–339, 1990.

179. Mizumoto A, Fujimura M, Iwanaga Y, et al: Anticholinesterase activity of histamine H_2-receptor antagonists in the dog: Their possible role in gastric motor activity. J Gastrointest Motility 2:273–280, 1990.

180. Humphries TJ: Famotidine: A notable lack of drug interactions. Scand J Gastroenterol Suppl 134:55–60, 1987.

181. Ueki S, Seiki M, Yoneta T, et al: Gastroprokinetic activity of nizatidine, a new H_2-receptor antagonist, and its possible mechanism of action in dogs and rats. J Pharmacol Exp Ther 264:152–157, 1993.

182. Spurling NW, Selway SA, Poynter D: An evaluation of the safety of ranitidine during seven years daily oral administration to beagle dogs. Hum Toxicol 8:23–32, 1989.

183. Johnson WS, Miller DR: Ranitidine and bradycardia. Ann Intern Med 108:493, 1988.

184. Spychal RT, Wickham NW: Thrombocytopenia associated with ranitidine. Br Med J (Clin Res Ed) 291:1687, 1985.

185. McEwan NA, et al: Drug eruption in a cat resembling pemphigus foliaceus. J Small Anim Pract 28:713, 1987.

186. Norwood J, Smith TM, Stein DS: Famotidine and hyperpyrexia. Ann Intern Med 112:632, 1990.

187. Slugg PH, Haug MT 3d, Pippenger CE. Ranitidine pharmacokinetics and adverse central nervous system reactions. Arch Intern Med 152:2325–2329, 1992.

188. Boulay JP, Lipowitz AJ, Klausner JS: Effect of cimetidine on aspirin-induced gastric hemorrhage in dogs. Am J Vet Res 47:1744–1746, 1986.

189. Silverstein FE, Graham DY, Senior JR, et al: Misoprostol reduces serious gastrointestinal complications in patients with rheumatoid arthritis receiving nonsteroidal anti-inflammatory drugs. A randomized, double-blind, placebo-controlled trial. Ann Intern Med 123:241–249, 1995.

190. Murtaugh RJ, Matz ME, Labato MA, et al: Use of synthetic prostaglandin E_1 (misoprostol) for prevention of aspirin-induced gastroduodenal ulceration in arthritic dogs. JAVMA 202:251–256, 1993.

191. Johnston SA, Leib MS, Forrester SD, et al: The effect of misoprostol on aspirin-induced gastroduodenal lesions in dogs. J Vet Intern Med 9:32–38, 1995.

192. Kornbluth A, Gupta R, Gerson CD: Life-threatening diarrhea after short-term misoprostol use in a patient with Crohn ileocolitis. Ann Intern Med 113:474–475, 1990.

193. Jenkins CC, DeNovo RC, Patton CS, et al: Comparison of effects of cimetidine and omeprazole on mechanically created gastric ulceration and on aspirin-induced gastritis in dogs. Am J Vet Res 52:658–661, 1991.

194. Coruzzi G, Adami M, Bertaccini G: Gastric antisecretory activity of lansoprazole in different experimental models: Comparison with omeprazole. Gen Pharmacol 26:1027–1032, 1995.

195. McCarthy DM: Sucralfate. N Engl J Med 325:1017–1025, 1991.

196. Slomiany BL, Piotrowski J, Tamura S, et al: Enhancement of the protective qualities of gastric mucus by sucralfate: Role of phosphoinositides. Am J Med 91:30S–36S, 1991.

197. Wallace JL, Morris GP, Beck PL, et al: Effects of sucralfate on gastric prostaglandin and leukotriene synthesis: Relationship to protective actions. Can J Physiol Pharmacol 66:666–670, 1988.

198. Danesh JZ, Duncan A, Russell RI, et al: Effect of intragastric pH on mucosal protective action of sucralfate. Gut 29:1379–1385, 1988.

199. Louw JA, Zak J, Lucke W, et al: Triple therapy with sucralfate is as effective as triple therapy containing bismuth in eradicating Helicobacter pylori and reducing duodenal ulcer relapse rates. Scand J Gastroenterol Suppl 191:28–31, 1992.

200. Parpia SH, Nix DE, Hejmanowski LG, et al: Sucralfate reduces the gastrointestinal absorption of norfloxacin. Antimicrob Agents Chemother 33:99–102, 1989.

201. Gasbarrini G, Andreone P, Baraldini M, et al: Antacids in gastric ulcer treatment: Evidence of cytoprotection. Scand J Gastroenterol Suppl 174:44–47, 1990.

202. Szelenyi I, Brune K: Possible role of sulfhydryls in mucosal protection induced by aluminum hydroxide. Dig Dis Sci 31:1207–1210, 1986.

203. Salim AS: Sulfhydryls protect patients against complications of erosive gastritis. Dig Dis Sci 35:1436–1437, 1990.

204. Washabau RJ, Hall JA: Cisapride. JAVMA 207:1285–1288, 1995.

205. Felts JF, Fox PR, Burk RL: Thread and sewing needles as gastrointestinal foreign bodies in the cat: A review of 64 cases. JAVMA 184:56–59, 1984.

206. Basher AW, Fowler JD: Conservative versus surgical management of gastrointestinal linear foreign bodies in the cat. Vet Surg 16:135–138, 1987.

207. Peeters ME: Pyloric stenosis in the dog: Developments in the surgical treatment and a retrospective study in 47 patients. Eur J Companion Anim Pract 2:37–40, 1991.

208. Van der Gaag I: Hypertrophic gastritis in 21 dogs. Zentralbl Veterinarmed [A] 31:161–173, 1984.

209. Walter MC, Matthiesen DT: Acquired antral pyloric hypertrophy in the dog. Vet Clin North Am Small Anim Pract 23:547–554, 1993.

210. Dennis R, Herrtage ME, Jefferies AR, et al: A case of hyperplastic gastropathy in a cat. J Small Anim Pract 28:491–504, 1987.

211. Walter MC, Goldschmidt MH, Stone EA, et al: Chronic hypertrophic pyloric gastropathy as a cause of pyloric obstruction in the dog. JAVMA 186:157–161, 1985.

212. Pearson H, Gaskell CJ, Gibbs C, et al: Pyloric and oesophageal dysfunction in the cat. J Small Anim Pract 15:487–501, 1974.

213. Biller DS, Partington BP, Miyabayashi T, et al: Ultrasonographic appearance of chronic hypertrophic pyloric gastropathy in the dog. Vet Radiol Ultrasound 35:30–33, 1994.

214. Leib MS, Saunders GK, Moon ML, et al: Endoscopic diagnosis of chronic hypertrophic pyloric gastropathy in dogs. J Vet Intern Med 7:335–341, 1993.

215. De Backer A, Bove T, Vandenplas Y, et al: Contribution of endoscopy to early diagnosis of hypertrophic pyloric stenosis. J Pediatr Gastroenterol Nutr 18:78–81, 1994.

216. Walter MC, Matthiesen DT, Stone EA: Pylorectomy and gastroduodenostomy in the dog: Technique and clinical results in 28 cases. JAVMA 187:909–914, 1985.

217. Papageorges M, Breton L, Bonneau NH: Gastric drainage procedures: Effects in normal dogs. I. Introduction and description of surgical procedures. Vet Surg 16:327–331, 1987.

218. Fossum TW, Rohn DA, Willard MD: Presumptive, iatrogenic gastric outflow obstruction associated with prior gastric surgery. J Am Anim Hosp Assoc 31:391–395, 1995.

219. Walter MC, Matthiesen DT: Gastric outflow surgical problems. Probl Vet Med 1:196–214, 1989.

220. Twaddle AA: Congenital pyloric stenosis in two kittens corrected by pyloroplasty. N Z Vet J 19:26, 1971.

221. Papageorges M, Bonneau NH, Breton L: Gastric drainage procedures: Effects in normal dogs. III. Postmortem evaluation. Vet Surg 16:341–345, 1987.

222. Barsanti JA: Miscellaneous fungal infections. In Greene CE (ed): Clinical Microbiology and Infectious Diseases of the Dog and Cat. Philadelphia, WB Saunders, 1984, p 738.

223. Troy GC: Canine phycomycosis: A review of twenty-four cases. Calif Vet 39:12–17, 1985.

224. Bowersox TS, Caywood DD, Hayden DW: Idiopathic, duodenogastric intussusception in an adult dog. JAVMA 199:1608–1609, 1991.

225. Hosgood G: Gastric dilatation-volvulus in dogs. JAVMA 204:1742–1747, 1994.

226. Glickman LT, Glickman NW, Perez CM, et al: Analysis of risk factors for gastric dilatation and dilatation-volvulus in dogs. JAVMA 204:1465–1471, 1994.

227. Glickman LT, Lantz GC, Schellenberg DB, et al: A prospective study of survival and recurrence following the acute gastric dilatation-volvulus syndrome in 136 dogs. J Am Anim Hosp Assoc 34:253–259, 1998.

228. Brockman DJ, Washabau RJ, Drobatz KJ: Canine gastric dilatation/volvulus syndrome in a veterinary critical care unit: 295 cases (1986–1992). JAVMA 207:460–464, 1995.

229. Brourman JD, Schertel ER, Allen DA, et al: Factors associated with perioperative mortality in dogs with surgically managed gastric dilatation-volvulus: 137 cases (1988–1993). JAVMA 208:1855–1858, 1996.

230. Elwood CM: Risk factors for gastric dilatation in Irish setter dogs. J Small Anim Pract 39:185–190, 1998.

231. Schellenberg D, Yi Q, Glickman NW, et al: Influence of thoracic conformation and genetics on the risk of gastric dilatation-volvulus in Irish setters. J Am Anim Hosp Assoc 34:64–73, 1998.

232. Schaible RH, Ziech J, Glickman NW, et al: Predisposition to gastric dilatation-volvulus in relation to genetics of thoracic conformation in Irish setters. J Am Anim Hosp Assoc 33:379–383, 1997.

233. Glickman LT, Glickman NW, Schellenberg DB, et al: Multiple risk factors for the gastric dilatation-volvulus syndrome in dogs: A practitioner/owner case-control study. J Am Anim Hosp Assoc 33:197–204, 1997.

234. Burrows CF, Bright RM, Spencer CP: Influence of dietary composition on gastric emptying and motility in dogs: Potential involvement in acute gastric dilatation. Am J Vet Res 46:2609–2612, 1985.

235. Hall JA, Twedt DC, Curtis CR: Relationship of plasma gastrin immunoreactivity and gastroesophageal sphincter pressure in clinically normal dogs and in dogs with previous gastric dilatation-volvulus. Am J Vet Res 50:1228–1232, 1989.

236. Braun L, Lester S, Kuzma AB, et al: Gastric dilatation-volvulus in the dog with histological evidence of preexisting inflammatory bowel disease: A retrospective study of 23 cases. J Am Anim Hosp Assoc 32:287–290, 1996.

237. Van Kruiningen HJ, Wojan LD, Stake PE, et al: The influence of diet and feeding frequency on gastric function in the dog. J Am Anim Hosp Assoc 23:145–153, 1987.

238. Hall JA, Willer RL, Seim HB, et al: Gastric emptying of nondigestible radiopaque markers after circumcostal gastropexy in clinically normal dogs and dogs with gastric dilatation-volvulus. Am J Vet Res 53:1961–1965, 1992.

239. Funkquist B, Garmer L: Pathogenetic and therapeutic aspects of torsion of the canine stomach. J Small Anim Pract 8:523–532, 1967.

240. van Sluijs FJ, van den Brom WE: Gastric emptying of a radionuclide-labeled test meal after surgical correction of gastric dilatation-volvulus in dogs. Am J Vet Res 50:433–435, 1989.

241. Leib MS, Monroe WE, Martin RA: Suspected chronic gastric volvulus in a dog with normal gastric emptying of liquids. JAVMA 191:699–700, 1987.

242. Hall JA, Solie TN, Seim HB, et al: Gastric myoelectric and motor activity in dogs with gastric dilatation-volvulus. Am J Physiol 265:G646–G653, 1993.

243. Hall JA, Willer RL, Seim HB, et al: Gross and histologic evaluation of hepatogastric ligaments in clinically normal dogs and dogs with gastric dilatation-volvulus. Am J Vet Res 56:1611–1614, 1995.

244. Stampley AR, Burrows CF, Ellison GW: The use of retrievable electrodes for recording gastric myoelectric activity after spontaneous gastric dilatation-volvulus in dogs. Cornell Vet 82:423–434, 1992.

245. Stampley AR, Burrows CF, Ellison GW, et al: Gastric myoelectric activity after experimental gastric dilatation-volvulus and tube gastrostomy in dogs. Vet Surg 21:10–14, 1992.

246. Millis DL, Nemzek J, Riggs C, et al: Gastric dilatation-volvulus after splenic torsion in two dogs. JAVMA 207:314–315, 1995.

247. Bredal WP, Eggertsdottir AV, Austefjord O: Acute gastric dilatation in cats: A case series. Acta Vet Scand 37:445–451, 1996.

248. Caywood D, Teague HD, Jackson DA: Gastric gas analysis in the canine gastric dilatation-volvulus syndrome. J Am Anim Hosp Assoc 13:459–462, 1977.

249. Orton EC: Gastric dilatation-volvulus. In Kirk RW (ed): Current Veterinary Therapy IX. Small Animal Practice. Philadelphia, WB Saunders, 1986, pp 856–862.

250. Fossum TW: Surgery of the stomach. In Fossum TW (ed): Small Animal Surgery. St. Louis, Mosby, 1997, pp 277–283.

251. Wingfield WE, Betts CW, Rawlings CA: Pathophysiology associated with gastric dilatation-volvulus in the dog. J Am Anim Hosp Assoc 12:136–141, 1976.

252. Merkely DF, Howard DR, Eyster GE, et al: Experimentally induced acute gastric dilatation in the dog: Cardiopulmonary effects. J Am Anim Hosp Assoc 12:143–148, 1976.

253. Lefer AM: Role of a myocardial depressant factor in shock states. Mod Concepts Cardiovasc Dis 42:59–64, 1973.

254. Lefer AM: Myocardial depressant factor and circulatory shock. Klin Wochenschr 52:358–370, 1974.

255. Olcay I, Kitahama A, Miller RH, et al: Reticuloendothelial dysfunction and endotoxemia following portal vein occlusion. Surgery 75:64–70, 1974.

256. Hathcock JT: Radiographic view of choice for the diagnosis of gastric volvulus: The right lateral recumbent view. J Am Anim Hosp Assoc 20:967–969, 1984.

257. Allen DA, Schertel ER, Muir WW, et al: Hypertonic saline/dextran resuscitation of dogs with experimentally induced gastric dilatation-volvulus shock. Am J Vet Res 52:92–96, 1991.

258. Schertel ER, Allen DA, Muir WW, et al: Evaluation of a hypertonic saline-dextran solution for treatment of dogs with shock induced by gastric dilatation-volvulus. JAVMA 210:226–230, 1997.

259. Matthiesen DT: The gastric dilatation-volvulus complex: Medical and surgical considerations. JAVMA 19:925–932, 1983.

260. Davidson JR, Lantz GC, Salisbury SK, et al: Effects of flunixin meglumine on dogs with experimental gastric dilatation-volvulus. Vet Surg 21:113–120, 1992.

261. Muir WW: Acid-base and electrolyte disturbances in dogs with gastric dilatation-volvulus. JAVMA 181:229–231, 1982.

262. Leib MS, Martin RA: Therapy of gastric dilatation-volvulus in dogs. Compend Contin Educ Pract Vet 9:1155–1165, 1987.

263. Whitney WO: Complications associated with the medical and surgical management of gastric dilatation-volvulus in the dog. Probl Vet Med 1:268–280, 1989.

264. Lantz GC, Bottoms GD, Carlton WW, et al: The effect of 360 degree gastric volvulus on the blood supply of the nondistended normal dog stomach. Vet Surg 13:189–196, 1984.

265. MacCoy DM, et al: Partial invagination of the canine stomach for treatment of infarction of the gastric wall. Vet Surg 15:237, 1986.

266. Ellison GW: Gastric dilatation volvulus. Surgical prevention. Vet Clin North Am Small Anim Pract 23:513–530, 1993.

267. Davidson JR: Acute gastric dilatation-volvulus in dogs: Surgical treatments. Vet Med 87:118–126, 1992.

268. Flanders JA, Harvey HJ: Results of tube gastrostomy as treatment for gastric volvulus in the dog. JAVMA 185:74–77, 1984.

269. Johnson RG, Barrus J, Greene RW: Gastric dilatation-volvulus: Recurrence rate following tube gastrostomy. JAVMA 20:33–37, 1984.

270. Fallah AM, Lumb WV, Nelson AW, et al: Circumcostal gastropexy in the dog. A preliminary study. Vet Surg 11:9–12, 1982.

271. Leib MS, Konde LJ, Wingfield WE, et al: Circumcostal gastropexy for preventing recurrence of gastric dilatation-volvulus in the dog: An evaluation of 30 cases. JAVMA 187:245–248, 1985.

272. Woolfson JM, Kostolich M: Circumcostal gastropexy: Clinical use of the technique in 34 dogs with gastric dilatation-volvulus. J Am Anim Hosp Assoc 22:825–830, 1986.

273. Leib MS, Konde LJ, Wingfield WE, et al: Circumcostal gastropexy for preventing recurrence of gastric dilatation-volvulus in the dog: An evaluation of 30 cases. JAVMA 187:245–248, 1985.

274. Fox SM, McCoy CP, Copper RC, et al: Circumcostal gastropexy versus tube gastrostomy: Histological comparison of gastropexy adhesions. J Am Anim Hosp Assoc 24:273–279, 1988.

275. Schulman AJ, Lusk R, Lippincott CL, et al: Muscular flap gastropexy: A new surgical technique to prevent recurrences of gastric dilation-volvulus syndrome. J Am Anim Hosp Assoc 22:339–346, 1986.

276. Whitney WO, Scavelli TD, Matthiesen DT, et al: Belt-loop gastropexy: Technique and surgical results in 20 dogs. J Am Anim Hosp Assoc 25:75–83, 1989.

277. MacCoy DM, Sykes GP, Hoffer RE, et al: A gastropexy technique for permanent fixation of the pyloric antrum. J Am Anim Hosp Assoc 18:763–768, 1982.

278. Meyer-Lindenberg A, Harder A, Fehr M, et al: Treatment of gastric dilatation-volvulus and a rapid method for prevention of relapse in dogs: 134 cases (1988–1991). JAVMA 203:1303–1307, 1993.

279. Waschak MJ, Payne JT, Pope ER, et al: Evaluation of percutaneous gastrostomy as a technique for permanent gastropexy. Vet Surg 26:235–241, 1997.

280. Greenfield CL, Walshaw R, Thomas MW: Significance of the Heineke-Mikulicz pyloroplasty in the treatment of gastric dilatation-volvulus. A prospective clinical study. Vet Surg 18:22–26, 1989.

281. Jennings PB Jr, Mathey WS, Ehler WJ: Intermittent gastric dilatation after gastropexy in a dog. JAVMA 200:1707–1708, 1992.

282. Granger DN: Role of xanthine oxidase and granulocytes in ischemia-reperfusion injury. Am J Physiol 255:H1269–H1275, 1988.

283. Moore RM, Muir WW, Granger DN: Mechanisms of gastrointestinal ischemia-reperfusion injury and potential therapeutic interventions: A review and its implications in the horse. J Vet Intern Med 9:115–132, 1995.

284. Lantz GC, Badylak SF, Hiles MC, et al: Treatment of reperfusion injury in dogs with experimentally induced gastric dilatation-volvulus. Am J Vet Res 53:1594–1598, 1992.

285. Badylak SF, Lantz GC, Jeffries M: Prevention of reperfusion injury in surgically induced gastric dilatation-volvulus in dogs. Am J Vet Res 51:294–299, 1990.

286. Muir WW, Bonagura JD: Treatment of cardiac arrhythmias in dogs with gastric distention-volvulus. JAVMA 184:1366–1371, 1984.

287. Muir WW: Gastric dilatation-volvulus in the dog, with emphasis on cardiac arrhythmias. JAVMA 180:739–742, 1982.

288. Horne WA, Gilmore DR, Dietze AE, et al: Effects of gastric distention-volvulus on coronary blood flow and myocardial oxygen consumption in the dog. Am J Vet Res 46:98–104, 1985.

289. Millis DL, Hauptman JG, Fulton RB Jr: Abnormal hemostatic profiles and gastric necrosis in canine gastric dilatation-volvulus. Vet Surg 22:93–97, 1993.

290. Hall JA, Washabau RJ: Gastrointestinal prokinetic therapy: Acetylcholinesterase drugs. Compend Contin Educ Pract Vet 19:615–621, 1997.

291. Hall JA, Solie TN, Seim HB, et al: Effect of metoclopramide on fed-state gastric myoelectric and motor activity in dogs. Am J Vet Res 57:1616–1622, 1996.

292. Eggertsdottir AV, Moe L: A retrospective study of conservative treatment of gastric dilatation-volvulus in the dog. Acta Vet Scand 36:175–184, 1995.

293. Eggertsdottir AV, Stigen O, Lonaas L, et al: Comparison of two surgical treatments of gastric dilatation-volvulus in dogs. Acta Vet Scand 37:415–426, 1996.

294. Hall JA, Willer RL, Solie TN, et al: Effect of circumcostal gastropexy on gastric myoelectric and motor activity in dogs. J Small Anim Pract 38:200–207, 1997.

295. Frendin J, et al: Gastric displacement in dogs without clinical signs of acute dilatation. J Small Anim Pract 29:775, 1988.

296. Boothe H, Ackerman N: Partial gastric torsion in two dogs. J Am Anim Hosp Assoc 12:27–30, 1976.

297. Hinder RA: Individual and combined roles of the pylorus and the antrum in the canine gastric emptying of a liquid and a digestible solid. Gastroenterology 84:281–286, 1983.

298. Kelly KA: Effect of gastric surgery on gastric motility and emptying. In Akkermans LMA, Johnson AG, Read NW (eds): Gastric and Gastroduodenal Motility. New York, Praeger, 1984, pp 241–262.

299. Muller-Lissner SA, Sonnenberg A, Schattenmann G, et al: Gastric emptying and postprandial duodenogastric reflux in pylorectomized dogs. Am J Physiol 242:G9–G14, 1982.

300. Lang IM, Sarna SK, Condon RE: Gastrointestinal motor correlates of vomiting in the dog: Quantification and characterization as an independent phenomenon. Gastroenterology 90:40–47, 1986.

301. Muller-Lissner SA, Fimmel CJ, Blum AL: Is there a relationship between duodenogastric reflux, gastric ulcer and gastritis? In Akkermans LMA, Johnson AG, Read NW (eds): Gastric and Gastroduodenal Motility. New York, Praeger, 1984, pp 282–291.

302. Muller-Lissner SA, Schattenmann G, Schenker G, et al: Duodenogastric reflux in the fasting dog: Role of pylorus and duodenal motility. Am J Physiol 241:G159–G162, 1981.

303. Sonnenberg A, Muller-Lissner SA, Schattenmann G, et al: Duodenogastric reflux in the dog. Am J Physiol 242:G603–G607, 1982.

304. MacEwen EG, Patnaik AK, Johnson GF, et al: Extramedullary plasmacytoma of the gastrointestinal tract in two dogs. JAVMA 184:1396–1398, 1984.

305. Gualtieri M, Monzeglio MG: Gastrointestinal polyps in small animals. Eur J Comp Gastro 1:5, 1996.

306. Alizadeh H, Castro GA, Weems WA: Intrinsic jejunal propulsion in the guinea pig during parasitism with Trichinella spiralis. Gastroenterology 93:784–790, 1987.

307. Fioramonti J, Bueno L: Gastrointestinal myoelectric activity disturbances in gastric ulcer disease in rats and dogs. Dig Dis Sci 25:575–580, 1980.

308. Malbert CH, Hara S, Ruckebusch Y: Early myoelectrical activity changes during gastric or duodenal ulceration in dogs. Dig Dis Sci 32:737–742, 1987.

309. Dubois A, Jacobus JP, Grissom MP, et al: Altered gastric emptying and prevention of radiation-induced vomiting in dogs. Gastroenterology 86:444–448, 1984.

310. Bueno L, Fargeas MJ, Gue M, et al: Effects of corticotropin-releasing factor on plasma motilin and somatostatin levels and gastrointestinal motility in dogs. Gastroenterology 91:884–889, 1986.

311. Bueno L, Fioramonti J: Effects of corticotropin-releasing factor, corticotropin and cortisol on gastrointestinal motility in dogs. Peptides 7:73–77, 1986.

312. Willard MD, Schall WD, McCaw DE, et al: Canine hypoadrenocorticism: Report of 37 cases and review of 39 previously reported cases. JAVMA 180:59–62, 1982.

313. Morgan KG, Schmalz PF, Go VL, et al: Effects of pentagastrin, G17, and G34 on the electrical and mechanical activities of canine antral smooth muscle. Gastroenterology 75:405–412, 1978.

314. Bauer AJ, Szurszewski JH: Effect of opioid peptides on circular muscle of canine duodenum. J Physiol (Lond) 434:409–422, 1991.

315. Kromer W: Endogenous and exogenous opioids in the control of gastrointestinal motility and secretion. Pharmacol Rev 40:121–162, 1988.

316. Edin R, Lundberg J, Terenius L, et al: Evidence for vagal enkephalinergic neural control of the feline pylorus and stomach. Gastroenterology 78:492–497, 1980.

317. Reynolds JC, Ouyang A, Cohen S: Evidence for an opiate-mediated pyloric sphincter reflex. Am J Physiol 246:G130–G136, 1984.

318. Reynolds JC, Ouyang A, Cohen S: Opiate nerves mediate feline pyloric response to intraduodenal amino acids. Am J Physiol 248:G307–G312, 1985.

319. Washabau RJ, Hall JA: Diagnosis and management of gastrointestinal motility disorders in dogs and cats. Compend Contin Educ Pract Vet 19:721–737, 1997.

320. McCallum RW, Fink SM, Lerner E, et al: Effects of metoclopramide and

GI

bethanechol on delayed gastric emptying present in gastroesophageal reflux patients. Gastroenterology 84:1573–1577, 1983.

321. Orihata M, Sarna SK: Contractile mechanisms of action of gastroprokinetic agents: Cisapride, metoclopramide, and domperidone. Am J Physiol 266:G665–G676, 1994.

322. de Ridder WJ, Schuurkes JA: Cisapride and 5-hydroxytryptamine enhance motility in the canine antrum via separate pathways, not involving 5-hydroxytryptamine 1,2,3,4 receptors. J Pharmacol Exp Ther 264:79–88, 1993.

323. Gue M, Fioramonti J, Bueno L: A simple double radiolabeled technique to evaluate gastric emptying of canned food meal in dogs. Application to pharmacological tests. Gastroenterol Clin Biol 12:425–430, 1988.

324. Hinder RA, San-Garde BA: Gastroduodenal motility—A comparison between domperidone and metoclopramide. S Afr Med J 63:270–273, 1983.

325. Hall JA, Washabau RJ: Gastrointestinal prokinetic therapy: Motilin-like drugs. Compend Contin Educ Pract Vet 19:281–288, 1997.

326. Peeters TL: Erythromycin and other macrolides as prokinetic agents. Gastroenterology 105:1886–1899, 1993.

327. Withrow SJ: Tumors of the Gastrointestinal System. E. Gastric Cancer. In Withrow SJ, MacEwen EG (eds): Small Animal Clinical Oncology. Philadelphia, WB Saunders, 1996, pp 244–248.

328. Morrison WB: Nonlymphomatous cancers of the esophagus, stomach, and intestines. In Morrison WB (ed): Cancer in Dogs and Cats: Medical and Surgical Management. Baltimore, Williams & Wilkins, 1998, pp 551–558.

329. Grooters AM, Johnson SE: Canine gastric leiomyoma. Compend Contin Educ Pract Vet 17:1485–1491, 1995.

330. Boari A, Barreca A, Bestetti GE, et al: Hypoglycemia in a dog with a leiomyoma of the gastric wall producing an insulin-like growth factor II–like peptide. Eur J Endocrinol 132:744–750, 1995.

331. Beaudry D, Knapp DW, Montgomery T, et al: Hypoglycemia in four dogs with smooth muscle tumors. J Vet Intern Med 9:415–418, 1995.

332. Cribb AE: Feline gastrointestinal adenocarcinoma: A review and retrospective study. Can Vet J 29:709–712, 1988.

333. Couto CG, Rutgers HC, Sherding RG, et al: Gastrointestinal lymphoma in 20 dogs. A retrospective study. J Vet Intern Med 3:73–78, 1989.

334. Kapatkin AS, Mullen HS, Matthiesen DT, et al: Leiomyosarcoma in dogs: 44 cases (1983–1988). JAVMA 201:1077–1079, 1992.

335. Brunnert SR, Dee LA, Herron AJ, et al: Gastric extramedullary plasmacytoma in a dog. JAVMA 200:1501–1502, 1992.

336. Zikes CD, Spielman B, Shapiro W, et al: Gastric extramedullary plasmacytoma in a cat. J Vet Intern Med 12:381–383, 1998.

337. Bortnowski HB, Rosenthal RC: Gastrointestinal mast cell tumors and eosinophilia in two cats. J Am Anim Hosp Assoc 28:271–275, 1992.

338. Bellah JR, Ginn PE: Gastric leiomyosarcoma associated with hypoglycemia in a dog. J Am Anim Hosp Assoc 32:283–286, 1996.

339. Couto CG: Gastrointestinal neoplasia in dogs and cats. In Kirk RW, Bonagura JD (eds): Kirk's Current Veterinary Therapy XI. Philadelphia, WB Saunders, 1992, pp 595–607.

340. Penninck DG, Moore AS, Gliatto J: Ultrasonography of canine gastric epithelial neoplasia. Vet Radiol Ultrasound 39:342–348, 1998.

341. Rivers BJ, Walter PA, Johnston GR, et al: Canine gastric neoplasia: Utility of ultrasonography in diagnosis. J Am Anim Hosp Assoc 33:144–155, 1997.

342. Elliott GS, Stoffregen DA, Richardson DC, et al: Surgical, medical, and nutritional management of gastric adenocarcinoma in a dog. JAVMA 185:98–101, 1984.

343. Sellon RK, Bissonnette K, Bunch SE: Long-term survival after total gastrectomy for gastric adenocarcinoma. J Vet Intern Med 10:333–335, 1996.

344. Oliveri M, Gosselin Y, Sauvageau R: Gastric adenocarcinoma in a dog: Six-and-one-half month survival following partial gastrectomy and gastroduodenostomy. J Am Anim Hosp Assoc 20:78–82, 1985.

CHAPTER 137

DISEASES OF THE SMALL INTESTINE

Edward J. Hall and Kenneth W. Simpson

The small intestine (SI) has opposing functions as both a barrier and an absorptive surface; it must digest and absorb nutrients, exclude antigens and bacteria, and eliminate fecal waste in an acceptable form. There may be changing dietary intake, yet it maintains a dynamic luminal microflora. It is not only a major organ for digestion and absorption but also a major immunologic organ. Furthermore, its activities must be integrated with the function of the entire gastrointestinal (GI) tract, and it must respond, through neuroendocrine mechanisms, to events in other organ systems. In view of the complexity of SI function, minor daily variations in stool quality are to be considered normal.

Diarrhea, a significant increase in frequency, fluidity, or volume of feces, is the cardinal sign of SI malfunction. However, diarrhea may be a manifestation of disease elsewhere in the GI tract or even in other organ systems (Table 137–1). Furthermore, diarrhea is not present in all cases of SI disease (Table 137–2). Understanding normal SI function and hence pathophysiologic mechanisms permits a logical approach to diagnosis and treatment. Through a detailed history, thorough physical examination, and relevant tests a definitive diagnosis should be reached and rational therapy prescribed.

STRUCTURE AND FUNCTION OF THE SMALL INTESTINE

NORMAL STRUCTURE

Gross Structure

The SI begins at the pylorus of the stomach and ends at the ileocolic valve. It is approximately 3 feet long in adult cats and varies from 3 to 15 feet in adult dogs.[1] It is divided anatomically into three arbitrary segments: the duodenum, jejunum, and ileum (Fig. 137–1A).

The *duodenum* is approximately 10 per cent of the length of the SI. The common bile duct and one pancreatic duct enter the duodenum via the major papilla, and in dogs an accessory pancreatic duct may enter at a minor papilla. The papillae are notable endoscopic landmarks (Fig. 137–2A). Except in cats and small dogs, the distal duodenal flexure is often at the limit of the reach of an endoscope (Fig. 137–2B). In dogs the antimesenteric side of the duodenum is marked by a line of mucosal depressions signifying the presence of Peyer's patches (Fig. 137–2C).

The *jejunum* arises as an indistinct structural and func-

TABLE 137–1. CAUSES OF DIARRHEA

Gastrointestinal disease
  Primary small intestinal disease
  Primary large intestinal disease
  Diet induced—food poisoning, gluttony, sudden change of diet
  Gastric disease
    Achlorhydria*
    Dumping syndromes*
  Pancreatic disease
    Exocrine pancreatic insufficiency
    Pancreatitis
    Pancreatic neoplasia
  Liver disease
    Hepatocellular failure
    Intrahepatic and extrahepatic cholestasis
Nongastrointestinal disease
  Polysystemic infections, for example, distemper, leptospirosis, infectious canine hepatitis in dogs; FIP‡, FeLV, FIV in cats
  Endocrine disease
    Hypoadrenocorticism
    Hyperthyroidism†
    Hypothyroidism
    APUDomas (gastrinoma or Zollinger-Ellison syndrome)*
  Renal disease
    Uremia
    Nephrotic syndrome
  Miscellaneous
    Toxemias—pyometra, peritonitis
    Congestive heart failure
    Autoimmune disease
    Metastatic neoplasia
    Various toxins and drugs

*Rare conditions.
†Rare in dogs only.
‡FIP = feline infectious peritonitis; FeLV = feline leukemia virus; FIV = feline immunodeficiency virus; APUD = amine precursor uptake and decarboxylation.

tional transition from the duodenum and forms the majority of the SI.

The *ileum* makes up approximately the last foot of the SI. It has some unique functional characteristics, such as the absorption of bile salts and cobalamin (cbl), but is not anatomically clearly demarcated from the jejunum. The ileum ends at ileocolic valve in close association with the cecocolic junction (Fig. 137–2D).

Microstructure

The SI is basically a tube in continuity with the external environment, proximally from the mouth via the esophagus

TABLE 137–2. CLINICAL SIGNS OF SMALL INTESTINAL DISEASE

Primary sign
  Diarrhea—an increase in frequency, volume, and consistency of bowel movements
Secondary signs
  Vomiting
  Weight loss and/or failure to thrive
  Hematemesis
  Melena
  Altered appetite—inappetence or anorexia
  Polyphagia, coprophagia, pica
  Abdominal discomfort, pain
  Abdominal distention
  Borborygmi and flatus
  Halitosis
  Dehydration
  Polydipsia
  Ascites and edema
  Shock

and stomach and distally to the anus via the large intestine (LI) (Fig. 137–1B). The basic cross-sectional structure of serosa, muscularis, submucosa, and mucosa is present throughout the length of the SI (Fig. 137–1C), but variations in proportions reflect varying functions of the proximal, middle, and distal regions, with the mucosa being thinnest in the ileum. The mucosal layer is responsible for secretion and absorption as well as being a barrier to the luminal environment.

The *mucosa* is the most clinically important layer of the intestine. It comprises the epithelium and the lamina propria and is modified by gross folds and finger-like processes, the villi (see Fig. 137–1C). The lamina propria contains aggregates of lymphoid tissue and nonaggregated immunocytes. Blood flow to a villus is from an arteriole that passes to its tip, where it arborizes and forms a subepithelial capillary network draining into veins. Crypts are supplied by independent arterioles. Mucosal capillaries are fenestrated and, in conjunction with a central villous lymphatic (lacteal), carry away protein-rich tissue fluid. Loss of epithelial integrity permits leakage of the protein-rich fluid and the development of a protein-losing enteropathy (PLE).

FUNCTIONAL ANATOMY

Surface Area of the Small Intestine

The surface area of the SI is increased vastly relative to the animal's size. An approximately 600-fold increase compared with a basic tubular structure is created by folds in the mucosal wall (~3-fold), cylindrical projections into the intestinal lumen called villi (~10-fold), and microscopic microvilli on the surface of each enterocyte (~20-fold) (see Fig. 137–1). Villous atrophy or even just microvillar damage is likely to produce profound malabsorption and diarrhea.

Crypt-Villus Unit

A villus and its associated crypts constitute the functional unit of the SI (Fig. 137–1D). Crypts are continually replenished by cell division, producing undifferentiated epithelial cells. There are between 4 and 40 stem cells per crypt in the adult intestine, with further division of daughter cells occurring as the cells pass up the crypt.[2] Cells pass through a maturation zone and undergo a final division, differentiating into immature enterocytes. A number of crypts supply the enterocytes to one villus, which consequently may represent a polyclonal cell population.[3]

Mucosal Epithelial Cells

The intestinal surface is covered by an epithelial cell monolayer. Enterocytes predominate in the epithelium, representing approximately 80 per cent of all cells, with interspersed mucus-secreting goblet cells. The epithelial basement membrane is permeable to nutrients and by expressing glycoproteins called laminins promotes enterocyte adhesion, growth, polarization, and differentiation through interaction with enterocyte integrins, transmembrane molecules involved in cell recognition. Enterocyte differentiation up the villus may be programmed and mediated by the expression of different integrins at different sites on the crypt-villus axis.[4] Crypt cells have a potent secretory capacity, but as enterocytes migrate to the villus tip, their maturation involves the loss of secretary activity and development of

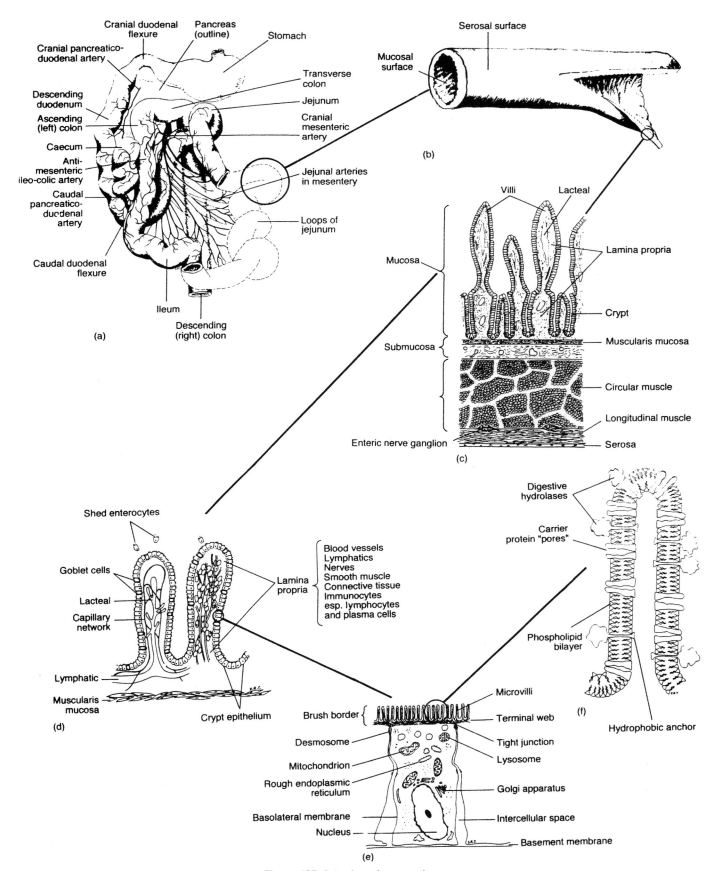

Figure 137-1 *See legend on opposite page*

GI

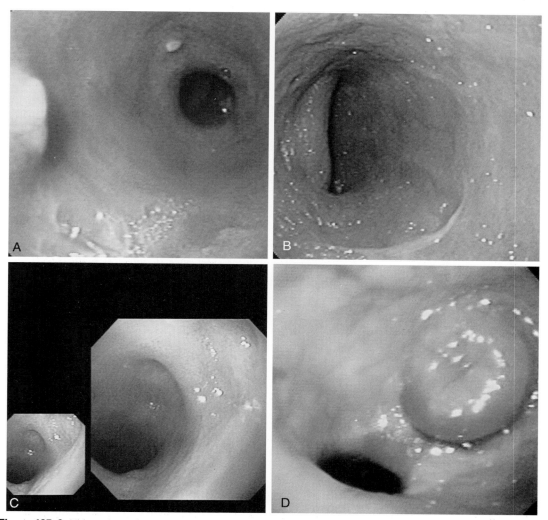

Figure 137–2. Videoendoscopic appearance of the upper small intestine. *A,* Major and minor duodenal papillae in a normal canine duodenum. *B,* The distal duodenal flexure as it bends to the left. *C,* Peyer's patches on the antimesenteric side of the duodenum appearing as a line of mucosal depressions. *D,* The mushroom-like appearance of the ileocolic valve, viewed from the ascending colon, and the opening to the cecum.

structural and functional elements associated with digestion and absorption. Some enterocytes undergo apoptotic or stochastic (random) cell death, but the majority are exfoliated at the tips of the villi. The duration of migration from crypt to villus tip is 3 to 5 days in dogs and cats.

Goblet cell density in the mucosa varies, being highest in the ileum. The cells secrete protective mucus and some novel cloverleaf-shaped peptides (trefoil peptides), which act as growth factors.[5] Endocrine and paracrine secreting cells in the mucosal surface layer also have important trophic activities,[6] as have a variety of other luminal and humoral growth regulatory factors (Table 137–3). Receptors for epi-

Figure 137–1. Functional anatomy of the small intestine. (a) Anatomic arrangement of the small intestine. (b) The small intestine is basically a tube with a serosal surface covered by visceral peritoneum and an inner absorptive and digestive surface, the mucosa. (c) Beneath the outer serosa, longitudinal and circular muscle layers produce peristaltic and segmental contractions for propelling and mixing the luminal contents. The submucosa is rich in blood and lymphatic vessels. The mucosa comprises the thin muscularis mucosae, the lamina propria, and the columnar epithelium and is thrown into folds and covered by finger-like villi to increase the digestive and absorptive surface area. (d) Enterocytes are shed from the villus tip but are continually replaced by division of crypt cells and are the site of nutrient digestion and absorption. Goblet cells secrete protective mucus. Water-soluble nutrients pass into the rich capillary network of the lamina propria, and fat is passed as chylomicrons into the lacteals. Immunocytes in the lamina propria are involved in maintaining tolerance to luminal antigens. (e) The luminal membrane of the enterocyte is thrown into processes called microvilli that increase the luminal surface area. Tight junctions between enterocytes maintain epithelial integrity. Absorbed nutrients are passed from the enterocyte into the intercellular space for distribution to the body. (f) Schematic representation of a microvillus showing digestive hydrolases anchored in the phospholipid cell membrane and protruding into the intestinal lumen. Carrier proteins within the membrane are believed to act as "pores," shuttling nutrients across the membrane by conformational changes in their structure often induced by sodium influx at the expense of energy utilization through an Na$^+$,K$^+$-ATPase on the basolateral membrane. (From Hall EJ: Small intestinal disease. *In* Gorman NT [ed]: Canine Medicine and Therapeutics, 4th ed. Oxford, Blackwell Science, 1998, p 488.)

TABLE 137–3. PHYSIOLOGICALLY ACTIVE GROWTH REGULATORY AGENTS IN THE SMALL INTESTINE

Mucosal factors
   Gastrointestinal peptides
     Epidermal growth factor
     Transforming growth factor-α (TGF-α)
     Trefoil peptides
   Prostaglandins
Luminal factors
   Alimentary secretions
     Acid
     Bile
     Pancreatic enzymes
     Epidermal growth factor (EGF)
     TGF-α
   Diet
     Sodium chloride
     Glucose
     Saturated fats
     Fiber
     Ingested carcinogens
   Intestinal flora
   Mesenchymal neurogenic influences
Humoral factors
   Systemic hormones
     Cortisol
     Growth hormone
     Insulin-like growth factors
     Thyroxine
     Prostaglandins

dermal growth factor (EGF) on the luminal and basolateral surfaces of enterocytes suggest that they respond to both blood-borne and luminal EGF secreted from salivary and pancreatic tissue or delivered in milk. Transforming growth factor-α (TGF-α) is expressed throughout the mucosa.[2] However, EGF and TGF-α are probably more important in repair of damaged epithelium, stimulating repair without fibroblast activity; TGF-β, which inhibits epithelialization, stimulates fibroplasia and is important in deeper wound repair.[7] In discrete areas, called Peyer's patches, enterocytes overlying lymphoid aggregates are modified into follicle epithelium and specialized M cells, probably in response to signals from the lymphoid cells themselves.[8]

Enterocytes

The *mucosal barrier* is formed by the epithelium, with tight junctions encircling the lateral aspects of enterocytes excluding antigens and bacteria. Effete enterocytes are shed from the villus tip (see Fig. 137–1D), but the integrity of tight junctions is probably loosest in the crypts, where fluid secretion occurs.

Enterocyte function dictates normal digestion and nutrient absorption and depends on the polarity of the enterocyte with a specialized portion of the cell membrane on the luminal surface, the microvillar membrane (MVM). The MVM is also called the brush border because of its microscopic appearance (Fig. 137–1 E and F): its surface consists of thousands of parallel cylindrical processes, the microvilli. The MVM is a phospholipid bilayer with specific proteins inserted in it. Digestive enzymes are anchored with an active site exposed to the intestinal lumen (see Fig. 137–1F), and specific carrier proteins traverse the MVM and, through conformational changes, shuttle nutrients into the enterocyte. Maximum brush border enzyme and transport activities are expressed in the midvillus region. As enterocytes migrate to the villus tip, enzyme activities are cleaved from the brush border by bacterial and pancreatic proteases and released into the lumen to form the *succus entericus,* which is thus not a true secretion.

Enterocyte metabolism is geared to the production of brush border proteins and the transfer of nutrients from the lumen to blood. Basolateral cell membranes transport sodium from inside the cell via an energy-dependent sodium-potassium adenosine triphosphatase (ATPase). Water can follow osmotically, or compensatory sodium influx at the luminal surface can drive carrier-mediated nutrient absorption. Isolated enterocytes can metabolize glucose, but inhibition of glycolysis in vivo facilitates transfer of glucose from the intestinal lumen to the blood.[9] Enterocytes can also utilize ketone bodies derived from luminal fermentation. However, in contrast to other cells, enterocytes have glutamine as their major energy source, which is largely derived from the intestinal lumen (Fig. 137–3). This helps explain the decline in villous structure, epithelial integrity, and absorptive function in starvation and anorexia and hence the clinical importance of trying to maintain enteral nutrition.[10]

Brush border activities are variable, tending to be highest in the proximal SI and declining in an abroad gradient.[11] Digestive enzymes, especially disaccharidases, and transport proteins may be inducible in response to the composition of the diet.[12] This has been shown in dogs[13] but could not be demonstrated in cats,[14] perhaps reflecting their carnivorous nature. A sudden change in diet in dogs may cause diarrhea through transient intolerance until either existing enterocytes up-regulate expression of specific enzymes and carriers or

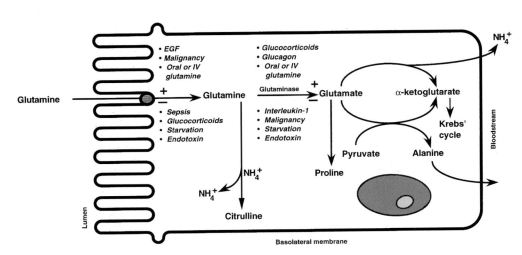

Figure 137–3. Metabolism of glutamine by enterocytes and the effects of various pathophysiologic stresses.

new enterocytes expressing induced proteins differentiate. The diarrhea thus becomes self-limiting.

DIGESTION

In order to facilitate absorption of nutrients in a usable form, major dietary constituents must be hydrolyzed from their initial polymeric structure to monomers that can be transported across the MVM. This is largely achieved in the SI by luminal enzymes. The majority are secreted by the pancreas and activated within the SI lumen. Thus, exocrine pancreatic insufficiency (EPI) is a major cause of malabsorption (see Chapter 146). The intestine provides the optimum environment in terms of solute, temperature, and pH for the actions of bile salts and pancreatic enzymes.

Normally, only terminal digestion need be performed by MVM enzymes. However, increases in enzyme activities can partially compensate for the lack of luminal enzymes in EPI and at least 40 per cent of dietary protein can still be hydrolyzed. Even with diffuse mucosal disease, there is usually sufficient reserve capacity to enable adequate digestion of starch. Capacity probably does not normally exceed twofold, being regulated according to physiologic demand, but can be modified in response to dietary change. The reserve capacity that is called into function after significant intestinal resection probably represents not only increases of brush border protein expression but also compensatory hypertrophy of the remaining tissue.

Carbohydrate Digestion

Starch is the major dietary carbohydrate and must be hydrolyzed completely to glucose for absorption (Fig. 137–4A). Digestion products of pancreatic alpha-amylase are hydrolyzed by brush border maltase (glucoamylase) and isomaltase (alpha-dextrinase). Sucrose is an unusual dietary constituent unless semimoist pet foods or human foods are fed. It is hydrolyzed directly at the MVM to glucose by sucrase, part of the sucrase-isomaltase brush border enzyme complex. Sucrase activity in cats is lower than in dogs (Table 137–4), probably reflecting the average composition of their diets. Lactose is found almost exclusively in dairy products, and its hydrolysis to glucose and galactose by brush border lactase is most important in the nursing animal. At weaning, activities of lactase decline, especially in cats,[14] and animals may become lactose intolerant. Congenital lactase deficiency has not been demonstrated.

Protein Digestion

Digestion of proteins follows a pattern similar to that of carbohydrate digestion (Fig. 137–4B). The amounts of pancreatic enzyme secreted and mucosal peptidase expressed are influenced by the protein content of the diet. Luminal proteolysis by gastric and pancreatic proteases results in a mixture of oligo-, tri-, and dipeptides as well as free amino acids. Oligopeptides are hydrolyzed by a number of brush border peptidases, which have some overlap in specificity. A reported selective deficiency of aminopeptidase N in dogs is of no clinical significance.[15] Tri- and dipeptides can also be absorbed intact on a brush border carrier.

Lipid Digestion

Partial fat digestion is begun by gastric lipase, secreted by gastric epithelial mucous cells. After solubilization by bile salt micelles, digestion of triglyceride to di- and monoglycerides and free fatty acids is completed by pancreatic lipase (Fig. 137–4C).[16] Maximal lipase activity is dependent on a protein cofactor, colipase, secreted by the pancreas as inactive pro-colipase. Reserve capacity for fat digestion exists, but neuroendocrine mechanisms, in response to fat in the duodenum and ileum, control the rate of gastric emptying and hence the rate of fat delivery and pancreatic lipase secretion. Pancreatic phospholipase A_2 hydrolyzes phospholipid to lysophospholipids, and pancreatic cholesterol esterase deesterifies cholesterol. After fat absorption, the bile salts may form further mixed micelles but ultimately are reabsorbed by a specific sodium-linked cotransporter in the ileum and recycled from portal blood back into bile.

ABSORPTION

Digested nutrients need to pass from the intestinal lumen across the mucosal barrier to enter the lymphatics or bloodstream. This uptake can occur via passive diffusion or by active or facilitated carrier-mediated transport. Endocytosis of small, antigenic peptides is of no nutritional significance but is crucial to the mucosal immune response. Receptor-mediated endocytosis enables the uptake of small amounts of a specific intact nutrient (e.g., cbl).

Carbohydrate Absorption

The main product of carbohydrate digestion, glucose, is absorbed by active transport. Glucose and sodium are co-transported, with energy expenditure by the basolateral

TABLE 137–4. JEJUNAL BRUSH BORDER DISACCHARIDASE ACTIVITIES (mU/mg PROTEIN) REPORTED IN DOGS AND CATS

ANIMALS AND SOURCE	SUCRASE	MALTASE	LACTASE	
Cats				
Hore & Messer[138]	2.8	20	0.6–1.2	(U/mg wet weight)
Kienzle[14]	17 ± 23	102 ± 58	7 ± 8	
Dogs				
Hore & Messer[138]	0.87	4.2	0.33	(U/mg wet weight)
Levanti et al[139]	~80	~400	~30	
Noon et al[140]	57 ± 2	240 ± 13	26 ± 1	
Kienzle[141]			33	
Batt et al[142]	67 ± 5	329 ± 25	33.5 ± 4	
Hall and Batt[13]				
Normal diet	78 ± 7	398 ± 26	23 ± 1	
Cereal-free diet	50 ± 8	252 ± 32	20 ± 2	

GI

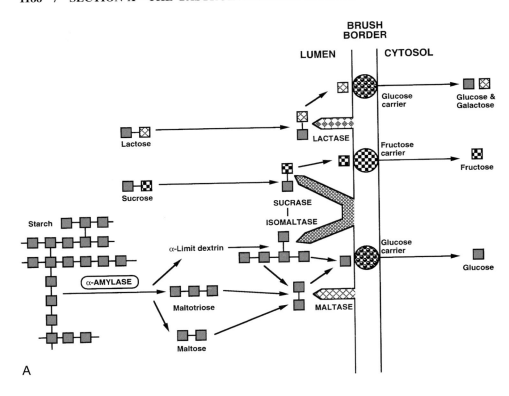

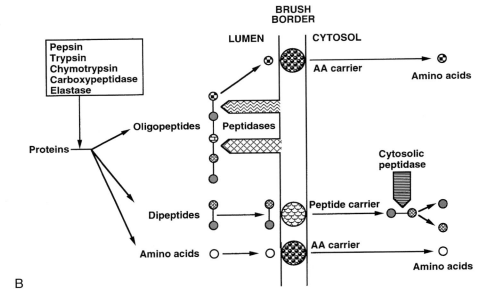

Figure 137–4. Diagrammatic representation of digestion and absorption of *(A)* carbohydrate, *(B)* protein, and *(C)* triglyceride. (Adapted from Batt RM: The molecular basis of malabsorption. J Small Anim Pract 21:555, 1980.)

Na$^+$,K$^+$-ATPase expelling sodium. The cotransporter molecule has been identified as the sodium-glucose cotransporter protein (SGLT1) in many species, including dogs and cats (Fig. 137–5).[17] This molecule has the highest affinity for glucose, but it is also the galactose carrier. Glucose and galactose may thus exhibit competitive inhibition, but glucose is the major substrate. Facilitated transport of glucose across mammalian cell membranes is performed by a family of facilitated glucose transporters (GLUTs); different isoforms are found in different tissues.[18] GLUT 2 is found on the basolateral membrane of enterocytes and shuttles glucose, galactose, and fructose out of the enterocyte by facilitated diffusion (Fig. 137–5). GLUT 2 is absent from the MVM. GLUT 5 is present, and shares homology with other GLUTs, but actually allows facilitated diffusion of fructose. GLUT 5 is also probably the site D-xylose absorption, as fructose and xylose absorption is unaffected in humans with a mutation in SGLT1 expression causing glucose-galactose malabsorption. However, the mechanism of D-xylose uptake is species dependent,[19] and evidence for facilitated diffusion in dogs and cats has been extrapolated. Fructose uptake in cats is low (as the feline diet is likely to be fructose deficient) and D-xylose absorption is equally low, perhaps explaining why the xylose absorption test is unhelpful in cats.[20]

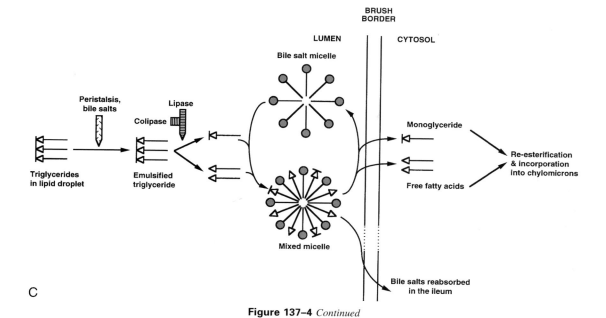

C

Figure 137-4 *Continued*

Protein Absorption

L-Amino acids are absorbed on stereospecific carriers. Sodium-linked active transport is responsible, with four carriers having selectivity for neutral (Gly, Ala), acidic (Asp, Glu), basic (Arg, Lys), and imino (Pro, HO-Pro) amino acids. Cats have a high rate of uptake of basic amino acids as they have an essential requirement for arginine. Peptide uptake has traditionally been considered to be by facilitated diffusion, with a single carrier for any oligopeptide, and the concentration gradient maintained by intracellular peptide hydrolysis, with only free amino acids being exported from enterocytes. However, in humans this peptide carrier, Pept-1, is involved in active influx of peptides, being linked to the influx of H^+ down an electrochemical gradient.[21] Protons are exchanged across the MVM with sodium, which is pumped out by the basolateral Na^+,K^+-ATPase (Fig. 137-6). A mixture of peptides and free amino acids is exported, but peptides are transported more readily than free amino acids. This has clinical significance, as the inclusion of dipeptides in elemental diets has a theoretical advantage over simple amino acid solutions. Pept-1 is also the carrier for peptidomimetic drugs (e.g., beta-lactams and angiotensin-converting enzyme inhibitors).

Lipid Absorption

The products of fat digestion are absorbed by passive diffusion from mixed micelles. The limiting factor, assuming normal pancreatic function, is the intestinal surface area, and diseases that cause villous atrophy are likely to cause fat malabsorption and steatorrhea. Generally, the products are reassembled within enterocytes to prevent back diffusion, being combined with synthesized lipoproteins for entry into the lymphatics as chylomicrons. However, medium-chain triglycerides (8 to 12 carbon atoms in length) can be absorbed directly into the portal blood and provide an alternative route for fat uptake when lymphatic flow is impaired.

Figure 137-5. Diagrammatic representation of the absorption of monosaccharides by enterocytes.

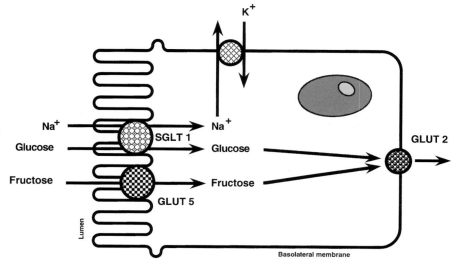

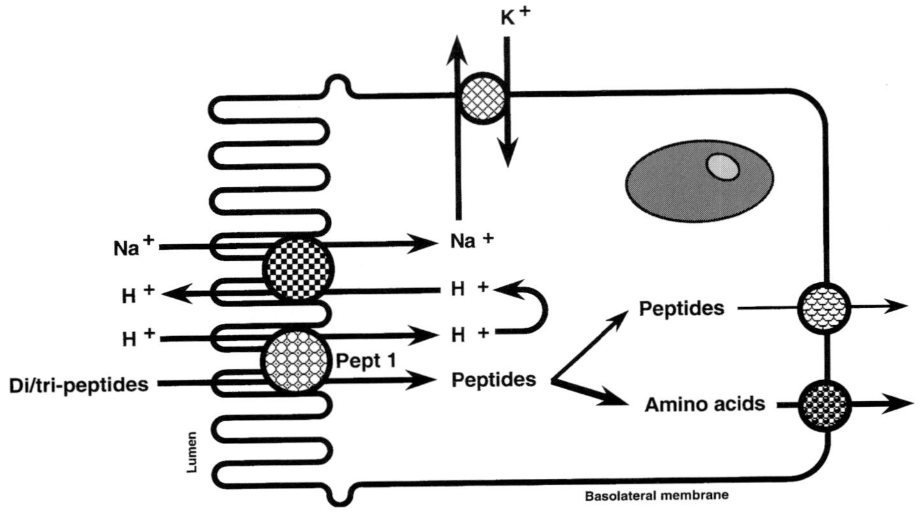

Figure 137–6. Diagrammatic representation of the absorption of di- and tripeptides by enterocytes.

Fat-Soluble Vitamins

Dietary fat-soluble vitamins A, D, E and K are solubilized in mixed micelles before passive diffusion across the brush border. Fat malabsorption associated with inadequate amounts of bile salts (e.g., biliary obstruction), lymphangiectasia, or severe villous atrophy may result in vitamin deficiency. This is clinically most important for vitamin K, as its body stores are not large, and, particularly in cats, can lead to vitamin K–dependent coagulation factor deficiencies and possible hemorrhage.

Water-Soluble Vitamins

Water-soluble B vitamins are absorbed by a mixture of passive diffusion (e.g., pyridoxine [B_6]), saturable facilitated transport (e.g., riboflavin [B_2]), or active and facilitated transport (e.g., thiamine [B_1]). The absorptive mechanisms for folic acid and vitamin B_{12} are more complicated (Fig. 137–7A) and important clinically as they may be helpful in determining the site and nature of the intestinal disease (Fig. 137–7B).[22]

Folic acid is present in adequate amounts in most commercial foods but is also produced by the enteric flora. It is usually conjugated in a poorly absorbable polyglutamate form and, before absorption, must be hydrolyzed by folate deconjugase, a brush border enzyme. Folate (pteroyl monoglutamate) is absorbed in the proximal SI by a carrier-mediated process at low luminal concentrations (see Fig. 137–7A) and by passive diffusion at high concentrations. After absorption, folate is methylated in the cell to methyltetrahydrofolate.

Cobalamin (vitamin B_{12}; cbl) is absorbed by receptor-mediated endocytosis in the ileum (see Fig. 137–7A), but the process is complex as intact cbl is absorbed while potentially harmful analogues are excluded. After ingestion, cbl is released from food in the stomach and then bound by R proteins (haptocorrins), nonspecific binding proteins of salivary and gastric origin. At acidic pH, cbl has high affinity for R proteins, but on entering the more alkaline environment of the SI, R proteins bind cbl less avidly and undergo proteolysis. Thus, cbl is transferred to another binding protein, intrinsic factor (IF), which promotes cbl absorption in the ileum. The source of IF is the stomach and pancreas in dogs and just the pancreas in cats.[23, 24] Intrinsic factor–bound

cbl complexes pass to the ileum until they bind specific receptors and are endocytosed. In portal blood cbl is bound to transcobalamin 2, enabling it to enter tissues or be reexcreted in bile. Cats and dogs have less capacity to store cbl than humans, and severe cbl malabsorption can deplete them within a month (see Fig. 137–7B).

INTESTINAL MOTILITY

Slow wave motion and segmental and peristaltic contractions are generated by the coordinated contraction of smooth muscle in response to spontaneous electrical activity modulated by coordinated neurohumoral and neurochemical input.[25] The majority of myenteric neurons are either excitatory or inhibitory, containing acetylcholine (ACh) and tachykinins or vasoactive intestinal polypeptide (VIP), the peptide histidine-isoleucine, and nitric oxide synthase, respectively. Norepinephrine, serotonin, gastrin, cholecystokinin (CCK), secretin, motilin, thyrotropin-releasing hormone (TRH), substance P, glucagon, gastric inhibitory polypeptide, histamine, and prostaglandins may also affect SI motility. Many of these molecules are also involved in regulating intestinal secretion and absorption and perhaps the mucosal immune system.[26]

Segmental contractions slow passage and ensure mixing of nutrients, whereas peristaltic contractions propel ingesta onward. In health, there is a balance between delaying the transit of food, to allow digestion and absorption, and keeping ingesta moving. Reduced segmental motility may lead to rapid transit, whereas decreased peristalsis delays transit. Clinical manifestations are diarrhea and ileus, respectively.

Intestinal motility in the fasted state in dogs is characterized by three phases. The first is a quiescent phase (about 1 hour), the second is characterized by minor contractile activity (15 to 40 minutes), and the third consists of the migrating myoelectric complex (MMC, 4 to 8 minutes). The MMC is short in duration and is a period of intense motor and contractile activity that sweeps undigested food, secretions, desquamated cells, and bacteria down the intestine. It is known as the intestinal "housekeeper" and is induced by motilin secretion. The three-phase fasting cycle is repeated approximately every 3 hours. The pattern of intestinal motility in cats appears different, with a migrating spike complex correlating with the MMC.[27]

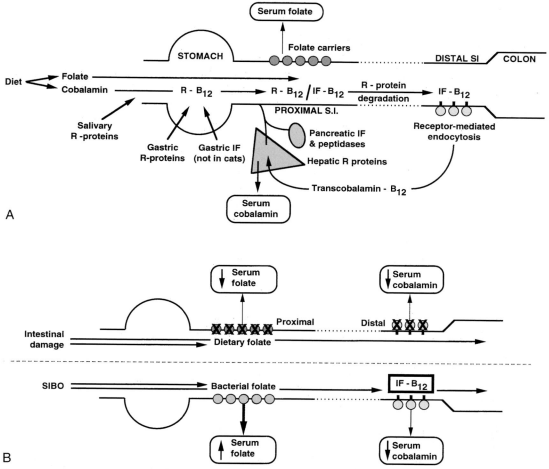

Figure 137–7. Diagrammatic representation of the absorption of folate and cobalamin. *A,* By normal intestine: folate is absorbed in the proximal SI by carrier-mediated diffusion and cobalamin in the ileum by receptor-mediated endocytosis. *B,* By diseased intestine: proximal and distal mucosal damage causes folate and cobalamin malabsorption, respectively, and bacterial overgrowth may cause increased folate uptake because of bacterial folate synthesis and decreased cobalamin uptake because of bacterial binding.

In the fed state the pattern of motility is more similar to phase 2 fasting motility and lasts from 3 to 12 hours. Its duration is determined by nature of the diet, with fats and fiber prolonging it.

FLUID BALANCE

The ability of the intestine to absorb fluid and electrolytes varies according to site, with water absorption becoming increasingly efficient distally. The net amount of fluid and electrolytes in the GI tract reflects a balance between absorption and secretion, with net absorption occurring in healthy intestine.

Absorption

In a 20-kg dog approximately 2.7 L of fluid (oral intake, stomach juice, saliva, pancreatic juice, and bile) is presented to the SI each day. About 1.35 L is absorbed in the jejunum, 1 L in the ileum, and 300 mL in the colon, leaving 50 mL in feces.[28] Thus, the jejunum absorbs 50 per cent, the ileum 75 per cent, and the colon 90 per cent of the fluid volume presented to it (Fig. 137–8). The gradient in absorptive ability is a function of enterocyte pore size, membrane potential difference, and the type of transport process associated with each intestinal segment (Fig. 137–9 and 137–10).[29] The site of the enterocyte on the villus is also important; villus enterocytes absorb whereas crypt cells secrete.

Transport Processes. The absorption of water is passive and follows transport of solutes across the GI epithelium by one of three processes: passive absorption, active absorption, and solvent drag. *Passive absorption* can be trans- or paracellular and is down an electrochemical gradient (e.g., passive transport of Na and Cl in the jejunum and ileum). *Active transport* is against a concentration gradient and requires an energy input (e.g., Na transport. by an Na^+,K^+-ATPase present in all enterocytes) (see Fig. 137–9, mechanism A). This maintains the electrochemical Na gradient required not only for net transepithelial Na movement but also for the transport of other solutes.[29] *Solvent drag* describes solute movement secondary to water flow (e.g., NaCl transport in the jejunum via the paracellular route).

Jejunum. With high permeability, passive transport provides the major contribution to Na and Cl movement in the jejunum. Although Na-nutrient– and Na-H–linked absorption is present, solvent drag–mediated sodium absorption (see Figs. 137–9, mechanism B, and 137–10), secondary to monosaccharide absorption, is the major mechanism for Na absorption in this segment.

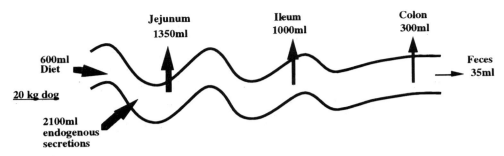

Mucosal resistance	Leaky	Mod. leaky	Tight
Potential difference (PD)	3mV	6mV	20mV

Absorptive Mechanism

Sodium	Na+/ nutrient Na+/ H+	Na+/ nutrient coupled Na+/Cl-	coupled Na+/Cl-
Potassium	Passive K+	Passive K+	Passive K+ Active K+
Chloride	PD-dependent Cl-	PD-dependent Cl- coupled Na+/Cl- HCO3- -dependent Cl-	PD-dependent Cl- coupled Na+/Cl- HCO3- -dependent Cl-

Figure 137–8. Fluid fluxes in the intestine. (Adapted from references 28, 29, and 137.)

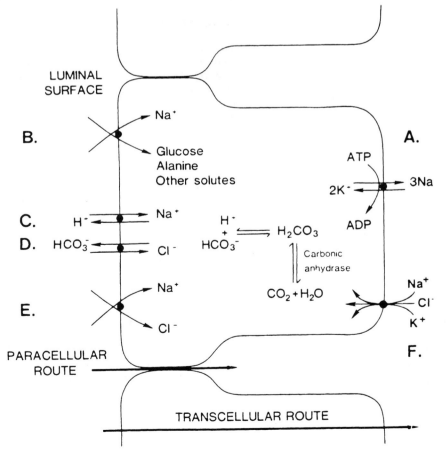

Figure 137–9. Membrane transport processes present in different regions of the SI. Absorptive mechanisms: all enterocytes *(A)*, jejunum *(B)*, and ileum *(B–E)*. Secretory mechanisms *(F)*. (From Moseley RH: Fluid and electrolyte disorders and gastrointestinal disease. *In* Kokko JP, Tannen RL [eds]: Fluids and Electrolytes, 3rd ed. Philadelphia, WB Saunders, 1996, p 675.)

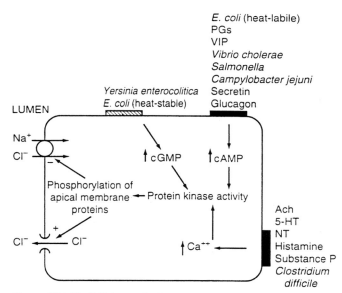

Figure 137–10. Cellular mechanisms controlling sodium chloride absorption and chloride secretion by enterocytes. (From Moseley RH: Fluid and electrolyte disorders and gastrointestinal disease. *In* Kokko JP, Tannen RL [eds]: Fluids and Electrolytes, 3rd ed. Philadelphia, WB Saunders, 1996, p 675.)

Ileum. Sodium is absorbed predominantly by neutral NaCl absorption (see Figs. 137–9 mechanism C, D, or E, and 137–10) with some contribution by Na-nutrient (see Fig. 137–9, mechanism B).

Colon. In the colon Na is absorbed against large electrochemical gradients (see Fig. 137–8). Mineralocorticoids (e.g., aldosterone) activate Na channels in the luminal membrane and increase Na^+,K^+-ATPase molecules in the basolateral membrane. A consequence of Na absorption in the colon is transfer of potassium into the lumen. Colonic absorption is important in SI disease, compensating for fluid losses. Furthermore, dogs and cats with SI disease may have signs of LI dysfunction as products from the SI, such as hydroxylated fatty acids or deconjugated bile acids, impair colonic absorption or stimulate secretion.

Intestinal Secretion

Intestinal secretion is a function of villous crypt cells. It is thought to be caused by the electrogenic transport of chloride across the basolateral membrane into the enterocyte (see Fig. 137–9, mechanism F) and chloride efflux through chloride channels in the MVM into the intestinal lumen (see Fig. 137–10). Passive flux of water follows chloride secretion.

Control of the Absorption and Secretion of Water and Electrolytes

Fluid balance is largely an autonomous process regulated by the neurocrine systems located in the submucosal plexus.[29] VIP and ACh are major mediators of secretion. At a cellular level they increase intracellular calcium and cyclic adenosine monophosphate (cAMP), inhibiting neutral sodium and chloride absorption and facilitating transcellular chloride efflux. Many bacterial agents exert their diarrheogenic effects by increasing intraenterocyte cAMP. The principal regulators of absorption, noradrenaline, somatostatin, and opioids, lower intracellular cAMP and calcium concentra-

tions, stimulate neutral NaCl absorption, and can have therapeutic antidiarrheal effects.

BACTERIAL FLORA

The bacterial flora of the SI increases in number from the duodenum to the colon. Factors maintaining this aboral gradient are luminal patency, intestinal motility, substrate availability, various bacteriostatic or bactericidal secretions (e.g., gastric acid, bile, and pancreatic secretions), and an intact ileocecocolic valve. Abnormalities of these control mechanisms may facilitate the overgrowth of SI bacteria. The normal SI flora is a diverse mixture of aerobic, anaerobic, and facultatively anaerobic bacteria. Common aerobic species include *Staphylococcus* spp., *Streptococcus* spp., Enterobacteriaceae, *Escherichia coli*, *Bacillus* spp., *Proteus* spp., *Pasturella* spp., *Corynebacterium* spp., *Lactobacillus* spp., and *Enterococcus* spp. Frequent anaerobes are *Clostridium* spp., and *Bacteroides* spp., Quantitative bacteriology using samples of undiluted intestinal juice has revealed that healthy dogs harbor up to 10^9 colony-forming units (CFU)/mL aerobic and anaerobic bacteria in the proximal SI.[30] Similarly, bacterial counts in healthy cats range from 10^2 to 10^8 aerobic and anaerobic bacteria.[31, 32] These numbers are considerably higher than those reported in healthy humans (less than 10^{3-5}) and indicate that "cutoff" values for normal flora in dogs and cats cannot be extrapolated from humans, despite the fact that reports describing small intestinal bacterial overgrowth (SIBO) in dogs used a cutoff value of 10^5.[33, 34]

The resident bacterial flora is an integral part of the healthy SI and influences a wide variety of parameters such as villous size, enterocyte turnover, enzyme turnover on the microvilli, and intestinal motility. The digestion and assimilation of fats, carbohydrates, and proteins; amino acids such as taurine; and vitamins such as cbl and folate are also influenced by bacteria. Certain bacterially derived short-chain fatty acids are substrates for enterocytes, and others can stimulate intestinal secretion. The presence of a stable enteric flora is important for preventing colonization by pathogens and stimulates the development of the enteric immune system. Indeed, the host response to a bacterium is likely to be as important as the intrinsic pathogenicity of the bacterium. Loss of tolerance for the normal bacterial flora may precipitate abnormal intestinal function, intestinal inflammation, and possibly neoplasia.

The SI flora is relatively resistant to dietary changes. Studies utilizing different diets or the addition of fructooligosaccharides to the diet of dogs demonstrated no effects on the number or type of bacteria in the proximal SI but some effects on the colonic flora.[35, 36] Given the intimate interrelationship of the healthy intestine with its flora, the indiscriminate use of antibiotics in dogs and cats with diarrhea or gastroenteritis is ill advised and may enhance antibiotic resistance. Although the consequences of inappropriate antibiotic therapy are often mild, postantibiotic salmonellosis has had fatal consequences in cats.[37]

MUCOSA-ASSOCIATED LYMPHOID TISSUE

The barrier function of the intestinal mucosa protects the animal against luminal pathogens or antigens. A number of nonspecific mechanisms are involved (Table 137–5), but the barrier is underpinned by the mucosa-associated lymphoid

TABLE 137-5. COMPONENTS OF THE INTESTINAL MUCOSAL BARRIER

Protein denaturation by gastric acid
Protein degradation by proteolytic enzymes and bacteria
Clearance of waste by peristalsis
Unstirred water layer
Surface mucus layer
Secretory immunoglobulin A
Enterocyte microvillous membrane
Epithelial tight junctions
Mucosa-associated lymphoid tissue

tissue (MALT). The MALT constitutes approximately 25 per cent of the mucosal mass, and is estimated to contain more immunocytes than any other organ system. In addition to the synthesis of immunoglobulin (IgA), the major immunoglobulin secreted by the mucosa, the MALT plays a crucial role in defending against potential pathogens while maintaining tolerance against harmless dietary and bacterial antigens. Tolerance is a state of local responsiveness and systemic hyporesponsiveness.

Antigen Presentation

Small amounts of antigen are perpetually crossing the mucosal barrier; an estimated 0.002 per cent of dietary antigen is absorbed intact, and this can invoke an immune response.

Peyer's Patches. Major sites of antigen uptake are phagocytic M cells found in the follicle-associated epithelium overlying Peyer's patches, which are approximately 20 discrete, macroscopic aggregates of lymphoid tissue found along the SI. Isolated lymphoid nodules found throughout the gut probably function in the same way as Peyer's patches. M cells possess surface receptors for some pathogenic organisms, such as salmonella and rotavirus, and may offer a route for invasion. More important, their lack of significant microvilli and minimal glycocalyx and the paucity of goblet cells and IgA secretion at Peyer's patches essentially create a break in barrier function. M cells sample luminal antigens and transfer them to subepithelial macrophages, dendritic cells, and lymphocytes in the underlying lymphoid follicle with which they are in intimate contact (Fig. 137–11). The macrophages act as antigen-presenting cells (APCs). They express major histocompatibility complex (MHC) class II molecules, surface glycoproteins that enable processed antigen to be presented to lymphocytes (Fig. 137–12).[38, 39]

Enterocytes. As well as M cells, enterocytes can endocytose luminal antigen. Soluble macromolecules are likely to be degraded in lysosomes. However, membrane-bound antigens are internalized and, although probably modified intracellularly, ultimately do pass out through the basolateral membrane.[40] Gut-processed antigen that has been absorbed into the serum has distinct characteristics and can transfer tolerance experimentally. Because macromolecules appear to bind more readily to immature enterocytes, this mechanism may be more important in young animals. Enterocytes can also express MHC class II molecules, just as APCs in Peyer's patches do, and are capable of presenting antigen. However, the importance of this potential is uncertain, as the distribution of MHC class II molecules on such "nonprofessional APCs" varies considerably between species. In dogs the majority are expressed on crypt cells but particularly in the distal SI (Fig. 137–13).[41] Antigen presentation by nonprofessional APCs such as enterocytes may be important in the induction of tolerance.

Paracellular Uptake. Entry of antigen may also occur normally through tight junctions, but uptake is likely to be increased if the mucosa is damaged, especially if intercellular permeability is increased by cytokines such as interferon-γ (IFN-γ) and the passage of neutrophils. Entry of antigen in such an abnormal way and escape from the normal APC

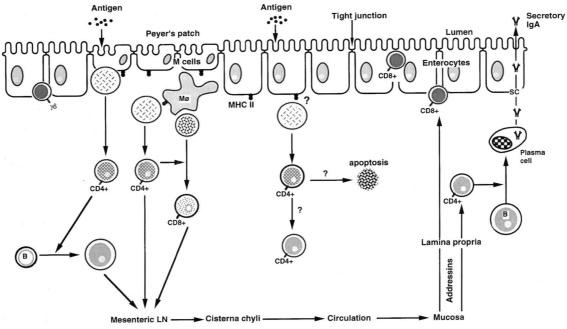

Figure 137-11. Diagrammatic representation of the mucosa-associated lymphoid tissue showing M cells in a Peyer's patch sampling luminal antigen, presentation of the antigen to the associated lymphoid tissue, priming of B and T cells, and their circulation to the lamina propria, with subsequent immunoglobulin A secretion.

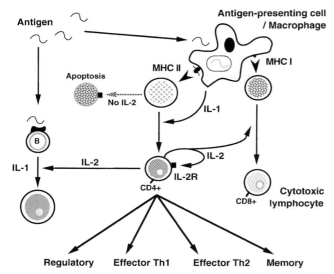

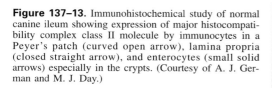

Figure 137–12. Activation of mucosal CD4⁺ T cells by antigen presentation in association with MHC class II molecules with subsequently either clonal expansion into memory and effector cells or apoptosis, depending on the synthesis of IL-2 receptor and IL-2. CD8⁺ T cells are activated by antigen presentation in association with MHC class I molecule and under the influence of CD4⁺ T cell–derived cytokines develop into intraepithelial lymphocytes. γδT cells also form a part of the intraepithelial cell compartment. IL-2 = interleukin-2; MHC = major histocompatibility complex.

mechanisms is a potential route by which sensitization and hypersensitivity may develop.

B-Cell Responses

Antigen presentation in Peyer's patches results in clonal expansion of B and T cells. Primed B cells proliferate, stimulated by interleukin-1 (IL-1) from APCs and IL-2 from T cells, and undergo class switching to form activated B cells that secrete a specific immunoglobulin class. They migrate via mesenteric lymph nodes, cisterna chyli, and thoracic duct to the circulation and return to the intestine, "homing" to the lamina propria (see Fig. 137–11), by recognition of specific receptors (addressins) in the tissue.[42]

The density and class of B cells vary both along the gut and up the villus, but the majority are IgA cells, and ulti-

mately, under the influence of cytokines such as TGF-β, they mature into plasma cells secreting dimeric IgA.[43] This IgA combines with secretory component, a receptor on the basolateral membrane of enterocytes, is internalized by the enterocyte, and is then secreted onto the luminal surface, where it remains trapped in the surface mucous layer as a protective barrier. IgA is also secreted in large quantities in bile.[44] This directed IgA response literally "paints" the intestinal surface with protective antibody tailored to act against luminal antigens and pathogens.

Although IgA is an important barrier mechanism, other immunoprotective mechanisms are present. B cells producing IgM and IgG are normally present at a lower density in the lamina propria, but, with IgA, their respective antibodies can bind antigens in the lumen. Immune complexes formed with any antigens that enter the lamina propria are cleared to the reticuloendothelial cells of the liver. Increased numbers of cells secreting antibodies, especially IgG and IgM, in the lamina propria are seen in inflammatory disease and are part of the pathologic process. IgE-secreting B cells may be present in response to intestinal parasites and are important in the "self-cure" that may be seen in nematode infestations, but their role in dietary hypersensitivities is clearly pathologic. Other cells such as neutrophils and macrophages are recruited to the lamina propria by proinflammatory cytokines and bacterial chemotactic oligopeptides. The role of eosinophils and mast cells in normal and inflamed intestine in dogs and cats has not been adequately studied.

T-Cell Responses

The role of T cells in the lamina propria is crucial in the maintenance of tolerance and the development of appropriate immune responses in the intestine. It is underpinned by the unique spatial arrangement of the different T-cell phenotypes in the intestinal mucosa. CD4-positive T cells predominate in the lamina propria, and in the intestinal epithelium CD8-positive T cells predominate. This distribution has now been demonstrated in many species including dogs[45] and cats[46] and is probably programmed by the integrins each cell subset expresses. In the normal gut, naive CD8⁺T cells can be primed by antigen presentation in association with MHC class I molecules and proliferate with help from CD4⁺ T

GI

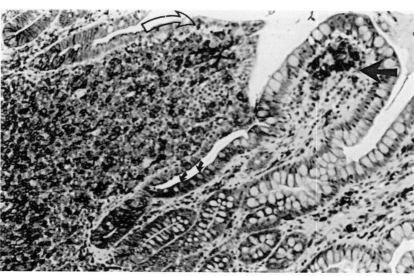

Figure 137–13. Immunohistochemical study of normal canine ileum showing expression of major histocompatibility complex class II molecule by immunocytes in a Peyer's patch (curved open arrow), lamina propria (closed straight arrow), and enterocytes (small solid arrows) especially in the crypts. (Courtesy of A. J. German and M. J. Day.)

cells secreting IL-2. They may be cytotoxic cells that principally respond to antigen expressed on virus-infected or neoplastic cells. However, the role of CD8+ intraepithelial lymphocytes (IELs) is uncertain.[47, 48]

Th Lymphocyte Subsets. The concept that CD4+ and CD8+ T cells correspond to "helper" and "suppressor" cells, respectively, is outdated. In fact, the induction and maintenance of oral tolerance appear to reside within the CD4+ T cell population. Priming and activation of CD4+ T cells require presentation of antigen in association with MHC class II on APCs (see Fig. 137–12). Subsequent expression of IL2-receptor and IL2 secretion by the lymphocytes autoactivate them and lead to clonal expansion, with the development of memory and effector cells. Pathogen-specific memory cells in the mucosa have been demonstrated.[49]

Upon priming, CD4+ effector T cells can differentiate into one of two mutually exclusive subsets, so-called Th1 and Th2 cells, and it appears to be the balance between the subsets that is important. Each subset has its own characteristic cytokine profile: Th1 cells express IL-2, IFN-γ, and tumor necrosis factor (TNF); Th2 cells express IL-4, IL-5, IL-6, IL-10, and IL-13.[50] The factors involved in driving CD4+ T cells down Th1- or Th2-like pathways include the nature and amount of antigen, the local cytokine environment, the affinity of the T-cell receptor for the antigen, and the MHC ligand density on the APC.[51] Within a Th-subset, the characteristic cytokines tend to self-amplify cell differentiation while inhibiting the other subset (Fig. 137–14). In general, Th1 cells regulate cell-mediated immunity, and Th2 cells regulate humoral responses, although such a clear-cut division is too simplistic. Nevertheless, Th1-like differentiation tends to be initiated by activated macrophages, dendritic cells, and T cells through the release of IL-12, and their cytokine response enhances phagocytic and T cell–mediated cytotoxicity. In contrast, Th2-like differentiation tends to be initiated by alternative cellular sources through IL-4 production, and their cytokine response induces neutralizing IgG production, IgE-dependent mast cell and eosinophil activation, and, ultimately, inhibition of acute inflammatory responses through IL-10 production (see Fig. 137–14). IL-10 appears to be a major inhibitor of the inflammatory response and is a major product of lamina propria T cells (especially Th2 cells) and macrophages.[52] Although the balance between two T-cell subsets is an attractive mechanism for explaining oral tolerance, the actual situation is undoubtedly more complex. It is unlikely that a single mechanism could be sufficient to maintain tolerance to the vast array of antigens to which the mucosa is exposed.

Oral Tolerance. It has been suggested that there are two main mechanisms of tolerance: active suppression and clonal deletion or anergy.[53] Exposure to low doses of antigen leads to induction of TGF-β–secreting active suppressor cells, whereas exposure to high doses may cause anergy or apoptosis. The lamina propria microenvironment and the nature of the APC probably play an important role in deciding whether an active immune response or tolerance to an antigen develops. Antigen presentation by nonprofessional APCs may favor induction of tolerance, whereas professional APCs (dendritic cells) favor immune responsiveness.[54] IL-10 and TGF-β production, which also induces class switching to IgA secretion, may lead to active suppression or anergy or apoptosis of cell-mediated responses and production of protective immunoglobulin.

In summary, in normal animals, the MALT is arranged anatomically and functionally to help exclude and clear harmless antigen without invoking an inflammatory response while still being able to respond to potential pathogens. In view of its complexity, it may be surprising that breakdown of tolerance and development of food allergy are not more common.

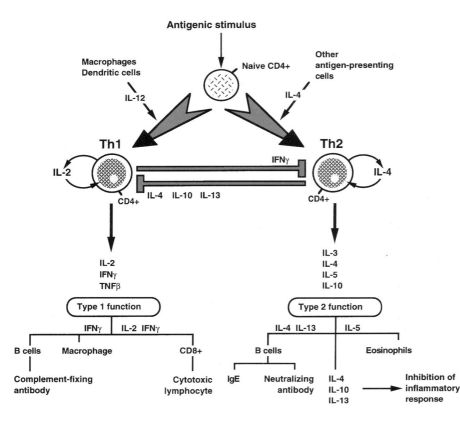

Figure 137–14. Diagrammatic representation of the effector functions of Th1 and Th2 CD4+ T cells and their mutual interaction, mediated by their secretion of cytokines.

PATHOPHYSIOLOGIC MECHANISMS IN INTESTINAL DISEASE

LUMINAL DISTURBANCES

Lack of pancreatic enzymes in EPI and increased destruction of enzymes because of SIBO result in failure of digestion. Bacteria may also compete for nutrients (e.g., binding of cbl in SIBO). Interruption of enterohepatic circulation and lack of bile salt micelles result in fat malabsorption and can be caused by portosystemic shunting, intra- or extrahepatic cholestasis, bacterial deconjugation of bile salts in the gut lumen, or ileal disease. Surgical resection of the ileum (e.g., after ileocolic intussusception) and infiltrative bowel disease affecting the distal SI cause both bile salt and cbl malabsorption.

VILLOUS ATROPHY

Villous atrophy results in loss of intestinal surface area and malabsorption. Despite some reserve capacity in the distal SI, fat absorption is impaired. Also, with a finite number of nutrient transporters, carrier-mediated uptake is rate limiting, and the loss of carriers is crucial to carbohydrate and protein digestion. Finally, the epithelial damage may lead to a breach of the mucosal barrier and development of intestinal inflammation.

Atrophy of the villi is caused by either a decrease in production of enterocytes or an increased rate of loss. Infectious agents that damage enterocytes may infect the tip of the villus (e.g., rotavirus) or the midvillus (e.g., coronavirus) and cause just cell loss and a mild to moderate diarrhea. Increased loss through immune-mediated mechanisms, as is suspected in gluten sensitivity in Irish setters, is associated with partial villous atrophy. Persistent abnormal loss of mature enterocytes is usually associated with compensatory crypt hyperplasia and an increased crypt cell proliferation rate. If the cell loss is matched by the increased proliferation, villous atrophy does not occur but enterocytes are immature and not fully functional. However, sometimes enterocyte loss outpaces increased proliferation rates, and villous atrophy results. Nevertheless, if the loss can be halted the villus should regain its normal dimensions; in most situations villus atrophy is completely reversible if the initiating cause can be removed. Finally, cytotoxic drugs (e.g., vincristine) and diseases (e.g., parvovirus infection) that cause crypt arrest or destruction, respectively, can be even more devastating, causing complete villus and crypt collapse and severe diarrhea. Assuming that some stem cells survive the insult, regeneration is possible but it is likely to take several days.

ENTEROCYTE DYSFUNCTION

If enterocytes are damaged, the loss of brush border proteins is probably most important. Interference with enterocyte function can occur without histologic damage through the action of various secretagogues produced by bacteria. Bacterial deconjugation of bile salts and hydroxylation of fatty acids stimulate secretion and impair absorptive function. Malnutrition and ischemia also impair function and increase epithelial permeability.

MICROVILLAR MEMBRANE DAMAGE

The MVM is obviously damaged in diseases with overt histologic damage to the villus, but even without light microscopic changes, there can be massive impairment of mucosal function if the microvilli are damaged. Such damage is seen with enteropathogenic *E. coli* infection or lectins, causing a loss of surface area and secondary deficiencies of brush border enzymes and carriers.

BRUSH BORDER MEMBRANE DISEASE

Primary brush border membrane diseases are biochemical abnormalities that occur in the absence of histologic damage. Congenital absence of specific enzymes or transport proteins is well characterized in humans (Table 137–6), and defects affecting amino acid transport often involve identical renal tubular defects.[55] Equivalent defects in dogs and cats have rarely been demonstrated. Relative lactase deficiency does occur in dogs and particularly in cats.[14] For example, kittens can tolerate lactose at 100 g/kg/day, but adults can hydrolyze only a maximum of 2 g/kg/day without adverse effects. Trehalase absence in cats is of little significance as their carnivorous diet usually does not contain trehalose. A lack of aminopeptidase N in dogs[15] is of no clinical significance because of the overlap in specificity with other peptidases. A specific defect in the ileal receptor for cbl-IF complexes has been documented in giant schnauzers[56] and causes cbl deficiency with inappetence, failure to thrive, neutropenia, and anemia but no specific GI signs. Lethal acrodermatitis in bull terriers is associated with zinc malabsorption.[57]

The MVM is also susceptible to secondary damage by luminal factors even without histologic changes. Bacterial overgrowth is associated with subtle but specific damage to the membrane. Obligate anaerobes are effective at degrading or releasing brush border enzymes, an effect seen in EPI. In idiopathic anaerobic overgrowth there is a marked fall in the MVM density suggestive of degradation of membrane glycoproteins. In contrast, aerobic overgrowth results in loss of alkaline phosphatase by damaging the hydrophobic part of the MVM associated with it (Fig. 137–15).

GI

TABLE 137–6. BRUSH BORDER MEMBRANE DISEASES IDENTIFIED IN HUMANS

Carbohydrate digestion and absorption
  Lactase deficiency
    Congenital
    Adult onset (lactase expression switched off)
  Sucrase-isomaltase deficiency
  Trehalase deficiency
  Glucose-galactose malabsorption
Defects of protein digestion and absorption
  Enterokinase deficiency
  Hartnup's disease (monoamino-monocarboxyl amino acid
    transporter defects)
Specific amino acid malabsorption and urinary absorption defects
  Cystine (cystinuria)
  Lysine (lysinuria)
  Tryptophan
  Methionine
  Imino acids and glycine
Defects of electrolyte transporters
  Congenital chloridorrhea (chloride-bicarbonate exchange in
    ileum and colon)
  Cystic fibrosis (mutation of regulated chloride channel in
    intestine and other tissues)
  Primary hypomagnesemia
Vitamin-mineral malabsorption
  Imerslund-Gräsbeck syndrome (cobalamin malabsorption)
  Congenital folate malabsorption
  Acrodermatitis enteropathica (zinc malabsorption)
Miscellaneous defects
  Primary bile salt malabsorption

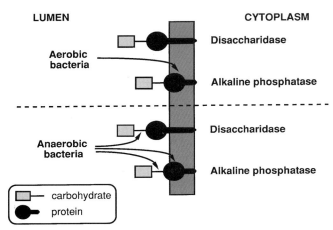

Figure 137–15. Effects of bacterial overgrowth on microvillar membrane proteins. (From Barrows CF, Batt RM, Sherding RG: Diseases of the small intestine. *In* Ettinger SJ, Feldman EC: Textbook of Veterinary Internal Medicine, 4th ed. Philadelphia, WB Saunders, 1995, p 1216.)

MUCOSAL BARRIER DISRUPTION

The mucosal barrier is crucial in maintaining oral tolerance and excluding pathogens. Barrier damage may lead to entry of antigens, subsequent allergic and/or inflammatory reactions, and even translocation of bacteria into the circulation. Leakage of protein-rich tissue fluid in the opposite direction is of clinical significance too. Causes of increases in permeability include luminal aggressive factors and endogenous inflammatory mediators such as IFN-γ (Table 137–7). In animal models, malnutrition is associated with villous atrophy; with loss of intestinal weight, protein, and RNA content; and with increased macromolecule transepithelial absorption, abnormal mucin, and reduced IgA secretion.[58]

HYPERSENSITIVITY

Sensitization of an animal to a dietary antigen may provoke an IgE-mediated allergic reaction and may actually enhance transfer of antigens through enterocytes by increasing the rapidity of the response. The release of numerous mast cell mediators (e.g., histamine, serotonin, heparin, interleukins) may have remote effects (e.g., pruritus, urticaria)

TABLE 137–7. EXAMPLES OF AGENTS THAT CAN DAMAGE THE MUCOSAL BARRIER

Luminal aggressive factors
  Enteric infections
  Endotoxin
  Ethanol
  Nonsteroidal anti-inflammatory drugs
  Cytotoxic drugs
  Bile salts
Endogenous factors
  Malnutrition—starvation, malabsorption
  Ischemia
  Reperfusion injury
  Nitric oxide
  Remote inflammatory disease and burns
  Intestinal inflammation
  Interferon-γ
  Neutrophil migration
  Mast cell mediators (e.g., histamine, bradykinin)

and even generalized systemic effects (i.e., anaphylaxis). They also have local effects on the intestine, acting directly on epithelium, muscle, and endothelium and indirectly via fibroblast and nerve activity.[59] They induce rapid changes in absorption and secretion, mucus secretion, epithelial and endothelial permeability, and gut motility, causing vomiting and diarrhea.

MUCOSAL INFLAMMATION

Inflammation is a cellular and vascular response to a number of inciting causes that include infection, ischemia, trauma, toxins, neoplasia, and immune-mediated reactions. It occurs in the intestine by processes similar to those elucidated in other tissues. The normal mucosa is continually bombarded by bacteria and luminal antigens and can be considered to be in a state of "controlled inflammation." However, anything that damages the mucosal barrier is likely to trigger uncontrolled inflammation. Once initiated, the inflammation may be self-perpetuating, particularly if there is immune dysregulation. In IBD in humans, TNF is one of the major proinflammatory cytokines, and anti-TNF antibody treatment has shown early promise as a therapeutic modality.[60]

NEOPLASIA

Solitary tumors can cause diarrhea, probably through the effects of partial obstruction, stasis of ingesta, and secondary bacterial overgrowth. More commonly, tumors are associated with signs of intestinal obstruction (i.e., vomiting, abdominal pain, absence of feces), bleeding, cancer-associated anorexia, and so forth. Mast cell tumors may cause duodenal perforation and peritonitis through histamine-mediated gastric acid hypersecretion. Diffuse tumors, such as lymphoma, infiltrating the mucosa cause diarrhea. Malignant cells may simply obstruct blood and lymphatic flow, but enterocyte function is also impaired or the whole epithelium may be eroded.

NUTRIENT DELIVERY BLOCKADE

Primary lymphatic obstruction (lymphangiectasia) may be idiopathic or associated with lymphangitis. Secondary lymphangiectasia is seen with lymphatic obstruction. These conditions and chronic liver disease causing portal hypertension impair absorption and lead to exudation of fluid.

INTESTINAL PROBLEMS

DIARRHEA

Diarrhea is due to an increase in fecal mass caused by an increase in fecal water and/or solid content. It is accompanied by an increase in the frequency and/or fluidity and/or volume of feces, and by this definition, even the frequent passage of bulky stools would be recognized as diarrhea. It must be remembered that the absence of recognizable diarrhea does not preclude the possibility of significant SI disease. Any disturbance of normal intestinal electrolyte, nutrient, and water transport may result in diarrhea and can be caused by many diseases of the GI tract, other organ systems, and systemic diseases. There are several ways to classify diarrhea (Table 137–8); they are not mutually exclusive

TABLE 137–8. CLASSIFICATIONS OF DIARRHEA

Mechanistic
    Osmotic
    Secretory
    Permeability (exudative)
    Dysmotility
    Mixed
Temporal
    Acute
    Chronic
Anatomic
    Extraintestinal
    Small intestinal
    Large intestinal
    Diffuse
Pathophysiologic
    Biochemical
    Allergic
    Inflammatory
    Neoplastic
Etiologic, for example, diet, bacterial, viral, parasitic
Causal, for example, exocrine pancreatic insufficiency,
    salmonellosis, lymphoma
Clinical
    Acute, nonfatal, self-limiting
    Acute, potentially fatal
    Acute systemic disease
    Chronic

TABLE 137–9. CAUSES OF SECRETORY DIARRHEA

Bacterial enterotoxins and endotoxins, *Clostridium perfringens*, *Escherichia coli*, *Salmonella* spp., *Shigella* spp., *Yersinia enterocolitica*
Unconjugated bile acids from bacterial fermentation
Hydroxylated fatty acids from bacterial fermentation
Giardia
Hyperthyroidism?
Laxatives (castor oil, dioctyl sodium sulfosuccinate, bisacodyl)
Cardiac glycosides
APUD* neoplasms: excess vasoactive intestinal polypeptide, serotonin, prostaglandins, substance P
Intestinal inflammation

*APUD = amine precursor uptake and decarboxylation.

and they allow the problem to be viewed from different perspectives, facilitating diagnosis and choice of appropriate treatment. A mechanistic approach is a simple way to classify diarrhea but can aid understanding of the pathophysiology, although typically an individual case is more complex. Many SI diseases in dogs and cats have a component of osmotic diarrhea, but even in a situation as simple as lactase deficiency, other mechanisms become involved (Fig. 137–16). Osmotic diarrhea in lactose malabsorption causes intestinal distention, which induces peristalsis and rapid transit, and bacterial fermentation products in the colon cause secretion. Indeed, bacterial fermentation of unabsorbed solutes is often a complicating factor in malabsorption. The fecal pH is often low because of the production of volatile fatty acids, and some products of fermentation (e.g., hydroxylated fatty acids, unconjugated bile acids) can cause colonic inflammation and secretion, so that signs of LI diarrhea frequently accompany prolonged SI disease.

Osmotic Diarrhea

Excess water-soluble molecules in the intestinal lumen retain water osmotically. Diarrhea occurs when the resulting fluid volume overwhelms the absorptive capacity of the SI and colon. Osmotic diarrhea is particularly common when dietary nutrients are unabsorbed (e.g., with a sudden diet change, overeating, or malabsorption) or when osmotic laxatives, such as lactulose, are given. The diarrhea typically resolves when food or laxatives are withheld.

Secretory Diarrhea

In the normal SI the amount of fluid absorbed approximately matches the amount ingested and secreted. The remainder is absorbed by the colon or excreted in feces. Stimulation of SI secretion so that the reserve absorptive capacity is overwhelmed results in diarrhea, even though the absorptive ability of the SI and colon may not actually be impaired. Treatment with oral rehydration fluids containing glucose and amino acids such as glycine to increase water absorption is appropriate if there is no histologic damage and the enterocytes are still functioning.

Typically, secretory diarrhea does not resolve with fasting but does not cause weight loss unless there is anorexia, vomiting, or additional SI damage. Morbidity or even mortality is associated with the dehydration that results from excessive fluid loss. Secretory diarrhea is typically caused by chemical toxins and toxins elaborated by enteric bacteria (Table 137–9). Heat-labile and heat-stable toxins are secreted by enterotoxigenic *E. coli* and are potent inducers of secretion through stimulation of enterocyte adenylate and guanylate cyclase, respectively.

Permeability (Exudative) Diarrhea

Intestinal inflammation can stimulate increased fluid and electrolyte secretion and impair absorption, but leakage of tissue fluid, serum proteins, blood, and mucus may also occur from sites of inflammation, ulceration, or infiltration.

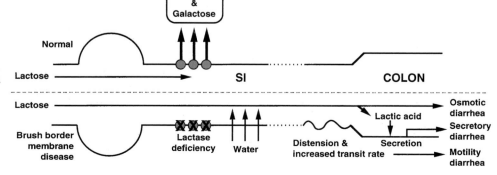

Figure 137–16. Diagrammatic representation of the mechanisms of diarrhea caused by lactase deficiency.

Exudates can also be lost through portal hypertension associated with right-sided heart failure or hepatic disease and lymphatic obstruction. Increased permeability severe enough to cause loss of plasma proteins in excess of their rate of synthesis results in a protein-losing enteropathy (PLE).

Dysmotility

Alterations of normal intestinal motility as a primary cause of diarrhea are probably rare and largely misunderstood. However, secondary alterations in motility often occur in many diarrheal diseases: unabsorbed solute may decrease transit time as the osmotically retained fluid causes intestinal distention and hypermotility. Hyperthyroidism decreases transit time in cats and causes diarrhea, and rapid waves of contractions have been demonstrated in enterotoxigenic diarrhea. However, in most instances diarrhea is actually associated with hypomotility of the intestine.

Ileus. Abnormal dilatation of the intestine, termed ileus, may be due to hypomotility or obstruction. Adynamic ileus is a transient and reversible functional obstruction of the intestine with a number of causes (Table 137–10). In enteric viral infections, for example, ileus is common, promoting diarrhea as stasis allows bacterial fermentation.

Irritable Bowel Syndrome. This enigmatic problem, in which LI signs usually predominate, probably involves the SI. Disordered intestinal motility is considered to be of primary importance as no other cause can be discerned. Whether any of the proposed mechanisms for IBS in humans (Table 137–11)[61] are responsible for the signs of recurrent, usually acute, episodes of abdominal pain, borborygmi, and diarrhea is unknown. A variety of treatments including antispasmodics (anticholinergics, smooth muscle relaxants), anxiolytics (e.g. diazepam), and dietary modification (low-fat diet, increased fiber) have been tried with no consistent results.

MALABSORPTION

Failure of food digestion and absorption is sometimes classified as primary failure to digest (*maldigestion*) and primary failure to absorb (*malabsorption* or *malassimilation*). Such a classification is misleading because digestive and absorptive functions are inextricably linked and failure of absorption is an inevitable consequence of failure to digest. The preferred use of the term *malabsorption* is as a global one meaning defective absorption of a dietary constituent resulting from interference with the digestive and/or absorptive phases in the processing of that molecule.

Within the broad definition of malabsorption, the site of the primary abnormality may be premucosal (i.e., intralumi-

TABLE 137–10. CAUSES OF ILEUS

Physical	Functional
Intestinal obstruction	Abdominal surgery
Overdistention by aerophagia	Ischemia
Neuromuscular	Inflammatory
Anticholinergic drugs	Peritonitis
Dysautonomia	Pancreatitis
Spinal cord injury	Parvovirus
Visceral myopathies	
Metabolic	
Hypokalemia	
Uremia	
Endotoxemia	

TABLE 137–11. CAUSES OF IRRITABLE BOWEL SYNDROME

Primary motility disorders	Food intolerance
Visceral hyperalgesia	Undiagnosed inflammatory disease
Psychosomatic disorders	

nal), mucosal, or postmucosal (i.e., hemolymphatic), although there may be considerable overlap (Table 137–12). Although there is usually malabsorption of a number of nutrients and consequent diarrhea, malabsorption of a single micronutrient may occur with no gastrointestinal signs (e.g., cbl). Also, the reserve capacity of the distal SI and colon may prevent overt diarrhea despite significant malabsorption and weight loss.

The clinical manifestations of malabsorption are largely a result of the lack of nutrient uptake and the losses in feces (Table 137–13). Animals are often systemically healthy with an increased appetite unless there is an underlying neoplastic or severe inflammatory condition. It is only when the animal is quite malnourished or develops hypoproteinemia that it becomes ill.

MELENA

The presence of dark, tarry, oxidized blood in feces is termed melena and reflects either swallowed blood or GI

TABLE 137–12. PATHOPHYSIOLOGIC MECHANISMS OF MALABSORPTION

MECHANISM	EXAMPLE
Premucosal (luminal)	
Dysmotility	
Rapid intestinal transit	Hyperthyroidism
Defective substrate hydrolysis	
Enzyme inactivation	Gastric hypersecretion
Lack of pancreatic enzymes	Exocrine pancreatic insufficiency
Fat maldigestion	
Decreased bile salt delivery	Cholestatic liver disease, biliary obstruction
Increased bile salt loss	Ileal disease
Bile salt deconjugation	Bacterial overgrowth
Fatty acid hydroxylation	Bacterial overgrowth
Impaired release of cholecystokinin, secretin	Severe small intestinal disease impairs pancreatic secretion
Cobalamin malabsorption	
Intrinsic factor deficiency	Exocrine pancreatic insufficiency
Competition for cobalamin	Bacterial overgrowth
Mucosal	
Brush border enzyme deficiency	
Congenital	Trehalase (cats)
Acquired	Relative lactose deficiency
Brush border transport protein deficiency	
Congenital	Intrinsic factor receptor
Acquired	Secondary to diffuse small intestinal disease
Enterocyte defects	
Enterocyte processing defects	Abetalipoproteinemia
Reduction in surface area	Villous atrophy
Immature enterocytes	Increased enterocyte turnover
Mucosal inflammation	Inflammatory bowel disease
Postmucosal (hemolymphatic)	
Lymphatic obstruction	
Primary	Lymphangiectasia
Secondary	Obstruction by neoplasia, infection, or inflammation
Vascular compromise	
Vasculitis	Infection, immune mediated
Portal hypertension	Hepatopathy, right-sided heart failure, cardiac tamponade

TABLE 137–13. CLINICAL SIGNS OF MALABSORPTION

Often systemically well	Altered appetite
Diarrhea	Polyphagia, coprophagia, pica
Weight loss	Anorexia
	Edema and/or ascites if hypoproteinemic

bleeding, which is usually proximal to the LI (Table 137–14). It has been estimated that the loss of 350 to 500 mg/kg hemoglobin into the GI tract is required for melena to be detected.[62] Blood lost proximal to the colon can sometimes appear as fresh blood if transit time is short, whereas prolonged retention of blood after colonic bleeding can result in as melena. Medication with ferrous sulfate or bismuth subsalicylate (Pepto-Bismol) can impart a black color to the feces. An increased blood urea nitrogen (BUN)/creatinine ratio resulting from bacterial digestion of blood is evidence for GI bleeding.

The general approach to melena is to rule out ingestion of blood, coagulopathies, and underlying metabolic disorders before pursuing primary GI causes. A thorough examination of the nares and oral cavity is required. A history of nonsteroidal anti-inflammatory drug administration is important as NSAIDs are a frequent cause of GI ulceration. Physical findings may suggest the cause (e.g., jaundice) or the consequences (e.g., pallor) of blood loss into the GI tract. The presence of melena and abdominal pain should prompt consideration of GI perforation or ischemia.

A complete blood count, biochemistry panel, urinalysis, and coagulation screen help to define the cause, severity, and chronicity of melena. The presence of microcytosis with or without thrombocytosis is suggestive of iron deficiency secondary to chronic blood loss. Inappropriate lymphocytosis and eosinophilia, with or without alterations in the Na/K ratio, may suggest hypoadrenocorticism. Hypoproteinemia may indicate significant blood loss or the presence of a PLE.

When other causes of melena have been ruled out, abdominal radiography and ultrasonography can be used to evaluate GI bleeding further. Ultrasonography is particularly useful for detecting gastrointestinal masses and thickening, and Doppler evaluation of vessels can demonstrate infarction. The next step for investigating upper GI blood loss is endoscopy to examine the esophagus, stomach, and duodenum. If the source of GI bleeding is still undetermined, tagged red blood cell scintigraphy, exploratory laparotomy, angiography, and enteroscopy are methods that can be used to localize the site of GI bleeding.

BORBORYGMI AND FLATULENCE

Borborygmus is defined as a rumbling noise caused by the propulsion of gas through the intestines. Swallowed air and bacterial fermentation of ingesta are the main causes of borborygmi and flatulence. Homemade diets such as low-fat cottage cheese and rice (1:2), or highly assimilable commercial diets effect a cure in many instances. Feeding a diet that is highly digestible and has a low fiber content should leave little material present in the intestine for bacterial fermentation.

If borborygmi or flatulence continues, despite dietary modification, the animal may be excessively aerophagic or have malabsorption, especially if diarrhea or weight loss is also present. Medical management with charcoal or simethicone may be indicated as an adjunct to diet when aerophagia is the problem.

WEIGHT LOSS OR FAILURE TO THRIVE

General causes of weight loss are reduced nutrient intake, increased nutrient loss, and increased catabolism or ineffective metabolism (Table 137–15). The history should reveal whether the type and amount of diet fed are adequate and whether anorexia, dysphagia, or vomiting is a potential cause. Weight loss or failure to thrive accompanied by diarrhea is often a feature of malabsorption, and the diagnostic approach is the same as for chronic diarrhea. However, diarrhea does not invariably accompany intestinal causes of weight loss or failure to thrive, as it is manifest only when the colonic reserve for water absorption is exceeded and may be absent in PLEs. For animals without diarrhea that have weight loss or failure to thrive, numerous nonintestinal causes must be considered.

PROTEIN-LOSING ENTEROPATHY

When SI disease is so severe that protein leakage into the gut lumen exceeds protein synthesis, hypoproteinemia develops. The source of intestinal protein loss is either the vasculature or the mucosal interstitial space. Causes of intestinal protein loss are summarized in Table 137–16. Chronic diarrhea associated with hypoproteinemia usually requires intestinal biopsy to define the cause of the PLE. Nonintestinal diseases that may potentially be associated with intestinal

TABLE 137–14. CAUSES OF MELENA

Ingestion of blood	Oral, nasal, pharyngeal, pulmonary bleeding
Coagulopathies	Thrombocytopenia, factor deficiencies, disseminated intravascular coagulopathy
Gastrointestinal erosion or ulceration	
Metabolic	Uremia, liver disease
Inflammatory	Gastritis, enteritis, hemorrhagic gastroenteritis
Neoplastic	Leiomyoma, adenocarcinoma, lymphosarcoma
Paraneoplastic	Mastocytosis, hypergastrinaemia, and other APUDomas
Vascular	Arteriovenous fistula, aneurysms, angiodysplasia
Ischemia	Hypovolemic shock, hypoadrenocorticism, thrombosis or infarction, reperfusion
Drug induced	Nonsteroidal and steroidal antiinflammatories
Foreign objects	

TABLE 137–15. CAUSES OF WEIGHT LOSS OR FAILURE TO THRIVE

Low dietary intake	Quality, quantity, anorexia, inappetence, oral dysphagia
Vomiting or regurgitation	
Malabsorption	Intestinal or exocrine pancreatic disease
Excessive catabolism or ineffective metabolism	Renal, hepatic or cardiac failure; neoplasia; infection, parasites; immune disorders; endocrinopathies—thyroid, adrenal, pancreatic, pituitary
Neuromuscular disease	

TABLE 137–16. PROTEIN-LOSING ENTEROPATHIES

Lymphangiectasia	Primary lymphatic disorder
	Venous hypertension, for example, right-sided heart failure, hepatic cirrhosis
Infectious	Parvovirus, salmonellosis, histoplasmosis, phycomycosis
Structural	Intussusception
Neoplasia	Lymphosarcoma
Inflammation	Lymphocytic-plasmacytic, eosinophilic, granulomatous
Endoparasites	*Giardia, Ancylostoma*
Gastrointestinal hemorrhage	Hemorrhagic gastroenteritis, neoplasia, ulceration

protein loss include congestive heart disease, caval obstruction, and portal hypertension. These animals usually have ascites rather than diarrhea. Hypoproteinemia associated with GI disease is much less common in cats than in dogs and most often appears to accompany GI lymphoma.

Clinical Presentation

Breeds that appear to be predisposed to PLE are the basenji, Lundehund, soft-coated wheaten terrier, Yorkshire terrier, and Shar Pei. Clinical signs associated with PLE include weight loss, diarrhea, vomiting, edema, ascites, and pleural effusion. Weight loss is frequently the predominant feature and diarrhea is not invariably present, particularly with lymphangiectasia or focal intestinal neoplasia. Physical findings may include edema, ascites, emaciation, thickened intestines, and melena. Thromboembolic disease may occur as a consequence of the loss of anticoagulants in excess of procoagulants.[63]

Diagnosis

The serum concentrations of both albumin and globulin are reduced in most animals with PLEs. Exceptions are raised globulins with hypoalbuminemia found in immunoproliferative SI disease of the basenji and in histoplasmosis. Renal and hepatic causes of hypoalbuminemia should also be pursued, especially when diarrhea is absent and globulin concentrations are normal or elevated, by assay of serum bile acids and urinary protein loss. Hypocholesterolemia, hypocalcemia, and lymphopenia are also common in PLEs. Preliminary investigations suggest that the measurement of fecal loss of alpha$_1$-protease inhibitor may be useful for documenting PLEs.[64]

Survey abdominal radiographs are often normal in patients with PLE, but ultrasonography may reveal intestinal thickening, mesenteric lymphadenopathy, or abdominal effusion. Thoracic radiographs may show pleural effusion, metastatic neoplasia, or evidence of histoplasmosis. Intestinal function tests are usually bypassed in favor of intestinal biopsy. As many intestinal causes of PLE are diffuse, endoscopy is a safer way to obtain biopsy specimens, but surgical biopsy may be required for a definitive diagnosis of lymphoma and diseases causing secondary lymphangiectasia.

Treatment

Plasma transfusion may be indicated during the perioperative period and diuretics may reduce ascites. Spironolactone (1 to 2 mg/kg by mouth twice a day) may be more effective than furosemide for treating ascites. Thromboembolism is a feature of some patients with PLE (see Chapter 180).

DIAGNOSIS OF SMALL INTESTINAL DISEASE

Most dogs and cats with diarrhea have an acute, nonfatal, and self-limiting condition. They require only symptomatic support. However, any animal with diarrhea has the potential to have a life-threatening condition, be an infectious risk to other animals, or have a zoonosis. The extent of any diagnostic investigation is a clinical judgment reflecting this potential. Acute diarrhea that is severe or bloody, that is accompanied by systemic signs, or that does not respond to symptomatic treatment needs more detailed investigations. Chronic diarrhea also requires investigation. Diagnostic approaches to acute and chronic diarrhea are shown in Figure 137–17 and Figure 137–18, respectively. Treatment with fluids and electrolytes, as needed, must be given while the diagnostic effort is in progress.

History and physical examination are crucial steps toward a diagnosis. Their importance cannot be overemphasized, and indeed they may be all that is required. Preliminary investigations may also include collection of baseline data: hematology, serum biochemistry, urinalysis, and fecal examination. Diagnostic imaging may be indicated, especially if there is a likelihood of surgical disease. In acute diarrhea that fails to respond to symptomatic treatment or chronic diarrhea, an etiologic diagnosis is usually required to enable specific treatment. The dog or cat should be tested for EPI. Indirect tests of intestinal function and damage may be indicated, and, ultimately, direct examination of the SI by endoscopy or surgery with histologic examination of biopsy specimens may be necessary.

HISTORY

An appropriate and thorough history should identify all pertinent background information and characterize the clinical signs to indicate the location, nature, severity, and possible causes of the disease. Diarrhea as a manifestation of extra-GI disease may be identified by a characteristic constellation of signs. Differentiation of SI from LI disease may be possible on the basis of information about the nature of the diarrhea and defecation habits (Table 137–17). However, in some animals it is not possible to categorize the disease neatly as of small or large bowel origin. This may be because it is a truly diffuse disease or because prolonged SI disease has produced secondary disease in the colon.

Information About the Patient

The animal's age, sex, and breed may alert the clinician to certain differential diagnoses; a number of breed predispositions have been noted (Table 137–18).

Environmental History

Whether the pet is kept indoors or outdoors and whether it is free to roam and scavenge are important questions. Access to parasite-contaminated ground, possible contact with infected animals, or a history of a change of environment or of ever having lived in known specific endemic disease areas may be relevant.

Past Medical History

Vaccination status and worming status are particularly relevant. A history of previous abdominal surgery or cutane-

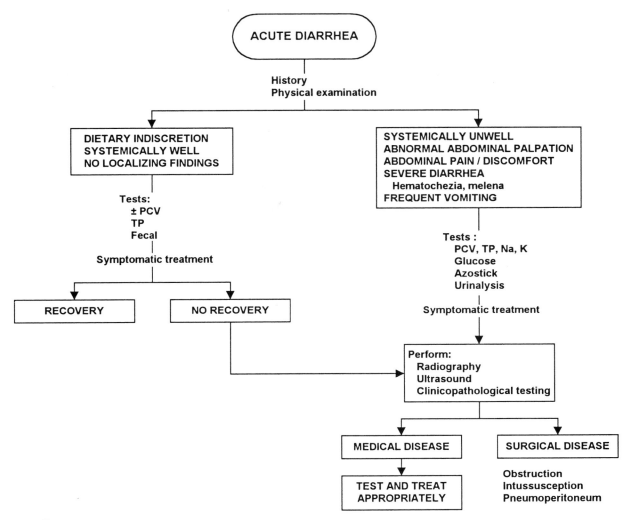

Figure 137–17. Algorithm showing a diagnostic approach to acute diarrhea. PCV = packed cell volume; TP = total protein; Fecal = Fecal examination for parasites.

ous mast cell tumor excision should be noted. A history of recurrent episodes of illness may be an indicator of IBD. Administration of drugs may be important: NSAIDs can damage the mucosal barrier, and antibiotics may cause diarrhea.

TABLE 137–17. CLINICAL SIGNS ASSOCIATED WITH SMALL OR LARGE BOWEL DISEASE

SIGNS	SMALL INTESTINE	LARGE INTESTINE
Feces		
Stool volume	Large	Small
Mucus	Rare	Common
Blood (if present)	Melena	Fresh blood
Fat	Sometimes	Absent
Color	Variable	Normal
Defecation		
Tenesmus	Rare	Common
Undigested food	Occasionally	Absent
Frequency	2–3 × normal per day	>3 × normal per day
Urgency	Uncommon	Common
Other signs		
Vomiting	Sometimes	Uncommon
Gas	Sometimes	Absent
Weight loss	Common	Rare

CLINICAL SIGNS

A systems review should determine whether non-GI disease is present; a checklist can help (Table 137–19). Clinical signs of intestinal disease are listed (see Table 137–2), and signs that help localize the problem to the SI are given in Table 137–17. As well as the sign, its nature and progression may also be important (Table 137–20). Intermittent signs may suggest functional rather than organic disease, and diarrhea that progressively worsens and is accompanied by vomiting, bleeding, or ascites is suggestive of severe disease. Any treatments given previously that may have either improved or worsened the condition are noted.

Reported Signs

Body Condition. Loss of body weight or failure to thrive is suggestive of chronic disease but is not specific for intestinal disease.

Appetite. Malabsorption typically causes weight loss and increased appetite, but hyperthyroidism can do the same. A ravenous appetite may include depravity. Coprophagy and pica are seen most commonly in EPI and SIBO. In general,

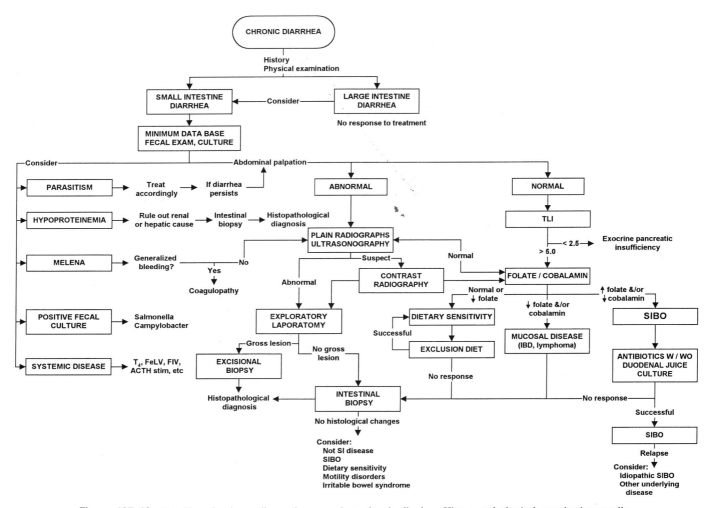

Figure 137–18. Algorithm showing a diagnostic approach to chronic diarrhea. History and physical examination usually identify an SI problem, but failure of specific therapy for an apparent LI problem should also make the clinician consider SI disease. A minimum database may provide evidence of systemic disease (leading the investigation away from the SI) or a protein-losing enteropathy. Fecal examination identifies GI parasites, but they may not necessarily be the cause of the problem. If abdominal palpation is abnormal, plain radiographs and ultrasonography are indicated. Contrast radiography is rarely helpful, especially in cases of diffuse mucosal disease, and exploratory laparotomy with mandatory biopsy is usually preferred. TLI (trypsin-like immunoreactivity) should probably be measured in all cases in which there are no abnormalities on abdominal palpation, as the signs of EPI (exocrine pancreatic insufficiency) are not always typical and serum folate and/or cobalamin concentrations are altered. Serum folate and cobalamin concentrations may give clues to the most likely diagnosis, although intestinal biopsy provides more definitive evidence. However, in a number of cases there is no histologic diagnosis and, if folate and cobalamin concentrations are suggestive and the nature of the case permits, empirical trials of antibiotics and exclusion diets at this stage are an acceptable pragmatic approach. SIBO = small intestinal bacterial overgrowth; w/wo = with or without; IBD = infiltrative or inflammatory bowel disease; SI = small intestine.

anorexia is a sign of systemic, surgical, severe inflammatory, or malignant disease.

Thirst. Polydipsia is sometimes seen in animals with malabsorption, especially EPI, but usually indicates extraintestinal disease.

Halitosis. This may be normal in dogs fed a high-protein diet and is usually a result of oropharyngeal disease or perianal licking. It can indicate malabsorption and/or coprophagia.

Vomiting. There are numerous extraintestinal causes of vomiting in dogs and cats, as well as primary gastric disease. However, intestinal obstruction or inflammation can also cause vomiting, and in cats it is a major presenting sign of IBD. Reportedly, approximately 30 percent of dogs with idiopathic colitis vomit intermittently, but evidence ruling out concurrent SI disease is not always obtained.

Gas. Borborygmi and/or flatulence may merely indicate dietary indiscretion but can signal excessive motility or bacterial fermentation of malabsorbed food.

Abdominal Discomfort or Pain. Intestinal inflammation, ischemia or distention, mesenteric stretching, and peritonitis can all cause abdominal pain.

Ascites and Edema. Hypoproteinemia associated with PLEs can result in ascites and/or ventral and limb edema.

Nature of Feces

The physical appearance of the feces confirms the existence of diarrhea and can provide clues to the nature of the disease. However, it is impossible to make a definitive diagnosis from the color and odor of the feces. A case that "smells like parvo" has merely the smell of fermenting hemorrhagic diarrhea with one of many causes.

Color. Changes in fecal color are typical of SI disease

TABLE 137–18. SOME SUSPECTED AND CONFIRMED BREED SUSCEPTIBILITIES TO INTESTINAL DISEASE IN DOGS AND CATS

BREED	CONDITION
Basenji	Lymphocytic-plasmacytic enteritis (synonymous with immunoproliferative small intestinal disease)
Beagle	Idiopathic SIBO* (usually asymptomatic)
German shepherd dog	Idiopathic (antibiotic-responsive) SIBO
	Inflammatory bowel disease (lymphocytic-plasmacytic, eosinophilic)
	Intestinal volvulus
Giant schnauzer	Defective cobalamin absorption
Irish setter	Gluten-sensitive enteropathy
Lundehund	Lymphangiectasia
Retrievers	Dietary allergy†
Rottweiler	Susceptibility to parvovirus
Soft-coated wheaten terrier	Protein-losing enteropathy or nephropathy
Shar Pei	Lymphocytic-plasmacytic enteritis
Toy breeds	Hemorrhagic gastroenteritis
Yorkshire terrier	Lymphagiectasia

*SIBO = small intestinal bacterial overgrowth.
†Suspected.

but are not pathognomonic, as they merely reflect the completeness of digestion and bacterial metabolism of bile pigments. Malabsorption and alterations in the rate of transit and bacterial flora can all alter fecal color. Feces are typically pale in EPI and may appear more orange in animals with fast SI transit or those given antibiotics. Some medications (e.g., metronidazole, bismuth) themselves cause dark stools.

Odor. Hemorrhagic diarrhea has a characteristic sickly odor, and in malabsorption the odor is often acrid and foul because of bacterial fermentation of undigested food.

Mucus and Blood. Fresh blood and mucus are typical of LI diarrhea (see Table 137–17). The presence of dark tarry stools suggests digested blood (melena).

Consistency. Feces are likely to be voluminous and watery in SI disease because of the osmotic effect of unabsorbed solutes and stimulation of secretion.

Steatorrhea. The presence of fat in feces indicates malabsorption and is particularly notable in EPI and lymphangiectasia.

Physical Examination

The examination of dogs or cats with diarrhea should include all body systems, as it is important to identify nonintestinal causes of diarrhea; for example, palpation of the cervical region for thyroid nodules is mandatory in cats with intestinal signs. However, it is not unusual for there to be no overt physical abnormalities in primary SI disease; poor body condition may be all that is noted. The mouth and rectum are the only parts of the GI tract that the clinician can examine directly, and palpation and auscultation of the abdomen require patience and experience. Palpation should

TABLE 137–19. CHECKLIST FOR PERFORMING SYSTEMS REVIEW

Appetite	Exercise tolerance
Defecation	Changes in weight and muscle mass
Vomiting or regurgitation	Changes in hair coat and pruritus
Water intake and urination	Changes in behavior
Coughing or sneezing	Collapse and seizure
Oculonasal discharge	Sexual activity

TABLE 137–20. QUESTIONS ABOUT THE NATURE AND PROGRESSION OF CLINICAL SIGNS

Severity
Duration
Frequency
Continuous or intermittent
Length of sign-free intervals
Moderating influences (improve or worsen signs), for example, treatments, diets
Order of appearance of signs

always be repeated if an animal has been sedated or anesthetized, because abdominal wall relaxation makes it much easier.

Oropharynx. Examination of the mucous membranes helps assessment of hydration, cardiovascular status, anemia, and icterus. The base of the tongue should be carefully checked for strings indicating a linear foreign body, especially in cats.

Abdominal Palpation and Auscultation. The aim of palpation is to identify abdominal effusions, masses, bunching of intestinal loops, foreign bodies, abnormal accumulations of ingesta, and any associated pain. The presence of fecal material in the colon can be confirmed by gentle squeezing, but in cats the cecum feels firm and may be mistaken for a mass. Any abnormality on palpation should be followed by radiographic and ultrasonographic examination to confirm the need for exploratory surgery. Auscultation of the abdomen is useful in identifying ileus, particularly after abdominal surgery.

Rectal Examination. Digital rectal examination is mandatory in all animals with intestinal disease, not only when rectal or anal disease is suspected. Rectal examination can provide a sample of stool and reveal previously unreported melena. A dry, tacky rectal mucosa can be found with intestinal obstruction. After examination, rectal cytology can be performed (see later).

Cutaneous Examination. Cutaneous changes in GI disease generally reflect any malnutrition, but occasionally evidence of concurrent pruritus and intestinal signs may be suggestive of food allergy. Infection with *Uncinaria stenocephala* may also cause diarrhea and pedal pruritus because of larval migration.

MINIMUM DATABASE

A fecal examination can be diagnostic and should always be performed in animals with diarrhea, but extensive use of other tests is not always necessary. In acute diarrhea, an initial database of packed cell volume (PCV), total protein, and urine specific gravity may be adequate. In chronic diarrhea more tests are indicated, starting with a minimum database of a hemogram, serum chemistries, and urinalysis. Results are rarely diagnostic but assess hydration status and permit extra-GI disease to be ruled out. In young dogs with GI signs, an adrenocorticotropic hormone (ACTH) stimulation test should be performed if hypoadrenocorticism is possible. In cats, virologic tests for feline leukemia virus (FeLV) and feline immunodeficiency virus (FIV) are performed, not because these infections are necessarily the cause of the signs but because they are important factors in the overall prognosis.

Hematology

An increase in PCV in conjunction with increased serum total protein is a marker for dehydration. Anemia may indicate intestinal blood loss or chronic inflammation associated with intestinal disease. Microcytosis, decreased red blood cell hemoglobin, and thrombocytosis are seen in dogs with iron deficiency anemia secondary to chronic intestinal blood loss. A mild neutrophilia with or without a left shift may be seen in IBD, but rarely are there marked changes. Leukemoid responses are rarely seen. An eosinophilia may be associated with parasitism and is an inconsistent marker of eosinophilic gastroenteritis. Leukopenia in acute gastroenteritis is suggestive of parvovirus infection and lymphopenia is characteristic in lymphangiectasia.

Serum Biochemistries

Sodium and Potassium. Electrolyte abnormalities may be a feature of persistent vomiting, intestinal obstruction, and secretory diarrhea and should be noted when choosing fluid replacement therapy. Hyponatremia and hyperkalemia are suggestive of hypoadrenocorticism. Rarely, similar electrolyte changes are noted in dogs with secretory diarrhea, especially with whipworm infection, and therefore an ACTH stimulation test should be performed for confirmation.

Albumin and Globulin. Panhypoproteinemia is seen in PLEs and should be distinguished from the hypoalbuminemia of liver failure and protein-losing nephropathies. Globulins may be increased if there is an intense inflammatory condition (often noted in basenji enteropathy).

Liver Enzymes. Mild to moderate increases in liver enzymes may be seen in primary SI disease, presumably because portally delivered antigens, endotoxins, and bacteria have crossed an impaired mucosal barrier and cause secondary liver damage.

Cholesterol. Low serum cholesterol may be a feature of fat malabsorption and is notable in lymphangiectasia.

Fecal Examination

Fecal examinations should be included in the evaluation of any pet with GI disease. Tests such as quantification of 72-hour fecal fat excretion are unsuitable for practice and bacteriologic culture is sometimes of questionable value, but identification of parasites is important.

Direct Smear. Staining of smears for undigested starch granules (Lugol's iodine), fat globules (Sudan stain), and muscle fibers (Wright's or Diff-Quik stain) may indicate malabsorption but is unreliable. Sudan staining before and after heating the sample on a slide with acetic acid can help identify split and unsplit fat but is of little diagnostic value. Fungal elements and sporulating clostridia may be seen, but rectal cytology is more useful. Unstained wet mounts may be used to identify protozoal trophozoites, such as *Giardia* sp., *Pentatrichomonas* sp., *Balantidium* sp., and *Entamoeba* sp. However, for the detection of most parasites fecal concentration methods are more rewarding.

Enterotoxin production by *Clostridium perfringens* is a potential cause of diarrhea. The presence of large numbers of clostridial endospores (more than five per oil field) on

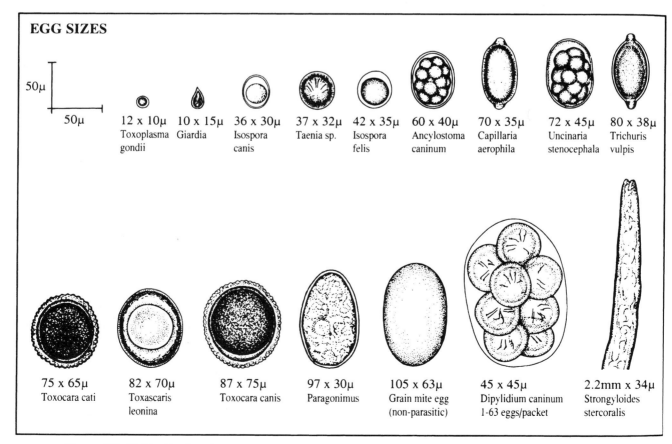

EGG SIZES

50μ

50μ

| 12 x 10μ Toxoplasma gondii | 10 x 15μ Giardia | 36 x 30μ Isospora canis | 37 x 32μ Taenia sp. | 42 x 35μ Isospora felis | 60 x 40μ Ancylostoma caninum | 70 x 35μ Capillaria aerophila | 72 x 45μ Uncinaria stenocephala | 80 x 38μ Trichuris vulpis |

| 75 x 65μ Toxocara cati | 82 x 70μ Toxascaris leonina | 87 x 75μ Toxocara canis | 97 x 30μ Paragonimus | 105 x 63μ Grain mite egg (non-parasitic) | 45 x 45μ Dipylidium caninum 1-63 eggs/packet | 2.2mm x 34μ Strongyloides stercoralis |

Figure 137–19. Identification of protozoan cysts and worm eggs that may be found in the feces of dogs and cats. (By kind permission of Hoechst-Roussel-Agri Vet Company, USA.)

TABLE 137–21. METHODOLOGY FOR PERFORMING FECAL FLOTATION FOR EXAMINATION FOR PARASITES

2–3 g feces in 15 mL of solution*
Mix thoroughly
Strain through tea strainer or cheesecloth†
Place in 15-mL polypropylene centrifuge tube
Centrifuge at 1500 rpm for 5 minutes
Place coverslip on top touching the mensicus for 3–4 minutes
    (alternatively, use bacteriologic loop)
Place coverslip on microscope slide and examine‡

*Sugar solution (454 g of sugar + 355 mL of water) or 33 per cent zinc sulfate solution (33 g of zinc sulfate in 100 mL of distilled water, specfic gravity 1.18).
†If there is excess fat after filtering, the sample can be mixed with 2–3 mL of ethyl acetate or ether, centrifuged, and the supernatant discarded.
‡Stain with Lugol's iodine for zinc sulfate flotation, if desired.

Diff-Quik–stained smears may be suggestive, but a positive fecal enterotoxin assay (enzyme-linked immunosorbent assay [ELISA] or reverse passive latex agglutination) is more significant.

Fecal Concentration Methods. Fecal flotation with sugar solution (Table 137–21) or sedimentation with formol-ether is suitable for screening for metazoan ova (roundworms, hookworms, and whipworms) (Fig. 137–19). In tropical climates a direct smear, sedimentation, or the Baermann technique can identify larvae of *Strongyloides* spp. Examination of three fecal samples by zinc sulfate flotation (see Table 137–21) is recommended for detecting *Giardia* oocysts. Coccidia and *Cryptosporidium* spp. are best identified by sugar flotation.

Bacteriologic Examination. Culture of feces is indicated for animals with bloody diarrhea, pyrexia, an inflammatory leukogram, or the presence of neutrophils on rectal cytology and probably for all diarrheic young animals. Identification of potential pathogens such as *Salmonella* spp., *Campylobacter jejuni*, and *Clostridium difficile* may be helpful, but these organisms can be present in normal animals. Furthermore, the colonic flora does not necessarily reflect what is happening in the SI and cannot be used to diagnose SIBO. Some strains of *E. coli* isolated are undoubtedly pathogenic, but molecular probes for pathogenicity markers in small animal medicine are not generally available yet.[65] Feces can be cultured for fungi, such as *Histoplasma capsulatum*, using Sabouraud's medium, but isolation is difficult and takes at least 2 weeks.

Virologic Examination. Viral diarrhea is usually acute and self-limiting with no need for a positive diagnosis. Electron microscopy can be used to identify the characteristic viral particles of rotavirus, coronavirus, and parvovirus. A fecal ELISA for parvovirus is also available and gives rapid answers compared with serology. However, virus is best detected early in the disease.

***Giardia* Antigen.** This can be detected in feces by a commercially available ELISA. However, results suggest that the sensitivity is not as good as that of three consecutive zinc sulfate flotations.

Occult Blood. These tests are used to search for intestinal bleeding from ulcerated mucosa and benign or malignant tumors. Unfortunately, all test nonspecifically for hemoglobin and are sensitive, reacting with any meat diet and not just the patient's blood. Therefore, the patient must be fed a meat-free diet for at least 72 hours for a positive result to have any reliability.[62]

Alpha₁-Protease Inhibitor. This test assays the fecal appearance of a naturally occurring, endogenous serum protein that is resistant to bacterial degradation if it is lost into the intestinal lumen. Three fresh fecal samples must be assayed. Preliminary work suggests that it is useful for diagnosing PLEs.[66]

Rectal Cytology. At the end of the rectal examination, the rectal wall is mildly abraded, the gloved finger rolled on a microscope slide, and the smear stained. Although the test is often negative and probably more suggestive of large intestinal disease when abnormal, increased numbers of neutrophils (Fig. 137–20A) may be suggestive of a bacterial problem and indicate the need for fecal culture. Occasionally, malignant lymphocytes are seen, reflecting alimentary lymphoma (Fig. 137–20B). Clostridial endospores and fungal elements (*Histoplasma, Aspergillus, Pythium, Candida*) may be identified. The test is fast and simple, but in all cases confirmatory tests are indicated.

IMAGING

In the past, imaging of the intestinal tract was limited to plain and contrast radiographs. This has been dramatically altered by the use of ultrasonography and endoscopy. Scintigraphy, computed tomography (CT), and magnetic resonance imaging (MRI) scanning are beginning to be adopted, and "virtual" endoscopy by helical CT holds promise for the future.

Radiography

Survey Radiographs. Plain radiographs are most useful in the investigation of primary vomiting, vomiting associated

GI

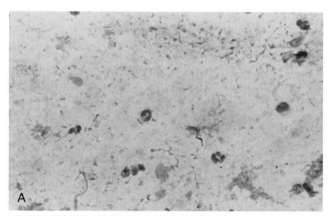

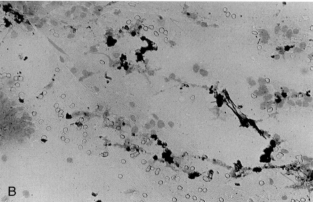

Figure 137–20. Rectal cytology specimens showing (A) polymorphonuclear leukocytes suggestive of an inflammatory enteropathy and (B) malignant lymphocytes suggestive of alimentary lymphoma.

with diarrhea, abdominal pain, and palpable abnormalities. Generally, the aim is the detection of (acute) surgical disease; they enable detection of foreign bodies, masses, obstructions, decreased serosal detail, free peritoneal gas, and ileus (Table 137–22). Ileus is an abnormal dilatation of an immotile segment of intestine, and the differential diagnosis depends on whether it is localized or generalized and whether there is accumulation of gas or fluid (Table 137–23). The usefulness of plain radiographs in malabsorption is minimal.

Contrast Radiography. Contrast studies are still of value in evaluating esophageal and gastric disease. However, since the introduction of endoscopy, they have fallen from favor for the investigation of SI disease, as they are low yield procedures.

Barium Follow-Through Examinations. Studies using microfine barium suspensions can identify ulcers and irregular mucosal detail if lesions are severe. They can be helpful for confirmation of a radiolucent foreign body. Their use to identify mural masses is limited, and they offer little beyond the information that can be gleaned from a good-quality survey radiograph (Fig. 137–21). Intestinal inflammation may delay gastric emptying, leading to an erroneous diagnosis of gastric disease, and the administration of barium may interfere with the ability to perform endoscopy for at least 24 hours.

Barium-Impregnated Polyethylene Spheres (BIPSs). BIPSs have been introduced as a more convenient way of performing contrast studies. The BIPSs are radiopaque and are administered with food. Small spheres (1.5 mm in diameter) are markers of gastric emptying and intestinal transit, and large spheres (5 mm in diameter) may identify partial obstructions (see Fig. 137–21). The transit time of BIPSs is highly variable, and there is a poor correlation with the passage of barium meals or the more physiologic scintigraphic techniques.[67]

Enteroclysis. This is a double-contrast method for identifying SI mucosal lesions. First the duodenum is infused with barium suspension, followed by a water infusion. Intubation of the duodenum and observation of the infusions are performed with sedation and fluoroscopic guidance. The need for fluoroscopy and the degree of expertise required have severely limited the use of a method that has the potential to help diagnose enteritis, villous atrophy, ulcers, intussusceptions, foreign bodies, strictures, and neoplasms.

TABLE 137–22. HELPFUL FINDINGS IN SURVEY ABDOMINAL RADIOGRAPHS IN PATIENTS WITH INTESTINAL DISEASE

Radiopaque foreign bodies	Visible on survey films
Ileus	Either adynamic-paralytic or obstructive (see Table 137–10)
Abnormal soft tissue shadow	Abdominal mass
Displacement of viscera	Abdominal mass, enlargement of intra- or retroperitoneal organ, rupture, or hernia
Bunching of intestines	Excess intra-abdominal fat, large mass, adhesions, linear foreign body
Bowel wall thickness	Edema, infiltrative (inflammatory, neoplastic) disease
Bowel wall irregularity	Enteritis, neoplasia, ulcers
Loss of serosal detail	Emaciation and immaturity
	Peritoneal effusion (ascites in hypoproteinemia and/or portal hypertension, peritonitis, carcinomatosis)

TABLE 137–23. DIFFERENTIAL DIAGNOSIS OF ILEUS

Generalized gas ileus	Localized gas ileus
Aerophagia	Localized peritonitis (e.g., pancreatitis)
Smooth muscle paralyzing drugs	Early stage bowel obstruction
	Disruption of mesenteric arterial supply
Generalized peritonitis	Localized fluid ileus
Enteritis	Foreign body
Generalized fluid ileus	Tumor causing obstruction
Enteritis	Intussusception
Diffuse intestinal neoplasia	

Ultrasonography

Transabdominal ultrasonographic examination of the SI is now a routine part of the investigation of intestinal disease.[68] In the future endoscopic ultrasonography will offer the ability to examine the mucosal wall and adjacent viscera (e.g., pancreas) in more detail. Conventional ultrasonographic examination can detect layering of the wall, peristalsis, and luminal contents and measure intestinal thickness and luminal diameter. It is helpful for detecting lesions such as intussusceptions, masses, and radiolucent foreign bodies but can also be used to identify intestinal wall thickening and associated lymphadenopathy in chronic inflammatory and neoplastic enteropathies (Fig. 137–22). The normal SI wall is less than 3 mm thick. Disruption of the normal five-layered sonographic appearance (mucosal surface, mucosa, submucosa, muscularis, serosa) is typical of neoplasia. Ultrasound-guided fine-needle aspiration for cytologic examination is possible.

Scintigraphy

A gamma camera can be used to follow the passage of technetium 99m–labeled food through the intestine. Such studies can be used to measure the rate of gastric emptying and intestinal transit time. Indium 111–labeled transferrin has been used to investigate PLEs.

SPECIAL TESTS

In cases of malabsorption, intestinal biopsy is usually necessary to obtain a definitive diagnosis. However, EPI should be ruled out before biopsy as clinical signs of malabsorption are not specific (see Fig. 137–18). It is also well recognized that biopsies of up to 50 per cent of patients with malabsorption are considered normal by light microscopy.[69, 70] Therefore, usually before biopsy, a number of indirect tests are performed to assess intestinal damage and function.

Diagnosis of Exocrine Pancreatic Insufficiency

The signs of EPI cannot readily be distinguished from those of many primary SI causes of malabsorption. EPI must be ruled out before invasive testing is considered. EPI can be confirmed by assay of serum trypsin-like immunoreactivity (TLI) (see Chapter 146).

Serum Folate and Cobalamin Concentrations

The assay of serum folate and vitamin B_{12} (cbl) concentrations can be performed using the serum sample taken for the TLI test and can be a helpful screening test in the initial

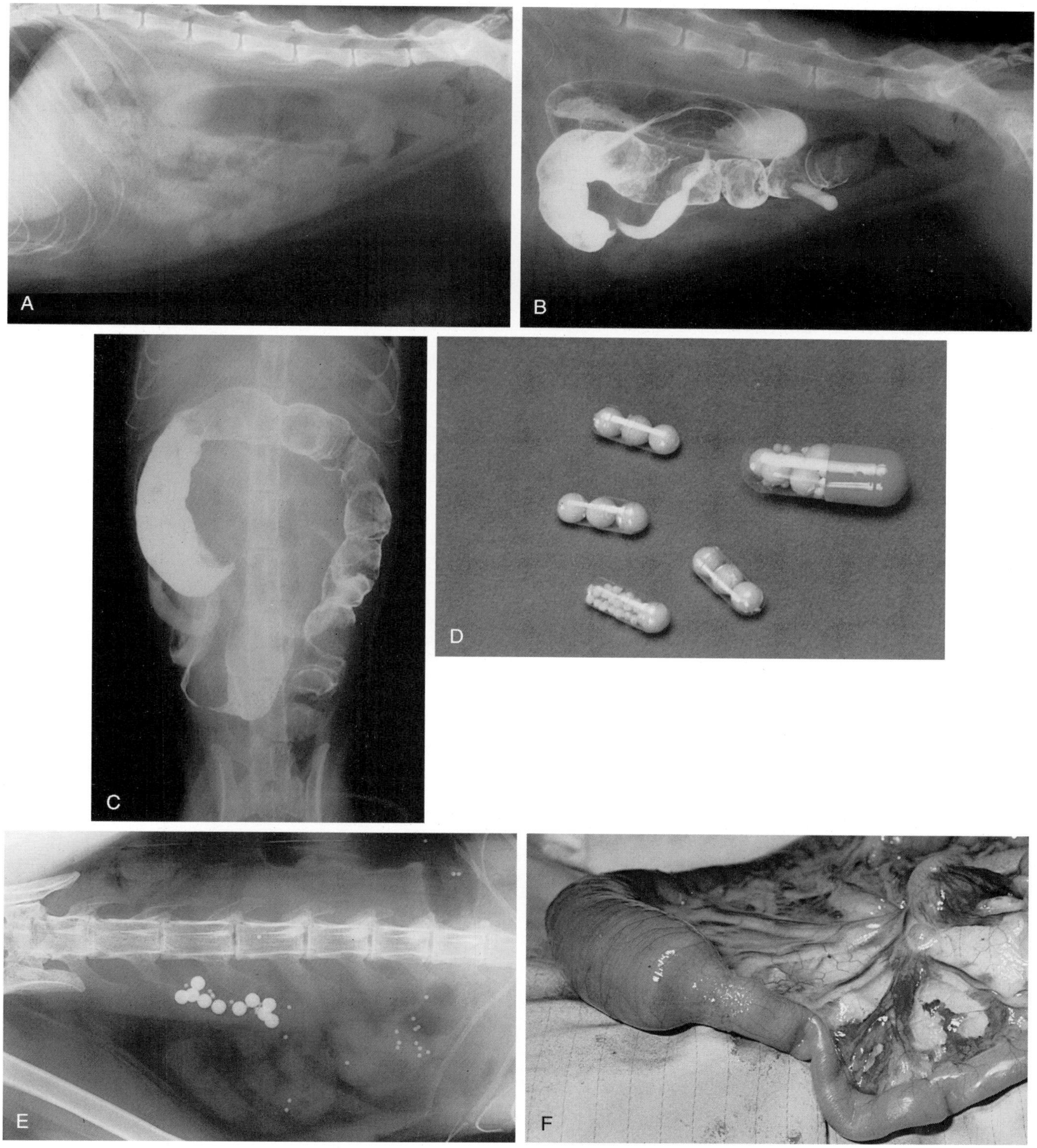

Figure 137–21. Identification of an intestinal mass in a Siamese cat. *A*, Plain lateral radiograph showing a dilated loop of bowel associated with a possible caudal abdominal mass. *B*, Lateral radiograph after the oral administration of barium suspension showing a dilated loop as well as colonic filling. *C*, Ventrodorsal radiograph after oral administration of barium suspension showing a dilated loop of SI in the midline as well as colonic filling and possible narrowing of the intestinal lumen connecting SI and LI. *D*, Barium-impregnated polyethylene spheres (BIPSs) of two sizes in gelatin capsules. *E*, Ventrodorsal radiograph after oral administration of BIPS showing accumulation of the larger markers at the site of partial obstruction. *F*, The annular adenocarcinoma in the ileum demonstrated at laparotomy. (Courtesy of A. H. Sparkes.)

GI

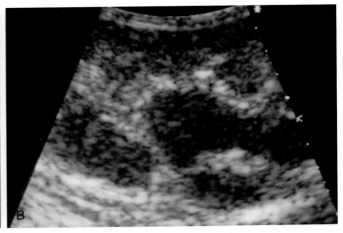

Figure 137–22. Abdominal ultrasonography. *A,* Cylindrical small intestinal mass in a dog with a chronic intussusception. The characteristic double-layered structure has been lost because of the prolonged presence of the condition and the associated tissue inflammation, necrosis, and adhesions. *B,* Mesenteric lymphadenopathy in a cat with alimentary lymphoma. (Courtesy of H. Rudorf.)

assessment of canine patients.[22] The test also appears to be useful in cats, although reference ranges differ from those for the dog. The test is based on the absorption of folate by the proximal jejunum and cbl by the ileum (see Fig. 137–7A). Low serum concentrations may be caused by folate and cbl malabsorption, which reflects proximal and distal SI disease, respectively, and diffuse disease is likely to affect both analytes (see Fig. 137–7B). The finding of a low serum folate and/or cbl often seems to correlate well with severe IBD in both cats and dogs, especially Shar Peis. Severe cbl deficiency in giant schnauzers and Border collies has been linked to an IF-cbl receptor deficiency.[71, 72]

In SIBO, the bacteria synthesize folate and bind cbl, so that serum folate concentrations tend to increase and cbl decreases. Unfortunately, these findings have a low sensitivity (5 per cent) but a reported 100 per cent specificity.[33] Using just a high folate or a low cbl alone improves sensitivity but at the expense of specificity. Folate and cbl concentrations are influenced by various factors (Table 137–24).

Indirect Assessment of Intestinal Absorption

Attempts to assess intestinal function by measuring the mediated absorption of numerous substrates (glucose, lactose, starch, fat) have largely been discarded.

TABLE 137–24. FACTORS INFLUENCING SERUM CONCENTRATIONS OF COBALAMIN AND FOLATE IN DOGS

	DECREASED	INCREASED
Folate	Dietary deficiency	High dietary intake
	Proximal or diffuse SI disease	Parenteral supplementation
		Intestinal bacteria
	Drugs (e.g., sulfasalazine)	Low intestinal pH
	Widespread malignancy	Exocrine pancreatic insufficiency
		Artifact: hemolysis, increased laboratory temperature
Cobalamin	Dietary deficiency	High dietary intake
	Ileal disease	Parenteral supplementation
	Intestinal bacteria	Release of hepatic stores?
	Exocrine pancreatic insufficiency	
	Artifact: excess light exposure	

D-Xylose Absorption Test. The principle of the test is the measurement blood xylose or its urinary excretion after oral administration. This test fails to meet the expectations of a sensitive and specific test in dogs or cats and it is now rarely used.

Xylose and 3-*O*-Methyl-D-Glucose Test. The differential absorption of these two sugars eliminates the nonmucosal effects that blight the xylose test, and initial results suggest that the test may be of value in dogs and cats. However, the assay of the sugars is technically demanding and the test is not readily available.[73]

Intestinal Permeability

Intestinal permeability is an index of mucosal integrity, or intestinal "leakiness," and is assessed by the measurement of unmediated uptake of nondigestible probe markers. Permeation is believed to be by passive diffusion through paracellular channels in tight junctions and is not carrier mediated. Increased permeability may simply be a nonspecific marker for damage to the mucosal barrier, but it may be important in the pathogenesis of IBD and food allergy, perhaps being the pathway by which antigen enters the mucosa and evades the normal APC-driven immune response. A probe marker that is not metabolized after permeation and is subsequently rapidly excreted in the urine offers a practicable, noninvasive approach to assessing intestinal permeability.

Errors related to nonmucosal factors can be eliminated by measuring the unmediated absorption of two different-sized, nondigestible probes that are absorbed by different routes across the mucosa; calculation of their excretion ratio eliminates these errors, as both probes should be affected equally (Fig. 137–23). There are a number of candidates for the probe molecules and a mixture of one large (e.g., lactulose, cellobiose, raffinose) and one small (e.g., rhamnose, arabinose, mannitol) simple sugar can be chosen. After advances in high-performance liquid chromatographic (HPCL) assays, the lactulose-rhamnose test will probably become the standard test of SI permeability. It can be combined with the xylose, 3-*O*-methyl-D-glucose test and has even been adapted to a blood test.[73, 74]

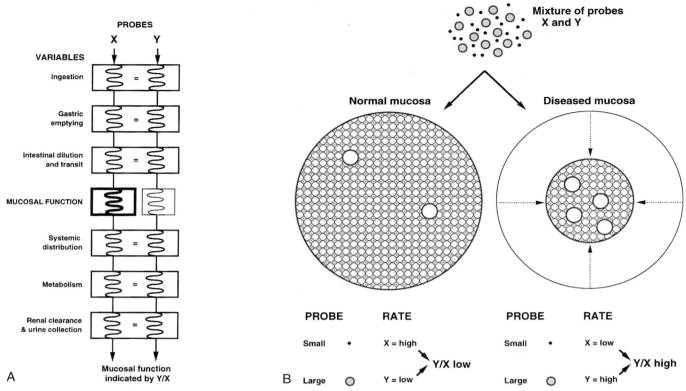

Figure 137–23. The principle of differential permeability testing. *A,* Simultaneous administration of two probes selected to respond identically to each variable except mucosal permeability. The Y/X ratio provides a specific index of mucosal permeability. *B,* Differential permeation of two probes of different sizes through the mucosal epithelium. Normal mucosa has a high incidence of small pores permitting entry of the smaller probe X and a low incidence of larger pores accommodating the larger probe Y. Diseased mucosa has a decreased surface area and decreased numbers of small pores, but damage increases the number of large pores. In the diseased state the Y/X ratio is increased. (From Hall EJ: Small intestinal disease—is endoscopic biopsy the answer? J Small Anim Pract 35:408, 1994.)

Tests for Protein-Losing Enteropathy

Historically, intestinal protein loss has been detected by measuring the fecal loss of chromium 51–labeled albumin. The test is unpleasant to perform, is potentially hazardous, and has largely been discarded. Assay of fecal alpha$_1$-protease inhibitor appears to be a promising option (see earlier).[64]

Breath Tests

Breath tests are used to assess bacterial metabolism within the GI tract. The bacteria synthesize a gas that is absorbed and excreted in breath. Breath hydrogen tests have been used most extensively because mammalian cells cannot produce hydrogen, so any measured must be bacterial in origin. Breath hydrogen tests have been used for the assessment of carbohydrate malabsorption, bacterial colonization of the SI, and orocecal transit time in animals.[75, 76]

Breath collection from dogs is simple using a face mask and modified anesthetic bag, and the hydrogen content is stable if the sample is kept airtight. Assay by a hydrogen monitor is also simple, but monitors were once prohibitively expensive. Cheaper handheld monitors are now available, although their performance is variable. Cats do not tolerate the face mask as well as dogs, and an alternative collection system is preferred; cats can be enclosed in a Perspex box through which air is passed, and cumulative hydrogen excretion is calculated.[77]

Analysis of sequential breath samples after oral administration of a substrate allows the site and amount of intestinal hydrogen production to be inferred. If a substrate such as xylose or a meal is used, hydrogen production should begin only if any residue reaches the colon. If there is carbohydrate malabsorption, significant amounts of substrate do reach the colon and are fermented, with hydrogen production.[75, 76] Equally increased breath hydrogen could represent SIBO with fermentation occurring in the SI, and sometimes an early SI and a later colonic peak are discernible.[74] Administration of a nondigestible substrate such as lactulose or feeding of a meal that is not completely digested causes hydrogen production when the substrate enters the colon. The time to the increase in breath hydrogen can therefore be a measure of orocecal transit time.[77]

However, various factors can alter breath hydrogen excretion. Indeed, the protocol and interpretation of breath hydrogen testing have not yet been properly validated in veterinary medicine and it would be prudent to consider the test currently to be experimental.[78]

Unconjugated Bile Salts

Intestinal bacterial deconjugation of bile salts is likely to be increased in SIBO. Separation and assay of unconjugated serum bile acids may become a useful test.[79]

Miscellaneous Tests

A number of tests for intestinal bacterial metabolites have been devised in the hope of being able to detect SIBO.

Measurement, by the nitrosonaphthol test, of urinary *p*-hydroxyphenylacetic acid, which is synthesized from tyrosine by intestinal bacteria, has been reported.[80] Bacterial release of sulfapyridine from sulfasalazine or *p*-aminobenzoic acid (PABA) from a bile salt conjugate (PABA–ursodeoxycholic acid) and measurement of serum sulfapyridine or PABA, respectively, may be used to assess SIBO or intestinal transit time.

ENDOSCOPY

The ability to pass a flexible endoscope into the SI and examine the mucosa for gross abnormalities and collect mucosal biopsy specimens without surgery has revolutionized both human and veterinary gastroenterology in the past 25 years. The only limitations to endoscopy are the length and diameter of the endoscopes and the expertise of the operator.[81] Visualization of the ileocolic valve by rectum should always be possible after adequate cleansing, and if the endoscope cannot be passed into the ileum, blind biopsies may be performed by passing the biopsy forceps through the valve. Only the jejunum cannot be satisfactorily examined by routine endoscopy. As most cases of malabsorption involve diffuse disease, this limitation may not be a problem, but searching for localized masses or sources of bleeding may be impossible. Push enteroscopy, developed in humans and using a much narrower and thinner endoscope, may enable examination of most of the jejunum.[82]

Videogastroscopes are now considered essential for teaching endoscopy (Fig. 137–24) but are expensive, and in practice a good-quality fiber-optic gastroscope is satisfactory. Most important is a narrow tip diameter (9 mm or less), four-way tip flexibility, and the ability to retroflex the tip in at least one plane. A satisfactory endoscope also has channels for air insufflation, washing, and biopsy.

INTESTINAL BIOPSY

In most cases of acute diarrhea, a tissue diagnosis is not needed and intestinal biopsy is never performed. In chronic

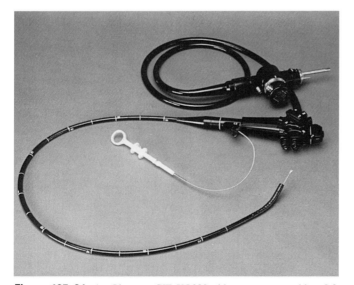

Figure 137–24. An Olympus GIF XQ230 videogastroscope with a 9.2-mm-diameter tip and a 2.8-mm channel suitable for duodenal intubation, with biopsy forceps inserted through the channel.

TABLE 137–25. CRITERIA FOR HISTOLOGIC ASSESSMENT OF INTESTINAL BIOPSIES

Crypt villus unit	Lamina propria
Villus height and width	Immune cell density
Villus clubbing or fusion	Predominant cell type
Crypt depth	Lymphangiectasia
Mitotic index	Miscellaneous
Crypt abscessation	Hyperemia or congestion
Crypt-villus ratio	Edema
Epithelium	Fibrosis
Erosions	Infective agents
Enterocyte height	Neoplasia
Intraepithelial lymphocyte density	
Goblet cell number or size	

diarrhea a definitive diagnosis often depends on histologic examination of intestinal tissue. Yet it must be remembered that in almost 50 per cent of cases biopsy specimens are normal by light microscopy.[83] What constitutes normal intestinal morphology, particularly with respect to the normal density of immunocytes in the lamina propria, is only now being determined,[41] and the recognition of subtle abnormalities is challenging. Although a number of criteria can be applied in the examination of biopsy specimens (Table 137–25), the interpretation by the histopathologist is by necessity somewhat subjective.[70] Discrepancies between biopsies and postmortem findings are surprisingly common.[84] Nevertheless, there are a number of conditions in which a normal biopsy is to be expected (Table 137–26).

Biopsy specimens are usually collected either by endoscopy or by surgical biopsy. The clear advantages of endoscopy to the patient and client are balanced by a number of drawbacks (Table 137–27), and the client should always be warned that surgical biopsy may ultimately be needed for full-thickness tissue or biopsy from the distal SI. If there is any concern about extraintestinal disease or a focal lesion, surgery is the preferred option. Biopsies are always done even if everything looks grossly normal as there may be microscopic changes. Multiple endoscopic biopsies should be done as the size of the specimens, crush artifacts, and fragmentation can make interpretation difficult.

Biopsy specimens of the duodenum and proximal jejunum (if possible) are routinely obtained by endoscopy; ileal biopsy specimens may be obtained via colonoscopy. Surgical biopsy specimens are usually taken from at least three sites: duodenum, jejunum, and ileum. A full-thickness longitudinal elliptical incision is made and tissue removed. Care must be taken to include mucosa in the biopsy specimen as it has a tendency to roll away from the incision line, and use of a

TABLE 137–26. CAUSES OF CHRONIC DIARRHEA WHERE SMALL INTESTINAL BIOPSY MAY BE NORMAL*

Small intestinal bacterial overgrowth
Dietary indiscretion
Food intolerance
Type I hypersensitivity to food (if dog starved before biopsy)
Toxigenic or secretory diarrheas
Motility disorders or irritable bowel syndrome
Brush border membrane disease (e.g., hypolactasia)
Patchy mucosal disease not sampled
Intestinal sclerosis if biopsies not full thickness
Undiagnosed exocrine pancreatic insufficiency or colonic or systemic disease

*Detection of histologic abnormalities depends on the size and quality of the biopsy specimen, quality of processing, and expertise of the pathologist.

TABLE 137–27. RELATIVE ADVANTAGES OF ENDOSCOPIC AND SURGICAL INTESTINAL BIOPSY

TECHNIQUE	ADVANTAGES	DISADVANTAGES
Endoscopy	Minimally invasive Visualize and obtain biopsies of focal lesions Multiple biopsies Minimal adverse reactions Can start steroids early	Requires general anesthetic Only duodenum (distal ileum) accessible Small, superficial (and crushed) biopsies Expensive equipment Technically demanding
Laparotomy	Biopsies of multiple sites Large full-thickness biopsies Inspect other organs Potential for corrective surgery	Requires general anesthetic Surgical risk Convalescence Delay before starting steroids

4-mm sterile skin punch may be preferred. The enterotomy site can be closed longitudinally or transversely (Fig. 137–25). Surgical biopsy of the colon is not generally recommended, unless there is a focal lesion, because of the risk of fecal contamination. Colonic biopsy specimens are more safely collected with a flexible or rigid endoscope (see Chapter 138).

Examination of Biopsy Specimens

Squash preparations of endoscopic biopsy specimens and cytologic examination can be performed and may give clues to an inflammatory, infectious, or neoplastic disease, but histologic examination is necessary for a definitive diagnosis. Criteria for the description of histologic changes are listed in Table 137–25, but some diseases involve no significant histologic changes, and even descriptions of marked inflammatory changes may not reveal an etiologic agent.

DUODENAL JUICE

Duodenal juice can be collected during duodenoscopy through a sterile polyethylene tube passed down the biopsy channel or by needle aspiration through the intestinal wall at laparotomy. However, collection of a sufficient sample can be difficult and contamination by air, gastric juice, bile, or blood may invalidate results. The sample can be examined for *Giardia* trophozoites and subjected to quantitative and qualitative, aerobic and anaerobic culture. Rapid delivery of the sample to the bacteriology laboratory and plating out under anaerobic conditions are important for achieving accurate results, and this places the test out of reach of most practitioners.

ACUTE SMALL INTESTINAL DISEASE

The extent to which a diagnosis is pursued and therapy is instituted is based largely on the nature of historical and physical problems. Dogs and cats with acute diarrhea that are bright, alert, and not dehydrated may require no further investigation as signs often resolve on their own or after short-term symptomatic therapy (see Fig. 137–17). Causes of acute diarrhea are listed in Table 137–28. Further investigations of acute diarrhea are indicated when

- The dog or cat is dull or depressed, febrile, dehydrated, tachycardic, or bradycardic or has abdominal discomfort, melena, bloody mucoid stools, or frequent vomiting.
- Obvious physical abnormalities such as intestinal masses, thickening, or plication localize the problem to the SI, and diagnostic imaging, noninvasive biopsy, or surgery can define the cause.
- Systemic abnormalities are present as defined by a minimum database and other clinicopathologic tests.

An initial database comprising PCV, total protein, electrolytes, urea, glucose, and urine specific gravity and dipstick enables rapid detection of systemic problems such as azotemia, anemia, hypoproteinemia, hypokalemia, hyperkalemia, hyponatremia, hypernatremia, and hypoglycemia. An electrocardiogram is obtained if a dysrhythmia is suspected.

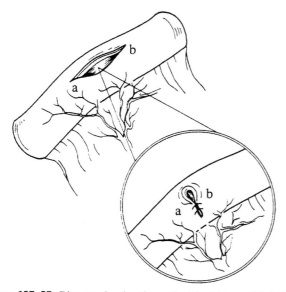

Figure 137–25. Diagram showing the method for taking a full-thickness biopsy specimen from the SI at laparotomy. (From Williams JW: Surgical management of conditions of the gastrointestinal tract and associated glands. *In* Simpson JW, et al [eds]: BSAVA Manual of Canine and Feline Gastroenterology. BSAVA, Cheltenham, UK, 1996, p 238.)

TABLE 137–28. CAUSES OF ACUTE DIARRHEA

Dietary	Hypersensitivity (allergy), intolerance, sudden diet change Food poisoning—poor-quality spoiled foods, bacterial
Toxic	Food or other
Infectious	Parvovirus, coronavirus, paramyxovirus, adenovirus, ±FeLV or FIV* related *Salmonella, Campylobacter, Clostridium?, Escherichia coli?*
Parasites	Helminths, Coccidia, *Giardia*
Acute pancreatitis	
Anatomic	Intussusception
Metabolic	Hypoadrenocroticism

*FeLV = feline leukemia virus; FIV = feline immunodeficiency virus.

These data form the basis for fluid therapy and other investigations. Amylase and lipase or TLI can be submitted to screen for pancreatitis if vomiting or abdominal pain is a problem. For young or unvaccinated animals with bloody diarrhea, vomiting, or abdominal pain, a fecal ELISA for parvovirus is warranted. Hematochezia or diarrhea associated with fever or septicemia is an indication to culture for *Salmonella*. Radiography and ultrasonography help to detect intussusception, foreign object, peritonitis, intestinal masses, and acute pancreatitis. Symptomatic therapy is usually initiated while the results of the initial database and further tests are pending. It is important to reevaluate the patient regularly to monitor response to therapy and to detect new abnormalities that arise.

ACUTE DIARRHEA INDUCED BY DIET, DRUGS, OR TOXINS

Diet is probably the most common cause of acute self-limiting diarrhea in dogs. Potential causes include rapid diet change, dietary indiscretion, dietary intolerance and hypersensitivity, and food poisoning. Dietary hypersensitivity (food allergy) is probably rare. Ingestion of drugs (e.g., NSAIDs) antibacterials, or toxins (e.g., insecticides) may also cause diarrhea and vomiting. The history may enable a more specific presumptive diagnosis of diet-, drug-, or toxin-associated diarrhea to be made, especially if accompanied by other more specific signs. However, the exact cause in many cases is never determined because these dogs and cats respond to symptomatic therapy. The prognosis for acute diarrhea that is not associated with systemic abnormalities is usually excellent. If the diarrhea does not respond or the animal deteriorates, further investigation is necessary.

INFECTIOUS AND PARASITIC CAUSES OF ACUTE DIARRHEA

Diarrhea caused by infectious and parasitic agents is particularly common in animals that are young, immunologically naive or immunocompromised, or housed in large numbers or in unsanitary conditions. Parvovirus, *Giardia, Salmonella, Campylobacter*, and helminths are significant causes of diarrhea. The importance of coronavirus, *C. perfringens*, and *E. coli* as causes of diarrhea has still to be defined. Other viruses, such as paramyxoviruses, adenoviruses, and feline leukemia and immunodeficiency viruses may cause diarrhea but can also affect many other organ systems.

HEMORRHAGIC GASTROENTERITIS

Hemorrhagic gastroenteritis (HGE) is the term given to a syndrome that is characterized by acute hemorrhagic diarrhea accompanied by marked hemoconcentration. The cause of the syndrome is unknown. It may represent an intestinal type I hypersensitivity reaction or could potentially be a consequence of *C. perfringens* enterotoxin production.

Clinical Findings

Small breed dogs such as toy and miniature poodles and miniature schnauzers are most frequently affected. Clinical signs are acute bloody diarrhea, which has often been described as resembling raspberry jam. Fever is unusual, but vomiting, depression, and abdominal discomfort are common. The syndrome often occurs so acutely and is associated with such marked fluid shifts into the SI that signs of shock appear before signs of dehydration.

Diagnosis

A diagnosis of HGE is initially suspected on the basis of appropriate clinical findings associated with a PCV of 55 to 60 or more. Total protein is often normal or is not as high as would be expected with the PCV, probably because of protein loss into the intestine. Radiographs and clinicopathologic tests are usually unremarkable apart from ileus and hemoconcentration, respectively. The absence of leukopenia and presence of hemoconcentration help to distinguish HGE from parvovirus. Positive fecal tests for *C. perfringens* spores or enterotoxin may support a diagnosis of clostridiosis.

Treatment

Intravenous fluids are essential in treating dogs with HGE. Fluid therapy is usually started before all clinicopathological tests and diagnostic imaging have been performed and is based on the results of clinical findings and a minimum database. Many dogs with HGE become hypoproteinemic and may require support with colloids or plasma. Rapid improvement is usually noted within a few hours, although diarrhea may take several days to resolve. Parenteral antibiotics such as ampicillin or a first- or second-generation cephalosporin should be administered because of the high risk of sepsis. A combination of a cephalosporin or amoxycillin with a fluroquinolone or amikacin can be used in dogs with shock; aminoglycosides should not be given until rehydration is accomplished. Monitoring the patient is essential. Those that have not responded within 24 hours should be reevaluated for the presence of parvovirus, intussusception, or foreign objects. Standard dietary therapy for acute diarrhea is given as outlined in the following. The prognosis for most animals with HGE is good. When HGE is complicated by severe hypoproteinemia or sepsis, the prognosis is more guarded.

TREATMENT OF ACUTE DIARRHEA

The initial management of acute diarrhea associated with systemic illness is symptomatic, supportive, and based on clinical findings and an initial database. Treatment options are fluid therapy, diet modification, adsorbents and protectants, secretion or motility modifiers, antibiotics, and immunosuppressive drugs.

Fluid Therapy

Dogs and cats with diarrhea and mild dehydration who are not vomiting or are vomiting infrequently may benefit from oral electrolyte replacement.[85] When diarrhea is accompanied by vomiting and dehydration parenteral fluids should be administered at a rate that replaces deficits, supplies maintenance needs, and compensates for ongoing losses. The type of fluid and requirement for potassium supplementation are best judged by obtaining a minimum database and blood gas analysis. Parenteral fluids are usually best given intravenously. In puppies or kittens the intraosseus route can be used.

Dogs and cats with signs of decreased perfusion require more aggressive support and the volume deficit can be replaced with crystalloids (usually lactated Ringer's solution) at an initial rate of 60 to 90 mL/kg for the first hour or so. Fluid therapy is then tailored to maintain perfusion and hydration. Please see Chapter 78 for a complete discussion of fluid therapy.

Diet

There is a paucity of studies of the role of diet in the treatment of diarrhea in dogs and cats. Current recommendations are largely based on "common sense" and anecdotal evidence rather than controlled trials. It is generally considered that acute diarrhea is best treated by giving no food by mouth for 24 to 48 hours and then offering a bland diet, fed in small amounts and often, for 3 to 5 days. The original diet is then gradually reintroduced over the next 3 to 5 days by mixing it with the bland one. For animals with no other significant clinical findings, this may be the only therapy required. Common choices of a bland, fat-restricted, diet for dogs are home-prepared chicken and low-fat cottage cheese and boiled rice. Cats seem to have a lower tolerance for dietary starch and may benefit from a diet with a higher fat content than dogs, and poultry-based diets are used. Nutritional adequacy of home-prepared bland diets is not critical when they are fed for a short time.

The concept of intestinal rest has been challenged by studies demonstrating that feeding human infants through diarrhea decreases bacterial translocation across the mucosa and promotes recovery. The success of feeding through diarrhea depends on the cause, with most benefit in diarrhea caused by bacterial endotoxins and least in that caused by viral infections. The inclusion of enterocyte "fuels" such as glutamine in feeding regimens may also promote recovery and decrease bacterial translocation.

Protectants and Adsorbents

Bismuth subsalicylate, kaolin-pectin, activated charcoal, and magnesium-, aluminum-, and barium-containing products are often administered in acute diarrhea to bind bacteria and their toxins and to coat and protect the intestinal mucosa. Although efficacy has not been proved for most common small animal GI diseases, these products are probably safer and more efficacious than anticholinergics or antibiotics. Care should be taken when considering administering bismuth subsalicylate to cats, as elimination is prolonged. Therapy for dogs with acute diarrhea (1 mL per 5 kg by mouth three times a day) should probably not exceed 5 days.

Motility- and Secretion-Modifying Agents

Anticholinergics and opiate or opioid analgesics are frequently employed for the symptomatic management of acute diarrhea. Anticholinergic agents can potentiate ileus and are not recommended. Opiate analgesics were thought to exert their effects by stimulating segmental motility, but they actually act mainly by decreasing intestinal secretion and promoting absorption. Opiates and opioids (loperamide 0.1 mg/kg by mouth three times a day, diphenoxylate 0.05 mg/kg by mouth three times a day) can be used in the symptomatic management of acute diarrhea in dogs. They should probably not be given for more than 5 days and are potentially contraindicated when infectious causes of diarrhea are sus-

pected. Adverse reactions and lack of safe dosing information restrict their use in cats.

Antibiotics

Antibiotics should be given only when there is a clear indication that animals have a bacterial or protozoal infection or are at risk for sepsis. Leukopenia, neutrophilia, fever, bloody stools, and shock are indications for prophylactic antibiotics in animals with diarrhea. Initial choices in these situations include ampicillin or a cephalosporin (effective against gram-positive and some gram-negative and anaerobic bacteria), which can be combined with an aminoglycoside (effective against gram-negative aerobes) when sepsis is present and hydration status is adequate. Enrofloxacin is a suitable alternative to an aminoglycoside in skeletally mature dogs and cats at risk for nephrotoxicity through volume depletion. Intravenous quinolones have been shown to reach therapeutic concentrations within the canine gut lumen and be effective against enterococci, *E coli*, and anaerobes.[86] Specific infections that are amenable to antibiotics are those with *Salmonella, Campylobacter, Clostridium,* and *Giardia.* Oxytetracycline, tylosin, and metronidazole are suitable for the treatment of SIBO.

VIRAL ENTERITIDES

Most viral enteritides of dogs and cats, especially parvovirus infections, cause an acute and usually self-limiting diarrhea. In cats, however, some viruses have been associated with chronic diarrhea.

CANINE PARVOVIRUS

Canine parvovirus type 2 (CPV-2) is a highly contagious cause of acute enteritis.[87] CPV-2 emerged as a pathogen in the late 1970s and is related to feline panleukopenia and mink enteritis viruses. Infection is acquired via the fecal-oral route. Infected animals shed massive quantities of virus particles in feces during the acute illness and for about 8 to 10 days after it. CPV-2 is extremely stable and can remain infectious for many months in the environment. It has an affinity for rapidly dividing cells, and, after initial replication in the lymph nodes of the pharynx and tonsils, a viremia develops. Virus then localizes to the intestine (crypt cells), bone marrow, and lymphoid tissues, causing intestinal crypt necrosis, severe diarrhea, leukopenia and lymphoid depletion. Clinical signs of diarrhea typically occur 4 to 7 days after infection.

Clinical Findings

Anorexia, depression, fever, vomiting, diarrhea (often profuse and hemorrhagic), and dehydration are common. Hypothermia, jaundice, and disseminated intravascular coagulopathy are associated with terminal bacterial sepsis or endotoxemia. Infection is most common in the summer months. Dogs of any age can be affected but the incidence of clinical disease is highest in puppies between weaning and 6 months. Puppies younger than 6 weeks are often protected by maternal antibody. In dogs older than 6 months, males are more likely than females to become infected.[88] Overcrowding; intestinal parasitism; and concurrent infections with distemper virus, coronavirus, *Giardia, Salmonella,* or *Campylobacter* can increase the severity of illness.

GI

Death can occur in severe cases, especially in young puppies and susceptible breeds such as rottweilers, Dobermans, English springer spaniels, and American pitt bull terriers.[88] Puppies infected in utero or shortly after birth, when maternal antibody is ineffective, may develop myocarditis and either die suddenly or develop cardiomyopathy. However, death is usually attributed to dehydration, electrolyte imbalances, endotoxic shock, or overwhelming bacterial sepsis related to mucosal barrier disruption and leukopenia. Endotoxemia, TNF activity, coliform septicemia, and proliferation of enteric *C. perfringens* determine morbidity and mortality.[88]

Diagnosis

Parvovirus should be suspected in young dogs with sudden onset of vomiting and diarrhea, especially if they are also depressed, febrile, or leukopenic or have been in contact with infected dogs. Leukopenia may be detected in up to 85 per cent of field cases. In the absence of leukopenia, clinical signs are indistinguishable from those in other bacterial or viral enteritides. Acute salmonellosis, bacterial sepsis, GI foreign bodies with peritonitis, and intussusception cause similar clinical signs.

Definitive diagnosis requires the demonstration of CPV-2 virus (or viral antigens) in the feces. Leukopenia (often 500 to 2000 white blood cells/μL) associated with neutropenia and lymphopenia, caused by loss of neutrophils through the damaged gut and impaired bone marrow production, is suggestive. The degree of neutropenia usually correlates with clinical severity. Biochemical abnormalities often include hypokalemia, hypoglycemia, prerenal azotemia, and increased bilirubin or liver enzymes. Abdominal radiographs may reveal intestinal gas, fluid, and ileus that must be distinguished from foreign bodies and intussusception. Fecal ELISA (Cite-Parvo test: IDEXX) is regarded as an accurate and specific diagnostic test. Single anti-CPV antibody determination in serum is not useful for diagnosis. Serum IgM analysis by hemagglutination inhibition of 2-mercaptoethanol–treated and –untreated serum may provide evidence of recent infection.

Treatment

Treatment is supportive and is similar to regimens used for most animals with severe gastroenteritis.[89] Intravenous fluid therapy is usually indicated and is continued until vomiting stops and oral intake resumes. A balanced electrolyte solution (e.g., lactated Ringer's solution) supplemented with potassium and 2.5 per cent glucose is often used. The intraosseous route can be used if venous access is impossible, but subcutaneous administration of fluids is likely to be inadequate and may be complicated by a high incidence of cellulitis and skin sloughs in leukopenic patients. Plasma or whole blood infusion is used to treat severe hypoproteinemia or anemia.

Antibiotics are used to control potentially fatal sepsis and are given parenterally. A cephalosporin or ampicillin is often combined with an aminoglycoside (gentamicin, amikacin) in neutropenic dogs. Adequate hydration must be ensured when using aminoglycosides. Fluoroquinolones are a less nephrotoxic alternative to aminoglycosides, but there are potential adverse effects on cartilage development in young dogs. Antiendotoxin therapy has been useful in some patients, but the timing of antiendotoxins in relation to antibiotic therapy may be important. As endotoxin liberation may be increased by antibiotics, it may be better to administer antiendotoxin serum before antibiotics.

Traditionally, oral intake is discontinued until vomiting has ceased for at least 24 hours; this may take 3 to 5 days in severe cases. It may be better to trickle feed small amounts of glutamine-containing solutions to decrease bacterial translocation rather than avoid the oral route completely. When vomiting is under control, small amounts of a bland diet are fed initially and a gradual transition is made back to a normal diet. Frequent or persistent vomiting caused by parvovirus can be managed with metoclopramide (0.5 mg/kg subcutaneously three times a day or continuous infusion of (1 to 2 mg/kg per 24 hours diluted in intravenous fluids) as long as intussusception is ruled out. Phenothiazines (e.g., chlorpromazine) can be used if metoclopramide is ineffective and the animal has been rehydrated.

The administration of corticosteroids is of unproven benefit and is probably best limited to dogs with severe endotoxic shock. Flunixin meglumine is best avoided because of its adverse effects on the GI tract and kidneys. Administration of recombinant human granulocyte colony-stimulating factor to neutropenic patients may raise neutrophil counts but appears to be of no clinical benefit.[90]

Prognosis

Most dogs with parvovirus recover if dehydration and sepsis are treated appropriately. Complications include hypoglycemia, hypoproteinemia, anemia, intussusception, and secondary bacterial or viral infections. Severe infection and leukopenia are associated with a high mortality rate.

Prevention

Prevention is achieved by limiting exposure to virus, adequate disinfection (1:32 dilution of sodium hypochlorite bleach), and vaccination.[87] Vaccination is an effective means of preventing and controlling CPV-2, but maternal antibody interference is a problem. Maternally derived antibodies can persist for up to 18 weeks and interfere with vaccination. Modified live CPV-2 vaccines are usually used; killed vaccines provide less duration of immunity but may be recommended in pregnant dogs and puppies younger than 5 weeks. Commercially produced vaccines may differ considerably in efficacy; it is considered that low-passage, high-titer vaccines are most effective, and only one injection after 12 weeks may be needed.[91] In susceptible breeds and dogs in high-risk areas, vaccination usually begins at 6 to 8 weeks of age and is repeated every 3 to 4 weeks until they are 18 weeks of age. Unvaccinated dogs older than 16 weeks are usually given two doses 2 to 4 weeks apart. There is a good correlation between antibody titer and resistance to infection with CPV. Annual revaccination is currently recommended.

FELINE PARVOVIRUS (FELINE PANLEUKOPENIA)

Feline panleukopenia is a highly contagious parvoviral infection of cats that causes severe acute diarrhea and death. It has become an uncommon disease because of routine vaccination. Outbreaks are occasionally seen in unvaccinated animals, particularly in feral populations and catteries. Transmission and pathogenesis are similar to those of CPV (see Chapter 92).

CANINE CORONAVIRUS

Canine coronavirus (CCV) is closely related to feline enteric coronavirus, feline infectious peritonitis virus (FIPV), and transmissible gastroenteritis of swine and has been implicated as a cause of diarrhea in dogs. Transmission is by the fecal-oral route. The virus invades enterocytes at the villus tips, causing diarrhea of variable severity. The incubation period is 1 to 4 days and infected dogs may shed virus intermittently for months after clinical recovery (see Chapter 88).

FELINE ENTERIC CORONAVIRUS

Feline enteric coronavirus (FECV) is related to FIP-producing strains of coronavirus and is ubiquitous in the cat population. Like canine coronavirus, FECV invades the epithelial cells at villus tips. Inapparent infection is common in normal cats, many of which shed FECV in feces and are seropositive. Transmission is thought to be fecal-oral and young kittens (4 to 12 weeks old) are most susceptible. FECV infection is important because enteric coronaviruses may mutate to FIPV (see Chapter 92).

INTESTINAL FELINE INFECTIOUS PERITONITIS

An unusual manifestation of FIP of isolated mural intestinal lesions has been reported in 26 of 156 cats with FIP.[92] Predominant clinical signs were diarrhea and vomiting for 3 months or less before biopsy. All cats had a palpable neoplastic-like mass in the colon or ileocecocolic junction. Affected intestine was markedly thickened, nodular, firm, and white, with multifocal pyogranulomas extending through the intestinal wall, and associated lymph nodes were large. FIPV was demonstrable by immunohistochemistry. Most cats were euthanatized or died within 9 months of biopsy, many with signs of multisystemic FIP (see Chapter 91).

FELINE IMMUNODEFICIENCY VIRUS

Infection is associated with a 10 to 20 per cent incidence of chronic enteritis. Although secondary and often opportunistic infectious agents such as coccidia, *Cryptosporidium, Giardia, Candida, Salmonella,* and *Yersinia* may be responsible for signs, sometimes no other etiologic agent can be identified. Anorexia, chronic diarrhea, and emaciation are typical. Thickened bowel loops reflect a chronic enteritis characterized by villous atrophy and fusion with transmural granulomatous inflammation. High mortality is seen (see Chapter 90).

FELINE LEUKEMIA VIRUS

This retrovirus found in approximately 20 per cent of alimentary lymphomas in cats. Its role in other cases is uncertain. It can also cause a fatal peracute enterocolitis and induce a lymphocytic ileitis (see Chapter 89).

TOROVIRUS

A torovirus or torovirus-like agent has been isolated from the feces of a number of cats afflicted with a characteristic self-limiting syndrome of chronic diarrhea and protruding nictitating membrane.[93]

BACTERIAL ENTERITIDES

Most GI infections by pathogenic bacteria are associated with acute diarrhea, but sometimes these organisms may be isolated from animals with chronic diarrhea. Confusion exists about the significance of such organisms. Enteroinvasive bacteria such as *Campylobacter* spp., *Salmonella* spp., *Shigella* spp., and *Yersinia enterocolitica* can all be pathogenic and may be isolated from animals with chronic diarrhea. Yet they can also be isolated from clinically healthy animals. The incidence of infection is greatest in young, kenneled animals or immunocompromized patients. Dogs may become asymptomatic carriers of *Shigella* spp. after exposure to infected human feces. Although there is no doubt that some of these organisms represent a zoonotic risk, their attempted eradication with antibiotics may be unhelpful and unnecessary and may even induce a carrier state.[94] Furthermore, an underlying enteropathy that predisposes the patient to persistent infection may be the primary problem.

CAMPYLOBACTER

Campylobacter jejuni and *C. upsaliensis* are gram-negative microaerophilic bacteria that have been associated with intestinal disease in dogs and cats. Natural transmission is by the fecal-oral route. Most infections are asymptomatic, and carriage rates in healthy dogs and cats are up to 50 per cent. Dogs younger than 1 year old that had diarrhea were twice as likely as asymptomatic adults to have *Campylobacter* infection (see Chapter 85).

SALMONELLA

Salmonella spp. are gram-negative motile rods that can cause significant clinical signs in dogs and cats. Transmission is by the fecal-oral route. Asymptomatic carriage is common, and *Salmonella* has been isolated from the feces of up to 30 per cent of healthy dogs and 18 per cent of healthy cats. Certain *Salmonella* spp. have zoonotic potential (see Chapter 85).

Clinical Findings

Clinically significant disease is uncommon and is most often encountered in young, parasitized, kenneled, or immunocompromised animals. Outbreaks in hospital kennels may result from nosocomial infection or increased susceptibility in previously asymptomatic carriers. Glucocorticoids, anticancer chemotherapy, and antibiotic administration may precipitate salmonellosis. The three scenarios after infection are gastroenteritis, bacteremia and endotoxemia, and asymptomatic carriage. Significant infection usually causes acute diarrhea, ranging from mild to severe and bloody; anorexia; fever; abdominal pain; and vomiting. In severe cases clinical signs may resemble those of parvovirus infection. Mesenteric lymphadenopathy may be present. Bacterial translocation from the gut lumen may result in septicemia, with endotoxemia, disseminated intravascular coagulopathy, multi-organ failure, and death in some susceptible animals. Cats with *Salmonella* infection may exhibit only vague signs such as fever, leukocytosis, and conjunctivitis without gastrointestinal signs.

Diagnosis

Diagnosis is based on the isolation of *Salmonella* from feces or from blood in septicemic patients. Clinicopathologic features are nonspecific and range from leukocytosis to leukopenia and evidence of multi-organ involvement. Hyperkalemia and hyponatremia, suggestive of hypoadrenocorticism, may occur.

Treatment

When *Salmonella* is isolated in feces from healthy animals or stable animals with acute diarrhea, it is usually not treated with antibiotics. Antibiotics may promote bacterial resistance and a carrier state. In animals with severe bloody diarrhea, marked depression, shock, persistent fever, or sepsis, a parenteral antibiotic should be administered. In animals with chronic diarrhea and *Salmonella,* care should be taken to determine whether an underlying enteropathy is allowing colonization. Antibiotic therapy is warranted in patients with chronic diarrhea with sepsis or a high risk of sepsis (e.g., severe bloody diarrhea, PLE, neutropenia). The choice of antibiotic should be governed by sensitivity testing when possible. Fluoroquinolones (enrofloxacin, 5 mg/kg twice a day) appear to be effective against many *Salmonella* spp.[95] Antibiotic therapy should initially be given for 10 days and the feces then recultured. Prolonged therapy may be required, and feces should be recultured on several future occasions to ensure that the infection (or shedding) has been eliminated. Owners of infected animals should be advised to take suitable hygienic precautions.

Prognosis

The prognosis for diarrhea associated with *Salmonella* in most cases is good. A guarded prognosis should be given in patients with septicemia. Negative prognostic indicators include peracute onset, high fever (temperature above 104°F), hypothermia, severe bloody diarrhea, degenerative left shift, and hypoglycemia (see Chapter 85).

CLOSTRIDIUM

Clostridium perfringens and *C. difficile* are anaerobic gram-positive bacilli that are part of the normal resident intestinal microflora of dogs and cats. They are suspected causes of diarrhea as a consequence of sporulation and enterotoxin production. However, as enterotoxin has been detected in the feces of healthy dogs and dogs with diarrhea, a causal relationship between *Clostridium* spp. and diarrhea remains to be demonstrated (see Chapter 85).

MISCELLANEOUS BACTERIAL INFECTIONS

Enteropathogenic Escherichia coli

The role of enteropathogenic and enterotoxigenic *E. coli* as a cause of diarrhea in dogs and cats is unresolved. Although many strains are normal commensals, some are a significant cause of acute diarrhea and other isolates may cause chronic diarrhea. Identification of pathogenic strains requires specialized assays such as bioassays for toxins and genome probes for identification of pathogenicity markers. Research studies have shown that approximately 25 per cent of dogs with suspected idiopathic SIBO actually carry enteropathogenic *E. coli* (EPEC).[65] The significance of this finding is uncertain, but EPECs have been associated with chronic diarrhea in cats and dogs. EPECs attach to the mucosa, cause effacement of microvilli, and produce profound malabsorption and diarrhea without causing marked changes on light microscopy (Fig. 137–26; see Chapter 85).

Enteroadherent Organisms

Enteroadherent *E. coli* exist, and adherent organisms, thought to be *Streptococcus* spp., have been reported to cause chronic diarrhea in dogs.[96]

Yersinia enterocolitica

This organism has been cultured from the stools of clinically normal dogs and cats and those with large bowel diarrhea. It is important because of its public health significance (see Chapter 85).

Yersinia pseudotuberculosis

Y. pseudotuberculosis can be ingested when cats eat rodents or birds. It affects the GI tract, liver, and lymph nodes. Clinical findings are marked weight loss, diarrhea, inappetence, lethargy, jaundice, and mesenteric lymphadenopathy. Diagnosis is based on isolation of the organism from biopsy specimens of affected organs. The disease is usually progressive and fatal. Treatment may be attempted with oxytetracycline or trimethoprim-sulfa. *Y. pseudotuberculosis* is of public health significance.

Bacillus piliformis (Tyzzer's Disease)

This is a rare disease causing acute, fatal diarrhea in puppies and kittens. The organism is harbored by rodents and causes severe enterocolitis and hepatic necrosis. Clinical signs include diarrhea and depression, and death usually

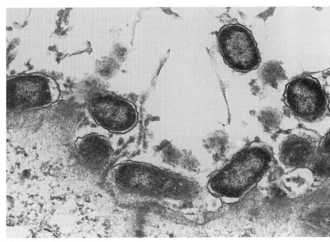

Figure 137–26. Electron micrograph showing attaching and effacing *Escherichia coli* organisms on the luminal surface of an enterocyte and causing widespread microvillus damage. (Courtesy of R. J. Higgins and G. R. Pearson.)

ensues within 48 hours. No effective treatment has been described.

Tuberculosis

Mycobacterium spp. are rare infectious agents in dogs and cats, causing multisystemic granulomatous reactions that may include the GI tract. Cats are typically infected with *Mycobacterium bovis,* presumably by drinking infected cow's milk. Localization to the GI tract occurs more commonly in cats than in dogs and is associated with vomiting, small bowel diarrhea, weight loss, mesenteric lymphadenopathy, and peritonitis.

Actinomyces

Gram-positive, branching filamentous organisms such as *Actinomyces* and *Nocardia* can produce a fibrinous peritonitis, sometimes with characteristic sulfur granules (see Chapter 93). Extension of the inflammation to involve the intestine can produce marked adhesions and vomiting and diarrhea as well as pyrexia and abdominal effusion.

RICKETTSIAL DIARRHEA (SALMON POISONING)

Neorickettsia helminthoeca and *N. elokominica* are found in the metacercarieae of the fluke *Nanophyetus salmonicola,* which is present in salmon in the western regions of the Cascade Range from northern California to central Washington. About a week after the ingestion of infected salmon by dogs, the rickettsiae emerge from the mature fluke and cause a disease characterized by high fever, hemorrhagic gastroenteritis, vomiting, lethargy, anorexia, polydipsia, nasal-ocular discharge, and peripheral lymphadenopathy. Cervical and presecapular lymphadenopathy can be detected as early as 5 days after infection. Clinical signs can resemble those of parvovirus infection. Mortality is extremely high in untreated patients. Diagnosis is based on a history of ingestion of raw fish in an endemic area, the detection of operculated fluke eggs in feces, and the presence of intracytoplasmic inclusion bodies in macrophages from lymph node aspirates. Oxytetracycline (7 mg/kg intravenously three times a day) is the treatment of choice and should be continued for at least 5 days. The trematode vector is eradicated with praziquantel (10 to 30 mg/kg by mouth of subcutaneously once) (see Chapter 86).

ALGAL INFECTIONS

Toxic algal blooms can lead to acute gastroenteritis and death in animals that drink contaminated water. Blue-green algae can cause hepatorenal toxicity and can synthesize an anticholinesterase that induces vomiting, diarrhea, ataxia, and rapid death in dogs. *Prototheca* spp. are achlorophyllous algae that cause protothecosis. Typically a cutaneous infection in cats, in dogs infection can involve the intestine. Large intestinal disease is more common (see Chapter 87), but fatal disseminated disease affecting the SI and the eyes has been reported.

FUNGAL INFECTIONS

Low numbers of fungi are found in the normal intestinal microflora and are generally not pathogenic. However, in the right circumstances, such as immunosuppression, they may invade the intestinal mucosa and even disseminate throughout the body. The incidence of these diseases varies worldwide; some are ubiquitous, some are localized to tropical and subtropical areas, and some are endemic in restricted areas. Intestinal infection with a variety of poorly septate molds and fungi is called phycomycosis. Of all cases, infection with *Pythium* spp. (pythiosis) is by far the most common, with 60 of 63 cases of GI fungal infections being pythiosis in one study.[97]

PYTHIOSIS

Pythium is a member of the Oomycetes and differs from other fungi and molds in not having ergosterol in its cell membrane. *Pythium insidiosum* is the only member of the genus known to cause disease in mammals and may be a primary pathogen. Pythiosis is either a cutaneous-subcutaneous or an intestinal infection. *P. insidiosum* is water borne and animals may develop intestinal infection by ingesting zoospore-contaminated water. Intestinal disease is seen most commonly from fall to spring after infection in late summer, when environmental conditions of warm, swampy water favor fungal growth. Pythiosis occurs sporadically throughout the world in tropical and subtropical climates. In the United States it is most common in the states bordering the Gulf of Mexico, namely Texas, Louisiana, and Florida, although it has been recorded in other southern states. Although the disease is a potential zoonosis, there are no reports of spread of infection between hosts.[98]

History and Clinical Signs

Infection is more common in dogs; rare cutaneous infections in cats are reported. Pythiosis is typically seen in young, large-breed dogs 3 years of age or younger. Hunting dogs working in swampy environments are likely to be exposed to infection. The organism can infect any part of the GI tract, but SI infection causes chronic intractable diarrhea that is sometimes bloody. Vomiting, anorexia, depression, and progressive weight loss are usually noted. Infection is characterized by regions of diffuse or multifocal transmural pyogranulomatous inflammation and necrosis within the intestinal wall, with variable areas of mucosal ulceration. The bowel wall becomes greatly thickened and this may eventually result in partial or complete obstruction. Similar pyogranulomatous lesions may occur in the stomach, colon, and adjacent mesentery and lymph nodes and may spread to other intra-abdominal organs.

Diagnosis

On physical examination the most consistent findings in dogs with intestinal pythiosis are emaciation with one or more palpable abdominal mass(es) and a thickened irregular segment of bowel incorporating adjacent mesentery and lymph node. These lesions should be obvious on radiographic and ultrasonographic examination of the abdomen. Mild to moderate nonregenerative anemia and a mild neutrophilia with or without a left shift are typical. Definitive diagnosis can only be made by demonstration of the organism. Grossly the mass(es) can resemble neoplasia at laparotomy, and the differentiation from lymphoma and other granulomatous intestinal diseases is possible only by identification of branching, poorly septate or nonseptate hyphae in

GI

the tissues. The organisms stain poorly with hematoxylin and eosin or periodic acid–schiff (PAS) but are evident with Gomori's methenamine silver stain; they are easiest to find within necrotic areas in the submucosa and muscularis (see Chapter 93).

Treatment and Prognosis

The prognosis for phycomycosis is grave; less than 5 per cent of animals survive for 3 months after diagnosis. Conventional treatment is by surgical excision followed by antifungal treatment. However, lack of ergosterol in the cell membrane suggests that azole derivatives are unlikely to be effective. Euthanasia is often necessary either because radical surgical excision is not possible or because of recurrence and wound dehiscence. Amphotericin B and iodide treatments are unsuccessful, but ketoconazole has shown some efficacy. Itraconazole (10 mg/kg by mouth every 24 hours) has been shown to be effective in two cases of pythiosis, but generally itraconazole and fluconazole have limited success and they are expensive.[99] A combination of itraconazole and terbinafine has been successful in human infection. The prognosis remains poor (see Chapter 93).

ZYGOMYCOSIS

Other organisms have been isolated sporadically from cases of phycomycosis. They are from the Zygomycetes class (zygomycosis) and include members of the Entomophthoraceae (e.g., *Basidiobolus* spp., *Conidiobolus* spp.) and Mucoraceae (e.g., *Absidia* spp., *Rhizopus* spp., *Mucor* spp., *Mortierella* spp.). These organisms are widespread in nature and are opportunistic pathogens. Immune suppression may be important in the development of the infections (see Chapter 93).

HISTOPLASMOSIS

The cause, many manifestations, and treatment of this disease are discussed in Chapter 93. *Histoplasma capsulatum* usually causes a mild, self-limiting respiratory infection. It can disseminate throughout the body to other tissues including the GI tract. The condition is more common in dogs than cats.

MISCELLANEOUS MYCOSES

Apart from histoplasmosis and phycomycosis, fungi are rarely associated with intestinal disease and diarrhea. Opportunistic fungi that are normal commensals may infect young animals already compromized by preexisting bacterial or parvovirus infection, parasitism, or prolonged antibiotic usage (see Chapter 93).

HELMINTHS

Helminth infestation is common in dogs and cats. Some species are pathogenic in large numbers, and some live in virtual symbiosis with the host.

ROUNDWORM ASCARIDS

Toxocara canis and *Toxascaris leonina* are found in dogs;[100] *Toxocara cati* and *Toxascaris leonina* are found in cats.[101] *T. canis* can be transmitted across the placenta and *T. canis* and *T. cati* via the milk. Infection is also caused by ingesting the ova or hosts such as rodents containing the ova. Adult roundworms live in the SI. Migrating juvenile *T. canis* can cause hepatic and pulmonary damage. *T. canis* presents a public health problem, visceral larval migrans.

Clinical Findings

Roundworms most often cause disease in young animals and common signs are diarrhea, weight loss, and failure to thrive. A poor haircoat and a potbelly may be evident in puppies or kittens. Intestinal obstruction and perforation have been described in severe cases.

Diagnosis

Almost all puppies can be presumed to have *T. canis* infection. Diagnosis is by fecal flotation (see Table 137–21 and Fig. 137–19).

Treatment

A wide range of anthelmintics are effective against roundworms (Table 137–29). Treatment should be repeated at 2- to 3-week intervals in affected animals. Young animals should be routinely wormed at 2, 4, 6, 8, 12, and 16 weeks of age and then at 6-month intervals. It is important to ensure proper hygiene to stop reinfection or spread. *T. canis* can be controlled by administering fenbendazole to pregnant bitches at a dose of 50 mg/kg daily from day 40 to 2 days after whelping. Monthly administration of milbemycin or ivermectin plus pyrantel pamoate is approved for the prevention and control of ascarid infections in dogs.

Prognosis

The prognosis for all but the most severely affected patients is excellent.

HOOKWORMS

Ancylostoma caninum is the most important hookworm of dogs and is associated with blood loss and hemorrhagic enteritis. *A. tubeforme* is the most common hookworm in cats but is less pathogenic. *A. braziliense* occurs in dogs in the southern United States. *Uncinaria stenocephala* is the hookworm of dogs in the United Kingdom but does occur in the northern United States and Canada. Infection is most commonly reported in kenneled dogs, particularly greyhounds, and can be acquired prenatally, during lactation, by ingesting larvae, by migration of larvae through the skin, and by ingestion of a paratenic host.

Clinical Findings

Diarrhea, weakness, pallor, vomiting, dehydration, poor growth, and anemia are common in puppies with *A. caninum* infection. The infection can cause a rapid and fatal anemia or a more chronic iron deficiency anemia. *U. stenocephala* do not suck large quantities of blood and cause anemia, although severe infestations may be associated with diarrhea. The most noticeable clinical sign associated with *U. stenocephala* is interdigital dermatitis caused by larval migration.

TABLE 137–29. ANTHELMINTICS FOR INTESTINAL PARASITES

DRUG	SPECTRUM*	DOSAGE	SPECIES*
Treatment			
Febantel plus praziquantel	R, H, W, C	10 mg/kg PO sid 3 days	D, C
		15 mg/kg for puppies younger than 6 months	
Fenbendazole	R, H, W, C	50 mg/kg PO sid 3 days	D, C
Mebendazole	R, H, W, C	22 mg/kg PO sid 3 days	D
Niclosamide	C	125 mg/kg	D
Nitroscanate	R, H, C	50 mg/kg	D
Oxfendazole	R, H, W, C	10 mg/kg PO sid 3 days	D
Piperazine	R	55 mg/kg PO	D, C
Praziquantel	C	5–12.5 mg/kg PO or SC	D, C
Pyrantel pamoate	R, H	5 mg/kg PO dog, 20 mg/kg cat	D, C
Thiabendazole	S	50–75 mg/kg PO sid 3 days	D
Prevention			
Milbemycin oxime	R, H, W	0.5 mg/kg once monthly PO	D
Ivermectin (I) + pyrantel pamoate (P)	R, H	0.006 mg/kg I, 5 mg/kg P, monthly	D
Diethylcarbamazine (DEC) + oxibendazole (O)	R, H, W	6.6 mg/kg DEC, 5 mg/kg O PO sid	D

*R = roundworm; H = hookworm; W = whipworm; C = cestode; S = strongyloides; D = dog.
Compiled from Reinemeyer CR: Canine gastrointestinal parasites. *In* Bonagura JD (ed): Kirk Current Veterinary Therapy XII. Philadelphia, WB Saunders, 1995, p 711; Reinemeyer CR: Feline gastrointestinal parasites. In Bonagura JD (ed): Kirk Current Veterinary Therapy XI. Philadelphia, WB Saunders, 1992, p 626.

Diagnosis

Diagnosis is achieved by demonstrating eggs in feces (see Table 137–21 and Fig. 137–19).

Treatment

Appropriate anthelmintics are shown in Table 137–29. Pyrantel pamoate has been suggested as the treatment of choice for anemic puppies as it acts rapidly and is comparitively safe in debilitated animals. Anemic puppies may require blood transfusion and supportive care. Hookworm disease can be prevented by treating puppies at 2, 4, 6, and 8 weeks of age. Monthly administration of milbemycin or ivermectin plus pyrantel pamoate is approved for the prevention or control of hookworm in dogs. Control is also dependent on adequate kennel hygiene, with fecal material being collected and runs disinfected.

TAPEWORMS

Dipylidium caninum is the most common tapeworm infecting dogs and cats in the United States and Europe. Fleas are the intermediate host. *Echinococcus granulosus* is a tapeworm that uses dogs as definitive hosts and humans and sheep as intermediate hosts. *E. granulosus* is most frequently encountered in areas of extensive sheep farming and is an important zoonosis. Various other *Taenia* spp. are also common in dogs and cats.

Clinical Findings

Heavy infestations of *D. caninum* are only rarely associated with diarrhea, weight loss, and failure to thrive. Usually, no clinical signs are noted except "rice grains" (proglottids) in the perineal area or feces. *E. granulosus* is not associated with clinical signs in dogs but is important because of its zoonotic potential.

Diagnosis

A diagnosis of *D. caninum* is usually made by finding the characteristic egg capsules contained in proglottids obtained from the feces or perineal area (see Fig. 137–19). *E. granulo-* *sus* is not reliably detected in the feces and definitive diagnosis may require arecoline purging and fecal analysis for adult worms.

Treatment

Treatment of *D. caninum* involves adequate flea control (the animal and the environment) and administration of an appropriate anthelmintic (see Table 137–29). *E. granulosus* and other *Taenia* spp. are best controlled by routine administration of an effective anthelmintic such as praziquantel (see Table 137–29).

STRONGYLOIDES

Strongyloides stercoralis is a small nematode that may cause hemorrhagic enteritis in young puppies and can also infect people. Infective larvae are ingested or can penetrate the skin, and after a migration through the lung they develop in the SI. *S. tubefasciens* has been associated with nodules in the large intestine.

Diagnosis

Fecal evaluation using the Baermann procedure or demonstration of motile first-stage larvae in smears of fresh feces (see Table 137–21 and Fig. 137–19) helps differentiate larvae from *Filaroides* and mature hookworms.

Treatment

Treatment is with thiabendazole or potentially fenbendazole or ivermectin (see Table 137–29).

PROTOZOA

COCCIDIA

Isospora

Isospora are the most common coccidial parasites of dogs (*I. canis, I. ohioensis*) and cats (*I. felis, I. rivolta*). Transmission is by ingestion of ova or paratenic hosts. Sporozoites

GI

are liberated in the SI and enter cells to begin development. The prepatent period ranges from 4 to 11 days, depending on the species. *Isospora* are rarely associated with clinical signs. Puppies and kittens kept in unhygienic conditions or immunosuppressed animals may develop heavy infestations that can be associated with diarrhea, which is often mucoid but occasionally may be bloody.

Isospora oocysts are found on direct examination of a fecal smear or by flotation. Cryptosporidial oocysts are directly infective, and it has been recommended that feces be mixed with formalin (one part 38% formaldehyde to nine part fluid feces) before fecal analysis. Infection with *Isospora* is often self-limiting, but sulfadimethoxine (50 mg/kg by mouth once a day for 10 days) or sulfonamide-trimethoprim (15 to 30 mg/kg by mouth once a day for 5 days) can be used where clinical signs warrant treatment. The prognosis for recovery from *Isospora* infection is good.

Cryptosporidium

Cryptosporidium parvum has been associated with diarrhea in dogs and cats. Immunocompromised animals may develop severe bloody diarrhea. Anti-*Cryptosporidium* antibodies have been demonstrated in healthy and sick domestic and feral cats.[102] *Cryptosporidium* sp. can also affect cats and dogs. Transmission is by the fecal-oral route and humans may become infected. Cryptosporidial oocysts are extremely small (about one tenth the size of *Isospora*) and require evaluation by fecal flotation and oil immersion microscopy. *Cryptosporidium* can also be observed in intestinal biopsies. Paromomycin (165 mg/kg by mouth for 5 days) was effective against *Cryptosporidium* sp. in one cat, but consistently effective treatment has not been described. Fortunately, the disease is usually self-limiting in immunocompetent animals. The prognosis for recovery from *Cryptosporidium* in immunocompromised animals is poor.

Giardia

Giardia sp. can affect both dogs and cats. The prevalence of infection in dogs ranges from about 10 per cent in well-treated dogs to 100 per cent in kennels. Cats are less commonly infected than dogs. The parasite is spread by the fecal-oral route. Ingested oocysts excyst in the upper SI and trophozoites attach to the intestinal mucosa from the duodenum to the ileum. After multiplication of trophozoites, oocysts are passed in the feces 1 to 2 weeks after infection. *Giardia* may be a potential zoonotic risk.[103]

Clinical Findings

Most infections of dogs and cats are probably not associated with clinical signs. Clinical signs range from mild, self-limiting acute diarrhea to severe or chronic small bowel diarrhea associated with intestinal protein loss and weight loss.

Diagnosis

Giardia can be diagnosed by demonstrating motile trophozoites in a fresh fecal smear or cysts after zinc sulfate flotation. Shedding of cysts is intermittent and repeated fecal analysis is often required to confirm a diagnosis. *Giardia* trophozoites can also be visualized in samples of intestinal juice and antigen detected by ELISA in feces. The best detection method is examination by zinc sulfate flotation of three fecal samples collected over a 3- to 5-day period.

Treatment

Metronidazole is the drug most commonly used to treat *Giardia* in small animals. The standard dosage recommended is 25 mg/kg by mouth twice a day for 5 days for dogs and 10 to 25 mg/kg by mouth twice a day for 5 days for cats. The drug is effective in eliminating *Giardia* in two thirds of infected dogs. Metronidazole may cause vomiting, anorexia, hypersalivation, and neurologic signs at these high doses.[103] Trials in dogs indicate that albendazole (25 mg/kg by mouth twice a day for 2 days) and fenbendazole (50 mg/kg by mouth once a day for 3 days) also eliminate *Giardia*. Fenbendazole has the advantage over albendazole that it is not believed to be teratogenic and has not been associated with bone marrow toxicosis. A combination of praziquantel, pyrantel pamoate, and febantel has also been shown to be an effective treatment for *Giardia* in dogs.[104] Quinacrine (6.6 mg/kg by mouth twice a day for 5 days) and furazolidone (4 mg/kg by mouth twice a day for 5 to 10 days) are two other alternative treatments that may be effective, although they have not been extensively evaluated, do have adverse side effects, and should not be administered to pregnant animals. Decontamination of the patient's habitat by steam cleaning or use of quaternary ammonium compounds is required to prevent reinfection. Attempts are being made to produce a vaccine.

Prognosis

The prognosis is usually good. Some pets may require several treatments to eliminate infection.

CHRONIC IDIOPATHIC ENTEROPATHIES

Definitions

Chronic enteropathies associated with malabsorption have historically been defined by histologic descriptions of tissue. However, such an approach gives little information about the nature of the intestinal dysfunction or its etiology.[105] Furthermore, a significant proportion of animals with SI disease have no obvious histologic changes.[70] Application of new methods of investigation and a change in emphasis toward understanding the pathophysiologic mechanisms involved have led to identification and characterization of a number of conditions. However, there remain a number of idiopathic enteropathies, not least those grouped under the umbrella term *inflammatory bowel disease* (IBD), for which morphologic classification is the only criterion we currently have for making a diagnosis.

Management

The treatment of idiopathic enteropathies is symptomatic. Inflammatory diseases are treated with immunosuppressive drugs, bacterial overgrowth with antibiotics, and dietary sensitivities with exclusion diets. Withholding food and gradually reintroducing bland food have no role to play in the treatment of chronic diarrhea. However, a "controlled" diet can play a part in the symptomatic management of idiopathic enteropathies.

The ideal controlled diet is of good quality, highly digestible, and gluten free and may be considered "hypoaller-genic." If it also contains only a single protein source, it is a true exclusion diet. It should moderately low in fat and lactose free and not markedly hypertonic. It should contain generous quantities of water and fat-soluble vitamins, and essential minerals; potassium supplementation is probably important, especially in cats. Inclusion of a moderately fermentable fiber, such as psyllium and ispaghula, is usually recommended, particularly for colonic health. Good palatability is essential if a sick animal is to eat it, and because no other source of food is likely to be given, it must be nutritionally balanced. Feeding the daily requirement in two or three divided meals reduces the load on a compromised intestine.

Supplementation of a restricted fat diet with medium-chain triglycerides (MCTs) is one way to try to increase the caloric density of canine diets; MCT oils are contraindicated in cats because of the danger of encephalopathy. MCTs are found naturally in coconut milk, but supplementation is more easily accomplished with a pharmaceutical preparation (MCT oil, Mead Johnson). Each milliliter provides 8 kcal, and the total given should not exceed 20 per cent of the animal's daily energy intake. A dose of 1 to 2 ml/kg can be used in dogs. Gradual introduction is necessary as initial tolerance is poor.

SMALL INTESTINAL BACTERIAL OVERGROWTH

Normally, the bacterial population of the SI is controlled by a number of mechanisms (see earlier). Bacterial overgrowth is an uncontrolled proliferation of the bacteria within the SI. Affected dogs reportedly have numbers of bacteria several orders of magnitude greater than those of normal dogs, in which the upper SI is supposedly relatively sterile. Although SIBO is best considered a sign of intestinal disease rather than a diagnosis, as it can be secondary to a number of conditions, in some animals no underlying disease process can be identified. This so-called idiopathic SIBO is most frequently recognized in young, large-breed dogs, especially German shepherd dogs, and is well known to practitioners by its antibiotic-responsive nature and its tendency to recur. It has not been demonstrated in cats.[31]

Definition

SIBO is defined by the absolute number of bacteria in the upper SI during the fasted state, that is, the number of colony-forming units cultured per milliliter of duodenal juice (CFU/mL). This definition was extrapolated to dogs from values in humans; the normal upper SI was thought to be relatively sterile between meals, and culture of more than 10^5 total or more than 10^4 anaerobic bacterial colonies per mL was considered diagnostic of SIBO. However, evidence in the veterinary literature has left this supposed "gold standard" open to question. The original values were established using few animals and questionable bacteriologic techniques. Changes in collection methodology and improvements in anaerobic culture techniques have led to results that suggest that the accepted numbers for defining SIBO are too low, as numbers as high as 10^7 CFU/mL have been found commonly in asymptomatic dogs.[31, 106]

An alternative view is that clinically healthy animals can have SIBO (by the numeric definition) but its clinical significance depends on other factors. It may be better to call this condition "idiopathic antibiotic-responsive diarrhea" until a better definition of the problem is obtained.

Etiology

The cause of idiopathic antibiotic-responsive diarrhea is, by definition, unknown. Altered intestinal motility that prevents clearance of bacteria is a possibility, but spontaneous achlorhydria has been ruled out. Studies have demonstrated bacterial counts higher than 10^5 CFU/mL with local IgA deficiency, but the deficiency is not absolute.[107] Thus, reduced serum IgA concentrations may be only a marker for a more fundamental immune dysfunction, as German shepherds are predisposed to aspergillosis and anal furunculosis as well. The frequent lack an inflammatory mucosal response in SIBO is surprising if bacterial numbers are actually so high.

Proliferation of bacteria in the upper SI can also be secondary to diseases that either leave increased substrate in the intestinal lumen (EPI, motility disorder, blind loop) or inhibit the clearance of bacteria by the normal interdigestive housekeeping waves of peristalsis (e.g., partial obstruction, abnormal motility) or by the mucosal immune response (e.g., IBD) (Table 137–30). Work suggests that primary pathogenic *E. coli* may be present in some dogs.[65]

Pathogenesis

Increased numbers of bacteria in the upper SI could cause malabsorption and diarrhea by a number of mechanisms. First, bacteria compete for nutrients. For example, they use cbl, make it unavailable for absorption, and consequently cause the low serum cbl concentration that can be a marker of the condition. In cats, luminal bacteria may be involved in making taurine unavailable for absorption, predisposing to deficiency. Second, bacteria also modify certain nutrients, making them unavailable for absorption and potential causes of diarrhea; for example, hydroxylation of fatty acids and deconjugation of bile salts cause fat malabsorption and their products (deconjugated bile salts, hydroxy fatty acids) can cause diarrhea by stimulation of colonocyte secretion. Finally, the bacterial flora has a deleterious effect on the mucosal brush border. Subtle changes in the enzyme activity of the brush border that can be detected biochemically are reversible with antibiotic treatment but are rarely associated with significant histologic changes.

The flora present in idiopathic antibiotic-responsive diarrhea may consist predominantly of either aerobic or anaero-

TABLE 137–30. CAUSES OF SECONDARY SMALL INTESTINAL BACTERIAL OVERGROWTH

Achlorhydria
  Spontaneous: atrophic gastritis
  Acid blockers
Exocrine pancreatic insufficiency
Partial intestinal obstruction
  Chronic intussusception
  Stricture
  Tumor
Abnormal anatomy
  Surgical resection of ileocolic valve
  Blind loop
Motility disorder
  Primary
  Hypothyroidism
Mucosal disease
  Latent primary pathogens?
  Inflammatory bowel disease (cause or effect?)
  Chronic giardiasis
Dietary sensitivity?

bic bacteria, but it tends to be a mixed population, with staphylococci, streptococci, coliforms, enterococci, corynebacteria, and anaerobes such as *Bacteroides, Fusobacterium,* and *Clostridium.* These bacteria are generally commensals found normally in the oropharynx and the SI and LI. A colonic-type flora tends to predominate in an anaerobic overgrowth, and coprophagia probably reinforces this type of flora. However, culture of fecal bacteria cannot be correlated with SI bacterial numbers and cannot be used to diagnose this condition.

Clinical Presentation

Idiopathic Antibiotic-Responsive Diarrhea. This condition is most commonly recognized in young German shepherd dogs, with signs often abating in adult life, but presumed SIBO has now been reported in a number of other dog breeds, although not cats.[33] Affected dogs show signs of chronic intermittent diarrhea accompanied by failure to thrive, weight loss, and/or stunted growth. Intermittent watery diarrhea, often associated with excessive gas production (manifested as borborygmi and flatus), is seen most frequently. However, vomiting and signs of colitis are sometimes reported, and occasionally dogs are stunted but do not have diarrhea. Many dogs have normal activity levels and an increased appetite. Indeed, they may show polyphagia, pica, and coprophagia. However, a minority of dogs have a decreased appetite. A positive response to antibiotics is expected, and the animal's condition often deteriorates if it is given corticosteroids. The major differential diagnoses are EPI and IBD, both of which are common in German shepherd dogs.

Secondary SIBO. The syndrome of SIBO may be secondary to a number of primary conditions listed in Table 137–30. Bacterial numbers in blind loops often exceed 10^9 CFU/mL. The link between SIBO and IBD is not clear. Antibiotic-responsive intestinal inflammation has been reported. However, idiopathic IBD could predispose to secondary SIBO.[33] The presence of chronic *Giardia* infection is sometimes associated with SIBO, and again it is not clear whether there is an underlying mucosal defect that permits continued infection and SIBO or whether mucosal damage by *Giardia* predisposes to SIBO.

Diagnosis

Whatever method is used to diagnose SIBO, it is important that the clinician rule out causes of secondary overgrowth. Systemic disease is ruled out by the minimum database and EPI by serum TLI assay. Fecal examination for parasites is mandatory. Radiographs and ultrasonography may be necessary to rule out a partial obstruction.

Duodenal Juice Culture. Quantitative aerobic and anaerobic culture of duodenal juice with more than 10^5 total or more than 10^4 anaerobic bacterial CFU/mL has been the accepted diagnostic criterion sine qua non. However, the proposed numbers are probably too low, as 10^7 CFU/mL are found commonly and numbers as high as 10^9 CFU/mL are found occasionally in asymptomatic dogs[106] and cats.[31] Some of the discrepancies may reflect difficulties and differences in the methodology (Table 137–31), as numbers vary widely when individual animals are repeatedly sampled. Culture of endoscopic biopsy specimens has not been shown to be of greater diagnostic significance.[108]

Use of a low cutoff value leads to overdiagnosis of SIBO and probably explains why it has been reported to be present

TABLE 137–31. POSSIBLE EXPLANATIONS FOR DIFFERENCES REPORTED IN NORMAL SMALL INTESTINAL BACTERIAL NUMBERS

Technical factors	Patient-related factors
Method of collection	Natural variability
Dilution by nonintestinal secretions	Immunoglobulin A status
Anaerobic technique	Diet
Bacteriologic method	Coprophagy
	Pet dog versus kenneled dog

in 50 per cent of dogs with chronic intestinal disease.[33] The relatively high numbers of bacteria in SI of dogs and cats may also have important consequences for the application of intestinal function tests. For example, bacterial deconjugation of bile acids, production of folate, utilization of cbl, intestinal permeability, and breath hydrogen production may be greater in healthy dogs and cats than would be anticipated on the basis of findings in healthy people.

Serum Folate and Cobalamin Concentrations. Bacteria synthesize folate, tending to increase serum folate, and bind cbl, causing vitamin B_{12} malabsorption. Thus, classically, SIBO is associated with increased serum folate and decreased cbl.[22] Unfortunately, although it has high specificity, this combination of changes has low sensitivity and approximately 95 per cent of cases of SIBO, as defined by culture, would be missed.[33] Raised folate or decreased cbl alone have better sensitivity (51 and 24 per cent, respectively) but poorer specificity (79 and 87 per cent, respectively). There are also difficulties in interpretation, as diet, concurrent disease, and drugs can all affect serum vitamin concentrations. Nevertheless, this is the most convenient test available to practitioners, although in interpreting results one should consider the whole clinical picture.

Breath Hydrogen Excretion. Fermentation by intestinal bacteria releases H_2, which is absorbed and can be measured when excreted in the breath. Theoretically, SIBO is associated with either a high resting breath H_2 or an early (or double) H_2 peak after ingestion of a test meal (food, xylose, lactulose). However, increased breath H_2 is also seen if there is carbohydrate malabsorption or decreased orocecal transit time.

Biochemical Tests. Measurement of increased amounts of a bacterial product produced either naturally or after oral administration of a test substance could be used to diagnose SIBO, but none of the previously discussed tests has been shown to be reliable. Serum unconjugated bile acids hold the most promise for a noninvasive test for SIBO.[79]

Intestinal Permeability. Intestinal permeability measured by chromium 51–labeled ethylenediaminetetracetic acid (EDTA) and differential sugar absorption can be abnormal in SIBO and improve after antibiotic treatment.

Lack of Histologic Changes on Intestinal Biopsy. Usually, no or minimal histologic changes are seen in cases of idiopathic SIBO, but that cannot be considered diagnostic. Furthermore, SIBO may be seen in cases of IBD, in which it may be a primary cause or secondary effect.

Empirical Response to Antibiotics. Such a pragmatic approach can be helpful in confirming the antibiotic responsiveness of the diarrhea, but it cannot help distinguish between idiopathic and secondary SIBO, and undiagnosed bacterial pathogens.

Treatment

If an underlying cause such as a chronic intussusception can be identified, its specific treatment may be all that is required to resolve SIBO. Treatment of EPI with pancreatic extracts may reduce bacterial numbers, as the proteases have antibacterial activity, but recalcitrant cases often need antibiotic therapy as well.

Antibiotics. There is no cure for idiopathic antibiotic-responsive diarrhea, but signs can be controlled with antibiotics. A broad-spectrum antibiotic is indicated, and in the first instance a 4- to 6-week course is tried, although the antibiotic should be changed after 2 weeks if there has been no response. Prolonged treatment is recommended as premature cessation frequently leads to relapse, often within 24 hours. In the United Kingdom, oxytetracycline (10 to 20 mg/kg by mouth three times a day) seems efficacious, whereas in the United States metronidazole (10 to 20 mg/kg by mouth three times a day) and tylosin (20 mg/kg by mouth two or three times a day) are the preferred choices.

Oxytetracycline has the advantages that it is inexpensive, safe, and can be given with food. It cannot be used before permanent tooth eruption because of staining of tooth enamel. When an antibiotic fails, an underlying cause of SIBO or another diagnosis should be considered, but occasionally other antibiotics work where the first fails. However, whether this is an effect on SIBO or whether a susceptible primary pathogenic bacterium is present is uncertain.

Some animals suffer relapse several months after cessation of antibiotics. They are best treated with repeated antibiotic courses. However, immediate relapse when antibiotics are withdrawn indicates a need to search again for an underlying cause; an exclusion diet trial may be worth pursuing at this stage. Judicious use of corticosteroids is indicated if there is intestinal inflammation on biopsy. If there is no obvious cause of relapse, antibiotics can be continued indefinitely. Resistance does not appear to be a problem and efficacy can be maintained for years. Furthermore, efficacy may be maintained if the dosage is reduced from thrice to even once daily. Thus, whether oxytetracycline acts as an antibiotic or has a direct effect on the intestinal mucosa has yet to be determined. Dogs also appear to outgrow this problem with age, perhaps simply because of a decrease in their caloric intake or because of the maturity of the intestinal immune system.

Ancillary Treatments. Dietary manipulation can be a useful adjunct in treating the syndrome of SIBO. In general, a highly digestible, low-fat diet is desired to reduce the substrate available for bacterial use. Addition of fructo-oligosaccharide may decrease the numbers of harmful bacteria,[35] although proof of efficacy is lacking. Administration of probiotics (Lactobacillus preparations, live yogurt) seem unlikely to work as the primary problem is considered to be already increased numbers of a mixed flora. Dogs with SIBO may be cbl deficient, and parenteral administration of vitamin B_{12} is indicated.

INFLAMMATORY BOWEL DISEASE

Inflammatory bowel disease is a collective term describing a group of disorders characterized by histologic evidence of intestinal inflammation and associated with persistent or recurrent GI signs.[109, 110] However, indiscriminate use of the term IBD to describe GI disease is no more useful than a dermatologist making a diagnosis of chronic dermatitis. Whereas a number of recognized diseases are associated with chronic intestinal inflammation (Table 137–32), the cause of idiopathic IBD is by definition unknown. Variations in the histologic appearance of the inflammation suggest that

TABLE 137–32. CAUSES OF CHRONIC SMALL BOWEL INFLAMMATION

Chronic infection
  Giardia
  Histoplasma
  Toxoplasma
  Mycobacteria
  Prototothecosis
  Pythiosis
  Pathogenic bacteria (*Campylobacter*, *Salmonella*, pathogenic
    Escherichia coli)
Food allergy
Associated with other primary gastrointestinal diseases
  Lymphoma
  Lymphangiectasia
Idiopathic
  Lymphocytic-plasmacytic enteritis (LPE)
  Eosinophilic (gastro)-entero-(colitis) (EGE)
  Granulomatous enteritis (same as regional enteritis?)

idiopathic IBD is not a single disease entity (Fig. 137–27). The nomenclature reflects the predominant cell type present. Lymphocytic-plasmacytic enteritis (LPE) is the form most commonly reported, eosinophilic (gastro-)enteritis (EGE) is less common, and granulomatous enteritis is rare. Neutrophils are a feature of human IBD but are seen infrequently in idiopathic IBD.

Clinical Presentation

Idiopathic IBD is probably the most common cause of chronic vomiting and diarrhea in dogs and cats. There is no apparent sex predisposition, and the disease is seen most frequently in middle-age dogs and cats. There is often a history of intermittent signs, controlled at least in part by dietary manipulation, from an earlier age. Certain breeds are predisposed to certain types of IBD (see Table 137–18).

Ultimately, IBD is a histologic diagnosis. The nature and severity of the signs can be crudely correlated with the region affected within the GI tract, the histologic type of inflammation, and its severity. The signs of IBD may wax and wane, sometimes with obvious precipitating events, such as stress or dietary change. Vomiting and diarrhea are most common, but an individual dog or cat may show some or all of the signs in Table 137–33.[109] Gastric signs are seen more commonly if there is gastric or upper SI inflammation, and in cats vomiting may be the predominant sign. LI-type diarrhea may be due to colonic inflammation but can also be secondary to prolonged SI diarrhea; alternatively, both SI and LI may be inflamed. The presence of blood in the vomit or diarrhea is associated with more severe disease, especially eosinophilic inflammatory infiltrates. Severe disease may be associated with weight loss, protein-losing enteropathy (PLE), hypoproteinemia and ascites. Appetite is variable; it may be increased if there is significant malabsorption or decreased with severe inflammation. Mild inflammation may not affect appetite, but postprandial pain can be a significant problem even in the absence of other signs and chronic pancreatitis is one differential diagnosis.

Etiology

The infiltration of the lamina propria in idiopathic IBD may reflect an immune response to dietary, microbial, or self-antigens. Most dogs or cats require treatment with immunosuppressive drugs, suggesting that there is an underly-

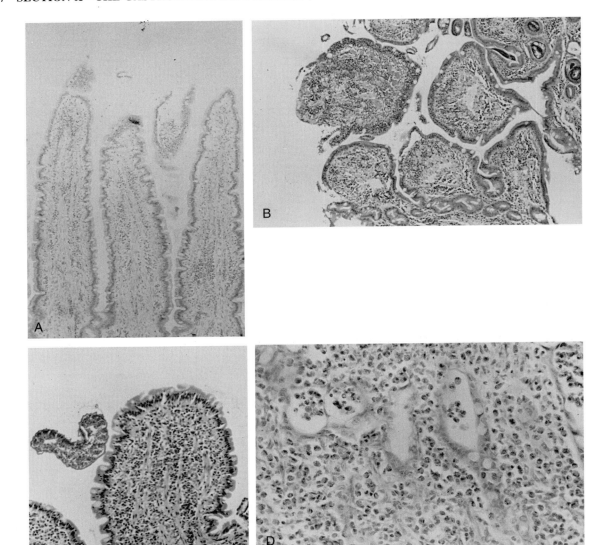

Figure 137–27. Histological appearance. *A,* Normal jejunum showing long slender villi and minimal numbers of cells in the lamina propria. *B,* Idiopathic lympho-plasmacytic enteritis in a dachshund showing stunted villi and a lympho-plasmacytic infiltrate. *C,* Lympho-plasmacytic intestinal inflammation associated with a *Strongyloides* infection. A worm is actually visible in the section on the mucosal surface. *D,* Eosinophilic enteritis in a German shepherd dog showing a massive infiltration of the crypt area with eosinophils. (Courtesy of G. R. Pearson.)

ing immune defect that causes intestinal inflammation but that luminal antigens may exacerbate the problem.

Diagnosis

Intestinal biopsy is necessary for a definitive diagnosis of IBD, but the clinical signs and physical findings are often suggestive (see Table 137–33). Palpably thickened bowel loops are sometimes noted but intestinal inflammation must be confirmed by biopsy. Endoscopy is the easiest method of biopsy but has limitations, particularly the inaccessibility of the jejunum (and ileum). In some cases, exploratory laparot-

omy and full-thickness biopsy are preferred. Before intestinal biopsy is undertaken, laboratory tests and imaging examinations should be performed. They do not confirm a diagnosis of idiopathic IBD, but they should rule out anatomic intestinal disease (e.g., tumor, intussusception), extraintestinal disease (e.g., pancreatitis), and known causes of intestinal inflammation.

Hematology. A neutrophilia and occasionally a mild left shift in LPE are seen. Eosinophilia is not diagnostic of EGE and is not invariably present. Anemia may reflect chronic inflammation or chronic blood loss.

Serum Biochemistry. There are no pathognomonic

TABLE 137–33. CLINICAL SIGNS ASSOCIATED WITH INFLAMMATORY BOWEL DISEASE

Vomiting bile ± hair in cats and grass in dogs
Hematemesis
Small intestinal–type diarrhea
    Large volume
    Watery
    Melena
Thickened bowel loops
Large intestinal–type diarrhea
    Hematochezia
    Mucoid stool
    Frequency and tenesmus
Abdominal discomfort or pain
Excessive borborygmi and flatus
Weight loss
Altered appetite
    Polyphagia
    Decreased appetite or anorexia
    Eating grass
Hypoproteinemia or ascites

changes in IBD, but diseases of other organ systems can be recognized. Hypoalbuminemia and hypoglobulinemia are characteristic of PLE, and hypocholesterolemia is suggestive of malabsorption. Mild elevations in liver marker enzymes (alanine aminotransferase, alkaline phosphatase) may reflect secondary liver reaction to intestinal inflammation and are of no consequence. However, in cats there is a recognized association between IBD, chronic pancreatitis, and lymphocytic cholangitis.

Fecal Examination. Ideally, three consecutive samples should be checked for hookworms, whipworms, and *Giardia*. In reality, it is usually easier to treat empirically with fenbendazole. The isolation of *Salmonella* or *Campylobacter* may be significant.

Folate and Cobalamin. Proximal inflammation may cause folate malabsorption, whereas distal inflammation may lower serum cbl. Although they are not reliable indicators, severe reductions of folate and cbl usually correlate with severe, diffuse intestinal inflammation.

Imaging. Plain radiographs are used to look for anatomic abnormalities. Contrast studies rarely add further information in IBD unless there is severe mucosal disease. Ultrasound examination permits evaluation of the thickness of any mucosal infiltrate and mesenteric lymphadenopathy. Guided fine-needle aspiration can be attempted.

Treatment

Dietary Modification. Intestinal inflammation is sometimes actually a manifestation of a dietary sensitivity, and in view of the side effects of immunosuppression, an exclusion diet trial is probably indicated in mild cases of apparent IBD before administration of corticosteroids. "Hypoallergenic" diets limit the antigenic load to the intestine. A hydrolyzed soya diet theoretically should limit the antigenicity further, but rice is the preferred carbohydrate source because of its high digestibility. Potato, corn starch, and tapioca are also gluten free. Fat restriction is useful in reducing clinical signs as fat malabsorption may be present. Modification of the n-3/n-6 fatty acid ratio may also modulate the inflammatory response. Supplementation with oral folate and parenteral cbl is indicated if serum concentrations are subnormal.

Antibacterials. Mucosal damage in IBD can affect an animal's ability to control its intestinal flora and secondary SIBO has been reported.[33] Antibiotics are not often needed

in IBD despite immunosuppressive therapy. However, treatment with antibiotics may reduce inflammation, whereas steroids may actually make the signs worse. Metronidazole is often used in mild to moderate IBD, especially in cats, although it is not clear whether its antibacterial activity or its effect on cell-mediated immunity is beneficial.

Immunosuppressive Drugs. The mainstay of treatment of idiopathic IBD is immunosuppression.

Glucocorticoids are generally used for immunosuppression. Prednisolone is the drug of first choice; dexamethasone has some deleterious effects on enterocytes. In severe IBD, parenteral prednisolone can given initially. A dosage of 2 to 4 mg/kg by mouth divided twice a day is given for 2 to 4 weeks and then tapered slowly over weeks to months until it is completely withdrawn or at least reduced to an alternate-day schedule. Cushingoid side effects are common but transient as the dosage is reduced. If, however, dosages cannot be reduced without relapse, alternative drugs are required in the long term. Oral administration may be difficult in cats and depot preparations of methylprednisolone acetate (10 mg/kg subcutaneously every 2 to 4 weeks initially) may be an effective alternative.

Azathioprine (2 mg/kg in dogs and 0.3 mg/kg in cats by mouth once a day) has good steroid-sparing properties, and maintenance with alternate-day steroids is often successful. Azathioprine is potentially myelosuppressive, especially in cats, and regular monitoring of the hemogram is prudent. Cyclophosphamide and cyclosporine are potent immunosuppressives but are rarely used in IBD.

Anti-Inflammatories. Derivatives of 5-aminosalicylic acid (e.g., sulfasalazine, olsalazine, mesalazine) are anti-inflammatory and are reserved for local control of colonic inflammation. Their absorption from the SI is potentially nephrotoxic. Experimentally, human Crohn's disease has been controlled with anti–TNF-α antibody.[60] Oxpentifylline (pentoxifylline) is a phosphodiesterase inhibitor of TNF-α transcription and has in vitro activity in inflamed intestine. Its efficacy in IBD in vivo has yet to be proved.[111]

LYMPHOCYTIC-PLASMACYTIC ENTERITIS

The most common form of idiopathic intestinal inflammation, LPE is characterized by the predominant cell type found in the mucosal infiltrate, namely lymphocytes and plasma cells (see Fig. 137–27B).[109, 110] There are many other causes of lymphocytic-plasmacytic infiltration in the SI (see Table 137–32 and Fig. 137–27C). In particular, associations with enteric parasites, bacteria in dogs and *Toxoplasma* in cats, have been noted.

Etiology and Pathogenesis

Idiopathic LPE is believed to reflect an abnormal MALT response to luminal bacterial, dietary, or self-antigens. There is a spectrum from mild inflammation to severe infiltration, sometimes called immunoproliferative disease, as reported in basenjis.[112] Complete or partial villous atrophy may or may not be present, and villous fusion and crypt abscessation may be noted in severe cases.[70] The distinction between severe LPE and alimentary lymphoma is sometimes difficult. Comparisons of endoscopic biopsies and postmortem examinations of the same patient revealed frequent disparities in the histologic diagnosis.[84] However, it is possible to have both conditions present in adjacent areas of gut and some consider there to be a spectrum ranging from mild inflammation through severe to immunoproliferative changes and ultimately lymphoma.

Attempts have been made to establish histologic criteria by which the severity of LPE can be graded.[110] However, there is not a good correlation between severity of histologic changes and clinical signs; interpretation of the degree of inflammation is quite subjective, and there are often discrepancies between observations by the endoscopist and the histologist.[69] Changes may be patchy and proximal endoscopic biopsies may not be representative. The inflammation may not even be uniform within the lamina propria, with perhaps just villi or crypts affected, and if hypoproteinemia and edema are present it may be difficult to assess the true cell density. Immunohistochemistry has suggested an increase in IgA-containing cells relative to T cells, but T-cell subset phenotypes were not assessed.[113]

Clinical Signs

The signs of LPE do not particularly distinguish it from other histologic forms of IBD. Weight loss and SI diarrhea are typical, and severe cases may manifest as PLE. Frequently in cats and sometimes in dogs, cycles of chronic vomiting are the predominant sign. Thus, diagnosis depends on biopsy-proven lymphocytic-plasmacytic intestinal inflammation in the absence of an underlying cause. Severe LPE (immunoproliferative disease), which often causes PLE, is recognized in basenjis, and there is a clinical impression that LPE is prevalent in German shepherd dogs, Shar Peis, pure-bred cats, and soft-coated wheaten terriers. LPE typically affects older animals, but affected kittens 16 weeks of age and puppies 20 weeks of age have been reported.

Diagnosis

The approach to diagnosing LPE is the same as that for any chronic diarrhea case (see Fig. 137–18), although definitive diagnosis ultimately depends on biopsy after ruling out known causes of intestinal inflammation.

Treatment and Prognosis

The treatment of LPE is that already outlined for idiopathic IBD.

BASENJI ENTEROPATHY

A severe hereditary form of LPE has been well characterized in basenjis.[112] The disease may have a hereditary basis, although the mode of inheritance is unclear. It has been likened to immunoproliferative small intestinal disease (IPSID) of humans as both involve intense intestinal inflammation. However, IPSID is characterized by an associated gammopathy (alpha heavy-chain disease). Affected basenjis often have hyperglobulinemia but not alpha heavy-chain disease, but they may be predisposed to lymphoma.[114] The intestinal lesions in basenjis are characterized by an increase in CD4$^+$ and CD8$^+$ T cells.

Clinical Signs

Signs are of chronic intractable diarrhea and emaciation. Concurrent involvement of the stomach is often seen, with a lymphocytic-plasmacytic gastritis, hypergastrinemia, and mucosal hyperplasia. The enteropathy is frequently a PLE

with attendant hypoalbuminemia, but edema and ascites are not common, presumably because of the osmotic effect of the hyperglobulinemia. Signs are usually progressive and intestinal perforation may occur.

Treatment

Treatment is generally unsuccessful, and dogs die within months of diagnosis, but aggressive combination treatment with prednisolone, antibiotics, and dietary modification may achieve remission if started early.

CANINE SPRUE

This is a severe enteropathy in dogs that resembles tropical sprue of humans, a severe malabsorption associated with villous atrophy seen in tropical countries.[115] In humans the condition is oxytetracycline responsive and has been considered to be a chronic form of SIBO. The condition in dogs has been reported mainly in German shepherd dogs but it does not respond to conventional antibiotic treatment, although it might still be the long-term result of prolonged SIBO. Sprue has not been well characterized histologically; the presence of villous atrophy and a variable inflammatory infiltrate suggests that this is best considered a form of LPE. However, treatment with immunosuppressive agents usually fails. Signs of intractable diarrhea, weight loss, and general deterioration are noted and the prognosis is very poor.

EOSINOPHILIC ENTERITIS

Eosinophilic enteritis is the second most common form of idiopathic IBD and frequently involves the stomach and/or colon in EGE and/or colitis.[116] It is characterized by a mixed mucosal inflammatory infiltrate in which eosinophils predominate (see Fig. 137–27D). Some eosinophils may be a minor component of the infiltrate in LPE but they are the predominant cell in EGE. The degree of infiltration may vary from mild to severe and variable villus atrophy is present. The condition is seen in dogs of any breed and age, although there is perhaps a tendency to younger animals. It is quite common in Boxers, Dobermans, and German shepherd dogs.

Clinical Signs

The signs in EGE tend to depend on the area of GI tract involved: vomiting, SI diarrhea, and LI diarrhea may all be seen in various combinations. Segmental eosinophilic enteritis has been reported. There is a tendency for any eosinophilic infiltrate to be associated with mucosal erosion or ulceration. Hematemesis, or melena, and/or hematochezia may be seen. Severe EGE has been associated with PLE and hypoproteinemia and, rarely, perforation.

Pathogenesis

An eosinophilic mucosal infiltrate may be indicative of a diet-induced, type I hypersensitivity, although most dogs with EGE do not respond simply to an exclusion diet. A response to parasites may be the cause, and empirical treatment with fenbendazole is appropriate. However, most veterinary cases are probably truly idiopathic, reflecting immune dysregulation. In cats, EGE may be one manifestation of the hypereosinophilic syndrome and may also be associated with mast cell tumors.

Diagnosis

The diagnosis of EGE is made by biopsy after exclusion of parasites, food allergy, and so forth. Eosinophilia is not invariably present, and even when present it does not prove the presence of EGE. Eosinophilia is also a marker for parasitism, hypoadrenocorticism, allergic cutaneous or respiratory disease, and mast cell tumor.

Treatment

Treatment of EGE is with hypoallergenic diets and immunosuppression. The prognosis is guarded, even with a good initial response to treatment, as recurrence is common.

GRANULOMATOUS ENTERITIS

This rare form of IBD is characterized by mucosal infiltration with macrophages forming granulomas.[117] The distribution of inflammation can be patchy, and this condition is probably the same as "regional enteritis," in which ileal granulomas have been reported. Histologically it can resemble human Crohn's disease, but obstructive granulomas, abscessation, and fistula formation are not noted in dogs. Conventional IBD therapy does not appear to be effective in this condition and the prognosis is guarded. In cats, a pyogranulomatous transmural inflammation has been associated with FIPV infection.

LYMPHANGIECTASIA

Definition and Cause

Intestinal lymphangiectasia is characterized by marked dilatation and dysfunction of intestinal lymphatics. Abnormal lymphatics leak protein-rich lymph into the intestinal lumen, and the condition is an example of PLE, with hypoproteinemia being a common sequel. Lymphangiectasia may be a primary disorder or secondary to lymphatic obstruction.[118]

Primary lymphangiectasia is usually limited to the intestine, although it may be part of a more widespread lymphatic abnormality. Concurrent lymphatic abnormalities, such as chylothorax, lend support to that argument. It may be a congenital abnormality, but signs are not usually present from birth. However, the development of associated lipogranulomatous lymphangitis superimposed on congenital abnormalities might lead to progressive disease. Alternatively, it may be an idiopathic acquired disease. The disease is most commonly seen in small terrier breeds (e.g., Yorkshire, Maltese) and the Norwegian Lundehund (Fig. 137–28), suggesting some genetic predisposition.

Secondary lymphangiectasia is caused by intestinal lymphatic obstruction and can be produced experimentally by obstruction of all mesenteric lymphatics but, surprisingly, not by obstruction of the thoracic duct. It may be seen with (1) infiltration or obstruction of lymphatics by an inflammatory, fibrosing, or neoplastic process; (2) perhaps obstruction of the thoracic duct; and (3) right-sided heart failure resulting from congestive heart failure or cardiac tamponade from pericardial effusion or restrictive pericarditis. Lipogranulo-

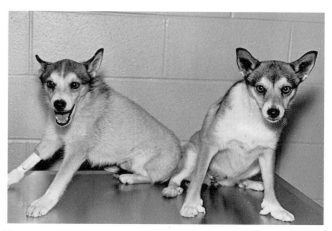

Figure 137–28. A normal Lundehund (left) and one affected with lymphangiectasia, showing abdominal distention because of hypoproteinemic ascites. (Courtesy of D. A. Williams.)

matous lymphangitis is sometimes reported in association with lymphangiectasia, but it is not clear which is the primary event; lymphangitis could cause lymphatic obstruction or leakage of lymph could cause granuloma formation.

History and Clinical Signs

The clinical manifestations of lymphangiectasia are largely attributable to the effects of the enteric loss of lymph. Other intestinal functions remain largely intact, and hypoproteinemia in the absence of diarrhea may occur. More typically, diarrhea, steatorrhea, profound weight loss, and an increased appetite are present. However, the signs are often insidious in onset and may fluctuate, with chronic intermittent diarrhea. Vomiting, lethargy, and anorexia are reported occasionally. Ascites and/or edema may be the result of hypoproteinemia and is usually seen when the serum albumin concentration approaches 10 g/L. The ascitic fluid is likely to be a pure transudate. However, if right-sided heart failure causes secondary lymphangiectasia, a modified transudate develops because of portal hypertension. Lymphangiectasia has been associated with a granulomatous hepatopathy and in Lundehunds with chronic gastritis and gastric carcinoma.[119, 120]

Diagnosis

Clinical signs of PLE, panhypoproteinemia, hypocholesterolemia, and lymphopenia are characteristic of lymphangiectasia. Hypocalcemia, when present, is probably due to hypoalbuminemia and perhaps vitamin D and calcium malabsorption. Indirect markers of enterocyte dysfunction such as xylose absorption, folate, and cbl are likely to be normal. Intestinal protein loss can be documented by measuring leakage of chromium 51-labeled albumin or fecal excretion of alpha$_1$-protease inhibitor. Endoscopically, the tips of the villi may appear distended with chyle, characterized by the presence of white lipid droplets, and prominent mucosal blebs. Endoscopic biopsies may be supportive of the diagnosis, but full-thickness biopsies may be needed for definitive diagnosis. The problem is that true lymphangiectasia (Fig. 137–29A) must be distinguished from normal postprandial dilatation of lacteals and from secondary dilatation of lacteals sometimes noted in IBD (Fig. 137–29B). The true disease is probably rare. Failure to recognize IBD may explain the

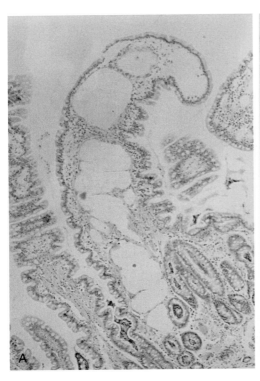 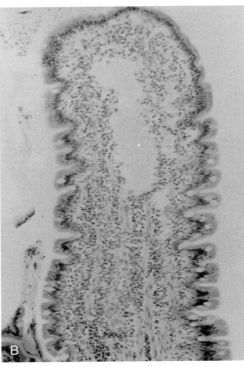

Figure 137–29. Histologic appearance of jejunal biopsy specimens. *A,* From a Jack Russell terrier with a protein-losing enteropathy. Markedly dilated lacteals consistent with a diagnosis of lymphangiectasia are present. *B,* From a retriever with moderate lympho-plasmacytic enteritis and mild secondary ectasia of lacteals.

success of steroid treatment in some cases. Assessment of the degree of inflammatory cell infiltrate in the lamina propria is subjective, and if there is edema, the density of cells may be underestimated. For a definitive diagnosis, ballooning dilatation of lymphatics must be evident not only in the mucosa but also in the submucosa, and full-thickness intestinal biopsies are needed.

At laparotomy, a prominent web of dilated lymphatics may be obvious in the mesentery and on the serosal surface of the gut. Mesenteric lymph nodes may be enlarged, but frequently yellow-white nodular masses 1 to 3 mm diameter are observed in and around the mesenteric and serosal lymphatics. These spots are lipogranulomas consisting of accumulations of lipid-laden macrophages. They may be the result of extravasation of chyle into perilymphatic tissue or be associated with a lymphangitis.

Treatment

Secondary lymphangiectasia is managed by specific treatment of underlying disease such as pericardiocentesis or pericardectomy for cardiac tamponade. The goal in treating primary lymphangiectasia is to decrease enteric loss of plasma protein, stop intestinal or lymphatic inflammation, and control edema or effusions. Dietary manipulation and corticosteroids are the mainstays of treatment.

A severely fat-restricted diet would theoretically be ideal. The diet should be calorie dense and highly digestible; a weight reduction diet, although low in fat, is unsuitable. Some fat can be given in the form of MCTs, which are absorbed directly into the portal blood. Supplementation with fat-soluble vitamins is advised, and there are anecdotal reports of improvement with glutamine supplementation. Glucocorticoid therapy (prednisolone, 1 to 2 mg/kg by mouth divided daily) to exert an anti-inflammatory and immunosuppressive effect may be beneficial, especially if there are associated lymphangitis, lipogranulomas, and a lympho-

plasmacytic infiltrate in the lamina propria. Antibiotics such as tylosin or metronidazole have been tried with no obvious success. Diuretics are used in the management of effusions. The response to treatment is unpredictable but cessation of clinical signs may be achieved temporarily, with remissions of months to several years. However, the long-term prognosis is poor.

DIETARY SENSITIVITY

A repeatable adverse or unpleasant reaction to food can be a manifestation of either an immunologic reaction to a dietary antigen (i.e., a true food allergy) or a nonimmunologic reaction (i.e., an intolerance). Although both mechanisms may produce similar clinical signs and can be treated by exclusion of the offending food, the distinction is not just semantic. Food intolerances may be associated with just one ingredient of a prepared food (e.g., lactose, preservative) that may be present in immunologically unrelated foods. Similarly, confirmed allergy to a specific food may impart allergy to related foods. In humans, food intolerance is numerically more important than allergy, but its true prevalence in small animals is unknown.

FOOD ALLERGY

Food allergy is rare; other causes of GI and/or dematologic signs are more common and some may also respond (for nonallergic reasons) to dietary manipulation (Table 137–34). The management of food allergy is simple; feed any food that does not contain the allergen and the animal is normal. The difficulty for the clinician lies in the recognition of food allergy and the identification of foods that must be excluded.

TABLE 137–34. CONDITIONS THAT MAY IMPROVE CLINICALLY IN RESPONSE TO DIETARY MODIFICATION

Food allergy	Pancreatitis
Food intolerance	Chronic gastritis
Small intestinal bacterial overgrowth	Gastroesophageal reflux
Inflammatory bowel disease	Gastric emptying disorders
Lymphangiectasia	Portosystemic shunt
Exocrine pancreatic insufficiency	

Mechanisms

A food allergy is a repeatable immunologically mediated adverse reaction to a dietary component. Current hypotheses about food allergy propose one or a combination of mechanisms leading to breakdown of oral tolerance: an inadequate mucosal barrier, abnormal presentation of dietary antigens to the MALT, or dysregulation of the MALT (see earlier). Such hypotheses could explain both genetic susceptibility to the development of allergy and development of allergies after a primary GI insult.

Clinical Signs

A temporal association between ingestion of a particular food and signs is suggestive of an immediate (type I), IgE-mediated hypersensitivity, but acquired sensitivities to foods that have been in the normal diet for years also occur, and mixed or delayed reactions are probably more common. Then the inevitable delay between food ingestion and onset of signs obscures any causative link, particularly if repeated ingestion causes chronic disease.

Clinical signs of food allergy generally involve the skin and GI tract (Table 137–35). Most case studies have focused on the dermatologic signs, with few reports of food allergic GI disease.[121] Systemic signs (anorexia, lethargy) are poorly recorded, and urticaria-angioedema and even anaphylaxis seem rare. Concurrent skin and GI signs probably occur but have been reported rarely.

Food Allergic Skin Disease. The major sign is pruritus; most other signs are the result of self-trauma. The pruritus is nonseasonal and has no characteristic distribution, although pedal pruritus, facial pruritus, and otitis externa may be noted. Excoriation, crusting, scaling, and lichenification arise as self-traumatic lesions and may predispose to secondary pyoderma. In cats, food allergy is sometimes the cause of miliary dermatitis, eosinophilic granuloma complex, and symmetric alopecia.

TABLE 137–35. CLINICAL SIGNS RECOGNIZED AS MANIFESTATIONS OF FOOD ALLERGY

Systemic signs	Gastrointestinal signs
Anorexia	Vomiting
Lethargy	Hematemesis
Peripheral lymphadenopathy (cats)	Diarrhea
Urticaria-angioedema	Small intestinal–like
Anaphylaxis	Colitis-like
Cutaneous signs	Abdominal pain, "colic"
Primary papules	Weight loss and/or stunting
Erythroderma	Altered appetite
Pruritus and self-trauma	
Secondary pyoderma	
Scaling	
Otitis externa	
Miliary dermatitis (cats)	
Eosinophilic granuloma complex (cats)	

Food Allergic Gastrointestinal Disease. Signs are not pathognomonic and include vomiting, diarrhea, abdominal pain, and weight loss or failure to thrive.

Diagnosis

The cornerstone of the diagnosis of a food allergy is the response to dietary manipulation: remission with exclusion of a specific dietary component and relapse when challenged with that particular food must be proved. Unfortunately, there is frequently a lack of objective criteria by which to judge the response, (see Table 137–34).

Indirect Tests. The difficulties of diet trials have led to attempts to devise indirect tests for food allergy. None have been shown to be reliable in veterinary medicine. *Low serum folate* appears to be a poor marker of food allergy and *antigen-specific serum antibodies* measured in vitro are of little relevance. *Skin testing* has proved unreliable in the diagnosis of food allergic skin disease. *Food-specific IgE* can be measured by radioallergosorbent (RAST) and ELISA assays but results have been disappointing. *Gastroscopic food sensitivity testing* (GFST), in which dietary antigens are instilled directly onto the gastric mucosa in an anesthetized patient, is likely to give more specific results. However, only 50 per cent correlation was noted between the results of GFST and results of clinical challenge trials.[122] The method is tedious, technically demanding, prone to artifact, and detects only immediate hypersensitivities. Using the colonic mucosa as the testing surface may be easier in the future.[123, 124]

Diet Trial. This remains the only certain method of confirming food allergy. Objectivity in assessing the response to diet change can be enhanced by noting changes in intestinal permeability or repeated biopsy. No pathognomonic histologic changes are recognized on skin or gut biopsy (Table 137–36).

Diet Trials

Preliminary Investigations. After evaluation of a minimum database, specific investigations of the skin and GI tract should be performed. Ectoparasites and skin infections as causes of pruritus should be diagnosed and treated before considering a food trial. After three fecal examinations or empirical fenbendazole treatment and perhaps empirical antibiotics for idiopathic SIBO, intestinal biopsy should be performed to look for intestinal inflammation. However, many of the histologic changes seen in idiopathic IBD can also be seen with food allergies (see Table 137–36).

Exclusion. The principle of an exclusion (elimination) diet is to feed a diet comprising food not found in the patient's staple diet. This must be the only thing fed until it is certain that remission has or has not been achieved. Complete owner compliance is essential, and any treats and even vitamin supplements must be withheld. An *exclusion*

TABLE 137–36. HISTOLOGIC CHANGES IN GASTROINTESTINAL BIOPSIES THAT ARE SOMETIMES SUSPECTED OF BEING MANIFESTATIONS OF FOOD ALLERGY BUT ARE ALSO SEEN IN OTHER GASTROINTESTINAL DISEASES

Intraepithelial lymphocyte infiltration	Lympho-plasmacytic gastritis
Villus atrophy, partial or subtotal	Lympho-plasmacytic enteritis
Decreased enterocyte height	Eosinophilic gastroenteritis

diet is composed of single protein and carbohydrate sources. Because the exclusion diet is fed for a short time period, it need not be nutritionally balanced. Lamb or chicken and rice have been the standard choices for years. However, the increased diversity of commercial pet foods has led to the need to use more esoteric food sources. Commercial exclusion diets containing chicken, soya, fish, catfish, venison, and duck with rice, corn (maize), tapioca, or potato are all marketed.

Hypoallergenic diets are marketed for food allergies as well as IBD. They are highly digestible, so the antigenic load is rapidly lowered during digestion, and some also have a restricted fat content. Although some are true exclusion diets (i.e., single protein source) and can be used for an exclusion trial, some do not have a restricted antigen source and are not suitable.

Palatability can be a problem during food trials. Although most dogs eat chicken or fish, cats are more fastidious. Lamb and rice baby foods have been recommended, although they are not nutritionally complete for cats. Home-cooked diets have been preferred to commercial diets because of reports of relapse when patients are switched to a commercial equivalent of the diet. However, such instances seem rare and the theoretic advantages may be outweighed by the increased owner compliance seen with commercial diets.

Challenge. When remission is achieved, challenge with the original diet should be performed to confirm the diagnosis. Some clients refuse, particularly if relapse is likely to bring diarrhea, and lifelong maintenance with the exclusion diet is acceptable provided the diet is nutritionally balanced. However, it is preferable, through a series of provocation tests, to identify the offending food(s) so that, ultimately, a safe but regular diet can be fed. Some animals may not have relapses either because of misdiagnosis or because restoration of the mucosal barrier prevents further antigen access and/or there is waning of hypersensitivity.

Rescue and Provocation. After relapse with challenge, remission is regained by "rescue" with the exclusion diet. Single foodstuffs are then introduced sequentially as provocation tests. If there is no relapse, the food is identified as "safe" and the next food tested; if there is a relapse, rescue is repeated and the food identified as "unsafe."

Maintenance. When all the offending foods have been identified or at least sufficient safe ones are recognized to permit the choice of a normal diet, the animal should be maintained with a safe commercial version.

Protocol. A standardized protocol for food trials has not been established. The optimal duration for an exclusion diet trial is unknown, and 3 weeks has been chosen arbitrarily. Challenge trials and provocation tests are usually conducted for up to 14 days. They are halted earlier if signs recur on two consecutive days.

Treatment

A number of gluten-free proprietary diets based on lamb, fish, or chicken are often suitable as maintenance diets, and they are preferred to home cooking as they are nutritionally balanced. Assuming a correct diagnosis, dietary management should be all that is required. Treatment failure should lead to reevaluation of the diagnosis.

GLUTEN-SENSITIVE ENTEROPATHY

SI disease induced by the presence of wheat gluten in food has been clearly documented in Irish setter dogs.[13] The disease is familial with an association with MHC genes *DQA* and *DQB*.[125] Gluten-sensitive enteropathy probably affects other breeds of dogs, but it has not yet been reported in cats. Gluten sensitivity has been demonstrated in soft-coated wheaten terriers with PLE and/or nephropathy, but there is probably an underlying immunologic disease because gluten restriction does not necessarily resolve clinical signs.[126]

Pathogenesis

It is presumed that the wheat protein gluten or one of its digestion products is either directly toxic to the intestinal mucosa or induces an immune reaction. In humans, binding of gluten peptides to an enzyme, tissue transglutaminase, and induction of autoantibodies has been proposed, but the exact mechanism remains controversial.[127] Altered $CD4^+$ and $CD8^+$ T-cell populations have been shown in affected setters, but serum antibody responses to gluten and endomysial antigens, which are markers for human celiac disease, have not been demonstrated.

Remission and relapse of signs and histologic and biochemical changes have been demonstrated in Irish setters on feeding both wheat flour and crude gluten extract. An amount of gluten equivalent to eating a thick slice of wholemeal bread a day was sufficient to induce changes. An abnormal 90-kilodalton serum protein is found in affected setters, although its nature and significance are unclear.[128] The age of introduction of gluten and the dose may modulate the expression of the disease. Similarly, introduction of gluten to littermates of affected dogs that had been reared with a cereal-free diet for a year reduced the severity of changes observed with gluten challenge. Irish setters fed large doses of gluten from weaning developed more severe and more rapid changes initially but appeared ultimately to develop tolerance.[129] This is consistent with the previously discussed concept of oral tolerance and the influence of dose and timing of antigen presentation affecting Th1-Th2 balance.

Clinical Signs

Affected Irish setters typically have poor weight gain and chronic intermittent diarrhea in the months after weaning. Serum folate is variably reduced but cbl is normal and SIBO is not present on duodenal juice culture. Histologic changes in jejunal biopsies show partial villous atrophy and intraepithelial lymphocyte infiltration, with a variable lamina propria infiltrate. Superficially, the histology appears typical of idiopathic IBD, but the changes have been shown to resolve when dogs are fed a gluten-free diet and relapse with wheat and gluten challenge.[13] Electron microscopic studies show significant MVM damage.[129]

Treatment

Clinical signs in affected setters usually diminish as they become mature, but successful treatment depends on exclusion of gluten from the diet. There is confusion over what constitutes a gluten-free diet. The gliadin proteins in wheat gluten are a group of related proteins rich in prolamine. All have the potential to elicit mucosal damage in gluten sensitivity in humans. Other cereals contain similar proteins that are often collectively termed gluten, but only the proteins in rye (secalins), barley (hordeins), and oats (avenins) are immunologically similar to gliadins. Thus, gluten sensitivity in humans usually encompasses sensitivity to wheat, rye, and barley. From an antigenic viewpoint, rice and corn (maize) are gluten free.

FOOD INTOLERANCE

Polyphagia, scavenging, and food poisoning are seen quite commonly and may be considered examples of food intolerance. However, all of these tend to be isolated incidents and are not repeatable. True intolerances are repeatable. Responses may be predictable because unsafe food is eaten accidentally, food contaminants affect any animals that eat normal quantities of the food, or foods are eaten in excessive quantities. Alternatively, responses may be unpredictable (although repeatable in a susceptible individual) because of idiosyncratic reactions. Reasons for idiosyncrasies include differences that may be under genetic control such as intestinal enzyme activities, intestinal permeability, postabsorption metabolism, and mast cell stability, as well as differences in the intestinal flora.

Mechanisms

Most nonimmunologic mechanisms in intolerances are complex, have not been demonstrated in dogs or cats, and have been adopted by extrapolation from humans.

Food Poisoning. This is an effect of a toxin present in a food or released by contaminating organisms.

Pharmacologic Intolerances. These are caused by active compounds in food. For example, chocolate poisoning caused by excessive intake of methyxanthines is well recognized in dogs.

Pseudoallergic Mechanisms. These imply histamine-mediated adverse reactions, including anaphylaxis, produced by nonimmunologic mechanisms. A high histamine content naturally present in some foods (e.g., in tuna and mackerel) or present because of histamine-producing bacteria (e.g., cheese or canned fish contaminated by *Proteus* or *Klebsiella*) can produce signs. Alternatively, some foods (e.g., shellfish, strawberries) and food additives (e.g., tartrazine) can cause histamine release from mast cells without IgE mediation.

Clinical Signs

The clinical signs expected in food intolerance are generally related to the GI tract: vomiting, diarrhea, and abdominal discomfort. Pruritus and even anaphylaxis are possible if histamine release is involved.

Diagnosis

The only reliable means of diagnosing food intolerance is by monitoring the response to withholding the suspected food and relapse with rechallenge. Such studies are rare in veterinary medicine.

Treatment

Treatment is simple when a diagnosis has been made. Avoidance of the offending food prevents the occurrence of signs.

SURGICAL DISEASE

INTESTINAL OBSTRUCTION

Intestinal obstruction can be classified as acute or chronic, partial or complete, and simple or strangulated. Obstruction is caused by extraluminal compression, intramural thickening, or an intraluminal mass. The most common extraluminal cause of obstruction is intussusception. Intestinal neoplasia is the most common intramural cause, with hematomas, focal FIP granulomas, IBD, stricture, and phycomycosis less common. Foreign objects such as peach stones, toys, and fishhooks are common causes of intraluminal obstruction in dogs, whereas linear string and thread (which are frequently anchored under the tongue) are more common in cats. Adverse effects of intestinal obstruction are a consequence of fluid losses into the intestine, proliferation of intestinal bacteria, and inflammation of the intestine. Intestinal perforation may ultimately occur, especially with linear foreign objects and intestinal neoplasia.

Clinical Findings

Younger animals are more likely to develop intussusception, particularly after gastroenteritis or intestinal surgery. Intestinal neoplasia is more frequent in middle-aged and older animals.

Vomiting might be expected to be a major feature of intestinal obstruction. However, complete obstruction in dogs is frequently not associated with vomiting. Clinical signs are more often related to marked loss of fluid and electrolytes into the intestine. With complete obstruction of the ileum there is a gradual increase in the secretion of sodium, potassium, and water into the obstructed bowel. Overgrowth of bacteria and endotoxin production proximal to the obstruction may exacerbate fluid losses and precipitate potentially fatal septicemia or endotoxemia. Partial obstruction, particularly of the distal small bowel, can be associated with chronic diarrhea and weight loss (caused by intestinal stasis) and may initially respond to antibiotics.

Physical findings are variable and depend on the severity of fluid losses, fluid shifts, and intestinal compromise caused by obstruction. Findings range from mild dehydration to those of septic shock. Shock and abdominal pain are the major findings with strangulated obstructions such as intestinal volvulus, incarcerated obstructions, and intussuception. A thorough oral examination should not be neglected, particularly in cats, in which linear foreign objects may be anchored under the tongue.[130] Localized discomfort may be evident with foreign objects, intussusceptions, and tumors, and palpation may be resented or impossible if intestinal inflammation or perforation is present. Focal increases in intestinal thickness suggest tumors, intussusceptions, or foreign objects, and a sausage-shaped mass is suggestive of an intussusception. Plication of intestinal loops occurs with linear foreign bodies. Mesenteric lymphadenopathy is often present in animals with inflammatory and neoplastic intestinal disease.

Diagnosis

Intestinal obstruction should be considered in the differential diagnosis of dogs and cats with acute vomiting, chronic diarrhea, weight loss, failure to thrive, or an acute abdomen. A minimum database and clinicopathologic tests help to characterize the fluid losses and inflammation. Hypochloremia and hypokalemia are common in pets with intestinal obstruction. Metabolic alkalosis with or without aciduria may occur with upper duodenal obstruction.

Animals with palpable abnormalities or signs of dehydration or shock should undergo immediate radiographic and/or ultrasonographic examination. Radiographic features of obstruction are obvious foreign bodies, variation in intestinal diameter related to the accumulation of fluid or gas, and accumulation of ingested food (gravel sign). Displacement, bunching, or plication of the intestine may also be evident. Decreased serosal detail and free abdominal gas indicate peritonitis and intestinal perforation, respectively. Survey radiographs are often unremarkable in chronic partial obstruction and ileocecocolic intussusception. Contrast radiography is useful in detecting complete or partial obstruction. Ultrasonography is valuable for detecting nonpalpable causes of obstruction and ascertaining the appearance of palpable lesions and other organ involvement.[131] Ultrasound-guided needle aspiration enables investigation of masses.

Treatment

Mechanical obstruction by foreign objects, intussusception, or intramural masses is usually treated surgically. Fluid therapy should be initiated on the basis of clinical findings and a minimum database. Fluid shifts can be severe, and aggressive monitoring of central venous blood pressure, PCV, total protein, urine output, and acid-base and electrolyte status is often necessary to detect and correct abnormalities. Fluid balance and electrolyte abnormalities should be corrected as much as possible before surgery. Broad-spectrum antibiotics effective against gram-negative and gram-positive aerobic and anaerobic bacteria should be administered to pets with signs of sepsis of intestinal compromise and can be administered prophylactically before surgery.

Prognosis

The prognosis depends on the cause of obstruction and the severity of associated abnormalities. It ranges from good for simple foreign bodies to grave for metastatic intestinal neoplasia.

ADYNAMIC ILEUS AND INTESTINAL PSEUDO-OBSTRUCTION

Adynamic ileus is a common sequela of parvoviral enteritis, abdominal surgery, pancreatitis, peritonitis, endotoxemia, and hypokalemia.[132] It is also a feature of dysautonomia: feline dysautonomia is seen most commonly in the United Kingdom but is rare in dogs. Intestinal pseudo-obstruction is a term used when there is clinical evidence of an obstruction without evidence of physical obstruction. It has been most frequently associated with idiopathic sclerosing enteropathy in the dog. Management of adynamic ileus and intestinal pseudo-obstruction is initially aimed at distinguishing them from mechanical obstruction and then identifying and treating the underlying cause. Prokinetic agents such as the 5-hydroxytryptamine type 4 receptor agonist cisapride, the D_2 dopaminergic antagonist metoclopramide and motilin-like drugs such as erythromycin can be used to stimulate intestinal motility.[133] In dogs and cats cisapride appears likely to be the most effective agent, but clinical trials are required to determine the comparative efficacy of various prokinetics.

INTESTINAL NEOPLASIA

Lymphosarcoma (LSA), adenocarcinoma, and mast cell tumor are the most common GI tumors in cats, whereas adenocarcinoma and leiomyoma are most common in

dogs.[134] Fibrosarcoma, carcinoid, and plasma cell tumors are rare. LSA can infiltrate the bowel diffusely, whereas other tumors are usually more discrete. Clinical signs usually include weight loss. Diarrhea, anorexia, melena, vomiting, abdominal discomfort, abdominal effusion, and anemia may also occur. Intussusception and intestinal perforation may occur as a consequence of the tumor.

Intestinal Lymphosarcoma

LSA is characterized by mucosal and submucosal infiltration of neoplastic lymphocytes, which cause malabsorption. Focal forms of LSA may cause obstruction (Fig. 137–30). They are thought to be related to FeLV in cats, although the majority of patients are FeLV negative at the time of diagnosis. In most animals alimentary LSA is diffuse (see Chapter 98).

Clinical Findings. Weight loss, chronic diarrhea, and progressive inappetence are common. Vomiting and melena may also be noted. Diffusely thickened or nodular intestines with or without mesenteric lymphadenopathy may be palpable, and abdominal pain may indicate intestinal perforation. Concurrent hepatosplenomegaly and generalized lymphadenopathy are suggestive of multicentric LSA.

Diagnosis. Middle-aged or older dogs and cats are most commonly affected. Routine biochemistry may reveal panhypoproteinemia in dogs and cats with diffuse LSA. Anemia, which is either normocytic, normochromic, and nonregenerative or microcytic and hypochromic, and neutrophilia may also be present. Low serum concentrations of cbl may support diffuse ileal involvement or the presence of partial obstruction. Ultrasonography is useful for evaluating intestinal thickness and detecting mesenteric lymphadenopathy. Diagnosis can be made by demonstrating neoplastic lymphocytes in aspirates or biopsy specimens from enlarged intestinal or peripheral lymph nodes but is more often made by intestinal biopsy (see Fig. 137–30). Endoscopic biopsies may miss the lesion or show lymphocytic-plasmacytic enteritis.

Treatment and Prognosis. Dogs with diffuse LSA usually respond poorly to therapy (see Chapter 98).

Intestinal Adenocarcinoma

Adenocarcinoma is a relatively common intestinal tumor in middle-aged to older dogs and cats. They occur most frequently in the duodenum in dogs and the jejunum and ileum in cats (see Fig. 137–21). Siamese cats seem to be overrepresented.

Clinical Findings. Adenocarcinomas are locally infiltrative and clinical signs tend to be those of partial obstruction or peritonitis where perforation has occurred. Palpation may reveal focal thickening of the intestine. Ulceration is frequent and melena and pallor may be apparent.

Diagnosis. Anemia may be normocytic, normochromic or hypochromic and microcytic, suggesting iron deficiency. Occasionally the anemia is Coombs positive. Radiography or ultrasonography helps to reveal nonpalpable masses. Diagnosis is made by percutaneous aspiration or surgical biopsy.

Treatment. Surgical resection is the treatment of choice.

Prognosis. The prognosis is usually poor to grave because of the advanced stage of tumors at the time of diagnosis. Remissions of up to 2 years or so have been reported but the remission is usually less than 6 months. Chemotherapy has not been demonstrated to be effective.

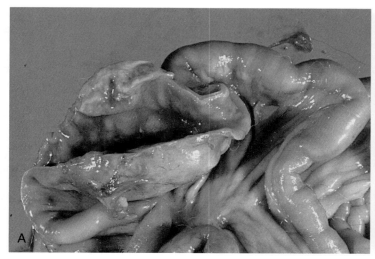

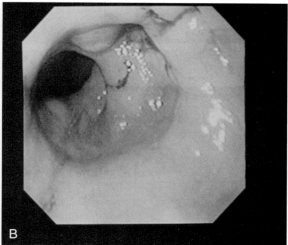

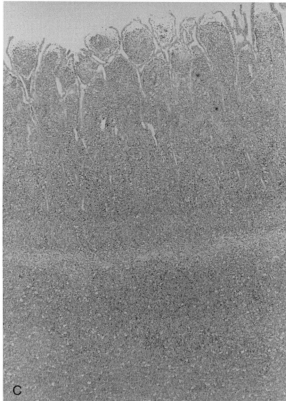

Figure 137–30. Intestinal lymphosarcoma. *A,* Nodular mass in the jejunum of a 10-year-old Pekingese dog cut open to demonstrate the mucosal wall thickening caused by focal lymphoma. *B,* Endoscopic image of the duodenum of a 6-year-old retriever showing bulging of the mucosa caused by diffuse infiltration of lymphoma. *C,* Histologic appearance of lymphoma showing loss of the normal epithelium and infiltration of all layers with malignant lymphocytes. (Courtesy of G. R. Pearson.)

GI

APUDomas

See Chapter 156.

Other Neoplasms

Leiomyomas, fibrosarcomas, mast cell tumors, and nonfunctional carcinoid tumors tend to be focally invasive. Clinical signs, diagnosis, and treatment are similar to those for intestinal adenocarcinoma. Diagnosis is based on histologic confirmation of the tumor type. Adenomatous polyps affecting the SI have been reported in middle-aged cats.[135] Clinical signs were vomiting, hematemesis, and diarrhea. Anemia was severe and life threatening in some. Upper GI endoscopy or contrast radiography is most useful in detecting these lesions, which range in size from 0.5 to 1.5 cm and are usually located in the proximal duodenum. Surgery is the treatment of choice and can be curative.

SHORT-BOWEL SYNDROME

Short-bowel syndrome is the name given to the syndrome that results when large amounts (more than two thirds) of the SI are absent because of resection or, rarely, a congenital anomaly.[136] Too little SI remains to allow adequate absorption of nutrients and electrolytes and diarrhea results. The degree of malabsorption depends on the amount resected and the site of resection. Resection of the jejunum causes malabsorption of food, water, and electrolytes. Resection of the ileum causes malabsorption of cbl and bile acids. Massive resection of the SI also precipates changes in GI hormonal regulation, such as hypergastrinemia and increased acid secretion. The syndrome may be transient after resection because of the ability of the remainder to undergo adaptive hyperplasia. In experimental studies, dogs have tolerated resection of up to 85 per cent of the SI.

Clinical Findings

Diagnosis is usually based on a history of intestinal resection associated with diarrhea and weight loss. Where a congenital lesion is suspected, the diagnosis is made by ruling out other causes of diarrhea and demonstrating an abnormally short bowel with contrast radiography.

Treatment

Initially, after massive resection, parenteral fluids and total parenteral nutrition may be required. Oral feeding is restricted but not withheld completely, as food, bile, and pancreatic secretions within the gut are important stimuli for intestinal adaptation. An isotonic, oligomeric fat-restricted liquid diet could be fed initially, with a gradual transition first to a polymeric liquid diet and then to an easily assimilable, fat- and fiber-restricted diet if well tolerated. Malabsorption of fat and water-soluble vitamins, zinc, copper, and calcium may also occur and dietary or parenteral supplementation may be required. Parenteral cbl supplementation is required if the ileum has been resected. Antacids (H_2 receptor antagonists) may be employed postoperatively to counteract possible hypergastrinemia. Antimicrobial agents may be necessary if the ileocecocolic valve has been resected or if SIBO is suspected. If the response to diet and antibiotics is poor, antisecretory agents (loperamide, diphenoxylate) or octreotide may be required. Bile salt binding resin (e.g., cholestyramine) may help reduce colonic secretion caused by bile salts malabsorbed after ileal resection.

Prognosis

The prognosis depends on the amount of intestine left and the response to therapy. Some animals undergo remarkable adaptive hyperplasia and may return to a normal diet, whereas others never respond adequately.

REFERENCES

1. Kararli TT: Comparison of the gastrointestinal anatomy, physiology and biochemistry of humans and commonly used laboratory animals. Biopharm Drug Dispos 16:351, 1995.
2. Jankowski JA, et al: Maintenance of normal intestinal mucosa: function, structure, and adaptation. Gut 41(Suppl 1):S1, 1992.
3. Griffiths DFR, et al: Demonstration of somatic mutation and colonic crypt clonality by X-linked enzyme histochemistry. Nature 333:461, 1988.
4. Basora N et al: Relation between integrin $\alpha_7\beta_1$ expression in human intestinal cells and enterocytic differentiation. Gastroenterology 113:1510, 1997.
5. Otto W, Wright N: Trefoil peptides: Coming up clover. Curr Biol 4:835, 1994.
6. Kitamura N, et al: Endocrine cells in the gastrointestinal tract of the cat. Biomed Res 3:612, 1982.
7. Konturek PC, et al: Epidermal growth factor in protection, repair, and healing of gastroduodenal mucosa. J Clin Gastroenterol 13(Suppl):S88, 1991.
8. Kernéis S, et al: Conversion by Peyer's patch lymphocytes of human enterocytes into M cells that transport bacteria. Science 277:949, 1997.
9. Newsholme EA, Carrié A-L: Quantitative aspects of glucose and glutamine metabolism by intestinal cells. Gut 41(Suppl 1):S13, 1992
10. Souba WW: Glutamine: A key substrate for the splanchnic bed. Annu Rev Nutr 11:285, 1991.
11. Lagnière S, et al: Digestive and absorptive functions along dog small intestine: Comparative distributions in relation to morphological parameters. Comp Biochem Physiol A Physiol 79:463, 1984.
12. Rodolosse A, et al: Glucose-dependent transcriptional regulation of the human sucrose-isomaltase (SI) gene. Biochimie 79:119, 1997.
13. Hall EJ, Batt RM: Development of a wheat-sensitive enteropathy in Irish setters: Biochemical changes. Am J Vet Res 51:983, 1990.
14. Kienzle E: Carbohydrate metabolism of the cat. 4. Activity of maltase, isomaltase, sucrase and lactase in the gastrointestinal tract in relation to age and diet. J Anim Physiol Anim Nutr 70:89, 1993.
15. Pemberton PW, et al: An aminopeptidase N deficiency in dog small intestine. Res Vet Sci 63:195, 1997.
16. Van Tilbeurgh H, et al: Structure of the pancreatic lipase-procolipase complex. Nature 359:159, 1992.
17. Wright EM: The intestinal Na$^+$/glucose cotransporter. Annu Rev Physiol 55:575, 1993.
18. Thorens B: Facilitated glucose transporters in epithelial cells. Annu Rev Physiol 55:591, 1993.
19. Ohkohchi N, Himukai M: Species difference in mechanisms of D-xylose absorption by the small intestine. Jpn J Physiol 34:669, 1984.
20. Hawkins EC, et al: Digestion of bentiromide and absorption of xylose in healthy cats and absorption of xylose in cats with infiltrative bowel disease. Am J Vet Res 47:567, 1986.
21. Adibi SA: The oligopeptide transporter (Pept-1) in human intestine: Biology and function. Gastroenterology 113:332, 1997.
22. Batt RM, Morgan JO: Role of serum folate and vitamin B$_{12}$ concentrations in the differentiation of small intestinal abnormalities in the dog. Res Vet Sci 32:17, 1982.
23. Simpson KW, et al: Cellular localization and hormonal regulation of pancreatic intrinsic factor secretion in dogs. Am J Physiol 265:178, 1993.
24. Fyfe JC: Feline intrinsic factor (IF) is pancreatic in origin and mediates ileal cobalamin absorption. J Vet Intern Med 7:133, 1993.
25. Makhlouf GM: Neuromuscular function of the small intestine. In Johnson LR (ed): Physiology of the Gastrointestinal Tract. New York, Raven Press, 1994, p 977
26. O'Dorisio MS: Neuropeptides and gastrointestinal immunity. Am J Med 81:74, 1986.
27. Roussel AJ: Intestinal motility. Compend Contin Educ Pract Vet 16:1433, 1994.
28. Strombeck DR: Small and large intestine: Normal structure and function. In Guilford WG, et al (eds): Strombeck's Small Animal Gastroenterology. Philadelphia, WB Saunders, 1996, p 318.
29. Sellin JH: Intestinal electrolyte absorption and secretion. In Felman F, et al (eds): Sleisenger and Fordtran's Gastrointestinal and Liver Disease. Philadelphia, WB Saunders, 1998, p 1461.
30. Uchida K, Ogami E: Intestinal microflora of dogs. Nippon Vet Zootech Coll Bull 17:42, 1969.
31. Johnston K, et al: An unexpected bacterial flora in the proximal small intestine of normal cats. Vet Rec 132:362, 1993.
32. Papasouliotis K, et al: Assessment of the bacterial flora of the proximal part of the small intestine in healthy cats, and the effect of sample collection method. Am J Vet Res 59:48, 1998.
33. Rutgers HC, et al: Small intestinal bacterial overgrowth in dogs with chronic intestinal disease. JAVMA 206:187, 1995.
34. Rutgers HC, et al: Intestinal permeability and function in dogs with small intestinal bacterial overgrowth. J Small Anim Pract 37:428, 1996.
35. Willard MD, et al: Effect of dietary supplementation of fructo-oligosaccharides on small intestinal bacterial overgrowth in dogs. Am J Vet Res 55:654, 1994.
36. Papasouliotis K, et al: The effect of dietary supplementation with fructoolgosaccharides on the faecal flora of healthy cats (abstract). Proceedings of the 41st BSAVA Congress, Birmingham, 1998, p 293.
37. McDonough PL, Simpson KW: Diagnosing emerging bacterial infections: Salmonellosis, campylobacteriosis, clostridial toxicosis and helicobacteriosis. Semin Vet Med Surg 11:1, 1996.
38. Hogenesch H, Felsburg PJ: Isolation and phenotypic and functional characterisation of cells from Peyer's patches in the dog. Vet Immunol Immunopathol 31:1, 1992.
39. Amerongen M, et al: M-cell mediated transport and monoclonal IgA antibodies for mucosal immune protection. Ann Res N Y Acad Sci 664:18, 1992.
40. Terpend K, et al: Protein transport and processing by human HT29-19A intestinal cells: Effect of interferon γ. Gut 42:538, 1998.
41. German AJ, et al: Expression of major histocompatibility complex class II antigens in the canine intestine. Vet Immunol Immunopathol 61:171, 1998.
42. Springer TA: Traffic signals for lymphocyte recirculation and leukocyte emigration: The multistep paradigm. Cell 76:301, 1994.
43. Stavnezer J: Regulation of antibody production and class switching by TGF-β. Immunol Today 17:57, 1995.
44. German AJ, et al: Measurement of IgG, IgM and IgA concentrations in canine serum, saliva, tears and bile. Vet Immunol Immunopathol 64:107, 1998.
45. Elwood CM, et al: Quantitative and qualitative immunohistochemistry of T cell subsets and MHC class II expression in the canine small intestine. Vet Immunol Immunopathol 58:195, 1997.
46. Roccabianca P, et al: Mucosal-associated lymphoid tissue: Morphological and phenotypic characterisation of feline normal small intestine. Proceedings of the Feline Immunology Workshop, University of California at Davis, 1997, p 2.
47. Abreu-Martin MT, Targan SR: Regulation of immune responses to dietary antigens: Oral tolerance. Immunol Today 19:173, 1996.
48. Williams N: T cells on the mucosal frontline. Science 280:198, 1998.
49. Molberg Ø, et al: CD4$^+$ T cells with specific reactivity against astrovirus isolated from normal human small intestine. Gastroenterology 114:115, 1998.

50. Abbas AK, et al: Functional diversity of helper T lymphocytes. Nature 383:787, 1996.
51. Murray JS: How the MHC selects Th1/Th2 immunity. Immunol Today 19:157, 1998.
52. Braunstein J, et al: T cells of the human intestinal lamina propria are high producers of interleukin-10. Gut 41:215, 1997.
53. Strober W, et al: Oral tolerance. J Clin Immunol 18:1, 1998.
54. Matzinger P: Tolerance, danger and the extended family. Annu Rev Immunol 12:991, 1994.
55. Harries JT, et al: Congenital and inherited defects of the enterocyte. In Booth CC, Neale G (eds): Disorders of the Small Intestine. Oxford, Blackwell, 1985, p 52.
56. Fyfe JC, et al: Defective brush-border expression of intrinsic factor–cobalamin receptor in canine inherited intestinal cobalamin malabsorption. J Biol Chem 266:4489, 1991.
57. Jezyk PF, et al: Lethal acrodermatitis in bull terriers. JAVMA 188:833, 1986.
58. Welsh FKS, et al: Gut barrier function in malnourished patients. Gut 42:396, 1998.
59. Crowe SE, Perdue MH: Gastrointestinal food hypersensitivity: Basic mechanisms of pathophysiology. Gastroenterology 103:1075, 1992.
60. Van Deventer SJH: Tumour necrosis factor and Crohn's disease. Gut 40:443, 1997.
61. Naliboff B, Mayer EA: Commentary: Sensational developments in the irritable bowel. Gut 39:770, 1996.
62. Gilson SD, et al: Evaluation of two commercial test kits for detection of occult blood in feces of dogs. Am J Vet Res 51:1385, 1990.
63. Conlan MG, et al: Prothrombotic abnormalities in inflammatory bowel disease. Dig Dis Sci 34:1089, 1989.
64. Williams DA, et al: Evaluation of fecal alpha$_1$-protease inhibitor concentration as a test for canine protein-losing enteropathy. J Vet Intern Med 5:133, 1991.
65. Sancak AA, et al: Role of Escherichia coli in dogs with small intestinal bacterial overgrowth. Proceedings of the 6th Annual ESVIM Congress, Lyon, 1996, p 44.
66. Melgarejo T, et al: Enzyme-linked immunosorbent assay for canine alpha 1-protease inhibitor. Am J Vet Res 59:127, 1998.
67. Sparkes AH, et al: Reference ranges for gastrointestinal transit of barium-impregnated polyethylene spheres in healthy cats. J Small Anim Pract 38:340, 1997.
68. Penninck DG: Ultrasonography of the gastrointestinal tract. In Nyland TG, Mattoon JS (eds): Veterinary Diagnostic Ultrasound. Philadelphia, WB Saunders, 1995, p 125.
69. Roth L, et al: Comparisons between endoscopic and histologic evaluation of the gastrointestinal tract in dogs and cats: 75 cases (1984–1987). JAVMA 196:635, 1990.
70. van der Gaag I, Happé RP: The histological appearance of peroral small intestinal biopsies in clinically healthy dogs and dogs with chronic diarrhea. J Vet Med A 37:401, 1990.
71. Fyfe JC, et al: Inherited selective intestinal cobalamin malabsorption and cobalamin deficiency in dogs. Pediatr Res 29:24, 1991.
72. Outerbridge CA, et al: Hereditary cobalamin deficiency in collie dogs (abstract). J Vet Intern Med 10, 1996.
73. Elwood CM, et al: A novel method of assessing canine intestinal permeability and function using a multiple sugar test. J Vet Intern Med 7:131, 1993.
74. Sørensen SH, et al: A blood test for intestinal permeability and function: A new tool for the diagnosis of chronic intestinal disease in dogs. Clin Chim Acta 264:103, 1997.
75. Washabau RJ, et al: Evaluation of intestinal carbohydrate malabsorption in the dog by pulmonary hydrogen gas excretion. Am J Vet Res 47:1402, 1986.
76. Washabau RJ, et al: Use of pulmonary hydrogen gas excretion to detect carbohydrate malabsorption in dogs. JAVMA 189:674, 1986.
77. Muir P, et al: Evaluation of carbohydrate malassimilation and intestinal transit time in cats by measurement of breath hydrogen excretion. Am J Vet Res 52:1104, 1991.
78. Ludlow CL: Breath hydrogen testing: Can it be useful in small animal medicine? Proceedings of the 14th ACVIM Forum, San Antonio, 1996, p 355.
79. Melgarejo T and Williams DA: Serum total unconjugated bile acids (TUBA) in dogs with small intestinal bacterial overgrowth (abstract). Proceedings of the 15th ACVIM Forum, San Diego, 1997, p 661.
80. Burrows CF, Jezyk PF: Nitrosonaphthol test for screening small intestinal diarrheal disease in the dog. JAVMA 183:318, 1983.
81. Simpson KW: Gastrointestinal endoscopy in the dog. J Small Animl Pract 34:180, 1993.
82. Landi B, et al: Diagnostic yield of push-type enteroscopy in relation to indication:. Gut 42:421, 1998.
83. Hall EJ: Small intestinal disease—Is endoscopic biopsy the answer? J Small Anim Pract 35:408, 1994.
84. van der Gaag I, Happé RP: Follow-up studies by peroral small intestinal biopsies and necropsy in dogs with chronic diarrhea. J Vet Med A 37:561, 1990.
85. Johnson SE: Fluid therapy for gastrointestinal, pancreatic, and hepatic disease. In DiBartola SP (ed): Fluid Therapy in Small Animal Practice. Philadelphia, WB Saunders, 1992, p 507.
86. Thadepalli H, et al: Antimicrobial activity of intravenous quinolones on the intestinal microflora in dogs. Chemotherapy, 31:6, 1991.
87. Smith Carr S, et al: Canine parvovirus. 1. Pathogenesis and vaccination. Compend Contin Educ Pract Vet 19:125, 1997.
88. Houston DM, et al: Risk factors associated with parvovirus enteritis in dogs: 283 cases (1982–1991). J Vet Med [A] 208:542, 1996.
89. Macintire DK, et al: Canine parvovirus. II. Clinical signs diagnosis and treatment. Compend Contin Educ Pract Vet 19:291, 1997.
90. Rewerts JM, et al: Effect of rhG-CSF administration on the clinical outcome of neutropenic, parvovirus infected puppies (abstract). Proceedings of the AC-VIM Forum, San Antonio, 1996, p 120.
91. Larson LJ, Schultz RD: Comparison of selected canine vaccines for their ability to induce protective immunity against canine parvovirus infeceion. Am J Vet Res 58:360, 1997.
92. Harvey CJ, et al: An uncommon intestinal manifestation of feline infectious peritonitis: 26 cases (1986–1993). JAVMA 209:1117, 1996.
93. Muir PA, et al: A clinical and microbiological study of cats with protruding nictitating membranes and diarrhoea: Isolation of a novel virus. Vet Rec 127:324, 1990.
94. Cookson SL, et al: Treatment of gastrointestinal infections. Curr Opin Gastroenterol 10:105, 1994.
95. Rutgers, HC, et al: Enrofloxacin treatment of gram-negative infections. Vet Rec 135:357, 1994.
96. Jergens AE, et al: Adherent gram-positive cocci on the intestinal villi of two dogs with gastrointestinal disease. JAVMA 198:1950, 1991.
97. Miller RI: Gastrointestinal phycomycosis in 63 dogs. JAVMA 186:473, 1985.
98. Thomas RC, Lewis DT: Pythiosis in dogs and cats. Compend Contin Educ Pract Vet 20:63, 1998.
99. Taboada J, et al: Successful management of gastrointestinal pythiosis with itraconazole in two dogs. J Vet Intern Med 8:176, 1994.
100. Reinemeyer CR: Canine gastrointestinal parasites. In Bonagura JD (ed): Kirk Current Veterinary Therapy XII. Philadelphia, WB Saunders, 1995, p 711.
101. Reinemeyer CR: Feline gastrointestinal parasites. In Bonagura JD (ed): Kirk Current Veterinary Therapy XI. Philadelphia, WB Saunders, 1992, p 626.
102. Lappin MR, et al: Enzyme-linked immunosorbent assay for the detection of Cryptosporidium parvum IgG in the serum of cats. J Parasitol 83:957, 1997.
103. Barr SC, Bowman DD: Giardiasis in dogs and cats. Compend Contin Educ Pract Vet 16:603, 1994.
104. Barr SC, et al: Efficacy of a drug combination of praziquantel, pyrantel pamoate, and febantel against giardiasis in dogs. Am J Vet Res 59:1134, 1998.
105. Batt RM, Hall EJ: Chronic enteropathies in the dog. J Small Anim Pract 30:3, 1989.
106. Batt RM, et al: Small intestinal bacterial overgrowth and enhanced intestinal permeability in clinically healthy beagle dogs. Am J Vet Res 53:1935, 1992.
107. Batt RM, et al: Relative IgA deficiency and small intestinal bacterial overgrowth in German shepherd dogs. Res Vet Sci 50:106, 1991.
108. Delles EK, et al: Comparison of species and numbers of bacteria in concurrently cultured samples of proximal small intestinal fluid and endoscopically obtained duodenal mucosa in dogs with intestinal bacterial overgrowth. Am J Vet Res 55:957, 1994.
109. Jergens AE, et al: Idiopathic inflammatory bowel disease in dogs and cats: 84 cases (1987–1990). JAVMA 201:1603, 1992.
110. Dennis JS, et al: Lymphocytic/plasmacytic gastroenteritis in cats: 14 cases (1985–1990). JAVMA 200:1712, 1992.
111. Bauditz J, et al: Treatment with tumour necrosis facor inhibitor oxpentifylline does not improve corticosteroid dependent chronic active Crohn's disease. Gut 40:470, 1997.
112. MacLachlan NJ, et al: Gastroenteritis of basenji dogs. Vet Pathol 25:36, 1988.
113. Jergens AE, et al: Morphometric evaluation of immunoglobulin A–containing cells and T cells in duodenal mucosa from healthy dogs and from dogs with inflammatory bowel disease or non-specific gastroenteritis. Am J Vet Res 57:697, 1996.
114. De Buysscher EV, et al: Elevated serum IgA associated with immunoproliferative enteropathy of basenji dogs: Lack of evidence for alpha heavy-chain disease or enhanced intestinal IgA secretion. Vet Immunol Immunopathol 20:41, 1988.
115. Batt RM, et al: Subcellular biochemical studies of a naturally occurring enteropathy in the dog resembling chronic tropical sprue in human beings. Am J Vet Res 44:1492, 1983.
116. Van der Gaag I, et al: Regional eosinophilic coloproctitis, typhlitis and ileitis in a dog. Vet Q 12:1, 1990.
117. Barker I, et al: VI. The intestine. J. Malassimilation and protein loss in the small intestine. In Jubb KVF et al (eds): Pathology of Domestic Animals. San Diego, Academic Press, 1993, p 124.
118. Suter MM, et al: Primary intestinal lymphangiectasia in three dogs: A morphological and immunological investigation. Vet Pathol 22:123, 1985.
119. Chapman BL, et al: Granulomatous hepatitis in dogs—9 cases (1987–1990). JAVMA 203:680, 1993.
120. Kolbjornsen O, et al: Gastropathies in the Lundehund. 1. Gastritis and gastric neoplasia associated with intestinal lymphangiectasia. APMIS 102:647, 1994.
121. Paterson S: Food hypersensitivity in 20 dogs with skin and gastrointestinal signs. J Small Anim Pract 36:529, 1995.
122. Vaden SL, et al: Gastroscopic food sensitivity testing and oral challenge in soft-coated wheaten terriers with protein-losing enteropathy and/or nephropathy. J Vet Intern Med 12:202, 1998.
123. Bischoff SC, et al: Colonoscopic allergen provocation (COLAP): A new diagnostic approach for gastrointestinal food allergy. Gut 40:745, 1997.
124. Puhl S, et al: Colonoscopic allergen provocation (COLAP) test in dogs (abstract). Proceedings of the 2nd Annual Conference of the European Society of Veterinary and Comparative Nutrition, Vienna, 1998, p 71.
125. Polvi A, et al: Canine major histocompatibility complex genes DQA and DQB in Irish setter dogs. Tissue Antigens 49:236, 1997.
126. Vaden SL, et al: Gluten administration provokes mucosal mononuclear cell

GI

infiltration, but does not increase intestinal permeability in soft-coated wheaten terriers (SCWT). J Vet Intern Med 12:202, 1998.

127. Sollid LM, et al: Autoantibodies in coeliac disease: Tissue transglutaminase—Guilt by association. Gut 41:851, 1997.

128. Pemberton PW, et al: Gluten-sensitive enteropathy in Irish setter dogs: Characterisation of jejunal microvillar proteins by two-dimensional electrophoresis. Res Vet Sci 62:191, 1997.

129. Manners HK, et al: Effect of a high dose of dietary gluten on the development of a gluten-sensitive enteropathy in Irish setter dogs (abstract). Gastroenterology 106:A620, 1994.

130. Felts JF, et al: Thread and sewing needles as gastrointestinal foreign bodies in the cat. A review of 64 cases. JAVMA 184:45, 1984.

131. Tidwell AS, Penninck DG: Ultrasonography of gastrointestinal foreign bodies. Vet Radiol 33:160, 1992.

132. Cullen JJ, et al: Pathophysiology of adynamic ileus. Dig Dis Sci 42:731, 1997.

133. Washabau RJ, Hall JA: Gastrointestinal motility disorders of dogs and cats. Eur J Comp Gastroenterol 2:9, 1997.

134. Straw RC: Tumors of the intestinal tract. In Withrow SJ, MacEwen EG (eds): Small Animal Clinical Oncology. Philadelphia, WB Saunders, 1996, p 252.

135. MacDonald JM, et al: Adenomatous polyps of the duodenum in cats: 18 cases (1985–1990). JAVMA 202:647, 1993.

136. Yanoff SR, Willard MD: Short bowel syndrome in dogs and cats. Semin Vet Med Surg (Small Anim) 4:226, 1989.

137. Chang EB, Rao MC: Intestinal water and electrolyte transport: Mechanisms of physiological and adaptive responses. In Johnson LR (ed): Physiology of the Gastrointestinal Tract. New York, Raven Press, 1994, p 2027.

138. Hore P, Messer M: Studies on disaccharidase activities of the small intestine of the domestic cat and other carnivorous mammals. Comp Biochem Physiol 24:717, 1968.

139. Levanti G, et al: Distribution le long de l'intestin du chien des enzymes de la bordure en brosse des entérocytes. Ann Biol Anim Biochim Biophys 18:1155, 1978.

140. Noon KF, et al: Detection and definition of canine intestinal carbohydrases, using a standard method. Am J. Vet Res 38:1063, 1977.

141. Kienzle E: Enzyme-activity in pancreatic tissue, intestinal-mucosa and chyme of dogs in relation to age and diet. J Anim Physiol Anim Nutr 60:276, 1988.

142. Batt RM, et al: Biochemical changes in the jejunal mucosa of dogs with a naturally occurring enteropathy associated with bacterial overgrowth. Gut 25:816, 1984.

CHAPTER 138

DISEASES OF THE LARGE INTESTINE

Albert E. Jergens and Michael D. Willard

NORMAL STRUCTURE AND FUNCTION

GROSS AND MICROSCOPIC STRUCTURE

Anatomically, the large bowel is divided into the cecum, colon, and rectum. The cecum exists as a blind diverticulum associated with the proximal colon by means of the cecocolic orifice. This opening lies approximately 1 cm from the ileocolic orifice (Fig. 138–1). The large intestine varies in length, measuring 0.3 to 0.9 m in the dog and up to 0.45 m in the cat.[1] It begins at the ileocolic valve where the short ascending colon courses cranially and turns from right to left at the right colic (hepatic) flexure to become the transverse colon. Both the cecum and ascending colon lie to the right of the median plane. From the right colic flexure, the transverse colon runs cranial to the mesenteric root to the left colic (splenic) flexure, and becomes the descending colon. The descending colon, the longest colonic segment, continues caudally along the left abdominal wall through the pelvic canal to the anus as the rectum.

Blood supply to the large bowel is from the cranial and caudal mesenteric arteries. Venous drainage is essentially the same as arterial supply. The vagus and pelvic nerves supply the colon with parasympathetic innervation. Sympathetic innervation arises from the paravertebral sympathetic trunk via the sympathetic ganglia.

Histologically, the large bowel contains mucosal, submucosal, muscular, and serosal layers. The mucosa of the cecum and colon lack villi, although ridges or folds on the mucosal surface increase its surface area. The single layer of surface epithelia has more sparse and less regular microvilli in comparison with small intestinal absorptive cells.[2] Numerous colonic glands (e.g., crypts of Lieberkühn) extend from the absorptive surface down to the muscularis mucosae. These

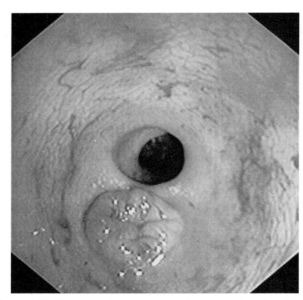

Figure 138–1. Endoscopic appearance of the normal canine ileocolic region. The button-like protuberance is the ileocolic valve, and the opening above it is the cecocolic orifice.

structures contain both epithelial cells and mature mucus-producing cells near their surface, and primarily undifferentiated cells in the lower one half of the glands. Crypt cells multiply and differentiate as they migrate up gland walls to replace surface absorptive epithelia. Colonic lamina propria is minimal between tightly packed colonic glands. Proprial cell populations are diffusely distributed, and leukocyte populations consist predominately of lymphocytes and plasma cells. General guidelines for histologic interpretation of colonic tissues are reported elsewhere.[3, 4]

Mucosal Immunity: The Basics

The natural "self-defenses" of the gastrointestinal tract comprise mechanical and immunologic mechanisms.[5] Mechanical factors include an effective mucosal barrier of epithelial cells; normal peristalsis, which serves to clear the lumen of debris; mucus secretion by goblet cells, which traps pathogens and precludes mucosal penetration; and a luxuriant resident microflora, which prevents colonization by pathogenic bacteria.

The colonic immune system is an extension of the gut-associated lymphoid tissue (GALT) consisting of aggregated (lymphoid nodules and Peyer's patches) and nonaggregated (luminal, intraepithelial, and lamina propria lymphocytes) lymphoid components. The GALT contains an impressive array of B and T lymphocytes and antigen-processing cells, which include macrophages and dendritic cells. Specialized epithelial cells overlying Peyer's patches, termed membranous or M cells, function to "sample" and process intact luminal antigens to evoke an appropriate immune response.[6] Following antigen presentation to GALT, the immune system produces clones responsible for cell-mediated immunity, humoral immunity, immune regulation, and the phenomenon of oral tolerance. Immune responses are largely dominated by T-cell suppression, which renders the immune system tolerant to ingested antigens and microbial flora. The cell-mediated response of GALT produces activated effector T cells that differentiate into memory cells and cytotoxic cells and can synthesize numerous biologically active lymphokines. In contrast to systemic lymphoid tissues, most GALT B cells are preferentially committed to differentiate into clones of IgA-secreting plasma cells. Secretory IgA (sIgA) and other mechanical factors exclude mucosal antigenic uptake.[7]

Intraepithelial lymphocytes (predominantly CD8$^+$ T cells) and a diffuse population of mucosal B and T cells contribute prominently to mucosal immunity. Recent morphometric and phenotypic studies indicate that IgA-containing cells and CD3$^+$ T cells are the most numerous immune cell types in normal colonic mucosa (Table 138–1).[8, 9] Imbalances of mucosal immune cell populations are a salient feature of specific colonic disorders, such as canine inflammatory bowel disease.[10]

In summary, the colonic immune system protects the host through antigen exclusion (primarily sIgA), immune regulation (via suppressor T cells), antigen elimination (antibody secretion, cell-mediated immunity, inflammatory response), and development of oral tolerance.

Colonic Microflora

The canine large bowel contains the greatest number of bacteria in the gastrointestinal tract, up to 10^{11} organisms per gram of feces. Anaerobic bacteria (e.g., *Bacteroides*, bifidobacteria, clostridia, and lactobacilli) comprise the majority (>90 per cent) of colonic microflora.[11] Enterobacteria and streptococci are the predominant aerobic bacteria found in the large bowel. Little published data exist on the normal feline colonic microflora; however, one investigation[12] suggests a more equitable distribution of aerobic bacteria (predominantly *E. coli* and lactobacilli) to anaerobic bacteria (predominantly *Clostridium perfringens* and *Bacteroides* spp.) within the lumen.

Physiologic regulation of this normal flora is required to prevent bacterial overgrowth by normal residents and colonization by single, pathogenic microorganisms. Factors contributing to colonic microbial homeostasis include normal motility, maintenance of a mucosal barrier that prevents bacterial adherence and invasion, bacterial interactions favoring the growth of normal microflora, oxygen availability, and dietary nutrients.[11, 13, 14] The administration of antibacterial agents and the overproduction of endogenous substances (e.g., bile salts) may affect colonic function and bacterial numbers.[15]

The colonic microflora plays pivotal roles in the digestion of undigested carbohydrates and proteins. Luminal microflora degrade these nutrients to short-chain fatty acids (SCFA), especially acetate, propionate, and butyrate.[16] Acetate and propionate are preferentially utilized by the liver for cholesterol or triglyceride synthesis, or metabolized by hepatocytes and used as energy sources. Butyrate is the primary source of metabolic fuel used by colonocytes, and is crucial for maintenance of epithelial growth and repair.[17] The SCFA produced additionally function as intraluminal cations serving to maintain an acidic luminal pH.[18] This acidification helps prevent formation of colonic irritants (such as free ammonia, ionized long-chain fatty acids, and bile acids) that may contribute to colonic disease.

Normal Motility

Motor activity is similar to that of the small intestines, consisting of both rhythmic segmentation and propulsive movements.[19] Segmentation, originating in the circular smooth muscle, mixes and slows the passage of colonic contents to ensure completeness of digestion and absorption.

TABLE 138–1. DISTRIBUTION OF IMMUNE CELLS IN COLONIC MUCOSA OF HEALTHY DOGS

REGION	IgA	IgG	IgM	CD3$^+$	CD4$^+$	CD8$^+$
Ascending colon	87.0 ($\pm$5.3)	26.4 ($\pm$5.3)	44.2 ($\pm$5.3)	226.7 ($\pm$12.4)	72.0 ($\pm$13.1)	149.8 ($\pm$12.4)
Transverse colon	76.6 ($\pm$5.3)	28.4 ($\pm$5.3)	46.5 ($\pm$5.3)	213.0 ($\pm$12.4)	70.8 ($\pm$12.6)	159.3 ($\pm$12.6)
Descending colon	99.9 ($\pm$5.2)	22.7 ($\pm$5.2)	44.8 ($\pm$5.2)	233.1 ($\pm$12.4)	76.1 ($\pm$12.4)	153.4 ($\pm$12.4)

Data are expressed as mean $\pm$ SEM. Cell counts enumerated as number of cells per millimeter of mucosal length.

Adapted from Jergens AE, et al: Immunohistochemical characterization of immunoglobulin-containing cells and T cells in the colonic mucosa of healthy dogs. Am J Vet Res 59:552, 1998.

TABLE 138–2. SOME FACTORS AFFECTING COLONIC MOTILITY

Luminal distention (+)	Sympathetic stimulation (−)
Dietary fiber (+)	Enteric neurotransmitters (±)
Parasympathetic stimulation (+)	Nitric oxide, VIP, enkephalins, CCK, substance P, somatostatin, bombesin
Cholinergic drugs (+)	Anticholinergic drugs (−)
Prostaglandins (+)	Narcotic analgesics (±)
Morphine (+)	Inflammation (−)

(+) = stimulatory; (−) = inhibitory; (±) = stimulatory and inhibitory.

Peristalsis, performed by the longitudinal smooth muscle, serves to drive colonic contents aborally. Variable motility patterns are found in the different colonic regions. The cranial colon exhibits retrograde peristalsis that mixes food and enhances mucosal absorption of fluid and electrolytes. The midportion of the colon shows coordinated peristalsis as contents are propelled toward the rectum. The caudal colon shows strong peristaltic contractions (migrating spike bursts or mass movements) that move caudally and empty the colon.

Control of peristalsis and rhythmic segmentation is determined by slow wave activity, an inherent myoelectric function of smooth muscle. The frequency of slow wave activity determines the rate of contractions, and slow waves are essential for spike potentials that initiate muscular contractions. Slow waves arise in the circular muscle and are generated by ion fluxes across the membranes of the smooth muscle cell. A single pacemaker in the proximal colon propagates slow waves in an orad direction, while other colonic pacemakers stimulate segmentation to move contents aborally toward the rectum. The principal stimulus for colonic motility is luminal distention. Distension stimulates segmentation by local reflexes mediated through the intrinsic nervous system. A variety of other myogenic, neural, and hormonal factors affect colonic motility (Table 138–2).

FLUID AND ELECTROLYTE TRANSPORT

Colonic water absorption is a passive process directly related to the absorption of solute (e.g., sodium). Most colonic sodium absorption appears linked (coupled) to chloride secretion.[20] Sodium entry into the colonic epithelia is driven by an electrochemical gradient, where sodium diffuses "downhill" from a high concentration in the lumen to very low concentrations intracellularly. A Na^+/K^+-ATPase actively transports sodium from within colonic epithelial cells, across their basolateral membranes, to the circulation. Glucocorticoids, mineralocorticoids, and catecholamines stimulate this transport.[20]

The movement of potassium, bicarbonate, and chloride occurs by varying means. In the colon, potassium may be secreted or absorbed. Under most circumstances, net secretion of potassium occurs through an active conductance mechanism on the apical membrane.[21] Bicarbonate is secreted by colonic epithelia and neutralizes acids produced by colonic bacteria. In vivo, most chloride absorption probably occurs through diffusion.

Relatively minor dysfunction in either the colon's reservoir function or its absorptive capacity can have profound effects on fecal water content, causing large bowel diarrhea. General causes for altered electrolyte and water transport include increased secretion (via bacterial toxins, deconjugated bile acids, and hydroxylated fatty acids) and increased mucosal permeability to water and ions caused by invasive bacteria, bacterial toxins, and/or cellular infiltration.

DIAGNOSTIC EVALUATION OF THE COLON

HISTORY AND CLINICAL SIGNS

Most colonic diseases cause signs such as hematochezia, fecal mucus, tenesmus, and increased frequency of defecation, but usually without systemic signs of illness (e.g., weight loss). General causes for hematochezia in dogs and cats are listed in Table 138–3. Other signs (e.g., abdominal pain, anal pruritus, flatulence) are reported less frequently. Most animals are alert, active, and well fleshed with normal appetites on presentation. Some diseases (alimentary neoplasia, inflammatory bowel disease, mycotic enterocolitis) may cause concurrent small intestinal disease.

One should search for dietary, environmental, parasitic, and infectious causes of large bowel dysfunction. Dietary and parasitic causes may constitute up to 50 per cent of clinical cases.[1] Salient dietary considerations include the diet, recent dietary changes (which might impugn responsible nutrients), the amount and frequency of feeding, and the administration of dietary supplements or medications (e.g., antibiotics, narcotics, motility modifiers) that might alter colonic function. Resolution of clinical signs when the patient is fed a controlled (hypoallergenic or elimination) diet is suggestive of food intolerance or allergy. Similarly, previous response to glucocorticoid therapy may indicate benign cellular infiltrates (e.g., inflammatory bowel disease). Animals that roam freely are more likely to develop parasitic, toxic, and infectious disorders. Multiple fecal examinations appropriate for specific parasites, as well as empiric therapy, are reasonable. Lastly, the animal's travel history may suggest an increased risk of diseases with a regional incidence (e.g., histoplasmosis[22] and intestinal parasites).

Physical examination in most animals with colonic disease is normal. However, general examination may detect abnormalities suggestive of mycotic infections, metastatic neoplasia, and metabolic disease (uremia). Abdominal palpation is important in assessing for prostatomegaly, genitourinary disorders, fecal impaction, and intussusception that can cause tenesmus/dyschezia. A carefully performed digital rectal examination should be performed to search for rectal masses, foreign objects, stricture (rare), and perianal diseases. Roughened colonic mucosa may be palpable with infiltrative (i.e., inflammatory, neoplastic) processes. Additionally, rectal evaluation may confirm the presence of hematochezia or fecal mucus and provide valuable exfoliative specimens for cytologic interpretation.

TABLE 138–3. COMMON CAUSES OF HEMATOCHEZIA

Colitis	Parasites
Inflammatory bowel disease	*Trichuris vulpis*
Bacterial infection	Hookworms
Fungal infection	Coccidia
Neoplasia	Colonic trauma
Colorectal adenocarcinoma	Foreign objects
Lymphosarcoma	Automotive induced
Rectal polyp	Intussusception
Coagulopathy	Dietary hypersensitivity
Clotting defects	"Irritable bowel syndrome"
Thrombocytopenia	

DIAGNOSTIC TESTS

Diagnostic strategies for diseases of the large intestine vary considerably, depending on etiology, chronicity of signs, presence of systemic illness, and historical or likely response(s) to symptomatic therapy (Fig. 138–2).

Admission Laboratory Tests. A complete blood count (CBC), serum biochemistry profile, and urinalysis are especially important in patients having systemic signs (anorexia, weight loss, pyrexia) of illness. These tests also serve as a general health screen prior to general anesthesia and colonoscopy with mucosal biopsy. The CBC may provide important clues of anemia (anemia of chronic disease), inflammation (leukocytosis, increased globulins), or parasitism (absolute eosinophilia). A platelet count or estimation is recommended in patients with hematochezia. Serum biochemistries identify incidental problems in other organ systems and evaluate for electrolyte disturbances (hypokalemia, hypercalcemia of malignancy) seen with some of the colonic disorders. Hypoalbuminemia is seen with severe infiltrative disorders (e.g., histoplasmosis, pythiosis, colonic lymphosarcoma). Urinalysis is required to evaluate renal function. Serologic tests for FeLV and FIV are warranted in cats.

Fecal Parasitic Evaluation. Intestinal parasites must be ruled out (especially in puppies and kittens) by fecal flotation for parasitic ova and direct fecal smears for protozoa. Zinc sulfate fecal flotation is a useful and sensitive means of detecting most nematode ova and *Giardia* spp. cysts.[23] Some parasites (*Trichuris vulpis* and *Giardia* spp.) intermittently shed small numbers of ova or cysts and are notoriously difficult to diagnose, even on serial fecal flotations. Direct fecal examination is not as sensitive as flotation techniques for the detection of colonic parasites. However, a fresh fecal saline smear may occasionally identify motile trophozoites of *Giardia, Trichomonas, Balantidium,* or *Entamoeba,* or eggs of *Heterobilharzia* or *Trichuris.*[24]

Bacterial Fecal Culture. Fecal cultures are reasonable in animals suspected of having infectious diarrhea. Animals at risk include very young animals, those involved in kennel outbreaks, animals recently obtained from shelters or pet stores, and households where more than one animal has diarrhea.[25] The pathogens most likely to be cultured from feces in these patients are *C. perfringens, Salmonella* spp., *Campylobacter jejuni,* and occasionally *Yersinia enterocolitica.* Verotoxin-producing strains of *Escherichia coli* may be a potential cause of infectious diarrhea as well. Accurate interpretation of culture results should include some description as to the relative amounts of said pathogen cultured in relation to other bacterial flora. Culture results should be interpreted in light of clinical signs, cytology/histology of colonic mucosa, elimination of other causes, and confirmation of enterotoxin production (if applicable).

Fecal specimens for culture must be fresh, of adequate quantity (1 to 3 g weight), and transported rapidly to the laboratory for inoculation into enrichment media.[26, 27] If inoculation is to be delayed, specific fecal transport solutions should be used.

Fecal Cytologic Examination. Exfoliative rectal or endoscopic cytology specimens are used to identify etiologic agents and inflammatory cells. Rectal smears are made by insertion of a moistened cotton-tipped applicator into the rectum, rolling the swab against the rectal mucosa, withdrawing the swab from the rectum, and gently rolling the swab with exfoliated cells onto glass slides. Alternatively, a flat, platinum conjunctival spatula may be used to obtain rectal scraping specimens. The slides are then air-dried and stained. Increased numbers of leukocytes indicate inflammatory or infectious colonic disease. Histoplasmosis may occasionally be identified. Finding increased numbers of spore-forming bacteria has been suggested to support clostridial colitis. However, recent work has shown that the presence of spores or *C. perfringens* enterotoxin is not specific for clostridial colitis; and that healthy dogs may have excessive spores and/or produce enterotoxin as well.[28]

Critical evaluation of endoscopic exfoliative cytologic specimens obtained from dogs and cats with colonic disease has been described.[29] Excellent correlation between exfoliative cytology and histology was observed. Using objective grading criteria (Table 138–4), brush and touch cytologic preparations were found to be sensitive and specific for the detection of normal mucosa, benign mucosal inflammation (e.g., lymphocytic-plasmacytic colitis), and lymphoid malignancy (Figs. 138–3 to 138–5). Cytologic discordance was rare and generally associated with mild inflammatory disease. Additionally, endoscopic cytology was safe, required little time to procure specimens, and could be performed concurrently with mucosal biopsy. These results indicate that gastrointestinal exfoliative cytology is a useful and reliable adjunct to endoscopic biopsy.

RADIOGRAPHIC IMAGING

Radiographic findings are infrequently diagnostic in animals with colonic disease. Survey abdominal radiographs

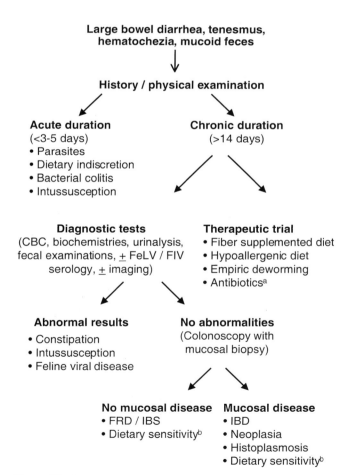

Figure 138–2. Simplified approach to diagnosis of large intestinal diseases. FRD/IBS = fiber-responsive diarrhea/irritable bowel syndrome; IBD = inflammatory bowel disease. [a]Only used if suspicious of clostridial colitis. [b]Includes food intolerance or food allergy.

TABLE 138–4. GRADING CRITERIA FOR GASTROINTESTINAL CYTOLOGY

CATEGORY	SCORE	
Inflammatory cells	0	
Epithelial cells[a]	1	} Mild
	2	} 1–2/oil
Atypical cells	3	} Moderate
Bacteria[b]	4	} 3–4/oil
Hemorrhage	5	} Severe
Debris/ingesta	6	} 5–7/oil
Mucus	7	}

The assigned numbers 0–7 correspond to the number/amount of cells or debris per ten 50× oil immersion fields.
[a]The grade for epithelial cells corresponds to the number of clusters observed per 10× field.
[b]Includes both gastric spirillar organisms and intestinal flora.
Adapted from Jergens AE, et al.: Cytologic examination of exfoliative specimens obtained during endoscopy for diagnosis of gastrointestinal tract disease in dogs and cats. JAVMA 213:1755, 1998.

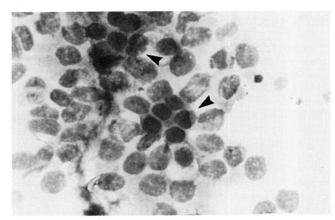

Figure 138–4. Endoscopic exfoliative cytologic specimen. Example of LP colitis. (Courtesy of Dr. Claire B. Andreasen, Iowa State University.)

may identify radiopaque foreign objects, fecal impaction, and extraluminal obstruction (e.g., pelvic canal stenosis, prostatomegaly, regional lymphadenopathy). Ileocolic or cecocolic intussusception may appear as a tubular, soft tissue opacity if contrasted with air. In the absence of endoscopy, barium enemas may provide evidence of mucosal irregularities and luminal compromise. Pneumocolon can be performed as a simple alternative to barium enema to highlight luminal masses or when location of the colon must be determined (Fig. 138–6).

Colonic ultrasonography is less commonly performed as a result of the technical difficulties caused by luminal gas accumulation. Nevertheless, various abnormalities (e.g., mass lesions, intussusception, regional lymphadenopathy, bowel wall thickening) may be diagnosed ultrasonographically (Fig. 138–7).[30] Fine-needle aspiration of mural thickenings, luminal masses, or pericolonic structures can be performed with the assistance of a skilled sonographer.

COLONOSCOPY

Colonoscopy is indicated in pets with chronic large bowel disease unresponsive to empiric therapies, and in some animals with obstipation. Therapeutic monitoring of mucosal

disease (inflammatory or neoplastic) may also be performed. Colonic biopsies and exfoliative cytologies are particularly useful in the diagnosis of idiopathic (lymphocytic-plasmacytic) colitis.

Either flexible endoscopy or rigid proctoscopy may be performed. Diffuse colonic diseases may be diagnosed by rigid proctoscopy, which allows one to obtain larger (and potentially more diagnostic) mucosal specimens from the descending colon alone. Advantages of flexible endoscopy include excellent visualization of the entire colon and cecum, and targeted biopsies may be obtained from all colonic regions. Desirable features of a flexible endoscope appropriate for use in most dogs and cats include four-way tip deflection capability, an outside diameter less than 10 mm, an operating channel diameter of 2.8 mm, and a working length of at least 100 cm.[31] Serrated jaw pinch biopsy forceps without a central needle and guarded cytology brushes are preferred by the authors.

Patient preparation for endoscopy varies.[27, 32] Food should be withheld for at least 24 to 36 hours. Complete evacuation of colonic contents is needed to adequately visualize mucosal surfaces. Use a colonic lavage solution (e.g., GoLYTELY given orally in two doses of 14 mL/lb 6 to 12 hours apart) plus two tepid water enemas (10 mL/lb) the evening prior

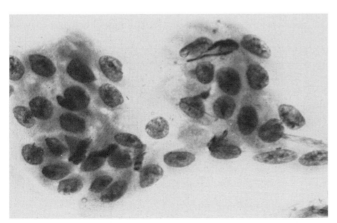

Figure 138–3. Endoscopic exfoliative cytologic specimen. Normal colonic epithelium. (Courtesy of Dr. Claire B. Andreasen, Iowa State University.)

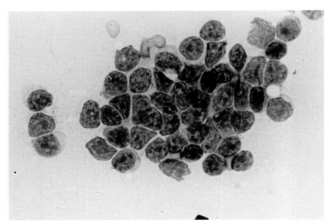

Figure 138–5. Endoscopic exfoliative cytologic specimen. Diffuse lymphoblasts are observed within a colonic touch cytology specimen. The histologic diagnosis was malignant lymphoma. (Courtesy of Dr. Claire B. Andreasen, Iowa State University.)

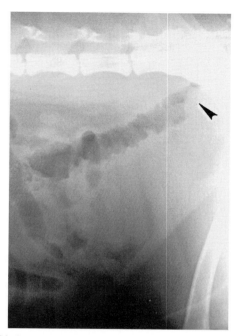

Figure 138–6. Lateral abdominal radiograph demonstrating pneumocolon in a dog. Air contrast outlines a soft tissue mass in the descending colon (arrow). Endoscopic biopsy confirmed the mass to be a focal adenocarcinoma. (Courtesy of Dr. Kristina G. Miles, Iowa State University.)

to and the morning of the procedure. It may also be used in cats.

Endoscopic mucosal examination of the colon has been described previously.[33–35] Abnormal findings may include erythema, increased mucosal granularity, increased mucosal friability, ulceration (rare), and erosions (common) (Table 138–5). Mass lesions (e.g., granulomatous, inflammatory, or neoplastic) are predominantly observed in the descending colon and rectum. Decreased wall distensibility is observed with infiltrative diseases. Loss of submucosal vascularity is a significant endoscopic observation and may be caused by mucosal edema, the accumulation of exudate (blood, mucus,

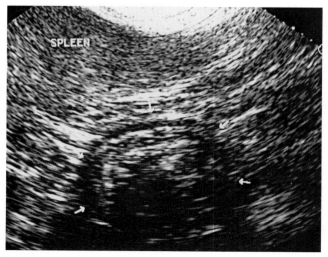

Figure 138–7. Ultrasonographic image (transverse view) of intussusception in a dog (arrows). Colonoscopy confirmed this to be a cecocolic intussusception, and typhlectomy was curative. (Courtesy of Dr. Kristina G. Miles, Iowa State University.)

TABLE 138–5. DESCRIPTIVE CRITERIA OF MUCOSAL ASSESSMENT

ENDOSCOPIC TERM	MUCOSAL ABNORMALITY
Erythema	Redness or hyperemia
Granularity	Increased surface texture
Friability	Ease of damage or bleeding
Ulcer	Focal, deep crateriform defect
Erosions	Multiple, superficial defects
Mass	Sessile or pedunculated lesion
Stricture	Circumferential narrowing of lumen

necrotic debris), or mucosal infiltration by inflammatory or neoplastic cells.

Colonic mucosal biopsy specimens are always obtained, regardless of endoscopic appearance. Focal lesions are biopsied directly. Masses are biopsied repeatedly to obtain deeper biopsy material. In the absence of gross mucosal abnormalities, obtain three to four biopsy specimens from each of the mid-ascending, mid-transverse, and mid-descending colonic regions. Overdistention of the colon with air causes colonic folds to flatten, making adequate tissue samples difficult to obtain. After obtaining mucosal samples, brush/touch cytologic specimens should be obtained and interpreted by a pathologist competent in gastrointestinal cytology.

INFECTIOUS DISORDERS

BACTERIAL COLITIS

Clostridial Colitis. *Clostridium perfringens* is a spore-forming, gram-positive, obligate anaerobic rod-shaped bacteria. It occurs in feces of normal and diarrheic dogs and cats.[36] Under appropriate environmental influences (e.g., diet[37]), *C. perfringens* sporulates. Sporulation of toxigenic strains causes enterotoxin A (also known as CPE) production and release.[38] Enterotoxin A may cause mucosal damage and colonic fluid secretion.[39] Clostridial colitis is a major cause of acute, nosocomial[40] as well as chronic large bowel diarrhea.[41, 42] It seems more common in dogs than in cats. Acute nosocomial diarrhea typically occurs within 1 to 5 days of being boarded; the dog suddenly begins defecating loose stools, often with obvious frank blood. Affected patients typically are otherwise normal, although some vomit or have mild lethargy. Clinical pathology abnormalities are rare. Acute nosocomial clostridial colitis typically resolves within 1 to 3 days, with or without therapy. Chronic clostridial colitis typically causes stools varying from soft and mucoid to bloody, which may wax and wane for years.

Definitive diagnosis can be difficult. Many normal animals have *C. perfringens* residing in the colon, and it is difficult to distinguish toxigenic from non-toxigenic strains. Finding excessive numbers (i.e., >3 to 5/oil immersion field) of rod-shaped bacteria with spores has been suggested to be supportive of clostridial colitis; however, one might not find spores in feces from affected dogs if colonic conditions are not conducive to spore formation at the time that the feces are examined. Reexamination 12 to 18 hours later may reveal numerous spores. Furthermore, normal dogs may have numerous spores without clinical disease.[28] Assaying for enterotoxin A, although supposedly more specific for diagnosing clostridial colitis, also has false-negative results (for the same reason that spores may be absent) and may be positive in clinically normal animals.[28] Mucosal biopsy typi-

GI

cally reveals a normal or near-normal colonic mucosa, although occasional animals have grossly abnormal colons (i.e., mucosal bleeding) and obvious histopathologic changes (e.g., catarrhal or suppurative changes).

Therapeutic trials may allow tentative diagnosis; however, apparent response to therapy does not guarantee that the patient had clostridial disease. Likewise, failure to respond to therapy does not eliminate clostridial colitis because there may be an underlying disease (e.g., dietary intolerance) permitting secondary clostridial colitis. Tylosin and amoxicillin are typically effective against *C. perfringens*. Metronidazole is inconsistently effective,[37] possibly because it does not always achieve adequate fecal concentrations.[43] Therapy probably does not eliminate *C. perfringens* from the colon; rather, it suppresses numbers of bacteria and/or prevents sporulation. If antibiotic therapy appears effective for a protracted time (which helps ensure that the patient did respond to the therapy and did not experience a spontaneous, transient remission), one may slowly decrease the dose and frequency to find the lowest effective dose (something not done for other bacterial infections because the goal here is to suppress toxin production, not eliminate the bacteria). Some patients respond to high-fiber diets, possibly because fiber changes the colonic microenvironment, making conditions unfavorable for sporulation. We often begin antibiotic therapy and a high-fiber diet simultaneously, hoping that the antibiotics may eventually be withdrawn and resolution maintained with high-fiber diet alone. Most animals with chronic clostridial colitis need to eat high-fiber diets or receive antibiotics for much of their life.

Affected animals usually respond within days to appropriate therapy. Prognosis for control is excellent. Multiple animals in one household can be affected[44]; clostridial spores are resistant to the environment and easily transmitted between animals. Anecdotally, there are reports of clostridial colitis affecting dogs and people in the same household.

Salmonellosis. *Salmonella* spp. are predominately motile, gram-negative facultative anaerobic rod-shaped bacteria found in normal and diarrheic animals. Reported prevalence rates in normal dogs vary from 1 per cent to greater than 30 per cent.[36, 45–47] *S. typhimurium* DT104 is reportedly the species most commonly grown from diarrheic dogs and cats.[48, 49] Transmission is probably via the fecal-oral route, including food, water, and fomites. There might be an association between exposure to birds and feline salmonellosis. If adequate numbers of *Salmonella* spp. are ingested and/or host defenses are compromised (e.g., antibiotics altering normal alimentary flora, other diseases), they may invade the intestines (especially at mucosal lymphoid aggregates) and produce diarrhea secondary to subsequent inflammation. Acute enterocolitis (with or without vomiting) is probably the most common sign, systemic inflammation or septicemia occurring occasionally. Overwhelming septicemia may cause neutropenia, resembling parvoviral enteritis. Salmonellosis may be acute or chronic.

Diagnosis requires growing *Salmonella* spp., eliminating other causes, plus an appropriate history and clinical picture. Fecal culture should consist of fresh feces being promptly submitted to a laboratory or using Amies transport media with charcoal.[36] Enrichment media and multiple cultures are recommended. Polymerase chain reaction techniques have also been used to demonstrate *Salmonella* spp. in feces.[50, 51] Culturing food may be useful in determining the source of infection.[47]

Mild cases usually require only symptomatic therapy (e.g., intestinal protectants, fluids). Antibiotics are believed to cause carrier states in animals with mild disease; however, evidence supporting this happening in dogs is meager. If culture results are unavailable, trimethoprim-sulfamethoxazole, ampicillin, chloramphenicol, and enrofloxacin are usually efficacious; however, *S. typhimurium* DT104 is often resistant to multiple drugs.[49, 52] Prognosis for recovery is good in non-septicemic patients. Salmonellosis is transmissible to people.[53] Infected cats can shed *Salmonella* in feces for greater than 14 weeks[54]; therefore, careful hygiene and appropriate disinfection are indicated. Children are at particular risk of being infected because of their characteristically poor hygiene.

Colibacillosis. *Escherichia coli* is a gram-negative, facultative anaerobic rod-shaped bacteria. It can be grown from almost all dogs' and cats' feces, but is also a major potential cause of diarrhea in people and animals. *E. coli* causes diarrhea by several mechanisms (e.g., enterotoxin, invasion, attaching/effacing). Verotoxin (VT)–producing *E. coli* (i.e., enterohemorrhagic *E. coli*) have been isolated from cats and dogs with and without diarrhea.[55–57] Canine isolates producing VT2 and heat-stable toxin were associated with diarrhea, whereas those only producing VT1 were not.[55] Signs usually consisted of acute diarrhea. The presence of VT-producing *E. coli* was not obviously associated with diarrhea in cats in one study,[57] while diarrheic cats had a higher incidence of VT-producing *E. coli* than non-diarrheic cats in another study.[56] In another study, attaching and effacing *E. coli* (which have the *eae*A gene) were found in 44 of 122 dogs dying of diarrhea. Approximately 45 per cent of these dogs had bacteria adhering to their colonic mucosa,[58] suggesting a possible causal relationship. Diagnosis requires isolating *E. coli*, demonstrating virulence factor(s) (which requires genetic probe or cell culture assay), and eliminating other causes. Treatment should probably be supportive. Antibiotics have not shortened the clinical course in affected people, although they may lessen shedding. Transmission from pets to people may occur,[59] but is not well documented.

Campylobacteriosis. *Campylobacter jejuni* is a motile, curved, gram-negative facultative anaerobic rod-shaped bacteria. It has been grown from up to 49 per cent of normal dogs, even being reported in 100 per cent of asymptomatic dogs in a colony.[36, 60–62] It is probably transmitted via the fecal-oral route including contaminated food and water. Poultry may be a common source. If ingested, it can colonize the mid to lower alimentary tract, especially the colon, invading the mucosa and/or elaborating toxins. It typically causes acute or chronic large bowel diarrhea in animals less than 6 months of age.[62] Fecal mucus and blood are common, and systemic illness and cholecystitis occasionally occur. Most infections are self-limiting. Diagnosis requires demonstrating the organism (i.e., culture or fecal cytology), eliminating other causes, and having an appropriate response to therapy. Cytologically, *C. jejuni* often appears as S- and W-shaped (i.e., "seagull wings") rods. It may be necessary to stain fecal smears for extended periods of time to demonstrate these rods well. Successful culture requires appropriate transport media (e.g., Cary-Blair held at 4°C) plus enrichment and/or selective media. Erythromycin (especially stearate) is the drug of choice, although tetracycline, aminoglycosides, clindamycin, and quinolones are usually effective.[63] Prognosis for recovery is excellent if there is no systemic involvement. *C. jejuni* is transmissible to people and other animals.[61]

Yersiniosis. *Yersinia enterocolitica* is a motile, gram-negative facultative anaerobic coccobacillus-shaped bacteria that is rarely found in dogs.[64, 65] More common in cold environments (especially around pigs), the organism is primarily spread via the fecal-oral route and ingestion of contaminated food and water. After being ingested, it may invade the mucosa and/or produce enterotoxins. Acute or chronic diarrhea may result. People often experience colic. Diagnosis requires growing the organism and eliminating other causes. Successful culture often requires cold enrichment and selective media. Tetracycline, trimethoprim-sulfamethoxazole, and cephalosporins are usually effective. Prognosis is unknown because so few canine and feline cases have been reported. The risk of transmission from pets to people is unknown but probably small; however, there are reports suggesting it has happened.[66]

Antibiotic-Associated Diarrhea and Antibiotic-Associated Colitis. Diarrhea associated with antibiotic administration occurs in people[67] and apparently dogs. In dogs, it occurs not infrequently, penicillins and first-generation cephalosporins often being incriminated. These diarrheas are typically mild, rarely containing blood. Stopping the antibiotic or switching to a different antibiotic usually resolves signs. Sometimes symptomatic therapy (e.g., Kaopectate, bismuth subsalicylate, withholding food) is necessary. Severe colonic disease (i.e., copious hematochezia, mucosal destruction) is probably rare in dogs and cats,[68] but may be due to overgrowth of particularly damaging bacteria (e.g., *Clostridium difficile, Pseudomonas aeruginosa*). Concurrent use of opioid antidiarrheals might make severe disease more likely, but this is uncertain. Excessive depression, copious blood in scant stools, and marked neutrophilic leukocytosis with a left shift suggest severe disease. If severe antibiotic-associated diarrhea is suspected, aerobic and anaerobic fecal cultures and assaying for *C. difficile* toxin are appropriate. One may perform colonoscopy in nonsedated animals; severe colonic mucosal disease is usually obvious. It is best to prevent severe antibiotic-associated diarrhea by changing antibiotics.

***Clostridium difficile*–Associated Disease.** *Clostridium difficile* causes severe, even fatal, antibiotic-associated colitis in people.[69] The bacterium has been found in diarrheic dogs[70] as well as asymptomatic dogs and cats.[71, 72] One may culture the organism (requires fresh feces and selective/enrichment media)[72] or detect its toxin in the feces.[73] If *C. difficile* appears to be causing diarrhea, oral vancomycin or metronidazole is a reasonable therapy.[74] Prognosis is uncertain, as is the risk of transmission to people.

Intestinal Spirochetosis. Large numbers of motile spirochetes are found in the feces of some dogs with large bowel diarrhea.[75, 76] The pathogenicity of these organisms is not well defined, and some consider their presence to be due to being washed out of colonic crypts by copious colonic secretions. However, spirochetes are suspected pathogens in diarrheic primates.[77]

PARASITIC COLITIS

Whipworms. *Trichuris vulpis* is a common cause of canine large bowel disease in parts of the United States. Up to 50 per cent of dogs are infected in some areas.[78] Cats are occasionally infected with *T. serrata* and *T. campanula*.[79] Whipworms have a direct life cycle. Eggs usually embryonate 30 days after being shed.[80] Ingested eggs hatch in the small intestine, and larvae migrate to the cecum and sometimes the large intestine where they burrow into the mucosa, feeding on tissue fluid and blood. Host response varies from mild, localized inflammation to mucosal hyperplasia and granulomatous inflammation.

Clinical signs vary from none to intermittent diarrhea to soft stools with specks of blood to copious diarrhea with obvious blood, depending upon the number of worms and host response. Eosinophilia, anemia, and hypoalbuminemia are possible, although uncommon. Some dogs develop a constellation of signs and laboratory findings suggestive of hypoadrenocorticism (i.e., hyponatremia, hyperkalemia, metabolic acidosis, and prerenal azotemia) that resolve after worms are eliminated.[81] Perityphilitis with adhesion of the cecum to the body wall may occur, causing some dogs to constantly lick their sides.[78]

Diagnosis is made by finding eggs in feces or parasites during colonoscopy. Eggs (Fig. 138–8) are tan colored, have a plug on both ends, and are usually longer than 75 μm.[78] They may be shed intermittently, and negative fecal flotation examinations do not eliminate trichuriasis. The eggs are relatively heavy, and fecal flotation solutions should be appropriately dense (i.e., specific gravity $\geq$ 1.200) to ensure they float. It is usually reasonable to treat empirically; most dogs with symptomatic whipworm infections improve after appropriate therapy.

Fenbendazole, febantel, milbemycin oxime,[82, 83] and oxibendazole[84] are usually effective in infested dogs. Dogs should be retreated at monthly intervals for 3 months.[80] Prognosis for cure is excellent. *Trichuris* eggs are resistant to environmental influences and disinfectants, making reinfection easy. Prolonged sunlight and desiccation may kill the eggs,[78] and concrete surfaces may be disinfected with fire. However, it is almost impossible to kill eggs in soil[78] without killing all vegetation. There is minimal risk of people being infected with *T. vulpis*.

Trichomoniasis. *Pentatrichomonas hominis* is found in dogs[85] and cats.[86] It is probably a normal commensal and has a direct life cycle, being passed between animals by the fecal-oral route. Identification of motile trophozoites on direct fecal examination is diagnostic. Motile *Pentatrichomonas* trophozoites (5 to 20 × 3 to 14 μm)[87] are easy to confuse with *Giardia lambia* trophozoites (12 to 17 × 7 to 10 μm) if one does not see the undulating membrane found on *Pentatrichomonas*. Occasionally present in large numbers in diarrheic animals, there is no good evidence that the organism is pathogenic. Diarrheic animals with large numbers of *P. hominis* seemingly often have other causes of diarrhea.[80] Metronidazole typically eliminates the organism, although reinfection may occur.

Amebiasis. *Entamoeba histolytica* is rarely found in dogs. Dogs[88] are infected when they ingest infective cysts,

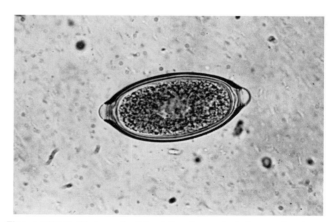

Figure 138–8. Photograph of fecal flotation analysis from a dog demonstrating a characteristic ovum from whipworms.

and ameba invade colonic mucosa causing ulcers and erosions. Pathogenicity depends upon the numbers of organisms, colonic bacteria, and the host's immune response. Signs vary from none to bloody diarrhea and dysentery. Finding trophozoites in the stool (usually liquid stools) or colonic mucosa is diagnostic. Alternatively, cysts may be found (usually in formed feces). Ameba trophozoites cytologically resemble leukocytes. Therapy usually consists of metronidazole.[80] Prognosis is uncertain because there have been so few reported cases.

There is minimal human health risk from infected dogs because they do not generally shed infective cysts. Dogs are more likely to be infected by people than people are to be infected by dogs.

Balantidiasis. *Balantidium coli* is a large (up to 150 μm long), ciliated protozoan primarily found in pigs. Dogs are rarely infected,[89] and those that harbor the parasite usually have contact with pigs. After an animal swallows infective cysts, organisms may invade cecal or colonic mucosa. Signs vary from none to ulcerative colitis. Concurrent presence of *T. vulpis* seemingly worsens signs.[90] Finding motile trophozoites and/or cysts is suggestive; however, trophozoites in canine feces may be passing through the dog after it has eaten infected pig feces (i.e., they indicate coprophagia, not infection).[78] Treating whipworms, if present, often alleviates clinical signs. *B. coli* may be eliminated with metronidazole or tetracycline. Prognosis is excellent with treatment. There is minimal human health risk.

Heterobilharziasis. *Heterobilharzia americana* rarely occurs in dogs.[91] Raccoons, nutria, bobcats, rabbits, and mice are common sources, and dogs are infected when motile cercaria from snails penetrate their skin.[78] Resulting schistosomes migrate to the liver and eventually to mesenteric veins, where there they start releasing eggs 66 to 77 days after infection. The eggs lodge in the bowel and produce a granulomatous response. Clinical signs vary from none to large bowel diarrhea plus anorexia. Hypoalbuminemia, anemia, hyperglobulinemia, eosinophilia, and hypercalcemia[92] may occur in severe cases. Diagnosis is made by finding eggs in feces or biopsied tissue. The eggs are 60 to 80 × 74 to 113 μm and have a thin non-operculated shell (Fig. 138–9).[78] Direct fecal smears or flotation with 0.85 per cent saline are preferred means of finding the eggs. Fenbendazole, especially when used sequentially with praziquantel, may be effective.[78, 93] It is reasonable to check or treat asymptomatic dogs in the same environment as the infected dog. There is

no human health risk for being directly infected by a dog shedding the eggs.

Ancylostomiasis. Hookworms may rarely occur in the colon if there is an overwhelming infestation. Therapy with pyrantel or fenbendazole should be curative. Repeat treatment in 3 weeks is recommended.

FUNGAL/ALGAL COLITIS

Histoplasmosis. *Histoplasma capsulatum* is a dimorphic fungus affecting dogs and cats.[94] Infection occurs after inhaling spores from the environment. Some infections remain localized, while others disseminate. Colonic disease typically predominates in dogs with disseminated disease,[95] whereas colonic involvement is rare in cats,[96] usually only occurring in advanced cases. Signs in affected dogs vary from mild, chronic large bowel diarrhea to severe disease causing fecal mucus, hematochezia, tenesmus, fever, and weight loss. Labored breathing, thrombocytopenia, and/or anemia indicates extra-alimentary involvement. Small bowel involvement occurs infrequently. Hypoalbuminemia[97] associated with large bowel disease is suggestive of such colonic fungal infections (as well as neoplasia).

Diagnosis requires finding the yeast; current serologic tests looking for antibodies to *H. capsulatum* are unreliable.[94] Colonic or rectal mucosal cytology (not fecal cytology) is often diagnostic, especially if the mucosa is thickened or rough. If mucosal cytology is negative, colonoscopy and multiple mucosal biopsies are required. Special stains (e.g., PAS) are indicated, especially if there is any mention of neutrophilic, histiocytic, or granulomatous infiltrates, however minor. It is easy to miss the organisms if only hematoxylin and eosin stains are applied.[94]

Any dog with large bowel diarrhea, especially but not limited to those from endemic areas, may have colonic histoplasmosis. Therefore, it is imperative that dogs with chronic large bowel disease not be given a therapeutic trial with corticosteroids for suspected lymphocytic-plasmacytic colitis. Such administration may cause clinical deterioration and possibly death.[97] Therapy usually consists of itraconazole[98] or liposomal amphotericin B. Prognosis depends upon how advanced the disease is. Widespread disease, especially with pulmonary involvement causing dyspnea or tachypnea, carries a guarded to poor prognosis. There is minimal risk of dog-person transmission. It is more likely that a person would become infected from the same source as the infected dog.[99]

Pythiosis. *Pythium insidiosum* is an aquatic oomycete primarily affecting dogs in the southeastern United States, although it also occurs in the Midwest.[100] Motile zoospores are probably ingested from the environment and penetrate alimentary mucosa. There is debate as to whether preexisting alimentary disease is necessary for spore penetration. Any area of the alimentary tract may be affected. Infections may involve the colon, ileocolic,[101] or rectal areas; cats are seldom affected. *P. insidiosum* typically causes marked thickening of the bowel wall as a result of submucosal disease, although overlying mucosa may be hemorrhagic and ulcerated. If the large bowel or ileum is involved, signs may include large bowel diarrhea with or without hypoalbuminemia and weight loss. If the rectal area is involved, the lesion may mimic perianal fistulas or rectal adenocarcinoma. Cutaneous infections also occur.

Diagnosis requires demonstrating the organism. Hyphae with rare septae are primarily found in the submucosa, along

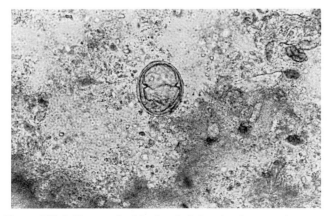

Figure 138–9. Photograph of fecal analysis in a dog demonstrating an egg from *Heterobilharzia americana*.

with marked fibrosis; therefore, surgical biopsy or biopsy using rigid forceps is usually needed. The abundant fibrosis makes it difficult to adequately biopsy the submucosa with flexible endoscopic biopsy forceps. Flexible biopsy forceps obtain overlying mucosa that typically has secondary inflammation and necrosis but seldom contains organisms. Cytology may be diagnostic if one scraps the thickened submucosa with a scalpel blade to obtain material. However, the hyphae do not take up typically used stains, but appear as "ghosts"; special stains are required to demonstrate organisms.[102] Finding hyphae with rare septa allows presumptive diagnosis. Eosinophilic infiltrates are common but not a consistent finding. Regional lymph nodes may be involved. Vascular involvement with thrombosis occasionally occurs. Immunohistochemical staining and culture allow definitive diagnosis. Freezing may kill the organism.

Surgical resection may be curative. If total resection is impossible (e.g., rectal lesions, lesions involving the mesenteric root), prognosis is poor. Itraconazole and liposomal amphotericin B may help or cure occasional animals, but most respond poorly. There is no evidence of animal-animal transmission,[102] but people could be infected from the same source responsible for infecting the dog.

Prototthecosis. *Prototheca zopfii* and *P. wickerhamii* are unicellular achlorophyllous algae[103] that rarely cause disease in dogs and cats. They probably are ingested from the environment, the site of colonization depending upon the species of *Prototheca*. Colonic involvement may cause mild inflammation, granulomatous responses, or ulceration/hemorrhage. Collies seem to be predisposed. Clinical signs are typically bloody large bowel diarrhea with or without weight loss.[104] Extracolonic involvement may cause blindness or CNS signs.[103] Diagnosis requires demonstrating the organism cytologically or histopathologically, or growing it from tissue. There is no consistently effective therapy. Anecdotally, liposomal amphotericin B may sometimes be effective. The prognosis is guarded at best, and poor for widely disseminated cases. There is no known animal-animal transmission.

INFLAMMATORY/IMMUNE-MEDIATED DISORDERS

ACUTE COLITIS

Acute large bowel diarrhea is generally self-limiting. Causes may include diet (e.g., allergy, intolerance, bacterial toxins, foreign material, hair), bacteria and/or their toxins, viral agents, and/or parasites. Diarrhea may be the initial sign, or vomiting that progresses to diarrhea may occur as a toxin or irritant proceeds from the stomach to the small and then the large intestines. Acute colitis typically causes multiple defecations per day, often with fecal mucus, hematochezia, tenesmus, and/or secondary anal excoriation. Some animals evidence depression, although most are normal except for diarrhea. Some resent rectal examination, probably because of accompanying proctitis.

Typically a self-limiting problem, underlying causes are seldom defined. History, physical examination, and elimination of other causes of hematochezia (e.g., parvoviral enteritis, hemorrhagic gastroenteritis) permit tentative diagnosis. Nosocomial, acute colitis suggests a bacterial cause (e.g., clostridial colitis). Multiple animal involvement suggests bacterial, parasitic, and dietary causes. Multiple direct and fecal flotation examinations are always appropriate; parasites may contribute to the problem even when they are not the

primary cause. Supportive care and reduced oral intake for 1 to 2 days to minimize the amount of stool passing through the colon usually suffice. If a bacterial cause is suspected, appropriate antibiotics are reasonable. Motility modifiers (e.g., loperamide) are seldom needed. If diarrhea continues for more than 3 to 5 days despite such therapy or if the patient has systemic signs (e.g., fever, anorexia, severe depression, weakness), a more thorough diagnostic approach is recommended, (e.g., CBC, serum chemistries, fecal culture).

IDIOPATHIC INFLAMMATORY BOWEL DISEASES: OVERVIEW

Inflammatory bowel disease (IBD) denotes a spectrum of chronic, inflammatory disorders of the gastrointestinal tract of unknown cause and pathogenesis.[105, 106] Interest in IBD stems from the incidence of the clinical disease syndrome in companion animals and some similarities to idiopathic IBD (e.g., ulcerative colitis and Crohn's disease) in humans.[107] Histologic lesions are characterized by mucosal epithelial/glandular alterations and a variably increased mucosal cellular infiltrate that suggests an immunologic pathogenesis.[105, 106, 108, 109]

Despite extensive investigations in people, no clearly defined causes have emerged. Studies involving animal models have identified interactions between the mucosal immune system, host genetic susceptibility, and environmental factors (e.g., normal microflora).[110] Two general hypotheses have been proposed. First, the disease is due to an abnormal immune response (e.g., precipitated by increased intestinal permeability, defective suppressor function of GALT, and/or other, yet to be defined, primary immunologic events); and second, the disease is initiated by an appropriate immune response to an enteric pathogen.[111] With either paradigm, both cellular components (clonal expansion of activated intestinal B and T lymphocytes) and molecular elements (complement fragments, prostanoids, leukotrienes, proinflammatory cytokines, leukocyte proteases, nitric oxide, and oxygen-derived free radicals) likely contribute to mucosal inflammation.[112] Clinical signs are attributed to mucosal cellular infiltrates and inflammatory mediators.[113]

Objective criteria for diagnosis of canine and feline IBD are described.[108] It is *essential* that clinical signs be correlated with histologic evidence of gastroenteritis, and that other causes for chronic mucosal inflammation be excluded by appropriate diagnostic testing. Classification of IBD is based on the mucosal cellular infiltrate and the area(s) of the gastrointestinal tract that are inflamed.

Lymphocytic-Plasmacytic Colitis. Lymphocytic-plasmacytic colitis (LPC) is the most common IBD of canine[113] and feline[114] colon. The etiology for LPC is unknown, but many of the immunologic factors implicated above are probably important. Dogs with LPC have increased numbers of mucosal IgA- and IgG-containing cells and CD3[+] T cells in comparison with control dogs (Table 138–6).[10] Furthermore, overproduction of nitric oxide in dogs with LPC is suggested by increased colonic luminal nitrite levels and increased mucosal expression and concentrations of inducible nitric oxide synthase (iNOS) in endoscopic biopsy specimens.[115, 116]

Breeds seemingly at increased risk for LPC include Boxers, German shepherds, and, perhaps, purebred cats.[117] Most affected animals are middle aged or older, although a distinct subset of patients will manifest signs at an early age.[108] Clinical signs in dogs are often classic for large bowel dysfunction, with frequent passage of small quantities of

GI

TABLE 138–6. COMPARISON OF COLONIC IMMUNE CELLS IN HEALTHY DOGS AND DOGS WITH IBD

GROUP	IgA	IgG	IgM	CD3+
Healthy dogs (n = 10)	99 (±6)	23 (±2)	42 (±4)	137 (±17)
IBD dogs (n = 11)	179 (±15)*	38 (±2)*	41 (±4)	179 (±10)†

Data are expressed as mean ± SEM.
*$P < .01$ compared with healthy dogs.
†$P < .05$ compared with healthy dogs.
From Jergens AE, et al.: Colonic immune cell populations in canine inflammatory bowel disease: An immunohistochemical and morphometric study. Am J Vet Res, in press.

diarrhea, hematochezia, and/or tenesmus reported by most clients. Systemic signs (anorexia, weight loss, vomiting) are uncommon except with concurrent small intestinal involvement. Physical examination is often unremarkable. Laboratory abnormalities are usually mild and nonspecific.

Histologic evaluation of biopsy specimens is essential for diagnosis. Abnormalities observed during colonoscopy may include increased mucosal friability, increased mucosal granularity, loss of submucosal vascularity, and erosions (Figs. 138–10 and 138–11).[108, 118] Absence of these observations does not eliminate LPC. Histologic assessment of mucosal specimens by a pathologist familiar with IBD is required to differentiate LPC from other causes of lymphocytic-plasmacytic inflammation. Biopsy interpretation is notoriously subjective from one pathologist to the next, and is further hampered by the technical constraints of specimen size and procurement/processing artifacts inherent in evaluation of endoscopic specimens. No standard microscopic grading system of IBD lesions has been established. The senior author (AEJ) utilizes a grading system based upon the presence of cellular infiltrates *and* the extent of architectural disruption and mucosal epithelial changes (Table 138–7).[108, 119] Other histologic grading schemes to assess the degree of mucosal inflammation have been published.[109, 117]

Eosinophilic Colitis. It is debatable whether eosinophilic colitis (EC) represents a true variant of IBD or whether it is an allergic manifestation to dietary or parasitic antigens.[113, 114] In the authors' experience, EC is considerably less common (more frequent in dogs than in cats) than LPC, although the true prevalence is unknown. Eosinophilic colitis may occur alone, as a component of eosinophilic enterocolitis, or in association with the hypereosinophilic syndrome in cats.[120] Granulomatous eosinophilic inflammation is a rare feature in some dogs with EC.[121] The etiopathogenesis of EC is unknown, but similar immune mechanisms as for LPC are suspect.

There are no apparent sex or breed predispositions for EC. As with LPC, middle-aged animals are affected most frequently. Clinical signs in pets with EC may include bloody, mucoid diarrhea and tenesmus. Cats with hypereosinophilic syndrome may show general malaise, bloody diarrhea, coughing, and dermatologic abnormalities.[122] Physical examination may detect palpably thickened intestinal loops in both dogs and cats. Peripheral lymphadenopathy and hepatosplenomegaly are also reported in cats with hypereosinophilic syndrome. Laboratory testing reveals eosinophilia in some dogs and most cats. As with LPC, mucosal biopsy is required for diagnosis. The endoscopic findings are similar to those described for LPC. Histologic lesions are characterized by a diffuse infiltration of eosinophils within the mucosa; however, lesser numbers of other immune cell types may also be present.[4] Cats with the hypereosinophilic syndrome may have transmural eosinophilic inflammation detectable on full-thickness excisional specimens.[122]

Variants of Colonic IBD. A variety of IBD variants, including chronic histiocytic ulcerative colitis (CHUC), suppurative colitis, and granulomatous enterocolitis, are occasionally diagnosed. Like LPC and EC, most animals present

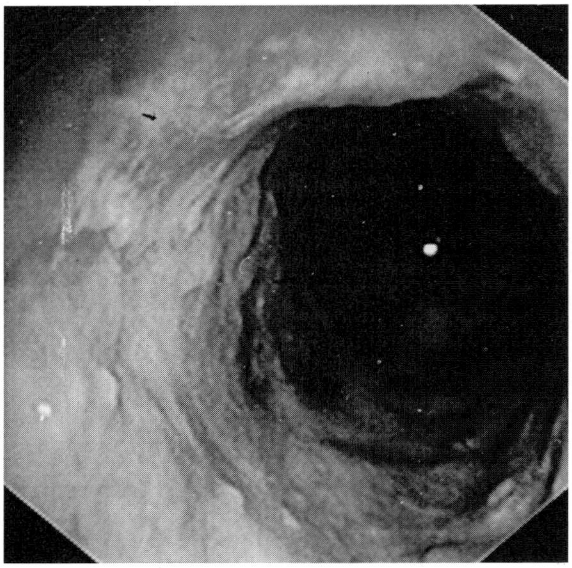

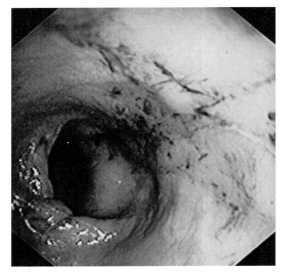

Figure 138–10. Endoscopic appearance of the descending colon in a dog with chronic tenesmus. Note the increased mucosal granularity, which is suggestive of infiltrative disease. Histologic review of endoscopic biopsy specimens confirmed a diagnosis of severe lymphocytic-plasmacytic colitis.

Figure 138–11. Endoscopic appearance of the canine transverse colon. Multiple erosions are observed along the lateral wall of this structure. Histologic review of endoscopic biopsy specimens confirmed a diagnosis of neutrophilic and lymphocytic-plasmacytic colitis.

TABLE 138–7. PROPOSED HISTOLOGIC GRADING SYSTEM FOR INFLAMMATORY BOWEL DISEASE (IBD)

HISTOLOGIC LESION	SEVERITY OF IBD		
	Mild	*Moderate*	*Severe*
Cellular infiltrate	+	+	+
Epithelial immaturity		+	+
Focal epithelial necrosis		+	+
Multifocal epithelial necrosis			+
Architectural distortion*			+

*Denotes the presence of significant villus or glandular atrophy, mucosal edema, and/or lamina propria fibrosis.

with intractable large bowel diarrhea, hematochezia, and tenesmus of variable severity.

Histiocytic ulcerative colitis is the most frequently diagnosed IBD variant. Histologically, lesions are characterized by a mixed inflammatory infiltrate with PAS-positive histiocytes. Boxers are predisposed to CHUC, and the disease is diagnosed most frequently in male dogs less than 1 year of age.[123, 124] Lethargy, anorexia, and weight loss are commonly observed. Colonoscopy usually reveals increased mucosal granularity, friability, and diffuse erosions (Fig. 138–12). Other forms of IBD and non–PAS-positive histiocytic colitis must be ruled out before CHUC can be diagnosed. Prognosis is generally poor.

Neutrophils are usually a minor component of the inflammatory response in IBD and are primarily seen with erosive lesions of the alimentary tract. However, suppurative colitis occurs especially in cats.[125] Histologic lesions include dense infiltrates of lymphocytes, plasma cells, and neutrophils. The cause is unknown. Suppurative colitis has also been associated with bacterial colitis (*Clostridium* spp. and *Campylobacter jejuni*).

Granulomatous enterocolitis (regional enteritis) is an uncommon but serious IBD variant primarily reported in dogs.[4, 126] Most dogs have been males less than 4 years of age.[127] Clinical signs include chronic colitis, weight loss, and vomiting associated with distal alimentary tract (ileocolic)

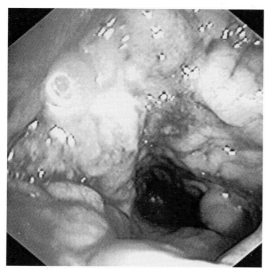

Figure 138–12. Endoscopic appearance of the canine descending colon in a 7-month-old Boxer with chronic hematochezia. Note the severe, increased granularity to the colonic mucosa. Histologic review of biopsy specimens was diagnostic of histiocytic ulcerative colitis.

obstruction. Diagnostic work-up is identical as for other forms of colonic IBD. Transmural infiltrates of non–PAS-positive histiocytes (with a significant eosinophilic infiltrate) are the salient histologic lesion.

Management of Colonic IBD. Management of colonic IBD may include controlled diets, dietary fiber supplementation, and administration of anti-inflammatory and immunosuppressive drugs. Well-designed therapeutic trials have not been performed, and therapy remains largely empiric, being influenced by the rapidity of clinical remission, the severity of adverse effects, the acceptability by patients and clients, and drug costs.

Dietary Therapy. Because dietary antigens are implicated as causing IBD, dietary modification is typically prescribed. Nutritional therapy likely augments clinical improvement through nutrient repletion and reduction in the mucosal inflammatory response to dietary antigens or additives. The benefits of dietary therapy (alone or in conjunction with pharmacologic therapy) in the management of canine, feline, and human colonic IBD are well documented.[117, 128–132]

The most convenient means of dietary manipulation in veterinary patients is with controlled (hypoallergenic) diets. These diets are defined as those in which the clinician has control over all or most of the dietary ingredients. General characteristics of a controlled diet usually include highly digestible protein and carbohydrate sources; relative hypoallergenicity; gluten-free foods; foods low in lactose and fat; a regimen nutritionally balanced; and high palatability.[113] These diets should be formulated with ingredients that the animal has not been fed before (e.g., novel protein source) or that are unlikely to evoke allergic responses (e.g., potatoes). Thus, suitable hypoallergenic diets will vary among patients depending on their previous dietary history. A variety of commercial controlled diets are available. Homemade recipes are preferred by some clinicians but are nutritionally incomplete for long-term use (Table 138–8). Controlled diets probably have to be fed at least 6 to 10 weeks to assess their efficacy. Furthermore, some clinicians advocate changing the novel protein source after 6 weeks of therapy to prevent acquired hypersensitivity and delayed recovery of IBD.[113] The controlled diet should be fed for several months beyond remission of signs before attempting to wean the animal onto its regular ration.

Fiber Supplementation. Fiber-enriched diets are recommended to mitigate signs of large bowel diarrhea and tenesmus. Dietary fiber may increase fecal consistency, bind potential colonic irritants, improve abnormal colonic motility, and produce beneficial short-chain fatty acids (e.g., butyrate), which positively influence large bowel structure and function.[133–135] Commercial high-fiber diets or appropriate hypoallergenic diets supplemented with moderately fermentable fiber (e.g., psyllium or oat bran) may be fed. Dosages are empiric but generally range from 1 to 6 teaspoons per meal, depending on the animal's body weight.

TABLE 138–8. EXAMPLES OF HOMEMADE, HYPOALLERGENIC DIETS

1 part skinless chicken or turkey to 2 parts boiled or baked potato (no skin)
1 part boiled/broiled white fish to 2 parts boiled or baked potato (no skin)
1 part boiled skinless mutton or venison or rabbit to 2 parts boiled or baked potato (no skin)
1 part low-fat cottage cheese to 2 parts boiled or baked potato (no skin)

From Willard MD: General therapeutic principles. *In* Nelson RW, Couto CG (eds): Small Animal Internal Medicine. St. Louis, CV Mosby, 1998, p 390.

GI

Dietary therapy with fiber supplementation is continued indefinitely, even after the completion of drug therapy.

Pharmacologic Therapy. In the senior author's experience, dietary management alone for moderate to severe IBD is seldom successful and most animals will require pharmacologic therapy. Effective modulation of mucosal inflammation is at present achieved with drugs (e.g., corticosteroids, sulfasalazine, 5-aminosalicylic acid) that inhibit or decrease the formation of a variety of inflammatory mediators or block their specific receptors (see IBD overview).

Corticosteroids. The efficacy of corticosteroids for acute IBD in humans is well established.[136, 137] Steroids have systemic effects plus the potential for topical activity via poorly absorbable or rapidly metabolized preparations. They may inhibit the release of arachidonic acid from cell membranes (thereby reducing the formation of proinflammatory eicosanoids such as leukotriene [LT] B$_4$) and reduce lymphoid proliferation.[138, 139]

Oral corticosteroids are reasonable first-choice agents for induction therapy of IBD colitis in some dogs and most cats. Prednisone or prednisolone are used most frequently because they have short durations of action, are cost-effective, and are widely available. As previously noted, the dosage of prednisone used is empirically chosen as a compromise between clinical effectiveness and liability to adverse effects. Beneficial responses are usually observed when dosages of 0.5 to 1 mg/lb body weight/day are used in conjunction with dietary therapy. Induction therapy of 2 to 4 weeks (depending on severity of signs and type of histologic lesion) is generally recommended. Higher doses (2 to 3 mg/lb/day) of corticosteroids may be required to control signs in cats with eosinophilic colitis or hypereosinophilic syndrome.[140] Combination drug therapy (e.g., steroids combined with metronidazole, azathioprine, or sulfasalazine) allows a reduced steroid dose for maintenance therapy. Once the desired clinical response is achieved, the dose of oral glucocorticoid may be judiciously reduced by 25 per cent at 1- to 2-week intervals while maintaining remission with use of a controlled diet.

Alternative glucocorticoid preparations characterized by high topical anti-inflammatory activity and first-pass hepatic metabolism have been used in human patients with IBD.[141–143] They were developed to attain maximal therapeutic effect of conventional steroids while minimizing deleterious systemic effects. These medications are administered rectally (tixocortol pivilate, beclomethasone dipropionate) or orally (budesonide). The efficacy (and potential toxicity) of these new preparations in dogs and cats remains to be proven, although anecdotal evidence suggests that budesonide may be of value in some dogs with LPC.[144]

Sulfasalazine. Sulfasalazine (SASA) has been the stalwart of therapy for human IBD as demonstrated by well-controlled studies. It has an established role in the treatment of acute mild and moderate ulcerative colitis (UC), it maintains UC in remission, and is used in the symptomatic treatment of Crohn's ileitis and ileocolitis.[145–147] Similar studies have not been performed in companion animals, but clinical impressions indicate that it may be the first-choice drug for canine LPC.

SASA consists of mesalamine (5-aminosalicylate or 5-ASA) linked by an azo bond to sulfapyridine.[148] Following oral administration, the drug undergoes partial (30 per cent) small intestinal absorption and is delivered relatively intact to the colon. Bacteria in the distal small bowel and colon cleave the azo bond, releasing both components. Most of the cleaved sulfapyridine is absorbed by the colon, metabolized

in the liver, and excreted by the kidneys. Sulfapyridine has no therapeutic effect and acts only as a carrier molecule to deliver 5-ASA to the large bowel. The 5-ASA moiety is poorly absorbed and has potent topical anti-inflammatory activity on the colonic mucosa. Much experimental work has shown that mesalamine inhibits lipoxygenase (which causes decreased leukotriene levels), acts as a scavenger of oxygen-derived free radicals, and inhibits autoantibody formation.[149, 150]

The recommended dosage range for SASA in dogs is 9 to 22 mg/lb up to a maximum of 1.0 g q8h in refractory patients or those having severe disease.[151, 152] The senior author has had considerable success using an initial dosage of 5.7 mg/lb q8h. It is important to continue induction therapy for a minimum of 4 weeks before modifying drug dosage. With resolution of signs, SASA dosages are gradually decreased by 25 per cent at 2-week intervals and eventually discontinued while maintaining dietary management. Caution is advised in using SASA in cats because of their sensitivity to salicylates. Nevertheless, safe and effective feline dosages have been reported (4.5 to 9 mg/lb q24h) by others.[140] The most common side effects of SASA in small animals include anorexia, vomiting, anemia (cats), and transient or permanent keratoconjunctivitis sicca (KCS).[153] Dogs undergoing long-term SASA treatment should have tear production periodically assessed to identify KCS early. The hypothesis that toxicity of SASA could be ascribed to sulfapyridine and clinical efficacy to 5-ASA has resulted in the development of newer 5-ASA agents.

Newer 5-ASA Preparations. Topical and oral 5-ASA preparations are now used for treatment of human IBD.[154–156] Two oral preparations of potential use in dogs include olsalazine and mesalamine. Olsalazine (Dipentum) consists of two molecules of mesalamine linked by an azo bond.[157] Various enteric-coated preparations of mesalamine (Pentasa, Asacol) release active drug (5-ASA) in the distal small intestine and colon, respectively.[157] The use of these agents for treatment of canine and feline IBD has not been critically evaluated, but there are substantial anecdotal reports of their efficacy. The proposed dose is approximately one half that of SASA.

Metronidazole. Anecdotal reports suggest that metronidazole has beneficial effects in the therapy of canine and feline IBD.[113, 119] Metronidazole has been shown to be superior to placebo and equal to sulfasalazine in the treatment of active Crohn's disease by controlled trials.[158] Its mechanisms of action might include antiprotozoal action, inhibition of cellular immunity, and bactericidal spectrum of activity against anaerobes (e.g., *Bacteroides* spp).[119, 159, 160] The recommended dosage of metronidazole used in dogs and cats for IBD is 4.5 to 9 mg/lb q8–12h. Metronidazole is most often combined with corticosteroids or sulfasalazine in patients having moderate-to-severe clinical signs or histologic lesions. It is also effective as a sole agent in animals having mild disease. Uncommon side effects include anorexia and vomiting in cats and CNS toxicity (at high doses) in dogs and cats.[161]

Azathioprine. Azathioprine (AZA) is a potent cytotoxic drug occasionally used as adjunctive therapy in *severe and refractory* IBD. This drug is metabolized in the body to 6-mercaptopurine (6-MP), its active metabolite, which functions to interfere with antigenic triggering of lymphocytes.[139] Controversy exists concerning the efficacy and safety of AZA and 6-MP in the treatment of human IBD.[162] The suggested dosage is 1 mg/lb q24h in dogs and 0.14 mg/lb q48h in cats.[113, 140] A lag time of 3 to 5 weeks is expected before clinical improvement may be observed. Side effects seen in dogs and cats include leukopenia, hepatic disease, and acute pancreatitis.[113] A complete blood count should be performed every 2 weeks in animals receiving AZA therapy.

Miscellaneous Immunomodulating Drugs. A variety of other drugs (e.g., cyclophosphamide, chlorambucil, cyclosporine, tylosin) are occasionally of value in treating refractory IBD. Cyclosporine acts primarily by inhibiting interleukin-2 release from helper T cells, which prevents T-cell recruitment/amplification and inhibits the release of gamma-interferon.[163] Preliminary observations in humans with IBD suggest that cyclosporine may act synergistically with corticosteroids and produce a more rapid response than classic immunosuppressants.[164]

Dietary Sensitivity. Dietary sensitivity may manifest as either *food intolerance* (e.g., a non–immune-mediated reaction to a dietary component) or *food allergy* (e.g., an immune-mediated hypersensitivity to a dietary component). Dietary sensitivity is an important contributing factor in canine and feline large bowel diarrhea. The inciting food may cause direct toxicity or trigger mucosal inflammation and the generation of clinical signs.[165–167] Various colonic disorders, including LPC and EC, have been attributed to dietary sensitivity, and management of these diseases is frequently more successful when dietary therapy is included.[113, 114]

Historically associating a certain diet with gastrointestinal signs suggests dietary sensitivity. However, dietary sensitivity can only be diagnosed by elimination-challenge trials.[165] Practically speaking, this may be difficult to accomplish because clients often fail to adhere to recommended diets. Furthermore, a diagnosis of food allergy requires that the adverse reaction be immunologically mediated.[168]

Treatment of the food-sensitive animal is most conveniently achieved by using commercially prepared hypoallergenic diets (see dietary therapy of IBD). Patients with food allergy associated with gastrointestinal inflammatory disorders (e.g., such as IBD) can be fed diets based on protein hydrolysates to minimize the risk of acquired sensitivities to the therapeutic diet.[165]

THERAPEUTIC MANAGEMENT OF CHRONIC COLITIS

Because most dogs and cats with chronic large bowel diarrhea have dietary, parasitic, and/or bacterial causes (all of which can be hard to diagnose with endoscopy/biopsy), and because these patients often are otherwise healthy (i.e., they are not losing weight and can afford to have diagnosis and therapy delayed), therapeutic trials are often a reasonable initial approach instead of major diagnostic work-ups that include endoscopy and biopsy. However, digital rectal examination and multiple fecal examinations for parasites and ova should always be performed. When designing a therapeutic trial, you should select a disease that is reasonably likely and then use a therapy that is extremely effective for that disease. Thus, if the therapeutic trial fails, you may at least eliminate that disease as being a cause and move on to another. It is important (1) to perform the trial long enough so that a response to therapy will be obvious and (2) continue the trial for much longer than you believe is necessary so that you can distinguish the patient that fortuitously got better about the same time that you started the therapy from the patient that is truly responding to your therapy. Many large bowel diseases wax and wane, and it is easy to mistake spontaneous improvement for response to medication. If the

diarrhea recurs while the therapeutic trial is ongoing, that is usually a sign that the therapeutic trial never really worked in the first place (or that the owners have broken the therapeutic trial). The biggest disadvantage of therapeutic trials is that a patient may have more than one disease occurring simultaneously (e.g., clostridial colitis and food intolerance), making it easy to decide that a disease is not present when in fact it is.

Clostridial colitis usually responds promptly to therapy with amoxicillin or tylosin. If the patient has not responded within 5 to 8 days of initiating therapy, it is very doubtful that clostridial colitis is the sole cause of the animal's diarrhea. If you believe that one of these antibiotics eliminated the diarrhea, treat for at least another 2 weeks before you stop or change therapy. Likewise, a 3-day course of fenbendazole is usually very effective against whipworms, although retreatment may be needed.

Dietary trials may include fiber-supplemented diets or hypoallergenic (elimination) diets. Most animals that respond to a fiber-supplemented diet do so within 1 to 2 weeks of starting the diet. If the patient appears to respond to a fiber-supplemented diet, it should be continued for at least another 4 weeks (or indefinitely). Hypoallergenic diets are hard to design and may need to be fed for 6 to 10 weeks before a response is seen. Absolutely *NOTHING* else should be fed during this time, including flavored chewable tablets. If a hypoallergenic diet appears to be effective in eliminating the diarrhea, one should continue to feed it for another 2 to 3 months to be sure that the diarrhea does not recur while the patient is still eating it.

Corticosteroids are often used as a trial for inflammatory bowel disease of the colon. This is a potentially dangerous thing to do in dogs. Dogs can have smoldering histoplasmosis for long periods of time that behaves much like any mild, benign colonic disease. Administering steroids to such a dog can result in severe disseminated histoplasmosis and death. Colonic histoplasmosis is rare in cats but has occurred.

DISORDERS AFFECTING MOTILITY

INTUSSUSCEPTIONS

Ileocolic. Ileocolic intussusceptions are the most common type and are usually found in young dogs, although cats are rarely affected.[169] They are usually secondary to other disease (e.g., parvoviral enteritis). Acute intussusceptions classically cause scant bloody diarrhea[170] and vomiting. Abdominal pain sometimes is seen. Most affected cats do not have diarrhea.[169] Palpation of a markedly thickened loop of bowel (i.e., a "sausage") is suggestive; however, it is easy to fail to palpate short intussusceptions. Occasional intussusceptions "slide" in and out, making it possible to palpate the abdomen when the intussusception is absent. Chronic intussusceptions may cause diarrhea without mucus, hematochezia, vomiting, or abdominal pain. Protein-losing enteropathy (PLE) in young, diarrheic dogs is suggestive of chronic intussusception, which typically causes protein loss despite lack of hemorrhage.

Plain abdominal radiographs are seldom diagnostic. Barium enemas are often diagnostic, but ultrasonography is the preferred diagnostic technique. Flexible colonoscopy often finds the intussusceptum filling the colonic lumen. Some intussusceptions protrude from the rectum, mimicking a rectal prolapse. Therefore, it is important to perform a digital rectal examination in animals with "rectal prolapse" to

GI

distinguish prolapse (i.e., with a fornix) from intussusception (i.e., without a fornix).

Therapy involves either resection or reduction of the intussusception. If possible, the ileocolic valve should be preserved. Intestinal plication helps prevent re-intussusception.

Cecocolic. Cecocolic intussusceptions are infrequent. The cause is uncertain, but whipworms have been suggested as a potential reason. The major sign is hematochezia,[171] caused by congestion of cecal mucosa. Diarrhea is less common, anemia and hypoproteinemia occasionally occurring.

Diagnosis requires finding the intussuscepted cecum. Abdominal palpation and plain radiographs are seldom diagnostic. Barium enema is diagnostic, if performed correctly. Abdominal ultrasonography and flexible colonoscopy are the preferred tests (Fig. 138–13). Surgical removal is curative.

FIBER-RESPONSIVE DIARRHEA AND "IRRITABLE BOWEL SYNDROME"

These two diagnoses probably reflect a plethora of diseases. "Fiber-responsive diarrhea" (FRD) refers to large bowel diarrhea that is ameliorated by dietary fiber supplementation. Signs are generally mild to moderate large bowel diarrhea with or without mucus and hematochezia. "Irritable bowel syndrome" (IBS) in people refers to a functional gut disorder typically characterized by abdominal pain, abdominal distention, diarrhea, constipation, and/or fecal mucus.[172–174] IBS has often been used in veterinary medicine to refer to a somewhat different syndrome: idiopathic large bowel diarrhea without a discernable organic cause that usually responds to dietary fiber supplementation. Using this latter definition, IBS and FRD are essentially synonymous. However, some clinicians understand IBS to refer to "excitable" animals that may have apparent psychologic reasons for alimentary signs including vomiting and/or abdominal discomfort.

Diagnosis of FRD requires resolution of diarrhea after beginning dietary fiber supplementation, whereas diagnosis of IBS requires excluding all known causes of diarrhea, including inflammatory mucosal infiltrates. Canine IBS is often characterized by a positive response to supplementing dietary fiber, although it may also require administration of antispasmodics or motility modifiers.

There are different fiber types, and some patients respond to one fiber type but not to another. Separating fiber into soluble and insoluble categories is overly simplistic. Many factors influence the effects of dietary fiber (e.g., size, processing), and apparently similar fibers can have different effects upon viscosity, production of short-chain fatty acids, fecal pH, and gas production.[175] In general, the fermentable fibers (usually the soluble types, such as pectins, gums, and some hemicelluloses) are metabolized by colonic bacteria to short-chain fatty acids, which may provide nutrition for colonocytes. Because the fiber serves as a bacterial food source, bacterial numbers increase, which increases fecal bulk and affects colonic motility.[176, 177] Some fiber types help retain water in the feces. Psyllium (i.e., Metamucil) is a commonly supplemented fiber that has soluble and insoluble characteristics. Too much psyllium can cause excessive fecal water retention and soft, voluminous stools. Occasionally, a patient not responding to psyllium supplementation responds to another fiber, or vice versa. There is currently some thought that using a mixture of soluble and insoluble fiber may be more "physiologic"; however, its clinical value is currently unknown.

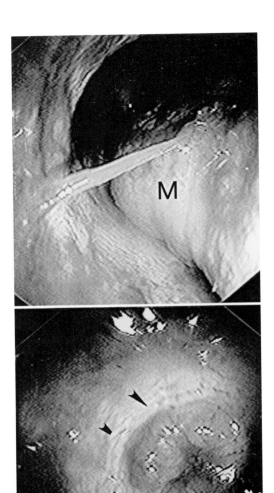

Figure 138–13. Endoscopic appearance of cecocolic intussusception in a dog. *A,* View of the transverse colon showing a large tubular structure (M) within the lumen extending orally toward the ileocolic region. *B,* View of the ileocolic region showing the unaffected ileocolic valve (black arrows) and the structure traversing obliquely through the cecocolic orifice (white arrows).

Motility modifiers (e.g., loperamide, diphenoxylate) benefit some patients that do not fully recover with a fiber-supplemented diet. Colonic spasms are sometimes alleviated with Librax or anticholinergics (e.g., propantheline, dicyclomine). Changing the patient's environment may be useful. Most patients with FRD or IBS require lifelong therapy. Fortunately, weight loss is rare, meaning that an effective therapy can usually be found, if the clinician and client persist.

CONSTIPATION

Hypothyroidism. Hypothyroidism may cause diminished colonic motility[178] and gradual accumulation of fecal material. Affected patients do not always have classic signs of hypothyroidism. Measuring serum free T_4 concentrations and administering thyroxine are reasonable in dogs with suspected hypothyroid-associated constipation. Four or more weeks of appropriate thyroxine supplementation may be needed before clinical improvement occurs.

Megacolon. Megacolon is marked, generalized colonic distention. One must distinguish a colon that is filled and slightly distended with feces from megacolon, in which the large intestine is typically distended at least twice its normal diameter. This is accomplished by abdominal palpation or radiographs. Megacolon may be caused by obstruction or motility deficits, cats being affected more commonly than dogs. Malaligned healing of pelvic fractures is relatively common in cats,[179] while rectal tumors are more common in dogs.[180] Rarely, congenital defects are responsible (e.g., Manx cats). Many cases of feline megacolon are idiopathic.[181] There may be unproductive efforts to defecate, or the patient may not even attempt to expel stool. Scant amounts of liquid stool with mucus or blood may be passed from around the fecal mass. Anorexia, weight loss, vomiting, and weakness may occur secondary to severe constipation. Digital rectal examination is performed to detect pelvic canal obstruction; radiographs may be needed in animals too large to be adequately examined digitally. Clinical pathology is used to look for electrolyte changes (i.e., hypokalemia, hypercalcemia) causing muscular weakness. Rarely, endoscopy is needed to find obstructions beyond reach of the digit. If a cause cannot be found, idiopathic megacolon is diagnosed.

Management involves removing impacted feces and eliminating causes of constipation.[179] Initial management of idiopathic megacolon should usually be medical, although surgery for massive, prolonged feline colonic distention is reasonable. Medical management first involves removing all feces, typically with multiple warm water enemas (avoid using large amounts of soap). Sometimes a rigid colonoscope and rigid alligator forceps are helpful. Hypertonic phosphate enemas should never be used.[182] After the feces are removed, strategies to prevent recurrence may include moderate dietary fiber supplementation, stool softeners (e.g., dioctyl sodium sulfosuccinate), osmotic cathartics (e.g., lactulose), and prokinetic drugs (i.e., cisapride).[183] If medical management is unsuccessful in a cat, subtotal colectomy is often performed.[184] Cats receiving subtotal colectomies typically have soft, tarry stools for weeks to months after surgery, but most eventually produce normal stools. Dogs seldom tolerate colectomies as well as cats.

COLORECTAL NEOPLASIA

Although gastrointestinal tract tumors are rare (comprising only 1 per cent of all malignancies), the colon and rectum may be affected by various benign and malignant growths. Malignant tumors predominate in the canine large bowel, with adenocarcinoma (AC) diagnosed most frequently, followed by lymphosarcoma (LSA) and leiomyosarcoma.[185, 186] Adenomas (e.g., adenomatous polyps) are the most common benign colonic growth, but leiomyomas may also occur.[187] Extramedullary plasmacytomas have also been reported in the dog.[188] The majority of large bowel neoplasms are located in the descending colon and rectum, although leiomyosarcomas are often located in the cecum.[186] Metastasis of canine colorectal AC and leiomyosarcoma to regional lymph nodes or lungs is relatively uncommon.[189, 190]

Adenocarcinoma and LSA are the most common malignant colonic neoplasms in cats, followed by mast cell tumors.[191, 192] Malignant feline tumors usually arise in the ileocolic and descending colon.[191, 192] In contrast to dogs, metastasis occurs to the peritoneum, mesentery, and regional lymph nodes in approximately 50 per cent of cats with AC.[193]

Most malignant tumors occur in older dogs and cats. Clinical signs seen with colorectal neoplasia are often indistinguishable from other causes of chronic colitis or large bowel obstruction. Signs range from changes in stool diameter (caused by annular constriction), to tenesmus and hematochezia (caused by mucosal cellular infiltration), to constipation (caused by obstruction). Lethargy, anorexia, and weight loss may accompany any malignant tumor, especially in cats. Dogs with smooth muscle tumors may be asymptomatic for extended periods, presumably owing to the slow growth of these neoplasms.[194]

Physical examination may reveal cachexia, palpable abdominal mass, mesenteric lymphadenopathy, ascites (with carcinomatosis), or stricture, rectal mass, or mucosal irregularity on digital examination.[180, 186, 189, 191, 192, 195] Routine laboratory tests are generally unremarkable. Most cats with alimentary LSA are FeLV-negative. Survey and contrast abdominal radiography (e.g., pneumocolon) may provide additional information concerning the presence/extent of colonic lesions. Ultrasonography is the staging method of choice for detection of regional metastasis to sublumbar lymph nodes. Thoracic radiographs are performed to identify pulmonary metastasis.

Rigid or flexible colonoscopy with mucosal biopsy is the preferred diagnostic modality. Endoscopic abnormalities may include increased mucosal friability, increased granularity, erosions, the presence of an intraluminal mass, and/or nondistensible, circumferential luminal narrowing seen with submucosal infiltrative lesions (Fig. 138–14). Multiple biopsy specimens of both abnormal and normal appearing mucosa should be obtained.[34, 35] Cytologic specimens should also be obtained during endoscopy to enhance the diagnostic yield for LSA.[29]

Treatment of colorectal neoplasia is variable depending on tumor type, its location, and extent of metastasis. Complete surgical excision is recommended for focal AC, cecal leiomyosarcoma, and, possibly, obstructive LSA. Radiation therapy may be palliative for recurrent distal rectal AC.[195] Diffuse colonic LSA is best treated with multiple-agent chemotherapy.

The prognosis for most malignant neoplasms is guarded. Surgical resection alone results in a 22- and 15-month aver-

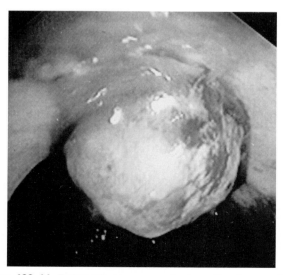

Figure 138–14. Endoscopic appearance of a 1-cm-diameter smooth, encapsulated colorectal mass in a dog. Endoscopic biopsy specimens from this mass were histologically interpreted as an adenocarcinoma.

GI

age survival in dogs and cats with AC, respectively; and some cats may live more than 2 years.[180, 196] The presence of metastatic disease in cats with intestinal AC is not necessarily a poor prognostic factor.[196] In dogs with AC, annular mass lesions carry a poorer prognosis with an average survival of 1.6 months.[180] Only limited survival analysis data in animals with colonic LSA have been reported. Median survival times of 3 to 4 months were observed in cats with LSA, regardless of surgical procedure (e.g., mucosal biopsy versus resection) performed or administration of chemotherapy.[191] The prognosis is good with leiomyomas[194] and guarded to good with leiomyosarcomas following tumor resection.[186]

Benign (adenomatous) polyps may appear as friable, sessile or pedunculated masses originating from the distal rectal mucosa (Fig. 138–15). These masses are grossly indistinguishable from malignant growths, necessitating biopsy for diagnosis. Surgical resection is recommended, with a good to excellent prognosis. Local recurrence may occur with incomplete excision.

COLONIC DISORDERS ASSOCIATED WITH OTHER DISEASES

PANCREATITIS

Severe pancreatitis sometimes causes diarrhea[197] that may be bloody. The ostensible reason is the close proximity of the left limb of the pancreas to the transverse colon. Diarrhea typically resolves as the pancreatitis resolves.

NEUROLOGIC DYSFUNCTION

Dogs being treated for severe spinal cord disease sometimes evidence colonic problems such as bloody diarrhea, especially after administration of large doses of dexamethasone. The colon rarely perforates, causing overwhelming septic peritonitis. Causes of perforation might involve fecal retention (due to altered colonic motility secondary to spinal cord disease), increased catecholamines decreasing colonic blood flow, and adverse effects of steroids on the colonic mucosa. Most perforations are on the antimesenteric border

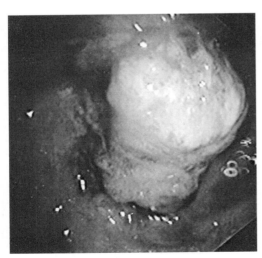

Figure 138–15. Endoscopic appearance of a 2.5-cm friable colorectal mass in a dog. Histologic review of biopsy specimens procured from this mass confirmed a diagnosis of rectal polyp.

of the proximal descending colon, occurring 3 to 8 days after surgery.[198, 199]

REFERENCES

1. Leib MS, Matz ME: Diseases of the large intestine, In Ettinger SJ, Feldman EC (eds): Textbook of Veterinary Internal Medicine, 4th ed. Philadelphia, WB Saunders, 1995, p 1232.
2. Barker IA, et al: The alimentary system. In Jubb KVF, et al (eds): Pathology of Domestic Animals. New York, Academic Press, 1993, p 1.
3. Spinato MT, et al: A morphometric study of the canine colon: Comparison of control dogs and cases of colonic disease. Can J Vet Res 54:477, 1990.
4. Wilcox B: Endoscopic biopsy interpretation in canine or feline enterocolitis. Semin Vet Med Surg 7:162, 1992.
5. Willard MD: Normal immune function of the gastrointestinal tract. Semin Vet Med Surg 7:107, 1992.
6. Kawanishi H: Recent progress in immune responses in gut. Dig Dis 7:113, 1989.
7. Doe WF: The intestinal immune system. Gut 30:1679, 1989.
8. Willard MD, et al: Number and distribution of IgM cells and IgA cells in colonic tissue of conditioned sex- and breed-matched dogs. Am J Vet Res 43:688, 1982.
9. Jergens AE, et al: Immunohistochemical characterization of immunoglobulin-containing cells and T cells in the colonic mucosa of healthy dogs. Am J Vet Res 59:552, 1998.
10. Jergens AE, et al: Colonic immune cell populations in canine inflammatory bowel disease: An immunohistochemical and morphometric study. Am J Vet Res, in press.
11. Smith HW: Observations on the flora of the alimentary tract of animals and factors affecting its composition. J Path Bact 89:95, 1965.
12. Sparkes AH, et al: Effect of dietary supplementation with fructooligosaccharides on fecal flora of healthy cats. Am J Vet Res 59:436, 1998.
13. Sumners RK, Kent TH: Effects of altered propulsion on rat small intestinal flora. Gastroenterology 59:740, 1970.
14. Rowley D: Specific immune antibacterial mechanisms in the intestines of mice. Am J Clin Nutr 27:1417, 1974.
15. Isikawa H, et al: Studies on bacterial flora of the alimentary tract of dogs. III. Fecal flora in clinical and experimental cases of diarrhea. Jpn J Vet Sci 44:343, 1982.
16. Macfarlane GT, Gibson GR: Microbiological aspects of the production of short-chain fatty acids in the large bowel. In Cummings JH, et al (eds): Physiological and Clinical Aspects of Short Chain Fatty Acids. Cambridge, Cambridge University Press, 1995, p 87.
17. Roediger WEW: Utilization of nutrients by isolated epithelial cells of the rat colon. Gastroenterology 83:424, 1982.
18. Newmark HL, Lupton JR: Determinants and consequences of colonic luminal pH. Nutr Canc 14:161, 1990.
19. Christensen J: Motility of the colon. In Johnson LR (ed): Physiology of the Gastrointestinal Tract. New York, Raven Press, 1987, p 665.
20. Powell DW: Intestinal water and electrolyte transport. In Johnson LR (ed): Physiology of the Gastrointestinal Tract. New York, Raven Press, 1987, p 1267.
21. Binder HJ, Sandle GI: Electrolyte absorption and secretion in the mammalian colon. In Johnson LR (ed): Physiology of the Gastrointestinal Tract. New York, Raven Press, 1987, p 1389.
22. Sherding RG, Johnson SE: Intestinal histoplasmosis, In Kirk RW, Bonagura JD (eds): Current Veterinary Therapy XI. Philadelphia, WB Saunders, 1992, p 609.
23. Zajac AM: Giardiasis. Comp Contin Ed Pract Vet 14:604, 1992.
24. Zimmer JF, Burrington DB: Comparison of four techniques of fecal examination for detecting canine giardiasis. J Am Anim Hosp Assoc 22:161, 1986.
25. Tams T: Gastrointestinal symptoms. In Tams T (ed): Handbook of Small Animal Gastroenterology. Philadelphia, WB Saunders, 1996, p 1.
26. Dow SW: Acute medical diseases of the small intestine. In Tams T (ed): Handbook of Small Animal Gastroenterology. Philadelphia, WB Saunders, 1996, p 245.
27. Willard MD: Diagnostic tests for the alimentary tract. In Nelson RW, Couto CG (eds): Small Animal Internal Medicine. St. Louis, CV Mosby, 1998, p 368.
28. Marks SL, et al: Critical appraisal of methods to diagnose Clostridium perfringens–associated diarrhea in dogs (abstract). J Vet Intern Med 12:204, 1998.
29. Jergens AE, et al: Cytologic examination of exfoliative specimens obtained during endoscopy for diagnosis of gastrointestinal disease in dogs and cats. JAVMA 213:1755, 1998.
30. Penninck DG: Ultrasonography of the gastrointestinal tract. In Nyland TG, Mattoon JS (eds): Veterinary Diagnostic Ultrasound. Philadelphia, WB Saunders, 1995, p 125.
31. Tams TR: Gastrointestinal endoscopy: Instrumentation, handling technique, maintenance. In Tams TR (ed): Small Animal Endoscopy. St. Louis, CV Mosby, 1990, p 31.
32. Burrows CF: Evaluation of a colonic lavage solution to prepare the colon of the dog for colonoscopy. JAVMA 195:1719, 1989.
33. Jones BD: Endoscopy of the lower gastrointestinal tract. Vet Clin North Am Small Anim Pract 20:1229, 1990.
34. Leib MS: Colonoscopy. In Tams TR (ed): Small Animal Endoscopy. St. Louis, CV Mosby, 1990, p 211.
35. Leib MS: Gastrointestinal endoscopy. In August JR (ed): Consultations in Feline Internal Medicine. Philadelphia, WB Saunders, 1994, p 119.

36. McDonough PL, et al: Diagnosing emerging bacterial infections: Salmonellosis, campylobacteriosis, clostridial toxicosis, and helicobacteriosis. Semin Vet Med Surg 11:187, 1996.

37. van der Steen I, et al: Futterungseinflusse auf das vorkommen und die enterotoxin-bildung von *Clostridium perfringens* im darmkanal des hundes. Kleintierpraxis 42:855, 1997.

38. Lindsay JA: *Clostridium perfringens* Type A enterotoxin (CPE): More than just explosive diarrhea. Crit Rev Microbiol 22:257, 1996.

39. Twedt DC: Canine *Clostridium perfringens* diarrhea. Proceed Waltham/OSU Sympos 17:28, 1993.

40. Kruth SA, et al: Nosocomial diarrhea associated with enterotoxigenic *Clostridium perfringens* infection in dogs. JAVMA 195:331, 1989.

41. Twedt DC: *Clostridium perfringens* associated diarrhea in dogs. Proc Am Coll Vet Int Med 11:121, 1993.

42. Carman RJ, et al: Recurrent diarrhoea in a dog associated with *Clostridium perfringens* type a. Vet Rec 112:342, 1983.

43. Johnson S, et al: Treatment of asymptomatic *Clostridium difficile* carriers (fecal excretors) with vancomycin or metronidazole. Ann Intern Med 117:297, 1992.

44. Foley J, et al: An outbreak of *Clostridium perfringens* enteritis in a cattery of Bengal cats and experimental transmission to specific pathogen free cats. Fel Pract 24:31, 1996.

45. Cantor GH, et al: Salmonella shedding in racing sled dogs. J Vet Diagn Invest 9:447, 1997.

46. Kawashima K, et al: Salmonella carriers among cats derived from Kanagawa prefecture. J Jpn Vet Med Assoc 43:679, 1990.

47. Anonymous: Salmonellosis. J Small Anim Pract 38:375, 1997.

48. Weber A, et al: Occurrence of Salmonella in fecal samples of dogs and cats in northern Bavaria from 1975 to 1994. Berl Munch Tierarztl Wochenschr 108:401, 1995.

49. Wall PG, et al: Multiresistant *Salmonella typhimurium* DT104 in cats: A public health risk. Lancet 348:471, 1996.

50. Cohen ND, et al: Comparison of polymerase chain reaction and microbiological culture for detection of Salmonellae in equine feces and environmental samples. Am J Vet Res 57:780, 1996.

51. Stone GG, et al: Detection of *Salmonella typhimurium* from rectal swabs of experimentally infected beagles by short cultivation and PCR-hybridization. J Clin Microbiol 33:1292, 1995.

52. Low JC, et al: Multiple-resistant *Salmonella typhimurium* DT104 in cats. Lancet 348:1391, 1996.

53. Morse EV, et al: Canine salmonellosis: A review and report of dog to child transmission of *Salmonella enteritidis*. Am J Public Health 66:82, 1976.

54. Wall PG, et al: Chronic carriage of multidrug resistant *Salmonella typhimurium* in a cat. J Small Anim Pract 36:279, 1995.

55. Hammermueller J, et al: Detection of toxin genes in *Escherichia coli* isolated from normal dogs and dogs with diarrhea. Can J Vet Res 59:265, 1995.

56. Abaas S, et al: Cytotoxin activity on Vero cells among *Escherichia coli* strains associated with diarrhea in cats. Am J Vet Res 50:1294, 1989.

57. Smith KA, et al: A case-control study of verocytotoxigenic *Escherichia coli* infection in cats with diarrhea. Can J Vet Res 62:87, 1998.

58. Turk J, et al: Examination for heat-labile, heat-stable, and Shiga-like toxins and for the eaeA gene in *Escherichia coli* isolates obtained from dogs dying with diarrhea: 122 cases (1992–1996). JAVMA 212:1735, 1998.

59. Trevena WB, et al: Vero cytotoxin producing *Escherichia coli* O157 associated with companion animals. Vet Rec 138:400, 1996.

60. Torre E, et al: Factors influencing fecal shedding of *Campylobacter jejuni* in dogs without diarrhea. Am J Vet Res 54:260, 1993.

61. Altekruse SF, et al: Food and animal sources of human *Campylobacter jejuni* infection. JAVMA 204:57, 1994.

62. Anonymous: Campylobacter infection. J Small Anim Pract 39:99, 1998.

63. Allos BM, et al: *Campylobacter jejuni* and the expanding spectrum of related infections. Clin Infect Dis 20:1092, 1995.

64. Fantasia M, et al: Characterization of Yersinia species isolated from a kennel and from cattle and pig farms. Vet Rec 132:532, 1993.

65. Papageorges M, et al: *Yersinia enterocolitica* enteritis in two dogs. JAVMA 182:618, 1983.

66. Wilson HD, et al: *Yersinia enterocolitica* infection in a 4-month-old infant associated with infection in household dogs. J Pediat 89:767, 1976.

67. Moulis H, et al: Antibiotic-associated hemorrhagic colitis. J Clin Gastroenterol 18:227, 1994.

68. Dvorak J, et al: Pan-fibrinonecrotic colitis in a dog treated by colectomy. JAVMA 198:264, 1991.

69. Kelly CP, et al: *Clostridium difficile* colitis. N Engl J Med 330:257, 1994.

70. Berry AP, et al: Chronic diarrhoea in dogs associated with *Clostridium difficile* infection. Vet Rec 118:102, 1986.

71. Madewell BR, et al: *Clostridium difficile*: Fecal carriage in cats. Proc Am Coll Vet Int Med 16:717, 1998.

72. Struble AL, et al: Fecal shedding of *Clostridium difficile* in dogs: A period prevalence survey in a veterinary medical teaching hospital. J Vet Diagn Invest 6:342, 1994.

73. Gerding DN, et al: Optimal methods for identifying *Clostridium difficile* infections. Clin Infect Dis 16(S4):439, 1993.

74. Wenisch C, et al: Comparison of vancomycin, teicoplanin, metronidazole, and fusidic acid for the treatment of *Clostridium difficile* associated diarrhea. Clin Infect Dis 22:813, 1996.

75. Lee JI, et al: The prevalence of intestinal spirochaetes in dogs. Aust Vet J 74:466, 1996.

76. Duhamel GE, et al: Intestinal spirochetosis and giardiasis in a Beagle pup with diarrhea. Vet Pathol 33:360, 1996.

77. Duhamel GE, et al: Colonic spirochetal infections in nonhuman primates that were associated with *Brachyspira aalborgi*, *Serpulina pilosicoli* and unclassified flagellated bacteria. Clin Infect Dis 25(S2):186, 1997.

78. Georgi JR, et al: *In* Canine Clinical Parasitology. Philadelphia, Lea & Febiger, 1992.

79. Hass DK, et al: *Trichuris campanula* infection in a domestic cat from Miami, Florida. Am J Vet Res 39:1553, 1978.

80. Bowman DD, et al: *In* Georgis' Parasitology for Veterinarians. Philadelphia, WB Saunders, 1995.

81. Graves TK, et al: Basal and ACTH-stimulated plasma aldosterone concentrations are normal or increased in dogs with Trichuris-associated pseudohypoadrenocorticism. J Vet Intern Med 8:287, 1994.

82. Blagburn BL, et al: Efficacy of milbemycin oxime against naturally acquired or experimentally induced *Ancylostoma* spp and *Trichuris vulpis* infections in dogs. Am J Vet Res 53:513, 1992.

83. Horii Y, et al: Anthelmintic efficacy of milbemycin oxime against *Trichuris vulpis* in dogs. J Vet Med Sci 60:271, 1998.

84. Overgaauw PAM, et al: Anthelmintic efficacy of oxibendazole against some important nematodes in dogs and cats. Vet Quart 20:69, 1998.

85. Narayana GS: Intestinal trichomoniasis in a pup—a case report. Ind Vet J 53:477, 1976.

86. Romatowski J: An uncommon protozoan parasite (*Pentatrichomonas hominis*) associated with colitis in three cats. Fel Pract 24:10, 1996.

87. Soulsby EJL: *In* Helminths, Arthropods and Protozoa of Domesticated Animals. Philadelphia, Lea & Febiger, 1982.

88. Wittnich C: *Entamoeba histolytica* infection in a German shepherd dog. Can Vet J 17:259, 1976.

89. Hayes FA: Canine helminthiasis complicated with Balantidium species. JAVMA 129:161, 1956.

90. Ewing SA, et al: Severe chronic canine diarrhea associated with Balantidium-Trichuris infection. JAVMA 149:519, 1966.

91. Edwards J, et al: Canine colonic heterobilharziasis from south Texas. Tex Vet Med J April:20, 1995.

92. Troy GC, et al: *Heterobilharzia americana* infection and hypercalcemia in a dog: A case report. J Am Anim Hosp Assoc 23:35, 1987.

93. Ronald NC, et al: Fenbendazole for the treatment of *Heterobilharzia americana* infection in dogs. JAVMA 182:172, 1983.

94. Wolf AM: Histoplasmosis. *In* Greene CE (ed): Infectious Diseases of the Dog and Cat. Philadelphia, WB Saunders, 1990, p 679.

95. Clinkenbeard KD, et al: Canine disseminated histoplasmosis. Compend Contin Educ Pract Vet 11:1347, 1989.

96. Clinkenbeard KD, et al: Disseminated histoplasmosis in cats: 12 cases (1981–1986). JAVMA 190:1445, 1987.

97. Clinkenbeard KD, et al: Disseminated histoplasmosis in dogs: 12 cases (1981–1986). JAVMA 193:1443, 1988.

98. Hodges RD, et al: Itraconazole for the treatment of histoplasmosis in cats. J Vet Intern Med 8:409, 1994.

99. Davies SF, et al: Concurrent human and canine histoplasmosis from cutting decayed wood. Ann Intern Med 113:252, 1990.

100. Fischer JR, et al: Gastrointestinal pythiosis in Missouri dogs: Eleven cases. J Vet Diag Invest 6:380, 1994.

101. Miller RI: Gastrointestinal phycomycosis in 63 dogs. JAVMA 186:473, 1985.

102. Thomas RC, et al: Pythiosis in dogs and cats. Compend Contin Educ Pract Vet 20:63, 1998.

103. Tyler DE: Prototheosis. *In* Greene CE (ed): Infectious Diseases of the Dog and Cat. Philadelphia, WB Saunders, 1990, p 742.

104. Migaki G, et al: Canine protothecosis: Review of the literature and report of an additional case. JAVMA 181:794, 1982.

105. Sherding RG: Diseases of the small bowel. *In* Ettinger SJ (ed): Textbook of Veterinary Internal Medicine. Philadelphia, WB Saunders, 1982, p 1278.

106. Strombeck DR: Chronic inflammatory bowel disease. *In* Strombeck DR (ed): Small Animal Gastroenterology. Davis, CA, Stonegate Publishing, 1979, p 240.

107. Barkin R, Lewis JH: Overview of inflammatory bowel disease in humans. Semin Vet Med Surg 7:117, 1992.

108. Jergens AE, Moore FM, Haynes JS, et al: Idiopathic inflammatory bowel disease in dogs and cats: 84 cases (1987–1990). JAVMA 201:1603, 1992.

109. Roth L, Walton AM, Leib MS, et al: A grading system for lymphocytic plasmacytic colitis in dogs. J Vet Diagn Invest 2:257, 1990.

110. Sartor RB: Insights into the pathogenesis of inflammatory bowel diseases provided by new rodent models of spontaneous colitis. Inflam Bowel Dis 1:64, 1995.

111. Podolsky D: Inflammatory bowel disease. N Engl J Med 325:928, 1991.

112. MacDermott RP: Alterations in the mucosal immune system in ulcerative colitis and Crohn's disease. Med Clin North Am 78:1207, 1994.

113. Guilford WG: Idiopathic inflammatory bowel diseases. *In* Guilford WG, et al (eds): Strombeck's Small Animal Gastroenterology. Philadelphia, WB Saunders, 1996, p 451.

114. Willard MD: Disorders of the intestinal tract. *In* Nelson RW, Couto CG (eds): Small Animal Internal Medicine. St. Louis, CV Mosby, 1998, p 433.

115. Gunawardana SC, et al: Colonic nitrite and immunoglobulin G concentrations in dogs with inflammatory bowel disease. JAVMA 211:318, 1997.

116. Jergens AE, et al: Molecular detection of inducible nitric oxide synthase in canine inflammatory bowel disease (abstract). J Vet Intern Med 12:205, 1998.

GI

117. Dennis JS, et al: Lymphocytic/plasmacytic colitis in cats: 14 cases (1985–1990). JAVMA 202:313, 1993.
118. Roth L, et al: Comparisons between endoscopic and histologic evaluation of the gastrointestinal tract of dogs and cats: 75 cases (1984–1987). JAVMA 196:635, 1990.
119. Jergens AE: Feline idiopathic inflammatory bowel disease. Compend Contin Educ Pract Vet 14:509, 1992.
120. Moore RP: Feline eosinophilic enteritis. In Kirk RW (ed): Current Veterinary Therapy VIII. Philadelphia, WB Saunders, 1981, p 791.
121. Johnson SE: Canine eosinophilic gastroenteritis. Semin Vet Med Surg 7:145, 1992.
122. Hendricks M: A spectrum of hypereosinophilic syndromes exemplified by six cats with eosinophilic enteritis. Vet Pathol 18:188, 1981.
123. Van Kruiningen HJ: Granulomatous colitis of boxer dogs: Comparative aspects. Gastroenterology 53:114, 1967.
124. Hall EJ, et al: Boxer colitis. Vet Rec 130:148, 1991.
125. Leib MS, et al: Suppurative colitis in a cat. JAVMA 188:739, 1986.
126. Van Kruiningen HJ: Clinical efficacy of tylosin in canine inflammatory bowel disease. J Am Anim Hosp Assoc 12:498, 1976.
127. DiBartola SP, et al: Regional enteritis in two dogs. JAVMA 181:904, 1982.
128. Nelson RW, et al: Nutritional management of idiopathic chronic colitis in the dog. J Vet Intern Med 2:133, 1988.
129. Richter KP: Lymphocytic-plasmacytic enterocolitis in dogs. Semin Vet Med Surg 7:134, 1992.
130. Leib MS, et al: Plasmacytic lymphocytic colitis in the dog. Semin Vet Med Surg 4:241, 1989.
131. Hodgson HJF: Inflammatory bowel disease and food intolerance. J Royal College Physicians 20:45, 1986.
132. Jones VA: Comparison of total parenteral nutrition and elemental diet in induction of remission of Crohn's disease. Long term maintenance of remission by personalized food exclusion diets. Dig Dis Sci 32:100S, 1987.
133. Jenkins DJA: Carbohydrates. In Schils ME, Young VR (eds): Modern Nutrition in Health and Disease. Philadelphia, Lea & Febiger, 1988, p 52.
134. McIntyre A, et al: Butyrate production from dietary fibre and protection against large bowel cancer in a rat model. Gut 34:386, 1993.
135. Reinhart D, Lebenthal E: Intestinal mucosal energy metabolism: A new approach to therapy of gastrointestinal disease. J Pediatr Gastroenterol Nutr 10:1, 1990.
136. Hanauer SB: Inflammatory bowel disease revisited: Newer drugs. Scand J Gastroenterol 25(S175):97, 1990.
137. Ogorek CP, Fisher RS: Current drug therapy for inflammatory bowel disease. Comp Ther 17:31, 1991.
138. Lennard-Jones JE: Inflammatory bowel disease: Medical therapy revisited. Scand J Gastroenterol 27(S192):110, 1992.
139. Hawthorne AB, Hawkey CJ: Immunosuppressive drugs in inflammatory bowel disease: A review of their mechanisms of efficacy and place in therapy. Drugs 38:267, 1989.
140. Tams TR: Chronic feline inflammatory bowel disorders. II. Feline eosinophilic enteritis and lymphosarcoma. Compend Contin Educ Pract Vet 8:464, 1986.
141. Danielsson A, et al: A controlled randomized trial of budesonide versus prednisolone retention enemas in active distal ulcerative colitis. Scand J Gastroenterol 22:987, 1987.
142. Lofberg R, et al: Oral budesonide in active ileocecal Crohn's disease: A pilot trial with a topically acting steroid (abstract). Gastroenterology 100:A226, 1991.
143. Halpern Z, et al: A controlled trial of beclomethasone versus betamethasone enemas in distal ulcerative colitis. J Clin Gastroenterol 13:38, 1991.
144. Stewart A, Bolineck J: The use of a novel formulation of budesonide as an improved treatment over prednisone for inflammatory bowel disease (abstract). J Vet Intern Med 11:115, 1997.
145. Misiewicz JJ, et al: Controlled trial of sulfasalazine in maintenance therapy for ulcerative colitis. Lancet 1:185, 1965.
146. Summers RW, et al: National cooperative Crohn's disease study: Results of drug treatment. Gastroenterology 77:847, 1979.
147. Miner PB, Biddle WL: Modern treatment of ulcerative colitis. Compr Ther 15:38, 1989.
148. Schroder H, et al: Metabolism of salicylazosulfapyridine in healthy subjects and in patients with ulcerative colitis. Clin Pharm Ther 14:802, 1973.
149. Selby W: Current management of inflammatory bowel disease. J Gastroenterol Hepatol 8:70, 1983.
150. Hanauer SB: Medical therapy of ulcerative colitis. Lancet 342:412, 1993.
151. Leib MS, et al: Management of chronic large bowel diarrhea in dogs. Vet Med 86:922, 1991.
152. Burrows CF: Canine colitis. Compend Contin Educ Pract Vet 14:1347, 1992.
153. Morgan RV, Bachrach A: Keratoconjunctivitis sicca associated with sulfonamide therapy in dogs. JAVMA 180:432, 1982.
154. Azad K, et al: An experiment to determine the active therapeutic moiety of sulfasalazine. Lancet 2:292, 1977.
155. Rasmussen SN, et al: Treatment of Crohn's disease with peroral 5-aminosalicylic acid. Gastroenterology 85:1350, 1983.
156. Selby WS, et al: Olsalazine in active ulcerative colitis. Br Med J 291:1373, 1985.
157. Ruderman WB: Newer pharmacologic agents for the therapy of inflammatory bowel disease. Med Clin North Am 74:133, 1990.
158. Ursing B, et al: A comparative study of metronidazole and sulfasalazine for active Crohn's disease: The cooperative Crohn's disease study in Sweden. Gastroenterology 83:550, 1982.
159. Miller JJ: The imidazoles as immunosuppressive agents. Transplant Proc 12:300, 1980.
160. Willard MD: Inflammatory bowel disease: Perspectives on therapy. J Am Anim Hosp Assoc 28:27, 1992.
161. Dow SW, et al: Central nervous system toxicosis associated with metronidazole treatment of dogs: 5 cases (1984–1987). JAVMA 195:365, 1989.
162. Lennard-Jones JE, Singleton JW: The azathioprine controversy. Dig Dis Sci 26:364, 1981.
163. Bunjes D, et al: Cyclosporin A mediates immunosuppression of primary cytotoxic T-cell responses by impairing the release of interleukin-1 and interleukin-2. Eur J Immunol 11:657, 1981.
164. Stange EF, et al: Cyclosporin A treatment in inflammatory bowel disease. Dig Dis Sci 34:1387, 1989.
165. Guilford WG: Adverse reactions to food. In Guilford WG, et al (eds): Strombeck's Small Animal Gastroenterology. Philadelphia, WB Saunders, 1996, p 436.
166. Heyman MB: Food sensitivity in eosinophilic gastroenteropathies. In Sleisinger MH, Fordtram JS (eds): Gastrointestinal Disease. Philadelphia, WB Saunders, 1989, p 1113.
167. Guilford WG: Development of a model of food allergy in the dog. J Vet Intern Med 6:128, 1992.
168. Bahna SL: Practical considerations in food challenge testing. Immunol Allergy Clin North Am 11:845, 1991.
169. Bellenger CR, et al: Intussusception in 12 cats. J Small Anim Pract 35:295, 1994.
170. Wilson GP, et al: Intussusception in the dog and cat: A review of 45 cases. JAVMA 164:515, 1974.
171. Miller WW, et al: Cecal inversion in eight dogs. J Am Anim Hosp Assoc 20:1009, 1984.
172. Thompson WG: Irritable bowel syndrome: Pathogenesis and management. Lancet 341:1569, 1993.
173. Andrews PL: Irritable bowel syndrome: Just a pain in the butt? Gastroenterology 107:1886, 1994.
174. Francis CY, et al: The irritable bowel syndrome. Postgrad Med J 73:1, 1997.
175. Tomlin J: Which fibre is best for the colon. Scand J Gastroenterol S129:100, 1987.
176. Burrows CF, et al: Influence of alpha-cellulose on myoelectric activity of proximal canine colon. Am J Physiol 245:G301, 1983.
177. Burrows CF, et al: Effects of fiber on digestibility and transit time in dogs. J Nutr 112:1726, 1982.
178. Feldman EC, et al: Hypothyroidism. In Feldman EC, et al (eds): Canine and Feline Endocrinology and Reproduction, 2nd ed. Philadelphia, WB Saunders, 1996, p 68.
179. Schrader SC: Pelvic osteotomy as a treatment for obstipation in cats with acquired stenosis of the pelvic canal: Six cases (1978–1989). JAVMA 200:208, 1992.
180. Church EM, et al: Colorectal adenocarcinoma in dogs: 78 cases (1973–1984). JAVMA 191:727, 1987.
181. Washabau RJ, et al: Alterations in colonic smooth muscle function in cats with idiopathic megacolon. Am J Vet Res 57:580, 1996.
182. Atkins CE, et al: Clinical, biochemical, acid-base, and electrolyte abnormalities in cats after hypertonic sodium phosphate enema administration. Am J Vet Res 46:980, 1985.
183. Guilford WG, et al: Miscellaneous disorders of the bowel, abdomen, and anorectum. In Guilford WG, et al (eds): Strombeck's Small Animal Gastroenterology. Philadelphia, WB Saunders, 1996, p 503.
184. Rosin E, et al: Subtotal colectomy for treatment of chronic constipation associated with idiopathic megacolon in cats: 38 cases (1979–1985). JAVMA 193:850, 1988.
185. Brodey RS, Cohen D: An epizootiologic and clinicopathologic study of 95 cases of gastrointestinal neoplasms in the dog. Chicago, Proceedings 101st Annual Meeting of the AVMA, 1964, p 167.
186. Kapatkin AS, et al: Leiomyosarcaroma in dogs: 44 cases (1983–1988). JAVMA 201:1077, 1992.
187. White RAS, Gorman NT: The clinical diagnosis and management of rectal and pararectal tumours in the dog. J Small Anim Pract 28:87, 1987.
188. Trevor PB, et al: Metastatic extramedullary plasmacytoma of the colon and rectum in a dog. JAVMA 203:406, 1993.
189. Birchard SJ, et al: Non-lymphoid intestinal neoplasia in 32 dogs and 14 cats. J Am Anim Hosp Assoc 22:533, 1986.
190. Patnaik AK, et al: Canine intestinal adenocarcinoma and carcinoid. Vet Pathol 17:149, 1980.
191. Slawienski MJ, et al: Malignant colonic neoplasia in cats: 46 cases (1990–1996). JAVMA 211:878, 1997.
192. Mahony OM, et al: Alimentary lymphoma in cats: 28 cases (1988–1993). JAVMA 207:1593, 1995.
193. Patnaik AK, et al: Feline intestinal adenocarcinoma: A clinicopathologic study of 22 cases. Vet Pathol 13:1, 1976.
194. McPherron MA, et al: Colorectal leiomyomas in seven dogs. J Am Anim Hosp Assoc 28:43, 1992.
195. Turrel JM, Theon AP: Single high-dose irradiation for selected canine rectal carcinomas. Vet Radiol 27:141, 1986.
196. Kosovsky JE, et al: Small intestinal adenocarcinoma in cats: 32 cases (1978–1985). JAVMA 192:233, 1988.
197. Simpson KW: Diagnosis and treatment of acute pancreatitis in the dog. The 17th Annual Waltham/OSU Symposium 17:117, 1993.
198. Toombs JP, et al: Colonic perforation in corticosteroid-treated dogs. JAVMA 188:145, 1986.
199. Bellah JR: Colonic perforation after corticosteroid and surgical treatment of intervertebral disk disease in a dog. JAVMA 183:1002, 1983.

CHAPTER 139

RECTO-ANAL DISEASE

Robert C. DeNovo, Jr., and Ronald M. Bright

The pelvic canal and anorectum consist of smooth and striated muscles and the intrinsic and extrinsic neurons that innervate them. The normal actions of these muscles retain and expel feces voluntarily. The ability to retain fecal content, to perceive that the rectum is full, and to determine a suitable time for defecation is termed fecal continence. Neuromuscular dysfunction of the anorectum causes constipation or fecal incontinence. Disease of the anorectal mucosa generally causes signs of inflammation or obstruction, observed clinically as tenesmus, hematochezia, mucoid feces, or frequent defecation.

ANATOMY

The rectum is a continuation of the descending colon, beginning at the pelvic inlet and ending at the anal canal.[1] The longitudinal muscles of the colon form the continuous longitudinal muscle layer of the rectum that surrounds an inner circular muscle layer. The rectal mucosa is columnar epithelium with abundant goblet cells. Prominent circular folds caused by contractions of the circular muscle and numerous solitary lymph follicles that appear as diffuse, slightly raised and punctate depressions can be visualized endoscopically. The most distal part of the rectum narrows at the juncture of the rectum and anal canal, where there is an abrupt transition to squamous epithelium. This junction is formed by the distal extent of the rectum and the proximal border of the internal and external anal sphincters. The internal anal sphincter is the thickened distal continuation of the circular smooth muscle of the rectum. The external anal sphincter is a circular band of striated muscle located more distal to and partially surrounding the internal anal sphincter. Dorsally, the external anal sphincter attaches mainly to the fascia of the tail. Ventrally, fibers from the external anal sphincter decussate and blend with the muscles of the external genitalia.

The short anal canal extends from the rectum to the anus, which is the terminal opening of the alimentary canal.[1] The anal canal is surrounded by both smooth muscle of the internal anal sphincter and striated muscle of the external anal sphincter. The action of the anus is therefore determined by both involuntary smooth muscle and voluntary striated muscle. The mucosa of the anal canal is divided into three zones. The most caudal is the cutaneous zone, composed of an outer hairless and keratinized area peripheral to the anus and an inner portion where the ducts of the anal sac terminate. The anus is located in the plane separating the two portions of the cutaneous zone. A narrow scalloped fold that encircles the anal canal is the intermediate zone, joining the stratified squamous epithelium of the cutaneous zone and the mucosa of the columnar zone. The columnar zone is composed of longitudinal ridges of columnar mucosa that merge with the mucosa of the rectum.

Two spherical anal sacs are located ventrolateral to the anus and interposed between the inner smooth and outer striated muscle of the anal sphincters.[1] The ducts from the anal sacs cross the caudal boarder of the internal sphincter and open into the anal canal near the junction of the inner cutaneous and intermediate zones. Three types of glands are located in the anal area. Circumanal "hepatoid" glands are nonsecretory sebaceous glands located subcutaneously around the anus. These glands are responsive to androgens and can grow throughout life in the intact male, sometimes resulting in adenomas in old male dogs. Anal glands are microscopic tubuloalveolar sweat glands located craniolateral to the circumanal glands and open into the intermediate zone of the anal canal. They produce a fatty secretion, the function of which is not known. Glands of the anal sac are located in the wall of the anal sac. These coiled tubular glands have apocrine and sebaceous components that secrete a serous to pasty liquid that accumulates in the anal sac along with desquamated epithelium and bacteria. The anal sacs are of clinical importance because they frequently become enlarged with accumulated secretions, sometimes leading to infection and abscess formation.

Blood is supplied to the structures of the anal canal and the anal sphincters from the right and left caudal rectal arteries. Venous drainage occurs via the cranial rectal and caudal mesenteric veins to the portal system and via the caudal rectal and perineal veins to the systemic venous system.[1] Lymphatics drain into the internal iliac lymph nodes.

Innervation of the rectum is similar to that of the colon.[1] A well-defined enteric nervous system exists, consisting of a myenteric and a submucosal plexus that contain many sensory, integrative, and motor neurons. These neurons integrate movements of the colon and rectum to ensure well-coordinated storage and transit of feces. In addition, these neurons regulate mucus secretion by goblet cells in the rectal mucosa and react to distention of the rectal wall by transmitting such information to the brain. Innervation of the anus is somewhat more complex and different from that of the rest of the digestive tract.[1,2] The internal anal sphincter and rectum are innervated by autonomic fibers from the pelvic plexuses. The parasympathetic portion comes from the sacral level of the spinal cord (S1-3) via the pelvic nerve and is excitatory to the rectum and inhibitory to the internal anal sphincter, causing it to relax. Sympathetic nerve fibers arise from the lumbar spinal cord; postganglionic fibers reach the internal anal sphincter via the hypogastric nerves from the caudal mesenteric ganglion. Sympathetic stimulation inhibits rectal motility and is excitatory to the internal anal sphincter, causing it to contract. The internal anal sphincter is also innervated by the myenteric plexus of the rectum, which helps to ensure coordinated rectal and anal function. The external anal sphincter and surrounding pelvic muscles are innervated via the pudendal nerves, which leave from the sacral level of the spinal cord.

The pelvic diaphragmatic musculature supports the rectum

GI

and anal canal and participates in the functions of fecal continence and defecation. Paired rectococcygeal muscles originate on each side of the rectum and attach dorsally to the base of the tail. These smooth muscles are innervated by autonomic fibers from the pelvic plexus and shorten the rectum during defecation to assist evacuation of feces. Laterally, the paired levator ani and the coccygeus muscles surround the rectum. These striated muscles are innervated by the third sacral and first caudal nerves and help to compress the rectum during defecation.

NORMAL FUNCTION OF THE RECTUM AND ANUS

In the normal resting state, the rectum is empty and intraluminal rectal pressure is low.[2] Higher pressure is generated in the anal canal by the internal anal sphincter and to a lesser extent by the external anal sphincter, which are normally contracted, thus maintaining fecal continence.[2] The external anal sphincter further contributes to fecal continence by generating increased pressure in response to a sudden increase of intra-abdominal pressure such as occurs with coughing, in response to a sudden increase in rectal filling, and in response to conscious squeezing of the anal sphincter. The primary stimulus for defecation is rectal distention. Feces from the colon intermittently arrive in the rectum, where stretch receptors detect changes in filling. As the rectum fills, the internal anal sphincter relaxes and the external anal sphincter contracts involuntarily, a reflex known as the rectoanal inhibition reflex.[2] As the rectum is stretched by a volume of feces, relaxation of the internal anal sphincter allows contact between receptors in the anal mucosa and the feces. This contact is thought to result in conscious perception of rectal filling, with sensory information transmitted via sacral afferent fibers to the cerebral cortex. The rectoanal inhibition reflex allows accumulation of feces until defecation is appropriate. If the volume of stretch is small or if defecation is not appropriate, internal anal sphincter relaxation is brief and fecal material is transported back to the colon. This process is repeated until the rectum is distended by larger volumes, which cause more stretch of rectal receptors, prolonged relaxation of the internal anal sphincter, and more contact between the anal mucosa and feces, thus stimulating a stronger urge to defecate. When defecation is initiated, colorectal distention activates parasympathetic efferents in the colon and rectum and inhibits excitatory somatic input to the external anal sphincter and pelvic musculature. Parasympathetic activation causes contraction primarily of colonic smooth muscle, resulting in mass movement of the distal colon, which provides the main propulsive force to move feces in the aboral direction. The rectum produces small contractions that are not propulsive.[3] The rectum therefore acts as a passive conduit for passage of feces during defecation. Inhibition of motor input to the external anal sphincter and pelvic musculature allows relaxation of these striated muscles for passage of feces. Defecation is facilitated by proper posture and generation of increased abdominal pressure by closure of the glottis, fixation of the diaphragm, and contraction of the abdominal wall musculature. If defecation is suppressed, descending impulses to sacral nerves and the pudendal nerve mediate conscious contraction of the levator ani and external anal sphincter muscles to maintain fecal continence.

HISTORY AND PHYSICAL EXAMINATION

Diseases of the anus and rectum are typically characterized by signs of inflammation or abnormal motility. Hematochezia, mucoid feces, tenesmus, dyschezia, frequent defecation, constipation, and fecal incontinence are common signs of both colonic and anorectal disease in dogs and cats. Systemic signs, diarrhea, and weight loss are not usually observed. A careful history and thorough physical examination can help determine whether disease involves the colon or is confined to the anorectal segment.

Hematochezia is the presence of bright red blood in the feces, a common sign of colonic and rectal disease.[4] Hematochezia, fresh blood dripping from the rectum, or excess fecal mucus in the presence of normally formed feces is often indicative of rectal disease such as proctitis, polyps, or malignant tumors. Anal sacculitis or perianal fistula can also cause bleeding onto normal feces as they are passed. Tenesmus or straining to defecate, often characterized by urgent, frequent, and unproductive attempts to defecate, is a hallmark of colonic and rectal disease. Dyschezia, which is more characteristic of rectoanal disease, refers to painful defecation and is difficult to differentiate from tenesmus. Tenesmus and dyschezia are usually caused by inflammatory disease of the colon, rectum, or anus that stimulates the defecation reflex, resulting in frequency, urgency, and straining. These are common signs of proctitis, polyps, rectal foreign body, and malignant tumors. Tenesmus and dyschezia can also be caused by anal sacculitis, anal sac abscess, perianal fistula, or perineal hernia. Constipation, obstruction, and motility disorders cause ineffective straining, often with production of small amounts of hard dry feces or without production of any feces. Some owners confuse tenesmus with dysuria. A careful history must be obtained to determine whether straining is associated with defecation or with urination and whether other clinical signs such as hematuria, urinary incontinence, or a distended urinary bladder are present. Observation of the animal during defecation is helpful in further localizing and defining the clinical signs. Causes of tenesmus and dyschezia in the dog and cat are listed in Table 139–1.

TABLE 139–1. CAUSES OF TENESMUS AND DYSCHEZIA

Colorectal disease
  Constipation
  Colitis-proctitis
    Inflammatory bowel disease
    Histoplasma capsulatum (histoplasmosis)
    Clostridium perfringens (enterotoxicosis)
    Prototheca zopfii (protothecosis)
  Rectal stricture
  Neoplasia-polyps
  Foreign material
  Irritable bowel syndrome
Perineal-perianal disease
  Anal sacculitis, impaction, abscess
  Anal sac neoplasia
  Perianal fistula
  Perineal hernia
Urogenital disease
  Cystitis-urethritis-vaginitis
  Cystic-urethral calculi
  Prostatitis-prostatic abscess
  Parturition
  Neoplasia of urethra, bladder, prostate, vagina
Miscellaneous
  Caudal abdominal cavity mass
  Pelvic fracture–neoplasia

Physical examination should begin with a close inspection of the perineum for inflammation, fistulas, herniation, prolapse, or tumors. Digital palpation of the anus and rectum is done to determine anal sphincter contractility, size and consistency of the anal sacs, size of the anorectal lumen, texture of the rectal mucosa, integrity of the bony pelvis and pelvic diaphragmatic musculature, and size and shape of the prostate and to identify the presence of blood, mucus, or foreign material in the feces. Animals with severe proctitis or anal sac abscess often cannot be palpated without sedation because of extreme pain. Thorough abdominal palpation is necessary to detect associated colonic or intestinal disease as well as to evaluate the urinary bladder and prostate. Distention of a colon and rectum with hard feces indicates that constipation is the cause of tenesmus. Detection of a thickened colon by abdominal palpation or a thickened irregular rectal mucosa by rectal palpation is typical of inflammatory or infiltrative bowel disease such as lymphocytic-plasmacytic colitis-proctitis, lymphosarcoma, or histoplasmosis. A firm or distended urinary bladder may indicate that straining is urinary in origin.

Routine hematology and biochemical tests are seldom of diagnostic value in the diagnosis of rectoanal disease but help to identify complicating conditions that might influence the choice of additional diagnostic tests and treatments. Acute tenesmus, dyschezia, and hematochezia are often caused by dietary changes, by ingestion of foreign material, or by parasites. In this instance, fecal flotations for nematode ova, particularly *Trichuris vulpis;* zinc-sulfate flotations for *Giardia* cysts; and rectal cytology to detect large numbers *Clostridium perfringens* spores should be part of the initial database. Dietary restriction for 24 to 72 hours and anthelmintic treatment for occult trichuriasis are a good approach to acute disease.

Radiographic examination does not usually contribute to the diagnosis of most rectoanal diseases but may identify foreign bodies, neoplastic or granulomatous masses, or sublumbar lymphadenopathy. Gas within the lumen of the bowel helps to identify intramural masses or a thickened bowel wall such as occurs with diffuse colorectal disease.[5] A dilated feces-filled colon occurs in dogs and cats with constipation caused by idiopathic megacolon or by extraluminal compression from pelvic fractures. Contrast radiographs are seldom needed to evaluate rectoanal disease but can be useful in the evaluation of rectal strictures and tumors, especially if colonoscopy is not available or if luminal narrowing prohibits passage of an endoscope. Ultrasonography is likewise seldom useful in the diagnosis of most rectoanal diseases. Intrarectal ultrasonography using endoscopic ultrasound probes is useful for determining the depth of tumor penetration and involvement of pararectal structures; however, availability of this relatively new technology is limited to human use.[6]

DISEASES OF RECTUM

PERINEAL HERNIA

A perineal hernia is a peritoneum-lined sac that protrudes through the weakened musculature of the pelvic diaphragm. Associated with this are stretching and deviation of the rectal wall. Pelvic and abdominal contents may move caudally between the rectum and the pelvic diaphragm. Perineal hernias were first recognized clinically in the dog in 1892.

History and Physical Examination

Most animals with perineal hernias are older intact male dogs. This condition is rarely seen in cats or in female dogs. A reducible ventrolateral perineal swelling is usually seen unilaterally, with occasional bilateral involvement. Most unilateral hernias occur on the right side.[7] Constipation and tenesmus are common signs associated with a perineal hernia. In cats with megacolon, constipation and tenesmus often precede the perineal herniation. Dysuria and stranguria accompany other signs in dogs that have retroflexion of the bladder into the ischiorectal fossa. With bladder entrapment, signs of azotemia are common. On occasion, urinary incontinence can be a problem. Rectal examination reveals a weakness or defect in the pelvic diaphragm and prostatomegaly.

Diagnosis

The diagnosis of a perineal hernia is based on the history, signalment, clinical signs (a reducible perineal swelling and tenesmus), rectal examination (a palpable defect of the pelvic diaphragm musculature and the presence of impacted feces in a rectal sacculation), and a barium enema, which demonstrates rectal contents within the hernia. A retrograde urethrocystogram may outline the bladder in the ischiorectal fossa. Rarely, signs of endotoxemia may be seen as a complication of a loop of bowel becoming strangulated after its entrapment within the hernia. Differential diagnoses of a perineal hernia should include a rectal diverticulum, neoplasia, prostatic or paraprostatic cyst, seroma, or hematoma.

Pathogenesis

The pelvic diaphragm is composed of the external anal sphincter, coccygeus musculature (including the levator ani), and fascial coverings. When the muscles undergo atrophy and weaken, abdominal and pelvic organs can herniate into the perineum. Contents of the hernia can include the prostate gland, prostatic or paraprostatic cysts, fat, urinary bladder, and a deviated segment of rectum. Perineal hernia can occur in both dogs and cats and in the dog is a male-related condition. Intact male dogs are 2.7 times more likely than castrated dogs to have a perineal hernia.[8] Hormonal imbalance (androgen deficiency theory) or derangement of the serum testosterone–estradiol-17β concentrations may cause relaxation and weakening of the pelvic diaphragm musculature, although the latter may be more dependent on the affinity or number of hormonal receptors than the hormone levels per se.[9] Tenesmus caused by constipation secondary to prostatomegaly in the dog, or megacolon in the cat,[10] may contribute to weakness of the perineal musculature. In cats, a perineal hernia may also be seen as a complication after a perineal urethrostomy. Degenerative changes of the levator ani muscle have been implicated as well. In the dog, the levator ani muscle is thinner and narrower in the male and has a weaker fascial attachment to the external anal sphincter and rectal wall.[11] Some of the atrophied muscles, especially the levator ani, may rupture, thus removing some of the rectal wall support. Herniation is seen most commonly between the external anal sphincter and the levator ani muscle.

In cats, perineal hernias are associated primarily with tenesmus and constipation. Approximately 50 per cent of perineal hernias in cats were classified as idiopathic.[10] The remaining cats had some factor that was thought to predispose to the development of a hernia. These factors included a megacolon, perianal mass, chronic fibrosing colitis, and a previous perineal urethrostomy.

GI

Therapy

Dietary management may be tried in dogs with minimal signs or when the anesthetic risk is too great for surgical correction. Medical management is also an adjunct to surgery. Use of a low-residue food to reduce fecal volume may be helpful. Stool softeners or enemas are necessary to promote evacuation of the bowel. Digital removal of feces is done in the severely impacted cases. If the bladder is retroflexed, catheterization should be attempted immediately. If this is unsuccessful, a cystocentesis is necessary. Immediately after decompression of the bladder, the hernia should be reduced and the bladder pushed cranially into the abdominal cavity. Whether this is successful or not, another try at placing a transurethral catheter should be made. If it is successful, the catheter should be attached to a closed urinary collection system until a herniorrhaphy is performed.

Definitive treatment with surgery is preferred in most instances. The aim of surgical repair is to replace the support lost by the muscles constituting the pelvic diaphragm. Preoperatively, the geriatric patient should have a complete evaluation of organ status with a complete blood count, chemistry panel, and urinalysis. An electrocardiogram is obtained when indicated. Abdominal and pelvic radiography may be indicated. Fecal softeners and a low-residue diet can be started 3 to 5 days before surgery. Food is withheld for 24 hours before the operation. Feces are manually removed from the rectum after the dog is anesthetized, followed by the placement of a purse-string suture. A preoperative antibiotic (second-generation cephalosporin) is given 20 to 30 minutes before surgery. Enteric coliforms and anaerobes are the targeted microbes.

A standard herniorrhaphy essentially closes the triangular area bounded by the coccygeus, external anal sphincter, levator ani, and obturator muscles.[12] Because of the severe muscle atrophy, the sacrotuberous ligament is sometimes used for lateral support. In the cat, this structure is not present and therefore cannot be used to provide this support. Superficial and deep fasciae are closed over the apposed muscles. Unfortunately, with the conventional method there is a high rate of recurrence (10 to 46 per cent).[12] Postoperative complications (besides recurrence) are varied and are unacceptably high with conventional repair.[7, 12, 13]

Transposition of the superficial gluteal muscle is an alternative to the conventional technique. A low recurrence rate was initially reported with this technique but a later study showed a higher recurrence rate than with the standard herniorrhaphy.[12]

Early and Kolata have described the obturator transposition technique.[13] This technique was used to address the problems associated with the high recurrence rate with previously reported techniques. It was also thought to help overcome the problem of excess tension on the sutures apposing the external anal sphincter muscle to the coccygeus and obturator muscles and the sacrotuberous ligament. The ventral component of a perineal hernia often breaks down with the standard repair. This area of weakness is reinforced by transposition of the obturator muscle. The recurrence rate has decreased with the use of the obturator technique.[13]

A combination of the obturator and superficial gluteal muscle techniques has been reported with a success rate of 94 per cent.[14] A ventral hernia, however, may still continue to be a problem with this technique because two of the three failures in this report were ventral in location.

The ventral defect may also benefit from use of the semitendinosus muscle. This muscle is severed from its insertion and brought to lie ventrally along the floor of the pelvis.[14]

Adjunct surgical procedures can be employed in special circumstances. These include colopexy or fixation of the vas deferens in combination with a herniorrhaphy or as the only procedure in cases in which there is severe sacculation or prolapse of the rectum and retroflexion of the bladder, respectively. These procedures were originally done for large hernias or those with which recurrence had been a problem.[15] Because of the simplicity of this technique, it should also be considered for older dogs at risk in longer surgical procedures such as a herniorrhaphy. In one report, these procedures effectively resolved rectal prolapse and reduced signs of stranguria when retroflexion of the urinary bladder occurred. Tenesmus was resolved in approximately 44 per cent of the cases in which these techniques were used without a concurrent herniorrhaphy.[15]

Cats with megacolon often have a concurrent uni- or bilateral perineal hernia. In these cases, a subtotal colectomy may be indicated initially. Herniorrhaphy is done if the subtotal colectomy fails to relieve the signs of constipation and tenesmus.

Food is withheld for 24 hours postoperatively. A low-residue diet and stool softeners are used indefinitely to decrease straining. Local perianal swelling is common for 24 to 48 hours postoperatively. Hot compresses to the perineum are indicated in these cases.

Prognosis

Recurrence rates are related to the skill of the surgeon and the type of surgical repair utilized. There is universal agreement that in the hands of a skilled surgeon, the obturator transposition technique combined with the conventional repair or with a superficial gluteal muscle repair is probably the best surgical option available at present. Regardless of the technique employed, however, recurrence is higher in dogs with worse signs preoperatively and those with bilateral involvement.[15] Postoperative complications, other than recurrence, include infection, seroma, fecal incontinence, mild rectal prolapse (especially when bilateral repair is done), straining, sciatic nerve paralysis, and pain associated with injury to the nerve. Urinary-related complications include incontinence or urethral obstruction caused by the placement of sutures through or around the urethra.

RECTAL TUMORS

The large intestine is the second most common site of alimentary neoplasia in dogs and cats, with tumors of the oral cavity being most common. Several studies found that primary tumors of the colon and rectum account for 36 to 60 per cent of all canine and 10 to 15 per cent of all feline alimentary tumors.[16] In the dog, most tumors of the large intestine occur in the distal third of the colon or in the rectum.[17] Benign polyps, most of which occur in the rectum, account for approximately 50 per cent of all large intestinal tumors in the dog.[16] Adenocarcinoma is the most common malignant rectal tumor diagnosed in dogs, followed by lymphosarcoma. Rectal carcinomas, leiomyosarcomas, leiomyoma, carcinoids, anaplastic sarcomas, and extramedullary plasmacytomas occur less frequently.[16–19] Lymphosarcoma is the most commonly diagnosed large intestinal tumor in cats, followed by adenocarcinoma, which rarely affects the rectum. In the cat, most adenocarcinomas occur near the ileocecal junction. Rectal polyps are uncommon in cats.

Adenoma

Adenoma, or rectal polyp, is the most common benign colorectal tumor found in the dog. Polyps can be single or multiple and are most often located in the distal rectum, where they intermittently protrude from the anus. Most rectal polyps in the dog are benign. However, some polyps invade the lamina propria and submucosa and are considered by some authors to be precancerous.[20] Malignant transformation to adenocarcinoma and tendency to metastasize are more likely to occur with larger polyps.

Adenocarcinoma

Rectal adenocarcinomas occur predominantly in middle-aged to older dogs, with a mean age of 9 years, and in older cats, with a mean age of 16 years.[20, 21] Male dogs and cats are more frequently affected than females. Most cats with intestinal adenocarcinoma are feline leukemia virus (FeLV) negative.[22] Rectal adenocarcinomas can appear as a single pedunculated mass or as multiple nodular masses protruding into the lumen, as a diffusely infiltrative tumor causing mural thickening or as an annular stricture, or as an ulcerative lesion with raised and proliferative margins.

Intestinal adenocarcinoma is an aggressive tumor that spreads through the bowel wall, invades the lymphatics, and metastasizes to regional lymph nodes, omentum, liver, and lungs. Metastasis has often occurred before diagnosis has been made.[20, 21] Metastasis has been found at necropsy in 75 per cent of cats with intestinal adenocarcinoma. In contrast, metastasis of colorectal adenocarcinoma appears to be considerably less common. In one study of 78 dogs with colorectal adenocarcinoma, no evidence of metastasis was found, even after long survival times after surgical resection of the primary tumor.[23] Dogs with annular colorectal adenocarcinomas were reported to have an average survival of 1.6 months after surgical resection, whereas dogs with multiple nodules had an average survival of 12 months and those with a single pedunculated polyp had a survival of 32 months after surgery.[23]

Lymphosarcoma

Lymphosarcoma of the colon and rectum is the most common large bowel tumor of the cat and the second most common large bowel tumor in the dog. Middle-aged male dogs and older cats have a higher incidence of colorectal lymphosarcoma, which can occur as a primary gastrointestinal malignancy or be secondary to multicentric lymphosarcoma.[20, 24, 25] Although lymphosarcoma in cats is caused by FeLV, most cats with colorectal lymphosarcoma are reported to have a negative FeLV enzyme-linked immunosorbent assay at the time of diagnosis.[25] Virus neutralization is thought to occur after FeLV-induced malignant transformation of cells. Colorectal lymphosarcoma can occur as a discrete mass, as multiple masses, or as a diffuse mucosal infiltrate that causes a corrugated and thickened mucosa. Annular strictures occur infrequently.

History and Physical Examination

Clinical signs of rectal tumor are initially subtle. Tumors have usually been present for several weeks to months before the animal is evaluated. As the tumor develops, signs of ulceration or rectal obstruction become apparent. Tenesmus, dyschezia, hematochezia, mucoid stool, and rectal hemor-

rhage not associated with defecation are common signs.[23, 26] Feces are usually formed but may be abnormally shaped. Severe constipation accompanied by continual posturing to defecate and occasional rectal prolapse may occur. Anorexia, depression, lethargy, weight loss, and debilitation can result from fecal impaction or an advanced malignancy with metastasis. Diffuse colorectal lymphosarcoma can cause chronic diarrhea and malabsorption syndrome, similar to that caused by inflammatory bowel disease or by fungal colitis. Dogs with rectal leiomyomas may be asymptomatic, presumably because of slow growth, until the tumor becomes large.[27]

Dogs with rectal polyps seldom have signs of systemic illness as occurs with malignant disease. Tenesmus and hematochezia are common signs; some animals have a dark red mass, often misinterpreted by the owner as a "hemorrhoid," intermittently protruding from the anus. Cats with colorectal tumors are often debilitated by chronic constipation or advanced malignancy. Owners report hematochezia or chronic constipation, sometimes misinterpreted as stranguria.

Physical examination findings depend on tumor type and duration of disease. Animals with malignant tumors are often depressed, dehydrated, and in poor body condition. Abdominal palpation may reveal a grossly enlarged and painful colon impacted with hard feces. Digital rectal examination often elicits pain and reveals a firm, thickened, and irregular rectal wall, rectal stenosis, or a discrete mass.[23, 27] Rectal polyps can often be exteriorized digitally and appear as a pedunculated, dark red to purple friable mass. Animals with polyps and benign tumors usually have no other physical abnormalities.

Diagnosis

Rectal tumors can be identified by visualization, palpation, or during endoscopy. Thoracic and abdominal radiographs and ultrasonography should be used in an attempt to identify metastases. Plain abdominal radiographs occasionally identify a colorectal mass but more frequently reveal other abnormalities such as sublumbar lymphadenopathy, fecal impaction, or fluid- and gas-filled loops of bowel suggestive of obstruction. Pneumoperitoneum and ascites, uncommon findings with tumors confined to the rectum, can occur with colonic involvement and indicate that colonic or rectal perforation and septic peritonitis have probably occurred. Contrast radiography is seldom necessary to identify rectal tumors; filling defects and segmental strictures are typical findings. Thoracic radiographs are usually negative for metastasis at the initial diagnosis of colorectal tumors. Ultrasonography is the method of choice for staging abdominal metastasis and can be used as a guide for obtaining biopsy specimens.[28] Intrarectal ultrasonography using endoscopic ultrasound probes is useful for accurately determining tumor depth in the bowel wall and assessing regional lymph node involvement.

Endoscopy can be used to assess the extent of disease and to obtain biopsy specimens. Endoscopy of the entire large bowel should be done in dogs and cats with rectal tumors to identify additional proximal tumors that could otherwise go undetected; such staging is particularly important if surgical treatment is anticipated. Multiple biopsy specimens should be obtained from any lesions observed. Biopsy specimens obtained via flexible endoscopy are small and may not provide adequate tissue to identify neoplasia deep to the mucosa. Ulcerated tumors frequently have overlying necrotic and inflammatory tissue that obscures the tumor. Rigid uterine or rectal cup-type biopsy forceps passed through a rigid proctoscope provide larger tissue samples that improve diagnostic accuracy. Impression smears of biopsy samples should be examined cytologically for neoplastic cells and to rule out infectious causes of diffuse proctitis such as *Histoplasma* or *Prototheca*. Submucosal tumors such as lymphosarcoma might require needle aspiration of rectal lesions from a pararectal approach or incisional biopsy for diagnosis.

Treatment

Most rectal polyps are located distally and are accessible through the anus by traction and eversion of the rectal mucosa. Polyps can be removed by submucosal resection or by electrocautery.[29] Polyps located more proximally in the rectum can be removed with an electrocautery snare passed through a rigid or flexible endoscope. The prognosis for rectal polyps is good, even when submucosal invasion is present. New polyps may occur and animals should be reexamined at 6- to 12-month intervals after surgical resection.

Surgical excision, radiation therapy, and cryosurgery have been used to treat colorectal tumors.[23, 27, 30] Colorectal adenocarcinomas in dogs have a low rate of metastasis and surgical resection is usually associated with long survival times. Of multiple treatment modalities evaluated, local excision resulted in the longest average survival (22 months) with the lowest complication rate.[23] In contrast, radical surgical excision of annular colorectal adenocarcinoma resulted in wound dehiscence and septic peritonitis in all four dogs treated.[23] These observations indicate that surgical success and overall prognosis are related to the ease with which surgical excision can be done. Various surgical techniques, including rectal prolapse and pull-through procedures for distal tumors and pelvis splitting for tumors located more proximally in the rectum, have been described.[17, 29] Radiation therapy using a single high dose (15 to 25 Gy) of orthovoltage teletherapy has been reported to provide control for small distal rectal adenocarcinoma.[30] In six dogs, the median duration of tumor control was 6 months without significant complication. In another report,[23] one dog developed a perforated rectum and fatal septic peritonitis 2 months after radiation therapy. Cryosurgery has also been reported to prolong survival in dogs with colorectal adenocarcinoma; however, complications of rectal stricture, rectal prolapse, and perineal hernia were common.[23] Results of chemotherapy for treatment of colorectal adenocarcinoma have not been reported.

Prognosis

The prognosis for animals with colorectal adenocarcinoma is guarded. Mean survival times of 6 to 12 months after treatment have been reported in dogs.[20, 23] Survival is reported to be longer in dogs with single masses and much shorter in dogs with annular lesions.[23] The prognosis for adenocarcinoma in cats is more guarded, with a mean survival time of 20 weeks postoperatively.[31] The prognosis for lymphosarcoma is generally poor, but occasional cases respond to treatment with long-term remission.[31] Mean survival time in dogs and cats treated with chemotherapy has been reported to be 4.5 to 6.5 months.[20] Focal rectal or colonic lymphosarcoma treated with chemotherapy after surgical resection of the affected site has a better prognosis.[31]

RECTAL PROLAPSE

Rectal prolapse is an eversion of one or more layers of the rectum through the anus. In a complete rectal prolapse, all layers are prolapsed, whereas a partial prolapse involves the eversion of the mucosa alone.

History and Physical Examination

Rectal prolapse can occur in any breed of dog or cat and at any age. However, it is most prevalent in the younger animals (usually younger than 4 months of age) because of its association with colitis, typhlitis, and proctitis secondary to endoparasites.[31] There appears to be a predilection in Manx cats.[32] Other predisposing factors would include neoplasia of the distal colon or rectum, rectal deviation, dystocia, urolithiasis, prostatic disease, and foreign bodies. It can also be a sequela of perineal herniorrhaphy in the dog or perineal urethrostomy in the cat.[31] On physical examination, rectal tissue is everted, edematous, and hyperemic. Some degree of ulceration or necrosis may be evident. The prolapsed mass is usually cylindrical in shape with a depression (bowel lumen) in the end. Tenesmus or pain is sometimes noted when gently palpating the prolapsed segment.

Diagnosis

The presence of an elongated portion of everted rectum is usually sufficient to make a diagnosis of rectal prolapse. However, small or large intestinal intussusceptions must be differentiated from rectal prolapse because therapy is different. Signs of partial or complete obstruction usually accompany an intussusception. In addition, a blunt lubricated probe can be passed between the rectal wall and the prolapsed tissue in an intussusception. This is not possible in a rectal prolapse because the prolapsed tissue converges with the mucocutaneous junction of the anus.[31]

Anal prolapse is similar to rectal prolapse and often accompanies the repair of bilateral perineal hernias in dogs. In this condition there is a limited amount of protruding mucosa, which appears to worsen after defecation. It is usually a self-limiting and temporary problem when it occurs as a sequela of perineal herniorrhaphy.

Pathogenesis

Rectal prolapse can be associated with dystocia, proctitis, or colitis. However, there may be no predisposing factor. Contributing factors may include weakness or laxity of the perirectal or perianal connective tissues or musculature. Others include inflammation and edema of the rectal mucosa.[32]

Therapy

The primary goal is to eliminate the underlying cause of the rectal prolapse if it can be identified. If the prolapse is mild, of short duration, and the tissue is healthy, then a conservative approach is indicated. A warm isotonic solution should be applied to the mucosa. The mucosa is gently manipulated and massaged in an attempt to decrease any edema. Application of a thin layer of water-soluble gel is followed immediately by an attempt to reduce the prolapse. If this is successful, a loose purse-string suture is placed in the anus. A narcotic epidural can be given before recovery from anesthesia to reduce rectal straining.[29] A low-residue diet is fed and a stool softener is given for 10 to 12 days while the purse-string suture is in place. After removal of the purse-string suture, stool softeners are continued for another 2 to 3 weeks. Concurrent correction of the underlying problem is done while the purse-string suture is in place.

If conservative management fails, a colopexy is indicated. This procedure fixes the descending colon to the left abdominal wall while placing the colon under a slight amount of cranial traction. Four to six nonabsorbable mattress sutures are used. If the prolapsed tissue is devitalized, lacerated, or irreducible, amputation is necessary. Excision of the prolapsed tissue is followed by a full-thickness anastomosis of the remaining rectal segments.[33] Postoperative management should consist of a low-residue diet and stool softeners for 2 to 3 weeks.

Prognosis

Partial prolapses and those occurring the first time have a better prognosis.[31] A complete prolapse or those that recur after the purse-string suture technique often respond to a colopexy.[32, 33] Rectal amputation involves a worse prognosis because of the technical demands of this surgery and the potential for leakage during the early postoperative period or a stricture at a later time.

RECTAL AND ANAL STRICTURE

Narrowing of the rectal lumen or anus occurs infrequently and is usually the result of fibrosis caused by inflammatory disease or trauma or of proliferative neoplastic disease. Deformity of the pelvic canal resulting from pelvic fracture causes extramural narrowing of the rectum that is clinically indistinguishable from rectal stricture.

History and Clinical Signs

Older dogs tend to be affected more frequently, presumably because of an increased incidence of rectal neoplasia and chronic anorectal disease.[29] Affected animals usually have chronic constipation or a history of progressive difficulty defecating. Persistent tenesmus, prolonged posturing to defecate, and frequent attempts to defecate with production of a narrow ribbon of feces or no feces are typical observations. Hematochezia, mucoid feces, or diarrhea might occur with inflammatory disease. Nonspecific signs such as lethargy, decreased appetite, vomiting, or weight loss occur as the duration and severity of constipation worsen. A history of recent rectal or anal surgery, chronic inflammatory bowel disease, or chronic ingestion of bones or other nondigestible materials is a clue to the existence of a stricture.

Palpation of the caudal abdomen usually reveals a distended and firm colon impacted with feces. Digital rectal examination is usually adequate to identify a narrow and tight lumen of the rectum or anus. Fibrotic strictures are firm, thick, and annular, whereas proliferative neoplastic strictures tend to be asymmetric mass-like lesions. Rectal adenocarcinomas are usually indistinguishable from benign fibrotic strictures.

Diagnosis

History and physical examination are usually adequate to identify the presence of a rectal or anal stricture. Palpation of the caudal abdomen usually reveals a distended and firm colon impacted with feces. Digital rectal examination is adequate to identify a firm, thick, and annular stricture. Rectal adenocarcinomas, however, are often indistinguishable from benign fibrotic strictures.

Diagnostic efforts should be directed to determining whether the stricture is malignant or benign. Survey radiographs of the pelvis and caudal abdomen help to determine whether pelvic fracture, prostatomegaly, caudal abdominal masses, or lymphadenopathy is the cause of the clinical signs. Barium contrast radiographs are seldom necessary to identify the presence of a stricture but are useful in defining the extent of the stricture. Biopsy should be done to differentiate neoplastic, inflammatory, and benign causes of the stricture. Proctoscopy using either a rigid or flexible endoscope helps to determine the severity of the stricture and allows biopsy; however, limitations of this procedure exist. The endoscope often cannot be passed through the stricture and the lesion may be difficult to visualize because of nondistensibility of the rectum. If neoplasia is suspected but not confirmed with endoscopic biopsy, surgical biopsy is necessary.

Treatment

Rectal strictures can be managed by surgical techniques, by bougienage, or by balloon dilatation. Most reports of treatment of rectal stricture recommend surgical correction involving resection and anastomosis, rectal pull-through procedures, or rectal myotomy.[29] Strictures of moderate severity may respond to bougienage, but results are often temporary.[53] We have successfully treated several dogs with benign rectal and anal strictures using balloon dilatation (Rigiflex Colonic Dilatation Balloons, Microvasive Inc., Milford, MA). Balloon dilatation requires general anesthesia and is preferably done with endoscopic and fluoroscopic assistance. The diameter of balloon to use and the number of dilations necessary to create a sustained luminal diameter depend on the severity and chronicity of the stricture and on the size of the animal being treated. Table 139–2 provides general guidelines for choice of balloon diameter. Balloon placement can be done under endoscopic observation or by digital guidance of the balloon through the stricture lumen. Radiographic or fluoroscopic monitoring during dilatation helps to center the balloon in the stricture and allows comparison of the magnitude of dilation with the size of the nonstrictured rectal lumen.

Strictures of moderate severity without excessive fibrosis, such as those that have occurred within a few weeks postoperatively, can often be successfully dilated with one or two dilatation procedures. Severe strictures characterized by greater than 75 per cent reduction of lumen diameter and by significant thickening of the rectal wall might require four to six balloon dilatations to achieve a functional rectal lumen. In our experience, a series of four dilatations done at 4- to 5-day intervals provides a good result and decreases the need for repeated dilatations at a later time. The purpose of multiple dilatations done several days apart is to increase the lumen diameter progressively, preferably until the stric-

TABLE 139–2. GUIDELINES* FOR BALLOON DILATATION OF RECTAL STRICTURES

PATIENT WEIGHT	BALLOON DIAMETER (mm)
Cats	10–15
Dogs ≤10 pounds	
Dogs 10–20 pounds	12–18
Dogs 20–35 pounds	20–30
Dogs ≥35 pounds	30–40

*Size of balloon used for initial dilatation varies, depending on the severity of the stricture. Smaller diameter balloons may be required for initial dilatations.

GI

ture "waist" is eliminated, and to prevent restricture. Because restricture often occurs within 7 to 10 days, we do not recommend long intervals between treatments. Depending on the severity of the stricture, the first dilatation is used to open the stricture partially and to assess the extent of damage caused by the procedure. Superficial mucosal tears and mild hemorrhage are expected to occur. If minimal mucosal tearing is noted endoscopically, the procedure can be repeated using a larger diameter balloon. The procedure should be stopped if deep tears or significant hemorrhage occurs. Broad-spectrum antibiotics targeting anaerobes and coliforms should be given before and for 48 hours after each dilation. Feeding can resume the day after each dilation. Supplementation of the diet with psyllium or lactulose or feeding a high-fiber diet helps to produce a softer consistency stool, which should improve the patient's comfort and increase the frequency of defecation. The use of corticosteroids in an attempt to decrease fibrosis and subsequent restricture has not been evaluated.

Prognosis

In general, benign rectal strictures and those caused by inflammatory disease have a guarded prognosis. Surgical techniques to correct strictures are often complicated by infection, dehiscence, restricture, and fecal incontinence. Results of limited experience in our practice indicate that aggressive balloon dilatation might be a more successful treatment with less risk of complication. Prognosis for neoplastic strictures is poor; the reader is referred to the discussion of rectal neoplasia.

DISEASES OF THE ANUS

ATRESIA ANI

Atresia ani is an condition in puppies and kittens that affects the anal opening and terminal rectum, resulting in closure of the anal outlet and/or abnormal routing of feces through the vagina or urethra. Atresia ani has several anatomic variations and the classification scheme is as follows.[29] Type I (imperforate anus) occurs when a membrane over the anal opening persists, with the rectum ending as a blind pouch just cranial to the closed anus. In type II, the anus is closed, as in type I, but the rectal pouch is located somewhat cranial to the membrane overlying the anus. In type III, the rectum ends as a blind pouch cranially within the pelvic canal (rectal atresia) and the terminal rectum and anus are normal. Type IV exists in female animals and is a persistent communication between the rectum and vagina (rectovaginal fistula) or between the rectum and urethra (rectourethral fistula). This rerouting of feces can occur with or without concurrent atresia ani.

History and Physical Examination

Signs usually begin to be noticed when a puppy or kitten is 2 to 6 weeks of age. Type I, II, and III defects are associated with tenesmus, bulging of the perineum, absence of feces, no visible opening of the anus, abdominal distention, and some abdominal or perineal discomfort. Type IV may be associated with some degree of tenesmus, passage of a small amount of watery feces via the vagina or urethra, and perivulvar erythema.[34]

Diagnosis

The diagnosis of atresia ani is based on the signalment (young animal) and a history of tenesmus, lack of feces (except type IV), and restlessness. Physical examination reveals the perineum to be bulging, although this is not always apparent in type III. Absence of an anal opening is observed in types I and II. Abdominal distention and discomfort on abdominal palpation are sometimes seen in types I, II, and III.

Horizontal beam abdominal radiography may help distinguish type I from type II. The animal should be held by its hind feet and placed upside down. Colonic gas migrates to the distal colon and rectum, thereby defining the limits of the rectal pouch.

Differential diagnoses include anogenital clefts in the female dog or cat. These anomalies occur when the mucosa of the anus or rectum or vagina is continuous along the perineal midline. In the male cat, a similar communication can exist between the rectum and urethra, allowing a common opening for both.[34]

Therapy

Surgical correction depends on the type of anomaly present. Some procedures may require staging. An atresia ani can be corrected as a first stage of repair and any other associated anomalies, such as a rectovaginal or rectourethral fistula, can be repaired at a later date when the animal is a better anesthetic risk. Animals with type I atresia ani usually require only a small incision through the membrane overlying the anal opening followed by gentle bougienage. Failure to respond to this more conservative approach may require partial or complete removal of the stenosed segment and a 360-degree anoplasty.[29] Types II and III require a more technically demanding procedure. In all cases, the preservation of the external anal sphincter is of major concern. Type IV lesions require closure of the rectal and vaginal or urethral defects. If atresia ani is present concurrently, the anus is opened and the mucosa of the rectum is sutured to the surrounding skin.

Prognosis

Younger and weaker animals are less likely to survive any type of surgical procedure regardless of the anomaly. Prognosis for complete return of function to the anorectal region after surgery for any of the atresia ani anomalies is fair to poor because of the likelihood of injury to the external anal sphincter or its innervation. If sphincter dysfunction occurs after surgery, it sometimes resolves several weeks postoperatively. Constipation related to secondary development of a megacolon may be irreversible and require aggressive medical management indefinitely or a subtotal colectomy. Stricture of the anus is always a concern after any type of surgery to the anorectal area.

PERIANAL FISTULA

Perianal fistulas or anal furunculosis is a debilitating disease characterized by multiple draining tracts surrounding the anus. These lesions are chronic, usually progressive in nature, ulcerative in appearance, and malodorous. One or more draining tracts are commonplace and, in severe cases, the entire perianal tissue is involved. In untreated cases, fecal incontinence or anal stricture may result. This condition has not been reported in cats.

History and Physical Examination

This disease can be insidious in nature and clinical signs may go unnoticed. Owners of animals often cite frequent licking of the perianal area as an early sign. Gross lesions are often overlooked because of the long hair surrounding the perianal area and base of the tail. Additional signs include one or more of the following: diarrhea, dyschezia, hematochezia, foul-smelling mucopurulent discharge from ulcerated draining tracts, perianal bleeding, constipation, and tenesmus. Some dogs may have weight loss secondary to anorexia, which presumably results from the animal's pain and discomfort. Sometimes personality changes are noted. Fistulas are seen primarily in large-breed older dogs with broad-based tails and a tail carriage that may predispose to an environment that encourages contamination of perianal structures. German shepherd dogs and Irish setters are two of the most commonly affected breeds.[35]

Physical examination may require heavy sedation because of the pain associated with inspection of the perianal area while lifting the tail. Clipping of the hair and gentle cleansing of the area are necessary to assess the extent of the involvement visually. Multiple ulcerated draining tracts are seen, which, in severe cases, can extend around the entire circumference of the anus. At times these tracts can extend onto the underside of the tail head. Rectal examination often reveals various degrees of thickened granulation tissue extending cranially along the anus and distal rectum. A rectal examination also helps define any decreased anal tone or stricture that may coexist with the fistulation. Palpation and expression of the anal sacs should be done to see if they are involved secondarily with fistulas.

Diagnosis

The signalment, history, and physical examination findings are usually sufficient to make a diagnosis of perianal fistula. Chronic anal sac abscessation with fistulas leading from these sacs is an important differential diagnosis. Perianal tumors (especially adenocarcinoma), caustic or thermal injury, and trauma (dog bite) are other important considerations. Probing the fistulous tracts while the dog is heavily sedated or anesthetized helps to confirm the diagnosis. In the German shepherd dog, a concurrent colitis may exist and can be confirmed by performing proctoscopy and collecting biopsy specimens.[35]

Pathogenesis

Middle-aged (5 to 9 years of age) male German shepherd dogs constitute the majority of dogs with this disease.[36] Anatomic predisposition has long been considered a major factor associated with the formation of perianal fistulous tracts. A broad-based tail in this breed and in Irish setters, a low tail carriage,[37] and an increased density of apocrine sweat glands in the zona cutanea are all factors that may increase the risk of perianal fistulas in certain breeds. The broad tail base and low tail carriage are thought to allow the accumulation of fecal material and glandular secretions and create a poorly ventilated moist environment.

A relationship between perianal fistulas and an immunologic defect or thyroid disorder has been proposed. A study evaluating 33 dogs with fistulas was not helpful in implicating these factors.[38] However, an immune-mediated basis for this disease was later supported by a clinical trial that demonstrated a positive response to immunosuppressive doses of prednisone in German shepherd dogs with perianal fistulas and colitis.[35]

Chronic inflammation of the perianal area followed by infection and necrosis of one of several structures in the perianal region (circumanal glands, sebaceous glands, hair follicles, or anal sacs) has been investigated as a cause of fistulas.[39] Perianal fistulas are thought to be initially an inflammatory process with bacterial infection secondary to epidermal ulceration. A mixed aerobic infection is common, causing the malodorous condition as well.

Therapy

A mild condition with one or two fistulous tracts may be successfully managed with hair removal and perianal cleansing using an antiseptic solution (chlorhexidine or povidone-iodine) and hydrotherapy. Prednisone (1 mg/lb daily) for 2 weeks in combination with antibiotics has had some success in managing this problem in German shepherd dogs.[35] This is followed by a maintenance dose (0.44 mg/lb daily) of prednisone for 4 more weeks. Prednisone is then given at a dose of 0.44 mg/lb every 48 hours and adjusted as necessary to keep the fistulation at a minimum. Alternative protein diets are given concurrently. The combination of high-dose prednisone and dietary alteration resulted in complete resolution in approximately one third of the cases reported, improvement in another one third of the dogs, and no change in the remaining dogs.[35] Immunosuppression using cyclosporine for 4 weeks in combination with a first-generation cephalosporin has shown some promise in one study.[40] Topical application of cyclosporine may be of some value as well after the initial 4 weeks of oral cyclosporine.

Severe cases of perianal fistulas or those responding poorly to medical management may require some form of surgery. Deroofing is recommended in dogs with less than one half of the anal circumference involved and superficial lesions.[41] A bilateral anal sacculectomy is initially done, followed by the probing of all fistulous tracts and deroofing, which is the process of removing the skin covering each tract. Once the lining of the tracts is exposed, they are meticulously electrofulgurated. An alternative is to use electrocoagulation with a ball-tipped electrode and charring of the tissue.[41] Although this procedure usually preserves anal sphincter function, recurrence is common. Cryosurgery has been used, but the success rate varies considerably and anal stenosis is a common sequela.[41]

Surgical excision of all diseased tissue has been described as an acceptable alternative for moderate to severe cases of fistula.[41] Anal sacculectomy may be indicated if the fistulous tracts are overlying the anal sacs. In severe cases, a complete 360-degree excision of tissue is removed, followed by a modified rectal pull-through procedure.[29] This is a salvage procedure and is indicated when there is anorectal stricture. Tail amputation has been suggested as a means of eliminating the unfavorable environment surrounding the perianal tissues. Although successful in 80 per cent of dogs in one study, its use alone in severely affected cases is probably ineffective unless it is combined with surgical excision.[37, 41]

Laser excision has met with some success in a limited number of cases,[42] although fecal incontinence as a sequela is still a major concern. The authors of this report cited an overall success rate of 95 per cent in 20 dogs treated with laser surgery.

GI

Prognosis

The prognosis should be considered guarded to fair for most dogs with perianal fistulas. All methods of medical and surgical management have met with some degree of success. Recurrence and incontinence still remain major concerns with the various surgical options outlined. The success reported with prednisone and cyclosporine makes medical management of perianal fistulas a more attractive option for a significant population of affected dogs. In instances in which medical management is not completely successful, it is likely that less extensive surgery would be required and the serious complication of incontinence would occur less frequently.[40]

ANAL SAC IMPACTION, SACCULITIS, ABSCESSATION

Anal sac disease is common in dogs (affecting approximately 12 per cent of the canine population) but is rarely diagnosed in cats.[43]

History and Physical Examinations

Licking and biting at the tail head region and "tail chasing" are usually early signs of anal sac inflammation or impaction. Discomfort when sitting or reluctance to sit is often reported by the owner. Rubbing the anus on the ground or "scooting" signifies discomfort related to anal sac disease. Tenesmus or not wanting to defecate is sometimes due to extreme pain. Draining tracts from an anal sac are typical of a rupture of an abscessed anal sac.

The anal sacs are usually swollen and more easily palpated when diseased. Anal sac contents vary from a thick pasty brown or grayish brown secretion seen with an impaction to a foul-smelling purulent exudate associated with anal sacculitis.[29] Occasionally, when the anal sac contents are inspissated, it is difficult to express the sacs and irrigating them with warm saline or mineral oil may be necessary to help evacuate the contents. The presence of pus and/or blood draining from a unilateral tract located ventrolaterally from an anal sac is a common sequela of an anal sac abscess.

Diagnosis

Clinical signs localize the problem to the perianal region. Closer examination reveals a slight bulge of the skin overlying the anal sac(s). Rectal examination, sometimes requiring heavy sedation because of pain, confirms anal sac involvement and allows the anal sacs to be emptied. Impaction is confirmed by noting the presence of a thick gray-brown material upon expression of the sacs. Anal sacculitis is diagnosed after demonstrating pain during palpation and attempted expression of the anal sacs and the presence of expressed material that is greenish yellow or cream colored and sometimes mixed with flecks of blood.[31] Fever may be associated with anal sacculitis and is almost always present when there is an abscess. Differential diagnoses should include anal sac or perianal neoplasia, perianal fistulas, trauma (especially bite wounds), and a perivulvular infection in the bitch.

Pathogenesis

Inflammatory conditions involving the anal sac are almost always related to some degree of obstruction of the duct resulting in stasis of secretions and an opportunity for a secondary infection to develop.[31] Animals producing a large amount of thick secretions and having a small duct system or anal irritation are considered at increased risk of developing anal sac disease, with small-breed dogs likely have a higher incidence of anal sac disease. Changes in anal muscle tone, a loose stool, or a recent estrus have all been cited as predisposing factors.[29, 31] Bacteria cultured from diseased anal sacs include organisms such as *Escherichia coli, Streptococcus faecalis, Clostridium welchii,* and *Proteus* species.

If anal sacculitis is chronic and the duct becomes obstructed, the skin overlying the anal sac often becomes edematous, erythematous, indurated, and painful.[29] This occurs just before rupture of an abscess and is associated with a great deal of pain. An anal sac abscess in a cat must be differentiated from an abscess caused by a bite wound.

Therapy

A simple anal sac impaction requires expression of the anal sacs by externally squeezing the skin overlying the anal sacs or by internal compression with a finger in the rectum. If the material is too thick to express, flushing the sac with saline or mineral oil softens the material and assists in evacuation.[31] After emptying of the sacs, an antibiotic solution can be instilled into each sac. Manual expression may need to be repeated one or more times at weekly intervals. In cases of chronic impaction, some owners can be taught to express the anal sacs periodically. An alternative is to perform an anal sacculectomy.

Anal sacculitis usually responds to gentle expression of the anal sacs with the animal under heavy sedation, followed by flushing of the sacs with a warm antiseptic solution using 0.5 per cent chlorhexidine solution or 10 per cent povidone-iodine solution. After irrigation, an antibiotic solution can be placed into each sac. Owners can help alleviate some discomfort by applying hot compresses to the area. Oral broad-spectrum antibiotics should be prescribed for 10 to 14 days. The process of expressing, flushing, and instilling antibiotics can be repeated every 10 to 14 days for one or two more treatments. Rarely is surgical intervention necessary for cases of anal sacculitis. An alternative therapy for chronic anal sacculitis using electrocoagulation and instillation of 80 per cent phenol has been reported.[44] There is some concern, however, that inappropriate use of this agent may create severe local sloughing of tissues surrounding the anus. An anal sac abscess should be initially managed by placing the animal under heavy sedation or anesthesia and lancing the ventral aspect of the abscess. Some abscesses may rupture spontaneously and drain. In either case, the opening to the abscess cavity should be vigorously flushed with an antiseptic solution for about 3 days. Systemic antibiotics are recommended for 10 to 14 days. Application of hot compresses for 3 to 5 days speeds the healing process. If there is recurrence of an abscess, a sacculectomy is indicated. Surgery is best delayed, however, until the abscess has completely responded to medical therapy and is healed.

Prognosis

Anal sac impactions and anal sacculitis usually respond to conservative therapy, with only a few animals requiring surgical intervention. Anal sac abscessation requires more vigorous medical therapy and is probably associated with a higher number of dogs requiring a sacculectomy. Surgery for any of the anal sac diseases should be approached cautiously because of the risk of causing fecal incontinence. This is of greater concern in older dogs, which may already have some degree of decreased tone to the external anal sphincter.

ANAL SAC TUMORS

Tumors that develop from the glandular epithelium of the anal sac are almost always malignant adenocarcinomas, sometimes causing paraneoplastic hypercalcemia. The incidence of these tumors in the dog is low and occurrence in the cat has not been reported.

History and Physical Examination

Anal sac adenocarcinoma occurs predominantly in old female dogs, both intact and neutered.[45, 46] Affected dogs are usually 5 to 17 years of age. Dyschezia, tenesmus, ribbon-like stools, and perineal swelling are the most frequent client complaints. Tenesmus may be caused by either the primary tumor or sublumbar lymphadenopathy. Frequently, the owner does not detect any clinical abnormality and the tumors are detected as an incidental finding during routine physical examination.[45] In other instances, tumors are not detected until after hypercalcemia or problems related to hypercalcemia such as polyuria, polydipsia, anorexia, vomiting, constipation, or muscular weakness have been identified.[45]

Anal sac tumors are usually between 1 and 10 cm in diameter; however, smaller tumors occur that can easily be missed during rectal examination. Most are unilateral. Anal sac adenocarcinomas have often metastasized by the time of diagnosis, most commonly to the external iliac lymph nodes and less frequently to the liver, spleen, and lung. Small tumor size does not correlate with metastatic or paraneoplastic potential.

Diagnosis

Definitive diagnosis is made by biopsy, although a high index of suspicion for this disease should exist if a perianal or anal sac mass is found in an older female dog with hypercalcemia. Thorough digital palpation of both anal sacs is necessary, especially to detect small tumors. Because an estimated 25 to 50 per cent of dogs with anal sac adenocarcinoma are hypercalcemic and hypophosphatemic, all dogs with a palpable mass of the anal sac should have a complete blood count, urinalysis, and serum biochemical profile.[46] Likewise, if hypercalcemia is detected on routine blood chemistry, palpation of the anal sacs for presence of a tumor should be done (see Chapter 149). Because of the high incidence of metastasis at the time of examination, abdominal radiography and ultrasonography, particularly of regional lymph nodes, should be done; pulmonary metastasis is uncommon.

Pathophysiology

Humoral hypercalcemia of malignancy can be caused by anal sac adenocarcinoma and results from the expression of the gene for parathyroid hormone–related protein, a peptide with effects similar to those of parathyroid hormone.[45, 47] In most studies, a majority of affected dogs have been hypercalcemic.[45–47] Hypophosphatemia occurs in some but not all dogs that are hypercalcemic. Hypercalcemia can be severe enough to cause renal failure. Tumor resection results in normocalcemia; however, local recurrence of the tumor or metastasis can result in recurrence of the hypercalcemia.

Anal sac adenocarcinomas tend to metastasize early in the course of disease, especially to the external iliac lymph nodes. In most studies, 50 to 90 per cent of the dogs had metastasis to regional lymph nodes (see Chapter 97). Much less frequent sites of metastasis are the lungs, lumbar vertebrae, liver, and kidneys.

Treatment

Surgical excision of the primary tumor is the treatment of choice, but this can be difficult if the tumor is large. Postsurgical complications include wound dehiscence and infection, sepsis, and permanent fecal incontinence. Local recurrence occurs in approximately 25 per cent of affected dogs after removal of the primary tumor.[46] Removal of enlarged sublumbar lymph nodes is advocated by some; however, this can be a difficult procedure with significant risk of complications.[48] Enlarged nodes frequently involve adjacent vessels and nerves, which increases the risk for hemorrhage and transient urinary incontinence after lymph node surgery. One retrospective study failed to demonstrate improved survival with excision of regional metastasis.[46] The efficacy of chemotherapy as an adjuvant to surgery has not been determined. Surgical excision of the primary tumor and sublumbar nodes followed by chemotherapy with cisplatin and radiation therapy has been suggested as a treatment.[48]

Prognosis

Average postoperative survival has been reported to be about 8 months, with a range of 2 weeks to 39 months.[47, 48] Early detection of a tumor without evidence of metastasis and with complete surgical excision of the primary tumor warrants a good prognosis. Large or nonresectable tumors and the presence of metastasis indicate a poor prognosis for long-term survival.

ANAL AND PERIANAL TUMORS

Benign Perianal Tumors

Perianal adenomas (circumanal gland or "hepatoid cell" adenomas) are the most common tumors of the anal region in dogs but are rare in cats. These benign tumors of the circumanal glands are usually located subcutaneously at the outer cutaneous zone of the anus. Occasionally, these tumors are found in the prepuce, inguinal area, thighs, and ventral skin near the base of the tail. Approximately 85 per cent of these commonly diagnosed tumors have been in old, intact male dogs, and these are among the most common tumors found in male dogs.[49] Cocker spaniels, English bulldogs, Samoyeds, and beagles are breeds predisposed to develop perianal adenomas. Other types of tumors including benign lipomas, fibromas, trichoepitheliomas, and leiomyomas are infrequently found in the anal and perianal region.

History and Physical Examination. Perianal adenomas cause few clinical signs. Most are firm, single or multiple nodular masses located near the subcutaneous junction of the anus. Tumors vary in size from less than 1 cm to 10 cm in diameter. Some dogs persistently lick the perianal area or have difficulty with defecation. Larger lesions tend to ulcerate and bleed.

Diagnosis. Diagnosis of perianal adenoma is often made by fine-needle aspiration cytology, which reveals clusters of hepatoid epithelial cells with discrete nuclei. Diagnosis is confirmed with excisional biopsy.

GI

Pathophysiology. Perianal adenomas are slow-growing tumors whose development and growth are closely related to plasma androgen levels. Androgenic stimulation causes proliferation of the circumanal hepatoid glands, although the function of these glands is unknown. These tumors are minimally invasive and are not metastatic.

Treatment and Prognosis. These tumors are effectively treated by surgical excision; however, cryosurgery and radiation therapy are reported to be effective.[29, 49] Castration causes regression of existing tumor and reduces the risk of new tumor growth.[29, 49] Estrogen therapy to decrease tumor growth is not recommended because of the myelosuppressive effects of this hormone. Surgical removal of the primary tumor and castration of intact males are curative.

Malignant Perianal Tumors

Malignant tumors occur infrequently and include perianal adenocarcinoma, squamous cell carcinoma, and melanoma.[50] German shepherds, Arctic Circle breeds, and dogs over 35 kg in body weight are reported to be predisposed to develop adenocarcinomas, which often metastasize to sublumbar lymph nodes.[50] Constipation and tenesmus occur as the tumor enlarges; however, growth of perianal adenocarcinomas does not appear to be influenced by androgens. Diagnosis is confirmed by fine-needle aspiration or by surgical biopsy. Treatment for adenocarcinoma requires surgical excision, although complete removal is difficult in many cases. Castration does not cause these tumors to regress.[50] Prognosis for adenocarcinoma is guarded to poor, especially if metastasis is present. Squamous cell carcinoma of the cutaneous portion of the anus occurs rarely and can appear as a small ulcer or as a proliferative-ulcerative mass with irregular margins. Metastasis to sublumbar lymph nodes occurs rapidly. Early detection and surgical removal might be curative. Rarely, malignant melanomas occur as flat to round nodules on the anus. Most are pigmented, but unpigmented melanomas that resemble perianal gland adenomas occur. These also tend to metastasize rapidly.

FECAL INCONTINENCE

Fecal incontinence refers to inability to control defecation and retain feces until defecation is consciously initiated; the result is involuntary passage of feces. Fecal incontinence can be caused by neurologic disorders that affect function of the anal sphincter (neurogenic sphincter incontinence), primary disorders of the external anal sphincter (non-neurogenic sphincter incontinence), or diseases that affect the normal reservoir function of the colon or rectum (reservoir incontinence). Specific causes of fecal incontinence are listed in Table 139–3. Loss of voluntary control of defecation accompanied by urgency to defecate, tenesmus, hematochezia, or mucoid feces is usually caused by inflammatory colorectal disease, treatment of which usually resolves the incontinence. Incontinence characterized by lack of conscious posture to defecate and uncontrolled passage of feces is suggestive of a neurologic or muscular abnormality of the anal sphincter. In general, animals with sphincter incontinence have more severe symptoms and are likely to be irreversibly affected.

History and Physical Examination

Animals with fecal incontinence intermittently eliminate feces involuntarily without assuming a normal posture to

TABLE 139–3. CAUSES OF FECAL INCONTINENCE

Neurologic disease	
Sacral spinal cord	Congenital vertebral malformation
	Meningomyelocele
	Sacrococcygeal hypoplasia of Manx cats
	Sacral fracture
	Sacrococcygeal subluxation
	Lumbosacral instability
	Viral meningomyelitis
	Discospondylitis
	Degenerative myelopathy
	Neoplasia
Peripheral neuropathy	Trauma
	Repair of perineal hernia
	Perianal urethrostomy
	Penetrating wounds
	Dysautonomia
	Hypothyroidism
	Diabetes mellitus
Non-neurologic disease	
Colorectal	Inflammatory bowel disease
	Neoplasia
	Constipation
Anorectal	Trauma
	Surgery—anal sac, perineal hernia, rectal resection
	Perianal fistula
	Neoplasia
Miscellaneous	Severe diarrhea
	Irritable bowel syndrome
	Decreased mentation
	Old age

defecate. Fecal material accumulates around the anus, and some animals have constant dribbling of feces. A detailed history can help to determine the cause of fecal incontinence. Previous spinal disease, pelvic trauma, dystocia, chronic constipation, and anorectal surgery are conditions that can damage mechanisms of fecal continence. Some owners misinterpret urgency to defecate as fecal incontinence. Frequent and conscious defecation with normal posturing is usually caused by loss of reservoir function of the colon and rectum. Inflammatory, infectious, and neoplastic diseases can decrease compliance and disrupt normal motility. Severe or chronic diarrhea, especially that caused by colitis, can cause fecal incontinence, whereas the presence of normal feces is consistent with neurogenic or non-neurogenic sphincter incontinence. The animal's ability to urinate should be evaluated because micturition and defecation share common neural pathways, and the anal sphincter works in synchrony with skeletal muscle of the urethral sphincter mechanism.[51] Concurrent fecal incontinence with abnormal micturition characterized by dribbling urine, incomplete voiding, or inability to void suggests the presence of neurologic dysfunction.

Careful inspection of the perineum and digital palpation of the anorectum for abscess, fistulas, perineal hernia, rectal mass, stricture, or fecal impaction should be done. Decreased anal sphincter tone during digital examination is present in most cases of neurogenic and non-neurogenic sphincter incontinence. Palpation of the caudal abdomen is done to determine whether constipation is present and to evaluate the bladder. A distended and flaccid bladder from which urine is easily expressed is consistent with a lesion of the sacral spinal cord, the sacral nerves, or the pudendal nerve.

Dogs with neurogenic sphincter incontinence may have other neurologic deficits such as an abnormal posture, hindlimb gait abnormalities, depressed myotatic reflexes, or an abnormal pudendal-anal reflex.[52] A complete neurologic examination, including observation of gait and posture and evaluation of myotatic and postural responses, and evaluation for lumbosacral pain should be done. Perianal sensation and sacral spinal cord function are mediated through the pudendal nerve and are best assessed by the anal reflex and the pudendal-anal (bulbocavernosus) reflex. The anal reflex is tested by pinching the perianal skin which normally causes a brisk contraction of the anus. Both right and left sides of the anus should be tested. The pudendal-anal reflex is tested by squeezing the penis or vulva while observing for normal anal contraction. Lesions of the perineal afferent nerves, the sacral spinal cord, or the pudendal efferent nerves can abolish these reflexes and cause a dilated anal sphincter, loss of sensation to coccygeal dermatomes, and loss of micturition control.[52]

Diagnosis

Fecal incontinence associated with diarrhea, frequency of defecation, and a normal posture to defecate is most consistent with loss of colorectal reservoir function. A diagnostic plan that includes proctoscopy or colonoscopy with biopsy is usually indicated to identify the primary disease. Diagnosis of sphincter incontinence is usually apparent from history and physical examination, and neurologic examination differentiates neurogenic from non-neurogenic sphincter incontinence. Sphincter incontinence can be confirmed with anal sphincter electromyography or manometry,[53] although use of these techniques is seldom necessary. Vertebral radiographs and special imaging using myelography, epidurography, computer-assisted tomography, magnetic resonance imaging, and cerebral fluid analysis should be considered to identify lesions affecting the lumbosacral spinal cord or cauda equina.[52, 54]

Pathophysiology

Fecal continence is maintained by several essential structures including the rectum, the internal and external anal sphincters, and the coccygeus and levator ani muscles. These structures are innervated by the pelvic, hypogastric, pudendal, and sacral nerves. Motor and sensory impulses are integrated in the sacral spinal cord to coordinate normal function of these structures to maintain fecal continence. Sacral spinal cord lesions such as cauda equina syndrome, somatic nerve disease such as polyneuropathy, autonomic nerve disease such as dysautonomia, or trauma to the pudendal nerve causes neurogenic sphincter incontinence. Occasionally, central nervous system disease such as distemper encephalomyelitis has been associated with neurogenic incontinence.[54] Perianal surgery, such as anal sacculectomy and perineal herniorrhaphy, is a common cause of non-neurogenic sphincter incontinence. Severe inflammatory and infiltrative diseases of the colon and rectum occasionally impair rectal accommodation and anal sphincter function enough to cause fecal incontinence.

Treatment

Prognosis and treatment of fecal incontinence depend on the primary cause. Incontinence caused by loss of reservoir function secondary to inflammatory colorectal disease usually resolves with treatment of the primary disease. Neurogenic and non-neurogenic sphincter incontinence is usually permanent and not treatable. Fecal incontinence caused by compressive spinal cord lesions or by sacrococcygeal verte-

bral subluxation may improve after spinal surgery. Incontinence caused by trauma or surgical injury to the anorectum may be transient.

Symptomatic management of non-neurogenic and mild neurogenic sphincter incontinence can be attempted, but results are usually unrewarding. Frequent small meals of a low-fiber diet help to decrease fecal volume, thereby diminishing the amount and frequency of defecation. Opiates such as diphenoxylate or loperamide increase anal canal function and slow intestinal transit, thereby allowing absorption of more water from the fecal mass. However, these drugs do not improve anal sphincter function. Daily warm-water enemas and frequent exercise may help to stimulate defecation at desired times.

Surgical techniques using an implanted perianal Silastic sling or autogenous muscle graft to augment muscles of continence and to improve anorectal angulation have been described.[29] The success rate with these techniques is not satisfactory.

The prognosis for return to normal or acceptable sphincter function is poor in most cases. Many pets are eventually euthanized because of unacceptable sanitary and social consequences of this condition.[55]

REFERENCES

1. Evans HE: Miller's Anatomy of the Dog. Philadelphia, WB Saunders, 1993, pp 486–491.
2. Smout AJ, Akkermans LM: Innervation of the gastrointestinal tract. In Normal and Disturbed Motility of the Gastrointestinal Tract. Hampshire, UK, Wrightson Biomedical Publishing, 1992, pp 25–38.
3. Karaus M, Sarna SA: Giant migrating contractions during defecation in the dog colon. Gastroenterology 92:925–933, 1987.
4. Leib MS, Codner EC, Monroe WE: A diagnostic approach to chronic large bowel diarrhea in dogs. Vet Med (Praha) 86:892–899, 1991.
5. Kleine LJ, Lamb CR: Comparative organ imaging: The gastrointestinal tract. Vet Radiol 30:133–141, 1989.
6. Senagore A, et al: A comparison between intrarectal ultrasound and CT scanning and staging of experimental rectal tumors. J Surg Res 44:522, 1988.
7. Bellenger CR, Canfield RB: Perineal hernia. In Slatter D (ed): Textbook of Small Animal Surgery, 2nd ed. Philadelphia, WB Saunders, 1985, pp 471–627.
8. Hayes MH, Wilson G, Tarme RE: The epidemiologic features of perineal hernia in 771 dogs. J Am Anim Hosp Assoc 14:703–707, 1978.
9. Mann FA, Boothe HW, Amoss MS, et al: Serum testosterone and estradiol 17-beta concentrations in 15 dogs with perineal hernia. JAVMA 194:1578–1580, 1989.
10. Welches CD, Scavelli TD, Aronsohn MG, et al: Perineal hernia in the cat: A retrospective study of 40 cases. J Am Anim Hosp Assoc 28:431–438, 1992.
11. Desai R: An anatomical study of the canine male and female pelvic diaphragm and the effect of testosterone on the status of levator ani of male dogs. J Am Anim Hosp Assoc 18:95–202, 1982.
12. Weaver AD, Omamegbe JO: Surgical treatment of perineal hernia in the dog. J Small Anim Pract 22:749–758, 1981.
13. Early TJ, Kolata RJ: Perineal hernia in the dog: An alternative method of correction. In Bojrab MJ (ed): Current Techniques in Small Animal Surgery, 2nd ed. Philadelphia, Lea & Febiger, 1983, pp 405–407.
14. Raffan PJ: A new surgical technique for repair of perineal hernia in the dog. J Small Anim Pract 34:13–19, 1993.
15. Huber DJ, Seim HB, Goring RL: Cystopexy and colopexy for management of large or recurrent perineal hernia in the dog: 9 cases (1994–1996). Proceedings of the Sixth Annual Scientific Meeting of the European College of Veterinary Surgeons, June 27–29, 1997, p 156.
16. Crow SE: Tumors of the alimentary tract. Vet Clin North Am 15:577–596, 1985.
17. White RAS: The alimentary system. In White RAS (ed): Manual of Small Animal Oncology. Cheltenham, UK, British Small Animal Veterinary Association, 1991, pp 237–263.
18. Rakich PM, et al: Mucocutaneous plasmacytomas in dogs: 75 cases (1980–1987). JAVMA 194:803, 1989.
19. Trevor PB, Saunders GK, Waldron DR, et al: Metastatic extramedullary plasmacytoma of the colon and rectum in a dog. JAVMA 203:406–409, 1993.
20. White RAS, Gorman NT: The clinical diagnosis and management of rectal and pararectal tumours in the dog. J Small Anim Pract 28:87–107, 1987.
21. Carpenter JL, Andrews LK, Holzworth J: Tumors and tumor-like lesions. In Holzworth J (ed): Diseases of the Cat. Medicine and Surgery. Philadelphia, WB Saunders, 1987, pp 406–596.
22. Kosovsky JE, Matthiesen DT, Patnaik AK: Small intestinal adenocarcinoma in cats: 32 cases (1978–1985). JAVMA 192:233–235, 1988.
23. Church EM, Mehlhaff CJ, Patnaik AK: Colorectal adenocarcinoma in dogs: 78 cases (1973–1984). JAVMA 191:727–730, 1987.

GI

24. Couto CG, Rutgers HC, Sherding RG, et al: Gastrointestinal lymphoma in 20 dogs: A retrospective study. J Vet Intern Med 3:73–78, 1989.

25. Davenport DJ: Gastrointestinal lymphosarcoma. *In* August JR (ed): Consultations in Feline Internal Medicine. Philadelphia, WB Saunders, 1991, pp 419–423.

26. Birchard SJ, Couto CG, Johnson S: Nonlymphoid intestinal neoplasia in 32 dogs and 14 cats. J Am Anim Hosp Assoc 22:533–537, 1986.

27. McPherron MA, Withrow SJ, Seim HB III, et al: Colorectal leiomyomas in seven dogs. J Am Anim Hosp Assoc 28:43–46, 1992.

28. Penninck DG, Crystal MA, Matz ME, et al: The technique of percutaneous ultrasound guided fine-needle aspiration biopsy and automated microcore biopsy in small animal gastrointestinal diseases. Vet Radiol Ultrasound 34:433–436, 1993.

29. Matthiesen DT, Marretta SM: Diseases of the anus and rectum. *In* Slatter D (ed): Textbook of Small Animal Surgery, 2nd ed, Vol 1. Philadelphia, WB Saunders, 1993, pp 627–645.

30. Turrel JM, Theon AP: Single high-dose irradiation for selected canine rectal carcinomas. Vet Radiol 27:141–145, 1986.

31. Washabau RJ, Brockman DJ: Recto-anal disease. *In* Ettinger SJ, Feldman EC (eds): Textbook of Veterinary Internal Medicine, 3rd ed, Vol 2. Philadelphia, WB Saunders, 1995, pp 1398–1409.

32. Bright RM: Surgery of the digestive system. *In* Sherding RG (ed): The Cat: Diseases and Clinical Management, 2nd ed, Vol 2. New York, Churchill Livingstone, 1994, pp 1353–1401.

33. Eugen MH: Management of rectal prolapse. *In* Bojrab MJ (ed): Current Techniques in Small Animal Surgery, 4th ed. Baltimore, Williams & Wilkins, 1998, pp 254–258.

34. Bright RM: Diseases of the anus and perineal area. *In* Morgan RV (ed): Handbook of Small Animal Practice, 2nd ed. New York, Churchill Livingstone, 1992, pp 473–482.

35. Harkin KR, Walshaw R, Millaney TP: Association of perianal fistula and colitis in the German shepherd dog: Response to high-dose prednisone and dietary therapy. J Am Anim Hosp Assoc 32:515–520, 1996.

36. Budsberg SC, Spurgeon TL, Liggett HD: Anatomic predisposition to perianal fistulae formation in the German Shepherd Dog. Am J Vet Res 46:1468–1472, 1985.

37. Van Ee RT, Palminteri A: Tail amputation for treatment of perianal fistulas in dogs. J Am Anim Hosp Assoc 23:95–100, 1987.

38. Killingsworth CR, Walshaw R, Remman HA, et al: Thyroid and immunologic status of dogs with perianal fistula. Am J Vet Res 49:1742–1746, 1988.

39. Day MJ, Weaver BMQ: Pathology of surgically resected tissue from 305 cases of anal furunculosis in the dog. J Small Anim Pract 33:583–589, 1992.

40. Matthews KA, Sukhiani HR: Randomized controlled trial of cyclosporine for treatment of perianal fistulas in dogs. JAVMA 211:1249–1253, 1997.

41. Ellison GW: Treatment of perianal fistulas in dogs. JAVMA 206:1680–1682, 1995.

42. Ellison GW, Bellah JR, Stubbs WP: Treatment of perianal fistulas with ND/YAG laser—Results of 20 cases. Vet Surg 24:140–147, 1997.

43. Van Duijkeren E: Disease conditions of canine anal sacs. J Small Anim Pract 36:12–16, 1995.

44. Lowenstein C, Lowenstein MD, Bertling J: Electrocoagulation—A method of treatment for chronic anal sac inflammation and its morphological changes. Kleintierpraxis 33:483–488, 1988.

45. Rosol TJ, Capen CC, Danks JA, et al: Identification of parathyroid hormone–related protein in canine apocrine adenocarcinoma of the anal sac. Vet Pathol 27:89–95, 1990.

46. Ross JT, Scavelli TD, Matthiesen DT, et al: Adenocarcinoma of the apocrine glands of the anal sac in dogs: A review of 32 cases. J Am Anim Hosp Assoc 27:349–355, 1991.

47. Weir EC, et al: Isolation of 16,000-dalton parathyroid hormone–like proteins from two animal tumors causing humoral hypercalcemia of malignancy. Endocrinology 123:2744, 1988.

48. Olgilvie GK, Moore AS: Adenocarcinoma of the apocrine glands of the anal sac in dogs. *In*: Managing the Veterinary Cancer Patient. Trenton, NJ, Veterinary Learning Systems, 1995, pp 357–360.

49. Wilson G, Hayes HM: Castration for treatment of perianal gland neoplasms in the dog. JAVMA 174:1301–1303, 1979.

50. Vail DM, Withrow SJ, Schwarz PD, et al: Perianal adenocarcinoma in the canine male: A retrospective study of 41 cases. J Am Anim Hosp Assoc 26:329–334, 1990.

51. Gonella J, et al: Extrinsic nervous control of motility of small and large intestines and related sphincters. Physiol Rev 67:902, 1987.

52. Kornegay JN: Paraparesis, tetraparesis, urinary/fecal incontinence. Probl Vet Med 3:363, 1991.

53. Strombeck DR, Harrold D: Anal sphincter pressure and the rectosphincteric reflex in the dog. Am J Vet Res 49:191, 1988.

54. Guilford WG: Fecal incontinence in dogs and cats. Compend Contin Educ 12:313, 1990.

55. Chapman BL, Voith VL: Behavioral problems in old dogs: 26 cases (1984–1987). JAVMA 196:944, 1990.

SECTION XI

DISEASES OF THE LIVER AND PANCREAS

CHAPTER 140

HISTORY, PHYSICAL EXAMINATION, AND SIGNS OF LIVER DISEASE

Jan Rothuizen and Hein P. Meyer

HISTORY OF ANIMALS WITH LIVER DISEASE

To understand the clinical signs encountered in dogs and cats with diseases of the liver, the portal vasculature, or the biliary system, it is important to keep some basic rules in mind. First, for most of its functions the liver has a huge (about 80 percent) reserve capacity and a fantastic potential to regenerate.[1] Clinical signs occur only when the reserve is exhausted by progressive disease. In many cases a disease may remain chronically subclinical. Often, signs are relatively mild and nonspecific because the liver reserve prevents overt abnormalities. Thus, some apathy, occasional vomiting, or mild polyuria and polydipsia may alert the clinician that a liver disorder could be developing. When more serious signs develop, much of the reserve may be lost. The onset of signs may be acute, but they may be the end result of a chronic disease that has been present for many weeks or months.

Because there are no specific physical abnormalities with most liver diseases, it is important to keep the possibility of liver disease in mind when signs of illness are unexplained or nonspecific. Such liver diseases may easily be detected by sensitive and specific laboratory tests. A second feature is that most of the different liver diseases cause similar signs (Table 140–1). There are only a few exceptions to this rule. One is that acholic feces occur nearly exclusively in dogs with extrahepatic obstruction of the common bile duct.[2] The light-grey appearance of stool may be noted by the owner, and in combination with jaundice, it is virtually diagnostic for extrahepatic cholestasis. Otherwise, different combinations of signs may occur in any liver disease. Statistically, one disease may be associated with a typical pattern of signs in dogs and cats. However, the overlap noted in these patterns is so great that it is useless to try to identify the exact disease based on clinical signs alone (see Table 140–1). Clinical signs associated with liver diseases of cats are similar, except for polyuria and dysuria, which are not seen in cats. Hepatic encephalopathy causes a variety of neurologic signs with certain liver diseases. These signs, in different stages of the syndrome, are listed in Table 140–2.[3] It is noteworthy that the neurologic signs associated with hepatic encephalopathy fluctuate. As a result, any medication given seems to be effective because of the natural resolution of signs. Therefore, the fact that the signs may be of hepatic origin may be missed. Seizures alone are never due to hepatic encephalopathy; they are rarely associated with it, and if seizures do occur, they are in combination with other signs seen with this syndrome.

It is usually not possible to use clinical signs to differentiate between liver diseases and diseases of other organs. The signs associated with liver diseases are not specific; similar problems may occur in diseases of many other organ systems. This is apparent from the signs listed in Table 140–1. A rare sign, not included in the table, is an ulcerative form of dermatosis. This so-called superficial necrolytic dermatitis or hepatodermal syndrome is a rare finding in dogs with liver cirrhosis and nodular hyperplasia and is not understood pathogenetically.[4] This and the more common symptoms of apathy, vomiting, inappetence, diarrhea, weight loss, polyuria/polydipsia, and neurologic signs are frequently associated with disease of other organs. Therefore, the history often reveals signs that may indicate liver disease but may also be caused by other disorders. There are two main reasons for the nonspecificity of liver-related clinical signs. First, the liver is the central organ for many metabolic and detoxifying pathways in the body; therefore, failing liver function may cause dysfunction of other organs. One of many examples is hepatic encephalopathy, when neurotransmitter dysfunctions of the brain, caused by metabolic dysfunctions of the liver, result in neurologic signs.[5] Second, the liver is often secondarily affected by toxic factors resulting from diseases of other organ systems, especially from the intestinal tract. Examples are hepatic lipidosis in diabetes mellitus, steroid hepatopathy in Cushing's syndrome, reactive hepatitis in gastrointestinal diseases, and centrolobular liver necrosis in acute, severe anemia. Therefore, signs of liver disease may be hidden within signs of other organ dysfunction, and vice versa. Because the clinical signs and physical examination findings may be compatible with liver disease, and because the laboratory tests to detect liver disease are also abnormal with primary and secondary hepatopathies, it is often necessary to make a histologic diagnosis of the liver disorder to resolve this dilemma.[6]

Another factor that may prevent recognition of a primary liver disease is the lack of specific findings on physical examination. Most dogs with illnesses causing the clinical signs listed in Table 140–1 are candidates for having a primary hepatopathy. In all such cases, a laboratory test should be performed to confirm or exclude the presence of a liver disease, as summarized in Figure 140–1.

Some hepatopathies have a distinct predisposition with respect to breed, sex, or age or may be drug-induced. The presence of a high risk factor can be a stimulus for further diagnostic work-up, and absence of such suspicions may result in investigation for other diseases. The most common drug-induced liver disease is destructive cholangiolitis, which is caused by hypersensitivity to sulfonamides.[7] A

TABLE 140–1. COMMON CLINICAL SIGNS IN DOGS WITH LIVER DISEASE

LIVER DISEASE WITH RELATIVE FREQUENCY (%)	Percentage of Dogs With Sign												
	Apathy, Depression	Inappetence	Reduced Endurance	Vomiting	Diarrhea	Weight Loss	Hepatic Encephalopathy	Polyuria/ Polydipsia	Dysuria	Anesthesia Intolerance	Acholic Feces	Distended Abdomen	Retarded Growth
Acute hepatitis (3)	44	49		61	21	12		11					
Chronic hepatitis (10)	18	29	14	43	33	39		49					
Cirrhosis (7)	25	53	39	61	37	58		56					
Lobular dissecting hepatitis (2)	58	21	29	32	20	45	9	39				55	
Reactive hepatitis (25)	10	34		48	77	39	22	9				65	
Destructive cholangiolitis (1)	76	82		68	21	66		49					
Portosystemic shunt (16)	99	68	62	31	12	81	91	52			9	8	39
Portal vein thrombosis (1)	25	10		38	44	15	5	32		9		33	
Portal vein hypoplasia (4)	49	13	22	16	21	14	38	45	3			60	8
Liver cell carcinoma (4)	15	26	18	74	14	32		19				25	
Metastatic tumor (10)	24	54	17	67	27	60		38				14	
Malignant lymphoma (14)	18	75	32	70	21	85		55					
Cholecystitis/stones (1)		65		93	19	30						5	
Extrahepatic cholestasis (2)	10	72		81	37	54		46			16		

Figures are from the Utrecht University Clinic population. The relative frequencies are based on 2500 referred cases.

LIV

TABLE 140–2. NEUROLOGIC SIGNS SEEN WITH HEPATIC ENCEPHALOPATHY IN DOGS AND CATS

CLINICAL SIGN	STAGE	DOG	CAT
Depression, listlessness	I	2	2
Slight behavioral changes	I	2	1
Involuntary movements: circling, head pressing	II	2	0
Ataxia	II	2	1
Apparent blindness	II	1	0
Abnormal swallowing, salivation	II–III	1	2
Stupor, reduced response to stimuli	III	1	1
Seizures	II–IV	1	0
Coma, nonresponsiveness to stimuli	IV	1	1

Characteristically, these signs occur in episodes. Seizures are never the only sign of hepatic encephalopathy but are associated with a number of other problems. The frequency in dogs and cats is semiquantitatively given as 0 (absent) to 2 (common).

history of recent medication with such a drug in combination with jaundice makes this condition likely and should prompt immediate discontinuation of the medication. Breed associations may occur when a disease is (in part) determined by genetic factors. Familial selection by breeders may by chance increase the incidence of such a disease in the breed. Because dog breeds may represent more or less closed populations in a country, breed predispositions may vary among countries. Therefore, we mention only generally applicable predispositions; locally, there may be other breed associations. First, chronic hepatitis and cirrhosis, both of which are, as a rule, different stages of one disease, occur more frequently in certain breeds.[8] Associated breeds are Doberman pinschers, American and English cocker spaniels, Bedlington terriers, and West Highland white terriers. The specific Doberman hepatitis is sex-linked, confined to females, and aggressive.[9] In contrast to other forms of hepatitis, it does not respond to medication and terminates in micronodular cirrhosis. This form of cirrhosis is also different from other forms, because dogs usually develop macronodular cirrhosis with large hyperplastic nodules. We have found that hepatitis is overrepresented in female Dobermans by a factor of 10. A recent study in Finland showed that about 10 per cent of Dobermans may be affected.[10] Spaniels have the more common form of chronic hepatitis and develop macronodular cirrhosis when left untreated. There is no sex predisposition, but there seems to be a worldwide overrepresentation of hepatitis in these breeds. Hepatitis may develop at any age, but typically not before 2 years of age. Only lobular dissecting hepatitis tends to occur at young age, often before 1 year of age.[11] Inherited copper toxicosis is a liver disease of Bedlington terriers all over the world and of West Highland white terriers in the United States.[12] Both sexes may be affected, and owing to the gradual accumulation of copper, clinical signs usually develop at after 4 years of age.

Congenital portosystemic shunts are inherited diseases of both sexes that have certain breed predispositions as well. Intrahepatic shunts predominate in large breeds and extrahepatic shunts in small and toy breeds. Worldwide predispositions occur in Irish wolfhounds, Labrador retrievers, dachshunds, Yorkshire terriers, Cairn terriers, Maltese terriers, and miniature schnauzers.[3] In the United States, an increased prevalence of shunts has also been reported in German shepherds, Doberman pinschers, and golden retrievers. Clinical signs are usually seen in young dogs and cats (<1 year old) with congenital shunts.

PATHOGENESIS OF COMMON SIGNS OF PRIMARY LIVER DISEASES

Vomiting. Vomiting is one of the most common clinical signs seen in dogs and cats with liver disease and may be induced via a number of pathways. Vomiting may be caused by direct stimulation of the vomiting center via the chemoreceptor trigger zone in the fourth ventricle by (endo)toxins that are not cleared by the liver.[13] This occurs most commonly when the liver is bypassed in its guardian function between the gastrointestinal tract and the rest of the organism. Therefore, vomiting is a frequent sign in all conditions with the combination of portosystemic shunting and liver dysfunction, such as in congenital shunts and in acquired shunts due to hepatitis, fibrosis, cirrhosis, and portal vein hypoplasia or thrombosis. Dislocation of the upper gastrointestinal tract by an abnormal liver shape may induce nausea and vomiting by vagal stimulation. This may result from

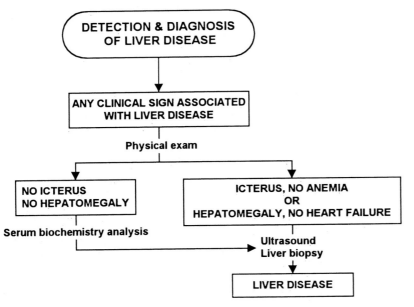

Figure 140–1. Algorithm for the detection and diagnosis of liver disease.

tumors of the liver, especially liver cell carcinomas, but also from unilateral collapse and contralateral hypertrophy, as may occur with thrombosis of one main branch of the portal vein. Finally, the gallbladder and larger bile ducts have a rich sympathetic innervation, and dilatation (extrahepatic cholestasis), cholecystitis, or cholelithiasis may be suspected in vomiting dogs and cats.

Vomiting is also one of the major signs of upper gastrointestinal disease. In many such diseases, there is an increased absorption of endotoxins, which has the potential to cause secondary, nonspecific, reactive hepatitis.[14] This is one of the most frequent liver abnormalities in dogs but is rare in cats. Reactive hepatitis is characterized by intrahepatic canalicular cholestasis, liver cell necrosis, and an exudative inflammatory reaction. Both the signs and the laboratory results associated with primary liver disease and reactive hepatitis are similar, and only further diagnostic work-up may reveal the primary cause.

Diarrhea. Small-intestinal diarrhea is a frequent sign associated with liver disease (see Table 140–1). There are two main mechanisms by which diarrhea as a symptom of liver disease can be explained. First, in cholestatic diseases (either intrahepatic or extrahepatic caused by common bile duct obstruction), the normal enterohepatic cycle of bile acids is disrupted.[13] Therefore, less bile reaches the duodenum in these conditions. The result may be a decreased resorption of dietary fat, causing hyperosmotic intestinal contents and diarrhea. Another mechanism for diarrhea in liver disease is an increased resistance to the portal blood flow, resulting in portal hypertension and congestion of the splanchnic organs. Congestion of the intestinal vasculature reduces intestinal water resorption and increases the volume of intestinal contents. This is the predominant mechanism underlying diarrhea in diseases such as chronic hepatitis, cirrhosis, lobular dissecting hepatitis, portal vein thrombosis, and portal vein hypoplasia. Of course, a combination of these mechanisms occurs in many liver diseases. Alternatively, when the primary cause of diarrhea is intestinal disease, the liver may be secondarily affected. In those cases, the increased absorption of (endo)toxins or bacteria by the affected intestinal wall should be removed by the hepatic macrophage system. An increased exposure, however, can lead to secondary, nonspecific, reactive hepatitis. Endotoxins are known to be effective inhibitors of bile formation and flow, leading to cholestasis. It is therefore common to find increased plasma liver enzymes and bile acid levels in cases of reactive hepatitis; clinical jaundice may be apparent. The cause of diarrhea can be determined only by further diagnostic methods, including histologic evaluation of a liver biopsy. Reactive hepatitis resolves rapidly when the primary disease is treated successfully. One may therefore elect to follow liver values after treatment of the intestinal disease and perform a liver biopsy only if the liver parameters do not improve within a few weeks.

Hepatic Encephalopathy. Hepatic encephalopathy is a complex of neurologic signs (see Table 140–2) resulting from portosystemic shunting of blood in combination with a reduction of the functional liver mass.[5] It may therefore occur in animals with congenital portosystemic shunts or in those with acquired portosystemic collaterals due to portal hypertension. Diseases associated with the latter form are chronic hepatitis, cirrhosis, portal vein hypoplasia, lobular dissecting hepatitis, and portal vein thrombosis.[15] Cats, owing to their dependence on some essential amino acids, may also develop hepatic encephalopathy without portosystemic

shunting, especially when they have a severe form of hepatic lipidosis.[16]

Hepatic encephalopathy is caused by derangement of neurotransmitter systems due to defective metabolic processes in the liver.[17] Inadequate metabolism of ammonia and aromatic amino acids by the liver may lead to a reduction of the excitatory glutamate and monoaminergic neurotransmitter systems, respectively.[18, 19] In addition, there is an increased tone of the inhibitory gamma-aminobutyric acid (GABA) system.[20] It is the presence of these neurotransmitter derangements that makes anesthesia risky in certain animals with liver disease.

Polyuria and Polydipsia. The combination of polyuria and polydipsia is one of the most frequent signs in dogs with liver disease but is uncommon in cats. Polyuria and polydipsia are most common in diseases associated with congenital or acquired portosystemic shunting and, therefore, with hepatic encephalopathy. It has been well documented that in such dogs the abnormal neurotransmitters lead to an overstimulation of the anterior and intermediate pituitary lobes to form and secrete adrenocorticotropic hormone.[21] Such dogs have an increased level of free cortisol, and chronic hypercortisolism affects the posterior lobe of the pituitary. The main effect is that the antidiuretic hormone (ADH)–secreting cells develop an increased threshold for the osmotic stimulation of ADH release. Thus, a little higher osmolality of the plasma is required to stimulate the antidiuresis through ADH, and before reaching that threshold, such dogs become thirsty and start drinking.[22] When the dog feels ill and does not drink, the threshold is reached, and ADH release and urinary concentration start, so that real dehydration does not occur easily. Another possible but undocumented mechanism that may play a role in such diseases is the reduced formation of urea in the liver. The kidneys thus have insufficient urea available to build up an osmotic gradient in the medulla. Apart from this mechanism, polydipsia also occurs in liver diseases not associated with hepatic encephalopathy, such as extrahepatic cholestasis and liver tumors. In these dogs, the mechanism is unclear. Nausea with an emotional impulse to drink and the compensation of water loss by vomiting and diarrhea may play a role.

Dysuria. Dysuria may occur as a result of insufficient liver function when nonmetabolized uric acid is excreted by the kidneys and precipitates to form uroliths. Such calculi are seen in dogs but not in cats. There are two main categories of liver dysfunction causing this symptom. Most frequently it is caused by congenital portosystemic shunting, by which the liver is underdeveloped and fails to metabolize uric acid into allantoin. In the urine, uric acid flocculates easily in the presence of high ammonia concentrations to form ammonium urate. These dogs usually have clinical signs related to shunting and liver dysfunction, such as hepatic encephalopathy, polydipsia, or vomiting. In the other category, the enzyme uricase, which forms allantoin, is inactive due to an inborn error by which only this function is affected. This is common in Dalmatians but may also occur in other breeds.[23] Such dogs only have signs related to urolithiasis.

Anesthesia Intolerance. Anesthesia intolerance is sometimes noticed by chance when an animal with unknown liver disease is anesthetized. The liver is the site of inactivation of many anesthetics, and the unforeseen delay of recovery from anesthesia may put the pieces of the puzzle of nonspecific clinical signs together in the recognition of an underlying liver disease. This occurs especially in dogs and cats with portosystemic shunting, either congenital or acquired. Apart of the reduced clearance of anesthetics, these drugs exert their action via the neurotransmitter systems in the brain, which may already be functioning abnormally due to hepatic encephalopathy.[17] This is especially true of drugs that act via the GABA-benzodiazepine pathway. That pathway is already overstimulated and may provoke an exaggerated and prolonged anesthetic effect.

Acholic Feces. Acholic feces are one of the few signs that may be noted by an owner that can provide a direct clue to the underlying diagnosis. Fat-loaded feces that do not contain normal bile pigment are seen only when there is complete disruption of bile flow into the intestinal tract, usually due to extrahepatic obstruction of the common bile duct.[2] The only intrahepatic process so severe that the bile flow is completely abolished is destructive cholangiolitis. The latter disease is caused by a hypersensitivity reaction to sulfonamide-containing drugs, by which the smaller bile ductuli become necrotic and the liver lobuli may be disconnected from the biliary tree. Such dogs have a history of recent medication with sulfonamides. Acholic feces contain excess fat because resorption is impaired and lack the normal black-brown fecal pigments because their precursor, bilirubin, does not reach the duodenum. The feces are grey-white and soft. Animals with this condition are icteric. The icterus reduces the liklihood of exocrine pancreatic insufficiency.

Abdominal Distention. Abdominal distention may occur in dogs and cats with liver disease for a number of reasons. First, ascites is a frequent finding associated with liver disease in dogs but is less common in cats. Abdominal distention may also result from organ enlargement, which in the case of liver disease may include the liver and, when there is portal hypertension, the spleen. In contrast to dogs, cats often have hepatomegaly with liver disease.

Other Clinical Signs. A number of other clinical signs frequently encountered in liver diseases are nonspecific, such as apathy, reduced appetite or anorexia, and weight loss. Retarded growth is common in young animals. These problems reflect the central role of the liver in many metabolic and detoxifying functions. In addition, nausea, inappetence, vomiting, and diarrhea can result in a catabolic state, which in turn contributes to development or aggravation of hepatic encephalopathy. Signs of early hepatic encephalopathy include depression and other nonspecific problems. Anemia, another common finding in liver disease (see later), can cause general malaise. Dogs with liver cell carcinoma often have hypoglycemia,[24] which may be the primary problem underlying apathy and weakness. This is thought to result from the production of insulin-like growth factors by the tumor.

PHYSICAL EXAMINATION AND SIGNS OF LIVER DISEASES

Physical examination is informative in only a minority of dogs with liver disease but is more often useful in cats. Possible findings are icterus, hepatomegaly, splenomegaly, ascites, and pale mucous membranes. Petechiae of the skin or mucous membranes are extremely infrequent. Of all these possible findings, only icterus and hepatomegaly are specific for liver diseases; the other physical abnormalities occur more frequently with diseases of other organ systems. Ascites and hepato- and splenomegaly may have been noted by the owner as abdominal enlargement.

Icterus. Icterus is the most frequent specific physical abnormality in dogs and cats with liver disease. However, in our referral clinic, this accounts for only about 20 percent of the dogs with hepatobiliary diseases and 30 to 40 per cent of the cats. Therefore, most of the animals with liver disease do not have icterus. Jaundice is the result of bilirubin accumulation in the blood and in the extravascular space due to increased production, reduced clearance, or impaired conjugation by the liver and/or impairment of the bile flow. In most cases, it results from a combination of all these factors, with cholestasis being predominant and therefore conjugated bilirubin being the highest bilirubin fraction. Hemolysis alone does not result in jaundice when the liver functions normally. When hemolysis is severe, however, it may result in such a degree of portal hypoxia that the centrolobular zones of the liver lobules become necrotic. In those cases, it is the combination of increased production and reduced liver function and cholestasis that results in icterus.[25] Therefore, if hemolysis is the primary cause of jaundice, it must be severe, and the mucous membranes will be extremely pale. Primary liver diseases that may cause icterus are commonly accompanied by hemolysis. Whereas the erythrocyte lifetime is reduced to 6 to 10 days in dogs with severe primary hemolytic disease, it is 20 to 60 days (normally 100 days) in hepatobiliary disease. Therefore, increased production of bilirubin and liver dysfunction with cholestasis result in a combined conjugated and unconjugated hyperbilirubinemia in dogs and cats with primary hepatic or hemolytic disease.[26] Icterus due to hemolytic disease is characterized by pale mucous membranes, whereas the mucous membranes in animals with primary liver disease are normal or only slightly pale. Therefore, the combined evaluation of icterus and the color of the mucous membranes immediately reveals the nature of the underlying process.

Pale Mucous Membranes. As previously discussed, most hepatobiliary diseases are accompanied by an increased degradation of red blood cells. The mechanisms behind hemolysis in liver disease are not completely clear. Hypersplenism and reduced portal blood flow due to portal hypertension may drastically prolong the transit time of erythrocytes through the spleen, with a greater chance that they will be trapped when they are slightly abnormal. Increased fragility of the red cell membranes may be due to the high bile acid levels in most liver diseases, whereas a reduced clearance of enteral endotoxins and bacteria by the liver may also induce immune-mediated hemolysis. Apart from hemolysis, nonregenerative anemia may also occur as part of the syndrome of anemia of chronic disease as an expression of catabolism and slight deficiencies of iron and B vitamins. Although common in liver diseases,[6] anemia, in contrast to jaundice, is nonspecific.

Hepatomegaly. Liver enlargement is a distinct sign of an abnormal liver. In dogs, most liver diseases do not cause hepatomegaly. Exceptions include tumors of the liver, liver congestion, and secondary liver involvement in metabolic diseases. Examples of the latter conditions are glycogen accumulation in the liver in Cushing's disease, fatty liver with diabetes mellitus, and rare cases of amyloidosis of the liver. The more chronic liver diseases of dogs tend to reduce liver size, and acute diseases cause little change in size. Liver enlargement due to congestive heart disease can, in most cases, be recognized easily by physical examination of the circulatory system. In case of doubt, measurement of the central venous pressure is diagnostic. The exception is liver congestion by a thrombus in the caudal vena cava proximal to the liver, which has to be assessed by other methods. When the liver is distinctly enlarged owing to congestion, there is usually ascites as well, which has the typical slightly hemorrhagic appearance of congestive fluid. Dogs with enlarged livers and no signs of congestive disease often have liver cancer, which may be primary, metastatic, or part of a form of malignant lymphoma. With most tumors, the liver is diffusely enlarged, but primary hepatocellular carcinomas or adenomas may cause enlargement of the affected lobe only. Bile duct carcinomas disseminate easily over the biliary system and usually cause pronounced icterus in combination with hepatomegaly. Most cats with liver disease develop more or less pronounced enlargement of the liver. In cats, liver enlargement occurs with cholangiohepatitis, hepatic lipidosis, amyloidosis, tumors of the liver (mostly malignant lymphoma), and congestive disease. When the liver is involved in feline infectious peritonitis, it may not be enlarged. Cats with congenital portosystemic shunts have small livers.

Splenomegaly and Ascites. Splenomegaly and ascites in association with liver disease are nonspecific findings. They occur especially with liver diseases causing portal hypertension. Both findings are frequent in dogs and rare in cats. There is a positive undulation test with distinct ascites; slight ascites can be found with ultrasonography rather than physical examination. When there are central causes of venous congestion, the liver may be enlarged as well. Canine liver diseases associated with portal hypertension are chronic hepatitis and cirrhosis, portal vein hypoplasia, and lobular dissecting hepatitis; in cats, it is sometimes seen in cirrhosis due to advanced cholangiohepatitis. In these diseases, hepatic encephalopathy is also common. Portal vein thrombosis is a prehepatic cause of portal hypertension usually causing ascites. Although as a rule the liver is small in these cases, a unilateral obstruction of a main branch of the portal vein may cause hypertrophy of the rest of the liver, which may be palpable.

REFERENCES

1. Fausto N, Webber EM: Liver regeneration. In Arias M, Boyer JL, Fausto N, et al (eds): The Liver: Biology and Pathobiology, 3rd ed. New York, Raven Press, 1994, pp 1059–1084.
2. van den Ingh TSGAM, Rothuizen J, van den Brom WE: Extrahepatic cholestasis in the dog and the differentiation of extrahepatic and intrahepatic cholestasis. Vet Q 8:150, 1986.
3. Center SA, Magne ML: Historical, physical examination and clinicopathological features of portosystemic vascular anomalies in the dog and cat. Semin Vet Med Surg (Small Anim) 5:75, 1991.
4. Jacobson LS, Kirberger RM, Nesbit JW: Hepatic ultrasonography and pathological findings in dogs with hepatocutaneous syndrome: New concepts. J Vet Intern Med 9:399, 1995.
5. Conn HO, Bircher J: Hepatic Encephalopathy: Management With Lactulose and Related Carbohydrates. East Lansing, MI, Medi-Ed Press, 1988.
6. Dial SM: Clinicopathologic evaluation of the liver. Vet Clin North Am Small Anim Pract 25:257, 1995.
7. van den Ingh TSGAM, Rothuizen J, van Zinnicq Bergman HMS: Destructive cholangiolitis in seven dogs. Vet Q 10:240, 1988.
8. Andersson M, Sevelius E: Breed, sex and age distribution in dogs with chronic liver disease—a demographic study. J Small Anim Pract 32:1, 1991.
9. Crawford MA, Schall WD, Jensen RK, Tasker JB: Chronic active hepatitis in 26 Doberman pinschers. JAVMA 12:1343, 1985.
10. Speeti M, Ihantola M, Westermarck E: Subclinical versus clinical hepatitis in the Doberman: Evaluation of changes in blood parameters. J Small Anim Pract 37:465, 1996.
11. van den Ingh TSGAM, Rothuizen J: Lobular dissecting hepatitis in juvenile and young adult dogs. J Vet Intern Med 8:217, 1994.
12. Rolfe DS, Twedt DC: Copper-associated hepatopathies in dogs. Vet Clin North Am Small Anim Pract 25:399, 1995.
13. Batt RM, Twedt DC: Canine gastrointestinal disease. In Wills JM, Simpson KW (eds): Waltham Book of Clinical Nutrition of the Dog & Cat, 1st ed. Pergamon Press, 1994.
14. Dillon R: The liver in systemic disease: An innocent bystander. Vet Clin North Am Small Anim Pract 15:97, 1985.
15. van den Ingh TSGAM, Rothuizen J, Meyer HP: Circulatory disorders of the liver in dogs and cats. Vet Q 17:70, 1995.
16. Center SA, Crawford MA, Guida L, et al: A retrospective study of 77 cats with severe hepatic lipidosis, 1975–1990. J Vet Intern Med 7:349, 1993.
17. Butterworth RF: Hepatic encephalopathy. In Arias IM (ed): Liver: Biology and Pathobiology, 3rd ed. New York, Raven Press, 1994, pp 1193–1208.
18. Lavoie J, Giguere JF, Layrargues GP, Butterworth RF: Amino acid changes in autopsied brain tissue from cirrhotic patients with hepatic encephalopathy. J Neurochem 49:692, 1987.
19. Fischer JE, Baldessarini RJ: False neurotransmitters and hepatic failure. Lancet 2:75, 1971.
20. Jones EA, Schafer DF, Ferenci P, Pappas SC: The GABA hypothesis of the pathogenesis of hepatic encephalopathy: Current status. Yale J Biol Med 57:301, 1984.
21. Rothuizen J, Mol JA: The pituitary-adrenocortical system in canine hepatoencephalopathy. In van Wimersma Greidanus TB (ed): Frontiers of Hormone Research. Basel, Karger, 1987, pp 28–36.
22. Rothuizen J, Biewenga WJ, Mol JA: Chronic glucocorticoid excess and impaired osmoregulation of vasopressin release in dogs with hepatic encephalopathy. Domest Anim Endocrinol 12:13, 1995.
23. Sorenson JL, Ling GV: Metabolic and genetic aspects of urate urolithiasis in Dalmatians. JAVMA 203:857, 1993.
24. Leifer CE, Peterson ME, Matus RE, Patnaik AK: Hypoglycemia associated with nonislet cell tumor in 13 dogs. JAVMA 186:53, 1985.
25. Rothuizen J, van den Brom WE, Fevery J: The origins and kinetics of bilirubin in dogs with hepatobiliary and haemolytic diseases. J Hepatol 15:17, 1992.
26. Rothuizen J, van den Brom WE: Bilirubin metabolism in canine hepatobiliary and haemolytic disease. Vet Q 9:235, 1987.

LIV

CHAPTER 141

LABORATORY DIAGNOSIS OF HEPATOBILIARY DISEASE

Cynthia R. Leveille-Webster

The liver plays a central role in carbohydrate, lipid, and protein metabolism; detoxification of metabolites and xenobiotics; storage of vitamins, trace metals, fat, and glycogen; fat digestion; and immunoregulation. An appreciation of these varied functions is valuable for understanding the clinicopathologic abnormalities that accompany hepatic disease, because in large part, these abnormalities reflect deficiencies in one or more of these functions (Table 141–1). Laboratory assessment of hepatobiliary disease is especially important, because clinical signs associated with these disorders are

TABLE 141–1. CLINICAL AND LABORATORY ABNORMALITIES ASSOCIATED WITH DEFICITS IN MAJOR HEPATOBILIARY FUNCTIONS

FUNCTION	LABORATORY ABNORMALITY	CLINICAL CONSEQUENCE
Glucose homeostasis	Hypoglycemia Hyperglycemia	CNS disturbances Diabetes mellitus

Lipid metabolism
  Cholesterol synthesis and excretion
  Triglyceride metabolism and storage
  Lipoprotein synthesis
  Fatty acid oxidation
	Hypocholesterolemia, hypercholesterolemia
	Hypertriglyceridemia
	Abnormal circulating lipoproteins: lipoprotein X
	↑ Serum fatty acids
		Alterations in cellular plasma membranes
		Aberrations in triglyceride storage, lipoprotein formation and/or release or impaired fatty acid oxidation associated with the development of hepatic lipidosis

Protein metabolism
  Albumin synthesis
  Coagulation factor synthesis, activation, and clearance
  Nonimmunoglobulin synthesis: acute phase reactants
 	
  Urea synthesis
 	
  Amino acid regulation
  Ammonia detoxification
	Hypoalbuminemia
	↑ PT, ↑ APTT
	
	Hyperglobulinemia, hypoglobulinemia, hyper- or hypofibrinogenemia
	
	↓ Serum urea nitrogen
	
	↓ BCAA/AAA
	Hyperammonemia
		Ascites, edema
		Bleeding tendencies
		
		Early inflammatory disease associated with ↑ globulins and late end-stage disease associated with ↓ globulins
		↓ Renal medullary interstitial gradient: polyuria/polydipsia
		Hepatic encephalopathy
		Hepatic encephalopathy

Bile acid synthesis and enterohepatic circulation
  Fat digestion and absorption
 	
  Stimulation of bile flow
	Vitamin K deficiency: ↑ PT, ↑ APTT, ↑ PIVKAs
	Retention of hepatotoxic substances (e.g., bile acids, leukotrienes, copper, and bilirubin)
		Bleeding tendencies, steatorrhea
		
		Progression of hepatic injury

Detoxification and biliary excretion
  Bilirubin
  Xenobiotics (e.g., barbiturates, metronidazole, diazepam, chloramphenicol, lidocaine, theophylline)
  Copper
	Hyperbilirubinemia
	↑ Serum drug concentrations
	
	↑ Hepatic copper concentrations
		Icterus
		Enhanced drug toxicity
		
		Oxidant liver injury

Immunoregulation
  Kupffer cells: phagocytic function, endotoxin clearance, humoral immune responsiveness
  Complement synthesis and metabolism
	Endotoxemia, bacteremia
	
	Complement deficiency
		Increased susceptibility to infection
		
		Increased susceptibility to infection

Storage
  Water-soluble vitamins
  Fat-soluble vitamins
  Iron
  Triglycerides
  Glycogen
	Vitamin B deficiency
	Vitamin K deficiency: ↑ PT, ↑ APTT
	↑ Hepatic iron
	↑ Hypertriglyceridemia
	↑ Hypoglycemia
		CNS disturbance (thiamine deficiency in cats)
		Bleeding tendencies
		Oxidant liver injury
		Hepatic lipidosis
		Glycogen storage disease

CNS = central nervous system; PT = prothrombin time; APTT = activated partial thromboplastin time; BCAA = branched chain amino acid; AAA = aromatic amino acid; PIVKAs = proteins induced by vitamin K absence or antagonists.

often quite nonspecific. The liver's tremendous reserve capacity, its ability to regenerate, and its sensitivity to secondary injury complicate the interpretation of hepatic clinicopathology.

The primary reason to pursue laboratory evaluation of hepatobiliary function is to detect the presence of hepatobiliary disease. The value of an individual laboratory test in determining the presence of hepatobiliary disease is measured by its sensitivity and specificity. Sensitivity is a measure of a test's ability to detect animals with hepatobiliary disease, and specificity is a test's ability to exclude individuals without hepatobiliary disease. Ideally, every test would have 100 per cent sensitivity and specificity, but in reality, this seldom occurs. Screening tests evaluate a random cross section of the hospital population in order to identify individuals with occult hepatobiliary disease. Screening tests should have high sensitivity so that few animals with hepatobiliary disease escape detection and a reasonably high specificity so that time and expense are not invested in pursuing false-positive tests. Diagnostic tests are used to confirm disease in animals that are already suspected of having hepatobiliary disease. These tests should have high specificity.

Clinicopathologic evaluation of the hepatobiliary function is also used to assess disease severity, establish a prognosis, define potential complications, and monitor disease progression (Fig. 141–1).

CLINICAL ENZYMOLOGY

Clinical enzymology is commonly used to screen for the presence of hepatobiliary disease, because consistent increases in the serum concentration of several enzymes occur following hepatobiliary injury.[1] A number of factors contribute to the accumulation of hepatobiliary enzymes in the serum. Normal serum enzyme concentration is proportional to tissue enzyme concentration, which in turn represents the product of cellular enzyme concentration times the total mass of cells that contain the enzyme. A second determinant of serum enzyme concentration is serum enzyme half-life. An enzyme must have a serum half-life of sufficient duration to permit accumulation. Serum enzyme concentration is also dependent on intracellular localization, because enzymes must have access to the vascular compartment before they can accumulate. In general, cytosolic enzymes gain access to the serum easier than enzymes that are within organelles or membrane bound.

Following hepatobiliary injury, the serum concentration of

hepatobiliary enzymes increases for several reasons. Cytosolic enzymes, such as the aminotransferases and arginase, leak from hepatobiliary cells following plasma membrane damage. The serum concentration of membrane-bound enzymes, such as alkaline phosphatase (ALP) and gamma-glutamyl transpeptidase (GGT), increases owing to de novo synthesis as well as elution from membranes.

Although increases in serum enzyme activities are valuable screening tests for hepatobiliary disease, they have several limitations. First, they are not specific predictors of hepatobiliary disease. The liver's central role in metabolism and high blood flow make it uniquely sensitive to secondary injury. Thus there are several clinical conditions in which liver enzyme abnormalities may not be associated with significant hepatobiliary disease (Table 141–2). Although the magnitude of serum enzyme activity increase is usually proportional to the severity of active hepatobiliary damage, it is not predictive of hepatobiliary functional capacity. Marked increases may indicate substantial hepatobiliary injury but, owing to the tremendous regenerative capacity of the liver, are not necessarily indicative of a poor prognosis. Alternatively, in severe end-stage chronic liver disease, serum enzymes may be normal or only mildly increased because replacement of hepatocytes by fibrosis and/or prolonged enzyme leakage has resulted in depletion of total liver enzyme content. A single serum enzyme determination, therefore, should never be used to establish a prognosis. The prognostic value of serum enzymology can be improved by following sequential determinations, especially in conjunction with a hepatic function test or hepatic biopsy.

ALANINE AMINOTRANSFERASE

Alanine aminotransferase (ALT) is a liver-specific cytosolic enzyme in the dog and cat.[1] The largest increases in serum ALT are seen with acute hepatocellular necrosis and inflammation.[2] ALT is a leakage enzyme, and the magnitude of elevation is roughly proportional to the number of injured hepatocytes. The serum half-life in dogs is 2.5 days.[1, 3] There are no published values for the serum ALT half-life in cats. In the dog, increases in serum ALT occur with muscle necrosis, but examination of specific muscle enzymes, such as creatine phosphokinase, easily differentiates elevations due to muscle damage from those associated with hepatic injury.

In experimental acute cytotoxic liver injury, serum ALT increases up to 100-fold within 24 to 48 hours.[4] Values peak by day 5 and gradually return to normal in two to three weeks if the toxic insult does not continue. In canine acute liver disease, the finding of a 50 per cent decrease in sequential serum ALT determinations over several days is considered a good prognostic sign. In dogs, but not cats, anticonvulsants (phenobarbital, primidone, and phenytoin) and corticosteroids increase serum ALT.[4, 5] In most dogs, drug induction causes a mild increase in ALT (fourfold), but in some individuals, increases approach those seen with acute hepatocellular injury. Once inducing drugs are stopped, serum ALT gradually returns to normal over several weeks.

Serum ALT may increase with primary or metastatic hepatic neoplasia.[4, 6, 7] Mild to moderate increases in serum ALT are seen in 70 to 80 per cent of dogs with hepatocellular or bile duct carcinoma. Increased serum ALT likely reflects hepatocellular injury secondary to compression of normal tissue and/or lysis of necrotic tumor cells. Metastatic neoplasia in the liver is invariably associated with mild increases in serum ALT. Occasionally, nodular hyperplasia results in increased serum ALT. These elevations may be associated with impairment of bile and blood flow owing to distortion of the hepatic architecture by the regenerative nodules.

ASPARTATE AMINOTRANSFERASE

Aspartate aminotransferase (AST) is not liver-specific in dogs or cats, as it is also present in cardiac and skeletal muscle, kidneys, and brain.[1] There are two liver isoenzymes: cytosolic and mitochondrial. The half-life of serum AST is 5 to 12 hours in the dog and 77 minutes in the cat. In dogs and cats, serum AST is more sensitive than serum ALT in the detection of hepatobiliary disease, although it is considerably less specific. In general, increases in serum AST in the dog and cat parallel increases in serum ALT and, like ALT, are associated with leakage following altered membrane permeability.[1, 3, 4, 6] If serum AST is much higher than serum ALT, a muscle source for the increase should be suspected. In dogs, serum AST is mildly increased by corticosteroids and anticonvulsants. Increases in serum AST may be more sensitive than ALP or ALT in the detection of hepatic metastasis.

ARGINASE

Arginase, a liver-specific enzyme in the dog and cat, is located in the mitochondria.[1, 8] It has a short serum half-life

TABLE 141–2. CONDITIONS IN WHICH INCREASES IN SERUM HEPATOBILIARY ENZYME CONCENTRATIONS MAY OCCUR IN THE ABSENCE OF PRIMARY LIVER DISEASE

Drug induction
   Corticosteroids (dogs): ↑ ↑ ↑ALP, ↑ ↑GGT, ↑ALT, ↑AST
   Anticonvulsants (phenobarbital, phenytoin, primidone): ↑ALT, ↑ALP, ↑AST, ↑GGT
Endocrinopathies
   Hyperthyroidism (cats): ↑ALP, ↑ALT
   Hypothyroidism (dogs): ↑ALP
   Diabetes mellitus: ↑ALP
   Hyperadrenocorticism (dogs): ↑ ↑ ↑ALP, ↑ALT, ↑GGT, ↑AST
Hypoxia/hypotension: ↑ ↑ALT, ↑ALP, ↑GGT, ↑AST
   Congestive heart failure
   Severe acute blood loss
   Status epilepticus
   Hypotensive crisis
     Surgery
     Septic shock
     Hypoadrenocorticism
     Circulatory shock
Muscle injury: ↑ALT, ↑AST
   Acute muscle necrosis/trauma
   Malignant hyperthermia
   Myopathies
Neoplasia
   Adenocarcinomas: pancreatic, intestinal, adrenocortical, mammary
   Sarcomas: hemangiosarcoma, leiomyosarcoma
   Hepatic metastasis: ↑AST, ↑ALT, ↑ALP
   Unique enzyme induction: ↑ ↑ALP, ↑ ↑GGT
Miscellaneous
   Systemic infections
   Pregnancy (cats): ↑placental ALP
   Colostrum-fed neonates (dogs): ↑GGT
Bone disorders: ↑ALP
   Young animals (up to 7 months)
   Osteosarcoma
   Osteomyelitis

ALP = alkaline phosphatase; ALT = alanine aminotransferase; AST = aspartate aminotransferase; GGT = gamma-glutamyl transpeptidase.

LIV

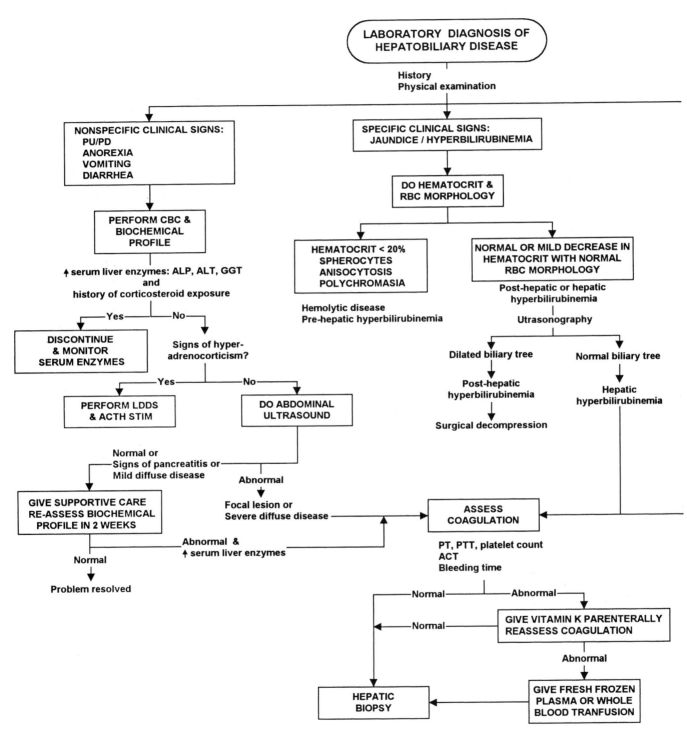

Figure 141–1 *See legend on opposite page*

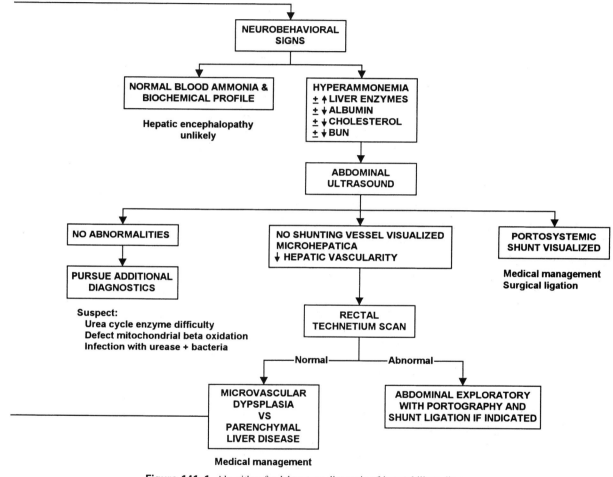

Figure 141–1. Algorithm for laboratory diagnosis of hepatobiliary disease.

LIV

(<12 hours) but is present in large amounts in hepatocytes. Following acute hepatocellular injury, serum arginase increases within hours by 500 to 1000 times orders of magnitude. Owing to the short serum half-life, in the absence of ongoing injury, serum arginase decreases rapidly within two to three days. At the same time, serum transaminases are typically still increased. Thus in acute liver injury, a rapid rise and decline of serum arginase may be an early indicator of recovery. Although serum arginase is easily and reliably determined, the test is not routinely evaluated in veterinary medicine. Dogs treated with corticosteroids develop transient, mild (five to eightfold) increases in serum arginase.[1, 9]

ALKALINE PHOSPHATASE

The clinical utility of serum ALP arises from its sensitivity in detecting hepatobiliary disease,[1, 3, 4, 10–13] whereas confusion in interpretation is due to its low specificity for hepatobiliary disease. ALP's low specificity is associated with the presence of several isoenzymes[14–17] and its unique sensitivity to drug induction.[5, 9, 18–22] Isoenzymes of ALP are present in the liver, kidney, intestine, bone, and placenta.[1, 14, 15] The intestinal, kidney, and placental isoenzymes do not contribute to serum ALP owing to their extremely short half-lives in both the dog (< six minutes) and the cat (< two minutes). An exception is late-term pregnancy in cats, where the placental isoenzyme represents a significant source of the serum enzyme. The bone isoenzyme, B-ALP, contributes about one third of total serum ALP. Increased osteoblastic activity associated with growing bones in young animals or with pathologic conditions such as osteomyelitis or osteosarcoma can mildly increase total serum ALP.

Two liver isoenzymes contribute to the serum ALP in dogs: a liver (L-ALP) and corticosteroid-induced isoenzyme (C-ALP). In the cat, there is only one liver isoenzyme. In the dog and cat, L-ALP is a membrane-bound enzyme found on the hepatocyte canalicular membrane and the luminal surface of biliary epithelial cells.[16] Canine C-ALP is actually a hyperglycosylated form of the intestinal isoenzyme.[1] It is also located on the hepatocyte canalicular membrane.[16] The serum half-life of both L-ALP and C-ALP in the dog is 70 hours. The serum half-life of the feline liver isoenzyme is only six hours. Increases in serum ALP in the dog and cat are the result of increased de novo synthesis and/or elution of the enzyme from cellular membranes.

In dogs with hepatobiliary disease, focal or diffuse intrahepatic or extrahepatic cholestasis results in the largest increases in serum ALP.[4, 11] Partial bile duct obstructions can cause large increases in serum ALP.[9] After acute diffuse hepatocellular necrosis, serum ALP values rise slowly. Within three to four days, two- to fivefold increases in serum ALP are seen, which gradually decline over a two- to three-week period. Canine bile duct and hepatocellular carcinomas are frequently accompanied by moderate to marked increases in serum ALP.[4, 7] Several nonhepatic tumors may also be associated with increases in serum ALP activity (see Table 141–2). It is unsure whether these increases are due to the presence of hepatic metastasis or associated with induction of a unique ALP isoenzyme.

In a series of 270 dogs with histologically confirmed hepatic disease, the highest serum ALP activities were seen with cholestasis (median 10-fold increase), followed by chronic hepatitis, corticosteroid-induced hepatopathy, and hepatic necrosis (all approximately sixfold).[11] Whereas the specificity of serum ALP determination for hepatobiliary

disease was only 51 per cent, the sensitivity was quite high (approximately 80 percent).

Exposure of dogs to excess endogenous or exogenous corticosteroids causes increases in serum ALP.[4, 9, 18–22] In experimental studies, dogs given prednisone (4 mg/kg intramuscularly once a day) had increases in serum ALP within three days, which continued to rise (Fig. 141–2).[16, 18, 21, 22] Similar, though quantitatively smaller, increases in ALP (10-fold) were seen in dogs given parenteral dexamethasone (3 to 4 mg/kg).[19] Oral anti-inflammatory doses of prednisone (0.55 mg/kg twice a day for five weeks) failed to cause a significant overall increase in ALP, although some individuals did have increases.[23]

Serum ALP elevations in corticosteroid-treated dogs are accompanied by changes in hepatic morphology.[18, 21, 24, 25] Morphologic changes consist of ballooning enlargement of hepatocytes and development of intracytoplasmic hepatic vacuolation due to glycogen accumulation. In some studies, focal areas of hepatocyte necrosis have been described. In dogs treated with prednisone, these morphologic changes begin by day 2 and gradually progress in severity as corticosteroid treatment continues.

The contribution of individual canine ALP isoenzymes to total serum ALP can be determined by several methods.[1, 14, 15, 17] Presently, the most widely used technique is levamisole inhibition,[14] which is based on the fact that levamisole inhibits L-ALP and B-ALP but not C-ALP. In dogs with normal total serum ALP, C-ALP represents from 5 to 20 per cent of total serum ALP.[16, 22]

One of the challenges in the interpretation of canine serum ALP elevations is distinguishing between increases associated with cholestatic hepatic disease and those secondary to exposure to corticosteroids. In theory, analysis of serum ALP isoenzyme distribution should separate the two groups, because hepatobiliary disease should be associated with increases in L-ALP and corticosteroid exposure associated with increases in C-ALP. In reality, several studies have demonstrated considerable overlap between isoenzyme distribution in these two conditions. Isoenzyme analysis of total serum ALP in dogs treated with prednisone (4 mg/kg once a day) demonstrated that the initial rise in serum ALP is

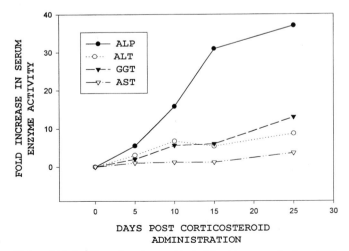

Figure 141–2. Effect of corticosteroid administration on canine hepatobiliary serum enzyme concentrations. The magnitude of increase in the serum concentration of alkaline phosphatase (ALP), alanine aminotransferase (ALT), aspartate aminotransferase (AST), and gamma-glutamyl transpeptidase (GTT) in dogs given prednisone (4.4 mg/kg intramuscularly) is illustrated. The data from three separate studies are summarized.[16, 21, 22]

actually associated with induction of L-ALP.[16, 22] It is only after several days of treatment that C-ALP becomes the prominent isoenzyme. Chronic corticosteroid exposure due to hyperadrenocorticism or iatrogenic hypercortisolism from parenteral, oral, or topical corticosteroid administration is consistently associated with increases in C-ALP.[4, 14] In fact, increases in serum C-ALP have a sensitivity of greater than 95 per cent for the detection of chronic exposure to corticosteroids.[17] The specificity of C-ALP, however, is low, because many dogs with hepatobiliary disease also have significant increases in serum C-ALP.[14, 17] In addition, serum C-ALP increases in chronically ill animals, apparently from long-term endogenous cortisol excess.[13, 14]

Anticonvulsants (phenobarbital, phenytoin, and primidone) induce mild (two- to sixfold) increases in serum ALP.[4, 5] Phenobarbital may induce L-ALP and/or C-ALP.[15] Interpretation of serum ALP elevations in dogs on anticonvulsants is complicated by the fact that these drugs are known hepatotoxins.[5] Because ALT, AST, and GGT are also induced by anticonvulsants, they are of no value in differentiating serum ALP increases due to microsomal induction from those associated with morphologic injury. Dogs on chronic anticonvulsant therapy with enzyme induction should have determination of serum albumin, bilirubin, and bile acids to monitor hepatobiliary function.

Because feline ALP is not susceptible to drug induction, elevations in serum ALP are more specific for feline hepatobiliary disease.[10] The magnitude of serum ALP elevations in feline hepatobiliary disease, however, is not as great as that in canine disease, owing to the short serum half-life of feline ALP and the fact that hepatic stores of ALP are less in the cat than in the dog. Thus serum ALP is a less sensitive indicator of hepatic disease in the cat than in the dog.[1, 10] Clinically, the largest increases in feline ALP are seen in hepatobiliary conditions associated with intrahepatic or extrahepatic cholestasis, particularly idiopathic hepatic lipidosis, cholangiohepatitis, and common bile duct obstruction.[4]

GAMMA-GLUTAMYL TRANSPEPTIDASE

GGT is present in the kidney, pancreas, gallbladder, liver, spleen, lung, skeletal muscle, and erythrocytes.[1] Although the highest concentrations are in the kidney and pancreas, serum GGT is derived primarily from the liver. Renal GGT is located on the brush border of the proximal tubules and excreted into the urine. Pancreatic GGT is located on the apical surface of the acinar cells and secreted into the duodenum. In the dog and cat, hepatic GGT is located on the hepatocyte canalicular membrane. Serum elevations of GGT are most common with cholestatic disorders and are associated with increased de novo synthesis as well as elution from membranes.

In dogs, increases in GGT are seen with intrahepatic and extrahepatic cholestasis.[4, 11] In acute hepatocellular injury, the magnitude of increase of serum GGT is mild (one- to twofold). In a series of dogs with histologically confirmed hepatic disease,[11] serum GGT was more specific (87 per cent) than serum ALP (51 per cent) in the detection of hepatobiliary disease, but less sensitive (50 per cent) than ALP (80 per cent). When serum GGT and ALP were used in series, their specificity for the detection of hepatobiliary disease increased to 94 per cent. Serum GGT cannot be used to differentiate serum ALP elevations caused by hepatobiliary damage from those due to drug induction, because serum GGT is also increased by corticosteroids and anticonvul-

sants.[5, 9, 16, 22, 26] Parenteral administration of corticosteroids results in four- to sevenfold increases in serum GGT after the first week and up to 10-fold in two weeks (see Fig. 141–1). Anticonvulsants cause mild (two- to threefold) increases in serum GGT.

In a series of 36 dogs with primary or metastatic hepatic neoplasia, 39 per cent had high serum GGT values.[4, 7] In humans, a fetal form of GGT has been associated with hepatocellular carcinomas. It is unknown whether this isoenzyme is present in canine neoplasia.

In a series of 69 cats with hepatobiliary disease, the largest increases in serum GGT were associated with bile duct obstruction and cholangiohepatitis.[10] Serum GGT had a higher sensitivity than serum ALP (86 vs. 50 per cent) but a lower specificity (67 vs. 93 per cent) for the detection of hepatobiliary disease. In some cats with cirrhosis, bile duct obstruction, or cholangitis, serum GGT may be considerably greater than serum ALP values. A notable exception is in idiopathic hepatic lipidosis, where serum GGT values may be normal or only mildly increased (two- to sixfold), while serum ALP values are markedly increased (10-fold).[4]

LACTATE DEHYDROGENASE

Lactate dehydrogenase (LDH) has a wide tissue distribution, with the highest concentrations in skeletal and cardiac muscle. Lesser amounts are present in kidney, intestine, liver, lung, pancreas, and bone.[1] Five different LDH isoenzymes have been characterized. The predominant isoenzymes produced by the liver in the dog and cat are LDH5 and LDH4. LDH1 is the predominant isoenzyme in cardiac muscle. LDH2 and LDH5 predominate in skeletal muscle, and LDH3 is the pancreatic isoenzyme. In the dog, the liver isoenzyme supplies the major component of the total serum LDH. Owing to its wide tissue distribution, however, determination of total LDH is of little diagnostic value.

MISCELLANEOUS CAUSES OF HEPATIC SERUM ENZYME ELEVATION

CORTICOSTEROIDS

The pattern of serum enzyme activity increase in normal dogs given daily intramuscular injections of prednisone (4.4 mg/kg) is illustrated in Figure 141–2.[16, 21, 22] The magnitude of induction is ALP >> GGT > ALT > AST. Several studies have shown that hepatic concentrations of ALP and GGT increase following corticosteroid administration, confirming that serum increases in these serum enzyme activities are due to induction.[21, 22, 24] Studies have failed to demonstrate increases in the hepatic concentrations of AST or ALT.[22] Increases in the concentration of these serum enzyme activities may be secondary to the focal necrosis and/or cholestasis that has been reported to accompany the vacuolar hepatopathy induced by corticosteroids.[18, 21] Consistent with this idea is the observation that corticosteroid excess can result in abnormal hepatic function testing (mild to moderate increases in total serum bile acids).[4, 9]

The degree of corticosteroid-induced enzyme induction in individual dogs depends not only on the dose, method of administration, and type of corticosteroid administered but also on individual sensitivity. Some dogs develop profound increases in serum enzyme activities at doses that barely affect other dogs. It is uncertain whether the magnitude of serum enzyme elevations reflects the severity of morphologic changes in the liver. Some studies have suggested that there is no association.

FELINE HYPERTHYROIDISM

Increases in serum ALT and ALP activities are seen in most cases of feline hyperthyroidism.[4, 6] Isoenzyme analysis has shown increased B-ALP and L-ALP activity, as well as the presence of one unique isoenzyme. Serum enzyme abnormalities are not typically associated with hepatic dysfunction and resolve with treatment. The presence of hepatic morphologic changes in cats with hyperthyroidism has been poorly documented. In humans, hyperthyroidism may be accompanied by mild changes on hepatic biopsy, such as centrilobular lipidosis and mild focal necrosis.

METABOLIC DISORDERS

Increases in serum GGT and ALP activities frequently accompany canine and feline pancreatitis. These increases are associated with the intrahepatic or extrahepatic cholestasis that may accompany this disorder. Mild increases in serum ALP (two- to threefold) are seen with canine hypothyroidism and in canine and feline diabetes mellitus. The latter is associated with the development of hepatic lipidosis. Severe hypoxia or hypotension can result in ischemic hepatitis (see Table 141–2).

PLASMA PROTEINS IN HEPATIC DISEASE

The liver synthesizes many plasma proteins and detoxifies ammonia, the major breakdown product of protein metabolism. The clinical consequences of disruptions in hepatic protein metabolism are decreases in plasma oncotic pressure due to hypoalbuminemia, bleeding tendencies associated with coagulation protein deficiencies, and the development of hepatic encephalopathy due to ammonia retention.

ALBUMIN

Albumin is synthesized exclusively in the liver. Because synthesis occurs at 33 per cent of maximum capacity and the serum half-life of albumin is eight to nine days, serum hypoalbuminemia is most often seen in chronic hepatic disorders such as cirrhosis and portosystemic vascular anomalies (PSVAs).[3, 6, 27, 28] In cirrhotic dogs, the decrease in plasma oncotic pressure due to serum hypoalbuminemia is frequently accompanied by ascites. Because portal hypertension and avid sodium and water retention also play important roles in ascites development, serum hypoalbuminemia may reflect third-part sequestration of albumin as well as hepatic synthetic failure.

Serum hypoalbuminemia is not specific for hepatic disease. Pathologic processes associated with increased albumin loss, such as protein-losing enteropathies, protein-losing nephropathies, or exudative cutaneous lesions, can also result in serum hypoalbuminemia. Inadequate nutrition can curtail hepatic albumin synthesis. Systemic inflammatory disease may shut down hepatic albumin synthesis in favor of the production of acute-phase proteins. In this sense, albumin is a negative acute-phase reactant.

GLOBULINS

Total serum globulins represent the sum of immunoglobulins and nonimmunoglobulins. Many nonimmunoglobulins are synthesized and stored in the liver, including 75 per cent of the alpha globulins and 50 per cent of the beta globulins. Many nonimmunogloblins are acute-phase reactants whose hepatic production is increased in response to systemic inflammatory disease. The acute-phase alpha globulins produced by the liver include alpha$_1$-antitrypsin, alpha$_1$–acidic glycoprotein, alpha$_2$-macroglobulin, ceruloplasmin, protein C, and haptoglobin. Acute-phase beta globulins synthesized by the liver include fibrinogen, complement, C-reactive protein, and ferritin. In early canine chronic inflammatory liver disease, serum electrophoresis of plasma proteins demonstrates an increase in alpha globulin concentrations.[29] As hepatic disease progresses, decreases in alpha globulins, in particular, alpha$_1$-antitrypsin and haptoglobin, are detected.[29] Hypoglobulinemia is likely the result of hepatic synthetic failure.

Immunoglobulins are not synthesized in the liver but may be increased in chronic inflammatory hepatic disease. A polyclonal increase in gamma globulins has been documented in chronic canine hepatic disease.[12] Serum hypergammaglobulinemia exists in 50 per cent of cats with cholangiohepatitis. In some of these cats, this increase is due to elevations in serum IgG.[30]

Hypergammaglobulinemia in chronic liver disease may be associated with enhanced systemic immunoreactivity due to abnormal Kupffer's cell processing of portal antigens or secondary to autoantibody production. Low titers of antinuclear antibodies have been detected in 50 per cent of dogs with chronic inflammatory hepatic disease.[31] In a series of dogs with chronic inflammatory hepatic disease, 48 per cent had antibodies that reacted with canine liver membrane preparations.[32] Although dogs with positive titers tended to have higher serum ALT and bilirubin values and more severe histopathologic lesions than dogs without antibody responses, it remains to be determined whether these autoantibodies have any role in disease progression.

PLASMA AMINO ACIDS

Plasma amino acid profiles in dogs with experimentally induced and naturally occurring liver disease have been examined.[26, 33, 34] Experimentally induced acute hepatic necrosis results in marked hyperaminoacidemia associated with lysis of necrotic liver tissue and/or hyperglucagonemia-stimulated release of amino acids from muscle.[34] An exception to the general increase in plasma amino acids is a decrease in the urea cycle intermediates arginine and citrulline. These decreases may reflect disruption of the urea cycle secondary to mitochondrial damage. In naturally occurring canine chronic hepatitis or PSVA, decreases in alanine and threonine and increases in serine, glutamic acid, and alpha-amino-N butyric acid occur.[33]

One consistent change noted in canine hepatic disease is a decrease in the molar ratio of branched chain amino acids (BCAA; valine, isoleucine, leucine) to aromatic amino acids, (AAA; phenylalanine, tryptophan).[26, 33, 34] Whereas normal dogs have BCAA-AAA ratios of about 4.1, dogs with naturally occurring PSVA or chronic hepatitis have ratios of about 0.9 or 1.3, respectively. Increases in AAA may reflect decreased hepatic extraction and degradation. Decreased BCAA may be due to increased utilization of these amino acids by muscle and adipose tissue for energy metabolism.

Alterations in the BCAA-AAA ratio are clinically significant, in that they may contribute to the development of hepatic encephalopathy. Because BCAA and AAA normally compete for transport across the blood-brain barrier, the net result of a reduction in the BCAA-AAA ratio is increased brain uptake of AAA. In the brain, AAA are used to synthesize inhibitory and/or false neurotransmitters that contribute to hepatic encephalopathy.

ALPHA-FETOPROTEIN

Alpha-fetoprotein (AFP), a protein produced by the yolk sac and fetal liver, is increased in experimentally induced and naturally occurring hepatic neoplasia in dogs.[35] In one study, determination of serum AFP was capable of differentiating primary hepatic tumors (lymphoma and hepatocellular and biliary adenocarcinoma) from non-neoplastic or metastatic liver disease. The clinical utility of serum AFP for this purpose awaits further studies.

COAGULATION PROTEINS

The liver plays an important role in hemostasis. Hepatocytes synthesize all coagulation factors, except Factor VIII, as well as critical inhibitors of coagulation and fibrinolysis (antithrombin III, antiplasmin) and fibrinolytic proteins (plasminogen). In addition, the liver is responsible for clearance and catabolism of activated coagulation factors, plasminogen activators, and breakdown products of fibrinolysis such as fibrin degradation products (FDPs). The liver is also the site of vitamin K–dependent activation of Factors II, VII, IX, and X and protein C.

Assessment of coagulation status is important in animals suspected of having liver disease, because altered hemostasis can contribute to clinical signs and complicate invasive diagnostic procedures. The complexity and overlap of the liver's synthetic and clearance functions, however, make the interpretation of hemostatic testing difficult. The commonly used tests to assess coagulation include determination of prothrombin time (PT), activated partial thromboplastin time (APTT), fibrinogen, and FDPs. Abnormalities in these coagulation tests in hepatobiliary disease may be indicative of hepatic synthetic failure, vitamin K deficiency, or the presence of a consumption coagulopathy such as disseminated intravascular coagulation (DIC).

Abnormalities in coagulation tests are quite common in dogs and cats with hepatobiliary disease. In one study of dogs with naturally occurring hepatic disease, 50 and 75 per cent had an abnormal PT and APTT, respectively.[36] Specific factor analysis revealed that greater than 90 per cent of the dogs had at least one abnormality.[37] The most common abnormalities were decreases in Factors X, XI, VIII:C, and VII and increases in Factor VIIIR:Ag. Because factor depletion must be greater than 70 per cent to show prolongation of coagulation times, it is not surprising that many more dogs had abnormalities in the concentration of coagulation factors than had prolongation of PT or APTT. In 82 per cent of cats with naturally occurring hepatobiliary disease, at least one coagulation abnormality was present. The most common abnormalities were an increase in PT (16 of 22) and low Factor VII activity (15 of 22).[38]

Vitamin K is a cofactor in the carboxylation of glutamic acid residues in Factors II, VII, XI, and X and protein C, a modification required for activation of these proteins. During activation, vitamin K is oxidized to its epoxide form, which must then be regenerated by sequential enzymatic reduction. Vitamin K deficiency may develop during hepatobiliary disease for several reasons. Prolonged bile duct obstruction interrupts the enterohepatic circulation of bile acids, resulting in intestinal bile acid deficiency and resultant fat-soluble vitamin K malabsorption. Oral antibiotics may alter the intestinal flora, resulting in the destruction of vitamin K–generating bacteria. Inadequate dietary consumption of vitamin K, although rarely a primary cause of vitamin K deficiency, may be contributory, especially in disorders such as feline idiopathic hepatic lipidosis, which are marked by prolonged anorexia. Prolongation of PT is the first coagulation abnormality seen with vitamin K deficiency, because Factor VII has the shortest plasma half-life. In vitamin K deficiency, vitamin K–dependent factors circulate in an inactive form. The concentration of these inactive factors can be measured and is referred to as proteins induced by vitamin K absence or antagonists (PIVKAs). The presence of increased PIVKAs is more sensitive than changes in PT for detecting vitamin K deficiency. Failure to activate vitamin K–dependent factors may occur in the presence of adequate vitamin K stores if the animal is incapable of rejuvenating vitamin K owing to hepatic synthetic failure. Parenteral administration of vitamin K readily (within 24 to 48 hours) corrects coagulation abnormalities due to vitamin K deficiency but has little to no effect on coagulation abnormalities due to hepatic synthetic failure. In a study of cats with naturally occurring hepatobiliary disease, 50 per cent had coagulation abnormalities compatible with vitamin K deficiency (increased PT and APTT, low Factor VII, and normal thrombin time). A normal thrombin time was used to differentiate vitamin K deficiency from hepatic synthetic failure in these cats.[38] The study did not monitor response to vitamin K therapy.

Owing to the liver's central role in coagulation and fibrinolysis, it can be quite challenging to differentiate coagulation abnormalities associated with a consumptive coagulopathy from those due to severe liver disease. Typically, the presence of DIC is recognized by prolongation of PT and APTT, decreased fibrinogen, thrombocytopenia, and increased FDPs, all of which may accompany hepatic failure. Increases in PT and APTT may accompany hepatic synthetic failure or vitamin K deficiency. Interpretation of fibrinogen levels in hepatic disease is complicated by the fact that it is an acute-phase reactant. In early liver disease, fibrinogen concentrations may be normal to increased, and as hepatic function deteriorates, concentrations may decrease due to synthetic failure. Mild hypofibrinogenemia in dogs with chronic inflammatory hepatic disease have been observed. This occurs in the absence of other coagulation test abnormalities and likely represents hepatic synthetic failure rather than excessive consumption due to compensated DIC. Increases in FDPs have been detected in 14 per cent of dogs with chronic hepatic disease[12] and in 30 per cent of cats with idiopathic hepatic lipidosis.[13] These increases may represent impaired hepatic clearance of FDPs and/or the presence of DIC.

Despite the presence of abnormalities in coagulation tests, spontaneous hemorrhage in animals with hepatic disease is rare. Hemorrhage is more likely to occur following a challenge to hemostasis such as venipuncture, hepatic biopsy, or gastric ulceration. Coagulation tests are poor predictors of an individual's tendency to bleed. One should assume that animals with hepatobiliary disease have a higher than normal

LIV

risk of bleeding following provocative procedures, regardless of the results of coagulation testing.

Assessment of coagulation has prognostic significance in hepatic disease. In dogs with chronic inflammatory liver disease, prolongation of PT and APTT to 1.3 to 1.4 times normal was associated with survival of less than one week.[34] In humans with acute liver failure, prolongation of the PT to more than 50 seconds indicates the need for hepatic transplantation. Although prognostic and useful in managing and predicting the complications of hepatic disease, PT and APTT are not sensitive or specific indicators of hepatic disease and should not be used as screening or diagnostic tests.

Both quantitative and qualitative platelet defects accompany hepatobiliary disease. Many dogs with chronic hepatic disease have mild thrombocytopenia (120,000 to 180,000). Thrombocytopenia is rare in cats with hepatobiliary disease unless DIC is present.[38] Studies in dogs with hepatobiliary disease have demonstrated the presence of qualitative defects in platelet aggregation.[39]

BLOOD AMMONIA

The liver is responsible for the majority of ammonia detoxification. Ammonia is generated primarily in the gastrointestinal tract by bacterial degradation of amines, amino acids, and purines by the action of bacterial urease on urea and by intestinal catabolism of glutamine (Fig. 141–3). Ammonia readily diffuses through the intestinal mucosa and into the portal circulation, where it travels to the liver. After uptake by hepatocytes, ammonia is detoxified either by conversion to urea in the Krebs-Henseleit cycle or by consumption in the synthesis of glutamine. The mitochondrial urea cycle converts ammonia to urea by a series of sequential reactions. The urea that is generated undergoes renal excretion. Ammonia that escapes hepatic metabolism enters the systemic circulation, where other tissues, including the kidney, muscle, brain, and intestines, detoxify it by the formation of glutamine.

Hepatic synthetic failure or shunting of portal blood away from the liver results in hyperammonemia. Because the urea cycle operates at only 60 per cent capacity, hepatic synthetic failure must be fairly advanced for blood ammonia concentrations to rise. Because intrahepatic and extrahepatic shunting of portal blood directly deposits ammonia in the systemic circulation, blood ammonia concentrations are more sensitive in the detection of hepatobiliary disorders associated with shunting. Hyperammonemia also occurs in animals with urea cycle enzyme deficiencies and with pathologic conditions that result in decreased availability of urea cycle substrates. Hyperammonemia has been described in two dogs with a deficiency of the urea cycle enzyme arginosuccinate synthetase,[40] and in cats fed a diet deficient in arginine, an essential substrate in the urea cycle.[41]

The biggest obstacle in the clinical use of blood ammonia determinations is the difficulty in obtaining an accurate measurement. Samples for blood ammonia must be drawn into cold heparinized tubes and immediately transferred to an appropriate laboratory on ice for refrigerated centrifugation and assay, preferably within one hour of collection. Feline, but not canine, plasma samples may be frozen at −20°C for 48 hours without sacrificing accuracy. Because erythrocytes contain two to three times the amount of ammonia in plasma, if they are not separated from the plasma immediately or if there is hemolysis in the sample, spurious increases will be detected. During venous sampling, overzealous occlusion of a vein for prolonged periods of time or vigorous muscle activity may also increase venous blood ammonia.

Technical limitations aside, blood ammonia determination is of value in hepatobiliary disease. Hyperammonemia is an important, although not exclusive, cause of hepatic encephalopathy and is the only toxin implicated in this condition that can be measured clinically. The presence of hyperammonemia can be used to verify the presence of hepatic encephalopathy (HE). Not all animals with HE, however, have abnormal blood ammonia concentrations, and such abnormalities may occur with any disorder associated with significant shunting of portal blood away from the liver. Thus 80 per cent of dogs and 90 per cent of cats with PSVA

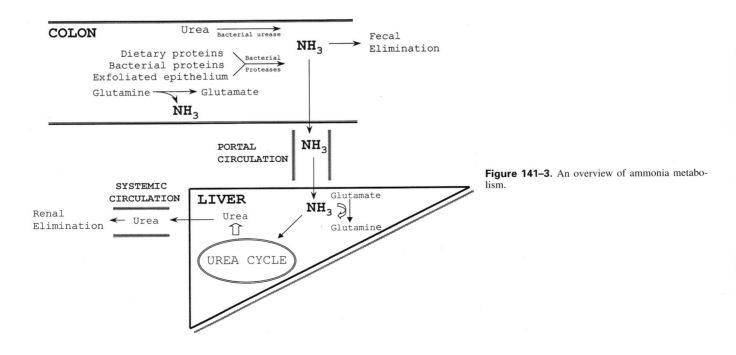

Figure 141–3. An overview of ammonia metabolism.

demonstrate fasting hyperammonemia.[27] Fasting hyperammonemia occurs less often with chronic parenchymal disease, being abnormal in approximately 50 per cent of dogs with chronic hepatitis.[12] Elevations in blood ammonia are unusual with acute hepatic disease, unless it is fulminant.

The diagnostic value of determining the blood ammonia concentration can be improved by performing an ammonia tolerance test (ATT).[4, 42] In an ATT, a baseline blood ammonia value should be determined after a 12-hour fast, and then ammonium chloride (NH_4Cl_2) should be given orally or rectally and blood ammonia determined again. In the oral ATT, NH_4Cl_2 is given at a dose of 100 mg/kg in a dilute solution (not to exceed a concentration of 20 mg/mL and a total dose of 3 g) and blood ammonia determined 30 minutes later. Because vomiting can be a major problem after oral administration of NH_4Cl_2 and the bitter taste of the salt makes stomach tubing of the solution necessary, NH_4Cl_2 is better given in a gelatin capsule. The oral test is subject to variations in small-intestinal absorption and gastric emptying. In the rectal ATT, a warm water enema is given 12 hours before the administration of 2 mL/kg of 5 per cent NH_4Cl_2 via a catheter inserted into the rectum. The solution must be given far enough into the colon to prevent premature evacuation of the solution and to prevent absorption of ammonia by vessels in the distal colon, because this area is not drained by the portal circulation. Samples for blood ammonia are taken at 20 and 40 minutes after challenge. The rectal ATT does not provide as great a challenge to ammonia clearance as the oral tolerance test and is not as sensitive in detecting liver disease. In normal animals, after oral or rectal challenge, blood ammonia should not increase more than two-fold. In animals with hepatic insufficiency or PSVA, ammonia values generally increase three- to 10-fold. Virtually all dogs and cats with PSVA and 90 per cent of dogs with chronic hepatitis have an abnormal ATT.[12, 27] Rarely an ATT precipitates hepatic encephalopathy.

Approximately 65 per cent of dogs and cats with PSVA have a decreased serum urea nitrogen (SUN).[28] Decreases in SUN are thought to arise secondary to decreased urea production in the atrophied liver. Because many of these animals also have a low serum creatinine and low urine specific gravity, fluid diuresis secondary to primary polyuria or polydipsia may also contribute to the low SUN. Decreased SUN has a very low sensitivity for the detection of parenchymal liver disease. It is also not specific for liver disease, because hydration status, dietary protein content, gastrointestinal hemorrhage, glomerular filtration rate, and fluid or solute diuresis can influence SUN.

BILIRUBIN

Bilirubin is a yellow pigment derived from the breakdown of heme (Fig. 141–4). Most of the heme pigment metabolized to bilirubin is derived from the hemoglobin of senescent erythrocytes, with smaller amounts derived from the catabolism of non-hemoglobin sources, including myoglobin and cytochromes. In reticuloendothelial system (RES) cells, heme pigment is degraded to biliverdin by heme oxygenase. Biliverdin is further reduced via the action of bilirubin reductase to bilirubin. Bilirubin released from RES cells is not water-soluble and is transported in plasma reversibly bound to albumin. The liver extracts bilirubin by a carrier-mediated transport mechanism. Once within the hepatocyte, bilirubin is conjugated by esterification with glucuronic acid in a reaction catalyzed by glucuronyl transferase. This water-

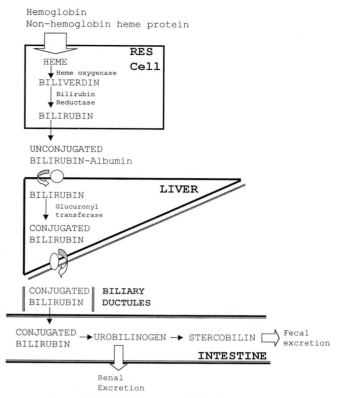

Figure 141–4. An overview of bilirubin metabolism.

soluble conjugated bilirubin is actively secreted against a concentration gradient into the bile. Bilirubin secreted into the bile eventually enters the intestinal tract, where it is either excreted unchanged in the feces or converted to urobilinogen by the action of enteric bacteria. Most of the urobilinogen is further degraded into the brown pigmented stercobilins. The absence of stercobilins in the feces results in pale-colored acholic stools. Small amounts of urobilinogen enter the portal venous system and undergo enterohepatic circulation. The majority is re-excreted into the bile, but a small amount undergoes urinary excretion.

Icterus is the clinical manifestation of bilirubin retention within tissues.[3] Although less sensitive than serum liver enzymes for the detection of hepatobiliary disease, serum hyperbilirubinemia is more specific. Hyperbilirubinemia occurs when an abnormality in the processing of bilirubin exists, and it can be divided into three categories: prehepatic, hepatic, and posthepatic. Prehepatic hyperbilirubinemia is associated with increased production of bilirubin owing to the need to process large amounts of heme, such as occurs during severe hemolytic anemia. It is readily differentiated from hepatic and posthepatic causes by determining hematocrit. Hepatic hyperbilirubinemia is associated with impaired hepatic uptake, conjugation, or excretion of bilirubin. It is seen in hepatic disorders in which severe intrahepatic cholestasis develops, such as idiopathic feline hepatic lipidosis and some canine and feline inflammatory hepatopathies. Hepatic hyperbilirubinemia may also accompany severe extrahepatic infections.[43] In this condition, referred to as the cholestasis of sepsis, circulating cytokines, in particular interleukin-6 and tumor necrosis factor, directly inhibit hepatocyte bilirubin transport. Posthepatic hyperbilirubinemia is associated with interruption of flow within the extrahepatic bile ducts, such as may occur with choleliths, pancreatitis, or biliary neoplasia.

The van den Bergh bilirubin fractionation was developed to facilitate differentiation of prehepatic from hepatic or posthepatic icterus but has proved to be of little clinical value in veterinary patients.[3, 4, 44] The basis of fractionization is that it permits determination of the amount of unconjugated and conjugated bilirubin constituting the total bilirubin. In the van den Bergh reaction, conjugated (direct) bilirubin directly reacts with diazotized sulfanilic acid, whereas unconjugated (indirect) bilirubin will not react until an alcohol accelerator is added. An excess of indirect bilirubin should accompany prehepatic hyperbilirubinemia, whereas posthepatic disease should result in an excess of direct bilirubin. In reality, the two forms of bilirubin most often equilibrate so that similar amounts of both fractions are measured.[44]

The differentiation of hepatic and posthepatic icterus can be quite challenging clinically yet is extremely important because these conditions demand different interventional strategies. Posthepatic hyperbilirubinemia usually requires surgical decompression of the biliary tract, whereas hepatic hyperbilirubinemia is typically a medical condition. It has been proposed that the presence of urobilinogen in the urine be used as an indicator of bile duct patency because in a normal animal, a small fraction of urobilinogen undergoes renal elimination. Urine urobilinogen, however, is not a reliable indicator. False-negatives occur when urobilinogen is oxidized to urobilin, which does not react on the urine dipstick. This may occur upon prolonged storage or following exposure of urine to light. Urinary acidification promotes urobilinogen degradation and increases renal tubular reabsorption of urobilinogen. Alterations in intestinal flora, such as those associated with antibiotic therapy, bacterial overgrowth, or intestinal malabsorption, may decrease the formation of urobilinogen. False-positive results may occur with gastrointestinal bleeding. The clinical differentiation between hepatic and posthepatic hyperbilirubinemia is best made by ultrasound evaluation of the biliary system, combined with careful consideration of clinical history, physical examination, and ancillary laboratory testing.

During prolonged cholestasis, excess conjugated bilirubin may become irreversibly bound to albumin. These so-called biliproteins are clinically significant in that they are measured as direct reacting bilirubin, but their serum half-life approximates that of albumin. Their presence can result in persistently increased serum bilirubin weeks after resolution of the underlying cholestatic liver disorder. In one study of icteric dogs, biliproteins were present in 34 of 35 dogs.[45] The fraction of biliprotein varied from 2 to 94 per cent of total bilirubin. Biliprotein determination is possible with special methodologies but is not routinely available in most veterinary laboratories.

BILE ACIDS

Total serum bile acids (TSBAs) are synthesized exclusively in the liver from cholesterol. Bile acids represent a family of detergent-like compounds that have in common a steroid nucleus hydroxylated at the 3 position.[46, 47] Additional hydroxylation at the 7 position creates the dihydroxy bile acid chenodeoxycholate, and addition of another hydroxyl group at the 12 position creates the trihydroxy bile acid cholic acid. Bile acids are conjugated to glycine or taurine. The cat is an obligate taurine conjugator; dogs preferentially conjugate to taurine but are able to switch to glycine conjugation, if needed. Hydroxylation and conjugation of bile acids improve their water solubility, enabling them to form micelles, which facilitates their role in intestinal fat digestion and absorption.

Bile acids undergo efficient enterohepatic circulation that typically operates at 95 per cent efficacy (Fig. 141–5). Conjugated bile acids are excreted across the hepatocyte canicular membrane into bile by an adenosine triphosphate (ATP)–dependent transporter. They traverse the biliary ducts and eventually reach the gallbladder, where they are stored. Ingestion of a meal stimulates the release of cholecystokinin, resulting in gallbladder contraction and release of bile acids into the duodenum. When bile acids reach the ileum, a sodium-coupled transporter deposits them into the portal circulation. The bile acids travel back to the hepatic sinu-

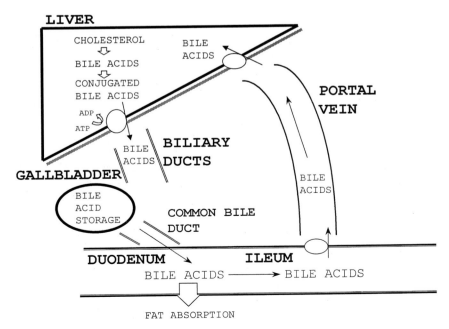

Figure 141–5. The enterohepatic circulation of bile acids.

soids, where another sodium-coupled transporter on the sinusoidal surface of the hepatocyte efficiently recaptures them. Bile acids move through the hepatocyte cytosol and after arrival at the canalicular membrane are re-excreted into bile. The net result of this movement of bile acids through the hepatocyte is to supply the osmotic driving force for the majority of bile flow.

In normal animals, TSBA concentrations are determined by the spillover of bile acids that escape from the enterohepatic circulation. During fasting, when the enterohepatic circulation of bile acids is low, TSBAs are low. After a meal, bile acids are released into the intestines and subsequently absorbed into the portal circulation. Increased portal vein bile acid concentrations are reflected in a transient elevation in TSBAs. This endogenous challenge to the enterohepatic circulation of bile acids is used clinically. In a typical bile acid test, TSBAs are determined after a 12-hour fast, a test meal is fed, and then postprandial TSBAs are determined two hours later.

The most commonly used method for the determination of TSBAs is an enzymatic method that relies on the reaction of 3-hydroxy bile acids with bacterial 3-hydroxysteroid dehydrogenase and subsequent generation of a spectrophotometric end point after reaction with a diformazan dye.[46] Normal values for fasting TSBA concentrations using this method are 1.7 ± 0.3 μM in cats and 2.3 ± 0.4 μM in dogs. Two-hour postprandial values are 8.3 ± 0.3 μM in cats and 8.3 ± 2.2 μM in dogs. Sample collection for this assay is easy, because serum bile acids are stable even at room temperature. Care must be taken to avoid hemolysis, because the absorption spectrum of the spectrophotometric end point is in the range absorbed by hemoglobin. Lipemia also interferes with end-point evaluation. This can be particularly problematic in postprandial samples. If necessary, clarification of the lipemia by centrifugation may be required.

Disruption of the enterohepatic circulation of bile acids results in increases in the concentration of TSBAs. Numerous studies have demonstrated the efficacy of fasting and postprandial TSBAs in the diagnosis of feline and canine hepatobiliary disease and PSVA.[46] In a series of 108 cats with hepatobiliary disease, when cutoff values of greater than 15 μM were used as abnormal, fasting TSBAs were more specific (96 per cent) than increases in serum ALP, ALT, or GGT in predicting the presence of hepatobiliary disease. The sensitivity at this cutoff value (54 per cent) was about the same as for serum enzyme determination. The determination of postprandial TSBAs using a cutoff of greater than 20 μM as abnormal improved both the sensitivity (100 per cent) and the specificity (80 per cent) of bile acid testing in the detection of feline hepatobiliary disease. Postprandial TSBAs had a greater sensitivity than fasting TSBAs for the detection of all categories of feline hepatobiliary disease except hepatic necrosis.

In a series of 107 dogs with histologically confirmed hepatic disease, the specificity of fasting TSBAs using a cutoff of greater than 5 μM as abnormal was 80 per cent. Using a cutoff of greater than 15 μM as abnormal, postprandial TSBAs had a specificity of 89 per cent. When cutoff values for abnormal fasting and postprandial TSBAs were increased to greater than 20 μM and greater than 25 μM, respectively, the specificity of both tests was 100 per cent. The sensitivity for fasting TSBA determination using greater than 5 μM as a cutoff for abnormal was 83 per cent. Sensitivity decreased to 59 per cent when a cutoff value of greater than 20 μM was used. The sensitivity for postpran-

dial TSBAs using a cutoff of greater than 15 μM as abnormal was 82 per cent, with a decrease to 74 per cent at a cutoff of greater than 25 μM. At the higher cutoff values, neither fasting nor postprandial TSBAs outperformed the other. A notable exception was improved performance of postprandial TSBAs in the detection of inactive cirrhosis or PSVA.

Maltese dogs may have elevated postprandial TSBAs in the absence of hepatobiliary disease.[48] In a screening of 200 Maltese dogs, 79 per cent had postprandial TSBAs above the reference range using the enzymatic method. Several had confirmation of postprandial increases by high-performance liquid chromatography. Nine dogs with abnormal postprandial TSBAs and normal rectal ATT had no evidence of hepatobiliary disease on hepatic biopsy. Two dogs with abnormal postprandial TSBAs and ATT had PSVA. The etiology of increased postprandial TSBA values in these Maltese dogs remains undetermined.

A number of factors that influence the enterohepatic circulation of bile acids in normal animals can affect TSBA values.[46] These include the completeness of gallbladder emptying, the rate of gastric emptying, the intestinal transit rate, the efficiency of ileal bile acid reabsorption, and the frequency of enterohepatic cycling. Inadequate fat or amino acid content in the test meal or consumption of an insufficient amount of food can result in failure of cholecystokinin release and gallbladder contraction. In general, it is recommended that the animal eat a regular meal of dog or cat food, although 2 teaspoons of food for animals less than 10 pounds and 2 tablespoons for larger animals has been reported to be adequate. Visual confirmation of meal consumption is mandatory. In some animals, force-feeding may be necessary. The presence of any concurrent disease that delays gastric emptying may result in failure to stimulate gallbladder contraction. Alterations in intestinal transit time so that the movement of conjugated bile acids to the ileum is delayed can result in less than optimal timing for determination of the postprandial values. Severe ileal disease can result in decreased bile acid reabsoption and inadequate challenge to the enterohepatic circulation. The presence of small-bowel overgrowth leads to bacterial deconjugation of bile acids and decreased ileal absorption of bile acids. Occasionally, fasting TSBA concentrations are higher than postprandial values. This happens when interdigestive gallbladder contraction occurs during the course of the fast preceding the test. It may also be associated with individual variations in gastric emptying, response to cholecystokinin release, and intestinal transit time.

The interpretation of abnormal TSBAs is subject to a number of limitations. First, TSBAs are not capable of discriminating one hepatobiliary disease from another. Some general patterns of response, however, do emerge when comparing pre- and postprandial TSBAs. Animals with significant extrahepatic (PSVA) or intrahepatic (cirrhosis) shunting often have normal or mildly elevated fasting TSBAs. In these conditions, a 12-hour fast may provide sufficient time for the liver to extract most of the bile acids. When the enterohepatic circulation is challenged with a meal, however, TSBAs increase dramatically. In animals with posthepatic obstruction, fasting TSBAs usually exceed 250 μM and there is little, if any, change after endogenous challenge. The determination of TSBAs is usually not indicated in the presence of jaundice, because these animals will have hyperbilirubinemia, and increases in bile acids are expected. The only time TSBA determination is warranted in icteric animals is when hemolysis cannot be ruled out.

LIV

Because bilirubin and bile acids do not share hepatic transport systems, in hemolytic disease, TSBAs should be normal.

A second limitation of TSBA determination is that there is little, if any, correlation between the severity of histologic disease or the degree of portosystemic shunting and the extent of TSBA elevation. When evaluating serial determinations of TSBAs to monitor disease progression or response to therapy, only a return to normal can be used as a reliable indicator of clinical remission.

EXCRETION OF ORGANIC DYES AS INDICATORS OF HEPATIC FUNCTION

The water-soluble cholephilic dyes sulfobromophthalein and indocyanine green have been used to evaluate hepatobiliary perfusion and function in veterinary patients. Many variables other than the presence of hepatobiliary dysfunction can influence plasma clearance of these dyes, such as the presence of hypoalbuminemia, systemic hypotension, congestive heart failure, fever, and hyperbilirubinemia. Owing to these limitations and the availability of alternative testing procedures for hepatic function (TSBAs and ATT), the use of these dyes in veterinary medicine is considered obsolete.

CARBOHYDRATE METABOLISM

The major function of the liver in carbohydrate metabolism is to maintain glucose homeostasis during the fasting state. The liver responds to hormonal cues to break down or synthesize glycogen and/or to synthesize glucose. Hepatic glycogenolysis and gluconeogenesis are stimulated by glucagon, epinephrine, and corticosteroids and inhibited by insulin. The functional consequences of deranged glucose homeostasis in liver disease are hypoglycemia or postprandial hyperglycemia.

The liver has a large reserve for maintaining glucose homeostasis so that more than 70 per cent of hepatic function must be lost before hypoglycemia occurs. Hypoglycemia is a rare complication of end-stage chronic inflammatory liver disease. It occurs more often in acute fulminant hepatic failure and in small breed dogs with PSVA. In severe acute hepatocellular injury, hypoglycemia may be a relatively early indicator of hepatic failure. Up to 35 per cent of dogs with congenital PSVA exhibit hypoglycemia.[28] In these dogs, hypoglycemia may be due to impaired hepatic glucose production, decreased hepatic glycogen stores, and/or reduced responsiveness to glucagon. Inadequate glycogen stores may reflect immaturity of the carbohydrate metabolizing enzyme systems or be a consequence of chronic stimulation of glycogenolysis.

Hypoglycemia has been reported as a paraneoplastic syndrome in dogs with hepatic neoplasia.[4, 7] Proposed mechanisms for the hypoglycemia include increased glucose utilization by the tumor or secretion of an insulin-like substance that inhibits gluconeogenesis and promotes glycogenolysis. Serum insulin concentrations, however, are usually normal.

Glycogen storage diseases may cause hypoglycemia.[13] In dogs, congenital deficiencies in lysosomal α-1,4-glucosidase or glucose-6-phosphate have been associated with fasting hypoglycemia and the development of hepatomegaly due to glycogen accumulation. These diseases are diagnosed by provocative testing with glucagon and tissue-specific enzyme assays.

The presence of glucose intolerance has not been well documented in dogs and cats with hepatic disease. Although mild hyperglycemia is common in feline hepatobiliary disease, this may be related to catecholamine-induced stress hyperglycemia and not be a result of hepatic disease. Glucose intolerance may accompany the vacuolar hepatopathy reported in dogs with necrolytic migratory erythema.[13] These dogs, which have an ulcerative dermatopathy, have laboratory testing suggestive of hepatic disease, including marked elevations in serum enzymes and abnormal TSBAs. All dogs studied have decreased plasma amino acid concentrations, and several have been shown to have hyperinsulinemia. Fifty per cent develop diabetes mellitus.

CHOLESTEROL AND LIPID METABOLISM

The liver has several functions in lipid metabolism. Plasma fatty acids released from adipose tissue are extracted by the hepatocytes, after which they either are converted to triglycerides or undergo mitochondrial beta oxidation. Triglycerides are either stored or packaged as very low-density lipoproteins and released into the vasculature. The liver also extracts chylomicron remnants and low-density lipoproteins from plasma. This is the major route by which cholesterol enters into the liver, although the liver is also capable of cholesterol synthesis. Hepatic cholesterol can be esterified and then packaged and secreted in lipoproteins or stored in the liver. The majority of unesterified (free) cholesterol in the liver undergoes biliary excretion.

In the dog and cat, posthepatic obstruction is accompanied by increases in serum cholesterol.[4] Hypercholesterolemia is associated with increased hepatic synthesis and/or decreased biliary excretion of cholesterol. Hypertriglyceridemia is less common with obstruction but may occur secondary to an accumulation of triglyceride-rich chylomicron remnants in the plasma.

In dogs, the appearance in the blood of a novel lipoprotein, lipoprotein X, accompanies obstructive jaundice.[4] Lipoprotein X is a complex of unesterified cholesterol and phospholipid bound to albumin. The presence of lipoprotein X is due to regurgitation of biliary lipids into the plasma. Its presence may also be related to a deficiency in lecithin-cholesterol acyltransferase (LCAT), an enzyme synthesized in the liver, which is responsible for cholesterol esterification. LCAT deficiency may contribute to the excess of unesterified cholesterol in the serum of animals with hepatobiliary disease.

Hypocholesterolemia occurs in approximately 62 per cent of dogs and 67 per cent of cats with congenital PSVA.[28] The mechanism for the low serum cholesterol is unknown but may involve decreased cholesterol synthesis or increased incorporation of cholesterol into bile acids. Hypocholesterolemia is less common with parenchymal liver disease. Progressive hepatopathy in dogs receiving chronic anticonvulsant therapy may be accompanied by marked hypocholesterolemia.[4]

URINALYSIS

A highly variable, but often predominant, clinical sign in animals with chronic hepatobiliary disease or PSVA is the presence of polyuria and/or polydipsia. Urinalysis may reveal isosthenuria or hyposthenuria. The mechanism for the polyuria and/or polydipsia is unknown, but the following have been hypothesized: (1) psychogenic polydipsia; (2)

alterations in portal vein osmoreceptors; (3) decreased hepatic urea production, resulting in disruption of the renal medullary concentration gradient; (4) potassium depletion; (5) stimulation of thirst centers due to hepatic encephalopathy, and (6) increased endogenous cortisol levels associated with increased adrenal production or decreased hepatic degradation.[3, 4, 28]

About 44 per cent of dogs and 12 per cent of cats with PSVA present with isosthenuria or hyposthenuria.[28] Most dogs in which this has been studied have been able to partially concentrate their urine following water deprivation. After surgical correction of the shunt, urine concentrating ability returns.

Between 40 and 74 per cent of dogs and 15 per cent of cats with PSVA have ammonia biurate crystalluria.[28] Repeated examination of fresh urine specimens may be necessary to document the presence of these crystals. Uric acid, a by-product of purine nucleotide catabolism, is normally converted to allantoin by hepatic urate oxidase. In hepatic disease, a deficiency of this enzyme may lead to hyperuricemia. In the presence of concurrent hyperammonemia, increased concentrations of both ions appear in the urine, resulting in the precipitation of ammonia biurate. Abdominal ultrasonography of the urinary system should be performed in animals with ammonium biurate crystalluria to look for the presence of ammonia biurate uroliths. Animals with uroliths may have hematuria and pyuria.

Bilirubinuria is the presence of conjugated bilirubin in the urine. Bilirubinuria in the dog is not abnormal, because dogs have a low renal threshold for bilirubin, and their renal tubular epithelium is capable of bilirubin production.[3] Feline bilirubinuria is always abnormal and suggests the presence of a hepatobiliary or hemolytic disorder.[49] Cats have a high renal threshold for bilirubin, and feline kidneys do not make bilirubin. Because bilirubinuria may be evident before hyperbilirubinemia, it may be used as a screening test for feline hepatobiliary disease.

HEMATOLOGIC ABNORMALITIES

Qualitative and quantitative abnormalities in erythrocytes may accompany hepatobiliary disease in dogs and cats. Anemia can be regenerative or nonregenerative. Regenerative anemia is most often associated with blood loss. Although bleeding associated with coagulopathies is rare in veterinary patients with hepatic disease, blood loss may occur following provocative procedures or secondary to gastrointestinal ulceration.

Nonregenerative anemia is a common finding in hepatic disease. In many instances, it is normocytic and normochromic and most likely associated with inefficient utilization of systemic iron stores (anemia of chronic disease). A microcytic, hypochromic nonregenerative anemia should prompt consideration of chronic gastrointestinal blood loss. From 29 to 80 per cent of dogs and 54 per cent of cats with congenital PSVA have erythrocyte microcytosis.[28] Microcytosis may also occur in dogs with acquired shunting secondary to cirrhosis and in some cats with idiopathic hepatic lipidosis.[12, 13] Studies investigating iron metabolism in dogs with PSVA have documented a relative iron deficiency that may be associated with impaired iron transport.[50, 51] Erythrocyte microcytosis resolves following complete shunt ligation.

Target cells and poikilocytes may be seen in dogs and cats with hepatic disease.[4, 52] The presence of feline poikilocytes should alert the clinician to the possibility of hepatic disease. These morphologic changes may be associated with alterations in the erythrocyte plasma membrane lipoprotein content, resulting in altered cell deformability.

DIAGNOSTIC IMAGING

RADIOGRAPHY

Radiography can be used to assess changes in the size and opacity of the liver.[53, 54] The determination of hepatic size by radiography is subjective and relatively insensitive. Diffuse hepatomegaly is indicated by rounding of the liver edges, extension of the hepatic shadow beyond the costal arch, and caudal-dorsal displacement of the stomach axis. Hepatomegaly may occur due to congestion, infiltrative disease (neoplasia, lipidosis, glycogen accumulation, amyloidosis), inflammatory disease, RES cell hyperplasia, or extramedullary hematopoiesis. Focal hepatomegaly can be discerned by observing displacement of the structures bordering the liver and may occur with cysts, granulomas, neoplasia, regenerative nodules, hematomas, or abscesses. Microhepatica is visualized radiographically by a decreased size of the hepatic shadow and a shift of the gastric axis to a more upright orientation with cranial displacement. Microhepatica is observed with hepatic atrophy and fibrosis.

Normally the liver is visualized as a homogeneous soft tissue opacity. Cholelithiasis or choledocholithiasis may be visualized as mineralization in the liver. The former is recognized as a discrete round opacity in the cranial right ventral liver shadow, and the latter is seen as diffuse mineralization. Focal mineralization may also be seen with chronic gallbladder infection or neoplasia, granulomatous lesions, abscesses, and resolving hematomas and within regenerative nodules.

Gas opacities in the liver may be associated with hepatic abscesses or emphysematous cholecystitis or following long-term bile duct obstruction. The finding of gas within the portal vessel indicates the entry of gastrointestinal gas or infection with gas-producing organisms and is a grave sign seen with gastric torsions or severe necrotizing gastroenteritis.

Radiographic contrast imaging of the portal venous system is used to localize PSVA. It can be accomplished via three methods. The first, cranial mesenteric arteriography, involves cannulation of the cranial mesenteric artery via the femoral artery and injection of iodinated contrast followed by rapid fluoroscopic imaging. This procedure is technically difficult and is seldom performed. The second method, splenoportography, involves injection of a contrast agent directly into the spleen either percutaneously or at the time of laparotomy. Complications include splenic infarction and hemorrhage. The third method to demonstrate PSVA is operative mesenteric portography. This involves intraoperative jejunal vein catherization and injection of iodinated contrast.

Cholecystography can be used to visualize the gallbladder and biliary tract but is rarely employed in small animals. Several techniques using oral, intravenous, or percutaneoous administration of iodinated contrast agents have been described.[53] These studies rarely yield information that is not obtainable by ultrasound examination of the biliary system.

Colorectal scintigraphy is employed in small animals for the detection of PSVA.[4, 54] A small amount of technetium 99m pertechnetate can be administered rectally, which is then absorbed via the colon into the portal venous system. In the normal dog, radioactivity is visualized in the liver within 10 to 22 seconds, and then it proceeds to the heart

LIV

and lungs. In animals with PSVA, radioactivity reaches the heart and lungs first or at the same time as the liver. Rectal technetium scans are abnormal in dogs with macroscopic PSVA and normal in dogs with microvascular dysplasia. Rectal technetium scans may underestimate shunting when gastrosplenic vessels are involved, because venous blood from the colon does not pass through these vessels. This may complicate the use of rectal scans in cats, because left gastric vein shunts are the most common feline PSVA.

ULTRASONOGRAPHY

Ultrasonography may differentiate focal from diffuse disease; evaluate alterations in hepatic parenchyma in diffuse disease, the biliary system, and the portal vasculature; and assist in procurement of tissue for hepatic histopathology.[53, 55–57] The normal liver has a homogeneous echogenicity that is isoechoic to slightly hyperechoic to the renal cortex. It has sharp, smooth edges and contains numerous variably sized circular and tubular anechoic structures that represent hepatic and portal veins. During hepatobiliary disease, changes in hepatic size, vascularity, and echogenicity may occur. It must be emphasized that few hepatic lesions have diagnostic sonographic features and that a normal hepatic ultrasound examination does not rule out the possibility of diffuse hepatic disease.

The determination of liver size by sonography is at best subjective. A large liver may be easily imaged and has rounded edges. There is a relatively large distance between the diaphragm and stomach. A small liver may be difficult to image, with a narrow distance identified between the diaphragm and stomach. Two studies have evaluated the sonosographic measurement of hepatic size by determining the distance from the ventral liver up to the craniodorsal diaphragm margins, with conflicting results.[53]

In diffuse hepatic disease, the liver may appear hyperechoic or hypoechoic.[55] The hyperechoic liver is brighter than the renal cortices. Portal vein margins become indistinct in the hyperechoic liver. Increased echogenicity may accompany fibrotic liver disease, lipidosis, corticosteroid hepatopathy, or hepatic neoplasia (lymphoma, bile duct adenocarcinoma). Fibrosis should be suspected when the liver is small, when regenerative nodules are present, and when ascites or splenomegaly is found. In a series of cats with various hepatobiliary disorders, the finding of a hyperechoic liver that was isoechoic to falciform fat was highly suggestive of the presence of hepatic lipidosis. A hypoechoic liver is less echogenic than the renal cortices and has enhanced visualization of portal vasculature. It may accompany moderate to severe suppurative hepatic disease, passive congestion, or hepatic lymphoma.

The sonographic appearance of hepatic lymphoma can be quite variable.[7, 53] The liver may be diffusely hyper- or hypoechoic. There may be focal or multifocal, poorly circumscribed hypoechoic masses or well-circumscribed hyperechoic nodules surrounded by areas of hypoechogenicity, so-called target lesions.

A variety of focal hepatic lesions can be recognized with ultrasonography. Hepatic cysts appear as round, smooth-walled, anechoic structures with acoustic enhancement. Biliary cysts appear as thin-walled, circular, anechoic structures. Hematomas have a variable appearance, depending on their state of resolution. Early hematomas are hyperechoic, progress to hypoechoic, and once they mature are anechoic. They may have areas of mineralization. Regenerative nodules also

have a variable appearance. They may be hypoechoic, isoechoic, or hyperechoic or have mixed echogenicity. They are most often variably sized multiple hypoechoic areas. They may appear anechoic if necrosis occurs within them. Abscesses or granulomas have a variable appearance, depending on their cellular composition and duration. Early abscesses are hyperechoic with poorly defined margins. As they mature, they become more hypo- to anechoic and may have mixed echogenicity. The presence of gravity-dependent hyperechoic cellular material may be demonstrated. Occasionally, they may contain gas or mineralization. Some posterior acoustic enhancement may occur. Primary hepatic neoplasia may have a variable appearance. It usually is a large, solitary, moderately circumscribed mass that bulges beyond the normal liver margins with an echo texture similar to that of normal liver. Metastatic neoplasia appears as one or more spherical lesions that may be hypoechoic, hyperechoic, or isoechoic. These areas may also appear as target lesions.

The gallbladder may be distended in anorexic animals and often contains a gravity-dependent layer of echogenic bile, i.e., biliary sludge. The wall is normally thin. A diffusely thickened gallbladder wall occurs with cholecystitis or secondary to abdominal fluid accumulation. Focal thickening of the gallbladder wall may represent benign cystic hyperplasia of the mucous glands or neoplasia. Choleliths are visualized as gravity-dependent hyperechoic foci within the gallbladder that produce strong acoustic shadowing.

Ultrasonography is important in determining the presence of posthepatic biliary obstruction.[56, 58] The first indication of obstruction is distention of the gallbladder with loss of tapering of the neck into the cystic duct.[53, 56] This occurs 24 hours after experimental bile duct ligation in the dog. The common bile duct distends by 48 hours after ligation. Extrahepatic bile ducts dilate by 72 hours and are visible as many tortuous anechoic structures at the hepatic portal between the gallbladder and the pancreas. Intrahepatic bile ducts distend by one week and are seen as tortuous, irregularly branching, anechoic structures with echogenic walls throughout the liver. Distention of the feline common bile duct to greater than 5 mm has been consistently associated with obstruction.[58] Ultrasonography also enables visualization of the cause of the obstruction, which may be associated with intraluminal (neoplasia, strictures, choleliths) or extraluminal (pancreatitis, neoplasia) disorders.

Abdominal ultrasonography can be used to identify the presence of PSVA. Animals with PSVA have small livers with a decrease in portal vascular structures. Vascular anomalies involving the portal vein and the systemic vasculature may be visualized. In general, intrahepatic shunts are easier to visualize than extrahepatic shunts. Doppler capabilities enhance the operator's ability to detect extrahepatic shunts. Portoazygos shunts are the most difficult to identify.

Hepatic arteriovenous fistulas can be seen as tortuous, tubular, anechoic structures within or adjacent to the liver. Doppler-assisted ultrasonography demonstrates areas of turbulent blood flow. The hepatic artery and portal vein branches may be dilated and tortuous. Celiac arteriography can be used to identify arteriovenous fistulas and to define the limits of surgical resection.

REFERENCES

1. Kramer JW, Hoffman WE: Clinical enzymology. In Kaneko J, Harvey J, Bruss, M (eds): Clinical Biochemistry of Domestic Animals. Boston, Academic Press, 1997, p 330.
2. Valentine BA, et al: Increased serum alanine aminotransferase activity associated with muscle necrosis in the dog. J Vet Intern Med 4:140, 1990.

3. Tennant BC: Hepatic function. *In* Kaneko J, Harvey J, Bruss M (eds): Clinical Biochemistry of Domestic Animals. Boston, Academic Press, 1997, p 327.
4. Center SA: Diagnostic procedures for evaluation of hepatic disease. *In* Guilford W, Center S, Strombeck D, et al (eds): Small Animal Gastroenterology. Philadelphia, WB Saunders, 1996, p 130.
5. Bunch S: Hepatotoxicity of pharmacological agents in dogs and cats. Vet Clin North Am Small Anim Pract 23:659, 1993.
6. Dial SM: Clinicopathologic evaluation of the liver. Vet Clin North Am Small Anim Pract 25:257, 1995.
7. Hammer AS, Sikkema D: Hepatic neoplasia in the dog and cat. Vet Clin North Am Small Anim Pract 25:419, 1995.
8. Noonan NE, Meyer DJ: Use of plasma arginase and γ-glutamyl transpeptidase as specific indicators of hepatocellular or hepatobiliary disease in the dog. Am J Vet Res 40:942, 1979.
9. DeNovo R, Prasse K: Comparison of serum biochemical and hepatic functional alterations in dogs treated with corticosteroids and hepatic duct ligation. Am J Vet Res 44:1703, 1983.
10. Center SA, et al: Diagnostic value of γ-glutamyl transferase and alkaline phosphatase activities in hepatobiliary disease in the cat. JAVMA 188:507, 1986.
11. Center SA, et al: Diagnostic efficacy of serum alkaline phosphatase and γ-glutamyltransferase in dogs with histologically confirmed hepatobiliary disease. JAVMA 201:1258, 1992.
12. Center SA: Chronic hepatitis, cirrhosis, breed specific hepatopathies, copper storage disease, suppurative hepatitis, granulomatous hepatitis and idiopathic hepatic fibrosis. *In* Guilford W, Center S, Strombeck D, et al (eds): Small Animal Gastroenterology. Philadelphia, WB Saunders, 1996, p 705.
13. Center SA: Hepatic lipidosis, glucocorticoid hepatopathy, vacuolar hepatopathy, storage disorders, amyloidosis and iron toxicosis. *In* Guilford W, Center S, Strombeck D, et al (eds): Small Animal Gastroenterology. Philadelphia, WB Saunders, 1996, p 766.
14. Hoffman W, et al: A technique for automated quantification of canine glucocorticoid induced isoenzyme of alkaline phosphatase. Vet Clin Pathol 17:66, 1991.
15. Kidney BA, Jackson ML: Diagnostic value of alkaline phosphatase isoenzyme separation by affinity electrophoresis in the dog. Can J Vet Res 52:106, 1988.
16. Sanecki RK, et al: Subcellular location of corticosteroid induced alkaline phosphatase in canine hepatocytes. Vet Pathol 24:296, 1987.
17. Wilson SM, Feldman EC: Diagnostic value of steroid induced isoenzyme of alkaline phosphatase in the dog. J Am Anim Hosp Assoc 28:245, 1992.
18. Badylak SF, Van Fleet J: Sequential morphologic and clinicopathologic alterations in dogs with experimentally induced glucocorticoid hepatopathy. Am J Vet Res 42:1310, 1981.
19. Dillon AR, et al: Prednisolone induced hematologic, biochemical and histologic changes in the dog. J Am Anim Hosp Assoc 16:831, 1980.
20. Dillon AR, et al: Effects of dexamethasone and surgical hypotension on hepatic morphologic features and enzymes in dogs. Am J Vet Res 44:1996, 1983.
21. Rutgers C, et al: Subcellular pathologic features of glucocorticoid hepatopathy in dogs. Am J Vet Res 56:898, 1995.
22. Solter P, et al: Hepatic total 3α-hydroxy bile acids concentration and enzyme activities in prednisone treated dogs Am J Vet Res 55:1086, 1994.
23. Moore GE, et al: Hematologic and serum biochemical effects of long-term administration of anti-inflammatory dosage of prednisone in dogs. Am J Vet Res 53:1033, 1992.
24. Badylak SF, Van Fleet JF: Tissue γ-glutamyl transpeptidase activity and hepatic ultrastructural alterations in dogs with experimentally induced glucocorticoid hepatopathy. Am J Vet Res 43:649, 1982.
25. Strombeck DR, et al: Effects of corticosteroid treatment on survival time in dogs with chronic hepatitis: 151 cases. JAVMA 193:1109, 1988.
26. Rutgers C, et al: Plasma amino acid analysis in dogs with experimentally induced hepatocellular and obstructive jaundice. Am J Vet Res 48:696, 1987.
27. Center SA: Liver function tests in the diagnosis of portosystemic vascular anomalies. Semin Vet Med Surg 5:94, 1990.
28. Center SA, Magne ML: Historical, physical examination and clinicopathologic features of portosystemic vascular anomalies in the dog and cat. Semin Vet Med Surg 5:83, 1990.
29. Sevelius E, Anderson M: Serum protein electrophoresis as a prognostic marker of chronic liver disease in dogs. Vet Rec 137:663, 1995.
30. Lucke IM, Davies JD: Progressive lymphocytic cholangitis in the cat. J Small Anim Pract 25:249, 1984.
31. Anderson M, Sevelius E: Circulating autoantibodies in dogs with chronic liver disease. J Small Anim Pract 33:389, 1992.
32. Weiss D, et al: Anti-liver membrane protein antibodies in dogs with chronic hepatitis. J Vet Intern Med 9:267, 1995.
33. Strombeck DR, Rogers Q: Plasma amino acid concentrations in dogs with hepatic disease. JAVMA 173:93, 1978.
34. Strombeck DR, et al: Plasma amino acid, glucagon and insulin concentrations in dogs with nitrosamine-induced hepatic disease. Am J Vet Res 44:2028, 1983.
35. Lowseth LA, et al: Detection of serum alpha-fetoprotein in dogs with hepatic tumors. JAVMA 199:735, 1991.
36. Badylak SF, Van Fleet JF: Alterations of prothrombin time and activated partial thromboplastin time in dogs with hepatic disease. Am J Vet Res 42:2053, 1981.
37. Badylak SF, et al: Plasma coagulation factor abnormalities in dogs with naturally occurring hepatic disease. Am J Vet Res 44:2336, 1983.
38. Lisciandro SC, et al: Coagulation abnormalities in 22 cats with naturally occurring liver disease. J Vet Intern Med 12:71, 1998.
39. Willis SE, et al: Whole blood platelet aggregation in dogs with liver disease. Am J Vet Res 50:1893, 1989.
40. Strombeck DR, et al: Hyperammonemia due to urea cycle enzyme abnormality in 2 dogs. JAVMA 166:1109, 1975.
41. Morris JG: Nutritional and metabolic responses to arginine deficiency in carnivores. J Nutr 115:524, 1985.
42. Rothuizen J, van den Ingh TSGAM: Rectal ammonia tolerance in the evaluation of portal circulation in dogs with liver disease. Res Vet Sci 33:22, 1982.
43. Taboada J, Meyer DJ: Cholestasis associated with extrahepatic bacterial infection in 5 dogs. J Vet Intern Med 3:216, 1989.
44. Rothuizen J, van den Brom E: Bilirubin metabolism in canine hepatobiliary and haemolytic disease. Vet Q 9:235, 1987.
45. Rothuizen J, van den Ingh T: Covalently protein-bound bilirubin conjugates in cholestatic disease of dogs Am J Vet Res 49:702, 1987.
46. Center SA: Serum bile acids in companion animal medicine. Vet Clin North Am Small Anim Pract 223:625, 1993.
47. Leveille-Webster CR: Bile acids—what's new. Semin Vet Med Surg 12:2, 1997.
48. Tisdall P, et al: Post-prandial serum bile acid concentrations and ammonia tolerance in Maltese dogs with and without hepatic vascular disease. Aust Vet J 72:121, 1995.
49. Lees GE, et al: Clinical implications of feline bilirubinuria. J Am Anim Hosp Assoc 20:765, 1984.
50. Bunch SE, et al: Characterization of iron status in young dogs with portosystemic shunt. Am J Vet Res 56:853, 1995.
51. Simpson KW, et al: Iron status and erythrocyte volume in dogs with congenital portosystemic vascular anomalies. J Vet Intern Med 11:14, 1997.
52. Christopher MM, Lee SE: Red cell morphologic alterations in cats with liver disease. Vet Clin Pathol 23:7, 1994.
53. Partington BP, Biller DS: Hepatic imaging with radiology and ultrasound. Vet Clin North Am Small Anim Pract 25:305, 1995.
54. Penninck D, Berry C: Liver imaging in the cat. Semin Vet Med Surg 12:10, 1997.
55. Biller DS: Ultrasonography of diffuse liver disease. J Vet Intern Med 6:71, 1992.
56. Nyland TG, Gillet NA: Sonographic features of experimental bile duct ligation in the dog. Vet Radiol 23:252, 1982.
57. Yeager AE, Muhammed H: Accuracy of ultrasonography in the detection of severe hepatic lipidosis in cats. Am J Vet Res 53:597, 1992.
58. Leveille R, et al: Sonographic evaluation of the common bile duct in cats. J Vet Intern Med 10:296, 1996.

LIV

CHAPTER 142

INDICATIONS AND TECHNIQUES FOR LIVER BIOPSY

Deborah G. Day

Liver disease is common in dogs and cats and is initiated by myriad agents or events. Determination of specific histologic abnormalities allows prognostication and suggests the proper treatment. Multiple methods are available for obtaining a liver biopsy, and the method used depends on the type of lesion present, the location of the lesion, the overall size of the liver being biopsied, and the clinical stability of the animal.

INDICATIONS

General indications for liver biopsy include moderately to markedly elevated serum bile acids, hepatic hyperbilirubinemia, generalized hepatic hypoechogenicity on ultrasound examination, unexplained hepatomegaly, presence of a solitary mass lesion, presence of multiple focal nodules within the hepatic parenchyma, and evaluation of response to therapy. Abnormalities of liver enzyme activities (ALT, ALP, GGT) in the absence of documented liver dysfunction or parenchymal changes do not warrant a liver biopsy, because these enzymes may be altered in the absence of primary liver disease.

CONTRAINDICATIONS

The only absolute contraindication for liver biopsy, regardless of the method used to obtain the sample, is severe coagulopathy. The presence of disseminated intravascular coagulation is a relative contraindication for hepatic biopsy, and the risks of hemorrhage must be carefully weighed against the proposed benefits of the procedure performed. If an abscess is suspected based on ultrasonography or the presence of hepatic gas on survey radiographs, exploratory laparotomy should be performed instead of blind or ultrasound-guided techniques.

PATIENT PREPARATION

A complete blood count and platelet count should be obtained and evaluated before hepatic biopsy. A buccal mucosal bleeding time evaluates platelet function and screens for the presence of von Willebrand's disease. It may be warranted in selected animals. Prothrombin time and partial thromboplastin time should be completed before needle biopsy or open wedge biopsy to evaluate the dog's or cat's clotting ability.

Animals undergoing liver biopsy are fasted for 12 to 24 hours before the procedure. The length of the fast should be determined by the type of sedation or anesthesia being used and the method of biopsy. The more invasive procedures using general anesthesia require longer fasting than the less invasive procedures using only mild sedation or local anesthesia. Feeding a fatty meal before biopsy was previously advocated as a means of causing gallbladder contraction. This practice is no longer recommended, because changes in gallbladder size using this technique have not been documented.[1] Additionally, recent feeding is likely to make ultrasound-guided procedures more difficult owing to gas interference that may obscure images of the liver.

BIOPSY METHODS

A diagnostic hepatic sample may be obtained using fine-needle aspiration, needle biopsy, or open wedge resection. Although several biopsy methods are available, not every method is suitable for each situation or animal (Fig. 142–1). The method of obtaining a liver biopsy must be tailored to the individual dog or cat to maximize yield while minimizing potential complications.

FINE-NEEDLE ASPIRATION

Fine-needle aspiration is a simple and easy technique for obtaining cells for cytologic evaluation of the liver. Cytology is often sufficient for the diagnosis of several diffuse hepatopathies, including hepatic lipidosis, steroid hepatopathy, diffuse neoplasia, or severe hepatic inflammation.[2] Fine-needle aspiration is performed using a 22- or 25-gauge 1.5-inch needle attached to a fluid extension tubing and a 10- or 12-mL syringe. The extension tubing allows for freedom of movement during aspiration and minimizes risk of hepatic laceration. Once the needle is advanced into the liver, suction is applied several times until bloody fluid appears in the needle hub. The suction is released, and the needle is immediately withdrawn. An assistant is useful for applying suction to the syringe, because it is difficult to apply adequate suction with one hand.

The syringe is removed from the extension tubing, and air is aspirated into the syringe. The syringe is immediately reattached to the tubing, and the plunger is pushed into the syringe to expel the contents of the needle onto a glass slide. "Pull" smears should then be made. Slides are air dried and stained using a commercially available stain (Diff Quik,

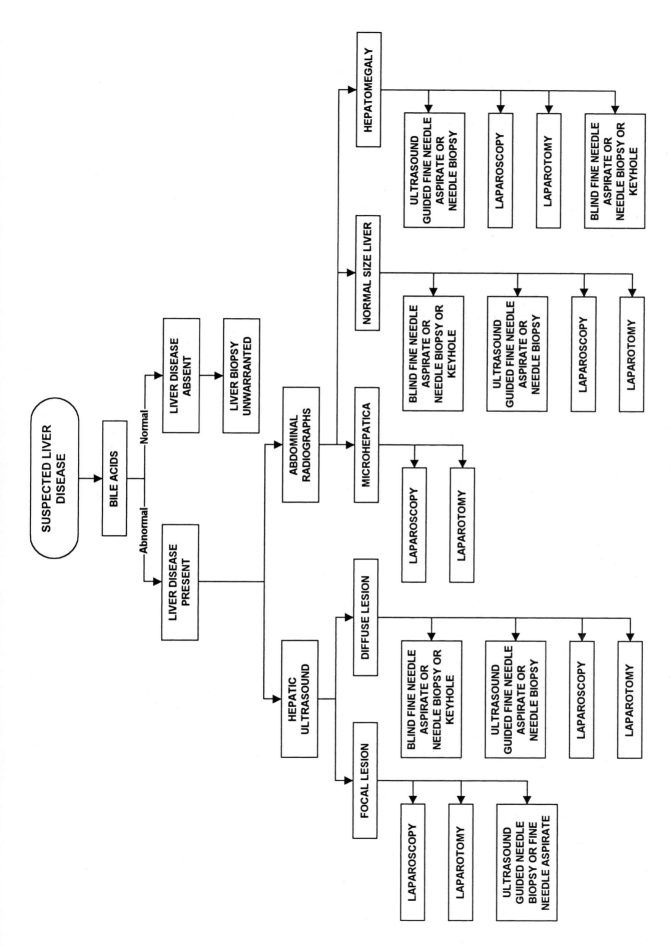

Figure 142–1. Algorithm for determining appropriate biopsy methods in animals with liver disease.

LIV

1295

TABLE 142–1. NEEDLES COMMONLY USED FOR HEPATIC BIOPSY

NEEDLE	SOURCE
Bauer Tenmo	Products Group International, Inc., Lyons, CO
Vet-Core	Cook Veterinary Products, Inc., Bloomington, IN
TruCut	Travenol Laboratories Inc., Deerfield, IL
Menghini	V. Mueller Co., Chicago, IL
Jamshidi	Kormed, Inc., St. Paul, MN
Franklin modified Vim-Silverman	Baxter, Deerfield, IL

Harleco, Gibbstown, NJ). If the slides are to be sent to a clinical pathologist for evaluation, several slides should be reserved unstained for processing at the laboratory using the staining procedure favored by the pathologist reviewing the slides.

The cost of this procedure is minimal, and complications are few. Sedation is rarely required, thus eliminating the need for anesthetic drugs that might harm an animal with severe liver failure. The sample size is small and may be nondiagnostic, particularly when focal disease is present and the aspirate is obtained blindly.

NEEDLE BIOPSY

Needle biopsy techniques obtain a larger hepatic sample than aspiration, allowing examination of hepatic architecture. This technique is most successful when diffuse hepatic disease is present, because focal lesions may be missed. Needle biopsies are performed using a 14-gauge biopsy needle to obtain the largest sample size, but smaller needles are available for very small animals. Several manufacturers make needles appropriate for liver biopsy (Table 142–1). Spring-loaded needles (Vet-Core, Cook Veterinary Products, Inc.; Bauer Tenmo, Products Group International, Lyons, CO) are preferred, are easy to operate, and can be fired using one hand. The following discussion pertains to the Vet-Core and Tenmo needles. For use of other types of biopsy needles, refer to the manufacturer's instructions. The Vet-Core and Tenmo needles are cocked by pulling back on the firing mechanism until the needle clicks. The biopsy notch of the inner obturator is exposed by gently pushing the firing mechanism forward. Continued pressure fires the needle. Before biopsy, the needle is cocked and fired to be certain that it is in good working condition. If the firing mechanism is sluggish, the needle is discarded and another needle is

selected. This is extremely important when reusing needles. This technique requires moderate to heavy sedation (Table 142–2) to prevent movement during biopsy and is more expensive than fine-needle aspiration to perform. These needles may be sterilized for reuse using ethylene oxide.

Upon removal of the needle from the abdominal cavity, the needle is cocked and the obturator is advanced to reveal the biopsy specimen. The tissue is gently teased from the biopsy channel using a sterile 25-gauge needle. The biopsy specimen may be gently rolled on a glass slide for cytologic examination before immersion in formalin if desired. The biopsy specimen should then be placed immediately in 10 per cent buffered formalin. An additional sample may be obtained for microbiologic culture and should be placed immediately in the appropriate transport medium.

OPEN WEDGE BIOPSY

The animal is prepared for exploratory laparotomy in an appropriate manner. If diffuse disease is present, a ligature amputation method may be used.[3, 4] Briefly, a loop of absorbable suture should be placed around the tip of a liver lobe and slowly tightened, crushing the hepatic parenchyma and ligating blood vessels. The sample is cut free distal to the ligature using a scalpel or cautery. Focal lesions may be biopsied using one of the biopsy needles described earlier. Several methods for liver lobectomy have been described.[3, 5, 6]

A portion of the biopsy specimen should be placed immediately in 10 per cent buffered formalin in a ratio of 1:10 (sample to formalin) for routine histopathology. Samples for microbiologic culture can be placed immediately in the appropriate transport medium. Contact the specific laboratory for instructions on sample handling for specimens obtained for copper analysis or special stains.

BIOPSY APPROACHES

BLIND PERCUTANEOUS APPROACH

This approach may be used for either fine-needle aspiration or needle biopsy. The animal can be positioned in oblique dorsal recumbency at a 30- to 45-degree angle with the right side toward the table. The table may be tilted at a 45-degree angle if desired to facilitate palpation of the liver margins and to move the other internal organs away from the liver. The hair is clipped over the tip of the xiphoid to the left costal arch and umbilicus, and this area is surgically

TABLE 142–2. ANESTHETIC PROTOCOLS APPROPRIATE FOR HEPATIC BIOPSY

BIOPSY METHOD	CLINICAL STATUS*	ANESTHETIC PROTOCOL
Fine-needle Aspirate	Poor to good	None or infiltration of 2% lidocaine at puncture site
Needle biopsy	Poor	1. Diazepam 0.2–0.4 mg/kg IV and butorphanol 0.2–0.4 mg/kg IV *or* 2. Diazepam 0.2–0.4 mg/kg and oxymorphone 0.05–0.1 mg/kg IV *or* (1) or (2) plus propofol 2 mg/kg IV if needed
	Good	3. Diazepam/ketamine 1 mL of 50:50 mixture/5–10 kg IV *or* 4. Propofol 2–6 mg/kg IV *or* (1) + (3) or (4) *or* (2) + (3) or (4)
Laparoscopy	Poor to good	Premedication with (1) or (2) IM Induction with (3) or (4) Maintenance with isofluorane in oxygen
Laparotomy	Poor to good	Same as laparoscopy

*Clinical status refers to the animal's disposition. The better the clinical status, the more likely that more sedation or general anesthesia will be required.

scrubbed. For additional analgesia when using light anesthetic protocols, the puncture site is infiltrated with 2 per cent lidocaine. A Number 11 blade is used to make a 2-mm incision through the skin and subcutaneous fat half the distance between the tip of the xiphoid and the left costal arch. The needle is aimed cranially and toward the left liver lobe about 20 degrees in dogs.[1, 7–9] The needle is kept more perpendicular in cats until the needle enters the abdominal cavity; then it is aimed slightly left. Upon entering the peritoneal cavity with the needle tip, the needle is advanced 1 to 2 cm toward the left of midline and the spine. The biopsy notch is then advanced into the liver, and the needle is fired. The needle must be checked after each biopsy attempt to determine whether tissue has been obtained. Multiple attempts may be made in medium to large size dogs if the initial attempt is unsuccessful. The biopsy needle may penetrate deeper on subsequent attempts to a maximum penetration of 5 cm. Repeated attempts should be performed cautiously in small dogs and cats, because the risk of lacerations to the liver and other organs is higher in small animals. The needle should be removed immediately if any changes in respiration are noted during the biopsy procedure.

KEYHOLE APPROACH

The animal is prepared in a manner identical to the blind percutaneous approach, except that instead of making a 1- to 2-mm incision, an incision large enough to admit one sterilely gloved finger is made.[7, 10, 11] The operator stabilizes the liver lobe for insertion of the biopsy needle and guides the needle into the liver lobe. This technique requires heavy sedation with a local block or general anesthesia (see Table 142–2).

ULTRASOUND-GUIDED APPROACH

Some animals with liver disease are seriously ill, and the stress of general anesthesia and laparotomy may cause decompensation. Ultrasound-guided percutaneous hepatic biopsy is often possible with minimal restraint and light sedation (see Table 142–2), making this technique preferable in many situations. Because the hepatic architecture can be visualized, the type of hepatic lesion present may be determined before biopsy[12–15] and may aid in the selection of a biopsy technique. The presence of a small fibrotic liver, highly vascular liver, abscess, or cyst would preclude a closed biopsy technique. Ultrasound is extremely useful for guiding the needle into focal lesions.

The animal is positioned as for blind percutaneous approaches. The abdomen is clipped for ultrasound examination. Upon completion of the ultrasound examination, the needle puncture site is prepared aseptically. The ultrasound transducer is covered with a sterile sleeve, and sterile coupling gel is used to visualize the lesion and needle path. A small stab incision is made in the skin using a Number 11 blade to allow smooth passage of the biopsy needle. The biopsy needle is passed parallel or slightly perpendicular to the path of the transducer. The needle is advanced to the edge of the liver lobe or lesion. The needle biopsy notch is then advanced into the selected area and fired. The needle is withdrawn, and the sample is retrieved using a sterile 25-gauge needle. The liver is scanned for evidence of hemorrhage, which will appear hyperechoic in the area of biopsy. Because the needle path is visualized, the risk of puncturing

organs other than the liver is reduced. Hepatic vessels and biliary ducts may be lacerated if the biopsy needle penetrates too deeply into the hepatic parenchyma.

LAPAROSCOPIC APPROACH

The benefits of laparoscopy include good visualization of the liver and other abdominal organs, ability to direct the needle into focal lesions, and ability to biopsy small livers using a small incision. This technique requires expensive equipment, considerable operator experience, and general anesthesia. This technique is not appropriate if the animal is known or suspected to have surgically correctable disease, and it is technically more difficult in the presence of moderate to severe abdominal effusion. Laparoscopy has been described elsewhere.[10, 16] Complications include air embolism and CO_2-induced acid-base imbalances. A modified laparoscopic procedure using a sterile otoscope has been described.[17]

SURGICAL APPROACH

Open wedge biopsy can be performed during exploratory laparotomy in any clinic without the need for special equipment. This technique allows good visualization of the liver being biopsied, direct observation and control of hemorrhage, and primary repair of some lesions. General anesthesia is required, which may decompensate an apparently stable animal in liver failure (see Table 142–2). This procedure is more invasive, time consuming, and costly than closed methods of liver biopsy. Exploratory laparotomy should be performed when the liver is small, abscess or cyst is suspected, biliary obstruction or rupture is suspected, or extrahepatic disease requiring surgical correction is present. Complications that may occur include hemorrhage, poor recovery from general anesthesia, poor wound healing (especially when hypoalbuminemia is present), and incisional dehiscence.

AFTERCARE

All animals should be monitored for signs of hemorrhage for several hours after biopsy. Mucous membrane color, heart rate, pulse character, and mentation should be monitored carefully. Animals should be placed in sternal recumbency so that the weight of the liver helps to compress the biopsy site and control hemorrhage.

POTENTIAL COMPLICATIONS

Specific complications have been discussed with each technique. The most serious complications regardless of technique used include hemorrhage and puncture of stomach, intestine, or biliary system. Steps should be taken before biopsy to manage complications as they develop. Packed red blood cells or whole blood should be available if needed for serious hemorrhage.

SUMMARY

Liver biopsy is required for the identification of specific pathologic abnormalities of liver disease in dogs and cats.

LIV

Once the specific etiology is identified, prognosis and treatment options can be given. Numerous biopsy techniques are available, and the appropriate technique is selected based on the animal's clinical status, liver size, location of lesion, operator experience, and equipment available.

REFERENCES

1. Hardy RM: Hepatic biopsy. *In* Kirk RW (ed): Current Veterinary Therapy VIII: Small Animal Practice. Philadelphia, WB Saunders, 1983, p 813.
2. Kristensen AT, et al: Liver cytology in cases of canine and feline hepatic disease. Compend Contin Educ Pract Vet 12:797, 1990.
3. Breznock EM: Surgery of the hepatic parenchymal and biliary tissues. *In* Bojrab MJ (ed): Current Techniques in Small Animal Surgery II. Philadelphia, Lea & Febiger, 1983, p 212.
4. Putnam CW, Starzl TE: Simplified biopsy of the liver in dogs. Surg Gynecol Obstet 144:759, 1977.
5. Kosovsky J, et al: Results of partial hepatectomy in 18 dogs with hepatocellular carcinoma. J Am Anim Hosp Assoc 25:203, 1989.
6. Lewis D, et al: Hepatic lobectomy in the dog: A comparison of stapling and ligation techniques. Vet Surg 19:221, 1990.
7. Kerwin SC: Hepatic aspiration and biopsy techniques. Vet Clin North Am Small Anim Pract 25:275, 1995.
8. Hardy RM: Liver biopsy the percutaneous approach. Vet Med Report 2:192, 1990.
9. Hitt ME, et al: Percutaneous transabdominal hepatic needle biopsies in dogs. Am J Vet Res 53:785, 1992.
10. Jones BD, et al: Hepatic biopsy. Vet Clin North Am Small Anim Pract 15:39, 1985.
11. Osborne CA, et al: Needle biopsy of the liver. JAVMA 155:1605, 1969.
12. Feeney DA, et al: Two-dimensional, gray-scale ultrasonography for assessment of hepatic and splenic neoplasia in the dog and cat. JAVMA 184:68, 1984.
13. Wrigley RH: Radiographic and ultrasonographic diagnosis of liver diseases in dogs and cats. Vet Clin North Am Small Anim Pract 15:21, 1985.
14. Biller DS, et al: Ultrasonography of diffuse liver disease: A review. J Vet Intern Med 6:71, 1992.
15. Yeager AE, Mohammed H: Accuracy of ultrasonography in the detection of severe hepatic lipidosis in cats. Am J Vet Res 53:597, 1992.
16. Wildt D, et al: Laparoscopy for direct observation of internal organs of the domestic cat and dog. Am J Vet Res 38:1429, 1977.
17. Bunch SE, et al: A modified laparoscopic approach for liver biopsy in dogs. JAVMA 187:1032, 1985.

CHAPTER 143

CHRONIC HEPATIC DISORDERS

Susan E. Johnson

CANINE CHRONIC HEPATITIS, FIBROSIS, AND CIRRHOSIS

OVERVIEW OF DIAGNOSIS AND TREATMENT

Definition and Etiology

Chronic hepatitis is a heterogeneous group of inflammatory-necrotizing diseases of the liver. Lymphocytes and plasma cells are the predominant inflammatory infiltrate. Although there are many potential causes of chronic hepatitis in dogs (Table 143–1), with few exceptions, the cause, pathogenesis, natural history, and optimal treatment of these disorders in dogs are unknown.

The terminology for chronic hepatitis in human and veterinary medicine is confusing.[1, 2] Originally, the term "chronic active hepatitis" was used for humans, not as a specific disease entity but as a morphologic description of chronic hepatitis with features suggesting that progression to cirrhosis was likely. A variety of etiologies including viral hepatitis, chronic drug therapy, copper accumulation, and an autoimmune (or steroid-responsive) disorder could cause chronic active hepatitis. A distinction was made between the progressive chronic active hepatitis and the nonprogressive "chronic persistent hepatitis," even though in some cases the same etiology (e.g., viral) could cause both lesions. Because of the confusing terminology, a classification system for chronic liver injury in humans has been proposed that is based on etiology, grade of inflammation and necrosis, and stage of progression (fibrosis).[1] The term "chronic active hepatitis" is considered obsolete.[1]

In the veterinary literature, many different terms have been used for canine chronic inflammatory liver disease including chronic active hepatitis, chronic persistent hepati-

TABLE 143–1. CAUSES OF CANINE CHRONIC HEPATITIS

Familial predisposition
    Bedlington terrier
    Cocker spaniel (American and English)
    Doberman pinscher
    Labrador retriever
    Skye terrier
    West Highland white terrier
    Standard poodle
Infectious
    Infectious canine hepatitis
    Acidophil cell hepatitis
    Leptospirosis
        Serogroup Grippotyphosa (serovar *grippotyphosa*)
        Serogroup Australis (serovars *australis, bratislava, muenchen*)
Drug-induced
    Anticonvulsants
    Oxibendazole-diethylcarbamazine
    Carprofen?
Lobular dissecting hepatitis
Idiopathic chronic hepatitis

tis, chronic lobular hepatitis, chronic progressive hepatitis, and chronic cholangiohepatitis. For the purpose of this chapter, the term *idiopathic chronic hepatitis* is used when chronic hepatocellular necrosis and inflammation are detected and known causes of chronic hepatitis have been excluded (see Table 143–1). If the inflammation is targeted at the biliary tract (inflammatory cells within or around the bile ducts) rather than hepatocytes, the term *cholangiohepatitis* is more appropriate.[3]

A familial predisposition to develop chronic hepatitis has been suggested by demographic studies, pathologic surveys, and clinical case series. Breeds of dogs at increased risk for chronic hepatitis include the Bedlington terrier,[4, 5] West Highland white terrier[6, 7] Doberman pinscher,[8, 9] American and English cocker spaniel,[10–12] Skye terrier,[13] Labrador retriever,[10] and standard poodle[14, 15] Unfortunately, with the exception of hereditary hepatic copper accumulation in Bedlington terriers,[4] information is lacking for most of the breed-related disorders. Chronic hepatitis occurs equally in male and female dogs[16] although some sex differences have been noted within particular breeds (female Doberman pinschers, female Labrador retrievers, male cocker spaniels).[8–10] The mean age is 5 to 7 years, but adult dogs of any age (or breed) can be affected.[10, 16]

Pathophysiologic mechanisms of chronic hepatitis in dogs are poorly understood. Some dogs with chronic hepatitis appear to respond to corticosteroid therapy and thus their condition may correspond to the autoimmune form of chronic active hepatitis in humans.[16] Several studies have evaluated the role of immune mechanisms in dogs with chronic hepatitis. Twenty-four dogs with chronic inflammatory liver disease were evaluated for circulating autoantibodies (against cell nuclei, smooth muscle, liver membrane, and mitochondria) by indirect immunofluorescence.[17] Antibodies to cell nuclei and liver membranes were detected but were also found in dogs with other types of hepatic disease, suggesting a nonspecific secondary response.[17] In another study, serum anti–liver membrane protein antibody–positive dogs (1:40 to more than 1:1600) had higher alanine aminotransferase (ALT) activity, a higher total bilirubin concentration, and more severe hepatic lesions than anti-liver membrane protein antibody–negative dogs, but it was not determined whether autoantibodies were primary or secondary.[18] Dogs with chronic inflammatory liver disease have also been found to have higher peripheral blood mononuclear cell proliferation in response to liver membrane protein than with non-inflammatory liver disease, supporting the involvement of immune-mediated processes in canine chronic hepatitis.[19] Whether this occurs as a primary (autoimmune) event or is secondary to liver destruction remains to be determined.[19] Accumulation of alpha$_1$-antitrypsin in hepatocytes, a well-recognized cause of cirrhosis in humans, may be important in the pathogenesis of chronic hepatitis in some dogs.[12]

Copper accumulation in the liver can be associated with significant hepatic injury resulting in acute hepatitis, chronic hepatitis, and cirrhosis.[20] It is one of the few well-documented causes of chronic hepatitis in dogs. The severity of hepatic injury is related to the amount of accumulated copper. The hepatic copper concentration in normal dogs is less than 400 ug/g dry weight (parts per million).[20] Hepatic damage does not consistently occur until the copper concentrations exceed 2000 ug/g dry weight.[21] Copper metabolism has been reviewed in detail elsewhere.[21] Copper accumulation in the liver may be a cause or a consequence of chronic hepatitis. Bedlington terriers develop chronic hepatitis as a result of an inherited metabolic defect in biliary copper excretion caused by abnormal binding of copper with metallothionein in the liver.[4, 5, 20] Hepatic copper concentrations in affected Bedlingtons range from 850 to 12,000 ug/g. Inherited copper-associated liver disease is also described in West Highland white terriers, Doberman pinschers, and Skye terriers, but in these breeds the hepatic copper levels are much lower. The pathophysiology of copper accumulation and the relationship to chronic liver disease in these breeds are poorly understood. Specific features of these breed-related disorders are discussed in the following section (Table 143–2).

Hepatic copper accumulation could also theoretically occur with any cholestatic hepatobiliary disorder that impairs bile flow, because copper is normally excreted in the bile. Secondary copper accumulation rarely exceeds 2000 ug/g.[20] Increased hepatic copper content was identified in 49 per cent of 130 canine liver biopsy samples that were submitted to a veterinary diagnostic laboratory.[20] Copper levels in most dogs ranged from 500 to 1000 ug/g, and copper accumulation was considered to be a secondary event.[20] Whether secondary copper accumulation can further contribute to hepatic injury is unclear but is an important question because of the implications for the use of copper chelator therapy.

Chronic hepatitis can progress to hepatic cirrhosis (end-stage liver disease).[3, 22] Hepatic cirrhosis is characterized by fibrosis and regenerative nodules that result in disorganization of the hepatic architecture (Fig. 143–1A and B). These are important features because even if the underlying cause can be identified and reversed, cirrhosis is an irreversible change. If clinical signs of liver failure are already present, the long-term prognosis is poor. Hepatic fibrosis and regenerative nodules cause increased hepatic vascular resistance and portal hypertension, resulting in ascites, multiple acquired portosystemic shunts, and hepatic encephalopathy (HE). The incidence of cirrhosis in dogs is unknown, although in one survey cirrhosis accounted for 15 per cent of the cases of liver disease in which biopsies were obtained.[22]

History and Clinical Findings

Signs are often initially vague and nonspecific, such as anorexia, lethargy, depression, weight loss, vomiting, diarrhea, polyuria, and polydipsia. With increased severity of hepatic dysfunction, signs of overt liver failure develop, such as ascites, jaundice, and HE. Ascites was the most consistent finding in dogs with cirrhosis, whereas icterus occurred in only 4 of 33 dogs.[3] Melena associated with gastroduodenal ulceration or coagulopathy may also occur.[3] Because of the large functional reserve capacity of the liver, the onset of

LIV

TABLE 143–2. BREEDS WITH INCREASED HEPATIC COPPER AND HEPATIC DISEASE

Airedale terrier	Keeshond
Bedlington terrier*	Kerry blue terrier
Boxer	Labrador retriever
Bulldog	Norwich terrier
Bull terrier	Old English sheepdog
Cocker spaniel	Pekingese
Collie	Poodle
Dachshund	Samoyed
Dalmatian	Schnauzer
Doberman pinscher*	Skye terrier*
German shepherd dog	West Highland white terrier*
Golden retriever	Wire fox terrier

*Hereditary mechanism for increased hepatic copper.
From Rolfe DS, Twedt DC: Copper-associated hepatopathies in dogs. Vet Clin North Am Small Anim Pract 25:399, 1995.

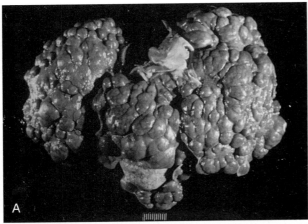

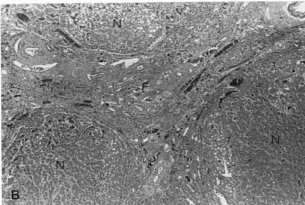

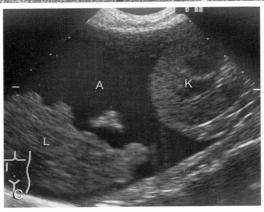

Figure 143–1. Hepatic cirrhosis in a 9-year-old neutered male cocker spaniel with signs of chronic liver failure. *A,* Variable-sized regenerative nodules are seen grossly throughout the liver at necropsy. *B,* Microscopic evaluation reveals tracts of fibrosis (F) and parenchymal nodules (N) that disrupt the normal hepatic architecture (42×). *C,* Abdominal ultrasonography performed before the dog's death reveals the nodular margin of a liver lobe (L) adjacent to the right kidney (K). The irregular margins of the liver are easily seen because of the presence of ascitic fluid. (*A,* Courtesy of Dr. D. S. Biller.)

signs may appear recent, initially suggesting an acute rather than chronic hepatic disorder. Clinicopathologic features that support chronicity include poor body condition, ascites, microhepatica, hypoalbuminemia, and histologic evidence of fibrosis.

Laboratory Evaluation

Dogs with chronic inflammatory liver disease usually have persistent increases in liver enzyme activity. Serum ALT activity is often 4 to 25 times normal, reflecting ongoing hepatic injury (inflammation and necrosis). Serum alkaline phosphatase (ALP) activity is usually 2 to 40 times normal, reflecting variable degrees of intrahepatic cholestasis. Dogs with chronic cholangiohepatitis have higher ALT and ALP activities than those with other types of chronic inflammatory liver disease.[3] When cirrhosis occurs, increases in liver enzyme activity may not be dramatic and these values are occasionally normal, indicating absence of significant ongoing inflammation or intrahepatic cholestasis or decreased viable parenchymal mass.[22]

Other potential biochemical findings include hyperbilirubinemia, hypoalbuminemia, hyperglobulinemia, decreased blood urea nitrogen (BUN), and hypoglycemia. Hypoalbuminemia is a consistent feature of cirrhosis.[3] Hematologic findings include mild nonregenerative anemia and microcytosis. Tests of liver function such as fasting and postprandial serum bile acid (SBA) concentrations, sulfobromophthalein (BSP) dye excretion, or ammonia tolerance are frequently abnormal, reflecting the degree of liver dysfunction. Abnormal hemostatic parameters (prolonged activated partial thromboplastin time [APTT] and prothrombin time [PT]) are indicative of severe hepatic dysfunction or disseminated intravascular coagulation (DIC). Analysis of ascitic fluid reveals a transudate or modified transudate.

Liver Imaging

Abdominal radiographs are unremarkable except when advanced stages of disease are accompanied by microhepatica or ascites. Microhepatica is a common radiographic finding in dogs with hepatic fibrosis or cirrhosis, because parenchymal tissue is replaced by fibrous tissue. When ascites is present, liver size can be difficult to evaluate on survey films.

Ultrasonography of the liver may be normal in the early stages of chronic hepatitis, or nonspecific changes in echogenicity may be detected.[23] Potential ultrasonographic findings with cirrhosis include microhepatica, irregular hepatic margins, focal lesions representing regenerative nodules, increased parenchymal echogenicity associated with increased fibrous tissue, and ascites (Fig. 143–1C).[23] Splenomegaly and acquired portosystemic shunts may also be detected. Ultrasonography is also helpful in evaluating for other causes of chronic hepatic disease such as extrahepatic biliary tract disorders or mass lesions of the liver.

Liver Biopsy

Histopathologic features of chronic hepatitis in dogs are similar regardless of the underlying cause. Wedge biopsies are preferred to needle biopsies because they provide more tissue and are more likely to represent the pathologic process in the liver.[2] When cirrhosis is present, laparotomy or laparoscopy often provides a better appreciation of the gross nodularity of the liver than blind percutaneous needle biopsy.

Histopathologic evaluation of the liver is required to differentiate chronic hepatitis from other chronic hepatopathies (e.g., hepatic neoplasia, vacuolar hepatopathy); to document the presence, severity, and location of inflammation and necrosis; to characterize specific features of chronic hepatitis (e.g., copper accumulation); and to evaluate for progression to cirrhosis. Chronic hepatitis is characterized by moderate to severe inflammation (usually combinations of lymphocytes and plasma cells) associated with piecemeal necrosis (necrosis involving the layer of hepatocytes adjacent to the portal tract or "limiting plate"). The term "bridging necrosis" is used when necrosis and inflammation dissect across the hepatic lobule from portal areas to central veins or to adjacent hepatic lobules and suggests a severe form of chronic hepatitis.[2, 24] When neutrophils are a significant component of the inflammation, a bacterial component should be considered, especially if features of cholangiohepatitis are detected. Granulomatous inflammation is not a typical histologic feature of chronic hepatitis; a search for infectious etiologies such as systemic mycoses or mycobacteria that incite this type of response is warranted.

Histochemical stains, such as rubeanic acid and rhodanine, can be used to evaluate semiquantitatively for copper in the liver. These stains consistently detect copper in liver biopsy specimens when amounts exceed 400 ug/g dry weight.[21] Quantitative analysis for copper is the definitive method for documenting increased hepatic copper content. Quantitative copper analysis by atomic absorption analysis is best performed on fresh hepatic tissue. Values obtained by quantitative copper analysis have a strong correlation with the number and size of granules seen with histochemical stains within the range of 400 to 1000 µg copper per gram of liver tissue.[21]

When chronic hepatitis has been confirmed, a careful consideration of known causes of chronic hepatitis is essential (see Table 143–1). A history of chronic drug therapy should be sought, especially long-term anticonvulsant therapy or heartworm preventative with oxibendazole-diethylcarbamazine. The disorders capable of causing lesions of chronic hepatitis are discussed in more detail in the following sections.

General Therapy

Recommendations for treatment of chronic hepatitis are empirical at best, because of the lack of controlled therapeutic studies of a well-defined population of dogs with this disorder. If a probable cause or category of injury can be determined, then specific treatment is directed at removing the primary etiology, for example, discontinuing anticonvulsants, treating for leptospirosis with antibiotics, or chelating hepatic copper with penicillamine. In most cases, specific therapy is unavailable. When end-stage cirrhosis is diagnosed, treatment is mainly supportive, because cirrhosis itself is essentially irreversible. Treatment is directed at general symptomatic and supportive therapy of hepatic failure (Table 143–3). Measures should also be instituted to control the complications of chronic liver failure, such as ascites, HE, gastroduodenal ulcers, coagulopathy, and infection (see Table 143–3). Additional therapies that have been empirically recommended for dogs with chronic hepatitis are described in the following subsections.

Modulate Inflammation

Treatment of chronic hepatitis in dogs has traditionally centered around the use of corticosteroids, presuming that, as in humans with the autoimmune form of chronic active hepatitis, immunologic mechanisms contribute to hepatic inflammation and progression to cirrhosis. Controlled prospective trials of glucocorticoid therapy in a well-defined population of dogs with chronic hepatitis are lacking. A large retrospective study suggested that corticosteroid therapy improved survival in dogs with chronic hepatitis.[16] However, many concurrent drugs were given and a heterogeneous group of disorders were undoubtedly, included in the diagnosis of "chronic hepatitis."

Corticosteroids have anti-inflammatory, antifibrotic, and choleretic effects that may be beneficial in chronic hepatitis.[25] They also stimulate appetite and promote an overall feeling of well-being. Corticosteroid therapy is probably indicated in dogs with persistent clinical and biochemical evidence of hepatic dysfunction and histologic features as described earlier (piecemeal and bridging necrosis, moderate to severe mononuclear inflammation, and bridging fibrosis) and for which known causes of chronic hepatitis have been excluded.[16] Glucocorticoid therapy is not indicated for treatment of chronic hepatitis caused by drug therapy, primary hepatic copper accumulation, or infectious agents.

Oral prednisolone (or prednisone) is given at 1.0 mg/lb/day by mouth for 2 to 4 weeks.[25] The dose is then tapered to 0.5 mg/lb for another 2 weeks and then to the lowest effective dose (or 0.3 mg/lb) on a daily or alternate-day basis. Optimal duration of therapy is unknown. Because glucocorticoids increase liver enzyme activity (especially serum ALP activity), response to therapy is best evaluated by follow-up liver biopsy performed 3 to 6 months after starting therapy. Complications of corticosteroid therapy include gastrointestinal bleeding (which can precipitate HE), secondary infections, iatrogenic Cushing's disease, and worsening of ascites. Dexamethasone (0.1mg/lb by mouth once a day) may be preferred in dogs with ascites or edema, because it lacks mineralocorticoid activity, which could exacerbate these signs. If glucocorticoid therapy is eventually discontinued, clinical and biochemical parameters should be periodically monitored to detect a relapse.

If side effects of prednisolone become objectionable, combination therapy using both azathioprine (Imuran), and prednisolone should be considered. Azathioprine is an antimetabolite with anti-inflammatory and immune-modulating effects. Azathioprine is given at 0.5 to 1 mg/lb/day by mouth once a day for induction therapy; for maintenance therapy, the same dose is given once every other day. Prednisolone (0.25 to 0.5 mg/lb/day) is given on the alternate days. Because azathioprine may cause bone marrow suppression, a complete blood count (CBC) should be monitored every 2 to 3 weeks for the first 2 months and every other month thereafter. Hepatotoxicity of azathioprine has been described in humans but has not been reported in veterinary medicine.

Reduce Hepatic Copper

The copper chelator penicillamine is used to chelate hepatic copper and promote its urinary excretion (Table 143–4). Penicillamine therapy is indicated in dogs with chronic hepatitis when hepatic copper concentrations approach 2000 µg/g. It usually requires months to years of treatment to produce significant decreases in hepatic copper (approximately 900 µg/g per year in Bedlington terriers and a more rapid response in Doberman pinschers and other breeds). Subjective clinical improvement may occur in Bedlington terriers after a few weeks of therapy, suggesting that penicillamine has other protective effects besides depletion of hepatic copper. Penicillamine induces hepatic metallothionein, which may bind and sequester copper in a nontoxic form.[20] Additional effects of penicillamine that may be beneficial include inhibition of collagen deposition, stimulation of collagenase activity, immunosuppression, and immunomodulation. Treatment of dogs affected with hereditary copper accumulation who are asymptomatic may prevent acute hepatitis, chronic hepatitis, and progression to cirrhosis. Trientine hy-

LIV

drochloride, an alternative copper chelator, also appears to be a safe and effective therapy for reducing hepatic copper concentrations (see Table 143–4).

Zinc salt therapy has been evaluated as an alternative to copper chelators, because zinc decreases intestinal copper absorption.[20, 26] Dietary zinc induces the intestinal copper-binding protein metallothionein within intestinal epithelial cells. Metallothionein binds dietary copper and prevents its

TABLE 143–3. GENERAL THERAPY OF HEPATIC FAILURE

THERAPEUTIC GOALS	THERAPEUTIC REGIMEN
Fluid therapy	
Maintain hydration	Use 0.9% NaCl or lactated Ringer's solution IV.* Use 0.45% NaCl in chronic disease.
Prevent hypokalemia	Add 20–30 mEq KCl to each liter of maintenance fluid. Monitor serum potassium daily and adjust as necessary.
Maintain acid-base balance	Avoid alkalosis in HE. Give $NaHCO_3$ rather than lactated fluids for treatment of severe metabolic acidosis.
Prevent or control hypoglycemia	To treat hypoglycemia, give 50% dextrose (0.5–1 mL/kg) IV to effect. To maintain normoglycemia, add dextrose to fluids to achieve 2.5–5.0% solution.
Nutritional support	
Maintain caloric intake	Provide 60 to 100 kcal/kg/day good-quality diet.
Provide adequate vitamins and minerals	Add B vitamins to fluids of anorexic cats. For long-term therapy, give oral vitamin-mineral (especially B vitamin) supplement. Give parenteral vitamin K_1 (3 mg/kg q12h, IM or SC [dogs]; 1 mg/kg q12h, IM or SC [cats]) in biliary obstruction or severe cholestastic liver disease.
Modify diet to control complications	See specific complications (e.g., HE, ascites).
Control HE	
Modify diet	Give NPO in initial stages of HE. For long-term management, provide a reduced-protein (dairy or vegetable source protein preferred; avoid meat or egg protein), easily digested, high-CHO diet. Recommend moderate protein restriction of 18–22% dry matter (dogs) or 30–35% dry matter (cats). Increase dietary soluble fiber (psyllium 1 to 3 tsp/day).
Prevent formation and absorption of enteric toxins	In hepatic coma, give warm water cleansing enema initially (10–25 mL/kg) until fluid is clear, followed by retention enema, 5–10 mL/kg, q8–12h containing: lactulose† (30% lactulose with 70% water) and neomycin (22 mg/kg) and held for 20–30 minutes or povidone iodine solution (diluted 1:10 with water; 50–200 mL total; flush out within 10 minutes). For maintenance therapy, give neomycin (22 mg/kg q8–12h, PO) or metronidazole (7.5 mg/kg q12h, PO) or amoxicillin (22 mg/kg PO q12h) and lactulose† (0.25–0.5 mL/kg q8–12h, PO to achieve two to three soft stools a day). When lactulose is used in combination with antibiotics, check the fecal pH after 7–14 days. If pH < 6, lactulose is being adequately degraded by enteric bacteria. If pH > 7, increase lactulose dose or discontinue antibiotic.
Control gastrointestinal hemorrhage	Correct coagulopathy; treat GI parasites; treat gastric ulcer (famotidine and sucralfate‡); avoid drugs that exacerbate GI hemorrhage (e.g., aspirin and other NSAIDS, glucocorticoids).
Correct metabolic imbalances (e.g., dehydration, azotemia, hypokalemia, alkalosis, hypoglycemia)	See fluid therapy above.
Avoid drugs or therapies that exacerbate HE.	When possible, avoid sedatives, tranquilizers, anticonvulsants, analgesics, anesthetics, methionine-containing products, diuretics, stored blood, or commercial protein hydrolysates.
Control seizures	Use intravenous phenobarbital (monitor serum concentrations to adjust the dose) or oral loading doses of bromide (60–100 mg/kg q6h for 24 hours, then 20–40 mg/kg q24h) for refractory seizures and status epilepticus. Avoid benzodiazepines. General anesthesia with pentobarbital or propofol may be required to control seizures. Intubate and use mechanical respirator to maintain PO_2 and PCO_2. Give mannitol (0.5–1 g/kg by rapid IV bolus) for suspected cerebral edema. For chronic, stable seizure management or long-term therapy, give bromide (20–40 mg/kg q24h, PO in food). Monitor serum concentrations to adjust the dose.
Control infection	Give systemic antibiotics (see below).
Control ascites and edema	Give low-sodium diet; spironolactone (1–2 mg/kg q12h, PO),§ spironolactone-hydrochlorothiazide (Aldactazide¶ 2 mg/kg q12h, PO), or furosemide (1–2 mg/kg q12h, PO)§; paracentesis for relief of dyspnea or extreme abdominal distention; plasma transfusion or colloids such as hetastarch (10–20 mL/kg IV given over 6–8 hours; two doses, 12–24 hours apart) or dextrans (10–20 mL/kg/day to effect).
Control coagulopathy and anemia	Give vitamin K_1 (3 mg/kg q12h, IM or SC [dogs]; 1 mg/kg q12h, IM or SC [cats]); fresh plasma or blood transfusion. For DIC, give heparin (50–75 IU/kg q8–12h, SC).
Control gastrointestinal ulceration	Give famotidine (0.5–1.0 mg/kg q12–24h, PO or IV) or nizatidine (2.5–5.0 mg/kg q24h, PO); sucralfate‡ (1-g tablet per 25 kg q8h, PO).
Control infection and endotoxemia	Give systemic antibiotics (e.g., amoxicillin, ampicillin, penicillin, cephalosporins, aminoglycosides, metronidazole**).

*May be given subcutaneously if animal is mildly dehydrated and is not vomiting.
†Crystalline lactulose (powder) will soon be commercially available as 10 or 20 gm packets (syrup concentration is 10g/15ml) and distributed by Mylan Pharmaceuticals, Morgantown, WV 26505.
‡Beware of drug-associated constipation which may worsen HE.
§Dose may be doubled if there is no effect in 4–7 days.
¶GD Searle & Co, Chicago, IL.
**Partially metabolized by liver. Use reduced dose (7.5 mg/kg q12h, PO) in animals with liver failure.
HE = hepatic encephalopathy; NPO = nothing per os; GI = gastrointestinal; DIC = disseminated intravascular coagulation; CHO = carbohydrate; NSAID = nonsteroidal anti-inflammatory drug.
Adapted from Johnson SE: Liver and biliary tract. *In* Anderson NV (ed): Veterinary Gastroenterology, 2nd ed. Philadelphia, Lea & Febiger, 1992, p 504.

TABLE 143–4. TREATMENT OF HEPATIC COPPER ACCUMULATION

PRODUCT	FORMULATION	DOSE	SIDE EFFECTS	COMMENTS
Chelate systemic copper (Cu)				
Penicillamine (Cuprimine, Merck & Co.; Depen, Wallace)	Cuprimine: 125- and 250-mg caps Depen: 250-mg tabs	10–15 mg/kg q12h, PO given on an empty stomach to improve absorption; do not give concurrently with any medication, including zinc* or vitamin-mineral supplement.	Anorexia and vomiting† are common; dermatologic drug eruption or autoimmune-like vesicular lesions of mucocutaneous junctions‡; reversible renal disease.‡	Causes systemic Cu chelation and urinary excretion. Indicated when hepatic Cu > 2000 μg/g. Takes months to years to produce significant decrease in hepatic Cu concentration. Not effective for treatment of Cu-associated hemolysis.
Trientine dihydrochloride§ (Syprine, Merck & Co.)	250-mg caps	10–15 mg/kg q12h, PO; give 1 hour before meals; do not give concurrently with any medication, including zinc* or vitamin/mineral supplement.	None noted as yet.	Use as an alternative to penicillamine if vomiting occurs; may be useful for treatment of hemolysis by chelating Cu in blood; more expensive than penicillamine.
2,3,2-Tetramine	Not commercially available	15 mg/kg PO	None noted as yet.	Derivative of trientine that is four to nine times as potent; thus, lowers hepatic Cu concentrations more rapidly than penicillamine or trientine.
Decrease intestinal copper absorption				
Zinc acetate, sulfate, gluconate, or methionine	Many available	5–10 mg elemental zinc per kg q12h. Use high end of dose for 3 months, then 50 mg PO q12h for maintenance. Separate administration from meals by 1–2 hours.	Vomiting,¶ zinc-induced hemolysis at plasma levels > 1000 μg/dL.	Induces intestinal metallothionein, which binds Cu and prevents absorption takes 3–6 months to obtain therapeutic zinc plasma levels. Do not use zinc alone in dogs with active hepatitis (add Cu chelator). Monitor plasma zinc every 2–3 months to maintain level >200 but <400 μg/dL by adjusting dose.
Decrease copper intake				
Low-copper diet	None commercially available	< 0.5 ppm Cu in diet		Low-copper diet may slow further Cu accumulation but does not "decopper" the liver. Most commercial diets exceed National Research Council requirements for copper. Even Cu-restricted diets such as Hill's Prescription Diet u/d (4 ppm) are not low enough. Homemade low-Cu diet most beneficial for managing young dogs with inherited hepatic Cu metabolism defect to slow hepatic Cu accumulation. Avoid high-Cu foods such as liver, shellfish, organ meats, chocolate, nuts, mushrooms, cereals, mineral supplements.
Antioxidant therapy*				
Vitamin E	Many available	400–600 IU/day, PO	None noted as yet.	Oxidative damage occurs in Cu-associated liver disease. Vitamin E protects the liver against oxidant damage.

*Penicillamine and trientine theoretically chelate zinc (and decrease its absorption) when given concurrently. Staggered oral administration is recommended.

†Often resolves after several weeks; start at reduced dose and increase to maintenance after a few days. Giving with food decreases absorption, but a small amount of milk, cheese, or bread given concurrently may decrease vomiting.

‡Rare complications; renal compromise more likely with Depen.

§Availability limited, may require a special order direct from manufacturer.

¶Zinc acetate or methionine may be less irritating to the stomach than other formulations. To minimize vomiting, open capsule and mix contents with small amount of tuna or hamburger.

**Although vitamin C has antioxidant effects, it should be avoided in dogs with Cu accumulation because it may increase Cu's oxidative damage to the liver.

Adapted from Johnson SE, Sherding RG: Diseases of the liver and biliary tract. In Birchard SJ, Sherding RG (eds): Saunders Manual of Small Animal Practice. Philadelphia, WB Saunders, 1994, p 746.

absorption. Eventually, the intestinal cell is sloughed, causing copper bound to metallothionein to be lost in the stool. Theoretically, zinc should not be effective in "decoppering" a liver. However, zinc therapy decreased the hepatic copper content in six Bedlington and West Highland white terriers with hepatic copper accumulation and chronic hepatitis when used as the sole therapeutic agent for 2 years.[26] The decrease in hepatic copper content was associated with decreased hepatic inflammation and improved liver function.[26] Zinc therapy may be added to chelator therapy but should not be used alone in dogs with severe copper accumulation and signs of liver dysfuction.[20]

LIV

Feeding a low-copper diet may slow further copper accumulation but is of little value when hepatic copper accumulation has occurred. Most commercial diets meet or exceed the National Research Council (NRC) requirements for copper.[20] Yet these guidelines appear high for breeds of dogs that accumulate copper. A homemade low-copper diet would be most beneficial for managing young asymptomatic, affected Bedlington terriers to slow copper accumulation (see Table 143–4).

Modulate Fibrosis

Hepatic fibrosis results in altered hepatic architecture and impaired liver function. A comprehensive review of hepatic fibrogenesis and therapeutic strategies has been published.[27] Many drugs have potential antifibrotic effects, including colchicine, prednisolone, azathioprine, penicillamine, zinc, prostaglandin E, interferon, and antioxidants such as vitamin E.[27–29]

Colchicine is an inhibitor of microtubule assembly that interferes with transcellular movement of procollagen, and increases collagenase activity, which may promote collagen degradation.[30] An apparent clinical benefit in dogs has been suggested.[25, 31] Colchicine therapy should probably be reserved for dogs with extensive hepatic fibrosis as the primary lesion. A dose of 0.014 mg/lb/day has been suggested. Side effects in dogs include vomiting and diarrhea. The author has also seen reversible neutropenia with use of this drug.

Corticosteroids and azathioprine have antifibrotic properties.[27] Penicillamine is used primarily for copper chelation but has potential antifibrotic and immune-modulating effects. Zinc therapy is used to decrease intestinal copper absorption but also has antifibrotic and hepatoprotective properties.

Vitamin E

Increased production of free radicals has been implicated in a variety of experimentally induced hepatic diseases, including hepatic copper and iron accumulation, ethanol consumption, cholestasis, ischemia-reperfusion injury, and drug-induced hepatic injury.[29] Free radicals may contribute to oxidative hepatocellular injury if not counteracted by cytoprotective mechanisms. Antioxidants, such as Vitamin E, are important in scavenging free radicals and preventing oxidative injury.[29] Oxidant injury to hepatic mitochondria occurs in Bedlington terriers with copper toxicosis.[32] On the basis of this information, vitamin E therapy (400 to 600 IU/day) may be warranted in dogs with hepatic copper accumulation. In light of its safety and lack of expense, vitamin E is also used empirically in dogs with other types of chronic hepatitis. Because absorption of fat-soluble vitamins, including vitamin E, may be decreased in cholestatic hepatobiliary disorders, a water-soluble form of vitamin E (Nutr-E-Sol) may be preferable.

Ursodeoxycholic Acid

Ursodeoxycholic acid (Actigall) is a synthetic hydrophilic bile acid that is used in the treatment of cholestatic hepatobiliary disorders and chronic hepatitis in humans.[33] Ursodeoxycholic acid is believed to be beneficial by expanding the bile acid pool and displacing potentially hepatotoxic hydrophobic bile acids that may accumulate in cholestasis. It also stimulates bile flow, stabilizes hepatocyte membranes, and has cytoprotective and immunomodulatory effects on the liver. Use of ursodeoxycholic acid in the treatment of a dog with chronic hepatitis and cholestasis was recently described.[34] Clinical and biochemical improvement was noted over a 6-month period with ursodeoxycholic acid treatment. Evaluation of individual bile acid profiles revealed a decrease in potentially hepatotoxic endogenous bile acids.[34]

Ursodeoxycholic acid is believed to be useful as adjunctive therapy in cholestatic hepatic disorders of dogs and is safe when used at a dose of 4.4 to 7 mg/lb by mouth once a day.[25] Ursodeoxycholic acid therapy is contraindicated in dogs with biliary obstruction. It is prohibitively expensive to use in large breed dogs.

Prognosis

The response to treatment of chronic hepatitis is variable. The long-term prognosis for dogs with fibrosis and cirrhosis is usually poor. In one study, survival time of dogs with cirrhosis was 1 week.[3]

COPPER-ASSOCIATED HEPATOPATHIES

Bedlington Terriers

Bedlington terriers develop chronic hepatitis as a result of an inherited metabolic defect in biliary copper excretion caused by abnormal binding of copper with metallothionein in the liver.[4, 5, 20] The disorder is transmitted by autosomal recessive inheritance. With progressive accumulation of copper, hepatic injury becomes significant. Hepatic injury associated with copper accumulation in Bedlington terriers involves oxidant damage to hepatic mitochondria.[32] Affected dogs can be asymptomatic or show signs of acute hepatic necrosis, chronic hepatitis, or cirrhosis. This disease has been recognized in Bedlington terriers around the world but occurs primarily in the United States, where the prevalence may be as high as 66 per cent. The disease is similar but not identical to Wilson's disease in humans.

Biochemical findings vary with the stage of disease. Increased serum ALT activity is the most sensitive laboratory indicator, although up to a third of affected dogs have a normal value. These are mostly younger dogs that are in the early stages of the disease. Acute release of copper from necrotic hepatocytes occasionally causes hemolytic anemia. During episodes of hemolysis, plasma copper levels are increased; other findings include low packed cell volume (PCV), hemoglobinemia, and hemoglobinuria.

Liver biopsy is indicated for definitive diagnosis, for staging of the disease, and in dogs considered for breeding. Dogs should be older than 1 year of age to be sure adequate time for copper accumulation has occurred. The liver can be grossly normal or swollen and smooth with accentuation of the lobules. As cirrhosis develops, the liver decreases in size and has a mixture of fine and coarse nodules. Histologically, hematoxylin and eosin–stained hepatic tissue reveals dark granules in hepatocyte cytoplasm. These granules are lysosomes that contain copper. In the early stages, centrilobular hepatocytes are most affected, but later the distribution is diffuse. Histochemical stains for copper such as rhodanine and rubeanic acid are positive. Associated histologic hepatic damage is variable. In the most mildly affected dogs, only copper granules are detected. Over time, additional findings include focal hepatitis, chronic hepatitis, and eventually cirrhosis (Fig 143–2A and B).

Most affected dogs that are older than 1 year have a quantitative copper concentration that is greater than

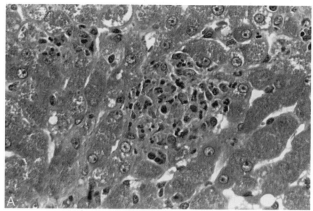

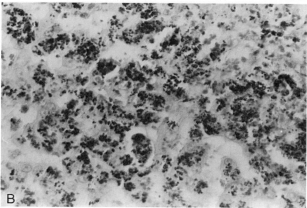

Figure 143–2. Copper-associated hepatitis in a Bedlington terrier. *A,* Focal hepatic necrosis and inflammation are detected on a hematoxylin-eosin–stained liver biopsy. *B,* Rhodanine stain reveals large numbers of dark-staining granules that represent copper-containing hepatic lysosomes (168×). The quantitative hepatic copper concentration was 12,000 μg/g (normal = less than 400 μg/g).

1000 μg/g dry weight and may be as high as 12,000 μg/g. The lowest hepatic concentrations of copper are found in the youngest dogs and concentrations increase with age, peaking at around 6 years. Copper content usually declines thereafter in affected dogs, but not to normal. This decline may be due to replacement of copper-containing hepatocytes by fibrous tissue or to regenerative nodules that do not contain copper.

Treatment of hepatic copper accumulation has been discussed previously under General Therapy and is summarized in Table 143–4. Bedlington terriers who are affected but asymptomatic should have dietary copper restriction and zinc supplementation. Intermittent or long-term chelator therapy may be required. Decisions are based on periodic monitoring of quantitative hepatic copper content. Many Bedlington terriers receiving long-term penicillamine therapy do not develop hepatic failure despite continued elevated copper levels. Treatment of hemolytic anemia may require a blood transfusion. Trientine dihydrochloride (but not penicillamine) may be effective in chelating circulating copper during a hemolytic episode (see Table 143–4).

Elimination of this hereditary disease from Bedlington terriers requires identifying affected dogs and carriers of the recessive gene and removing them from breeding programs. A linked DNA marker (CO4107) for copper toxicosis in the Bedlington terrier has been identified.[35] For this approach to have widespread application for the detection of affected and carrier Bedlington terriers, a battery of an additional

three to five polymorphic markers closely linked to CO4107 needs to be developed.[35]

A liver registry has been formed for lifetime certification of Bedlington terriers who are unaffected as determined by a quantitative hepatic copper level of less than 400 μg/g dry weight in dogs 1 year of age or older (Canine Liver Registry, Veterinary Medical Data Base, 1235 SCC-A, Purdue University, West Lafayette, IN 47907-1235). A liver registry has also been started with the Orthopedic Foundation for Animals (2300 Nifong Blvd., Columbia, MO 65201).

West Highland White Terriers

West Highland white terriers are at increased risk of developing chronic hepatitis and cirrhosis.[6, 7, 10] An increased hepatic copper concentration (greater than 2000 μg/g) appears to be a factor in some but not most affected dogs.[7, 10] Numerous West Highland white terriers have increased hepatic copper levels (usually 200 to 1500 μg/g), but rarely does the value exceed 2000μg/g and clinical illness associated with excess hepatic copper accumulation is uncommon.[7] In those with chronic hepatitis who have hepatic copper concentrations less than 2000 μg/g, the copper may not contribute to hepatic injury.[7] Excess hepatic copper accumulation is a familial trait but the mode of inheritance has not been established.[7]

Quantitative copper analysis is necessary to determine whether copper accumulation is significant (greater than 2000 μg/g). Copper granules are found in centrolobular hepatocytes and are associated with foci of inflammation when levels exceed 2000 μg/g.[7]

If chronic hepatitis and cirrhosis are associated with increased hepatic copper content (greater than 2000 μg/g), treatment for hepatic copper accumulation should be instituted (see Table 143–4). Mature West Highland white terriers with chronic hepatitis and a copper level below 2000 μg/g may not require chelator therapy, because, as opposed to that in Bedlington terriers, hepatic copper accumulation is not continuous throughout life.

Doberman Pinschers

Doberman pinschers are at increased risk for developing chronic hepatitis and cirrhosis.[8, 9, 36–38] The underlying etiopathogenic mechanisms are unknown, but a genetic basis is suggested by the high frequency in this breed. Middle-aged female dogs are at increased risk.[8, 9] Hepatic copper concentrations are increased in many but not all affected dogs. The significance of the increased hepatic copper concentration in this breed remains controversial. In one study, 23 affected Dobermans had quantitative copper analysis performed on liver tissue.[38] One dog was normal (250 μg/g). Ten of 23 dogs had hepatic copper content greater than 2000 μg/g, with the three highest values being 4700, 3700, and 3390 μg/g.[38] Twelve of 23 dogs had elevated copper concentrations ranging from 650 to 1900 μg/g.[38] It was previously reported that normal Doberman pinschers (on the basis of clinical signs and liver biopsy) were one of several breeds that had hepatic copper concentrations higher than what was previously considered normal (less than 400 μg/g), with a mean value of 413 ± 298 μg/g and a range of 140 to 1500 μg/g.[21] Thus, increased hepatic copper may be an incidental finding in Doberman pinschers with chronic hepatitis.[38] Another consideration is that Doberman pinschers may develop hepatic injury at lower hepatic copper concen-

LIV

trations than Bedlington terriers or West Highland white terriers.

Most Doberman pinschers are diagnosed in the advanced stages of hepatic failure. Evidence of excessive bleeding (gingival bleeding, epistaxis, and melena) is common. Signs of HE often predominate in the terminal stages. Common findings on physical examination include ascites, jaundice, and weight loss. Splenomegaly (associated with portal hypertension) is common. Laboratory findings are consistent with a cholestatic hepatopathy. Coagulopathy and thrombocytopenia are common in the advanced stages. Concurrent von Willebrand's disease should also be considered in affected dogs with a bleeding disorder because of its prevalence in this breed.

The subclinical stage of hepatitis in Doberman pinschers has been described.[36, 37] Of 626 randomly selected, clinically healthy Doberman pinschers, 55 dogs (8.8 per cent) had persistently increased ALT activity. Of these 55 dogs, 23 underwent liver biopsy and 21 of them were found to have hepatitis (parenchymal and portal mononuclear inflammation and positive stains for copper).[37] When compared with Doberman pinschers with overt clinical signs of chronic hepatitis, the dogs with subclinical hepatitis had lower values for ALP activity and serum bilirubin.[36] The asymptomatic period lasted an average of 19 months.

Chronic hepatitis should be suspected in any Doberman pinscher (especially females) with clinical or biochemical evidence of hepatic disease. Definitive diagnosis requires liver biopsy. Other causes of chronic hepatitis should also be considered (See Table 143–1). Most dogs are diagnosed in the advanced stages when the disease has progressed to cirrhosis. Typical histologic lesions include portal inflammation (lymphocytes, plasma cells, and macrophages), piecemeal necrosis, bridging necrosis, bile duct proliferation, and portal fibrosis.[8, 9] A detailed description of the precirrhotic histopathology has been published.[38] Contrary to previous descriptions, the earliest pathologic change was inflammation and scar tissue deposition around small hepatic veins.[38] Progressive fibrosis, inflammation (lymphocytes and plasma cells), and hepatocyte loss were described. Portal inflammation was seen in the later stages of disease. When increased hepatic copper was detected the copper accumulation was contrilobular.[38]

Effective treatment for Doberman pinschers with chronic hepatitis has not been established. At present, therapy with immunosuppressant drugs such as prednisolone with or without azathioprine is often instituted (see General Therapy). The efficacy of this treatment remains to be determined, but generally the response is poor. In large part, this may be because most dogs are presented in advanced stages of liver failure. Dobermans with subclinical hepatitis treated with low doses of prednisolone (0.05 to 0.22 mb/lb/day) did not show significant improvement.[37]

The use of copper chelating agents in this disease remains controversial. Treatment of affected Dobermans with penicillamine can decrease hepatic copper concentrations to less than 400 μg/g after 3 to 12 months of therapy.[39] This is a notable difference from Bedlington terriers with copper accumulation, who may never achieve normal copper levels despite lifelong penicillamine therapy. However, even with a normalized hepatic copper content, anecdotal reports suggest that hepatitis in Doberman pinschers is progressive. These findings suggest that copper accumulation is not the cause of hepatic injury. Ursodeoxycholic acid is expensive for large breed dogs but may be beneficial in this disorder.

Treatment of copper-associated hepatitis in Doberman pinschers is usually unsuccessful. Most dogs die within weeks to months. The prognosis may be more favorable if the disease is detected in the early stages, but the optimal therapeutic regimen remains to be determined.

Skye Terriers

Chronic hepatitis and cirrhosis associated with hepatic copper accumulation (800 to 2200 μg/g) in genetically related Skye terriers has been described.[13] In the early stages, copper accumulation is absent, and biopsy findings indicate hepatocellular degeneration with cholestasis and mild inflammation. Chronic lesions are associated with intracanalicular cholestasis, chronic hepatitis, and cirrhosis. Skye terrier hepatitis is speculated to be a disorder of disturbed bile secretion with subsequent accumulation of copper.

CHRONIC HEPATITIS IN COCKER SPANIELS

American and English cocker spaniels have an increased incidence of chronic hepatitis and cirrhosis.[3, 10–12] The cause of chronic hepatitis and liver failure in cocker spaniels is unknown. Accumulation of alpha$_1$-antitrypsin in hepatocytes, a well-recognized cause of cirrhosis in humans, may be important in the pathogenesis.[12]

Young, male cocker spaniels are at increased risk.[10, 11] Despite the chronicity and severity of the underlying hepatic lesions, most affected dogs have a short duration of clinical illness, usually 2 weeks or less.[11] Ascites is the most consistent presenting complaint. Profound hypoalbuminemia occurs. Cholestasis is not a key feature of the disorder. Ascitic fluid analysis identifies a transudate or modified transudate.

On liver biopsy, hepatic lesions consist of chronic periportal hepatitis (lymphocytes, plasma cells, and smaller numbers of neutrophils) with micro- or macronodular cirrhosis.[11] Hepatic copper accumulation does not appear to be a consistent feature.

Treatment for cocker spaniels with chronic hepatitis consists of general supportive therapy for the complications of liver failure. Corticosteroid therapy before progression to cirrhosis may be beneficial.[11] The prognosis is poor and most dogs die within a month of diagnosis.

INFECTIOUS CAUSES OF CHRONIC HEPATITIS

Infectious Canine Hepatitis

Infectious canine hepatitis caused by canine adenovirus 1 (CAV-1) has long been recognized as a cause of acute hepatic necrosis in dogs.[40] CAV-1 antigen was demonstrated in formalin-fixed liver sections from 5 of 53 dogs with various hepatic inflammatory lesions, suggesting that CAV-1 may play a role in spontaneous chronic hepatitis.[41] Polymerase chain reaction and immunohistochemistry for detection of CAV-1 were negative for 45 dogs with chronic hepatitis or cirrhosis.[42] The possibility that the CAV-1 initiates the hepatic damage provoking a self-perpetuating hepatitis cannot be excluded.[42]

Acidophil Cell Hepatitis

Canine acidophil cell hepatitis, reported in Great Britain, is caused by a transmissible agent (most likely a virus) that is distinct from CAV-1.[43, 44] A spectrum of hepatic lesions ranging from acute and chronic hepatitis to cirrhosis and even hepatocellular carcinoma has been described. The disease is experimentally transmissible by bacteriologically sterile liver extracts from affected dogs. Most dogs with spontaneous disease are presented with signs of chronic hepatic failure. Increased liver enzyme activity is a consistent finding. Liver biopsy is required for diagnosis. The liver is enlarged and friable in the acute stages and becomes progressively smaller and nodular with chronicity. Acidophil cells scattered throughout the parenchyma are dying hepatocytes with an angular shape, acidophilic cytoplasm, and hyperchromatic nucleus.

Leptospirosis

Canine leptospirosis is classically associated with acute cholestatic hepatic disease and acute renal failure. However, chronic infection with serovar *grippotyphosa* has been incriminated as a cause of chronic hepatitis.[45] Sixteen young beagle dogs in a breeding colony who were vaccinated against leptospirosis (serogroups Canicola and Icterohaemorrhagiae) developed chronic hepatitis associated with leptospiral infection.[46] Spirochetes were identified within bile canaliculi and confirmed as *Leptospira* by immunohistochemical methods. Significant antibody titers were not detected in six dogs in which leptospires were isolated. However, serologic survey of kennelmates revealed high antibody titers to serogroup Australis, which was unlikely to have resulted from vaccination.[46]

DRUG-INDUCED CHRONIC HEPATIC DISEASE

Anticonvulsants

The anticonvulsants primidone, phenytoin, and phenobarbital, used alone or in combination, have been associated with chronic hepatic disease and cirrhosis in dogs.[47–49] Hepatic dysfunction develops in as many as 14 per cent of dogs treated with anticonvulsants for more than 6 months.[47] Chronic hepatic disease was described in 18 dogs administered phenobarbital for 5 to 82 months.[48] Concentrations exceeded 40 μg/mL (therapeutic range 15 to 40 μg/mL), for prolonged periods of time.[48] Other dogs required high oral doses of phenobarbital (4.4 to 8.8 mg/lb/day) to maintain effective blood levels. Phenobarbital-induced hepatotoxicity may represent an idiosyncratic reaction or the extreme of a spectrum of toxicosis.

Clinical signs are sedation and ataxia[48] as well as anorexia, weight loss, ascites, jaundice, and coagulopathy. A decreased seizure frequency was reported in the majority of dogs diagnosed with phenobarbital toxicosis, possibly because impaired hepatic metabolism of phenobarbital resulted in higher serum phenobarbital concentrations and less fluctuation of serum levels.[48]

Anticonvulsant-induced hepatic injury should be suspected in any dog with a history of chronic anticonvulsant therapy and clinical and biochemical evidence of hepatic dysfunction. Mild reversible increases in serum ALP activity (2 to 12 times normal) and serum ALT activity (2 to 5 times normal) are common in dogs treated with phenobarbital, primidone, or phenytoin because of microsomal enzyme induction. Mildly increased liver enzyme activity is not a reliable indicator of serious hepatic damage in dogs given anticonvulsant drugs. An increase in serum ALT activity that exceeds the increase in serum ALP activity may be a better

indication of hepatocellular injury but is not a consistent finding.[48] Increased fasting and postprandial SBA concentrations, prolonged BSP retention, increased total serum bilirubin concentration, and hypoalbuminemia are better indicators of hepatic damage. Severe hypocholesterolemia has been noted in some dogs with anticonvulsant-induced damage.[49] With chronic anticonvulsant-induced hepatic disease, radiographic and ultrasonographic hepatic abnormalities are detected.

The most consistent histologic lesion seen in dogs treated with phenobarbital is hepatocellular hypertrophy, which is caused by hyperplasia of the smooth endoplasmic reticulum caused by microsomal enzyme induction. This histologic finding is commonly identified in dogs without clinical or biochemical evidence of hepatic dysfunction and does not warrant a change in therapy.

Chronic hepatitis associated with anticonvulsant therapy is characterized by histologic bridging portal fibrosis, nodular regeneration, biliary hyperplasia, and mild inflammatory infiltrates.[48, 49]

Phenobarbital therapy should be modified or discontinued if possible in dogs with biochemical and histologic evidence of hepatic disease. Potassium bromide (10 to 18 mg/lb by mouth every 24 hours with food) may be considered as an anticonvulsant in these dogs. In dogs with phenobarbital-associated toxicosis, clinical, biochemical, and histologic improvement can occur if phenobarbital is discontinued or used at a reduced dosage before severe, end-stage liver disease.[48] Improvement in clinical signs can be noted within days to weeks of decreasing serum phenobarbital levels. The earlier hepatic damage is recognized and drug therapy is discontinued, the better the prognosis for recovery from hepatic injury. Unfortunately, by the time clinical signs are detected, severe irreversible hepatic disease or even cirrhosis may be present and drug withdrawal may not be beneficial. Supportive treatment is indicated (see Table 143–3).

Despite the evidence for hepatotoxicity, phenobarbital is still the drug of choice for long-term control of seizures in dogs.[50] To avoid possible hepatotoxicity, serum phenobarbital concentrations should not exceed 35 μg/mL.[48] Liver enzymes (ALP and ALT), total serum bilirubin concentration, and serum albumin concentration should be routinely monitored every 6 months in all dogs receiving chronic anticonvulsant therapy to detect early evidence of hepatic damage. If abnormalities other than mild increases in liver enzyme activity are detected, fasting and postprandial SBA should be determined. Significant hepatic damage is much less likely if SBA concentrations are normal.

Oxibendazole and Diethylcarbamazine

Oxibendazole, marketed in combination with diethylcarbamazine as a hookworm-heartworm preventative, has been associated with acute and chronic hepatic injury in dogs.[49, 51] Doberman pinschers in particular may be predisposed to develop oxibendazole-diethylcarbamazine hepatotoxicity.[49] With the chronic form of oxibendazole-diethylcarbamazine hepatic injury, hepatic disease is often not detected until the drug has been administered for 2 to 10 months.[49] Clinical signs include anorexia, lethargy, weight loss, ascites, seizures, behavioral changes, and jaundice.[49] Laboratory abnormalities include increased serum ALP and ALT activity, hypoalbuminemia, hyperbilirubinemia, hyperammonemia, prolonged BSP retention, microcytosis, and mild thrombocytopenia.[49] Some dogs may be asymptomatic, with increased serum liver enzyme activity as the only indication of hepatic

LIV

injury. If ascites is present, fluid analysis reveals a transudate.[49]

With the chronic form, histologic evidence of periportal hepatitis is accompanied by periportal fibrosis and biliary hyperplasia.[51] As with the acute hepatic reaction, clinical improvement is likely after discontinuing the drug. Histologic and biochemical abnormalities may improve but not totally resolve.[49]

Carprofen

Carprofen (Rimadyl), a nonsteroidal anti-inflammatory drug marketed for use in dogs with arthritis, has been associated with idiosyncratic hepatic injury and acute hepatic failure within 5 to 30 days after starting the drug.[52] Labrador retrievers are at increased risk. Liver biopsy findings include hepatocellular necrosis, ballooning degeneration, and cholestasis. Whether carprofen can cause subclinical chronic hepatotoxicosis is unknown.[52] However, one dog received carprofen for 54 days and was clinically normal when increased liver enzymes were detected.[52] Another dog was treated for 6 months before acute anorexia and vomiting occurred. On biopsy, in addition to acute hepatocellular necrosis, both dogs had increased fibrous tissue, indicating chronicity. It appears prudent to discontinue carprofen administration to any dog with acute or chronic hepatic disease and monitor for improvement in hepatic parameters.

LOBULAR DISSECTING HEPATITIS

Lobular dissecting hepatitis is a term used for a specific histologic form of chronic hepatitis.[14, 15, 53] It has been suggested that this is a reaction pattern of the liver that is unique in neonatal and juvenile dogs exposed to a wide variety of hepatic insults.[53] Standard poodles may be at increased risk.[14, 15] The median age of 21 affected dogs was 11 months, and 54 per cent of dogs were 7 months of age or younger.[53] Clinical features are those of advanced hepatic failure and portal hypertension. The most consistent clinical finding is ascites. Liver enzyme activities are typically increased. Hypoalbuminemia and increased SBA concentrations are common.

Inflammatory cells (lymphocytes, plasma cells, macrophages, and neutrophils) are scattered throughout the hepatic lobule rather than concentrated in periportal regions. Bands of collagen and reticulin fibers dissect around single or small groups of hepatocytes and disrupt the hepatic lobular architecture. Copper stains are negative to moderately positive, consistent with secondary copper accumulation. The liver is shrunken, pale to tan, with an almost smooth surface and occasional hyperplastic nodule. Multiple acquired portosystemic shunts are present.

CHRONIC CHOLANGIOHEPATITIS

Cholangiohepatitis is an inflammatory disorder that is targeted at the biliary tree rather than hepatocytes. It is one of the most common hepatobiliary disorders of cats but is recognized much less frequently in dogs.[3, 54, 55] Biliary tract inflammation (cholangitis, cholangiohepatitis, cholecystitis) in dogs can be caused by ascending biliary bacterial infections (especially gram-negative and anaerobic organisms), *Salmonella* sp., and *Campylobacter jejuni*.[55] Cholangiohepatitis may also occur in association with cholelithiasis, common bile duct obstruction, biliary tract surgery, and, rarely, intrahepatic biliary coccidiosis.[55]

Clinical features of canine cholangiohepatitis have not been described in detail. Icterus is common,[3] as are anorexia, depression, vomiting, diarrhea, polyuria, and polydipsia. With acute cholangiohepatitis, fever and abdominal pain may be present.[54] Laboratory findings reveal a cholestatic hepatopathy (hyperbilirubinemia, marked increases in ALP and gamma-glutamyltransferase [GGT] activity), and an inflammatory CBC.[3, 54] Diagnosis of cholangiohepatitis requires liver biopsy and aerobic and anaerobic cultures of bile and infected tissues. Histologic features of cholangiohepatitis include suppurative or mononuclear inflammation within and around bile ducts. When suppurative inflammation occurs, antibiotic therapy is indicated.

IDIOPATHIC HEPATIC FIBROSIS

Idiopathic hepatic fibrosis is a disease of unknown etiology that is associated with chronic hepatic failure and portal hypertension.[56] Young dogs are primarily affected but ages range from 4 months to 7 years. German shepherd dogs accounted for 9 of 15 dogs in one series.[56] The liver is small, firm, and irregular and multiple acquired portosystemic shunts are a consistent feature. Histologically, the key feature is hepatic fibrosis without evidence of inflammation. Various patterns of fibrosis are detected including diffuse pericellular, periportal ("hepatoportal fibrosis"), and periacinar fibrosis.[56] Portal fibrosis is a significant feature in some dogs with hypoplasia of the portal vein, and the authors speculated that these disorders may be related.[57]

Clinical signs including HE are attributed to portal hypertension and multiple acquired portosystemic shunts. In dogs with idiopathic hepatic fibrosis, serum ALP activity is usually increased (up to 20 times normal); increased ALT activity is a less consistent finding.[56] The prognosis is usually poor when overt signs of liver failure are present; however, some dogs lived up to 4 years.[56] Colchicine therapy may be beneficial.

FELINE CHRONIC INFLAMMATORY LIVER DISEASE

DEFINITION AND ETIOLOGY

Inflammatory diseases of the liver are the second most common type of feline liver disease, after hepatic lipidosis.[58, 59] The cause, pathogenesis, natural history, and optimal treatment of inflammatory liver disease in cats are largely unknown. Various terms have been used to describe these disorders, such as cholangitis-cholangiohepatitis syndrome, suppurative cholangiohepatitis, nonsuppurative cholangiohepatitis, lymphoplasmacytic cholangiohepatitis, lymphocytic cholangitis, progressive lymphocytic cholangitis, sclerosing cholangitis, and biliary cirrhosis. A retrospective review of the histologic features of feline inflammatory liver disease suggested that two types of histologically distinct inflammatory patterns can be identified: cholangiohepatitis (either acute or chronic) and lymphocytic portal hepatitis.[59] On the basis of this proposed classification, further attempts were made to correlate histopathologic and clinicopathologic features.[60] This classification scheme is used in the following discussion.

Acute and Chronic Cholangiohepatitis

Cholangiohepatitis is an inflammatory disorder that is targeted at the biliary tree rather than hepatocytes. The term cholangitis is used when inflammation is confined to the bile ducts; the term cholangiohepatitis implies secondary hepatocyte involvement. Cholangiohepatitis can be separated into acute and chronic forms. Acute cholangiohepatitis (also called suppurative cholangiohepatitis) is characterized by neutrophilic inflammation within the walls or lumen of bile ducts. Periportal hepatocellular necrosis occurs, with disruption of the limiting plate and extension of inflammatory infiltrate into the hepatic parenchyma. Bile duct epithelial degeneration is a common feature. Chronic cholangiohepatitis (also called lymphoplasmacytic or nonsuppurative cholangitis or cholangiohepatitis) is characterized by a mixed inflammatory response (equal numbers of neutrophils and lymphocytes or plasma cells) within portal areas and bile ducts (Fig 143–3).[59] Other features of chronicity include marked bile duct proliferation, bridging fibrosis, and pseudolobule formation.[59] Chronic cholangiohepatitis may progress to biliary cirrhosis.[58, 60]

Acute cholangiohepatitis is believed to be caused by ascending bacterial infection of the biliary tract, although this is unproved. Bacterial organisms isolated from bile or liver tissue are primarily gram-negative and anaerobic bacteria such as *Escherichia coli*, *Staphylococcus*, alpha-hemolytic *Streptococcus*, *Bacillus*, *Actinomyces*, *Bacteroides*, and *Clostridium* and are consistent with an enteric origin.[55, 60] However, bacteria are not always isolated from bile or tissue of cats with acute cholangiohepatitis, possibly because of prior antimicrobial therapy. Chronic bacterial infections elsewhere in the body (sinusitis, splenic abscess, pyelonephritis) and septicemia may also be associated with acute cholangiohepatitis.[55] Less frequent associations include toxoplasmosis, *Hepatozoon canis*–like infection, and liver flukes. Chronic cholangiohepatitis may represent a persistent bacterial infection or the lesion may have been initiated by bacteria but an immune-mediated response may result in a chronic self-perpetuating disorder.[60]

Concurrent abnormalities of the biliary tract are common in cats with acute and chronic cholangiohepatitis.[55, 61, 62] Congenital biliary tract malformations or biliary reconstructive surgery may predispose to ascending bacterial infection.[61, 63] Concurrent extrahepatic bile duct obstruction, sludging of bile, cholelithiasis, and cholecystitis may be a cause or a consequence of ascending bacterial infection and cholangitis. Cholangiohepatitis in cats is also commonly associated with chronic subclinical pancreatitis and inflammatory bowel disease.[64] Concurrent inflammation in the biliary tract and pancreas may be related to the anatomic arrangement of the common bile duct and pancreatic ducts, which, in the cat, anastomose as they approach the duodenal wall. Histologic features of hepatic lipidosis may accompany cholangiohepatitis in some cats, possibly related to anorexia and weight loss.[59]

A severe form of chronic cholangiohepatitis, called sclerosing cholangitis, is characterized by the disappearance of small bile ducts and replacement with an "onion skin" layering of connective tissue and marked periductal fibrosis.[55] This lesion is similar to primary sclerosing cholangitis in humans.

Lymphocytic Portal Hepatitis

Lymphocytic inflammation (with or without plasma cells) in portal areas has been referred to as nonsuppurative cholangitis or cholangiohepatitis, lymphocytic cholangitis or cholangiohepatitis, or lymphoplasmacytic cholangitis or cholangiohepatitis.[55, 65–67] A retrospective review of liver biopsies of cats with inflammatory liver disease identified a subset of cats with lymphocytic portal infiltrates who had histopathologic features distinct from those of acute or chronic cholangiohepatitis.[59] The term lymphocytic portal hepatitis was proposed.[59, 60] As opposed to findings in cholangiohepatitis, there was a lack of neutrophilic inflammation, bile duct involvement, infiltration of inflammatory cells into hepatic parenchyma, or periportal necrosis.[59] Lymphocytic portal hepatitis is not associated with inflammatory bowel disease or pancreatitis.[59, 64] Previous reports of progressive lymphocytic cholangitis or lymphocytic cholangitis[65, 66] referred to varying degrees of neutrophilic inflammation and the condition may actually have been a chronic form of cholangiohepatitis.[59] Lymphocytic portal hepatitis is a common finding in liver biopsies of old cats (older than 10 years), suggesting that it is a common aging change or that a subclinical form of disease is prevalent.[59, 60] Lymphocytic portal hepatitis appears to progress slowly with varying degrees of portal fibrosis and bile duct proliferation but no pseudolobule formation.[59] An immunologic pathogenesis is suspected.[60] Concurrent hepatic lipidosis is less likely than with cholangiohepatitis. In cats with marked lymphocytic infiltration, chronic inflammatory disease must be differentiated from hepatic lymphoma.

HISTORY AND CLINICAL FINDINGS

Clinical findings in cats with chronic inflammatory liver disease include anorexia, depression, weight loss, intermittent vomiting and diarrhea, icterus, fever, and dehydration. Signs may be acute or chronic, intermittent or persistent. Cats with acute cholangiohepatitis often have a short duration of illness (less than 5 days) and male cats appear to be at increased risk.[55] Fever and abdominal pain are more likely with acute cholangiohepatitis. With chronic cholangiohepatitis or lymphocytic portal hepatitis, a long-standing history over a period of weeks or months is more likely. Vomiting, icterus, and hepatomegaly are common findings. Hepatic encephalopathy, ascites, and excessive bleeding are uncommon unless severe end-stage liver disease is present. However, ascites was a common presenting sign of cats in

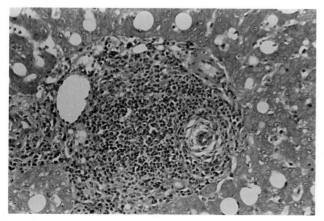

Figure 143–3. Microscopic appearance of chronic cholangiohepatitis in a cat, characterized by marked accumulation of lymphocytes and neutrophils around the bile duct within a portal tract (67×).

the United Kingdom with progressive lymphocytic cholangitis.[66, 67] Young cats and Persian cats appear to be at increased risk for this disorder.[66, 67]

LABORATORY EVALUATION

Laboratory findings with chronic inflammatory liver disease include hyperbilirubinemia, bilirubinuria, increased serum bile acids, and increased serum liver enzymes (ALT, aspartate aminotransferase [AST], ALP, GGT). Because ALP is an induced enzyme, it may be normal or only mildly increased in cats with acute cholangiohepatitis.[55] Hyperglobulinemia is found in approximately 50 per cent of cats with chronic cholangiohepatitis. The CBC may reveal neutrophilia and a left shift, especially with acute cholangiohepatitis. Lymphocytosis is present in some cats with chronic cholangiohepatitis. A mild nonregenerative anemia is also common. A coagulopathy may occur in cats with chronic inflammatory liver disease as a result of vitamin K malabsorption, hepatocyte failure, or DIC. Hypoalbuminemia, decreased BUN, and hyperammonemia suggest advanced disease. The feline trypsinogen assay (trypsin-like immunoreactivity [TLI] test) should be considered to identify cats with concurrent or underlying pancreatitis. In tropical locations, fecal examinations or a therapeutic trial of praziquantel should be considered to rule out liver flukes.

IMAGING

Abdominal radiographs may reveal a liver that is normal to increased in size. Radiopaque choleliths associated with chronic cholangiohepatitis may also be detected. Abdominal ultrasonography is useful in evaluating for hepatic disease in cats.[62] Most cats with cholangiohepatitis have no detectable parenchymal abnormalities or diffuse hepatic hypoechogenicity and prominent portal vasculature.[62] Concurrent abnormalities of the biliary tract and pancreas are common in cats with cholangiohepatitis, and ultrasonography is useful in evaluating for associated common bile duct obstruction, cholelithiasis, sludging of bile, cholecystitis, and pancreatic abnormalities.[55, 62]

LIVER BIOPSY

Definitive diagnosis requires liver biopsy to distinguish feline chronic inflammatory liver disease from other common hepatic disorders such as hepatic lipidosis, hepatic feline infectious peritonitis, and neoplasia. Percutaneous liver biopsy is adequate for diagnosis if extrahepatic obstruction and cholelithiasis are not evident ultrasonographically. An aerobic and anaerobic bacterial culture of liver tissue (or bile obtained by transhepatic cholecystocentesis) should be performed.[55] Cytologic evaluation of impression smears of bile or liver tissue has been recommended because bacteria are more easily detected cytologically than histopathologically.[55] Cats receiving antibiotics may have negative cultures but bacteria may be seen on cytology.[55]

Indications for surgical intervention to obtain a liver biopsy include (1) biliary decompression for extrahepatic biliary obstruction, (2) sludge removal and bile duct and gallbladder irrigation, (3) cholelith removal, and (4) cholecystectomy for necrotizing cholecystitis. A complete evaluation of the biliary system and pancreas should be performed. Duodenal and pancreatic biopsies should also be obtained to identify concurrent inflammatory bowel disease (IBD) and pancreatitis. With chronic cholangiohepatitis, the gallbladder and common bile duct are frequently thickened, firm, and distended. Inspissated bile and choleliths may be present. Aerobic and anaerobic cultures of liver and bile should be obtained. If biliary obstruction is detected, a cholecystojejunostomy should be performed.

TREATMENT

Antibiotics are the primary therapy for acute (suppurative) cholangiohepatitis. They are also used in the initial therapy of chronic cholangiohepatitis before starting glucocorticoid therapy, in order to eliminate any bacterial component. Antibiotics are given for a minimum of 6 to 8 weeks, especially in acute cholangiohepatitis. In some cats with persistent elevation of serum bilirubin and liver enzymes, antibiotic therapy should continue 3 to 6 months. If possible, the choice of drug should be based on culture and sensitivity testing results; otherwise, consider ampicillin, amoxicillin, amoxicillin-clavulanate, or a cephalosporin as an initial choice, combined with metronidazole for broader spectrum against anaerobes, as well as modulation of cell-mediated immunity and treatment of concurrent IBD. For refractory cases, enrofloxacin or a 1-week course of an aminoglycoside should be considered.

Because of its anti-inflammatory and immunosuppressive properties, prednisolone (prednisone) is used empirically in the treatment of (1) chronic cholangiohepatitis that does not respond to antibiotic therapy, (2) sclerosing cholangiohepatitis, and (3) lymphocytic portal hepatitis. The dose of prednisolone is 1 to 2 mg/lb/day until clinical remission, then tapered over 6 to 8 weeks. The side effects of glucocorticoid therapy may outweigh the potential benefits in cats with advanced hepatic disease and biliary cirrhosis. Corticosteroids are catabolic and may worsen signs of HE. Furthermore, exacerbation of ascites may occur because of sodium-retaining properties.

For cats that are resistant to prednisolone (especially those with sclerosing cholangitis), low-dose pulse oral methotrexate in combination with prednisolone, metronidazole, and ursodeoxycholic acid has been recommended.[55] A suggested total dose is 0.4 mg of methotrexate per cat divided into three doses over a 24-hour period (i.e., 0.13 mg at 0, 12, and 24 hours). This dose is repeated every 7 to 10 days. If there is no response after several months, consider increasing the dose to 0.26 mg at time 0 and continuing 0.13 mg at 12 and 24 hours. Potential side effects include leukopenia, vomiting, diarrhea, and hepatotoxicity.

Ursodeoxycholic acid is recommended in all cats with cholangiohepatitis when extrahepatic biliary obstruction has been eliminated. It is hepatoprotective (anti-inflammatory, immunomodulatory, and antifibrotic effects) and is a choleretic that promotes increased fluidity of biliary secretions to treat or prevent sludging.[55] It appears to be well tolerated and safe in cats.[68] Ursodiol (Actigall) comes as a 300-mg capsule that can be compounded into 30-mg capsules to aid in dosing cats.

Dietary protein restriction is not instituted unless overt signs of HE are present. If concurrent IBD is suspected, dietary modifications may include controlled or single-protein-source diets and fiber supplementation. Parenteral vitamin K_1 may be indicated with chronic severe cholestasis that interferes with vitamin K absorption (see Table 143–3).

The prognosis for cats with cholangiohepatitis is variable.

Complete recovery from acute cholangiohepatitis after antibiotic therapy is possible. Many cats with chronic cholangiohepatitis or lymphocytic portal hepatitis continue to have chronic smoldering disease requiring treatment for many months.

HEPATIC VASCULAR DISORDERS

CONGENITAL PORTOSYSTEMIC SHUNT

Portosystemic shunts (PSSs) are vascular communications between the portal and systemic venous systems that allow portal blood to reach the systemic circulation without first passing through the liver. Signs of HE dominate the clinical picture because of inadequate hepatic clearance of enterically derived toxins such as ammonia, mercaptans, short-chain fatty acids, gamma-aminobutyric acid, and endogenous benzodiazepines. Decreased hepatic blood flow and lack of hepatotropic factors such as insulin, glucagon, and nutrients result in hepatic atrophy. Urate urolithiasis, an important complication of PSSs, occurs because of increased urinary excretion of ammonia and uric acid. Renal, cystic, or urethral calculi may occur. Urolithiasis may be a complication in as many as 50 per cent of animals with congenital PSS.[69]

PSSs in dogs and cats can be either congenital or acquired. The congenital form is most commonly recognized. Congenital PSSs are anomalous embryonal vessels that usually occur as single shunts (either intrahepatic or extrahepatic) and are not associated with portal hypertension. The genetic basis for congenital PSS is unknown, although affected lines have been recognized in Miniature schnauzers, Irish wolfhounds, Old English sheepdogs, and Cairn terriers.[69–72] An autosomal polygenic mechanism is suspected in Irish wolfhounds.[71] Acquired PSSs, which form in response to portal hypertension, are typically multiple extrahepatic shunts that connect the portal system and the caudal vena cava (for further discussion, see the section on multiple acquired PSSs).[73]

Single intrahepatic PSSs provide a communication between the portal vein and the caudal vena cava. Intrahepatic shunts can be classified as left, central, or right divisional.[74] The morphology of the left divisional shunt (via the left hepatic vein) is consistent with failure of the fetal ductus venosus to close.[74] The ductus venosus, a fetal vessel that allows oxygenated blood to be shunted from the umbilical vein directly into the caudal vena cava, normally closes within the first few days after birth. The underlying mechanisms associated with failure of the ductus to close are unknown.[75] The pathogenesis of intrahepatic PSSs that occur in the right medial (central divisional) or right lateral (right divisional) liver lobes is unknown.[74] Single intrahepatic PSSs are most common in large breed dogs.[76]

Single extrahepatic PSSs usually connect the portal vein or one of its tributaries (often the left gastric or splenic vein) with the caudal vena cava cranial to the phrenicoabdominal veins. Less frequently, the anomalous vessel enters the azygos vein or other systemic vessel. Single extrahepatic PSSs represent a developmental abnormality of the vitelline system. Single extrahepatic PSSs are most common in cats and small breed dogs.[69, 76, 77]

In dogs and cats with congenital PSS, the liver is grossly small and often mottled in appearance. Liver biopsy most consistently reveals hepatocyte atrophy with small or absent portal veins and arteriolar hyperplasia, although biopsy abnormalities may be subtle.[58] Additional features may include sinusoidal congestion, periportal vacuolization, biliary hyperplasia, lipogranulomas, and increased periportal connective tissue. Biopsy findings are indistinguishable from those in hepatic microvascular dysplasia. Microscopic abnormalities of the central nervous system consist of polymicrocavitation of the brain stem and cerebellum and astrocytosis of the cerebral cortex.

Congenital PSSs occur more commonly in purebred than in mixed breed dogs.[70, 75] Breeds at increased risk include Miniature schnauzers, Yorkshire terriers, Irish wolfhounds, Cairn terriers, Maltese, Australian cattle dogs, Golden retrievers, Old English sheepdogs, and Labrador retrievers.[69–71, 74, 78] In contrast, mixed breed cats are affected more commonly than purebred cats.[79] Of the affected purebreds, Persian and Himalayan cats appear to be at increased risk.[79]

A slight predilection for male cats and female dogs has been suggested and affected male dogs and cats are commonly cryptorchid.[69, 70, 79] Age is an important diagnostic clue because most animals develop signs by 6 months of age.[69, 79] A congenital PSS should still be a diagnostic consideration in middle-aged or older dogs, because signs may be subtle and some dogs with congenital PSS go undiagnosed until as late as 10 years of age. This is especially true for dogs with urate urolithiasis who may not have an obvious history of HE.[80]

Clinical signs of congenital PSS are referable to the central nervous system, gastrointestinal system, or urinary tract.[69, 70, 75, 77, 79] Signs of HE usually predominate. The most consistent signs of HE are often subtle, such as anorexia, depression, and lethargy. Other common findings indicative of diffuse cerebral disease include episodic weakness, ataxia, head pressing, disorientation, circling, pacing, behavioral changes, amaurotic blindness, seizures, and coma. Bizarre aggressive behavior, seizures, and blindness appear more likely in cats.[69, 79] Hypersalivation is also a prominent sign in cats but also occurs in dogs.[69, 79] Clinical signs of HE tend to wax and wane and are often interspersed with normal periods, reflecting the variable production and absorption of enteric products that are neurotoxic. Signs of HE may be exacerbated by a protein-rich meal; gastrointestinal bleeding associated with parasites, ulcers, or drug therapy; or administration of methionine-containing urinary acidifiers or lipotropic agents. Clinical improvement of HE after fluid therapy is common and most likely attributed to correction of dehydration and promotion of urinary excretion of ammonia and other toxins. Improvement with broad-spectrum antibiotic therapy reflects the effect of antibiotics on the toxin-producing intestinal flora.

Gastrointestinal signs of intermittent anorexia, vomiting, and diarrhea are common nonspecific features of hepatic dysfunction and are not necessarily accompanied by overt signs of HE. Many affected animals have a history of stunted growth, failure to gain weight compared with unaffected littermates, or weight loss.[69, 79]

Polydipsia and polyuria are common in dogs but not in cats.[69, 79] Some dogs are able to concentrate their urine after water deprivation, suggesting a primary psychogenic polydipsia. Other dogs have partial or incomplete urine-concentrating ability, consistent with medullary washout secondary to polyuria and polydipsia or a primary renal concentrating defect.[69] Increased free cortisol levels have been documented in dogs with PSS and HE, suggesting an altered hypothalamic-pituitary-adrenal axis.[81] If urolithiasis is a complicating feature, pollakiuria, dysuria, and hematuria may occur. Some animals are presented primarily for evalua-

LIV

tion of urolithiasis without obvious HE or gastrointestinal signs.[80]

A history of prolonged recovery after general anesthesia or excessive sedation after treatment with tranquilizers, anticonvulsants, or organophosphates can be attributed to impaired hepatic metabolism of these substances. Other less consistent clinical findings include polyphagia, pica and foreign body ingestion, intermittent fever, recurrent upper respiratory signs in cats, and intense pruritus in dogs.[69, 79]

Physical examination may be unremarkable except for small body stature or weight loss. The neurologic examination is normal, or if overt signs of HE are present, neurologic findings are consistent with diffuse cerebral disease. Many affected cats have golden or copper-colored irises.[69] Heart murmurs have also been auscultated in some affected cats.[79] Ascites and edema are rare findings unless a congenital PSS is complicated by hypoalbuminemia (albumin less than 1.0 g/dL). Ascites is more likely with acquired hepatic disorders that cause portal hypertension and multiple acquired PSS (see the section on multiple PSSs).

In young animals with consistent clinical features of a congenital PSS but without a demonstrable shunt on portography or transcolonic portal scintigraphy, hepatic microvascular dysplasia should be considered (see later).[82] Rarely, a congenital urea cycle enzyme deficiency has been associated with hyperammonemia and HE in young animals (see later section on urea cycle enzyme deficiency). Other disorders that are associated with central nervous system signs in young dogs and cats that must be considered in the differential diagnosis include infectious diseases (canine distemper, FIP, toxoplasmosis, and feline leukemia virus [FeLV]– or feline immunodeficiency virus [FIV]–related diseases), toxicities, hydrocephalus, idiopathic epilepsy, and metabolic disorders such as hypoglycemia and thiamine deficiency.

Routine hematologic and biochemical findings are often unremarkable in dogs and cats with congenital PSS.[83] Hematologic findings include erythrocytic microcytosis, target cells, poikilocytosis (especially in cats), and mild nonregenerative anemia. These red blood cell changes can be subtle but important diagnostic clues in an otherwise normal CBC. The cause of microcytosis is not known; however, decreased serum iron concentration, normal to increased ferritin concentration, and accumulation of stainable iron in the liver suggest that microcytosis is associated with abnormal iron metabolism (impaired iron transport or sequestration of iron) rather than absolute iron deficiency.[84, 85] Decreased availability of iron for hemoglobin synthesis appears to occur despite adequate tissue iron stores.

Isosthenuria or hyposthenuria is frequently detected by urinalysis of dogs that are polyuric and polydipsic. Ammonium biurate crystals are a common finding on urine sediment examination and are an important clue to underlying liver disease in dogs and cats. If urolithiasis is a complication of congenital PSS, additional findings may include hematuria, proteinuria, and pyuria. Coagulation tests in dogs may show increased partial thromboplastin times and hypofibrinogenemia, but clinical evidence of a bleeding problem is rare.[83]

Hepatocellular dysfunction is suggested by hypoproteinemia, hypoalbuminemia, hypoglobulinemia, hypoglycemia, decreased BUN, and hypocholesterolemia. Hypoalbuminemia and hypoglobulinemia are common findings in dogs with congenital PSS but less so in affected cats.[69, 70] Hypoglycemia, especially after a prolonged fast, is most likely in affected toy breeds of dogs such as Yorkshire terriers.[70, 83] Potential mechanisms for hypoglycemia include decreased

hepatic glycogen stores, decreased insulin catabolism, and endotoxemia. The total serum bilirubin concentration is typically normal. The serum liver enzyme activity (ALP, ALT, and AST) is normal to mildly (two or three times) increased, consistent with a lesion of hepatic atrophy and minimal hepatocellular injury or intrahepatic cholestasis.

Serum bile acid concentrations should be determined to document hepatic dysfunction in dogs and cats suspected to have congenital PSSs. The fasting SBA is often increased but can be normal, because during prolonged fasting, the liver may eventually clear the bile acids from the systemic circulation.[83] Postprandial SBA is consistently abnormal and is a good screening test for animals suspected to have PSSs.[83] Postprandial SBA concentrations typically exceed 100 umol/L. If postprandial SBA concentrations are consistently in the normal range, a diagnosis of congenital PSS is unlikely. Hyperammonemia is a common finding in dogs and cats with PSSs, although the fasting blood ammonia concentration may be normal. The ammonia tolerance test is consistently abnormal and is equal in sensitivity to postprandial SBA in detecting hepatic dysfunction associated with congenital PSS.[83] Blood ammonia is not a suitable screening test for congenital PSS in young Irish wolfhounds because a transient metabolic hyperammonemia unassociated with liver disease occurs in this breed.[86] Prolonged BSP dye retention is a common but inconsistent finding in animals with congenital PSSs and its use has largely been replaced by measurement of SBA concentrations.[83]

Survey abdominal radiographs are often obtained for animals with suspected PSS to evaluate for microhepatica or presence of urinary calculi and to investigate other causes of gastrointestinal or urinary tract signs. Microhepatica, a common finding on survey abdominal radiographs of dogs with congenital PSS, is a less consistent finding in cats. In many animals, the size of the liver is difficult to evaluate because of the lack of intra-abdominal fat. Cranial displacement of the stomach is often an indirect indication of a small liver. Mild renomegaly is occasionally noted in dogs and cats with congenital PSS. Ammonium urate calculi are not usually visible on survey radiographs unless they also contain substantial amounts of magnesium and phosphate.

Additional radiographic imaging techniques, such as ultrasonography, contrast portography, or transcolonic portal scintigraphy, can provide important information about the presence, location, and type of PSS. Use of these techniques may be limited by equipment availability or operator experience. Although ultrasonography and transcolonic portal scintigraphy have the advantage of being noninvasive, contrast portography is still considered the "gold standard" for the anatomic evaluation of the portal vasculature. The advantages and disadvantages of each of the imaging techniques used for evaluation of PSS are discussed in more detail in the following. The experienced surgeon may elect to bypass further diagnostic imaging and go directly to an abdominal exploratory examination for diagnosis and treatment of a suspected PSS, especially in small dogs or cats (who are most likely to have an easily recognized extrahepatic shunt) with typical historical, clinical, and laboratory features.

Ultrasonography is a useful noninvasive method for evaluating animals with a suspected congenital PSS.[87] Intrahepatic PSSs are more reliably detected with this procedure than are extrahepatic PSSs.[87] It is a rapid technique that can be performed without sedation or anesthesia but is highly dependent on the experience of the operator. Ultrasonographically, the liver usually appears small, there is a consistent decrease in the number and size of intrahepatic veins, and the shunting vessel may be identified. The kidneys and bladder should also be routinely scanned to detect urate urolithiasis.

Positive-contrast portography is the procedure of choice for accurate characterization of the anatomic location of a PSS. Techniques described include mesenteric (or jejunal) portography, splenoportography, and cranial mesenteric or celiac arterial portography. Operative mesenteric portography is the preferred technique because it allows a high-quality study of the portal system, does not require special equipment, and results in few complications. Mesenteric portography is performed with general anesthesia. A loop of jejunum is isolated through a ventral midline incision. Two ligatures are placed around a jejunal vein and an over-the-needle catheter is positioned within the vessel. After the ligatures are tied and the catheter is secured to the vessel, the abdominal incision is temporarily closed. A water-soluble contrast agent (0.5 to 1 mL/lb body weight) is injected as a bolus into the catheter. If a rapid film changer is not available, a radiograph is taken as the final milliliter is injected. Lateral and ventrodorsal radiographs should be obtained, which requires a separate dye injection for each view.

In normal animals, the portal blood (and injected dye) flows to the liver, outlining the portal vein and its multiple intrahepatic branches (Fig. 143–4A). With a single congenital PSS, the shunting vessel is outlined as blood is diverted directly into the lower pressure systemic venous system (usually the caudal vena cava) (Fig. 143–4B). Intrahepatic portal vein branches may or may not be opacified. Opacification of the intrahepatic portal system during portography is a favorable prognostic factor. Failure to visualize the intrahepatic portal system is not a reliable indicator of portal atresia but may suggest higher intrahepatic vascular resistance and a greater likelihood of postoperative complications.[79, 88] Repeated portography performed after temporary occlusion of the shunt may provide additional information about the severity of intrahepatic portal atresia.[89]

Transcolonic portal scintigraphy using technetium 99m pertechnetate is a noninvasive alternative to mesenteric portography that does not require sedation or anesthesia.[90, 91] Technetium 99m pertechnetate, given by rectum, is rapidly absorbed from the colon into the portal blood, and in normal animals radioactivity is detected first in the liver and later in the heart. With portosystemic shunting, radioactivity reaches the heart before or at the same time as it reaches the liver. The shunt fraction, determined by computer analysis, represents the percentage of portal blood that bypasses the liver. This procedure does not provide reliable anatomic information, and the type and location of the shunt must be further determined at surgery. Potential causes of a false-negative study include shunts from the gastric vein to the caudal vena cava (a common type of shunt in cats), because portal blood from the colon does not typically pass through this vessel. In addition, if a shunt occurs adjacent to the liver, the degree of shunting may be underestimated if the shunting vessel is included in the liver region of interest.[91] Transcolonic portal scintigraphy is more likely to detect shunts from the distal portal system (e.g., colonic vein to caudal vena cava) than a mesenteric portogram. Transcolonic scintigraphy is especially useful for monitoring progressive postoperative closure of a shunt after partial suture ligation or ameroid constrictor placement.[91, 92] A period of isolation (usually 12 to 18 hours) is required after the procedure until radiation levels are reduced. Because of equipment expense, availability of transcolonic portal scintigraphy is limited to referral institutions.

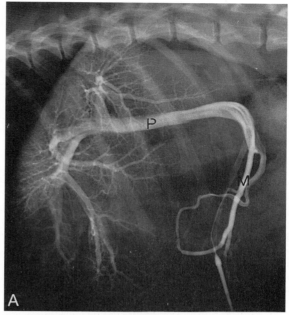

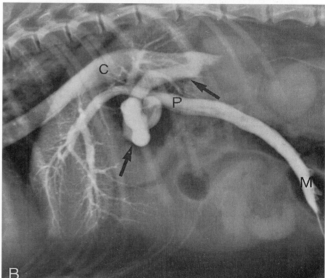

Figure 143–4. Mesenteric portography in a normal dog (A) and a dog with a single congenital extrahepatic portosystemic shunt (portal vein to caudal vena cava) (B). In both views, the catheter for contrast injection is positioned in a mesenteric vein (M). A, Contrast medium outlines the mesenteric vein as well as the portal vein (P) and its multiple branches within the liver. B, Contrast medium outlines the portal vein, intrahepatic portal branches, and a single large tortuous shunt (arrows) that communicates with the caudal vena cava (C).

LIV

Medical management of HE in dogs and cats with congenital PSS is indicated before anesthesia and definitive surgical correction. The cornerstone of therapy is a diet that is moderately protein restricted with the bulk of calories derived from carbohydrates and fat (see Table 143–3).[93] Vegetable (soy protein) and dairy (cottage cheese, yogurt) proteins are preferred. Meat and egg proteins are poorly tolerated. The recommended dietary protein intake on a dry matter basis for patients with HE is 18 to 22 per cent (dogs) and 30 to 35 percent (cats). The protein content of the diet should be increased to the maximum amount tolerated without signs of HE. Dietary supplementation with soluble fiber (psyllium l to 3 teaspoons per day) appears to be beneficial in managing HE by mechanisms similar to those with lactulose and may allow higher levels of dietary protein to be tolerated.[94, 95]

Lactulose, a nonmetabolizable disaccharide, acidifies colonic contents (causing ammonia trapping), shortens the intestinal transit time, alters colonic flora, promotes incorporation of ammonia into bacterial proteins, and reduces production of potentially toxic short-chain fatty acids (SCFA) by producing the nontoxic SCFA acetate.[96] The dose is 0.1 to 0.22 mL/lb by mouth every 8 to 12 hours to achieve two or three soft stools per day. It can be safely given on a long-term basis. It is currently available as a sweet syrup, but a crystalline form (powder) is to be marketed in 10- and 20-g packets. Antibiotics such as neomycin (10 mg/lb by mouth every 8 to 12 hours) or metronidazole (4 mg/lb by mouth every 12 hours) are commonly used on a short-term basis to alter the urease-producing intestinal bacterial population. Systemic antibiotics such as amoxicillin or ampicillin are also effective.

When severe CNS depression or coma prevents oral administration of lactulose and neomycin, these drugs are administered by enema. Acute decompensation of HE requires fluid therapy for correction of dehydration, correction of electrolyte and acid-base imbalances, and maintenance of blood glucose. Lactated Ringer's solution should be avoided. Precipitating causes of HE such as hypoglycemia, gastrointestinal bleeding, hypokalemia, and alkalosis should be identified and corrected whenever possible. Benzodiazepines, sedatives, and tranquilizers should be avoided. In addition to routine management of HE, control of seizures with anticonvulsant therapy (potassium bromide or phenobarbital) is indicated before general anesthesia and surgery.

The short-term response to therapy for HE in dogs with congenital PSS is often dramatic. Most dogs are clinically normal with therapy, even before surgical shunt ligation. The response of cats to medical management of HE may not be as rewarding. If surgical shunt correction is not feasible or is declined by the owner, long-term medical management can adequately control clinical signs for as long as 2 to 4 years in some dogs.[70, 75] However, most dogs managed medically on a long-term basis are not clinically normal and eventually have refractory neurologic signs. Medical therapy does not reverse the progressive hepatic atrophy and associated alterations in carbohydrate, lipid, and protein metabolism.

The treatment of choice for dogs and cats with a congenital PSS is surgical attenuation or ligation of the anomalous vessel.[75, 97, 98] Single intrahepatic shunts are technically more difficult to correct than single extrahepatic shunts. Total surgical ligation of a single congenital PSS is preferred; however, in many cases only partial (60 to 80 per cent) ligation of the shunt can be safely performed because of the risk of portal hypertension (PH). PH occurs because the intrahepatic vasculature cannot accommodate the additional volume of portal blood that is diverted back to the liver after total occlusion of the shunt vessel. Many animals with partial suture ligation of a single extrahepatic PSS eventually have complete closure of their shunt, as assessed by transcolonic scintigraphy.[91, 92] However, recurrence of clinical signs (41 to 50 per cent of dogs) is more likely if a partial rather than complete ligation has been performed.[99, 100] A liver biopsy specimen is also taken at the time of surgery.

Use of an ameroid constrictor for gradual occlusion of single extrahepatic PSS has been described.[101] The ameroid constrictor is a specialized device consisting of hydroscopic casein material in a stainless steel ring. The device is surgically placed around the shunt, and as fluid is absorbed the lumen of the ring becomes progressively smaller, causing shunt occlusion. Advantages of this procedure include gradual progressive occlusion of the shunt over a 30- to 60-day period (thus preventing acute postoperative PH), decreased surgical and anesthesia time, and lack of need to monitor portal pressures during surgery. This technique appears preferable to suture ligation for single extrahepatic PSS and makes the surgical issue of partial versus complete shunt ligation obsolete. Suture ligation is still indicated for most intrahepatic PSSs because ameroid constrictors may not be available in large enough sizes and surgical access to the shunt is more difficult. Successful use of transvenous coil embolization for gradual occlusion of a patent ductus venosus under radiographic guidance has also been described.[102]

When suture attenuation or ligation is performed, PH may occur 2 to 24 hours after surgery. Signs of acute severe PH include abdominal distention and pain, bloody diarrhea, ileus, endotoxic shock, and peracute cardiovascular collapse. If severe portal hypertension occurs, an emergency laparotomy is required to remove the ligature. However, most animals do not survive. Concurrent medical therapy consists of shock doses of intravenous fluids (0.45 per cent saline or Ringer's solution with 5 per cent dextrose), systemic antibiotics such as gentamicin combined with penicillin, and glucocorticoids. Because the associated gastrointestinal bleeding can exacerbate HE, lactulose enemas may also be beneficial. After emergency surgery, the animal should be stabilized medically for 2 to 3 weeks and then a second attempt at surgical shunt ligation can be performed.[98] Transient abdominal distention and ascites are signs of mild PH but are not usually an indication for ligature removal unless accompanied by other signs. In the postoperative period, ascites may be exacerbated by severe hypoalbuminemia or overzealous fluid therapy. Ascites usually resolves within 14 to 21 days after surgery.[103] Sustained PH that is not immediately life-threatening can result in the development of multiple acquired PSSs after 1 to 2 months.[75, 104]

On occasion, seizures and status epilepticus are a complication of surgical shunt ligation.[103, 105, 106] The use of an ameroid constrictor does not appear to prevent the likelihood of this complication. Dogs older than 18 months of age may be at increased risk.[105] The pathogenesis is obscure, but seizures do not appear to be caused by simple hypoglycemia or HE. It is possible that the brain may have adapted to an altered metabolism. Sudden withdrawal of the anticonvulsant effects of endogenous benzodiazepines (produced in the gut) after ligation of the PSS has been hypothesized.[107] Patients should be evaluated for hyperammonemia, hypoglycemia, hypoxia, electrolyte imbalances, acid-base imbalances, and systemic hypertension. In addition to routine management of HE and correction of underlying metabolic imbalances (including thiamine administration in cats), seizures should be managed with intravenous phenobarbital or oral loading doses of potassium bromide. If seizures cannot be controlled, intravenous propofol is recommended to induce general anesthesia for 12 to 24 hours. An endotracheal tube is placed and a respirator is used to maintain the partial pressures of oxygen and carbon dioxide. Anesthesia can be maintained by propofol drip or isoflurane gas anesthesia. Mannitol (0.44 g/lb intravenously) may be indicated for control of cerebral edema. The prognosis for recovery from this complication is poor. Other perioperative complications of shunt ligation include intraoperative hypothermia and hypoglycemia, anesthetic complications, fever and positive blood cultures, portal vein thrombosis, acute pancreatitis, cardiac arrythmias, and hemorrhage.[75, 103, 108]

Routine postoperative management consists of systemic antibiotics and fluid therapy. Oral lactulose and neomycin (or metronidazole) and a protein-restricted diet are usually continued for at least 4 to 8 weeks or longer, depending on the individual patient's clinical response. On a long-term basis, many dogs are clinically normal and do not require a protein-restricted diet or medications for HE, especially if total shunt ligation has been performed.[70, 79, 99] After shunt ligation, hepatic regeneration and an increase in liver blood flow result in liver enlargement and reversal of histopathologic abnormalities. Indicators of hepatic function such as SBA concentrations often improve but do not usually return to normal, even in dogs that become clinically normal.[109] Persistent hepatic dysfunction may be related to coexisting hepatic microvascular dyplasia and persistent microscopic shunting of portal blood (see following section). In one study, there was no correlation between follow-up SBA concentrations and the clinical response.[109]

Transcolonic scintigraphy is useful for assessing shunt closure after ameroid constrictor placement or partial suture ligation and should be performed 2 to 3 months after surgery to be sure complete occlusion has occurred.[92] A portogram should be obtained if there is persistent shunting on transcolonic scintigraphy or no improvement or only transient improvement in clinical signs. Potential findings include failure of the shunt to close, recanalization of the shunt, identification of a second previously undetected shunt, or development of multiple acquired PSSs secondary to surgically induced PH.

The prognosis in dogs for resolution of signs after total surgical ligation of the shunt is excellent if the dog survives the immediate postoperative period.[70, 99] In dogs with partial shunt ligation, the prognosis is not as good.[99, 100] Although clinical signs may resolve after surgery and the response appears favorable in the first few years, long-term follow-up (more than 3 years) suggests that signs recur in 40 to 50 percent of dogs with partial shunt ligations.[99, 100] On the basis of this information, dogs who have previously undergone a partial ligation should be reevaluated by transcolonic scintigraphy. If shunting persists, surgical exploration to perform complete suture ligation or ameroid constrictor placement is indicated.

The response to surgical correction of a congenital PSS in cats appears to be less encouraging than in dogs.[79, 89] With partial shunt ligation, clinical improvement is usually noted after surgery, but relapse of clinical signs is common. Persistent seizures and blindness are also more likely to occur when partial rather than total ligation is performed.[79] Total shunt ligation may not be possible because of the high likelihood of severe intrahepatic portal atresia and associated PH.[79, 89] The development of multiple acquired PSSs after surgery appears to be more likely in cats than in dogs.[89]

HEPATIC MICROVASCULAR DYSPLASIA

Hepatic microvascular dysplasia (HMD), also called microvascular portal dysplasia, is a congenital disorder of dogs that is associated with increased SBA concentrations and histologic vascular abnormalities of the liver that resemble those seen in dogs with congenital PSSs.[72, 82, 110–112] Indocyanine green (ICG) clearance is also delayed.[72] The disorder is often subclinical, but some dogs show signs similar to those of congenital PSS.[72, 82] It has been hypothesized that micro-

scopic intrahepatic vascular shunting is the cause of abnormal liver function, but this has not been proved.[72] An inborn error of organic anion metabolism is considered less likely because handling of bile acids and handling of ICG involve different mechanisms.[72] An ultrastructural abnormality that alters the ability to regulate plasma clearance of bile acids and ICG is another consideration.[72]

The histologic vascular abnormalities seen in dogs with HMD are also present in dogs with congenital PSSs and do not necessarily resolve after surgical ligation of the PSS.[110] Concurrent HMD may explain these findings and the failure to normalize SBA concentrations that sometimes occurs despite complete surgical shunt ligation. The relationship between HMD and congenital PSSs is unclear, but the increased incidence of HMD in breeds such as Cairn terriers and Yorkshire terriers that are also at increased risk for PSSs suggests that they may be varying expressions of a more general portal vascular malformation.[72, 110] A polygenic mechanism of inheritance for HMD is suspected in Cairn terriers.[72]

Yorkshire terriers and Cairn terriers are the breeds most commonly affected.[72, 110] However, HMD has been diagnosed in many other small breeds of dogs (especially terriers) such as Maltese, dachshund, poodle, Shih Tzu, Lhasa apso, cocker spaniel, and West Highland white terrier.[82, 110] Dogs with HMD tend to be older at presentation than dogs with congenital PSSs.[82]

Clinical signs are not consistently seen in affected dogs. This is especially true for Cairn terriers with HMD who are clinically normal.[72] In more severely affected dogs, signs are similar to those seen with congenital PSS and include anorexia, lethargy, vomiting, diarrhea, HE, and dysuria and hematuria related to urate urolithiasis.[82] Results of a physical examination are often within normal limits unless signs of HE are present.

Dogs with HMD consistently have increased SBA concentrations.[72, 82] A shunting pattern is typically seen: normal or low fasting SBA concentrations with moderate to markedly increased postprandial SBA concentrations. In one study, dogs with HMD had higher values for mean corpuscular volume, total protein, albumin, creatinine, blood urea nitrogen, glucose, and cholesterol when compared to dogs with congenital PSSs.[112] Dogs with PSSs had higher fasting SBA and postprandial SBA concentrations, white cell counts, and ALP and AST activities.[112] Hyperammonemia and ammonium biurate crystalluria rarely develop in dogs with HMD.[110]

The liver is usually normal in size but may be equivocally small in some cases. On ultrasonography, the liver may be subjectively decreased in size with decreased portal vasculature. Bladder or kidney calculi are uncommon. Results of transcolonic portal scintigraphy are usually normal or only mildly abnormal, as opposed to the increased shunt fractions seen with congenital PSSs. No large shunting vessel can be identified on a portogram. Cairn terriers with HMD have abnormal truncation of the terminal branches of the portal veins and delayed clearing of contrast material, which gives the parenchyma a "blush" appearance.[72]

A wedge biopsy of the liver is preferred to a needle biopsy for diagnosing HMD because it provides more hepatic lobules for evaluation. Grossly, the liver is normal in size and color, compared with the small liver seen with congenital PSSs. The histologic features of HMD are identical to those seen in dogs and cats with a congenital PSS or after experimental surgical creation of a PSS.[110] Findings include hepatic arteriolar hyperplasia, small portal triads, increased smooth muscle thickness of hepatic venules, and an increase in small vascular structures in the periportal area. Histologic lesions vary between liver lobes, with some lobes appearing abnormal and others appearing normal.[72] Thus, more than one lobe should be sampled.

Hepatic microvascular dysplasia should be considered in dogs with clinical features of congenital PSS, increased SBA concentrations, and consistent liver biopsy findings who do not have a demonstrable shunt. It is essential to pursue the diagnosis of congenital PSS in this setting, because the clinical and histologic features of HMD alone are similar to those of congenital PSS, and specific surgical correction is available if a shunt is identified. Transcolonic portal scintigraphy is a noninvasive method for ruling out a congenital PSS. A normal examination would make congenital PSS unlikely, but false-negative results are possible.

It is also important to consider the possibility that a dog with increased SBA concentrations may have HMD and be asymptomatic for the disorder (especially Cairn terriers). Presenting clinical signs may be due to a nonhepatic disease. Detection of increased SBA concentrations may focus diagnostic efforts on the liver, causing the clinician to miss the true cause of the clinical signs.

No treatment is indicated for dogs with subclinical findings. If signs of HE are present, they can often be successfully managed with a moderately protein-restricted diet.[82] Additional therapy for HE with lactulose and neomycin (or metronidazole) is sometimes warranted (see Table 143–3). Follow-up of 11 dogs for a mean period of 15 months (range of 1 week to 4.5 years) indicated a good clinical response to dietary therapy alone.[82] SBA concentrations remained unchanged in repeated tests. Whether dogs who are asymptomatic for HMD ever progress to have clinical signs remains to be determined.

MULTIPLE ACQUIRED PORTOSYSTEMIC SHUNTS AND ASSOCIATED DISORDERS

Multiple acquired PSSs are extrahepatic collateral vessels that develop as a compensatory response to PH.[73] These acquired shunts are rudimentary nonfunctional microvascular communications between the portal and systemic veins that are present in normal dogs and cats. With sustained PH, these vessels enlarge and function to shunt blood into the lower pressure systemic circulation, thus decreasing portal pressure. Multiple acquired PSSs typically connect the portal system and the caudal vena cava. Acquired PSSs usually appear as multiple tortuous vessels that communicate with the caudal vena cava in the area of the left kidney (Fig. 143–5). Multiple acquired PSSs are less commonly detected in cats than in dogs.

PH and multiple acquired PSSs are usually associated with chronic, severe diffuse intrahepatic disorders that cause increased intrahepatic resistance to portal blood flow. Examples include chronic hepatitis, lobular dissecting hepatitis, idiopathic hepatic fibrosis, and cirrhosis.[22, 56] Portosystemic shunting is probably a more common consequence of severe chronic liver disease than is usually appreciated, because angiography is not routinely performed and the observation of shunts at surgery or necropsy is overshadowed by the more marked primary hepatic disorder.

Hepatic arteriovenous fistulas, which are vascular communications between the hepatic artery and portal vein, are a rare but important cause of severe PH and multiple extrahepatic PSSs in young animals and are discussed in the next

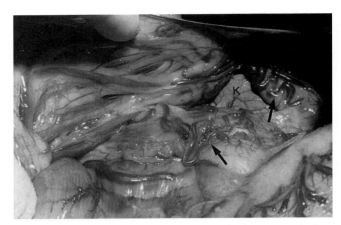

Figure 143–5. Gross appearance of multiple acquired portosystemic shunts (arrows) seen in the region of the left kidney (K) during exploratory laparotomy in a dog with cirrhosis and portal hypertension. (Courtesy of Dr. D. D. Smeak.)

section.[113] Veno-occlusive disease causing PH and multiple PSSs has been described in four young related American cocker spaniels.[114] Clinical signs were indicative of chronic liver disease. Liver biopsies revealed prominent smooth muscular sphincters, dilated central and portal veins, hepatocyte atrophy, and variable fibrosis. Similar histologic features are noted with portal vein hypoplasia and idiopathic noncirrhotic PH (see later) and these disorders may be related.

Portal vein hypoplasia (atresia) was diagnosed in 42 young dogs with PH, multiple PSSs, and signs of chronic liver disease, especially ascites and HE.[57] The extrahepatic portal vein was patent but underdeveloped in 13 of 42 dogs. Microscopically, all dogs had small portal veins. Other features included normal lobular architecture with hepatocyte atrophy, absence of inflammation, variable arteriolar hyperplasia, bile duct proliferation, and portal fibrosis (which was sometimes severe). Whether hypoplasia of the portal system is the primary event or a response of the portal system to decreased perfusion remains to be determined. The prognosis was poor because most dogs died or were euthanized within a few weeks of diagnosis.

Idiopathic noncirrhotic PH is a newly described syndrome of PH and multiple acquired PSSs in young dogs without an arteriovenous (AV) fistula, portal vein hypoplasia, or significant intrahepatic fibrosis or inflammation.[115, 116] The mean age in one study was 2 years.[116] Medium or large breed dogs appear to be at increased risk.[116] One study involved three related and one unrelated Doberman pinschers.[115] Common clinical findings included ascites, polydipsia, vomiting, and diarrhea. Signs of HE were uncommon.[116] Laboratory findings were consistent with hepatic dysfunction and included microcytosis, hypoalbuminemia, decreased BUN, increased SBA, and mild increases in ALP and ALT (two to three times normal). Findings on portography included multiple extrahepatic PSSs, patency of the extrahepatic portal vein, and presence of intrahepatic portal vascular branches. Findings on liver biopsy are similar to the changes seen in dogs with a single congenital PSS and dogs with portal vein hypoplasia and include hepatocellular atrophy, arteriolar hyperplasia, mild portal fibrosis, muscular hypertrophy of central veins, and inconspicuous portal venules in some cases.[116] The mechanism of PH in these dogs is unknown. PH could be caused by severe intrahepatic portal vascular hypoplasia. However, dogs with a single congenital PSS also have varying degrees of intrahepatic portal vascular atresia, yet PH and ascites are not typical features. The long-term prognosis is variable, but some dogs can live for years with a protein-restricted diet.[116]

Other rare causes of PH and multiple acquired PSSs include chronic partial occlusion of the portal vein caused by thrombosis, neoplasia, or extraluminal compression.[117, 118] Acquired PSSs also develop as a result of obstruction of the caudal vena cava or main hepatic veins, although because of the pressure gradient, these shunts communicate with the cranial rather than the caudal vena cava via the azygos, internal thoracic, esophageal or subcutaneous veins.[104] Multiple acquired PSSs may develop after surgical ligation of a congenital PSS.[75, 89]

The clinical and laboratory findings in animals with multiple acquired PSSs are nonspecific and reflect PH, portosystemic shunting, or the underlying hepatic disorder causing PH.[5, 56, 104] Because PH is the mechanism of secondary shunt formation, ascites is a common clinical sign. Microcytosis, a common finding in dogs and cats with congenital PSSs, is also seen in dogs with primary hepatic disorders accompanied by PH and multiple acquired PSSs.[56, 114] A pattern of normal to mildly increased fasting SBA concentrations accompanied by markedly increased postprandial SBA concentrations is consistent with portosystemic shunting regardless of the underlying mechanism of shunt formation. Additional clinical and laboratory findings reflect the underlying disorder.

Multiple acquired PSSs can be seen ultrasonographically, appearing as enlarged tortuous vessels caudal to the liver. Other features of PH such as dilated portal veins, ascites, or splenomegaly may also be detected. Additional ultrasonographic findings are dependent on the underlying cause of PH. Multiple acquired PSSs can be confirmed by contrast portography (Fig. 143–6) or at exploratory laparotomy (or necropsy). When multiple acquired PSSs are identified, further diagnostic efforts should be directed toward identifying the underlying cause of PH, because shunts are only a secondary phenomenon. Liver biopsy is essential in evaluating for primary intrahepatic disorders. Congenital hepatic AV fistulas can be diagnosed by celiac arteriography or exploratory laparotomy.[113] Portal vein obstruction or com-

pression can be demonstrated by ultrasonography, mesenteric portography, or at surgery or necropsy.[117, 118] The portal pressure can be measured to document PH (normal portal pressure is 6 to 13 cm H_2O).

Surgical ligation of multiple acquired PSSs is contraindicated. Ligation may result in fatal PH, because shunts form as a protective compensatory response to PH. Suture attenuation (banding) of the abdominal vena cava has been performed in dogs with multiple acquired PSSs to improve hepatic perfusion.[119] The goal of this procedure is to increase caudal vena cava pressure to a value slightly above portal pressure, thus redirecting portal blood flow (and hepatotropic factors) back through the liver to improve hepatic function. However, there was no significant increase in survival in dogs with multiple PSSs who had this surgery compared with dogs that had conservative medical management.[119]

HEPATIC ARTERIOVENOUS FISTULAS

Hepatic AV fistulas are vascular communications between the hepatic artery and the portal vein that allow blood to bypass the hepatic sinusoidal network and flow retrograde into the portal system.[113] The diversion of high-pressure arterial blood into the low-pressure portal system causes PH, ascites, and multiple acquired PSSs.

Most hepatic AV fistulas are macroscopic communications that appear as large, thin-walled, tortuous, pulsating vascular channels that distort the involved liver lobes and elevate the overlying hepatic capsule. One or more hepatic lobes can be involved. The right medial lobe is most commonly affected.[113] Histologically, fistulas consist of thick-walled arterial vessels and dilated venous vessels. Histologic changes in the adjacent liver tissue include bile duct proliferation, hepatocellular atrophy, sinusoidal congestion, portal vein collapse, dilation of hepatic artery branches, and proliferation of hepatic arterioles.[120] Hepatic parenchymal changes are similar to those seen in animals with congenital PSSs.[120, 121]

Hepatic AV fistulas can be either congenital or acquired. A congenital cause has been suspected in the few cases described, because of the young age at the time of diagnosis.[113] Congenital hepatic AV fistulas, also called hamartomas or hemangiomas, are caused by abnormal development of vessels before differentiation into arteries and veins. Potential causes of acquired hepatic AV fistulas include abdominal trauma, hepatic surgery, hepatic neoplasia, and rupture of a hepatic artery aneurysm. However, there are no reports in the veterinary literature documenting an acquired hepatic AV fistula in dogs or cats.

Hepatic AV fistulas are most frequently diagnosed in animals younger than 1.5 years of age, with a mean age of 6 months.[113] The most consistent clinical signs are acute-onset depression, lethargy, ascites, vomiting, and diarrhea. Other reported findings include signs of HE, failure to grow or weight loss, polyuria and polydipsia, and abdominal pain. Clinical signs are attributed to severe PH that leads to splanchnic vascular congestion, ascites, and multiple acquired PSSs.

A continuous murmur (bruit) may be auscultated through the abdominal wall over the area of the affected liver lobe(s).[113] Fever is a less frequent finding, possibly caused by escape of endotoxin or bacteria from the portal system through an acquired PSS.

Hepatic AV fistulas must be differentiated from other causes of ascites in young animals. Clinical features are

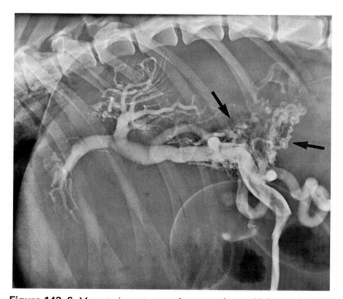

Figure 143–6. Mesenteric portogram demonstrating multiple acquired portosystemic shunts (arrows) in a 3-year-old male rottweiler with hepatic cirrhosis and portal hypertension.

LIV

1318 / SECTION XI—DISEASES OF THE LIVER AND PANCREAS

similar to those of congenital PSSs, except that ascites is an unusual finding in animals with a congenital PSS. Other differential diagnoses to consider include liver disorders such as idiopathic hepatic fibrosis, portal vein hypoplasia, lobular dissecting hepatitis, or idiopathic noncirrhotic PH; congenital heart defects causing right-sided congestive heart failure (e.g., cor triatriatum dexter); and other causes of hypoproteinemia besides liver disease, such as protein-losing enteropathy or protein-losing nephropathy.

Hematologic and biochemical findings are similar to those in animals with congenital PSSs and include mild anemia and hypoproteinemia; normal or mildly increased (less than twofold) liver enzyme activity; and hepatic dysfunction suggested by increased fasting and postprandial SBA concentrations, prolonged BSP dye retention, and ammonia intolerance. Leukocytosis was a consistent finding in one study and may be associated with escape of endotoxin or bacteria from the portal system through an acquired PSS.[113] Ascitic fluid is typically a transudate containing less than 2.5 g/dL protein. Chest radiographs are usually unremarkable and abdominal radiographs reveal severe fluid accumulation. On abdominal ultrasonography, hepatic AV fistulas appear as tortuous, anechoic tubular structures in the area of the liver.[122] Secondary PSSs may be detected as multiple extrahepatic vessels.

Celiac arteriography or a nonselective aortogram can confirm the diagnosis of hepatic AV fistulas.[113] Injected dye outlines the hepatic arteries, which appear as multiple, dilated, tortuous vessels in the area of the fistula and communicate directly with the portal vein. The normal arterial capillary phase is absent because of retrograde (hepatofugal) blood flow into the dilated portal vasculature. As filling of the portal system occurs, multiple acquired PSSs are often outlined. It is important to emphasize that, if a congenital PSS is initially suspected and a mesenteric portogram is obtained, only multiple acquired PSSs and not the underlying hepatic AV fistula are identified. Hepatic AV fistulas should be considered as an underlying cause of multiple extrahepatic PSSs in all young animals.

In most cases, the diagnosis of hepatic AV fistulas is made at the time of laparotomy (or necropsy). Hepatic AV fistulas are easily identified by their gross appearance. A fremitus is palpable over the area of the shunt, and compression of the hepatic artery supplying the affected hepatic lobe obliterates the fremitus and can result in bradycardia (Branham's sign). Mixing of bright red arterial blood with the darker portal blood may be observed through the thin-walled vessels. Increased portal blood flow causes distention of splanchnic vessels and congestion and edema of the intestines. Increased portal pressures ranging from 13 to 22 cm H_2O are a consistent finding.[113] Secondary PSSs are frequently visualized. The liver is usually small.

Partial hepatectomy is indicated for treatment of hepatic AV fistulas involving one liver lobe.[113, 123] Surgical techniques are described elsewhere.[113, 123] Despite resection of involved liver lobes, hepatic function may not return to normal because of persistent shunting of portal blood through acquired PSSs. Consequently, caudal vena cava banding has been recommended to improve hepatic perfusion and decrease portosystemic shunting of blood.[113, 123] Follow-up evaluation of dogs undergoing both partial hepatectomy and vena caval banding 1 to 2 years after surgery indicated persistent abnormalities of blood flow and hepatic function.[113] Medical management of HE with a low-protein diet, lactulose, and neomycin may be necessary (see Table 143–3).

HEPATIC VENOUS OUTFLOW OBSTRUCTION

Hepatic venous outflow obstruction, caused by functional or mechanical obstruction of hepatic venous return to the heart, results in passive venous congestion of the liver, hepatomegaly, PH, and ascites. Hepatic venous outflow obstruction is associated with posthepatic or, more specifically, "postsinusoidal" causes of PH. The site of increased resistance to portal blood flow occurs after the hepatic sinusoid, which corresponds anatomically to obstruction of the central veins, intralobular veins, hepatic veins, caudal vena cava, or heart. Regardless of the underlying cause, these disorders have in common features of sinusoidal congestion and hypertension, which are associated with hepatomegaly and ascites formation.

The most common causes of hepatic venous outflow obstruction are disorders involving the heart or caudal vena cava (Table 143–5).[104, 124–127] Rarely, obstruction occurs in the efferent venous system within the liver (central veins, intralobular veins, or hepatic veins).[128] In humans, the term Budd-Chiari syndrome is used to describe the clinical features associated with hepatic venous outflow obstruction caused by thrombosis of the main hepatic veins. In veterinary medicine, hepatic vein thrombosis is rare and the term has been used in a more general way to include other causes of postsinusoidal PH with similar clinical features.[125, 128] Disorders causing hepatic venous outflow obstruction are rare in cats; however, membranous obstruction of the caudal vena cava has been reported.[126]

With acute passive venous congestion, the liver is grossly swollen, dark, and bloody on cross section.[129] Histopathologic features include periacinar (centrilobular) congestion and sinusoidal dilation; lymphatic distention; and periacinar vacuolization, necrosis, and atrophy. With more chronic duration of passive venous congestion, the liver capsule is grossly irregular with patchy fibrosis and a reticulated acinar pattern known as "nutmeg" liver.[129] Microscopically, periacinar fibrosis ("cardiac cirrhosis") occurs in the chronic stages. Concomitant splenomegaly caused by PH and passive venous congestion of the spleen is a variable finding.

Ascites is a consistent clinical feature of PH associated with hepatic venous outflow obstruction. However, some species variations occur; for example, cats are less likely than dogs to have ascites under similar circumstances. Asci-

TABLE 143–5. CAUSES OF HEPATIC VENOUS OUTFLOW OBSTRUCTION

Heart
    Right-sided congestive heart failure
    Pericardial tamponade
    Constrictive pericarditis
    Intracardiac neoplasm
    Congenital anomaly—cor triatriatum dexter
Caudal vena cava
    Stenosis or fibrosis at junction of CVC* and right atrium
    Postcaval syndrome of heartworm disease
    Trauma-induced kinking of the CVC
    Posttraumatic adhesion of pericardium to CVC
    CVC thrombosis or neoplasia
    Diaphragmatic hernia with CVC compression
    Membranous obstruction of the CVC (congenital?)
Hepatic veins
    Tumor invasion or compression within the liver
    Liver lobe torsion
    Idiopathic postsinusoidal venous obstruction

*Caudal vena cava.

tes occurs because postsinusoidal obstruction results in hepatic sinusoidal hypertension, which increases production of hepatic lymph. Hepatic lymph is normally formed when sinusoidal pressure causes fluid to move between endothelial cells lining the sinusoids into the perisinusoidal space of Disse. Hepatic lymph is normally high in protein because of the marked permeability of the sinusoidal endothelium. With sinusoidal hypertension, there is increased production of high-protein hepatic lymph. When the capacity for lymph drainage via the thoracic duct is exceeded, hepatic lymph accumulates in the peritoneal cavity as high-protein ascites, characterized as a modified transudate with greater than 2.5 g/dL protein.

Another consequence of PH is the development of multiple acquired PSSs, which connect the portal and systemic venous systems. Acquired PSSs are not a consistent feature of all disorders associated with postsinusoidal PH, because acquired PSSs develop only if a pressure gradient exists between the portal and systemic veins. Thus, cardiac causes of postsinusoidal PH, such as right-sided congestive heart failure or pericardial disorders, are not associated with acquired PSSs. However, with caudal vena caval obstruction, decompression of the portal venous system can occur by shunting via the azygos, internal thoracic, esophageal, or subcutaneous veins into the cranial vena cava.[124] Collateral abdominal veins can sometimes be seen on physical examination.[125] Obstruction of hepatic veins can also be associated with development of collateral vessels.[130] Multiple acquired PSSs were not identified in a basenji dog with functional intrahepatic postsinusoidal venous obstruction.[128]

Animals with hepatic venous outflow obstruction are typically presented for persistent abdominal distention and ascites. Clinical signs of hepatic dysfunction are usually absent. Additional clinical findings are related to the underlying cause of venous outflow obstruction. For example, with primary cardiac disorders, there may be a history of cough and exercise intolerance and physical examination findings may include jugular venous distention, positive hepatojugular reflex, and muffled heart sounds. A history of trauma may be elicited for animals with kinking of the caudal vena cava or liver lobe entrapment in a diaphragmatic hernia.[124, 127]

Hepatic venous outflow obstruction should be considered in dogs and cats with high-protein ascites (modified transudate with greater than 2.5 g/dL protein) accompanied by hepatomegaly. The high protein content of the fluid can be an important diagnostic clue to the presence of previously unsuspected postsinusoidal obstruction, because ascitic fluid that accumulates with most primary hepatic disorders or hypoproteinemia usually has less than 2.5 g/dL protein. With passive venous congestion of the liver, serum liver enzyme activity is usually normal or only mildly (two- to threefold) increased. Fasting and postprandial SBA concentrations are typically normal, supporting the concept that with passive venous congestion, hepatic function is not significantly impaired. Prolonged BSP dye retention is a common finding and probably represents altered hepatic perfusion associated with congestion, dehydration, and hypovolemia rather than hepatic dysfunction. Mild to moderate hypoproteinemia is also a common biochemical finding. Other causes of hepatomegaly (but not necessarily ascites) such as hepatic neoplasia, steroid hepatopathy, and diffuse inflammation are more likely to be associated with increased liver enzyme activity or impaired liver function.

Thoracic radiographs should be obtained in the initial evaluation to detect obvious underlying disorders such as congestive heart failure, heartworm disease, intrathoracic masses, kinking of the caudal vena cava, or a diaphragmatic hernia. Widening of the caudal vena cava suggests that passive venous congestion of the liver may be present. However, survey radiographic findings of disorders such as intracardiac neoplasms, constrictive pericarditis, cor triatriatum dexter, and intraluminal obstruction of the caudal vena cava are less diagnostic. Cardiac ultrasonography and angiography are usually required to diagnose intracardiac masses, pericardial disease, and obstructive lesions of the right atrium such as cor triatriatum dexter.[125]

On abdominal radiographs, marked ascites may make it difficult to evaluate liver size. Hepatic ultrasonography is useful for confirming hepatomegaly in the presence of ascites. With passive venous congestion caused by lesions of the caudal vena cava or heart, the intrahepatic caudal vena cava and hepatic veins are usually dilated.[23] Hepatic biopsy is indicated to evaluate hepatomegaly, but only if the initial work-up does not identify an obvious cardiac or vena caval cause for passive venous congestion. When hepatic congestion is identified histologically, a more detailed search for causes of postsinusoidal obstruction is indicated (see Table 143–5).

Specialized diagnostic procedures such as cardiac catheterization, manometry, and angiography are indicated when routine radiographic and ultrasonographic evaluation does not identify a cause for hepatic venous congestion or to characterize further the pathophysiology of an obstructive lesion. Venous pressure measurements in the right side of the heart, thoracic caudal vena cava, and main hepatic veins may identify a pressure gradient at the site of obstruction. Dye studies are performed concurrently for anatomic delineation of the obstructive lesion. Lesions of the caudal vena cava and main hepatic veins are best evaluated with hepatic venography.

The treatment and prognosis depend on the underlying cause of hepatic venous outflow obstruction. The most common cause, congestive heart failure, is managed medically. Surgery is indicated for definitive diagnosis and for removal of obstructive or compressive lesions of the caudal vena cava and main hepatic veins, pericardial disease, intracardiac tumors, and cor triatriatum dexter.

HEPATIC NODULAR HYPERPLASIA, NEOPLASIA, CYSTS

NODULAR HYPERPLASIA

Nodular hyperplasia of the liver, an age-related phenomenon, is a common post-mortem finding in dogs older than 8 years of age.[129, 131] There is no breed or sex predilection. No specific etiology of nodular hyperplasia has been identified in dogs. Hyperplastic nodules are not a preneoplastic finding in dogs.

Nodular hyperplasia is not usually associated with clinical signs but can cause mild to moderate increases in serum ALP and ALT activity. Multiple hyperplastic nodules are often found in a random distribution throughout the liver lobes. The importance of nodular hyperplasia to the clinician is that when hepatic nodules are identified during ultrasonography, laparoscopy, or surgery, benign nodular hyperplasia should be considered in the differential diagnosis. The ultrasonographic appearance of hyperplastic nodules is quite variable, corresponding to the variety of histologic changes that can occur.[132] Some hyperplastic nodules are not detected ultrasonographically because they are similar in echogenicity to normal hepatic tissue. Other hyperplastic nodules appear as focal homogeneous hypoechoic masses or mixed hypoechoic to hyperechoic lesions. This ultrasonographic appearance is indistinguishable from that of primary and secondary neoplasia and a tissue biopsy must be performed to make this distinction. Histologically, it can be difficult to differentiate a hyperplastic nodule from hepatocellular adenoma or adenocarcinoma, especially when only a small sample is available via needle biopsy. Thus, a wedge biopsy sample obtained at surgery is usually necessary. Occasionally, single hyperplastic nodules can become quite large and mimic a hepatocellular adenoma both clinically and microscopically.

HEPATOBILIARY NEOPLASIA

Neoplasia involving the liver can be categorized as primary hepatic tumors, metastatic carcinomas and sarcomas, and hemolymphatic tumors (Table 143–6).[133] In dogs, metastatic tumors are most common and can originate from the pancreas, spleen, mammary glands, adrenal glands, bone, lungs, thyroid glands, and gastrointestinal tract. Common metastatic tumors include hemangiosarcoma, pancreatic carcinoma, and fibrosarcoma. Common metastatic tumors in cats include pancreatic carcinoma, intestinal carcinoma, and renal carcinoma.[133] Hemolymphatic tumors (especially lymphoma and myeloproliferative disease) are the most common type of neoplasia involving the liver of cats.[133] Hepatic lymphoma also occurs frequently in dogs.

Primary hepatic tumors are uncommon in dogs and cats.[133] They may be of epithelial or mesodermal origin and either benign or malignant (see Table 143–6). A benign tumor of the hepatocytes is called a hepatocellular adenoma (or hepatoma), and its malignant counterpart is called a hepatocellular carcinoma. Hepatocellular carcinoma is the most common primary hepatic tumor in dogs.[133]

TABLE 143–6. HEPATIC NEOPLASIA IN DOGS AND CATS

Primary hepatic neoplasia
  Epithelial origin
    Hepatocellular carcinoma
    Hepatocellular adenoma
    Biliary carcinoma (cholangiocarcinoma, biliary cystadenocarcinoma)
    Biliary adenoma (including biliary cystadenoma)
    Hepatic carcinoid
  Mesodermal origin
    Hemangiosarcoma
    Hemangioma
    Leiomyosarcoma
    Fibrosarcoma
    Fibroma
    Osteosarcoma
Metastatic hepatic neoplasia
  Hemangiosarcoma
  Islet cell carcinoma
  Pancreatic carcinoma
  Fibrosarcoma
  Osteosarcoma
  Transitional cell carcinoma
  Intestinal carcinoma
  Renal cell carcinoma
  Pheochromocytoma
  Thyroid carcinoma
  Mammary carcinoma
Hemolymphatic tumors
  Lymphoma
  Mast cell tumor
  Myeloproliferative disorders
  Myeloma
  Thymoma

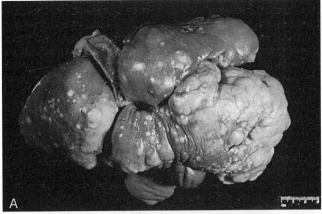

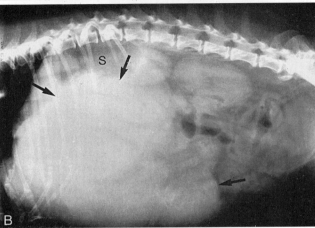

Figure 143–7. Bile duct carcinoma in a 7-year-old neutered female mixed breed dog. *A,* Necropsy specimen showing the massive form of bile duct carcinoma. *B,* Lateral abdominal radiograph of same dog in *A* before its death revealed marked hepatomegaly (arrows) with dorsal displacement of the body of the stomach (S). (From Johnson SE: Liver and biliary tract. *In* Anderson NV [ed]: Veterinary Gastroenterology, 2nd ed. Philadelphia, Lea & Febiger, 1992, pp 504–569.)

A benign tumor arising from the biliary epithelium is called a biliary adenoma. The malignant form is called a biliary carcinoma (Fig. 143–7A). Biliary carcinomas may be intrahepatic, extrahepatic, or within the gallbladder. The intrahepatic form is most common in dogs and cats. Biliary carcinomas and adenomas are the most common primary hepatic tumors in cats.[134, 135] Cystic forms of these tumors (cystadenocarcinoma, cystadenoma) have also been described, especially in cats.[136, 137] A cystadenoma is a slow-growing, benign cystic neoplasm that is most often an incidental finding in old cats at necropsy but may be associated with clinical signs if it becomes large.[136, 137] Malignant transformation is also possible.[135]

Hepatocellular carcinoma and biliary carcinoma occur as solitary mass lesions, multifocal nodular or diffuse infiltrations of large portions of the liver (see Fig. 143–7A). Involvement of more than one liver lobe is more likely in cats with primary hepatic tumors than in dogs.[135] The solitary mass form occurs in about 50 per cent of dogs with hepatocellular carcinoma and in approximately 33 per cent of dogs with biliary carcinoma.[133] Solitary masses are most likely to be successfully resected surgically. Extrahepatic metastases occur frequently with both of these tumors but are more common with biliary carcinoma. The hepatic lymph nodes, peritoneal cavity, and lungs are most frequently involved, but widespread metastases can occur.

Primary hepatic tumors of mesodermal origin (sarcomas) are much less common in dogs and cats than are tumors of epithelial origin (see Table 143–6). Hemangiosarcoma and leiomyosarcoma are most commonly described.[129, 133, 135]

The cause of spontaneous primary hepatic neoplasms in dogs and cats is not usually determined. Potential causes based on reports of experimental and spontaneous hepatic tumors include aflatoxins, nitrosamines, Aramite, liver flukes (*Clonorchis* spp., *Platynosomum concinnum*), and radioactive compounds such as strontium 90 and cesium 144. As opposed to findings in humans, no association with viral infections has been identified.[129, 134]

Primary hepatic neoplasms are most common in dogs and cats that are older than 10 years.[133, 134] Male dogs and cats may be at a slightly increased risk for hepatocellular carcinoma.[133] Male cats and female dogs may be at increased risk for biliary carcinoma.[133, 134, 138] Labrador retrievers were found to be disproportionately represented in one study of dogs with biliary carcinoma.[133] Domestic shorthair cats may have a higher rate of development of hepatic neoplasia than purebred cats.[134]

Dogs and cats with hepatic neoplasia usually show vague, nonspecific signs of hepatic dysfunction that often do not appear until the more advanced stages of hepatic disease.[133, 134, 139] The most consistent signs in dogs are anorexia, lethargy, weight loss, polydipsia, polyuria, vomiting, and abdominal distention. Other less frequent findings include jaundice, diarrhea, and excessive bleeding. Signs of central nervous system dysfunction such as depression, dementia, or seizures can be attributed to HE, hypoglycemia, or central nervous system metastases. Anorexia and lethargy are the most common presenting signs in cats; ascites and vomiting are uncommon in cats as opposed to dogs.[134] When the liver is secondarily involved with metastases, the clinical signs may reflect the primary tumor location or other metastatic sites rather than the hepatic involvement.

On physical examination, a cranial abdominal mass or marked hepatomegaly is commonly detected in dogs and cats with primary hepatic tumors.[133, 134] Hepatomegaly is less likely with metastatic tumors. Ascites or hemoperitoneum may contribute to abdominal distention. Tumor rupture and hemorrhage are most likely with hepatocellular adenoma, hepatocellular carcinoma, and hepatic hemangiosarcoma. Anemia and pale mucous membranes may be attributed to anemia of chronic disease or excessive hemorrhage from a ruptured neoplasm. Jaundice is uncommon in dogs unless the tumor mass causes obstruction of the common bile duct. In contrast, one third of cats with nonhematopoietic hepatic neoplasia were jaundiced.[134] Severe weight loss and cachexia are common but nonspecific findings. Weakness may be associated with paraneoplastic hypoglycemia or myasthenia gravis.[133, 140]

Hematologic and biochemical findings in dogs and cats with hepatic neoplasia are not specific and are indicative of hepatic disease and its complications. Potential hematologic findings include anemia and leukocytosis.[133, 134, 139] Anemia is usually nonregenerative but may be regenerative if associated with excess bleeding or tumor rupture. Although clinical evidence of impaired hemostasis is infrequent, prolongation of the prothrombin time and activated partial thromboplastin time may be identified in dogs with hepatic neoplasia. When hematopoietic or lymphoid malignancies secondarily involve the liver, abnormal cells or pancytopenia may be detected on peripheral blood smears because of concurrent bone marrow involvement. Analysis of abdominal fluid usually indicates a transudate or modified transudate; however, neoplastic cells or a bloody effusion is occasionally noted.

Mild to marked increases in serum liver enzyme (ALP and ALT) activity are common in dogs with hepatic neoplasia. In contrast, most cats with nonhematopoietic hepatic neoplasms have increased serum ALT or AST activity but serum ALP activity is usually normal.[134] Metastatic liver disease is more likely to be associated with increased serum AST activity and hyperbilirubinemia in dogs.[133] Hyperbilirubinemia was detected in one third of cats with primary liver tumors.[134]

Other biochemical findings are quite variable and include hypoalbuminemia, hyperglobulinemia, hypoglycemia, and increased SBA concentrations. The magnitude of increase in SBA concentrations in dogs with hepatic neoplasia can be quite small; SBA concentrations are often within normal limits. Hypoglycemia, sometimes severe, is occasionally noted in dogs with hepatocellular carcinoma and less frequently with hepatocellular adenoma, leiomyosarcoma, and hemangiosarcoma.[141] Serum insulin concentrations are normal to decreased.[141, 142] Potential mechanisms of hypoglycemia include excess utilization of glucose by the tumor, release of insulin-like factors from the tumor, release of other substances such as somatostatin from the tumor, and secondary hepatic parenchymal destruction with impaired glycogenolysis or gluconeogenesis. Increased serum alphafetoprotein concentrations (greater than 250 ng/mL by enzymetry) may be an indicator of hepatocellular carcinoma and biliary carcinoma[143] or of marked hepatic regeneration.

Abdominal radiographic findings in animals with hepatic neoplasia include symmetric or asymmetric hepatomegaly and ascites (Fig. 143–7B). In one study of 22 dogs with nonvascular, nonhematopoietic liver neoplasia, the most common radiographic appearance was that of a right cranial abdominal mass causing caudal and left gastric displacement.[138] Thoracic radiographs should be obtained to detect pulmonary metastases.

Ultrasonography is a useful technique for further evaluation of the liver when primary or metastatic hepatic neoplasia is suspected.[144, 145] Potential ultrasonographic findings include focal, multifocal, or diffuse changes in hepatic echo texture. Hepatocellular carcinoma usually appears as a focal hyperechoic mass.[144] Primary or secondary neoplasia and nodular hyperplasia often appear as focal or multifocal hypoechoic or mixed echogenic lesions.[146] "Target" lesions, consisting of an echogenic center surrounded by a more sonolucent rim, are often neoplastic.[146] The ultrasonographic appearance of hepatic lymphoma is quite variable: patterns described include normal to mild diffuse hyper- or hypoechogenicity, multifocal hypoechoic lesions, or mixed echogenic target lesions.[144, 146] The diagnosis of hepatic neoplasia cannot be made on the basis of ultrasonographic findings alone.

Definitive diagnosis of hepatic neoplasia requires liver biopsy and histopathologic evaluation. The procedure of choice for a single large hepatic mass is laparotomy, because excision of the mass can also be performed concurrently.[136, 139] Ultrasound-guided biopsy is useful for diagnosing focal or diffuse hepatic involvement, but the small size of the biopsy specimen can make differentiation of nodular hyperplasia versus primary hepatic neoplasia difficult. A surgical wedge biopsy is often necessary. Blind percutaneous needle biopsy or fine-needle aspiration biopsy is most useful for diagnosis of diffuse hemolymphatic tumors such as lymphoma, myeloproliferative disease, and mast cell tumor.

Surgical removal of the affected liver lobe is the treatment of choice for primary hepatic neoplasms such as hepatocellu-

LIV

lar adenoma or carcinoma that involve a single lobe.[139] In 18 dogs that underwent partial hepatectomy for removal of a solitary mass lesion of hepatocellular carcinoma, 10 dogs were still alive a mean of 1 year (range 195 to 1025 days) after surgery.[139] Thus, early detection before metastasis to other liver lobes affords the best chance for surgical control. A complete evaluation of the abdominal cavity for evidence of metastases should be performed and biopsy specimens of hepatic lymph nodes should always be obtained. When all lobes are affected, the prognosis is poor.

Chemotherapy is not currently an effective means of control for hepatocellular carcinoma or biliary carcinoma. Chemotherapy with vincristine, doxorubicin, and cyclophosphamide has induced remission and prolonged survival in dogs with primary or metastatic hepatic hemangiosarcoma.[133] Hemolymphatic hepatic neoplasms such as lymphoma, mast cell tumor, or myeloproliferative disease may also respond temporarily to chemotherapeutic intervention.

HEPATOBILIARY CYSTS

Single or multiple diffuse hepatic cysts are occasionally identified in the liver of dogs and cats, usually at necropsy but occasionally in the live animal.[58, 147–150] These cysts can be congenital or acquired, although the distinction is sometimes difficult to make. In general, acquired cysts are usually solitary and congenital cysts are often multiple.

Congenital polycystic disease of the liver and kidneys has been reported in Cairn terriers and West Highland white terriers.[147, 150] Concurrent hepatic cysts are an infrequent finding in cats with polycystic renal disease.[151] Acquired cysts may represent benign biliary adenomas or cystadenomas[136, 137] or may be secondary to trauma.[149] Most solitary hepatic cysts do not cause any clinical signs unless they compress or displace adjacent structures. Signs are more likely to occur when congenital polycystic disease is accompanied by obstruction of the extrahepatic biliary tract. Abdominal distention secondary to an enlarged cyst is a common presenting feature. Hepatic cysts should be considered in the differential diagnosis of any cavitated hepatic mass lesion detected on palpation, radiography, or ultrasonography (Fig. 143–8). Surgery can confirm the diagnosis and allow excision of large solitary cysts.[58, 136, 149]

INBORN ERRORS OF METABOLISM

GLYCOGEN STORAGE DISORDERS

Glycogen storage disorders are inherited disorders resulting from deficiency of specific enzymes required for normal glycogen metabolism.[152] Enzyme deficiency results in impaired glycogen mobilization and subsequent visceral glycogen accumulation. Impaired hepatic glycogen mobilization is usually associated with fasting hypoglycemia, because maintenance of normal blood glucose concentration during fasting depends on release of glucose from stored glycogen. Glycogen accumulation in the liver causes massive hepatomegaly. In humans, at least eight types of glycogen storage diseases have been described.[152] Three of these have been confirmed in dogs by enzymatic assay: type I (von Gierke's disease), type II (Pompe's disease), and type III (Cori's disease).

Glycogen storage disease type Ia is caused by a deficiency of the enzyme glucose-6-phosphatase, which is required to

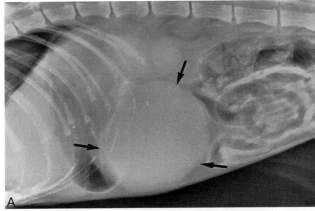

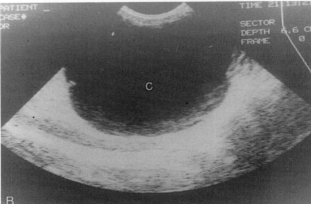

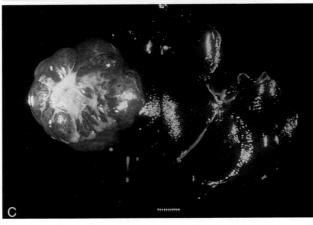

Figure 143–8. Benign hepatic cyst in a 16-year-old female domestic shorthair cat that was not associated with clinical signs. *A*, Lateral abdominal radiograph reveals a large, well-circumscribed mass (arrows) caudal to the stomach. *B*, Abdominal ultrasonography reveals a large hypoechoic cyst (C) originating from the liver. *C*, Gross appearance of the cyst at necropsy after the cat was euthanized for an unrelated problem. (Courtesy of Dr. D. S. Biller.)

release glucose from glycogen. It has been documented in two 7-week-old littermate Maltese puppies with a history of failure to thrive, mental depression, and poor body condition.[153] Necropsy findings revealed pale, friable, enlarged livers with marked diffuse vacuolization histologically. Hepatic vacuoles were periodic acid–Schiff positive and Sudan IV negative, consistent with glycogen rather than fat accumulation.[153] Glucose-6-phosphatase levels in the liver were markedly reduced. Molecular techniques were used to identify a mutation in glucose-6-phosphatase associated with markedly reduced activity.[154]

Type II glycogenosis, caused by deficiency of lysosomal alpha-1,4-glucosidase, has been described in Lapland dogs.[155] An autosomal recessive mechanism of inheritance is suspected. In type II glycogenosis, opposed to type I and type III, hepatic glycogen accumulation was minimal and hypoglycemia did not occur. Clinical signs were instead related to cardiac and skeletal muscle glycogenosis and included regurgitation (megaesophagus), systemic muscle weakness, and cardiac abnormalities. The prognosis is poor, and most dogs died by 1.5 years of age.

Type III glycogenosis, caused by a deficiency of debranching amyloclastic enzyme (amylo-1,6-glucosidase), has been described in related female German Shepherd dogs. Clinical signs included depression, weakness, failure to grow, and abdominal distention resulting from hepatomegaly. Hypoglycemia occurred, and only a marginal increase in blood glucose was observed after epinephrine administration. At necropsy, glycogen infiltration was found in the liver, myocardium, skeletal muscle, and central nervous system. Hepatic activity of amylo-1,6-glucosidase was 0 to 7 per cent of normal.

Hepatic glycogen storage disease, types I and III, should be considered in young dogs with persistent or recurrent fasting hypoglycemia. It must be differentiated from more common disorders causing hypoglycemia such as transient juvenile hypoglycemia associated with fasting, parvoviral enteritis with endotoxemia, and congenital PSS. Failure to increase blood glucose in response to glucagon or epinephrine supports the diagnosis of a glycogen storage disease. Hepatomegaly caused by massive glycogen accumulation is a consistent finding in types I and III in dogs and can be demonstrated on liver biopsy. Definitive diagnosis of these disorders requires enzyme assay performed on affected tissue that has been freshly frozen. The prognosis for all glycogen storage disorders is poor.

UREA CYCLE ENZYME DEFICIENCY

The urea cycle is the major pathway for ammonia detoxification and subsequent urea production. A congenital deficiency of a urea cycle enzyme results in hyperammonemia, protein intolerance, and HE. Urea cycle enzyme deficiency is rare in dogs but has been described.[156] Two young dogs with clinical signs of HE were diagnosed as having arginosuccinate synthetase deficiency by enzyme assay of hepatic tissue. Serum liver enzyme activity, BSP retention, and BUN were within normal limits. This diagnosis should be considered in young dogs and cats with hyperammonemia and HE in which primary hepatic disease, PSS, and hepatic microvascular dysplasia have been excluded. Treatment is symptomatic only (see Table 143–3).

HEPATIC AMYLOIDOSIS

Amyloidosis is a progressive systemic disease associated with extracellular deposition of insoluble fibrillar proteins, which results in organ dysfunction. Amyloidosis in dogs and cats is reactive and may be secondary to chronic infection, chronic inflammation, neoplasia, or an immune disorder. Amyloidosis is a familial disorder in the Chinese Shar Pei dog and in Abyssinian, Oriental, and Siamese cats.[157–159] In Chinese Shar Pei dogs, amyloidosis is associated with episodic fever and swollen hocks ("Shar Pei fever").[158, 160]

Although concurrent amyloid deposition in the kidneys, liver, spleen, and adrenal glands can occur, clinical manifestations of renal failure are most common. This is especially true for Abyssinian cats and Chinese Shar Pei dogs.[160, 161] Clinical and biochemical evidence of hepatic dysfunction occurs less frequently. Oriental and Siamese cats appear more likely to show clinical hepatic disease.[159] Occasionally, Chinese Shar Pei dogs present for signs associated with hepatic rather than renal amyloidosis.[157, 158] Clinical findings with hepatic involvement include anorexia, polyuria, polydipsia, vomiting, icterus, and hepatomegaly. When amyloidosis causes hepatic vascular fragility leading to hepatic rupture and hemoabdomen, findings include acute onset of lethargy, pale mucous membranes, and a hemorrhagic abdominal effusion.[158, 159]

Potential laboratory findings in dogs and cats with amyloidosis include azotemia and dilute urine (with renal involvement), proteinuria (with renal involvement in dogs), normal to increased ALP and ALT activity, hyperbilirubinemia, and increased SBA (with hepatic involvement). Anemia may be secondary to hepatic hemorrhage and rupture. Leukocytosis and left shift are common in Chinese Shar Pei dogs during a febrile episode. Coagulation tests are usually normal. Findings on abdominal radiographs may include hepatomegaly and possible abdominal effusion. Abdominocentesis reveals hemorrhagic abdominal effusion.

Diagnosis of hepatic amyloidosis requires liver biopsy with special stains (Congo red) to confirm its presence. In affected animals, the liver is pale, large, and friable with hemorrhages, hematomas, and capsular tears. Histologically, amyloid in the liver appears as a homogeneous, amorphous, eosinophilic material within the space of Disse and vessel walls.

Colchicine has been recommended for the treatment of amyloidosis because it may block formation of amyloid in the early phases. Dimethyl sulfoxide has been used experimentally in the treatment of amyloidosis to promote resorption of amyloid. A dose of 80 mg/kg as an 18 per cent solution in sterile water is given subcutaneously three times a week or 125 mg/kg by mouth twice a day. The unpleasant odor of dimethyl sulfoxide may limit owners' compliance.

REFERENCES

1. Batts KP, Ludwig J: Chronic hepatitis: An update on terminology and reporting. Am J Surg Pathol 19:1409, 1995.
2. Cullen JM: Hepatic histopathology for internists. Proceedings of the 15th ACVIM Forum, Lake Buena Vista, FL, May 1997, pp 39–41.
3. Sevelius E: Diagnosis and prognosis of chronic hepatitis and cirrhosis in dogs. J Small Anim Pract 36:521, 1995.
4. Hardy RM, et al: Chronic progressive hepatitis in Bedlington terriors associated with elevated liver copper concentrations. Minn Vet 15:13, 1975.
5. Twedt DC, et al: Clinical, morphologic, and chemical studies on copper toxicosis of Bedlington terriers. JAVMA 175:269, 1979.
6. Thornburg LP, et al: Hereditary copper toxicosis in West Highland white terriers. Vet Pathol 23:148, 1986.
7. Thornburg LP, et al: The relationship between hepatic copper content and morphologic changes in the liver of West Highland white terriers. Vet Pathol 33:656, 1996.
8. Johnson GF, et al: Chronic active hepatitis in Doberman pinschers. JAVMA 180:1438, 1982.
9. Crawford MA, et al: Chronic active hepatitis in 26 Doberman pinschers. JAVMA 187:1343, 1985.
10. Andersson M, Sevelius E: Breed, sex and age distribution in dogs with chronic liver disease: A demographic study. J Small Anim Pract 32:1, 1991.
11. Hardy RM: Chronic hepatitis in cocker spaniels—another syndrome? Proceedings of the 11th ACVIM Forum, Washington, DC, May 1993, pp 256–258.
12. Sevelius E, et al: Hepatic accumulation of alpha-1-antitrypsin in chronic liver disease in the dog. J Comp Pathol 111:401, 1994.
13. Haywood S, et al: Hepatitis and copper accumulation in Skye terriers. Vet Pathol 25:408, 1988.

LIV

14. Bennett AM, et al: Lobular dissecting hepatitis in the dog. Vet Pathol 20:179, 1983.
15. Jensen AL, Nielsen OL: Chronic hepatitis in three young standard poodles. J Vet Med A 38:194, 1991.
16. Strombeck DR, et al: Effects of corticosteroid treatment on survival time in dogs with chronic hepatitis: 151 cases (1977–1985). JAVMA 193:1109, 1988.
17. Andersson M, Sevelius E: Circulating autoantibodies in dogs with chronic liver disease. J Small Anim Pract 33:389, 1992.
18. Weiss DJ, et al: Anti–liver membrane protein antibodies in dogs with chronic hepatitis. J Vet Intern Med 9:267, 1995.
19. Poitout F, et al: Cell-mediated immune responses to liver membrane protein in canine chronic hepatitis. Vet Immunol Immunopathol 57:169, 1997.
20. Rolfe DS, Twedt DC: Copper-associated hepatopathies in dogs. Vet Clin North Am Small Anim Pract 25:399, 1995.
21. Thornburg LP, et al: Hepatic copper concentrations in purebred and mixed-breed dogs. Vet Pathol 27:81, 1990.
22. Twedt, DC: Cirrhosis: A consequence of chronic liver disease. Vet Clin North Am Small Anim Pract 15:151, 1985.
23. Biller DS, et al: Ultrasonography of diffuse liver disease. J Vet Intern Med 6:71, 1992.
24. Zawie DA, Gilbertson SR: Interpretation of canine liver biopsy. A clinician's perspective. Vet Clin North Am Small Anim Pract 15:67, 1985.
25. Center SA: Chronic hepatitis, cirrhosis, breed-specific hepatopathies, copper storage hepatopathy, suppurative hepatitis, granulomatous hepatitis, and idiopathic hepatic fibrosis. In Guilford WG, et al (eds): Strombeck's Small Animal Gastroenterology, 3rd ed. Philadelphia, WB Saunders, 1996, p 705.
26. Brewer GJ, et al: Use of zinc acetate to treat copper toxicosis in dogs. JAVMA 201:564, 1992.
27. Leveille CR, Arias IM: Pathophysiology and pharmacologic modulation of hepatic fibrosis. J Vet Intern Med 7:73, 1993.
28. Schuppan D, et al: Hepatic fibrosis—Therapeutic strategies. Digestion 59:385, 1998.
29. Britton RS, Bacon BR: Role of free radicals in liver diseases and hepatic fibrosis. Hepatogastroenterology 41:343, 1994.
30. Kershenobich D, et al: Colchicine in the treatment of cirrhosis of the liver. N Engl J Med 318:1709, 1988.
31. Boer HH, et al: Colchicine therapy for hepatic fibrosis in a dog. JAVMA 185:303, 1984.
32. Sokol RJ, et al: Oxidant injury to hepatic mitochondria in patients with Wilson's disease and Bedlington terriers with copper toxicosis. Gastroenterology 107:1788, 1994.
33. Saksena S, Tandon RK: Ursodeoxycholic acid in the treatment of liver diseases. Postgrad Med J 73:75, 1997.
34. Meyer DJ, et al: Use of ursodeoxycholic acid in a dog with chronic hepatitis: Effects on serum hepatic tests and endogenous bile acid composition. J Vet Intern Med 3:195, 1997.
35. Yuzbasiyan-Gurkan V, et al: Linkage of a microsatellite marker to the canine copper toxicosis locus in Bedlington terriers. Am J Vet Res 58:23, 1997.
36. Speeti M, et al: Subclinical versus clinical hepatitis in the Doberman: Evaluation of changes in blood parameters. J Small Anim Pract 37:465, 1996.
37. Speeti M, et al: Lesions of subclinical Doberman hepatitis. Vet Pathol 35:361, 1998.
38. Thornburg LP: Histomorphologic and immunohistochemical studies of chronic active hepatitis in Doberman pinschers. Vet Pathol 35:361, 1998.
39. Twedt DC: Copper chelator therapy. Proceedings of the 10th ACVIM Forum, San Diego, CA, May 1992, pp 53–55.
40. Gocke DJ et al: Experimental viral hepatitis in the dog: Production of persistent disease in partially immune dogs. J Clin Invest 46:1506, 1967.
41. Rakich PM et al: Immunohistochemical detection of canine adenovirus in paraffin sections of liver. Vet Pathol 23:478, 1986.
42. Chouinard L, et al: Use of polymerase chain reaction and immunohistochemistry for detection of canine adenovirus type I in formalin-fixed, paraffin-embedded liver of dogs with chronic hepatitis or cirrhosis. J Vet Diagn Invest 10: 320, 1998.
43. Jarrett WFH, O'Neil BW: A new transmissible agent causing acute hepatitis, chronic hepatitis and cirrhosis in dogs. Vet Rec 116:629, 1985.
44. Jarrett WFH, et al: Persistent hepatitis and chronic fibrosis induced by canine acidophil cell hepatitis virus. Vet Rec 120:234, 1987.
45. Bishop L, et al: Chronic active hepatitis in dogs associated with leptospires. Am J Vet Res 40:839, 1979.
46. Adamus C, et al: Chronic hepatitis associated with leptospiral infection in vaccinated beagles. J Comp Pathol 117:311, 1997.
47. Bunch SE, et al: Compromised hepatic function in dogs treated with anticonvulsant drugs. JAVMA 184:444, 1984.
48. Dayrell-Hart B, et al: Hepatotoxicity of phenobarbital in dogs: 18 cases (1985–1989). JAVMA 199:1060, 1991.
49. Bunch SE: Hepatotoxicity associated with pharmacologic agents in dogs and cats. Vet Clin North Am Small Anim Pract 23:659, 1993.
50. Podell M: Antiepileptic drug therapy. Clin Tech Small Anim Pract 13:185, 1998.
51. Hardy RM, et al: Periportal hepatitis associated with the use of a heartworm-hookworm preventative (diethylcarbamazine-oxibendazole) in 13 dogs. J Am Anim Hosp Assoc 25:419, 1989.
52. MacPhail CM, et al: Hepatocellular toxicosis associated with administration of carprofen in 21 dogs. JAVMA 212:1895, 1998.
53. van den Ingh TSGAM, Rothuizen J: Lobular dissecting hepatitis in juvenile and young adult dogs. J Vet Intern Med 8:217, 1994.
54. Forrester SD, et al: Cholangiohepatitis in a dog. JAVMA 200: 1704, 1992.
55. Center SA: Diseases of the gallbladder and biliary tree. In Guilford WG, et al (eds): Strombeck's Small Animal Gastroenterology, 3rd ed. Philadelphia, WB Saunders, 1996, p 860.
56. Rutgers HC, et al: Idiopathic hepatic fibrosis in 15 dogs. Vet Rec 133:115, 1993.
57. Van den Ingh TSGAM, et al: Portal hypertension associated with primary hypoplasia of the hepatic portal vein in dogs. Vet Rec 137:424, 1995.
58. Zawie DA, Garvey MS: Feline hepatic disease. Vet Clin North Am Small Anim Pract 14:1201, 1984.
59. Gagne JM, et al: Histopathologic evaluation of feline inflammatory liver disease. Vet Pathol 33:521, 1996.
60. Armstrong PJ, et al: Inflammatory liver disease. In August JR (ed): Consultations in Feline Internal Medicine—III. Philadelphia, WB Saunders, 1997, p 68.
61. Hirsch VM, Doige CE: Suppurative cholangitis in cats. JAVMA 182:1223, 1983.
62. Newell SM, et al: Correlations between ultrasonographic findings and specific hepatic diseases in cats: 72 cases (1985–1997). JAVMA 213:94, 1998.
63. Jackson MW, et al: Administration of vancomycin for treatment of ascending bacterial cholangiohepatitis in a cat. JAVMA 204:602, 1994.
64. Weiss DJ, et al: Relationship between inflammatory hepatic disease and inflammatory bowel disease, pancreatitis, and nephritis in cats. JAVMA 209:1114, 1996.
65. Prasse KW, et al: Chronic lymphocytic cholangitis in three cats. Vet Pathol 19:99, 1982.
66. Lucke VM, Davies JD: Progressive lymphocytic cholangitis in the cat. J Small Anim Pract 25:249, 1984.
67. Day MJ: Immunohistochemical characterization of the lesions of feline progressive lymphocytic cholangitis/cholangiohepatitis. J Comp Pathol 119:135, 1998.
68. Day DG, et al: Evaluation of total serum bile acid concentration and bile acid profiles in healthy cats after oral administration of ursodeoxycholic acid. Am J Vet Res 55:1474, 1994.
69. Center SA, et al: Historical, physical examination, and clinicopathologic features of portosystemic vascular anomalies in the dog and cat. Semin Vet Med Surg (Small Anim) 5:83, 1990.
70. Johnson CA, et al: Congenital portosystemic shunts in dogs: 46 cases (1979–1986). JAVMA 191:1478, 1987.
71. Meyer HP, et al: Increasing incidence of hereditary intrahepatic portosystemic shunts in Irish wolfhounds in the Netherlands (1984 to 1992). Vet Rec 136:13, 1995.
72. Schermerhorn T, et al: Characterization of hepatoportal microvascular dysplasia in a kindred of Cairn terriers. J Vet Intern Med 10:219, 1996.
73. Johnson SE: Portal hypertension. Part I. Pathophysiology and clinical consequences. Compend Contin Educ 9:741, 1987.
74. Lamb CR, White RN: Morphology of congenital intrahepatic portocaval shunts in dogs and cats. Vet Rec 142:55, 1998.
75. Martin RA: Congenital portosystemic shunts in the dog and cat. Vet Clin North Am Small Anim Pract 23:609, 1993.
76. Bostwick DR, et al: Intrahepatic and extrahepatic portal venous anomalies in dogs: 52 cases (1982–1992). JAVMA 206:1181, 1995.
77. Schunk CM: Feline portosystemic shunts. Semin Vet Med Surg (Small Anim) 12:45, 1997.
78. Tisdall PLC, et al: Congenital portosystemic shunts in Maltese and Australian cattle dogs. Aust Vet J 71:174, 1994.
79. Levy JK et al: Feline portosystemic vascular shunts. In Bonagura JD (ed): Kirk's Current Veterinary Therapy, Small Animal Practice XII. Philadelphia, WB Saunders, 1995, pp 743–748.
80. Harvey J, Erb HN: Complete ligation of extrahepatic congenital portosystemic shunts in nonencephalopathic dogs. Vet Surg 27:413, 1998.
81. Meyer HP, Rothuizen J: Increased free cortisol in plasma of dogs with portosystemic encephalopathy (PSE). Domest Anim Endocrinol 11:317, 1994.
82. Phillips L, et al: Hepatic microvascular dysplasia in dogs. Prog Vet Neurol 7:88, 1996.
83. Center SA, et al: Liver function tests in the diagnosis of portosystemic vascular anomalies. Semin Vet Med Surg (Small Anim) 5:94, 1990.
84. Bunch SE, et al: Characterization of iron status in young dogs with portosystemic vascular anomalies. Am J Vet Res 56:853, 1995.
85. Simpson KW, et al: Iron status and erythrocyte volume in dogs with congenital portosystemic vascular anomalies. J Vet Intern Med 11:14, 1997.
86. Meyer HP, et al: Transient metabolic hyperammonaemia in young Irish wolfhounds. Vet Rec 138:105, 1996.
87. Holt DE, et al: Correlation of ultrasonographic findings with surgical, portographic, and necropsy findings in dogs and cats with portosystemic shunts: 63 cases (1987–1993). JAVMA 207:1190, 1995.
88. Swalec KM, et al: Partial versus complete attenuation of single portosystemic shunts. Vet Surg 19:406, 1990.
89. Van Gundy TE, et al: Results of surgical management of feline portosystemic shunts. J Am Anim Hosp Assoc 26:55, 1990.
90. Koblik PD, Hornof WJ: Transcolonic sodium pertechnetate Tc 99m scintigraphy for diagnosis of macrovascular portosystemic shunts in dogs, cats, and potbellied pigs: 176 cases (1988–1992). JAVMA 207:729, 1995.
91. Forster-van Hijfte MA, et al: Per rectal portal scintigraphy in the diagnosis and management of feline portosystemic shunts. J Small Anim Pract 37:7, 1996.
92. Van Vechten BJ, et al: Use of transcolonic portal scintigraphy to monitor blood flow and progressive postoperative attenuation of partially ligated single extrahepatic portosystemic shunts in dogs. JAVMA 204:1770, 1994.
93. Bauer JE: Diet selection and special considerations in the management of hepatic diseases. JAVMA 210:625, 1997.

94. Morgan MY: The treatment of chronic hepatic encephalopathy. Hepatogastroenterology 38:377, 1991.

95. Garcia-Compeau D, et al: Fiber content rather than protein determines tolerance to nitrogen load in chronic portal systemic encephalopathy: A randomized trial. Hepatology 7:1034, 1987.

96. Clausen MR, Mortensen PB: Lactulose, disaccharides, and colonic flora. Drugs 53:930, 1997.

97. Butler LM, et al: Surgical management of extrahepatic portosystemic shunts in the dog and cat. Semin Vet Med Surg (Small Anim) 5:127, 1990.

98. Birchard SJ: Management of congenital portosystemic shunts. Proceedings of the 17th Annual OSU/Waltham Symposium, Columbus, OH, 1993, pp 51–55.

99. Hottinger HA, et al: Long-term results of complete and partial ligation of congenital portosystemic shunts in dogs. Vet Surg 24:331, 1995.

100. Komtebedde J, et al: Long-term clinical outcome after partial ligation of single extrahepatic vascular anomalies in 20 dogs. Vet Surg 24:379, 1995.

101. Vogt JC, et al: Gradual occlusion of extrahepatic portosystemic shunts in dogs and cats using the ameroid constrictor. Vet Surg 25:495, 1996.

102. Partington BP, et al: Transvenous coil embolization for treatment of patent ductus venosus in a dog. JAVMA 202:281, 1993.

103. Komtebedde J, et al: Intrahepatic portosystemic venous anomaly in the dog. Perioperative management and complications. Vet Surg 20:37, 1991.

104. Johnson SE: Portal hypertension. Part II. Clinical assessment and treatment. Compend Contin Educ 9:917, 1987.

105. Matushek KJ, et al: Generalized motor seizures after portosystemic shunt ligation in dogs: Five cases (1981–1988). JAVMA 196:2014, 1990.

106. Hardie EM, et al: Status epilepticus after ligation of portosystemic shunts. Vet Surg 19:412, 1990.

107. Aronson LR, et al: Endogenous benzodiazepine activity in the peripheral and portal blood of dogs with congenital portosystemic shunts. Vet Surg 26:189, 1997.

108. Roy RG, et al: Portal vein thrombosis as a complication of portosystemic shunt ligation in two dogs. J Am Anim Hosp Assoc 28:53, 1992.

109. Lawrence D, et al: Results of surgical management of portosystemic shunts in dogs: 20 cases (1985–1990). JAVMA 201:1750, 1992.

110. Center SA: Hepatic vascular diseases. In Guilford WG, et al (eds): Strombeck's Small Animal Gastroenterology, 3rd ed. Philadelphia, WB Saunders, 1996, p 802.

111. Baer KE, et al: Hepatic vascular dysplasia in dogs and cats (105 cases). Proceedings of the 42nd Annual Meeting of the American College of Veterinary Pathology, Orlando, FL, 1991, p 71.

112. Allen L, et al: Clinicopathologic features of dogs with hepatic microvascular dysplasia with and without portosystemic shunts: 42 cases (1991–1996). JAVMA 214:218, 1999.

113. Whiting PG, et al: Partial hepatectomy with temporary hepatic vascular occlusion in dogs with hepatic arteriovenous fistulas. Vet Surg 15:171, 1986.

114. Rand JS, et al: Portosystemic vascular shunts in a family of American cocker spaniels. J Am Anim Hosp Assoc 24:265, 1988.

115. DeMarco J, et al: A syndrome resembling idiopathic noncirrhotic portal hypertension in 4 young Doberman pinschers. J Vet Intern Med 12:147, 1998.

116. Bunch SE: Noncirrhotic portal hypertension in 27 dogs. In press.

117. Willard MD, et al: Obstructed portal venous flow and portal vein thrombus in a dog. JAVMA 194:1449, 1989.

118. Van Winkle TJ, Bruce E: Thrombosis of the portal vein in eleven dogs. Vet Pathol 30:28, 1993.

119. Booth HW, et al: Multiple extrahepatic portosystemic shunts in dogs: 30 cases (1981–1993). JAVMA 208:1849, 1996.

120. Moore PF, Whiting PG: Hepatic lesions associated with intrahepatic arterioportal fistulae in dogs. Vet Pathol 23:57, 1986.

121. Schermerhorn T, et al: Suspected microscopic hepatic arteriovenous fistulae in a young dog. JAVMA 211:70, 1997.

122. Bailey MQ, et al: Ultrasonographic findings associated with congenital hepatic arteriovenous fistula in three dogs. JAVMA 192:1099, 1988.

123. Whiting PG, Peterson SL: Portosystemic shunts. In Slatter D (ed): Textbook of Small Animal Surgery, 2nd ed, Vol I. Philadelphia, WB Saunders, 1993, p 660.

124. Cornelius LM, Mahaffey MB: Kinking of the intrathoracic caudal vena cava in five dogs. J Small Anim Pract 26:67, 1985.

125. Miller MW, et al: Budd-Chiari–like syndrome in two dogs. J Am Anim Hosp Assoc 25:277, 1989.

126. Macintire DK, et al: Budd-Chiari syndrome in a kitten, caused by membranous obstruction of the caudal vena cava. J Am Anim Hosp Assoc 31:484, 1995.

127. Fine DM, et al: Surgical correction of late-onset Budd-Chiari–like syndrome in a dog. JAVMA 212:835, 1998.

128. Cohn LA, et al: Intrahepatic postsinusoidal venous obstruction in a dog. J Vet Intern Med 5:317, 1991.

129. Kelly WR: The liver and biliary system. In Jubb KVF, et al (eds): Pathology of Domestic Animals, 4th ed, Vol 2. New York, Academic Press, 1993, pp 319–406.

130. Boyer TD: Portal hypertension and bleeding esophageal varices. In Zakim D, Boyer TD (eds): Hepatology, a Textbook of Liver Disease, 2nd ed, Vol 1. Philadelphia, WB Saunders, 1990, pp 572–615.

131. Bergman JR: Nodular hyperplasia in the liver of the dog: An association with changes in the Ito cell population. Vet Pathol 22:427, 1985.

132. Stowater JL, et al: Ultrasonographic features of canine hepatic nodular hyperplasia. Vet Radiol 31:268, 1990.

133. Hammer AS, Sikkema DA: Hepatic neoplasia in the dog and cat. Vet Clin North Am Small Anim Pract 25:419, 1995.

134. Post G, Patnaik AK: Nonhematopoietic hepatic neoplasms in cats: 21 cases (1983–1988). JAVMA 201:1080, 1992.

135. Patnaik AK: A morphologic and immunocytochemical study of hepatic neoplasms in cats. Vet Pathol 29:405, 1992.

136. Trout NJ, et al: Surgical treatment of hepatobiliary cystadenomas in cats: Five cases (1988–1993). JAVMA 206:505, 1995.

137. Adler R, Wilson DW: Biliary cystadenoma of cats. Vet Pathol 32:415, 1995.

138. Evans SM: The radiographic appearance of primary liver neoplasia in dogs. Vet Radiol 28:192, 1987.

139. Kosovsky JE, et al: Results of partial hepatectomy in 18 dogs with hepatocellular carcinoma. J Am Anim Hosp Assoc 25:203, 1989.

140. Krotje LJ, et al: Acquired myasthenia gravis and cholangiocellular carcinoma in a dog. JAVMA 197:488, 1990.

141. Liefer CE, et al: Hypoglycemia associated with nonislet cell tumor in 13 dogs. JAVMA 186:53, 1985.

142. Thompson JC, et al: Observations on hypoglycemia associated with hepatoma in a cat. N Z Vet J 43:186, 1995.

143. Lowseth LA, et al: Detection of serum alpha-fetoprotein in dogs with hepatic tumors. JAVMA 199:735, 1991.

144. Whiteley MB, et al: Ultrasonographic appearance of primary and metastatic canine hepatic tumors. A review of 48 cases. J Ultrasound Med 8:621, 1989.

145. Nyland TG: Ultrasonographic patterns of canine hepatic lymphosarcoma. Vet Radiol 25:167, 1984.

146. Nyland TG, Hager DA: Sonography of the liver, gallbladder, and spleen. Vet Clin North Am Small Anim Pract 15:6, 1985.

147. McKenna SC, Carpenter JL: Polycystic disease of the kidney and liver in the Cairn terrier. Vet Pathol 17:436, 1980.

148. Van Den Ingh TSGAM, Rothuizen J: Congenital cystic disease of the liver in seven dogs. J Comp Pathol 95:405, 1985.

149. Berry CR, et al: Iatrogenic biloma (biliary pseudocyst) in a cat with hepatic lipidosis. Vet Radiol Ultrasound 33:145, 1992.

150. McAloose D, et al: Polycystic kidney and liver disease in two related West Highland white terrier litters. Vet Pathol 35:77, 1998.

151. Eaton KA, et al: Autosomal dominant polycystic kidney disease in Persian and Persian-cross cats. Vet Pathol 34:117, 1997.

152. Ghishan FK, Greene HL: Inborn errors of metabolism that lead to permanent liver injury. In Zakim D, Boyer TD (eds): Hepatology, a Textbook of Liver Disease, 2nd ed, Vol 2. New York, WB Saunders, 1990, pp 1300–1348.

153. Brix AE, et al: Glycogen storage disease type Ia in two littermate Maltese puppies. Vet Pathol 32:460, 1995.

154. Kishnani PS, et al: Isolation and nucleotide sequence of canine glucose-6-phosphatase mRNA: Identification of mutation in puppies with glycogen storage disease type Ia. Biochem Mol Med 61:168, 1997.

155. Walvoort HC, et al: Canine glycogen storage disease type II: A clinical study of four affected Lapland dogs. J Am Anim Hosp Assoc 20:279, 1984.

156. Strombeck DR, et al: Hyperammonemia due to a urea cycle enzyme deficiency in 2 dogs. JAVMA 166:1109, 1975.

157. Loeven KO: Hepatic amyloidosis in two Chinese Shar Pei dogs. JAVMA 204:1212, 1994.

158. Loeven KO: Spontaneous hepatic rupture secondary to amyloidosis in a Chinese Shar Pei. J Am Anim Hosp Assoc 30:577, 1994.

159. van der Linde-Sipman JS, et al: Generalized AA-amyloidosis in Siamese and Oriental cats. Vet Immunol Immunopathol 56:1, 1997.

160. DiBartola SP, et al: Familial renal amyloidosis in Chinese Shar Pei dogs. JAVMA 197:483, 1990.

161. DiBartola SP, et al: Tissue distribution of amyloid deposits in Abyssinian cats with familial amyloidosis. J Comp Pathol 96:387, 1986.

LIV

CHAPTER 144

ACUTE HEPATIC DISORDERS AND SYSTEMIC DISORDERS THAT INVOLVE THE LIVER

Susan E. Bunch

ACUTE HEPATIC DISORDERS

Acute hepatic injury pertains to illness of generally less than or equal to 2 weeks' duration with no previous evidence of hepatobiliary disease. A partial list of recognized causes of acute hepatic injury associated with substantial liver-specific abnormalities in physical examination and laboratory test results in dogs and cats is given in Table 144–1; often a specific cause cannot be identified. In these condi-

TABLE 144–1. CLINICALLY RELEVANT ACUTE HEPATIC DISORDERS IN DOGS AND CATS

CATEGORY	EXAMPLE(S)
Toxic injury	Therapeutic agents
	Acetaminophen (cat)
	Carprofen (dog)*
	Tetracycline (cat and dog)
	Trimethoprim-sulfa (dog)*
	Diazepam (cat)*
	Methimazole, glipizide (cat)
	Mebendazole (dog)[8]*
	Thiacetarsamide (dog)[16, 17]
	Diethylcarbamazine-oxibendazole (dog)[18, 19]
	Diethylcarbamazine in dogs with microfilaria[20]*
	Methoxyflurane, halothane (dog)[21, 22]*
	Griseofulvin (cat)[23]
	Imidocarb dipropionate (dog)[24]*
	Closantel (dog)[25]*
	Iron-containing supplements[26]
	Plants, insects, and chemicals (primarily dogs)
	Mushrooms (*Amanita phalloides, A. verna*)*
	Cycad palm seeds (Cycadaceae sp.)*
	Chinaberry tree (*Melia azedarach*)*
	Heavy metals and industrial compounds
	Envenomation (Hymenoptera sp. [hornet stings])
	Aflatoxin[27, 28]
Metabolic disturbance	Lipidosis (cat)*
Traumatic injury	Automobile accident
	High-rise syndrome
	Horse kick
Thermal insult	Heatstroke[174, 175]
Vascular compromise	Liver lobe infarction resulting from torsion or entrapment
	Vena caval syndrome associated with heartworm disease[176, 177]
Cytopathic infectious agents	Infectious canine hepatitis*
	Canine acidophil hepatitis (Britain)*
	Helicobacter canis

*Reported to cause severe acute hepatic injury potentially resulting in death.

tions, it is clear that hepatic injury is a major contributor to, if not solely responsible for, the animal's illness.

The spectrum of acute hepatic injury can range widely. Multifocal single-cell hepatocyte necrosis associated with abnormal serum liver enzyme activity is usually clinically silent and is discovered during routine evaluation or pursuit of other problems, such as some of the disorders listed in Table 144–2. At the opposite end of the spectrum is *acute hepatic failure* (AHF), which occurs when there has been sudden, massive loss of previously normal hepatocyte mass sufficient to result in multiple function loss and potentially death before therapeutic intervention can occur.[1–4] The worst possible form of AHF in animals with naturally occurring disease probably resembles a rare but devastating form of hepatic failure in human patients, *fulminant hepatic failure* (FHF).[5, 6] In this condition, AHF is associated with the development of hepatic encephalopathy (HE) within 8 weeks of the onset of signs attributable to hepatocellular dysfunction.[5, 6] An alternative definition suggests that FHF is associated with the development of HE within 2 weeks of the onset of jaundice.[7] Although there are variations on this theme according to the duration of illness and country of origin in human medicine,[3, 6] such further subdivision into late-onset or hyperacute forms has not been considered for use in animals. There are numerous reviews of AHF in human medicine, but there is little original information in the veterinary literature about the overall incidence, common causes, and outcome of AHF in animals. Information about AHF in animals exists in the form of case descriptions of animals with a particular cause, such as mebendazole toxicity,[8] or in controlled laboratory investigations (e.g., using carbon tetrachloride[9, 10] or dimethylnitrosamine[11, 12]) conducted for the purpose of understanding the pathophysiology of AHF. Regardless of the cause, the predominant histologic lesion is necrosis. Of the causes listed in Table 144–1, toxic and thermal injuries are most likely to inflict sufficient damage to cause AHF and even death. Severe idiopathic hepatic lipidosis, although not causing widespread necrosis, could be considered another cause in cats. In addition to HE, other complications accompany widespread hepatocellular necrosis in human patients (Table 144–3), the most life threatening of which is cerebral edema and brain stem herniation, followed by coagulopathy.[5] Review of the clinical and experimental veterinary literature suggests that this is also generally true in cats and dogs. Because there is no preexisting hepatic compromise, the chance for complete recovery is good, assuming the pathogenetic insult has been removed, the patient survives the initial insult, there has been less than

TABLE 144–2. SYSTEMIC DISORDERS WITH CLINICALLY RELEVANT HEPATIC INVOLVEMENT

CATEGORY OF DISORDER	EXAMPLE(S)*
Extension of abdominal inflammation	Pancreatitis (cat, dog)
	Peritonitis of any kind (cat, dog)
	Inflammatory bowel disease (cat, dog), lymphangiectasia
Endocrine disease	Hyperthyroidism (cat)
	Hypercortisolism (Cushing's syndrome; dog)
	Glucocorticoid insufficiency (dog)
	Diabetes mellitus (cat, dog)
	Hypothyroidism (dog)
Secondary portal vein thrombosis	Severe immune-mediated hemolytic anemia (dog)
	Cushing's syndrome (dog)
	Pancreatic necrosis (cat, dog)
	Chronic hepatic disease with portal hypertension (dog)
	Peritonitis of any kind (cat, dog)
	Nonhepatobiliary neoplasia (dog)
Infectious disease[81]	Bacterial
	Cholestasis associated with extrahepatic infection (dog)
	Bacterial abscess(es) (dog)
	Leptospirosis (cat, dog)
	Tularemia (cat, dog)
	Brucellosis (dog)
	Tyzzer's disease (cat, dog)
	Fungal, algal
	Histoplasmosis (cat, dog)
	Blastomycosis (cat, dog)
	Disseminated aspergillosis (dog)
	Protothecosis (dog)
	Protozoal
	Toxoplasmosis (cat, dog)
	Neospora caninum (dog)
	Hepatozoon canis
	Leishmaniasis (dog)
	Cytauxzoonosis (cat)
	Viral and rickettsial
	Feline infectious peritonitis
	Herpesvirus (canine neonates)
	Canine ehrlichiosis
	Canine Rocky Mountain spotted fever
Other	Superficial necrolytic dermatitis
	Amyloidosis

*Listed in order of the "drama" of the hepatic involvement, considering the clinical signs, physical examination findings, laboratory features, and histopathologic changes.

50 per cent permanent loss of functional mass, and the liver has retained its capacity to regenerate.

CAUSES—HISTORY, PHYSICAL EXAMINATION, AND PRELIMINARY TEST RESULTS

Toxic Injury—Therapeutic Agents

Adverse hepatic reactions to *therapeutic agents* have been reviewed.[13–15] Information about acute drug reactions in dogs and cats has been accumulated from a mixture of single or a small number of case reports, reports of adverse reactions to drugs to the Center for Veterinary Medicine at the Food and Drug Administration, and the old literature. It is believed that most of these reactions occur as a result of individual idiosyncrasies in drug metabolism, yielding injurious metabolites, or accidental overdose. New information about known adverse hepatic reactions and several new adverse reactions associated with drugs currently in widespread clinical use are discussed in detail in the following. For information

about hepatotoxic reactions described previously, the reader is encouraged to consult earlier reviews[13–15] and the references provided in Table 144–1.[8, 16–28] Because the list of agents believed to cause acute hepatic injury in dogs and cats is long and the true prevalence of documented drug reactions is unknown, drugs should be suspected in any dog or cat with evidence of acute hepatic injury.

Acetaminophen (APAP) is likely to be found on the shelf in many homes because of its analgesic and antipyretic benefits in human medicine. Dogs and cats can tolerate single doses up to 45 mg/lb and 27 mg/lb, respectively, with minimal clinical and hematologic consequences and without changes in blood levels of glutathione. Overproduction of reactive metabolites of APAP rapidly depletes available liver and erythrocyte glutathione.[29, 30] Massive doses that resemble those taken by humans during suicide attempts (410 mg/lb) cause lethal AHF in dogs.[31] Toxicity results when glutathione stores are consumed to 30 per cent of normal, allowing reactive metabolites to bind covalently to vital cellular macromolecules.[29] The potentially lethal toxic effect of APAP overdose in both dogs and cats is cyanosis resulting from severe methemoglobinemia, which occurs 24 to 36 hours before hepatic injury. The blood from poisoned animals is brown in color, and there are large numbers of Heinz bodies. Overall, clinical toxicity is more severe in cats because they have a relative deficiency of hepatic glucuronyltransferase activity and are unable to accelerate excretion of excess APAP by forming glucuronide conjugates.[32] Seventeen cats with APAP intoxication were identified over a 12-year period and their cases reviewed.[33] Owners administered APAP (dosage range 4.5 to 182 mg/lb) to their mostly middle-aged cats because of perceived pain or illness. Most cats (more than 59 per cent) were depressed, dyspneic, and had pale or muddy mucous membranes; biochemical evidence of hepatic injury was detected in 35 per cent. All cats were treated supportively and received the recommended antidotal protocol (see Specific Treatment). Cats that were treated within 24 hours of APAP ingestion survived (12 of 17 cats) with no lasting consequences. The median dose for cats that survived (77 mg/lb) was higher than that for cats that died (45 mg/lb), underscoring the need for early therapeutic intervention regardless of dose.

In response to increasing demand for safe, effective, orally administered analgesic preparations for treatment of osteoarthritis and other painful musculoskeletal conditions, several new nonsteroidal anti-inflammatory drugs have been developed and approved for use in dogs. One such preparation, *carprofen*, was believed to be responsible for acute hepatic-

TABLE 144–3. COMPLICATIONS OF ACUTE HEPATIC FAILURE IN HUMAN PATIENTS

Hepatic encephalopathy
Cerebral edema, brain stem herniation
Coagulopathy
Cardiac dysrhythmias
Hypotension
Hypoxemia
Pulmonary edema
Refractory adult respiratory distress syndrome
Functional renal failure (hepatorenal syndrome)
Sepsis
Metabolic abnormalities
    Hypoglycemia
    Mixed acid-base disturbances
    Hypokalemia
    Hyponatremia

LIV

related illness in 21 dogs, 13 of which were Labrador retrievers.[34] Signs developed in 18 dogs within 30 days of initiation and in the Labrador retrievers after at least 14 days from administration. Forty per cent of the dogs received higher than recommended dosages. Predominant clinical signs and physical examination findings consisted of anorexia (17 dogs), vomiting (16 dogs), jaundice (15 dogs), lethargy (8 dogs), and diarrhea (8 dogs). Consistent clinicopathologic features were high serum liver enzyme activities (alanine transaminase [ALT], 21 of 21 dogs, 10 to 50 times high normal; aspartate transaminase [AST], 14 of 15 dogs, 1.4 to 21 times high normal; and alkaline phosphatase [AP], 20 of 21 dogs, 1.2 to 45 times high normal) and bilirubin concentration (18 of 21 dogs, 1.5 to 70 times high normal). Six of nine dogs also had evidence of acute renal injury (proteinuria, glucosuria, and cylindruria) by urinalysis. The liver was slightly enlarged in three dogs and somewhat smaller than normal in four dogs. Liver biopsy results for 18 dogs were consistent with mild multifocal to extensive hepatocellular necrosis, ballooning degeneration, and apoptosis. Bridging necrosis with lobular collapse was seen in most of the liver biopsy specimens, with secondary changes including mild mixed inflammatory cell infiltrates, bridging fibrosis, biliary hyperplasia, aggregates of debris-laden macrophages, accumulation of bile pigment, and extramedullary hematopoiesis. Seventeen dogs recovered completely with intensive supportive care (fluid therapy, antibiotics, antiulcer medications, vitamin supplementation) after up to 7 days in the hospital, and four dogs died or were euthanatized within the first 3 to 5 days after hospitalization because of clinical disease severity. Six dogs had biochemical evidence of residual mild hepatic dysfunction. Several dogs had received other potentially hepatotoxic drugs at some time in their lives, including primidone, diethylstilbestrol, and phenylbutazone. The actual role of these agents in the development of hepatotoxicity in these dogs is unclear, but the temporal relationships between initiation of carprofen administration, onset of illness attributable to acute hepatic injury, and recovery after drug discontinuation and supportive care were conspicuous. The frequency of side effects of carprofen administration was considered extremely low before its release, but the prevalence of deleterious reactions has increased in association with widespread use. Because of the lack of correlation between dosage and duration of administration, magnitude of clinicopathologic abnormalities, and histologic severity of the hepatic lesions, it is believed that in these 21 dogs, carprofen was responsible for an idiosyncratic cytotoxic hepatocellular reaction. Dogs with evidence of preexisting renal or hepatic compromise may be poor candidates for treatment with carprofen.

Certain antibiotics have also been reported to cause acute hepatic injury. Treatment with *tetracycline*[35] for a presumptive diagnosis of hemobartonellosis in a middle-aged cat resulted in a 7-fold elevation of serum ALT activity above pretreatment values after 3 days of administration and a 15-fold elevation after 10 days. Clinical signs at the time were anorexia and constant salivation. Centrilobular fibrosis, mild diffuse cholangiohepatitis, and mild lipidosis were the pertinent liver biopsy findings. Treatment in addition to discontinuing tetracycline included forced enteral nutrition via tube gastrostomy and vitamin E and selenium supplementation (given for treatment and prevention of tetracycline hepatotoxicity derived from experimental studies) for the initial 13 days. Recovery was considered complete by 45 days after tetracycline administration was suspended. Although the histologic lesions were not characteristic of most causes of acute hepatic injury (e.g., necrosis), they were, in part, compatible with changes ascribed to tetracycline hepatotoxicity in experimental investigations of microvesicular lipid accumulation,[36] and the time course of illness and relationship to drug administration were convincing. Two types of adverse hepatic reactions have been attributed to *trimethoprim-sulfonamide* administration. One, a seemingly reversible cholestatic hepatopathy described in three single case reports, developed after 2 weeks of trimethoprim-sulfadiazine administration.[37-39] One dog had been given the drug twice previously without incident and was receiving other medications concurrently (prednisone and cyclophosphamide) for treatment of myeloma. Each of the affected dogs had nonspecific signs of illness (i.e., lethargy, anorexia, and vomiting) followed soon after by jaundice and laboratory evidence of acute hepatic injury. One dog underwent liver biopsy; mixed inflammatory cell infiltrates primarily within portal triads, dilated bile canaliculi, and mild vacuolar changes in the hepatocytes surrounding the terminal hepatic venules were observed. All dogs recovered after drug administration was stopped and supportive care given. A more serious adverse hepatic reaction characterized by lethal AHF was described in five dogs, four of which had been given trimethoprim-sulfamethoxazole.[40, 41] Illness developed within 1 week in three of the four dogs; there did not appear to be a dose relationship. Submassive hepatocellular necrosis in the periacinar (periportal) and midzonal areas was seen histologically.

An alert regarding severe, usually fatal hepatotoxicity in seven apparently healthy cats treated with conventional dosages of *diazepam* for behavior modification was first made by the American Association of Feline Practitioners in 1993.[42] All cats became ill within 8 to 9 days of starting oral administration of diazepam (either generic or trademarked formulations), and most died despite aggressive medical care. Since then, 23 more cases have been recorded,[43] and an in-depth report on 11 cats has been published.[44] Adult to middle-aged neutered cats were given diazepam most often because of inappropriate urination or aggression. The dosage ranged from 1 mg once daily to 2.5 mg twice daily. Cats became ill after 5 days of treatment. Clinicopathologic features of most cats were consistent with severe acute hepatic injury and failure (indicated by coagulopathy, hypocholesterolemia, and hypoglycemia) and only 1 of the 11 cats survived. As expected, centrilobular to massive necrosis was found. In addition, suppurative cholangitis and moderate to marked biliary hyperplasia were noted, which remain unexplained. To understand why this devastating drug reaction had apparently gone unnoticed for years, a retrospective study of all feline necropsies performed at a university over a 9-year period was undertaken in an attempt to identify all cats with severe, acute centrilobular hepatic necrosis.[45] When cats with anemia were eliminated, nine cases were identified, eight of which had received diazepam or a relative, zolazepam. The clinical course of these cases was similar to those reported previously.

Adverse hepatic reactions to several medications used to control endocrine conditions in cats have also been reported. A small percentage (1.5 per cent) of hyperthyroid cats treated with *methimazole* developed a hepatopathy characterized by anorexia, vomiting, lethargy, and high serum liver enzyme activities (6 to 27 times high normal ALT, 3 to 6 times high normal AST, and 2 to 5 times high normal AP) and bilirubin concentration (3.5 to 8 mg/dL).[46] Illness is apparent within 2 months of treatment and resolves when treatment with methimazole is stopped, although it may take several weeks.

Liver biopsy of one cat showed hepatocellular degeneration and necrosis. Similar reactions can occur with similar infrequency (6 per cent) after administration of propylthiouracil.[47] Although not available in the United States at this time, carbimazole (a derivative of methimazole) is believed to cause fewer side effects than methimazole or propylthiouracil.[48] Insulin injection is the most common approach for treatment of diabetes mellitus in cats. Some cats, however, may respond to oral hypoglycemic agents, the most frequently prescribed of which is the sulfonylurea *glipizide*. High serum liver enzyme activities and jaundice have been reported to occur in 8 per cent[49] to 21 per cent[50] of diabetic cats within 2 to 4 weeks after starting glipizide treatment. Reactions ranged from asymptomatic mild increases in serum liver enzyme activities that did not warrant drug suspension,[49] to moderate to severe illness that resolved within 5 days after treatment was stopped.[50] In one study,[50] glipizide was successfully reintroduced beginning with a low dose (1.25 mg once daily) and the dose was gradually increased to that being given at the time the adverse hepatic reaction occurred (5 mg twice daily).

Toxic Injury—Plants, Insects, and Chemicals

It is not unusual for dogs to ingest a variety of plant products by accident and suffer only mild consequences of gastrointestinal irritation such as vomiting and diarrhea that remit rapidly with conservative treatment. Ingestion of as little as one bite-sized fragment of certain species of *mushrooms* (e.g., *Amanita phalloides, Amanita verna,* and *Gyromitra* sp.), however, can result in massive hepatic necrosis and death in adult humans and experimental animals.[51–53] These mushrooms are found throughout North America growing under trees; toxicities in human[52] and canine[54, 55] patients occur most often during the months of June through October. The toxic principle is a group of heat-stable cyclic octapeptides, which account for only 0.1 to 0.4 per cent of the mushroom's weight. One particular toxin, alpha-amanitin, is responsible for the most tissue injury, and the lethal dose is 0.045 mg/lb. Whereas most drug-induced hepatotoxicities occur as a result of individual idiosyncrasy, alpha-amanitin predictably causes hepatocellular death by inhibiting messenger ribonucleic acid (mRNA) synthesis. In experimental canine studies, gastrointestinal signs (vomiting and bloody diarrhea) were seen within about 16 hours after ingestion of mushroom extract.[56] These signs abated after about 48 hours, at which time the acute, severe hepatic effects became obvious (jaundice and coagulopathy). Although much of the ingested dose is excreted renally without repercussion in dogs, significant amounts of alpha-amanitin enter the enterohepatic circulation, which enhances hepatic toxicity.[56]

Dogs living in the southern United States or Hawaii that have a taste for seeds and other parts of the *cycad palm tree* are at risk for development of serious hepatic and neurologic sequelae.[57, 58] The plant is found naturally in Florida but is also available as a cultivated ornamental plant. The toxic agent responsible for hepatic and gastrointestinal disease is a by-product of cycasin (methylazoxymethanol), which is found in high concentration in seeds. The clinical course appears similar to that of amatoxicosis; persistent vomiting and diarrhea and abdominal pain are observed within 12 hours after seed ingestion, followed in 2 to 3 days by clinical and laboratory evidence of acute severe hepatic injury and failure (i.e., high serum liver enzyme activities, jaundice, coagulopathy, and encephalopathy). About 50 per cent of intoxicated dogs also develop neurologic signs such as ataxia, proprioceptive deficits, and seizures. It is not known whether these are a reflection of hepatic failure and HE or of direct neurotoxicity. Unlike dogs with amatoxicosis, most dogs ill because of cycad ingestion appear to recover after intensive supportive care.

Two separate instances in which a puppy became ill and died within 48 hours of ingestion of fallen fruit from the *chinaberry tree* have been reported.[59] The principal toxins are believed to be tetranortriterpene meliatoxins A_1, A_2, B_1, and B_2, which are enterotoxic and neurotoxic. Although the predominant clinical signs involved the gastrointestinal tract and nervous system, congestion, hemorrhage, and fatty degeneration were found in liver and kidney tissue sections.

In a study published over 30 years ago, more human fatalities were attributed to stings from *hymenopteran insects* (bees, wasps, and hornets) than to any other venomous bite.[60] Unique hypersensitivity accounts for severe systemic allergic reactions associated with any number of stings, but multiple stings usually result in toxic reactions.[61] Three dogs were believed to have suffered severe systemic reactions after multiple hornet or bee stings.[62] The owners of two of the dogs witnessed the insect swarm, and dead hornets were found in the haircoat of the third dog on physical examination. Inflammatory leukon (three of three dogs), azotemia (two of three dogs), and high serum ALT activity (three of three dogs; range, 444 to 16,484 IU/L) were typical laboratory findings. Two dogs survived; the third dog was presumed to have died with disseminated intravascular coagulopathy (DIC).

Metabolic Derangement—Lipidosis

In health, a balance is maintained between lipid mobilization to the liver from dietary sources or other metabolic processes such as fasting or new synthesis and lipid removal from the liver by mitochondrial oxidation or transport from the liver to other tissues in the form of very-low-density lipoproteins (VLDLs). Use of fat is regulated by complex interactions between blood glucose concentration and hormonal, nutritional, and neural factors.[63–65] In the clinical setting, an imbalance in input and egress that results in accumulation of lipid within hepatocytes could occur by several different mechanisms.[63, 64]

Increased deposition of triglyceride is associated with prolonged *starvation* (usually at least 2 weeks in experimental models[66, 67]) via heightened mobilization of fatty acids from fat stores and reduced synthesis of lipid-transporting proteins (lipoproteins). Protracted anorexia in toy breed puppies (32 hours or more) results in inadequate gluconeogenesis, hypoglycemia, ketogenesis associated with hypoinsulinemia and hyperglucagonemia, and diffuse microvesicular hepatic lipidosis.[68, 69] A *poorly balanced diet* (especially if markedly deficient in protein) given over a more extended time could produce similar effects, primarily because of altered lipoprotein synthesis and consequent disturbed dispersal of VLDLs from the liver. Depletion of certain nutrients important in lipoprotein synthesis, such as choline and its precursor methionine, or other substances such as carnitine, which is critical to mitochondrial function in processing fatty acids, further impairs lipid homeostasis. Fat stores are used as an energy source when there is *insufficient insulin* to preserve glucose homeostasis. The liver's response to certain endogenous and exogenous toxins is to accumulate lipid. Conditions in dogs and cats in which hepatic lipid accumulation occurs but is an expected response, is not inherently injurious, and

LIV

is usually clinically insignificant are given in Table 144–4. Mild degrees of abnormal serum liver enzyme activity may be found, but there is no evidence of hepatic dysfunction. It is important to know this for appropriate interpretation of diagnostic test results and liver biopsy specimens.

Lipid accumulation of proportion sufficient to cause hepatic compromise (usually over 50 per cent of hepatocytes affected) and clinical illness occurs most commonly in cats. Global surveys of feline hepatobiliary diseases have not been done lately, but it is generally agreed that, as with findings in an earlier study,[70] hepatic lipidosis (HL) has become the most common liver disease of cats. The exact pathogenesis remains unclear but most likely involves multiple factors in addition to obesity and prolonged anorexia. Obese cats that are otherwise healthy do have excess fat in their livers.[66, 71] Whether cats are fed a diet with energy content restricted to 25 per cent of normal requirements, as demonstrated by experimental studies,[66, 67] fast voluntarily,[72] are anorexic because of concurrent disease (secondary HL), or stop eating for unknown reasons (idiopathic HL),[63–65, 73–75] the result is the same: progressive accumulation of hepatic fat, intrahepatic cholestasis, and, without treatment, death.

Owners of cats with the naturally occurring disease often remark that a stressful event might have precipitated anorexia, such as a new pet in the household or a sudden change in diet. Vomiting may be reported. There is no breed predilection; most are middle-aged cats. Most studies of spontaneous HL found an equal gender predisposition, although in one study there was a female preponderance.[75] Typical physical examination findings include depression, jaundice, and weight loss to 25 to 40 per cent of the previous body weight. Generalized muscle wasting with preservation of intra-abdominal and inguinal fat stores is also characteristic. Hepatomegaly is an inconsistent finding, and few cats demonstrate overt signs of HE. Clinicopathologic features are generally compatible with cholestasis of any cause: hyperbilirubinemia (0.9 to 19.4 mg/dL); high serum AP (0.5 to 65.6 times high normal), ALT (0.4 to 22.7 times high normal), and AST (0.2 to 34.9 times high normal) activities; and high fasting or postprandial serum bile acids.[75] Unlike that in other cholestatic hepatopathies, serum gamma-glutamyltransferase (GGT) activity in cats with HL is minimally affected, and values are often normal to mildly elevated (0 to 2 times high normal).[75, 76] More severely affected cats also have coagulation disorders; prolonged prothrombin time is the most consistent finding.[75, 77] Blood glucose and serum cholesterol and triglyceride concentrations are variable. Common hematologic findings in cats with idiopathic HL are mild to moderate nonregenerative anemia and poikilocytosis. Leukon changes are consistent with stress in cats with idiopathic HL and with the concurrent disease process in cats

TABLE 144–4. CONDITIONS ASSOCIATED WITH MILD TO MODERATE HEPATIC LIPID ACCUMULATION IN DOGS AND CATS

DOGS	CATS
Diabetes mellitus	Diabetes mellitus
Hypothyroidism	Tetracycline toxicity
Congenital portosystemic shunt	Pancreatitis
Severe dietary protein restriction	Severe dietary protein restriction
Anorexia in toy breed puppies	Inflammatory bowel disease (?)
Chronic hypoxia from anemia or passive congestion	
Idiopathic hyperlipidemia in schnauzer dogs	

with secondary HL. Lipiduria was conspicuous in 85 per cent of cats with HL that had microscopic sediment examination as part of the urinalysis in one study.[75] Any other abnormalities are most likely consequences of anorexia and vomiting, such as dehydration, low serum urea nitrogen, hypokalemia, and prerenal azotemia.

Vascular Compromise

Abrupt loss of hepatic and/or portal venous blood flow to one or more liver lobes results in *infarction* (ischemic injury) and hepatocellular necrosis. Congenital absence, laxity of, or trauma-induced rent in the ligamentous supporting structures associated with the liver could allow a lobe to twist on its hilar attachment or become entrapped. This is a rare condition in dogs and cats. Three single case reports described illness in adult large-breed dogs characterized by acute signs of vomiting (2 days or less) or collapse, fever, abdominal pain, and septic peritonitis.[78–80] Abdominal radiographs disclosed a soft tissue mass containing multifocal gas opacities in the cranial abdomen in each case. Two dogs died or were euthanatized; the third dog recovered after surgical resection of the necrotic liver lobe. A different lobe was affected in each case: the quadrate, the papillary process of the caudate, and the left lobe. Hepatocellular necrosis and proliferation of resident clostridial organisms in an anaerobic environment created by lack of lobar portal blood flow were the factors most likely responsible for the severe clinical signs. A predisposing element was identified in only one of the three cases—two abdominal surgeries within the previous 5 days.

Infectious Agents

Infectious agents that cause acute liver injury have been reviewed.[81] *Infectious canine hepatitis* is caused by canine adenovirus type 1 (CAV-1).[82] Exposure to this environmentally resistant virus leads to viremia and rapid dissemination to lymphoid and other tissues and secretions including saliva, urine, and feces. Cytotoxic injury caused by direct viral infection of vascular endothelium and hepatocytes is responsible for the clinical features of this infection, which include uveitis, corneal edema, glomerulonephritis, and centrilobular hepatic necrosis. The degree of antibody response to infection determines the extent of hepatic injury, which, in the presence of low titers, is extensive and potentially fatal. Higher antibody titers are associated with sublethal hepatic necrosis and persistent inflammation and fibrosis. Because of widespread use of effective cross-reacting vaccines containing the relative adenovirus type 2 (CAV-2), CAV-1 infection is a rare clinical condition except in young dogs or unvaccinated dogs.[82]

Acute and chronic hepatic injuries were induced in young dogs by subcutaneous inoculation of bacteriologically sterile serum or liver homogenate from two dogs that died of chronic hepatitis in Scotland.[83] Although the clinical and laboratory features of the index cases were typical of progressive liver damage and development of irreversible changes including cirrhosis and regenerative nodule formation, a unique cell was discovered in the regenerative nodular tissue and termed an acidophil. It is believed to be a hepatocyte containing acidophilic granules in the cytoplasm that eventually coalesce as the cell is undergoing death, imparting a characteristic angular appearance. Because similar lesions developed in experimental animals on serial passage of serum or tissue, it was concluded that the cause was a nonbacterial infectious agent. Because the agent has not yet been identified, the disease is still called *canine acidophil cell hepatitis.* Similar reports of this unique hepatopathy have not been published in the United States.

As a result of new information on the participation of *Helicobacter* sp. in the development of gastrointestinal ulcer disease in human patients, the role of these organisms in various gastrointestinal disorders has been investigated in dogs and cats. Most reports have focused on the place of spiral bacteria in the gastrointestinal flora of normal animals and animals with inflammatory bowel disease and ulcer formation. The hepatobiliary system has received less attention, except under laboratory conditions, in which two novel species, *Helicobacter bilis* and *Helicobacter hepaticus,* have been identified and found to be responsible for chronic hepatitis in mice.[84, 85] Another new species was isolated from the liver of a 2-month-old puppy with a peracute illness characterized by weakness and vomiting for several hours before death.[86] Yellowish foci in the liver up to 1.5 cm in diameter consisted of necrotic hepatocytes with a mixed inflammatory cell infiltrate surrounded by sinusoidal leukocytosis. Application of Warthin-Starry silver stain revealed spiral bacteria in the areas of necrosis, between hepatocytes, and within the lumina of bile ducts that were ultimately determined to be a new urease-negative species called *Helicobacter canis.* The organism had been previously identified in the feces of a small number of dogs (4 per cent) and the blood of diarrheic children, but this was the first time it was associated with illness in companion animals.[86]

DEFINITIVE DIAGNOSIS

A presumptive diagnosis of acute hepatic injury is made from information gained from the history, physical examination findings, and preliminary laboratory testing. Survey abdominal radiographs are usually unremarkable; there may be mild generalized hepatomegaly. Gas opacities observed in the area of the liver on survey radiographs suggest liver lobe infarction and abscess formation. Generalized hypoechogenicity may be seen in the liver ultrasonographically,[87, 88] except in cats with hepatic lipidosis, in which the pattern is fine hyperechogenicity.[89]

For most *toxic* causes of hepatic injury, an effort is made to establish a temporal relationship between administration of a therapeutic agent or exposure to an environmental hazard and the onset of signs of illness attributable to acute hepatic injury such as vomiting, jaundice, or HE by thoroughly interviewing the owner. This usually provides sufficient evidence to arrive at a reasonable conclusion of cause and is further supported by recovery after drug discontinuation and supportive care. An adverse hepatic reaction to a drug or environmental toxin could be proved by reexposing the patient to the suspect substance and observing identical clinical consequences, as noted previously. This is unreasonable in most cases, and most owners would not agree to such a test. Examination of the vomitus of animals with suspected plant intoxication may give clues to the type of plant in question, such as pieces of mushroom, cycad palm leaves or seeds, or yellow-green, round to oval berry-like fruits from the chinaberry tree. Having the owner harvest specimens from plants or mushrooms that appeared to have been chewed and that can be identified by a trained botanist or mycologist would also be helpful.

The constellation of laboratory test abnormalities in cats with *hepatic lipidosis* could be confused with those in extrahepatic bile duct obstruction, except that serum GGT activity

is remarkably normal in cats with HL compared with other causes of severe cholestasis. Cats with severe HL that are cachectic and have a coagulopathy may have concurrent pancreatitis and a more guarded prognosis for recovery.[75, 77] Measurement of serum trypsin-like immunoreactivity may be a useful adjunct for detecting concurrent pancreatitis (see Chapter 146).[90] Abdominal ultrasonography is used to provide supporting evidence of HL (e.g., generalized hepatomegaly and hyperechogenicity), to rule out extrahepatic bile duct obstruction by examining the intrahepatic and extrahepatic biliary system, and to identify evidence for concurrent disease. For example, abdominal effusion and an enlarged pancreas suggest pancreatitis, whereas cats with cholangiohepatitis may have normal to hypoechoic hepatic parenchyma, prominent portal vasculature, and biliary tract abnormalities.[88] Specimens for cytologic or histologic examination are obtained at the same time. Fine-needle aspiration may provide preliminary evidence of micro- or macrovesicular lipid vacuolation; application of Oil Red O stain before any other fixation techniques confirms that the vacuoles are filled with lipid. Cytologic specimens may suffice in cats with idiopathic HL; there is no other evidence of necrosis or inflammation. In cats with diagnostic features of secondary HL, needle (14 or 16 gauge) or operative liver biopsy is required to obtain a large enough specimen to examine architecture and arrive at an accurate diagnosis.

In most other acute hepatic disorders, liver biopsy is not necessary unless the animal is not responding to treatment as expected. Biopsy is delayed until the animal is stable. The predominant histopathologic change is moderate to severe hepatic necrosis. Patterns of lesion distribution within the hepatic lobule have been described for some classic hepatotoxins in experimental settings.[15] Meliatoxin (chinaberry tree) intoxication results in fatty degeneration of hepatocytes.[59] Most other clinically relevant adverse hepatic reactions in companion animals have a similar distribution of necrosis (centrilobular to massive), so the pattern is unlikely to be useful in determining the causative agent. Because the role of *Helicobacter* sp. in canine and feline hepatobiliary disease is unclear, it may be prudent to apply Warthin-Starry silver stain to biopsy specimens from dogs or cats with unexplained acute hepatic injury.

SPECIFIC TREATMENT

The goals of treatment are to remove or reverse the inciting cause, to address the systemic derangements associated with hepatic dysfunction (see Table 144–3), and to facilitate hepatic regeneration. Owners should be instructed to discontinue drug administration immediately if their dogs or cats develop anorexia, vomiting, or jaundice during the course of treatment. If the owner saw the animal ingest a toxic substance, less than 2 hours have passed, and the substance is not caustic, administration of emetics and/or activated charcoal may be beneficial (see Chapters 80 & 81). For other potential causes of acute hepatic injury, nothing can be done until the animal is presented to a veterinarian. Animals with relatively mild clinical signs are managed as outpatients. Treatment of animals with severe acute hepatic injury caused by conditions in Table 144–1 is best provided in an intensive care unit to provide optimal opportunity for recovery.

Removal of the inciting cause is ideal but may be difficult or impossible for many causes of severe acute hepatic injury. *Specific antidotes* with clinically proven beneficial effects on

LIV

outcome are unavailable for most acute hepatotoxins except for acetaminophen. Replacement of depleted glutathione, if started early, prevents binding of reactive metabolites to essential macromolecules.[29, 30] If poisoning has occurred within 2 hours, vomiting should be induced, activated charcoal should be given, and a sodium sulfate cathartic should be administered (0.22 g/lb as a 20 per cent slurry by mouth).[30] If cyanosis is already present, oxygen should be given and stress minimized. Oral or intravenous administration of glutathione precursors such as *N*-acetylcysteine (NAC) is initiated as soon as possible: NAC, 64 mg/lb orally or intravenously as a 20 per cent solution for the first dose, regardless of time since poisoning, repeated in 6 hours, followed by 32 mg/lb every 6 hours for a total of seven treatments. Ascorbic acid (14 mg/lb orally) is given at the same time intervals as NAC.[30] Pretreatment with NAC (64 mg/lb IV) may also avert serious hepatotoxicity in dogs given thiacetarsamide.[91]

An antidote for *Amanita* mushroom toxicity has been developed and found to be protective experimentally in dogs if given at 5 and 24 hours after ingestion.[56, 92] This substance, silibinin (23 mg/lb in Ringer's solution, given intravenously over 1 hour), inhibits the uptake of amatoxins by hepatocytes, reduces their enterohepatic recirculation, and so enhances their renal excretion. It is not widely available and requires application to the Food and Drug Administration for an independent new drug registration. A less effective but more readily available antidote is penicillin G, which also blocks the uptake of amatoxins by hepatocytes. In experimental canine studies, the effective dose is 44 mg/lb (dissolved in Ringer's solution) at 5 hours after ingestion.[93] It is given to human patients as an intravenous infusion, 1×10^6 units/kg on the first day, followed by 0.5×10^6 units/kg daily for 2 subsequent days.[93] The combination of silibinin and penicillin is not believed to be more efficacious than either agent alone.

Other approaches for treatment of drug-induced hepatotoxicity have been examined in a laboratory setting and in human patients but are as yet untested in animals with naturally occurring disease. For example, some investigators have suggested that use of cimetidine to inhibit formation of injurious electrophilic metabolites by cytochrome P-450 enzymes may be beneficial in the treatment of human patients with acetaminophen- or halothane-associated hepatic injury.[94, 95]

SYMPTOMATIC TREATMENT

In cases of acute hepatic injury that have no specific treatment, as long as there has been only a single sublethal insult to the liver, recovery should occur with supportive care.

Fluid Therapy

Fluid, electrolyte, and acid-base abnormalities are addressed aggressively. Replacing, maintaining, and expanding vascular volume are critical steps in assisting tissue perfusion to speed recovery and discourage the development of DIC. Renal excretion of toxic metabolites may also be hastened. Metabolic disturbances such as metabolic alkalosis, hypokalemia, and hypoglycemia (see Table 144–3), which are among the conditions known to aggravate HE (Table 144–5), are corrected.

Standard methods are used to determine individual fluid

TABLE 144–5. CONDITIONS THAT MAY PRECIPITATE OR ACCENTUATE HEPATIC ENCEPHALOPATHY IN DOGS AND CATS

Increased generation of ammonia in the intestine
  High-protein diet (especially red meat)
  Gastrointestinal hemorrhage
  Azotemia (increased enterohepatic recirculation of urea)
  Constipation (increased dwell time)
  Infection (increased tissue catabolism and endogenous nitrogen load, decreased BCAA/AAA* ratio)
Movement of ammonia intracellularly in the brain
  Metabolic alkalosis (favors formation of readily diffusible form of the ammonia molecule: $NH_3 + H^+ \rightarrow NH_4^+$)
  Hypokalemia (increases renal ammonia production)
Increased release of ammonia during gluconeogenesis from extrahepatic sites
  Hyperglucagonemia secondary to hypoglycemia
Excess tranquilization (direct depressant action by heightened brain benzodiazepine and barbiturate receptor sensitivity)
Use of methionine-containing compounds (urinary acidifiers, "lipotrophic" agents)
Use of stored blood for transfusion (high ammonia content)

*AAA = aromatic amino acid; BCAA = branched-chain amino acid.

volume needs (rehydration, maintenance, continuing losses). Because most animals with acute hepatic injury are seriously ill, administration of fluids other than intravenously is inadequate. The ideal fluid for animals with AHF should be electrolyte balanced, limited in lactate content, and have a neutral or slightly acidic pH. Potassium supplementation is also recommended; 20 to 30 mEq of potassium chloride per liter of administered fluid is added until results of serum biochemical analysis are available, when standard guidelines for dosage adjustment may be used. Hypokalemia is more likely to be associated with chronic hepatic failure (see Chapter 145), but potassium supplementation is warranted to minimize signs of HE in animals with AHF. This is especially important in cats, in which severe potassium depletion may cause myopathy.[96, 97] A reasonable first choice to begin fluid administration before test results are available is Ringer's solution,[98–100] with B complex vitamins added (1 mL per liter of administered fluids).

Glucose is added to the fluid mixture if hypoglycemia is present. Hypoglycemia may be a reflection of sepsis and endotoxemia or overall diminished ability to mobilize hepatic glycogen stores. Hepatic glycogen depletion, associated with advanced liver dysfunction, and secondary hyperglucagonemia are known to occur in humans with cirrhosis.[101, 102] Whether massive loss of hepatic function develops abruptly or progressively, secondary hyperglucagonemia stimulates ammonia release,[101, 102] so maintaining euglycemia is important in relieving signs of HE. Infusions or boluses of 10% glucose or higher may be needed initially. A final concentration of 2.5 to 5% of glucose is adequate for maintenance in most cases.

Hepatic Encephalopathy

Treatment of HE is aimed at restoring and maintaining normal neurologic function. Because central nervous system dysfunction is directly related to contact with gut-derived encephalotoxins generated by protein degradation, treatment is focused on reducing the formation and absorption of these substances, correcting acid-base and electrolyte abnormalities that enhance their activity, and eliminating conditions that precipitate HE. Dietary protein restriction is usually combined with agents that reduce formation of or inhibit absorption of ammonia and other gut-derived encephalotoxins. Because animals with AHF may have central nervous system dysfunction that renders them unable or unwilling to eat, or they are vomiting, food and water are withheld for the first 48 to 72 hours.

Administration of locally acting agents that discourage formation of readily absorbable ammonia and hasten evacuation of the intestinal tract is indicated for animals with AHF. The semisynthetic disaccharide *lactulose* has important beneficial effects in animals with HE, including acidification of the intestinal contents to trap ammonium and discourage the formation of ammonia and promotion of osmotic diarrhea. It also provides a nonprotein substrate for bacteria, which diminishes synthesis of ammonia.[103] During the first 24 to 48 hours of management of an animal with AHF and HE, lactulose is delivered as a retention enema, using a solution of three parts lactulose to seven parts water at 9 mL/lb every 4 to 6 hours. The solution is instilled with a Foley catheter as far as possible into the colon and left in place for 15 to 20 minutes. The pH of the evacuated material should be 6 or less, indicating that lactulose has effectively acidified the intestinal contents. Because lactulose contains about 1 g/mL osmotically active sugars, dehydration and hypernatremia can occur if enemas are used too frequently (more often than every 4 to 6 hours) or the dwell time is prolonged[104] without careful attention to fluid intake and hydration status. If lactulose is not available, a solution of povidone iodine (10%) or neomycin sulfate liquid (10 mg/lb) in water may be used to decrease bacterial numbers.[105] If none of these additives is available, enemas are given using warm balanced electrolyte solution to remove colonic contents and prevent absorption of gut-derived encephalotoxins. When central nervous system integrity has returned, enteral feeding of a protein-restricted diet and medications can begin.

When animals with AHF feel well enough to eat, small portions of a protein-restricted diet are offered three to four times daily. The ideal *diet* for management of HE should be based primarily on carbohydrates as the energy source; contain highly digestible protein of high biologic value; contain low levels of aromatic amino acids (AAAs) and methionine and high levels of branched-chain amino acids (BCAAs) and arginine; have adequate vitamins A, B, C, D, E, and K; and be supplemented with potassium, calcium, and zinc.[106-108] Diets that meet these requirements are available commercially or can be prepared by owners using milk-based protein, such as low-fat cottage cheese (Table 144–6). Egg protein is a good source of arginine (especially for cats, which are unable to synthesize it) but also contains more methionine than milk protein, which may induce HE. Vegetables can also provide protein calories with less methionine content with the added benefit of more rapid intestinal transit,[108] but excess bulkiness precludes their use as the sole protein source. Soybean protein (tofu) is also a reasonable protein choice. Vegetables and fruits can be used to supplement existing diets to increase palatability and as treats. Formulation of homemade diets is tailored to the individual according to clinical signs and acceptance. For dogs, adding condiments such as garlic powder or salt-free seasoning and warming the food are ways to stimulate voluntary intake of both commercial and home-prepared protein-restricted diets.

Treatment of animals for HE continues after the initial hospitalization period until there is complete recovery or evidence that there is ongoing, persistent hepatic dysfunction. Many animals with HE require more than dietary protein restriction to control signs of encephalopathy satisfacto-

TABLE 144–6. HOME-PREPARED PROTEIN-RESTRICTED DIETS FOR TREATMENT OF HEPATIC ENCEPHALOPATHY IN DOGS AND CATS

ANIMAL	INGREDIENTS*	KCAL/LB AS FED
Feline	0.25 lb braised liver 2 large hard-boiled eggs 2 cups cooked rice (no added salt) 1 T vegetable oil 1 tsp calcium carbonate	635
Canine	0.25 lb braised ground beef 1 large hard-boiled egg 2 cups cooked rice (no added salt) 3 slices crumbled white bread 1 tsp calcium carbonate	750
	24% protein:† 　1.5 cup low-fat cottage cheese (1% fat) 　3 cups cooked rice (do not use instant rice) 　1 oz cooked beef liver 　1 tsp dicalcium phosphate 　1 tsp corn oil 　250 mg vitamin C 　1 capsule B complex vitamins plus iron 18% protein 　Same as above except use 1 cup low-fat cottage cheese	

*From Lewis LD, Morris ML Jr, Hand MS: Small Animal Clinical Nutrition III. Topeka, KS, Mark Morris Associates, 1987. A balanced vitamin-mineral supplement should accompany all of these diets. tsp = teaspoon; T = tablespoon.
†From Biourge V, Nutrition Support Service, School of Veterinary Medicine, University of California at Davis. Contains 1000 kcal of metabolizable energy. Calculate calorie requirements with the formula: $132[\text{body weight (kg)}]^{0.75}$.

rily. In such cases, *lactulose* (2.5 to 15 mL [dogs] or 1 to 3 mL [cats] by mouth every 8 hours) may be added to the treatment regimen. The dosage is adjusted until there are two or three soft stools per day; overdose results in watery diarrhea. There are no known complications of long-term use of lactulose at appropriate dosage in animals. Some animals strongly object to the sweet taste of lactulose. An attractive alternative is *lactitol*, a close relative. Although controlled studies of human patients with acute HE demonstrated that it was better tolerated than lactulose and equally effective,[110] it is available only as an investigational medication in Europe.

Another alternative to dietary therapy alone for management of HE is addition of *antibacterial drugs* that are effective for anaerobic (metronidazole, 3.4 mg/lb PO q12h; ampicillin, 10 mg/lb by mouth every 8 hours) and gram-negative urea-splitting (neomycin sulfate, 9 mg/lb by mouth every 8 to 12 hours) organisms. These organisms are known to be the major producers of ammonia, mercaptans (e.g., methanethiol, ethanethiol, dimethyldisulfide), and other gut-derived substances responsible for signs of HE. There are few serious adverse effects of long-term use of ampicillin or neomycin, although nephrotoxicity and malabsorption attributable to neomycin have been observed rarely in animal patients. Central nervous system dysfunction (ataxia, vertical and positional nystagmus) may be induced in dogs given metronidazole at dosages recommended for treatment of giardiasis or anaerobic infections (27 mg/lb by mouth daily) with presumably normal liver function.[111] Reduction of the dosage is recommended for human patients with hepatic failure, considering the extensive involvement of the liver in biotransformation of metronidazole.[112] It would seem prudent to follow the same suggestion in animals with hepatic failure

LIV

and use the dosage at the low end of the range (3.4 mg/lb by mouth every 12 hours).

Other medical approaches, such as use of *BCAA solutions* as dietary supplements or by intravenous infusion and use of benzodiazepine (BDZ) receptor antagonists (e.g., flumazenil; commercially available only in Europe), have been investigated in a laboratory setting and used in human patients with HE. Despite experimental and clinical evidence that parenteral administration of solutions containing BCAAs can reverse neurologic signs of HE, most large clinical trials have not demonstrated clear benefit over conventional treatments.[113, 114] Restoration of a normal BCAA-to-AAA serum ratio does not necessarily guarantee recovery from HE. Dogs with induced HE[115] and some human patients[113, 114] improved after BCAAs were given, but lack of controlled clinical trials in both dogs and cats and the cost of these solutions preclude their routine use at this time.

The discovery that increased BDZ receptors were associated with the gamma-aminobutyric acid receptor complex in laboratory animals with HE led to the hypothesis that BDZ receptor antagonists could relieve the depressed neurotransmission associated with HE.[116–118] This was observed in rats and rabbits with induced AHF that were given flumazenil, a prototype BDZ antagonist originally used to reverse the effects of BDZ during anesthesia and for BDZ overdose.[117, 119] Some human patients with cirrhosis and HE given flumazenil experienced a variable, but distinct, rapid improvement in mental status.[120] Because the onset of action of injected flumazenil is rapid and its duration is relatively short, it can also be used to differentiate other encephalopathies from HE.[119] Measurement of BDZ-like activity in the spinal fluid of dogs with HE associated with a congenital portosystemic shunt or a created portosystemic shunt with partial hepatectomy failed to detect these chemicals in either the natural or experimental state.[121] This implies that BDZ-receptor antagonists such as flumazenil have no role in the treatment of HE in dogs. Anecdotal reports have indicated, however, that a small number of dogs and cats with HE have responded favorably after administration of flumazenil (0.01 mg/lb intravenously).[2] Controlled investigations must still be done to determine a specific place for flumazenil in the management of HE in animals.

Cerebral Edema

Persistent central nervous signs in animals with AHF can be the result of uncontrolled HE and/or of increased intracranial pressure (ICP) and cerebral edema. If appropriate measures have been undertaken to control HE and the animal's neurologic status deteriorates, additional steps are taken to avoid brain stem herniation. The earliest indicator of increased ICP in human patients is increased muscle tone in the limbs, followed by decerebrate rigidity, hyperpronation, and adduction of the arms.[3] As ICP increases, pupillary dilation and slow pupillary light reflexes develop. Trismus and opisthotonos are noted immediately before brain herniation.[3, 122] Recommendations for treatment of human patients with raised ICP include elevation of the head and trunk to 20 to 30 degrees to the horizontal, strict bed rest to avoid excessive head movement, and mannitol (0.45 g/lb of 20% solution intravenously over 30 minutes, repeated every 4 hours if needed).[3–6] Corticosteroids have not been found to be beneficial compared with placebo in controlled trials of human patients with FHF, and serious side effects were noted.

Certain conditions, listed in order of frequency in clinical

TABLE 144–7. SUMMARY OF MEDICAL MANAGEMENT OF HEPATIC ENCEPHALOPATHY IN DOGS AND CATS

Acute (3 days)
  Nothing by mouth
  Fluids given intravenously
  1. 0.45% saline in 2.5% dextrose with added potassium (use 20–30 mEq KCl per liter of administered fluids) until serum electrolyte results are available.
  2. Add potassium according to serum electrolyte values using the following guidelines:

If serum K⁺ is:	Add:*	Maximum IV rate:†
3.1–3.5	7	7.3
2.6–3.0	10	5.5
2.1–2.5	15	3.6
<2.0	20	2.7

  Enemas every 6 hours
  1. Cleansing enemas using warm balanced electrolyte fluids
  2. Retention enemas (instill into the colon using a Foley catheter; leave in place for 15–20 minutes; evacuate the colon). Use one of the following solutions:
    a. Lactulose (3 parts lactulose to 7 parts water at 9 mL/lb)
    b. Povidone iodine (10%)
    c. Neomycin sulfate (10 mg/lb)
  Other (no clear consensus for use)
  1. Branched-chain amino acid solutions
  2. Benzodiazepine-receptor antagonists, such as flumazenil
Chronic (long term)
  Protein-restricted diets (commercial or homemade)
  Lactulose (starting dose for dogs: 2.5–15 mL PO q8–12h, cats: 1–3 mL PO q8–12h)
  Antibiotics (dosages are for either dog or cat)
  1. Metronidazole (3.4 mg/lb PO q12h)
  2. Neomycin sulfate (10 mg/lb PO q8h)
  3. Ampicillin (10 mg/lb PO q8h) or amoxicillin (10 mg/lb PO q12h)

*mEq KCl/250 mL fluid given.
†mL/lb/hr; do not exceed 0.23 mEq/lb/hr.

observations of animals with acute or chronic hepatic failure, are known to accentuate or precipitate HE and should be avoided (see Table 144–5). A summary of the steps in medical management of HE in animals is given in Table 144–7.

Nutritional Considerations

Adequate nutrition is important for recovery from any serious illness. For dogs or cats that remain anorexic after the initial 48 to 72 hours and that are not vomiting, a nasoesophageal feeding tube is placed. This enables enteral feeding of a liquid diet,*† with small boluses frequently or a continuous infusion device.[123] This approach can be used temporarily (for 4 to 7 days) until voluntary intake occurs or, if necessary, a more permanent feeding system such as esophagostomy,[124] gastrostomy,[125] or jejunostomy is chosen.[126]

Cats with severe hepatic lipidosis present a special challenge. The most important aspect of treatment for cats with hepatic lipidosis is complete nutritional support, along with treatment of known concurrent and possibly precipitating illness. Extending the period without food intake is contraindicated. Severely affected cats are stabilized (e.g., correct acid-base, electrolyte, and fluid imbalance, control of HE) before anesthesia is considered for hepatic biopsy and/or feeding tube placement. During the initial 3 days of hospital-

*Canine or Feline CliniCare liquid enteral diet, Pet-Ag. Inc., Hampshire, IL; each contains about 0.9 kcal/mL.
†Peptamen, Baxter Healthcare Corporation, Keerfield, IL; contains 1 kcal/mL.

ization, nutritional support is provided via nasoesophageal catheter with one of several available liquid enteral diets.[123,*,†] After calculating the total number of calories to be fed daily on the basis of the current weight of the cat,‡ one third of the daily requirement is administered in two or three meals on day 1, and this is increased to two thirds of the daily requirement on day 2. The full complement of feedings is administered by day 3 (total daily needs split into three or four feedings) and can be continued for 1 to 2 weeks. When the cat is stable, a more permanent feeding tube is placed (esophagostomy, gastrostomy, or jejunostomy) with the cat under general anesthesia. Use of blenderized diets with a normal protein content is recommended for cats with HL unless they have overt signs of HE. Earlier reports suggested that supplementation with taurine and carnitine (250 mg of each every 12 hours) may hasten the recovery process. Results of studies concerning the role of carnitine in the development of hepatic lipidosis in cats are conflicting.[127–129] Although absolute carnitine deficiency has not been demonstrated,[127] some investigators believe supplementation with this amino acid has resulted in improved clinical survival in cats with severe HL.[129] Arginine is an essential amino acid in the cat and is needed for normal processing of ammonia.[130] One study documented a plasma arginine deficiency in cats with severe HL,[131] so it seems wise to supplement with arginine (250 mg every 12 hours) in the early phase of tube feeding, especially when a liquid enteral diet is used.

Coagulopathy

Dogs and cats with severe hepatic dysfunction may have an *increased tendency to bleed.*[132–134] This may be noted as a generalized inclination (oozing from venipuncture sites, formation of ecchymoses in the skin with minimal trauma) or seem to be localized to the upper gastrointestinal tract (hematemesis, melena). In animals with AHF, this is most likely associated with massive endothelial injury and consequent DIC.

The effects of a substantial loss of functional hepatic mass that normally maintains homeostasis between synthesis of both procoagulant factors (all but factor VIII) and that of anticoagulant factors are likely to be present simultaneously and almost impossible to differentiate by use of standard coagulation tests (prothrombin time, activated partial thromboplastin time, concentration of fibrin degradation products, antithrombin III activity). Investigations have disclosed that dogs and cats with severe hepatic disease may have normal results of routine coagulation tests but have prolonged clotting times associated with proteins induced by vitamin K antagonism (PIVKA).[135, 136] The test is done by use of a fibrometer and a commercial kit (THROMBOTEST) using citrated plasma. When the PIVKA clotting time was over 18 seconds in dogs and over 25.5 seconds in cats, the animals benefited from administration of vitamin K_1 (2.5 mg subcutaneously every 12 hours for 3 days). No other particular treatment is indicated for subclinical coagulopathy. If there is obvious bleeding, administration of a blood component to provide factors temporarily should be started as soon as blood specimens for coagulation tests (including platelet

count and bleeding time) are drawn. Heparin may be added to either fresh whole blood or frozen plasma shortly before administration for management of DIC (see Chapter 180).

Additional treatment for gastrointestinal bleeding in animals with AHF consists primarily of histamine-receptor antagonists. Cimetidine (2.2 mg/lb subcutaneously or intravenously every 8 hours) is used if there is a specific indication to inhibit cytochrome P-450 drug-metabolizing enzyme systems, such as for some drug-associated hepatotoxicities. For routine antiulcer prevention to avoid adverse drug interactions, ranitidine (1 mg/lb intravenously every 8 hours for dogs and 1.2 mg/lb intravenously every 12 hours for cats) or famotidine (0.22 mg/kg intravenously every 24 hours for dogs) is preferred.

Susceptibility to Infection

Human patients with serious acute and chronic hepatocellular disease have a high frequency of *bacteremia* arising from infection in various tissues (e.g., skin, lung, urinary tract, intestine). Sepsis is a common cause of death in human patients with FHF; its diagnosis is complicated by lack of typical clinical indicators (e.g., fever, leukocytosis).[4, 5, 137–139] It was once thought that gram-negative organisms originating in the intestinal tract were the most common isolates, especially if there was evidence of gastrointestinal hemorrhage. Later studies also implicated gram-positive bacteria from a number of non–digestive tract sources, especially the skin, respiratory tract, and urinary tract, because of the need for intravenous and urinary catheters and ventilator therapy. In such patients, hepatic mononuclear-phagocytic system phagocytosis is decreased, neutrophil function is abnormal, and serum bactericidal and opsonic activities are defective.

Similar investigations of the immunocompetence of dogs and cats with acute hepatocellular disease have not been carried out. It is reasonable to suggest that these animals would be more susceptible to infection by similar mechanisms. If typical markers of sepsis are absent (e.g., fever, leukocytosis with a left shift, and toxic neutrophils) but there is general clinical deterioration, specimens for anaerobic and aerobic culture are collected. Treatment with a combination of antibiotics with bactericidal four-quadrant coverage and minimal nephrotoxicity is instituted.[140, 141] Amikacin (2.2 to 4.4 mg/lb intravenously, subcutaneously, or intramuscularly every 8 hours) or gentamicin in well-hydrated animals without renal compromise (1 to 2 mg/lb intravenously, subcutaneously or intramuscularly every 8 hours or 2.7 mg/lb intravenously every 24 hours) combined with ampicillin or cephazolin (10 mg/lb intravenously every 6 to 8 hours) is a good choice initially. Another acceptable combination effective for gram-negative and multidrug-resistant organisms and streptococci is enrofloxacin (1.1 mg/lb slowly intravenously every 12 hours; not approved for this route) and ampicillin (10 mg/lb intravenously every 6 to 8 hours).

Other, sometimes novel, treatment approaches that have not been found in large clinical trials to be of benefit to human patients with AHF include prostaglandin E_2 and prostacyclin, insulin-glucagon, hepatocyte growth factors, and corticosteroids. Currently, areas of emphasis in human medicine include development of the optimal system of prognostic indicators that could identify, as early as possible, candidates with AHF who are unlikely to survive without liver transplantation.[3–6] Companion to this is development of an extracorporeal liver-assist system that could be used until there is evidence of sufficient hepatic regeneration to permit recovery or that could act as a bridge to transplantation.[3–5]

---

*Canine or Feline CliniCare liquid enteral diet, Pet-Ag. Inc., Hampshire, IL; each contains about 0.9 kcal/mL.

†Peptamen, Baxter Healthcare Corporation, Keerfield, IL; contains 1 kcal/mL.

‡Maintenance energy requirement (MER, in calories) = 1.4[30(body weight in kg) + 70].

LIV

These options are not within reach for animal patients at this time.

ACUTE DECOMPENSATION OF CHRONIC HEPATOBILIARY DISEASE

It may be impossible to distinguish acute decompensation of chronic hepatic insufficiency from true AHF without the benefit of historical and clinicopathologic features consistent with preexisting hepatobiliary disease. At the time of the onset of acute illness, both may appear similar clinically, but true AHF has a potentially more favorable long-term prognosis. If the animal is icteric, medical causes of primary and secondary hepatobiliary disorders (see Tables 144–1 and 144–2) must be distinguished from disorders of the extrahepatic biliary system that require surgical intervention (see Chapter 145).

Common reasons for clinical deterioration of previously undetected chronic hepatobiliary disease include onset of HE associated with gastrointestinal bleeding or other cause (see Table 144–5) and/or sepsis. Less commonly, sudden elaboration of copper into the circulation from hepatocytes undergoing necrosis in dogs with familial copper hepatotoxicity could cause signs of a hemolytic crisis, as in copper poisoning in sheep.[142] Emergency treatment with ammonium tetrathiomolybdate has been advocated for humans with Wilson's disease and sheep with acute copper toxicosis but has not been attempted in dogs.[142]

SYSTEMIC DISORDERS THAT INVOLVE THE LIVER

Many of these conditions are systemic illnesses with relatively mild hepatic manifestations (e.g., high liver enzyme activities and/or hyperbilirubinemia) that do not require treatment, such as inflammatory bowel disease. In such cases, hepatobiliary consequences resolve with appropriate treatment of the primary illness, and there is no evidence of persistent hepatic disturbance. In some conditions, liver involvement may provide an avenue for diagnosis through histologic confirmation of the cause, as with histoplasmosis in cats. In other conditions, the liver component of the illness can be rather dramatic and can potentially lead to misdiagnosis, as in cholestasis associated with extrahepatic infection and glucocorticoid-deficient hypoadrenocorticism.

INTESTINAL DISEASE

Hepatobiliary disease associated with certain types of inflammatory bowel disease is common in human patients.[143, 144] Changes vary from asymptomatic periportal inflammatory cell infiltrates to severe and chronic parenchymal and biliary diseases, such as primary sclerosing cholangitis, chronic active hepatitis, cholelithiasis, cirrhosis, and granulomatous hepatitis. The precise relationships between the intestine and liver in these conditions remain obscure. On the basis of clinical experience, many clinicians have suspected that a similar relationship could exist in dogs and cats and could explain mild increases in serum liver enzyme activities in animals with intestinal disease. Granulomatous hepatitis was described in nine dogs with hepatomegaly, high serum liver enzyme activities, and jaundice associated with a variety of nonhepatic diseases.[145] Although previous reports had

suggested that systemic mycotic infection was the most common cause of this lesion, two of the nine dogs had intestinal lymphangiectasia. Two other reports have documented a rather high rate of concurrent inflammatory bowel and hepatic disease in cats (83 per cent in one study).[146, 147] That the main pancreatic duct joins the bile duct before entering the duodenum in cats is probably at least partly responsible for this finding.

GLUCOCORTICOID-DEFICIENT (ATYPICAL) HYPOADRENOCORTICISM

Dogs with an unusual form of naturally occurring adrenal insufficiency may have clinical features, laboratory test results, and ultrasonographic changes consistent with primary hepatobiliary disease. Two groups of dogs totaling 58 cases were described as having hypoalbuminemia, hypocholesterolemia, hypoglycemia, low blood urea nitrogen content, mild nonregenerative anemia, and microhepatia.[148, 149] Some of these abnormalities, more easily than others, are explained by lack of sufficient cortisol. Absence of classic serum electrolyte changes suggesting mineralocorticoid deficiency and adrenal hyporesponsiveness to adrenocorticotropic hormone were consistent with glucocorticoid deficiency. Most dogs responded completely to administration of glucocorticoids alone, but several dogs ultimately needed mineralocorticoid supplementation as well.

PORTAL VEIN THROMBOSIS

A retrospective necropsy study of animals with grossly visible portal vein thrombi identified 11 dogs in 9.5 years.[150] Inflammatory abdominal conditions, such as pancreatitis and peritonitis, and severe hepatic disease were believed to be responsible for creating circumstances (endothelial injury, changes in blood flow, and changes in blood coagulability) that favored portal vein thrombosis. Corticosteroids, administered to 10 of 11 dogs, may have contributed to thrombus formation in other locations, notably the pulmonary arteries, and in dogs without abdominal inflammation or altered blood flow.

CHOLESTASIS ASSOCIATED WITH EXTRAHEPATIC INFECTION

Cholestasis associated with sepsis of nonhepatobiliary origin is well recognized in human patients[151, 152] and has been described in five dogs.[153] Infection was believed to arise from several different locations, including the lungs, abdominal cavity, urinary tract, skin, and heart valves. Gram-negative organisms were cultured from two dogs, gram-positive organisms from two dogs, and one dog had a mixed infection. Serum liver enzyme activities were modestly abnormal; AP was 2 to 5 times high normal and ALT was 2 to 3.7 times high normal. The serum bilirubin concentration ranged from 3.5 to 33.5 mg/dL and the fasting serum bile acid concentration was high in the dog in which it was measured (259 μmol/L; normal less than 10). It was not possible to show that the hepatobiliary abnormalities resolved with antibacterial treatment because all five dogs died. However, clinical experience in other cases suggests that this is true. In the five reported cases, there was no histopathologic evidence of primary hepatobiliary disease; there was only marked accumulation of bile pigment in hepatocytes and bile canaliculi in all five dogs.

HEPATIC ABSCESSES

Hepatic abscesses are usually the result of septic embolization from an abdominal site of bacterial infection. Puppies with omphalophlebitis and adult dogs with inflammatory conditions of the pancreas or hepatobiliary system or conditions associated with an immunocompromised state (diabetes mellitus or hypercortisolism) are at risk. In three reports describing a total of 29 dogs with hepatic abscesses, aerobic bacteria were isolated in 24 of 25 cases in which material from the hepatic lesions was submitted for culture.[154–156] Although the most common isolates were gram-negative enteric organisms, *Staphylococcus* spp. were identified in six dogs. *Clostridium* sp. was the only isolate cultured anaerobically from abscess fluid in 4 of 15 dogs. Anorexia, lethargy, and vomiting were consistent presenting complaints. Physical examination findings referable to the presence of hepatic abscessation included fever, tachycardia, and abdominal pain. Hepatomegaly was detected in dogs with primary hepatobiliary disease, diabetes mellitus, and hypercortisolism.

Neutrophilic leukocytosis with a left shift and high serum AP and ALT activities were typical clinicopathologic abnormalities. One or more hypoechoic or anechoic hepatic masses, some with a hyperechoic rim, were characteristic ultrasonographic findings. Abscesses were found most often in the left liver lobes. In some cases, fine-needle aspiration was used to obtain material for cytology and aerobic and anaerobic bacterial culture from a representative lesion so that antibiotic treatment could be initiated preoperatively; no complications were reported. In other cases, specimens were obtained at surgery. Treatment consisted of surgical removal of infected tissue, administration of appropriate antibiotics, supportive care, and resolution of underlying predisposing conditions. Infected liver tissue was removed and submitted for histopathologic examination and, if not done previously, bacterial culture. Specific recommendations for duration of antibiotic treatment after surgery varied according to the underlying cause and amount of infected tissue that was removed. It seems reasonable to suggest that antibiotic treatment should continue past the time of clinicopathologic and ultrasonographic resolution.

LEPTOSPIROSIS

Classic leptospirosis, caused by the serovars *icterohemorrhagica* and *canicola* of the species *Leptospira interrogans,* is uncommon because of widespread use of vaccination programs.[157–160] Infections caused by other species and serovars have become more prevalent owing to lack of vaccine cross-protection and increased contact with nondomestic maintenance hosts such as skunks, opossums, and raccoons. The predominant manifestation of leptospirosis has been that of acute or subacute renal failure in dogs associated with serovars *grippotyphosa, pomona,* and *bratislava;* feline infection is rare.[157–162] Typical presenting signs include anorexia, depression, vomiting, fever, and abdominal pain. Coincident hepatic involvement appears to be a minor component in most cases, consisting primarily of modest abnormalities in serum liver enzyme activities (less than 3.5 times high normal for AP and ALT). Most dogs have high AP and normal ALT activities, and about 25 per cent have hyperbilirubinemia. (See Chapter 85.)

SUPERFICIAL NECROLYTIC DERMATITIS

This distinctive ulcerative crusting dermatosis in dogs with various concurrent diseases, including diabetes mellitus, glucagon-secreting pancreatic neoplasm, and severe hepatic disease, has been described extensively.[163–166] It is believed to resemble a human condition called necrolytic migratory erythema, which is associated with certain nutritional deficiencies; glucagonoma; several intestinal, pancreatic, and hepatic diseases; and diabetes mellitus. Most affected animals are male dogs of any breed and older than 10 years of age; one aged cat with pancreatic carcinoma has been reported.[167]

Animals are usually presented because of skin disease: erythematous crusting plaques; erosions; ulcerations; and alopecia involving the face and ears, mucocutaneous junctions, feet, and ventrum. Clinicopathologic test results include mild nonregenerative anemia, high serum liver enzyme activities, fluctuating hyperglycemia, hypoaminoacidemia, and hypoalbuminemia. Hepatic ultrasonography reveals an enlarged nodular liver and a unique echo pattern believed to be pathognomonic: a hyperechoic network surrounding hypoechoic areas, resulting in a Swiss cheese–like pattern.[168] This translates into a moderate to severe vacuolar hepatopathy (staining positively for lipid) and parenchymal collapse. Collagen deposition may also be observed in varying amounts interlobularly and pericellularly. The severity of the hepatic lesion seems to correlate positively with the stage of progression of the systemic illness. The cutaneous and hepatic lesions probably represent a repercussion of marked metabolic or hormonal disturbance rather than initiating events. Clarifying the pathogenesis has been extremely frustrating; the emphasis has largely been on measurement of glucagon in peripheral plasma. Spot values have not been consistently abnormal, but complex studies of glucagon dynamics have not been done.

Because the specific cause of this disorder remains elusive, treatment is based on symptomatic management. Rarely, an underlying cause can be removed (e.g., pancreatic tumor) and the disease remits.[169] More often, nutritional supplements (zinc, niacin, and fatty acids) are added to a good-quality protein diet, and topical medications are prescribed for the skin lesions (moisturizers, antibacterials, medicated shampoo). Overall, the prognosis is poor.

HEPATIC AMYLOIDOSIS

Reactive (secondary) hepatic amyloidosis was diagnosed in three young Chinese Shar Pei dogs.[170, 171] Two dogs had clinical features of cholestatic hepatic disease and one dog was presented for hemoperitoneum later determined to be associated with a ruptured liver lobe. All dogs had previous recurrent episodes of anorexia, fever, inflammatory leukon, and limb and abdominal pain consistent with the inherited familial Shar Pei febrile disorder.[172] Amyloid deposition in the liver was believed to be a consequence of recurrent episodes of inflammation associated with high levels of interleukin-6, which is characteristic of this condition. Although kidney biopsies were not obtained, renal involvement, as described previously,[173] was presumed on the basis of urinalysis results. The hepatic manifestations dominated the clinical course of illness, and treatment with colchicine (0.01 mg/lb [0.03 mg/kg] by mouth every 24 hours) appeared to deter progression in two dogs for at least 2 years.

LIV

REFERENCES

1. Johnson SE: Acute hepatic failure. *In* Kirk RW (ed): Current Veterinary Therapy IX. Philadelphia, WB Saunders, 1986, p 945.
2. Hughes D, King LG: The diagnosis and management of acute liver failure in dogs and cats. Vet Clin North Am Small Anim Pract 25:437, 1995.
3. Lee WM: Acute liver failure. Am J Med 95(Suppl 1A):1A-3S, 1994.
4. Caraceni P, Van Thiel DH: Acute liver failure. Lancet 345:163, 1995.
5. Riegler JI, Lake JR: Fulminant hepatic failure. Med Clin North Am 77:1057, 1993.
6. O'Grady JG, et al: Fulminant hepatic failure. *In* Schiff L, Schiff ER (eds): Diseases of the Liver, 7th ed. Philadelphia, JB Lippincott, 1993, p 1077.
7. Bernuau J, et al: Fulminant and subfulminant liver failure: Definitions and causes. Semin Liver Dis 6:97, 1986.
8. Polzin DJ, et al: Acute hepatic necrosis associated with the administration of mebendazole to dogs. JAVMA 179:1013, 1981.
9. Everett RM, et al: Alkaline phosphatase, leucine aminopeptidase, and alanine aminotransferase activities with obstructive and toxic hepatic disease in cats. Am J Vet Res 38:963, 1977.
10. Spano JS, et al: Serum γ-glutamyl transpeptidase activity in healthy cats and cats with induced hepatic disease. Am J Vet Res 44:2049, 1983.
11. Strombeck DR, et al: Plasma amino acid, glucagon, and insulin concentrations in dogs with nitrosamine-induced hepatic disease. Am J Vet Res 44:2028, 1983.
12. Boothe DM, et al: Dimethylnitrosamine-induced hepatotoxicosis in dogs as a model of progressive canine hepatic disease. Am J Vet Res 53:411, 1992.
13. Johnson SE: Diseases of the liver. *In* Ettinger SJ, Feldman EC (eds): Textbook of Veterinary Internal Medicine, 4th ed. Philadelphia, WB Saunders, 1995, p 1313.
14. Bunch SE: Hepatotoxicity associated with pharmacologic agents in dogs and cats. Vet Clin North Am Small Anim Pract 23:659, 1995.
15. Center SA: Acute hepatic injury: Hepatic necrosis and fulminant hepatic failure. *In* Guilford WG, Certer SA, Strombeck DR, Williams DA, Meyer DJ (eds): Strombeck's Small Animal Gastroenterology, 3rd ed. Philadelphia, WB Saunders, 1996, p 654.
16. Morgan JC, Rainey CT: Clinical aspects of canine heartworm disease. Proceedings of the First International Symposium on Canine Heartworm Disease. Gainesville, FL, 1970, p 76.
17. Rawlings CA, Calvert CA: Heartworm disease. *In* Ettinger SJ, Feldman EC (eds): Textbook of Veterinary Internal Medicine, 4th ed. Philadelphia, WB Saunders, 1995, p 1046.
18. Hardy RM, et al: Periportal hepatitis associated with the use of a heartworm-hookworm preventative (diethylcarbamazine-oxibendazole) in thirteen dogs. J Am Anim Hosp Assoc 25:419, 1989.
19. Vaden SL, et al: Hepatotoxicosis associated with heartworm/hookworm preventive medication in a dog. JAVMA 192:651, 1988.
20. Kume S: The use of diethylcarbamazine in prevention of the infection; pathogenesis of allergic shock from the use of diethylcarbamazine. Proceedings of the First International Symposium on Canine Heartworm Disease. Gainesville, FL, 1970, p 1.
21. Ndiritu CG, Weigel J: Hepatorenal injury in a dog associated with methoxyflurane. Vet Med Small Anim Clin 72:545, 1977.
22. Meuten DJ, Pecquet-Goad ME: Hepatic necrosis associated with use of halothane in a dog. JAVMA 184:478, 1984.
23. Helton KA, et al: Griseofulvin toxicity in cats: Literature review and report of seven cases. J Am Anim Hosp Assoc 22:453, 1986.
24. Kock N, Kelly P: Massive hepatic necrosis associated with accidental imidocarb dipropionate toxicosis in a dog. J Comp Pathol 104:113, 1991.
25. McEntee K, et al: Closantel intoxication in a dog. Vet Hum Toxicol 37:234, 1995.
26. Greentree WF, Hall JO: Iron toxicosis. *In* Bonagura JD, Kirk RW (eds): Kirk's Current Veterinary Therapy XII. Philadelphia, WB Saunders, 1995, p 240.
27. Chaffee VW, et al: Aflatoxicosis in dogs. Am J Vet Res 30:1737, 1969.
28. Liggett AD, et al: Canine aflatoxicosis: A continuing problem. Vet Hum Toxicol 28:428, 1986.
29. St. Omer VV, McKnight ED: Acetylcysteine for treatment of acetaminophen toxicosis in the cat. Am J Vet Res 176:911, 1980.
30. Cullison RF: Acetaminophen toxicosis in small animals: Clinical signs, mode of action, and treatment. Compend Contin Educ Pract Vet 6:315, 1984.
31. Ortega L, et al: Acetaminophen-induced fulminant hepatic failure in dogs. Hepatology 5:673, 1985.
32. Wilke JR: Idiosyncrasies of drug metabolism in cats: Effect on pharmacotherapeutics in feline practice. Vet Clin North Am Small Anim Pract 14:1345, 1984.
33. Aronson LR, Drobatz K: Acetaminophen toxicosis in 17 cats. J Vet Emerg Crit Care 6:65, 1996.
34. MacPhail DM, et al: Hepatocellular toxicosis associated with administration of carprofen in 21 dogs. JAVMA 212:1895, 1998.
35. Kaufman AC, Greene CE: Increased alanine transaminase activity associated with tetracycline administration in a cat. JAVMA 202:628, 1993.
36. Freneaux E, et al: Inhibition of the mitochondrial oxidation of fatty acids by tetracycline in mice and man: Possible role in microvesicular induced by this antibiotic. Hepatology 8:1056, 1988.
37. Toth DM, Derwelis SK: Drug-induced hepatitis in a dog. Vet Med Small Anim Clin 75:421, 1980.
38. Anderson WI, et al: Hepatitis in a dog given sulfadiazine-trimethoprim and cyclophosphamide. Mod Vet Pract 65:115, 1984.
39. Rowland PH, et al: Presumptive trimethoprim-sulfadiazine–related hepatotoxicosis in a dog. JAVMA 200:348, 1992.
40. Thomson GW: Possible sulfamethoxazole/trimethoprim-induced hepatic necrosis in a dog. Can Vet J 31:530, 1990.
41. Twedt DC, et al: Association of hepatic necrosis with trimethoprim sulfonamide administration in 4 dogs. J Vet Intern Med 11:20, 1997.
42. AAFP news: Drug reaction warnings. Feline Pract 21:31, 1993.
43. Levy JK, et al: Adverse reactions to diazepam in cats. JAVMA 205:156, 1994.
44. Center SA, et al: Fulminant hepatic failure associated with oral administration of diazepam in 11 cats. JAVMA 209:618, 1996.
45. Hughes D, et al: Acute hepatic necrosis and liver failure associated with benzodiazepine therapy in six cats, 1986–1995. J Vet Emerg Crit Care 6:13, 1996.
46. Peterson ME: Methimazole treatment of 262 cats with hyperthyroidism. J Vet Intern Med 2:150, 1988.
47. Peterson ME: Propylthiouracil treatment of feline hyperthyroidism. JAVMA 179:85, 1981.
48. Feldman EC, Nelson RW: Feline hyperthyroidism. *In* Feldman EC, Nelson RW (eds): Canine and Feline Endocrinology and Reproduction. Philadelphia, WB Saunders, 1996, p 118.
49. Feldman EC, et al: Intensive 50-week evaluation of glipizide administration in 50 cats with previously untreated diabetes mellitus. JAVMA 210:772, 1997.
50. Nelson RW, et al: Effect of an orally administered sulfonylurea, glipizide, for treatment of diabetes mellitus in cats. JAVMA 203:821, 1993.
51. Benjamin DR: Mushrooms: Poisons and Panaceas. A Handbook for Naturalists, Mycologists, and Physicians. New York, WH Freeman, 1995, p 422.
52. Mepartland JM, Vilgalys RJ: Mushroom poisoning. Am Fam Physician 55:1797, 1997.
53. Koppel C: Clinical symptomatology and management of mushroom poisoning. Toxicon 31:1513, 1993.
54. Kallet A, et al: Mushroom (*Amanita phalloides*) toxicity in dogs. Calif Vet 47(Jan/Feb): 9, 1988.
55. Liggett AD, Weiss R: Liver necrosis caused by mushroom poisoning in dogs. J Vet Diagn Invest 1:267, 1989.
56. Vogel G, et al: Protection by silibinin against *Amanita phalloides* intoxication in beagles. Toxicol Appl Pharmacol 73:355, 1984.
57. Senior DF, et al: Cycad intoxication in the dog. J Am Anim Hosp Assoc 21:103, 1985.
58. Albretsen JC, et al: Cycad palm toxicosis in dogs: 60 cases. JAVMA 213:99, 1998.
59. Hare WR, et al: Chinaberry poisoning in two dogs. JAVMA 210:1638, 1997.
60. Parrish HM: Analysis of 460 fatalities from venomous animals in the United States. Am J Med Sci 245:129, 1965.
61. Meerdink GL: Bites and stings of venomous animals. *In* Kirk RW (ed): Current Veterinary Therapy VIII. Philadelphia, WB Saunders, 1983, p 155.
62. Cowell AK, et al: Severe systemic reactions to *Hymenoptera* stings in three dogs. JAVMA 198:1014, 1991.
63. Center SA: Hepatic lipidosis, glucocorticoid hepatopathy, vacuolar hepatopathy, storage disorders, amyloidosis, and iron toxicity. *In* Guilford WB, Certer SA, Strombeck DR, Williams DA, Meyer DJ (eds): Strombeck's Small Animal Gastroenterology, 3rd ed. Philadelphia, WB Saunders, 1996, p 766.
64. Armstrong PJ: Hepatic lipidosis. Vet Prev 1:10, 1994.
65. Dimski DS: Feline hepatic lipidosis. Semin Vet Med Surg (Small Anim) 12:28, 1997.
66. Armstrong PJ: Feline hepatic lipidosis. Proceedings, 7th Annual Forum, American College of Veterinary Internal Medicine, San Diego, CA, 1989, p 335.
67. Biourge VC, et al: Experimental induction of hepatic lipidosis in cats. Am J Vet Res 55:1291, 1994.
68. van der Linde-Sipman JS, et al: Fatty liver syndrome in puppies. J Am Anim Hosp Assoc 26:9, 1990.
69. van Toor AJ, et al: Experimental induction of fasting hypoglycaemia and fatty liver syndrome in three Yorkshire terrier pups. Vet Q 13:16, 1991.
70. Zawie DA, Garvey MS: Feline hepatic disease. Vet Clin North Am Small Anim Pract 14:11201, 1984.
71. Dimski DS, et al: Serum lipoprotein concentrations and hepatic lesions in obese cats undergoing weight loss. Am J Vet Res 53:1259, 1992.
72. Biorge VC, et al: Spontaneous occurrence of hepatic lipidosis in a group of laboratory cats. J Vet Intern Med 7:194, 1993.
73. Jacobs G, et al: Treatment of idiopathic hepatic lipidosis in cats: 11 cases (1986–1987). JAVMA 195:635, 1989.
74. Hubbard BS, Vulgamott JC: Feline hepatic lipidosis. Compend Contin Educ Pract Vet 14:459, 1992.
75. Center SA, et al: A retrospective study of 77 cats with severe hepatic lipidosis: 1975–1990. J Vet Intern Med 7:349, 1993.
76. Center SA, et al: Diagnostic value of serum γ-glutamyl transferase and alkaline phosphatase activities in hepatobiliary disease in the cat. JAVMA 188:507, 1986.
77. Akol KG, et al: Acute pancreatitis in cats with hepatic lipidosis. J Vet Intern Med 7:205, 1993.
78. Tomlinson J, Black A: Liver lobe torsion in a dog. JAVMA 183:225, 1983.
79. McConkey S, et al: Liver torsion and associated bacterial peritonitis in a dog. Can Vet J 38:438, 1997.
80. Downs MO, et al: Liver lobe torsion and liver abscess in a dog. JAVMA 212:678, 1998.
81. Greene CE (ed): Infectious Diseases of the Dog and Cat, 2nd ed. Philadelphia, WB Saunders, 1998.
82. Greene CE: Infectious canine hepatitis and canine acidophil cell hepatitis. *In* Greene CE (ed): Infectious Diseases of the Dog and Cat, 2nd ed. Philadelphia, WB Saunders, 1998, p 22.

83. Jarrett WFH, O'Neil BW: A new transmissible agent causing acute hepatitis, chronic hepatitis and cirrhosis in dogs. Vet Rec 116:629, 1985.
84. Fox JG, et al: *Helicobacter hepaticus* sp. nov., a microaerophilic bacterium isolated from livers and intestinal mucosal scrapings from mice. J Clin Microbiol 32:1238, 1994.
85. Fox JG, et al: *Helicobacter bilis* sp. nov., a novel *Helicobacter* species isolated from bile, livers, and intestines of aged, inbred mice. J Clin Microbiol 33:445, 1995.
86. Fox JG, et al: *Helicobacter canis* isolated from a dog liver with multifocal necrotizing hepatitis. J Clin Microbiol 34:2479, 1996.
87. Biller DS, et al: Ultrasonography of diffuse liver disease. A review. J Vet Intern Med 6:71, 1992.
88. Newell SM, et al: Correlations between ultrasonographic findings and specific hepatic diseases in cats: 72 cases (1985–1997). JAVMA 213:94, 1998.
89. Yeager AE, Mohammed H: Accuracy of ultrasonography in the detection of severe hepatic lipidosis in cats. Am J Vet Res 53:597, 1992.
90. Bruner JM, et al: High feline trypsin-like immunoreactivity in a cat with pancreatitis and hepatic lipidosis. JAVMA 210:1757, 1997.
91. Hitt ME, et al: Hepatocellular cytoprotection against the hepatotoxic effects of thiacetarsamide using dextrose and *N*-acetyl-cysteine in the dog. Proceedings, Tenth Annual Forum, American College of Veterinary Internal Medicine, San Diego, CA, 1992, p 808.
92. Floersheim GL, et al: Effects of penicillin and silymarin on liver enzymes and blood clotting factors in dogs given a boiled preparation of *Amanita phalloides*. Toxicol Appl Pharmacol 46:455, 1978.
93. Faulstich H, Zilker TR: Amatoxins. *In* Spoerke DG, Rumack BH (eds): Handbook of Mushroom Poisoning, 2nd ed. Boca Raton, FL, CRC Press, 1994, p 233.
94. Nomura F, et al: Effects of anticonvulsant agents on halothane-induced liver injury in human subjects and experimental animals. Hepatology 6:952, 1986.
95. Black M: Hepatotoxic and hepatoprotective potential of histamine (H$_2$)-receptor antagonists. Am J Med 83(Suppl 6A):68, 1987.
96. Dow SW, et al: Potassium depletion in cats: Hypokalemic polymyopathy. JAVMA 191:1563, 1987.
97. Dow SW, et al: Hypokalemia in cats: 186 cases (1984–1987). JAVMA 194:1604, 1989.
98. Grauer GF, Nichols CER: Ascites, renal abnormalities, and electrolyte and acid-base disorders associated with liver disease. Vet Clin North Am Small Anim Pract 15:197, 1985.
99. Wolfsheimer KJ: Fluid therapy in the critically ill patient. Vet Clin North Am Small Anim Pract 19:361, 1989.
100. Johnson SE: Fluid therapy for gastrointestinal, pancreatic, and hepatic disease. *In* DiBartola SP (ed): Fluid Therapy in Small Animal Practice. Philadelphia, WB Saunders, 1992, p 507.
101. Kabadi UM, et al: Elevated plasma ammonia level in hepatic cirrhosis: Role of glucagon. Gastroenterology 88:750, 1985.
102. Kabadi UM: The association of hepatic glycogen depletion with hyperammonemia in cirrhosis. Hepatology 7:821, 1987.
103. Conn HO, et al: Comparison of lactulose and neomycin in the treatment of chronic portal systemic encephalopathy. A double blind controlled trial. Gastroenterology 72:573, 1977.
104. Nanji AA, Lanener RW: Lactulose-induced hypernatremia. Drug Intell Clin Pharm 18:70, 1984.
105. Hardy RM: Hepatic coma. Semin Vet Med Surg (Small Anim) 3:311, 1988.
106. Marks SL, et al: Nutritional support in hepatic disease: Part I. Metabolic alterations and nutritional considerations in dogs and cats. Compend Contin Educ Pract Vet 16:971, 1994.
107. Marks SL, et al: Nutritional support in hepatic disease: Part II. Management of common liver disorders in dogs and cats. Compend Contin Educ Pract Vet 16:1287, 1994.
108. Bauer JE: Diet selection and special considerations in the management of hepatic diseases. JAVMA 210:625, 1997.
109. Greenberger NJ, et al: Effect of vegetable and animal protein diets on chronic hepatic encephalopathy. Am J Dig Dis 22:845, 1977.
110. Morgan MY, Hawley KE: Lactitol vs. lactulose in the treatment of acute hepatic encephalopathy in cirrhotic patients: A double-blind, randomized trial. Hepatology 6:1278, 1987.
111. Dow SW, et al: Central nervous system toxicosis associated with metronidazole treatment of dogs: Five cases (1984–1987). JAVMA 195:365, 1991.
112. Melikian DM, Flaherty JF: Antimicrobial agents. *In* Schrier RW, Gambertoglio JG (eds): Handbook of Drug Therapy in Liver and Kidney Disease. Boston, Little, Brown, 1991, p 14.
113. Alexander WF, et al: The usefulness of branched chain amino acids in patients with acute or chronic hepatic encephalopathy. Am J Gastroenterol 84:91, 1989.
114. Sax HC, et al: Clinical use of branched-chain amino acids in liver disease, sepsis, trauma, and burns. Arch Surg 121:358, 1986.
115. Rossi-Fanelli F, et al: Induction of coma in normal dogs by the infusion of aromatic amino acids and its prevention by the addition of branched-chain amino acids. Gastroenterology 83:664, 1982.
116. Baraldi M, et al: Supersensitivity of benzodiazepine receptors in hepatic encephalopathy due to fulminant hepatic failure in the rat: Reversal by a benzodiazepine antagonist. Clin Sci 67:167, 1984.
117. Jones EA, et al: Flumazenil: Potential implications for hepatic encephalopathy. Pharmacol Ther 45:331, 1990.
118. Whitwam JG: Flumazenil: A benzodiazepine antagonist. Br Med J 218:797, 1988.
119. Bassett ML, et al: Amelioration of hepatic encephalopathy by pharmacologic antagonism of the GABA$_A$-benzodiazepine receptor complex in a rabbit model of fulminant hepatic failure. Gastroenterology 93:1069, 1987.
120. Bansky G, et al: Effects of the benzodiazepine receptor antagonist flumazenil in hepatic encephalopathy in humans. Gastroenterology 97:44, 1989.
121. Meyer HP, Rothuizen J: No benzodiazepine activity in cerebrospinal fluid of dogs with chronic hepatic encephalopathy (abstract). Proceedings, Sixteenth Annual Forum, American College of Veterinary Medicine, San Diego, CA, 1998, p 705.
122. Ede RJ, Williams R: Hepatic encephalopathy and cerebral edema. Semin Liver Dis 6:107, 1986.
123. Crowe DT, et al: The use of polymeric liquid enteral diets for nutritional support in seriously ill or injured small animals: Clinical results in 200 patients. J Am Anim Hosp Assoc 33:500, 1997.
124. Armstrong PJ, Hardie EM: Percutaneous endoscopic gastrostomy: A retrospective study of 54 clinical cases in dogs and cats. J Vet Intern Med 4:202, 1990.
125. Devitt CM, Seim HB III: Clinical evaluation of tube esophagostomy in small animals. Compend Contin Educ Pract Vet 33:55, 1997.
126. Swann HM, et al: Complications associated with use of jejunostomy tubes in dogs and cats: 40 cases (1989–1994). JAVMA 210:1764, 1997.
127. Jacobs G, et al: Comparison of plasma, liver, and skeletal muscle carnitine concentrations in cats with idiopathic hepatic lipidosis and in healthy cats. Am J Vet Res 51:1349, 1990.
128. Armstrong PJ, et al: L-Carnitine reduces hepatic fat accumulation during rapid weight reduction in cats (abstract). Proceedings, Tenth Annual Forum, American College of Veterinary Medicine, San Diego, CA, 1992, p 810.
129. Center SA: Feline hepatic lipidosis: Better defining the syndrome and its management. Proceedings, Sixteenth Annual Forum, American College of Veterinary Medicine, San Diego, CA, 1998, p 56.
130. Morris JG, Rogers QR: Arginine: An essential amino acid for the cat. J Nutr 108:1944, 1978.
131. Center SA, et al: Hepatic ultrastructural and metabolic derangements in cats with severe hepatic lipidosis. Proceedings, Ninth Annual Forum, American College of Veterinary Medicine, New Orleans, LA, 1991, p 193.
132. Badylak SF: Coagulation disorders and liver disease. Vet Clin North Am Small Anim Pract 18:87, 1988.
133. Green RA: Pathophysiology of antithrombin III deficiency. Vet Clin North Am Small Anim Pract 18:95, 1988.
134. Willis SE, et al: Whole blood platelet aggregation in dogs with liver disease. Am J Vet Res 50:1893, 1989.
135. Center SA, et al: PIVKA clotting times in dogs with suspected coagulopathies (abstract). Proceedings, Sixteenth Annual Forum, American College of Veterinary Medicine, San Diego, CA, 1998, p 704.
136. Center SA, et al: PIVKA clotting times in clinically ill cats with suspected coagulopathies (abstract). Proceedings, Sixteenth Annual Forum, American College of Veterinary Medicine, San Diego, CA, 1998, p. 704.
137. Rajkovic JA, Williams R: Mechanisms of abnormalities in the host defenses against bacterial infection in liver disease. Clin Sci 68:247, 1985.
138. Rolando N, et al: Prospective study of bacterial infection in acute liver failure: An analysis of fifty patients. Hepatology 11:49, 1990.
139. Rolando N, Wyke RJ: Infections. Gut 32(Suppl):S25, 1991.
140. Kirby R: Septic shock. *In* Bonagura JD, Kirk RW (eds): Kirk's Current Veterinary Therapy XII. Philadelphia, WB Saunders, 1995, p 139.
141. Vaden SL, Papich MG: Empiric antibiotic therapy. *In* Bonagura D, Kirk RW (eds): Kirk's Current Veterinary Therapy XII. Philadelphia, WB Saunders, 1995, p 276.
142. Rolfe DS, Twedt DC: Copper-associated hepatopathies in dogs. Vet Clin North Am Small Anim Pract 25:399, 1995.
143. Christophi C, Hughes ER: Hepatobiliary disorders in inflammatory bowel disease. Collective review. Surg Gynecol Obstet 160:187, 1985.
144. Harmatz A: Hepatobiliary manifestations of inflammatory bowel disease. Med Clin North Am 78:1387, 1994.
145. Chapman BL, et al: Granulomatous hepatitis in dogs: Nine cases (1987–1990). JAVMA 203:680, 1993.
146. Center SA, Rowland PH: The cholangitis/cholangiohepatitis complex in the cat. Proceedings, Twelfth Annual Forum, American College of Veterinary Medicine, San Francisco, CA, 1994, p 766.
147. Weiss DJ, et al: Relationship between inflammatory hepatic disease and inflammatory bowel disease, pancreatitis, and nephritis in cats. JAVMA 209:1114, 1996.
148. Lifton SJ, et al: Glucocorticoid deficient hypoadrenocorticism in dogs: 18 cases (1986–1995). JAVMA 209:2076, 1996.
149. Feldman EC, Nelson RW: Hypoadrenocorticism (Addison's disease). *In* Feldman EC, Nelson RW (eds): Canine and Feline Endocrinology and Reproduction, 2nd ed. Philadelphia, WB Saunders, 1996, p 266.
150. Van Winkle TJ, Bruce E: Thrombosis of the portal vein in eleven dogs. Vet Pathol 30:28, 1993.
151. Zimmerman HJ, et al: Jaundice due to bacterial infection. Gastroenterology 7:362, 1979.
152. Franson TR, et al: Frequency and characteristics of hyperbilirubinemia associated with bacteremia. Rev Infect Dis 7:1, 1985.
153. Taboada J, Meyer DJ: Cholestasis associated with extrahepatic bacterial infection in five dogs. J Vet Intern Med 3:216, 1989.
154. Grooters AM, et al: Hepatic abscesses associated with diabetes mellitus in two dogs. J Vet Intern Med 8:203, 1994.
155. Parrar ET, et al: Hepatic abscesses in dogs: 14 cases (1982–1994). JAVMA 208:243, 1996.

LIV

156. Schwarz LA, et al: Hepatic abscesses in 13 dogs: A review of the ultrasono-graphic findings, clinical data and therapeutic options. Vet Radiol Ultrasound 39:357, 1998.
157. Bolin CA: Diagnosis of leptospirosis: A re-emerging disease of companion animals. Semin Vet Med Surg (Small Anim) 11:166, 1996.
158. Brown CA, et al: *Leptospira interrogans* serovar *grippotyphosa* infection in dogs. JAVMA 209:1265, 1996.
159. Wohl JS: Canine leptospirosis. Compend Contin Educ Pract Vet 18:1215, 1996.
160. Levitan DM: Did you consider leptospirosis? Acute renal failure with or without jaundice can have this zoonotic etiology. Vet Forum 15:42, 1998.
161. Rentko VT, et al: Canine leptospirosis: A retrospective study of 17 cases. J Vet Intern Med 6:235, 1992.
162. Harkin KR, Gartrell CL: Canine leptospirosis in New Jersey and Michigan: 17 cases (1990–1995). J Am Anim Hosp Assoc 32:495, 1996.
163. Miller WH, et al: Necrolytic migratory erythema in dogs: A hepatocutaneous syndrome. J Am Anim Hosp Assoc 26:573, 1990.
164. Gross TL, et al: Glucagon-producing pancreatic endocrine tumors in two dogs with superficial necrolytic dermatitis. JAVMA 197:1619, 1990.
165. Gross TL, et al: Superficial necrolytic dermatitis (necrolytic migratory erythema) in dogs. Vet Pathol 30:75, 1993.
166. Taboada J, Merchant S: Superficial necrolytic dermatitis and the liver. Proceedings, Fifteenth Annual Forum, American College of Veterinary Medicine, Lake Buena Vista, FL, 1997, p 534.

167. Patel A, et al: A case of metabolic epidermal necrosis in a cat. Vet Dermatol 7:221, 1996.
168. Jacobson SL, et al: Hepatic ultrasonography and pathological findings in dogs with hepatocutaneous syndrome: New concepts. J Vet Intern Med 9:399, 1995.
169. Torres SMF, et al: Resolution of superficial necrolytic dermatitis following excision of a glucagon-secreting pancreatic neoplasm in a dog. J Am Anim Hosp Assoc 33:313, 1997.
170. Loeven KO: Hepatic amyloidosis in two Chinese Shar Pei dogs. JAVMA 204:1212, 1994.
171. Loeven KO: Spontaneous hepatic rupture secondary to amyloidosis in a Chinese Shar Pei. J Am Anim Hosp Assoc 30:577, 1994.
172. Rivas AL, et al: A canine febrile disorder associated with elevated interleukin-6. Clin Immunol Immunopathol 64:36, 1992.
173. DiBartola SP, et al: Familial renal amyloidosis in Chinese Shar Pei dogs. JAVMA 197:483, 1990.
174. Holloway SA: Heatstroke in dogs. Compend Contin Educ Pract Vet 12:1598, 1992.
175. Ruslander D: Heatstroke. *In* Kirk RW (ed): Current Veterinary Therapy XI. Philadelphia, WB Saunders, 1992, p 143.
176. Goggin JM, et al: Ultrasonographic identification of *Dirofilaria immitis* in the aorta and liver of a dog. JAVMA 210:1635, 1997.
177. Ware WA: Heartworm disease. *In* Nelson RW, Couto CG (eds): Small Animal Internal Medicine, 2nd ed. St. Louis, CV Mosby, 1998, p 162.

CHAPTER 145

DISEASES OF THE GALLBLADDER AND EXTRAHEPATIC BILIARY SYSTEM

Michael D. Willard and Theresa W. Fossum

ANATOMY

Bile is formed by hepatocytes and discharged into the canaliculi lying between the hepatocytes. Canaliculi unite to form interlobular ducts, which ultimately merge to form lobar or bile ducts. The gallbladder plus the hepatic, cystic, and common bile ducts constitute the extrahepatic biliary system. Bile drains from the bile ducts into the cystic and common bile ducts and is stored and concentrated in the gallbladder (Fig. 145–1). The gallbladder lies between the quadrate lobe of the liver medially and the right medial lobe laterally.[1] It is a pear-shaped organ that, in a medium-size dog, normally holds approximately 15 mL of bile. The rounded end of the gallbladder is the fundus. Between the neck of the gallbladder (i.e., the tapering end leading into the cystic duct) and the fundus is the body.

The cystic duct extends from the neck of the gallbladder to the junction with the first tributary from the liver.[1] From this point to the opening of the biliary system into the duodenum, the duct is termed the common bile duct. The common bile duct runs through the lesser omentum for approximately 5 cm and enters the mesenteric wall of the duodenum. The canine common bile duct terminates in the duodenum near the opening of the minor pancreatic duct. This combined opening of the minor pancreatic duct and common bile duct is the major duodenal papilla. The intramural portion of the common bile duct is termed the sphincter of Oddi in people. The feline common bile duct usually joins the major pancreatic duct before entering the duodenum.[1]

PHYSIOLOGY

Bile contains primarily water, conjugated bile acids, bile pigments, cholesterol, and inorganic salts. Greater than 90 per cent of bile salts are reabsorbed from the intestinal tract, transported back to the liver via the portal vein, and reexcreted—a process termed enterohepatic circulation. Bilirubin and biliverdin produce the typical yellow color of bile. Bile is continually secreted into the gallbladder, where it is stored and modified. Gallbladder emptying is normally in-

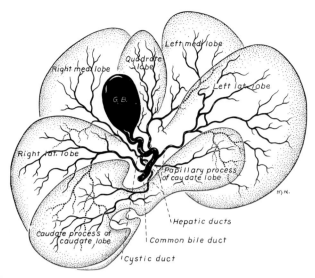

Figure 145–1. Anatomy of the canine gallbladder. (From Evans HE, Christensen GC: Miller's Anatomy of the Dog, 2nd ed. Philadelphia, WB Saunders, 1979, p 499.)

duced by neural (vagal parasympathetics) and humoral (cholecystokinin) stimuli. Parasympathomimetic drugs and magnesium sulfate[2] cause gallbladder contraction, whereas anticholinergic drugs and somatostatin inhibit contraction.[1]

DIAGNOSTIC TOOLS FOR EVALUATING THE GALLBLADDER AND BILE DUCTS

Icterus, vomiting, abdominal pain, and/or ascites are consistent with biliary tract dysfunction. If cholecystic or choledochal disease is suspected based on clinical pathology data or abdominal imaging, a complete history should be obtained and a physical examination performed, although they rarely definitively diagnose biliary tract disease.

Complete blood count (CBC), serum biochemistry profile, and urinalysis are indicated if biliary tract dysfunction is suspected. The CBC inconsistently reflects cholecystic inflammation. Increased alanine aminotransferase (ALT) is common if inflammation ascends into the hepatic parenchyma. Increased serum alkaline phosphatase (SAP) with or without hyperbilirubinemia is typical in extrahepatic biliary tract obstruction (EHBO)[3] and when inflammatory disease ascends from the biliary tract. Cats tend to have lesser elevations of SAP than dogs. Hypercholesterolemia may occur secondary to EHBO. Urinalysis may be helpful, because bilirubinuria occurs before hyperbilirubinemia. Imaging and/or surgery are usually required to differentiate icterus due to hepatic disease versus biliary tract disease.

Abdominal radiographs may reveal radiodense objects (e.g., gallstones) or air in the gallbladder. Animals with EHBO due to pancreatitis may have a soft tissue mass or poor serosal detail in the region of the pancreas. Contrast radiographs of the biliary tree are rarely useful in icteric animals. Endoscopic retrograde pancreatography and direct injection of contrast into dilated bile ducts via transabdominal placement of a "slim" needle are rarely performed.

Ultrasonography is the most useful nonsurgical technique to distinguish hepatic parenchymal from biliary tract disease. It can identify abnormalities within the lumen of the gallbladder (e.g., stones, tumors, flocculent material) and most biliary tract obstructions (Fig. 145–2).[3] Anorexic animals often have marked cholecystic enlargement, which can be misdiagnosed as obstruction. Dilatation of the gallbladder plus loss of the tapering of the gallbladder neck occur within 24 hours of ligation of the bile duct. This is followed by dilatation of the common duct at 48 hours and of the extrahepatic ducts at 72 hours. Similar changes occur in the intrahepatic bile ducts within a week.[4] The common bile duct is typically less than 3 mm in diameter in medium-size dogs[5] and less than 2.5 mm in cats.[3] One study found that 28 cats without EHBO had a common bile duct 4 mm or less in diameter, whereas a common bile duct greater than 5 mm in diameter meant EHBO in six of seven cats.[6] If the clinician is unsure whether EHBO is present after performing ultrasonography, repeating the examination in two to four days or after inducing gallbladder contraction (e.g., feeding a high-fat meal or administering prokinetic drugs such as sincalide[7]) is often definitive. However, loss of elasticity of the bile ducts may occur as a result of aging, inflammation, or chronic obstruction (especially in cats), and some ducts never return to their original diameter after obstruction.[4, 5]

Gallstones are typically identified ultrasonographically as hyperechoic foci or by the observation of acoustic shadowing originating from the gallbladder.[4] Sediment (sometimes referred to as "sludge") is occasionally noted in the gallbladder, but its significance is uncertain. Supposedly, bile becomes progressively thicker as water is absorbed during biliary stasis. Finally, soft tissue changes of the gallbladder (e.g., tumors, granulation tissue, and congenital defects) may be seen ultrasonographically. Cholecystitis may cause gallbladder wall thickening and/or edema, which can produce a layered or "double-wall" ultrasonographic appearance.[4, 8]

Bile (for culture or cytologic examination) can be aspirated from the gallbladder by ultrasound-guided fine-needle aspiration using a 22-gauge needle.[8] As much bile as possible is withdrawn to lessen the likelihood of subsequent bile leakage into the abdomen. This procedure appears to be relatively safe,[8] although vagal-induced severe bradycardia and other problems have occurred in people.[1] The value of culturing bile versus culturing hepatic parenchyma is unknown; however, aerobic and anaerobic cultures of bile (and hepatic parenchyma) are recommended if bacterial cholecystitis is suspected.

Nuclear scintigraphy is rarely used to define canine or

LIV

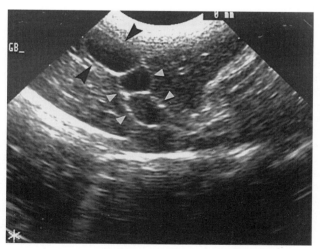

Figure 145–2. Distention and convolution of the gallbladder body (black arrowheads) and neck (white arrowheads) in a cat with common bile duct obstruction. (Courtesy of Dr. L. Homco, Texas A&M University.)

feline biliary disease owing to the need for specialized equipment and facilities. Scintigraphy has been used to study gallbladder function in cats[9] and dogs[10] and is an accurate indicator of canine EHBO.[11]

Exploratory laparotomy should be performed in animals with suspected leakage of bile into the abdomen, EHBO, and neoplasia, parasites, stones, infiltrates, and other mass lesions of or within the biliary tract. During exploration, patency of the common bile duct must be assured by compressing the gallbladder or catheterizing the duct. Readers are referred to surgery texts for detailed information regarding extrahepatic biliary tract surgery.[12]

SPECIFIC PROBLEMS SEEN WITH GALLBLADDER AND BILIARY TRACT DISEASE

Vomiting, icterus, and anorexia are common in animals with inflammatory or obstructive biliary tract disease.[3, 8, 13, 14] Fever and abdominal discomfort also occur, but not as consistently. Icterus (see Chapter 58) is particularly helpful for localizing the problem to the biliary tract. After hemolytic disease is eliminated, ultrasonography is used to distinguish hepatic parenchymal from biliary tract disease.

Ascites (see Chapter 39) may occur owing to leakage of bile into the peritoneal cavity. Bilious effusions are obvious because the fluid looks like bile. If one is unsure whether abdominal fluid is bilious or bile-stained, compare bilirubin concentrations in the serum and in the effusion. Bilious effusions have fluid bilirubin concentrations greater than serum concentrations.

Acute abdomen (i.e., shock, sepsis, and/or pain [see Chapter 39] due to abdominal disease) may be caused by leakage of bile into the peritoneal cavity, particularly if the bile is septic. Hematemesis is uncommon in animals with cholecystic disease. Intracystic bleeding may allow blood to exit into the duodenum, where it is refluxed into the stomach and vomited[15]; however, there are more common causes of hematemesis, and cholecystic disease should not be an early consideration.

SPECIFIC DISEASES OF THE GALLBLADDER

OBSTRUCTIVE DISEASE

Pancreatic disease is the most common cause of canine EHBO.[3] Scar formation may occur in or around the duct, or the duct may be compressed by inflamed pancreatic tissue, pancreatic abscesses, or cysts. Treatment of EHBO secondary to benign pancreatitis initially consists of medical management of the pancreatitis. If this is unsuccessful or if ascending bacterial infection is suspected, cholecystoduodenostomy or cholecystojejunostomy may be considered. In extremely ill animals with EHBO that cannot undergo surgical exploration, temporary decompression of the gallbladder with a Foley catheter or a self-retaining accordion catheter[16] may be warranted.

Neoplasia may cause EHBO. Surgery for pancreatic neoplasia causing EHBO is generally unrewarding, because most pancreatic tumors are malignant. Cholecystojejunostomy may be palliative if the intestinal lumen is patent. Pancreatic-duodenal resection (i.e., Billroth II) is possible, but surgical cures are unlikely. Biliary, intestinal, hepatic, or lymph node malignancy may also obstruct the bile ducts; biopsy is imperative to obtain a diagnosis. Surgical resection of these tumors is also difficult, and the prognosis is typically poor; however, chemotherapy benefits some animals with lymphosarcoma.

Choleliths (see later under Nonobstructive Disease) that obstruct the common bile duct should be removed. Cholecystectomy is the treatment of choice when clinical signs are secondary to cholelithiasis.[14] If stones are present in the common bile duct, the duct can be catheterized via the duodenum and the stones flushed into the gallbladder. Alternatively, enlarged bile ducts can be incised (choledochotomy) and the stones removed directly; however, care is needed when closing the common bile duct to avoid iatrogenic stricture formation. Clinical studies have found a 13-fold greater mortality in people with cholelithiasis when a choledochotomy is performed versus a cholecystectomy.[17]

Miscellaneous causes of EHBO include diaphragmatic hernia,[18] mucoceles,[19] and biliary pseudocysts.[20]

NONOBSTRUCTIVE DISEASE

Cholecystitis (i.e., inflammation of the gallbladder) usually involves the associated bile ducts. It is typically due to a bacterial infection caused by bacteria ascending from the intestine via the common bile duct or by hematogenous seeding, and it can often be cured with antibiotics. However, if cholecystitis recurs repeatedly despite appropriate use of antibiotics, cholecystectomy is usually curative. Cholecystitis may take one of several courses.

Bacterial cholangitis/cholangiohepatitis occurs if the infection ascends the biliary tree into the liver. This appears to be more common in cats than in dogs. Any bacteria may be responsible; *Escherichia coli* seems especially common, although numerous species, including anaerobic bacteria, have been reported.[8, 14, 21] These animals often present to veterinarians because of icterus, anorexia, and/or vomiting. Fever is uncommon. Increased serum ALT, SAP, and bilirubin are typical, but neutrophilia is inconsistent. Imaging is seldom diagnostic[8] but helps eliminate other diseases. Hepatic biopsy with aerobic and anaerobic culture of bile and hepatic parenchyma is indicated. The prognosis is variable, but good results are expected when the correct antibiotics are administered promptly. Enrofloxacin plus amoxicillin is reasonable until culture results are available. Vitamin K_1 should be administered if coagulopathy is suspected.

Necrotizing cholecystitis occurs when a bacterial infection severely damages the gallbladder wall, sometimes rupturing it (Fig. 145–3) and spilling bile into the abdomen.[22] This usually causes generalized septic peritonitis (see Chapter 39). If the bile is inspissated, rupture causes spillage of a

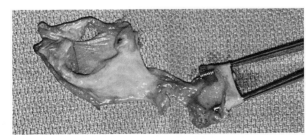

Figure 145–3. Photograph of a ruptured gallbladder that has been resected from a dog. The rupture was spontaneous and was due to necrotizing cholecystitis. The forceps are in the cystic duct.

relatively thick, gelatinous mass into the cranial abdomen, producing a localized peritonitis. These animals tend not to be as sick as those with diffuse peritonitis. Sometimes pain can be localized to the anterior abdomen. If diagnosed before the gallbladder ruptures, signs are similar to those of localized peritonitis. Adhesions or fistulous tracts around the gallbladder occasionally occur.[22] Diagnosis is usually made by ultrasonography or exploratory laparotomy. Ultrasonography can be followed by abdominocentesis and/or diagnostic peritoneal lavage. Surgical exploration should be performed once the animal is stable. Treatment consists of cholecystectomy, antibiotics, and appropriate therapy for peritonitis. Attempts to salvage the gallbladder by closing the defect are inappropriate, because the wall is typically necrotic. The common bile duct must not be ligated when the gallbladder is removed. The mortality rate was 39 per cent in a study of 23 dogs with necrotizing cholecystitis; delayed diagnosis probably contributed to this high mortality.[22]

Emphysematous cholecystitis occurs when gas-forming bacteria infect the gallbladder[23] and gas fills the lumen and/or invades the wall (tympanic and emphysematous cholecystitis, respectively). Once considered pathognomonic of diabetes mellitus, emphysematous cholecystitis can develop in any animal. Signs may be similar to those described for bacterial and necrotizing cholecystitis. Plain radiographs are diagnostic (Fig. 145–4), and treatment consists of antibiotics. Knowing that gas-forming bacteria (e.g., E. coli, Clostridium perfringens) must be responsible helps guide the selection of antibiotics (e.g., enrofloxacin plus amoxicillin).

Choleliths are often fortuitous findings at necropsy or during imaging.[1] They often cause no problems (Fig. 145–5); however, they may be associated with cholecystitis.[14] If found in an animal with biliary tract disease, they should be removed. Aged, female, small breed dogs (especially schnauzers and poodles) appear to be at increased risk.[1, 14] Whereas people commonly develop dietary-induced cholesterol gallstones, canine gallstones usually contain bilirubin, calcium, and mucin.[1] The rarity of canine cholelithiasis may be owing to decreased concentrations of cholesterol in canine bile; absorption of ionized calcium from the gallbladder, limiting the amount of free ionized calcium in bile[1]; and failure to diagnose them. Calcium salts are the major compo-

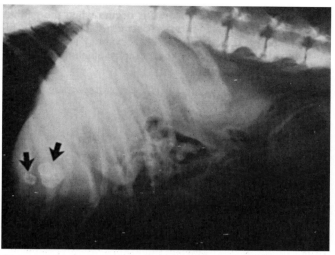

Figure 145–5. Lateral radiograph of a dog showing mineral densities in the region of the gallbladder (arrows). These were gallstones that were not causing clinical disease in this dog.

nents of pigment gallstones; thus, availability of ionized calcium may be important in canine gallstone formation. Pigment gallstones can be experimentally produced in dogs by feeding a methionine-deficient diet[24] or a taurine-deficient, high-cholesterol diet.[1]

Parasites of the gallbladder and/or bile ducts are seldom diagnosed. *Platynosomum fastosum* (previously *concinnum*) is a fluke principally found in animals from Florida, Hawaii, and the Caribbean. It typically infects cats that eat lizards or toads (i.e., a second intermediate host). The fluke may ultimately be found in the gallbladder and/or bile ducts, where it may be asymptomatic or cause fibrosis and/or obstruction. Signs of infection can be similar to those of cholecystitis. Diagnosis is by ultrasonography or by finding the ova by fecal sedimentation examination (not fecal flotation), assuming that there is not complete biliary tract obstruction. Therapy may be attempted with praziquantel (20 mg/kg subcutaneously, once a day for three days). Prognosis is uncertain, but severe hepatic disease warrants a guarded prognosis.[1] *Amphimerus pseudofelineus* has also been associated with cholangitis, cholangiohepatitis, and distention of the feline common bile duct.[25] High-dose (40 mg/kg) praziquantel therapy administered orally once a day for three days reportedly eradicated the infection. *Metorchis conjunctus* and *Eurytrema procyonis* may also be found in the feline biliary tract.[26]

Neoplasia of the gallbladder or extrahepatic biliary tract is rare. Bile duct carcinomas have been reported in cats and dogs.[23] Metastasis of bile duct carcinomas commonly occurs before clinical signs manifest; therefore, surgery is rarely curative. Surgical therapy of cholecystic tumors may be curative if there is no metastasis.[15]

RUPTURE OF THE GALLBLADDER OR EXTRAHEPATIC BILIARY DUCTS

Extrahepatic biliary duct or gallbladder rupture may be iatrogenic or associated with blunt abdominal trauma, cholecystitis, or obstruction secondary to stones, neoplasia, or parasites. Trauma usually causes rupture of bile ducts rather than the gallbladder. Ductal rupture probably occurs when a force is applied adjacent to the gallbladder sufficient to cause

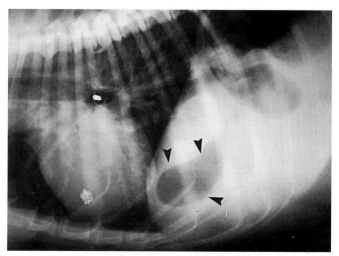

Figure 145–4. Lateral radiograph of a dog showing a pear-shaped, air-filled structure (arrows). This is the gallbladder of a dog with emphysematous, tympanic cholecystitis. (Courtesy of Dr. Robert Toal, College of Veterinary Medicine, University of Tennessee.)

LIV

a shearing force on the duct. The most common site of ductal rupture appears to be the common bile duct just distal to the entrance of the last hepatic duct[27]; however, rupture may occur in the distal common bile duct, cystic duct (rare), or hepatic ducts. Gallbladder rupture is more commonly associated with necrotizing cholecystitis or cholelithiasis, with or without obstruction of the common bile duct.[22]

Early diagnosis of biliary tract rupture is imperative. Leakage of infected bile causes clinical signs of bile peritonitis to develop quickly. In a study of 24 dogs and 2 cats with biliary tract rupture, there was 54 per cent mortality, which was limited to animals with infected bile. *E. coli* was the bacterium most commonly cultured from infected animals.[13] Ascites and icterus may be the only signs in dogs with sterile bile in the peritoneal cavity due to traumatic rupture; however, necrosis and changes in mucosal permeability secondary to the bile can lead to secondary bacterial infection of the effusion.[23] Delayed diagnosis of a ruptured biliary tract results in necrotic tissues and adhesions, which complicate surgical repair. Diagnostic peritoneal lavage may assist in the early diagnosis of sterile bile peritonitis.

Surgical treatment for a ruptured common bile duct involves repair of the duct or biliary diversion. Repair is often possible if the rupture is diagnosed early, but it becomes difficult once adhesions develop. In such cases, cholecystojejunostomy is generally easier and safer. Ruptured hepatic ducts are usually ligated. Gallbladder rupture secondary to infective processes should be treated by cholecystectomy.

MISCELLANEOUS FINDINGS

Cystic mucinous hypertrophy is occasionally found in older animals, either at necropsy or during ultrasonography. It is not clearly associated with disease, although progestational drugs may produce it.[1] Unless there is evidence of significant gallbladder dysfunction, this lesion does not warrant further evaluation. Congenital defects of the gallbladder are occasionally observed. Bifid gallbladders have been reported in cats, although their significance is unknown.[26] Gallbladder cysts have been reported in people with signs of acute abdomen,[28] and they may occur in dogs or cats. Non–biliary tract disorders may also produce cholecystic lesions. Gallbladder edema is reportedly common in infectious canine hepatitis. In other diseases, however, gallbladder lesions are seldom significant. Even in canine salmonellosis, the gallbladder is rarely important as a reservoir of infection.

REFERENCES

1. Center SA: Diseases of the gallbladder and biliary tree. *In* Strombeck's Small Animal Gastroenterology, 3rd ed. Philadelphia, WB Saunders, 1996, p 860.
2. Sterczer A, et al: Effect of cholagogues on the volume of the gallbladder of dogs. Res Vet Sci 61:44, 1996.
3. Fahie MA, Martin RA: Extrahepatic biliary tract obstruction: A retrospective study of 45 cases (1983–1993). J Am Anim Hosp Assoc 31:478, 1995.
4. Partington BP, Biller DS: Liver. *In* Green RW (ed): Small Animal Ultrasound. Philadelphia, Lippincott-Raven, 1996, p 105.
5. Raptopoulus V, et al: The effect of time and cholecystectomy on experimental biliary tree dilatation. Invest Radiol 20:276, 1985.
6. Leveille R, et al: Sonographic evaluation of the common bile duct in cats. J Vet Intern Med 10:296, 1996.
7. Finn ST, et al: Ultrasonographic assessment of sincalide-induced canine gallbladder emptying: An aid to the diagnosis of biliary obstruction. Vet Rec 32:269, 1991.
8. Rivers BJ, et al: Acalculous cholecystitis in four canine cases: Ultrasonographic findings and use of ultrasonographic guided percutaneous cholecystocentesis in diagnosis. J Am Anim Hosp Assoc 33:207, 1997.
9. Newell SM, et al: Hepatobiliary scintigraphy in the evaluation of feline liver disease. J Vet Intern Med 10:308, 1996.
10. Rothuizen J, van den Brom WE: Quantitative hepatobiliary scintigraphy as a measure of bile flow in dogs with cholestatic disease. Am J Vet Res 51:253, 1990.
11. Boothe HW, et al: Use of hepatobiliary scintigraphy in the diagnosis of extrahepatic biliary obstruction in dogs and cats: 25 cases (1982–1989). JAVMA 201:134, 1992.
12. Fossum TW: Surgery of the extrahepatic biliary system. *In* Fossum TW (ed): Small Animal Surgery. St. Louis, Mosby-Year Book, 1997, p 389.
13. Ludwig LL, et al: Surgical treatment of bile peritonitis in 24 dogs and 2 cats: A retrospective study 1987–1994 (abstract). Vet Surg 24:430, 1995.
14. Kirpensteijn J, et al: Cholelithiasis in dogs: 29 cases (1980–1990). JAVMA 202:1137, 1993.
15. Willard MD, et al: Neuroendocrine carcinoma of the gallbladder in a dog. JAVMA 192:926, 1988.
16. Lawrence D, et al: Temporary bile diversion in cats with experimental extrahepatic bile duct obstruction. Vet Surg 21:446, 1992.
17. Herzog U, et al: Surgical treatment for cholelithiasis. Surg Gynecol Obstet 175:238, 1992.
18. Cornell KK, et al: Extrahepatic biliary obstruction secondary to diaphragmatic hernia in two cats. J Am Anim Hosp Assoc 29:502, 1993.
19. Newell SM, et al: Gallbladder mucocele causing biliary obstruction in two dogs: Ultrasonographic scintigraphic and pathological findings. J Am Anim Hosp Assoc 31:467, 1995.
20. Hunt GB, et al: Successful management of an iatrogenic biliary pseudocyst in a dog. J Am Anim Hosp Assoc 33:166, 1997.
21. Oswald GP, et al: *Campylobacter jejuni* bacteremia and acute cholecystitis in two dogs. J Am Anim Hosp Assoc 30:165, 1994.
22. Church EM, Mattheisen DT: Surgical treatment of 23 dogs with necrotizing cholecystitis. J Am Anim Hosp Assoc 24:305, 1988.
23. Neer TM: Review of disorders of the gallbladder and extrahepatic biliary tract in the dog and cat. J Vet Intern Med 6:186, 1992.
24. Rege RV, Prystowski JB: Inflammatory properties of bile from dogs with pigment gallstones. Am J Surg 171:197, 1996.
25. Lewis DT, et al: Cholangiohepatitis and choledochectasia associated with *Amphimerus pseudofelineus* in a cat. J Am Anim Hosp Assoc 27:156, 1991.
26. Johnson SE: Liver and biliary tract. *In* Anderson NV (ed): Veterinary Gastroenterology, 2nd ed. Philadelphia, Lea & Febiger, 1992, p 504.
27. Parchman MB, Flanders JA: Extrahepatic biliary tract rupture: Evaluation of the relationship between the site of rupture and the cause of rupture in 15 dogs. Cornell Vet 80:267, 1990.
28. Jacobs E, et al: Cyst of the gallbladder. Dig Dis Sci 36:1796, 1991.

CHAPTER 146

EXOCRINE PANCREATIC DISEASE

David A. Williams

The major function of the exocrine pancreas is to secrete digestive enzymes.[1] The exocrine pancreas also fulfills several other functions (Table 146–1). Bicarbonate in pancreatic juice contributes to the neutralization of gastric acid,[2] and other factors in pancreatic juice play a role in the absorption of cobalamin (vitamin B_{12}),[3,4] zinc,[5] and perhaps other nutrients. The pancreatic coenzyme colipase facilitates the action of pancreatic lipase in the intestinal lumen.[6–8] Pancreatic secretions also influence the function of the small intestine by inhibiting bacterial proliferation in the lumen of the proximal small intestine, by contributing to the normal degradation of exposed brush border enzymes,[9,10] and, together with biliary secretions, by exerting a trophic effect on the mucosa.[9–11] Finally, the pancreas protects itself against autodigestion by several mechanisms, including the synthesis of a specific enzyme inhibitor that is stored and secreted together with the digestive enzymes.[12]

ANATOMY

The pancreas of dogs and cats consists primarily of right and left lobes with a small central body where the lobes join together (Fig. 146–1). It develops from ventral and dorsal bud-like primordia that arise from the embryonic small intestine and therefore represents an extension of the glandular mucosa of the duodenum, to which it remains connected by secretory ducts. Because either the dorsal or ventral primordium or its associated ducts may involute during development, there is marked species and, to a lesser extent, individual variation in the origin of the gland and the pattern of its duct system.[13,14]

In the dog, both primordia usually persist and fuse, and the two original ducts are retained. The duct of the ventral primordium is the pancreatic duct (Wirsung's duct), which opens adjacent to the bile duct on the major duodenal papilla. The duct of the dorsal primordium is the accessory pancreatic duct (Santorini's duct), which opens on the minor duodenal papilla a few centimeters distal to the major duodenal papilla. These two duct systems usually intercommunicate within the gland. In some dogs, only the accessory pancreatic

duct (the larger of the two) is present, and all pancreatic juice enters the duodenum through the minor duodenal papilla. In the cat, only the duct of the ventral primordium, the pancreatic duct, generally persists, and it fuses with the bile duct before opening on the major duodenal papilla. However, in approximately 20 per cent of cats, the accessory pancreatic duct is also present.[11,14,15]

Anatomically, the pancreas is closely associated with the stomach, liver, and duodenum (see Fig. 146–1). The body lies in the bend of the cranial part of the duodenum, where it is crossed dorsally by the portal vein on its way to the liver. The right lobe lies in the mesoduodenum and accompanies the descending duodenum, in some cases extending to the cecum. The left lobe lies in the deep wall of the greater omentum and accompanies the pyloric part of the stomach to the left.

Each microscopic pancreatic lobule is composed mainly of (1) cells that synthesize the digestive enzymes and store them in zymogen granules (acinar cells) and (2) a smaller number of cells that make up the branching duct system (intralobular, interlobular, and main pancreatic ducts).[16,17] The pancreas also contains endocrine tissue, the islets of Langerhans, but this accounts for only 1 to 2 per cent of the gland, whereas the exocrine tissue together with associated vessels and nerves accounts for more than 98 per cent of the pancreatic mass.[13,18,19]

BIOCHEMISTRY AND PHYSIOLOGY

DIGESTIVE ENZYMES

The acinar cells secrete a fluid rich in enzymes that degrade proteins, lipids, and polysaccharides (Table 146–2).

TABLE 146–1. FUNCTIONS OF THE EXOCRINE PANCREAS

Secretion of digestive enzymes
Secretion of colipase
Secretion of bicarbonate
Facilitation of cobalamin and zinc absorption
Secretion of antibacterial factors
Modulation of intestinal mucosal function
Protection against autodigestion

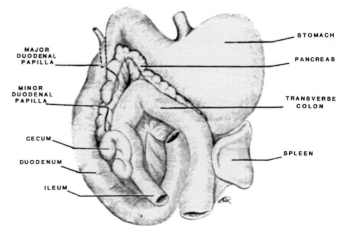

Figure 146–1. Anatomic associations of the canine pancreas.

TABLE 146–2. MAJOR SECRETORY PROTEINS OF THE EXOCRINE PANCREASE OF THE DOG

Enzymes secreted as inactive zymogens
  Trypsinogens [1 (anionic), 2 and 3 (cationic)] → trypsins
  Chymotrypsinogens (1, 2, and 3) → chymotrypsins
  Proelastases (1 and 2) → elastases
  Procarboxypeptidases (A1, A2, A3, and B) → carboxypeptidases
  Prophospholipase A_2 → phospholipase A_2
Coenzyme
  Procolipase → colipase
Enzymes
  Alpha-amylase
  Lipase
Inhibitor
  Pancreatic secretory trypsin inhibitor

Trypsins, chymotrypsins, and elastases are endopeptidases that cleave peptide bonds at specific sites within polypeptide chains; the carboxypeptidases are exopeptidases that cleave specific carboxy-terminal residues. Alpha-amylase hydrolyzes 4-glycosidic bonds in starches; phospholipase A_2 hydrolyzes fatty acid esters at the two position of some membrane phospholipids; and lipase, in the presence of the coenzyme colipase, hydrolyzes ester bonds in the one and three positions of triglycerides.[12]

DEFENSES AGAINST AUTODIGESTION

Several mechanisms exist that discourage autodigestion of the pancreas by the enzymes that it secretes.[12, 20] First, proteolytic and phospholipolytic enzymes are synthesized, stored, and secreted by the pancreas in the form of catalytically inactive zymogens (indicated by the addition of the prefix pro- or the suffix -ogen to the enzyme name) (see Table 146–2). These zymogens are activated by enzymatic cleavage of a small peptide, the activation peptide, from the amino-terminal of the polypeptide chain (Fig. 146–2).[12] Enzymes from several sources, including some lysosomal proteases, are capable of activating pancreatic zymogens, but, ordinarily, activation of zymogens does not occur until they are secreted into the small intestine. The enzyme enteropeptidase, which is synthesized by the enterocytes lining the duodenal mucosa, is particularly effective at cleaving the activation peptides from trypsinogens to form trypsins. Active trypsins subsequently cleave the activation peptides from other digestive zymogens (Fig. 146–3). Enteropeptidase therefore plays a crucial role in the activation of digestive enzymes.[12] Second, from the moment that synthesis of digestive enzymes begins, they are segregated, along with

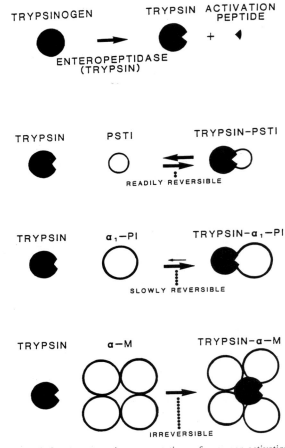

Figure 146–2. Diagrammatic representations of zymogen activation (trypsinogen) and the binding of proteases (trypsin) by major inhibitors.

potentially damaging lysosomal enzymes, into the lumen of the rough endoplasmic reticulum.[21] This is part of the cisternal space of the acinar cell, a compartment separate from the cell cytosol, which contains other enzymes with the potential to activate the zymogens. In the Golgi apparatus the lysosomal enzymes are then routed to lysosomes and the digestive enzymes to zymogen granules, thereby preventing activation of zymogens by lysosomal proteases (Fig. 146–4). Should any intrapancreatic activation of trypsinogen occur, there are at least two mechanisms that help prevent or limit cascade activation of other zymogens. Trypsin is quite effective at hydrolyzing itself, thereby limiting its activity so that activation of small amounts of trypsin tends not to

TABLE 146–3. MAJOR PROTEASE INHIBITORS IN CANINE PANCREAS AND PLASMA

INHIBITOR	PANCREATIC SECRETORY TRYPSIN INHIBITOR (PSTI)	ALPHA₁-PROTEINASE INHIBITOR (ALPHA₁-ANTITRYPSIN) (ALPHA₁-PI)	ALPHA-MACROGLOBULINS (ALPHA-M₁ AND ALPHA-M₂)
Principal locations	Pancreas, pancreatic juice	Plasma, intercellular space	Plasma
Approximate molecular weight	6000	59,000	750,000
Specificity	Trypsin only	Broad spectrum (serine proteases)	Broad spectrum (serine and other proteases)
Inhibition	Temporary (slowly degraded by trypsin)	Transient (transfers enzyme to α-M)	Irreversible (permanent trap for captured enzyme)
Function	Inhibits intrapancreatic autoactivation of trypsin	Readily diffusible inhibitor present in the intercellular space	Traps proteases prior to removal by monocyte-macrophage system

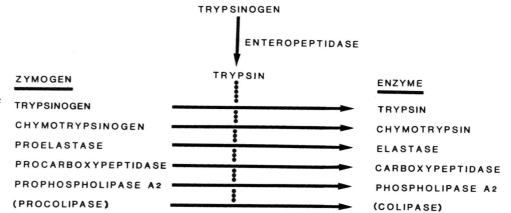

Figure 146–3. Activation of pancreatic proteases and phospholipase.

be catastrophic. Should significant activation occur, however, the acinar cells contain a specific trypsin inhibitor that is synthesized, segregated, stored, and secreted along with the digestive enzymes.[12] This low-molecular-weight pancreatic secretory trypsin inhibitor (PSTI) is distinct from the much larger plasma protease inhibitors (Table 146–3). It is believed that PSTI inhibits trypsin activity should there be significant activation of trypsinogen within the acinar cell or duct system, thereby limiting any tendency for further intrapancreatic activation of the digestive enzymes (see Fig. 146–2).[12]

REGULATION OF PANCREATIC SECRETION

The exocrine pancreas secretes juice into the duodenum both in the absence of food (basal or interdigestive secretion) and in response to a meal. The basal rate of secretion in dogs is about 2 per cent (bicarbonate) or 10 per cent (enzymes) of the maximal secretory rate in response to a meal,[2] but this rate increases transiently in association with the cyclic interdigestive contractile activity of the upper gastrointestinal tract.[22, 23] The response after feeding is biphasic: an initial phase that peaks at 1 to 2 hours and is rich in enzymes and a second, more voluminous phase that peaks at 8 to 11 hours and is rich in bicarbonate.[2, 23]

Pancreatic secretion related to feeding occurs as a response to cephalic stimulation, such as the anticipation and

smell of food, as well as gastric and intestinal stimulation by the presence of food in the stomach and small intestine.[22, 23] The response to these stimuli is mediated by a complex interplay of excitatory and inhibitory nervous and hormonal mechanisms; in dogs and cats the endocrine mechanisms are probably of particular importance.[23] Secretin and cholecystokinin, released into the blood from the proximal small intestine when acid and partly digested food are emptied from the stomach into the duodenum, stimulate the secretion of bicarbonate-rich and enzyme-rich components of pancreatic juice, respectively.[2, 22, 23] Secretion of cholecystokinin is regulated in part by monitor peptide, a trypsin-sensitive cholecystokinin-releasing peptide that in the rat is identical to PSTI. The presence of PSTI in the small intestinal lumen therefore signals release of cholecystokinin, and the completion of digestion of PSTI removes this stimulatory drive and helps switch off pancreatic secretion.[24–26]

PANCREATIC ENZYMES IN THE BLOOD

Amylase, lipase, and the zymogens of pancreatic proteases and phospholipase A_2 are present at low concentrations in the plasma of normal healthy animals. These pancreatic proteins are believed to leak directly from the gland into the bloodstream, from which they are cleared by glomerular filtration, with subsequent variable degradation by renal tubular epithelial cells.[20, 27]

DISEASES OF THE EXOCRINE PANCREAS

PANCREATITIS

Inflammatory disease of the human pancreas is usually divided into acute and chronic types on the basis of a combination of diagnostic criteria that may be loosely applied to cats and dogs (Table 146–4).[28] Acute pancreatitis may be defined as inflammation of the pancreas with a sudden onset. Recurrent acute disease refers to repeated bouts of inflammation with little or no permanent pathologic change. Chronic pancreatitis is a continuing inflammatory disease characterized by irreversible morphologic change and possibly leading to permanent impairment of function. Both acute pancreatitis and chronic pancreatitis may be further subdivided on the basis of etiology, if known, and severity. Diagnostic limitations often preclude the strict application of these criteria in veterinary medicine, and the true prevalence of each is not known, but acute disease and

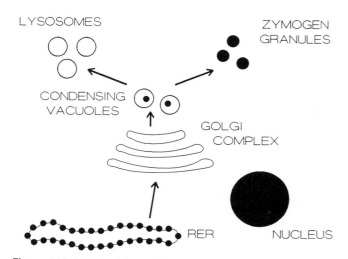

Figure 146–4. Normal intracellular routing of digestive and lysosomal enzymes by the pancreatic acinar cell.

TABLE 146–4. CLASSIFICATION OF PANCREATITIS

Acute
  Etiology—various
  Severity—mild
    No multisystem failure
    Uncomplicated recovery
  Severity—severe
    Multisystem failure
    Pancreatic complication (i.e., infected necrosis, pseudocyst, abscess)

Chronic
  Etiology—various
  Severity—mild
    Minimal morphologic change
    Subclinical loss of exocrine or exocrine function
  Severity—severe
    Severe morphologic damage
    Clinical exocrine pancreatic insufficiency or diabetes mellitus

TABLE 146–5. EXPERIMENTAL MODELS OF PANCREATITIS

Pancreatic duct obstruction
Intraductal bile injection
Intraductal enzyme injection
Intraductal fatty acid injection
Duodenal reflux (closed duodenal loop)
Pancreatic ischemia
Diet induced (ethionine supplemented, choline deficient)
Hyperstimulation induced (cerulein, bethanicol, cholecystokinin, scorpion venom)

recurrent acute disease are more commonly diagnosed than chronic pancreatitis.[20]

If an initial acute episode is not fatal, there may be complete resolution, or alternatively the inflammatory process may smolder continuously and asymptomatically. Extensive destruction of pancreatic tissue may reduce the gland to a few distorted lobules adjacent to where the ducts enter the duodenum (Fig. 146–5).[15] Reports have described acute necrotizing pancreatitis in cats similar to that seen in dogs,[29, 30] as well as a histologically distinct suppurative form.[29] Chronic mild interstitial pancreatitis, characterized by inflammation of interstitial tissue apparently spreading from the ducts, is the type of pancreatic inflammation traditionally reported in cats.[20, 31] The latter type of pancreatitis is often accompanied by cholangiohepatitis and sometimes by interstitial nephritis, either of which may be of greater clinical significance than the pancreatitis.[32]

Numerous experimental procedures and models have been used to develop pancreatitis (Table 146–5), often causing extremely severe and rapidly fatal pancreatitis, but their relevance to naturally occurring disease is questionable.[33] Alternative models based on dietary manipulation or hyperstimulation of the pancreas induce a mild to moderate inflammation that probably more closely mimics the natural disease.[34–37]

It is generally believed that pancreatitis develops when there is activation of digestive enzymes within the gland with resultant pancreatic autodigestion. The site of initiation of enzyme activation is likely to involve zymogen activation within acinar cells.[33, 34, 38] It has been shown that before the development of overt pancreatitis, abnormal fusion of lysosomes and zymogen granules occurs, probably owing to failure of normal secretory processes (Fig. 146–6).[34] It is known that lysosomal proteases, such as cathepsin B, are capable of activating trypsinogen and that the trypsin inhibitor present in zymogen granules is ineffective at the acid pH present in lysosomes.[12, 33, 39] Failure of normal subcellular mechanisms for effective segregation of zymogens and lysosomal proteases may well explain the development or progression of spontaneous and experimental pancreatitis with a variety of otherwise dissimilar causes.

Regardless of the cause of initiation of enzyme activation, a variety of inflammatory mediators and free radicals are important in the progression of pancreatitis. These mediators are mostly released from neutrophils and macrophages and include tumor necrosis factor-α (TNF-α), interleukin-1 (IL-1), IL-2, IL-6, IL-8, IL-10, interferon-α (INF-α), INF-γ, nitric oxide (NO), and platelet-activating factor (PAF).[40] Free radicals can damage cell membranes directly by peroxidation of lipids within the membrane. An important aspect of this injury is thought to be increased capillary permeability

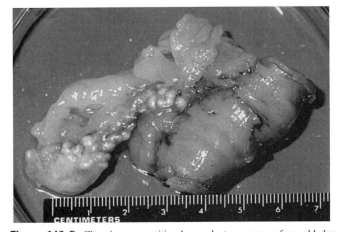

Figure 146–5. Chronic pancreatitis observed at necropsy of an old dog with a history of several bouts of severe acute pancreatitis. Acinar cells were restricted to a few residual nodular areas of relatively normal-looking tissue. The pancreatic pathology was not associated with any clinical signs at the time of euthanasia, although the serum concentration of trypsin-like immunoreactivity was subnormal. (From Williams DA: Exocrine pancreatic insufficiency. Waltham Int Focus 2:9, 1992.)

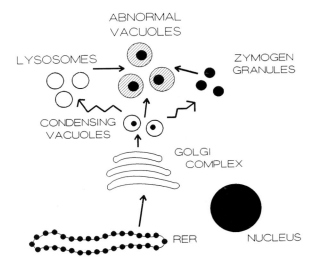

Figure 146–6. Abnormal intracellular routing of digestive enzymes destined for secretion results in mixing of zymogens and lysosomal proteases in abnormal intracellular vacuoles. Subsequent activation of zymogens by lysosomal proteases is currently considered to initiate development of pancreatitis.

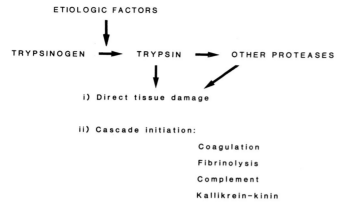

ETIOLOGIC FACTORS

TRYPSINOGEN → TRYPSIN → OTHER PROTEASES

i) Direct tissue damage

ii) Cascade initiation:

Coagulation

Fibrinolysis

Complement

Kallikrein–kinin

Figure 146–7. Local and systemic effects of trypsin in pancreatitis.

caused by endothelial cell membrane damage, with resultant pancreatic edema. Perfusion of the pancreas with free radical scavengers ameliorated the severity of pancreatitis induced by experimental ischemia, duct obstruction, and free fatty acid infusion in a canine model.[41–46] There is evidence that PAF may play a particularly important central role in mediating inflammation and that treatment with PAF antagonists such as lexipafant may be effective in decreasing mortality in severe acute pancreatitis.[40, 47, 48]

Once intracellular and intraductal activation of trypsinogens to trypsins takes place, further activation of all zymogens, particularly proelastase and prophospholipase, amplifies pancreatic damage. Experimental and clinical studies indicate that activation of progressively larger amounts of protease and phospholipase within the gland is associated with transformation of mild edematous pancreatic inflammation to hemorrhagic or necrotic pancreatitis with multisystem involvement and consumption of plasma protease inhibitors (Fig. 146–7 and Table 146–6).[11, 49–58]

Plasma protease inhibitors (see Table 146–3 and Fig. 146–2) are vital in protecting against the otherwise fatal effects of proteolytic enzymes in the vascular space.[53-56] Alpha-macroglobulins are particularly important in this regard. Dogs tolerate intravenous injection of trypsin or chy-

TABLE 146–6. THE ROLE OF ENZYMES IN THE PATHOPHYSIOLOGY OF PANCREATITIS

ENZYME OR PRODUCT	PATHOPHYSIOLOGIC ACTION
Trypsin	Activation of other proteases
	Coagulation and fibrinolysis (disseminated intravascular coagulation)
Phospholipase A₂	Hydrolysis of cell membrane phospholipids
	Pulmonary surfactant degradation
	Demyelination (cell necrosis and liberation of toxic substances such as myocardial depressant factor; respiratory distress; neurologic signs—pancreatic encephalopathy)
Elastase	Degradation of elastin in blood vessel walls (hemorrhage, edema, respiratory distress)
Chymotrypsin	Activation of xanthine oxidase and subsequent generation of oxygen-derived free radicals (membrane damage)
Kallikrein	Kinin generation from kininogens
Kinins	Vasodilatation, pancreatic edema (hypotension, shock)
Complement	Cell membrane damage, aggregation of leukocytes (local inflammation)
Lipase	Fat hydrolysis (local fat necrosis, hypocalcemia)

motrypsin without showing adverse effects provided free alpha-macroglobulins are available to bind the active proteases. When alpha-macroglobulins are no longer available, however, dogs die rapidly from acute disseminated intravascular coagulation and shock as the free proteases activate the kinin, coagulation, fibrinolytic, and complement cascade systems (see Fig. 146–7).[20, 54]

Binding of proteases by alpha-macroglobulin results in a change in conformation that allows the complex to be recognized and rapidly cleared from the plasma by the monocyte-macrophage system.[53, 59] This removal is important because alpha-macroglobulin–bound proteases retain catalytic activity, particularly against low-molecular-weight substrates (see Fig. 146–2)[12, 53]; normal functioning of the monocyte-macrophage system is an important factor determining survival in experimental pancreatitis.[20]

In experimental studies, 80 per cent of plasma alpha₁-proteinase inhibitor is still available to bind proteases when alpha-macroglobulins are saturated with trypsin, but the available alpha₁-proteinase inhibitor is not lifesaving.[20] The primary function of alpha₁-proteinase inhibitor is to inhibit neutrophil elastase during inflammation.[60] Although pancreatic proteases do bind to alpha₁-proteinase inhibitor and are effectively inhibited, the binding is reversible (see Fig. 146–2).[20] In pancreatitis, alpha₁-proteinase inhibitor probably serves as a transient inhibitor and an intermediary in the transport of protease to the protective alpha-macroglobulins, particularly in the extravascular spaces into which large alpha-macroglobulin molecules cannot permeate.[53]

Etiology

The inciting cause of naturally occurring canine and feline pancreatitis is usually unknown, but on the basis of causes documented in human patients, experimental studies, and clinical observations, the following potential factors should be considered.[20, 38, 61, 62]

Nutrition, Hyperlipoproteinemia, Genetic Factors

The exocrine pancreas is highly responsive to changes in nutritional substrates present in the diet, and it has been reported that pancreatitis is more prevalent in obese animals.[20] There is evidence that low-protein, high-fat diets induce pancreatitis and that pancreatitis is more severe when induced in dogs being fed a high-fat diet and less severe when induced in lean dogs.[20, 38] Malnutrition has also been reported to cause pancreatic inflammation and atrophy in human patients, and pancreatitis has been observed after refeeding after a prolonged fast, particularly in extremely malnourished individuals.[46] Finally, pancreatitis has been reported in association with idiopathic hepatic lipidosis in cats.[63]

Hyperlipoproteinemia, often grossly apparent, is common in dogs with acute pancreatitis and may be secondary to pancreatitis as a result of abdominal fat necrosis or may be a cause of the disease. Some familial hyperlipoproteinemias of human beings are associated with frequent episodes of pancreatitis that respond to control of serum triglyceride levels,[46, 64] and the clinical impression of a prevalence of pancreatitis in the miniature schnauzer dog in the United States may be related to underlying idiopathic hyperlipoproteinemia.[20] There is also anecdotal evidence that pancreatitis in dogs often develops after a fatty meal.[20] It is not known why hyperlipidemia might cause pancreatitis, but it has been suggested that toxic fatty acids are generated within the pancreas by the action of lipase on abnormally high concentrations of triglycerides in pancreatic capillaries.[46]

Hereditary pancreatitis is now well documented in human beings and is a particularly important cause of formerly idiopathic chronic pancreatitis in children and adults. Several mutations of the trypsinogen gene have been identified, the most prevalent being replacement of the arginine in position 117 of cationic trypsinogen with a histidine (R117H mutation). Once activated, trypsin is normally fairly rapidly degraded by other proteases, a process that must be facilitated by an initial conformational change that is secondary to a cleavage at the arginine in position 117 by trypsin itself. When this arginine is replaced by histidine, this cleavage cannot occur and the resulting "supertrypsin" is highly resistant to degradation. The trypsin therefore persists and can trigger cascade activation of other enzymes.[65, 66]

Drugs, Toxins, Hypercalcemia

A number of drugs may cause pancreatitis, although absolute proof of a causal relationship is often unavailable.[67] Suspect drugs commonly used in veterinary medicine include thiazide diuretics, furosemide, azathioprine, L-asparaginase, sulfonamides, and tetracyclines.[20, 46, 68] Considerable controversy exists about whether or not corticosteroids or H_2-receptor antagonists such as cimetidine may induce pancreatitis. High doses of glucocorticoids in association with spinal trauma (intervertebral disk disease and surgery) do seem to predispose to pancreatitis, but evidence that these drugs alone induce pancreatitis is weak.[20, 38] It is probably wise to discontinue use of these drugs in patients with pancreatitis of undetermined cause unless a specific indication for their use exists. Corticosteroids in particular may be contraindicated because they may inhibit clearance of enzyme–alpha-macroglobulin complexes by the monocyte-macrophage system and sensitize the pancreas to cholecystokinin-mediated stimulation.[20, 38]

Administration of cholinesterase inhibitor insecticides and cholinergic agonists has been associated with the development of pancreatitis, probably by causing hyperstimulation of the gland.[29, 69, 70] Scorpion stings are frequent causes of pancreatitis in human beings in Trinidad, and experimental administration of scorpion venom to dogs also elicits pancreatitis via a hyperstimulation-type mechanism.[61, 71] Hyperstimulation may also explain the possible association of pancreatitis with hypercalcemia related to hyperparathyroidism and other causes.[20, 38, 61, 72]

Duct Obstruction

Experimental obstruction of the pancreatic ducts produces atrophy and fibrosis, although inflammation and edema may develop when pancreatic secretion is stimulated.[34, 61, 73, 74] Clinical conditions that may lead to partial or complete obstruction of the pancreatic ducts include biliary calculi, sphincter spasm, edema of the duct or duodenal wall, tumor, parasites, trauma, and surgical interference. Biliary calculi are a major cause of pancreatitis in humans, but this has not been reported in dogs and cats, presumably because of their low prevalence of gallstones. Coexistent chronic interstitial pancreatitis, inflammatory bowel disease, and cholangiohepatitis have been observed in cats, and although the relationship between the changes in these organs is not clear, the convergence of the feline biliary and pancreatic ducts may be a factor.[20, 29, 31, 75] Congenital anomalies of the pancreatic duct system may predispose to pancreatitis in humans, and similar mechanisms may underlie some cases of pancreatitis in other species.[61]

Duodenal Reflux, Pancreatic Trauma, and Pancreatic Ischemia

Reflux of duodenal juice into the pancreatic ducts after surgical creation of a closed duodenal loop causes severe acute pancreatitis.[61] Enteropeptidase, activated pancreatic enzymes, bacteria, and bile present in the duodenal juice may all contribute to development of pancreatitis. Under normal circumstances such reflux is unlikely to occur because the duct opening is surrounded by a specialized compact, smooth mucosa over the duodenal papilla and is equipped with an independent sphincter muscle.[20] This antireflux mechanism may sometimes fail owing to abnormally high duodenal pressure, such as may occur with vomiting or after trauma to the duodenum.

Surgical manipulation, automobile accidents, and falls from high buildings are potential causes of pancreatic trauma, but reports of pancreatitis after such insults are rare, and in most cases of abdominal trauma, injury to the pancreas is probably mild or unrecognized.[20, 76] Pancreatitis is a rare complication of pancreatic biopsy performed by either wedge or needle technique and is also uncommon after resection of pancreatic neoplasms.[11, 61, 77, 78]

Experimental and clinical reports have indicated that ischemia is important in the pathogenesis of acute pancreatitis, either as a primary cause or as an exacerbating influence.[79–82] Pancreatic ischemia may develop during shock, secondary to hypotension during general anesthesia, or during temporary occlusion of venous outflow during surgical manipulations in the anterior abdomen and may explain some instances of postoperative pancreatitis when areas remote from the pancreas have undergone surgery.[61]

Miscellaneous

Viral, mycoplasmal, and parasitic infections may be associated with pancreatitis, although this is usually recognized as part of a more generalized disease.[20, 61] It is not known whether infection plays a role in the development of isolated pancreatitis in some instances, but concomitant bacterial infection does increase the severity of experimental pancreatitis and may act similarly in naturally occurring disease.[20, 83] Uremic pancreatitis may contribute to clinical signs of depression and anorexia in end stage renal disease, although severe acute pancreatitis clearly is not a common complication of renal failure in dogs and cats. It is likely that renal failure secondary to acute pancreatitis is encountered more frequently.[20, 84] Finally, evidence has been presented supporting an autoimmune mechanism in human patients with glucocorticoid-responsive pancreatitis.[85]

Diagnosis

History and Clinical Signs

Dogs with acute pancreatitis usually have depression, anorexia, vomiting, and, in some cases, diarrhea. Severe acute disease may be associated with shock and collapse; in other cases, there may be a history of less dramatic signs extending over several weeks. Some dogs demonstrate abdominal pain by assuming a "prayer" position with the forelimbs outstretched, the sternum on the floor, and the hindlimbs raised.

Signs of pain may be elicited by abdominal palpation, although some animals do not react even though they have severe acute pancreatitis. An anterior abdominal mass is palpable in some cases, and occasionally there is mild ascites. Most affected animals are mildly to moderately dehydrated and febrile. Uncommon systemic complications of pancreatitis that may be apparent on physical examination include jaundice, respiratory distress, bleeding disorders, and cardiac arrhythmias.[20, 86] Although dogs of any age may develop pancreatitis, affected animals are usually middle aged or older, sometimes obese, and the onset of signs may have followed ingestion of a large amount of fatty food.[20, 86] The clinical signs of chronic pancreatitis in dogs are poorly documented but are probably extremely variable and nonspecific, if the disease is clinically apparent at all.

Clinical signs of acute pancreatitis in cats are not well defined. In an experimental study, fever, tachycardia, and variable signs of abdominal pain were observed with only rare episodes of vomiting.[87] A survey of 40 cases of fatal pancreatitis in the cat revealed that nearly all the animals were severely lethargic and anorexic, more than 50 per cent were dehydrated or hypothermic, vomiting was noted in 35 per cent, and signs of abdominal pain or an abdominal mass were apparent in only 25 per cent.[29] Chronic pancreatitis is far more common in cats than acute pancreatitis (Figs. 146–8 and 146–9), and associated clinical signs may be hard to differentiate from those of concurrent inflammatory bowel disease that is often present.[32]

Radiographic Signs

History and clinical signs associated with pancreatitis are nonspecific and common to numerous gastrointestinal and metabolic disorders. Abdominal radiographs may provide evidence leading to one of these alternative diagnoses or support a tentative diagnosis of pancreatitis. Radiographic signs reported with pancreatitis include increased density, diminished contrast and granularity in the right cranial abdomen, displacement of the stomach to the left, widening of the angle between the pyloric antrum and the proximal duodenum, displacement of the descending duodenum to the right, presence of a mass medial to the descending duode-

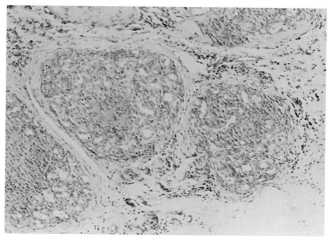

Figure 146–9. Microscopic appearance of a necropsy specimen from a cat with chronic pancreatitis. There are marked fibrosis and acinar cell atrophy associated with chronic inflammation. (Courtesy of Dr. Jörg Steiner, Texas A&M University.)

num, static gas pattern in or thickened walls of the descending duodenum, static gas pattern in or caudal displacement of the transverse colon, gastric distention suggestive of gastric outlet obstruction, and delayed passage of barium through the stomach and duodenum with corrugation of the duodenal wall indicating abnormal peristalsis.[20, 86] Unfortunately, definitive radiographic evidence supporting a diagnosis of pancreatitis is usually not present, the most common finding being a somewhat subjective loss of visceral detail ("ground glass" appearance) in the anterior abdomen.

Ultrasonic imaging is increasingly used to identify pancreatitis. Nonhomogeneous masses and loss of echo density have been noted in dogs with experimental and naturally occurring pancreatitis (Fig. 146–10), whereas ultrasonography may reveal cystic masses in dogs with pancreatic pseudocysts or abscesses and increased echo density when there

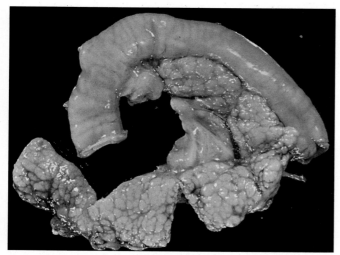

Figure 146–8. Gross appearance of a necropsy specimen from a cat with chronic pancreatitis. The pancreas is firm to the touch and has a coarse lobulated appearance. (Courtesy of Dr. John Edwards, Texas A&M University.)

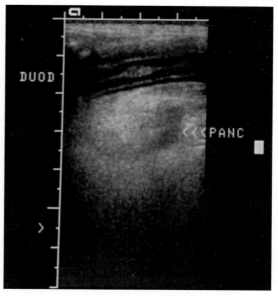

Figure 146–10. Ultrasonographic examination of the abdomen in pancreatitis may reveal areas of pancreas with loss of normal echo density (PANC) adjacent to areas of increased density, reflecting patchy areas of edema, hemorrhage, inflammation, and fibrosis.

are areas of fibrosis.[88-90] Computed tomography is currently the most useful modality for visualizing the pancreas and associated pathology (necrosis) in human patients. Serial examinations are particularly useful for identification and management of complications such as pancreatic abscess in patients that are not responding well to conservative therapeutic measures.[91, 92] A study of cats with macroscopically or microscopically confirmed pancreatitis showed that only 3 of 14 cases examined were detected by either ultrasonographic examination or computer-aided tomographic examination, perhaps reflecting the relative infrequency of severe inflammation and necrosis in the cat.[93]

Laboratory Aids to Diagnosis

Leukocytosis is a common hematologic finding in acute pancreatitis. The packed cell volume may be increased as a result of dehydration, although in some cases, particularly in cats after rehydration, anemia is observed.[20, 29, 87, 94] Azotemia is frequently present, usually the result of dehydration. Acute renal failure may be secondary to hypovolemia or to other mechanisms, such as circulating vasotoxic agents and plugging of the renal microvasculature by either fat deposits or microthrombi from the sites of disseminated intravascular coagulation.[11, 95, 96]

Liver enzyme activities are often increased, reflecting hepatocellular injury as a result of either hepatic ischemia or exposure of the liver to high concentrations of toxic products delivered from the pancreas in portal blood.[20, 29, 97, 98] In some cases, particularly in cats, there are hyperbilirubinemia and sometimes clinically apparent icterus, which may indicate severe hepatocellular damage and/or intrahepatic and extrahepatic obstruction of bile flow. Hyperglycemia may occur in dogs and cats with necrotizing pancreatitis, probably as a result of hyperglucagonemia and stress-related increases in the concentrations of catecholamines and cortisol. Some affected animals are diabetic after recovery from acute episodes of pancreatitis.[20, 29, 99] In contrast, cats with suppurative pancreatitis often develop hypoglycemia.[29] Hypocalcemia has often been reported but is usually mild to moderate and rarely associated with clinical sings of tetany.[20, 29, 87, 94] The mechanism leading to development of hypocalcemia is not clear, but deposition of calcium as soaps after excessive breakdown of fat by released pancreatic lipase is one potential explanation. Hypercholesterolemia and hypertriglyceridemia are common, and hyperlipemia is often grossly apparent even though food has not been recently ingested.[20, 29] Extreme hyperlipemia may prevent accurate determination of other serum biochemical values. Analysis of plasma lipids has not revealed any clear-cut abnormalities characteristic of acute pancreatitis.[100]

Assays of pancreatic enzymes and zymogens in serum may provide specific tests for pancreatitis.[20, 87, 94, 101] Numerous different assay methods exist, including conventional catalytic assays and newer highly specific immunoassays (Fig. 146–11), and it is important that an appropriate method for each species be utilized. Immunoassays are generally applicable only to the species for which they were developed. Clinical and experimental observations have involved primarily amylase and lipase, but phospholipase A_2 and serum trypsin-like immunoreactivity (TLI) have been investigated.[20, 51, 87, 94, 101]

Experimental studies in general indicate parallel changes in results of different enzyme determinations during the course of canine pancreatitis, except that serum TLI tends to increase proportionally more and sooner during the course

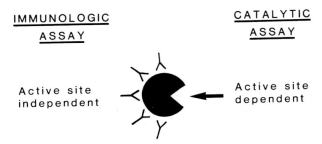

Active site independent

Active site dependent

Figure 146–11. Assay of pancreatic enzymes and zymogens in serum. Catalytic assays detect degradation of specific substrates exposed to the active site of the molecule and therefore measure enzyme activity. Immunoassays detect antigenic sites over the surface of the molecule and therefore measure enzyme or zymogen concentration.

of the disease than other enzymes. Serum TLI is pancreas specific in origin, whereas amylase, lipase, and phospholipase activities originate from pancreatic and extrapancreatic sources.[101] Diseases other than pancreatitis should be considered in patients with increases of one enzyme accompanied by minimal increases in another. Persistently normal activities are seen in some cases.[20] It is possible that by the time some clinical cases are investigated, the inflamed pancreas is depleted of stored enzymes, synthesis of new enzymes has been disrupted, and release into the bloodstream is therefore no longer increased.[102, 103] Similar reasoning may explain the lack of correlation between the magnitude of enzyme activities and clinical severity.

Increased concentrations of circulating pancreatic enzymes may also be secondary to reduced clearance from the plasma, as happens in renal failure. Because azotemia is common in acute pancreatitis, it is sometimes difficult to determine whether increased levels of pancreatic enzymes are due to pancreatic inflammation or renal disease. Increases more than four or five times above the upper limit of normal are unlikely to result from renal dysfunction alone, although there are exceptions.[20]

Amylase, lipase, and phospholipase originate from both pancreatic and extrapancreatic sources, including gastric and small intestinal mucosa, and serum activities may increase in dogs with hepatic, renal, or neoplastic disease in the absence of pancreatitis.[20, 104] Lipase activity has been reported to be a more reliable marker for the diagnosis of pancreatitis than that of amylase. However, dexamethasone administration has been shown to increase canine serum lipase activity up to fivefold without histologic evidence of pancreatitis, although parallel increases in amylase activity do not occur.[20] Moderate elevations of serum lipase in dogs receiving dexamethasone therefore should not be taken as strong evidence for pancreatitis unless amylase is also increased. In general, assay of lipase and TLI is most likely to identify affected dogs reliably.

Attempts to identify a pancreas-specific isoenzyme of canine amylase, as has been possible in human beings, have produced contradictory findings,[20, 105] although the persistence of all four canine isoenzymes both in dogs with acinar atrophy and in pancreatectomized dogs would seem to indicate that no such isoform exists in this species.[20, 104]

Methemalbumin is formed in humans with hemorrhagic pancreatitis as pancreatic enzymes degrade hemoglobin with subsequent binding of oxidized heme (hemin) to albumin.[106] Hemin does not bind to canine albumin, however, but rather to a variety of different serum proteins, so true methemalbuminemia cannot exist in dogs.[106] Although these protein-bound forms of hemin may also be formed in other conditions, such as hemolytic dyscrasias and intestinal infarctions, their presence in patients with other evidence of pancreatitis is highly suggestive of the hemorrhagic form of the disease and their concentration may be of prognostic value.[106]

There is increasing awareness of acute pancreatitis in cats, although there are still few clinical reports. Increases in serum amylase and lipase activities are usually not observed, and when they do occur the increases are much less than those reported in dogs, as are normal activities of these enzymes.[29, 30, 87, 99, 107] An experimental study demonstrated that although serum lipase increased significantly in cats after induction of pancreatitis, amylase activity was never increased above normal but rather decreased significantly during the course of the disease.[87] Specific immunoassay of feline TLI has shown that normal serum TLI concentrations in cats are higher than those in dogs. Several reports have documented increased serum TLI concentrations in cats with pancreatitis.[107–109] In one study serum TLI was increased in 17 of 21 cats with macroscopically or microscopically confirmed pancreatitis.[110]

Trypsin complexed with plasma alpha$_1$-proteinase inhibitor (see Fig. 146–2) and trypsinogen activation peptides (TAPs) in plasma or urine provide specific markers for pancreatitis, because in the absence of pancreatitis only free trypsinogen is present in the plasma (Table 146–7; see Fig. 146–2). Furthermore, the concentration of these markers correlates with the severity and clinical course of the disease.[49, 50, 53, 56–58, 71, 111–113] Technical complexities currently limit the usefulness of species-specific trypsin–alpha$_1$-proteinase inhibitor complex assay, but assays for the Asp-Asp-Asp-Asp-Lys peptide sequence common to TAPs in all vertebrates (see Table 146–7) may prove to be useful in dogs and cats. Unfortunately, TAP is quite labile, so sample submission requires special handling. There is also an interfering factor in urine from some normal dogs that creates false-positive test results.

Clearly, there is no widely available ideal test or combination of tests for the diagnosis of acute pancreatitis, and in the absence of direct examination of pancreatic tissue, the diagnosis can only be tentative. Nonetheless, careful evaluation of the entire clinical picture in many instances gives a high degree of confidence in the presumptive diagnosis. If gross or histopathologic confirmation of the diagnosis is required or the possibility of other abdominal disease is to be eliminated, it is important that attention be given to stabilization of fluid and electrolyte status before general anesthesia and surgical exploration of the abdomen.

Treatment

The classic basis for therapy of acute pancreatitis is maintenance of fluid and electrolyte balance while the pancreas is "rested" by withholding food and thereby allowed to recover from the inflammatory episode.[62, 114–116] Reports have challenged the logic and wisdom of this approach, however, and both parenteral nutrition and enteral nutrition have been well tolerated by patients with pancreatitis.[117, 118] There is also evidence in human patients that enteral nutrition may be superior to parenteral nutrition.[118] Oral intake should probably be limited only in patients with significant vomiting and then for as short a period as possible. It is probably particularly important to continue enteral nutrition in cats with pancreatitis and concurrent hepatic lipidosis, and parenteral nutrition should be utilized in cats and dogs only when there is severe protracted vomiting.

If drug-induced pancreatitis is suspected, any incriminated agents should be withdrawn and replaced by an unrelated alternative drug if necessary. Other potential etiologic factors (see earlier) should similarly be investigated and, if possible, eliminated. Sufficient balanced-electrolyte intravenous solution should be given to replace fluid deficits and provide maintenance requirements if oral intake is suspended or restricted. Mild cases of pancreatitis are probably self-limiting and may improve without therapy. Other dogs and cats require aggressive fluid therapy over several days to treat severe dehydration and ongoing fluid electrolyte loss with vomiting. Many animals become hypokalemic during such therapy, and serum potassium should be monitored and supplemented via the intravenous fluids. Serum creatinine or blood urea nitrogen should also be monitored to document resolution of azotemia. Although metabolic acidosis is probably common in acute pancreatitis, this may not always be the case, and vomiting patients may be alkalotic. "Blind" correction of suspected acid-base abnormalities therefore should not be attempted unless documentation is provided by appropriate tests.[115] Excessive bicarbonate administration may precipitate signs of hypocalcemia in individuals with subclinical hypocalcemia. It is common practice to give parenteral antibiotics during this supportive period, particularly when toxic changes are evident in the hemogram or when the dog or cat is febrile.[114, 115] Although antibiotic therapy is beneficial in human patients and in some experimental models of pancreatitis, any benefit in canine and feline patients, in which septic complications are extremely rare, would appear to be minimal.[119] Trimethoprim-sulfadiazine and enrofloxacin penetrate well into canine pancreas and are effective against many common pathogens isolated from human beings with pancreatitis.[120]

If abdominal pain is severe, analgesic therapy (meperidine hydrochloride or butorphanol tartrate) should be given to provide relief.[30, 121] Hyperglycemia is often mild and transient, but in some cases diabetes mellitus may develop, requiring treatment with insulin. Respiratory distress, neurologic problems, cardiac abnormalities, bleeding disorders, and acute renal failure are all poor prognostic signs. At-

LIV

TABLE 146–7. AMINO ACID SEQUENCES OF TRYPSINOGEN ACTIVATION PEPTIDES FROM A VARIETY OF SPECIES

SPECIES	SEQUENCES							
Dog—cationic trypsin	Phe-	Pro-	Ile-	Asp-	Asp-	Asp-	Asp-	Lys-
Dog—anionic trypsin	Thr-	Pro-	Thr-	Asp-	Asp-	Asp-	Asp-	Lys-
Cat	Phe-	Pro-	Ile-	Asp-	Asp-	Asp-	Asp-	Lys-
Cow			Val-	Asp-	Asp-	Asp-	Asp-	Lys-
Goat			Val-	Asp-	Asp-	Asp-	Asp-	Lys-
Pig	Phe-	Pro-	Thr-	Asp-	Asp-	Asp-	Asp-	Lys-
Horse	Ser-	Ser-	Thr-	Asp-	Asp-	Asp-	Asp-	Lys-
Dogfish		Ala-	Pro-	Asp-	Asp-	Asp-	Asp-	Lys-

tempts should be made to manage these complications by appropriate supportive measures, but recovery is unlikely unless the underlying pancreatitis resolves.

Some affected animals do not improve and some continue to deteriorate in spite of supportive care. Observations have indicated that in severe pancreatitis there is marked consumption of plasma protease inhibitors as activated pancreatic proteases are cleared from the circulation and that saturation of available alpha-macroglobulins is rapidly followed by acute disseminated intravascular coagulation, shock, and death.[11, 50, 53, 55, 56, 122–125] Transfusion of plasma or whole blood to replace alpha-macroglobulins may be lifesaving in these circumstances and has the additional benefit of maintaining plasma albumin concentrations.[124] Albumin is probably beneficial in pancreatitis because of its oncotic properties, which help to maintain blood volume and prevent pancreatic ischemia while limiting pancreatic edema formation.[79] Albumin also binds detergents that otherwise are available to help disrupt cell membranes.[126] Low-molecular-weight dextrans have also been used to expand plasma volume, but they may aggravate bleeding tendencies, contain no protease inhibitor, and provide no major advantages over plasma administration.[114] Hyperoncotic, ultrahigh-molecular-weight dextran solutions have been shown to reduce trypsinogen activation, prevent acinar necrosis, and lower mortality in rodent pancreatitis, perhaps by promoting pancreatic microcirculation.[127]

The use of corticosteroids in pancreatitis has been recommended because they stabilize lysosomal membranes, reduce inflammation, and alleviate shock, but they have not been shown to be of value in experimental studies.[20] Unless autoimmune pancreatitis is suspected, they should be given only on a short-term basis to animals in shock associated with fulminating pancreatitis and then in concert with fluids and plasma as described earlier.[115] Longer periods of administration may impair removal of alpha-macroglobulin–bound proteases from the plasma by the monocyte-macrophage system, with resultant complications related to systemic effects of circulating uninhibited enzymes.[20]

Indirect approaches to inhibition of pancreatic secretion that have been employed in addition to withholding food include suctioning of gastric secretions and inhibition of gastric secretion by use of antacids or cimetidine.[114] None of these methods has been consistently shown to be effective, and their use is not recommended. Attempts to rest the pancreas by use of direct inhibitors of secretion such as atropine, acetazolamide, glucagon, calcitonin, and somatostatin or its analogues have not yet been proved effective.[62, 114, 116, 128, 129] Pancreatic gamma irradiation is an effective if impractical method that reduces pancreatic secretion and lessens the severity of experimental pancreatitis.[20] Administration of a variety of naturally occurring and synthetic enzyme inhibitors with selective actions against individual pancreatic digestive enzymes has shown promise in experimental studies, but their value remains to be demonstrated in clinical trials.[114, 130, 131] Future clinical and experimental trials will probably be directed at the use of agents to modify events currently believed to be important in the pathobiology of pancreatitis, including inhibitors of inflammatory mediators such as PAF, free radical scavengers, enzyme synthesis and transport inhibitors, and factors that may stabilize lysosomal and other membranes.[20, 40, 131]

The use of peritoneal dialysis to remove toxic material accumulated in the peritoneal cavity is beneficial experimentally and is believed by many to be useful in human beings.[114] Although impractical in some veterinary hospitals,

peritoneal dialysis may be of value in some cases. Certainly, in patients in which acute pancreatitis is confirmed at exploratory laparotomy, removal of as much free fluid as possible by abdominal lavage is advisable. In some cases pancreatitis may be localized to one lobe of the gland, and surgical resection of the affected area may be followed by complete recovery.[20]

Utilization of ultrasonographic imaging has contributed to increased recognition of pancreatic masses (pseudocyst, abscess) and bile duct obstruction.[89, 132, 133] These lesions are usually sterile. There are a few reports of positive bacterial cultures in dogs and cats with pancreatitis. It is not clear whether these animals are best managed conservatively with supportive therapy or whether surgical intervention to débride necrotic tissue and allow drainage of affected areas facilitates recovery. Cholecystoduodenostomy was followed by recovery in six dogs with fibrotic obstructive masses.[133] In another study of seven dogs with pancreatic masses, one patient recovered spontaneously, but the remaining six dogs died within 9 days.[89] Three of six dogs with pancreatic abscesses recovered after open abdominal drainage and intensive care.[132] Given these mixed results and the risks, difficulties, and expense associated with anesthesia, surgery, and postoperative care, it is wise to avoid surgical intervention unless there is clear evidence of an enlarging mass and/or sepsis in a patient that is not responding well to medical therapy. Many patients that develop obstructive jaundice in association with acute pancreatitis recover spontaneously over 2 or 3 weeks with conventional supportive care alone (D. A. Williams, unpublished observations, 1993).

After vomiting has ceased to be a significant problem, small amounts of water should be offered, and if there is no exacerbation of clinical signs, food may be gradually reintroduced. The diet should preferably have a high carbohydrate content (rice, pasta, potatoes) because protein and fat are more potent stimulants of pancreatic secretion and are perhaps more likely to promote a relapse. If there is continued improvement, gradual introduction of a low-fat maintenance diet should be attempted. Another period of food deprivation should be instituted if signs of pancreatitis recur.[115, 134] Although the prognosis is poor for dogs and cats with repeated bouts of food intolerance, total or partial parenteral nutrition may be beneficial by sustaining them while the digestive system is rested for 7 to 10 days.[116, 117]

In many dogs and cats that suffer a single episode of pancreatitis, the only long-term therapy recommended is to avoid feeding meals with an excessively high fat content. In others, repeated bouts of pancreatitis occur, and it may be beneficial to feed a moderately or severely fat-restricted diet permanently. In spite of this, some animals experience recurrent disease.[134]

Oral pancreatic enzyme supplements may decrease the pain that accompanies chronic pancreatitis in human beings, probably by feedback inhibition of endogenous pancreatic enzyme secretion.[135] It is not known whether they are of similar value in dogs or cats, but because there is evidence for negative feedback of pancreatic secretion mediated by intraluminal pancreatic enzymes in dogs,[136] a trial period of enzyme therapy may be warranted in individuals with chronic or recurrent signs attributed to pancreatitis.

Prognosis

Pancreatitis is an unpredictable disease of widely varying severity, and it is difficult to give a prognosis even when a diagnosis is definitively established. Life-threatening signs accompanying acute fulminating pancreatitis are usually followed by death in spite of supportive measures, but some dogs recover fully after an isolated severe episode. In other cases, relatively mild or moderate chronic or recurrent pancreatitis persists despite all therapy, and the dog or cat either dies in an acute severe exacerbation of the disease or undergoes euthanasia because of failure to recover and the expense of long-term supportive care. Most animals with uncomplicated pancreatitis probably naturally recover after a single episode and do well as long as high-fat foods are avoided.

EXOCRINE PANCREATIC INSUFFICIENCY

Progressive loss of exocrine pancreatic acinar cells ultimately leads to failure of absorption because of inadequate production of digestive enzymes. The functional reserve of the pancreas is considerable, however, and signs of exocrine pancreatic insufficiency (EPI) do not occur until a large proportion of the gland has been destroyed. Steatorrhea and azotorrhea do not develop in dogs until more than 85 to 90 per cent of the secretory capacity of the pancreas has been lost.[20] The most common cause of such severe loss of exocrine tissue in the dog is pancreatic acinar atrophy (PAA) (Fig. 146–12). Pancreatic insufficiency is caused less commonly by chronic pancreatitis and rarely by pancreatic neoplasia.[20, 137] Although not yet documented, it is likely that congenital abnormalities of canine pancreatic exocrine function such as pancreatic hypoplasia, isolated deficiencies of individual pancreatic enzymes, and deficiency of enteropeptidase also occur.[138]

Although pancreatic enzymes perform essential digestive functions, alternative pathways of digestion for some nutrients do exist. After experimental exclusion of pancreatic secretion from the intestine, dogs can still absorb up to 63 per cent of ingested protein and 84 per cent of ingested fat. This residual enzyme activity probably originates from lingual and/or gastric lipases and gastric pepsins and also from intestinal mucosal esterases and peptidases.[20, 138, 139] Nonetheless, when exocrine pancreatic function is severely impaired, these alternative routes of digestion are inadequate, and clinical signs of malabsorption occur.

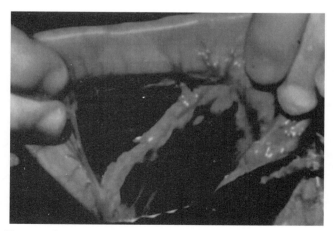

Figure 146–12. The duodenal limb of the pancreas of a dog with pancreatic acinar atrophy. Residual tissue contains islet (endocrine) cells and blood vessels, so diabetes mellitus is not a feature of this disease. (From Williams DA: Exocrine pancreatic insufficiency. Waltham Int Focus 2:9, 1992.)

Etiology

Pancreatic Acinar Atrophy

Atrophy of the acinar cells of the pancreas in the absence of a pronounced inflammatory response may occur in a variety of experimental circumstances. Spontaneous development of severe PAA in previously healthy adult animals appears to be uniquely common in the dog, although similar conditions occur sporadically in other species.[20] There is evidence that PAA in German shepherd dogs is preceded by patchy lymphocytic pancreatitis that is probably immune mediated (M.E. Wiberg, personal communication, 1998). Numerous nutritional deficiencies—such as amino acid imbalance and copper deficiency in the rat and protein-calorie malnutrition in humans—also cause atrophy of exocrine tissue.[20] Nutritional imbalance, acquired perhaps as a consequence of an underlying small intestinal mucosal abnormality, is an attractive alternative explanation for the development of pancreatic atrophy in dogs with previously normal exocrine pancreatic function. Although preexisting small intestinal disease in dogs with PAA has not been documented, it has been observed that affected dogs sometimes have a history of gastrointestinal disturbances long before the development of severe weight loss. Alternative explanations for development of canine PAA include (1) pancreatic duct obstruction, (2) a primary congenital abnormality in the pancreas itself, (3) toxicosis, (4) ischemia, (5) viral infection, and (6) defective secretory and/or trophic stimuli. Although PAA may occur at any age in a wide variety of breeds, a high prevalence in the young German shepherd is recognized. Investigations of family histories have suggested that predisposition to development of the disease is inherited in an autosomal recessive fashion in this breed.[140]

The pancreatic atrophy of CBA/J mice is the only naturally occurring disorder that resembles canine PAA.[20] Morphologic study of the pancreas from affected mice has implicated destabilization of zymogen granules as one of the earliest ultrastructural abnormalities, and biochemical studies indicate that premature activation of trypsinogen and chymotrypsinogen occurs within the zymogen granules. Progressive ultrastructural abnormalities of zymogen granules similarly preceded (by almost 2 years) development of overt PAA in a young German shepherd dog.[140]

Chronic Pancreatitis

Chronic pancreatitis resulting in progressive destruction of pancreatic tissue is a common cause of EPI in adult human beings, but gross and histologic examination rarely reveals end stage pancreatitis as the underlying cause of EPI in dogs. However, animals with EPI and coexistent diabetes mellitus probably fall into this category, the clinical signs reflecting damage to both exocrine and endocrine tissue as occurs in pancreatitis, in contrast to the selective acinar cell damage in PAA.[20] EPI is much less commonly diagnosed in cats than in dogs, but chronic pancreatitis has been the underlying cause in the majority of the few cases reported.[20, 141]

Hereditary, Congenital, and Miscellaneous Causes of Exocrine Pancreatic Insufficiency

Cystic fibrosis and Shwachman-Diamond syndrome are the most common causes of EPI in children, but these disorders differ from canine and feline EPI in that there are also abnormalities of organs other than the pancreas.[139] Other extremely rare causes of EPI in children include congenital deficiencies of individual pancreatic digestive enzymes or of intestinal enteropeptidase, but these have not been described in dogs or cats.[142] Occasionally, young dogs have both EPI and diabetes mellitus, with congenital pancreatic hypoplasia or aplasia as the underlying cause.[31, 143] There are also sporadic reports of apparently reversible EPI, which occurs in association with subtotal acinar atrophy and mild inflammation. This condition may reflect subclinical PAA.[144]

Finally, EPI has been reported as a complication of proximal duodenal resection and cholecystoduodenostomy in cats, a finding that probably reflects the absence of dual pancreatic ducts in this species so that damage to the major duodenal papilla blocks pancreatic secretion.[20]

Pathophysiology

Nutrient malabsorption in canine EPI does not arise simply as a consequence of failure of intraluminal digestion. Morphologic changes in the small intestine of some dogs with EPI have been reported, and studies of naturally occurring and experimental EPI in several species have revealed abnormal activities of mucosal enzymes and impaired function as indicated by abnormal transport of sugars, amino acids, and fatty acids.[20, 145, 146] The cause of this mucosal pathology is unknown, but the absence of the trophic influence of pancreatic secretions, bacterial overgrowth in the small intestine, and endocrine and nutritional factors may all be contributory.[10, 20]

Small Intestinal Mucosa

Exocrine pancreatic insufficiency in several species is associated with increased activities of jejunal brush border maltase and sucrase, as well as an increase in the proportion of microvillar membrane proteins of large molecular mass (>220 kDa).[10, 20, 146] These changes are attributed to reduced degradation of exposed brush border proteins as a consequence of decreased pancreatic protease activity within the gut lumen (Fig. 146–13). This explanation is supported by the reversal of the abnormalities in canine EPI after treatment with pancreatic enzymes.[146–148] The abnormal accumulation of these and other proteins on the surface of the brush border membrane may interfere with normal absorption. In contrast to the increased activities of maltase and sucrase, the activity of brush border peptidase (leucyl-2-naphthylamidase) is unchanged, whereas that of alkaline phosphatase is decreased in dogs with EPI.[147, 148] These proteins are relatively resistant to degradation by intraluminal proteases.[20]

Protein synthesis by jejunal mucosa is decreased in dogs with EPI but increases to normal after treatment.[147] Jejunal alkaline phosphatase activity also becomes normal after treatment, suggesting that the activity of this enzyme is particularly dependent on the rate of protein synthesis (see Fig. 146–13). The mechanism for the defect in protein synthesis is not known, but contributory factors may include malnutrition and intraluminal or humoral factors. Intraluminal pancreatic secretions and the products of digestion exert a trophic effect on the small intestine, and both are deficient in untreated dogs. Hormones and other regulatory peptides including gastrin, enteroglucagon, glucagon, insulin, and epidermal growth factor may mediate these trophic effects.[20]

Disturbances of glucose homeostasis are common in dogs with EPI, and in these dogs insulinopenia may be an additional factor affecting intestinal mucosal function. Insulin receptors are present on both basolateral and brush border membranes of enterocytes, and insulin has a stimulatory effect on DNA synthesis in the gastrointestinal tract.[20]

Small Intestinal Microflora

Bacterial overgrowth in the lumen of the small intestine is common in canine EPI.[10, 149, 150] Changes in the intestinal microflora may result from loss of the antibacterial properties of pancreatic juice[9] or as yet undefined abnormalities of intestinal immunity or motility. Achlorhydria may also predispose to bacterial overgrowth but is not a feature of canine EPI.[151]

The pathologic changes associated with bacterial overgrowth depend on the type of bacteria involved and probably on the chronicity of the overgrowth. In dogs with increases in aerobic and facultative anaerobic bacteria, changes are

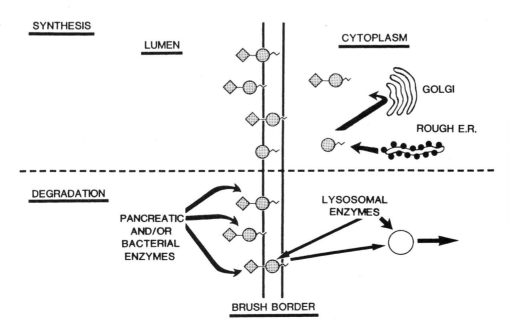

Figure 146–13. Factors influencing activities of jejunal brush border enzymes. The importance of degradation by intraluminal proteases depends at least in part on the location of the enzyme in the membrane and hence its susceptibility to proteolytic attack. (Modified from Alpers DH, Seetharam B: Pathophysiology of diseases involving intestinal brush-border proteins. N Engl J Med 296:1047, 1977.)

similar to those observed in dogs with EPI that do not have bacterial overgrowth.[10] In these dogs, activities of brush border enzymes other than alkaline phosphatase are either normal or increased. In contrast, when the overgrowth includes obligate anaerobic bacteria there is often an associated decrease in many enzyme activities and, in some cases, partial villous atrophy (Fig. 146–14).[10, 146] These findings are consistent with the known ability of some strains of obligate anaerobic bacteria to produce enzymes that release or destroy exposed brush border enzymes.[20, 152, 153] Even when bacterial overgrowth does not include large numbers of obligate anaerobes, the abnormal microflora may be of clinical significance because bacteria may indirectly impair absorption by competing for nutrients and by changing intraluminal factors such as the concentration of conjugated bile salts.[20, 153]

Pancreatic Regulatory Peptides

Histopathologic examination of pancreas from dogs with PAA reveals almost total atrophy of acinar tissue but plentiful, disorganized islet tissue, accompanied by numerous ganglia and patent exocrine ducts.[20] Immunohistochemical staining of the pancreas shows many insulin-, glucagon-, somatostatin-, and pancreatic polypeptide–immunoreactive cells scattered haphazardly throughout residual islet tissue.[20, 148] This differs from the more organized arrangement of cells in healthy canine pancreas, in which a central core of insulin- and scattered somatostatin-immunoreactive cells is surrounded by a halo of glucagon- (left lobe) or pancreatic polypeptide– (right lobe) immunoreactive cells.[154] In addition, enkephalin- and vasoactive intestinal polypeptide (VIP)–immunoreactive nerve fibers are extremely profuse in PAA islet tissue, accompanied by numerous enkephalin- and VIP-immunoreactive nerve cell bodies; in normal pancreas, enkephalin-immunoreactive fibers are rare, and VIP-immunoreactive innervation is moderate in acinar tissue but rarely present in islets.[20, 148] Enkephalin-like immunoreactivity in PAA pancreas is probably due to a precursor immunochemically related to proenkephalin.[155]

Disturbance of the morphologic relationships between cells in islet pancreatic tissue may impair intraislet and/or enteroislet homeostatic mechanisms and might account for subnormal basal plasma insulin concentrations in dogs with PAA.[156] The neuronal regulatory peptide abnormalities may represent a primary defect in canine PAA, or they may be secondary to the atrophy of acinar tissue, perhaps arising as a result of neuronal overgrowth in response to loss of target tissue.

Glucose Intolerance

In dogs and cats with EPI secondary to pancreatitis, diabetes mellitus may result from islet cell destruction. Oral and intravenous glucose tolerance is also abnormal in untreated dogs with PAA, although diabetes mellitus has not been reported in these dogs.[20, 156] The "incretin" effect is reduced in dogs with experimental pancreatic atrophy.[157] Incretin refers to insulinotropic factors released from the gut that are responsible for the augmentation of insulin secretion in response to orally administered glucose compared with that stimulated by the same dosage of intravenously administered glucose.[158] Gastric inhibitory polypeptide (GIP) is probably an important factor contributing to incretin activity, and feeding does not stimulate GIP release from the small bowel of dogs with PAA unless pancreatic enzymes are added to the food.[20, 158] Similar observations have been made in children with cystic fibrosis, and the failure of GIP secretion appears to arise because products of digestion (glucose, amino acids, fatty acids) are the stimuli for GIP release rather than the act of feeding or the undigested constituents of food itself.[20, 153] The relationship of plasma GIP responses to oral glucose intolerance in canine PAA and whether oral glucose tolerance returns to normal after treatment have not been reported.

Intravenous glucose tolerance testing in untreated dogs with PAA is associated with subnormal resting and stimulated insulin concentrations,[148, 156] abnormalities that are presumably independent of incretin. Similar abnormalities have been reported in dogs with experimental pancreatic atrophy.[20, 157] Treatment of PAA is followed by normalization of intravenous glucose tolerance, although basal plasma insulin concentrations remain subnormal.[148, 156]

It is probable that the abnormalities in glucose homeostasis are related at least in part to metabolic changes associated with the catabolic and undernourished state of many untreated dogs with EPI.[46] Withholding food from dogs for a period of 2 weeks produces a decrease in circulating insulin concentrations, and severely undernourished dogs develop

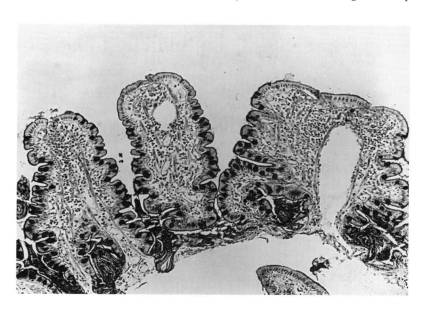

Figure 146–14. Partial villous atrophy in a jejunal biopsy specimen from a dog with exocrine pancreatic insufficiency related to pancreatic acinar atrophy. Villi are short and stumpy with a broadened plateau at the extrusion zone, and there is evidence of folding or fusion of villi. (From Williams DA, et al: Bacterial overgrowth in the duodenum of dogs with exocrine pancreatic insufficiency. JAVMA 191:201, 1987.)

LIV

markedly subnormal insulin responses to glucose.[20, 46] This probably represents an adaptation to reduced food intake because lower insulin levels facilitate enhanced lipolysis, leading to increased concentrations of plasma free fatty acids, which are available as an energy source.[20]

Nutritional Status

Many dogs with EPI suffer from malabsorption for a considerable period of time before a diagnosis is made. Thus the clinical and pathophysiologic features associated with EPI may, in some instances, be due to malnutrition. For example, malnutrition may have direct effects on the gastrointestinal mucosa, as well as produce systemic endocrine and immunologic changes, which may in turn have an effect on gastrointestinal function.[152, 159–161]

Protein-Calorie Malnutrition

In many cases, dogs with EPI are cachectic because of long-term protein-calorie malnutrition. In such malnourished individuals, alterations in circulating concentrations of insulin and other hormones may contribute to changes in glucose homeostasis and intestinal mucosal function.[20] Changes in small intestinal mucosal enzyme activities have been observed in severely malnourished children and may be a direct effect of nutrient deficiency impairing protein synthesis.[20, 160] Severe protein-calorie malnutrition may also affect the normal immune response, and this in turn may contribute to development of changes in the intestinal microflora.[20, 159] Furthermore, malnutrition in rats impairs the capacity to maintain a protective mucosal mucin content and accelerates the development of brush border enzyme deficiency in intraluminal bacterial overgrowth.[152, 161] Finally, protein-calorie malnutrition per se may contribute to EPI, perhaps through impairment of pancreatic protein synthesis, and this may worsen already impaired exocrine pancreatic function.[20, 46]

Trace Elements

Absorption of trace elements in EPI may be promoted or inhibited by loss of specific factors affecting absorption or a change in intraluminal pH.[20] Trace element deficiencies may potentially exacerbate exocrine dysfunction either directly or indirectly by impairing activities of metalloenzymes important in defenses against free radical injury.[46] However, assessment of serum copper and zinc concentrations in dogs with EPI did not reveal any evidence of deficiencies of these trace elements.[148]

Vitamins

Malabsorption of cobalamin (vitamin B_{12}) is well documented in association with EPI in human beings. Mildly subnormal serum cobalamin levels are often observed in dogs with EPI, and serum concentrations are usually undetectable in affected cats.[20, 141, 148, 162, 163] The mechanism for malabsorption of cobalamin in canine and feline EPI is not known, but potential contributory causes include overgrowth of cobalamin-binding bacteria in the proximal small bowel of dogs[10, 162]; deficiency of pancreatic intrinsic factor[4, 164]; and deficiency of pancreatic proteases that normally release cobalamin from salivary and/or gastric R proteins, thereby allowing successful transfer of cobalamin from R proteins to intrinsic factor in the intestinal lumen.[3, 162] Serum cobalamin concentrations rarely become normal and often decline after otherwise effective treatment with oral pancreatic enzymes, so cobalamin malabsorption is probably not due solely to lack of pancreatic enzymes in the gut lumen.[148, 162, 165, 166] Furthermore, in experimental canine EPI, exogenous pancreatic juice, but not bovine pancreatic enzyme replacement, enhances cobalamin absorption.[162] Cobalamin is essential for DNA synthesis, and severely subnormal serum cobalamin concentrations may adversely affect the normal proliferation of crypt cells in the intestinal mucosa and hence the specific activities of jejunal mucosal enzymes.[20] It is therefore possible that intestinal dysfunction secondary to persistent cobalamin deficiency may be a contributory factor in cases in which the response to treatment with enzyme replacement alone is suboptimal. Anorexia is the major clinical sign noted in inherited selective cobalamin deficiency in the dog,[167] potentially explaining the anorexia reported in a minority of dogs with EPI.[168]

Serum folate concentrations are often increased in dogs with EPI both before and after treatment,[148, 163, 166] perhaps reflecting overgrowth of bacteria in the small intestine.[148, 150] Intraluminal bacteria commonly synthesize and release folate, and overgrowth of such bacteria in the proximal small intestine, the site for folate absorption in the dog, may elevate serum concentrations.[20] Alternatively, folate absorption may be promoted by the decreased duodenal pH secondary to reduced pancreatic bicarbonate secretion.[20] However, this is perhaps a less likely explanation because pancreatic bicarbonate secretion is relatively well preserved in canine PAA, and the duodenum itself has a significant ability to neutralize acid.[20] The elevations of serum folate associated with canine EPI are probably of no functional significance. Serum folate concentrations in affected cats are rarely increased but in contrast are often decreased, reflecting malabsorption associated with concurrent small intestinal disease.[32]

Serum tocopherol (vitamin E) concentrations are often severely subnormal in canine EPI,[166] which is not surprising given the severe fat malabsorption that occurs. Overgrowth of bacteria may contribute to deficiencies of fat-soluble vitamins by exacerbating fat malabsorption. Serum tocopherol concentrations do not increase in response to treatment,[166] perhaps because treatment does not return fat absorption to normal even though clinical signs of EPI resolve or because intraluminal bacterial overgrowth persists.[20, 150] Tocopherol deficiency decreases the proliferative response of canine lymphocytes to mitogenic stimulants, and if this reflects an in vivo defect in immune function, tocopherol deficiency may be an additional factor predisposing to overgrowth of intestinal bacteria in dogs with EPI. Tocopherol deficiency may cause pathologic change in smooth muscle, central nervous system, skeletal muscle, and retina, and although not yet reported, similar changes may accompany chronic untreated tocopherol deficiency in dogs with EPI.[20]

Subnormal serum concentrations of vitamin A have also been observed in dogs with EPI, but no associated signs of deficiency have been reported.[20] Vitamin K–responsive coagulopathy has been reported in a cat with EPI.[141] The potential for selective chronic nutrient deficiencies in canine and feline EPI deserves further investigation.

Diagnosis

History

Animals with EPI usually have a history of weight loss despite a normal or increased appetite. Polyphagia is often severe, and owners may complain that dogs ravenously devour all food offered to them as well as scavenge from garbage. This is by no means always the case, however, and some dogs may even have periods of inappetence. Coprophagia and pica are also common, probably as manifestations of polyphagia but also perhaps as a consequence of specific nutritional deficiencies. Water intake may also increase in some dogs, and in chronic pancreatitis this may be due to diabetes mellitus.[20, 165, 168, 169]

Diarrhea often accompanies EPI but can be variable in character. Most owners report frequent passage of large volumes of semiformed feces, although some pets have intermittent or continuous explosive watery diarrhea; in other instances diarrhea is infrequent and is not considered a problem. Diarrhea generally improves or resolves in response to fasting. Introduction of a low-fat diet may also decrease or eliminate diarrhea. There may be a history of vomiting, and commonly there are marked borborygmus and flatulence. Owners sometimes report that affected dogs suffer from episodes of abdominal discomfort.[20, 168]

In some dogs there has been a protracted history of gastrointestinal disturbances before the final diagnosis of EPI, the significance of which is not clear but which may merely represent initial failure to diagnose EPI. Unless signs of vomiting, diarrhea, borborygmus, or flatulence are severe, many owners may not seek veterinary advice until weight loss is marked. When animals are presented early, the diagnosis may be missed because the "classic" signs have not yet appeared. Appropriate testing in such early cases allows the diagnosis of EPI to be made before severe deterioration of body condition occurs.

Pancreatic acinar atrophy is prevalent in young German shepherd dogs.[163] It must be emphasized, however, that even in young German shepherd dogs small intestinal disease is more prevalent than EPI and that PAA may occur in any breed at any age.[163, 170] Chronic pancreatitis is probably more common in older dogs, but the true prevalence of EPI related to chronic pancreatitis is not known. Whatever the underlying pathology, results based on radioimmunoassay of serum TLI indicate that numerous breeds are affected, and only 40 per cent of the cases are in German shepherd dogs.[170]

Clinical Signs

Mild to marked weight loss is usually seen in association with EPI. Some dogs are emaciated with severe muscle wasting and no palpable body fat. In the extreme, dogs may be physically weak owing to loss of muscle mass. The haircoat is often in poor condition, and some animals may give off a foul odor because of soiling of the coat with fatty fecal material and passage of excessive flatus.[20, 168]

Laboratory Aids to Diagnosis

The history and clinical signs of EPI are nonspecific, vary in severity, and do not distinguish the condition from other causes of malabsorption. Although replacement therapy with oral pancreatic enzymes is generally successful, response to treatment is not a reliable diagnostic approach. Not all dogs with EPI respond to treatment, and dogs with self-limiting small intestinal disease might improve naturally, giving the false impression of a response to enzyme supplementation. Furthermore, veterinarians often advise a change in diet when treating dogs with EPI, and this in itself can lead to clinical improvement in some dogs with small intestinal diseases. It is also possible that pancreatic extracts might have a favorable effect in the treatment of malabsorption with causes other than EPI.

In dogs with PAA, extreme atrophy of the pancreas is readily observed on gross inspection at either exploratory laparotomy or laparoscopy, although in dogs with chronic pancreatitis it may be impossible to gauge accurately the amount of residual exocrine pancreatic tissue because of severe adhesions and fibrosis. These procedures involve unnecessary anesthetic and surgical risks and therefore cannot be recommended as diagnostic procedures given the availability of reliable noninvasive tests.

Pancreatic juice secreted into the gut lumen can be collected after peroral intubation of the canine duodenum, and the enzyme activity of this intestinal juice can then be assayed in vitro. This technique has been used to investigate secretion of pancreatic amylase and bicarbonate by dogs with EPI in response to stimulation with exogenous secretin and cholecystokinin, but the value of this test as a diagnostic aid has not been assessed. Moreover, this procedure is technically difficult and therefore has limited clinical application.[20]

Routine laboratory test results are generally not helpful in establishing the diagnosis of EPI. Serum alanine aminotransferase levels are mildly to moderately increased and may reflect hepatocyte damage secondary to increased uptake of hepatotoxic substances through an abnormally permeable small intestinal mucosa. Other routine serum biochemical test results are unremarkable, except that total lipid, cholesterol, and polyunsaturated fatty acid concentrations are often reduced. Dogs with EPI display a remarkable ability to maintain normal serum protein concentrations even when severely malnourished. Mild lymphopenia and eosinophilia are occasionally seen in dogs with EPI, but complete blood count results are usually within normal limits.[20] Canine serum amylase, isoamylase, lipase, and phospholipase A_2 activities are generally normal or only slightly reduced in EPI, and these tests are not useful in the identification of affected dogs.[20, 104, 171] Nonpancreatic sources of these enzymes are clearly present in dogs, and although their activities may increase in inflammatory disease of the pancreas, they do not decrease proportionally as the mass of functional exocrine pancreatic tissue declines.

Many laboratory tests for the diagnosis of EPI have been described, but their sensitivities and specificities are often highly questionable.[20] The most reliable and widely used tests currently available are assay of serum TLI and assay of fecal proteolytic activity using a casein- or albumin-based substrate.

Serum Trypsin-like Immunoreactivity

Trypsinogen is synthesized exclusively by the pancreas and measurement of the serum concentration of this zymogen by species-specific radioimmunoassay* provides a good indirect index of pancreatic function in the dog.[172] This immunoassay detects both trypsinogen and trypsin, hence the use of the term trypsin-like immunoreactivity to describe the total concentration of these two immunoreactive species. Serum TLI concentration is both highly sensitive and specific for the diagnosis of canine EPI. Concentrations are dramatically reduced in dogs with EPI, whereas those in dogs with small intestinal disease are not significantly different from normal (Fig. 146–15).[172, 173] Marked reductions in

_____

*Canine TLI Assay, Diagnostic Products Corporation, 5700 West 96th Street, Los Angeles, CA 90045.

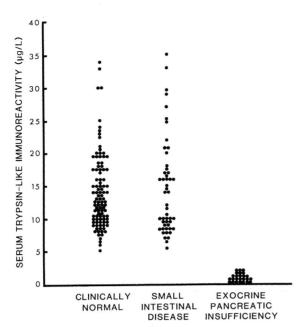

Figure 146–15. Serum trypsin-like immunoreactivity in 100 healthy dogs, 50 dogs with small intestinal disease, and 25 dogs with exocrine pancreatic insufficiency. (From Williams DA, Batt RM: Sensitivity and specificity of radioimmunoassay of serum trypsin-like immunoreactivity for the diagnosis of canine exocrine pancreatic insufficiency. JAVMA 192:195, 1988.)

serum TLI (to less than 2 μg/L) may even precede signs of weight loss or diarrhea, at a time when results of other tests (fecal proteolytic activity, bentiromide absorption) are still normal.[140, 143, 173]

Utilization of this test is simple in that analysis of a single serum sample obtained after food has been withheld for several hours is all that is required. Serum TLI is stable and samples can therefore be mailed to an appropriate laboratory for analysis. Administration of oral pancreatic extracts (usually of porcine origin) does not affect serum TLI concentration because trypsins from different species do not cross-react immunologically and little if any intact enzyme is absorbed intact from the gut lumen, so withdrawal from enzyme supplementation before testing of dogs that are already receiving treatment is unnecessary. Although it has not been documented, it can be predicted that serum TLI concentrations will be normal in the rare dogs with EPI related to tumors obstructing the pancreatic ducts or to congenital deficiencies of enzymes other than trypsinogen. Equivocal serum TLI concentrations in the range 2.5 to 5.2 μg/L sometimes reflect failure to withhold food before collecting blood. On retesting, serum TLI concentrations in many such cases are either clearly consistent with EPI or normal.[140] The few dogs with consistent "gray zone" serum TLI concentrations usually have poor responses to enzyme replacement therapy, may have subtotal acinar atrophy with degenerative ultrastructural changes, and may improve without therapy.[140, 144] Individual variation in extrapancreatic digestive capacity may explain the different and unpredictable responses and clinical courses in these pets.

Immunoassays for trypsin are usually species specific, and assays for human TLI do not detect canine TLI. Specific immunoassay of feline TLI is available through the author's laboratory.* There is no cross-reactivity between canine and

feline TLI, normal serum TLI values in cats range from 14 to 82 μg/L, and serum TLI is less than 8.5 μg/L in cats with EPI.[108, 174–176]

Fecal Proteolytic Activity

Fecal proteolytic activity has been used as an index of pancreatic enzyme activity for years, but the reliability of the test varies widely depending on the assay method employed as well as on the precautions taken to minimize autodegradation of the relatively labile proteases in the fecal sample during the interval between collection and assay.[177] The widely used x-ray film digestion test is certainly unreliable as performed in many laboratories. Gelatin digestion is difficult to evaluate with precision, and the test gives many false-negative and false-positive results, perhaps reflecting poor standardization of technique.[20] Proteolytic activity can be measured more precisely by using dyed protein substrates such as azocasein or by radial enzyme diffusion into agar gels containing casein substrate.[177, 178] Fecal proteolytic activity as assessed by these methods is consistently low in most dogs and cats with EPI, but because both dogs and cats with normal pancreatic function occasionally pass feces with low proteolytic activity, either repeated determinations must be made (Fig. 146–16) or, in dogs, the test can be performed on a single sample collected after feeding crude soybean meal for 2 days.[20, 172, 178] Some dogs with EPI have normal fecal proteolytic activity as assessed by this assay, but this is rare[172, 173]; it is likely that a similar situation exists in cats.

Synthetic substrates degraded only by enzymes with trypsin or chymotrypsin-like specificities and specific immunoassays have been used to investigate the value of assay of true fecal trypsin, chymotrypsin, or pancreatic elastase activities

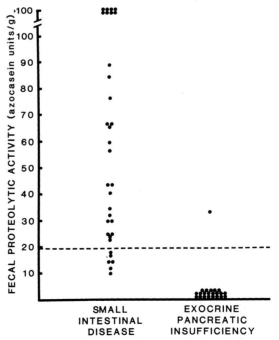

Figure 146–16. Fecal proteolytic activity determined by azocasein assay of 3-day collections from 34 dogs with small intestinal disease and 22 dogs with exocrine pancreatic insufficiency. The dashed line indicates the lower limit of the range of values in healthy dogs. (From Williams DA, Batt RM: Sensitivity and specificity of radioimmunoassay of serum trypsin-like immunoreactivity for the diagnosis of canine exocrine pancreatic insufficiency. JAVMA 192:195, 1988.)

---

*GI Laboratory, Small Animal Medicine and Surgery, Texas A&M University, College Station, TX 77843-4474. Telephone 409-862-2861, Fax 409-862-2864, E-mail gilab@cvm.tamu.edu, WWW cvm.tamu.edu/gilab.

or concentrations in the identification of patients with EPI.[20] These assays require expensive laboratory equipment and appear to offer no advantages over simple assays of general proteolytic activity based on azoproteins.

Other Tests

Chymotrypsin activity in the proximal small intestine may be assayed in vivo by the oral administration of the synthetic substrate bentiromide.[20, 179] Although several studies have shown the bentiromide test to be relatively reliable for diagnosis of EPI in dogs, it offers no advantages over assay of serum TLI or fecal proteolytic activity and has not found widespread use because of expense and technical constraints. Results of the bentiromide test in normal cats vary widely, but a markedly abnormal result has been reported in a cat with EPI.[141, 180] A potential advantage of the bentiromide test over serum TLI assay is that it should detect the rare cases of EPI involving obstruction of the flow of pancreatic juice, a situation in which release of trypsinogen into the blood, and hence the concentration of TLI, is normal.[137] However, assay of fecal proteolytic activity should also identify these individuals.

Microscopic examination of feces for evidence of undigested food (fat droplets, starch grains, muscle fibers) is subjective and imprecise, and interpretation is complicated by the variation in fecal characteristics that occurs with different diets and with changes in intestinal transit time.[20] Although EPI is usually associated with steatorrhea, this is often not apparent on examination of Sudan III–stained samples. Quantitative assessment of fecal fat output is a more sensitive and specific indicator of steatorrhea, but neither the qualitative nor quantitative tests reliably differentiate EPI from other causes of fat malabsorption (Fig. 146–17).[20] Microscopic evaluation of canine feces for the presence of

"split" (i.e., digested) and "neutral" (i.e., undigested) fat, although theoretically attractive, does not appear to be useful in differentiating pancreatic from nonpancreatic steatorrhea.[179]

Plasma turbidity (lipemia) after oral administration of fat is often diminished or absent in dogs with fat malabsorption. Theoretically, EPI can be distinguished from other causes of fat malabsorption by repeating the test after addition of pancreatic extract to the fat meal. However, some dogs with EPI develop visually detectable lipemia after a fatty meal without addition of pancreatic extract, because even when pancreatic enzymes are absent up to 80 per cent of fat in a meal may be absorbed. In addition, other poorly defined factors such as variations in gastrointestinal transit times and rates of lipid clearance from plasma make this test difficult to evaluate reliably. Finally, there is evidence that absorption of free fatty acids after oral administration of hydrolyzed fat is decreased in canine EPI; thus development of lipemia may be impaired even when affected dogs are given fat with pancreatic enzymes.[20]

In summary, assays of serum TLI or fecal proteolytic activity as described provide reliable tests for EPI in dogs and cats. Serum TLI assay is a more specific test, however, because assay of fecal proteolytic activity gives a higher proportion of abnormal results in patients with small intestinal disease. The bentiromide test is impractical in most clinical situations but is a serum test that offers sensitivity and specificity similar to those of assay of fecal proteolytic activity. Microscopic examination of feces for undigested food, assessment of fecal proteolytic activity by gelatin digestion, and plasma turbidity tests all give significant proportions of false-negative and false-positive results, and their use even as crude "screening" tests is not recommended. Assay of fecal proteolytic activity is the test of choice for use in cats, in the absence of an available feline TLI assay.

Treatment

Enzyme Replacement

Most dogs and cats with EPI can be successfully managed by supplementing each meal with pancreatic enzymes present in commercially available dried pancreatic extracts.[20] Numerous formulations of these extracts are available (tablets, capsules, powders, granules), some of which are enteric coated, and their enzyme contents and bioavailabilities vary widely.[20, 181–184] Addition of 2 teaspoons of powdered non–enteric-coated preparation with each meal per 20 kg of body weight is generally an effective starting dose. This can be mixed with a maintenance food immediately before feeding. Non-powdered preparations are not recommended. Two meals a day are usually sufficient to promote weight gain. Dogs generally gain 0.5 to 1.0 kg per week, and diarrhea resolves within 4 to 5 days. In some cases the reduction in frequency of defecation is dramatic, and other signs such as coprophagia and polyphagia often disappear within a few days. As soon as clinical improvement is apparent, owners can determine a minimum effective dose of enzyme supplement that prevents return of clinical signs. This varies slightly between batches of extract and also from patient to patient, probably reflecting individual variation in extrapancreatic digestive reserve. Most affected dogs require at least 1 teaspoon of enzyme supplement per meal, but lower doses are often adequate in cats and small dogs. One meal per day is sufficient in some dogs, but others continue to require two. Commercial dried pancreatic extracts are expensive

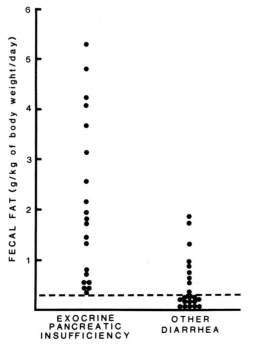

Figure 146–17. Fecal fat output in dogs with exocrine pancreatic insufficiency and dogs with chronic diarrhea of other causes. The dashed line indicates the upper limit of normal in healthy dogs. (Modified from Burrows CF, et al: Determination of fecal fat and trypsin output in the evaluation of chronic canine diarrhea. JAVMA 174:62, 1979.)

LIV

and, when available, substitution of 3 to 4 ounces per 20 kg of body weight of chopped raw ox or pig pancreas obtained from animals certified as healthy after appropriate post-mortem inspection is a more economical alternative. Pancreas can be stored frozen at −20°C for at least 3 months and enzyme activity is adequately maintained.

Measures to Increase the Effectiveness of Enzyme Supplementation

Although administration of pancreatic enzymes with food is generally successful, only a small proportion of the oral dose of each enzyme, particularly of lipase, is delivered functionally intact to the small intestine, and fat absorption does not return to normal.[20] Pancreatic lipase is rapidly inactivated at the acid pH encountered in the stomach, and trypsin and some other pancreatic proteases, although relatively acid resistant, are susceptible to degradation by gastric pepsins. In human beings only approximately 35 per cent of trypsin and 17 per cent of lipase ingested with a meal can be recovered intact from the duodenum.[184] In view of the expense of pancreatic enzyme preparations, attempts have been made to increase the effectiveness of enzyme supplementation. These include preincubation of enzymes with food before feeding, supplementation with bile salts, neutralization or inhibition of secretion of gastric acid, and use of enteric-coated preparations.[20]

Preincubation of food with enzyme powder for 30 minutes before feeding does not improve the effectiveness of oral enzyme treatment in promoting fat absorption in dogs with ligated pancreas ducts. This is not surprising because optimal activity is not achieved unless lipase is in solution at the appropriate pH and temperature and in the presence of appropriate concentrations of colipase and bile acids, conditions that are unlikely to be encountered in the feeding bowl.

There is no evidence that intraluminal bile acid concentrations are subnormal in patients with EPI, and addition of bile salts to enzyme supplement does not improve fat absorption over that obtained when enzymes alone are given with food to dogs with ligated pancreatic ducts. It is possible that bile salts may be precipitated in individuals with abnormally low small intestinal intraluminal pH, and although this may contribute to the development of steatorrhea related to a functional bile salt deficiency, supplementation with oral bile salts does not rectify such a situation.[20] Drastic reductions in duodenal intraluminal pH in canine EPI are unlikely, so functional bile salt deficiency is probably not of importance.

Gastric acid secretion may be reduced by administration of histamine type 2 receptor antagonists. Cimetidine at a dosage of 300 mg per 20 kg body weight given with food mixed with pancreatic enzymes does improve fat absorption in dogs with ligated pancreatic ducts but does not decrease fecal wet or dry weight. The routine use of cimetidine in the treatment of EPI is not recommended, given the expense of the drug and the fact that so many pets respond well when treated with enzymes alone. Indeed, it is possible that antacids may be detrimental in chronic EPI: although they may increase the quantity of orally administered pancreatic lipase reaching the small intestine, they may inhibit gastric lipase activity; the latter probably accounts for the considerable residual fat absorption in dogs with EPI but has an acid pH optimum.[8, 139, 185, 186] Oral antacids such as sodium bicarbonate and aluminum or magnesium hydroxide do not increase the effectiveness of enzyme therapy either in experimental canine EPI or in human patients with chronic pancreatitis.[20, 184]

Enteric-coated preparations have been formulated in an attempt to protect orally administered enzymes from gastric acid.[183] The formulation of these preparations (particle size, pH of disintegration of polymer coating) to release enzymes in the optimal locale is complex, and their efficacy is likely to vary both with different causes of EPI and in different species because of regional differences in the gastrointestinal milieu. In people these preparations have generally proved to be no more effective or less effective than non–enteric-coated extracts.[184] A survey of dogs with EPI showed that enteric-coated preparations were often ineffective or less effective than powdered pancreatic extract or fresh pancreas.[163] This may reflect selective retention of enteric-coated particles in the stomach or perhaps rapid intestinal transit such that adequate enzyme release does not occur.[183] Similar mechanisms may explain the ineffectiveness of an uncrushed tablet formulation of pancreatic enzymes in treating EPI in pancreatic duct–ligated dogs, whereas the same formulation was effective when crushed before feeding.[20]

It is possible that future enzyme preparations containing acid-resistant fungal lipase will prove useful.[187] However, in dogs with suboptimal weight gain in response to pancreatic enzymes alone, no advantage is seen on increasing the dose of enzymes above 2 teaspoons per meal or giving cimetidine, suggesting that factors other than enzyme delivery to the small intestine are involved.

Dietary Modification

Clinical studies in humans and experimental studies in dogs show that fat absorption does not return to normal despite appropriate enzyme therapy.[20, 184, 188] Dogs appear to compensate by eating slightly more than usual, and with any individual dog it is necessary to regulate the amount of food given in order to maintain ideal body weight. Feeding fat-restricted diets does not seem to be beneficial.[189]

Although therapy with regular maintenance dog food and appropriate enzyme replacement is usually effective, feeding of a highly digestible, low-fiber diet has been advocated.[190] A non-blinded clinical study found that owners considered that their dogs generally did better (reduced flatulence and borborygmi, decreased fecal volume and frequency of defecation) when fed a commercial highly digestible diet than when fed home-cooked or regular maintenance diets, but there was no difference in appetite, drinking, color or consistency of feces, or coprophagy.[191] Results of experimental studies to evaluate highly digestible diets have shown consistent reductions in fecal weight but have not shown consistent benefit with regard to fat digestibility, probably because different studies were not comparable with regard to variables such as feeding patterns and the use of gastric acid modifiers that might affect digestibilities of different diets.[166, 188] Some types of dietary fiber do impair pancreatic enzyme activity in vitro, and diets containing large amounts of insoluble or nonfermentable fiber probably should be avoided.[192] Highly digestible diets, particularly when they contain or are supplemented with medium-chain triglycerides, may be of particular value in promoting caloric uptake in dogs with EPI that do not regain normal body weight in response to other therapies. Some medium-chain triglycerides are absorbed intact, and they are hydrolyzed more readily by gastric lipase than are long-chain triglycerides.[8]

Vitamin Supplementation

Dogs and cats with EPI may have severely subnormal concentrations of serum cobalamin and tocopherol that usually do not increase in response to treatment with oral pancreatic enzymes, even in cases in which the clinical response in terms of weight gain and resolution of diarrhea is excellent.[20, 165, 166] Deficiencies of these vitamins may contribute to intestinal mucosal changes and perhaps cause systemic signs of deficiency, including anorexia, myopathy or myelopathy, and other abnormalities of nervous tissue, as reported in other species. It therefore seems prudent to supplement with these vitamins if serum concentrations are subnormal. Supplementation with large oral doses of tocopherol (30 IU for cats and 400 to 500 IU for dogs given once daily with food for 1 month) is effective in returning serum concentrations to normal (Table 146–8). In contrast, cobalamin must be given parenterally (125 to 500 μg by intramuscular or subcutaneous injection once a week for several weeks) to normalize serum concentrations. Subnormal serum folate concentrations in cats with EPI can be normalized by oral supplementation of folate (0.25 to 0.5 mg daily for 1 month).

Potential deficiencies of other vitamins in patients with EPI have not been investigated in detail, although vitamin K–responsive coagulopathy has been reported.[142] Malabsorption of fat-soluble vitamins is to be expected both before and after treatment in view of the failure of pancreatic replacement therapy to return fat absorption to normal, but malabsorption of vitamins A, D, and K may not be as marked as with tocopherol because tocopherol appears to be particularly sensitive to abnormalities in the intestinal lumen.[20] It should be noted that doses of individual vitamins in multivitamin preparations may be insufficient to normalize serum concentrations and that parenteral or high oral doses may be required for adequate supplementation.

Antibiotic Therapy

Dogs with PAA commonly have overgrowth of bacteria in the small intestine, but in most cases this is a subclinical abnormality and affected individuals respond satisfactorily to pancreatic enzyme without antibiotics.[10, 150, 166] Bacterial overgrowth can cause malabsorption and diarrhea, however, and in individuals that do not respond to oral enzyme supplementation alone, antibiotic therapy may be of value.[10] Oral

TABLE 146–8. DRUG INDEX

GENERIC	TRADE	DOSAGE	ROUTE*	FREQUENCY	BRIEF DESCRIPTION
Pancreatin	Pancrezyme Viokase-V	½–2 teaspoon	Oral	With each meal	Pancreatic digestive enzymes
Oxytetracycline		5–10 mg/lb (10–20 mg/kg)	Oral	q12h for 7–28 days	Antibiotic to treat bacterial overgrowth in small intestine
Metronidazole	Flagyl	5–10 mg/lb (10–20 mg/kg)	Oral	q12–24h for 7 days	Antibiotic to treat bacterial overgrowth in small intestine
Tylosin	Tylan	5 mg/lb (10 mg/kg)	Oral	With each meal as needed	Antibiotic to treat bacterial overgrowth in small intestine
Prednisolone or prednisone		½–1 mg/lb (1–2 mg/kg) initially	Oral	q12h for 7–14 days	Glucocorticoid to treat idiopathic inflammatory bowel disease or partial villous atrophy
Cimetidine	Tagamet	2–5 mg/lb (5–10 mg/kg)	Oral	With or 30 minutes before each meal	Histamine type 2 receptor antagonist; inhibits gastric acid secretion
Medium-chain triglyceride oil	MCT oil	0.5–4 teaspoons per day with food	Oral	Divided doses with meals	Readily absorbed caloric supplement (excess may cause diarrhea)
Cobalamin		125–250 μg (cat) 250–500 μg (dog)	IM or SQ	Weekly for 4–8 weeks, then q3–6 months as needed	To rectify cobalamin deficiency secondary to exocrine pancreatic insufficiency
Folic acid		0.25–0.5 mg (cat) 0.5–2.0 mg (dog)	Oral	Daily for 1 month, then q1–2 weeks as needed	To rectify folate deficiency in exocrine pancreatic insufficiency patients with concurrent folate malabsorption
Tocopherol		30 IU (cat) 100–400 IU (dog)	Oral	Daily for 1 month, then q1–2 weeks as needed	To rectify tocopherol deficiency secondary to exocrine pancreatic insufficiency
Vitamin K$_1$		1–2 mg/kg	SQ	q12h for 48 hours	To correct coagulopathy associated with vitamin K deficiency secondary to exocrine pancreatic insufficiency
Dopamine		5 μg/kg/min	IV		May ameliorate feline (and canine?) acute pancreatitis by maintaining vascular integrity
Meperidine	Demerol	0.5–2.5 mg/lb (1–5 mg/kg) (dog) 0.5–1.0 mg/lb initially (1–2 mg/kg) (cat)	IM or SQ	q0.5–6h as needed	Opioid agonist analgesic
Butorphanol	Torbugesic	0.1–0.5 mg/lb (0.2–1 mg/kg) (dog) 0.05–0.2 mg/lb (0.1–0.4 mg/kg) (cat)	IM, IV or SQ	q1–4h as needed	Opioid agonist-antagonist analgesic
Praziquantel	Droncit	20 mg/lb (40 mg/kg)	Oral	q24h for 3 days	Anthelmintic for treatment of hepatic fluke infection
Fenbendazole	Panacur	15 mg/lb (30 mg/kg)	Oral	q24h for 6 days	Anthelmintic for treatment of pancreatic fluke infection

*IM = intramuscular; IV = intravenous; SQ = subcutaneous.

LIV

oxytetracycline, metronidazole, or tylosin may be effective in improving the clinical response in some of the these dogs.[10, 150] Long-lasting untreated bacterial overgrowth may cause mucosal damage that is only partially reversible after even prolonged antibiotic therapy, and this may explain why some dogs fail to return to normal body weight.[20, 193] It is not clear whether a predisposition to recurrent development of overgrowth exists after antibiotic therapy.

Glucocorticoid Therapy

In the few pets that respond poorly to the preceding treatments, oral prednisolone (or prednisone) at an initial dosage of 1 to 2 mg/kg every 12 hours for 7 to 14 days is usually beneficial. In such cases lymphocytic-plasmacytic gastroenteritis usually coexists with EPI. Long-term glucocorticoid administration is generally unnecessary, however, and maintenance therapy with enzyme supplementation alone is usually sufficient (D. A. Williams, unpublished observations, 1993).

Prognosis

The underlying pathologic process leading to EPI is generally irreversible, and lifelong treatment is required. Pancreatic enzymes are expensive, and only in rare cases is the enzyme deficiency reversed. Therefore, in pets with consistently borderline pancreatic function test results or those in which chronic relapsing pancreatitis is suspected, it is reasonable to withdraw enzyme supplement for a trial period approximately every 6 months to determine whether treatment is necessary. Pancreatic acinar tissue does have some capacity to regenerate, and it is not inconceivable that after either pancreatitis or subtotal PAA residual acinar tissue might regenerate sufficiently to reverse clinical signs of EPI. In most cases, treatment is required for life, and the prognosis is good, although as many as 20 per cent of dogs have a suboptimal response.[164, 194] Some dogs may fail to regain normal body weight, but these animals usually have marked improvement of diarrhea and polyphagia and are acceptable as pets. A high prevalence of mesenteric torsion has been reported in German shepherd dogs with PAA in Finland,[194] but there is no evidence that this is a problem in dogs with EPI in other parts of the world. Long-term follow-up of large numbers of cats with EPI has not been reported, but most seem to respond well when treated as outlined earlier; correction of cobalamin deficiency appears to be a particularly important aspect of therapy in many affected cats.

Treatment of dogs and cats with both diabetes mellitus and EPI related to chronic pancreatitis is likely to be more troublesome and expensive. Diabetes mellitus is potentially more difficult to regulate in view of probably coexistent derangement in the secretion of glucagon and somatostatin. Inflammation in residual pancreatic tissue may cause anorexia, vomiting, or other signs of pancreatitis and this may further complicate treatment of diabetes mellitus.

NEOPLASIA OF THE EXOCRINE PANCREAS

Pancreatic adenocarcinomas may be acinar or duct cell in origin, but both are uncommon and they are particularly rare in cats. In both species they are seen in older animals. Pancreatic carcinoma may be more common in Airedale terriers than other breeds.[20, 31, 32, 169, 195, 196]

Adenocarcinomas are usually highly malignant tumors and have often metastasized to the duodenal wall, liver, and local lymph nodes, or less commonly to the lungs, at the time of presentation. Clinical signs are usually nonspecific: weight loss, anorexia, depression, and vomiting. Affected animals are often icteric because of associated obstruction of the bile ducts or widespread hepatic metastasis. Occasionally, dogs have characteristic signs of diabetes mellitus or EPI related to obstruction of the pancreatic ducts or beta-cell destruction.[137]

There are usually no specific findings on physical examination, but there may be abdominal tenderness because of associated pancreatitis, and occasionally an anterior abdominal mass is palpable. Abdominal radiographs may suggest pancreatitis or indicate the presence of an anterior mass, and thoracic radiographs may reveal pulmonary metastasis. Ultrasonographic examination may help further define pancreatic abnormalities, and cytologic examination of abdominal fluid or of material aspirated from suspect areas may reveal neoplastic cells.

There are no specific laboratory tests for pancreatic carcinoma, and results of routine tests may be misleading. Increased serum amylase and lipase activities are seen in some dogs with pancreatic carcinoma. Hepatic involvement is usually indicated by increased serum alkaline phosphatase and bilirubin, with lesser increases in alanine aminotransferase, suggestive of an obstructive hepatopathy.[20] In most cases, definitive diagnosis requires exploratory laparotomy. It is important to have a biopsy of abnormal pancreatic tissue because chronic pancreatitis may grossly resemble pancreatic carcinoma.

Given the frequency of metastasis at the time of diagnosis, the prognosis for animals with carcinomas of the exocrine pancreas is extremely poor[116]; survival for more than 1 year after diagnosis has not been reported. There are no reports of curative therapy, but, when possible, surgical excision of localized lesions, perhaps in combination with chemotherapy or radiation therapy, may be palliative.[116] Therapy with insulin and pancreatic enzymes may be required to treat associated diabetes mellitus and EPI.[137]

PANCREATIC FLUKES IN CATS

There are several reports of infection with pancreatic flukes, *Eurytrema procyonis* in the United States and *Opisthorchis felineus* in Europe, in domestic cats.[73, 197] Associated pathology generally includes pancreatic atrophy and fibrosis that in some cases, together with duct obstruction, may severely decrease exocrine pancreatic secretory capacity. In spite of marked loss of exocrine tissue, however, weight loss and diarrhea have not been reported, and the infection is usually subclinical.

Infection is often an incidental finding, with characteristic eggs observed in the feces. However, one report described a cat infected with *E. procyonis* that had marked inflammatory infiltrates in association with the parasites and a 2-year history of weight loss and intermittent vomiting, consistent with pancreatitis perhaps progressing to clinical EPI. Treatment with fenbendazole has been reported to be effective.[197]

The hepatic fluke *Amphimerus pseudofelineus* can also infect the pancreas of the cat and lead to pancreatitis. Diagnosis is made by fecal examination. Treatment with praziquantel has been successful.[32]

REFERENCES

1. Bernard C; Henderson J, trans: Memoir on the Pancreas and on the Role of Pancreatic Juice in Digestive Processes. Particularly in the Digestion of Neu-

tral Fat. Monographs of the Physiological Society, No 42. New York, Academic Press, 1985.

2. Case RM, Argent BE: Pancreatic duct cell secretion: Control and mechanisms of transport. In Go VLW, DiMagno EP, Gardner JD, et al (eds): The Pancreas: Biology, Pathobiology and Disease, 2nd ed. New York, Raven Press, 1993, p 301.

3. Herzlich B, Herbert V: The role of the pancreas in cobalamin (vitamin B_{12}) absorption. Am J Gastroenterol 79:489, 1984.

4. Batt RM, Horadagoda NU, McLean L, et al: Identification and characterization of a pancreatic intrinsic factor in the dog. Am J Physiol 256:G517, 1989.

5. Sturniolo GC, D'Incà R, Montino MC, et al: Citric acid corrects zinc absorption deficiency in chronic pancreatitis. J Trace Elem Exp Med 3:267, 1990.

6. Erlanson-Albertsson C: Pancreatic colipase. Structural and physiological aspects. Biochim Biophys Acta 1125:1, 1992.

7. Van Tilbeurgh H, Sarda L, Verger R, et al: Structure of the pancreatic lipase-procolipase complex. Nature 359:159, 1992.

8. Borgström B: Luminal digestion of fats. In Go VLW, DiMagno EP, Gardner JD, et al (eds): The Pancreas: Biology, Pathobiology and Disease, 2nd ed. New York, Raven Press, 1993, p 475.

9. Rubinstein E, Mark Z, Haspel J, et al: Antibacterial activity of the pancreatic fluid. Gastroenterology 88:927, 1985.

10. Williams DA, Batt RM, McLean L: Bacterial overgrowth in the duodenum of dogs with exocrine pancreatic insufficiency. JAVMA 191:201, 1987.

11. Williams DA: Exocrine pancreatic disease. In Ettinger SJ (ed): Textbook of Veterinary Internal Medicine, 3rd ed. Philadelphia, WB Saunders, 1989, p 1528.

12. Rinderknecht H: Pancreatic secretory enzymes. In Go VLW, DiMagno EP, Gardner JD, et al (eds): The Pancreas: Biology, Pathobiology and Disease, 2nd ed. New York, Raven Press, 1993, p 219.

13. Williams JA, Goldfine ID: The insulin-acinar relationship. In Go VLW, DiMagno EP, Gardner JD, et al (eds): The Pancreas: Biology, Pathobiology and Disease, 2nd ed. New York, Raven Press, 1993, p 789.

14. Slack JMW: Developmental biology of the pancreas. Development 121:1569, 1995.

15. Jubb KVF, Kennedy PC, Palmer N: The Pancreas. In Jubb KVF, Kennedy PC, Palmer N (eds): Pathology of Domestic Animals, 3rd ed. Orlando, FL, Harcourt Brace Jovanovich, 1985, p 313.

16. Bockman DE: Anatomy of the pancreas. In Go VLW, DiMagno EP, Gardner JD, et al (eds): The Pancreas: Biology, Pathobiology and Disease, 2nd ed. New York, Raven Press, 1993, p 1.

17. Kern HF: Fine structure of the human exocrine pancreas. In Go VLW, DiMagno EP, Gardner JD, et al (eds): The Pancreas: Biology, Pathobiology and Disease, 2nd ed. New York, Raven Press, 1993, p 9.

18. Bonner-Weir S: The microvasculature of the pancreas, with emphasis on that of the islets of Langerhans: Anatomy and functional considerations. In Go VLW, DiMagno EP, Gardner JD, et al (eds): The Pancreas: Biology, Pathobiology and Disease, 2nd ed. New York, Raven Press, 1993, p 759.

19. Holst JJ: Neural regulation of pancreatic exocrine function. In Go VLW, DiMagno EP, Gardner JD, et al (eds): The Pancreas: Biology, Pathobiology and Disease, 2nd ed. New York, Raven Press, 1993, p 381.

20. Williams DA: The pancreas. In Strombeck DR, Guilford WG, Center SA, et al (eds): Small Animal Gastroenterology, 3rd ed. Philadelphia, WB Saunders, 1996, p 381.

21. Scheele GA, Kern HF: Cellular compartmentation, protein processing, and secretion in the exocrine pancreas. In Go VLW, DiMagno EP, Gardner JD, et al (eds): The Pancreas: Biology, Pathobiology and Disease, 2nd ed. New York, Raven Press, 1993, p 121.

22. Chey WY: Hormonal control of pancreatic exocrine secretion. In Go VLW, DiMagno EP, Gardner JD, et al (eds): The Pancreas: Biology, Pathobiology and Disease, 2nd ed. New York, Raven Press, 1993, p 403.

23. Singer MV: Neurohormonal control of pancreatic enzyme secretion in animals. In Go VLW, DiMagno EP, Gardner JD, et al (eds): The Pancreas: Biology, Pathobiology and Disease, 2nd ed. New York, Raven Press, 1993, p 425.

24. Liddle RA: Regulation of cholecystokinin secretion by intraluminal releasing factors. Am J Physiol 269:G319, 1995.

25. Miyasaka K, Guan D, Liddle RA, et al: Feedback regulation by trypsin: Evidence for intraluminal CCK-releasing peptide. Am J Physiol 257:G175, 1989.

26. Uda K, Murata A, Nishijima J, et al: Elevation of circulating monitor peptide/pancreatic secretory trypsin inhibitor-I (PSTI-61) after turpentine-induced inflammation in rats: Hepatocytes produce it as an acute phase reactant. J Surg Res 57:563, 1994.

27. Levitt MD, Eckfeldt JH: Diagnosis of acute pancreatitis. In Go VLW, DiMagno EP, Gardner JD, et al (eds): The Pancreas: Biology, Pathophysiology and Disease, 2nd ed. New York, Raven Press, 1993, p 613.

28. Sarner M: Pancreatitis definitions and classification. In Go VLW, DiMagno EP, Gardner JD, et al (eds): The Pancreas: Biology, Pathobiology and Disease, 2nd ed. New York, Raven Press, 1993, p 575.

29. Hill RC, Van Winkle TJ: Acute necrotizing pancreatitis and acute suppurative pancreatitis in the cat. A retrospective study of 40 cases (1976–1989). J Vet Intern Med 7:25, 1993.

30. Schaer M, Holloway S: Diagnosing acute pancreatitis in the cat. Vet Med 1986:782, 1991.

31. Jubb KVF: The pancreas. In Jubb KVF, Kennedy PC, Palmer N (eds): Pathology of Domestic Animals, 4th ed. San Diego, Academic Press, 1993, p 407.

32. Steiner JM, Williams DA: Feline exocrine pancreatic disorders. Vet Clin North Am, in press.

33. Steer ML, Meldolesi J: The cell biology of experimental pancreatitis. N Engl J Med 316:144, 1987.

34. Steer ML, Saluja AK: Experimental acute pancreatitis: Studies of the early events that lead to cell injury. In Go VLW, DiMagno EP, Gardner JD, et al (eds): The Pancreas: Biology, Pathobiology and Disease, 2nd ed. New York, Raven Press, 1993, p 489.

35. Gorelick FS, Adler G, Kern HF: Cerulein-induced pancreatitis. In Go VLW, DiMagno EP, Gardner JD, et al (eds): The Pancreas: Biology, Pathobiology and Disease, 2nd ed. New York, Raven Press, 1993, p 501.

36. Reber HA, Adler G, Karanjia N, Widdison A: Permeability characteristics of the main pancreatic duct in cats: Models of acute and chronic pancreatitis. In Go VLW, DiMagno EP, Gardner JD, et al (eds): The Pancreas: Biology, Pathobiology and Disease, 2nd ed. New York, Raven Press, 1993, p 527.

37. Lerch MM, Adler G: Experimental animal models of acute pancreatitis. Int J Pancreatol 15:159, 1994.

38. Simpson KW: Current concepts of the pathogenesis and pathophysiology of acute pancreatitis in the dog and cat. Compend Contin Educ Pract Vet 15:247, 1993.

39. Rinderknecht H: Activation of pancreatic zymogens. Normal activation, premature intrapancreatic activation, protective mechanisms against inappropriate activation. Dig Dis Sci 31:314, 1986.

40. Norman J: The role of cytokines in the pathogenesis of acute pancreatitis. Am J Surg 175:76, 1998.

41. Sanfey H, Bulkley GB, Cameron JL: The pathogenesis of acute pancreatitis: The source and role of oxygen-derived free radicals in three different experimental models. Ann Surg 201:633, 1985.

42. Sanfey H, Bulkley GB, Cameron JL: The role of oxygen-derived free radicals in the pathogenesis of acute pancreatitis. Ann Surg 200:405, 1984.

43. Sanfey H, Cameron JL: Increased capillary permeability—An early lesion in acute pancreatitis. Surgery 96:485, 1984.

44. Niederau C, Schultz H-U, Letko G: Involvement of free radicals in the pathophysiology of chronic pancreatitis: Potential of treatment with antioxidant and scavenger substances. Klin Wochenschr 69:1018, 1991.

45. Schoenberg MH, Büchler M, Helfen M, et al: Role of oxygen radicals in experimental acute pancreatitis. Eur Surg Res 24(Suppl 1):74, 1992.

46. Pitchumoni CS, Scheele GA: Interdependence of nutrition and exocrine pancreatic function. In Go VLW, DiMagno EP, Gardner JD, et al (eds): The Pancreas: Biology, Pathobiology and Disease, 2nd ed. New York, Raven Press, 1993, p 449.

47. Kingsnorth AN: Platelet-activating factor. Scand J Gastroenterol Suppl 219:28, 1996.

48. McKay CJ, Curran F, Sharples C, et al: Prospective placebo-controlled randomized trial of lexipafant in predicted severe acute pancreatitis. Br J Surg 84:1239, 1997.

49. Borgström A, Lasson ÅA: Trypsin–alpha$_1$-protease inhibitor complexes in serum and clinical course of acute pancreatitis. Scand J Gastroenterol 19:1119, 1984.

50. Durie PR, Gaskin KJ, Ogilvie JE, et al: Serial alterations in the forms of immunoreactive pancreatic cationic trypsin in plasma from patients with acute pancreatitis. J Pediatr Gastroenterol Nutr 4:199, 1985.

51. Izquierdo R, Sandberg L, Nora MO, et al: Comparative study of protease inhibitors on coagulation abnormalities in canine pancreatitis. J Surg Res 36:606, 1984.

52. Lungarella G, Gardi C, De Santi MM, et al: Pulmonary vascular injury in pancreatitis: Evidence for a major role played by pancreatic elastase. Exp Mol Pathol 42:44, 1985.

53. Lasson ÅA: Acute pancreatitis in man. A clinical and biochemical study of pathophysiology and treatment. Scand J Gastroenterol Suppl 99:1, 1984.

54. Lasson ÅA, Ohlsson K: Acute pancreatitis. The correlation between clinical course, protease inhibitors, and complement and kinin activation. Scand J Gastroenterol 19:707, 1984.

55. Lasson ÅA, Ohlsson K: Protease inhibitors in acute human pancreatitis. Correlation between biochemical changes and clinical course. Scand J Gastroenterol 19:779, 1984.

56. Largman C, Reidelberger RD, Tsukamoto H: Correlation of trypsin–plasma inhibitor complexes with mortality in experimental pancreatitis in rats. Dig Dis Sci 31:961, 1986.

57. Gudgeon AM, Heath DI, Hurley P, et al: Trypsinogen activation peptide assay in the early prediction of severity of acute pancreatitis. Lancet 335:4, 1990.

58. Schmidt J, Fernandez-Del Castillo C, Rattner DW, et al: Trypsinogen-activation peptides in experimental rat pancreatitis: Prognostic implications and histopathologic correlates. Gastroenterology 103:1009, 1992.

59. Borth W: Alpha$_2$-macroglobulin, a multifunctional binding protein with targeting characteristics. FASEB J 6:3345, 1992.

60. Weiss SJ: Tissue destruction by neutrophils. N Engl J Med 320:365, 1989.

61. Steer ML: Etiology and pathophysiology of acute pancreatitis. In Go VLW, DiMagno EP, Gardner JD, et al (eds): The Pancreas: Biology, Pathobiology and Disease, 2nd ed. New York, Raven Press, 1993, p 581.

62. Leach SD, Gorelick FS, Modlin IM: New perspectives on acute pancreatitis. Scand J Gastroenterol Suppl 192:29, 1992.

63. Akol KG, Washabau RJ, Saunders HM, et al: Acute pancreatitis in cats with hepatic lipidosis. J Vet Intern Med 7:205, 1993.

64. Guzman S, Nervi F, Llanos O, et al: Impaired lipid clearance in patients with previous acute pancreatitis. Gut 26:888, 1985.

65. Bell SM, Bennett C, Markham AF, et al: Evidence for a common mutation in hereditary pancreatitis. J Clin Pathol Mol Pathol 51:115, 1998.

66. Dasouki MJ, Cogan J, Summar ML, et al: Heterogeneity in hereditary pancreatitis. Am J Med Genet 77:47, 1998.

LIV

67. Frick TW, Speiser DE, Bimmler D, et al: Drug-induced acute pancreatitis: Further criticism. Dig Dis 11:113, 1993.

68. Morrison WB: Pancreatitis associated with cytotoxic drug administration. In Morrison WB (ed): Proceedings of the Tenth Annual Veterinary Medical Forum of the ACVIM, San Diego, 1992, p 632.

69. Hsiao CT, Yang CC, Deng JF, et al: Acute pancreatitis following organophosphate intoxication. Clin Toxicol 34:343, 1996.

70. Weizman Z, Sofer S: Acute pancreatitis in children with anticholinesterase insecticide intoxication. Pediatrics 90:204, 1992.

71. Geokas MC, Baltaxe HA, Banks PA, et al: Acute pancreatitis. Ann Intern Med 103:86, 1985.

72. Frick TW, Spycher MA, Heitz PU, et al: Hypercalcaemia and pancreatic ultrastructure in cats. Eur J Surg 158:289, 1992.

73. Von Beust B, Freudiger U, Pfister K: Opisthorchiasis bei einer Katze. Schweiz Arch Tierheilkd 126:207, 1984.

74. Freudiger U: Krankheiten des exokrinen Pankreas bei der Katze. Berl Munch Tierarztl Wochenschr 102:37, 1989.

75. Weiss DJ, Gagne JM, Armstrong PJ: Relationship between inflammatory hepatic disease and inflammatory bowel disease, pancreatitis, and nephritis in cats. JAVMA 209: 1114, 1996.

76. Westermarck E, Saario E: Traumatic pancreatic injury in a cat—A case history. Acta Vet Scand 30:359, 1989.

77. Rodriguez J, Kasberg C, Nipper M, et al: CT-guided needle biopsy of the pancreas: A retrospective analysis of diagnostic accuracy. Am J Gastroenterol 87:1610, 1993.

78. Lutz TA, Rand JS, Watt P, et al: Pancreatic biopsy in normal cats. Aust Vet J 71:223, 1994.

79. Sanfey H, Broe PJ, Cameron JL: Experimental ischemic pancreatitis: Treatment with albumin. Am J Surg 150:297, 1985.

80. Bockman DE: Microvasculature of the pancreas: Relation to pancreatitis. Int J Pancreatol 12:11, 1992.

81. Kyogoku T, Manabe T, Tobe T: Role of ischemia in acute pancreatitis: Hemorrhagic shock converts edematous pancreatitis to hemorrhagic pancreatitis in rats. Dig Dis Sci 37:1409, 1992.

82. Waldner H: Vascular mechanisms to induce acute pancreatitis. Eur Surg Res 24(Suppl 1):62, 1992.

83. Isaji S, Suzuki M, Frey CF, et al: Role of bacterial infection in diet-induced acute pancreatitis in mice. Int J Pancreatol 11:49, 1992.

84. Padilla B, Pollak VE, Pesce A, et al: Pancreatitis in patients with end-stage renal disease. Medicine (Baltimore) 73:8, 1994.

85. Ito T, Nakano I, Koyanagi S, et al: Autoimmune pancreatitis as a new clinical entity. Three cases of autoimmune pancreatitis with effective steroid therapy. Dig Dis Sci 42:1458, 1997.

86. Pidgeon G: Exocrine pancreatic disease in the dog and cat. Part 2: Exocrine pancreatic insufficiency. Canine Pract 14:31, 1987.

87. Kitchell BE, Strombeck DR, Cullen J, et al: Clinical and pathologic changes in experimentally induced acute pancreatitis in cats. Am J Vet Res 47:1170, 1986.

88. Murtaugh RJ, Herring DS, Jacobs RM, et al: Pancreatic ultrasonography in dogs with experimentally induced acute pancreatitis. Vet Radiol 26:27, 1985.

89. Edwards DF, Bauer MS, Walker MA, et al: Pancreatic masses in seven dogs following acute pancreatitis. J Am Anim Hosp Assoc 26:189, 1990.

90. Hines BL, Salisbury SK, Jakovljevic S, et al: Pancreatic pseudocyst associated with chronic-active necrotizing pancreatitis in a cat. J Am Anim Hosp Assoc 32:147, 1996.

91. Moulton JS: The radiologic assessment of acute pancreatitis and its complications. Pancreas 6(Suppl 1):S13, 1991.

92. Meyer P, Clavien PA, Robert J, et al: Role of imaging technics in the classification of acute pancreatitis. Dig Dis 10:330, 1992.

93. Gerhardt A, Kramer S, Fuchs C, et al: Pankreasdiagnostik bei der Katze. DVG Meeting, Munich, 1998, in press.

94. Jacobs RM, Murtaugh RJ, DeHoff WD: Review of the clinicopathological findings of acute pancreatitis in the dog: Use of an experimental model. J Am Anim Hosp Assoc 21:795, 1985.

95. Wells AD, Schenk WG: Effectiveness of normal saline solution, dextran 40 or dextran 75, and aprotinin (Trasylol) on renal blood flow preservation during acute canine pancreatitis. Am J Surg 148:624, 1984.

96. Fabris C, Basso D, Naccarato R: Urinary enzymes excretion in pancreatic diseases: Clinical role and pathophysiological considerations (editorial). J Clin Gastroenterol 14:281, 1992.

97. Andrzejewska A, Dlugosz J, Kurasz S: The ultrastructure of the liver in acute experimental pancreatitis in rats. Exp Pathol 28:167, 1985.

98. Hirano T, Manabe T, Tobe T: Impaired hepatic energy metabolism in rat acute pancreatitis: Protective effects of prostaglandin E_2 and synthetic protease inhibitor ONO 3307. J Surg Res 53:238, 1992.

99. Garvey MS, Zawie DA: Feline pancreatic disease. Vet Clin North Am Small Anim Pract 14:1231, 1984.

100. Whitney MS, Boon GD, Rebar AH, et al: Effects of acute pancreatitis on circulating lipids in dogs. Am J Vet Res 48:1492, 1987.

101. Simpson KW, Batt RM, McLean L, et al: Circulating concentrations of trypsin-like immunoreactivity and activities of lipase and amylase after pancreatic duct ligation in dogs. Am J Vet Res 50:629, 1989.

102. Murayama KM, Drew JB, Nahrwold DL, et al: Acute edematous pancreatitis impairs pancreatic secretion in rats. Surgery 107:302, 1990.

103. Niederau C, Niederau M, Lüthen R, et al: Pancreatic exocrine secretion in acute experimental pancreatitis. Gastroenterology 99:1120, 1990.

104. Simpson KW, Simpson JW, Lake S, et al: Effect of pancreatectomy on plasma activities of amylase, isoamylase, lipase and trypsin-like immunoreactivity in dogs. Res Vet Sci 51:78, 1991.

105. Murtaugh RJ, Jacobs RM: Serum amylase and isoamylases and their origins in healthy dogs and dogs with experimentally induced acute pancreatitis. Am J Vet Res 46:742, 1985.

106. George JW: Methemalbumin: Reality and myth. Vet Clin Pathol 17:43, 1988.

107. Parent C, Washabau RJ, Williams DA, et al: Serum trypsin-like immunoreactivity, amylase and lipase in the diagnosis of feline acute pancreatitis (abstract). J Vet Intern Med 9:194, 1995.

108. Medinger TL, Burchfield T, Williams DA: Assay of trypsin-like immunoreactivity (TLI) in feline serum (abstract). J Vet Intern Med 7:133, 1993.

109. Bruner JM, Steiner JM, Williams DA, et al.: High feline trypsin-like immunoreactivity in a cat with pancreatitis and hepatic lipidosis. JAVMA 210:1757, 1997.

110. Gerhardt A, Kramer S, Fuchs C, et al: Diagnostic procedures for feline pancreatitis (abstract). British Small Animal Congress, 1999.

111. Williams DA, Moore M: Characterization of serum trypsin-like immunoassay (TLI) in dogs with naturally occurring fatal acute pancreatitis (AP) and severe chronic renal failure (CRF) (abstract). Proceedings 6th Annual Veterinary Medicine Forum, ACVIM, 1988, p 739.

112. Fernández-del Castillo C, Schmidt J, Rattner DW, et al: Generation and possible significance of trypsinogen activation peptides in experimental acute pancreatitis in the rat. Pancreas 7:263, 1992.

113. Karanjia ND, Widdison AL, Jehanli A, et al: Assay of trypsinogen activation in the cat experimental model of acute pancreatitis. Pancreas 8:189, 1993.

114. Lankisch PG: Acute and chronic pancreatitis: An update on management. Drugs 28:554, 1984.

115. Drazner FH: Diseases of the pancreas. In Jones BD, Liska WD (eds): Canine and Feline Gastroenterology. Philadelphia, WB Saunders, 1986, p 295.

116. Banks PA: Medical management of acute pancreatitis and complications. In Go VLW, DiMagno EP, Gardner JD, et al (eds): The Pancreas: Biology, Pathobiology and Disease, 2nd ed. New York, Raven Press, 1993, p 593.

117. Freeman LM, Labato MA, Rush JE, et al: Nutritional support in pancreatitis: A retrospective study. J Vet Emerg Crit Care 5:32, 1995.

118. Kalfarentzos F, Kehagias J, Mead N, et al: Enteral nutrition is superior to parenteral nutrition in severe acute pancreatitis: Results of a randomized prospective trial. Br J Surg 84:1665, 1997.

119. Sainio V, Kemppainen E, Puolakkainen P, et al: Early antibiotic treatment in acute necrotising pancreatitis. Lancet 346:663, 1995.

120. Bradley EL: Antibiotics in acute pancreatitis. Current status and future directions. Am J Surg 158:472, 1989.

121. Hansen B: Analgesics in cardiac, surgical, and intensive care patients. In Kirk RW, Bonagura JD (eds): Current Veterinary Therapy XI. Philadelphia, WB Saunders, 1992, p 82.

122. Murtaugh RJ, Jacobs RM: Serum antiprotease concentrations in dogs with spontaneous and experimentally induced acute pancreatitis. Am J Vet Res 46:80, 1985.

123. McMahon MJ, Bowen M, Mayer AD, et al: Relation of α_2 macroglobulin and other antiproteases to the clinical features of acute pancreatitis. Am J Surg 147:164, 1984.

124. Wendt P, Fritsh A, Schulz F, et al: Proteinases and inhibitors in plasma and peritoneal exudate in acute pancreatitis. Hepatogastroenterology 31:277, 1984.

125. Kimura T, Ito T, Sumii T, et al: Serum protease inhibitor capacity for elastase and the severity of pancreatitis. Pancreas 7:680, 1992.

126. Kimura W, Meyer F, Hess D, et al: Comparison of different treatment modalities in experimental pancreatitis in rats. Gastroenterology 103:1916, 1992.

127. Schmidt J, Fernandez-Del Castillo C, Rattner DW, et al: Hyperoncotic ultrahigh molecular weight dextran solutions reduce trypsinogen activation, prevent acinar necrosis, and lower mortality in rodent pancreatitis. Am J Surg 165:40, 1993.

128. Van Ooijen B, Tinga CJ, Kort WJ, et al: Effects of long-acting somatostatin analog (SMS 201-995) on eicosanoid synthesis and survival in rats with acute necrotizing pancreatitis. Dig Dis Sci 37:1434, 1992.

129. Gjorup I, Roikjær O, Andersen B, et al: A double-blinded multicenter trial of somatostatin in the treatment of acute pancreatitis. Surg Gynecol Obstet 175:397, 1992.

130. Balldin G, Lasson ÅA, Ohlsson K: Aprotinin turn-over studies in dog and in man with severe acute pancreatitis. Hoppe Seyler's Z Physiol Chem 365:1417, 1984.

131. Hermon-Taylor J, Heywood GD: A rational approach to the specific chemotherapy of pancreatitis. Scand J Gastroenterol 117:39, 1985.

132. Salisbury SK, Lantz GC, Nelson RW, et al: Pancreatic abscess in dogs: Six cases (1978–1986). JAVMA 193:1104, 1988.

133. Matthiesen DT, Rosin E: Common bile duct obstruction secondary to chronic fibrosing pancreatitis in the dog: Treatment by use of cholecystoduodenostomy in the dog. JAVMA 189:1443, 1986.

134. Pidgeon G: Exocrine pancreatic disease in the dog and cat. Part 1: Acute pancreatitis. Companion Anim Pract March:67, 1987.

135. Slaff J, Jacobson D, Tillman CR, et al: Protease-specific suppression of pancreatic exocrine secretion. Gastroenterology 87:44, 1984.

136. Shiratori K, Jo YH, Lee KY, et al: Effect of pancreatic juice and trypsin on oleic acid–stimulated pancreatic secretion and plasma secretin in dogs. Gastroenterology 96:1330, 1989.

137. Bright JM: Pancreatic adenocarcinoma in a dog with maldigestion syndrome. JAVMA 187:420, 1985.

138. Lerner A, Lebenthal E: Hereditary diseases of the pancreas. In Go VLW,

DiMagno EP, Gardner JD, et al (eds): The Pancreas: Biology, Pathobiology and Disease, 2nd ed. New York, Raven Press, 1993, p 1083.

139. Carrière F, Raphel V, Moreau H, et al: Dog gastric lipase: Stimulation of its secretion in vivo and cytolocalization in mucous pit cells. Gastroenterology 102:1535, 1992.

140. Westermarck E, Batt RM, Vaillant C, et al: Sequential study of pancreatic structure and function during development of pancreatic acinar atrophy in a German shepherd dog. Am J Vet Res 54:1088, 1993.

141. Perry LA, Williams DA, Pidgeon G, et al: Exocrine pancreatic insufficiency with associated coagulopathy in a cat. J Am Anim Hosp Assoc 27:109, 1991.

142. Lerner A, Heitlinger LA, Lebenthal E: Hereditary abnormalities of pancreatic function. In Go VLW et al (eds): The Exocrine Pancreas: Biology, Pathobiology and Diseases. New York, Raven Press, 1986, p 819.

143. Boari A, Williams DA, Famigli-Bergamini P: Observations on exocrine pancreatic insufficiency in a family of English setter dogs. J Small Anim Pract 35:247, 1994.

144. Westermarck E, Rimaila-Pärnänen E: Two unusual cases of canine exocrine pancreatic insufficiency. J Small Anim Pract 30:32, 1989.

145. Washabau RJ, Strombeck DR, Buffington CA, et al: Use of pulmonary hydrogen gas execretion to detect carbohydrate malabsorption in dogs. JAVMA 189:674, 1986.

146. Simpson KW, Morton DB, Sorensen SH, et al: Biochemical changes in the jejunal mucosa of dogs with exocrine pancreatic insufficiency following pancreatic duct ligation. Res Vet Sci 47:338, 1989.

147. Williams DA, Batt RM, McLean L: Reversible impairment of protein synthesis may contribute to jejunal abnormalities in exocrine pancreatic insufficiency. Clin Sci 68:37P, 1985.

148. Williams DA: Studies on the diagnosis and pathophysiology of canine exocrine pancreatic insufficiency. PhD thesis, University of Liverpool, Liverpool, England, 1985.

149. Simpson KW, Batt RM, Jones D, et al: Effects of exocrine pancreatic insufficiency and replacement therapy on the bacterial flora of the duodenum in dogs. Am J Vet Res 51: 203, 1990.

150. Westermarck E, Myllys V, Aho M: Effect of treatment on the jejunal and colonic bacterial flora of dogs with exocrine pancreatic insufficiency. Pancreas 8:559, 1993.

151. Williams DA, Batt RM, McLean L: Duodenal bacterial overgrowth may occur in canine exocrine pancreatic insufficiency but is not due to achlorhydria. Scientific Proceedings, American College of Veterinary Internal Medicine, Washington, DC, 1984, p 34.

152. Sherman P, Wesley A, Forstner G: Sequential disaccharidase loss in rat intestinal blind loops: Impact of malnutrition. Am J Physiol 248:G626, 1985.

153. Batt RM, McLean L: Comparison of the biochemical changes in the jejunal mucosa of dogs with aerobic and anaerobic bacterial overgrowth. Gastroenterology 93:986, 1987.

154. Orci L: Patterns of cellular and subcellular organization in the endocrine pancreas. J Endocrinol 102:3, 1984.

155. Vaillant C, Giraud A, Williams DA: Pancreatic enkephalin immunoreactivity in canine pancreatic acinar atropy. Dig Dis Sci 29:92S, 1984.

156. Williams DA, Batt RM: Reversible intravenous glucose intolerance in canine exocrine pancreatic insufficiency. Proceedings 4th Annual Forum ACVIM, Washington, DC, 1986, p 14.

157. Schwille PO, Engelhardt W, Gumbert E, et al: Long-term pancreatic duct occlusion impairs the entero-insular axis in the dog—Failure of plasma VIP to respond as "incretin." Peptides 4:445, 1984.

158. Creutzfeldt W, Ebert R: The enteroinsular axis. In Go VLW, DiMagno EP, Gardner JD, et al (eds): The Pancreas: Biology, Pathobiology and Disease, 2nd ed. New York, Raven Press, 1993, p 769.

159. Dowd PS, Heatley RV: The influence of undernutrition on immunity. Clin Sci 66:241, 1984.

160. Salazar de Sousa J: Malnutrition and small intestinal mucosa. J Pediatr Gastroenterol Nutr 3:321, 1984.

161. Sherman P, Forstner J, Roomi N, et al: Mucin depletion in the intestine of malnourished rats. Am J Physiol 248:G418, 1985.

162. Simpson KW, Morton DB, Batt RM: Effect of exocrine pancreatic insufficiency on cobalamin absorption in dogs. Am J Vet Res 50:1233, 1989.

163. Hall EJ, Bond PM, McLean C, et al: A survey of the diagnosis and treatment of canine exocrine pancreatic insufficiency. J Small Anim Pract 32:613, 1991.

164. Fyfe JC: Feline intrinsic factor (IF) is pancreatic in origin and mediates ileal cobalamin (CBL) absorption. J Vet Intern Med 7:133, 1993.

165. Williams DA: Exocrine pancreatic insufficiency. Waltham Int Focus 2:9, 1993.

166. Williams DA: The pancreas: Exocrine pancreatic insufficiency. In Anderson NV (ed): Veterinary Gastroenterology, 2nd ed. Philadelphia, Lea & Febiger, 1992, p 283.

167. Fyfe JC, Jezyk PF, Giger U, et al: Inherited selective malabsorption of vitamin B$_{12}$ in giant schnauzers. J Am Anim Hosp Assoc 50:533, 1989.

168. Raiha M, Westermarck E: The signs of pancreatic degenerative atrophy in dogs and the role of external factors in the etiology of the disease. Acta Vet Scand 30:447, 1989.

169. Dill-Macky E: Pancreatic diseases of cats. Compend Contin Educ Pract Vet 15:589, 1993.

170. Williams DA, Minnich F: Canine exocrine pancreatic insufficiency—A survey of 640 cases diagnosed by assay of serum trypsin-like immunoreactivity. J Vet Intern Med 4:123, 1990.

171. Westermarck E, Lindberg LA, Sandholm M: Quantitation of serum phospholipase A$_2$ by enzyme diffusion in lecithin agar gels. A comparative study in man and animals. Acta Vet Scand 25:229, 1986.

172. Williams DA, Batt RM: Sensitivity and specificity of radioimmunoassay of serum trypsin-like immunoreactivity for the diagnosis of canine exocrine pancreatic insufficiency. JAVMA 192:195, 1988.

173. Williams DA, Batt RM: Exocrine pancreatic insufficiency diagnosed by radioimmunoassay of serum trypsin-like immunoreactivity in a dog with a normal BT-PABA test result. J Am Anim Hosp Assoc 22:671, 1986.

174. Steiner JM, Williams DA: Validation of a radioimmunoassay for feline trypsin-like immunoreactivity (FTLI) and serum cobalamin and folate concentrations in cats with exocrine pancreatic insufficiency (EPI). J Vet Intern Med 9:193, 1995.

175. Steiner JM, Williams DA: Feline trypsin-like immunoreactivity in feline exocrine pancreatic disease. Compend Contin Educ Pract Vet 18:543, 1996.

176. Steiner JM, Medinger TL, Williams DA: Development and validation of a radioimmunoassay for feline trypsin-like immunoreactivity. Am J Vet Res 57:1417, 1996.

177. Williams DA, Reed SD: Comparison of methods for assay of fecal proteolytic activity. Vet Clin Pathol 19:20, 1990.

178. Williams DA, Reed SD, Perry LA: Fecal proteolytic activity in clinically normal cats and in a cat with exocrine pancreatic insufficiency. JAVMA 197:210, 1990.

179. Zimmer JF, Todd SE: Further evaluation of bentiromide in the diagnosis of canine exocrine pancreatic insufficiency. Cornell Vet 75:426, 1985.

180. Hawkins EC, Meric SM, Washabau RJ, et al: Digestion of bentiromide and absorption of xylose in healthy cats and absorption of xylose in cats with infiltrative intestinal disease. Am J Vet Res 47:567, 1986.

181. Morrow JD: Topics in clinical pharmacology: Pancreatic enzyme replacement therapy. Am J Med Sci 298:357, 1989.

182. Roberts IM: Enzyme therapy for malabsorption in exocrine pancreatic insufficiency. Pancreas 4:496, 1989.

183. Marvola M, Heinamaki J, Westermarck E, et al: The fate of single-unit enteric-coated drug products in the stomach of the dog. Acta Pharm Fenn 95:59, 1986.

184. DiMagno EP, Layer P, Clain JE: Chronic pancreatitis. In Go VLW, DiMagno EP, Gardner JD, et al (eds): The Pancreas: Biology, Pathobiology and Disease, 2nd ed. New York, Raven Press, 1993, p 665.

185. Balasubramanian K, Zentler-Munro PL, Batten JC, et al: Increased intragastric acid-resistant lipase activity and lipolysis in pancreatic steatorrhoea due to cystic fibrosis. Pancreas 7:305, 1992.

186. Carrière F, Moreau H, Raphel V, et al: Purification and biochemical characterization of dog gastric lipase. Eur J Biochem 202:75, 1991.

187. Griffin SM, Alderson D, Farndon JR: Acid-resistant lipase as replacement therapy in chronic pancreatic exocrine insufficiency: A study in dogs. Gut 30:1012, 1989.

188. Pidgeon G: Exocrine pancreatic disease in the dog and cat. Companion Anim Pract 1:67, 1987.

189. Westermarck E, Junttila J, Wiberg M: The role of low dietary fat in the treatment of dogs with exocrine pancreatic insufficiency. Am J Vet Res 56:600, 1995.

190. Lewis LD, Morris ML, Hand MS: Small Animal Clinical Nutrition. Topeka, KS, Mark Morris Associates, 1987.

191. Westermarck E, Wiberg M, Junttila J: Role of feeding in the treatment of dogs with pancreatic degenerative atrophy. Acta Vet Scand 31:325, 1990.

192. Dutta SK, Hlasko J: Dietary fiber in pancreatic disease: Effect of high fiber diet on fat malabsorption in pancreatic insufficiency and in vitro study of the interaction of dietary fibers with pancreatic enzymes. Am J Clin Nutr 41:517, 1985.

193. Wiberg ME, Lautala HM, Westermarck E: Response to long-term enzyme replacement treatment in dogs with exocrine pancreatic insufficiency. JAVMA 213:86, 1998.

194. Westermarck E, Rimaila-Pärnänen E: Mesenteric torsion in dogs with exocrine pancreatic insufficiency: 21 cases (1978–1987). JAVMA 195:1404, 1989.

195. Withrow SJ: Tumors of the gastrointestinal system: Exocrine pancreas. In Withrow SJ, MacEwen EG (eds): Clinical Veterinary Oncology, 1st ed. Philadelphia, JB Lippincott, 1989, p 192.

196. Steiner JM, Williams DA: Feline exocrine pancreatic disorders: Insufficiency, neoplasia, and uncommon conditions. Compendium 19:836, 1997.

197. Anderson WI, Georgi ME, Car BD: Pancreatic atrophy and fibrosis associated with Eurytrema procyonis in a domestic cat. Vet Rec 120:235, 1987.

LIV

SECTION XII

THE ENDOCRINE SYSTEM

CHAPTER 147

ACROMEGALY

Ad Rijnberk

Acromegaly is an insidious disease caused by excess secretion of growth hormone (GH), which leads to bony and soft tissue overgrowth. The condition is known to occur in middle-aged female dogs and middle-aged and elderly, predominantly male, cats.

GROWTH HORMONE

GH is a single-chain polypeptide. It contains two intrachain disulfide bridges and has a molecular weight of approximately 22,000 daltons. The amino acid sequence of canine GH has been elucidated and is identical to that of porcine GH.[1]

The release of GH is characterized by rhythmic pulses and intervening troughs. The GH pulses predominantly reflect the pulsatile delivery of GH-releasing hormone (GHRH) from the hypothalamus, whereas GH levels between pulses are primarily under somatostatin (= somatotropin-release inhibiting factor [SRIF]) control. The effects of GH can be divided into two main categories: (1) rapid or metabolic actions and (2) slow or hypertrophic actions. The acute catabolic responses are due to direct interaction of GH with the target cell and result in enhanced lipolysis and restricted glucose transport across the cell membrane due to insulin resistance. The slow anabolic effects are mediated by means of a growth factor that is synthesized in the liver and is known as insulin-like growth factor (IGF-I). In its chemical structure IGF-I (as well as IGF-II) has approximately 50 per cent sequence similarity with insulin, suggesting it and insulin have evolved from a common ancestral molecule. Contrary to insulin, the IGFs are bound to carrier proteins in plasma. As a result, they have a prolonged half-life, which is consistent with their long-term growth-promoting action. Insulin and IGF seem to complement each other, with insulin being the acute and IGF the long-term regulator of anabolic processes.

Circulating IGF-I is an important determinant in the regulation of body size. In dog breeds of widely differing body sizes, similar GH concentrations are usually found in plasma, but the total IGF-I levels are quite different and positively correlated with body size.[2] In addition, IGFs exert an inhibitory effect on GH release, most probably by stimulating the release of somatostatin and by a direct inhibitory influence at the pituitary level (Fig. 147–1).

However, evidence is increasing that the separation of the two opposing biologic actions is not as strict as suggested earlier. GH exerts its growth-promoting effect not only by means of IGF-I produced in the liver but also by a direct effect on cells in the growth plate. Here it stimulates cell differentiation directly and clonal expansion indirectly through the local production of IGF-I. This fits in with the recent observation suggesting that not circulating IGF-I but rather GH may be the major determinant of body size. It appears that young dogs of large breeds go through a period of GH excess.[3]

MAMMARY GROWTH HORMONE

In the 1970s and 1980s it was observed that administration of progestins to dogs could lead to physical changes reminiscent of acromegaly and increases in plasma concentrations of GH. Similar changes may occasionally be seen in middle-aged and elderly dogs during the natural rise in progesterone production in metestrus. These changes recede with the decline in the progesterone concentration, which is most pronounced after ovariohysterectomy.

In the search for the mechanism underlying this progestin-induced GH excess, it was found that supra-pituitary stimulants caused only minimal or no response. Administration of an analogue of somatostatin had no effect on the progestin-induced increases of GH concentration in plasma. It was concluded that the progestin-induced GH excess in dogs has characteristics of autonomous secretion.

This autonomy could not be attributed to neoplastic transformation because no pituitary tumors have been found in affected dogs. Moreover, the reversibility of the excess of GH on cessation of the progestin exposure was not consistent with the possibility of autonomous production of GH by a tumor, either ectopic or eutopic. The hypothesis that the progestin-induced GH excess could originate from a non-

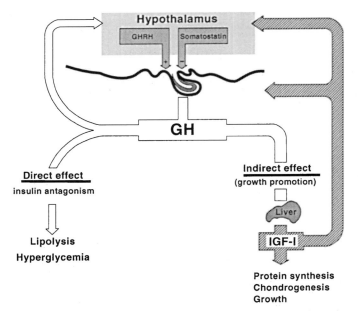

Figure 147–1. The secretion of GH is under inhibitory (somatostatin) and stimulatory (GHRH) hypothalamic control and is also modulated by a long-loop feedback control by IGF-I, a peptide formed in the liver under the influence of GH. The direct catabolic (diabetogenic) actions of GH are shown on the left side of the figure, and the indirect anabolic actions are shown on the right. (Redrawn from Rijnberk A [ed]: Clinical Endocrinology of Dogs and Cats. Dordrecht/Boston, Kluwer Academic Publishers, 1996.)

neoplastic extrapituitary site was then tested. The pituitary was excluded as a source of the GH excess when hypophysectomy was found not to influence the plasma concentration of GH.

Analysis of the GH content of various tissue homogenates revealed that the highest GH immunoreactivity was in extracts of the mammary gland. Progestin-induced GH excess was found to originate from foci of hyperplastic ductular epithelium of the mammary gland. By sequence analysis of the product obtained by reverse transcriptase-polymerase chain reaction (rT-PCR) it was demonstrated that the GH gene expressed in the mammary gland is identical to the gene in the pituitary gland.[4]

It is likely that the locally produced GH and the associated production of IGF and IGF-binding proteins participate in the cyclic development of the mammary gland. It may also promote mammary tumorigenesis by stimulating proliferation of susceptible, and sometimes transformed, mammary epithelial cells.[5, 6]

PATHOGENESIS

The pathogenesis of the GH excess is completely different in the dog and the cat. In female dogs either endogenous progesterone (metestrus) or exogenous progestagens (used in estrus prevention) may give rise to hypersecretion of mammary GH that results in acromegaly and glucose intolerance. In the cat, acromegaly is caused by primary pituitary tumors that secrete excessive amounts of GH.[7] Progestagens do not increase circulating GH levels in the cat as they do in the dog,[8] although it has been demonstrated that in cats with progestin-induced fibroadenomatous changes of the mammary gland the GH mRNA is also present in these tissues.[9] Apparently, unlike in dogs, this mammary GH does not seem to reach the systemic circulation. As a closing remark on the pathogenesis of acromegaly in dogs and cats it should be mentioned that the separation of the pathogeneses in dogs and cats may not be as strict as just indicated. A GH-producing adenoma has been reported in a dog.[10]

CLINICAL MANIFESTATIONS

Signs and symptoms of GH hypersecretion tend to develop slowly and are characterized initially in both the dog and the cat by soft tissue swelling of the face and the abdomen. These changes are readily appreciated when, fortunately, photographs taken 1 to 2 years apart can be compared (Fig. 147–2).

The soft tissue changes may be the reason for presentation, but more often they are so gradual that they do not impress the owners sufficiently to be mentioned spontaneously. Yet when asked, the owners may reply that the facial features and body dimensions have indeed increased. As the owner of a female golden retriever answered, "She almost looks like a male now."

In some dogs, severe hypertrophy of soft tissues of the mouth, tongue, and pharynx causes snoring and even inspiratory dyspnea. Those dogs in which the condition has developed during the luteal phase of the estrous cycle are usually presented with polyuria (and sometimes polyphagia) as the leading symptom. The polyuria is usually without glucosuria, but manifest diabetes mellitus can develop after repeated exposure to GH excess during metestrus.

In cats, the reason for suspicion of GH excess is almost

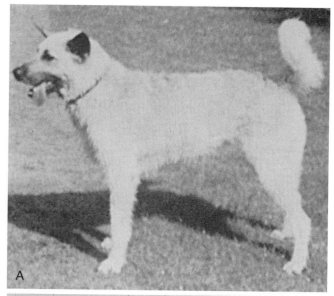
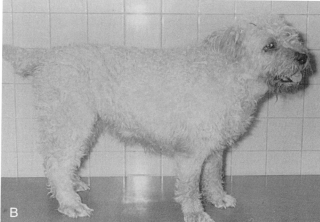

Figure 147–2. *A*, A female mongrel Belgian shepherd at the age of 3 years, photographed in the owner's garden. *B*, The same dog when presented 2 years later for examination because of decreased endurance, intolerance to warmth (frequent panting, preference for cool places), exaggerated growth of the coat, increase in abdominal size, and inspiratory stridor. The high GH concentrations in plasma ($\geq$45 μg/L) had been induced by thrice-yearly injections of medroxyprogesterone acetate for prevention of estrus. (From Rijnberk A [ed]: Clinical Endocrinology of Dogs and Cats. Dordrecht/Boston, Kluwer Academic Publishers, 1996.)

exclusively insulin-resistant diabetes mellitus. Cats with acromegaly that have been described thus far have had diabetes mellitus that could only be controlled with doses of insulin in excess of 30 U/d. Affected cats may also have dyspnea due to congestive heart failure.[7]

Physical examination in dogs reveals variable degrees of soft tissue and bony changes, including a heavy head and thick folds of skin, especially in the neck, and prognathism and wide interdental spaces (Fig. 147–3). Prolonged GH excess also leads to generalized visceromegaly involving the tongue, salivary glands, and abdominal organs. The latter causes abdominal enlargement. The increase in soft tissue mass in the pharyngeal and laryngeal area may give rise to stridor and even dyspnea.

The physical changes in cats tend to be less pronounced than in dogs. The head may also become somewhat massive and may have rather pronounced features, probably due in

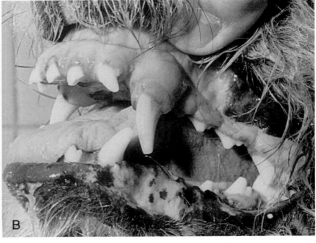

Figure 147–3. Same dog shown in Figure 147–2, after its coat had been clipped. *A*, The head, trunk, and limbs have a coarse and heavy appearance and the skin on the neck is thrown into folds. *B*, Note prognathism, wide spacing of the teeth, and a relatively large tongue. (From Rijnberk A [ed]: Clinical Endocrinology of Dogs and Cats. Dordrecht/Boston, Kluwer Academic Publishers, 1996.)

part to overgrowth of the bony structures bounding the paranasal sinuses (Fig. 147–4).

Routine laboratory investigations will often reveal hyperglycemia, especially in cats. In dogs, plasma levels of alkaline phosphatase may also be increased. This may be due in part to the glucocorticoid activity that is intrinsic to progestagens.[11, 12]

Radiographic examination of dogs will not enlarge on the physically observed signs of overgrowth of bone and soft tissue. In cats, the disease may be complicated by degenerative arthritis with periarticular periosteal reaction, which may require radiographic examination.[7]

DIFFERENTIAL DIAGNOSIS

In pronounced cases, the clinical features, including the specific medical history in both dogs and cats, are not easily confused with those of other diseases. However, in some dogs the metabolic changes lead to polyuria, polyphagia, and hyperglycemia. Together with the increase in abdominal size, the changes may mimic the signs of hyperadrenocorticism. The redundant folds of skin on the head may suggest the possibility of hypothyroidism, although there is usually no pronounced lethargy in acromegaly.

DIAGNOSIS

The diagnosis of GH excess can generally be established by measuring basal GH concentrations in plasma. Feline GH can also be measured in a homologous radioimmunoassay developed for the dog. The basal values in this condition often exceed the upper limit of the reference range (6 μg/L), and so a single measurement might be diagnostic. How-

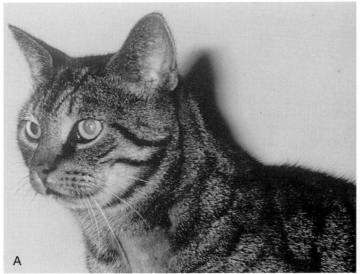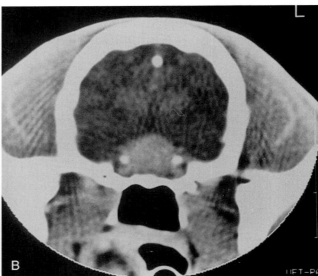

Figure 147–4. *A*, A 10-year-old castrated male cat with diabetes mellitus and acromegaly. This is a sturdy cat with possibly somewhat coarse facial features, although according to the owner its appearance had not changed. *B*, Contrast medium–enhanced CT scan through the pituitary fossa in this cat revealed a large pituitary tumor. (From Rijnberk A [ed]: Clinical Endocrinology of Dogs and Cats. Dordrecht/Boston, Kluwer Academic Publishers, 1996.)

ever, if the disease is mild or is just beginning, basal GH concentrations may be only slightly elevated. Conversely, a high value may be the result of a secretory pulse in a normal subject. There are also disease conditions associated with anorexia and malaise in which GH secretion may be increased. Especially in dogs, three to five repeated measurements at 10-minute intervals may be helpful, because plasma GH concentration does not fluctuate in acromegalic dogs as it does in healthy dogs. Non-responsiveness of normal or elevated GH levels to stimulation may also support the diagnosis in dogs; intravenous administration of 1 μg of GHRH per kilogram of body weight or 10 μg of clonidine normally causes the plasma GH concentration to rise to 10 ± 5 and 19 ± 6 μg/L, respectively (mean ± SEM).[1]

The measurement of IGF-I may also contribute to the diagnosis. As mentioned earlier, the IGF-I concentration in plasma is GH dependent. Being bound to transport proteins, it is much less subject to fluctuation than is GH. IGF concentrations are commonly higher in acromegalic dogs than in healthy control dogs of similar body size, but there is more overlap than for GH.

In cats, the excessive GH is secreted by a pituitary tumor. Thus, when GH hypersecretion has been demonstrated in a cat, the pituitary should be visualized by computed tomography, if possible. Documentation of the size and expansion of the pituitary tumor is of value for the prognosis and also for monitoring the response to treatment.

TREATMENT

Canine acromegaly can be treated easily and effectively by withdrawal of exogenous progestagens and/or ovariectomy/ovariohysterectomy. The animal may then change dramatically, owing to the reversal of the soft tissue changes. The size of the abdomen decreases, as does the thickening of soft tissues in the oropharyngeal region and hence the associated snoring. The bony changes, primarily prognathism and enlarged interdental spaces, appear to be irreversible but do not seem to cause problems to the animal. In cases in which the GH excess did not lead to complete exhaustion of the pancreatic beta cells, the elimination of the progesterone source by the ovariohysterectomy may prevent persistent diabetes mellitus (Fig. 147–5).

Serious problems can arise in dogs in which the progestagen causing the acromegaly has been administered only recently. Its action may persist for several months, and there is no alternative but to wait for the cessation of its effect. An alternative would be especially helpful in these cases, but thus far only the use of a synthetic anti-progestagen (RU 486) has proved to be effective.[13] There is as yet no experience with long-term administration of this drug; and, because it is a glucocorticoid antagonist as well, it should be used with caution. In the end, one may even decide for total mammectomy.

In cats, treatment should be directed at the pituitary tumor, and in principle there are three possibilities: hypophysectomy, irradiation, and medication. There is little experience with any of the three. From the limited number of reported cases one may conclude that medical treatments with drugs such as the dopamine agonist bromocriptine are not very effective in the cat. A long-acting somatostatin analogue* can lower circulating GH levels,[14] but it is questionable whether this will become applicable in clinical practice be-

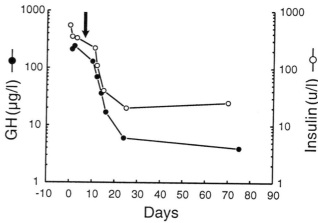

Figure 147–5. Plasma GH and insulin concentrations (log scales!) in an 8-year-old female beagle immediately before and after ovariohysterectomy (arrow). The dog was in the luteal phase of the sexual cycle and had developed persistent hyperglycemia. After elimination of the insulin resistance, that is, the progestin-induced GH excess, both the hyperinsulinemia and the hyperglycemia disappeared. (Redrawn from Rijnberk A [ed]: Clinical Endocrinology of Dogs and Cats. Dordrecht/Boston, Kluwer Academic Publishers, 1996.)

cause it has to be injected several times a day and is very expensive. Recently, a long-lasting somatostatin analogue* has been introduced for use in humans that only needs to be injected once per month. Nevertheless, at present, in humans, medical treatment of acromegaly is not an alternative to surgery. There are no reports on the use of this newer drug in cats. Cobalt irradiation has resulted in temporary improvement in one cat;[7] and in a recent abstract on five cats with diabetes mellitus and well-documented acromegaly it was reported that insulin therapy could be discontinued permanently in two cats and transiently in three cats.[15] Plasma GH concentrations decreased in three cats and IGF-I in one cat after pituitary irradiation. Hypophysectomy may become an option for the smaller pituitary tumors, but so far there are no reports to support this approach.

END

PROGNOSIS

In dogs with progestagen-induced GH excess the prognosis is good after elimination of the progestagen source. Diabetes mellitus resulting from the GH excess is sometimes reversible after reversal of the GH excess. Persistence of the GH excess is accompanied by insulin resistance, which can be quite severe.

In cats, the short-term prognosis may be relatively good without treatment of the GH excess. The insulin-resistant diabetes mellitus can generally be managed satisfactorily, although it requires large daily doses of insulin, at considerable expense. Complications such as congestive heart failure or an expanding pituitary tumor usually result in death or euthanasia within 1 to 2 years. The results of irradiation seem promising. Hypophysectomy in cats still needs to be developed.

REFERENCES

1. Mol JA, Rijnberk A: Pituitary function. *In* Kaneko JJ, Harvey JW, Bruss ML (eds): Clinical Biochemistry of Domestic Animals. San Diego, Academic Press, 1997, p 517.

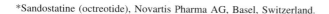

*Sandostatine (octreotide), Novartis Pharma AG, Basel, Switzerland.

*Sandostatin LAR, Novartis Pharma AG, Basel, Switzerland.

2. Eigenmann JE: Insulin-like growth factor I in the dog. Front Horm Res 17:161, 1987.

3. Nap RC, et al: Age-related plasma concentrations of growth hormone (GH) and insulin-like growth factor I (IGF-I) in great Dane pups fed different dietary levels of protein. Domest Anim Endocrinol 10:237, 1993.

4. Rijnberk A, Mol JA: Progestin-induced hypersecretion of growth hormone: An introductory review. J Reprod Fertil Suppl 51:335, 1997.

5. Mol JA, et al: The role of progestins, insulin-like growth factor (IGF) and IGF-binding proteins in the normal and neoplastic mammary gland of the bitch: A review. J Reprod Fertil Suppl 51:339, 1997.

6. Van Garderen E, et al: Expression of growth hormone in canine mammary tissue and mammary tumors: Evidence for a potential autocrine/paracrine stimulatory loop. Am J Pathol 150:1037, 1997.

7. Peterson ME, Randolph JF: Endocrine diseases. In Sherding RG (ed): The Cat: Diseases and Clinical Management. New York, Churchill Livingstone, 1989, p 1095.

8. Peterson ME: Effects of megestrol acetate on glucose tolerance and growth hormone secretion in the cat. Res Vet Sci 42:354, 1987.

9. Mol JA, et al: Growth hormone mRNA in mammary gland tumors of dogs and cats. J Clin Invest 95:2028, 1995.

10. Van Keulen LJM, et al: Diabetes mellitus in a dog with a growth hormone–producing acidophilic adenoma of the adenohypophysis. Vet Pathol 33:451, 1996.

11. Selman PJ, et al: Progestin treatment in the dog: II. Effects on the hypothalamic-pituitary-adrenocortical axis. Eur J Endocrinol 131:422, 1994.

12. Selman PJ, et al: Binding specificity of medroxyprogesterone acetate and proligestone for the progesterone and glucocorticoid receptor in the dog. Steroids 61:133, 1996.

13. Watson ADJ, et al: Effect of somatostatin analogue SMS 201-995 and antiprogestin agent RU 486 in canine acromegaly. Front Horm Res 17:193, 1987.

14. Rijnberk A: Hypothalamus-pituitary system. In Rijnberk A (ed): Clinical Endocrinology of Dogs and Cats. Dordrecht/Boston, Kluwer Academic Publishers, 1996, p 11.

15. Goossens M, et al: Pituitary tumor telecobalt irradiation in five cats with acromegaly. Abstract 75, 15th Annual ACVIM Forum. J Vet Intern Med 11:122, 1997.

CHAPTER 148

DIABETES INSIPIDUS

Ad Rijnberk

Diabetes insipidus refers to the passage of large quantities of dilute urine and is actually synonymous with polyuria. In central diabetes insipidus the polyuria results from a lack of sufficient vasopressin to concentrate urine. The disease is characterized by three primary findings: (1) dilute urine despite strong osmotic stimuli for vasopressin secretion, (2) absence of renal disease, and (3) a rise in urine osmolality after the administration of vasopressin.

VASOPRESSIN

Vasopressin is released by the posterior lobe or neurohypophysis, which is an extension of the ventral hypothalamus. Together with the other neurohypophyseal hormone oxytocin, vasopressin is synthesized in both the supraoptic and paraventricular nuclei in the hypothalamus, from which axons extend through the pituitary stalk to the posterior pituitary. The hormones vasopressin and oxytocin are formed by separate neurons and migrate down the axons as part of precursor proteins. They are stored in secretory granules within the nerve terminals in the neurohypophysis and are released by exocytosis into the bloodstream in response to appropriate stimuli. As in most mammals, in dogs and cats arginine-vasopressin (AVP) or antidiuretic hormone (ADH) (in pigs: lysine-vasopressin) plays a vital role in water conservation. Oxytocin stimulates uterine contractions and milk ejection.

The nonapeptide AVP is synthesized as part of a large precursor molecule that is composed of a signal peptide, the hormone, a carrier protein termed *neurophysin*, and a glycopeptide. The major determinant of the release of vasopressin is plasma osmolality. In addition, significant changes in circulating blood volume may influence the setting of the osmoregulation. Specialized neurons called osmoreceptors

are concentrated in the anterolateral hypothalamus, which is near but separate from the supraoptic nuclei. This area is supplied with blood by small perforating branches of the anterior cerebral arteries. The major role of vasopressin is to regulate body fluid homeostasis by affecting water reabsorption. The antidiuretic effect is achieved by promoting the reabsorption of solute-free water in the distal and collecting tubules of the kidney. The cellular mechanism of AVP activity in the renal tubule involves binding to specific contraluminal V_2-receptor sites, an adenylate cyclase response, and phosphorylation of membrane proteins that lead to transient insertion of water channels into the luminal membrane of the cell. In the presence of these channels water molecules can move passively along an osmotic gradient (i.e., from the distal and collecting tubules to the hypertonic renal medulla).

Cations, drugs, and hormones can influence the action of AVP, thereby causing polyuria. Calcium inhibits the adenylate cyclase response to vasopressin. Glucocorticoids also interfere with the action of AVP, although in dogs loss of reactivity of the osmoreceptor system also seems to contribute to the corticosteroid-induced polyuria (Fig. 148–1).[1] Even physiologic increases in cortisol inhibit basal vasopressin release in dogs.[2] Although much less pronounced than in the dog, in humans with hyperadrenocorticism there is also decreased ability to concentrate urine. Recently, interferences of glucocorticoids with vasopressin action, similar to those in dogs, have been reported in humans.[3]

PATHOGENESIS

Insufficient AVP release may be caused by defects at several functional sites in the chain of events that regulates discharge of the hormone into the blood. As a result, different forms of central diabetes insipidus can be distinguished.

CHAPTER 148—DIABETES INSIPIDUS / 1375

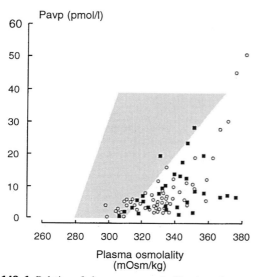

Figure 148–1. Relation of plasma vasopressin (Pavp) to plasma osmolality in nine dogs with pituitary-dependent hyperadrenocorticism (○) and six dogs with hyperadrenocorticism due to an adrenocortical tumor (■) during hypertonic saline infusion. The gray area represents the range in healthy dogs.[1] (Redrawn from Rijnberk A [ed]: Clinical Endocrinology of Dogs and Cats. Dordrecht/Boston, Kluwer Academic Publishers, 1996.)

In dogs and cats only two forms have been recognized: complete and partial central diabetes insipidus. In the first type, there is very little rise in urine osmolality with increasing plasma osmolality. These animals are essentially devoid of releasable AVP (Fig. 148–2). In the second type, AVP is released with increasing plasma osmolality but is subnormal in amount (Fig. 148–3). In some cases this moderate AVP release only starts at rather high plasma osmolality values and, therefore, it may be stated that not only is the secretory capacity limited but also there is a high setting of the osmoreceptor.

Among the lesions leading to impaired vasopressin release, an intracranial tumor is a likely cause in middle-aged and old animals. This is most often a primary pituitary neoplasm, but a craniopharyngioma or a meningioma may also be the causative lesion.[4-7] Metastatic, inflammatory, and parasitic lesions may also cause central diabetes insipidus.[8] Severe head injury, usually associated with fractures of the skull, is a rare cause in dogs and cats (see Fig. 148–2); spontanous remission may occur, probably because of regen-

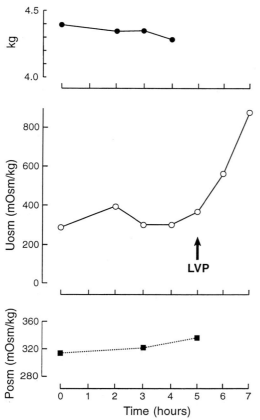

Figure 148–2. The effect of water deprivation on body weight, plasma osmolality (Posm), and urine osmolality (Uosm) in a 4-year-old castrated male cat with a history of head trauma. The arrow represents an injection of aqueous vasopressin (lysine-vasopressin [LVP]). In this case the dehydration-induced rise in Posm did not lead to an increase in Uosm. This in combination with the sharp rise in Uosm after vasopressin administration justified the diagnosis of complete central diabetes insipidus. (Redrawn from Rijnberk A [ed]: Clinical Endocrinology of Dogs and Cats. Dordrecht/Boston, Kluwer Academic Publishers, 1996.)

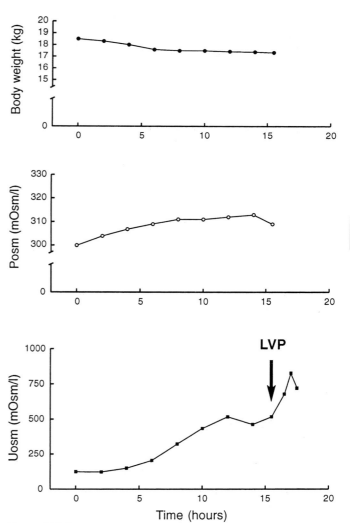

Figure 148–3. In a 5-month-old mongrel dog presented for polyuria, water deprivation led to a slow, subnormal rise in urine osmolality (Uosm). At maximal Uosm, that is, when a "plateau" was reached, vasopressin (lysine-vasopressin [LVP]) administration caused a 60 per cent increase in urine osmolality. These observations are compatible with partial central diabetes insipidus. (Redrawn from Rijnberk A [ed]: Clinical Endocrinology of Dogs and Cats. Dordrecht/Boston, Kluwer Academic Publishers, 1996.)

END

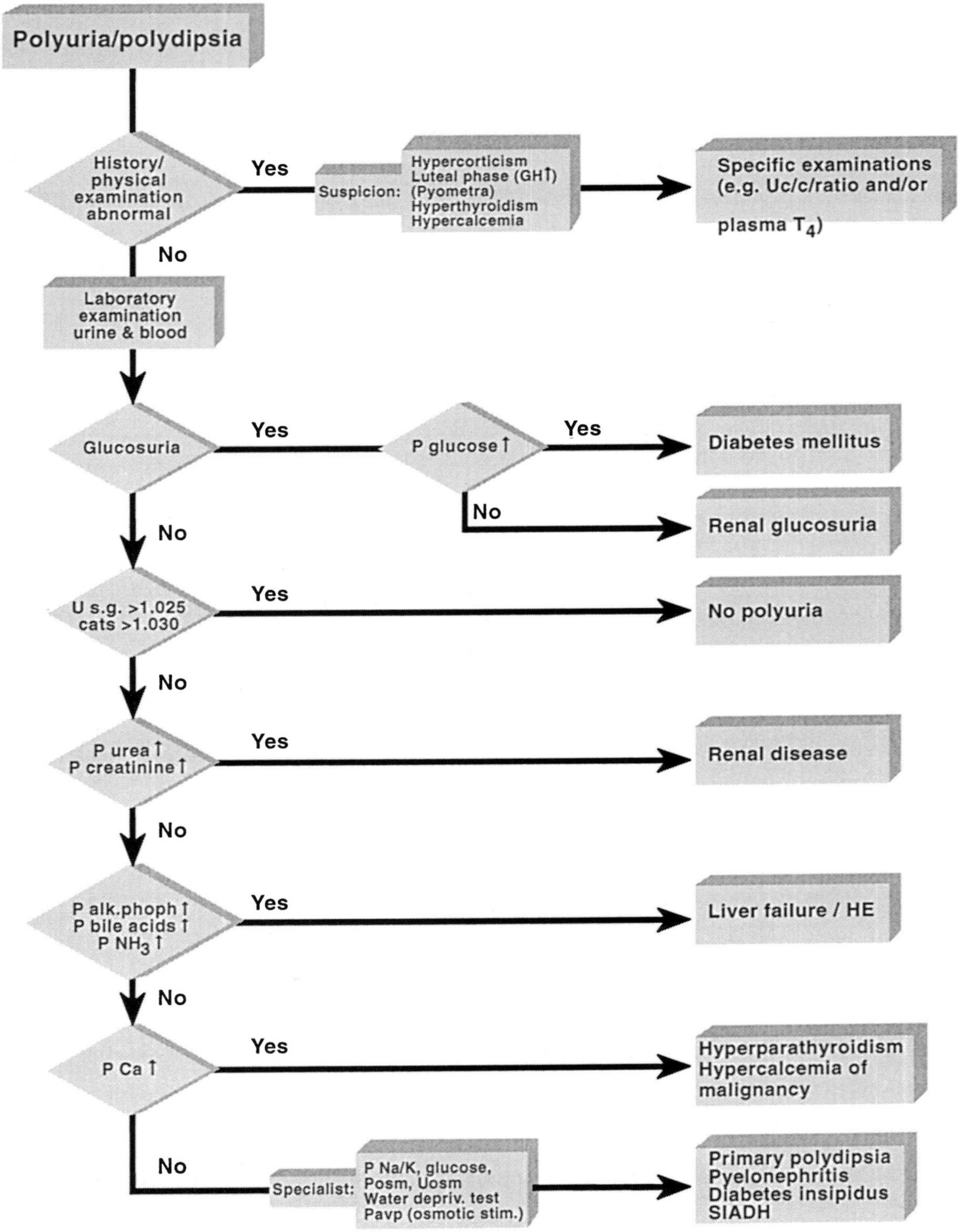

Figure 148–4. In the first part of this algorithm the approach to the problem polyuria/polydipsia (pu/pd) is based on the information from history. As a second step, urinalysis has been introduced because it may happen that an animal presented with a seemingly convincing history of polyuria/polydipsia has only polydipsia because the owner has changed the food to dry food. As indicated in the text, it may be advisable at this stage to ask the owner for urine collections at 2-hour intervals. When the routine clinical chemistry has not revealed a specific suspicion, tests such as water deprivation and hypertonic saline infusion with arginine-vasopressin measurements may be needed. (Redrawn from Rijnberk A [ed]: Clinical Endocrinology of Dogs and Cats. Dordrecht/Boston, Kluwer Academic Publishers, 1996.)

eration of disrupted axons in the pituitary stalk.[9] An increasing cause of central diabetes insipidus is pituitary surgery.[10] The diabetes insipidus develops immediately after surgery and is transient, resolving after a period of days to months. When the pituitary stalk is sectioned high enough to induce retrograde degeneration of the hypothalamic neurons, the central diabetes insipidus may be permanent. Finally, there is the possibility of the so-called idiopathic form. This term is used in cases of central diabetes insipidus in which no lesion in the hypothalamic and/or pituitary region can be demonstrated. This diagnosis is most common in young animals, although the course of the disease and/or the autopsy may eventually reveal a lesion that could not be identified initially.[11]

CLINICAL MANIFESTATIONS

The major manifestations are polyuria, polydipsia, and a near-continuous demand for water. These symptoms may be sudden in onset and the maximum urine flow reached in 1 or 2 days. In severe cases, water intake and urine volume may be immense, requiring micturition almost every hour throughout day and night. However, in the incomplete forms the urine volume may be only moderately increased. In severe cases, the enormous water intake may interfere with food intake and result in weight loss. Animals with a large neoplasm as the underlying cause may have additional neurologic signs.

The urine concentration will be below that of plasma (specific gravity [SG] < 1.010 and urine osmolality [Uosm] < 290 mOsm/kg), but in the mild cases higher osmolalities (up to 600 mOsm/kg) may be found. Blood examination usually does not reveal abnormalities except for a slight hypernatremia due to commonly inadequate replenishment of the excreted water. When water is withheld from animals with the complete form of the disease, they develop within a few hours a life-threatening hypertonic encephalopathy (plasma sodium concentration [PNa$^+$] > 170 mmol/L; plasma osmolality [Posm] > 375 mOsm/kg), initially characterized by ataxia and stupor. This situation may also be encountered when the causative lesion extends to the thirst center and adipsia develops.[12]

DIFFERENTIAL DIAGNOSIS

Apart from central diabetes insipidus there are in principle only two basic disorders that can account for the polyuria. These disorders are (1) primary polydipsia and (2) nephrogenic diabetes insipidus. Primary polydipsia is said to occur in hyperactive young dogs that are left alone during the day for many hours or have gone through significant changes in their environment. It has been observed that placing of the animal in a completely different environment may stop the problem. However, so far there are no convincing reports unequivocally documenting the occurrence of this condition.

There are a few individual case reports of congenital nephrogenic diabetes insipidus, the condition in which the kidney tubules are insensitive to the action of antidiuretic hormone. Familial occurrence has been documented in huskies, in which the defect could be ascribed to a mutation affecting the affinity of the V$_2$ receptor for ligand.[13]

However, in addition to these two basic and infrequently encountered differential diagnoses, a wide variety of conditions cause polyuria. In the young animal this may be con-

genital kidney disease, whereas at all ages acquired kidney disease may lead to polyuria. Especially in middle-aged and elderly animals, endocrine conditions such as diabetes mellitus, hyperadrenocorticism, hyperthyroidism, pyometra, progestin-induced (luteal phase) growth hormone excess, hyperparathyroidism, hypercalcemia of malignancy, and the syndrome of inappropriate vasopressin secretion have to be considered. In several of these conditions impaired release of vasopressin and/or interference with its action may play a role in the polyuria (see earlier and Fig. 148–1). This has been documented for conditions such as hyperadrenocorticism, hepatoencephalopathy, and polycythemia.[1, 14, 15] In polycythemia it is likely that increased blood volume causes the impairment of vasopressin release. This range of possibilities may make it a difficult task to come to a diagnosis in an animal with polyuria. The algorithm presented in Figure 148–4 may be helpful.

DIAGNOSIS

Urine osmolality (161 to 2830 mOsm/kg) and urine specific gravity (1.006 > 1.050) vary widely among healthy pet dogs.[16] In some dogs, urine osmolality fluctuates considerably during the day and values close to plasma osmolality may be reached (Fig. 148–5). There is experimental evidence that water consumption increases with food intake and exercise.[17] For example, with dry food, dogs consumed 40 per cent of the total daily water intake during 2 hours after food intake. After treadmill running for 30 minutes water intake was higher than the water losses during the exercise.[17] However, it is unlikely that the sometimes strong fluctuations in urine osmolality of pet dogs during the day can be explained solely as an effect of feeding. There may be individual differences in early satiation of thirst, as mediated through oropharyngeal receptors.[16]

Apparently in most pet dogs the low urine osmolalities are associated with sufficiently high urine osmolalities at other times of the day so that the owners do not perceive their dog to be polydipsic or polyuric. However, it may very well be that in other dogs the situation may be more

END

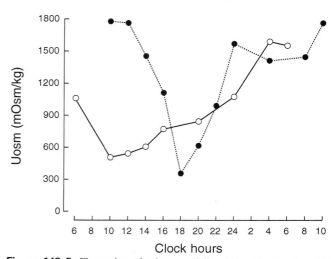

Figure 148–5. Fluctuation of urine osmolality during the day in a 9.5-year-old castrated male schnauzer (interrupted line) and a female 7.5-year-old Belgian shepherd (uninterrupted line). (Redrawn from Van Vonderen IK, et al: Intra- and interindividual variation in urine osmolality and urine specific gravity in healthy pet dogs of various ages. J Vet Intern Med 11:30, 1997.)

pronounced and the animals are brought to the veterinarian because of polyuria and polydipsia.[16] Some of these animals may be recognized as having primary polydipsia, although this has not been documented so far. Nevertheless it may be advisable to start the work-up of dogs with polyuria by repeated measurements of urine osmolality and/or urine specific gravity during the day. As in humans, this approach may limit further clinical studies.[18]

The water deprivation test combined with vasopressin administration,[19] as exemplified in Figures 148–2 and 148–3, is most commonly used for differentiating the causes of polyuria. The test is difficult to perform correctly, unpleasant for the animal, relies heavily on the emptying of the bladder, and is indirect because changes in urinary concentration are used as an index of vasopressin release. Furthermore, the stimulus to vasopressin release is a combination of hypertonicity and hypovolemia, especially toward the end of the period of dehydration.

Briefly the procedure is as follows: After 12 hours of fasting, water is withheld and plasma and urine are collected every hour or every 2 hours, depending on the severity of the polyuria. Osmolality is measured in both samples. At each collection, the animal is weighed. When the weight loss approaches 5 per cent of initial body weight, the test should be stopped. When, in the presence of an adequate osmotic stimulus (Posm > 305 mOsm/kg), urine concentration is maximal (less than 5 per cent increase in Uosm between consecutive collections), 2 U of lysine vasopressin is administered subcutaneously. Urine osmolality is measured again 1 hour later. In countries where lysine vasopressin is no longer available, an analogue such as desmopressin can also be used (see later).

In both nephrogenic diabetes insipidus and central diabetes insipidus, urine osmolality will remain low during water deprivation. In complete diabetes insipidus, urine osmolality will rise by 50 per cent or more after the injection of vasopressin, whereas in the partial forms of central diabetes insipidus the rise will be greater than or equal to 15 per cent, and in nephrogenic diabetes insipidus there will be very little or no rise in urine osmolality (see Figs. 148–2 and 148–3). Because of the indirect character of the test, the results may not always be conclusive.[20]

A more direct way to differentiate among the three basic causes of polyuria rests on the measurement of plasma vasopressin during osmotic stimulation by hypertonic saline infusion (see Figs. 148–1 and 148–6).[21] The euhydrated animal is infused for 2 hours through the jugular vein with 20 per cent NaCl solution at a rate of 0.03 mL/kg body weight per minute. Samples for plasma AVP and plasma osmolality are obtained at 20-minute intervals. Especially in the severely polyuric animal there is the risk of inducing critical hypertonicity. The test requires very close observation of the animal and monitoring of plasma osmolality. This, and the fact that vasopressin is very sensitive to proteolytic breakdown, makes it advisable that the test is performed in institutions that have developed experience with the test.[22]

As in humans this approach can improve the diagnostic accuracy. The advantage is not in the severe forms of central diabetes insipidus, because in these conditions the standard indirect test will give a correct diagnosis. In all other categories of polyuria (i.e., in animals that concentrate their urine to various degrees during dehydration), the indirect test may be less reliable. Dogs in which the polyuria had initially been attributed to renal disease or to primary polydipsia proved to have partial central diabetes insipidus in the direct test. However, with regard to primary polydipsia some reser-

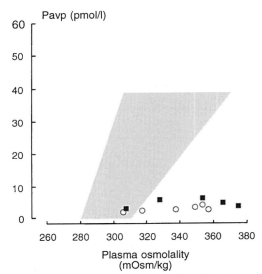

Figure 148–6. Relation of plasma vasopressin with plasma osmolality (Pavp) during hypertonic saline infusion in two dogs with central diabetes insipidus caused by pituitary tumor.[4] See also legend to Figure 148–1. (Redrawn from Rijnberk A [ed]: Clinical Endocrinology of Dogs and Cats. Dordrecht/Boston, Kluwer Academic Publishers, 1996.)

vation in the interpretation is needed, because it has been demonstrated for humans that this chronic overhydration downregulates the release of AVP in response to hypertonicity.[21]

The use of this direct approach has been limited so far, but it is worth considering in the few unresolved cases that remain after exclusion of the many other causes of polyuria (see Fig. 148–4). It is often a question of whether the animal must endure for many years a life hampered by thirst, a large bladder, and unwanted behavior.

TREATMENT

As for almost all peptides, orally administered vasopressin is ineffective. Aqueous (lysine) vasopressin may be administered subcutaneously in doses of 2 to 5 U. It will act for only about 3 hours. Nevertheless, a good response has been reported in one dog, which received 5 U each 48 hours.[6]

The vasopressin analogue desmopressin (DDAVP, 1-de-amino, 9-D-arginine vasopressin),* provides antidiuretic activity for about 8 hours. One drop (1.5 to 4 μg) placed twice daily in the conjunctival sac sufficiently controls the polyuria in most dogs with central diabetes insipidus. With the administration of three drops a day the urine production usually returns to normal, but some owners (in part for financial reasons) prefer to apply the drug only twice daily. In one report on a cat with partial diabetes insipidus the effect of conjunctivally administered desmopressin was described as poor, which might have been due to incorrect placement because of the cat's struggling.[23] With the injectable preparation (4 μg once a day or every 12 hours) of desmopressin the water consumption could be adequately controlled. The analogue can also be effective when administered as tablet: one-half tablet of 0.1 or 0.2 mg, two or three times per day, depending on the size of the animal and the effect.

---

*Minrin, Ferring AB, Malmö, Sweden (0.1 mg DDAVP/mL).

PROGNOSIS

In the absence of a neoplastic lesion the long-term prospects for diabetes insipidus are good. With appropriate treatment the animals become asymptomatic. Untreated animals with the complete form are especially always at risk of developing life-threatening dehydration when left without water for longer than a few hours. Animals with diabetes insipidus due to a pituitary tumor may lead acceptable lives for many months until the lesion has reached such size that neurologic signs develop.

REFERENCES

1. Biewenga WJ, et al: Osmoregulation of systemic vasopressin release during long-term glucocorticoid excess: A study in dogs with hyperadrenocorticism. Acta Endocrinol 124:583, 1991.
2. Papanek PE, Raff H: Physiological increases in cortisol inhibit basal vasopressin release in conscious dogs. Am J Physiol 266:R1744, 1994.
3. Knoepfelmacher M, et al: Resistance to vasopressin action on the kidney in patients with Cushing's disease. Eur J Endocrinol 137:162, 1997.
4. Biewenga WJ, et al: Persistent polyuria in two dogs following adrenocorticolysis for pituitary-dependent hyperadrenocorticism. Vet Q 11:193, 1989.
5. Goossens MMC, et al: Central diabetes insipidus in a dog with pro-opiomelanocortin-producing pituitary tumor not causing hyperadrenocorticism. J Vet Intern Med 9:361, 1995.
6. Harb MF, et al: Central diabetes insipidus in dogs: 20 cases (1986–1995). JAVMA 209:1884, 1996.
7. Bilzer T: Hypophysentumoren als gemeinsame Ursache von Morbus Cushing und Diabetes insipidus des Hundes. Tierärztl Prax 19:276, 1991.
8. Perrin IV, et al: Diabetes insipidus centralis durch Larva migrans visceralis in der Neuro-Hypophyse beim Hund. Schweiz Arch Tierheilkd 128:483, 1986.
9. Authement JM, et al: Transient, traumatically induced, central diabetes insipidus in a dog. JAVMA 194:683, 1989.
10. Meij BP, et al: Results of transsphenoidal hypophysectomy in 52 dogs with pituitary-dependent hyperadrenocorticism. Vet Surg 27:246, 1998.
11. Post K, et al: Congenital central diabetes insipidus in two sibling Afghan hound pups. JAVMA 194:1086, 1989.
12. DiBartola SP, et al: Hypodipsic hypernatremia in a dog with defective osmoregulation of antidiuretic hormone. JAVMA 204:922, 1994.
13. Luzius H, et al: A low affinity vasopressin V_2-receptor in inherited nephrogenic diabetes insipidus. J Receptor Res 12:351, 1992.
14. Rothuizen J, et al: Chronic glucocorticoid excess and impaired osmoregulation of vasopressin release in dogs with hepatic encephalopathy. Domest Anim Endocrinol 12:13, 1995.
15. Van Vonderen IK, et al: Polyuria and polydipsia and disturbed vasopressin release in 2 dogs with secondary polycythemia. J Vet Intern Med 11:300, 1997.
16. Van Vonderen IK, et al: Intra- and interindividual variation in urine osmolality and urine specific gravity in healthy pet dogs of various ages. J Vet Intern Med 11:30, 1997.
17. Meyer H, et al: Ein Beitrag zur Wasseraufnahme und Harnabgabe beim Hund. Wien Tierärztl Monatschr 81:163, 1994.
18. Mevorach RA, et al: Urine concentration and enuresis in healthy preschool children. Arch Pediatr Adolesc Med 149:259, 1995.
19. Mol JA, Rijnberk A: Pituitary function. In Kaneko JJ, Harvey JW, Bruss ML (eds): Clinical Biochemistry of Domestic Animals. San Diego, Academic Press, 1997, p 517.
20. Biewenga WJ, et al: Vasopressin in polyuric syndromes in the dog. Front Horm Res 17:139, 1987.
21. Moses AM, Clayton B: Impairment of osmotically stimulated AVP release in patients with primary polydipsia. Am J Physiol 265:R1247, 1993.
22. Rijnberk A: Protocols for function tests. In Rijnberk A (ed): Clinical Endocrinology of Dogs and Cats. Dordrecht/Boston, Kluwer Academic Publishers, 1996, p 205.
23. Pittari JM: Central diabetes insipidus in a cat. Feline Practice 24:18, 1996.

CHAPTER 149

DISORDERS OF THE PARATHYROID GLANDS

Edward C. Feldman

PRIMARY HYPERPARATHYROIDISM—HYPERCALCEMIA

ETIOLOGY

The essential disorder in primary hyperparathyroidism (PHPTH) is the excessive synthesis and secretion of parathyroid hormone (PTH) by abnormal, autonomously functioning parathyroid "chief" cells. The etiology of this hormonal excess is usually a solitary adenoma, but adenomatous hyperplasia of one or more parathyroid glands and parathyroid carcinomas have been identified in both dogs and cats. In contrast, other forms of hyperparathyroidism (e.g., renal or nutritional secondary hyperparathyroidism) are usually the result of non-endocrine alterations in calcium and phosphorus homeostasis. Such disturbances indirectly affect the parathyroid glands, causing diffuse hyperplasia. Depending on etiology, serum calcium concentrations in secondary disorders may range from low to normal to increased. PHPTH is almost always associated with hypercalcemia.

PATHOPHYSIOLOGY

Calcium-PTH Feedback System

Serum calcium is the major factor in regulation of PTH secretion. In normal animals, there is an inverse linear relationship between serum calcium and PTH levels.[1] The system functions as if there were a "calciostat" that operates at a set point of about 10.5 mg/dL. When the serum calcium concentration falls below this point, the rate of PTH secretion increases; when the serum calcium concentration exceeds the set point, PTH secretion is suppressed. In PHPTH, normal negative-feedback homeostatic control is lost, and PTH secretion is increased either autonomously or owing to a change in the set point. The autonomous secretion of PTH is not suppressible by the increased concentration of calcium perfusing the parathyroid glands. Conversely, in secondary hyperparathyroidism, secretion by the parathyroid glands is normally suppressible by increased concentrations of calcium.

Severe Hypercalcemia

Hypercalcemia develops when the entry of calcium into the extracellular fluid (regardless of the source) overwhelms the normal mechanisms that maintain normocalcemia. One of these mechanisms is suppressed secretion of PTH, a process obviously negated when the cause of the hypercalcemia is the autonomous secretion of PTH or a molecule with similar biologic activity. In cancer-associated hypercalcemia, the secretion of PTH is suppressed, but the humoral factor that activates osteoclasts is the autonomous secretion of a parathyroid hormone–related protein (PTHrP), a protein with a structure and biologic activity quite similar to that of PTH.[2]

In the setting of accelerated bone resorption, the kidney is the principal defense against hypercalcemia.[3] When renal and endocrine function is normal, any tendency for a rise in serum calcium is attenuated by increased urinary excretion of calcium. This process is inhibited by PTH in PHPTH or by PTHrP in hypercalcemia of malignancy. These hormones induce osteoclast-mediated bone resorption, intestinal absorption of calcium, and renal tubular reabsorption of calcium.[4] This impairs the ability of the kidneys to excrete the increased filtered load of calcium. Thus, animals with an excess of PTH lack the first lines of defense against hypercalcemia. The hypercalcemic state also interferes with renal mechanisms for reabsorption of sodium and water, leading to polyuria. This is due to an acquired inability to respond to antidiuretic hormone (ADH)—in essence, a reversible form of nephrogenic diabetes insipidus. In PHPTH, hypercalcemia is enhanced by the increased production of vitamin D and by a decrease in the amount of serum phosphate available to form complexes with serum ionized calcium. The result is a decreased tubular reabsorption of phosphate, hyperphosphaturia, and hypophosphatemia. These actions are responsible for the development of the biochemical triad classic for PHPTH: hypercalcemia, hypophosphatemia, and hyperphosphaturia.

SIGNALMENT

PHPTH is typically diagnosed in older dogs and appears to be much less common, or at least less frequently diagnosed, in cats. The mean age of dogs with PHPTH seen at our hospital is 10.5 years, with a range of 5 to 15 years. More than 95 per cent of the dogs are 7 years of age or older. There is no apparent sex predilection. More than 33 per cent of the dogs have been Keeshonds.

ANAMNESIS: CLINICAL SIGNS

Renal: Kidneys, Bladder, Urethra

Polydipsia and/or Polyuria. The most common clinical signs in dogs with PHPTH are polyuria, polydipsia, and/or urinary incontinence. Surprisingly, the polydipsia and polyuria are either not observed or thought to be mild by most owners. The specific gravity of a randomly obtained urine sample was 1.015 or less in most dogs and was almost always 1.028 or less.

Urinary Tract Calculi and/or Infections. One cause for owner concern in dogs with PHPTH is observation of clinical signs consistent with urinary tract infection and/or calculi. These signs include frequency, urgency, incontinence, hematuria, stranguria, or apparent urinary obstruction. Hypercalciuria resulting from PHPTH increases glomerular filtration of calcium and contributes to an increased incidence of urolithiasis and urinary tract infection.

General

Clinical signs due solely to hypercalcemia tend to be mild, insidious, and nonspecific. When signs are worrisome or severe, they are usually due to a concurrent problem (e.g., lymphosarcoma, Addison's). The most common gastrointestinal sign is decreased appetite. Vomiting, anorexia, and more worrisome signs are not common. Central nervous system signs include mental dullness. Listlessness has been observed in almost 50 per cent of dogs with PHPTH, and inappetence (poor appetite) has been observed in about 33 per cent. The latter problem is probably a result of hypercalcemia-induced decreased excitability of gastrointestinal smooth muscle or direct calcemic effects on the central nervous system. Less than 5 per cent of dogs in our series were uremic, which could also account for inappetence. Skeletal muscle weakness, primarily involving the proximal muscle groups, may result from a primary neuropathy, which ultimately causes mild muscle atrophy. Rarely, shivering, muscle twitching, and seizures have been observed.

Infrequent ocular abnormalities in dogs with PHPTH include band keratopathy and subconjunctival deposits of calcium. Band keratopathy results from the deposition of calcium phosphate in the cornea. It is seen as opaque material in parallel lines within the limbus of the eye, best visualized by slit-lamp examination.

PHYSICAL EXAMINATION

The physical examination is usually unremarkable in dogs with PHPTH. When abnormalities exist, they are typically related to the presence of uroliths. Other abnormalities (weakness, muscle atrophy) are usually subtle or nonspecific. Although an enlarged parathyroid gland (adenoma) has not been palpable in any of our dogs with PHPTH, palpable tumors have been identified in four of eight cats with this condition.

Although usually normal in dogs with PHPTH, a thorough physical examination is imperative in any animal with documented hypercalcemia. Several of the causes for hypercalcemia in dogs may be strongly suspected or considered less likely after examination. The most common cause of hypercalcemia in dogs is a manifestation of hypercalcemia of malignancy. Lymphosarcoma, apocrine gland carcinoma of the anal sac, mammary gland adenocarcinoma, vaginal sarcoma, and multiple myeloma are among the tumors capable of causing hypercalcemia that may be identified on physical examination. The diagnostic approach to a dog with confirmed hypercalcemia is to rule out the presence of these problems before pursuing the diagnosis of PHPTH (Fig. 149–1). Many of these tumors can be identified with careful palpation of all peripheral lymph nodes, the mammary glands, and perineal region. Rectal and vaginal examinations should always be included in the examination of a hypercal-

TABLE 149–1. SELECTED BIOCHEMICAL ABNORMALITIES FROM 104 DOGS WITH PRIMARY, NATURALLY OCCURRING HYPERPARATHYROIDISM

DOGS (No.)	SERUM CALCIUM (mg/dL)	SERUM PHOSPHATE (mg/dL)	BLOOD UREA NITROGEN (mg/dL)	SERUM CREATININE (mg/dL)	SERUM MAGNESIUM (mg/dL)	SERUM PARATHYROID HORMONE (pmol/L)
92	Range: 12.1–21.9	1.6–3.8	11–28	0.7–1.1	1.2–2.3	4–43
	Mean: 15.4	2.7	18	0.9	1.9	17
5	Range: 14.6–17.4	3.4–3.8	35–59	1.3–2.0	2.1 & 1.9	9–41
	Mean: 15.5	3.6	46	1.6		25
7	Range: 13.4–23.0	4.3–6.8	62–94	1.4–2.7	1.8–2.2	28–39
	Mean: 16.9	5.8	80	2.2	2.1	32
Normal ranges	8.9–11.4	3.0–4.7	12–28	0.8–1.5	1.8–2.4	1–8

Ninety-two of the 104 dogs had normal renal function test results, five had mild increases in blood urea nitrogen (BUN) but normal serum phosphate concentrations, and seven had increases in BUN *and* serum phosphate concentrations.

cemic animal. In addition to hypercalcemia of malignancy, other causes of hypercalcemia may be suspected after a thorough physical examination. In renal failure, the kidneys may be palpably abnormal. In Addison's disease, there may be bradycardia, weak femoral pulses, melena, or a bloody rectal discharge.

CLINICAL PATHOLOGY

Hemogram and Serum Biochemical Profile

There are no typical hemogram abnormalities in dogs with PHPTH. Owing to the various factors that can alter serum calcium concentration and keeping the differential diagnoses for hypercalcemia in mind, many parameters within the chemistry profile have importance. Specifically, the serum calcium concentration should be evaluated relative to the serum albumin concentration and correlated with the phosphorus, blood urea nitrogen (BUN), and serum creatinine concentrations.

Total Serum Calcium Concentration. Hypercalcemia is the hallmark feature of PHPTH (Fig. 149–2). In our series, the mean serum calcium concentration was 15.6 mg/dL, with a range of 12.1 to 23 mg/dL (Table 149–1). This mean value could be misleading, because the evaluation of hypercalcemia in our clinic is usually limited to those animals with serum calcium concentrations greater than 12 mg/dL.

Dehydration, lipemia, hemolysis, and excessive use of oral phosphate binders may cause the serum calcium concentration to increase. Young animals may have mild increases in serum calcium concentration, and postprandial samples may yield false increases. Alterations in plasma albumin or protein concentration (dehydration, blood loss, and so forth) may alter *total* serum calcium concentration, yet the ionized calcium concentration usually remains normal. Formulas have been developed that provide a more accurate assessment of total serum calcium concentration in dogs with hypoalbuminemia and/or panhypoproteinemia. The correction formula based on the serum albumin concentration is:

$$\text{Corrected total Ca (mg/dL)} = \text{total Ca (mg/dL)} - \text{albumin (g/dL)} + 3.5$$

Determination of ionized rather than total calcium concentration negates the effect that changes in serum albumin or total protein concentration may have on total serum calcium concentration. With ionized calcium assessment becoming readily available and relatively inexpensive through commer-

cial laboratories, formula-driven estimates become crude by comparison.

Serum Phosphorus Concentration. Low or low-normal serum phosphorus concentrations are typical of PHPTH (see Fig. 149–2). Hypophosphatemia develops following PTH-induced inhibition of renal tubular phosphorus resorption, resulting in excessive urinary losses. In our series of dogs with PHPTH, the mean serum phosphorus concentration was 3.1 mg/dL, with a range of 1.2 to 6.8 mg/dL. Typically, the phosphorus concentration is low (approximately one third of these dogs had hypophosphatemia) to low-normal, usually less than 4 mg/dL. Only in 7 of 104 dogs with both renal disease and PHPTH was the serum phosphate concentration greater than 3.8 mg/dL (see Table 149–1). The serum phosphorus concentration should always be evaluated relative to the serum calcium concentration and renal function. Hypophosphatemia, when dietary phosphate is adequate and oral phosphate-binding agents are not being given, is consistent with PHPTH and hypercalcemia of malignancy (see Fig. 149–2). Other causes for hypophosphatemia are less common (Table 149–2).

Hyperphosphatemia in the absence of azotemia suggests a non-parathyroid cause for hypercalcemia; if both hyperphosphatemia and azotemia exist, the clinician must rely on

END

TABLE 149–2. POTENTIAL CAUSES FOR HYPOPHOSPHATEMIA

Decreased Intestinal Absorption

Decreased dietary intake
Malabsorption/steatorrhea
Vomiting/diarrhea
Phosphate-binding antacids
Vitamin D deficiency

Increased Urinary Excretion

Primary hyperparathyroidism
Diabetes mellitus ± ketoacidosis
Hyperadrenocorticism (naturally occurring/iatrogenic)
Fanconi's syndrome (renal tubular defects)
Diuretic or bicarbonate administration
Hypothermia recovery
Hyperaldosteronism
Aggressive parenteral fluid administration
Hypercalcemia of malignancy (early stages)

Transcellular Shifts

Insulin administration
Parenteral glucose administration
Hyperalimentation
Respiratory alkalosis

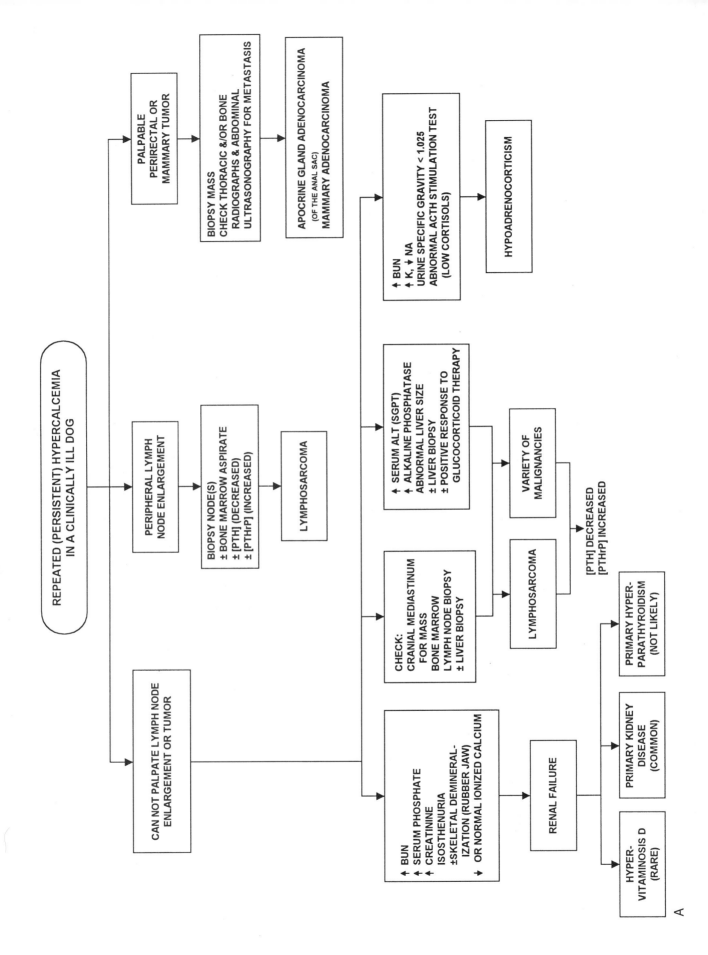

REPEATED (PERSISTENT) HYPERCALCEMIA IN A CLINICALLY ILL DOG

PALPABLE PERIRECTAL OR MAMMARY TUMOR

BIOPSY MASS
CHECK THORACIC &/OR BONE RADIOGRAPHS & ABDOMINAL ULTRASONOGRAPHY FOR METASTASIS

APOCRINE GLAND ADENOCARCINOMA
(OF THE ANAL SAC)
MAMMARY ADENOCARCINOMA

PERIPHERAL LYMPH NODE ENLARGEMENT

BIOPSY NODE(S)
± BONE MARROW ASPIRATE
± [PTH] (DECREASED)
± [PTHrP] (INCREASED)

LYMPHOSARCOMA

↑ SERUM ALT (SGPT)
↑ ALKALINE PHOSPHATASE
ABNORMAL LIVER SIZE
± LIVER BIOPSY
± POSITIVE RESPONSE TO GLUCOCORTICOID THERAPY

VARIETY OF MALIGNANCIES

CHECK:
CRANIAL MEDIASTINUM FOR MASS
BONE MARROW
LYMPH NODE BIOPSY
± LIVER BIOPSY

LYMPHOSARCOMA

↑ BUN
↑ K, ↓ NA
URINE SPECIFIC GRAVITY < 1.025
ABNORMAL ACTH STIMULATION TEST
(LOW CORTISOLS)

HYPOADRENOCORTICISM

CAN NOT PALPATE LYMPH NODE ENLARGEMENT OR TUMOR

↑ BUN
↑ SERUM PHOSPHATE
↑ CREATININE
ISOSTHENURIA
±SKELETAL DEMINERAL-IZATION (RUBBER JAW)
↓ OR NORMAL IONIZED CALCIUM

RENAL FAILURE

[PTH] DECREASED
[PTHrP] INCREASED

HYPER-VITAMINOSIS D (RARE)

PRIMARY KIDNEY DISEASE (COMMON)

PRIMARY HYPER-PARATHYROIDISM (NOT LIKELY)

A

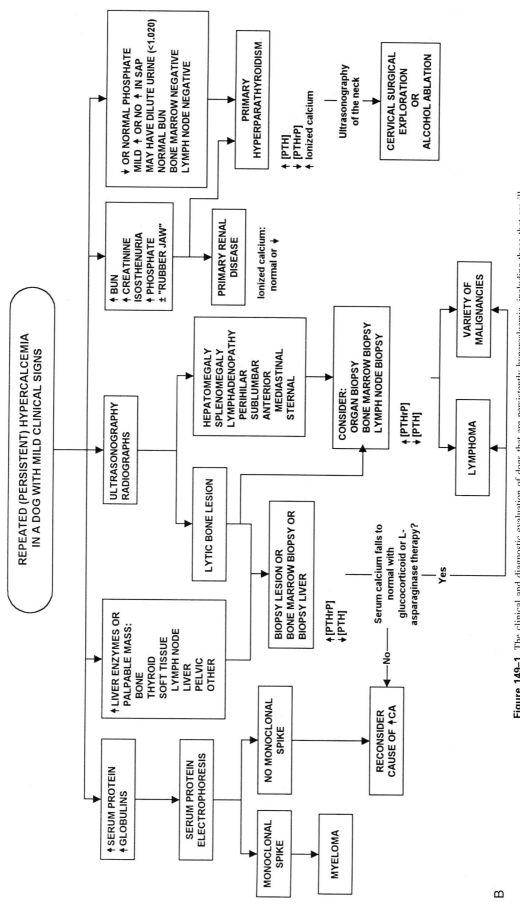

Figure 149–1. The clinical and diagnostic evaluation of dogs that are persistently hypercalcemic, including those that are ill (A) and those with subtle clinical signs (B).

B

END

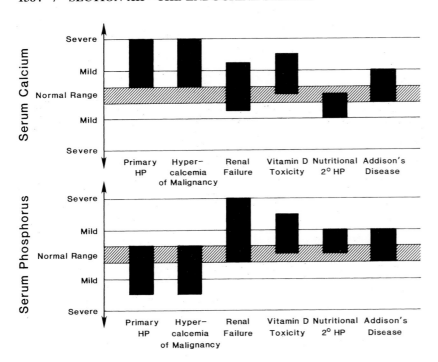

Figure 149–2. The range in serum calcium and phosphorus concentrations for the more common causes of hypercalcemia and/or hyperparathyroidism in the dog. HP = hyperparathyroidism; 2° HP = secondary hyperparathyroidism. (From Feldman EC, Nelson RW: Canine and Feline Endocrinology and Reproduction, 2nd ed. Philadelphia, WB Saunders, 1996.)

the history, physical examination, and other diagnostic tests to determine whether the primary problem is hypercalcemia with secondary renal failure or renal failure with secondary hypercalcemia. The differentiation remains a difficult diagnostic dilemma. However, determination of the serum ionized calcium concentration can be of value. Dogs with renal failure and increases in total serum calcium concentration usually have mild decreases in the ionized fraction, as op-

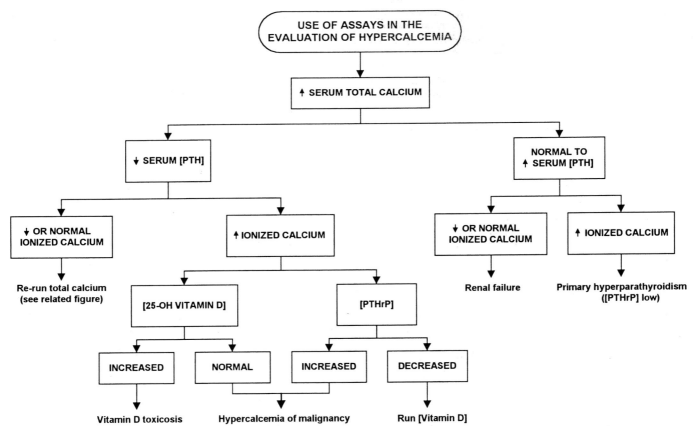

Figure 149–3. Algorithm demonstrating the potential value and use of various new assays in the evaluation of hypercalcemic dogs.

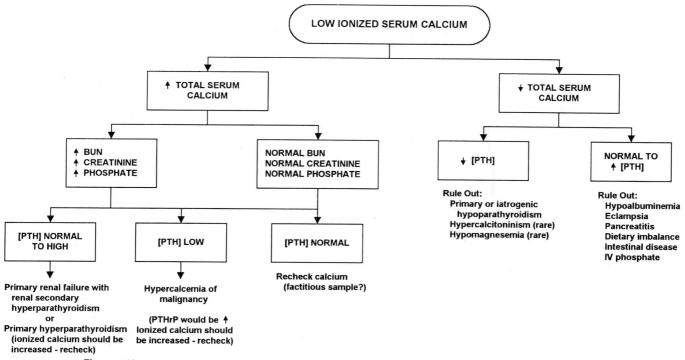

Figure 149–4. Algorithm for determining the cause of decreases in the ionized serum calcium concentration in dogs.

posed to those with PHPTH, in which both the total and the ionized fractions are increased.[5]

Blood Urea Nitrogen and Serum Creatinine. In dogs with uncomplicated PHPTH, serum renal parameters (BUN, creatinine) are usually normal. However, persistent and prolonged hypercalcemia has the potential to cause progressive nephrocalcinosis. Eleven per cent of dogs with PHPTH were azotemic at the time of initial examination, and only 4 per cent had hyperphosphatemia (see Table 149–2). The presence of azotemia in a hypercalcemic dog or cat is an indication for aggressive medical intervention to reduce the serum calcium concentration and improve renal perfusion. In addition, the combination of azotemia, hypercalcemia, and hyperphosphatemia represents a difficult diagnostic challenge, because these abnormalities may be identified in dogs with either primary renal failure or PHPTH. The availability of assays for ionized serum calcium and for PTH has diminished the difficulty associated with distinguishing between these disorders (Figs. 149–3 and 149–4).

Urinalysis

There are no specific abnormalities in the routine urinalysis suggestive of PHPTH. The urine specific gravity was less than 1.015 in about 80 per cent of randomly obtained urine samples from dogs with PHPTH and less than 1.028 in almost all—a result of hypercalcemia interfering with ADH action and renal concentrating ability. Many of these urine samples were isosthenuric (specific gravity of 1.008 to 1.012). Isosthenuria (or hyposthenuria) may develop from any cause of hypercalcemia and is nonspecific. However, confusion arises because progressive renal failure is a differential diagnosis for isosthenuria. Thus, a thorough review of the serum chemistry profile and other parameters may be necessary to determine the cause for isosthenuria or hyposthenuria. Hematuria, pyuria, bacteriuria, and crystalluria may

be found on examination of urine sediment. Hypercalciuria, proximal renal tubular acidosis with impaired bicarbonate resorption, and the production of alkaline urine may predispose dogs to the development of bacterial cystitis and cystic or renal calculi. Approximately 33 per cent of these dogs have calculi.

Serum PTH Concentration

Primary Parathyroid Disease. In dogs and cats with PHPTH, the serum PTH concentration is typically midnormal to exceedingly increased (Fig. 149–5). However, the serum PTH concentration must always be evaluated relative to the serum calcium concentration. In normal animals, as the serum calcium concentration increases, the serum PTH concentration decreases. Relative to their hypercalcemia (utilizing total or ionized calcium), virtually all dogs and cats with PHPTH have excessive concentrations of serum PTH (even though the PTH concentration may be within the normal range), consistent with a disease process associated with autonomous secretion of hormone (Fig. 149–6). Similarly, hypocalcemic animals with abnormally decreased serum PTH concentrations are most likely to be afflicted with primary hypoparathyroidism.

Malignancy-Associated Hypercalcemia. The serum PTH concentration in dogs with malignancy-associated hypercalcemia is typically low or undetectable, whereas PTHrP can be detected in the serum (see Fig. 149–5). PTH concentrations should not be viewed as a replacement for thoracic radiographs, abdominal ultrasonography, or any study used to identify neoplasia.

Chronic Renal Failure. In dogs with both renal disease and hypercalcemia, it may be difficult to understand whether the primary disorder resides in the parathyroid glands or in the kidneys. In either situation, both the serum PTH concentration and the serum calcium concentration may be

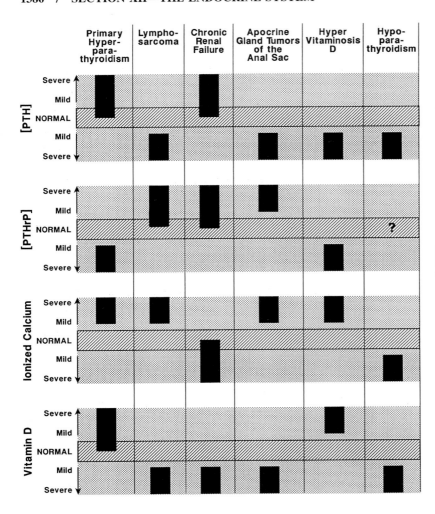

Figure 149–5. Graph illustrating the serum PTH, PTHrP, ionized calcium, and vitamin D concentrations in the most common causes of hypercalcemia in dogs.

increased. An ionized serum calcium concentration may also be useful (see Figs. 149–3 and 149–4).

Ionized Serum Calcium Concentration

The biologically active form of calcium within the circulation is its ionized fraction. Measurement of serum ionized calcium concentration has become more available and cost-effective (normal or reference concentrations for our laboratory are 1.02 to 1.32 mmol/L). In hypercalcemia due to PHPTH or secondary to malignancy, the serum ionized calcium concentration is increased. In dogs with chronic renal failure, less than 10 per cent had increased, 40 per cent had decreased, and greater than 50 per cent had normal serum ionized calcium values.[6] In hypocalcemia due to hypoalbuminemia, the serum ionized calcium concentration is normal.

Vitamin D Concentration

Serum 25 [OH] vitamin D and 1,25 [OH]$_2$ vitamin D assays are becoming available, but their clinical usefulness in veterinary medicine remains to be fully investigated.

Parathyroid Hormone–Related Proteins

The search for a PTH-like factor that causes the hypercalcemia of malignant disease led to the characterization of a novel class of peptide hormones. These peptides share marked N-terminal homology with PTH and have been referred to as PTH-related protein (PTHrP). This protein interacts with PTH receptors and has potent PTH-like bioactivity in vitro and in vivo. Many of the pathologic changes associated with malignant disease that resemble PHPTH are probably accounted for by this unique peptide.[7]

Simultaneous measurement of both PTH and PTHrP in the plasma may be especially valuable when attempting

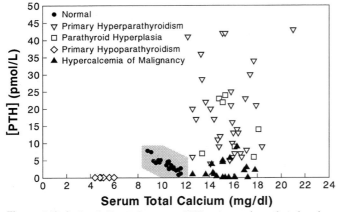

Figure 149–6. Graph illustrating serum PTH concentrations plotted against simultaneous serum calcium concentrations from normal dogs and those with abnormalities in calcium homeostasis. Note that the various groups are more distinguishable than would be the case if only the serum calcium or only the serum PTH concentrations were evaluated.

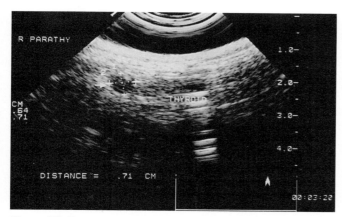

Figure 149–7. Cervical ultrasonogram of a dog with a functional parathyroid adenoma. Note the left thyroid lobe, in which a well-marginated, hypoechoic mass *(arrows)* is visible at the cranial pole of the thyroid. (Courtesy of Drs. Tom Nyland and Erik Wisner.)

to distinguish PHPTH from hypercalcemia of malignancy. Impaired renal function is associated with increased immunoreactivity to PTHrP fragments.[8] Several tumor cell types likely elaborate a PTHrP. The peptide is probably synthesized by transformed lymphocytes in hypercalcemic dogs with lymphosarcoma. The PTHrP-like factor has also been isolated from tumor cells obtained from hypercalcemic dogs with apocrine gland adenocarcinoma of the anal sac.[9–11]

ULTRASONOGRAPHY

The Neck

Normal parathyroid glands are not routinely visualized with ultrasonography.[12] Parathyroid nodules from most dogs with PHPTH were larger than 4 to 5 mm in diameter and were easily visualized.[13, 14] The masses may be round or oval, well marginated, and hypoechoic to anechoic compared with surrounding thyroid gland parenchyma (Fig. 149–7). The accuracy of cervical ultrasonography has been similar to that reported in humans, i.e., 80 to 95 per cent of parathyroid adenomas and a smaller percentage of hyperplastic parathyroid glands can be visualized. The experience of the operator and the sensitivity of the equipment are important factors.

The Abdomen

Ultrasonic scanning of the abdomen should also be a routine component of the diagnostic evaluation of hypercalcemic dogs and cats. If the liver, spleen, mesenteric lymph nodes, or other abdominal structures appear abnormal ultrasonographically, percutaneous aspiration or biopsy should be considered. The urinary tract, especially the bladder, should be evaluated for calculi, which are common in dogs with PHPTH.

ELECTROCARDIOGRAPHY

In our dogs with PHPTH, severe hypercalcemia has not been associated with significant changes in the electrocardiogram (ECG).

RADIOGRAPHY

Thoracic and abdominal radiographs should be obtained in an effort to identify occult neoplasia that is not readily demonstrable from physical examination. Abdominal ultrasonography may be more informative than abdominal radiography, although the two tests tend to complement each other. The cranial mediastinum and perihilar and sternal lymph nodes should be evaluated for a mass or lymphadenopathy—changes consistent with lymphoma. The skeleton can be evaluated for osteolytic areas due to myeloma or other metastatic tumors. The sublumbar area and mesenteric lymph nodes can be evaluated for enlargements that would support metastatic apocrine gland carcinoma of the anal sac or lymphoma. The liver and spleen can be evaluated for enlargement or irregularities associated with lymphoma. The urinary system should be evaluated for calculi. Lack of radiographic or ultrasonographic abnormalities in a hypercalcemic animal supports a diagnosis of PHPTH.

RADIONUCLIDE SCANS

In humans, technetium-99m-sestamibi radionuclide scans provide excellent results in localizing parathyroid adenomas.[15] This tool has been used successfully in a few dogs with PHPTH,[16, 17] although we have not had success with this procedure.

DIAGNOSTIC APPROACH TO THE HYPERCALCEMIC ANIMAL

Review of History and Physical Examination

The diagnostic approach to the hypercalcemic animal is straightforward (Tables 149–3 and 149–4; see Fig. 149–1). The first step should always be to confirm the presence of hypercalcemia by submitting a second blood sample for calcium and phosphorus determination. In addition, the calcium concentration should be corrected for alterations in serum protein and albumin concentrations. Review of the signalment, history, and physical examination often allows the clinician to identify the cause for hypercalcemia or to develop a list of high-priority possibilities. Both the history and the physical examination should be repeated following the serendipitous finding of hypercalcemia.

Signalment. Signalment (age, sex, breed) is emphasized,

TABLE 149–3. DIFFERENTIAL DIAGNOSES FOR HYPERCALCEMIA

Common

Lymphosarcoma
Chronic renal failure (mild hypercalcemia, when present)
Primary hyperparathyroidism
Hypoadrenocorticism

Less Common

Apocrine cell adenocarcinoma of the anal sac
Multiple myeloma
Other solid tumors
  Squamous cell carcinoma
  Thyroid adenocarcinoma
Hypervitaminosis D (rodenticide toxicosis)

Uncommon to Rare

Malignant mammary tumors
Nutritional secondary hyperparathyroidism
Acute renal failure
Blastomycosis
Septic bone disease
Hypothermia

TABLE 149–4. DIFFERENTIAL DIAGNOSIS FOR HYPERCALCEMIA OF MALIGNANCY

Hematologic Cancers

    Lymphosarcoma
    Lymphocytic leukemia
    Myeloproliferative disease
    Myeloma

Solid Tumors With Bone Metastasis

    Mammary adenocarcinoma
    Nasal adenocarcinoma
    Epithelial-derived tumors
    Pancreatic adenocarcinoma
    Lung carcinoma

Solid Tumors Without Bone Metastasis

    Apocrine gland adenocarcinoma of the anal sac
    Interstitial cell tumor
    Squamous cell carcinoma
    Thyroid adenocarcinoma
    Lung carcinoma
    Pancreatic adenocarcinoma
    Fibrosarcoma

in part, because of the remarkable incidence of PHPTH in the Keeshond. PHPTH is most common in dogs 8 years of age or older. Renal failure can occur at any age, but certain breeds are predisposed to familial renal problems. Young hypercalcemic dogs are more likely to suffer from renal failure, malignancy, or hypoadrenocorticism, whereas older females are more likely to have an apocrine gland tumor of the anal sac.

History. The owner should be questioned about the pet's diet, vitamin and mineral supplementation, and exposure to rat and mouse poisons or house plants that contain vitamin D analogues. One can attempt to determine whether the pet is in pain (lytic bone lesions). Questions regarding the presence of polydipsia, polyuria, appetite, and other general information are important. Generally, the more ill the pet appears, the less likely that it has PHPTH.

Physical Examination. After assessing hydration status and severity of illness, the physical examination should include careful palpation of peripheral lymph nodes and the mammary glands. Rectal, perirectal, and vaginal examinations are imperative in the identification of neoplasias, especially apocrine gland carcinoma of the anal sac. The veterinarian should gently palpate as much of the skeleton as possible, searching for an area of focal bone pain that could then be pursued with radiographs. The kidneys should be palpated in an attempt to assess size or irregularities.

Initial Database

Blood and Urine. The initial database should include a hemogram (complete blood count [CBC]), serum biochemical profile, urinalysis, and thoracic radiographs. The abdomen should be evaluated with ultrasonography and/or radiographs. If the serum phosphorus concentration is normal or low, renal failure and rodenticide toxicosis are unlikely. Dogs with hypoadrenocorticism usually have hyperkalemia, hyponatremia, uremia, and hyperphosphatemia. If the serum phosphorus concentration is increased and renal function is normal, bone osteolysis from metastatic disease should be considered. Low, low-normal, or normal serum phosphate concentrations are consistent with PHPTH and malignancy-associated hypercalcemia (see Fig. 149–2). Striking increases in total protein concentrations in hypercalcemic animals,

specifically due to a monoclonal spike, are classic for multiple myeloma.

Primary Parathyroid Disease Versus Primary Renal Disease. A diagnostic dilemma exists when hyperphosphatemia and hypercalcemia coexist with azotemia. The clinician must determine whether the hypercalcemia is the cause or the consequence of renal disease. Other abnormalities in the initial database may support renal failure as the primary problem. These abnormalities include nonregenerative anemia, isosthenuria, proteinuria, and/or palpably or radiographically small and irregular kidneys. If the hypercalcemia dissipates with aggressive fluid therapy and diuresis, PHPTH is less likely than primary renal failure. Serum ionized calcium concentrations tend to be normal or decreased in dogs with renal failure but are increased in PHPTH (see Figs. 149–4 and 149–5). Further, dogs with renal failure and hypercalcemia usually have total serum calcium concentrations less than 12.5 mg/dL. Dogs with PHPTH and secondary renal disease typically have total serum calcium concentrations in excess of 13 mg/dL.

Radiography and Ultrasonography. Radiographs of the thorax and ultrasonography of the abdomen should be evaluated for soft tissue masses, tissue calcification (most common with hypervitaminosis D or renal failure), evidence of fungal disease, organomegaly, osteolysis, and/or osteoporosis. The goal is to identify an abnormal area that could be biopsied to definitively explain the hypercalcemia. A cranial mediastinal mass is demonstrable radiographically in as many as 40 to 50 per cent of hypercalcemic dogs with lymphosarcoma.[18] Biopsy of an enlarged liver or spleen may be warranted. Adenocarcinomas derived from the apocrine glands of the anal sac may appear radiographically as sublumbar lymphadenopathy due to tumor metastasis.[19] Discrete lytic lesions in the vertebrae or long bones are consistent with either myeloma or malignancy-associated hypercalcemia. Radionuclide bone scans can be performed to help identify focal bone lesions not detected with plain radiographs. In either situation, biopsy provides the best opportunity of confirming the cause for hypercalcemia.

Ultrasonography of the cervical region is noninvasive and easily performed. Identification of a solitary mass within or near a thyroid gland would be supportive of a parathyroid adenoma.

Lymph Node and Bone Marrow Evaluation

Lymphosarcoma is the most common neoplasm associated with hypercalcemia. If the initial database has not established a diagnosis, evaluation of lymph nodes and/or bone marrow should be considered. If the dog or cat is relatively healthy, the CBC unremarkable, and the peripheral lymph nodes normal, lymph node aspirate or bone marrow aspirate is usually not warranted.

Specific Assays: PTH, PTHrP, Ionized Calcium

The availability of these relatively sensitive diagnostic tools improves our ability to identify the cause for hypercalcemia. Figures 149–4 and 149–5 review the expected results of these parameters for the various causes of hypercalcemia.

ACUTE MEDICAL THERAPY FOR THE HYPERCALCEMIC ANIMAL

The primary mode of therapy for severe hypercalcemia should be aimed at correcting the cause. In dogs and cats

TABLE 149–5. TYPICAL SERUM CALCIUM AND PHOSPHATE CONCENTRATIONS FOR VARIOUS CONDITIONS

CONDITION	TYPICAL SERUM CALCIUM (mg/dL)	TYPICAL SERUM PHOSPHATE (mg/dL)	TYPICAL CALCIUM X PHOSPHATE PRODUCT*
Normal dog	10	4.5	45
Primary hyperparathyroidism	15	3	45
Lymphosarcoma	15	3	45
Apocrine cell carcinoma of the anal sac	15	3	45
Chronic renal failure	11.5	10	115
Vitamin D toxicosis	11.5	10	115

*Aggressive therapy is recommended when the product of these two electrolytes exceeds 60 to 80. For most conditions causing hypercalcemia, emergency therapy is not necessary to reduce the serum calcium concentration.

with PHPTH, treatment involves surgical excision of the abnormal parathyroid gland or tumor. In these animals, however, the hypercalcemia is not an acute problem, and the calcium × phosphate product is usually well below 60. Products greater than 60 to 80 are likely to be associated with nephrotoxicity. Thus, the hypercalcemia caused by PHPTH, because it is associated with low or low-normal serum phosphate concentrations, is less worrisome and less dangerous than the hypercalcemia associated with renal failure or hypervitaminosis D. The latter two disorders are almost always accompanied by hyperphosphatemia, a problem that amplifies the potential for soft tissue calcification associated with hypercalcemia (Table 149–5). In dogs, saline, furosemide, and bicarbonate are the most commonly used and recommended agents in the management of hypercalcemia. If these therapies fail, glucocorticoids may be given.

SURGICAL THERAPY FOR PHPTH

Solitary Adenoma or Carcinoma. Eighty-eight of 104 dogs with PHPTH in our series had a solitary adenoma, four dogs had a solitary carcinoma, and five dogs had a solitary mass described as hyperplasia. Approximately half of the solitary tumors in our series were identified on the ventral surface of one thyroid lobe. If the tumor is not seen on the ventral surface, careful inspection of the dorsal surface of each thyroid lobe usually reveals the adenoma as a discrete structure on or within adjacent thyroid tissue (Fig. 149–8). "External" parathyroid adenomas have been easily removed without damage to surrounding tissue. In some dogs with "internal" parathyroid adenomas, surgeons have chosen to remove the entire thyroid-parathyroid complex from the affected side.

Enlargement of Multiple Parathyroid Glands. Only

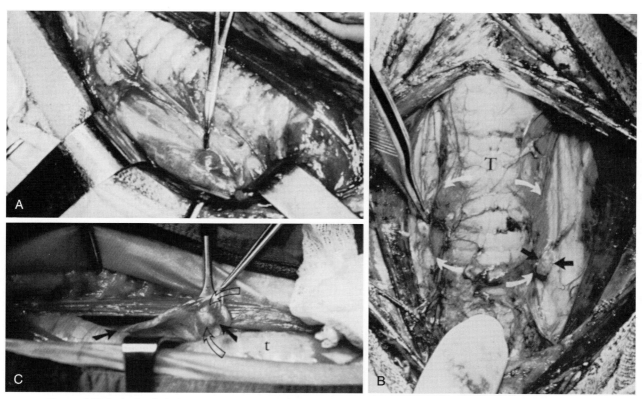

Figure 149–8. *A,* Surgical site during removal of a solitary parathyroid adenoma (tip of forceps). *B,* Surgical site during removal of a solitary parathyroid adenoma. T = trachea; white arrows delineate the cranial and caudal poles of the thyroid glands; black arrows point out the parathyroid adenoma. *C,* Surgical site during removal of an "internal" parathyroid adenoma. t = trachea; solid arrows delineate the cranial and caudal poles of the thyroid, which is being retracted from the trachea to reveal the parathyroid adenoma *(open arrows)* located on the dorsal surface of the thyroid. (From Feldman EC, Nelson RW: Canine and Feline Endocrinology and Reproduction, 2nd ed. Philadelphia, WB Saunders, 1996.)

seven of our 104 dogs with PHPTH (7 per cent) had enlargement of more than one gland. Two parathyroids from each of these dogs were described histologically as hyperplastic; in each of three dogs, two adenomas were removed during single surgeries. Only one of the seven, and therefore one of 104 dogs with PHPTH, had enlargement of all four glands.[20] These were diagnosed histologically as primary parathyroid hyperplasia. Enlargement of all four glands suggests either multiple adenomas or, more likely, parathyroid hyperplasia.

Recurrence of Primary Hyperparathyroidism. Four of 104 dogs with PHPTH had a solitary adenoma removed. Their hypercalcemia then resolved for a period of 12 to 19 months. Each then had recurrence of hypercalcemia caused by a second solitary, surgically removed parathyroid adenoma. Thus, it is possible for the disorder to recur, suggesting that periodic rechecks of the serum calcium concentration after stabilization are warranted. If these four dogs are added to the three dogs that each had two adenomas removed initially, seven of 104 dogs with PHPTH had two adenomas.

No Parathyroid Mass at Surgery. If an enlarged parathyroid gland is not found after thorough inspection of both thyroid areas by an experienced surgeon, the most likely diagnoses include hypercalcemia due to occult neoplasia, PTH production by a parathyroid tumor located in the cranial mediastinum, or the presence of a non-parathyroid tumor producing PTH (i.e., ectopic hyperparathyroidism). Careful exploration of the ventral neck should be completed, and any masses excised. Use of a new methylene blue infusion can also be considered,[21] although we have not tried this procedure.

POSTOPERATIVE MANAGEMENT OF HYPOCALCEMIA

Normal parathyroid glands atrophy if their function has been suppressed for prolonged periods. Physiologically, the long-term response to autonomous secretion of PTH by a parathyroid adenoma, carcinoma, or primary hyperplasia is atrophy of normal glands. Surgical removal of the autonomous source of PTH results in a rapid decline in circulating PTH concentrations (Fig. 149–9) and a corresponding decline in serum calcium concentrations (Fig. 149–10A). This process typically takes place over one to seven days. There is little doubt that postsurgical hypocalcemia is enhanced by the duration and severity of hypercalcemia before surgery.

Presurgical Serum Calcium Less Than 14 mg/dL.

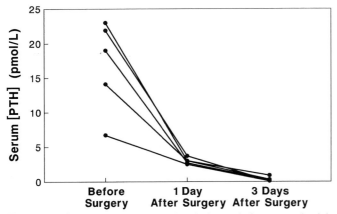

Figure 149–9. Serum PTH concentrations before and after surgery in eight dogs that had solitary functional parathyroid adenomas removed.

If the serum calcium concentration before surgery is less than 14 mg/dL, the risk of postsurgical hypocalcemia is relatively small. The recommendation is to hospitalize the dog for at least five days after surgery to monitor total and/or ionized serum calcium concentrations once or twice daily. Hospitalization also reduces activity by maintaining the dog in a cage or run. An active hypocalcemic dog is at much greater risk for clinical tetany than one kept quiet. If the serum calcium concentration remains above 8.5 mg/dL (ionized >0.9 mm/L), treatment is not recommended. If the serum calcium concentration declines below 7.5 to 8.5 mg/dL (ionized <0.8 mm/L) or if clinical signs of hypocalcemia are observed (Table 149–6), treatment with vitamin D (with or without calcium) is suggested.

Presurgical Serum Calcium Greater Than 14 mg/dL. The higher the presurgical serum calcium concentration and/or the more chronic the hypercalcemic condition, the more likely it is that a dog will become clinically hypocalcemic after surgical removal of a PTH-secreting mass. The recommendation is to prophylactically attempt to avoid hypocalcemia after surgery by beginning vitamin D (Hytakerol) with or without calcium therapy immediately following recovery from anesthesia. In some cases, we have begun vitamin D therapy 24 to 36 hours *before* surgery because of the known delay in onset of vitamin D action. This is important in dogs that are severely hypercalcemic before surgery (>18 mg/dL). Initiation of these treatments has not prevented decreases in serum calcium concentration to or below reference ranges. Postsurgical hypocalcemia has been seen in our patients as soon as 12 hours after surgery to as long as 20 days later. Most become hypocalcemic between the second and sixth days after surgery. The serum calcium concentration should be monitored once or twice daily. The goal of calcium and vitamin D therapy is to maintain the serum calcium concentration within the low to low-normal range (8 to 9.5 mg/dL) while preventing hypocalcemia and related clinical signs or the development of hypercalcemia.

Once the serum calcium concentration is stabilized and the dog has been returned to the owner, withdrawal of the supplements may be initiated. Vitamin D is usually withdrawn first, by gradually extending the time between administration (twice daily for two weeks, once daily for two weeks, and so forth). The serum calcium concentration should be checked before adjusting the dosing interval to ensure against development of occult hypocalcemia. If the total serum calcium concentration drops below 8 mg/dL, decreases in vitamin D supplementation should be delayed or the dose increased. The serum calcium concentration should remain above 8 mg/dL to minimize the risk of tetany. Once the vitamin D supplementation has been reduced to once weekly for a period of two to four weeks, it may be discontinued. If the serum calcium concentration remains within the normal range, the calcium supplements can then be gradually withdrawn. The entire withdrawal process for vitamin D and calcium usually takes three to four months. Because there is considerable individual variation in response to therapy, it is impossible to check the serum calcium concentration too frequently.

Vitamin D Resistance and Time Until an Effect Is Documented. We have encountered dogs, but more often cats, that seem resistant to vitamin D in tablet form. This problem has been quickly resolved by using the liquid form. It is not common for the drug to have an effect within the first 24 hours of therapy. Rather, vitamin D gradually takes effect during the first several days of therapy and almost always within seven days of the first dose.

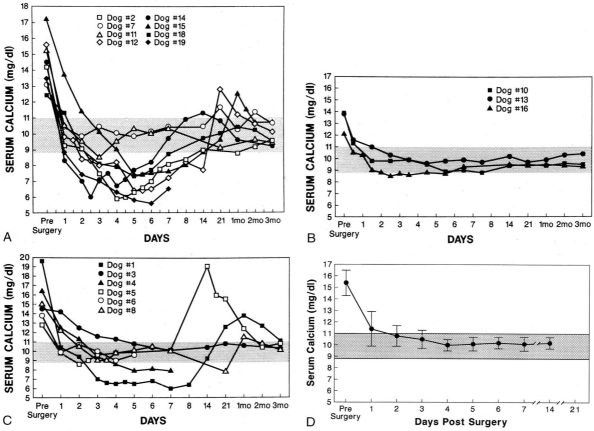

Figure 149–10. Serum calcium concentrations before and after removal of parathyroid tumors from dogs with primary hyperparathyroidism. *A*, These eight dogs were placed on vitamin D_2 and calcium supplementation after hypocalcemia was identified. *B*, These three dogs had mild hypercalcemia before surgery and were not treated with vitamin D or calcium after surgery. *C*, These six dogs began receiving vitamin D_2 and calcium immediately after recovery from anesthesia. *D*, These are the serum calcium concentrations from 34 dogs that began receiving dihydrotachysterol immediately after recovery from anesthesia.(*A–C* from Berger B, Feldman EC: Primary hyperparathyroidism in dogs. JAVMA 191:350, 1987.)

END

ALCOHOL INJECTION FOR TREATMENT OF PHPTH

We are currently investigating the treatment of PHPTH using an injection of ethanol into solitary parathyroid masses

TABLE 149–6. SIGNS NOTED BY OWNERS OF PRIMARY HYPOPARATHYROID HYPOCALCEMIC DOGS

SIGN	NUMBER OF DOGS (Total = 25)
Nervousness	25
Generalized seizure	20
Rear leg cramping or pain	25
Focal muscle fasciculations/twitching	15
Ataxia, stiff gait	14
Facial rubbing (intense)	14
Aggressive behavior	13
Panting	12
Weakness	10
Inappetence	7
Listlessness/depression	5
Biting/licking of paws (intense)	5
Polydipsia/polyuria	3
Weight loss	3
Vomiting	1
Diarrhea	1

Note that almost all these signs are "episodic."

identified on ultrasonography. This procedure requires a light plane of anesthesia for 10 to 15 minutes, involves no surgery, and has caused few side effects (in nine dogs treated, one developed a transient Horner's syndrome and one had a transient change in the sound of its bark). To date, this procedure has been an effective and permanent method of treating the condition. The response has been identical to surgical removal of a parathyroid tumor at less than half the cost, no surgical risk, and minimal anesthetic risk. The dogs are monitored and managed exactly as are those treated surgically.

PATHOLOGY

Histologic interpretation is subjective. Abnormal, autonomously functioning parathyroid glands from humans, dogs, and cats have been characterized histologically as adenoma, carcinoma, or hyperplasia. Unfortunately, controlled studies of histologic interpretations by pathologists have shown that it can be difficult to distinguish an adenoma from hyperplasia and that nonmalignant parathyroid tissue may, in some cases, have many of the histologic features of malignancy. Thus, histologic classification of parathyroid disease is dependent, to some degree, on gross features observed during surgery. The surgeon determines the number, size, and appearance of normal versus abnormal glands. The pathologist then determines whether removed tissue is parathyroid.

Single-gland involvement (adenoma) occurs in about 80 per cent of hyperparathyroid dogs and multiple-gland involvement (hyperplasia) in about 20 per cent. The diagnosis of carcinoma is based on a combination of gross appearance, histologic features, and, ultimately, biologic behavior of the lesion. Less than 2 per cent of autonomously secreting tumors in people are malignant, and a similarly small percentage has been seen in dogs.[22]

PROGNOSIS

The prognosis in PHPTH is dependent on the severity of secondary changes induced by hypercalcemia, specifically regarding renal function, and on the ability to prevent severe postoperative hypocalcemia. With proper monitoring and appropriate supplementation, hypocalcemia should not alter the prognosis. Of our dogs, 102 of 104 underwent surgery for removal of a parathyroid tumor. Only 28 (27 per cent) of these dogs developed clinically significant hypocalcemia. The routine use of vitamin D (dihydrotachysterol) and calcium supplementation has dramatically decreased the incidence of tetany. The presence of severe azotemia (BUN >70 mg/dL) is worrisome but relatively rare. Although normal renal function may return once hypercalcemia is corrected, some of these dogs require lifelong medical management for renal failure.

PHPTH IN CATS

Seven cats with hypercalcemia due to PHPTH have been described.[23] Their mean age was 12.9 years (range, 8 to 15 years); five were female, five were Siamese, and two were of mixed breeding. The most common clinical signs detected by their owners were anorexia and lethargy, in contrast to the polydipsia and polyuria seen in dogs. A parathyroid mass was palpable in three of the seven cats, and a fourth cat had a palpable mass that was not related to the parathyroids; an additional cat was recently described that had a palpable parathyroid tumor.[24] This is also in contrast to our experience with dogs.

The only consistent abnormality on CBC and serum biochemical profile from these eight cats was persistant hypercalcemia (12.1 to 22.8 mg/dL). One cat had multiple calcium oxalate uroliths. A systematic and logical search for causes of hypercalcemia was the focus of evaluation in each cat, just as in dogs. These problems were ruled out in each cat. The serum phosphorus concentration was low in two cats, normal in five cats, and slightly increased in one. Serum PTH concentrations were evaluated in two cats using the two-site "sandwich" assay. The preoperative PTH concentration was within reference limits in one cat and increased in one; both were abnormally increased relative to the concurrent hypercalcemia. The PTH concentrations decreased in both cats following surgery.

One cat did not have surgery, and necropsy demonstrated a parathyroid carcinoma. Solitary parathyroid adenomas were surgically removed from five cats, and bilateral cystadenomas were surgically resected in one cat. Serum calcium concentrations decreased into the reference range within 24 hours of surgery in all cats. None of the cats had clinical problems with hypocalcemia after surgery, although two cats became hypocalcemic. These two cats had the highest presurgical serum calcium concentrations and were treated with oral vitamin D and calcium. Both medications were tapered over a period of two to three months and discontinued. All six treated cats lived well beyond one year after surgery, although at 1.5 years one had recurrence of hypercalcemia and at necropsy was demonstrated to have both a parathyroid adenoma and a parathyroid carcinoma.

HYPOPARATHYROIDISM—HYPOCALCEMIA

Several historic landmarks in the understanding of parathyroid physiology, maintenance of homeostasis, and calcium regulation are significant with respect to our knowledge of hypocalcemia. Rickets (hypovitaminosis D) was first described in 1645. More than 200 years later (1884), an association was made between thyroidectomy in dogs and cats and the development of clinical hypocalcemia (tetany). In 1891, Gley proved that the parathyroids must be removed with the thyroids to produce tetany. Shortly thereafter, administration of calcium salts following parathyroidectomy was demonstrated to prevent tetany.

Primary hypoparathyroidism is an uncommon endocrine disorder. The condition develops as a result of an absolute or relative deficiency of PTH, which causes various physiologic problems. The final common pathway to clinical signs involves those neurologic and neuromuscular disturbances resulting from hypocalcemia. The signs of hypocalcemia are similar, regardless of the etiology (see Table 149–6).

PATHOPHYSIOLOGY

Initial Physiologic Alterations

Cessation of parathyroid function leads to a decrease in serum calcium concentration and an increase in plasma phosphate concentration. Urinary calcium and phosphate excretion diminishes. These changes are due to loss of PTH effects on mobilization of calcium and phosphate from bone, retention of calcium and enhanced excretion of phosphate by kidneys, and increased absorption of calcium and phosphate from intestine.

Neuromuscular Activity

Ionized calcium is involved in the release of acetylcholine during neuromuscular transmission. Calcium is essential for muscle contraction, and it stabilizes nerve cell membranes by decreasing their permeability to sodium. Calcium's role as a membrane stabilizer is most obvious during severe hypocalcemia. When the extracellular concentration of calcium ion declines to subnormal levels, the nervous system becomes progressively more excitable owing to increased neuronal membrane permeability. Nerve fibers begin to discharge spontaneously, initiating impulses to peripheral skeletal muscles, where they elicit tetanic contraction. Consequently, hypocalcemia causes tetany. Dogs with untreated hypoparathyroidism have serum calcium concentrations consistently below 6 mg/dL. The onset of clinical tetany, however, is not entirely predictable.

In hypocalcemic pet dogs, "latent" tetany probably occurs. Owners mention that sudden excitement, activity, or petting unpredictably causes muscle cramping, lameness, facial rubbing, pain, irritability, or aggressive behavior. These signs sporadically recur. The nontetanic, severely hypocalcemic pet is often described by the owner as having a change in personality. Such signs are vague, but after hypocalcemia is diagnosed, the clinical signs are consistent with those of an animal in latent tetany. The various disturbances are completely and quickly reversible with therapy.

CLINICAL FEATURES OF NATURALLY OCCURRING HYPOPARATHYROIDISM—DOGS

Signalment

In reviewing the records of dogs in our series with naturally occurring primary hypoparathyroidism, the youngest dog was diagnosed at 6 weeks of age and the oldest was 13 years (average was 4.8 years), and 65 per cent were female.[32] The breeds most frequently identified as having primary hypoparathyroidism were poodles, miniature schnauzers, retrievers, German shepherds, and terriers.

Anamnesis

Duration of Illness. The clinical course begins with an abrupt onset of intermittent neurologic or neuromuscular disturbances. In several dogs, signs were initiated or worsened by excitement or exercise. Signs associated with hypocalcemia had been observed for only one day in some dogs and as long as 12 months in others. Many had been diagnosed and treated for nonspecific seizure disorders without the benefit of pretreatment laboratory testing.

Most owners reported that their pets were tense or nervous. Intense facial rubbing with the paws or on the ground was commonly observed but not usually mentioned by owners until specifically questioned. Additional signs included cramping and tonic spasm of leg muscles. Focal muscle twitching, generalized tremors, fasciculations, or trembling was frequently observed, as was a stiff, stilted, hunched, or rigid gait.

Seizures. Grand mal convulsions have been observed in 80 per cent of dogs with primary hypoparathyroidism. Some of this seizure activity was atypical because there was no loss of consciousness and the dogs were not incontinent during the episode.[25] More than 80 per cent of these dogs were observed, by a veterinarian, to have seizures or to be "in tetany." This represents a much higher incidence of veterinarian-witnessed neuromuscular signs than expected with most seizure disorders. The neuromuscular problems became so severe that several dogs, although not having seizures, were not able to stand or walk. Seizure episodes were as brief as 20 to 90 seconds and rarely more than 30 minutes. Most, but not all, generalized seizures spontaneously abated.

Facial Rubbing. More than 60 per cent of the dogs in our series were observed to paw or rub violently at their muzzles, eyes, and ears, as well as rubbing their muzzles on the ground. These signs are thought to result from the pain associated with masseter and temporal muscle cramping caused by the hypocalcemia or from a "tingling" sensation around the mouth. Classic signs of hypocalcemia in humans include paresthesias—numbness and tingling that often occur around the mouth, in the tips of fingers, and sometimes in the feet.

Physical Examination

Other than signs related to hypocalcemia, dogs with primary hypoparathyroidism have no classic abnormalities on physical examination. A few dogs were thin, and several growled when examined. Retrospectively, the growling dogs were in pain or were anticipating that handling would result in pain, because after resolution of hypocalcemia, each became friendly. Cardiac abnormalities were apparent in about 40 per cent of dogs on initial examination. These abnormalities consisted of paroxysmal tachyarrhythmias and muffled heart sounds with weak pulses. About half of the dogs appeared to be extremely tense, with splinted abdomens and stiff gaits. A smaller number had generalized muscle fasciculations and/or fever. Almost 50 per cent had generalized seizures during their initial examination, and more than 80 per cent had at least one convulsion during the initial 48 to 96 hours of hospitalization.

CLINICAL FEATURES OF NATURALLY OCCURRING HYPOPARATHYROIDISM—CATS

The clinical features of eight cats reported in the literature to have naturally occurring hypoparathyroidism are much like those reported in dogs. The clinical course for each cat was characterized by an abrupt or gradual onset of intermittent neurologic or neuromuscular disturbances that included focal or generalized muscle tremors, seizures, ataxia, stilted gait, disorientation, and weakness. Other commonly observed abnormalities included lethargy, anorexia, panting, and raised nictitating membranes.

DIAGNOSTIC EVALUATION

Serum Values

Severe hypocalcemia was a serendipitous finding in each of our dogs and cats with primary natural hypoparathyroidism (Table 149–7). Because therapy for hypocalcemia was quickly instituted, each animal had its serum calcium concentration monitored three to five times during the first 72 hours of hospitalization. In no dog or cat was the serum calcium concentration greater than 6.5 mg/dL until the therapy began to have an effect. Each dog and cat also had a serum phosphorus concentration higher than its calcium concentration, and all had normal BUN. The absence of an *absolute* hyperphosphatemia in some of the dogs can be explained in part by the wide variation in what is considered "normal" by veterinary laboratories. No other laboratory findings were common.

Electrocardiogram

Hypocalcemia prolongs the duration of the action potential in cardiac cells. The findings most consistent with hypocalcemia included deep, wide T waves; prolonged Q-T intervals; and bradycardia. No obvious ECG findings could explain the arrhythmias, weak pulses, or muffled heart sounds that were noted on several physical examinations.

PTH Concentration

Undetectable serum PTH concentrations in animals that are severely hypocalcemic confirm the diagnosis of primary hypoparathyrodism, assuming that the assay used is reliable and validated. Serum PTH concentrations may be detectable or low-normal in some animals with hypoparathyroidism if the assay used is quite sensitive. However, a low-normal or low value would not be normal in a hypocalcemic animal that has healthy parathyroids.

END

TABLE 149–7. PERTINENT FINDINGS IN DOGS WTIH PRIMARY HYPOPARATHYROIDISM

DOG	AGE (YEARS)	GENDER	DURATION OF SIGNS (DAYS)	SERUM CALCIUM (mg/dL)	SERUM PHOSPHORUS (mg/dL)	SERUM MAGNESIUM (mg/dL)	BLOOD UREA NITROGEN (mg/dL)	SERUM ALBUMIN (mg/dL)	PARATHYROID HORMONE (pmol/L)	PARATHYROID HISTOLOGY
1	5	F/S	3	5.7	7.3	—	14	4.1	—	—
2	5	F/S	30	4.1	5.4	1.9	31	3.1	—	—
3	5	M	30	4.7	6.0	—	8	2.9	—	—
4	4	F	7	4.5	5.9	1.2	17	3.5	—	—
5	10	F/S	1	5.2	7.0	2.1	15	2.9	—	Lymphocytic parathyroiditis
6	11	F/S	3	5.6	8.9	—	4	3.7	—	—
7	1	F	14	4.2	9.8	—	20	3.6	—	—
8	5	M	180	5.7	10.2	—	12	3.1	—	—
9	10	F	3	5.5	7.2	1.9	9	3.5	—	—
10	1	M	1	5.2	7.8	—	19	3.2	—	—
11	10	M	11	4.9	5.9	1.8	10	3.1	1.0	Lymphocytic parathyroiditis
12	10	M	1	6.0	6.3	—	13	4.5	0.1	Lymphocytic parathyroiditis
13	4	F/S	14	3.9	4.9	1.9	16	3.5	1.0	—
14	7	F/S	10	6.0	8.3	2.3	12	3.1	1.0	Lymphocytic parathyroiditis
15	9	M	4	3.6	5.8	—	9	3.3	0.05	—
16	0.5	F/S	2	3.9	8.4	1.9	11	2.6	0.1	—
17	13	M	6	4.2	7.1	—	15	3.6	0.1	Lymphocytic parathyroiditis
18	1	F/S	7	5.1	8.7	1.2	14	2.9	0.1	Lymphocytic parathyroiditis
19	0.5	F/S	7	4.8	10.2	2.0	22	2.5	—	Lymphocytic parathyroiditis
20	2	M	45	4.4	7.4	2.1	16	3.4	0.1	—
21	3	F/S	9	5.1	6.8	—	25	4.1	0.5	—
22	6	M	360	5.1	8.8	2.2	23	3.8	0.1	Lymphocytic parathyroiditis
23	8	M	3	3.9	8.3	1.9	19	3.7	0.5	—
24	12	F/S	2	4.6	8.5	2.3	18	3.7	0.1	—
25	6	M	3	5.5	8.5	2.2	19	4.1	0.7	—
Mean	6	—	30	4.8	7.6	1.9	15.6	3.4	0.3	—
Reference range	—	—	—	8.9–11.4	3.0–4.7	1.8–2.4	12–28	2.3–4.3	2–13	—

M = male; F = female; S = spay/ovariohysterectomy.

DIFFERENTIAL DIAGNOSES FOR HYPOCALCEMIA

The differential diagnoses for hypocalcemia are presented in Table 149–8 and Figure 149–11.

Parathyroid-Related Hypocalcemia

Naturally occurring hypoparathyroidism is a rare condition in dogs and cats. Iatrogenic primary hypoparathyroidism has been recognized in dogs and cats following thyroid, parathyroid, or other surgeries of the neck.

Magnesium deficiency can cause hypocalcemia. Severe hypomagnesemia in humans can result in a condition characterized by being refractory to PTH or it inhibits synthesis or secretion of PTH.

Acute Renal Failure and Ethylene Glycol Toxicity

Acute renal failure, such as occurs with urethral obstruction or ethylene glycol poisoning, results in abrupt and severe increases in serum phosphate concentration. An acute increase in serum phosphate concentration causes a reduction in serum calcium concentration. This hypocalcemia may be exaggerated in acute renal failure, because the rapid progression of these disturbances blunts compensatory mechanisms. Cats with long-standing urethral obstruction and hyperphosphatemia often have associated hypocalcemia, hyperkalemia, azotemia, and sometimes seizures.[26] Ethylene glycol intoxication can cause severe renal failure, acidosis, and death. The metabolites of this toxin can chelate serum calcium ions and cause tetany.

Chronic Renal Failure, Hypoalbuminemia, Pancreatitis

Chronic renal failure is an extremely common disorder in dogs and cats, usually causing increased serum phosphate and normal serum calcium concentrations. However, either hypocalcemia or hypercalcemia may occur in animals with chronic renal failure. Serum ionized calcium concentrations from animals with renal failure are usually low-normal to low.[6] Reductions in total serum protein and/or albumin concentrations are encountered in a variety of disorders in veterinary medicine. Reductions in circulating albumin causes a decrease in the protein-bound fraction of circulating calcium. However, ionized calcium concentrations are typically normal. Hypocalcemia, when it occurs in dogs with acute pancreatitis, is usually mild and subclinical. Coexisting acidosis, which is commonly present, increases the amount of serum calcium that is ionized and further limits any chance of tetany.

Puerperal Tetany (Eclampsia)

Eclampsia is an acute life-threatening condition caused by extreme hypocalcemia in lactating bitches and queens. In most studies, eclampsic dogs are severely hypocalcemic (<6.5 mg/dL). Eclampsia is most common in small dogs,

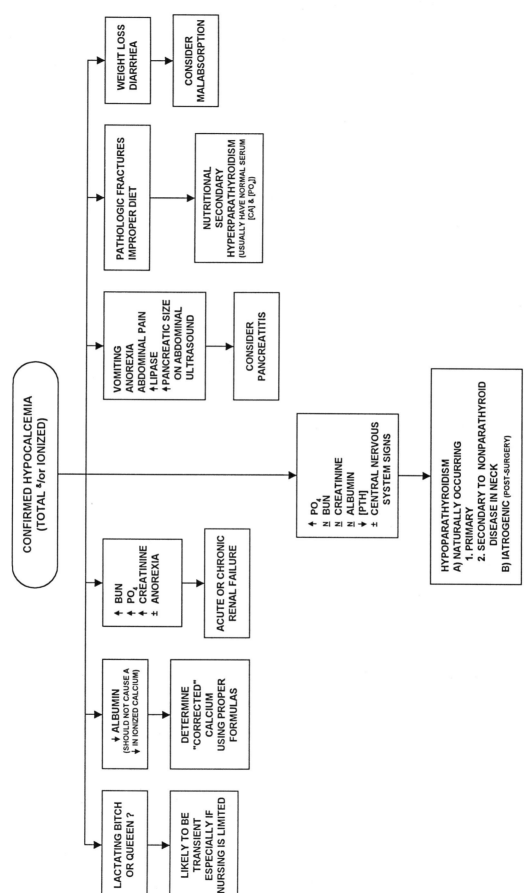

Figure 149–11. Algorithm illustrating the most common differential diagnoses for hypocalcemia and several features that help identify each syndrome.

END

TABLE 149–8. DIFFERENTIAL DIAGNOSIS OF HYPOCALCEMIA

Parathyroid-related hypocalcemia
  Primary hypoparathyroidism
    Destruction of glands
      Immune-mediated process
      Iatrogenic: surgical complication
      Any disease in neck causing damage
    Idiopathic atrophy (autoimmune process?)
  Pseudohypoparathyroidsm
Chronic renal failure
Hypoalbuminemia
Acute pancreatitis
Puerperal tetany (eclampsia)
Intestinal malabsorption syndromes
Nutritional secondary hyperparathyroidism (rare)
Anticonvulsant therapy
Acute renal failure
Ethylene glycol toxicity
Phosphate-containing enemas
Miscellaneous diagnoses
  Laboratory error
  Use of EDTA-anticoagulated blood
  Vitamin D deficiency
  Transfusion using citrated blood
  Soft tissue trauma
  Medullary carcinoma of the thyroid
  Primary and metastatic bone tumors
  Cancer chemotherapy

being less common in cats and large dogs. Neuromuscular signs in a lactating bitch or queen should be assumed to be caused by hypocalcemia unless proved otherwise.

Nutritional Secondary Hyperparathyroidism

Dogs and cats fed diets containing low calcium-to-phosphorus ratios, such as beef heart or liver, can develop severe mineral deficiencies. Dietary calcium deficiency results in transient decreases in serum calcium concentration, inducing increased PTH secretion, reduction in bone mass as calcium is removed from bone to replace that lacking in the diet, and diffuse skeletal disorders. These problems include bone pain and pathologic fractures. The skeletal disturbances are the result of an attempt to maintain serum mineral homeostasis.

Usually these animals have normal serum concentrations of both calcium and phosphorus. Rarely, an animal may be hypocalcemic. These dogs and cats are treated by providing balanced diets and restricting activity until skeletal remodeling is complete. Diagnosis is based on recognizing skeletal disorders in a dog or cat receiving an improper diet. Neuromuscular problems (tetany) are not a major component of the history.

Phosphate-Containing Enemas

Commercial phosphate-containing enemas may result in acute, marked hyperphosphatemia following colonic absorption of the enema solution, especially when administered to dehydrated cats with colonic atony and mucosal disruption.

Miscellaneous Causes of Hypocalcemia

These rare problems include laboratory error, vitamin D deficiency, use of citrated blood, trauma, medullary carcinoma of the thyroid, primary and metastatic bone tumors, and some forms of chemotherapy.

THERAPY FOR HYPOPARATHYROIDISM AND HYPOCALCEMIA

Emergency Therapy for Tetany

In the event that a practitioner is treating a seizing animal without a specific diagnosis, diazepam is the initial drug usually chosen to control the signs. However, if this treatment fails or if a diagnosis is still not obvious, blood should be drawn for glucose, calcium, and any other parameter that may lead to a definitive diagnosis.

Hypocalcemic tetany requires immediate replacement of calcium. Calcium should be administered intravenously, slowly, to effect. The dose is 1 to 1.5 mL/kg or 5 to 15 mg/kg, administered slowly over a 10- to 30-minute period. Calcium gluconate, as a 10 per cent solution (Table 149–9), is recommended because, unlike calcium chloride, calcium gluconate extravasating outside a vein is not caustic. Calcium chloride can cause not only tremendous tissue death

TABLE 149–9. CALCIUM PREPARATIONS

	PREPARATIONS AVAILABLE	APPROXIMATE CALCIUM CONTENT	DOSE
Oral			
Calcium carbonate/gluconate	Chewable tablets: 700 mg	250 mg Ca/tablet	Cats: 0.5–1 g/day
Calcium gluconate	Tablets: 325 mg	30 mg Ca/tablet	Dogs: 1–4 g/day
	500 mg	45 mg Ca/tablet	
	650 mg	60 mg Ca/tablet	
	1000 mg	90 mg Ca/tablet	
Calcium lactate	Tablets: 325 mg	42 mg Ca/tablet	
	650 mg	85 mg Ca/tablet	
Calcium carbonate	Capsules: 500 mg	145 mg Ca + 155 mg P/capsule	
	650 mg	190 mg Ca + 148 mg P/capsule	
	Tablets: 650 mg	190 mg Ca + 148 mg P/tablet	
	1000 mg	295 mg Ca + 228 mg P/tablet	
Calcium glubionate	Syrup: 360 mg/mL	20 mg Ca/mL	
Injectable			
Calcium gluconate (IV, SQ)	10% solution, 10-mL ampule	9.3 mg Ca/mL	1–1.5 mL/kg; 5–15 mg/kg; slowly
Calcium chloride (IV)	10% solution, 10-mL ampule	27.2 mg Ca.mL	Not recommended
Calcium gluceptate (calcium glucoheptonate) (IV, IM)	22% solution, 5 mL ampule	18 mg Ca/mL	—

Ca = calcium; P = phosphate; IV = intravenous; SQ = subcutaneous; IM = intramuscular.

and sloughing but also calcinosis cutis.[27] Electrocardiographic monitoring is advisable; if bradycardia, premature ventricular complexes, or shortening of the Q-T interval is observed, the intravenous infusion should be briefly discontinued.[28] This rapid emergency therapy is invariably successful, with a response noted within minutes of initiating the infusion. However, the final dose needed to control tetany is somewhat unpredictable. The recommendation is to use the suggested dose (in mg/kg) as a guideline and patient response as the definitive factor in determining the volume administered.

Infusion of calcium-rich fluids should proceed with caution in a dog or cat with hyperphosphatemia. This complication is extremely unusual. The additional calcium could result in mineralization of soft tissue. More importantly, further damage to the kidneys may occur in animals with coexisting renal insufficiency or failure.[26]

Fever

Fever frequently accompanies tetany. It is not unusual to have a dog or cat in tetany with a rectal temperature above 105°F. Veterinarians may be tempted to treat both the hypocalcemia and the fever (with ice or alcohol baths; parenteral drugs). It is recommended, however, that with institution of calcium therapy, one should monitor but not treat fever. Fever usually dissipates rapidly with control of tetany. Additional measures to lower body temperature may result in hypothermia and the development of shock.

Post-Tetany Short-Term Maintenance

Once signs of hypocalcemic tetany are controlled with intravenous calcium, the effects of the infusion persist for only 1 to 12 hours. Long-term maintenance therapy with oral vitamin D and oral calcium supplementation usually requires a minimum of 24 to 96 hours, or longer, before an effect is achieved. Hypocalcemic animals therefore need some calcium support during the initial post-tetany period.

Subcutaneous Calcium. Once tetany has been controlled with intravenous bolus calcium gluconate, administration of subcutaneous calcium is effective, simple, and inexpensive. The dose of calcium gluconate needed for the initial control of tetany can be given subcutaneouly every six to eight hours. The calcium gluconate should be diluted in an equal volume of saline. This protocol has effectively supported serum calcium concentrations while waiting for oral vitamin D and calcium to have effect. It is a procedure easily taught to owners, further decreasing their expenses.

After serum calcium concentrations have been maintained for 48 hours, the frequency of subcutaneous calcium administration should be decreased from every six to every eight hours. If serum calcium concentrations remain stable for the ensuing 48 to 72 hours, the calcium can be tapered to twice daily. This protocol is continued until parenteral calcium has been completely discontinued. Obviously, the tapering process in each animal may not be this smooth, as response to oral therapy is variable. Ideally, the serum calcium concentration should be maintained above 8 mg/dL. Serum calcium concentrations below 8 mg/dL indicate the need to increase the dose of parenteral calcium, serum calcium concentrations of 8 to 9 mg/dL suggest that the current dose should be maintained, and values greater than 9 mg/dL suggest the need to reduce the parenteral calcium dose.

Repeating Intravenous Bolus. One alternative to the management of hypocalcemia in the immediate post-tetany period would be intravenous calcium by bolus, as needed. This procedure is not recommended except as required in an emergency.

Calcium Supplementation in a Continuous Intravenous Solution. Calcium can be administered slowly, intravenously, via an infusion solution. Calcium gluconate is administered in the infusion to attain a dose of 60 to 90 mg/kg per day (approximately 2.5 mL/kg of 10 per cent calcium gluconate added to the infusion solution and administered every six to eight hours). The calcium cannot be added to a bicarbonate-containing solution because of precipitation problems. Serum calcium concentrations should be monitored once or twice daily, with the rate of infusion adjusted as needed.

Maintenance Therapy

Vitamin D

The need for vitamin D therapy is usually permanent in dogs and cats with primary naturally occurring parathyroid gland failure. Calcium supplementation, however, can often be tapered and then stopped, because dietary calcium is sufficient to meet the needs of the animal. Supplemental calcium in conservative doses, however, ensures that vitamin D, which raises serum calcium by promoting its intestinal absorption, has a substrate upon which to function. Iatrogenic hypoparathyroidism in cats that have had neck surgery is often transient, and lifelong therapy is not always needed. In contrast to treating tetany, when the immediate goal is to avoid recurrence of neuromuscular signs, the aim of long-term therapy is maintaining the serum calcium concentration at mildly low to low-normal concentrations (8 to 9.5 mg/dL). These calcium concentrations are above the level at risk for clinical hypocalcemia and below that which might be associated with hypercalciuria (risk of calculi formation) or severe hypercalcemia and hyperphosphatemia (risk of nephrocalcinosis and renal failure).

Vitamin D₂ (Ergocalciferol). Vitamin D_2 is a widely available, relatively inexpensive drug (Table 149–10). Initially, large doses are required to induce normocalcemia. Dogs and cats can be given 4000 to 6000 U/kg once daily. These doses are needed to offset the decreased biologic potency of this product in hypoparathyroid animals. Additionally, large doses are required to saturate fat depots quickly, because vitamin D is a fat-soluble vitamin. Effect of the medication is usually obvious 5 to 14 days after beginning therapy. Parenteral calcium can usually be discontinued 1 to 5 days after starting oral treatment.

Dogs and cats receiving vitamin D_2 are hospitalized, ideally, until the serum calcium concentration remains between 8 and 10 mg/dL without parenteral support. At this time, the pet is returned to the owner, and vitamin D is given every other day. Serum calcium concentrations should be monitored weekly, with the vitamin D dose adjusted to maintain a serum calcium concentration of 8 to 9.5 mg/dL. The aim of therapy is to avoid hypocalcemic tetany, but the most common problem with therapy is induction of hypercalcemia. Once the pet appears stable, monthly rechecks are strongly advised for six months and then every two to three months.

Dihydrotachysterol. The advantages of dihydrotachysterol versus vitamin D_2 are that it raises the serum calcium concentration more quickly (in one to seven days) and its effects dissipate faster when administration is discontinued. Therefore, the veterinarian has more control over the therapy.

END

TABLE 149–10. VITAMIN D PREPARATIONS

PREPARATION	DOSAGE FORM	COMMERCIAL NAME (MANUFACTURER)	DAILY DOSE	TIME REQUIRED FOR MAXIMAL EFFECT	TIME REQUIRED FOR TOXICITY RELIEF
Vitamin D$_2$ (ergocalciferol)	Capsules 25,000 U 50,000 U	Calciferol (Rorer) Drisdol (Winthrop-Breon) Deltalin (Lilly)	Initial: 4000–6000 U/kg/day	5–21 days	1–18 weeks
	Oral syrup 8,000 U/mL IM injectable 50,000 U/mL	Drisdol (Winthrop-Breon) Calciferol (Rorer) Vitadee (Gotham)	Maintenance: 1000–2000 U/kg once daily–once weekly		
Dihydrotachysterol	Tablets 0.125 mg 0.2 mg 0.4 mg	Dihydrotachysterol (Phillips-Roxane)	Initial: 0.02–0.03 mg/kg/day	1–7 days	1–3 weeks
	Capsules 0.125 mg Oral solution 0.25 mg/mL	Hytakerol (Winthrop-Breon) Hytakerol (Winthrop-Breon)	Maintenance: 0.01–0.02 mg/kg q24–48h		
Vitamin D$_1$ (calcitriol)	Capsules 0.25 μg 0.5 μg	Rocaltrol (Roche)	Approximate: 0.03–0.06 μg/kg/day	1–4 days	24 hours–2 weeks

Dihydrotachysterol is readily available and is more expensive than vitamin D$_2$ (see Table 149–10). This product is more potent than vitamin D$_2$, 1 mg of dihydrotachysterol being equivalent to 120,000 U of vitamin D$_2$.

Dihydrotachysterol is initially given at a dose of 0.03 mg/kg per day for two days or until effect is demonstrated, then 0.02 mg/kg per day for two days, and finally 0.01 mg/kg per day. As suggested with the less potent vitamin D, the pet should remain hospitalized until the serum calcium concentration remains stable between 8 and 9.5 mg/dL for several days. We have seen cats and dogs that appeared to be resistant to the tablet and capsule forms of this drug (0.125, 0.25, 0.4 mg) but responded readily to the liquid (0.25 mg/mL). Rechecks of the serum calcium concentration on a weekly basis allow dosage adjustment while avoiding prolonged hyper- or hypocalcemia. As with vitamin D$_2$, long-term rechecks at least every two to three months are strongly encouraged.

Hypercalcemia (>12 mg/dL) should be treated by discontinuing vitamin D therapy and, depending on the severity of the clinical signs and biochemistry abnormalities, possibly initiating intravenous fluids, furosemide, and/or corticosteroids. The lag period between stopping dihydrotachysterol and noting a fall in the serum calcium concentration is between 4 and 14 days, a much briefer period than that seen with vitamin D$_2$.

1,25-Dihydroxyvitamin D; Calcitriol. This drug offers the advantages of rapid onset of action (one to four days) and short half-life (less than one day). If hypercalcemia results from overdosage, it can be rapidly corrected by discontinuing the drug. Because 1,25-dihydroxyvitamin D does not require activation by the kidney, physiologic dosages should readily maintain normocalcemia in hypoparathyroidism, a state in which renal 1-alpha-hydroxylase activity is low. In contrast, pharmacologic doses of vitamin D$_2$ or dihydrotachysterol must be used to overcome this block in renal 1-hydroxylation. We have not used this drug for chronic maintenance therapy of dogs or cats with primary hypoparathyroidism.

Calcium

Initial Approach to Oral Calcium. Dietary calcium must be adequate when treating hypoparathyroidism, be-

cause the primary mode of therapy is the administration of vitamin D, which acts to increase absorption of calcium present in the intestinal lumen. There is usually sufficient calcium in commercial pet food to meet the needs of these dogs and cats. However, in order to avoid the catastrophic problems of hypocalcemia, especially early in the course of therapy, oral calcium supplementation is strongly recommended. Once tetany is controlled with parenteral calcium, oral calcium and vitamin D therapy should be started. After 24 to 96 hours, the parenteral calcium administration can often be discontinued, while oral therapy is maintained. In this manner, smooth, continuous control is achieved.

Calcium Supplements. Supplements can be provided by administering calcium as the gluconate, lactate, chloride, or carbonate salt. There are disadvantages of each. Calcium gluconate and lactate tablets contain relatively small quantities of elemental calcium, so that relatively large numbers of tablets must be given. Calcium chloride tablets contain large quantities of calcium but tend to produce gastric irritation. Calcium carbonate tablets also contain large quantities of calcium but tend to produce alkalosis, which may aggravate hypocalcemia. Calcium carbonate is 40 per cent calcium. One gram yields 20 mEq of calcium, and gastric acid converts the calcium carbonate to calcium chloride. Calcium lactate is 13 per cent calcium, and 1 g yields 6.5 mEq. Calcium gluconate contains 9 per cent calcium, and 1 g yields 4.5 mEq. Obviously, there are numerous calcium preparations available (see Table 149–10). Calcium carbonate is the preparation of choice in treating hypoparathyroid humans because of its high percentage of calcium, ready availability in drugstores in the form of antacids, low cost, and lack of gastric irritation.[29] No specific research is available to support recommendations for use of this drug in dogs and cats, although our success with calcium carbonate has been excellent.

Treatment Protocol. In cats, the dosage of calcium is approximately 0.5 to 1 g per day, in divided doses. In dogs, the dosage is usually 1 to 4 g per day, in divided doses. These recommendations are approximate, and the primary therapy that determines stability of the serum calcium concentration is the use of vitamin D. As the vitamin D dose reaches a steady level, the dose of calcium can be gradually tapered over two to four months. This method of treatment avoids unnecessary therapy, considering that dietary calcium should be sufficient to supply the needs of the pet and should decrease the demands of treatment placed on the owner. It must be emphasized that the ideal serum calcium concentration in these animals is 8 to 9.5 mg/dL. Concentrations above 10 are too high, are unnecessary in avoiding tetany, and increase the likelihood of unwanted hypercalcemia.

PARATHYROID HISTOLOGY IN HYPOPARATHYROIDISM

Animals have been classified as having idiopathic hypoparathyroidism when there is no evidence of trauma, malignant or surgical destruction, or other obvious damage to the neck or parathyroid glands. The glands are difficult to locate visually and are microscopically atrophied. Approximately 60 to 80 per cent of the glands are replaced by mature lymphocytes, occasional plasma cells, extensive degeneration of chief cells, and fibrous connective tissue. Chief cells are randomly isolated in multiple small areas or bands at the periphery. In the early stages, there is infiltration of the gland with lymphocytes and plasma cells, with nodular regenerative hyperplasia of remaining chief cells. Later, the parathyroid gland is completely replaced by lymphocytes, fibroblasts, and neocapillaries, with only an occasional viable chief cell. The final interpretation is one of lymphocytic parathyroiditis.[30, 31]

PROGNOSIS

The prognosis with primary hypoparathyroidism is dependent, for the most part, on the dedication of the owner and, to a lesser extent, on the experience of the veterinarian. With proper therapy, the prognosis is excellent. Twenty-one of our 25 dogs that have been observed have lived more than five years. However, proper management requires close monitoring of the serum calcium concentration, ideally once every one to three months once the pet is stabilized. The more frequent the rechecks, the better chance the pet has of avoiding extremes in serum calcium concentrations. The chance for a normal life expectancy is excellent with proper care.

REFERENCES

1. Aurbach GD, et al: Parathyroid hormone, calcitonin, and the calciferols. In Wilson JD, Foster DW (eds): Williams Textbook of Endocrinology, 7th ed. Philadelphia, WB Saunders, 1985, pp 1137–1217.
2. Harinck HIJ, et al: Role of bone and kidney in tumor-induced hypercalcemia and its treatment with bisphosphonate and sodium chloride. Am J Med 82:1133, 1987.
3. Bilezikian JP: Hypercalcemic states. In Coe FL, et al (eds): Disorders of Bone and Mineral Metabolism. New York, Raven Press, 1992, pp 493–521.
4. Mundy GR: Hypercalcemia of malignancy revisited. J Clin Invest 82:1, 1988.
5. Nachreiner RF, Refsal KR: The use of parathormone, ionized calcium and 25-hydroxy vitamin D assays to diagnose calcium disorders in dogs. Proceedings of the 4th Annual Meeting of the Society for Comparative Endocrinology, 1990, pp 27–30.
6. Chew DJ, Nagode LA: Renal secondary hyperparathyroidism. Proceedings: The Society for Comparative Endocrinology, 1990, pp 17–26.
7. Yates AJ, et al: Effects of a synthetic peptide of a parathyroid hormone–related protein on calcium homeostasis, renal tubular calcium reabsorption and bone metabolism in vivo and in vitro in rodents. J Clin Invest 81:932, 1988.
8. Budayr AA, et al: Increased serum levels of parathyroid hormone–like protein in malignancy-associated hypercalcemia. Ann Intern Med 111:807, 1989.
9. Weir EC, et al: Humoral hypercalcemia of malignancy in canine lymphosarcoma. Endocrinology 122:602, 1988.
10. Weir EC, et al: Adenyl cyclase stimulating, bone resorbing and B TGF-like activities in canine apocrine cell adenocarcinoma of the anal sac. Calcif Tissue Int 43:359, 1988.
11. Weir EC, et al: Isolation of 16,000-dalton parathyroid hormone like proteins from two animal tumors causing humoral hypercalcemia of malignancy. Endocrinology 123:2744, 1988.
12. Wisner ER, et al: Normal ultrasonographic anatomy of the canine neck. Vet Radiol 32:185, 1991.
13. Wisner ER, et al: Ultrasonographic evaluation of the parathyroid glands in hypercalcemic dogs. Vet Radiol Ultrasound 34:108, 1993.
14. Wisner ER, Nyland TG: Clinical vignette. J Vet Intern Med 8:244, 1994.
15. Taillefer R, et al: Detection and localization of parathyroid adenomas in patients with hyperparathyroidism using a single radionuclide imaging procedure with technetium-99m-sestamibi (double phase study). J Nucl Med 33:1801, 1992.
16. Wright KN, et al: Diagnostic and therapeutic considerations in a hypercalcemic dog with multiple endocrine neoplasia. J Am Anim Hosp Assoc 31:156, 1995.
17. Matwichuk C, et al: Double-phase parathyroid scanning with 99mTc-sestamibi for detection and localization of canine parathyroid adenoma (abstract). J Vet Intern Med 9:183, 1995.
18. Greenlee PG, et al: Lymphomas in dogs: A morphologic, immunologic and clinical study. Cancer 66:480, 1990.
19. Meuten DJ: Hypercalcemia. Vet Clin North Am Small Anim Pract 14:891, 1984.
20. DeVries SE, et al: Primary parathyroid gland hyperplasia in dogs: Six cases (1982–1991). JAVMA 202:1132, 1993.
21. Fingeroth JM, Smeak DD: Intravenous methylene blue infusion for intraoperative identification of parathyroid gland tumors in dogs. Part III: Clinical trials and results in three dogs. J Am Anim Hosp Assoc 24:673, 1988.
22. Berger B, Feldman EC: Primary hyperparathyroidism in dogs. JAVMA 191:350, 1987.
23. Kallet AJ, et al: Primary hyperparathyroidism in cats: Seven cases (1984–1989). JAVMA 199:1767, 1991.
24. Marquez GA, et al: Calcium oxalate urolithiasis in a cat with a functional parathyroid adenocarcinoma. JAVMA 206:817, 1995.
25. Peterson ME: Treatment of canine and feline hypoparathyroidism. JAVMA 181:1434, 1982.
26. Chew DJ, Meuten DJ: Disorders of calcium and phosphorus metabolism. Vet Clin North Am 12:411, 1983.
27. Schick MP, et al: Calcinosis cutis secondary to percutaneous penetration of calcium chloride in dogs. JAVMA 191:207, 1987.
28. Peterson ME: Hypoparathyroidism and other causes of hypocalcemia in cats. In Kirk RW, Bonagura JA (eds): Current Veterinary Therapy XI. Philadelphia, WB Saunders, 1992, pp 376–379.
29. Arnaud CD, Kolb FO: The calciotropic hormones and metabolic bone disease. In Greenspan FS (ed): Basic and Clinical Endocrinology. Los Altos, CA, Lange Medical Publications, 1991, pp 247–322.
30. Capen CC, Martin SL: Calcium-regulatory hormones and diseases of the parathyroid glands. In Ettinger SJ (ed): Textbook of Veterinary Internal Medicine, 2nd ed. Philadelphia, WB Saunders, 1983, pp 1581–1584.
31. Sherding RG, et al: Primary hypoparathyroidism in the dog. JAVMA 176:439, 1980.
32. Bruyette DS, Feldman EC: Primary hypoparathyroidism in the dog: Report of 15 cases and review of 13 previously reported cases. J Vet Intern Med 2:7, 1988.

END

CHAPTER 150

HYPERTHYROIDISM

Mark E. Peterson

HYPERTHYROIDISM IN CATS

Hyperthyroidism (thyrotoxicosis) is a multisystemic disorder resulting from excessive circulating concentrations of the thyroid hormones thyroxine (T^4) and triiodothyronine (T^3). First documented in the late 1970s to early 1980s, hyperthyroidism has become the most common endocrine disorder of cats and is one of the most frequently diagnosed disorders in small animal practice.[1, 2]

PATHOLOGIC FINDINGS AND POSSIBLE CAUSES

Functional thyroid adenomatous hyperplasia (or adenoma) involving one or both thyroid lobes is the most common pathologic abnormality associated with hyperthyroidism in cats.[1–4] In about 70 per cent of hyperthyroid cats, both thyroid lobes are enlarged, whereas the remaining cats have involvement of only one lobe.[1, 5, 6] On histologic examination, such enlarged thyroid lobes contain one or more well-discernible foci of hyperplastic tissue, sometimes forming nodules ranging in diameter from less than 1 mm to 3 cm.[2–4] Thyroid carcinoma, the primary cause of hyperthyroidism in dogs, rarely causes hyperthyroidism in cats, having a prevalence of approximately 1 to 2 per cent.[1, 2, 7] In addition, even when thyroid carcinoma is diagnosed in cats with hyperthyroidism, it tends not to be as highly malignant as the condition in dogs.

Although the thyroid pathologic abnormalities associated with hyperthyroidism in cats have now been well characterized, the pathogenesis of the adenomatous hyperplastic changes associated with the disorder remains unclear. A striking feature of hyperthyroidism in cats is that bilateral thyroid enlargement is observed in 70 per cent of cases.[1, 5, 6] Because there is no physical connection between two thyroid lobes in cats, it has been postulated that circulating factors (e.g., immunoglobulins), nutritional factors (e.g., iodine), or environmental factors (e.g., toxins or goitrogens) may interact to cause thyroid pathology in the cat.[4, 8–14] We undertook a case-control study to search for potential risk factors for this disease.[15] Owners of 379 hyperthyroid and 351 control cats were questioned about their cats' potential risk factors including breed, demographic factors, medical history, indoor environment, chemicals applied to the cat and environment, and diet. Two genetically related cat breeds (i.e., Siamese and Himalayan) were found to have a diminished risk of developing hyperthyroidism.[15] In addition, results suggested a two- to threefold increase in the risk of developing hyperthyroidism among cats eating a diet composed mostly of canned cat food and a threefold increase in risk among those using cat litter.[15] Thus, diet and other environmental factors may contribute to hyperthyroidism in cats, but further investigation is warranted.

Finally, studies also suggest that genetic factors may be involved in the pathogenesis of hyperthyroidism in both humans and cats.[16, 17] In human patients with toxic multinodular goiter (the human homologue of feline hyperthyroidism), the past few years have seen the discovery of mutations of the thyroid-stimulating hormone (TSH) receptor gene and, to a lesser extent, the alpha subunit of its associated G-protein that result in "gain of function." Such mutations result in continued stimulation of the cyclic adenosine monophosphate (cyclic AMP) pathway, which leads to both hyperthyroidism and hyperplastic or adenomatous changes of the thyroid gland.[16]

Only one group of investigators has looked for mutation of the TSH receptor gene among cats with naturally occurring hyperthyroidism but they failed to identify any mutations in the 13 cats examined.[18] However, in that study, they did not examine the entire receptor coding sequence for mutations, and therefore that study cannot exclude the possibility that such gain-of-function mutations of the cat TSH receptor gene occur in regions not examined.

Another study of hyperthyroid cats[17] demonstrated decreased expression (at the protein level) of a G-protein that is normally involved in inhibition of a wide range of G protein–dependent intracellular signaling processes, among them the signal to secrete thyroid hormone. The genetic basis of this finding and its possible role in the pathogenesis of hyperthyroidism are unclear, but it appears likely that altered G-protein expression may be involved.

CLINICAL FEATURES

Hyperthyroidism occurs in middle-aged to old cats; with a reported range of 4 to 22 years (median age, approximately 13 years). Only 5 per cent of hyperthyroid cats are younger than 10 years of age at the time of diagnosis. There is no breed or sex predilection.[1, 2, 6, 19, 20] Table 150–1 lists the most common historical and clinical signs recorded in 202 cats with hyperthyroidism that were diagnosed at The Animal Medical Center in the 1990s.[20] The clinical manifestations of hyperthyroidism in cats may be mild to severe and are affected by the duration of the condition, presence of concomitant abnormalities in various organ systems, and inability of a body system to meet the demands imposed by the disease. Because of the multisystemic effects of hyperthyroidism, most cats have clinical signs that reflect dysfunction of many organ systems. In some, however, clinical signs of one body system predominate and may obscure other features of hyperthyroidism. Because clinical signs of feline hyperthyroidism are so variable, the presence or absence of one sign can neither diagnose nor exclude hyperthyroidism. In addition, the condition may be misdiagnosed because of the resemblance of hyperthyroidism to many other diseases of the cat.

In most cats, the hyperthyroid state is slowly progressive. In addition, the fact that most cats maintain a good to excellent appetite and are active (or hyperactive) for their

TABLE 150–1. CLINICAL FINDINGS IN 202 CATS WITH HYPERTHYROIDISM

FINDING	NUMBER (%) OF CATS
Historical owner complaints	
Weight loss	177 (88%)
Polyphagia	99 (49%)
Vomiting	89 (44%)
Polydipsia and/or polyuria	73 (36%)
Increased activity	63 (31%)
Decreased appetite	32 (16%)
Diarrhea	30 (15%)
Decreased activity	24 (12%)
Weakness	24 (12%)
Dyspnea	20 (10%)
Panting	19 (9%)
Large fecal volume	17 (8%)
Anorexia	14 (7%)
Physical examination findings	
Large thyroid gland	167 (83%)
Thin	132 (65%)
Heart murmur	109 (54%)
Tachycardia	85 (42%)
Gallop rhythm	30 (15%)
Hyperkinesis	30 (15%)
Aggressive	20 (10%)
Unkempt	19 (9%)
Increased nail growth	13 (6%)
Alopecia	6 (3%)
Congestive heart failure	4 (2%)
Ventral neck flexion	2 (1%)

Data from Broussard JD, et al: Changes in clinical and laboratory findings in cats with hyperthyroidism from 1983 to 1993. JAVMA 206:302, 1995.

age usually makes the owner feel that the cat is in good health until obvious weight loss or other troublesome signs develop. On the other hand, as hyperthyroidism has become more commonly recognized, veterinarians are diagnosing it in more and more cats at an early stage of the disease even before most owners realize that their cats are ill.

General Appearance and Behavior

Most cats with hyperthyroidism show evidence of weight loss (see Table 150–1). Some have an unkempt haircoat, with excessive shedding and matting of hair. Cats with hyperthyroidism tend to be restless; may show a frantic, anxious expression; can be difficult to handle; and may become aggressive during the restraint of a physical examination.[1, 2, 19–21] Cats with hyperthyroidism tend to have impaired tolerance for stressful situations. In some cats, the stress of a car ride to the veterinary hospital together with the restraint of a physical examination may result in marked respiratory distress and weakness, with the development of cardiac arrhythmias (and even cardiac arrest) in a few cases. This decreased ability to cope with stress must be considered when planning diagnostic or therapeutic procedures.

Thyroid Gland

On physical examination, enlargement of one or both thyroid lobes can be detected in more than 80 per cent of cats with hyperthyroidism (see Table 150–1).[1, 2, 19, 20] The thyroid gland is not normally palpable. Finding enlargement of one or both thyroid lobes on physical examination cannot always be equated with hyperthyroidism, because gland enlargement can be detected in cats without clinical and laboratory evidence of the condition. Although some of these cats

may remain euthyroid (at least for prolonged periods of time), many cats with enlargement of one or both thyroid lobes eventually develop clinical and biochemical signs of hyperthyroidism as the thyroid nodules continue to grow and begin to oversecrete thyroid hormone.[22–24]

To palpate an enlarged thyroid gland, the cat's neck should be slightly extended with the head tilted backward. Using the thumb and index finger, one should gently pass the fingers over both sides of the trachea, starting at the laryngeal area and moving ventrally toward the thoracic inlet. The fingertips should remain within the jugular furrows; it is important to be gentle, because if one presses the muscle too hard, the nodule may be pressed into the muscle and difficult to feel. A thyroid nodule is usually felt as a somewhat movable, subcutaneous nodule or "blip" that slides or slips under the fingertips. Because thyroid lobes of the cat are loosely attached to the trachea, an enlarged lobe frequently descends ventrally from its normal location adjacent to the larynx. In hyperthyroid cats in which thyroid gland enlargement is not palpable, the possibility that the affected lobes have descended into the thoracic cavity should always be considered.[5]

Nervous System and Muscle

Increased circulating concentrations of thyroid hormone, presumably through a direct effect upon the nervous system, may cause behavioral changes in cats, including hyperactivity, restlessness, irritability, or aggression (see Table 150–1).[1, 2, 19–21] Even with careful questioning, however, such behavior may not be apparent to many owners. During physical examination, the hyperkinesis and aggression characteristic of cats with hyperthyroidism quickly become obvious to the veterinarian. Many of these cats cannot remain still even for the time it takes to complete a physical examination and become aggressive if restraint is attempted.

At home cats may aimlessly wander, pace, and circle, which may reflect a state of confusion, anxiety, and nervousness. Sleep may be abbreviated and cats may awaken easily. Although it is rare, a few hyperthyroid cats we have examined developed focal or generalized seizures characteristic of epilepsy; in all cats, the severity of seizures lessened or resolved after treatment of the hyperthyroidism.[21]

Weakness and fatigability, common complaints in humans with hyperthyroidism, are reported less frequently in cats (see Table 150–1). On questioning, owners may describe decreased ability to jump and fatigue associated with physical activity. In some cats, neck ventroflexion may be the only recognizable sign of weakness. With more advanced disease, cats may lie down or rest when moving from one place to another. In cats with severe hyperthyroidism, breathlessness is not uncommon, especially after exertion (see Table 150–1). In some of these cats with extreme weakness, thiamine deficiency and hypokalemia are possible complicating factors.[25] Although the biochemical basis for weakness in most hyperthyroid cats is unclear, the generalized muscle wasting that accompanies severe weight loss is likely to contribute.

Gastrointestinal System

Increased appetite and food intake are relatively common signs of hyperthyroidism in cats and occur in response to increased calorie utilization. In most cats, however, compensation is inadequate, and mild to severe weight loss develops (see Table 150–1).[1, 2, 19, 20] Although it is not always under-

END

stood, about 15 per cent of hyperthyroid cats also have periods of decreased appetite that usually alternate with periods of normal to increased appetite. Many of these cats that develop a poor appetite have concurrent problems, such as renal failure or cardiac disease (see Apathetic Hyperthyroidism).

Other gastrointestinal signs that occur in cats with hyperthyroidism include vomiting, diarrhea, and large volume of feces (see Table 150–1). Rapid overeating, common in the hyperthyroid cat, appears to contribute to vomiting which occurs shortly after eating. Intestinal hypermotility appears to be responsible for the increased frequency of defecation and diarrhea. Malabsorption with increased fecal fat excretion also develops in some cats with hyperthyroidism.[1, 6] Although the exact mechanism for steatorrhea is unknown, a reversible reduction in pancreatic exocrine secretion has been documented in humans with hyperthyroidism. In addition, it is likely that excessive fat intake resulting from polyphagia contributes to the increased fecal fat excretion that develops in some cats.[6]

Renal System

Thyroid hormones have a diuretic action, an effect that was reported in cats more than 50 years ago.[24] In accord with those experimental findings, polydipsia and polyuria are relatively frequent clinical signs among hyperthyroid cats (see Table 150–1). Although concurrent primary renal disease contributes to polyuria and polydipsia, these signs also occur in many cats without evidence of renal dysfunction in which resolution of polyuria and polydipsia usually occurs after treatment of hyperthyroidism. Although the precise cause of these signs in hyperthyroidism is unknown, the condition may impair urine concentrating ability by increasing total renal blood flow, thereby decreasing renal medullary solute concentration.[1, 26] This would cause polyuria and secondary polydipsia. Alternatively, in cats with normal renal concentrating ability, a hypothalamic disturbance caused by thyrotoxicosis may produce compulsive polydipsia with secondary polyuria.[1, 26]

Renal blood flow, glomerular filtration rate (GFR), and tubular reabsorptive and secretory capacities are increased in hyperthyroid humans and in animals given large doses of thyroid hormone.[1, 26–28] Results from one study of 13 hyperthyroid cats indicated that GFR decreased and serum creatinine concentrations increased 30 days after hyperthyroid cats were treated surgically by bilateral thyroidectomy.[29] Similar changes in GFR and creatinine have also been reported in eight cats with hyperthyroidism after medical treatment with methimazole for 6 weeks.[30] Another study found significant increases in serum creatinine and urea nitrogen in 22 hyperthyroid cats 30 days after treatment with radioiodine.[31] In that report, no significant decrease in GFR was found, but GFR was measured 6 days after treatment, possibly too soon for the GFR to fall. Those investigators did find that pretreatment determination of GFR was valuable in predicting which cats might develop renal failure after treatment.[31] Another study of 58 hyperthyroid cats found that the development of azotemia was not dependent on the treatment method used (i.e., methimazole, surgical thyroidectomy, or radioiodine), because serum creatinine and urea nitrogen concentrations rose to a similar degree in all three treatment groups.[32]

No specific renal pathology is associated with hyperthyroidism. Renal azotemia, although relatively common in the middle-aged to old cats that develop hyperthyroidism, does not appear to be caused by the hyperthyroid state. It is possible, however, that hyperthyroidism contributes to the development of chronic renal disease in older cats. Systemic hypertension accompanies hyperthyroidism. If failure of autoregulation occurs, systemic hypertension may result in intraglomerular hypertension and glomerular hyperfiltration. These factors are recognized as contributing to glomerular sclerosis and progression of renal disease. On the other hand, the increased renal hemodynamics associated with hyperdynamic circulation that accompanies untreated hyperthyroidism may be beneficial in maintaining sustainable renal function (and delaying the clinical and biochemical consequences of severe renal failure) in some cats with chronic renal failure.

The possible pathophysiologic relationship between hyperthyroidism and chronic renal disease raises important questions about the treatment of hyperthyroidism. It could be argued that reducing serum thyroid hormone concentrations in older cats with mild hyperthyroidism and chronic renal disease should be avoided because treatment may reduce GFR and allow emergence of azotemia and uremia. However, if increased GFR results in glomerular hyperfiltration in hyperthyroid cats, it may contribute to progression of renal disease. If so, hyperthyroidism may predispose cats to chronic renal disease, and early effective treatment of hyperthyroidism may be important to prevent pathophysiologic changes in the kidney that could lead to progressive renal disease.

Because chronic renal failure is common in aged cats, some cats with hyperthyroidism have underlying renal disease that is masked by the increased renal blood flow and GFR caused by the hyperthyroid state. In these cats, deterioration of renal function with development of clinical signs of renal failure could occur after successful treatment of the hyperthyroid state, even in cats that have normal (or only slightly increased) serum concentrations of urea nitrogen or creatinine before treatment. If underlying renal disease is suspected, treating the cats with methimazole until it can be determined whether correction of the hyperthyroid state would exacerbate the azotemia is prudent.

Respiratory System

Some cats with hyperthyroidism exhibit dyspnea, panting, or hyperventilation at rest (see Table 150–1).[1, 2, 19, 20] Such signs develop commonly after the stress of travel to the veterinary hospital and the restraint of a physical examination. The hyperthyroid condition can decrease vital capacity, decrease pulmonary compliance, and increase minute respiration.[33] These abnormalities in respiratory function probably result from a combination of respiratory muscle weakness and increased CO_2 production. In a few cats, thyrotoxic congestive heart failure also contributes to dyspnea and hyperventilation.[34–36]

Cardiovascular System

On physical examination, cardiovascular abnormalities, including systolic murmurs, tachycardia, and gallop rhythm, are fairly common in cats with hyperthyroidism (see Table 150–1). Less commonly, arrhythmias and signs of congestive heart failure (e.g., dyspnea, muffled heart sounds, ascites) may be detected.[6, 36] Radiographic findings may include mild to severe cardiomegaly, pleural effusion, and pulmonary edema.[6, 34, 36–38] Electrocardiographic abnormalities may include tachycardia, increased R-wave amplitude in lead II, various atrial and ventricular arrhythmias, and intraventricular conduction disturbances.[6, 37, 38] Echocardiographic abnormalities frequently found in cats with hyperthyroidism include left ventricular hypertrophy, thickening of the interventricular septum, left atrial and ventricular dilatation, and myocardial hypercontractility (manifested by increased shortening fraction and velocity of circumferential fiber shortening).[38, 39] Less commonly, echocardiographic evidence of a dilatative type of cardiomyopathy is observed with subnormal myocardial contractility and marked ventricular dilatation. These cats also usually have clinical and radiographic findings consistent with severe congestive heart failure.[36, 39] Postmortem examination has confirmed the presence of symmetrical hypertrophy of the left ventricular free wall and interventricular septum in most cats with either experimentally induced or naturally occurring hyperthyroidism.[34]

Although the exact pathogenesis of cardiac abnormalities associated with hyperthyroidism is unclear, cardiac changes may compensate for altered peripheral tissue function caused by thyrotoxicosis. Hyperthyroidism causes decreased vascular resistance and enhanced cardiac output because of increased tissue metabolism and oxygen requirements. Volume overload can be created by low peripheral vascular resistance coupled with reflex renal mechanisms that conserve fluid. The principal cardiac compensatory mechanisms in high-output states such as hyperthyroidism are dilatation (in response to volume overload) and hypertrophy (in response to dilatation). In addition, the direct action of thyroid hormones on heart muscle and interactions of T_4 and T_3 with the nervous system appear to be factors that influence cardiac function.

Studies of cats confirm that hyperthyroidism can induce a secondary form of cardiomyopathy—either a hypertrophic form of cardiomyopathy or, much less commonly, a dilatative type of cardiomyopathy. Either form of cardiomyopathy may result in congestive heart failure, but severe cardiac failure develops much more frequently in hyperthyroid cats with dilated cardiomyopathy.[38, 40] Cats with the hypertrophic cardiomyopathy and congestive heart failure often benefit from the judicious use of diuretics (e.g., furosemide) and beta-adrenergic blocking agents (e.g., propranolol).[38-40] Cats with the dilated form of congestive heart failure usually require therapeutic thoracocentesis, diuretics, antithyroid drugs, and inotropic therapy such as digoxin; because serious impairment in contractile strength exists in these cats with secondary dilated cardiomyopathy, beta-adrenergic blocking agents are usually contraindicated. In cats that fail to respond adequately, vasodilator therapy (e.g., captopril or enalapril) should be considered. After correction of the hyperthyroid state, the hypertrophic form of thyrotoxic cardiomyopathy is usually reversible.[39] In cats in which cardiomyopathy persists or worsens despite treatment, it is possible that the presence of excess thyroid hormone may cause irreversible cardiac structural damage, or underlying primary cardiomyopathy may be present.

Apathetic Hyperthyroidism

Apathetic or masked hyperthyroidism is a clinical form of thyrotoxicosis that develops in about 5 per cent of afflicted cats.[6, 19-21] In these cats, depression and weakness are the dominant clinical features. Weight loss remains a common clinical sign but is usually accompanied by anorexia rather than increased appetite. These cats also may have cardiac abnormalities, including arrhythmias and congestive heart failure. Ventroflexion of the neck, which may reflect severe

muscle weakness, may also be observed in these cats. Almost all cats with apathetic hyperthyroidism suffer from concurrent disease, such as renal failure, cardiac disease, or neoplasia.

SCREENING LABORATORY TESTS

Screening laboratory tests (e.g., complete blood count, serum biochemical profile, and analysis) should always be performed for a cat suspected of having hyperthyroidism (Table 150–2). Results of these tests may show alterations that aid in the diagnosis of hyperthyroidism. Even more important, however, results of such routine screening tests may reveal the presence of a concurrent disorder not directly related to the hyperthyroidism, a situation that should not be surprising considering the old age of most cats with hyperthyroidism. One must always remember to rule out concurrent disease, as well as disorders that mimic hyperthyroidism, such as diabetes mellitus, renal failure, cardiac disease, liver insufficiency, maldigestion and malabsorption, and neoplasia.

Complete Blood Count

Mature leukocytosis, eosinopenia, and lymphopenia are common hematologic findings in cats with hyperthyroidism and appear to reflect a stress response to thyroid hormone excess (see Table 150–2).[1, 2, 6, 20] The red blood cell (RBC) count, packed cell volume (PCV), and hemoglobin concentrations are usually in the high-normal to slightly high range in these cats. Although such erythrocytosis is generally mild to moderate in severity, a high PCV is found in approximately half of cats with hyperthyroidism. The erythrocytosis of hyperthyroidism appears to result from both a direct effect of thyroid hormones on erythroid marrow and increased production of erythropoietin.[41]

Serum Biochemical Tests

The most common serum biochemical abnormalities (which occur in approximately 50 to 85 per cent of cats

TABLE 150–2. ROUTINE LABORATORY FINDINGS ON 202 CATS WITH HYPERTHYROIDISM

FINDING	NUMBER (%) OF CATS
Complete blood count	
Erythrocytosis	106 (53%)
High MCV	63 (31%)
Leukocytosis	42 (21%)
Lymphopenia	81 (40%)
Eosinopenia	69 (34%)
Serum chemistry profile	
High ALT	167 (83%)
High AP	165 (58%)
High LDH	118 (58%)
High AST	86 (43%)
Azotemia	47 (23%)
Hyperglycemia	45 (22%)
Hyperphosphatemia	21 (10%)
Hyperbilirubinemia	7 (4%)
Complete urinalysis	
Specific gravity > 1.035	57/106 (52%)
Specific gravity < 1.015	3/106 (3%)

ALT = alanine aminotransferase; AST = aspartate aminotransferase; AP = alkaline phosphatase; LDH = lactate dehydrogenase; MCV = mean cell volume.
Data from Broussard JD, et al: Changes in clinical and laboratory findings in cats with hyperthyroidism from 1983 to 1993. JAVMA 206:302, 1995.

with hyperthyroidism) include increased enzyme activities of alanine aminotransferase (ALT), aspartate aminotransferase (AST), alkaline phosphatase (AP), and lactate dehydrogenase (LDH) (see Table 150–2).[1, 2, 6, 19, 20] More than 90 per cent of cats have at least mildly high activity of one of these enzymes.[1, 2, 6, 20] Histologic examination of liver usually reveals only modest and nonspecific changes, including centrilobular fatty infiltration and mild hepatic necrosis or degeneration. The cause of the high serum activities of these liver enzymes in cats with hyperthyroidism is not clear. Malnutrition, congestive heart failure, infection, hepatic hypoxia, and direct toxic effects of thyroid hormone on the liver may all contribute. Because only ALT is specific for hepatic necrosis in the cat, it is likely that other organs may also contribute to the elevations of AP, AST, and LDH concentrations. In accord with this, there is evidence that in cats, as in humans, both bone and liver isoenzymes of ALP are elevated in hyperthyroidism, with the bone isoenzyme being more consistently elevated.[42, 43] After successful treatment of hyperthyroidism, these high enzyme concentrations become normal within a few weeks.[44]

Evidence of concurrent renal dysfunction in untreated cats with hyperthyroidism is also fairly common, with mild to moderate elevations in serum creatinine and urea nitrogen concentrations being reported in over 20 to 40 per cent of cases.[1, 2, 6, 19, 20] Careful consideration should be given to the method of treatment selected for the hyperthyroid state in cats with concomitant azotemia. Deterioration of renal function with development of clinical signs of renal failure occurs in some cats after resolution of hyperthyroidism. In general, reversible medical therapy with methimazole (see Treatment) is usually favored as initial therapy for cats with concurrent azotemia. If no significant deterioration of renal function develops after medical control of the hyperthyroid state for at least 2 to 4 weeks, surgical thyroidectomy or radioiodine treatment for hyperthyroidism can be considered. If renal values worsen markedly with methimazole treatment, the dosage should be adjusted in small decrements to accommodate kidney malfunction as much as possible. In other words, patients are allowed to remain "somewhat" hyperthyroid. In occasional patients, treatment of hyperthyroidism must be discontinued because of worsening kidney failure.

THYROID FUNCTION TESTS

Resting Serum Thyroid Hormone Concentrations

High basal serum total thyroid hormone concentrations are the biochemical hallmark of hyperthyroidism. Resting serum concentrations of both T_4 and T_3 are abnormal in the majority of cats with hyperthyroidism.[6, 19, 20, 45] However, approximately 25 per cent of hyperthyroid cats have normal serum T_3 values despite clearly high serum T_4 concentrations,[20] making it clear that determination of serum T_4 is of greater diagnostic value than determination of serum T_3. Some cats with hyperthyroidism (reported range from 2 to 10 per cent of all hyperthyroid cats) have serum concentrations of both T_4 and T_3 that are within the high-normal range.[20, 46, 47] Because many hyperthyroid cats with normal serum concentrations of T_4 or T_3 have relatively early or mild clinical features of hyperthyroidism, it is likely that the normal thyroid hormone concentrations found in these cats would eventually increase into the thyrotoxic range if the disorder was allowed to progress untreated.

How can a cat develop clinical signs (albeit mild in many

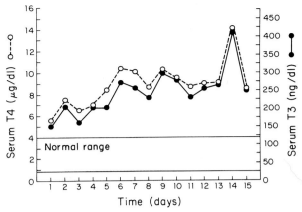

Figure 150–1. Serum T_4 and T_3 concentrations determined daily over a 15-day period in a cat with hyperthyroidism. To convert serum T_4 concentrations from nmol/L to μg/dL, divide the given values by 12.87. To convert serum T_3 concentrations from nmol/L to ng/dL, divide the given values by 0.0154. (From Peterson ME, et al: Serum thyroid hormone concentrations fluctuate in cats with hyperthyroidism. J Vet Intern Med 1:142, 1987.)

cases) of hyperthyroidism when serum thyroid hormone concentrations remain within the normal range? The finding of normal serum thyroid hormone concentrations in cats with clinical signs suggestive of hyperthyroidism can be problematic. Two explanations have been proposed to explain these findings: (1) fluctuation of T_4 and T_3 in and out of the normal range and (2) suppression of high serum T_4 and T_3 concentrations into the normal range because of concurrent nonthyroidal illness.

Thyroid hormone concentrations in cats with hyperthyroidism may fluctuate considerably.[48] In cats with thyroid hormone values well above the normal range, this fluctuation does not appear to be of clinical or diagnostic significance (Fig. 150–1). However, in some cats with mild hyperthyroidism, T_4 and T_3 fluctuation in and out of the normal range can occur (Fig. 150–2) suggesting that a diagnosis of hyper-

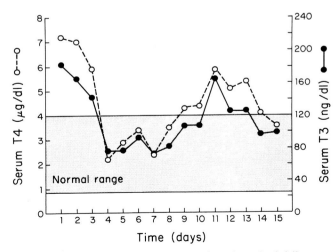

Figure 150–2. Serum T_4 and T_3 concentrations determined daily over a 15-day period in a cat with hyperthyroidism. Note the fluctuation in and out of the normal range for both serum T_4 and T_3 values. To convert serum T_4 concentrations from nmol/L to μg/dL, divide the given values by 12.87. To convert serum T_3 concentrations from nmol/L to ng/dL, divide the given values by 0.0154. (From Peterson ME, et al: Serum thyroid hormone concentrations fluctuate in cats with hyperthyroidism. J Vet Intern Med 1:142, 1987.)

thyroidism cannot be excluded on the basis of the finding of a single normal to high-normal serum T_4 or T_3 result alone. In cats with clinical signs consistent with hyperthyroidism (and especially in cats with a palpable thyroid gland), more than one serum T_4 determination could be required to confirm a diagnosis. This fluctuation in and out of the normal range may explain, at least in part, the finding of normal or high-normal serum concentrations of T_4 and T_3 in some cats with clinical hyperthyroidism.

In hyperthyroid cats with severe concurrent nonthyroidal illness (e.g., renal disease, diabetes mellitus, systemic neoplasia, primary hepatic disease, and other chronic illnesses), high-normal or only slightly high serum thyroid hormone concentrations may be found at the time of initial evaluation.[46, 47, 49] Because severe nonthyroidal illness would be expected to decrease serum thyroid hormone concentrations into the low to undetectable range in sick cats without concurrent hyperthyroidism,[47, 49] concomitant hyperthyroidism should be suspected in any middle-aged to old cat with severe nonthyroidal illness and high-normal serum T_4 and T_3 concentrations, especially if signs of hyperthyroidism are also present. In one study of the influence of systemic nonthyroidal illness on serum concentrations of T_4 in 110 cats with hyperthyroidism, nonthyroidal disease was diagnosed in 11 of the 14 cats with normal serum T_4 concentrations; of those, all but one cat had T_4 values in the high-normal range (between 30 and 50 nmol/L or between 2.5 and 4 μg/dL).[46] As opposed to the cats with mild hyperthyroidism that can show fluctuations of T_4 and T_3 into the reference range limits, some of these cats with severe nonthyroidal illness have moderate to severe hyperthyroidism. Upon stabilization of or recovery from the concurrent nonthyroidal disorder, serum thyroid hormone concentrations increase into the diagnostic thyrotoxic range.

When one suspects mild hyperthyroidism in a cat but the serum T_4 (and T_3) concentration is not high, the first step should always be to repeat the basal T_4 measurement and rule out nonthyroidal illness. Because there is greater variation in hormone concentrations over a period of days than over a period of hours,[48] we suggest that the second serum T_4 determination be made at least 1 to 2 weeks later. If the result is again in the normal to high-normal range and hyperthyroidism is still suspected, determination of a free T_4 concentration (by dialysis) or provocative testing with a T_3 suppression test or thyrotropin-releasing hormone (TRH) stimulation test is recommended.[47, 50–53]

Basal Free Thyroid Hormone Determinations

Circulating thyroid hormones can either be bound to carrier proteins or free (unbound) in the plasma. Most commercial T_4 and T_3 assays measure total concentrations, both free and protein bound. Because only the free fraction of thyroid hormone is available for entry into the cells, free T_4 determinations may provide a more consistent assessment of thyroid gland status than total T_4 concentrations.[54, 55] Also, free T_4 concentrations may not be as likely to be influenced by factors such as nonthyroidal illness or drug therapy that may falsely lower total T_4 concentrations. Free T_4 is most accurately determined by methods that include a dialysis step.[54, 55] In general, nondialysis techniques for free T_4 determination are less accurate, often underestimate the free T_4 concentration, and offer little advantage over the measurement of total T_4 concentration

The finding of a high free T_4 by dialysis is consistent with hyperthyroidism.[47, 56] Occasionally, however, cats with nonthyroidal illness that do not have hyperthyroidism have high free T_4 concentrations for reasons that are unclear.[47, 57] Therefore, to avoid a misdiagnosis of hyperthyroidism, free T_4 should always be evaluated in conjunction with the total T_4 concentration. In general, the combination of a high free T_4 value with a low total T_4 concentration (less than 20 nmol/L or 2.5 μg/dL) is indicative of nonthyroidal illness, whereas a high free T_4 value with a high-normal T_4 concentration (greater than 25 nmol/L or 3.0 μg/dL) is suggestive of hyperthyroidism.[47, 57]

Thyroid Hormone (Triiodothyronine) Suppression Test

Thyroid suppression testing is used to evaluate cats with suspected hyperthyroidism when simpler tests such as those of basal serum total T_4 and free T_4 concentrations are nondiagnostic. Inhibition of pituitary TSH secretion by high circulating concentrations of thyroid hormone is a characteristic feature of normal pituitary-thyroid regulation.[58] Normally, administration of thyroid hormone decreases TSH secretion; when exogenous T_3 is given to normal cats, this can be detected by a decrease in serum T_4 concentrations. In contrast, when thyroid function is autonomous (i.e., independent of TSH secretion), administration of thyroid hormone has little or no effect on thyroid function, because TSH secretion has already been chronically suppressed. This is invariably true with feline hyperthyroidism.

The protocol for the T_3 suppression test in cats begins with a blood sample drawn for determination of basal serum concentrations of total T_4 and T_3.[50, 51, 53, 56] This blood sample should be centrifuged and the serum removed and kept refrigerated or frozen. Owners are instructed to administer T_3 orally (liothyronine [Cytomel], Jones Medical Industries) beginning the following morning at a dosage of 25 μg three times daily for 2 days. On the morning of the third day, a seventh and final 25-μg dose of liothyronine is given and the cat returned to the veterinary clinic within 2 to 4 hours for serum T_4 and T_3 determinations. Both the basal (day 1) and postliothyronine serum samples should be submitted to the laboratory together to eliminate the effect of interassay variation in hormone concentrations.

When the T_3 suppression test is performed in normal cats, there is a marked decrease in serum T_4 concentrations after exogenous T_3 administration (Fig. 150–3). In contrast, when the test is performed in cats with hyperthyroidism, even in cats with only slightly high or high-normal resting serum T_4 concentrations, minimal, if any, suppression of serum T_4 concentrations is seen.

Regarding the interpretation of T_3 suppression test results, we find that the absolute serum T_4 concentration after liothyronine administration is the best means of distinguishing hyperthyroid cats from normal cats or cats with nonthyroidal disease.[50] Cats with hyperthyroidism have postliothyronine serum T_4 values greater than 20 nmol/L (about 1.5 μg/dL), whereas normal cats and cats with nonthyroidal disease have T_4 values less than 20 nmol/L (see Fig. 150–3B). There may be a great deal of overlap of the per cent decrease in serum T_4 concentrations after liothyronine administration in the three groups of cats, but suppression of 50 per cent or more occurs only in cats without hyperthyroidism (Fig. 150–4).

Serum T_3 concentrations, as part of the T_3 suppression test, are not useful in the diagnosis of hyperthyroidism per se. However, these basal and postliothyronine serum T_3 determinations can be used to monitor owner compliance with giving the drug. If inadequate T_4 suppression is found

END

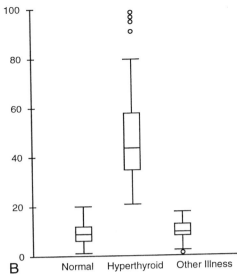

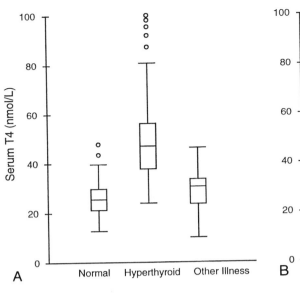

Figure 150–3. Box plots of the serum T_4 concentrations before (A) and after (B) administration of liothyronine to 44 clinically normal cats, 77 cats with hyperthyroidism, and 22 cats with nonthyroidal disease. The "box" represents the interquartile range from the 25th to 75th percentile (represents the middle one half of the data). The horizontal bar through the box is the median. The "whiskers" represent the main body of data, which in most cases is equal to the range. Outlying data points are represented by open circles. To convert serum T_4 concentrations from nmol/L to µg/dL, divide the given values by 12.87. (From Peterson ME, et al: Triiodothyronine (T_3) suppression test: An aid in the diagnosis of mild hyperthyroidism in cats. J Vet Intern Med 4: 233, 1990.)

but serum T_3 values do not increase after treatment with liothyronine, problems with owner compliance should be suspected and the test result considered questionable.

Overall, the T_3 suppression test is useful for diagnosis of mild hyperthyroidism in cats, but the disadvantages are that it is a relatively long test (3 days), owners are required to give multiple doses of liothyronine, and cats must swallow the tablets.[50, 51] If the liothyronine is not administered properly, circulating T_3 concentrations do not rise to decrease pituitary TSH secretion, and the serum T_4 value is not suppressed, even if the pituitary-thyroid axis is normal. Failure of a cat to ingest the liothyronine could result in a false-positive diagnosis of hyperthyroidism in a normal cat or cat with nonthyroidal disease.

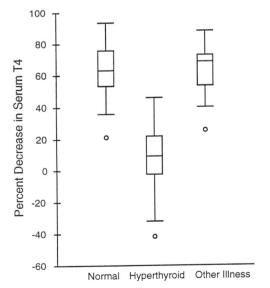

Figure 150–4. Box plots of the per cent decrease in serum T_4 concentrations (compared with pretreatment values) after administration of liothyronine to 44 clinically normal cats, 77 cats with hyperthyroidism, and 22 cats with nonthyroidal disease. Data are plotted (i.e., box plots) as described in the legend of Figure 150–3. To convert serum T_4 concentrations from nmol/L to µg/dL, divide the given values by 12.87. (From Peterson ME, et al: Triiodothyronine (T_3) suppression test: An aid in the diagnosis of mild hyperthyroidism in cats. J Vet Intern Med 4: 233, 1990.)

Thyrotropin-Releasing Hormone Stimulation Test

The TRH stimulation test measures the serum T_4 response to administration of TRH. In clinically normal cats, the administration of TRH causes an increase in TSH secretion and serum T_4 concentrations, whereas in cats with hyperthyroidism, the TSH and serum T_4 response to TRH is blunted or totally absent.[52] The lack of response is caused by the chronic suppression of TSH in cats with hyperthyroidism.

The protocol for the TRH stimulation test involves collecting blood for serum T_4 determination before and 4 hours after intravenous administration of 0.1 mg/kg TRH (Relefact TRH, Hoechst-Roussel Pharmaceuticals; Thypinone, Abbott Diagnostics).[52] Cats with mild hyperthyroidism show little, if any, rise in serum T_4 values after administration of TRH, whereas a consistent rise of serum T_4 concentrations (approximately twofold rise) occurs after TRH administration in both clinically normal cats and cats with nonthyroidal disease (Fig. 150–5). The serum T_3 response to TRH was less helpful in separating normal from hyperthyroid cats, because normal cats have either a small or inconsistent rise in serum T_3 concentrations after TRH administration.[52]

Regarding interpretation of the TRH stimulation test results, the relative rise (per cent increase) in serum T_4 concentration after administration of TRH was the best (most sensitive) criterion for determining whether cats are hyperthyroid (see Fig. 150–6). A rise in serum T_4 of less than 50 per cent is consistent with mild hyperthyroidism, whereas a value greater than 60 per cent is seen in normal cats and cats with nonthyroidal illness; values between 50 and 60 per cent should be considered equivocal (see Fig. 150–6).[52]

Studies have shown a close relationship between the presence (or absence) of suppressed serum T_4 concentrations in response to T_3 suppression and stimulated T_4 values in response to TRH stimulation.[52] Therefore, although the two tests evaluate the pituitary-thyroid axis in different ways, our findings indicate that the two screening tests provide similar information and can probably be used interchangeably for diagnosing mild hyperthyroidism in cats.

Advantages of the TRH stimulation test over the T_3 suppression test include the shorter time needed to perform the test (4 hours versus 3 days) and the fact that the TRH stimulation test is not dependent on the owner's ability to

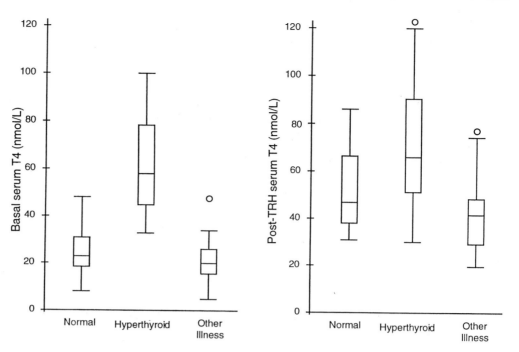

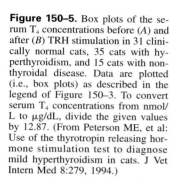

Figure 150–5. Box plots of the serum T_4 concentrations before (A) and after (B) TRH stimulation in 31 clinically normal cats, 35 cats with hyperthyroidism, and 15 cats with nonthyroidal disease. Data are plotted (i.e., box plots) as described in the legend of Figure 150–3. To convert serum T_4 concentrations from nmol/L to μg/dL, divide the given values by 12.87. (From Peterson ME, et al: Use of the thyrotropin releasing hormone stimulation test to diagnose mild hyperthyroidism in cats. J Vet Intern Med 8:279, 1994.)

administer oral medication. The major disadvantages of the TRH stimulation test in cats are the side effects (e.g., salivation, vomiting, tachypnea, and defecation) that almost invariably occur immediately after administration of the TRH. It has been reported that TRH evokes these effects in cats via activation of central cholinergic and catecholaminergic mechanisms, as well as by a direct neurotransmitter effect of TRH itself on specific central TRH binding sites.[59–61] Fortunately, all of the adverse side effects associated with TRH administration are transient and resolve completely by the end of the 4-hour test period. Therefore, at the discretion of the veterinarian, owners need not be exposed to the occurrence of these side effects in their cats.

Thyroid-Stimulating Hormone Response Test

In 1983, we reported that cats with moderate to severe hyperthyroidism were less responsive to administration of exogenous TSH than normal cats.[6] In that study, the cats with hyperthyroidism showed little, if any, rise in serum T_4 values after the administration of TSH, whereas a consistent rise of serum T_4 concentrations (doubling to tripling of basal values) was observed in clinically normal cats. On the basis of those findings, it has been suggested that the finding of a subnormal response to TSH administration may be helpful in confirming a diagnosis of hyperthyroidism in cats when the serum T_4 concentrations are within the normal range.

Mooney and colleagues[62] subsequently reported that hyperthyroid cats that have basal serum T_4 concentrations within the normal range respond to the administration of TSH with a rise in serum T_4 indistinguishable from that of normal cats. Therefore, although TSH response tests are useful for diagnosing hypothyroidism in cats,[24] the TSH test cannot be recommended for confirming the diagnosis of hyperthyroidism in cats with normal T_4 concentrations. In addition, TSH preparations are expensive and can be difficult to obtain.

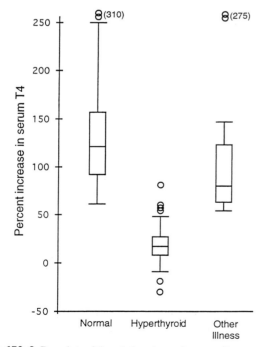

Figure 150–6. Box plots of the relative change in serum T_4 concentrations after TRH administration (per cent increase) in 31 clinically normal cats, 35 cats with hyperthyroidism, and 15 cats with nonthyroidal disease. Data are plotted (i.e., box plots) as described in the legend of Figure 150–3. To convert serum T_4 concentrations from nmol/L to μg/dL, divide the given values by 12.87. (From Peterson ME, et al: Use of the thyrotropin releasing hormone stimulation test to diagnose mild hyperthyroidism in cats. J Vet Intern Med 8:279, 1994.)

THYROID RADIONUCLIDE UPTAKE AND IMAGING

Thyroid imaging (scanning) is useful in the evaluation of hyperthyroidism because it delineates functioning thyroid tissue.[5, 63, 64] Although radioiodine (^{131}I, ^{123}I) and pertechnetate (^{99m}Tc) produce similar thyroid images in both normal cats and cats with hyperthyroidism (Figs. 150–7 to 150–10),[5]

END

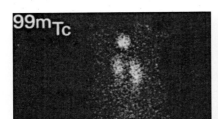
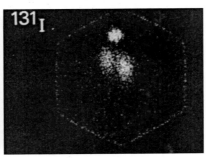

Figure 150–7. Thyroid scans of a normal cat obtained with $^{99m}TcO_4$ and ^{131}I. With either isotope, the thyroid lobes are symmetric in both position and size, with uniform distribution of radioactivity throughout the gland. A 2-cm² marker placed over the larynx is visible at the top of the scan. (From Peterson ME, Becker DV: Radionuclide thyroid imaging in 135 cats with hyperthyroidism. Vet Radiol 25:23, 1984.)

Figure 150–8. $^{99m}TcO_4$ and ^{131}I thyroid scans of a hyperthyroid cat with adenomatous hyperplasia of both thyroid lobes. Note that with both radionuclides the distribution of activity is heterogeneous, with defects in tracer uptake into the enlarged gland. (From Peterson ME, Becker DV: Radionuclide thyroid imaging in 135 cats with hyperthyroidism. Vet Radiol 25:23, 1984.)

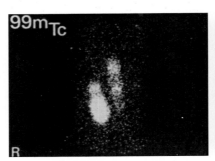
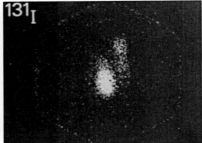

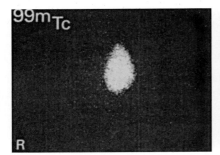
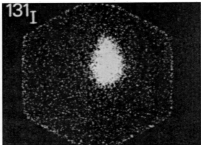

Figure 150–9. $^{99m}TcO_4$ and ^{131}I thyroid scans of a hyperthyroid cat with an adenoma (adenomatous hyperplasia) of one thyroid lobe. The left lobe is enlarged and has descended ventrally toward the thoracic inlet. Note that the uninvolved lobe cannot be visualized on either scan. (From Peterson ME, Becker DV: Radionuclide thyroid imaging in 135 cats with hyperthyroidism. Vet Radiol 25:23, 1984.)

TABLE 150–3. ADVANTAGES AND DISADVANTAGES OF TREATMENT MODALITIES FOR CATS WITH HYPERTHYROIDISM

FINDING	METHIMAZOLE OR CARBIMAZOLE	SURGERY	RADIOIODINE
Persistent hyperthyroidism	Low (dose related)	Rare	Low (dose related)
Complications			
Hypoparathyroidism	Never	Common	Never
Permanent hypothyroidism	Never	Intermediate	Rare (dose related)
Anorexia, vomiting	Common	Rare	Never
Hematologic effects	Rare (thrombocytopenia, agranulocytosis, serum antinuclear antibody)	Never	Rare (only with extremely high doses)
Neurologic damage	Never	Rare (vocal cord paralysis, Horner's)	Never
Hospitalization time required	None	1–3 days	1–4 weeks
Time until euthyroid	1–3 weeks	1–2 days	1–12 weeks
Relapse or recurrence	High	Intermediate	Low
Ease of treatment	Simple	Most difficult	Intermediate (not readily available)

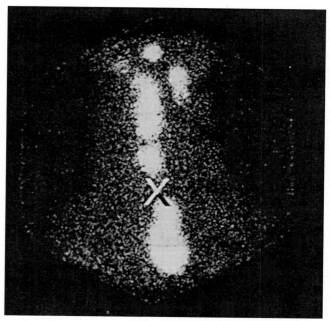

Figure 150–10. Thyroid scan of a hyperthyroid cat with thyroid adenocarcinoma. Note the multiple thyroid nodules that accumulate radioactivity and extension of the tumor into the thoracic cavity. X = thoracic inlet. (From Peterson ME, Becker DV: Radionuclide thyroid imaging in 135 cats with hyperthyroidism. Vet Radiol 25:23, 1984.)

there are several advantages of using ^{99m}Tc instead of radioiodine. Because of the rapid uptake of ^{99m}Tc, the imaging procedure can begin only 20 minutes after administration, as opposed to 4 and 24 hours for ^{123}I and ^{131}I, respectively. In addition, because higher doses of ^{99m}Tc can be safely administered without delivering a high radiation dose, thyroid scanning with ^{99m}Tc can be completed more rapidly than with radioiodine. Finally, the quality of ^{99m}Tc thyroid scans is consistently equal or superior to that of radioiodine scans.[5, 63]

Thyroid imaging can be a useful adjunct in diagnosing hyperthyroidism in cats. With pertechnetate thyroid scanning, a one-to-one ratio usually exists between the size and intensity of the salivary glands and the two thyroid lobes. In contrast, most cats with hyperthyroidism have obvious enlargement of one or both thyroid lobes, together with increased uptake of pertechnetate into the abnormal thyroid tissue as compared with the salivary glands.[64, 65] The per cent thyroidal ^{99m}Tc uptake can also be calculated for additional diagnostic value.[66]

The major usefulness of thyroid imaging, however, is in determining the extent of thyroid gland involvement and in detecting possible metastasis. In about 70 per cent of hyperthyroid cats, thyroid imaging reveals enlargement of and increased radionuclide accumulation in both lobes (see Fig. 150–8), whereas involvement of only one lobe is seen in the remaining cats (see Fig. 150–9).[5, 6, 63] With unilateral thyroid lobe involvement, the normal contralateral lobe is completely suppressed and cannot be visualized. Thyroid imaging is also helpful in the hyperthyroid cat in which no enlargement of the thyroid gland can be palpated; in many of these cats, thyroid imaging demonstrates that an affected lobe has descended into the thoracic cavity. Finally, scanning is of value in detecting regional or distant metastasis of functional thyroid carcinoma causing feline hyperthyroidism (see Fig. 150–10).[4, 5, 7, 63]

TREATMENT

The underlying cause of the thyroid adenomatous hyperplasia associated with feline hyperthyroidism is not known. Spontaneous remission of the disorder does not occur, and the aim of treatment is to control the excessive secretion of thyroid hormone from the adenomatous thyroid gland. In cats, hyperthyroidism can be treated in three ways—surgical thyroidectomy, radioactive iodine (^{131}I), or chronic administration of an antithyroid drug. Antithyroid drug therapy is also extremely useful as short-term treatment (3 to 6 weeks) in the preparation of the hyperthyroid cat before thyroidectomy. The advantages and disadvantages of each form of treatment, summarized in Table 150–3, should always be considered when selecting the most appropriate treatment.

The treatment of choice for an individual cat depends on several factors, including the age of the cat, presence of associated cardiovascular diseases or other major medical problems (e.g., renal disease), availability of a skilled surgeon or nuclear medicine department, and owner's willingness to accept the form of treatment advised. Of the three forms of treatment available, it must be emphasized that only surgery and radioactive iodine remove and destroy the adenomatous thyroid tissue, respectively, and thereby "cure" the hyperthyroid state. Use of an antithyroid drug (e.g., methimazole) blocks thyroid hormone synthesis; however, because antithyroid drugs do not destroy adenomatous thyroid tissue, relapse of hyperthyroidism invariably occurs within 24 to 72 hours after the medication is discontinued.[44, 45]

Antithyroid Drugs and Other Medical Treatments

Methimazole

Administration of methimazole (Tapazole, Jones Medical Industries), which lowers high circulating thyroid hormone concentrations by blocking thyroid hormone synthesis, is an effective and relatively safe alternative for both short-term (preoperative) and long-term management of hyperthyroidism in cats.[1, 2, 24, 45, 67] Methimazole is better tolerated and associated with fewer severe and milder adverse reactions than propylthiouracil[68, 69] and is the antithyroid drug of choice for the medical management of cats with hyperthyroidism.

Methimazole is actively concentrated in the thyroid tissue and acts there to block thyroid hormone synthesis at several steps.[70] Iodine uptake and the release of previously synthesized and stored hormone are not prevented. Unlike surgery or radioiodine, methimazole does not ablate the adenomatous thyroid glands. As a result, circulating thyroid hormone invariably returns to high concentrations 24 to 72 hours after discontinuation of the drug and continued daily administration is necessary to control the hyperthyroid state effectively.[1, 2, 24, 45, 67]

Management of hyperthyroid cats with methimazole has several advantages. It is a practical treatment choice for many practitioners as no advanced surgical skills, 24-hour monitoring, special facilities, or government licensing is needed (see Table 150–3). Hypothyroidism and hypoparathyroidism do not occur as a result of methimazole administration.[1, 24, 45] Compared with treatment with surgery or radioiodine, start-up costs are considerably less and, in addition, hospitalization is not necessary.

Methimazole administration may be an especially suitable

END

choice of therapy for hyperthyroid cats with concurrent disorders such as cancer, heart failure, or chronic renal failure.[67] Thyroid hormone increases renal blood flow and GFR, and studies have shown that treatment of hyperthyroidism decreases GFR.[29–32] Treatment of hyperthyroidism can lead to a worsening of chronic renal disease or an "unmasking" of the condition in some cats.[71]. Unlike the effect of thyroidectomy or radioiodine therapy, normalization of thyroid hormone concentrations with methimazole is reversible, allowing the clinician to balance the treatment of concurrent hyperthyroidism and chronic renal disease to maximize the benefit to the patient.

Methimazole is initially administered at a dosage of 5 to 15 mg/day in divided doses for 2 to 3 weeks depending on the degree of hyperthyroidism (Fig. 150–11). In most cats, this protocol lowers serum T_4 concentrations into or below reference range limits. If there is little to no fall in serum T_4 concentrations after this initial 2- to 3-week period, the methimazole dosage should be increased by 2.5–to 5-mg increments when poor owner compliance has been excluded. Rarely, a cat may require as much as 25 mg/day to control the hyperthyroid state.[1, 24, 45] Because most serious side effects associated with methimazole administration occur during the first 3 months of therapy, it is important to monitor the cat closely during this period. Therefore, cats should be examined every 2 to 3 weeks during the first 3 months of treatment to monitor for adverse reactions. Complete blood and platelet counts, serum biochemical profile, and serum T_4

concentration should also be evaluated at the time of each examination (see Fig. 150–11).

Methimazole should be administered as a preoperative preparation before thyroidectomy, as control of the hyperthyroid state significantly improves the anesthetic and surgical risk. Methimazole should be administered for 2 to 4 weeks before surgery. A serum T_4 concentration, serum biochemistry panel, and complete blood and platelet counts should be checked before surgery. The last dose of methimazole should be administered the morning of surgery.

During long-term therapy, the lowest daily dose of methimazole that maintains serum T_4 concentrations within the low-normal range should be given. This may reduce the frequency of some side effects.[1, 24, 45, 67] If subnormal serum T_4 concentrations are found during therapy, the daily methimazole dose should be decreased by 2.5 to 5 mg and serum T_4 determinations repeated at 2- to 4-week intervals until the lowest effective daily dose is found (see Fig. 150–11). In most cases, cats with hyperthyroidism can be controlled with a daily dose of 5 to 10 mg/day. Few cats can be effectively managed with dosages less than 2.5 mg/day, whereas some continue to require 15 to 25 mg/day to maintain euthyroidism. Subnormal serum T_4 concentrations are not infrequent during methimazole administration. However, clinical signs of hypothyroidism generally do not develop, probably because serum T_3 concentrations remain normal in these cats.[45, 72]

Despite a serum half-life of less than 3 hours,[73] methima-

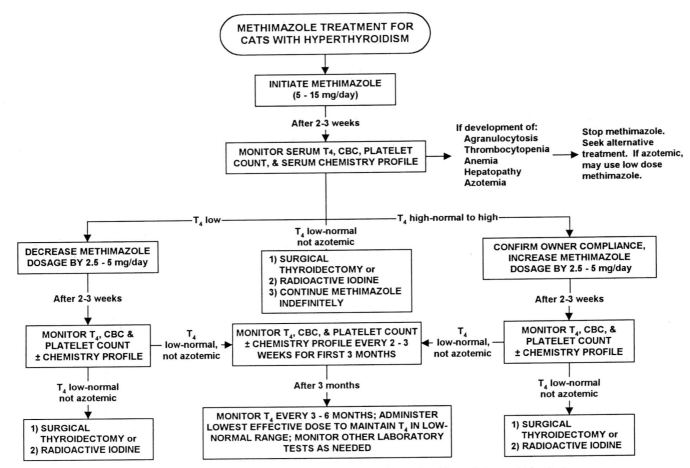

Figure 150–11. Algorithm for the treatment and monitoring of hyperthyroid cats during methimazole therapy.

TABLE 150–4. ADVERSE REACTIONS ASSOCIATED WITH METHIMAZOLE TREATMENT IN CATS WITH HYPERTHYROIDISM

ADVERSE REACTION	PER CENT OF CATS TREATED
Clinical findings	
Anorexia	10–20
Vomiting	10–20
Lethargy	10–20
Facial excoriations	2–5
Bleeding diathesis	2–3
Hepatopathy (icterus)	1–2
Myasthenia gravis	<0.5
Cold agglutinin–like disease	<0.5
Laboratory findings	
Thrombocytopenia	2–3
Agranulocytosis	1–2
Leukopenia	5
Eosinophilia	10
Lymphocytosis	7
Positive ANA titer	20
High hepatic enzyme activity (ALT, AST, SAP, bilirubin)	1.5
Positive Coombs' test	1.5
Hemolytic anemia	<0.5

ALT = alanine aminotransferase; ANA = antinuclear antibody; AST = aspartate aminotransferase; SAP = serum alkaline phosphatase.

zole is effective in many cats when given only once daily. Because methimazole is concentrated in the thyroid gland, the intrathyroidal residence time is considerably longer than the serum half-life and as a result once-daily administration is often effective.[1, 67] Owner compliance during long-term methimazole administration is likely to be significantly better with a treatment schedule of once-daily medication. After the first 3 months of therapy, serum T_4 concentrations should be determined at 3- to 6-month intervals to monitor dosage requirements and response to treatment (see Fig. 150–11). Other laboratory parameters should be monitored if adverse reactions are suspected.

Adverse effects associated with methimazole administration can occur at any time but most commonly occur during the first 3 months of therapy.[1, 2, 24, 45, 67] Mild and common clinical side effects include anorexia, vomiting and lethargy. These problems are seen in approximately 10 to 20 per cent of cats (Table 150–4), are usually transient, and commonly resolve despite continued methimazole administration. Occasionally, however, these adverse signs are severe or persistent and require stopping methimazole administration. Serious hematologic side effects, including thrombocytopenia, agranulocytosis (leukopenia with total granulocyte count less than 250 cells/mm³), and hemolytic anemia, can develop during methimazole administration (see Table 150–4).[1, 2, 24, 45, 67] Adverse signs should resolve within a week of cessation of methimazole and institution of supportive care. Hepatopathy is a serious reaction characterized by dramatic increases in serum activities of ALT, AST, AP, and total bilirubin, usually associated with severe depression, anorexia, and vomiting. Clinical improvement is often evident within a few days of discontinuing methimazole but jaundice and increased serum enzyme activities may take several weeks to resolve. A few cats have an apparent idiosyncratic drug reaction characterized by self-induced facial excoriations (see Table 150–4). This dermatopathy is partially glucocorticoid responsive but requires discontinuation of methimazole for complete resolution. Rare complications of methimazole administration in-

clude bleeding diathesis, hemolytic anemia, cold agglutinin–like disease (associated with necrosis of tips of ears), and acquired myasthenia gravis (see Table 150–4).[45, 71, 74] Although serious reactions are each seen in less than 3 per cent of cats treated with methimazole, their occurrence necessitates immediate cessation of therapy. These serious adverse reactions usually recur quickly after reinstitution of methimazole; therefore, alternative therapy must be sought for such cats.

Development of positive serum antinuclear antibody (ANA) titers is not uncommon during methimazole administration.[45] This phenomenon seems to increase with the duration of therapy and is present in approximately half of cats treated longer than 6 months. Development of ANA appears to be directly related to dosage of methimazole because most cats that develop ANA are receiving at least 15 mg/day, and ANA resolves in most cats if the dosage is lowered. Despite the relatively high rate of ANA during methimazole administration, occurrence of a lupus-like syndrome has not been well documented although the potential still exists. Therefore, the daily methimazole dose should be decreased to the lowest dose that maintains serum T_4 concentrations in the low-normal range (see Fig. 150–11).

In cats treated for months to years with methimazole, the thyroid nodule(s) continues to enlarge because methimazole blocks thyroid hormone secretion but does nothing to inhibit tumor growth. In these cats, it is not uncommon for the daily dose requirement to increase progressively as a result of this continued thyroid growth. Some of these cats may no longer respond adequately to methimazole treatment and may require other forms of therapy (e.g., thyroidectomy).

Carbimazole

Carbimazole is a carbethoxy derivative of methimazole currently used in Europe (where methimazole is not available).[44, 75, 76] It is not currently available in the United States. In cats, humans and rats carbimazole is rapidly converted to methimazole after oral administration, which is responsible for the antithyroid activity of the preparation.[77] Carbimazole should be initially administered at a dosage of 5 mg every 8 hours for 2 to 3 weeks, depending on the degree of hyperthyroidism.[44, 75, 76] Euthyroidism is established in 1 to 2 weeks in most cats, and noticeable clinical improvement typically takes 2 to 3 weeks. In less than 10 per cent of cats, there is little to no fall in serum T_4 concentrations after this initial 2- to 3-week period. In such cases (when poor owner compliance has been excluded), a longer duration of therapy or an increased dose (in 5-mg increments) should be effective in establishing euthyroidism.

Like methimazole, carbimazole can be administered as a preoperative preparation before thyroidectomy, as control of the hyperthyroid state significantly improves the anesthetic and surgical risk. Carbimazole should be given for 2 to 4 weeks before surgery. A serum T_4 concentration, serum biochemistry, and complete blood and platelet counts should be assessed before surgery. The last dose of carbimazole is administered on the morning of surgery.

Carbimazole appears to be as effective as methimazole for the long-term medical management of hyperthyroidism. In most cats a carbimazole dosage of 5 mg given at 12-hour intervals is necessary to maintain euthyroidism.[44, 75, 76] Subnormal serum T_4 concentrations may occur during long-term carbimazole administration, but serum T_3 concentrations typically remain normal and clinical signs of hypothyroidism are absent. Nonetheless, it would be prudent to

END

monitor serum T_4 concentrations at 3-to 6-month intervals during long-term carbimazole administration and administer the lowest daily dose (divided) of carbimazole that maintains serum T_4 concentrations within the low-normal range.

Adverse reactions are reported to be less common during carbimazole administration than with methimazole. Most side effects are seen during the first few weeks of therapy, are usually mild and transient, and rarely necessitate discontinuing therapy. Vomiting, sometimes associated with anorexia and lethargy, is seen in approximately 10 per cent of cats. Transient leukopenia or lymphocytosis occurs in approximately 5 per cent of cats.[44, 75, 76] Serious side effects such as agranulocytosis, thrombocytopenia, and hepatopathy have not been reported. Nonetheless, the possibility of such adverse reactions remains, and it is recommended that cats be examined to monitor for adverse reactions and that serum biochemistry and complete blood and platelet counts be evaluated every 2 to 3 weeks during the first 3 months of therapy. Thereafter these laboratory parameters are monitored if adverse reactions are suspected.

Ipodate

Ipodate is an iodine-containing oral cholecystographic contrast agent that has antithyroid effects.[75, 76, 78] Ipodate blocks conversion of T_4 to T_3 by inhibiting outer-ring deiodinase, resulting in decreasing serum T_3 concentrations. At higher dosages, serum T_4 concentrations may also decrease (although not necessarily become normal) as a result of inhibition of thyroid hormone production by the inorganic iodide released during the metabolism of ipodate. This effect of iodide on thyroid hormone production is usually transient, however. The recommended starting dose of ipodate is 100 mg/day, administered either as a single dose or divided every 12 hours.[78] The daily dosage can be increased to 200 to 300 mg for cats that do not demonstrate an adequate response to therapy by 1 month. For these dose sizes, the ipodate must be compounded by a licensed pharmacy service.

In one study, 8 of 12 hyperthyroid cats treated with ipodate had a fair to good response to therapy, whereas 4 failed to show a response.[78] In the cats that had a good response to ipodate, the serum T_3 concentration became normal, heart rates decreased, and weight gain was noted. Cats whose serum T_3 concentration does not return to the reference range are unlikely to have an adequate improvement in clinical signs. Cats with severe hyperthyroidism are less likely to demonstrate an adequate response to ipodate administration than those with moderate or mild disease. Even in cats that do show a response to therapy, however, ipodate is usually not effective for long-term management because of the ultimate escape from inhibition of thyroid hormone synthesis. Adverse clinical signs or hematologic abnormalities attributable to ipodate treatment have not been reported in hyperthyroid cats.

Ipodate is especially useful in management of cats with severe hyperthyroidism that require rapid, short-term control of their disease (e.g., in preparation for surgical thyroidectomy). Ipodate may also be a feasible alternative to methimazole for medical treatment of hyperthyroidism in cats, particularly those that cannot tolerate methimazole and are not candidates for surgery or radiotherapy.

Beta-Adrenoceptor Blocking Agents

Propranolol (Inderal, Wyeth-Ayerst) and atenolol (Tenormin, ICI Pharma) are the most commonly used beta-adrenergic blocking agents for hyperthyroid cats. Propranolol and atenolol have no direct effect on the thyroid gland but are useful in controlling the tachycardia, polypnea, hypertension, and hyperexcitability associated with hyperthyroidism.[1, 2, 75, 76] In addition, treatment with a beta-adrenergic blocker helps prevent arrhythmias that commonly develop during anesthesia in cats with hyperthyroidism.[79] These agents are used when rapid control of clinical effects is required and are usually combined with methimazole (or carbimazole) or stable iodine. Because propranolol and atenolol do not block uptake of radioactive iodine into the thyroid gland, they may be helpful for cats awaiting radiation therapy or those that have a delayed return to euthyroidism after treatment.

Propranolol is a nonselective beta-adrenergic blocking agent and is therefore contraindicated for cats with uncontrolled, overt congestive cardiac failure or cats with reactive airway disease (e.g., asthma) that are dependent on chronic beta-adrenergic stimulation. Atenolol offers some distinct advantages over propranolol, including selective beta or cardiac beta-receptor blocking action and a longer duration of activity.[1, 75, 76] Propranolol is administered at a dosage of 2.5 to 5 mg every 8 to 12 hours as required to decrease the heart rate to the normal resting range. Atenolol is administered at a dosage of 6.25 mg/per cat once to twice daily.[75, 76, 80]

Stable Iodine

Although the exact mechanism is unclear, large doses of stable iodine (^{127}I) inhibit thyroid hormone synthesis (Wolff-Chaikoff effect) and release and also reduce the size and vascularity of the adenomatous thyroid tissue.[81] These effects are not consistent, and serum thyroid hormone concentrations, although they often decrease may never became completely normal during stable iodine administration. In addition, the antithyroid effects are typically transient and escape from inhibition usually ensues within a few weeks.[75, 76, 81]

Therefore, iodine is not indicated for the long-term medical management of cats with hyperthyroidism but has been used (in combination with beta-adrenergic blockers) for the preoperative preparation of cats unable to tolerate methimazole.[75, 76] Oral iodine is generally administered in aqueous solution either as a saturated solution of potassium iodide (SSKI; 100 g potassium iodide per 100 mL solution, yielding a concentration of 38 mg iodine per drop) or as Lugol's solution (5 g iodine with 10 g potassium iodide per 100 mL solution, yielding a concentration of 6.3 mg iodine per drop).[81] The parenteral solution of sodium iodide (10 per cent solution) has an iodine content of 85 mg/mL.[81] In addition, many iodine-rich products, such as kelp (0.15 mg/tab), are also available in natural food stores. Whatever preparation is used, iodine should be administered at a dosage of 30 to 100 mg/day (in single or divided doses) for 10 to 14 days before surgery.[75, 76] Common side effects of oral treatment with SSKI or Lugol's solution include excessive salivation and decreased appetite; such adverse signs appear to result from the unpleasant taste of iodine. To prevent this adverse effect, the dose can be placed within a small gelatin capsule and immediately administered.

Surgery

Surgical thyroidectomy is a highly effective treatment for hyperthyroidism in cats. Although thyroidectomy is most often successful, it can be associated with significant morbidity and mortality, especially in cats with severe hyperthyroidism. The antithyroid drugs methimazole or carbimazole can be used to improve the condition of a hyperthyroid cat before surgery. After methimazole (or carbimazole) treatment has maintained euthyroidism for 1 to 3 weeks, most systemic complications associated with hyperthyroidism have improved or resolved. The anesthetic and surgical complications are, therefore, greatly minimized. The last dose of methimazole (or carbimazole) should be administered on the morning of surgery. In hyperthyroid cats that cannot tolerate antithyroid drug treatment, alternative preoperative preparation with beta-adrenergic blocking drugs (e.g., propranolol or atenolol), ipodate, or stable iodine, alone or in combination, should be used.[75, 76, 78]

Techniques for unilateral and bilateral thyroidectomy have been reported for cats with hyperthyroidism.[82–86] Both intracapsular and extracapsular methods designed for removal of thyroid tissue while preserving parathyroid function have been used. With the intracapsular technique for thyroidectomy, however, it can be difficult to remove the entire thyroid (and therefore all abnormal tissue) while concurrently preserving parathyroid function. Small remnants of thyroid tissue that remain attached to the capsule may regenerate and produce recurrent hyperthyroidism.[82, 84] The main advantage of the extracapsular, as compared with the intracapsular, technique is that the incidence of relapse is lower because all thyroid tissue is removed.[84]

Many potential complications are associated with thyroidectomy, including hypoparathyroidism, Horner's syndrome, and laryngeal paralysis (most commonly voice change).[82–86] The most serious complication is hypocalcemia, which develops after the parathyroid glands are injured, devascularized, or inadvertently removed in the course of bilateral thyroidectomy.[87, 88] Because only one parathyroid gland is required for maintenance of normocalcemia, hypoparathyroidism is a complication associated with bilateral thyroidectomy. If the surgeon recognizes that all parathyroid glands have been inadvertently removed, parathyroid autotransplanted into a muscle belly at the surgical site has been shown to have excellent potential for function.[89]

After bilateral thyroidectomy, the serum calcium concentration should be monitored on a daily basis until it has stabilized within the normal range. In most cats with iatrogenic hypoparathyroidism, clinical signs associated with hypocalcemia develop within 1 to 3 days of surgery.[87, 88] Mild hypocalcemia (6.5 to 7.5 mg/dL) is a common finding during this immediate postoperative period, and laboratory evidence of hypocalcemia alone does not mean that treatment is required. However, if accompanying signs of muscle tremors, tetany, or convulsions develop, therapy with vitamin D and calcium is indicated (see Chapter 149).[24, 87, 88] Although hypoparathyroidism may be permanent in some cats, recovery of parathyroid function may occur days to months after surgery. In most cases, transient hypocalcemia probably results from reversible parathyroid damage and ischemia incurred during surgery. Alternatively, accessory parathyroid tissue may secrete parathyroid hormone (PTH) and compensate for the damaged parathyroid glands to maintain normocalcemia, or accommodation of calcium-regulating mechanisms in the absence of PTH may occur.[90]

Serum thyroid hormone concentrations fall to subnormal levels for 2 to 3 months after hemithyroidectomy for unilateral involvement of the thyroid gland. However, L-thyroxine supplementation is rarely required during this period. If bilateral thyroidectomy has been performed, L-thyroxine (0.1 to 0.2 mg/day) should be started 24 to 48 hours after surgery. Although T_4 supplementation at this dosage can be safely continued indefinitely, the low serum concentrations of T_4

and T_3 that develop 24 to 48 hours after bilateral thyroidectomy may begin to increase naturally without supplementation in the weeks to months postoperatively.[84] If that occurs, thyroxine administration can be discontinued.

Because of the potential for recurrence of hyperthyroidism,[84, 91] all cats undergoing surgical thyroidectomy should have their serum thyroid hormone concentration monitored once or twice a year. In cases of recurrent thyrotoxicosis after bilateral thyroidectomy, treatment with either antithyroid drugs (methimazole or carbimazole) or radioiodine is favored over repeated surgery. Nonsurgical management is recommended because the incidence of surgical complications (especially permanent hypoparathyroidism) is considerably higher in cats undergoing more than one surgery.[84]

Radioactive Iodine

Radioactive iodine provides a simple, effective, and safe treatment for cats with hyperthyroidism and is regarded by many as the treatment of choice for most hyperthyroid cats. Treatment with radioiodine avoids the inconvenience of daily oral administration of an antithyroid drug and also avoids the side effects commonly associated with these drugs. Use of radioiodine also avoids the risks and perioperative complications associated with anesthesia and surgical thyroidectomy.

Thyroid hormones are the only iodinated organic compounds in the body. Therefore, the only function of ingested iodine (stable iodine, ^{127}I) is the incorporation into thyroid hormone. Indeed, the thyroid gland is the only tissue in the body that takes up stable iodine from the circulation and concentrates it. The basic principle behind treatment of hyperthyroidism with radioiodine is that thyroid cells do not differentiate between stable and radioactive iodine; therefore, radioiodine, like stable iodine, is concentrated by the thyroid gland.[92] In cats with hyperthyroidism, radioiodine is concentrated primarily in the hyperplastic or neoplastic thyroid cells, where it irradiates and destroys the abnormal tissue (whether in the normal cervical area or in ectopic sites). Normal thyroid tissue, however, tends to be protected from the effects of radioiodine, because normal thyroid tissue tends to be atrophied and receives only a small dose of radiation (unless large doses are administered).

The radioisotope used to treat hyperthyroidism is ^{131}I. Iodine 131 has a half-life of 8 days and emits both beta particles and gamma radiation.[92, 93] The beta particles, which cause 80 per cent of the tissue damage, travel a maximum of 2 mm in tissue and have an average path length of 400 μm. Therefore, beta particles are locally destructive but spare adjacent hypoplastic thyroid tissue, parathyroid glands, and other cervical structures.

Ideally, administering a single dose of radioiodine restores euthyroidism without inducing hypothyroidism. Although radioiodine treatment of hyperthyroid cats has been the subject of several studies,[94–101] the optimal method for determining the amount of radioactivity required for effective treatment remains somewhat controversial. Whatever method is used, the radiation dose delivered to the thyroid gland is determined by three factors: the fraction of administered radioiodine taken up by the gland, the rate of release of radioiodine from the gland, and the mass (weight) of the gland.[92]

One method for determining proper ^{131}I dose is to calculate the amount required by using tracer kinetic studies to estimate the percentage of iodine uptake and rate of disappearance from the gland together with thyroid imaging to esti-

END

mate the weight of the gland.[94–96] Although this method of dose determination works well and theoretically should produce the best results, a major disadvantage is the time and expense required to perform tracer thyroid gland kinetic studies and thyroid imaging. Also, these studies often require repeated tranquilization of cats. Because of the time and expense involved in determining thyroid kinetics and because results have not been domnstrated to be superior to those with other methods, most centers that treat hyperthyroid cats with radioiodine no longer use this method of dose determination.

A second method of treating hyperthyroid cats is to administer a fixed, relatively high dose of radioiodine to all cats (i.e., 4 or 5 mCi), regardless of the severity of hyperthyroidism or size of thyroid tumor.[97, 98] Although this method is the simplest, use of this approach results in undertreatment of a few cats with severe disease and, more commonly, overtreatment of a number of cats with mild disease.

In the third method of dose determination, the dose of radioiodine administered to hyperthyroid cats is determined on the basis of a scoring system that takes into consideration the severity of clinical signs, the size of the cat's thyroid gland, and the serum T_4 concentration.[99–101] Using this scoring system, a low, medium, or relatively high ^{131}I dose (e.g., 2 to 6 mCi) is selected without utilizing thyroid gland kinetics. For example, cats with mild clinical signs, small thyroid tumors, and only slightly increased serum T_4 concentrations would receive smaller doses of radioiodine (e.g., 3 mCi); cats with severe clinical signs, large thyroid tumors, and markedly high serum T_4 concentrations would receive high doses of radioiodine (e.g., 5 mCi); and cats in between these extremes would receive intermediate doses of radioiodine (e.g., 4 mCi). This approach has been shown to provide treatment results comparable to those obtained when thyroid kinetics were determined (i.e., the first method of dose determination).[99–101] The major advantages of this method are that nuclear medicine equipment is not needed, the time required to determine thyroid kinetics is eliminated, and sedation of the cat is not required. In addition, in contrast to the fixed-dose method, the total radiation dose delivered to cats with mild hyperthyroidism is minimized because lower doses are given to these cats.

The ideal goal of ^{131}I therapy is to restore euthyroidism with a single dose of radiation without producing hypothyroidism. Indeed, most hyperthyroid cats treated with radioactive iodine are cured by a single dose. In our survey of 524 hyperthyroid cats in which the therapeutic dose of ^{131}I was determined by the third method, serum thyroid hormone concentrations were normal within 2 weeks of therapy in approximately 85 per cent of cats and within 3 months in 95 per cent (Fig. 150–12).[101] Approximately 5 per cent of cats, however, fail to respond completely and remain hyperthyroid after treatment with radioiodine. In our study, most cats with persistent hyperthyroidism had large thyroid tumors, severe hyperthyroidism, and extremely increased serum T_4 concentrations.[101] One explanation for persistent hyperthyroidism in these cats with large tumors and severe hyperthyroidism is that a greater number of adenomatous cells must be destroyed than in cats with small tumors and mild disease. In cats that remain hyperthyroid 3 months after initial treatment, retreatment is generally recommended because virtually all cats that remain hyperthyroid after the first treatment can be cured by a second treatment.

After treatment with radioiodine, it is common to see a transient decrease in serum T_4 concentrations to subnormal levels for a few weeks, but associate clinical signs of hypo-

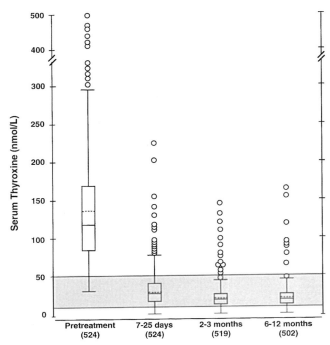

Figure 150–12. Box plots of serum T_4 concentrations in 524 cats before and at various times after administration of radioiodine for treatment of hyperthyroidism. Data are plotted (i.e., box plots) as described in the legend of Figure 150–3. Shaded area indicates normal ranges for T_4 concentration for cats. To convert serum T_4 concentrations from nmol/L to μg/dL, divide the given values by 12.87. (From Peterson ME, Becker DV: Radioiodine treatment of 524 cats with hyperthyroidism. JAVMA 207: 1422, 1995.)

thyroidism do not develop and treatment is almost never required. In most of these cats, free T_4 concentrations remain within reference range limits. In contrast, a few (less than 5 per cent) cats treated with radioiodine develop permanent hypothyroidism, with clinical signs developing 2 to 4 months after treatment. Clinical signs associated with iatrogenic hypothyroidism in these cats may include lethargy, nonpruritic seborrhea sicca, matting of hair, and marked weight gain. Bilateral symmetric alopecia does not develop.[72, 101] If hypothyroidism develops (diagnosis based on clinical signs, subnormal serum total and free T_4 concentrations, and response to replacement therapy), lifelong thyroid hormone supplementation is generally needed (i.e., 0.1 mg L-thyroxine per day).

In cats with thyroid carcinoma (incidence less than 2.5 per cent of all hyperthyroid cats[7]), radioiodine offers the best chance for successful cure of the tumor because it concentrates in all hyperactive thyroid cells, that is, carcinomatous tissue located in the typical cervical area as well as in metastatic sites. However, thyroid carcinomas concentrate and retain iodine less efficiently than thyroid adenomas (adenomatous hyperplasia) and carcinomas are usually much larger: in size; therefore, extremely high doses of radioiodine (10 to 30 mCi) are almost always needed to achieve destruction of all malignant tissue.[2, 102] The combination of surgical debulking and then administration of high-dose radioactive iodine has also been reported to be successful in cats with thyroid carcinoma.[101, 102] Longer periods of hospitalization are required with such high-dose radioiodine administration because of the prolonged time needed for radioiodine excretion. However, if the malignant cells are less efficient in "trapping" iodine, the iodine may be quickly excreted. Rapid excretion of radioactivity allows cats to be quickly released from the hospital, but the prognosis for destroying all malignant cells is poorer.

Regardless of the method of dose determination selected, certain radiation safety restrictions and procedures must be followed. The cats are discharged from the hospital or treatment facility when the radiation dose rate has decreased to a safe level that has been determined by the state radiation control office (usually after a 7- to 10-day period). Upon discharge, the cats are still excreting a small amount of radioiodine in their urine and feces. The remaining radioactivity is gradually eliminated from the cat over the next 2 to 4 weeks through radioactive decay and excretion into the urine and feces. Because of this, most authorities recommend restricting the cats to the owner's home; avoiding close (i.e., less than 3 to 6 feet), prolonged contact with the cat for the first 2 weeks after release; and carefully disposing of litter box waste. Hands should be thoroughly cleansed after the cat or the litter is handled.

Percutaneous Ethanol Injection

Infusion of ethanol into tissue can cause coagulation necrosis and vascular thrombosis. Therefore, if tissue is exposed to enough ethanol, that tissue dies. Percutaneous chemical ablation of tumors was first utilized in people with primary hyperparathyroidism.[103, 104] The same procedure has been successfully applied to dogs with primary hyperparathyroidism[105] (also see Chapter 149) and is currently being evaluated in hyperthyroid cats. The protocol utilizing this form of treatment for cats with hyperthyroidism involves placing a needle into the thyroid lobe to be treated using ultrasound guidance, via a 10-MHz transducer, while the cat is anesthetized. Ethanol (100 per cent) is then slowly injected until it is seen to diffuse throughout the lobe. The entire procedure requires approximately 10 minutes and the volume injected usually ranges from 25 to 100 per cent of the calculated mass volume. A pilot study of four cats with unilateral hyperthyroidism was completed. The unilateral nature of their disease was confirmed with nuclear scintigraphy and the thyroid mass had been visualized by ultrasonography before anesthesia. Each cat became clinically and biochemically euthyroid within a week of injection and each remained normal for at least 6 months after percutaneous ethanol injection (PEI).[106]

Pilot studies of the use of PEI for treatment of cats with bilateral hyperthyroidism have also begun. The first cat with bilateral hyperthyroidism reported to have been treated with PEI was injected four times over a period of 6 weeks, developed laryngeal paralysis that required surgical correction, and remained mildly hyperthyroid for several months after treatment.[107] Another group has also evaluated PEI for the treatment of cats with bilateral disease. One cat died within 12 hours of having both thyroid masses injected. Since then, five additional cats with bilateral disease have been treated. These five had the larger of the two thyroid lobes injected in a prospective trial of staging at least two injection procedures. Each cat became euthyroid within days of the first injection. Two of the five became hyperthyroid 2 and 6 weeks later, respectively, and had the second lobe injected. The other three remain euthyroid 2 months after PEI.[108]

Several worrisome side effects have been caused by ethanol leaking from the target tissue into the surrounding area. These have included transient voice changes, recurrent gagging, and Horner's syndrome. The voice changes and gagging may be caused by iatrogenic laryngeal paralysis. This may have been the cause of the one fatality after bilateral PEI. Before the staged injections, the larygeal area is being evaluated for paralysis.

PEI is a therapeutic modality that is still being evaluated. This form of treatment has the potential for providing permanent resolution of hyperthyroidism without the need for surgery with its inherent risks. It would also be easier and less expensive and would require less hospitalization than treatment with radioactive iodine.

THYROID NEOPLASIA AND HYPERTHYROIDISM IN DOGS

Thyroid tumors in dogs are relatively common, representing approximately 1 to 4 per cent of all canine neoplasms.[109–111] As opposed to the relatively small, noninvasive thyroid tumors (i.e., adenomatous hyperplasia) associated with hyperthyroidism in cats,[6, 19, 24] most clinically detected thyroid tumors in dogs are large, nonfunctioning, invasive carcinomas (i.e., do not produce hyperthyroidism). More than 90 per cent of clinically detected thyroid tumors in dogs are carcinomas, probably because thyroid adenomas are too small to be easily palpated and, unlike those in cats, these adenomas almost never produce signs of hyper- or hypothyroidism. In dogs with thyroid carcinoma, both local invasion of tumor into adjacent structures (e.g., esophagus, trachea, cervical musculature, nerves, and thyroid vessels) and distant metastasis (e.g., pulmonary metastasis) are common. Thyroid carcinomas in dogs are usually large, easily palpable, and result in clinical signs caused by invasion or compression of local tissue that can be recognized by the owner. Because many of these tumors are malignant and have reached an advanced state at the time of diagnosis, the prognosis is often poor.[109–111]

CLINICAL FEATURES

Signalment

Most dogs with thyroid tumors are middle aged or older (older than 5 years).[111] There is no sex predilection. Breeds reported to be at increased risk of developing thyroid neoplasia include boxers, beagles, and golden retrievers.[112, 113]

Clinical Signs

Many dogs with thyroid tumors are examined because the owner has noticed an enlargement of the neck.[109–113] In more than 75 per cent of dogs diagnosed in one survey,[111] either the cervical swelling was the only reason for seeking veterinary care or the thyroid mass was detected by the veterinarian during an examination for another problem. Unlike the relatively small, freely movable thyroid tumors of the cat,[6, 19, 24] most thyroid tumors in dogs are large, easily palpable, and fixed to the soft tissues of the neck. Because of the large tumor volume and high incidence of metastasis, clinical signs such as dyspnea, cough, hoarseness, dysphagia, vomiting, anorexia, and weight loss may be reported, especially in dogs with nonfunctional thyroid tumors.[109–116]

Of all thyroid tumors in dogs, approximately 10 per cent are autonomous and hyperfunctional, leading to signs of hyperthyroidism; in these dogs, the hyperthyroid state is usually the major reason for examination.[110, 111, 113–116] As in dogs with nonfunctional tumors, the vast majority of these hyperthyroid dogs have thyroid carcinoma, although thyroid adenoma causing hyperthyroidism has rarely been reported.[117] In general, hyperfunctional tumors causing hyperthyroidism are usually smaller than the nontoxic tumors and therefore have less of a compressive effect on adjacent structures. Polydipsia and polyuria are usually the earliest and most predominant signs associated with hyperthyroidism in dogs. Weight loss, despite an increase in appetite, is also common. Compared with most cats with hyperthyroidism, however, dogs usually have much less severe weight loss. Other signs that may develop in dogs with hyperthyroidism (usually in proportion to the severity and duration of the hyperthyroid state) include weakness and fatigue, heat intolerance, nervousness or restless behavior, and more frequent defecation with semiformed feces. Cardiac signs may include a more forceful apex beat and arterial pulse, and the electrocardiogram may show high voltage in all leads.

DIAGNOSIS

Thyroid neoplasia should be suspected in any dog with an enlarging mass in the ventral cervical region. The differential diagnosis for a mass in the ventral cervical region should include inflammatory conditions (e.g., abscess, granuloma) and nonthyroid neoplasia (e.g., regional soft tissue sarcomas, lymphoma, metastatic oral tumors), as well as thyroid tumors. Fine-needle aspiration cytology (using a 21- to 23-gauge needle) may be helpful in differentiating a thyroid tumor from an abscess, salivary mucocele, or enlarged lymph node, although these masses are typically quite vascular and one may retrieve only blood. In addition, cytologic examination of fine-needle aspirates can be a useful aid in the preoperative differential diagnosis of benign or malignant thyroid disease. However, a definitive diagnosis usually requires an excisional biopsy and histopathology.

Screening laboratory tests (e.g., complete blood count, serum biochemical profile, urinalysis) should always be performed for a dog with suspected thyroid neoplasia. Results of such pretreatment screening tests may reveal the presence of a concurrent disorder not directly related to the thyroid tumor that may influence subsequent surgical and anesthetic management or use of chemotherapy. Chest radiographs should always be reviewed because about a third of these dogs have pulmonary metastasis at the time of diagnosis.[112] It is important to realize, however, that small metastatic nodules may not be visible radiographically. In addition, electrocardiography, echocardiography, or other studies may also be warranted in dogs with hyperfunctional thyroid tumors, especially if signs of thyrotoxic congestive heart failure are present.

Pertechnetate (^{99m}Tc) thyroid imaging can also be performed to help determine the extent of thyroid invasion or metastasis in dogs with thyroid neoplasia.[116, 118] Pertechnetate thyroid scans do not provide information regarding thyroid function, but such imaging procedures do aid in demonstrating the location of abnormal thyroid tissue. Thyroid uptake can be considered normal if the radioactivity in the thyroid area is similar in size and density to that seen in the parotid salivary gland. In one study, all dogs with thyroid neoplasia had abnormal pertechnetate scans.[118]

As in cats with hyperthyroidism, high serum concentrations of total and free T_4 would be expected in dogs with hyperfunctional thyroid neoplasia causing hyperthyroidism.[115, 117] When endogenous serum TSH concentrations were measured in these dogs, low to low-normal concentrations were reported.[115] One of the major differential diagnoses for

hyperthyroidism in dogs is the presence of autoantibodies to T_4, T_3, or both.[119] These autoantibodies produce spurious results when serum or plasma T_4 or T_3 is measured by radioimmunoassay, often resulting in an elevated apparent concentration of the thyroid hormones in affected dogs. Not uncommonly, these values are markedly increased, causing the veterinarian to consider the possibility that the dog has hyperthyroidism. These dogs with thyroid hormone autoantibodies, however, do not have either a palpably large thyroid gland or typical signs of hyperthyroidism (e.g., polyuria, weight loss). In contrast, they commonly have clinical and laboratory evidence of hypothyoidism and, in many cases, are indeed found to be hypothyroid and respond to thyroid hormone supplementation.[119]

Most dogs (approximately 90 per cent) with thyroid tumors remain euthyroid. In general, the severity of the hyperthyroid state (based on both the degree of elevation of serum thyroid hormone concentrations and severity of clinical signs) is usually milder in dogs than in most hyperthyroid cats. Once the thyroid tumor is recognized, diagnostic studies for the hyperthyroid state are largely academic because the fundamental (and more life-threatening) problem is the malignant tumor.

TREATMENT

Treatment of thyroid neoplasia in dogs is not often curative, in large part because of the highly malignant nature of this disease. Nevertheless, an attempt at some treatment should be considered for most dogs because palliative relief can usually be achieved. Surgery, chemotherapy, cobalt radiation, and use of radioactive iodine therapy may be indicated, depending on the individual condition. In general, however, an attempt at surgical removal or debulking of the thyroid tumor should be the first step, followed by additional treatment as indicated or desired by the owner.

Surgery

For most dogs with thyroid tumors (with or without associated hyperthyroidism), the initial treatment of choice is attempted surgical resection. Small, well-encapsulated, movable (i.e., not attached to underlying tissue) thyroid tumors are relatively easy to remove, and surgery alone might be curative, especially in the rare dog with a thyroid adenoma that was palpated on physical examination.[120]

On the other hand, complete excision of large, invasive carcinomas is usually difficult and may be impossible. In one study, 17 of 38 dogs with thyroid carcinoma (45 per cent) had unresectable tumors.[121] However, even in the latter cases, debulking of the tumor mass may be beneficial in preparation for other treatment as well as in making the dog more comfortable (e.g., relief of dyspnea, dysphagia). In some dogs, however, the thyroid carcinoma may be too large, invasive, and vascular for consideration of a debulking procedure. In these dogs, biopsy of the thyroid mass should provide definitive confirmation of thyroid carcinoma, and other treatment should be undertaken to attempt to reduce the tumor volume. Some dogs with unresectable tumors might benefit from cobalt irradiation 2 to 3 months before surgery to reduce the tumor volume.

Dogs with distant metastasis should not be treated with surgery alone, but debulking of the primary thyroid mass may improve the effectiveness of adjunct chemotherapy or radiotherapy. Although debulking of the tumor can be helpful in treatment of thyroid cancer, aggressive attempts to remove all malignant thyroid tissue can do more harm than help, because recurrent laryngeal nerves, parathyroid glands, and major blood vessels may be seriously damaged in the process of surgical removal. Even if complete excision of the thyroid carcinoma is not possible, attempted thyroidectomy allows the excisional biopsy (and subsequent histopathologic examination) of the tumor needed to confirm the diagnosis.

Additional treatment should be considered for all dogs with confirmed thyroid carcinoma after surgery. For dogs that remain euthyroid or have developed hypothyroidism as a result of their thyroid carcinoma, treatment with external cobalt radiation directed at the cervical tumor tissue or chemotherapy with doxorubicin, or both, should be considered. This is true regardless of apparent surgical success. Dogs with hyperthyroidism are best treated with radioactive iodine, doxorubicin, or both after surgical debulking.

Chemotherapy

Although surgery should resolve a thyroid adenoma, total removal of all malignant thyroid tissue is not usually possible, especially in dogs with large, invasive carcinomas. Therefore, chemotherapy becomes an important adjunctive mode of therapy after surgery when distant metastatic lesions are identified or when the primary tumor is so large (more than 4 cm in diameter) that metastasis is likely even though it cannot be identified with thoracic radiographs or other routine diagnostic tests.

Doxorubicin (Adriamycin, Adria Laboratories) has been the most effective chemotherapeutic agent for thyroid carcinoma in dogs, but the response is variable.[110, 111, 122] The dose of doxorubicin recommended is generally 30 mg/m² body surface area intravenously every 3 to 6 weeks until total remission of the tumor occurs or adverse reactions (e.g., cardiac toxicity) to the chemotherapy develop.[122] For most dogs, this drug may prevent further growth of the tumor and sometimes results in reduction of tumor size; however, chemotherapy is rarely associated with total remission of the thyroid carcinoma. Alternative agents, such as cisplatin (Platinol, Bristol-Myers), may also be useful in dogs with thyroid carcinoma.[123] Combination chemotherapy with cyclophosphamide (Cytoxan, Mead Johnson) and viscristine (Oncovin, Eli Lilly) in combination with doxorubicin or cisplatin may be used when doxorubicin alone is not effective.[111]

External Beam Irradiation

External beam (cobalt) irradiation also appears to be useful as adjunct therapy for thyroid carcinoma in dogs, especially animals with thyroid tumors that do not concentrate radioiodine. Such radiation therapy is often successful in reducing tumor volume in dogs with large, unresectable thyroid tumors.[111] Side effects (e.g., skin changes, esophagitis, pharyngitis, laryngitis) are uncommon.

Thyroid neoplasia, however, is fairly resistant to the dose of external beam radiation that can be safely delivered. Because of this radiation resistance, together with the aggressive biologic behavior of these tumors, a combination of surgical debulking (either before or after external beam irradiation) and postoperative chemotherapy is sometimes recommended for treatment of thyroid carcinoma in dogs.

Radioiodine

Most thyroid carcinomas in dogs, especially the tumors that are hyperfunctional and result in hyperthyroidism, retain the ability to concentrate radioiodine. Therefore, a favorable response to treatment of these tumors with large doses of ¹³¹I might be expected, especially in dogs that are hyperthyroid and have a high degree of radioiodine uptake by the tumor. Results of ¹³¹I treatment for functioning thyroid carcinoma have been reported for only a few dogs. Whereas cats respond extremely well to relatively low doses of ¹³¹I, high doses (e.g., 50 to 150 mCi) are required in dogs with thyroid carcinomas.[124, 125] As in humans, it appears that radioiodine treatment alone can result in palliation of clinical signs in dogs that have large unresectable primary tumors or massive thyroid metastasis. However, large, repetitive ¹³¹I doses may be required for an adequate response. Therefore, although radioiodine therapy may prolong survival, this therapy is not nearly as successful as might be expected. Because of the lengthy hospitalization that is required (for the large administered ¹³¹I doses), as well as the need for proper collection and disposal of all waste material, this treatment is prohibitively expensive for most owners.

REFERENCES

1. Peterson ME: Hyperthyroid diseases. In Ettinger SJ (ed): Textbook of Veterinary Internal Medicine: Diseases of the Dog and Cat, 4th ed. Philadelphia, WB Saunders, 1995, pp 1466–1487.
2. Feldman EC, Nelson RW: Feline hyperthyroidism (thyrotoxicosis). In Feldman EC, Nelson RW (eds): Canine and Feline Endocrinology and Reproduction. Philadelphia, WB Saunders, 1996, pp 118–166.
3. Carpenter JL, et al: Tumors and tumor-like lesions. In Holzworth J (ed): Diseases of the Cat: Medicine and Surgery. Philadelphia, WB Saunders, 1987, pp 406–596.
4. Peter HJ, et al: Autonomy of growth and of iodine metabolism in hyperthyroid feline goiters transplanted onto nude mice. J Clin Invest 80 : 491, 1987.
5. Peterson ME, Becker DV: Radionuclide thyroid imaging in 135 cats with hyperthyroidism. Vet Radiol 25:23, 1984.
6. Peterson ME, et al: Feline hyperthyroidism: Pretreatment clinical and laboratory evaluation of 131 cases. JAVMA 183 : 103, 1983.
7. Turrel JM, et al: Thyroid carcinoma causing hyperthyroidism in cats: 14 cases (1981–1986). JAVMA 193 : 359, 1988.
8. Peterson ME, et al: Lack of circulating thyroid stimulating immunoglobulins in cats with hyperthyroidism. Vet Immunol Immunopathol 16 : 277, 1987.
9. Kennedy RL Thoday KL: Lack of thyroid stimulatory activity in the serum of hyperthyroid cats (letter). Autommunity 3 : 317, 1989.
10. Brown RS, et al: Thyroid growth immunoglobulins in feline hyperthyroidism. Thyroid 2 : 125, 1992.
11. Tarttelin MF, et al: Serum free thyroxine levels respond inversely to changes in levels of dietary iodine in the domestic cat. N Z Vet J 40 : 66, 1992.
12. Scarlett JM, et al: Feline hyperthyroidism: A descriptive and case-control study. Prev Vet Med 6 : 295, 1988.
13. Scarlett JM: Epidemiology of thyroid diseases of dogs and cats. Vet Clin North Am Small Anim Pract 24 : 477, 1994.
14. Gerber H, et al: Etiopathology of feline toxic nodular goiter. Vet Clin North Am Small Anim Pract 24 : 541, 1994.
15. Kass PH, et al: Evaluation of environmental, nutritional, and host factors in cats with hyperthyroidism. J Vet Intern Med, in press.
16. Paschke R, Ludgate M: The thyrotropin receptor in thyroid diseases. N Engl J Med 337 : 1675, 1997.
17. Ward CR, et al: Altered G protein expression in thyroid adenomas from hyperthyroid cats. J Vet Intern Med 12 : 212, 1998.
18. Pearce SH, et al: Mutational analysis of the thyrotropin receptor gene in sporadic and familial feline thyrotoxicosis. Thyroid 7 : 923, 1997.
19. Thoday KL, Mooney CT: Historical, clinical and laboratory features of 126 hyperthyroid cats. Vet Rec 131 : 257, 1992.
20. Broussard JD, et al: Changes in clinical and laboratory findings in cats with hyperthyroidism from 1983 to 1993. JAVMA 206 : 302, 1995.
21. Joseph RJ, Peterson ME: Review and comparison of neuromuscular and central nervous system manifestions of hyperthyroidism in cats and humans. Prog Vet Neurol 3 : 114, 1993.
22. Graves TK, Peterson ME: Diagnosis of occult hyperthyroidism in cats. Probl Vet Med 2 : 683, 1990.
23. Graves TK, Peterson ME: Occult hyperthyroidism in cats. In Kirk RW, Bonagura JD (eds): Current Veterinary Therapy XI. Philadelphia, WB Saunders, 1992, pp 334–337.
24. Peterson ME, et al: Endocrine diseases. In Sherding RG (ed): The Cat: Diagnosis and Clinical Management. New York, Churchill Livingstone, 1994, pp 1404–1506.
25. Nemzek JA, et al: Acute onset of hypokalemia and muscular weakness in four hyperthyroid cats. JAVMA 205 : 65, 1994.
26. Mackovic-Basic M, Kleeman CR: The kidneys and electrolyte metabolism in

END

thyrotoxicosis. *In* Braverman LE, Utiger RD (eds): The Thyroid: A Fundamental and Clinical Text, 6th ed. Philadelphia, JB Lippincott, 1991, pp 771–779.

27. Graves TK: Hyperthyroidism and the kidney. *In* August JR (ed): Consultations in Feline Internal Medicine 3. Philadelphia, WB Saunders, 1997, pp 345–348.
28. Adams WH, et al: Investigation of the effects of hyperthyroidism on renal function in the cat. Can J Vet Res 61 : 53, 1997.
29. Graves TK, et al: Changes in renal function associated with treatment of hyperthyroidism in cats. Am J Vet Res 55 : 1745, 1994.
30. Becker TJ, et al: Effects of methimazole in renal function in cats with hyperthyroidism. J Vet Intern Med 12 : 212, 1998.
31. Adams WH, et al: Changes in renal function in cats following treatment of hyperthyroidism using ¹³¹I. Vet Radiol Ultrasound 38 : 231, 1997.
32. DiBartola SP, et al: Effect of treatment of hyperthyroidism on renal function in cats. JAVMA 208 : 875, 1996.
33. Ingbar DH: The respiratory system in thyrotoxicosis. *In* Braverman LE, Utiger RD (eds): The Thyroid: A Fundamental and Clinical Text, 6th ed. Philadelphia, JB Lippincott, 1991, pp 744–758.
34. Liu SK, et al: Hypertrophic cardiomyopathy and hyperthyroidism in the cat. JAVMA 185 : 52, 1984.
35. Bond BR: Hyperthyroid heart disease in cats. *In* Kirk RW (ed): Current Veterinary Therapy IX. Philadelphia, WB Saunders, 1986, pp 399–402.
36. Jacobs G, et al: Congestive heart failure associated with hyperthyroidism in cats. JAVMA 188 : 52, 1986.
37. Fox PR, et al: Electrocardiographic and radiographic changes in cats with hyperthyroidism: Comparison of populations evaluated during 1992–1993 vs 1979–1982. J Am Anim Hosp Assoc 35 : 27, 1999.
38. Fox PR, et al: Hyperthyroidism and other high cardiac output states, *In* Fox PR (ed): Canine and Feline Cardiology, 2nd ed. New York, Churchill Livingstone, in press.
39. Bond BR, et al: Echocardiographic findings in 103 cats with hyperthyroidism. JAVMA 192 : 1546, 1988.
40. Jacobs G Panciera D: Cardiovascular complications of feline hyperthyroidism. *In* Kirk RW, Bonagura JD (eds): Current Veterinary Therapy XI. Philadelphia, WB Saunders, 1992, pp 756–759.
41. Ansell JE: The blood in thyrotoxicosis. *In* Braverman LE, Utiger RD (eds): The Thyroid: A Fundamental and Clinical Text, 6th ed. Philadelphia, JB Lippincott, 1991, pp 785–792.
42. Horney BS, et al: Agarose gel electrophoresis of alkaline phosphatase isoenzymes in the serum of hyperthyroid cats. Vet Clin Pathol 23 : 98, 1994.
43. Archer FJ, Taylor SM: Alkaline phosphatase bone isoenzymes and osteocalcin in the serum of hyperthyroid cats. Can Vet J 37 : 735, 1996.
44. Mooney CT, et al: Carbimazole therapy of feline hyperthyroidism. J Small Anim Pract 33 : 228, 1992.
45. Peterson ME, et al: Methimazole treatment of 262 cats with hyperthyroidism. J Vet Intern Med 2 : 150, 1988.
46. McLoughlin MA, et al: Influence of systemic nonthyroidal illness on serum concentrations of thyroxine in hyperthyroid cats. J Am Anim Hosp Assoc 29 : 227, 1993.
47. Peterson ME, et al: Measurement of serum concentrations of total and free T₄ in hyperthyroid cats and cats with nonthyroidal disease. J Vet Intern Med 12 : 211, 1998.
48. Peterson ME, et al: Serum thyroid hormone concentrations fluctuate in cats with hyperthyroidism. J Vet Intern Med 1 : 142, 1987.
49. Peterson ME, Gamble DA: Effect of nonthyroidal disease on serum thyroxine concentrations in cats: 494 cases (1988). JAVMA 197 : 1203, 1990.
50. Peterson ME, et al: Triiodothyronine (T₃) suppression test. An aid in the diagnosis of mild hyperthyroidism in cats. J Vet Intern Med 4 : 233, 1990.
51. Refsal KR, et al: Use of the triiodothyronine suppression test for diagnosis of hyperthyroidism in ill cats that have serum concentration of iodothyronines within normal range. JAVMA 199 : 1594, 1991.
52. Peterson ME, et al: Use of the thyrotropin releasing hormone stimulation test to diagnose mild hyperthyroidism in cats. J Vet Intern Med 8 : 279, 1994.
53. Graves TK, Peterson ME: Diagnostic tests for feline hyperthyroidism. Vet Clin North Am Small Anim Pract 24 : 567, 1994.
54. Ferguson DC: Free thyroid hormone measurements in the diagnosis of thyroid disease. *In* Bonagura JD, Kirk RW (eds): Current Veterinary Therapy XII. Philadelphia, WB Saunders, 1995, pp 360–364.
55. Kapstein EM: Clinical application of free thyroxine determinations. Clin Lab Med 13 : 653, 1993.
56. Nichols R, Peterson ME: Laboratory diagnosis of hyperthyroidism in cats. Monograph on Hyperthyroidism in Cats, Daniels Pharmaceuticals, 1998, pp 2–7.
57. Mooney CT, et al: Effect of illness not associated with the thyroid gland on serum total and free thyroxine concentrations in cats. JAVMA 208 : 2004, 1996.
58. Utiger RD: Tests of thyroregulatory mechanisms. *In* Ingbar SH, Braverman LE (eds): The Thyroid: A Fundamental and Clinical Text. Philadelphia, JB Lippincott, 1986, pp 511–523.
59. Holtman JR, et al: Central respiratory stimulation produced by thyrotropin-releasing hormone in the cat. Peptides 7 : 207, 1986.
60. Beleslin DB, et al: Nature of salivation produced by thyrotropin-releasing hormone (TRH). Brain Res Bull 18 : 463, 1987.
61. Beleslin DB, et al: Studies of thyrotropin-releasing hormone (TRH)–induced defecation in cats. Pharmacol Biochem Behav 26 : 639, 1987.
62. Mooney CT, et al: Serum thyroxine and triiodothyronine responses of hyperthyroid cats to thyrotropin. Am J Vet Res 57 : 987, 1996.

63. Kintzer PP, Peterson ME: Thyroid scintigraphy in small animals. Semin Vet Med Surg (Small Anim) 6 : 131, 1991.
64. Mooney CT, et al: Qualitative and quantitative thyroid imaging in feline hyperthyroidism using technetium-99m pertechnetate. Vet Radiol 33 : 313, 1992.
65. Beck KA, et al: The normal feline thyroid: Technetium pertechnetate imaging and determination of thyroid to salivary gland radioactivity ratios in 10 normal cats. Vet Radiol 26 : 35, 1985.
66. Nap AM, et al: Quantitative aspects of thyroid scintigraphy with pertechnetate ⁹⁹ᵐTcO₄⁻ in cats. J Vet Intern Med 8 : 302, 1994.
67. Kintzer PP: Considerations in the treatment of feline hyperthyroidism. Vet Clin North Am Small Anim Pract 24 : 577, 1994.
68. Peterson ME, et al: Propylthiouracil-associated hemolytic anemia, thrombocytopenia, and antinuclear antibodies in cats with hyperthyroidism. JAVMA 184 : 806, 1984.
69. Aucoin DP, et al: Propylthiouracil-induced immune-mediated disease in cats. J Pharmacol Exp Ther 234: 13, 1985.
70. Taurog A: Hormone synthesis: Thyroid iodine metabolism. *In* Braverman LE, Utiger RD (eds): The Thyroid: A Fundamental and Clinical Text, 6th ed. Philadelphia, JB Lippincott, 1991, pp 51–97.
71. Graves TK: Complications of treatment and concurrent illness associated with hyperthyroidism in cats. *In* Bonagura JD, Kirk RW (eds): Current Veterinary Therapy XII. Philadelphia, WB Saunders, 1994, pp 369–372.
72. Peterson ME Feline hypothyroidism. *In* Kirk RW, Bonagura JD (ed): Current Veterinary Therapy X. Philadelphia, WB Saunders, 1989, pp 1000–1001.
73. Trepanier LA, et al: Pharmacokinetics of methimazole in normal cats and cats with hyperthyroidism. Res Vet Sci 50 : 69, 1991.
74. Shelton GD, et al: Acquired myasthenia gravis in hyperthyroid cats on tapazole therapy. J Vet Intern Med 2 : 120, 1997.
75. Thoday KL, Mooney CT: Medical management of feline hyperthyroidism. *In* Kirk RW, Bonagura JD (eds): Current Veterinary Therapy XI. Philadelphia, WB Saunders, 1992, pp 338–345.
76. Mooney CT: Update on the medical management of hyperthyroidism. *In* August JR (ed): Consultations in Feline Internal Medicine 3. Philadelphia, WB Saunders, 1997, pp 155–162.
77. Peterson ME Aucoin DP: Comparison of the disposition of carbimazole and methimazole in clinically normal cats. Res Vet Sci 54 : 351, 1993.
78. Murray LAS, Peterson ME: Ipodate treatment of hyperthyroidism in cats. JAVMA 211 : 63, 1997.
79. Peterson ME: Considerations and complications in anesthesia with pathophysiologic changes in the endocrine system. *In* Short CE (ed): Principles and Practice of Veterinary Anesthesiology. Philadelphia, Williams & Wilkins, 1987, pp 251–270.
80. Ware WA: Current uses and hazards of beta blockers. *In* Kirk RW, Bonagura JD (eds): Current Veterinary Therapy XI. Philadelphia, WB Saunders, 1992, pp 676–684.
81. Roti E, Vagenakis AG: Effect of excess iodide: Clinical aspects. *In* Braverman LE, Utiger RD (eds): The Thyroid: A Fundamental and Clinical Text. Philadelphia, JB Lippincott, 1991, pp 390–402.
82. Birchard SJ: Surgical treatment of feline hyperthyroidism: Results of 85 cases. J Am Anim Hosp Assoc 20 : 705, 1984.
83. Flanders JA, et al: Feline thyroidectomy. A comparison of postoperative hypocalcemia associated with three different surgical techniques. Vet Surg 16 : 362, 1987.
84. Welches CD, et al: Occurrence of problems after three techniques of bilateral thyroidectomy in cats. Vet Surg 18 : 392, 1989.
85. Birchard SJ: Thyroidectomy and parathyroidectomy in the dog and cat. Probl Vet Med 3 : 277, 1991.
86. Flanders JA: Surgical therapy of the thyroid. Vet Clin North Am Small Anim Pract 24 : 607, 1994.
87. Peterson ME; Hypoparathyroidism. *In* Kirk RW (eds): Current Veterinary Therapy IX. Philadelphia, WB Saunders, 1986, pp 1039–1045.
88. Peterson ME: Hypoparathyroidism and other causes of hypocalcemia in cats. *In* Kirk RW, Bonagura JD (eds): Current Veterinary Therapy XI. Philadelphia, WB Saunders, 1992, pp 376–379.
89. Padgett SL, et al: Efficacy of parathyroid gland autotransplanation in maintaining serum calcium concentrations after bilateral thyroparathyroidectomy in cats. J Am Anim Hosp Assoc 34 : 219, 1998.
90. Flanders JA, et al: Functional analysis of ectopic parathyroid activity in cats. Am J Vet Res 52 : 1336, 1991.
91. Swalec KM, Birchard SJ: Recurrence of hyperthyroidism after thyroidectomy in cats. J Am Anim Hosp Assoc 26 : 433, 1990.
92. Solomon DH: Radioiodine. Iodine-131. *In* Ingbar SH, Braverman LE (eds): The Thyroid. Philadelphia, JB Lippincott, 1986, pp 1001–1003.
93. Links JM, Wagner HN: Radiation physics. *In* Braverman LE, Utiger RD (eds): The Thyroid: A Fundamental and Clinical Text, 6th ed. Philadelphia, JB Lippincott, 1991, pp 405–420.
94. Turrel JM, et al: Radioactive iodine therapy in cats with hyperthyroidism. JAVMA 184 : 554, 1984.
95. Broome MR, et al: Predictive value of tracer studies for ¹³¹I treatment in hyperthyroid cats. Am J Vet Res 49 : 193, 1988.
96. Theon AP, et al: Prospective randomized comparison of intravenous versus subcutaneous administration of radioiodine for treatment of hyperthyroidism in cats. Am J Vet Res 55 : 1734, 1994.
97. Meric SM, Rubin SI: Serum thyroxine concentrations following fixed-dose radioactive iodine treatment in hyperthyroid cats: 62 cases (1986–1989). JAVMA 197:621, 1990.

98. Craig A, et al: A prospective study of 66 cases of feline hyperthyroidism treated with a fixed dose of intravenous [131]I. Aust Vet Pract 23 : 2, 1993.

99. Jones BR, et al: Radio-iodine treatment of hyperthyroidism in cats. N Z Vet J 39:71, 1991.

100. Mooney CT: Radioactive iodine therapy for feline hyperthyroidism: Efficacy and administration routes. J Small Anim Pract 35 : 289, 1994.

101. Peterson ME, Becker DV: Radioiodine treatment of 524 cats with hyperthyroidism. JAVMA 207 : 1422, 1995.

102. Guptill L, et al; Response to high-dose radioactive iodine administration in cats with thyroid carcinoma that had previously undergone surgery. JAVMA 207 : 1055, 1995.

103. Karstrup S, et al: Acute change in parathyroid function in primary hyperparathyroidism following ultrasonically guided ethanol injection into solitary parathyroid adenomas. Acta Endocrinol 129 : 377, 1993.

104. Verges B, et al: Results of ultrasonically guided percutaneous ethanol injection into parathyroid adenomas in primary hyperparathyroidism. Acta Endocrinol 129 : 381, 1993.

105. Long C, et al: Ultrasound guided chemical parathyroidectomy in 4 dogs with primary hyperparathyroidism. Proceedings, Annual Meeting of the American College of Veterinary Radiology, Banff, Alberta, Canada, 1998,

106. Goldstein R, et al: Ultrasound guided percutaneous ethanol injection for the treatment of 4 cats with unilateral hyperthyroidism. Proceedings, American College of Veterinary Internal Medicine, Chicago, 1999.

107. Walker MC, Schaer M: Percutaneous ethanol treatment of hyperthyroidism in a cat. Feline Pract 26 : 10, 1998.

108. Wells A, et al: Ultrasound guided percutaneous ethanol injection for the treatment of 6 cats with bilateral hyperthyroidism. Proceedings, American College of Veterinary Internal Medicine, Chicago, 1999.

109. Birchard SJ, et al: Neoplasia of the thyroid gland in the dog: A retrospective study of 16 cases. J Am Anim Hosp Assoc 17 : 369, 1981.

110. Loar AS: Canine thyroid tumors. In Kirk RW (ed): Current Veterinary Therapy IX. Philadelphia, WB Saunders, 1986, pp 1033–1039.

111. Feldman EC, Nelson RW: Canine thyroid tumors and hyperthyroidism. In Feldman EC, Nelson RW (ed): Canine and Feline Endocrinology and Reproduction. Philadelphia, WB Saunders, 1996, pp 166–185.

112. Harari J, et al: Clinical and pathologic features of thyroid tumors in 26 dogs. JAVMA 188 : 1160, 1986.

113. Verschueren CP: Clinico-pathological and endocrine aspects of canine thyroid cancer. Ph.D. thesis, Utrecht, The Netherlands, 1992.

114. Weller RE, et al: Thyroid carcinoma in two dogs. Mod Vet Pract 67 : 116, 1986.

115. Melian C, et al: Horner's syndrome associated with a functional thyroid carcinoma in a dog. J Small Anim Pract 37 : 591, 1996.

116. Rijnberk A: Thyroids. In Rijnberk A (ed): Clinical Endocrinology of Dogs and Cats. Dordrecht, The Netherlands, Kluwer Academic, 1996, pp 35–59.

117. Lawrence D, et al: Hyperthyroidism associated with a thyroid adenoma in a dog. JAVMA 199 : 81, 1991.

118. Marks SL, et al: ^{99m}Tc-pertechnetate imaging of thyroid tumors in dogs: 29 cases (1980–1992). JAVMA 204 : 756, 1994.

119. Kemppainen RJ, Young DW: Canine triiodothyronine autoantibodies. In Kirk RW, Bonagura JD (ed): Current Veterinary Therapy. Philadelphia, WB Saunders, 1992, pp 327–330.

120. Klein MK, et al: Treatment of thyroid carcinoma in dogs by surgical resection alone: 20 cases (1981–1989). JAVMA 206 : 1007, 1995.

121. Carver JR, et al: A comparison of medullary thyroid carcinoma and thyroid adenocarcinoma in dogs: A retrospective study of 38 cases. Vet Surg 24 : 315, 1995.

122. Ogilvie GK, et al: Phase II evaluation of doxorubicin for treatment of various canine neoplasms. JAVMA 195 : 1580, 1989.

123. Fineman LS, et al: Cisplatin chemotherapy for treatment of thyroid carcinoma in dogs: 13 cases. J Am Anim Hosp Assoc 34:109, 1998.

124. Peterson ME, et al: Radioactive iodine treatment of a functional thyroid carcinoma producing hyperthyroidism in a dog. J Vet Intern Med 3 : 20, 1989.

125. Adams WH, et al: Treatment of differentiated thyroid carcinoma in 7 dogs utilizing [131]I. Vet Radiol Ultrasound 36 : 417, 1995.

CHAPTER 151

HYPOTHYROIDISM

J. Catharine R. Scott-Moncrieff and Lynn Guptill-Yoran

END

Hypothyroidism is the result of decreased production of thyroxine (T_4) and triiodothyronine (T_3) by the thyroid gland. Naturally occurring hypothyroidism is common in dogs but rare in cats.

PHYSIOLOGY AND METABOLISM

Thyroid hormones are iodine-containing amino acids synthesized in the thyroid gland (Fig. 151–1). All circulating T_4, but only 20 per cent of T_3, is derived from the thyroid gland. The majority of T_3 is derived from extrathyroidal enzymatic 5'-deiodination of T_4.

In the blood, more than 99 per cent of T_4 and T_3 is bound to plasma proteins, with T_4 more highly bound than T_3. In the dog, the thyroid binding proteins are thyroid hormone–binding globulin (TBG), transthyretin, albumin, and apolipoproteins, with most T_4 bound to TBG. Dogs have lower avidity of thyroid hormone binding to serum proteins than do humans, resulting in lower total serum concentrations of T_4 and T_3, higher free hormone concentrations, and more rapid clearance rates.

Only free hormone enters cells to produce a biologic effect and have a negative feedback effect on the pituitary and hypothalamus. T_3 enters cells more rapidly, has a more rapid onset of action, and is three to five times more potent than T_4. Thyroid hormones bind to receptors in the nuclei; the hormone receptor complex binds to DNA and influences the expression of a variety of genes coding for regulatory enzymes.

Thyroid hormone synthesis and secretion are regulated primarily by changes in the circulating concentration of pituitary thyrotropin (TSH) (Fig. 151–2). Thyroid hormones are metabolized by progressive deiodination of the molecule. Outer-ring deiodination of T_4 produces T_3, whereas inner-ring deiodination results in formation of biologically inactive reverse T_3 (rT_3). Deiodination is regulated by the relative activity of different deiodinase enzymes and is an important regulatory step in thyroid hormone metabolism. L-Thyroxine and T_3 are both concentrated in the liver and secreted in the bile.

Thyroid hormones have a wide variety of physiologic effects. Thyroid hormones increase the metabolic rate and oxygen consumption of almost all tissues, with the exception of the adult brain, testes, uterus, lymph nodes, spleen, and anterior pituitary. Thyroid hormones have positive inotropic and chronotropic effects on the heart. They increase the

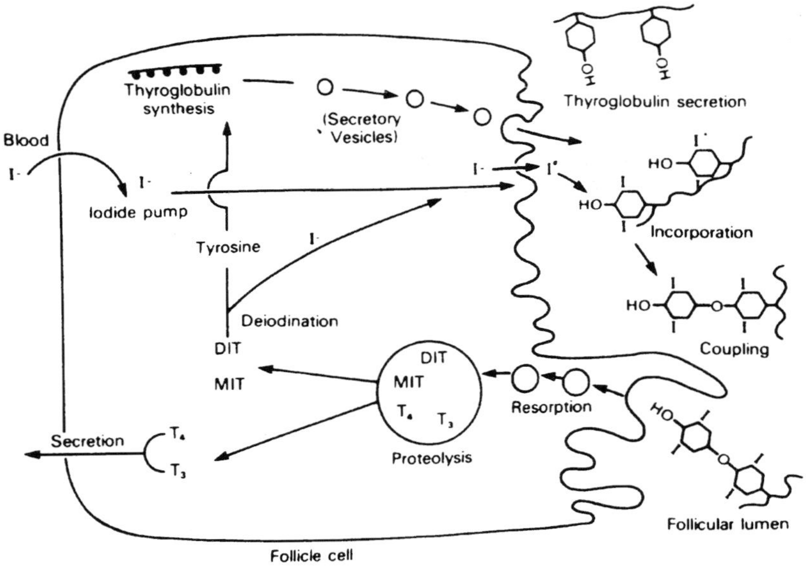

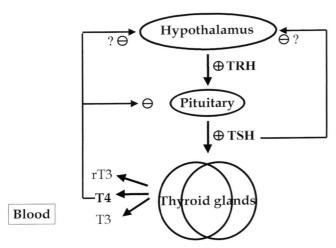

Figure 151–1. Synthesis of thyroid hormones. The follicular cells of the thyroid gland concentrate iodide, which diffuses down a gradient into the colloid. Thyroglobulin is synthesized within thyroid follicular cells and secreted into the colloid. Iodide is oxidized and bound to tyrosine residues on the thyroglobulin molecule by thyroid peroxidase. Iodinated tyrosine residues (monoiodotyrosine [MIT] and diiodotyrosine [DIT]) within the thyroglobulin molecule then undergo oxidative condensation to form the iodothyronines (T_3 and T_4), which remain bound to thyroglobulin until secreted. Thyroglobulin is ingested by endocytosis from the colloid; the peptide bonds between the iodinated residues and the thyroglobulin are hydrolyzed; and MIT, DIT, T_4, and T_3 are released into the cytoplasm. MIT and DIT are deiodinated and the iodine is recycled, while T_4 and T_3 are released into the bloodstream. (From Mountcastle VB: Medical Physiology, 14th ed, vol 2. St. Louis, CV Mosby, 1980.)

number and affinity of beta-adrenergic receptors, enhance the response to catecholamines, and increase the proportion of alpha myosin heavy chain. Thyroid hormones have catabolic effects on muscle and adipose tissue, stimulate erythropoiesis, and regulate both cholesterol synthesis and degradation. Thyroid hormones are also essential for the normal growth and development of the neurologic and skeletal systems.

CANINE HYPOTHYROIDISM

PATHOGENESIS

Hypothyroidism may occur owing to dysfunction of any part of the hypothalamic-pituitary-thyroid axis (see Fig.

Figure 151–2. Regulation of thyroid hormone concentrations. Thyroid hormone concentrations are controlled by the hypothalamic-pituitary-thyroid axis, which operates as a negative feedback loop. Thyrotropin (TSH) causes synthesis and release of T_4 and lesser amounts of T_3 from the thyroid gland. Intracellular T_3, derived from deiodination of T_4 within the pituitary gland, causes decreased TSH synthesis and secretion and is the main determinant of TSH concentration. Thyrotropin-releasing hormone (TRH), secreted by the hypothalamus, modulates TSH release from the pituitary gland. Increased thyroid hormone and TSH concentrations are also believed to decrease TRH synthesis and secretion. Hormones that inhibit TSH secretion include dopamine, somatostatin, serotonin, and glucocorticoids. Prostaglandins and alpha-adrenergic agonists increase TSH secretion.

151–2). Most cases of acquired canine hypothyroidism are caused by primary hypothyroidism due to lymphocytic thyroiditis or idiopathic thyroid atrophy.

Approximately 50 per cent of cases of primary hypothyroidism are due to lymphocytic thyroiditis.[1] Grossly, the thyroid gland may be normal or atrophic.[2] Histologically, there is multifocal or diffuse infiltration of the thyroid gland by lymphocytes, plasma cells, and macrophages. Remaining follicles are small, and lymphocytes, macrophages, and degenerate follicular cells may be found within vacuolated colloid. As thyroiditis progresses, parenchyma is destroyed and replaced by fibrous connective tissue.

Canine thyroiditis is believed to be immune-mediated,[3] and antithyroglobulin antibodies are present in 42 to 59 per cent of hypothyroid dogs.[4–7] Current evidence suggests that follicular cell destruction is due to binding of thyroid autoantibodies to the plasma membrane of follicular cells and subsequent antibody-dependent cell-mediated cytotoxicity. Thyroiditis is heritable in the beagle and the Borzoi.[2, 8, 9] Golden retrievers, Great Danes, Irish setters, Doberman pinschers, and Old English sheepdogs have an increased prevalence of antithyroglobulin antibodies.[5, 6, 10]

In idiopathic follicular atrophy, there is loss of thyroid parenchyma and replacement by adipose connective tissue.[1] Degeneration of individual follicular cells occurs, with exfoliation of cells into the colloid. Follicular atrophy may be the final result of thyroiditis, but the absence of fibrosis or inflammation suggests that idiopathic thyroid atrophy is a distinct syndrome.

Less commonly, bilateral thyroid neoplasia or invasion of the thyroid by metastatic neoplasia can result in hypothyroidism. Because hypothyroidism does not occur until at least 75 per cent of the thyroid parenchyma has been destroyed, most dogs with thyroid neoplasia are euthyroid.[11] Lymphocytic thyroiditis has been identified as a risk factor for thyroid neoplasia.[2]

A rare cause of primary hypothyroidism is adenomatous hyperplasia, in which the thyroid glands are composed of orderly clusters of follicular cells and fewer numbers of oxyphilic cells arranged in a compact follicular pattern.[12] The cause of adenomatous hyperplasia may be an intrathyroidal metabolic defect.

Secondary hypothyroidism (deficiency of TSH) is rarely

described in dogs, probably because a validated assay for canine TSH has been unavailable until recently. Causes of acquired secondary hypothyroidism include pituitary malformations and pituitary neoplasia. Histologic changes observed in secondary hypothyroidism include flattening of follicular epithelial cells and distention of thyroid follicles with colloid.[12] Tertiary hypothyroidism (deficiency of thyrotropin releasing hormone [TRH]) has yet to be documented in the dog.

Congenital hypothyroidism (cretinism) is rarely diagnosed in dogs. Reported causes of congenital primary hypothyroidism include iodine deficiency, thyroid dysgenesis, and dyshormonogenesis.[13, 14] Secondary congenital hypothyroidism due to apparent isolated TSH or TRH deficiency has been reported in a family of young giant schnauzers and in a young Boxer.[13, 15] In both reports, central hypothyroidism was suspected because of increased T_4 secretion and increased uptake of ^{99m}Tc-pertechnetate after repeated administration of TSH. Congenital secondary hypothyroidism is also a feature of panhypopituitarism.

Iatrogenic causes of hypothyroidism include ^{131}iodine treatment, administration of antithyroid drugs, and surgical thyroidectomy. Because of the presence of accessory thyroid tissue, permanent hypothyroidism is rare after thyroidectomy.

EPIDEMIOLOGY

The prevalence of canine hypothyroidism in a recent study was 0.2 per cent.[16] Mean age at diagnosis was 7.2 years, with a range of 0.5 to 15 years. Golden retrievers and Doberman pinschers are at higher risk for hypothyroidism.[16–18] Spayed female and castrated male dogs are at increased risk for developing hypothyroidism compared with sexually intact animals.

CLINICAL SIGNS

Because clinical signs of hypothyroidism may be vague, diffuse, and insidious in onset, hypothyroidism is considered in the differential diagnosis of a wide range of problems and is frequently misdiagnosed (Table 151–1). Lethargy, mental dullness, weight gain, unwillingness to exercise, and cold intolerance are the result of a decreased metabolic rate. Weakness or lethargy occurs in 20 per cent of hypothyroid dogs.[16] Obesity occurs in 41 per cent of hypothyroid dogs, but most obese dogs suffer from overnutrition rather than hypothyroidism.

Dermatologic changes occur in 60 per cent of hypothyroid

TABLE 151–1. CLINICAL MANIFESTATIONS OF CANINE HYPOTHYROIDISM

COMMON	UNCOMMON	UNKNOWN*
Lethargy	Neurologic	Male infertility
Weight gain	dysfunction	Coagulopathies
Alopecia	Female infertility	Cardiovascular disorders
Pyoderma	Myxedema	Gastrointestinal disorders
Seborrhea	Ocular disorders	Behavioral disorders
	Cretinism	

The information in this table was the consensus of participants in the international symposium on canine hypothyroidism held in Davis, California, in August 1996.
*There is no current proof that these disorders are caused by hypothyroidism in dogs.
Modified from Clinical Manifestations. Canine Pract 22:36, 1997.

dogs. Common findings include dry scaly skin, changes in haircoat quality or color, alopecia, seborrhea (sicca or oleosa), and superficial pyoderma. Hyperkeratosis, hyperpigmentation, comedone formation, hypertrichosis, ceruminous otitis, poor wound healing, increased bruising, and myxedema may also occur.

Alopecia is usually bilaterally symmetric and is first evident in areas of wear, such as the lateral trunk, ventral thorax, and tail. The head and extremities tend to be spared. The hair is often brittle and easily epilated, and loss of undercoat or primary guard hairs may result in a coarse appearance or a puppylike haircoat. Fading of coat color may also occur, and failure of hair regrowth after clipping is common. Occasionally, hair retention rather than alopecia occurs. Signs of decreased metabolic rate together with dermatologic abnormalities should increase the suspicion for hypothyroidism.

Hypothyroid dogs are predisposed to recurrent bacterial infections of the skin such as folliculitis, pyoderma, and furunculosis. *Malassezia* infections and demodicosis have also been associated with hypothyroidism. Pruritus may occur due to concurrent infection.

Myxedema is a rare manifestation of hypothyroidism characterized by a nonpitting thickening or puffiness of the skin, especially of the eyelids, cheeks, and forehead. It is caused by deposition of hyaluronic acid in the dermis.[19]

Reproductive problems associated with hypothyroidism in females include decreased libido, prolonged interestrous interval, silent heats, failure to cycle, spontaneous abortion, small or low-birth-weight litters, uterine inertia, and weak or stillborn puppies. Inappropriate galactorrhea apparently due to hyperprolactinemia has also been reported in sexually intact hypothyroid bitches.[20] Male reproductive problems that have been attributed to hypothyroidism include low libido, testicular atrophy, hypospermia, and azoospermia. Thyroiditis and orchitis in a colony of beagles were associated with decreased testicular size, subfertility, or sterility.[21] Subnormal fertility and poor semen quality were also reported in a colony of Borzois with thyroiditis, but testicular biopsies were not evaluated.[22] A prospective study of nine male beagles with ^{131}iodine-induced hypothyroidism showed no decrease in libido or sperm quality over a two-year period.[22]

The peripheral and central nervous systems may be affected by hypothyroidism. Peripheral neuropathy is the best documented neurologic manifestation of hypothyroidism.[23, 24] Affected dogs have exercise intolerance, weakness, ataxia, quadriparesis or paralysis, and decreased spinal reflexes. Clinical signs resolve after thyroid hormone supplementation. A subclinical myopathy also occurs in canine hypothyroidism.[25] Unilateral lameness reported in hypothyroid dogs may be a manifestation of generalized neuromyopathy.[26]

Dysfunction of multiple cranial nerves (facial, trigeminal, vestibulocochlear) and abnormal gait and postural reactions have been reported in hypothyroidism.[24, 27] Dogs with vestibular deficits have abnormal brain stem auditory-evoked responses. Clinical signs resolve after L-thyroxine supplementation. Because dogs with vestibular disease may have resolution of clinical signs owing to compensation, a causal relationship is less clear.[24] Although laryngeal paralysis and megaesophagus have been reported in association with hypothyroidism, treatment of hypothyroidism does not consistently result in resolution of clinical signs, and a causal relationship has not been confirmed. Myasthenia gravis has been reported to occur in association with hypothyroidism.[28] Concurrent hypothyroidism may exacerbate clinical signs of myasthenia gravis such as muscle weakness and mega-esophagus.

Rarely, cerebral dysfunction may occur in hypothyroidism due to myxedema coma, atherosclerosis, or the presence of a pituitary tumor causing secondary hypothyroidism. Seizures, disorientation, and circling may occur due to severe hyper-lipidemia or cerebral atherosclerosis.[29] In myxedema coma, profound mental dullness or stupor is accompanied by non-pitting edema, hypothermia, bradycardia, and inappetence.[30]

Abnormalities of the cardiovascular system such as sinus bradycardia, weak apex beat, low QRS voltages, and in-verted T waves may occur in hypothyroid dogs.[16] Reduced left ventricular pump function has also been documented, and hypothyroidism may exacerbate clinical signs in dogs with underlying cardiac disease.[31] Hypothyroidism alone rarely causes clinically significant myocardial failure in dogs. Although canine dilated cardiomyopathy and hypothyroid-ism may occur together, there is little evidence that the two diseases are causally related. Ocular abnormalities reported in canine hypothyroidism include corneal lipidosis, corneal ulceration, uveitis, lipid effusion into the aqueous humor, secondary glaucoma, lipemia retinalis, retinal detachment, and keratoconjunctivitis sicca.[32]

Clinical signs of secondary hypothyroidism are similar to those of primary hypothyroidism, but clinical signs related to a deficiency of other pituitary functions may predominate, particularly if a pituitary neoplasm is present.

Congenital hypothyroidism results in mental retardation and stunted, disproportionate growth due to epiphyseal dys-genesis and delayed skeletal maturation (Fig. 151–3).[33] Af-fected dogs are mentally dull and have large, broad heads, short limbs, macroglossia, hypothermia, delayed dental erup-tion, ataxia, and abdominal distention.[13, 15] Dermatologic findings are similar to those seen in the adult hypothyroid dog. Other clinical signs may include gait abnormalities and constipation. Affected puppies are often the largest in the litter at birth but start to lag behind their littermates within three to eight weeks. It is likely that many severely affected puppies die in the first few weeks of life.

CLINICOPATHOLOGIC CHANGES

Results of a hemogram, biochemical panel, and urinalysis may support a diagnosis of hypothyroidism and rule out other disorders. A mild nonregenerative anemia occurs in 30 per cent of hypothyroid dogs. Fasting hypercholesterolemia occurs in about 75 per cent of hypothyroid dogs, owing to increased concentrations of high-density lipoproteins (HDL$_1$). Hypertriglyceridemia due to increased low-density lipoproteins (LDL), very low-density lipoproteins (VLDL), and hyperchylomicronemia may also occur in some dogs and can cause atherosclerosis. Less common abnormalities include mild increases in alkaline phosphatase, alanine ami-notransferase, and creatine kinase. Mild hypercalcemia may occur in congenital hypothyroidism.

HEMOSTASIS

Decreased plasma von Willebrand factor antigen (vWf:Ag) concentration has been reported in hypothyroid dogs; however, other studies have failed to demonstrate a relationship between vWf:Ag or Factor VIII activity and thyroid hormone status.[34–36] Canine hypothyroidism is rarely associated with clinical bleeding, and platelet function and bleeding times are normal. Concentrations of vWf:Ag do not consistently increase during treatment of hypothyroid dogs with L-thyroxine.[35] There is no evidence to support thyroid supplementation of euthyroid dogs with von Willebrand's disease.

POLYENDOCRINOPATHIES

Canine hypothyroidism may occur in association with other immune-mediated endocrine disorders such as hypoad-renocorticism and diabetes mellitus.[37, 38] Hypothyroidism causes insulin resistance[39] and may mask electrolyte changes in hypoadrenocorticism.

DIAGNOSIS

Patient Selection

Appropriate patient selection is important when evaluating thyroid function. The positive predictive value of diagnostic

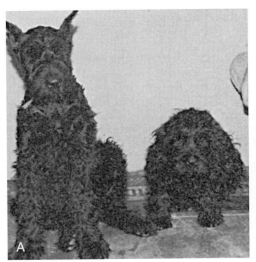
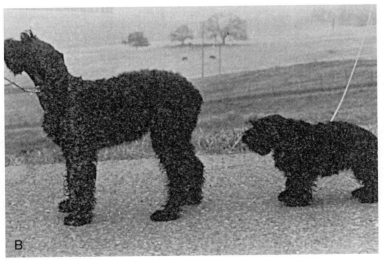

Figure 151–3. *A* and *B*, Eight-month-old female giant schnauzer littermates. The dog on the left is normal, while the smaller dog on the right has congenital hypothyroidism (cretinism). Note the small stature; disproportionate body size; large, broad head; wide, square trunk; and short limbs in the cretin. (From Feldman EC, Nelson RW: Canine and Feline Endocrinology and Reproduction, 2nd ed. Philadelphia, WB Saunders, 1996, p 83.)

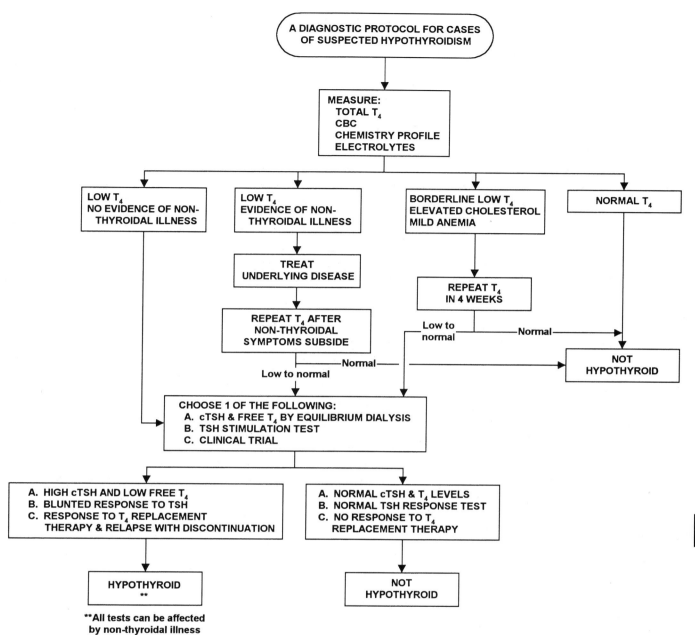

Figure 151–4. Algorithm for diagnosis of hypothyroidism.

tests is highest when the prevalence of the disease tested for is high. An adequate minimum database aids in identifying other diseases and determining whether thyroid dysfunction is likely. Testing of healthy dogs prior to breeding or of obese dogs with no other clinical signs of thyroid disease increases the chance of false-positive test results (Fig. 151–4).

Basal Thyroid Hormone Concentrations

Thyroid hormones commonly measured include total T_4 (TT_4), total T_3 (TT_3), and free T_4 (fT_4). Assays for free T_3 (fT_3) and reverse T_3 (rT_3) are less commonly used. Assays must be validated for the dog, and because canine thyroid hormone concentrations are lower than human concentrations, the assays must have adequate sensitivity. Serum anti-

bodies directed against T_3 and T_4 may interfere with thyroid hormone assays because they compete for hormone with antibodies used in the assay. These antibodies may cause spuriously high or low results, depending on the assay used. Hemolysis and lipemia do not change thyroid hormone concentrations measured by radioimmunoassay.[40, 41] Thyroid hormones are stable at 37°C for five days, provided the samples are stored in plastic rather than glass, and at 22°C for eight days.[42] They are also very stable when frozen, even with repeated freezing and thawing. Samples should be shipped to outside laboratories in plastic tubes.

Total T₄ Concentration

Total T_4 concentration is an excellent screening test for canine thyroid dysfunction (see Fig. 151–4). A dog with a

TT_4 concentration well within the reference range may be assumed to be euthyroid, unless anti-T_4 antibodies are causing a spurious increase in the TT_4 value. This is uncommon, because anti-T_4 antibodies are detected in only 0.8 per cent of canine serum samples.[10] A decreased TT_4 concentration is not specific for a diagnosis of hypothyroidism. Decreased TT_4 may be normal for that individual, result from nonthyroidal illness, or be secondary to drug administration. The reference range for TT_4 concentration depends on the laboratory but is usually 1.5 to 3.5 μg/dL. Time of day, age, breed, and ambient temperature may affect serum TT_4 concentration. In healthy euthyroid dogs, TT_4 concentration may decrease below the reference range as much as 20 per cent of the time, but there is no predictable diurnal pattern.[43] Serum TT_4 concentrations in neonates are similar to those in adult dogs; they then increase to more than two to five times the adult concentration by 3 weeks of age. Total T_4 concentrations return to those of the adult dog by 12 weeks of age, then gradually decline with age.[44] Total T_4 concentrations do not differ significantly between males and females but are higher in small dogs than in medium and large breed dogs.[44] Greyhounds and Scottish deerhounds have lower TT_4 concentrations than other breeds of dog. During diestrus and pregnancy, TT_4 concentrations are increased owing to changes in thyroid hormone protein binding. Mild increases in TT_4 concentrations may also occur in obesity.

Free T_4 Concentration

Protein-bound hormone acts as a reservoir to maintain concentrations of free hormone in the plasma despite fluctuations in release or metabolism of T_3 and T_4 or in plasma protein concentrations. Thus free hormone concentrations are less affected by changes in protein concentration and binding than are measurements of total hormone. Because only free hormone can enter cells and bind to receptors, measurement of fT_4 should give a more accurate representation of thyroid function (see Fig. 151–4). In humans, fT_4 concentration often remains normal during nonthyroidal illness, but this does not always occur in dogs. The standard method for measuring fT_4 is equilibrium dialysis. Because this is expensive and time consuming, single-stage solid-phase (analog) radioimmunoassays for human fT_4 are commonly used for measurement of canine fT_4. These assays depend on the dominance of thyroid hormone binding by TBG, concentrations of which are lower in dogs than in humans. Canine fT_4 concentrations measured by analog methods are lower than those measured by equilibrium dialysis and have no diagnostic advantage over measurement of TT_4.[45, 46] A commercial fT_4 assay that uses an equilibrium dialysis step is more accurate than analog methods and is more specific for canine hypothyroidism than is measurement of TT_4.[45, 47] This assay is also unaffected by anti-T_4 antibodies.

Total T_3 Concentration

Measurement of TT_3 concentrations is less accurate than TT_4 measurement for distinguishing euthyroid from hypothyroid dogs, because T_3 concentrations fluctuate out of the normal range even more than T_4 concentrations in euthyroid dogs.[43] Spurious results may occur owing to anti-T_3 antibodies.

Reverse T_3 and Free T_3 Concentrations

In humans, one mechanism for the euthyroid sick syndrome is decreased 5′-deiodinase activity. This results in a reciprocal relationship between T_3 and rT_3 concentrations. Although this change has been documented experimentally in dogs,[48] it does not occur predictably in all dogs with nonthyroidal illness. The clinical utility of measurement of rT_3 or fT_3 in dogs has not been demonstrated.

Effect of Drugs on Thyroid Hormone Concentrations

Drug administration can change thyroid hormone concentrations in dogs. The effect of corticosteroid administration is dependent on the dose and specific preparation. Administration of prednisone at a dose of 1.1 mg/kg every 12 hours for one month had no effect on TT_4 concentrations but decreased TT_3 concentrations.[49] Prednisolone at the same dose for 21 days decreased TT_4, fT_4, and TT_3 concentrations.[50]

Sulfonamides block iodination orally of thyroglobulin.[51] Trimethoprim-sulfadiazine (15 mg/kg every 12 hours) had no effect on thyroid function,[52] but trimethoprim-sulfamethoxazole at a dose of 30 mg/kg orally every 12 hours decreased TT_4 and TT_3 concentrations, increased canine TSH, and decreased response to TSH administration.[51, 53]

Phenobarbital administration decreases TT_4 and fT_4 concentrations and increases TSH concentration in normal dogs.[54] Other drugs that decrease thyroid hormone concentrations in humans and may have the same effect in dogs include androgens, dopamine, penicillin, phenothiazines, phenylbutazone, mitotane, phenytoin, primidone, propranolol, salicylates, diazepam, furosemide, and heparin.

Effect of Systemic Illness on Thyroid Hormone Concentrations

In nonthyroidal illness, thyroid hormone concentrations are often decreased. Changes in hormone binding to serum carrier proteins (e.g., decreased protein concentration, reduced binding affinity, circulating inhibitors of binding), changes in peripheral hormone distribution and metabolism (e.g., reduced 5′-deiodinase activity), inhibition of TSH secretion, and inhibition of thyroid hormone synthesis may occur. Cytokines such as interleukin-1, interleukin-2, interferon gamma, and tumor necrosis factor alpha decrease TT_4, TT_3, and fT_4 concentrations.[55] In dogs, TT_4 concentration is more frequently decreased than is TT_3 concentration. The magnitude of decrease depends on disease severity and is a predictor of mortality.[56] Thyroid hormone supplementation does not improve survival in humans with decreased thyroid hormone concentrations. Conditions reported to decrease basal T_4 concentrations in dogs include hyperadrenocorticism, diabetic ketoacidosis, hypoadrenocorticism, renal failure, hepatic disease, peripheral neuropathy, generalized megaesophagus, heart failure, critical illness or infection, and surgery or anesthesia.[56–58] In 59 euthyroid dogs with concurrent illness, 20 per cent had low TT_4 concentrations and 17 per cent had low fT_4 concentrations.[46] In 67 critically ill euthyroid animals, 61 per cent had low T_4 concentrations and 56 per cent had low T_3 concentrations.[56] In 42 dogs with hyperadrenocorticism, 38 per cent had low TT_4, 24 per cent had low fT_4, and 39 per cent had low TT_3 concentrations.[58] Dogs with chronic weight loss had decreased TT_4 and TT_3 concentrations regardless of the cause of weight loss.[59]

Basal Thyrotropin Concentration

A commercial assay for canine TSH (cTSH) has recently been validated and evaluated for the diagnosis of canine hypothyroidism.[60] The assay is specific for cTSH but is not sensitive enough to differentiate normal from decreased concentrations of TSH.

Measurement of an increased concentration of cTSH is specific for a diagnosis of hypothyroidism if the TT_4 or fT_4 is also decreased (see Fig. 151–4).[47, 61] Serum cTSH concentrations are increased in 7 to 12 per cent of dogs with normal TT_4 concentrations. In early thyroid failure, TT_4 is maintained in the normal range by an increase in the cTSH concentration. Other reasons for an increased cTSH with a normal TT_4 include effects of drugs and recovery from nonthyroidal illness. Measurement of cTSH has poor sensitivity for the diagnosis of canine hypothyroidism. Eighteen to 38 per cent of hypothyroid dogs have a cTSH concentration within the reference range.[47, 61–63] Possible reasons for a normal cTSH concentration in hypothyroidism include secondary or tertiary hypothyroidism, fluctuations in cTSH concentration, and effect of drugs or concurrent illness. In addition, the cTSH assay may not detect all isoforms of circulating cTSH. Although some hypothyroid dogs with normal or low cTSH concentrations have secondary or tertiary hypothyroidism, it is unlikely that this accounts for most hypothyroid dogs with normal cTSH concentrations. Serum cTSH concentrations in hypothyroid dogs can fluctuate into the normal range, but there is no predictable pattern.[64] In humans, concurrent illness and drugs can decrease TSH concentration toward or into the high-normal range. Whether this also occurs in dogs has not been investigated.

TSH Response Test

The TSH response test is a test of thyroid gland reserve and is considered the criterion standard for the diagnosis of canine hypothyroidism (see Fig. 151–4). The clinical use of this test is limited by the expense and availability of bovine TSH. The cost of the test may be decreased by storing reconstituted TSH either refrigerated for up to three weeks or frozen at −20°C for up to six months.[65–67] Numerous protocols have been published; the most widely accepted protocol is measurement of TT_4 followed by intravenous administration of bovine TSH at 0.1 units/kg (maximum 5 units). A second sample for measurement of TT_4 is collected six hours later. Other protocols use a fixed dose of 1 to 5 units per dog; however, lower TSH doses result in smaller and less prolonged increases in TT_4 concentration and more borderline responses in clinical patients. There have been occasional reports of anaphylactic responses after bovine TSH administration.[65] A diagnosis of hypothyroidism is likely if both the pre- and the post-TSH serum TT_4 concentrations are below the reference range (<1.5 µg/dL). A post-TSH T_4 concentration greater than 3 µg/dL indicates euthyroidism.[68–70] Interpretation of intermediate results is more difficult and should take into consideration the clinical signs and the severity of concurrent systemic disease. Changes in TT_3 before and after TSH administration are smaller and more variable and of little diagnostic utility. The TSH response test cannot be used to evaluate thyroid function in dogs receiving L-thyroxine, because treatment causes thyroid atrophy. Supplementation must be discontinued six to eight weeks before testing.

TRH Response Test

The TRH response test is used in humans to differentiate primary from secondary hypothyroidism. In people with primary hypothyroidism, response of TSH to TRH adminis-

tration is exaggerated, whereas in secondary hypothyroidism there is no response. In dogs, the test has been used in place of the TSH response test, and change in TT_4 has usually been measured. The most commonly used protocol is 0.1 mg/kg of TRH administered intravenously, with blood collected before and four to six hours after TRH administration. Side effects such as salivation, vomiting, urination, defecation, miosis, tachycardia, and tachypnea may be observed at this dose. Recent studies suggest that a lower fixed dose of 100 to 600 µg TRH intravenously, with samples collected at zero and four hours, is as reliable as the higher dose and is less likely to result in side effects.[68] A diagnosis of hypothyroidism is supported if the post-TRH TT_4 concentration is below the reference range (<1.5 µg/dL). Euthyroidism is likely if the concentration is greater than 2 µg/dL. Unfortunately, the change in serum TT_4 after TRH administration is smaller and more variable from dog to dog than is the change after TSH administration.[70] Some euthyroid dogs have a decreased response to TRH; therefore, the TRH response test is less reliable than the TSH response test in the diagnosis of canine hypothyroidism. Freshly reconstituted TRH may be frozen at −20°C for at least a week without a loss in potency.[71] Change in cTSH concentration after TRH administration has recently been evaluated in dogs. The maximal cTSH response occurs 10 to 30 minutes after intravenous TRH administration.[72] In contrast to the exaggerated response seen in humans with primary hypothyroidism, the majority of hypothyroid dogs have a smaller increase in cTSH concentration after TRH administration compared with euthyroid dogs. The TRH response test is therefore not useful for differentiation of primary and secondary hypothyroidism in dogs.

Antithyroglobulin Antibody

Antithyroglobulin antibodies (ATA) are found in 42 to 59 per cent of hypothyroid dogs and are believed to be the result of leakage of thyroglobulin into circulation owing to lymphocytic thyroiditis. A commercially available enzyme-linked immunosorbent assay (ELISA) for ATA is a sensitive and specific indicator of thyroiditis, with false-positive results occurring in less than 5 per cent of dogs with other endocrine disorders.[73] It is important to recognize that a positive ATA titer is not an indicator of abnormal thyroid function. Whether all dogs with ATA ultimately develop hypothyroidism is unknown. Measurement of ATA has been advocated for screening breeding stock, with the aim of ultimately eliminating heritable forms of thyroiditis. Whether this is an effective approach has yet to be demonstrated.

Anti-T_3 and -T_4 Antibodies

Antibodies directed against T_3 and T_4 also occur in canine thyroiditis, although they are less prevalent than ATA. Because T_3 and T_4 alone are small molecules, these antibodies probably develop against T_3- and T_4-containing epitopes of thyroglobulin. Anti-T_3 antibodies alone are found in approximately 4 per cent of samples submitted for thyroid testing, whereas anti-T_4 antibodies alone are found in 0.2 per cent of samples. Both anti-T_3 and anti-T_4 antibodies are found in 0.7 per cent of samples.[10] There is a higher prevalence of antithyroid antibodies in hypothyroid than in euthyroid dogs, and antibodies are most prevalent in younger dogs and in breeds with a high prevalence of hypothyroidism. Because dogs with thyroiditis may still have adequate thyroid reserve, antithyroid antibodies are not indicators of hypothyroidism.

END

Antibodies directed against T_3 and T_4 may interfere with hormone assays, leading to a spurious increase or decrease in the measured hormone concentration.

Scintigraphy

There are few studies evaluating the use of scintigraphy for the diagnosis of thyroid dysfunction in the dog. Dogs with normal thyroid function have a median thyroid-salivary (T:S) ratio of approximately 1 at both 20 and 60 minutes after injection of ^{99m}Tc-pertechnetate; however, the range of T:S values was greater than that which occurs in cats.[74] Decreased thyroid uptake of pertechnetate has been reported in hypothyroid dogs, but we have documented increased uptake of pertechnetate in a hypothyroid dog with thyroiditis. Further evaluation of scintigraphic findings in canine hypothyroidism is necessary. Scintigraphy is useful to identify the underlying cause in puppies with congenital hypothyroidism. In puppies with thyroid agenesis, minimal uptake of pertechnetate in the area of the thyroid gland is detected, whereas in those with iodination defects, thyroid lobes are large, with normal or increased T:S ratios. Scintigraphy may also help identify central hypothyroidism. Administration of TSH for three days does not alter the thyroid image in dogs with primary hypothyroidism but does result in increased thyroid uptake in dogs with central hypothyroidism.[13]

Thyroid Biopsy

Lymphocytic thyroiditis and thyroid atrophy are readily identified histopathologically, but it may be more difficult to determine thyroid function. A surgical approach is necessary for collection of thyroid tissue, and thyroid biopsy is rarely indicated for the clinical diagnosis of hypothyroidism.

Therapeutic Trial

A therapeutic trial may be necessary to establish a diagnosis of hypothyroidism in dogs when the results of diagnostic tests are equivocal and other nonthyroidal causes of clinical signs cannot be identified. A positive response to therapy should be interpreted with caution, because clinical signs may also improve in euthyroid animals treated with L-thyroxine. A diagnosis of hypothyroidism based on response to therapy should be confirmed by recurrence of clinical signs after withdrawal of supplementation. If clinical signs do not respond to a therapeutic trial, therapeutic monitoring should be performed to confirm that appropriate serum TT_4 levels were achieved.

TREATMENT AND THERAPEUTIC MONITORING

Hypothyroidism

The initial treatment of choice is synthetic L-thyroxine, because it results in normalization of both T_4 and T_3 concentrations. Risk of iatrogenic hyperthyroidism is low, because physiologic regulation of conversion of T_4 to T_3 is preserved.[75] Bioavailability may vary greatly from one product to another, so it is advisable to use a brand-name product for initial treatment. Although T_3 is the active hormone at the cellular level, treatment with synthetic L-triiodothyronine or combinations of T_3 and T_4 is not recommended. Treatment with T_3 may be indicated if poor gastrointestinal absorption of T_4 is suspected. L-triiodothyronine would also be indicated

in T_4 to T_3 conversion defects, but this has not been documented in dogs. The use of thyroid extracts is not recommended because the bioavailability and T_4:T_3 ratio of these compounds are variable, making consistent dosing difficult.

Optimal dose and frequency of supplementation vary among dogs because of variability in L-thyroxine absorption and serum half-life.[75-77] Treatment should be initiated at a dose of 0.02 mg/kg orally every 12 hours (Fig. 151–5), and then the dose should be adjusted based on results of therapeutic monitoring. Using twice-daily treatment initially improves the likelihood of response to treatment in all dogs.

Improvement in activity should occur after one to two weeks of treatment, and improvement in haircoat, body weight, and clinicopathologic abnormalities should be evident in four to six weeks. The haircoat may initially appear worse as telogen hairs are shed. Reversal of skin hyperpigmentation, myocardial changes, and neurologic abnormalities may take several months.

Blood samples for therapeutic monitoring should be collected beginning four to eight weeks after starting supplementation with L-thyroxine. Serum TT_4 concentrations should be within the reference range immediately before administration of a dose and should be at the high end or slightly above the reference range four to six hours after administration of a dose. Serum cTSH concentrations should also normalize with appropriate therapy, but the assay cannot distinguish between dogs that are adequately supplemented and those that are oversupplemented. Serum TT_4 concentrations should be measured at six- to eight-week intervals during the first six to eight months of treatment, because metabolism of T_4 will change when the metabolic rate normalizes, and dosage adjustments may be necessary. Once adequate serum TT_4 concentrations are documented, frequency of measurement of serum TT_4 may be decreased to once or twice a year. If the brand of supplement is changed, particularly if a generic product is substituted for a name-brand product, serum TT_4 concentration should be measured after four to eight weeks on the new product. The majority of dogs can be maintained on 0.02 mg/kg thyroxine given orally once daily if clinical signs resolve and TT_4 concentrations are within the therapeutic range.[76]

Myxedema Coma

In myxedema coma, L-thyroxine should initially be administered intravenously (5 µg/kg every 12 hours) because of poor gastrointestinal absorption.[30] Other supportive care includes appropriate fluid therapy, passive rewarming with blankets, and ventilatory support if necessary.

Concurrent Nonthyroidal Illness

Hyperadrenocorticism. Although dogs with hyperadrenocorticism commonly have low TT_4 concentrations and a diminished response to TSH or TRH, they rarely require thyroid hormone replacement therapy. Serum TT_4 concentrations usually normalize after treatment of hyperadrenocorticism.

Cardiomyopathy. In hypothyroid dogs with cardiac disorders, initial doses of thyroid hormone replacement should be 25 to 50 per cent of the usual starting dose. The dose may then be increased incrementally based on the results of therapeutic monitoring and reevaluation of cardiac function. Initiation of thyroid hormone supplementation increases myocardial oxygen demand and may cause cardiac decompensation. Because dogs with cardiac disease may have

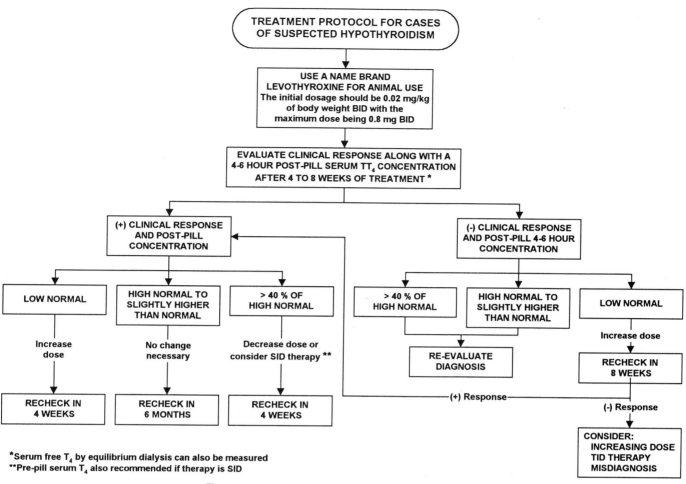

Figure 151–5. Algorithm for treatment of hypothyroidism.

decreased thyroid hormone concentrations, it is important to adequately document hypothyroidism to avoid inappropriate treatment with thyroid hormone.

Hypoadrenocorticism. Replacement of mineralocorticoid and glucocorticoid deficiency should be initiated before treatment with L-thyroxine, because the increased basal metabolic rate may exacerbate electrolyte disturbances in addisonian animals.

TREATMENT FAILURE

An incorrect diagnosis of hypothyroidism is the most common reason for treatment failure. Other causes include insufficient absorption from the gastrointestinal tract or poor owner compliance. A conversion defect in metabolism of T_4 to T_3 and tissue resistance to thyroid hormone have not been documented in dogs. Triiodothyronine is more consistently absorbed from the digestive tract in human beings and possibly in dogs as well, so T_3 may be substituted for L-thyroxine (4 to 6 μg/kg every eight hours) if poor absorption is suspected.[75, 78]

PROGNOSIS

Prognosis for return to normal function following treatment is excellent in most adult hypothyroid dogs. Prognosis

in myxedema coma is dependent on early recognition. Resolution of clinical signs in puppies with congenital hypothyroidism is dependent on the age at which treatment is initiated.

FELINE HYPOTHYROIDISM

Naturally occurring hypothyroidism is rare in cats. The most common cause of low serum TT_4 in cats is nonthyroidal illness. Iatrogenic hypothyroidism occasionally occurs following treatment for hyperthyroidism. Clinical signs of hypothyroidism in cats are similar to those reported for dogs. Causes of spontaneous feline hypothyroidism include congenital hypothyroidism in domestic shorthair cats and Abyssinian cats[79–81] and lymphocytic thyroiditis reported in a single 5-year-old cat and in young kittens.[82, 83]

Diagnosis of feline hypothyroidism is confirmed by physical examination, history, measurement of serum TT_4 concentration, and results of TSH or TRH stimulation tests. A feline TSH assay is not currently available. For a TSH stimulation test, TSH is administered at 1 IU/cat intravenously or 2.5 to 5 IU/cat intramuscularly. Blood samples should be collected before injection and 4 to 7 hours after intravenous injection or 8 to 12 hours after intramuscular injection. Serum TT_4 concentration should double after TSH administration. The dose of TRH is 0.1 mg/kg given intravenously, with blood collected before and four to six hours after injection. Serum TT_4 concentration should increase by greater than 50 per cent after TRH administration. Immediate transient side effects following TRH administration include salivation, vomiting, tachypnea, and defecation.

Hypothyroid cats may be treated with L-thyroxine supplementation at a dosage of 0.05 to 0.1 mg/cat given orally once daily. Therapeutic monitoring and dosage adjustments should be performed as recommended for dogs.

REFERENCES

1. Gosselin SJ, et al: Histologic and ultrastructual evaluation of thyroid lesions associated with hypothyroidism in dogs. Vet Pathol 18:299, 1981.
2. Benjamin SA, et al: Associations between lymphocytic thyroiditis, hypothyroidism, and thyroid neoplasia in beagles. Vet Pathol 33:486, 1996.
3. Gosselin SJ, et al: Induced lymphocytic thyroiditis in dogs: Effect of intrathyroidal injection of thyroid autoantibodies. Am J Vet Res 42:1565, 1981.
4. Gosselin SJ, et al: Biochemical and immunological investigations on hypothyroidism in dogs. Can J Comp Med 44:158, 1980.
5. Haines DM, et al: Survey of thyroglobulin autoantibodies in dogs. Am J Vet Res 45:1493, 1984.
6. Beale KM, et al: Prevalence of antithyroglobulin antibodies detected by enzyme-linked immunosorbent assay of canine serum. JAVMA 196:745, 1990.
7. Thacker EL, et al: Prevalence of autoantibodies to thyroglobulin, thyroxine, or triiodothyronine and relationship of autoantibodies and serum concentrations of iodothyronines in dogs. Am J Vet Res 53:449, 1992.
8. Fritz TE, et al: Pathology and familial incidence of thyroiditis in a closed beagle colony. Exp Mol Pathol 12:14, 1970.
9. Conaway DH, et al: Clinical and histological features of primary progressive, familial thyroiditis in a colony of Borzoi dogs. Vet Pathol 22:4439, 1985.
10. Refsal KR, Nachreiner RF: Thyroid hormone autoantibodies in the dog: Their association with serum concentrations of iodothyronines and thyrotropin and distribution by age, sex, and breed of dog. Can Pract 22:16, 1998.
11. Marks SL, et al: Tc-pertechnetate imaging of thyroid tumors in dogs: 29 cases (1980–1992). JAVMA 204:756, 1994.
12. Manning PJ: Thyroid gland and arterial lesions of beagles with familial hypothyroidism and hyperlipoproteinemia. Am J Vet Res 40:820, 1979.
13. Greco DS, et al: Congenital hypothyroid dwarfism in a family of giant schnauzers. J Vet Intern Med 5:57, 1991.
14. Chastain CB, et al: Congenital hypothyroidism in a dog due to an iodide organification defect. Am J Vet Res 44:1257, 1983.
15. Mooney CT, Anderson TJ: Congenital hypothyroidism in a Boxer dog. J Small Anim Pract 34:31, 1993.
16. Panciera DL: Hypothyroidism in dogs: 66 cases (1987–1992). JAVMA 204:761, 1994.
17. Nesbitt GH, et al: Canine hypothyroidism: A retrospective study of 108 cases. JAVMA 177:1117, 1980.
18. Milne KL, Hayes HM: Epidemiologic features of canine hypothyroidism. Cornell Vet 71:3, 1981.
19. Doliger S, et al: Histochemical study of cutaneous mucins in hypothyroid dogs. Vet Pathol 32:628, 1995.
20. Chastain CB, Schmidt B: Galactorrhea associated with hypothyroidism in intact bitches. J Am Anim Hosp Assoc 16:851, 1980.
21. Fritz TE, et al: Pathology and familial incidence of orchitis and its relation to thyroiditis in a closed beagle colony. Exp Mol Pathol 24:142, 1976.
22. Johnson CA, et al: Reproductive manifestations of hypothyroidism. Can Pract 22:29, 1997.
23. Indrieri RJ, et al: Neuromuscular abnormalities associated with hypothyroidism and lymphocytic thyroiditis in three dogs. JAVMA 190:544, 1987.
24. Jaggy A, et al: Neurological manifestations of hypothyroidism: A retrospective study of 29 dogs. J Vet Intern Med 8:328, 1994.
25. Braund KG, et al: Hypothyroid myopathy in two dogs. J Vet Pathol 18:589, 1981.
26. Budsberg SC, et al: Thyroxine-responsive unilateral forelimb lameness and generalized neuromuscular disease in four hypothyroid dogs. JAVMA 202:1859, 1993.
27. Bichsel P, et al: Neurologic manifestations associated with hypothyroidism in four dogs. JAVMA 192:1745, 1988.
28. Dewey CW, et al: Neuromuscular dysfunction in five dogs with acquired myasthenia gravis and presumptive hypothyroidism. Prog Vet Neurol 6:117, 1996.
29. Liu S-K, et al: Clinical and pathologic findings in dogs with atherosclerosis: 21 cases (1970–1983). JAVMA 189:227, 1986.
30. Kelly MJ, Hill JR: Canine myxedema stupor and coma. Compendium 6:1049, 1984.
31. Panciera DL: An echocardiographic and electrocardiographic study of cardiovascular function in hypothyroid dogs. JAVMA 205:996, 1994.
32. Kern TJ, Riis RC: Ocular manifestations of secondary hyperlipidemia associated with hypothyroidism and uveitis in a dog. J Am Anim Hosp Assoc 16:907, 1980.
33. Greco DS: Congenital canine hypothyroidism. Can Pract 22:23, 1997.
34. Avgeris S, et al: Plasma von Willebrand factor concentration and thyroid function in dogs. Am J Vet Res 196:921, 1990.
35. Panciera DL, Johnson GS: Plasma von Willebrand factor antigen concentration in dogs with hypothyroidism. JAVMA 205:1550, 1994.
36. Panciera DL, Johnson GS: Plasma von Willebrand factor antigen concentration and buccal mucosal bleeding time in dogs with experimental hypothyroidism. J Vet Intern Med 10:60, 1998.
37. Melendez LD, et al: Concurrent hypoadrenocorticism and hypothyroidism in 10 dogs. J Vet Intern Med 10:182, 1996.
38. Hargis AM, et al: Relationship of hypothyroidism to diabetes mellitus, renal amyloidosis, and thrombosis in purebred beagles. Am J Vet Res 42:1077, 1981.
39. Ford SL, et al: Insulin resistance in three dogs with hypothyroidism and diabetes mellitus. JAVMA 202:1478, 1993.
40. Lee DE, et al: Effects of hyperlipemia on radioimmunoassays for progesterone, testosterone, thyroxine, and cortisol in serum and plasma samples from dogs. Am J Vet Res 52:1489, 1991.
41. Reimers TJ, et al: Effects of hemolysis and storage on quantification of hormones in blood samples from dogs, cattle, and horses. Am J Vet Res 52:1075, 1991.
42. Behrend EN, et al: Effect of storage conditions on cortisol, total thyroxine, and free thyroxine concentrations in serum and plasma of dogs. JAVMA 212:1564, 1998.
43. Miller AB, et al: Serial thyroid hormone concentrations in healthy euthyroid dogs, dogs with hypothyroidism, and euthyroid dogs with atopic dermatitis. Br Vet J 148:451, 1992.
44. Reimers TJ, et al: Effects of age, sex, and body size on serum concentrations of thyroid and adrenocortical hormones in dogs. Am J Vet Res 51:454, 1990.
45. Scott-Moncrieff JC, Nelson R, Ferguson D, et al: Measurement of serum free thyroxine by modified equilibrium dialysis in dogs (abstract). J Vet Intern Med 8:164, 1994.
46. Nelson RW, et al: Serum free thyroxine concentration in healthy dogs, dogs with hypothyroidism, and euthyroid dogs with concurrent illness. JAVMA 198:1401, 1991.
47. Peterson ME, et al: Measurement of serum total thyroxine, triiodothyronine, free thyroxine, and thyrotropin concentrations for diagnosis of hypothyroidism in dogs. JAVMA 211:1396, 1997.
48. Yu AA, et al: Effect of endotoxin on hormonal responses to thyrotropin and thyrotropin-releasing hormone in dogs. Am J Vet Res 59:186, 1998.
49. Moore GE, et al: Effects of oral administration of anti-inflammatory doses of prednisone on thyroid hormone response to thyrotropin-releasing hormone and thyrotropin in clinically normal dogs. Am J Vet Res 54:130, 1993.
50. Torres SM, et al: Effect of oral administration of prednisolone on thyroid function in dogs. Am J Vet Res 52:416, 1991.
51. Hall IA, et al: Effect of trimethoprim/sulfamethoxazole on thyroid function in dogs with pyoderma. JAVMA 202:1959, 1993.
52. Panciera DL, Post K: Effect of oral administration of sulfadiazine and trimethoprim in combination on thyroid function in dogs. Can Vet J 56:349, 1992.
53. Campbell KL, et al: Effects of trimethoprim/sulfamethoxazole on thyroid physiology in dogs. Proceedings of the 11th annual meeting of the Society for Comparative Endocrinology, 1997, pp 21–22.
54. Muller PB, et al: Effect of long-term phenobarbital treatment on the thyroid axis in dogs. J Vet Intern Med 12:234, 1998.
55. Panciera DL, et al: Acute effects of continuous infusions of human recombinant interleukin-2 on serum thyroid hormone concentrations in dogs. Res Vet Sci 58:96, 1995.
56. Elliott DA, et al: Thyroid hormone concentrations in critically ill canine intensive care patients. J Vet Emerg Crit Care 5:17, 1998.
57. Panciera DL, Refsal KR: Thyroid function in dogs with spontaneous and induced congestive heart failure. Can J Vet Res 58:157, 1994.
58. Ferguson DC, Peterson ME: Serum free and total iodothyronine concentrations in dogs with hyperadrenocorticism. Am J Vet Res 53:1636, 1992.
59. Vail DM, et al: Thyroid hormone concentrations in dogs with chronic weight loss, with special reference to cancer cachexia. J Vet Intern Med 8:122, 1994.
60. Williams DA, et al: Validation of an immunoassay for canine thyroid-stimulating hormone and changes in serum concentration following induction of hypothyroidism in dogs. JAVMA 209:1730, 1996.
61. Scott-Moncrieff JC, et al: Serum thyrotropin concentrations in healthy dogs, hypothyroid dogs, and euthyroid dogs with concurrent disease. JAVMA 212:387, 1998.
62. Dixon RM, et al: Serum thyrotropin concentrations: A new test for canine hypothyroidism. Vet Rec 15:594, 1996.
63. Ramsey IK, et al: Thyroid-stimulating hormone and total thyroxine concentrations in euthyroid, sick euthyroid, and hypothyroid dogs. J Small Anim Pract 38:540, 1997.
64. Bruner JM, et al: Effect of time of sample collection on serum thyroid-stimulating hormone concentrations in euthyroid and hypothyroid dogs. JAVMA 212:1572, 1998.
65. Bruyette DS: Effect of thyrotropin storage on thyroid-stimulating hormone response testing in normal dogs. J Vet Intern Med 1:91, 1987.
66. Kobayashi DL, et al: Serum thyroid hormone concentrations in clinically normal dogs after administration of freshly reconstituted vs previously frozen and stored thyrotropin. JAVMA 197:597, 1990.
67. Paradis M, et al: Effects of administration of a low dose of frozen thyrotropin on serum total thyroxine concentrations in clinically normal dogs. Can Vet J 35:367, 1994.
68. Sparkes AH, et al: Assessment of dose and time responses to TRH and thyrotropin in healthy dogs. J Small Anim Pract 36:245, 1995.
69. Beale KM, et al: Comparison of two doses of aqueous bovine thyrotropin for thyroid function testing in dogs. JAVMA 197:865, 1990.
70. Frank LA: Comparison of thyrotropin-releasing hormone (TRH) to thyrotropin (TSH) stimulation for evaluating thyroid function in dogs. J Am Anim Hosp Assoc 32:481, 1996.

71. Rosychuk RAW, et al: Serum concentrations of thyroxine and 3,5,3′-triiodothyronine in dogs before and after administration of freshly reconstituted or previously frozen thyrotropin-releasing hormone. Am J Vet Res 49:1722, 1988.
72. Meij BP, et al: Thyroid-stimulating hormone responses after single administration of thyrotropin-releasing hormone and combined administration of four hypothalamic releasing hormones in beagle dogs. Domest Anim Endocrinol 13:465, 1996.
73. Nachreiner RF, et al: Prevalence of autoantibodies to thyroglobulin in dogs with non-thyroidal illness. Am J Vet Res 59:951, 1998.
74. Adams WH, et al: Quantitative 99mTc-pertechnetate thyroid scintigraphy in normal beagles. Vet Radiol Ultrasound 38:323, 1997.
75. Kaptein EM, et al: Thyroid hormone metabolism. Vet Clin North Am 24:431, 1994.
76. Nachreiner RF, Refsal KR: Radioimmunoassay monitoring of thyroid hormone concentrations in dogs on thyroid replacement therapy: 2,674 cases (1985–1987). JAVMA 201:623, 1992.

77. Ferguson DC, Hoenig M: Re-examinationof dosage regimens for L-thyroxine (T₄) in the dog: Bioavailability and persistance of TSH suppression. J Vet Intern Med 11:121, 1997.
78. Panciera DL: Canine hypothyroidism. Part II. Thyroid function tests and treatment. Compend Contin Educ 12:843, 1990.
79. Tanase H, et al: Inherited primary hypothyroidism with thyrotrophin resistance in Japanese cats. J Endocrinol 129:245, 1991.
80. Arnold U, et al: Goitrous hypothyroidism and dwarfism in a kitten. J Am Anim Hosp Assoc 20:753, 1984.
81. Jones BR, et al: Preliminary studies on congenital hypothyroidism in a family of Abyssinian cats. Vet Rec 131:145, 1992.
82. Rand JS, et al: Spontaneous adult-onset hypothyroidism in a cat. J Vet Intern Med 7:272, 1993.
83. Schumm-Draeger PM, et al: Spontaneous Hashimoto-like thyroiditis in cats. Verh Dtsch Ges Pathol 80:297, 1996.

CHAPTER 152

INSULIN-SECRETING ISLET CELL NEOPLASIA

Richard W. Nelson

ETIOLOGY

Functional tumors of the beta cells of the pancreatic islets secrete insulin or proinsulin independent of the negative feedback effects caused by hypoglycemia. Beta-cell tumors, however, are not completely autonomous, because these neoplastic cells respond to provocative stimuli (e.g., glucagon or glucose) by secreting insulin, often in excessive amounts. Immunohistochemical analysis of beta-cell tumors frequently reveals multihormonal production, including pancreatic polypeptide, somatostatin, glucagon, serotonin, and gastrin.[1, 2] Insulin has been the most common product demonstrated within the neoplastic cells, and clinical signs are a result of hyperinsulinemia.

The malignant potential of beta-cell tumors is difficult to predict using subjective phenotypic features such as increased nuclear size, pleomorphism, and proliferation index and is often underestimated in the dog.[3] Virtually all beta-cell tumors in dogs are malignant, and most have microscopic or grossly visible metastases at the time of surgery. The most common sites of tumor spread include lymphatics and lymph nodes (duodenal, mesenteric, hepatic, splenic), liver, mesentery, and omentum. Pulmonary metastasis is rare. Differentiating malignant from benign neoplasia is usually based on identification of metastasis at surgery or necropsy or on recurrence of hyperinsulinism weeks to months after surgical removal of a "solitary" pancreatic mass.

SIGNALMENT

Insulin-secreting tumors typically occur in middle-aged or older dogs. The median age at time of diagnosis of an insulin-secreting tumor in 71 dogs in our series was 10 years, with a range of 3 to 14 years (Fig. 152–1). There is no sex predilection, and insulin-secreting tumors are diagnosed in a wide variety of dog breeds (Table 152–1).

PATHOPHYSIOLOGY

Insulin-secreting tumors and the associated hyperinsulinemia interfere with glucose homeostasis by decreasing the

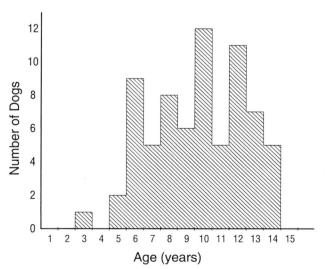

Figure 152–1. Age of 71 dogs at the time of initial diagnosis of an insulin-secreting islet-cell tumor.

TABLE 152–1. BREED DISTRIBUTION OF 63 DOGS WITH ISLET-CELL TUMORS

BREED	NO. OF DOGS	PERCENTAGE
Labrador retriever	8	12
German shepherd	7	11
German shepherd-X	2	3
Irish setter	6	10
Golden retriever	6	10
Collie	5	8
Terriers (fox, kerry blue, West Highland white)	5	8
Poodle	4	6
Doberman pinscher	3	5
Samoyed	2	3
Cocker spaniel	2	3
Other breeds (1 dog each)	13	21

X = mixed breed dog.

rate of glucose release from the liver and increasing the uptake of glucose via insulin-sensitive tissues. Insulin interferes with mechanisms that promote hepatic glucose output by limiting circulating concentrations of substrates needed for gluconeogenesis. This effect is accomplished by inhibiting enzymes necessary for mobilizing amino acids from muscle and glycerol from adipose tissue. In addition, insulin decreases the activity of hepatic enzymes used in gluconeogenesis and glycogenolysis.[4] Insulin also lowers blood glucose concentrations by stimulating glucose uptake and utilization in liver, muscle, and adipose tissue. Thus insulin increases tissue utilization of glucose that is already present within the extracellular space while interfering with hepatic production of glucose. The net effect is decreasing blood glucose concentrations.

Glucose is the primary fuel used by the central nervous system (CNS). Carbohydrate reserves in neural tissue are quite limited, and function of these cells depends on a continuous supply of glucose from sources outside the CNS. Glucose entrance into the neurons of the CNS occurs primarily by diffusion and is not insulin-dependent. Therefore, blood insulin concentrations do not affect neuronal glucose utilization. However, if hyperinsulinemia results in an inadequate glucose supply for intracellular oxidative processes within neurons, cellular changes typical of hypoxia occur, neuron death from anoxia follows, and signs of nervous system dysfunction develop. In acute hypoglycemia, histologic alterations are most marked in the cerebral cortex, basal ganglia, hippocampus, and vasomotor centers.[4] Although most of the damage from hypoglycemia occurs in the brain, peripheral nerve degeneration and demyelination are sometimes encountered.[5] Other major organ systems, such as the heart, kidneys, and liver, also depend on glucose. However, an acute decrease in blood glucose concentration results in clinical signs that involve the CNS before signs of other major organ system dysfunction become apparent.

Prolonged, severe hypoglycemia may result in irreversible brain damage; however, it is uncommon for a dog to die during a hypoglycemic episode. Hypoglycemia is a potent stimulus for release of the counterregulatory hormones that function to antagonize the effects of insulin and stimulate an increase in blood glucose concentrations. The temporal relation between secretion of these hormones and reversal of the effects of insulin on glucose kinetics suggests that catecholamines and glucagon exert the major counterregulatory influence.[6] Under normal circumstances, both adrenal medullary secretion and sympathetic nervous system activity are stimulated and are responsible, in part, for the reversal of acute hypoglycemia.

The clinical manifestations of hypoglycemia are believed to result from both a lack of glucose supply to the brain (neuroglycopenia) and stimulation of the sympathoadrenal system. The neuroglycopenic signs common to dogs include lethargy, weakness, ataxia, bizarre behavior, convulsions, and coma (Table 152–2). The signs resulting from stimulation of the sympathoadrenal system consist of muscle tremors, nervousness, restlessness, and hunger. In humans, the symptoms related to release of catecholamines often precede those of neuroglycopenia and act as an early warning sign of an impending hypoglycemic attack. This illustrates the rapid response of catecholamine secretion to hypoglycemia and, in part, explains why dogs with insulin-secreting tumors do not always progress to generalized seizure activity during a fast.[4]

Clinical manifestations depend on the duration, as well as the severity, of hypoglycemia. Animals with chronic and/or recurring fasting hypoglycemia appear to tolerate low blood glucose levels (i.e., 20 to 30 mg/dL) for prolonged periods without exhibiting clinical signs. Only relatively slight reductions in blood glucose then produce symptomatic episodes. The mechanism, or "adaptation process," whereby some dogs tolerate exceedingly low blood glucose concentrations without clinical signs is not well understood.

ANAMNESIS

Most dogs with insulin-secreting tumors are symptomatic for one to six months before being brought to a veterinarian. Clinical signs typically are related to neuroglycopenia (hypoglycemia) and an increase in circulating catecholamine concentrations (see Table 152–2). One characteristic of hypoglycemic signs, regardless of the cause, is their episodic nature. Signs are generally observed intermittently for only a few seconds to minutes because of the compensatory counterregulatory mechanisms that usually increase the blood glucose concentration after development of hypoglycemia. If these mechanisms are inadequate, syncope, seizures, or coma may occur as the blood glucose concentration continues to decrease. Seizure activity is common and appears to be self-limited, typically lasting from 30 seconds to 5 minutes. The seizure may stimulate further catecholamine secretion and

TABLE 152–2. CLINICAL SIGNS ASSOCIATED WITH INSULIN-SECRETING TUMORS IN 65 DOGS

CLINICAL SIGN	NO. OF DOGS	PERCENTAGE
Seizures	39	60
Weakness	29	45
Collapse	18	28
Ataxia	14	22
Posterior weakness	13	20
Muscle fasciculations	11	17
Depression, lethargy	10	15
Bizarre behavior	9	14
Polyphagia	6	9
Polyuria, polydipsia	6	9
Weight gain	6	9
Diarrhea	4	6
Syncope	3	5
Nervousness	2	3
Head tilt	2	3
Anorexia	2	3
Urinary incontinence	2	3
Blindness	1	2

other counterregulatory mechanisms that increase the blood glucose above critical concentrations.

There is a strong association between developing clinical signs of hypoglycemia and fasting, excitement, exercise, or eating. Exercise normally results in an increased demand for glucose production and stimulation of the sympathetic nervous system, which in turn inhibits insulin secretion and enhances hepatic release of glucose. Thus increased glucose utilization is balanced by increased hepatic glucose production. The balance between glucose utilization and production maintains the circulating blood glucose concentration, allowing the brain to continue to function. The exercising dog with an insulin-secreting tumor has continuing glucose utilization not just by muscle but by all tissues, owing to the autonomous and continuing secretion of insulin.[4] In addition, hepatic release of glucose is impaired. The potential for hypoglycemia is great, and this fact is supported by the number of owners who associate symptoms in their pets with jogging, play, or long walks. A similar pathophysiology is thought to explain the development of symptoms during periods of excitement.

Insulin-secreting tumors are usually responsive to increases in the blood glucose concentration. Food consumption can stimulate excessive insulin secretion and result in postprandial hypoglycemia two to six hours later.

PHYSICAL EXAMINATION

The physical examination of dogs with insulin-secreting tumors is surprisingly unremarkable. Afflicted dogs are usually free of visible or palpable abnormalities. Weight gain is evident in some dogs and is probably a result of insulin's potent anabolic effects.

Peripheral neuropathies have been reported in dogs with insulin-secreting tumors, which may produce detectable alterations on physical examination, including proprioception deficits, depressed reflexes, and muscle atrophy.[5,7,8] The pathogenesis of the polyneuropathy is not known. Proposed theories include metabolic defect in peripheral nerves making them susceptible to the effects of hypoglycemia, metabolic derangements of the nerves induced by the hyperinsulinemia, or an immune-mediated reaction as a result of shared antigens between tumor and nerves.[9] Improvement in peripheral neuropathy is variable after surgical removal of the insulin-secreting tumor and has been reported in one dog treated with frequent feedings and glucocorticoids.[10]

CLINICAL PATHOLOGIC ABNORMALITIES

Most dogs with insulin-secreting tumors are intially brought to a veterinarian for episodic weakness or seizures. The minimal diagnostic evaluation for dogs with these signs should include a complete blood count (CBC), serum biochemical panel, and urinalysis. Results of the CBC and urinalysis from dogs with insulin-secreting tumors are usually normal. Results of the serum biochemical profile, aside from the blood glucose, are also usually normal. Hypoalbuminemia, hypophosphatemia, hypokalemia, and increased activities in alkaline phosphatase and alanine aminotransferase have been reported.[11] These latter findings, however, are considered uncommon, nonspecific, and not helpful in achieving a definitive diagnosis. No correlation has been established between increased liver enzyme activities and obvious metastasis of pancreatic tumors to the liver.

The only consistent abnormality identified in serum biochemistry profiles is hypoglycemia. The mean initial blood glucose concentration in 71 of our dogs with insulin-secreting tumors was 46 mg/dL, with a range of 15 to 78 mg/dL. The median blood glucose concentration was 39 mg/dL. Sixty-two of the 71 dogs (87 per cent) had an initial random blood glucose concentration less than 60 mg/dL. Dogs with insulin-secreting tumors may occasionally have a normal blood glucose concentration on random testing. Such a finding does not eliminate hypoglycemia as a cause of episodic weakness or seizure activity. Fasting with hourly evaluations of blood glucose should be performed in dogs suspected of hypoglycemia. A fast of eight hours or less was successful in demonstrating hypoglycemia in 33 of 35 trials in 31 dogs with insulin-secreting tumors.[12] Longer fasts are reportedly needed in some dogs; however, it is rare that fasts exceeding 12 hours would fail to produce hypoglycemia in dogs with insulin-secreting tumors.

RADIOGRAPHY AND ULTRASONOGRAPHY

Insulin-secreting tumors are usually quite small. Thus it is not surprising that abdominal radiographs from afflicted dogs are routinely interpreted as normal. Displacement of viscera or a visible mass in the right cranial quadrant of the abdominal cavity is considered extremely rare. Thoracic radiographs are of limited help in documenting metastatic disease, primarily because beta-cell tumors rarely metastasize to the lungs.

Ultrasonic detection of a mass lesion in the region of the pancreas helps confirm the suspicion of beta-cell tumor in a dog with appropriate clinical signs and clinical pathologic abnormalities (Fig. 152–2). However, failure to identify a mass lesion in the region of the pancreas is common and does not rule out presence of a beta-cell tumor. Ultrasonic evaluation of the cranial abdomen may also be useful in detecting mass lesions within the hepatic parenchyma or peripancreatic tissues. Such a finding suggests metastatic disease and is an indication for hepatic biopsy, which, if positive for neoplasia, would support medical rather than surgical treatment for the dog.

DIFFERENTIAL DIAGNOSIS

Once fasting hypoglycemia is confirmed, careful evaluation of the history, physical examination findings, and routine clinical pathology usually provides clues regarding the underlying cause (Fig. 152–3). Hypoglycemia in a puppy is usually caused by idiopathic hypoglycemia, starvation, liver insufficiency (i.e., portal shunt), or sepsis. In a young adult dog, hypoglycemia is usually caused by liver insufficiency, hypoadrenocorticism, or sepsis. In an older dog, liver insufficiency, beta-cell neoplasia, extrapancreatic neoplasia, hypoadrenocorticism, and sepsis are the most common causes for hypoglycemia.

Hypoglycemia tends to be mild (i.e., >45 mg/dL) and is often an incidental finding in dogs with hypoadrenocorticism or liver insufficiency. Additional alterations in clinical pathology (e.g., hyponatremia and hyperkalemia in Addison's disease or increased alanine aminotransferase activity, hypoproteinemia, hypocholesterolemia, and decreases in blood urea nitrogen in liver insufficiency) are usually present. A corticotropin (ACTH) stimulation test or liver function test may be required to confirm the diagnosis. Severe hypoglyce-

END

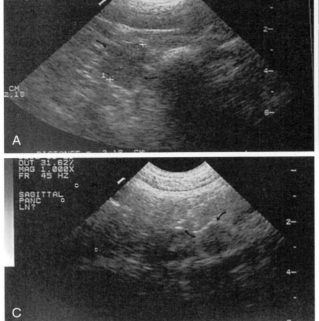

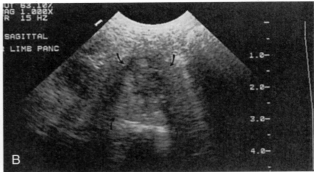

Figure 152–2. Ultrasonograms of the pancreas, illustrating islet beta-cell tumor *(arrows)* in a 13-year-old Borzoi *(A)* and in a 14-year-old miniature poodle *(B)*, and of the peripancreatic tissue, illustrating a metastatic beta-cell tumor *(arrows)* in a 5-year-old golden retriever *(C)*. (From Feldman EC, Nelson RW: Canine and Feline Endocrinology and Reproduction, 2nd ed. Philadelphia, WB Saunders, 1996, p 433.)

mia (<35 mg/dL) may develop in neonates and juvenile puppies (especially toy breeds) and with sepsis, beta-cell neoplasia, and extrapancreatic neoplasia, most notably hepatocellular carcinoma. Sepsis is readily identified by physical findings and abnormalities on a CBC, including a neutrophilic leukocytosis (typically >30,000/μL), a shift toward immaturity, and signs of toxicity. Extrapancreatic neoplasia can usually be identified on physical examination, abdominal or thoracic radiographs, and abdominal ultrasonography. Dogs with beta-cell neoplasia typically have a normal physical examination and a lack of abnormalities other than hypoglycemia on other diagnostic tests. Measurement of baseline serum insulin concentration when the blood glucose is less than 60 mg/dL is necessary to confirm a beta-cell tumor.

CONFIRMING AN INSULIN-SECRETING BETA-CELL TUMOR

Confirmation of an insulin-secreting beta-cell tumor requires identification of hypoglycemia, followed by documentation of inappropriate insulin secretion for that degree of hypoglycemia and identification of a pancreatic mass via ultrasonography or exploratory celiotomy. Considering the potential differential diagnoses (Table 152–3), a tentative diagnosis of insulin-secreting neoplasia can often be made on the basis of history, physical examination, and lack of abnormalities other than hypoglycemia on routine blood work.

Documenting inappropriate insulin secretion requires evaluation of serum insulin concentration at a time when hypoglycemia is present. Hypoglycemia suppresses insulin secretion in normal animals, the degree of suppression being directly related to the severity of the hypoglycemia. Hypoglycemia fails to have the same suppressive effect on insulin secretion when the insulin is synthesized and secreted from autonomous neoplastic cells. Invariably, a dog with an insulin-secreting tumor has excessive serum insulin concentra-

tion relative to that needed for a particular blood glucose concentration. This relative excess in insulin concentration is consistently more reliable if the simultanously obtained blood glucose concentration is less than 60 mg/dL. If the blood glucose concentration is below normal and the insulin

TABLE 152–3. CLASSIFICATION OF FASTING HYPOGLYCEMIA

I. Endocrine
  A. Excess insulin or insulin-like factors
    1. Insulin-producing islet-cell tumors
    2. Extrapancreatic tumors producing and secreting insulin-like substances
    3. Iatrogenic insulin overdose
  B. Growth hormone deficiency
    1. Hypopituitarism affecting several tropic hormones (e.g., ACTH, GH)
    2. Monotropic GH deficiency
  C. Cortisol deficiency
    1. Hypopituitarism
    2. Isolated ACTH deficiency
    3. Hypoadrenocorticism
II. Hepatic
  A. Congenital
    1. Vascular shunts
    2. Glycogen storage diseases
  B. Acquired
    1. Vascular shunts
    2. Chronic fibrosis (cirrhosis)
    3. Hepatic necrosis: toxins, infectious agents
III. Substrate
  A. Extrapancreatic tumors that use large quantities of glucose
  B. Fasting hypoglycemia of pregnancy
  C. Puppy hypoglycemia = ketonemia (alanine deficiency?)
  D. Uremia
  E. Severe malnutrition
  F. Severe polycythemia
IV. Miscellaneous
  A. Artifact
  B. Iatrogenic insulin overdose

ACTH = corticotropin; GH = growth hormone.

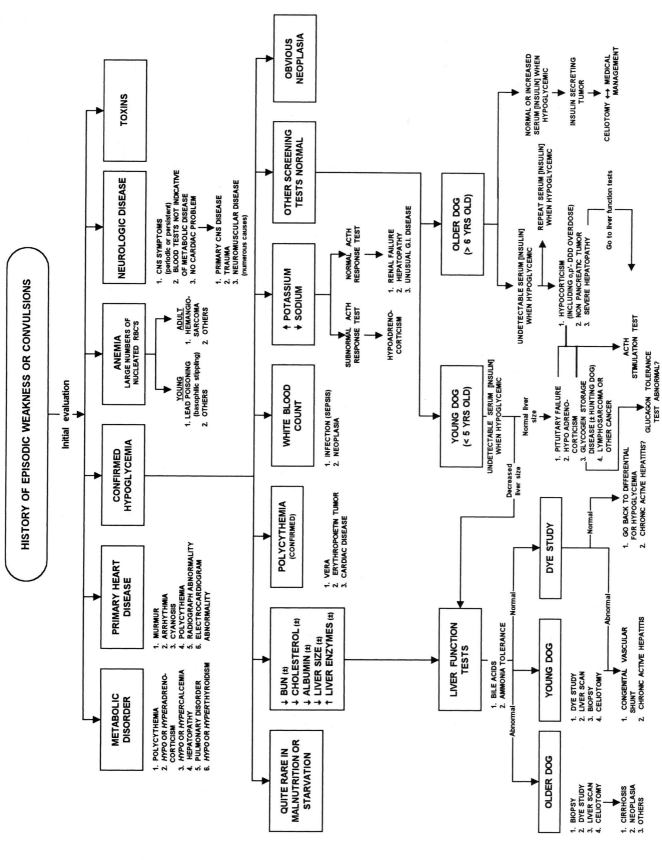

Figure 152–3. Flowchart for the diagnosis of episodic weakness and, more completely, hypoglycemia. (From Feldman EC, Nelson RW: Canine and Feline Endocrinology and Reproduction, 2nd ed. Philadelphia, WB Saunders, 1996, p 431.)

END

TABLE 152–4. PROTOCOL FOR OBTAINING BLOOD FOR GLUCOSE AND INSULIN DETERMINATION TO CONFIRM ISLET BETA-CELL TUMOR

8:00 A.M.	Blood glucose concentration is checked with Chemstrip bG
Every 60 minutes	Check blood glucose concentration with Chemstrip until blood glucose level is approximately 40 mg/dL
When 40 mg/dL is attained	Obtain blood for a laboratory blood glucose determination
	Obtain blood for an insulin determination by radioimmunoassay
	Feed dog several small meals over next few hours

concentration is within the normal range or increased, the animal has a relative or absolute excess of insulin that can be explained only if an insulin-secreting tumor, insensitive to hypoglycemia, is present.

Most dogs with insulin-secreting neoplasia are persistently hypoglycemic. If the blood glucose is less than 60 mg/dL, serum should be submitted to a commercial veterinary endocrine laboratory for insulin determination. If the dog is euglycemic, a 4- to 12-hour fast may be necessary to induce hypoglycemia. Blood glucose concentrations should be evaluated hourly during the fast with glucose reagent strips (e.g., Chemstrip bG, Biodynamics) and an in-house glucose meter (Table 152–4). When the "strip" glucose concentration is approximately 40 mg/dL, a blood sample should be assayed for both glucose and insulin by standard laboratory methods. The dog can then be fed several small meals over the next one to three hours to avoid dramatic fluctuations in blood glucose concentration and the potential postprandial reactive hypoglycemia that could follow a single large meal.

Serum insulin concentrations must be examined in relation to the simultaneous blood glucose concentration. Serum insulin and glucose concentrations in a healthy fasted dog are usually between 5 and 20 μU/mL and 70 and 100 mg/dL, respectively. Documenting a serum insulin concentration greater than 20 μU/mL in a dog with a corresponding blood glucose concentration less than 60 mg/dL and appropriate clinical signs and clinicopathologic findings strongly supports the diagnosis of an insulin-secreting tumor. An insulin-secreting tumor is also probable with a serum insulin concentration in the high-normal range (10 to 20 μU/mL). Insulin values in the low-normal range (5 to 10 μU/mL) may be found with other causes of hypoglycemia as well as insulin-secreting tumors. Careful assessment of the history, physical findings, clinical pathology, ultrasonography, and possibly repeated serum glucose and insulin values will usually identify the cause of hypoglycemia. Any serum insulin concentration that is below the normal range (typically <5 μU/mL) is consistent with insulinopenia and inconsistent for an insulin-secreting tumor.

Several ratios, including the insulin-glucose ratio, the glucose-insulin ratio, and the amended insulin-glucose ratio, have been recommended to evaluate the interrelationship between blood glucose and insulin concentrations and to help establish the diagnosis of insulin-secreting tumor when the laboratory results are ambiguous (e.g., hypoglycemia is marginal and serum insulin concentrations remain in the normal range).[4] We no longer use insulin-glucose ratios as part of our diagnostic evaluation of dogs with hypoglycemia and suspected beta-cell neoplasia. Rather, we rely on history, physical findings, results of clinicopathologic tests, abdominal ultrasonography, and interpretation of baseline serum insulin concentration during hypoglycemia to establish the diagnosis.

SURGICAL THERAPY

Surgical exploration is the best diagnostic, therapeutic, and prognostic tool for insulin-secreting tumors. The surgical intent should be to remove as much abnormal tissue as possible, including resectable sites of metastases. Surgery offers a chance to "cure" dogs with resectable solitary masses. With nonresectable tumors or those with obvious metastases, removal or debulking as much abnormal tissue as possible frequently results in remission of, or at least reduction in, clinical signs and improved response to medical therapy. Despite these benefits, surgery remains a relatively aggressive mode of diagnosis and treatment because of the high incidence of metastatic disease, the older age of many dogs, and the unpredictable improvement in prognosis compared with medical therapy. As a general rule, we are less inclined to recommend surgery in aged dogs, dogs with widespread metastatic disease identified on ultrasonography, and dogs with concurrent disease that significantly enhances anesthetic risk. Euthanasia is not recommended regardless of the findings at surgery. Many dogs with metastatic disease can be managed medically with minimal complications for several months to more than a year.

Until surgery is performed, a dog with an insulin-secreting tumor must be protected from episodes of severe hypoglycemia. This can usually be accomplished with frequent feeding of small meals and glucocorticoid therapy (Table 152–5). A continuous intravenous infusion of a balanced electrolyte solution containing 2.5 to 5 per cent dextrose before, during, and immediately after surgery provides adequate substrate for CNS function and helps ensure sufficient circulation to the pancreas, thereby minimizing the development of postoperative pancreatitis. The goal of a dextrose infusion is to maintain the blood glucose concentration greater than

TABLE 152–5. CHRONIC MEDICAL THERAPY FOR BETA-CELL NEOPLASIA

Step 1. Dietary Therapy

a. Feed canned or dry food in 3 to 6 small meals daily.
b. Avoid soft-moist foods.
c. Avoid foods containing monosaccharides or disaccharides.
d. Limit exercise.

Step 2. Glucocorticoid Therapy

a. Continue step 1.
b. Give prednisone or prednisolone, 0.5 mg/kg divided twice daily initially.
c. Gradually increase dose and frequency of administration as needed.
d. Goal is to control signs, not reestablish euglycemia.
e. Go to step 3 when signs of iatrogenic hypercortisolism become severe or glucocorticoids become ineffective.

Step 3. Diazoxide Therapy

a. Continue steps 1 and 2; reduce glucocorticoid dose to minimize adverse signs.
b. Diazoxide, 5 mg/kg twice daily initially.
c. Gradually increase dose as needed, not to exceed 60 mg/kg/day.
d. Goal is to control signs, not reestablish euglycemia.
e. Go to step 4 when step 3 becomes ineffective.

Step 4. Somatostatin Therapy

a. Continue steps 1, 2, and 3.
b. Give octreotide 10 to 40 μg subcutaneously two to three times a day.

From Nelson RW, Couto CG: Essentials of Small Animal Internal Medicine. St. Louis, Mosby–Year Book, 1992, p 584.

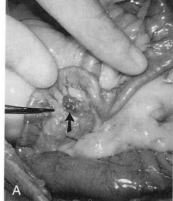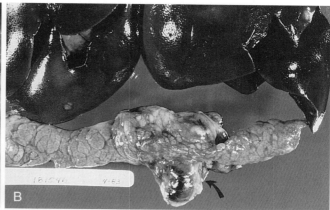

Figure 152–4. *A* and *B*, Photographs of pancreatic insulin-secreting islet-cell tumors *(arrows).*

35 mg/dL; infusion of dextrose-containing solutions rarely restores euglycemia. Concentrations of dextrose in excess of 5 per cent should be avoided to prevent overstimulation of the pancreatic tumor and rebound hypoglycemia, which is sometimes fatal. The blood glucose concentration should be monitored once or twice during surgery to help identify severe hypoglycemia (blood glucose <35 mg/dL). Alterations can then be made in the rate of administration of the dextrose-containing fluids to prevent severe hypoglycemia, or dexamethasone can be added to the infusion (Table 152–6).

A complete inspection of the abdominal contents is imperative to identify unsuspected abnormalities as well as sites of metastasis. The most common sites of tumor spread include the lymphatics and lymph nodes (duodenal, mesenteric, hepatic, splenic), liver, mesentery, and omentum. There appears to be little correlation between tumor size or shape and its malignant potential; failure to identify metastatic disease is common during surgery. As much of the pancreas as possible should be visually examined, and a complete, *gentle* digital inspection should be performed. Most dogs with insulin-secreting tumors have masses that are visible to the surgeon inspecting the pancreas (Fig. 152–4). In a smaller group of dogs, the tumor is not visible but is palpable. Multiple pancreatic masses may also occur, emphasizing the need for a thorough digital examination of the pancreas.

There is no predisposition for tumor location within the pancreas (Fig. 152–5). A mass located in the right (duodenal) or left (splenic) lobe of the pancreas is usually amenable to removal. A mass located in the central region of the pancreas is often intertwined with the pancreatic vessels and ducts and is more difficult to remove without causing severe postoperative pancreatitis. Many centrally located masses are considered inoperable because of the high probability of severe postoperative complications. If the surgeon fails to recognize a mass and the diagnosis has been confirmed by glucose and insulin measurements, the surgeon should attempt to remove at least half of the pancreas in the hope of removing the portion that contains the tumor. In theory, 90 per cent of the pancreas could be removed without causing overt diabetes mellitus or exocrine pancreatic insufficiency.

Postoperative complications include pancreatitis, hyperglycemia, and hypoglycemia. Intravenous polyionic fluids with 5 per cent dextrose (80 to 100 mL/kg every 24 hours) and nothing by mouth just prior to, during, and for 24 to 48 hours after surgery, followed by appropriate dietary therapy during the ensuing week, can help minimize the risk of developing pancreatitis. Serum electrolytes and blood glu-

END

TABLE 152–6. MEDICAL THERAPY FOR HYPOGLYCEMIC SEIZURES CAUSED BY AN INSULIN-SECRETING BETA-CELL TUMOR

Seizures at Home

Step 1. Rub or pour sugar solution on pet's gums.
Step 2. Once pet is sternal, feed a small, high-protein meal.
Step 3. Call the veterinarian.

Seizures in the Hospital

Step 1. Administer 1 to 5 mL of 50% dextrose intravenously *slowly* over 10 minutes.
Step 2. Once pet is sternal, feed a small meal.
Step 3. Initiate chronic medical therapy (see Table 152–5).

Intractable Seizures in the Hospital

Step 1. Administer 2.5 to 5% dextrose in water intravenously at 1.5 to 2 times maintenance fluid rate.
Step 2. Add 0.5 to 1 mg of dexamethasone/kg to intravenous fluids and administer over 6 h; repeat every 12–24h as necessary.
Step 3. Administer octreotide (Sandostatin) 20 to 40 μg subcutaneously two to three times per 24 h.
Step 4. If above fails, anesthetize pet with pentobarbital for 4 to 8 h while continuing therapy. Consider surgery to debulk functional tumor.

From Nelson RW, Couto CG: Essentials of Small Animal Internal Medicine. St. Louis, Mosby–Year Book, 1992, p 585.

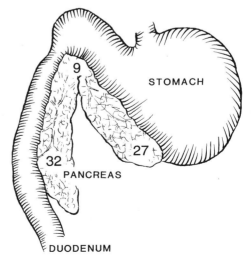

Figure 152–5. Diagram of tumor location in 68 dogs with islet beta-cell tumors. (From Feldman EC, Nelson RW: Canine and Feline Endocrinology and Reproduction, 2nd ed. Philadelphia, WB Saunders, 1996, p 435.)

cose concentration should be measured twice a day during treatment with intravenous fluids, and appropriate adjustments should be made in the electrolyte or dextrose composition of the fluids. One must rely heavily on physical examination findings in determining when to initiate water and a bland diet. Circulating pancreatic enzyme concentrations (e.g., lipase and amylase) are rarely determined after surgery. Arbitrarily treating the dog for pancreatitis without determining serum pancreatic enzyme concentrations beforehand has provided excellent results.

Some dogs develop diabetes mellitus after surgical removal of an insulin-secreting tumor. Diabetes mellitus is believed to result from inadequate insulin secretion by atrophied normal beta cells. Removal of all or a majority of the neoplastic cells can acutely deprive the dog of insulin. Until the atrophied normal cells regain their secretory capabilities, the dog will be hypoinsulinemic and may require exogenous insulin injections to maintain euglycemia. Postsurgical insulin therapy is initiated only if hyperglycemia and glucosuria persist for longer than two or three days after all dextrose-containing intravenous fluids have been discontinued or if ketones appear in the urine. Initial insulin therapy should be conservative (i.e., 0.25 to 0.5 U of NPH or Lente Insulin/kg of body weight given once daily). Subsequent adjustments in insulin therapy should be based on clinical response and serial blood glucose determinations. Diabetes mellitus is usually transient, lasting from a few days to several months. Evaluation of urine glucose in the home environment is helpful in identifying when insulin therapy is no longer needed. Persistent negative urine glucose results, especially with low daily insulin requirements, is an indication to attempt discontinuation of insulin therapy. If hyperglycemia and glucosuria recur, insulin therapy can be reinstituted. Most dogs that require exogenous insulin after surgery ultimately require medical management for an exacerbation of an insulin-secreting tumor several weeks to months after the need for insulin therapy dissipates.

Dogs that remain hypoglycemic after surgical removal of an insulin-secreting tumor are assumed to have functional metastases. Medical therapy should be initiated, beginning with feeding small meals frequently (see the later discussion). If the frequent feedings succeed in keeping the dog in clinical remission, other medical approaches to therapy can be set aside for potential future use. If the dog remains symptomatic for hypoglycemia despite the frequent feedings, additional medical therapy should be attempted before recommending euthanasia.

MEDICAL THERAPY FOR ACUTE HYPOGLYCEMIC CRISIS

The acute onset of clinical signs caused by hypoglycemia typically occurs after the dog has been returned to the owner or immediately after surgery in any dog with functioning metastases or inoperable neoplasia. Therapy is dependent on the severity of clinical signs and the location of the dog (i.e., home vs. hospital) and involves the administration of glucose, either as food or sugar water by mouth or as a 50 per cent dextrose solution intravenously.

If an owner contacts a veterinarian by telephone and reports that the pet is having a hypoglycemic seizure, the owner is instructed to pour a sugar solution (e.g., Karo syrup) over the fingers and rub the syrup on the pet's buccal mucosa. Hypoglycemic dogs usually respond in 30 to 120 seconds. The owner should never place a hand into the animal's mouth during a seizure because it might be bitten; nor should a sugar solution be poured directly into the animal's mouth. However, use of a 6-cc syringe into which Karo syrup has been poured is a safe means of administering sugar in small increments. Once the dog responds to glucose administration, it should be fed a small high-protein meal and be kept as quiet as possible (see Table 152–6). Veterinary attention can then be sought.

In the hospital, clinical signs of hypoglycemia can usually be alleviated with the intravenous administration of 50 per cent dextrose (see Table 152–6). It is imperative to avoid overstimulation of the tumor when administering dextrose intravenously. Overstimulation of the tumor can result in massive release of insulin into the circulation and severe rebound hypoglycemia. A vicious circle can result, with the clinician "chasing" the hypoglycemia with larger and larger amounts of 50 per cent dextrose and the resultant rebound hypoglycemia becoming more and more severe. This can result in persistent convulsions, cerebral edema, and eventual death of the animal. Hyperglycemia-hypoglycemia cycles can be avoided by minimizing dramatic fluctuations in blood glucose concentration. Dextrose should be administered in small amounts slowly rather than in large boluses rapidly. The goal of therapy is to control the clinical signs, not correct hypoglycemia. Once the signs are controlled with judicious administration of intravenous dextrose, diet and glucocorticoids can be initiated (see Table 152–5).

MEDICAL THERAPY FOR CHRONIC HYPOGLYCEMIA

Medical therapy for chronic hypoglycemia should be initiated when an exploratory celiotomy is not performed or when metastatic or inoperable neoplasia results in recurrence of clinical signs. The goals of chronic therapy are to reduce the frequency and severity of clinical signs and to avoid an acute hypoglycemic crisis. Specific chemotherapy that is effective against neoplastic beta cells and does not cause serious adverse reactions has not been reported. Medical therapy, therefore, revolves around nonspecific antihormonal therapy. Antihormonal therapy is palliative and is designed to minimize hypoglycemia by increasing absorption of glucose from the intestinal tract, increasing hepatic gluconeogenesis and glycogenolysis, or inhibiting the synthesis, secretion, or peripheral cellular actions of insulin. Antihormonal therapy consists primarily of frequent feedings and glucocorticoids (see Table 152–5). Surgical debulking of functional masses often enhances the effectiveness of medical therapy.

FREQUENT FEEDINGS

Dogs with insulin-secreting tumors have a persistent absolute or relative excess of circulating insulin. If a constant source of calories is provided as a substrate for this insulin, hypoglycemic episodes can be reduced in frequency or avoided. Diets that are high in proteins, fats, and complex carbohydrates are recommended. If dog food is used, a combination of canned and dry food, fed in three to six small meals daily, is recommended. Exercise should be limited to short walks on a leash. Simple sugars (including semimoist dog foods) may stimulate insulin secretion by neoplastic beta cells and should be avoided. Any signs of hypoglycemia should prompt the owner to feed the pet immediately. As long as the dog can eat, honey, maple syrup, corn syrup, and other sugar solutions should be avoided; they may delay one hypoglycemic episode but predispose the animal to another, more severe episode within 30 to 120 minutes.

GLUCOCORTICOID THERAPY

Glucocorticoids should be initiated when dietary manipulations are no longer effective in preventing signs of hypoglycemia. Glucocorticoids antagonize the effects of insulin at the cellular level, which decreases tissue utilization of glucose and indirectly increases the blood glucose concentration. Glucocorticoids also increase blood glucose concentrations directly by stimulating hepatic glycogenolysis and indirectly by providing the necessary substrates for hepatic gluconeogenesis.[4]

Prednisone is the glucocorticoid most often used. The initial dose is 0.5 mg/kg per day given in divided doses. If this controls the signs of hypoglycemia, the medication should be continued without adjusting the dose. Hypoglycemic signs commonly recur within months of instituting glucocorticoid therapy, presumably owing to tumor growth. When this happens, or if signs are not controlled at the initial dose of prednisone, the dose should gradually be increased in a stepwise manner until signs of hypoglycemia abate or signs of iatrogenic hyperadrenocorticism become intolerable to the owner. If the latter occurs, the dose of prednisone should be reduced (not stopped) and other medications (see Table 152–5) or surgical debulking of the tumor and its metastases should be considered.

DIAZOXIDE THERAPY

Diazoxide is a benzothiadiazide diuretic that inhibits insulin secretion, inhibits tissue use of glucose, and stimulates hepatic gluconeogenesis and glycogenolysis.[4] The net effect is the development of hyperglycemia. Diazoxide has been effective in controlling clinical signs of hypoglycemia in dogs with insulin-secreting tumors when used at 10 to 60 mg/kg, divided into two doses daily. Although diazoxide is currently available as an oral suspension (50 mg/mL; Baker-Norton), it is cost prohibitive for most clients.

SOMATOSTATIN THERAPY

Octreotide (Sandostatin), an analogue of somatostatin, has a relatively long duration of action, increased potency, and excellent bioavailability when administered subcutaneously. It inhibits the synthesis and secretion of insulin by normal and neoplastic beta cells. Intravenous administration of octreotide can rapidly decrease serum insulin concentration in some dogs with insulin-secreting neoplasia (Fig. 152–6). Its inhibitory actions on insulin secretion can be maintained for several hours after subcutaneous administration. The responsiveness of insulin-secreting tumors to the suppressive effects of octreotide is variable, being dependent on the presence of membrane receptors for somatostatin on the tumor cells.[13, 14] Some dogs also become refractory to octreotide treatment.[15] Adverse reactions have not been seen at dosages recommended for the treatment of insulin-secreting tumors (see Table 152–5).

CHEMOTHERAPY

Chemotherapeutic drugs directed against neoplastic beta cells have not been adequately evaluated in the dog. Strepto-

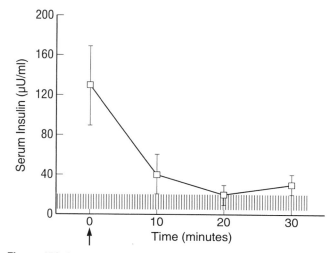

Figure 152–6. Mean ($\pm$SD) serum insulin concentration before and after the intravenous administration of 100 µg of octreotide per dog to six dogs with insulin-secreting islet-cell tumors. *Arrow*, octreotide administration; *hatched area*, normal range for fasting serum insulin concentration. (From Feldman EC, Nelson RW: Canine and Feline Endocrinology and Reproduction, 2nd ed. Philadelphia, WB Saunders, 1996, p 439.)

zotocin and alloxan have been used for the treatment of human insulin-secreting tumors, but their use has been reported only sporadically in the veterinary literature.[4] Acute renal failure is a serious complication associated with both of these drugs. Acute respiratory distress syndrome has also developed in dogs treated with alloxan.

PROGNOSIS

Because of the extremely high likelihood of metastasis in a dog with an insulin-secreting tumor, the long-term prognosis, at best, is guarded to poor. In our hospital, survival time is longer for dogs undergoing surgical debulking of insulin-secreting tumors and metastases at the time of diagnosis followed by medical therapy than for dogs treated only medically. Approximately 10 per cent of dogs undergoing surgery die or are euthanized during the perioperative period because of severe metastatic disease, uncontrollable postoperative hypoglycemia, or complications related to pancreatitis. Mean and median survival times of dogs surviving the perioperative period are 350 and 300 days, respectively, and approximately 15 per cent of dogs survive more than two years. In contrast, mean and median survival times of dogs treated only medically are 90 and 60 days, respectively, and very few dogs survive a year. Differences in survival between dogs treated surgically and those treated medically are due, in part, to our aggressive approach in treating dogs with insulin-secreting tumors and to the more severe metastatic disease in dogs not subjected to surgery. Death or euthanasia is usually due to recurrence of clinical hypoglycemia that is not responsive to medical treatment.

INSULIN-SECRETING ISLET CELL NEOPLASIA IN CATS

Insulin-secreting beta-cell tumors are rare in cats and have been identified only in aged cats, 12 to 17 years old.[16, 17] Clinical signs are caused by hypoglycemia and include seizures, weakness, ataxia, and muscle twitching. Blood glu-

END

cose concentration less than 60 mg/dL has been documented in all affected cats. The diagnosis is confirmed by documenting inappropriate serum insulin concentration despite the presence of hypoglycemia, as discussed previously for dogs. Not all commercially available radioimmunoassays for measuring insulin are valid in cats[18]; it is imperative that the radioimmunoassay used to measure insulin is validated for cats. Surgical exploration should be the initial treatment of choice for beta-cell neoplasia in the cat. Frequent feedings and glucocorticoid therapy have been effective in controlling clinical signs of hyperinsulinism and should be the mainstay of medical therapy for chronic hypoglycemia.[17]

REFERENCES

1. O'Brien TD, et al: Canine pancreatic endocrine tumors: Immunohistochemical analysis of hormone content and amyloid. Vet Pathol 24:308, 1987.
2. Hawkins KL, et al: Immunocytochemistry of normal pancreatic islets and spontaneous islet cell tumors in dogs. Vet Pathol 24:170, 1987.
3. Minkus G, et al: Canine neuroendocrine tumors of the pancreas: A study using image analysis techniques for the discrimination of metastatic versus nonmetastatic tumors. Vet Pathol 34:138, 1997.
4. Feldman EC, Nelson RW: Canine and Feline Endocrinology and Reproduction, 2nd ed. Philadelphia, WB Saunders, 1996.
5. Braund KG, et al: Insulinoma and subclinical peripheral neuropathy in two dogs. J Vet Intern Med 1:86, 1987.
6. Cryer PE, Gerich JE: Glucose counterregulation, hypoglycemia, and intensive insulin therapy in diabetes mellitus. N Engl J Med 313:232, 1985.
7. Shahar R, et al: Peripheral neuropathy in a dog with functional islet B-cell tumor and widespread metastasis. JAVMA 187:175, 1985.
8. Bergman PJ, et al: Canine clinical peripheral neuropathy associated with pancreatic islet cell carcinoma. Prog Vet Neurol 5:57, 1994.
9. Kudo M, Noguchi T: Immunoreactive myelin basic protein in tumor cells associated with carcinomatous neuropathy. Am J Clin Pathol 84:741, 1985.
10. Van Ham L, et al: Treatment of a dog with an insulinoma-related peripheral polyneuropathy with corticosteroids. Vet Rec 141:98, 1997.
11. Leifer CE, et al: Insulin-secreting tumor: Diagnosis and medical and surgical management in 55 dogs. JAVMA 188:60, 1986.
12. Kruth SA, et al: Insulin-secreting islet cell tumors: Establishing a diagnosis and the clinical course of 25 dogs. JAVMA 181:54, 1982.
13. Simpson KW, et al: Evaluation of the long-acting somatostatin analogue octreotide in the management of insulinoma in three dogs. J Small Anim Pract 36:161, 1995.
14. Robben JH, et al: In vitro and in vivo detection of functional somatostatin receptors in canine insulinomas. J Nucl Med 38:1036, 1997.
15. Lothrop CD: Medical treatment of neuroendocrine tumors of the gastroenteropancreatic system with somatostatin. In Kirk RW (ed): Current Veterinary Therapy X. Philadelphia, WB Saunders, 1989, p 1020.
16. O'Brien TD, et al: Pancreatic endocrine tumor in a cat: Clinical, pathological, and immunohistochemical evaluation. J Am Anim Hosp Assoc 26:453, 1990.
17. Hawks D, et al: Insulin-secreting pancreatic (islet cell) carcinoma in a cat. J Vet Intern Med 6:193, 1992.
18. Lutz TA, Rand JS: Comparison of five commercial radioimmunoassay kits for the measurement of feline insulin. Res Vet Sci 55:65, 1993.

CHAPTER 153

DIABETES MELLITUS

Richard W. Nelson

The endocrine pancreas is composed of the islets of Langerhans, which are dispersed as "small islands" in a "sea" of exocrine-secreting acinar cells. Four distinct cell types have been identified within these islets on the basis of staining properties and morphology: alpha cells, which secrete glucagon; beta cells, which secrete insulin; delta cells, which secrete somatostatin; and F cells, which secrete pancreatic polypeptide. Dysfunction involving any of these cell lines ultimately results in either an excess or a deficiency of the respective hormone in the circulation. In the dog and cat, the most common disorder of the endocrine pancreas is diabetes mellitus, which results from an absolute or relative insulin deficiency due to deficient insulin secretion by the beta cells. The incidence of diabetes mellitus is similar for the dog and cat, with a reported frequency varying from 1 in 100 to 1 in 500.[1]

CLASSIFICATION AND ETIOLOGY

OVERVIEW OF CLASSIFICATION

Diabetes mellitus is classified as type 1 and type 2 based on the pathophysiologic mechanisms and pathogenic alterations affecting the beta cells.[2] Type 1 diabetes mellitus is characterized by destruction or loss of beta cells with progressive and eventual complete insulin insufficiency.[3, 4] Dogs and cats acquiring type 1 diabetes mellitus may have a sudden and complete absence of insulin secretion and require insulin treatment from the time of diagnosis (i.e., insulin-dependent diabetes mellitus [IDDM]). Alternatively, dogs and cats may gradually lose insulin secretion as beta cells are destroyed slowly. These animals may have an initial period in which hyperglycemia can be controlled with treatments other than insulin (i.e., non–insulin-dependent diabetes mellitus [NIDDM]); however, with time, insulin secretion is lost and IDDM develops. Type 2 diabetes mellitus is characterized by insulin resistance and "dysfunctional" beta cells.[5, 6] Total amounts of insulin secreted may be increased, decreased, or normal as compared with the *normal* fasting animal. Regardless, that amount of insulin is insufficient to overcome insulin resistance in peripheral tissues. Insulin secretion prevents ketoacidosis in most type 2 diabetic patients.

Diabetes in dogs and cats is usually classified as either IDDM or NIDDM based on the animal's need for insulin treatment. This can be confusing because some diabetic animals, especially cats, can initially appear to have NIDDM progressing to IDDM, or fluctuate back and forth between IDDM and NIDDM as severity of insulin resistance and

TABLE 153–1. POTENTIAL FACTORS INVOLVED IN THE ETIOPATHOGENESIS OF DIABETES MELLITUS IN DOGS AND CATS

DOG	CAT
Genetics	Islet amyloidosis
Immune-mediated insulitis	Obesity
Pancreatitis	Infection
Obesity	Concurrent illness
Infection	Drugs (e.g., megestrol acetate)
Concurrent illness	Pancreatitis
Drugs (e.g., glucocorticoids)	Genetics (?)
Islet amyloidosis (?)	Immune-mediated insulitis (?)

impairment of beta cell function waxes and wanes. Apparent changes in the diabetic state (i.e., IDDM and NIDDM) are understandable when one realizes that islet pathology may be mild to severe and progressive or static; that the ability of the pancreas to secrete insulin depends on the severity of islet pathology and can decrease with time; that responsiveness of tissues to insulin varies, often in conjunction with the presence or absence of concurrent inflammatory, infectious, neoplastic, or hormonal disorders; and that all these variables affect the need for insulin, insulin dosage, and ease of diabetic regulation.

INSULIN-DEPENDENT DIABETES MELLITUS

The most common clinically recognized form of diabetes mellitus in the dog and cat is IDDM. In our hospital, virtually all dogs and 50 to 70 per cent of cats have IDDM. Insulin-dependent diabetes mellitus is characterized by permanent hypoinsulinemia and vital necessity for exogenous insulin therapy. The etiology of IDDM has been poorly characterized in dogs and cats but is undoubtedly multifactorial (Table 153–1). Severe islet-specific amyloidosis (cats; see section on non–insulin-dependent diabetes mellitus), beta cell vacuolation and degeneration (dogs and cats), and chronic pancreatitis (dogs and cats) are common histologic abnormalities with IDDM (Fig. 153–1).[7–10] Less commonly, a simple reduction in the number of pancreatic islets and the number of insulin-containing beta cells within islets is identified histologically in the absence of amyloidosis, inflammation, or degeneration of pancreatic islets.

Immune-mediated destruction of the islets may play a role in the development of IDDM in some dogs and cats. Islet cell autoantibodies and anti–beta cell antibodies have been identified in some dogs with IDDM.[11, 12] Immune-mediated insulitis has also been described.[13] Lymphocytic infiltration of islets, in conjunction with islet amyloidosis and vacuolation, has been uncommonly described in diabetic cats and suggests the possibility of immune-mediated insulitis.[14]

NON–INSULIN-DEPENDENT DIABETES MELLITUS

Clinical recognition of NIDDM is more frequent in the cat than the dog, accounting for as many as 30 to 50 per cent of diabetic cats seen at our hospital. The etiopathogenesis of NIDDM is undoubtedly multifactorial. Obesity-induced carbohydrate intolerance represents one potential causative factor in dogs and cats.[1, 15, 16] Obesity causes a reversible insulin resistance due to "downregulation" of insulin receptors, impaired receptor binding affinity for insulin, and postreceptor defects in insulin action.[17] Impaired glucose tolerance and an abnormal insulin secretory response after intravenous (IV) glucose infusion has been documented in obese cats,[16] abnormalities that improve when cats lose weight.[18]

Islet-specific amyloid deposition in the islets represents another potential causative factor in cats.[19, 20] Islet-amyloid polypeptide (IAPP), or amylin, is the principal constituent of amyloid isolated from the pancreatic tissue of humans with NIDDM and some adult cats with diabetes.[8] The amino acid sequence of human and feline islet-amyloid polypeptide (IAPP) is similar. The observations that IAPP is present in beta cells, is co-secreted with insulin, and can antagonize insulin action in vivo raise interesting possibilities that IAPP might be excessively secreted in NIDDM, contributing to or representing the sole cause of insulin resistance that characterizes this syndrome.[21–26] The severity of islet amyloidosis would determine whether an individual cat has IDDM or NIDDM (Fig. 153–2).

Clinical recognition of NIDDM is uncommon in the dog. A juvenile form of canine diabetes mellitus that closely resembles human maturity-onset diabetes of the young, a subclassification of NIDDM, has been described.[27] Increased plasma C-peptide concentrations have been identified in a small percentage of diabetic dogs and suggest either a severe form of type 2 diabetes mellitus or residual beta cell function in dogs with type 1 diabetes mellitus.[28] C-peptide is the Connecting peptide found in the proinsulin molecule and is secreted into the circulation in equimolar concentrations as insulin. Despite clinical characteristics of juvenile canine

END

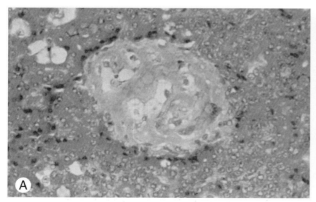 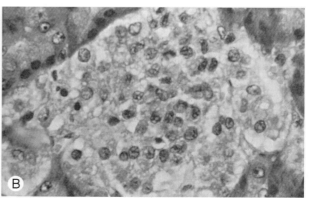

Figure 153–1. Pancreatic islet cell histology. *A,* Severe islet amyloidosis from a cat with IDDM. (H&E, ×100). *B,* Severe islet cell degeneration and vacuolation from a cat with IDDM. (H&E, ×200). (From Feldman EC, Nelson RW: Canine and Feline Endocrinology and Reproduction, 2nd ed. Philadelphia, WB Saunders, 1996, p 341.)

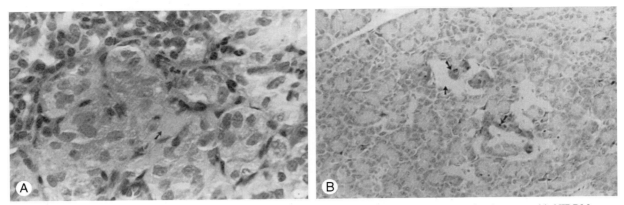

Figure 153–2. Pancreatic amyloidosis. *A,* Mild islet amyloidosis (arrow) and vacuolar degeneration in a cat with NIDDM treated with diet and glipizide. (H&E, ×200). *B,* Severe islet amyloidosis (straight arrow) in a cat with initial NIDDM that progressed to IDDM. Pancreatic biopsy specimen was obtained during IDDM state. Residual beta cells containing insulin (curved arrows) are also present. (Immunoperoxidase stain, ×100). (From Feldman EC, Nelson RW: Canine and Feline Endocrinology and Reproduction, 2nd ed. Philadelphia, WB Saunders, 1996, p 342.)

NIDDM and other dogs with some C-peptide secretory capabilities, all are treated with insulin to manage hyperglycemia.

TRANSIENT CLINICAL DIABETES MELLITUS

Transient clinical diabetes mellitus is extremely uncommon in dogs and usually occurs after correction of concurrent insulin antagonistic disease (e.g., diestrus in the bitch). In contrast, transient clinical diabetes mellitus occurs in approximately 20 per cent of diabetic cats. Some diabetic cats may never require insulin therapy once an initial period of insulin-requiring diabetes mellitus has dissipated, whereas others become permanently insulin dependent weeks to months after resolution of a prior diabetic state. Results of a recent study identified pancreatic islet pathology, decreased beta cell density, and presumably impaired insulin secretory response to insulin antagonism in a group of cats with transient overt diabetes mellitus,[29] which are abnormalities that may pre-dispose the cat to developing hyperglycemia if concurrent insulin-antagonistic drugs are administered or insulin-antagonistic disease (most notably chronic pancreatitis) or obesity develops. Hyperglycemia may further suppress beta cell function and initiate or perpetuate a clinical diabetic state as a result of glucose-induced desensitization or toxicity. *Glucose-induced desensitization* refers to a temporary, readily induced, and reversible state of beta cell refractoriness that is probably expressed at the level of insulin exocytosis, either by depleting insulin stores or making refractory the exocytotic mechanisms responsible for glucose-induced insulin release.[30, 31] *Glucose toxicity* indicates irreversible changes in beta cell function after long-term exposure to chronic hyperglycemia. Glucose toxicity may result from damage to the regulatory processes responsible for normal insulin gene transcription.[32–34] Treatment of diabetes and concurrent disorders results in improved beta cell function, re-establishment of euglycemia, and a transition from a clinical to subclinical diabetic state that does not require insulin or glipizide treatment (Fig. 153–3). Future recurrence of clinical diabetes is possible but unpredictable.

DIAGNOSIS OF IDDM VERSUS NIDDM

Dogs and cats are not typically brought to a veterinarian until clinical signs of diabetes become obvious and worri-some to an owner. For this reason, at the time of diagnosis, all diabetic dogs and cats have fasting hyperglycemia and glycosuria, regardless of the type of diabetes mellitus that may be present. Once the diagnosis of diabetes is established, the clinician must then consider the possibility of NIDDM and the need for insulin treatment. Dogs should

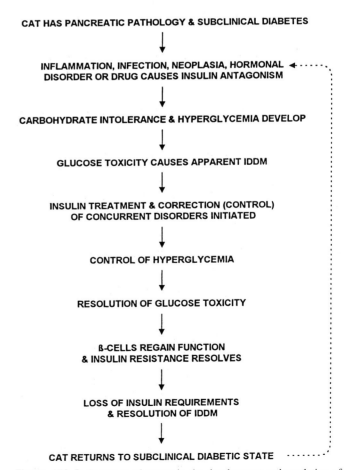

Figure 153–3. Sequence of events in the development and resolution of an insulin-requiring diabetic episode in cats with transient diabetes. (From Feldman EC, Nelson RW: Canine and Feline Endocrinology and Reproduction, 2nd ed. Philadelphia, WB Saunders, 1996, p 344.)

uniformly be considered to have IDDM, and treatment with insulin should be initiated unless there is a strong suspicion for diabetes mellitus secondary to a concurrent insulin-antagonistic disorder (e.g., intact bitch in diestrus).

Because of the significant incidence of NIDDM and transient diabetes in cats and the successful treatment of some diabetic cats with diet and oral hypoglycemic drugs, it would be advantageous to be able to prospectively differentiate IDDM from NIDDM in cats. Unfortunately, measurement of pre-treatment serum insulin concentration or serum insulin concentrations after administration of an insulin secretagogue have not been consistent aids in differentiating IDDM and NIDDM in the cat.[2, 35] A fasting serum insulin concentration greater than the normal mean concentration (> 12 μU/mL in our laboratory) or any post-secretagogue insulin concentration greater than 1 SD above the reference mean (> 18 μU/mL in our laboratory) suggests the existence of functional beta cells and the possibility for NIDDM. Most cats subsequently identified as having IDDM and many of those with NIDDM have a low baseline serum insulin concentration and do not respond to a glucose or glucagon challenge.[2, 35] This apparent insulin deficiency in cats subsequently identified with NIDDM is presumably due to concurrent glucose-induced desensitization of beta cells (see section on transient overt diabetes mellitus). The ultimate differentiation between IDDM and NIDDM is often made retrospectively, after the clinician has had several weeks to assess the response of the cat to therapy and to determine its need for insulin. The initial decision between insulin treatment versus oral hypoglycemic drugs is based on the severity of clinical signs, presence or absence of ketoacidosis, general health of the cat, and owner wishes.

PATHOPHYSIOLOGY

NON-KETOTIC DIABETES MELLITUS

Diabetes mellitus results from a relative or absolute deficiency of insulin secretion by the beta cells. Insulin deficiency, in turn, causes decreased tissue utilization of glucose, amino acids, and fatty acids. Glucose obtained from the diet or from hepatic gluconeogenesis, which occurs at a modest rate with hypoinsulinemia, accumulates in the circulation, causing hyperglycemia. As the blood glucose concentration increases, the ability of the renal tubular cells to resorb glucose from the glomerular ultrafiltrate is exceeded, resulting in glycosuria. This occurs when the blood glucose concentration exceeds 180 to 220 mg/dL in the dog. The renal threshold for glucose may be more variable in the cat, ranging from 200 to 320 mg/dL. The reported mean threshold for normal cats is 290 mg/dL. Glycosuria creates an osmotic diuresis, causing polyuria. Compensatory polydipsia prevents dehydration. The diminished peripheral tissue utilization of glucose results in breakdown of muscle and fat for liver production of glucose as the body attempts to compensate for perceived "starvation." This catabolic condition causes weight loss.

The amount of glucose entering cells in the satiety center in the ventromedial region of the hypothalamus directly affects the feeling of hunger; the more glucose that enters these cells, the less the feeling of hunger and vice versa.[36] The ability of glucose to enter the cells in the satiety center is mediated by insulin. In diabetics with a relative or absolute lack of insulin, glucose does not enter cells composing the satiety center. Thus, these individuals become polyphagic

despite hyperglycemia. Therefore, the four classic signs of diabetes mellitus are polyuria, polydipsia, polyphagia, and weight loss. As these signs become obvious to the owner, the pet is brought to the veterinarian for care.

KETOACIDOSIS

Unfortunately, some cats and dogs are not identified by their owners as having signs of disease, and these untreated diabetics may ultimately develop diabetic ketoacidosis (DKA). The etiopathogenesis of ketoacidosis in diabetes mellitus is complex and usually affected by concurrent clinical disorders. Virtually all dogs and cats with DKA have a relative or absolute deficiency of insulin. Some diabetic dogs and cats develop DKA despite receiving daily injections of insulin, and circulating insulin concentrations may even be increased.[37] In this group, a "relative" insulin deficiency is present. Presumably because of an increase in circulating diabetogenic hormones (i.e., epinephrine, glucagon, cortisol, growth hormone) and an altered metabolic milieu (e.g., increased plasma free fatty acids [FFAs] and amino acids, metabolic acidosis), these dogs and cats have insulin resistance. The ability to maintain normal glucose homeostasis represents a balance between the body's sensitivity to insulin and the amount of insulin secreted by the beta cell or injected exogenously. With the development of insulin resistance, the need for insulin may exceed the daily injected insulin dose, and this leads to a predisposition for the development of DKA.

Circulating concentrations of diabetogenic hormones are increased in humans with DKA and presumably in dogs and cats as well.[38] The body increases its production of diabetogenic hormones in response to a wide variety of infectious and inflammatory disorders. This response is usually beneficial. In DKA, however, the net effect of these hormonal disturbances is accentuation of insulin deficiency through the development of insulin resistance, stimulation of lipolysis leading to ketogenesis, and gluconeogenesis, which worsens hyperglycemia. It is rare for the dog or cat with DKA not to have some co-existing disorder, such as pancreatitis, infection, gastroenteritis, or congestive heart failure.[37] These disorders have the potential for increasing diabetogenic hormone secretion. The recognition and treatment of disorders that co-exist with DKA is critically important for successful management of DKA.

Insulin deficiency, insulin resistance, and increased circulating concentrations of counter-regulatory hormones work in concert to stimulate ketogenesis. Enhanced synthesis of ketone bodies (i.e., acetoacetic acid and β-hydroxybutyric acid) requires two major alterations in intermediary metabolism: (1) enhanced mobilization of FFAs from triglycerides stored in adipose tissue and (2) a shift in hepatic metabolism from fat synthesis to fat oxidation and ketogenesis.[39, 40] Insulin is a powerful inhibitor of lipolysis and FFA oxidation.[41] A relative or absolute deficiency of insulin "allows" increased rates of lipolysis, thus increasing the availability of FFAs to the liver and, in turn, promoting ketogenesis. As ketones continue to accumulate in the blood, the body's buffering system becomes overwhelmed, causing progressively worsening metabolic acidosis. As ketones accumulate in the extracellular space, they eventually surpass the renal tubular threshold for complete reabsorption and spill into the urine, contributing to the osmotic diuresis caused by glycosuria and enhancing the excretion of solutes (e.g., sodium, potassium, magnesium). Insulin deficiency per se also con-

END

tributes to the excessive renal losses of water and electrolytes. The result is an excessive loss of electrolytes and water, leading to volume contraction, underperfusion of tissues, and pre-renal azotemia. The increasing blood glucose concentration raises the plasma osmolality and the osmotic diuresis by causing water losses in excess of salt, further aggravating the rise in plasma osmolality. The increase in plasma osmolality causes a shift of water out of cells, leading to cellular dehydration. The severe metabolic consequences of DKA, which include severe acidosis, hyperosmolality, obligatory osmotic diuresis, dehydration, and electrolyte derangements, become life threatening.

SIGNALMENT

Diabetes mellitus typically occurs in older dogs and cats, with a peak prevalence at 7 to 9 years of age in dogs and 9 to 11 years in cats.[1, 9] Juvenile-onset diabetes occurs in dogs and cats younger than 1 year of age but is uncommon. In dogs, females are affected about twice as frequently as males, whereas in cats, diabetes occurs predominately in neutered males.[1, 9] Genetic predispositions to the development of diabetes have been suggested by familial associations in dogs and by pedigree analysis of keeshonden. Pulik, Cairn terriers, and miniature pinschers are breeds at higher risk than explained by breed popularity, which reflects a definite probability of genetic predisposition. Poodles, miniature schnauzers, Labrador retrievers, Lhasa apsos, Siberian huskies, and Yorkshire terriers are frequently affected breeds seen at our hospital. Diabetes is also commonly diagnosed in mixed-breed dogs. There is no apparent breed predisposition in cats.

ANAMNESIS

The history in virtually all diabetics includes the classic polydipsia, polyuria, polyphagia, and weight loss. Owners will often bring a dog to the veterinarian because they notice it urinating in the home. A common owner complaint for cats is the constant need to change the litter. Occasionally, an owner brings a dog to the veterinarian due to sudden blindness caused by cataract formation or brings a cat due to rear limb weakness and a plantigrade posture (Fig. 153–4).

The classic signs of diabetes mellitus may have gone unnoticed or been considered irrelevant by the owner. If the clinical signs associated with uncomplicated diabetes are not observed by the owner, and cataracts or rear limb weakness do not develop, a diabetic dog or cat is at risk for developing systemic signs of illness (i.e., lethargy, anorexia, vomiting, weakness) as progressive ketonemia and metabolic acidosis develop. The time sequence from onset of initial clinical signs to development of DKA is unpredictable and ranges from a few days to several months. Once ketoacidosis develops, however, the duration of severe illness before the pet is brought to the veterinarian is usually less than 1 week.

PHYSICAL EXAMINATION

Because concurrent disorders (e.g., infection, pancreatitis) are common, a thorough physical examination is imperative on any suspected or known diabetic before treatment or hospital admission. The findings on physical examination will depend on the presence and severity of DKA and the nature of any concurrent disorder. In the non-ketotic diabetic there are no classic physical findings. Many diabetic dogs and cats are obese but otherwise in good physical condition. Dogs and cats with prolonged untreated diabetes may have lost weight but are rarely emaciated, unless concurrent disease (e.g., exocrine pancreatic insufficiency, hyperthyroidism) is present. Hepatomegaly induced by hepatic lipidosis is common. Cataracts are another common clinical finding in canine diabetics. Diabetic cats often stop grooming, develop a poor hair coat with seborrhea and scales, and may develop a plantigrade posture (i.e., the hocks touch the ground when the cat walks) caused by diabetic neuropathy (see Fig. 153–4).

In the ketoacidotic diabetic dog or cat, physical examination findings include dehydration, depression, weakness, tachypnea, vomiting, and sometimes a strong odor of acetone on the breath. With severe metabolic acidosis, slow, deep breathing (i.e., Kussmaul respiration) may be observed. Gastrointestinal signs of vomiting, abdominal pain, and distention are common in DKA and must be differentiated from similar signs associated with pancreatitis, peritonitis, or other intra-abdominal disorders. Dogs and cats that develop severe hyperosmolarity are often extremely lethargic and may be comatose.

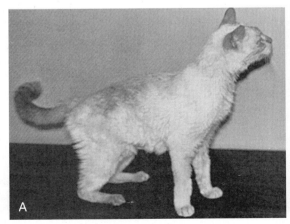
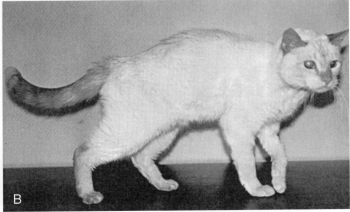

Figure 153–4. *A*, Plantigrade posture in a cat with diabetes mellitus and exocrine pancreatic insufficiency. *B*, Resolution of hind-limb weakness and plantigrade posture after improving glycemic control by adjusting insulin therapy and initiating pancreatic enzyme replacement therapy. (From Feldman EC, Nelson RW: Canine and Feline Endocrinology and Reproduction, 2nd ed. Philadelphia, WB Saunders, 1996, p 348.)

ESTABLISHING THE DIAGNOSIS OF DIABETES MELLITUS

A diagnosis of diabetes mellitus requires the presence of appropriate clinical signs (i.e., polyuria, polydipsia, polyphagia, weight loss) and documentation of persistent fasting hyperglycemia and glycosuria. In-hospital measurement of blood and urine glucose with appropriate blood (Chemstrip bG [Bio-Dynamics]) and urine (Keto-Diastix [Ames Division, Miles Laboratories]) reagent test strips allows rapid confirmation of diabetes mellitus in both dogs and cats. The concurrent documentation of ketonuria establishes DKA.

It is important to document both hyperglycemia and glycosuria when establishing a diagnosis of diabetes mellitus. Hyperglycemia differentiates diabetes mellitus from primary renal glycosuria, whereas glycosuria differentiates diabetes mellitus from other causes of hyperglycemia (Table 153–2), most notably epinephrine-induced stress hyperglycemia that may develop at the time of blood sampling. Hyperglycemia in the range of 300 to 400 mg/dL may occur in stressed cats. However, "stress" is subjective; it cannot be objectively measured, is not always easily recognized, and may evoke inconsistent responses. Glycosuria usually does not develop with stress hyperglycemia because the increase in blood glucose is mild, below renal threshold, or so transient that it prevents urine glucose from accumulating to a detectable concentration. If in doubt, the "stressed" cat can be sent home with instructions for the owner to monitor urine glucose concentration. Alternatively, blood glycosylated hemoglobin or serum fructosamine concentration can be measured. Stress-induced hyperglycemia has not been documented in dogs.

Mild hyperglycemia (i.e., 130 to 180 mg/dL) is clinically silent and is usually an unexpected and unsuspected finding. If the dog or cat with mild hyperglycemia is examined for polyuria and polydipsia, a disorder other than clinical diabetes mellitus should be sought. Mild hyperglycemia can occur up to 2 hours post prandial in some dogs and cats, in "stressed" cats, in early diabetes mellitus, and with disorders causing insulin antagonism. A diagnostic evaluation for disorders causing insulin ineffectiveness is indicated if mild hyperglycemia persists in the fasted, unstressed dog or cat. Insulin therapy is not indicated in these animals, because clinical diabetes mellitus is not present.

PATIENT EVALUATION

NON-KETOTIC DIABETIC

A thorough clinicopathologic evaluation is recommended once the diagnosis of diabetes mellitus has been established.

TABLE 153–2. CAUSES OF HYPERGLYCEMIA IN THE DOG AND CAT

Diabetes mellitus*
"Stress" (cat)*
Postprandial (soft moist foods)
Hyperadrenocorticism*
Acromegaly (cat)
Diestrus (bitch)
Pheochromocytoma (dog)
Pancreatitis
Exocrine pancreatic neoplasia
Renal insufficiency
Drug therapy,* most notably glucocorticoids, progestagens, and megestrol acetate
Glucose-containing fluids (esp. total parenteral nutrition mixtures)
Laboratory error

*Common.

TABLE 153–3. CLINICOPATHOLOGIC ABNORMALITIES COMMONLY FOUND IN DOGS AND CATS WITH UNCOMPLICATED DIABETES MELLITUS

Complete Blood Cell Count

Typically normal
Neutrophilic leukocytosis, toxic neutrophils if pancreatitis or infection present

Biochemistry Panel

Hyperglycemia
Hypercholesterolemia
Hypertriglyceridemia (lipemia)
Increased alanine aminotransferase activity (typically < 500 IU/L)
Increased alkaline phosphatase activity (typically < 500 IU/L)

Urinalysis

Urine specific gravity typically > 1.025
Glycosuria
Variable ketonuria
Proteinuria
Bacteriuria

Ancillary Tests

Hyperlipasemia
Hyperamylasemia
Serum trypsin-like immunoreactivity usually normal
  May be increased if pancreatitis present
  May be decreased if pancreatic exocrine insufficiency present
Variable baseline serum insulin concentration
  IDDM: low, normal
  NIDDM: low, normal, increased
  Insulin resistance induced: low, normal, increased

IDDM, Insulin-dependent diabetes mellitus; NIDDM, non–insulin-dependent diabetes mellitus.

The clinician must be aware of any disease that might be causing or contributing to carbohydrate intolerance (e.g., hyperadrenocorticism), that may result from carbohydrate intolerance (e.g., bacterial cystitis), or that may force modification of therapy (e.g., pancreatitis). The minimum laboratory evaluation in any diabetic dog or cat should include a complete blood cell count, serum biochemical panel, serum lipase or trypsin-like immunoreactivity (TLI) concentration, serum thyroxine (cat), and urinalysis with bacterial culture. Measurement of baseline serum insulin concentration is not routinely recommended, although it may be considered in cats before treatment with oral hypoglycemic drugs (see Diagnosis of IDDM Versus NIDDM, earlier). Additional tests may be warranted after obtaining the anamnesis, performing the physical examination, or identifying ketoacidosis. Potential clinical pathologic abnormalities are listed in Table 153–3. The reader is referred to the work of Feldman and Nelson (1996)[42] for a complete discussion of the clinical pathologic abnormalities associated with diabetes mellitus in dogs and cats.

KETOACIDOTIC DIABETIC

The laboratory evaluation of apparently healthy dogs and cats with both glucose and ketones present in urine is similar to that for the non-ketotic diabetic. "Healthy" here is defined as an animal that is eating, is drinking, and has no vomiting or diarrhea. These dogs and cats are hydrated and can usually be managed conservatively, without fluid therapy or intensive care. In contrast, sick ketoacidotic diabetic dogs and cats are often critically ill, representing metabolic emergencies that require a much more aggressive therapeutic plan. To aid in the formulation of an appropriate treatment protocol, a

END

group of vitally important studies must be performed, including urinalysis, hematocrit, total plasma protein concentration, blood glucose, venous total carbon dioxide or arterial acid-base evaluation, blood urea nitrogen or serum creatinine, serum electrolytes (Na^+, K^+, Ca^{2+}, PO_4^{-2}), and an electrocardiogram. Knowing the results of these tests allows proper choice of fluid therapy as well as for corrections that must be made with respect to electrolyte alterations, acidosis, and renal function. Additional data, such as from radiographs, abdominal ultrasonography, or further clinical pathologic studies, may be needed depending on results of the history, physical examination, and nature of concurrent disorders.

THERAPY

ILL DIABETIC KETOACIDOTIC

An aggressive therapeutic plan (Table 153–4) is indicated if the dog or cat has systemic signs of illness (i.e., lethargy, anorexia, vomiting); a physical examination reveals dehydration, depression, weakness, and/or Kussmaul respiration; blood glucose concentration is greater than 500 mg/dL; or severe metabolic acidosis is noted as diagnosed by a total venous CO_2 or arterial bicarbonate concentration less than 12 mEq/L. The goals in the treatment of the severely ill ketoacidotic diabetic pet are to (1) provide adequate amounts of insulin to normalize intermediary metabolism, (2) restore water and electrolyte losses, (3) correct acidosis, (4) identify precipitating factors for the present illness, and (5) provide a carbohydrate substrate when required by the insulin treatment. Proper therapy does not imply forcing as rapid a return to normal as possible. Because osmotic and biochemical problems can be created by overly aggressive therapy as well as by the disease process itself, rapid changes in various vital parameters can be as harmful as, or more harmful than, no change. If all abnormal parameters can be slowly returned toward normal (i.e., over a period of 36 to 48 hours), there is better likelihood of success in therapy.

Fluid Therapy

Correction of fluid deficiencies is important to ensure adequate cardiac output, blood pressure, and blood flow to all tissues. Improvement of renal blood flow is especially critical. The type of parenteral fluid initially used will depend on the animal's electrolyte status, blood glucose concentration, and osmolality. Most dogs and cats with DKA have severe deficits in total body sodium, regardless of the measured serum concentration. Unless serum electrolyte concentrations dictate otherwise, the initial IV fluid of choice is 0.9 per cent sodium chloride with appropriate potassium and phosphate supplementation. Most dogs and cats with severe DKA are usually sodium depleted and not suffering from dramatic hyperosmolality despite elevations in both the plasma glucose and the blood urea nitrogen concentrations. Hypotonic fluids must be used with caution in the dog or cat with DKA. Patients rarely die of hypertonicity, but they may die of the effects of volume contraction caused by infusion of too much free water (i.e., hypotonic fluids). Hyperosmolality is readily corrected during the initial 24 to 36 hours of treatment with appropriate fluid and insulin therapy.

The initial volume and rate of fluid administration are

TABLE 153–4. INITIAL MANAGEMENT OF THE DOG OR CAT WITH SEVERE DIABETIC KETOACIDOSIS

Fluid Therapy

Type: 0.9% saline (0.45% saline if plasma osmolality >350 mOsm/kg; use with caution)
Rate: 60 to 100 mL/kg/24 hr initially; adjust based on hydration status, urine output, persistence of fluid losses.
Potassium Supplement: based on serum K^+ concentration; if unknown, initially add 20 mEq KCl and 20 mEq KPO_4 to each liter of fluids.
Phosphate Supplement: based on K^+ supplement—provide one half of K^+ supplement as KPO_4.
Dextrose Supplement: not indicated until blood glucose level less than 250 mg/dL, then begin 5% dextrose infusion.

Bicarbonate Therapy

Indication: administer if plasma bicarbonate <12 mEq/L or total venous CO_2 <12; if not known, do not administer unless patient is severely ill and then only once.
Amount: mEq HCO_3^- = body weight (kg) × 0.4 × (12 − patient's HCO_3^-) × 0.5; if patient's HCO_3^- or total CO_2 unknown, use 10 in place of (12 − patient's HCO_3^-).
Administration: add to IV fluids and give over 6 hr; do not give as bolus infusion.
Retreatment: only if plasma bicarbonate remains less than 12 mEq/L after 6 hr of therapy.

Insulin Therapy

Type: regular crystalline insulin.
Administration Technique:
Intermittent IM technique: initial dose, 0.2 U/kg IM; then 0.1 U/kg IM hourly until blood glucose level < 250 mg/dL, then switch to SC regular insulin q6–8h.
Low-dose IV infusion technique: initial rate, 0.05 to 0.1 U/kg/hr diluted in 0.9% NaCl and administered via infusion or syringe pump in a line separate from that used for fluid therapy; adjust infusion rate based on hourly blood glucose measurements; switch to SC regular insulin q6–8h once blood glucose approaches 250 mg/dL.
Goal: gradual decline in blood glucose level, preferably around 75 mg/dL/hr until blood glucose approaches 250 mg/dL.

Ancillary Therapy

Concurrent infections are common in diabetic ketoacidosis; use of broad-spectrum, parenteral antibiotics usually indicated.
Additional therapy may be needed depending on concurrent disorders.

Patient Monitoring

Blood glucose every 1 to 2 hr initially; adjust insulin therapy and begin dextrose infusion when blood glucose drops below 250 mg/dL.
Hydration status, respiration, pulse every 2 to 4 hr; adjust fluids accordingly.
Serum electrolytes and total venous CO_2 every 6 to 12 hr; adjust fluid and bicarbonate therapy accordingly.
Urine output, glycosuria, ketonuria every 2 hr; adjust fluid therapy accordingly.
Body weight, packed cell volume, temperature, and blood pressure daily.
Additional monitoring depending on concurrent disease.

determined by assessing the degree of shock, the dehydration deficit, the patient's maintenance requirements, the plasma protein concentration, and the presence or absence of cardiac disease. Fluid administration should be directed at gradually correcting all deficits over a period of 24 to 48 hours. Rapid replacement of fluids is rarely indicated except if the dog or cat is in shock. Once out of this critical phase, fluid replacement should be decreased in an effort to correct the fluid imbalance in a slow but steady manner. A fluid rate of one and one-half to two times maintenance (i.e., 60 to 100 mL/kg/24 hr) is typically chosen initially, with subsequent adjustments based on frequent assessment of hydration status, urine output, severity of azotemia, and persistence of vomiting and diarrhea.

Potassium Supplementation

Most dogs and cats with DKA initially have either normal or decreased serum potassium concentrations. During therapy for DKA the serum potassium concentration will decrease because of rehydration (dilution), correction of acidemia (shift of hydrogen ions out of cells in exchange for potassium), insulin-mediated cellular uptake of potassium (with glucose), and continued urinary losses. Dogs and cats with hypokalemia require aggressive potassium replacement therapy to replace deficits and to prevent worsening, life-threatening hypokalemia after initiation of insulin therapy. The exception to potassium supplementation of fluids is hyperkalemia associated with oliguric renal failure. Potassium supplementation should initially be withheld in these dogs and cats until glomerular filtration is restored, urine production is ensured, and hyperkalemia is resolving.

Ideally the amount of potassium required should be based on actual measurement of the serum potassium concentration. If an accurate measurement of serum potassium is not available, potassium should initially be added at a quantity sufficient to create a concentration of 40 mEq/L of IV fluids. Fifty per cent of added potassium should be as potassium chloride and 50 per cent as potassium phosphate (see Phosphate Supplementation). Subsequent adjustments in potassium supplementation should be based on measurement of serum potassium concentration, preferably done every 6 to 8 hours until the dog or cat is stable and serum electrolyte concentrations are in the normal range.

Phosphate Supplementation

Phosphate shifts between the intracellular and extracellular compartment in a manner similar to that of potassium. The metabolic acidosis of DKA results in a shift of phosphorus from the intracellular to the extracellular compartment. Consequently, hypophosphatemia may not be identified at initial presentation, even though total body phosphorus may be severely deficient because of excess renal losses. Initiation of insulin therapy and correction of the metabolic acidosis may result in a marked shift in extracellular phosphorus into the intracellular compartment, causing potentially severe hypophosphatemia (< 1.5 mg/dL) within 12 to 24 hours. Life-threatening hemolytic anemia is the most common problem caused by severe hypophosphatemia. Weakness, ataxia, and seizures may also be observed. Severe hypophosphatemia may be clinically silent.

Phosphate therapy is indicated if clinical signs or hemolysis are identified or if the serum phosphorus concentration is less than 1.5 mg/dL. We routinely supplement IV fluids with phosphorus during the initial 24 to 48 hours of treatment of DKA to prevent development of severe hypophosphatemia during therapy. The recommended dose for phosphate supplementation in the dog is 0.01 to 0.03 mmol of phosphate/kg of body weight per hour, preferably administered in calcium-free IV fluids (e.g., 0.9 per cent sodium chloride).[43] An alternative approach is to determine the amount of potassium supplementation required in the dog or cat and then supplement with 50 per cent as potassium chloride and 50 per cent as potassium phosphate. Adverse effects from overzealous phosphate administration include iatrogenic hypocalcemia and its associated neuromuscular signs, hypernatremia, hypotension, and metastatic calcification. Phosphorus supplementation is contraindicated in dogs and cats with hypercalcemia, hyperphosphatemia, oliguria, or suspected tissue necrosis.

Bicarbonate Therapy

The clinical presentation of the dog or cat, in conjunction with the plasma bicarbonate or total venous CO_2 concentration, should be used to determine the need for bicarbonate therapy. Bicarbonate supplementation is not recommended when plasma bicarbonate (or total venous CO_2) is 12 mEq/L or greater, especially if the patient is alert. An alert dog or cat probably has a normal or near-normal pH in the cerebrospinal fluid. The acidosis in these patients is corrected through insulin and fluid therapy. Improvement in renal perfusion enhances the urinary loss of ketoacids, and insulin therapy markedly diminishes the production of ketoacids. Acetoacetate and beta-hydroxybutyrate are also metabolically usable anions, and 1 mEq of bicarbonate is generated from each 1 mEq of ketoacid metabolized.

When the plasma bicarbonate concentration is 11 mEq/L or less (total venous CO_2 is below 12), bicarbonate therapy should be initiated. Many of these dogs and cats have severe depression that may be a result of concurrent severe central nervous system acidosis. Metabolic acidosis should be corrected slowly, thereby avoiding major alterations in the pH of the cerebrospinal fluid. Only a portion of the bicarbonate deficit is given initially over a 6-hour period. The bicarbonate deficit (i.e., the milliequivalents of bicarbonate initially needed to correct acidosis to the critical level of 12 mEq/L over a period of 6 hours) is calculated as follows:

$$\text{mEq bicarbonate} = \text{body weight (kg)} \times 0.4 \times (12 - \text{patient's bicarbonate}) \times 0.5$$

or if the serum bicarbonate is not known:

$$\text{mEq bicarbonate} = \text{body weight (kg)} \times 2$$

The difference between the patient's serum bicarbonate concentration and the critical value of 12 mEq/L represents the treatable base deficit in DKA. If the patient's serum bicarbonate concentration is not known, the number 10 can be used for the treatable base deficit. The factor 0.4 corrects for the extracellular fluid space in which bicarbonate is distributed (40 per cent of body weight). The factor 0.5 provides one half of the required dose of bicarbonate in the IV infusion. In this manner, a conservative dose is given over a 6-hour period. Bicarbonate should never be given by bolus infusion. After 6 hours of therapy, the acid-base status should be re-evaluated and a new dose calculated. Once the plasma bicarbonate level is greater than 12 mEq/L, further bicarbonate supplementation is not needed.

END

Insulin Therapy

Insulin protocols for the treatment of DKA include the intermittent intramuscular (IM) technique, the continuous low-dose IV infusion technique, and the initial IM injection followed by intermittent subcutaneous (SC) technique. All three routes of insulin administration are effective in decreasing plasma glucose and ketone concentrations. Successful management of DKA is *not* dependent on route of insulin administration. Rather, it is dependent on proper treatment of each disorder associated with DKA.

Intermittent IM Regimen

Dogs and cats with severe DKA should receive an initial regular crystalline insulin loading dose of 0.2 U/kg followed by 0.1 U/kg every hour thereafter. This dose can initially be reduced by 25 to 50 per cent in dogs and cats with severe hypokalemia (K^+ < 2.5 mEq/L) to help prevent worsening hypokalemia. The insulin should be administered into the muscles of the rear legs to ensure that the injections are IM and not going into fat or subcutaneous tissue. Diluting regular insulin 1:10 with sterile saline and using 0.3 mL of U-100 insulin syringes are helpful when small doses of insulin are required. The blood glucose concentration should be measured every hour with glucose reagent strips or an in-house glucometer and the insulin dose adjusted accordingly. The goal of initial insulin therapy is to *slowly* lower the blood glucose concentration to the range of 200 to 250 mg/dL, preferably over a 6- to 10-hour period, thereby avoiding large shifts in osmolality. A declining blood glucose concentration also ensures that lipolysis and the supply of free fatty acids for ketone production have been effectively turned off. Glucose concentrations, however, decrease much more rapidly than do ketone levels. In general, hyperglycemia is corrected in 4 to 8 hours but ketosis takes 12 to 48 hours to resolve.

Once the blood glucose concentration approaches 250 mg/dL, hourly administration of regular insulin should be discontinued, and regular insulin should then be given every 6 to 8 hours SC. The initial dose is usually 0.1 to 0.4 U/kg, with subsequent adjustments based on blood glucose concentrations. The blood glucose concentration should be maintained between 150 and 300 mg/dL until the dog or cat is stable and eating. Fifty per cent dextrose added to the IV infusion solution to create a 5 per cent dextrose solution (100 mL of 50 per cent dextrose added to each liter of fluids) is necessary. If the blood glucose concentration decreases below 150 mg/dL or rises above 300 mg/dL, the insulin dose can be lowered or raised accordingly.

Constant Low-Dose Insulin Infusion Technique

The initial rate of regular crystalline insulin infusion is 0.05 to 0.1 U/kg per hour and is given in an IV line that is separate from that used for fluid therapy. This infusion rate can initially be reduced by 25 to 50 per cent in dogs and cats with severe hypokalemia (K^+ < 2.5 mEq/L) to help prevent worsening hypokalemia. An infusion or syringe pump should be used to ensure a constant rate of insulin infusion. Regular crystalline insulin needs to be diluted before administration simply because of the small amounts of insulin being infused into the patient. If a syringe pump is used, regular crystalline insulin can be diluted with sterile saline. Assuming U-100 regular crystalline insulin is used, the insulin should be diluted 10- to 100-fold, depending on the size of the dog or cat. If an infusion pump is used, regular crystalline insulin can be added to 250 mL of 0.9 per cent saline or Ringer's solution. Because insulin adheres to glass and plastic surfaces, 50 mL of the insulin-containing fluid should be run through the drip set before it is administered to the patient.

Adjustments in the infusion rate are based on hourly measurements of blood glucose concentration; an hourly decline of 50 to 100 mg/dL in the blood glucose concentration is ideal. Once the blood glucose concentration approaches 250 mg/dL, the insulin infusion can be discontinued and regular insulin given every 6 to 8 hours subcutaneously as discussed for the intermittent IM protocol. Alternatively, the insulin infusion can be continued (at a decreased rate to prevent hypoglycemia) until the insulin preparation is exchanged for a longer-acting product. Dextrose should be added to the IV fluids once the blood glucose level approaches 250 mg/dL, as discussed in the section on intermittent IM insulin technique.

Intermittent High-Dose IM/SC Technique

The high-dose IM followed by intermittent SC insulin technique is less labor intensive than the other techniques for insulin administration; however, the decrease in blood glucose can be rapid and the risk of hypoglycemia greater with the high-dose IM technique. The initial regular crystalline insulin dose is 0.25 to 0.5 U/kg IM every 4 hours. Usually, insulin is administered IM only once or twice. Once the patient is rehydrated, SC administration is substituted for IM administration and insulin is administered subcutaneously every 6 to 8 hours. Subcutaneous administration is not recommended initially because of problems with insulin absorption from subcutaneous sites of deposition in a dehydrated dog or cat. The IM or SC dose of insulin should be adjusted according to blood glucose concentrations, which initially should be measured hourly. Dextrose should be added to the IV fluids once the blood glucose approaches 250 mg/dL, as discussed in the section on intermittent IM insulin technique.

Initiating Longer-Acting Insulin

Longer-acting insulin (e.g., NPH, Lente, Ultralente, PZI) should not be administered until the dog or cat is stable (i.e., eating and drinking), maintaining fluid balance without any IV infusions, and no longer acidotic, azotemic, or electrolyte deficient. The initial dose of these longer-acting insulins is similar to the regular insulin dose being used just before switching to the longer-acting insulins. Subsequent adjustments in the longer-acting insulin dose should be based on measurement of serial blood glucose concentrations.

Concurrent Illness

Therapy for DKA frequently involves the management of concurrent, often serious illness. Common concurrent illnesses in dogs and cats with DKA include bacterial infection, pancreatitis, congestive heart failure, renal failure, and insulin antagonistic disorders, most notably hyperadrenocorticism and diestrus. Modifications in therapy for DKA (e.g., fluid therapy with concurrent heart failure) and/or additional therapy (e.g., antibiotics) may be required, depending on the concurrent illness. Insulin therapy, however, should never be delayed or discontinued. Resolution of ketoacidosis can only be obtained through insulin therapy. If nothing is to be given orally, insulin therapy should be continued and the blood glucose concentration maintained with a 5 per cent dextrose infusion. If concurrent insulin-antagonistic disease is present, treatment of that disease while the patient is still ill may be necessary to improve insulin effectiveness and resolve the ketoacidosis.

Complications of Therapy for DKA

Complications induced by therapy for DKA are common and usually result from overly aggressive treatment, inadequate patient monitoring, and failure to re-evaluate biochemical parameters in a timely manner. DKA is a complex disorder that carries a high mortality rate if improperly managed. To minimize the occurrence of therapeutic complications and improve the chances of successful response to therapy, all abnormal parameters should be *slowly* returned toward normal (i.e., over a period of 36 to 48 hours), the physical and mental status of the patient must be evaluated frequently (at least three to four times daily), and biochemical parameters (e.g., blood glucose, serum electrolytes, blood gases) must be evaluated frequently. During the initial 24 hours, blood glucose concentrations should be measured every 1 to 2 hours and serum electrolytes and blood gases measured every 4 to 6 hours. Fluid, insulin, and bicarbonate therapy typically require modification three or four times during the initial 24 hours of therapy. Failure to recognize changes in the status of DKA and to respond accordingly will potentially cause serious complications. The more common complications are hypoglycemia, central nervous system signs secondary to cerebral edema, severe hypernatremia and hyperchloremia, severe hypokalemia, and hemolytic anemia from hypophosphatemia.

HEALTHY DIABETIC KETOACIDOTIC

If systemic signs of illness are absent or mild, serious abnormalities are not readily identifiable on physical examination, and metabolic acidosis is mild (i.e., total venous CO_2 or arterial bicarbonate concentration > 16 mEq/L), short-acting regular crystalline insulin can be administered subcutaneously three times daily until ketonuria resolves. The insulin dose should be adjusted based on blood glucose concentrations. To minimize hypoglycemia, the dog or cat should be fed one third of its daily caloric intake at the time of each insulin injection. The blood glucose and urine ketone concentrations, as well as the patient's clinical status, should be monitored. If the blood glucose concentration is well controlled, ketone concentrations will decrease, although this may take a few days. Prolonged ketonuria is suggestive of a (significant) concurrent illness. Once the ketoacidotic state has resolved and the dog or cat is stable (eating and drinking), insulin regulation may be initiated utilizing the longer-acting insulin preparations.

NON-KETOTIC DIABETIC

Goals of Therapy

The primary goal of therapy is the elimination of owner-observed signs that occur secondary to hyperglycemia and glycosuria. Persistence of clinical signs (i.e., polyuria, polydipsia, polyphagia, weight loss) and the development of chronic complications (Table 153–5) is directly correlated with the severity and duration of hyperglycemia. Limiting

TABLE 153–5. COMPLICATIONS ASSOCIATED WITH DIABETES MELLITUS IN THE DOG AND CAT

COMMON	UNCOMMON
Iatrogenic hypoglycemia	Peripheral neuropathy (dog)
Persistent polyuria, polydipsia, weight loss	Glomerulonephropathy, glomerulosclerosis
Cataracts (dog)	Retinopathy
Bacterial infections, especially in the urinary tract	Exocrine pancreatic insufficiency
Pancreatitis (dog and cat)	Gastric paresis
Ketoacidosis	Diabetic diarrhea
Hepatic lipidosis	Diabetic dermatopathy (dog) (i.e., superficial necrolytic dermatitis)
Peripheral neuropathy (cat)	

blood glucose concentration fluctuations and maintaining near-normal glycemia will help minimize clinical signs and prevent the complications associated with poorly controlled diabetic patients. This goal can be accomplished through proper insulin administration, diet, exercise, oral hypoglycemic medications, and/or the avoidance or control of concurrent inflammatory, infectious, neoplastic, and hormonal disorders. Which therapeutic regimen is ultimately successful is dependent, in part, on the number of functional beta cells remaining in the pancreas and individual variation of response to treatment.

Although it is worthwhile attempting to normalize the blood glucose concentration, the veterinarian must also guard against the development of hypoglycemia, a serious and potentially fatal complication of therapy. Hypoglycemia is most likely to occur with overzealous insulin therapy. The veterinarian must balance the possible benefits of "tight" glucose control obtainable with insulin therapy against the risks of inducing hypoglycemia.

Dietary Therapy

Appropriate dietary therapy should be initiated in all diabetic dogs and cats, regardless of the type of diabetes present (Table 153–6). Dietary therapy should be directed at correcting obesity, maintaining consistency in the timing and caloric content of the meals, and furnishing a diet that minimizes postprandial fluctuations in blood glucose. Fluctuations in postprandial blood glucose concentration can be controlled to some degree by feeding diets that contain more fiber than typically found in most commercial foods. Fiber decreases postprandial blood glucose fluctuations by delaying gastric emptying of nutrients and delaying intestinal absorption of nutrients. These effects are most likely caused by delayed diffusion of glucose toward the brush border of the intestine and possibly by affecting release of regulatory gut hormones into the circulation.[44] Improvement in glycemic control is dependent, in part, on the type of fiber consumed, that is, insoluble fiber (e.g., lignin, cellulose) versus soluble fiber (e.g., gums, pectins). Consumption of soluble fiber is more effective in improving variables of glycemic control than is consumption of insoluble fiber. However, studies in diabetic dogs and cats have documented glycemic improvement with consumption of diets containing increased amounts of insoluble fiber.[45–47] Current commercial high-fiber diets contain a predominance of insoluble fiber. The amount of insoluble fiber varies considerably among products, ranging from 3 to 25 per cent of dry matter (normal diets contain < 2 per cent fiber on a dry matter basis). In general, the diets likely to be most effective for the correction of excess body weight and

TABLE 153–6. DIETARY RECOMMENDATIONS FOR TREATMENT OF DIABETES MELLITUS IN DOGS AND CATS

Dietary Composition

Increased fiber content (≥8% dry matter [DM])
Increased digestible carbohydrate content (>50% [DM]—dogs only)
Decreased fat content (< 17% DM)
Adequate protein content (dog: 15–20% DM; cat: 28–40% DM)

Product

Feed canned and/or dry kibble foods; avoid diets containing mono- and disaccharides and propylene glycol

Caloric Intake and Obesity

Average daily caloric intake in geriatric pet: 40–60 kcal/kg
   Adjust daily caloric intake on individual basis
Correct obesity, if present, by:
   Increasing daily exercise (dogs)
   Decreasing daily caloric intake
   Feeding low-calorie dense, low-fat, high-fiber (preferred in diabetics) or low-calorie dense, low-fat, low-fiber diet designed for weight loss

Feeding Schedule

Maintain consistent caloric content of the meals.
Maintain consistent timing of feeding schedule.
Feed within time frame of insulin action.
Feed at time of each insulin injection if twice-daily insulin therapy; at time of and 8 to 10 hours after insulin injection if once-daily insulin therapy.
Let "nibbler" cats and dogs continue to nibble throughout day and night.

improvement of glycemic control are those that contain the most fiber.

Susceptibility to complications associated with eating high-fiber diets depends, in part, on the animal's body weight, condition, and presence of concurrent disease (e.g., pancreatitis, renal failure). The diet that has the greatest therapeutic value ultimately dictates which, if any, fiber diet is recommended. Common clinical complications from feeding high-fiber diets include excessive frequency of defecation, constipation and obstipation, hypoglycemia 1 to 2 weeks after increasing the fiber content of the diet, and refusal to eat the diet. If firm stools or constipation become a problem, soluble fiber (e.g., canned pumpkin, sugar-free Metamucil) can be added to the diet to soften the stool. Refusal to consume a high-fiber diet may occur initially or develop after several months of eating the diet. If palatability is a problem initially, a gradual switch from the regular diet to one containing small amounts of fiber can be tried, followed by a gradual increase in the amount of fiber offered. Refusal to consume high-fiber diets months after their initiation is usually a result of boredom with the food. Periodic changes in types of high-fiber diets and mixtures of diets have been helpful in alleviating this problem.

Diets containing increased fiber content should not be fed to thin or emaciated diabetic dogs or cats. High-fiber diets have a low caloric density that can interfere with weight gain and may cause further weight loss. For thin diabetic dogs and cats, weight gain usually requires re-establishment of glycemic control through insulin therapy and the feeding of a higher calorie–dense, but lower-fiber diet designed for maintenance. Once normal body weight has been attained, a diet containing an increased fiber content can be gradually substituted.

Acarbose

Acarbose (Precose) is a complex oligosaccharide of microbial origin that competitively inhibits the α-glucosidases present in the brush border of the small intestinal mucosa and pancreatic α-amylase. Inhibition of carbohydrate digestive enzymes delays digestion of complex carbohydrates and disaccharides to monosaccharides, resulting in increased carbohydrate digestion within the ileum and, to a lesser extent, the colon. It also delays absorption of glucose from the intestinal tract and decreases post-prandial blood glucose and insulin concentrations. Placebo-controlled clinical studies completed in healthy and diabetic dogs have documented a decrease in post-prandial total glucose absorption and total insulin secretion when healthy dogs were treated with acarbose (compared with placebo) and a decrease in daily insulin dose, mean blood glucose per 8 hours, blood glycosylated hemoglobin, and serum fructosamine in diabetic dogs treated with acarbose (compared with placebo).[48] Results of these studies suggest that acarbose may be beneficial in improving control of glycemia in some dogs with IDDM. However, diarrhea and weight loss as a result of carbohydrate malassimilation are common adverse effects, occurring in approximately 35 per cent of dogs. Diarrhea is more prevalent at higher doses of acarbose (i.e., 100 and 200 mg/dog) and typically resolves within 2 to 3 days of discontinuing the medication.

More extensive studies using larger numbers of dogs are required before the role of acarbose in the treatment of diabetes in dogs is known. Currently, we consider using acarbose in diabetic dogs whose diabetes is poorly controlled with insulin and dietary therapy and for which another reason for the poor control cannot be identified. The initial dose is 25 mg/dog orally every 12 hours. The benefit of this drug is dependent on its interaction with the meal; it should only be given at the time of feeding. A stepwise increase to 50 mg/dog and, in large dogs (> 25 kg), a further increase to 100 mg/dog can be considered in dogs that fail to show improvement at lower doses. However, adverse reactions (especially diarrhea) are more likely to occur at these higher doses.

Exercise

Exercise can have value in helping to maintain glycemic control of the diabetic patient. Exercise helps promote weight loss and correct insulin resistance induced by obesity. Exercise also has a glucose-lowering effect, primarily as a result of increased mobilization of insulin from its injection site, presumably because of increased blood and lymph flow and increased blood flow (and therefore insulin delivery) to exercising muscles.[49, 50] The daily routine for diabetic dogs should include exercise, preferably at the same time each day. Strenuous and sporadic exercise can cause severe hypoglycemia and should be avoided.

The insulin dose should be decreased in dogs that undergo periods of sporadic, strenuous exercise (e.g., hunting dogs during hunting season) on those days when the dog undergoes more than its normal amount of exercise. The reduction in insulin dose required to prevent hypoglycemia is variable and requires trial and error. We recommend reducing the insulin dose by 50 per cent initially and making adjustments in subsequent insulin doses based on occurrence of symptomatic hypoglycemia and severity of polyuria and polydipsia that develops during the ensuing 24 to 48 hours. In addition, the owner must be aware of the signs of hypoglycemia and have a source of glucose (e.g., Karo syrup, candy, food) readily available should any of these signs develop in the dog.

Oral Hypoglycemic Drugs

Oral hypoglycemic drugs are indicated for the treatment of NIDDM in cats. In our experience, oral hypoglycemic drugs have been ineffective in improving glycemic control in dogs with diabetes mellitus; this undoubtedly reflects the extremely low incidence of NIDDM in dogs.

Sulfonylureas

Glipizide and glyburide are the most commonly used sulfonylureas for treating NIDDM. The primary effect of these drugs is the direct stimulation of insulin secretion from the pancreas.[51] Some pancreatic insulin secretory capability must exist for sulfonylureas to be effective in improving glycemic control. Clinical response to glipizide and glyburide treatment in diabetic cats is variable, ranging from excellent (i.e., blood glucose concentrations decreasing to < 200 mg/dL) to partial response (i.e., clinical improvement but failure to resolve hyperglycemia) to no response.[35, 52] Presumably, the population of functioning beta cells dictates the clinical response; that is, variation from no functioning beta cells (severe IDDM) to near-normal population of beta cells (mild NIDDM) results in a response range from none to excellent. Cats with a partial response to glipizide have some functioning beta cells but not enough to decrease blood glucose concentration to less than 200 mg/dL. These cats may have severe NIDDM or the early stages of IDDM.

No parameters have been identified that consistently allow the clinician to prospectively identify cats that will respond to glipizide or glyburide therapy. Identifying a high preprandial serum insulin concentration or an increase in serum insulin concentration during an insulin secretagogue test supports the diagnosis of NIDDM, but failure to identify these changes does not rule out the potential for a beneficial response to glipizide or glyburide. Selection of diabetic cats for treatment with glipizide must rely heavily on the veterinarian's assessment of the cat's health, severity of clinical signs, presence or absence of ketoacidosis, other diabetic complications (e.g., peripheral neuropathy), and owner's desires.

Glipizide. We administer glipizide (Glucotrol), 2.5 mg orally twice daily in conjunction with a meal, to those diabetic cats that are non-ketotic and relatively healthy on physical examination (Fig. 153–5). A history, complete physical examination, body weight determination, urine glucose/ketone measurement, and several blood glucose concentrations are evaluated 2 weeks after initiating glipizide. If adverse reactions (Table 153–7) have not occurred after 2 weeks of treatment, the glipizide dosage should be increased to 5.0 mg twice daily and the cat re-evaluated 2 weeks later. Therapy is continued as long as the cat is stable. If euglycemia or hypoglycemia develops, the glipizide dosage may be tapered or discontinued and blood glucose concentrations re-evaluated 1 week later to assess the need for the drug. If hyperglycemia recurs, the dosage is increased or glipizide is reinitiated, with a reduction in dosage in those cats previously developing hypoglycemia. Glipizide is discontinued and insulin therapy initiated if clinical signs continue to worsen, the cat becomes ill or develops ketoacidosis, blood glucose concentrations remain greater than 300 mg/dL after 1 or 2 months of therapy, or the owner becomes dissatisfied with the treatment. In some cats, glipizide becomes ineffective weeks to months later and exogenous insulin is ultimately required to control the diabetic state. Presumably, the transition from glipizide responsiveness to lack of response and a need for insulin treatment is due to progression of the underlying pathophysiologic mechanisms (e.g., islet-specific amyloid deposition) responsible for the development of diabetes in the cat. The more rapid the rate of progression, the shorter the beneficial response to glipizide.

Glyburide. Glyburide (DiaβBeta, Micronase) is another second-generation sulfonylurea with similar actions as glipizide. Glyburide has a longer duration of action than glipizide and is usually administered once a day, versus twice a day for glipizide. Most studies in human diabetics have reported similar responses in comparisons of glyburide and glipizide.[53, 54] We have minimal experience with glyburide for the treatment of diabetes in cats. However, in countries where glipizide is not available, treatment with glyburide should be considered at an initial dosage of 0.625 mg (one half of a 1.25-mg tablet) per cat once daily. Response to therapy and adverse reactions to glyburide are similar to those described for glipizide.

Biguanides

The most commonly used drug in this class of oral hypoglycemic agents is metformin (Glucophage). Unlike sulfo-

TABLE 153–7. ADVERSE REACTIONS ASSOCIATED WITH GLIPIZIDE TREATMENT IN DIABETIC CATS

ADVERSE REACTION	RECOMMENDATION
Vomiting within 1 hour of administration	Vomiting usually subsides after 2 to 5 days of glipizide therapy; decrease dose or frequency of administration if vomiting is severe; discontinue if vomiting persists > 1 week.
Increased serum hepatic enzyme activities	Continue treatment and monitor enzymes every 1 to 2 weeks initially; discontinue glipizide if cat becomes ill (lethargy, inappetence, vomiting) or alanine aminotransferase exceeds 500 IU/L.
Icterus	Discontinue glipizide; start glipizide at lower dose and frequency of administration once icterus resolves (usually within 2 weeks); discontinue glipizide permanently if icterus recurs.
Hypoglycemia	Discontinue glipizide; re-check blood glucose in 1 week; begin glipizide at lower dose or frequency of administration if hyperglycemia recurs.

END

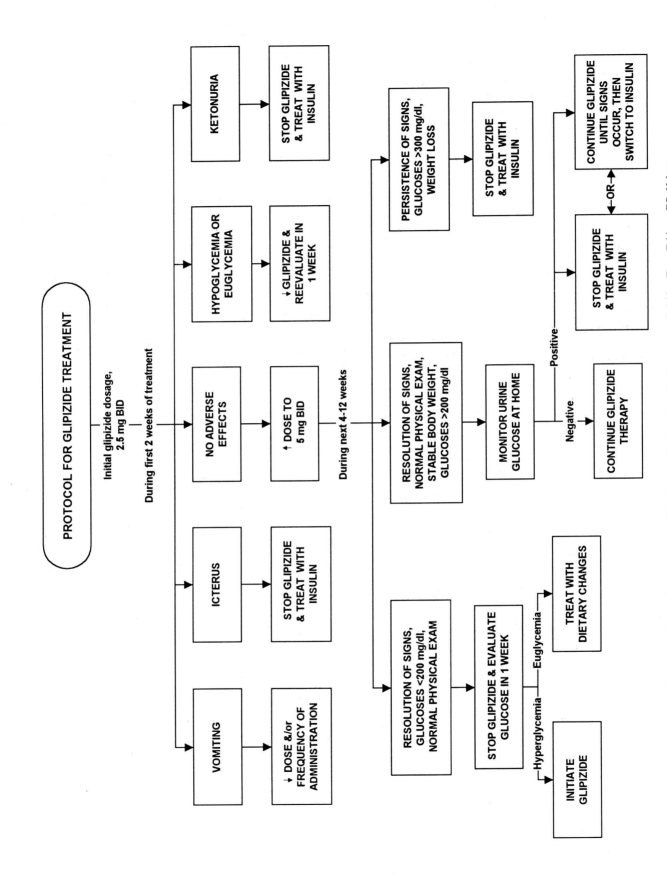

Figure 153–5. Algorithm for treating diabetic cats with the oral sulfonylurea drug, glipizide. (From Feldman EC, Nelson RW: Canine and Feline Endocrinology and Reproduction, 2nd ed. Philadelphia, WB Saunders, 1996, p 359.)

nylureas, metformin does not cause hypoglycemia or lower blood glucose concentrations in non-diabetic individuals, and only metformin has direct beneficial effects on serum lipid and lipoprotein concentrations.[55] The mechanism of action of metformin is poorly understood but does not involve stimulation of insulin secretion. Proposed actions include reduced gastrointestinal absorption of glucose, inhibition of hepatic glucose production, stimulation of tissue glucose uptake, and increased insulin-receptor binding.[56, 57] The major effect of the drug appears to be on promoting peripheral glucose utilization, primarily by increasing glucose transporters in cell membranes, thereby increasing glucose movement across the cell membrane.[55] Metformin has been reported to be as effective in controlling blood glucose concentrations as sulfonylureas in humans with NIDDM and to produce satisfactory results in approximately 50 per cent of diabetic humans in which sulfonylureas failed. Metformin's most common adverse effects are gastrointestinal and lactic acidosis. Unfortunately, vomiting within 2 hours of metformin administration is common in cats, even at 125 mg (one-fourth tablet)/cat. There are no reports on the efficacy of metformin for the treatment of NIDDM in cats.

Vanadium

Vanadium is a ubiquitous trace element that exerts insulin-like effects in vitro.[58] These effects may involve enhanced phosphorylation of the insulin receptor and/or mechanisms distal to the receptor but do not result from a rise in circulating insulin levels. In healthy cats, 4 weeks of oral vanadium administered in the drinking water resulted in a significant reduction in mean daily water consumption and occasional vomiting and diarrhea but was otherwise well tolerated.[59] Blood glucose concentrations decreased and clinical signs of diabetes resolved in one diabetic cat treated with orthovanadate in the drinking water for 4 weeks.[59]

Insulin Therapy

Types of Insulin

Commercial insulin is categorized by promptness, duration, and intensity of action after SC administration into short-acting (Regular crystalline), intermediate-acting (NPH, Lente), and long-acting (Ultralente, PZI) types. NPH and PZI insulin preparations contain the fish protein protamine and zinc to delay insulin absorption and prolong the duration of insulin effect. The Lente family of insulins rely on alterations in zinc content and the size of zinc-insulin crystals to alter the rate of absorption from the subcutaneous site of deposition. The larger the crystals, the slower the rate of absorption and the longer the duration of effect. Lente insulins contain no foreign protein (i.e., protamine). Stable mixtures of NPH and regular crystalline insulin (e.g., 70 per cent NPH/30 per cent Regular and 50 per cent NPH/50 per cent Regular) are also available (e.g., Humulin 70/30, Mixtard HM 70/30). In our experience, these premixed preparations are quite potent, causing a rapid decrease in blood glucose concentration within 60 to 90 minutes of SC administration. In addition, the duration of effect has usually been short (less than 8 hours).

Species of Insulin

For each type of insulin (e.g., NPH, Lente), the clinician must also choose the species of insulin to be administered.

Currently available species of insulin include recombinant human (e.g., Humulin), beef/pork combination (e.g., PZI), and purified pork (e.g., Iletin II Pork) insulin. Recombinant human insulin preparations are readily available and typically used to treat diabetes in dogs and cats. Although all species of insulin are generally effective in treating diabetes in dogs and cats, sufficient insulin antibodies to interfere with insulin action may uncommonly develop in some dogs and cats, necessitating a change in the species of insulin administered (see Complications of Insulin Therapy). Problems caused by insulin antibodies are more prevalent with beef/pork than human recombinant insulin in dogs.[60] To avoid problems with insulin effectiveness, use of recombinant human insulin is initially preferred in diabetic dogs, recognizing that the probability of having to administer insulin twice each day is high. The prevalence of insulin antibodies causing problems with glycemic control is uncommon in cats treated with recombinant human insulin.[61]

Initial Insulin Treatment for Diabetic Dogs

Intermediate-acting insulins (i.e., NPH, Lente) are the initial insulins of choice for glycemic regulation of the diabetic dog. We begin insulin therapy with Lente or NPH insulin of human recombinant origin at an approximate dosage of 0.5 U/kg twice a day. Dietary therapy is initiated concurrently. Because the vast majority of our diabetic dogs require recombinant human Lente or NPH insulin twice a day, we begin with a twice-daily protocol. In our experience, glycemic regulation is easier and problems with hypoglycemia are avoided when low-dose, twice-daily insulin therapy is initiated. Glycemic regulation is more problematic and development of hypoglycemia is more likely to occur when insulin is initially administered once a day followed by increases in the insulin dose over the ensuing 4 to 8 weeks and then switching to twice-a-day insulin therapy in an attempt to obtain better control of glycemia.

Initial Insulin Treatment for Diabetic Cats

Problems may occur with long-acting (Ultralente) and intermediate-acting (Lente, NPH) insulins in diabetic cats. Inadequate absorption of Ultralente insulin resulting in poor glycemic control despite insulin doses of 8 to 10 U per injection is a problem in approximately 20 per cent of diabetic cats. For these cats, a switch to Lente or NPH insulin at an initial dosage of 1 to 2 U twice a day is often effective in establishing better glycemic control. Unfortunately, duration of effect of Lente and NPH insulin can be considerably shorter than 12 hours, and problems with persistence of clinical signs because of short duration of effect are common with intermediate-acting insulins. For these cats, a switch to Ultralente insulin at an initial dosage of 1 to 2 U twice a day is often effective in establishing better glycemic control. It is not possible to predict which type of insulin will work best in individual diabetic cats. The initial insulin of choice ultimately is based on personal preference and experience. We usually begin insulin therapy with Ultralente insulin of recombinant human origin at a dosage of 1 to 2 U per cat administered twice daily. Dietary therapy is initiated concurrently.

Protamine zinc insulin is a long-acting insulin that historically was the insulin of choice for treatment of diabetes in cats. The Food and Drug Administration has approved the sale of PZI insulin for compassionate use only in diabetic cats. The intention is to provide PZI insulin for use in those diabetic cats that fail to respond to Ultralente, Lente, and NPH insulin and for which another cause of poor control of glycemia cannot be identified. PZI insulin has been effective in improving glycemic control in approximately 50 per cent of our diabetic cats when used under these guidelines. As with the other types of insulin, response to PZI insulin is unpredictable.

Initial Adjustments in Insulin Therapy

Newly diagnosed diabetic dogs and cats are typically hospitalized for no more than 24 to 48 hours to finish the diagnostic evaluation of the patient and to begin insulin therapy. Blood glucose concentrations are determined at the time insulin is administered and at 11 A.M., 2 P.M., and 5 P.M. The intent is to identify hypoglycemia (blood glucose < 80 mg/dL) in those dogs and cats that are unusually sensitive to the actions of insulin. If hypoglycemia occurs, the insulin dosage is decreased before sending the dog or cat home. The insulin dose is not adjusted in those dogs and cats that remain hyperglycemic during these first few days of insulin therapy. The objective during this first visit is *not* to establish perfect glycemic control before sending the dog or cat home. Rather, it is to begin to reverse the metabolic derangements induced by the disease, allow the patient to adapt to the insulin and change in diet, teach the owner how to administer insulin, and give the owner a few days to become accustomed to treating the diabetic dog or cat at home. Adjustments in insulin therapy are made on subsequent evaluations, once the owner and pet have become accustomed to the treatment.

We routinely re-evaluate dogs and cats once weekly until an insulin treatment protocol that maintains reasonable glycemic control of the patient has been identified. It typically takes approximately 1 month to establish a satisfactory insulin treatment protocol, assuming unidentified insulin antagonistic disease is not present. During this month, changes in insulin dose, type, and species, and possibly frequency of administration, are common and should be anticipated by the owner. At each evaluation, the owner's subjective opinion of water intake, urine output, and overall health of the pet is discussed; a complete physical examination is performed; any change in body weight is noted; and serial blood glucose measurements obtained from 7 to 9 A.M. until 4 to 6 P.M. are assessed. Adjustments in insulin therapy are based on this information, the pet is sent home, and an appointment is scheduled for the next week to re-evaluate the response to any change in therapy. Glycemic control is attained when clinical signs of diabetes have resolved, the pet is healthy and interactive in the home, its body weight is stable, the owner is satisfied with the progress of therapy, and, if possible, the blood glucose concentrations range between 100 and 250 mg/dL (dog) or 100 and 300 mg/dL (cat) throughout the day.

Monitoring the Diabetic Dog and Cat

The basic objective of insulin therapy is to eliminate the clinical signs of diabetes mellitus while avoiding the common complications associated with the disease (see Chronic Complications of Diabetes). We rely on owner observation for recurrence of clinical signs in conjunction with periodic physical examinations and assessment of body weight, serial evaluations of blood glucose concentrations, and blood glycosylated hemoglobin and serum fructosamine concentrations to evaluate control of the diabetic state. Most important

is the owner's subjective opinion of severity of clinical signs and overall health of their pet, findings on physical examination, and stability of body weight. If the owner is happy with results of treatment, the physical examination is supportive of good glycemic control, and the body weight is stable, the diabetes in the diabetic dog or cat is usually adequately controlled. Once glycemic control is established, the insulin dosage is re-evaluated every 3 to 6 months by physical examination, body weight, blood glycosylated hemoglobin and serum fructosamine concentrations, and, if necessary, evaluation of serial blood glucose concentrations in the hospital. Adjustments in insulin therapy are made accordingly (see Adjustments in Insulin Therapy). These evaluations are performed earlier if clinical signs of diabetes recur or other complications develop.

The insulin dosage required to maintain glycemic control typically changes (increase or decrease) with time. Initially, a fixed dosage of insulin is administered at home and changes in insulin dosage are made only after the owner consults with the veterinarian. As the insulin dosage range required to maintain glycemic control becomes apparent and as confidence is gained in the owner's ability to recognize signs of hypoglycemia and hyperglycemia, the owner is eventually allowed to make *slight* adjustments in insulin dosage at home based on clinical observations of the pet's well-being. However, the owner is instructed to stay within the agreed-on insulin dosage range. If the insulin dosage is at the upper or lower end of the established range and the pet is still symptomatic, the owner is instructed to call us before making further adjustments in the insulin dosage.

Occasional monitoring of urine for glycosuria and ketonuria is helpful (1) in those diabetic cats and dogs in whom "stress" may be affecting blood glucose measurements and the clinician is trying to determine if the diabetic is responsive to insulin in the home environment, (2) in cats with transient diabetes to identify if and when glycosuria recurs, (3) in cats treated with oral hypoglycemic drugs to determine if glycosuria resolves with treatment, and (4) in previously ketoacidotic or currently ill diabetics to determine if ketonuria is present. We do not have the owner adjust daily insulin dosages based on morning urine glucose measurements in diabetic dogs. Although this approach to the home management of the diabetic dog works in some, the vast majority of dogs develop complications as a result of owners being misled by morning urine glucose concentrations. If urine monitoring is done, the well-controlled diabetic pet should have urine that is free of glucose for most or all of each 24-hour period. Persistent glycosuria throughout the day and night suggests a problem that may require evaluation by means of in-hospital blood glucose determinations.

Glycosylated Hemoglobin and Fructosamine

Glycosylated hemoglobin (GHb) and fructosamine are glycated proteins found in blood of normal and diabetic individuals that are used to monitor glycemic control. GHb is formed by means of an irreversible, non-enzymatic, insulin-independent binding of glucose to hemoglobin in red blood cells.[62, 63] Fructosamines are serum proteins that have undergone non-enzymatic, insulin-independent glycation in a manner similar to Ghb.[64] The extent of glycosylation of hemoglobin and serum proteins is directly related to the blood glucose concentration; the higher the GHb and serum fructosamine concentrations, the poorer the glycemic control of the patient, and vice versa. Because serum proteins have a shorter half-life than hemoglobin, measurement of serum

TABLE 153–8. SAMPLE HANDLING, METHODOLOGY, AND INTERPRETATION OF BLOOD GLYCOSYLATED HEMOGLOBIN AND SERUM FRUCTOSAMINE CONCENTRATIONS MEASURED IN OUR LABORATORY

	GLYCOSYLATED HEMOGLOBIN		FRUCTOSAMINE	
Blood sample	2 mL whole blood in EDTA		1–2 mL serum	
Sample handling	Refrigerate and assay within 1 week		Freeze until assayed	
Methodology	Affinity chromatography—measures total GHb concentration (i.e., HbA_1)		Automated colorimetric assay using nitroblue tetrazolium chloride	
Factors affecting results	Anemia (decreased), polycythemia (increased)		Hypoalbuminemia (decreased), hypertriglyceridemia (?)	

Normal values	*Dog:* Mean, 3%
	          Upper limit, 4%
	Cat: Mean, 1.7%
	          Upper limit, 2.6%
			Dog: Mean, 310 µmol/L
			          Upper limit, 370 µmol/L
			Cat: Mean, 260 µmol/L
			          Upper limit, 340 µmol/L	

Interpretation in diabetics	DOG	CAT	DOG	CAT
Excellent control	< 5%	< 2%	< 400 µmol/L	< 400 µmol/L
Good control	5–6%	2.0–2.5%	400–475 µmol/L	400–475 µmol/L
Fair control	6–7%	2.5–3.0%	475–550 µmol/L	475–550 µmol/L
Poor control	> 7%	> 3.0%	> 550 µmol/L	> 550 µmol/L

fructosamine concentration provides an index of the average blood glucose concentration over the preceding 2 to 3 weeks, versus 4 to 8 weeks for GHb. This shorter period for change in serum fructosamine concentration may be advantageous in detecting improvement or deterioration of glycemic control more quickly than if GHb is monitored.

Information regarding sample handling, assay technique, factors affecting results, and reference ranges for our laboratory are given in Table 153–8. Blood GHb concentrations are lower in cats versus dogs because of species differences in red cell membrane permeability to glucose; the red blood cell membrane is more permeable to glucose in dogs than in cats.[65] Although GHb and serum fructosamine concentrations are typically increased in newly diagnosed, untreated diabetic dogs and cats, values may be normal in some diabetic dogs and cats, suggesting diabetes has only been present for a short time before diagnosis.[65, 66] Thus, increased blood GHb and serum fructosamine concentrations support the diagnosis of diabetes mellitus but normal values do not rule out diabetes.

Blood GHb and serum fructosamine concentrations correlate with severity and chronicity of hyperglycemia; that is, GHb and fructosamine concentrations increase when glycemic control of the diabetic dog or cat worsens and decrease when glycemic control improves (Table 153–8).[65–67] In addition, GHb and serum fructosamine concentrations are not affected by stress-induced hyperglycemia. Blood GHb and/or serum fructosamine concentrations can be measured during the routine evaluation of glycemic control performed every 3 to 6 months; to clarify the impact of stress on results of blood glucose measurements; to clarify discrepancies between the history, findings on physical examination, and results of serial blood glucose measurements; and to assess the effectiveness of changes in insulin therapy. For the latter, if changes in insulin therapy are appropriate, a decrease in serum fructosamine and blood GHb concentration should occur. Increased blood GHb or serum fructosamine concentrations suggest poor glycemic control and a need for insulin adjustments; however, GHb and fructosamine concentrations do not identify the underlying problem. Evaluation of serial measurements of blood glucose concentration is required to determine how to adjust insulin therapy.

Adjustments in Insulin Therapy

Indications

The need for adjustments in insulin therapy is based on presence or absence of clinical signs of diabetes (i.e., poly-

uria, polydipsia, polyphagia, weight loss), development of chronic complications indicative of poor glycemic control (e.g., rear limb weakness in cats), physical examination findings, changes in body weight, glycosylated hemoglobin and serum fructosamine concentrations, and owner satisfaction with the treatment. If an adjustment in insulin therapy is deemed necessary after reviewing this information, then a serial blood glucose curve must be generated to provide guidance in making the adjustment. Evaluation of a serial blood glucose curve is mandatory during the initial regulation of the diabetic patient, is periodically of value to assess glycemic control despite the fact that a dog or cat may appear to be doing well in the home environment, and is necessary to re-establish glycemic control in the patient in which clinical manifestations of hyperglycemia or hypoglycemia have developed.

Protocol for Generating the Serial Blood Glucose Curve

When assessing glycemic control, the insulin and feeding schedule used by the owner should be followed and blood should be obtained every 1 to 2 hours throughout the day for glucose determination. The owner should feed the pet at home, *not* at the hospital. If insulin is usually given within 1 hour before the pet's presentation to the clinic, insulin is given by the owner (using the owner's insulin and syringe) in the hospital *after* an initial blood glucose determination is obtained. The entire insulin administration procedure should be closely evaluated by a veterinary technician. If the owner usually administers insulin before 6 A.M., we recommend that the owner give the insulin at 6 A.M. and bring the pet to the hospital at the first appointment of the day. It is more important to maintain the pet's daily routine than to risk inaccurate blood glucose results caused by inappetence in the hospital or insulin administration at an unusual time. The exception is those instances in which the veterinarian wants to evaluate the owner's technique of administration of insulin rather than physiologic saline.

Blood glucose concentrations can be determined in a clinical chemistry laboratory or with glucose reagent strips (e.g., Chemstrip bG [Bio-Dynamics]) and a glucometer (e.g., Accuchek III [Bio-Dynamics]). Blood glucose concentrations are lower when determined by glucometers versus benchtop methodologies (e.g., glucose oxidase). This is due, in part, to the use of venous blood on these strips rather than capillary blood for which the units are designed. Failure to

END

consider this "error" could result in insulin underdosage and the potential for persistence of clinical signs despite "acceptable" blood glucose results.

By evaluating serial blood glucose measurements every 1 to 2 hours throughout the day, the veterinarian will be able to determine if the insulin is effective and to identify the glucose nadir, time of peak insulin effect, duration of insulin effect, and severity of fluctuation in blood glucose concentrations in a particular dog or cat. Obtaining only one or two blood glucose concentrations has not been reliable for evaluating the effect of a given insulin dose.

The *ideal* goal of insulin therapy is to maintain the blood glucose concentration between 100 and 200 mg/dL throughout the day and night for the diabetic dog without cataracts, between 100 and 300 mg/dL for diabetic dogs blind from cataract formation, and between 100 and 300 mg/dL in diabetic cats. If glucose test strips are used, the blood glucose level should remain more than 80 mg/dL. These goals can be difficult to achieve, and in some diabetic dogs and cats they may be impossible to attain. The ultimate decision on whether to adjust insulin therapy must always take into consideration the owner's perception of how the pet is doing at home, findings on physical examination, changes in body weight, glycosylated hemoglobin and serum fructosamine concentrations, as well as results of serial blood glucose measurements. Many diabetic dogs and cats do well despite blood glucose concentrations consistently in the high 100s to low 300s.

Interpreting the Serial Blood Glucose Curve

Insulin effectiveness, glucose nadir, and duration of insulin effect are the critical determinations from the serial blood glucose curve. The effectiveness of insulin is the first parameter to assess. Is the insulin effective in lowering the blood glucose concentration? The insulin dosage, highest blood glucose concentration, and the difference between the highest and lowest blood glucose concentration (i.e., blood glucose differential) must be considered simultaneously when assessing insulin effectiveness. For example, a blood glucose differential of 50 mg/dL is acceptable if the blood glucose level ranges between 120 and 170 mg/dL but is unacceptable if the blood glucose level ranges between 350 and 400 mg/dL. Similarly, a blood glucose differential of 100 mg/dL indicates insulin effectiveness if the patient receives 0.4 U of insulin/kg but suggests insulin resistance if the patient receives 2.2 U of insulin/kg.

If the insulin is not effective in lowering the blood glucose concentration, the clinician must consider insulin underdosage and the differentials for insulin ineffectiveness and resistance (see Recurrence of Clinical Signs). In general, insulin underdosage should be considered if the insulin dosage is less than 1.5 U/kg per injection in the diabetic dog and less than 6 to 8 U/injection for the diabetic cat. Insulin ineffectiveness and resistance should be considered if the insulin dosage exceeds these guidelines.

If insulin is effective in lowering the blood glucose concentration, the next parameter to assess is the lowest blood glucose (i.e., glucose nadir). The glucose nadir should ideally fall between 100 and 125 mg/dL (80 mg/dL if using glucose test strips). If the glucose nadir is greater than 150 mg/dL, the insulin dosage may need to be increased; and if the nadir is less than 80 mg/dL, the insulin dosage should be decreased. For the latter, the reduction in insulin dosage is dependent on the amount of insulin given at the time the

glucose curve is generated (see Insulin Overdosing and Glucose Counter-Regulation).

Duration of insulin effect can be assessed if the glucose nadir is greater than 100 mg/dL (80 mg/dL if using glucose test strips). Assessment of duration of insulin effect may not be valid when the blood glucose decreases to less than 80 mg/dL because of the potential induction of the Somogyi phenomenon, which could falsely decrease the apparent duration of insulin effect. The duration of effect is roughly defined as the time from the insulin injection through the lowest glucose level and until the blood glucose concentration exceeds 200 to 250 mg/dL. Ideally, insulin action should last 22 to 24 hours. Unfortunately, for most dogs and cats treated with recombinant human insulin, the duration of intermediate- and long-acting insulin effect is typically 10 to 14 hours, which is why twice-daily insulin protocols are recommended when insulin therapy is initiated. In a small percentage of diabetic dogs and cats, duration of insulin effect is less than 10 hours. This short duration of effect may cause recurrence or persistence of clinical signs of hyperglycemia, necessitating an adjustment in the type of insulin (e.g., Ultralente or PZI insulin) or frequency of insulin administration (e.g., every 8 hours) to establish better glycemic control. Measuring blood glucose concentrations every 1 to 2 hours for 8 to 12 hours after insulin administration will usually identify short duration of insulin effect.

Problems With Serial Blood Glucose Curves

The results of serial blood glucose determinations can be affected by many variables, including stress, inappetence, and the prolonged insulin antagonistic effects of the counter-regulatory hormones. Stress is difficult to define in dogs and cats and should be considered whenever results of a serial blood glucose curve suggest insulin ineffectiveness while owner observations, urine glucose determinations, physical findings, body weight, and glycosylated hemoglobin and serum fructosamine concentrations suggest good glycemic control. Stress may be a factor at the time of initial evaluation or become a factor weeks to months later, as the dog or cat develops an aversion to hospitalization and multiple venipunctures. Typical serial blood glucose curves in stressed dogs and cats will have the lowest blood glucose concentration at the first blood sampling and subsequent blood glucose concentrations progressively increase throughout the day, or blood glucose concentrations are initially increased (i.e., > 300 mg/dL) and remain increased throughout the day. Differentials for the latter type of serial blood glucose curve include stress-induced hyperglycemia, insulin underdosage, and all the causes for recurrence of clinical signs of diabetes.

Diabetic dogs and cats frequently refuse to eat in the veterinary hospital, which can profoundly alter the results of a serial blood glucose curve. To counter the effects of inappetence, the owner should feed the dog or cat before bringing the animal to the hospital. Blood samples can then be obtained until the next scheduled meal. The information gained in this manner will more reliably reflect what is happening at home.

The reproducibility of serial blood glucose curves varies from patient to patient. In some dogs and cats, serial blood glucose curves may vary dramatically from day to day or month to month, depending, in part, on the actual amount of insulin administered and absorbed from the subcutaneous site of deposition and on the interaction of insulin, diet, exercise, and counter-regulatory hormone secretion. In other dogs and cats, serial blood glucose curves are reasonably consistent from day to day and month to month. Generally, information gained from a prior serial blood glucose curve should never be assumed to be reproducible on subsequent curves, especially if several weeks to months have passed or the dog or cat has developed recurrence of clinical signs.

Insulin Therapy During Surgery

Generally, surgery should be delayed in diabetic dogs and cats until their clinical condition is stable and the diabetic state controlled with insulin. The exception are those situations in which surgery is required to correct insulin resistance (e.g., ovariohysterectomy in a diestrus bitch) or to save the animal's life (e.g., intestinal obstruction). The surgery itself does not pose a greater risk in a stable diabetic versus a non-diabetic dog or cat. The concern is the interplay between insulin therapy and lack of food intake during the perioperative period. The "stress" of anesthesia and surgery causes the release of diabetogenic hormones that, in turn, promote ketogenesis. Insulin must be administered during the perioperative period to prevent severe hyperglycemia and ketone formation. To compensate for lack of food intake, the amount of insulin administered during the perioperative period is decreased to prevent hypoglycemia.

The day before surgery the patient receives the normal dose of insulin and is fed as usual. Food is withheld after 10 P.M. On the morning of surgery, a blood glucose concentration is measured before giving insulin. If the blood glucose concentration is less than 100 mg/dL, insulin is not given and an IV infusion of 5 per cent dextrose is initiated. If the blood glucose concentration is between 100 and 200 mg/dL, one fourth of the usual morning dose of insulin is given and an IV infusion of dextrose is initiated. If the blood glucose is more than 200 mg/dL, one half of the usual morning dose of insulin is given but the IV dextrose infusion is withheld until the blood glucose concentration is less than 150 mg/dL. For all three situations, the blood glucose concentration is monitored every 30 to 60 minutes during the procedure, which should be started within 1 to 2 hours of the time that insulin is given. The goal is to maintain the blood glucose level between 150 and 300 mg/dL during the perioperative period. Intravenous 5 per cent dextrose infusion and intermittent regular crystalline insulin administration are done as needed to correct and prevent hypoglycemia and severe hyperglycemia, respectively. For the latter, regular crystalline insulin is administered IM or SC and is repeated at 4- to 6-hour intervals as needed. The initial dose of regular crystalline insulin is approximately 20 per cent of the dose of long-acting insulin being used in the home environment. Subsequent adjustments in the dose of regular crystalline insulin are based on results of blood glucose measurements. Once the dog or cat is eating regularly, it can be returned to its normal insulin and feeding schedule.

COMPLICATIONS OF INSULIN THERAPY

HYPOGLYCEMIA

Hypoglycemia is a common complication of insulin therapy. Signs of hypoglycemia are most likely to occur after increases in the insulin dose, with excessive overlap of insulin action in dogs and cats receiving insulin twice a day, during strenuous exercise, after prolonged inappetence, and in insulin-treated cats that have reverted to a non–insulin-

dependent state. In these situations, severe hypoglycemia may occur before the diabetogenic hormones (i.e., glucagon, cortisol, epinephrine, and growth hormone) are able to compensate for and reverse low blood glucose concentrations. Signs of hypoglycemia include lethargy, weakness, head tilting, ataxia, and seizures. Occurrence of clinical signs is dependent on the rate of blood glucose decline as well as on the severity of hypoglycemia. Hypoglycemia is treated with glucose administered as food, sugar water, or dextrose IV. Whenever signs of hypoglycemia occur, adjustments in insulin therapy need to be made. The owner should be instructed to decrease each insulin dose by 25 to 50 per cent, continue that dose for 2 to 3 days, and then return to the veterinarian for the dog or cat to be evaluated with serial blood glucose determinations.

Impaired Counter-Regulation

Secretion of the diabetogenic hormones, most notably epinephrine and glucagon, stimulates hepatic glucose secretion and helps counter severe hypoglycemia. An impaired counter-regulatory response to hypoglycemia has been documented in some dogs with IDDM.[68] As a consequence, when the blood glucose concentration approaches 60 mg/dL, there is no compensatory response to increase blood glucose, and prolonged hypoglycemia ensues. Impaired counter-regulation should be considered in a diabetic dog or cat exquisitely sensitive to small doses of insulin or with problems of prolonged hypoglycemia after administration of an acceptable dosage of insulin.

RECURRENCE OF CLINICAL SIGNS

Recurrence or persistence of clinical signs (i.e., polyuria, polydipsia, polyphagia, weight loss) is perhaps the most common "complication" of insulin therapy in diabetic dogs and cats. Recurrence or continuing clinical signs suggest problems with owner technique in administering insulin; insulin therapy as it relates to insulin activity, type, dosage, species or frequency of administration; or insulin resistance caused by concurrent inflammatory, infectious, neoplastic, or hormonal disorders. Documenting increased blood glucose concentrations does not, by itself, confirm a problem with insulin therapy. Stress can cause marked hyperglycemia that does not reflect the patient's responsiveness to insulin and can lead to the erroneous belief that the diabetes in the dog or cat is poorly controlled. When evaluating a diabetic dog or cat for suspected insulin ineffectiveness, it is important that all parameters used to assess glycemic control be evaluated, including owner observations of how the dog or cat is doing in the home environment, findings on physical examination, changes in body weight, and blood glycated protein concentrations.

If the history, physical examination, change in body weight, and blood glycated protein concentrations suggest poor control of the diabetic state, a thorough evaluation for causes of insulin ineffectiveness should be undertaken (Table 153–9). Whenever insulin ineffectiveness is suspected, problems with insulin activity or administration technique should be ruled out and insulin therapy critically assessed before an extensive diagnostic evaluation for insulin resistance is undertaken. Failure to administer an appropriate dosage of biologically active insulin can mimic insulin resistance because of unrecognized insulin underdosage. Insulin underdosage can result from administration of biologically inac-

TABLE 153-9. RECOGNIZED CAUSES OF INSULIN INEFFECTIVENESS OR INSULIN RESISTANCE IN THE DIABETIC DOG AND CAT

CAUSED BY INSULIN THERAPY	CAUSED BY CONCURRENT DISORDER
Inactive insulin	Diabetogenic drugs
Diluted insulin	Hyperadrenocorticism
Improper administration technique	Diestrus (bitch)
	Acromegaly (cat)
Inadequate dose	Infection (esp. oral cavity and urinary tract)
Somogyi effect	
Inadequate frequency of insulin administration	Hypothyroidism (dog)
	Hyperthyroidism (cat)
Impaired insulin absorption (esp. Ultralente insulin)	Renal insufficiency
	Liver insufficiency
Anti-insulin antibody excess	Cardiac insufficiency
	Glucagonoma (dog)
	Pheochromocytoma
	Chronic inflammation (esp. pancreatitis)
	Pancreatic exocrine insufficiency
	Severe obesity
	Hyperlipidemia
	Neoplasia

tive insulin (e.g., outdated, overheated, mixed by shaking), administration of diluted insulin, use of inappropriate insulin syringes for the concentration of insulin (e.g., U-100 syringe with U-40 insulin), or problems with insulin administration technique (e.g., misunderstanding on how to read the insulin syringe, inappropriate injection technique). These problems are identified by having the clinician administer new, undiluted insulin and measuring several blood glucose concentrations throughout the day. If an insulin-resistant type of serial blood glucose curve persists, a diagnostic evaluation to identify the cause may be warranted.

Problems With Insulin Therapy

Insulin therapy should be critically evaluated for possible insulin underdosage or overdosage, poor absorption of Ultralente insulin, short duration of insulin effect, inappropriate species of insulin, and insulin antibody formation. Changes in insulin therapy should be tried to improve insulin effectiveness, especially if the history and physical examination do not suggest a concurrent disorder causing insulin resistance.

Diluted Insulin. Diluted insulin should be replaced with full-strength insulin. In some dogs and cats, insufficient amounts of insulin are administered when diluted insulin is used, despite appropriate dilution and insulin administration techniques, inadequacies that are corrected when full-strength insulin is used. Small insulin syringes (U-100, 0.3 mL) can be used with full-strength U-100 insulin for cats and small dogs receiving small amounts of insulin.

Insulin Overdosing and Glucose Counter-Regulation. A high dose of insulin may cause overt hypoglycemia, glucose counter-regulation (Somogyi phenomenon), or insulin resistance. The Somogyi phenomenon results from a normal physiologic response to impending hypoglycemia induced by excessive insulin. When the blood glucose concentration declines to less than 65 mg/dL (less than 80 mg/dL if using glucose test strips) or when the blood glucose concentration decreases rapidly regardless of the glucose nadir, direct hypoglycemia-induced stimulation of hepatic glycogenolysis and secretion of diabetogenic hormones raises the glucose concentration. The hormones most responsible for this are epinephrine and glucagon. They increase the blood glucose concentration, minimize signs of hypoglycemia, and can cause marked hyperglycemia within 12 hours.[69]

Diagnosis of insulin-induced hyperglycemia requires demonstration of hypoglycemia (< 65 mg/dL) followed by hyperglycemia (> 300 mg/dL) within one 24-hour period after insulin administration. Therapy involves reducing the insulin dose. If the diabetic dog or cat is receiving an "acceptable" dose of insulin (i.e., ≤ 1.5 U/kg/injection in the dog; ≤ 5 U/injection in the cat), the insulin dose should be decreased 10 to 25 per cent. If the insulin dose exceeds these amounts, glycemic regulation should be started over again using the insulin dose recommended for the initial regulation of the diabetic dog or cat. Blood glucose concentrations should be re-evaluated approximately 7 days after initiating the new dose of insulin. Further adjustments in the insulin dose should be made after reviewing these results.

Secretion of diabetogenic hormones during the Somogyi phenomenon may induce insulin resistance, which can last 24 to 72 hours after the hypoglycemic episode. If serial blood glucose concentrations are evaluated on the day of hypoglycemia, the Somogyi phenomenon will be identified and the insulin dose lowered accordingly. However, if blood glucose concentrations are monitored after secretion of the diabetogenic hormones, insulin resistance may be diagnosed and the insulin dose increased, further exacerbating the Somogyi phenomenon. A cyclic history of one or two days of good glycemic control followed by several days of poor control should raise suspicion for insulin resistance caused by glucose counter-regulation. This is one of the most common causes of insulin resistance in cats. It can be induced with insulin doses of 2 to 3 units per injection and can result in cats receiving 10 to 15 units of insulin per injection. Establishing the diagnosis may require several days of hospitalization and determination of serial blood glucose curves. An alternative approach that we prefer is to arbitrarily reduce the insulin dose 1 to 3 units for diabetic dogs or cats and have the owner evaluate the patient's response (based on clinical signs) over the ensuing 2 to 5 days. If clinical signs of diabetes worsen after a reduction in the insulin dose, another cause for the insulin resistance should be pursued. However, if the owner reports no change or improvement in clinical signs, continued gradual reduction of the insulin dose should be pursued. Alternatively, glycemic regulation of the diabetic dog or cat could be started over, using insulin doses recommended for the initial management of the diabetic.

Short Duration of Insulin Effect. For most dogs and cats treated with recombinant human insulin, the duration of intermediate- and long-acting insulin effect is typically 10 to 14 hours. Twice-daily insulin administration is effective in controlling blood glucose concentrations. In a small percentage of diabetic dogs and cats, duration of insulin effect is less than 10 hours. As a result, hyperglycemia (> 250 mg/dL) occurs for several hours each day and owners of these pets usually mention continuing problems with polyuria and polydipsia or with weight loss. A diagnosis of short duration of insulin effect is made by demonstrating hyperglycemia (> 250 mg/dL) within 6 to 10 hours of the insulin injection, while the lowest blood glucose concentration is maintained above 80 mg/dL (see Interpreting the Serial Blood Glucose Curve). Treatment involves changing the type of insulin (e.g., switching to Ultralente or PZI insulin) or the frequency of insulin administration (e.g., initiating three-times-a-day therapy).

Inadequate Insulin Absorption. Slow or inadequate absorption of subcutaneously deposited insulin is most commonly observed in diabetic cats receiving Ultralente insulin, a long-acting insulin that has a slow onset and prolonged duration of effect. In approximately 20 per cent of cats in our hospital, Ultralente insulin is absorbed from the subcutaneous site of deposition too slowly for it to be effective in maintaining acceptable glycemic control. In these cats, the blood glucose concentration may not decrease until 6 to 10 hours after the injection or, more commonly, it decreases minimally despite insulin doses of 8 to 12 U given every 12 hours. As a consequence, the blood glucose concentration remains greater than 300 mg/dL for most of the day. We have had success in these cats by switching from Ultralente to Lente or NPH insulin given twice a day.

When changing type of insulin, a more potent insulin should be substituted for the previous one (Fig. 153–6). We generally switch to the next most potent insulin and reduce the insulin dose (usually to amounts initially used to regulate the diabetic dog or cat) to avoid hypoglycemia. For example, cats treated with Ultralente insulin are switched to Lente insulin at 2 to 3 U per injection, dogs treated with Lente insulin are switched to NPH insulin at 0.5 U/kg, and so forth. The duration of effect of the insulin becomes shorter as the potency of the insulin increases, which may create problems with short duration of insulin effect.

Circulating Insulin-Binding Antibodies

Insulin antibodies result from repeated injections of a foreign protein (i.e., insulin). The more divergent the insulin molecule being administered from the species being treated, the greater the likelihood that significant or worrisome amounts of insulin antibodies will be formed. The amino acid sequences of canine, porcine, and recombinant human insulin are similar, and the amino acid sequences of feline and bovine insulin are similar.[36, 70] Preliminary studies using

an enzyme-linked immunosorbent assay to detect insulin antibodies in insulin-treated diabetic dogs suggests that the prevalence of insulin antibodies is common in dogs treated with beef/pork insulin and is associated with erratic glycemic control in some dogs.[60] In these dogs, blood glucose concentrations typically fluctuate between 200 and 400 mg/dL, the status of glycemic control vacillates from day to day, but overt insulin resistance (i.e., blood glucose concentrations consistently > 400 mg/dL) is not evident. Excessive insulin-binding antibodies causing insulin resistance characterized by blood glucose concentrations consistently greater than 400 mg/dL are uncommon. Insulin-binding antibodies can also cause erratic fluctuations in the blood glucose concentration, with no correlation between the timing of insulin administration and changes in blood glucose concentration. Fluctuations in blood glucose concentration presumably result from changes in circulating free insulin concentration as antibody binding affinity for insulin changes.[71] In contrast, insulin antibody formation is infrequent in dogs treated with recombinant human insulin and glycemic control often improves when the source of insulin is changed from beef/pork to recombinant human. To avoid problems with insulin effectiveness, we prefer to use recombinant human insulin in diabetic dogs initially, recognizing that the probability of having to administer insulin twice each day is high.

Insulin antibody titers developed with approximately equal frequency in diabetic cats treated with beef insulin, compared with recombinant human insulin.[61] However, titers were weakly positive in most cats, prevalence of persistent titers was low, and insulin antibodies did not appear to affect glycemic control. These results suggest that the prevalence of insulin antibodies causing problems with glycemic control similar to those identified in dogs is uncommon in cats treated with recombinant human insulin.

Concurrent Disorders Causing Insulin Resistance

There are many disorders that can interfere with insulin action (see Table 153–9). Obtaining a complete history and performing a thorough physical examination is the most important step in identifying these concurrent disorders. Abnormalities identified on a thorough physical examination may suggest a concurrent insulin-antagonistic disorder or infectious process, which will give the clinician direction in the diagnostic evaluation of the patient (Table 153–10). If the history and physical examination are unremarkable, a complete blood cell count, serum biochemical analysis, serum thyroxine determination (cat), abdominal ultrasonography, and urinalysis with bacterial culture should be ordered to further screen for concurrent illness. Additional tests will depend on the results of the initial screening tests (see Table 153–10). The reader is referred to the work of Feldman and Nelson (1996)[42] for a complete discussion of causes of insulin resistance in diabetic dogs and cats.

CHRONIC COMPLICATIONS OF DIABETES MELLITUS

Complications resulting from the diabetic state (e.g., cataracts) or from therapy (e.g., insulin-induced hypoglycemia) are common in dogs and cats (see Table 153–5). The most common complications in the dog are blindness due to cataract formation, chronic pancreatitis, and recurring infections of the urinary tract, respiratory system, and skin. The

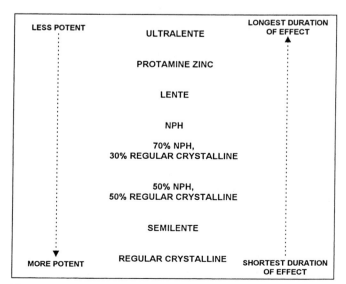

INSULIN POTENCY

Figure 153–6. Categorization of types of commercial insulin based on potency and duration of effect. Note the inverse relationship between potency and duration of effect. (From Feldman EC, Nelson RW: Canine and Feline Endocrinology and Reproduction, 2nd ed. Philadelphia, WB Saunders, 1996, p 380.)

END

TABLE 153–10. DIAGNOSTIC TESTS TO CONSIDER FOR THE EVALUATION OF INSULIN RESISTANCE IN THE DIABETIC DOG AND CAT

Complete blood cell count, serum biochemistry panel, urinalysis
Bacterial culture of the urine
Serum lipase and amylase concentration (pancreatitis)
Serum trypsin–like immunoreactivity (exocrine pancreatic insufficiency, pancreatitis)
Adrenocortical function tests
  ACTH stimulation test (spontaneous or iatrogenic hyperadrenocorticism)
  Low-dose dexamethasone suppression test (spontaneous hyperadrenocorticism)
  Urine cortisol/creatinine ratio (spontaneous hyperadrenocorticism)
Thyroid function tests
  Baseline serum thyroxine and free thyroxine (hypo- or hyperthyroidism)
  Baseline serum cTSH (dog—hypothyroidism)
  TSH stimulation test (hypothyroidism)
  TRH stimulation test (hypo- or hyperthyroidism)
  T_3 suppression test (hyperthyroidism)
Serum progesterone concentration (diestrus in intact bitch)
Plasma growth hormone or serum insulin–like growth factor-I concentration (acromegaly)
Serum insulin concentration 24 hours after stopping insulin therapy (insulin antibodies)
Serum triglyceride concentration (hyperlipidemia)
Abdominal ultrasound (adrenomegaly, adrenal mass, pancreatic mass)
Thoracic radiographs (cardiomegaly, neoplasia)
Computed tomography or magnetic resonance imaging (pituitary mass)

ACTH = adrenocorticotropic hormone; TSH = thyroid-stimulating hormone; cTSH = canine TSH; TRH = thyroid-releasing hormone; T_3 = triiodothyronine.

most common complications in the cat are weight loss, chronic pancreatitis, and peripheral neuropathy of the hind limbs, causing weakness and ataxia. Diabetic dogs and cats are also at risk for developing hypoglycemia and ketoacidosis. The devastating chronic complications of human diabetes (e.g., nephropathy, vasculopathy, coronary artery disease) require 10 to 20 years or longer to develop and, as such, are uncommon in diabetic dogs and cats.

CATARACTS AND LENS-INDUCED UVEITIS

Cataract formation is the most common and one of the most important long-term complications associated with diabetes mellitus in the dog but is rare in the cat. The pathogenesis of diabetic cataract formation is thought to be related to altered osmotic relationships in the lens, which result from glucose metabolism through the sorbitol pathway to sorbitol and fructose.[10] Sorbitol and fructose are not freely permeable to the cell membrane and act as potent hydrophilic agents, causing an influx of water into the lens, leading to swelling and rupture of the lens fibers and the development of cataracts. Cataract formation is an irreversible process once it begins. Clinically, dogs may progress from having normal vision to being blind over a period of days to months. Good glycemic control slows development of cataracts, whereas blindness due to cataracts reduces the need for stringent blood glucose control.

Blindness may be corrected by removing the abnormal lens. Vision is restored in 75 to 80 per cent of diabetic dogs undergoing cataract removal. Factors that affect the success of surgery include the status of glycemic control, concurrent retinal disease, and presence of lens-induced uveitis. Uveitis associated with a resorbing, hypermature cataract must be controlled before surgery. Treatment of lens-induced uveitis is designed to decrease inflammation and prevent further intraocular damage and includes topical ophthalmic corticosteroids and non–steroidal anti-inflammatory agents (e.g., 0.03 per cent flurbiprofen [Ocufen]). Although not as potent anti-inflammatory agents as corticosteroids, non–steroidal anti-inflammatory drugs do not interfere with glycemic control.

DIABETIC RETINOPATHY

Diabetic retinopathy is an uncommon clinical complication in the dog and cat. In diabetic people, there is a close correlation between diabetic retinopathy and suboptimal glycemic control.[72] Microaneurysms, hemorrhages, and varicose and shunt capillaries may be observed with an ophthalmoscope.[73, 74] Histologic changes include an increased thickness of the capillary basement membrane, loss of pericytes, capillary shunts, and microaneurysms. The histologic changes are believed to result from retinal ischemia.[75] Involvement of polyol pathway activity is controversial, although studies in diabetic dogs suggest the development of retinopathy is not critically dependent on excessive polyol production or accumulation.[76] Because of the high incidence of cataract formation, the retinas should always be evaluated in the dog with newly diagnosed diabetes to ensure normal function and lack of grossly visible disease, should cataract formation and subsequent lens removal become necessary in the future. An electroretinogram can also be used to evaluate the function of the retina before cataract surgery.

DIABETIC NEUROPATHY

Diabetic neuropathies are rarely reported in the dog and cat.[77–79] Clinical signs supportive of a co-existent neuropathy in the diabetic dog or cat include weakness, knuckling, muscle atrophy, depressed limb reflexes, and deficits in postural reaction testing. Cats often develop a plantigrade posture with the hocks touching the ground when the cat walks (see Fig. 153–4). A distal polyneuropathy primarily develops in the dog and is characterized by segmental demyelination and remyelination and axonal degeneration and regeneration.[10] Electrophysiologic testing may reveal fibrillation potentials and positive sharp waves, suggesting denervated muscle, and occasionally fasciculation potentials and bizarre high-frequency discharges.[80] In addition, there is a decrease in motor and sensory nerve conduction velocities.

The cause of diabetic neuropathy is not known. Three hypotheses that have received the most attention in human diabetics include ischemic disease of arterioles (vascular hypothesis), early functional changes followed by structural degeneration of axons (axonal hypothesis), and increased polyol pathway activity, with accumulation of sorbitol and fructose and corresponding decrease in myoinositol content in Schwann cells and axons (metabolic hypothesis).[75, 81, 82] There is no specific therapy for diabetic neuropathy. Aggressive glucoregulation with insulin may improve nerve conduction and, in cats, reverse the posterior weakness and plantigrade posture (see Fig. 153–4).[83] However, response to therapy is variable.

DIABETIC NEPHROPATHY

Although diabetic nephropathy has occasionally been reported in the dog, its clinical recognition appears to be low. In contrast, renal insufficiency occurs commonly in diabetic cats, being identified in approximately 20 per cent of diabetic cats in one study.[9] Histopathologic findings are dependent on the duration of disease and degree of glycemic control and include membranous glomerulonephropathy with fusion of the foot processes, glomerular and tubular basement membrane thickening, an increase in the mesangial matrix material, the presence of subendothelial deposits, glomerular fibrosis, and glomerulosclerosis.[9, 84, 85] The pathogenic mechanism of diabetic nephropathy is unknown but probably multifactorial.[75, 86]

Clinical signs depend on the severity of glomerulosclerosis and the functional ability of the kidney to excrete metabolic wastes. Initially, diabetic nephropathy is manifested as severe proteinuria (primarily albuminuria) as a result of glomerular dysfunction. As glomerular changes progress, glomerular filtration becomes progressively impaired, resulting in the development of azotemia and eventually uremia. With severe fibrosis of the glomeruli, oliguric and then anuric renal failure develops. There is no specific treatment of diabetic nephropathy apart from meticulous metabolic control of the diabetic state, conservative medical management of the renal insufficiency, and control of systemic hypertension. The progression of glomerulosclerosis is related to the degree of glycemic control. There appears to be a definite decrease in the incidence of glomerular microvascular changes with improved glycemic control.[87, 88]

PROGNOSIS

The prognosis for diabetic dogs and cats is dependent, in part, on owner commitment to treating the disorder, ease of glycemic regulation, presence and nature of concurrent disorders, and avoidance of chronic complications associated with the diabetic state (see Table 153–5). In general, diabetes mellitus carries a guarded long-term prognosis. In recent retrospective studies, median survival time from the time diabetes was diagnosed was 2.7 and 1.4 years in dogs and cats, respectively.[9, 89] Survival time increased considerably if the dog or cat survived the initial few months of treatment. Although most of our diabetic dogs and cats live less than 5 years from the time of diagnosis, this survival time must be tempered with the realization that many of our diabetic dogs and cats are older than 10 years of age at the time of diagnosis. With proper care by the owners, timely evaluations by the veterinarian, and good client-veterinarian communication, many diabetic dogs and cats can live relatively normal lives for several years.

In general, death shortly after diagnosing diabetes is usually due to severe ketoacidosis, concurrent illness (e.g., renal failure), or owner unwillingness to treat the disease. Death weeks to months after initiating therapy for diabetes is usually because of an inability to establish glycemic control with resultant persistence of clinical signs, development of chronic complications of diabetes (e.g., blindness due to cataracts), or from unrelated problems. Inability to establish glycemic control is usually due to problems with insulin therapy or insulin resistance caused by concurrent insulin antagonistic disorders. The latter may not be evident until weeks or months after diagnosing diabetes.

REFERENCES

1. Panciera DL, et al: Epizootiologic patterns of diabetes mellitus in cats: 333 cases (1980–1986). JAVMA 197:1504, 1990.
2. Kirk CA, et al: Diagnosis of naturally acquired type-I and type-II diabetes mellitus in cats. Am J Vet Res 54:463, 1993.
3. Eisenbarth GS. Type I diabetes mellitus: A chronic autoimmune disease. N Engl J Med 314:1360, 1986.
4. Palmer JP, McCulloch DK: Prediction and prevention of IDDM—1991. Diabetes 40:943, 1991.
5. Leahy JL: Natural history of B-cell dysfunction in NIDDM. Diabetes Care 13:992, 1990.
6. Reaven GM: Role of insulin resistance in human disease. Diabetes 37:1595, 1988.
7. O'Brien TD, et al: Immunohistochemical morphometry of pancreatic endocrine cells in diabetic, normoglycaemic glucose-intolerant and normal cats. J Comp Pathol 96:357, 1986.
8. Johnson KH, et al: Islet amyloid, islet amyloid polypeptide and diabetes mellitus. N Engl J Med 321:513, 1989.
9. Goossens M, et al: Response to insulin treatment and survival in 104 cats with diabetes mellitus (1985–1995). J Vet Intern Med 12:1, 1998.
10. Feldman EC, Nelson RW: Canine and Feline Endocrinology and Reproduction. Philadelphia, WB Saunders, 1987.
11. Haines DM, Penhale WJ: Autoantibodies to pancreatic islet cells in canine diabetes mellitus. Vet Immunol Immunopathol 8:149, 1985.
12. Hoenig M, Dawe DL: A qualitative assay for beta cell antibodies: Preliminary results in dogs with diabetes mellitus. Vet Immunol Immunopathol 32:195, 1992.
13. Alejandro R, et al: Advances in canine diabetes mellitus research: Etiopathology and results of islet transplantation. JAVMA 193:1050, 1988.
14. Nakayama H, et al: Pathological observations in six cases of feline diabetes mellitus. Jpn J Vet Sci 52:819, 1990.
15. Mattheeuws D, et al: Diabetes mellitus in dogs: Relationship of obesity to glucose tolerance and insulin response. Am J Vet Res 45:98, 1984.
16. Nelson RW, et al: Glucose tolerance and insulin response in normal weight and obese cats. Am J Vet Res 51:1357, 1990.
17. Truglia JA, et al: Insulin resistance: Receptor and post-binding defects in human obesity and non-insulin-dependent diabetes mellitus. Am J Med 979(Suppl 2B):13, 1985.
18. Biourge V, et al: Effect of weight gain and subsequent weight loss on glucose tolerance and insulin response in healthy cats. J Vet Intern Med 11:86, 1997.
19. Yano BL, et al: Feline insular amyloid: Incidence in adult cats with no clinicopathologic evidence of overt diabetes mellitus. Vet Pathol 18:310, 1981.
20. Yano BL, et al: Feline insular amyloid: Association with diabetes mellitus. Vet Pathol 18:621, 1981.
21. Westermark P, et al: Islet amyloid in type 2 human diabetes mellitus and adult diabetic cats is composed of a novel putative polypeptide hormone. Am J Pathol 127:414, 1987.
22. Westermark P, et al: Islet amyloid polypeptide-like immunoreactivity in the islet B cells of type 2 (noninsulin-dependent) diabetic and non-diabetic individuals. Diabetologia 30:887, 1987.
23. Johnson KH, et al: Immunolocalization of islet amyloid polypeptide (IAPP) in pancreatic beta cells using peroxidase antiperoxidase (PAP) and protein A-gold techniques. Am J Pathol 130:1, 1988.
24. Leighton B, Cooper GJS: Pancreatic amylin and calcitonin gene–related peptide cause resistance to insulin in skeletal muscle in vitro. Nature 335:632, 1988.
25. Molina J, et al: Induction of insulin resistance in vivo by amylin and calcitonin gene–related peptide. Diabetes 39:260, 1990.
26. Kassir AA, et al: Lack of effect of islet amyloid polypeptide in causing insulin resistance in conscious dogs during euglycemic clamp studies. Diabetes 40:998, 1991.
27. Atkins CE, Chin H: Insulin kinetics in juvenile canine diabetics after glucose loading. Am J Vet Res 44:596, 1983.
28. Montgomery TM, et al: Basal and glucagon-stimulated plasma C-peptide concentrations in healthy dogs, dogs with diabetes mellitus, and dogs with hyperadrenocorticism. J Vet Intern Med 10:116, 1996.
29. Nelson RW, et al: Transient clinical diabetes mellitus in cats: 10 cases (1989–1991). J Vet Intern Med 1998 (in press).
30. Robertson RP, et al: Differentiating glucose toxicity from glucose desensitization: A new message from the insulin gene. Diabetes 43:1085, 1994.
31. Anello M, et al: Fast reversibility of glucose-induced desensitization in rat pancreatic islets: Evidence for an involvement of ionic fluxes. Diabetes 45:502, 1996.
32. Robertson RP, et al: Preservation of insulin mRNA levels and insulin secretion in HIT cells by avoidance of chronic exposure to high glucose concentrations. J Clin Invest 90:320, 1992.
33. Olson LK, et al: Chronic exposure of HIT cells to high glucose concentrations paradoxically decreases insulin gene transcription and alters binding of insulin gene regulatory protein. J Clin Invest 92:514, 1993.
34. Olson LK, et al: Reduction in insulin gene transcription in HIT-T15 β cells chronically exposed to a supraphysiologic glucose concentration is associated with loss of STF-1 transcription factor expression. Proc Natl Acad Sci U S A 92:9127, 1995.
35. Nelson RW, et al: Effect of an orally administered sulfonylurea, glipizide, for treatment of diabetes mellitus in cats. JAVMA 203:821, 1993.
36. Ganong WF: Review of Medical Physiology, 15th ed. San Mateo, CA, Appleton & Lange, 1991.
37. Bruskiewicz KA, et al: Diabetic ketosis and ketoacidosis in cats: 42 cases (1980–1995). JAVMA 211:188, 1997.
38. DeFronzo RA, et al: Diabetic ketoacidosis: A combined metabolic-nephrologic approach to therapy. Diabetes Rev 2:209, 1994.
39. McGarry JD, et al: Regulation of ketogenesis and the renaissance of carnitine palmitoyltransferase. Diabetes Metab Rev 5:271, 1989.
40. Zammit VA: Regulation of ketone body metabolism: A cellular perspective. Diabetes Rev 2:132, 1994.

END

41. Groop LC, et al: Effect of insulin on oxidative and non-oxidative pathways of glucose and FFA metabolism in NIDDM: Evidence for multiple sites of insulin resistance. J Clin Invest 84:205, 1989.
42. Feldman EC, Nelson RW: Canine and Feline Endocrinology and Reproduction, 2nd ed. Philadelphia, WB Saunders, 1996.
43. Willard MD, et al: Severe hypophosphatemia associated with diabetes mellitus in six dogs and one cat. JAVMA 190:1007, 1987.
44. Nuttall FQ: Dietary fiber in the management of diabetes. Diabetes 42:503, 1993.
45. Nelson RW, et al: Effects of dietary fiber supplementation on glycemic control in dogs with alloxan-induced diabetes mellitus. Am J Vet Res 52:2060, 1991.
46. Nelson RW, et al: Effect of dietary insoluble fiber on control of glycemia in dogs with naturally acquired diabetes mellitus. JAVMA 212:380, 1998.
47. Nelson RW, et al: Dietary insoluble fiber and glycemic control of diabetic cats (abstract). J Vet Intern Med 8:165, 1994.
48. Robertson J, et al: Effect of α-glucosidase inhibitor acarbose in healthy and diabetic dogs (abstract). J Vet Intern Med 12:211, 1998.
49. Fernqvist E, et al: Effects of physical exercise on insulin absorption in insulin-dependent diabetics: A comparison between human and porcine insulin. Clin Physiol 6:489, 1986.
50. Ferrannini E, et al: Effects of bicycle exercise on insulin absorption and subcutaneous blood flow in normal subjects. Clin Physiol 2:59, 1982.
51. Miller AB, et al: Effect of glipizide on serum insulin and glucose concentrations in healthy cats. Res Vet Sci 52:177, 1992.
52. Feldman EC, et al: Intensive 50-week evaluation of glipizide administration in 50 cats with previously untreated diabetes mellitus. JAVMA 210:772, 1997.
53. Groop LC: Sulfonylureas in NIDDM. Diabetes Care 15:737, 1992.
54. Birkeland KI, et al: Long-term randomized placebo-controlled double-blind therapeutic comparison of glipizide and glyburide. Diabetes Care 17:45, 1994.
55. Klip A, Leiter LA: Cellular mechanism of action of metformin. Diabetes Care 13:696, 1990.
56. Bailey CJ: Metformin revisited: Its actions and indications for use. Diabet Med 5:315, 1988.
57. Gerich JE: Oral hypoglycemic agents. N Engl J Med 321:1231, 1989.
58. Brichard SM, et al: Long term improvement of glucose homeostasis by vanadate in obese hyperinsulinemic *fa/fa* rats. Endocrinology 125:2510, 1989.
59. Plotnick AN, et al: Oral vanadium compounds: Preliminary studies on toxicity in normal cats and hypoglycemic potential in diabetic cats (abstract). J Vet Intern Med 9:181, 1995.
60. Harb-Hauser M, et al: Prevalence of insulin antibodies in diabetic dogs (abstract). J Vet Intern Med 12:213, 1998.
61. Harb-Hauser M, et al: Prevalence of insulin antibodies in diabetic cats (abstract). J Vet Intern Med 12:245, 1998.
62. Hasegawa S, et al: Glycated hemoglobin fractions in normal and diabetic dogs measured by high performance liquid chromatography. J Vet Med Sci 53:65, 1991.
63. Hasegawa S, et al: Glycated hemoglobin fractions in normal and diabetic cats measured by high performance liquid chromatography. J Vet Med Sci 54:789, 1992.
64. Kawamoto M, et al: Relation of fructosamine to serum protein, albumin, and glucose concentrations in healthy and diabetic dogs. Am J Vet Res 53:851, 1992.
65. Elliott DA, et al: Glycosylated hemoglobin concentration for assessment of glycemic control in diabetic cats. J Vet Intern Med 11:161, 1997.
66. Elliott DA, et al: Glycosylated hemoglobin concentrations in the blood of healthy dogs and dogs with naturally developing diabetes mellitus, pancreatic β-cell neoplasia, hyperadrenocorticism, and anemia. JAVMA 211:723, 1997.
67. Crenshaw KL, et al: Serum fructosamine concentration as an index of glycemia in cats with diabetes mellitus and stress hyperglycemia. J Vet Intern Med 10:360, 1996.
68. Duesberg C, et al: Impaired counterregulatory response to insulin-induced hypoglycemia in diabetic dogs (abstract). J Vet Intern Med 9:181, 1995.
69. Feldman EC, Nelson RW: Insulin-induced hyperglycemia in diabetic dogs. JAVMA 180:1432, 1982.
70. Hallden G, et al: Characterization of cat insulin. Arch Biochem Biophys 247:20, 1986.
71. Bolli GB, et al: Abnormal glucose counterregulation after subcutaneous insulin in insulin-dependent diabetes mellitus. N Engl J Med 310:1706, 1984.
72. Engerman RL, Kern TS: Progression of incipient diabetic retinopathy during good glycemic control. Diabetes 36:808, 1987.
73. Herrtage ME, et al: Diabetic retinopathy in a cat with megestrol acetate–induced diabetes. J Small Anim Pract 26:595, 1985.
74. Ono K, et al: Fluorescein angiogram in diabetic dogs. Jpn J Vet Sci 48:1257, 1986.
75. Unger RH, Foster DW: Diabetes mellitus. In Wilson JD, Foster DW (eds): Williams Textbook of Endocrinology, 8th ed. Philadelphia, WB Saunders, 1992, p 1255.
76. Engerman RL, Kern TS: Aldose reductase inhibition fails to prevent retinopathy in diabetic and galactosemic dogs. Diabetes 42:820, 1993.
77. Braund KG, Steiss JE: Distal neuropathy in spontaneous diabetes mellitus in the dog. Acta Neuropathol (Berl) 57:263, 1982.
78. Katherman AE, Braund KG: Polyneuropathy associated with diabetes mellitus in a dog. JAVMA 182:522, 1983.
79. Johnson CA, et al: Peripheral neuropathy and hypotension in a diabetic dog. JAVMA 183:1007, 1983.
80. Steiss JE, et al: Electrodiagnostic analysis of peripheral neuropathy in dogs with diabetes mellitus. Am J Vet Res 42:2061, 1981.
81. Greene DA: Pathogenesis and prevention of diabetic neuropathy. Diabetes Metab Rev 4:201, 1988.
82. Winegrad AI: Banting lecture 1986: Does a common mechanism induce the diverse complications of diabetes? Diabetes 36:396, 1987.
83. Kennedy WR, et al: Effects of pancreatic transplantation on diabetic neuropathy. N Engl J Med 322:1031, 1990.
84. Jeraj K, et al: Immunofluoresence studies of renal basement membranes in dogs with spontaneous diabetes. Am J Vet Res 45:1162, 1984.
85. Steffes MW, et al: Diabetic nephropathy in the uninephrectomized dog: Microscopic lesions after one year. Kidney Int 21:721, 1982.
86. Clark CM, Lee DA: Prevention and treatment of the complications of diabetes mellitus. N Engl J Med 332:1210, 1995.
87. Nyberg G, et al: Impact of metabolic control in progression of clinical diabetic nephropathy. Diabetologia 30:82, 1987.
88. Wiseman MJ, et al: Effect of blood glucose control on increased glomerular filtration rate and kidney size in insulin-dependent diabetes. N Engl J Med 312:617, 1985.
89. Graham PA, Nash AS: Survival data analysis applied to canine diabetes mellitus (abstract). J Vet Intern Med 11:142, 1997.

CHAPTER 154

HYPERADRENOCORTICISM

Edward C. Feldman

CANINE CUSHING'S SYNDROME

In 1932 Dr. Harvey Cushing described 12 humans with a disorder that he suggested was "the result of pituitary-basophilism." Careful study of these and other individuals diagnosed years ago suggests that there are multiple causes of this syndrome, with chronic excesses in serum cortisol concentration representing the final common denominator in all the illnesses. The eponym Cushing's syndrome is an umbrella term referring to the constellation of clinical and chemical abnormalities resulting from chronic exposure to excessive concentrations of glucocorticoids. A pathophysiologic classification of causes of canine Cushing's syndrome include a pituitary tumor synthesizing and secreting excess adrenocorticotropic hormone (ACTH) with secondary adrenocortical hyperplasia (pituitary-dependent hyperadrenocorticism [PDH]); pituitary hyperplasia and, secondarily, adrenocortical hyperplasia caused by excesses in corticotropin-releasing hormone (CRH) secretion due to a hypothalamic disorder (also PDH); primary excesses in adrenal cortisol, autonomously secreted by an adrenocortical carcinoma or adenoma; and iatrogenic causes of excessive ACTH administration (rare) or excessive glucocorticoid medication (common). A tumor outside the hypothalamus or pituitary producing excessive ACTH has been described in humans but not in dogs or cats.

REGULATION OF GLUCOCORTICOID SECRETION

The hypothalamus controls secretion of ACTH by the anterior pituitary via CRH, a polypeptide containing 41 amino acid residues. ACTH, in turn, exerts control over adrenocortical secretion of cortisol. ACTH is a 39–amino acid peptide hormone (molecular weight 4500) processed from a large precursor molecule, proopiomelanocortin (molecular weight 28,500). Cortisol, in part, completes the circle by affecting the control exerted by hypothalamic and pituitary hormones.

The major hormones secreted by the adrenal cortex are cortisol and aldosterone. Histologically, the adrenal cortex is composed of three zones. The outer *zona glomerulosa* produces aldosterone and is deficient in 17α-hydroxylase activity, rendering this zone incapable of synthesizing cortisol or androgens. Glomerulosa cells have the ability to dehydrogenate 18-hydroxycorticosterone, allowing the synthesis of aldosterone. Aldosterone secretion is regulated primarily by renin, angiotensin, and serum potassium concentrations. The middle *zona fasciculata* is the thickest of the three adrenocortical layers. This zone, together with the narrow, inner *zona reticularis,* produces cortisol and a minor amount of androgens. Cells within these two layers of the adrenal cortex have 17α-hydroxylase activity and can synthesize 17α-hydroxypregnenolone and 17α-hydroxyprogesterone, precursors of cortisol. These zones are regulated primarily by ACTH, which acts to stimulate conversion of cholesterol to pregnenolone, the rate-limiting step in adrenal steroidogenesis.[1]

PATHOPHYSIOLOGY

Pituitary-Dependent Hyperadrenocorticism

Pituitary Control and Feedback. In normal individuals (human beings and animals), ACTH secretion appears random and episodic. This appearance is misleading, however, because ACTH functions exquisitely in maintaining plasma cortisol concentrations at levels required for homeostasis. The most common abnormality in PDH is that the frequency and amplitude of ACTH secretory "bursts" are chronically excessive. Chronic excesses in ACTH secretion result in excess cortisol secretion and, eventually, adrenocortical hyperplasia. The excessive secretion of cortisol is not readily appreciated by assaying a basal cortisol concentration. Most dogs and cats with hyperadrenocorticism have plasma cortisol concentrations within the normal range at any given moment. These animals, however, are exposed to more cortisol on a total daily basis than normal.

Pars Distalis Versus Pars Intermedia. The pathogenesis of PDH in dogs is complicated because this species has a pars distalis and a discrete pars intermedia. Further, the pars intermedia has been demonstrated to have two distinct cell types.[2] The predominant cells (A cells) immunostain intensely for α-MSH (melanocyte-stimulating hormone) but only weakly for ACTH. The second population of pars intermedia cells (B cells) stains strongly for ACTH and only weakly for α-MSH. The intense ACTH staining of pars intermedia B cells is similar to the staining characteristics of ACTH-producing pars distalis cells.[3] Pars distalis proopiomelanocortin and, therefore, ACTH secretion are regulated primarily by the interaction of the stimulatory hypothalamic peptides (CRH) and the inhibitory adrenocortical glucocorticoids. The pars intermedia, however, is under negative regulation by dopamine, secreted from the arcuate nucleus, as well as by serotonin and CRH. Dogs with PDH may have an adenoma of the pars distalis, an A cell pars intermedia adenoma, or a B cell pars intermedia adenoma. A small percentage of dogs with PDH has been diagnosed with pituitary hyperplasia, and there are also individuals with functional pituitary carcinomas. Even more confusing are individual dogs with two pituitary adenomas, each tumor apparently arising from a different pituitary lobe, and those with both a tumor and hyperplasia of the pituitary. As is quickly appreciated, pituitary hyperadrenocorticism is a syndrome with the potential for multiple etiologies.[4] The final common pathway for these disorders remains similar, however. There is chronic systemic cortisol excess due to adrenocortical hyperplasia resulting from chronic and excessive secretion of pituitary ACTH. We have not been able to distinguish these etiologies antemortem.[5] It is safe to propose that PDH may result from several different physiopathogenic mechanisms, but a hypothalamic etiology has not yet received strong scientific support.

Effect of Glucocorticoid Excess on Pituitary Function. In addition to the systemic effects of excess glucocorticoids, they inhibit other pituitary and hypothalamic functions, including thyrotropin (TSH), growth hormone (GH), and gonadotropin (luteinizing hormone [LH] and follicle-stimulating hormone [FSH]) release. Inhibition of the secretion of these trophic hormones results in reversible secondary hypothyroidism (TSH), failure to cycle in females or testicular atrophy in males (FSH and LH), and short stature in growing puppies (GH).

Adrenal Tumors

In approximately 15 per cent of dogs with naturally occurring Cushing's syndrome, primary adrenocortical tumors, both adenomas and carcinomas, develop autonomously and secrete excessive quantities of cortisol independent of pituitary control. Thus, the steroid products of these tumors suppress hypothalamic CRH and circulating plasma ACTH concentrations. The result of this chronic negative feedback is cortical atrophy of the uninvolved adrenal and atrophy of all normal cells in the involved adrenal (Fig. 154–1). Virtually all these tumors respond to exogenous ACTH, but they are unresponsive to dexamethasone. There have been no consistent features that aid in distinguishing dogs or cats with functioning adrenal adenomas from those with adrenal carcinomas.[6] Rarely, dogs with bilateral functioning adrenocortical tumors have been diagnosed.[7] We have also diagnosed dogs with pheochromocytoma in one adrenal and adrenocortical tumor in the contralateral gland. This can be confusing, because ultrasonography may reveal bilateral adrenomegaly, and endocrine testing suggests adrenocortical tumor.

Ectopic ACTH Syndrome

This syndrome has not been diagnosed in dogs or cats.

Adrenocortical Nodular Hyperplasia

Macronodular hyperplasia of the adrenals (grossly enlarged with multiple nodules) occurs in about 20 per cent of

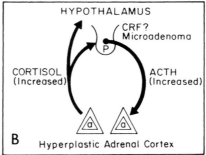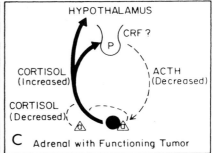

Figure 154–1. The pituitary-adrenal axis in normal dogs *(A)*, in dogs with pituitary-dependent hyperadrenocorticism *(B)*, and in dogs with functioning adrenocortical tumor *(C)*. a = adrenal; P = pituitary; CRF = corticotropin-releasing factor.

people with adrenocortical hyperplasia. Some of these people are thought to have autonomous (ACTH-independent) cortisol-secreting adrenals. Approximately 5 to 10 per cent of dogs and cats with PDH have bilateral adrenal nodular hyperplasia.

PATHOLOGY

The Pituitary

Microadenomas. Approximately 40 to 45 per cent of dogs with PDH have pituitary tumors less than 3 mm in diameter at the time of diagnosis. This means that the mass would not be visible with computed tomography (CT) or magnetic resonance imaging (MRI) scans. At the time of diagnosis, a majority (55 to 60 per cent) of PDH dogs without central nervous system (CNS) signs had tumors 3 to 12 mm in diameter.[8] Most ACTH-secreting pituitary tumors are defined as microadenomas because they are less than 1 cm in diameter. They are not usually encapsulated but may be surrounded by a rim of compressed normal pituitary cells. With routine histologic stains, these tumors are typically found to be composed of compact sheets of well-granulated basophilic cells in a sinusoidal arrangement. ACTH-secreting adenomas show Crooke's changes (a zone of perinuclear hyalinization that results from chronic exposure of corticotroph cells to hypercortisolism).

Macroadenomas. A significant percentage of dogs with PDH (15 to 20 per cent) develop large (>1 cm) pituitary tumors.[9] Most dogs with macro tumors are diagnosed 4 to 36 months after treatment for PDH has started. These tumors have the potential of compressing or invading adjacent structures as they expand dorsally from the sella turcica into the hypothalamus, often causing signs. Because the canine sella turcica is shaped like a saucer rather than like a cup (as in human beings), destruction of the bone making up the walls of the sella has not been observed. Such tumors may appear chromophobic on routine histology, but they typically contain ACTH and its related peptides. Malignant pituitary tumors occur but are uncommon.

Pituitary Hyperplasia. Diffuse hyperplasia of corticotroph cells has been reported in a small percentage of dogs with PDH. Most dogs with pituitary hyperplasia also have pituitary tumors. The experience in humans is no different. With surgical removal of the tumor in afflicted people, signs of hyperadrenocorticism typically resolve, negating the significance of histologically observed hyperplasia.[10]

Adrenocortical Hyperplasia

The histologic observation of typical bilateral hyperplasia usually occurs secondary to PDH. Combined adrenal weight is usually modestly increased. Histologically, there is equal hyperplasia of the compact cells of the zona reticularis and the clear cells of the zona fasciculata; the width of the cortex is increased.

Adrenal Tumors

Endocrine tissue often presents diagnostic challenges to pathologists. Pathologists may have difficulty distinguishing between normal and hyperplasia, hyperplasia and adenoma, and some adenomas and carcinomas. It can also be challenging to distinguish an adrenocortical tumor from an adrenal medullary tumor (pheochromocytoma).

Adenomas. Adrenal adenomas are encapsulated and grossly visible and usually range in size from 1 to 6 cm. They are usually three fourths the size of a normal kidney or smaller. Microscopically, clear cells of the zona fasciculata type predominate, although cells typical of the zona reticularis may also be seen. Approximately 50 per cent of adrenocortical adenomas are partially calcified.[6]

Carcinomas. Adrenal carcinomas tend to be larger than half the size of a normal kidney and are often equal in size or larger than a normal kidney. Grossly, they may not be encapsulated; vascularity, necrosis, hemorrhage, and cystic degeneration are common. Partial calcification is identified in approximately 50 per cent of carcinomas.[6] The histologic appearance of adrenocortical carcinomas varies considerably; they may appear to be benign or may exhibit considerable pleomorphism. Vascular or capsular invasion is predictive of malignant behavior, as is local extension. Adrenocortical carcinomas can invade local structures (kidney, liver, vena cava, aorta, and retroperitoneum) and metastasize hematogenously to liver and lung.

SIGNALMENT

Age and Sex

Dogs with PDH are usually older than 6 years of age, more than 75 per cent are older than 9, and their median age is 11 years.[6] We have seen only four dogs with Cushing's syndrome younger than 2 years of age at the time of diagnosis. Dogs with hyperadrenocorticism caused by functioning adrenocortical tumors tend to be older than those with pituitary-dependent disease. Most of these dogs, at the time of diagnosis, are 6 to 16 years of age, with a median age of 11.3 years. Fifty-five to 60 per cent of dogs with Cushing's syndrome are female.[6]

Breed and Body Weight

Pituitary-Dependent Hyperadrenocorticism. Poodles (various poodle breeds), Dachshunds, various terrier breeds, beagles, and German shepherd dogs were most commonly represented among the huge number of breeds and mixed breeds afflicted with PDH. Approximately 75 per cent of the dogs with PDH weigh less than 20 kg.[6]

Adrenocortical Tumor. Toy poodles (and other poodle breeds), German shepherd dogs, dachshunds, Laborador retrievers, and various terrier breeds were most commonly represented among dogs with functioning adrenocortical tumors. Forty-five to 50 per cent of these dogs are larger than 20 kg in body weight.

HISTORY

Most dogs with Cushing's have signs that slowly progress and are not alarming to owners. Dogs with this syndrome are rarely believed to be critically or even seriously ill. For example, these dogs rarely have anorexia, weight loss, vomiting, diarrhea, pain, seizures, or bleeding. Therefore, it is likely that most dogs with Cushing's will have obvious clinical signs by the time an owner realizes that a problem exists.

Adult-Onset Hyperadrenocorticism. Chronic exposure to excess cortisol often results in development of a classic combination of dramatic clinical signs and lesions (Table 154–1). These signs are insidious in onset and progressive. They include polydipsia, polyuria, polyphagia, abdominal enlargement (or obesity), alopecia (sparing the head and distal extremities), thin haircoat, failure to regrow shaved hair, pyoderma, panting, muscle weakness, and lethargy. Less common signs include heat intolerance, seborrhea, comedones, bruising, calcinosis cutis, skin hyperpigmentation, testicular atrophy, failure to cycle in females, facial paralysis, and a rare muscle stiffness condition called myotonia. It must be remembered that not all dogs with hyperadrenocorticism develop the same signs. From this list of potential signs, most dogs exhibit several (but not all) of these problems. Hyperadrenocorticism is a clinical disorder, and animals with this disease have some clinical signs. The signs are the sequelae of the combined gluconeogenic, immune-suppressive, anti-inflammatory, protein catabolic,

TABLE 154–1. INITIAL HISTORY FOR DOGS WITH HYPERADRENOCORTICISM

Polydipsia/polyuria
Polyphagia
Abdominal enlargement
Decreased exercise tolerance (muscle weakness)
Increased respiratory rate or panting
Lethargy
Obesity
Alopecia (sparing head and distal extremities)
Calcinosis cutis
Anestrus
Testicular atrophy
Heat intolerance
Acne (skin infection, comedones)
Cutaneous hyperpigmentation

TABLE 154–2. PHYSICAL EXAMINATION FINDINGS IN DOGS WITH HYPERADRENOCORTICISM

Thin skin	Muscle wasting of extremities
Bilaterally symmetric alopecia	Hepatomegaly
Acne (skin infection, comedones)	Panting
Cutaneous hyperpigmentation	Bruising
Calcinosis cutis	Testicular atrophy
Abdominal enlargement	Clitoral hypertrophy

and lipolytic effects of glucocorticoids on various organ systems.

Because these changes are quite gradual in onset and are often believed by the client to be a result of simple aging, it is only when the signs become intolerable or severe that veterinary advice is sought. Alternatively, abnormalities may be pointed out by people who see the pet infrequently (objectively noting changes that have developed so slowly that the owners do not observe them). Some owners have reported a rapid onset of signs and progression of illness. This is more likely the result of an owner not noticing earlier changes rather than the signs truly being acute in onset. The duration of clinical signs and the type of signs noticed have not been reliable aids in distinguishing pituitary-dependent from adrenal-dependent hyperadrenocorticism.

Hyperadrenocorticism in Young Dogs. Cushing's syndrome is most commonly diagnosed in dogs that are 6 to 8 years of age and older, with the mean age at the time of diagnosis older than 10 years. We have diagnosed only a few dogs with hyperadrenocorticism during the first 6 to 9 *months* of life. As in children and adolescents, the signs in these young dogs are usually weight gain and growth retardation. The dogs also had other more typical signs (polyuria, polydipsia, alopecia).

PHYSICAL EXAMINATION

It should first be noted that the physical examination of a typical Cushing's dog reveals an animal that is stable and hydrated, has good mucous membrane color, and is not in distress. Veterinarians typically observe many of the signs seen by owners. Among these abnormalities are abdominal enlargement, increased panting, truncal obesity, bilaterally symmetric alopecia, skin infections, and comedones (hair follicles filled with keratin and debris, usually black in color and easily expressed). Hyperpigmentation, testicular atrophy, and hepatomegaly are common. Ectopic calcification, clitoral hypertrophy, and easy bruisability are much less common (Table 154–2). There is, however, a remarkable variation in the number and severity of these signs. These dogs may have a single dominant sign or 10 signs (Figs. 154–2 and 154–3).

An enlarged liver is typical of hyperadrenocorticism, contributing to the abdominal enlargement previously discussed. The liver is typically swollen, large, pale, and friable. Hepatomegaly is easily palpated because of the weak abdominal muscles. The liver may be so large in some dogs that the veterinarian may become suspicious of a large abdominal tumor or ascites.

The negative feedback effects of hypercortisolism result in decreased pituitary gonadotropin secretion, causing testicular atrophy, decreased libido, and depressed plasma testosterone concentrations in male dogs. In females, the negative feedback effects of hypercortisolism result in prolonged anestrus and, in a small number of dogs, clitoral hypertrophy.

Sudden acquired retinal degeneration syndrome (SARDS)

END

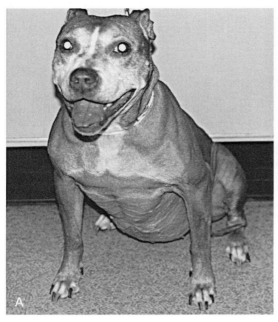

Figure 154–2. Poodle with pituitary-dependent hyperadrenocorticism, illustrating the potbellied appearance and diffuse alopecia sparing the head and distal extremities. (From Feldman EC, Nelson RW: Canine and Feline Endocrinology and Reproduction, 2nd ed. Philadelphia, WB Saunders, 1996, p 199.)

is a disorder of unknown etiology that causes sudden and permanent blindness in adult dogs. The syndrome is characterized by noninflammatory degeneration and loss of retinal photoreceptors. An association has been suggested between SARDS and hyperadrenocorticism.[11] Strong evidence has yet to be presented that confirms the presence of hyperadrenocorticism in a significant number of dogs with SARDS.

IN-HOSPITAL EVALUATION

General Approach

Any dog or cat suspected of having hyperadrenocorticism should be thoroughly evaluated before specific endocrine procedures are undertaken. These initial tests should include clinicopathologic studies (complete blood count [CBC]; urinalysis with culture; and a serum chemistry profile including liver enzymes, renal function tests, calcium, phosphorus, sodium, potassium, cholesterol, blood glucose, total plasma protein, plasma albumin, and total bilirubin). In addition to

blood and urine testing, abdominal ultrasonography (preferred over radiography) should be completed in these dogs and cats.

Routine Database

Finding a large percentage of abnormalities on initial screening tests that are consistent with hyperadrenocorticism allows the veterinarian to establish a presumptive diagnosis (Table 154–3). More expensive and sophisticated studies to confirm a diagnosis and localize the cause of the syndrome can then be recommended to the client. The initial results not only ensure that the veterinarian is pursuing the correct diagnosis but also can alert the clinician to any concomitant medical problems. These problems may be common for hyperadrenocorticism (urinary tract infection) or unexpected (congestive heart failure), but in either case they should not be ignored.

Excessive production of cortisol results in neutrophilia and monocytosis due to steroid-enhanced capillary demargination of these cells and the subsequent prevention of normal egress of cells from the circulation. Lymphopenia is most likely the result of steroid lympholysis, and eosinopenia results from bone marrow sequestration. These changes in the white blood cell differential are termed a stress response. Approximately 80 per cent of hyperadrenal dogs have reduced lymphocyte and eosinophil counts, and 20 to 25 per cent have increased total white blood cell numbers. The red blood cell count is usually normal, although mild polycythemia may occasionally be noted, especially in females.

Dogs and cats with hyperadrenocorticism occasionally have mild increases in fasting plasma glucose concentrations and, less commonly, overt diabetes mellitus. Polyuria is common and probably due to a reversible form of central diabetes insipidus in most dogs. One differential diagnosis for polyuria and polydipsia in any older dog would be renal insufficiency. Because a large percentage of Cushing's dogs have normal to *decreased* blood urea nitrogen and creatinine concentrations, this concern can be quickly dismissed. The alanine aminotransferase (ALT) activity is usually mildly increased (<400 IU/L) secondary to liver damage caused by

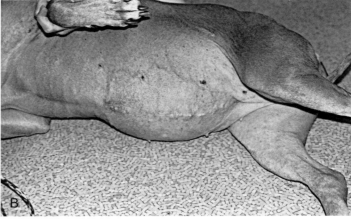

Figure 154–3. *A,* Ten-year-old dog with pituitary-dependent hyperadrenocorticism. *B,* Same dog as in *A;* note the potbellied appearance and thin skin.

TABLE 154–3. HEMATOLOGIC, SERUM BIOCHEMICAL, URINE, AND RADIOGRAPHIC ABNORMALITIES TYPICAL OF HYPERADRENOCORTICISM

TEST	ABNORMALITY*
Complete blood count	Mature leukocytosis Neutrophilia Lymphopenia Eosinopenia Erythrocytosis; mild (females)
Serum chemistries	Increased alkaline phosphatase (sometimes extremely elevated) Increased ALT (SGPT) Increased cholesterol Increased fasting blood glucose Increased or normal insulin Abnormal bile acids Decreased BUN Lipemia
Urinalysis	Urine specific gravity <1.015, often <1.008 Urinary tract infection Glycosuria (<10% of cases)
Radiography/ ultrasonography	Hepatomegaly Excellent abdominal contrast Potbelly Distended bladder Osteoporosis Calcinosis cutis/dystrophic calcification Adrenal calcification (usually adrenal tumor) Congestive heart failure (rare) Pulmonary thromboembolism (rare) Calcified trachea and main stem bronchi Pulmonary metastasis of adrenal carcinoma
Miscellaneous	Low T_4/T_3 concentrations Response to TSH that parallels normal, but both pre and post values may be decreased Hypertension

*It would be unusual for an individual animal to have all these abnormalities.
ALT = alanine aminotransferase; SGPT = serum glutamate pyruvate transaminase; BUN = blood urea nitrogen; T_4 = thyroxine; T_3 = triiodothyronine; TSH = thyroid-stimulating hormone.

swollen hepatocytes, glycogen accumulation, or interference with hepatic blood flow. Hepatocellular necrosis, a minor but significant feature of "steroid hepatopathy," is seen with enough frequency to account for mild increases in serum ALT.[12]

An increase in the serum alkaline phosphatase (SAP) activity is the most common routine laboratory abnormality in canine hyperadrenocorticism.[13] Approximately 85 per cent of hyperadrenal dogs have SAP activities that exceed 150 IU/L, and values in excess of 1000 IU/L are common. There is no correlation between SAP concentration and severity of Cushing's syndrome, response to therapy, or prognosis. Glucocorticoid stimulation of lipolysis causes an increase in blood lipid and cholesterol concentrations. Approximately 10 per cent of Cushing's dogs have serum cholesterol concentrations less than 250 mg/dL (normal), 15 per cent have concentrations of 250 to 300 mg/dL; and 75 per cent have values greater than 300 mg/dL. Lipemia (i.e., hypertriglyceridemia) is at least as frequent. Although of little diagnostic or clinical significance, mild abnormalities in the serum sodium (increased) and potassium (decreased) concentrations are seen in a small percentage of dogs with Cushing's. Assessment of serum electrolyte concentrations becomes extremely important if a dog with hyperadrenocorticism develops anorexia, vomiting, or diarrhea, because exaggeration of mild abnormalities in the serum electrolyte concentrations may become life-threatening.

Pancreatitis is uncommon in dogs with Cushing's syndrome. If pancreatitis occurs, it is likely secondary to lipemia or to the fact that these dogs are polyphagic and may eat garbage or large quantities of fat. In these instances, serum lipase and amylase concentrations may be increased. Serum lipase and amylase concentrations are not routinely measured, and measurement is not recommended unless signs of pancreatitis are present.

Bile acid test results in dogs with hyperadrenocorticism are usually within normal limits. Other liver function test results have been shown to be frequently abnormal in dogs with Cushing's. The liver pathology causing the abnormal test results is usually mild and reversible with successful treatment of Cushing's. Liver function test results do not aid in separating dogs with primary liver disorders from dogs with hyperadrenocorticism.

Urinalysis

The urinalysis is one of the most important initial studies in the evaluation of any animal with a history of urinary frequency or polydipsia and/or polyuria. It is strongly recommended that owners obtain a urine sample by clean-catch before bringing the pet to the hospital or that a urine sample be collected at the time of initial examination. The most frequent abnormality is the finding of dilute urine (specific gravity <1.015–1.020), which is documented in 85 per cent of dogs. Others have found dilute urine in a smaller percentage of dogs, perhaps because samples were obtained after they had been hospitalized for a number of hours. Dogs with Cushing's syndrome may not consume large quantities of water in a frightening environment (veterinary hospital). Some dogs with specific gravities at home that are consistently less than 1.007 consume much less water in the hospital, with specific gravities then reaching 1.025 to 1.035. It may therefore be unreliable to measure water intake in the hospital, and this practice is not encouraged.

In addition to determining specific gravity, the veterinarian should assess urine for glucose. Such a finding has been noted in 5 to 10 per cent of dogs and indicates that overt diabetes mellitus is present. Diabetes mellitus requires therapy regardless of whether the dog has hyperadrenocorticism. A large majority of Cushing's dogs have proteinuria. This proteinuria does not usually cause hypoproteinemia or hypoalbuminemia, but it may be associated with hypertension.

The previously mentioned outpatient urinalysis is used to check the specific gravity and for urine cortisol-creatinine ratio (see later section). Because urinary tract infection is a common sequela to Cushing's, urine for culture should also be obtained by cystocentesis. Approximately 40 to 50 per cent of dogs with Cushing's have a urinary tract infection at the time of initial examination. There are several potential explanations for this worrisome incidence of infection. Glucocorticoid excess results in immune suppression. Urine retention is common among dogs with severe polyuria and muscle weakness, predisposing them to infection. It has also been demonstrated that dilute urine increases susceptibility to lower urinary tract infection.[14]

Hypertension and Glomerulopathies

More than 50 per cent of dogs with Cushing's syndrome are hypertensive on random testing of blood pressure. Normal dogs have systolic, diastolic, and mean arterial blood pressures of approximately 150, 90, and 105 mmHg, respectively. Dogs with Cushing's had mean blood pressures of

162, 116, and 135 mmHg, respectively.[15] Multiple factors have been implicated in the development of hypertension, including excessive secretion of renin, enhanced vascular sensitivity to catecholamines and adrenergic agonists, reduction of vasodilator prostaglandins, and increased secretion of non–zona glomerulosa mineralocorticoids. Hypertension tends to resolve following successful management of the Cushing's.

Hypertension-induced blindness may be due to intraocular hemorrhage and/or retinal detachment.[16] Hypertension may exacerbate left ventricular hypertrophy or congestive heart failure. It may also cause glomerulopathies, which may lead to renal protein loss. Seventy-five per cent of dogs with Cushing's syndrome have urine protein-creatinine ratios greater than 1.0, with a mean of 2.3 (normal is <1.0).[15] Specifically, proteins important in coagulation (e.g., antithrombin III) may be lost, which could predispose the Cushing's patient to thromboembolism. Although direct arterial blood pressure measurements are the most reliable and are relatively easy to obtain, the equipment for indirect monitoring is becoming more reliable and more widely utilized.

Thyroid Function Tests

Thyroid function testing of dogs with hyperadrenocorticism is important because of the overlap in some clinical signs of hypothyroidism and Cushing's (e.g., listlessness, bilateral symmetric nonpruritic alopecia, apparent weight gain, hypercholesterolemia). Chronic hypercortisolism (iatrogenic or naturally occurring) suppresses pituitary secretion of TSH, leading to secondary hypothyroidism.[17] Hypercortisolism may also alter thyroid hormone binding to plasma proteins, enhance the metabolism of thyroid hormone, and decrease peripheral deiodination of thyroxine (T_4) to triiodothyronine (T_3). Approximately 70 per cent of dogs with naturally occurring hyperadrenocorticism have decreases in basal serum T_4 and/or T_3 concentrations.

Radiographs

Radiographs of the chest and the abdomen, if abdominal ultrasonography is not available, should be examined in dogs with suspected or proven Cushing's syndrome. In addition to looking for changes consistent with the diagnosis, the veterinarian should remember that these dogs are usually older and that they may have other serious concurrent (perhaps subclinical) diseases.

Abdominal Radiographs. Good contrast owing to abdominal fat deposition is usually observed in dogs and cats with Cushing's. Eighty to 90 per cent of dogs with Cushing's have mild to severe hepatomegaly. There is no obvious association between the duration of illness and the degree of hepatomegaly.[18] Distention of the urinary bladder may be seen radiographically, because many of these dogs are not capable of voiding completely. Perhaps the most important but least common finding on abdominal radiographs is visualization of an adrenal mass. Positive identification of such a mass occurs infrequently, because only 10 to 20 per cent of dogs with Cushing's syndrome have an adrenocortical tumor, and only approximately 50 per cent of these tumors are calcified, allowing them to be visualized radiographically. Approximately 50 per cent of both adenomas and carcinomas are calcified.[6]

Thoracic Radiographs. Thoracic radiographs should be evaluated for evidence of pulmonary metastases of an adrenocortical carcinoma. Because dogs with Cushing's syndrome are immune suppressed, evaluation of the pulmonary parenchyma for infection is important, and because the dogs are geriatric, the thoracic radiographs can be evaluated for other problems. Calcification of tracheal rings and osteoporosis (most obvious in the spine), although occasionally observed, are nonspecific abnormalities.

Ultrasonography

The ability to visualize normal adrenal glands in almost all dogs and cats has progressively improved over the last 10 years owing to the experience gained by radiologists as well as improvements in equipment. Perhaps more than any other tool, the value of ultrasonography directly correlates with the skill of the operator. Transverse, longitudinal, and oblique scanning from the ventral abdomen must be performed to thoroughly evaluate the adrenals.[19] We currently visualize almost all normal dog and cat adrenals, the limiting factors being interference by intestinal gas and willingness of the animal to lie still for several minutes. Normal maximum length and width of the left adrenal are 33 and 7.5 mm, respectively; 31 and 7 mm represent normal maximum length and width of the right adrenal.[20]

In dogs and cats suspected of having Cushing's, abdominal ultrasonography serves three major functions. First, it is part of the routine database used to evaluate the abdomen for any unexpected abnormalities (e.g., urinary calculi, masses, cysts). Second, if an adrenal tumor is identified, ultrasonography is an excellent screening test for hepatic or other organ metastasis, tumor invasion of the vena cava or other structures, and compression of adjacent tissues by a tumor. Third, the study is used to evaluate the size and shape of the adrenals. If both adrenals are visualized and are relatively equal in size—normal size or large—in a dog or cat otherwise diagnosed as having Cushing's, this is considered strong evidence in favor of adrenal hyperplasia due to pituitary-dependent disease (Table 154–4). A unilateral abnormally enlarged and shaped adrenal mass with an abnormally small or nonvisible contralateral adrenal is evidence of an adrenocortical tumor. Adrenal size is best determined using the width of the left adrenal. This parameter had a sensitivity of 81 per cent and a specificity of 100 per cent in detecting adrenal enlargement in dogs with hyperadrenocorticism.[20] However, adrenal ultrasonography should never be used as a diagnostic test for Cushing's syndrome; rather, it is a tool to aid in discriminating PDH from adrenocortical tumor (Fig. 154–4).

If a dog or cat with an adrenal mass has no historical, physical examination, or routine clinicopathologic findings suggestive of Cushing's, endocrine evaluation is not recommended. When Cushing's is not suspected, decisions need to be made regarding an identified mass and whether it should be evaluated and/or removed. Some adrenal masses are normal tissue. Other differential diagnoses include adrenal cyst, myelolipoma, hemorrhage, nonfunctioning (non-hormone-producing) primary tumor, pheochromocytoma, metastatic tumor, and granuloma.

SPECIFIC EVALUATION OF THE PITUITARY-ADRENOCORTICAL AXIS

Endocrine Testing

Generally, the evaluation of an animal suspected of having hyperadrenocorticism proceeds through three basic steps

TABLE 154–4. COMPARISON OF SIGNALMENT AND ADRENAL GLAND SIZE BY ABDOMINAL ULTRASONOGRAPHY

VARIABLE	HEALTHY DOGS (N = 20)			DOGS WITH NONENDOCRINE DISEASE (N = 20)			DOGS WITH PDH (N = 22)		
	Mean	Range	SD	Mean	Range	SD	Mean	Range	SD
Age (years)	5.2	0.6–13.2	4.1	11.7	7.6–15.4	2.4	10.2	7–13.3	1.6
Weight (kg)	19.6	4.4–38.8	9	18	2.4–40	9.8	17.3	3.8–43	13
Aortic diameter (mm)	9.3	6.1–12.4	1.8	9	4.9–12.4	2.1	8.9	5.2–13	2.3
Kidney length (mm)	58.5	36.8–80.5	12	57.7	26.8–76.7	11	58.1	37.5–82.7	12.5
Left adrenal gland									
Length (mm)	24.9	14.5–33.4	6	23	15.6–30.5	4.5	27.1	13.4–40.3	6.7
Maximum diameter (mm)	6.2	5.1–7.4	0.8	6.9	3.8–10.6	1.9	9.2	4.9–13.2	2.4
Minimum diameter (mm)	5.2	3–6.5	0.9	5.5	3.7–9	1.5	8	4.8–12.6	2
Right adrenal gland									
Length (mm)	22.4	14–31.1	5.2	22	12.2–28.1	4.3	26	2.8–34.6	5.4
Maximum diameter (mm)	5.7	3.6–8.1	1.2	6.5	3.8–11	1.9	8.6	3.9–13.9	2.4
Minimum diameter (mm)	4.1	1.8–6.7	1.2	5.2	3.4–9	1.4	6.8	3.4–12.1	2

From Barthez PY, et al: Ultrasonographic evaluation of the adrenal glands in dogs. JAVMA 207:1180, 1995.

(Fig. 154–5). The first is to understand that Cushing's syndrome is a clinical disorder with clinical signs. If a dog or cat has no clinical signs, we do not recommend treatment. This concept gains importance when it is understood that none of the screening tests is correct all the time (i.e., sensitivity and specificity are not 100 per cent for any test).[21] The second step is attempting to confirm the clinical impression with a positive endocrine screening test result, and the third step is attempting to differentiate dogs with PDH from those with adrenocortical tumors.

Screening Tests to Confirm the Diagnosis of Hyperadrenocorticism

The decision to treat a dog or cat for Cushing's syndrome should never be based solely on results of endocrine testing. Many dogs with nonadrenal disease have false-positive test results for hyperadrenocorticism if tested with the commonly employed pituitary-adrenal function tests. Because false-positive test results have been observed with all the commonly used screening tests (ACTH stimulation test, low-dose dexamethasone test, urine cortisol-creatinine ratio), the definitive diagnosis of hyperadrenocorticism should never be based on the results of one or more of these screening tests alone, especially in dogs without clinical signs of the disease or in those with known nonadrenal disease.[21]

Urinary Corticosteroids

Twenty-four-Hour Collection and Assay. Traditionally, measurement of cortisol concentration from an aliquot of urine collected over a 24-hour period provides an integrated assessment of the amount of hormone produced over time. Problems of episodic release of cortisol, present with

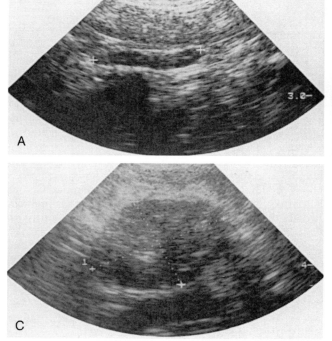

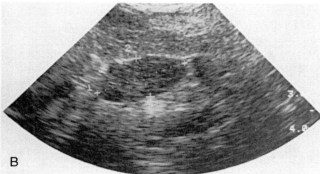

Figure 154–4. *A,* Sagittal view of the left adrenal in a normal dog (2.40 cm length). *B,* Sagittal view of the right adrenal in a dog with pituitary-dependent hyperadrenocorticism (1 = 2.41 cm length, 2 = 1.15 cm width). *C,* Left adrenal tumor in a dog with Cushing's syndrome (1 = 4.48 cm length, 2 = 3.26 cm width). (Courtesy of Drs. Paul Barthez and Tom Nyland.)

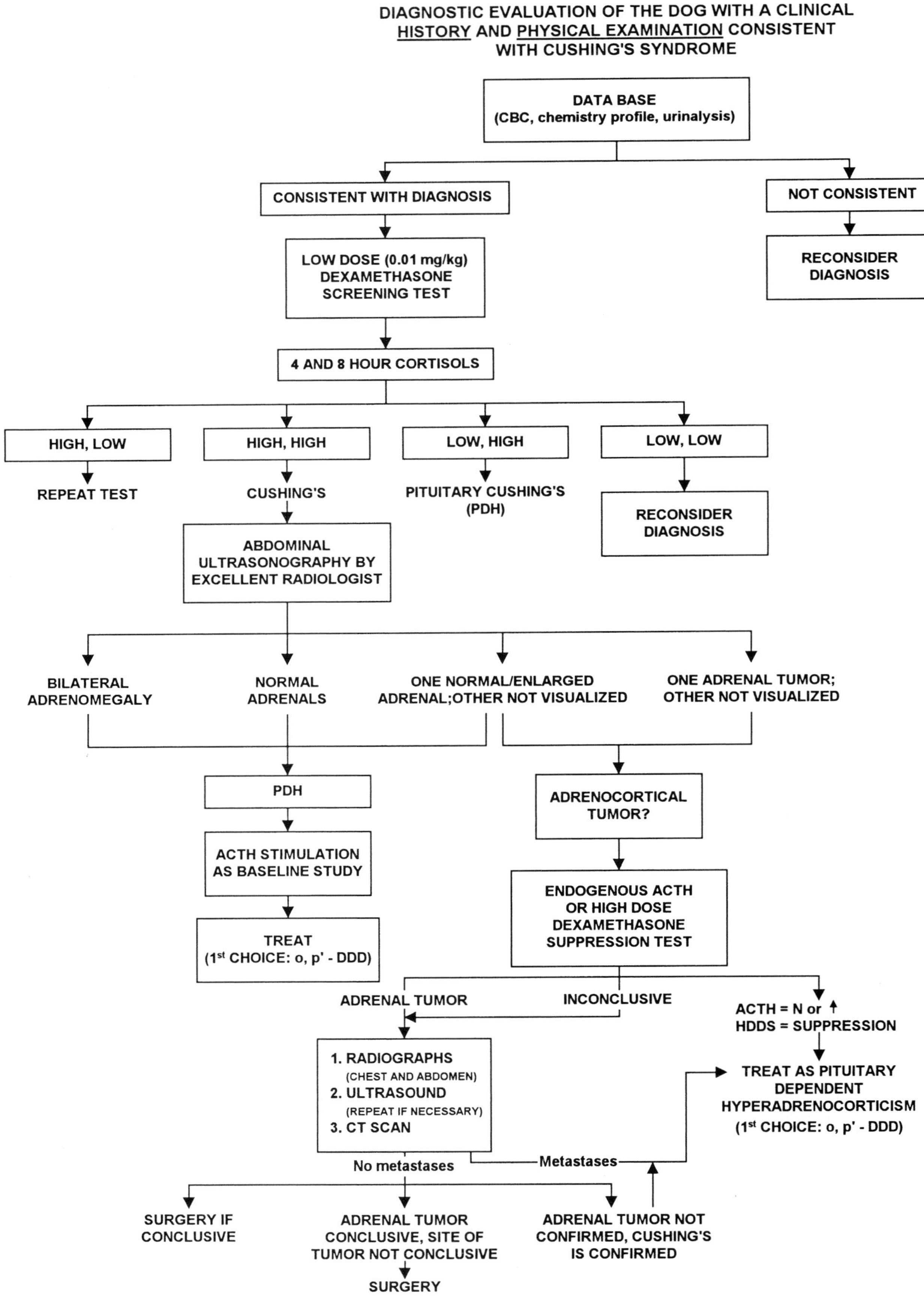

DIAGNOSTIC EVALUATION OF THE DOG WITH A CLINICAL
HISTORY AND PHYSICAL EXAMINATION CONSISTENT
WITH CUSHING'S SYNDROME

DATA BASE
(CBC, chemistry profile, urinalysis)

CONSISTENT WITH DIAGNOSIS

NOT CONSISTENT

RECONSIDER
DIAGNOSIS

LOW DOSE (0.01 mg/kg)
DEXAMETHASONE
SCREENING TEST

4 AND 8 HOUR CORTISOLS

HIGH, LOW

HIGH, HIGH

LOW, HIGH

LOW, LOW

REPEAT TEST

CUSHING'S

PITUITARY CUSHING'S
(PDH)

RECONSIDER
DIAGNOSIS

ABDOMINAL
ULTRASONOGRAPHY BY
EXCELLENT RADIOLOGIST

BILATERAL
ADRENOMEGALY

NORMAL
ADRENALS

ONE NORMAL/ENLARGED
ADRENAL;OTHER NOT VISUALIZED

ONE ADRENAL TUMOR;
OTHER NOT VISUALIZED

PDH

ADRENOCORTICAL
TUMOR?

ACTH STIMULATION
AS BASELINE STUDY

ENDOGENOUS ACTH
OR HIGH DOSE
DEXAMETHASONE
SUPPRESSION TEST

TREAT
(1st CHOICE: o, p' - DDD)

ADRENAL TUMOR

INCONCLUSIVE

ACTH = N or ↑
HDDS = SUPPRESSION

1. RADIOGRAPHS
(CHEST AND ABDOMEN)
2. ULTRASOUND
(REPEAT IF NECESSARY)
3. CT SCAN

TREAT AS PITUITARY
DEPENDENT
HYPERADRENOCORTICISM
(1st CHOICE: o, p' - DDD)

No metastases

Metastases

SURGERY IF
CONCLUSIVE

ADRENAL TUMOR
CONCLUSIVE, SITE OF
TUMOR NOT CONCLUSIVE

ADRENAL TUMOR NOT
CONFIRMED, CUSHING'S
IS CONFIRMED

SURGERY

Figure 154–5. Flowchart for the diagnostic evaluation of a dog or cat with suspected hyperadrenocorticism.

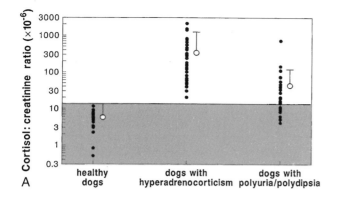

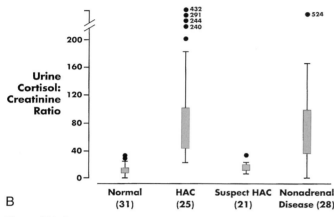

Figure 154–6. *A,* Urine cortisol-creatinine (C:C) ratios from healthy dogs, dogs with naturally occurring hyperadrenocorticism, and dogs with polyuria and polydipsia due to disorders other than hyperadrenocorticism. These values illustrate that the C:C ratio is a sensitive test for Cushing's syndrome but is not specific and should not be used as the sole test in confirming a diagnosis. *B,* Box plots of the urine C:C ratios found in normal dogs, dogs with hyperadrenocorticism (HAC), dogs in which hyperadrenocorticism was initially suspected but that did not have the disease (suspect HAC), and dogs with a variety of severe nonadrenal diseases. The number of dogs in each group is shown in parentheses. The box represents the interquartile range from the 25th to 75th percentiles (representing the middle half of the data). The horizontal bar through the box is the median. The "whiskers" represent the main body of data, which in most cases is equal to the range. Outlying data points are represented by the circles (exact values are given for these cases). These data illustrate that the urine C:C ratio is sensitive for the diagnosis of Cushing's syndrome but is not specific. (*A* from Feldman EC, Mack RE: Urine cortisol:creatinine ratio as a screening test for hyperadrenocorticism in dogs. JAVMA 200:1637, 1992; *B* from Smiley LE, Peterson ME: Evaluation of a urine cortisol:creatinine ratio as a screening test for hyperadrenocorticism in dogs. J Vet Intern Med 7:163, 1993.)

plasma assays, can be avoided. This has been and continues to be the gold standard used in the diagnosis of humans suspected of having hyperadrenocorticism.[22] Although it is reliable, because of the cumbersome nature of collecting 24-hour urine samples, it is rarely used in dogs and cats.

Urine Cortisol-Creatinine Ratio. Measurement of the cortisol-creatinine ratio from a randomly obtained urine sample (ideally a free-catch collection by an owner when the dog is in its home environment) is a relatively sensitive test (dogs with hyperadrenocorticism have an abnormal result). However, the test is not specific (many dogs with nonadrenal illnesses also have an abnormal result). Therefore, the test should not be used as the sole study to confirm a diagnosis. Two studies demonstrated that 79 and 76 per cent of dogs with moderate to severe nonadrenal disease had urine cortisol-creatinine ratios consistent with Cushing's.[21, 23] In our

studies, the urine cortisol-creatinine ratio was also demonstrated to be sensitive but nonspecific; that is, it was abnormal in dogs with Cushing's, but it was also abnormal in dogs with diabetes mellitus, diabetes insipidus, pyometra, hypercalcemia, and liver failure (Fig. 154–6).[23, 24]

Resting (Basal) Plasma Cortisol Concentrations

Basal, randomly obtained plasma cortisol determinations are of no diagnostic value.

ACTH Stimulation Test

Naturally Acquired Hyperadrenocorticism. Dogs and cats with hyperplastic or neoplastic adrenals have the capacity to synthesize excessive (abnormal) amounts of cortisol and the potential for an exaggerated response to ACTH stimulation. Numerous reliable protocols for the ACTH stimulation test have been published (Table 154–5). The test can begin at any time of day with plasma samples (heparinized blood) obtained before and one or two hours after injection of ACTH (depending on the ACTH used). Both natural (gel) and synthetic ACTHs are reliable.[25] Normal values for baseline cortisol concentrations usually range from 0.5 to 6.0 μg/dL, and post-stimulation values are 6 to 17 μg/dL (Fig. 154–7). Post-stimulation values between 17 and 22 μg/dL are usually considered borderline, and those of 22 μg/dL or greater are consistent with a diagnosis of Cushing's. It is important to emphasize that ratio or percentage change—comparing the basal with the post-stimulation cortisol—is not informative; only the absolute values should be evaluated. The ACTH response test is neither 100 per cent sensitive nor 100 per cent specific (dogs with nonadrenal illness can have abnormal results). No endocrine test can replace a history and physical examination for reliability in establishing a diagnosis.

Test results from dogs with PDH are not distinguishable from those that have functioning adrenocortical tumors. Thus the ACTH response test is a screening test in the diagnostic evaluation for hyperadrenocorticism. ACTH stimulation test results are abnormal in about 60 to 70 per cent of dogs with PDH, making the test useful but not absolutely reliable.

END

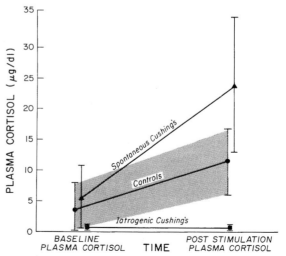

Figure 154–7. Mean RIA plasma cortisol concentrations (± 2 SD) determined before and one hour after administration of synthetic ACTH in control dogs, dogs with spontaneous hyperadrenocorticism, and those with iatrogenic hyperadrenocorticism.

TABLE 154–5. ACTH STIMULATION TEST PROTOCOLS FOR ASSESSING ADRENOCORTICAL GLUCOCORTICOID RESERVE

ACTH PREPARATION	DOSE	ROUTE OF ADMINISTRATION	PREINJECTION CORTISOL	TIMING OF POSTINJECTION CORTISOL	BEGIN TEST
Synthetic ACTH (Cortrosyn*)	0.25 mg/dog	IM	Yes	1 hour	8–9 A.M.
Synthetic ACTH (Cortrosyn*)	0.125 mg/cat	IM or IV	Yes	30 and 60 minutes	8–9 A.M.
Porcine ACTH (Cortigel-40†)	2.2 IU/kg (1 IU/lb) (dog)	IM	Yes	2 hours	8–9 A.M.
Porcine ACTH (Cortigel-40†)	2.2 IU/kg (cat)	IM	Yes	1 and 2 hours	8–9 A.M.

*Cortrosyn (cosyntropin), Organon Pharmaceuticals, West Orange, NJ 07052.
†Cortigel-40 (repositol corticotropin injection, USP), Savage Laboratories, Melville, NY 11747.
IM = intramuscular; IV = intravenous.
From Feldman EC, Nelson RW: Canine and Feline Endocrinology and Reproduction, 2nd ed. Philadelphia, WB Saunders, 1996, p 224.

Similar results are obtained from dogs with functioning adrenocortical tumors; 55 to 60 per cent have abnormally exaggerated ACTH stimulation test results. A significant percentage (30 to 40 per cent) have normal response tests.

Iatrogenic Cushing's Syndrome. One of the advantages of using the ACTH stimulation test as a screening test for dogs with suspected Cushing's syndrome is its ability to readily identify animals with iatrogenic disease. Dogs chronically receiving glucocorticoid therapy can develop all the clinical features typical of the naturally occurring condition. This concept is valuable, because some owners do not realize that their pets have been receiving glucocorticoid medications. A dog with clinical signs and routine laboratory test results suggestive of Cushing's syndrome, a low-normal baseline cortisol concentration, and little or no response to exogenous ACTH is quite likely to have iatrogenic Cushing's syndrome (Fig. 154–7). No other screening test differentiates naturally occurring hyperadrenocorticism from iatrogenic Cushing's syndrome.

o,p'-DDD Therapy. o,p'-DDD (Mitotane, Lysodren) is used commonly and ketoconazole (Nizoral) uncommonly in the treatment of hyperadrenocorticism. The most reliable means of monitoring either therapy is with ACTH stimulation, which is also reliable within 24 hours of surgery for ensuring that an adrenocortical tumor has been successfully removed. The test is easier to interpret if results can be compared with those obtained before treatment.

Anticonvulsant Medication. Primidone, phenytoin, and phenobarbital can cause polydipsia, polyuria, polyphagia, lethargy, increased serum liver enzyme values, and abnormal plasma cortisol concentrations. Although studies have not demonstrated obvious abnormalities in endocrine test results from dogs treated with anticonvulsants, it is possible that these studies were not carried out for a long enough time.[26, 27] One must be cautious when trying to establish a diagnosis of Cushing's syndrome in dogs on these medications. The diagnosis must first be based on careful evaluation of the history and physical examination.

Dexamethasone Screening Test (Low-Dose Dexamethasone Test)

Protocol. Obtain a morning baseline plasma sample for cortisol determination and then administer dexamethasone 0.01 mg/kg intravenously. If one uses a 0.15 mg/kg dosage, the test results are virtually identical, and dexamethasone sodium phosphate or dexamethasone in polyethylene glycol (Azium) may be used.[28] Samples for cortisol determination should be taken four and eight hours after dexamethasone administration.[29, 30]

Normal. Administering small doses of dexamethasone can inhibit pituitary secretion of ACTH and, in turn, cortisol

secretion within two to three hours. The duration of the effect is as long as 24 to 48 hours.[31] Dexamethasone, a synthetic glucocorticoid, is potent but does not cross-react with cortisol assays, allowing documentation of its effect. Therefore, function of the normal pituitary-adrenal axis can be demonstrated by administering dexamethasone and noting, within two to three hours, a reduction in plasma cortisol concentration (plasma cortisol <1.4 μg/dL) that persists longer than eight hours (Fig. 154–8). The low-dose dexamethasone test has been extremely reliable in differentiating normal dogs from those with hyperadrenocorticism. In compiling the data from recent reports, this test identified more than 98 per cent of dogs with Cushing's syndrome.

Adrenocortical Tumor. Functioning adrenocortical tumors secrete excess cortisol autonomously, suppress endogenous ACTH, and cause clinical signs of Cushing's. Therefore, ACTH is already inhibited by the autonomously secreting adrenocortical tumor, and dexamethasone administration to a dog with an adrenocortical tumor does not affect plasma cortisol concentration (Fig. 154–8B). Concentrations are persistently greater than 1.4 μg/dL, with only slight fluctuation in results.

Pituitary-Dependent Hyperadrenocorticism. ACTH secretion from functioning pituitary tumors causes adrenocortical hyperplasia owing to chronic and excessive stimulation. The abnormal pituitary must be somewhat resistant to cortisol negative feedback, or the hyperadrenocorticism would never develop. Administration of a low dose of dexamethasone to a dog with PDH causes variable transient suppression of cortisol at four hours (<1.4 μg/dL), but by eight hours, the plasma cortisol concentration is typically greater than 1.4 μg/dL. Several response patterns to low-dose dexamethasone have been identified in dogs with PDH. The plasma cortisol concentration may not vary in approximately 20 per cent of dogs with PDH, results that are similar to those in dogs with adrenocortical tumors (see Fig. 154–8). The plasma cortisol concentration may decrease slightly at four hours and return to basal concentrations at eight hours in approximately 20 per cent of PDH dogs (see Fig. 154–8C). The plasma cortisol concentration may decrease to levels less than 50 per cent of baseline at four and/or eight hours but never below 1.4 μg/dL in approximately 30 to 40 per cent of dogs with PDH (see Fig. 154–8D). The plasma cortisol concentration decreases to less than 1.4 μg/dL at four hours but increases to concentrations greater than 1.4 μg/dL at eight hours in approximately 25 per cent of PDH dogs (see Fig. 154–8E).[30]

Misleading Results. As with the ACTH stimulation test, dexamethasone screening test results can be misleading. Of 59 dogs with nonadrenal illness, 22 (38 per cent) and 33 (56 per cent) failed to demonstrate normal cortisol suppres-

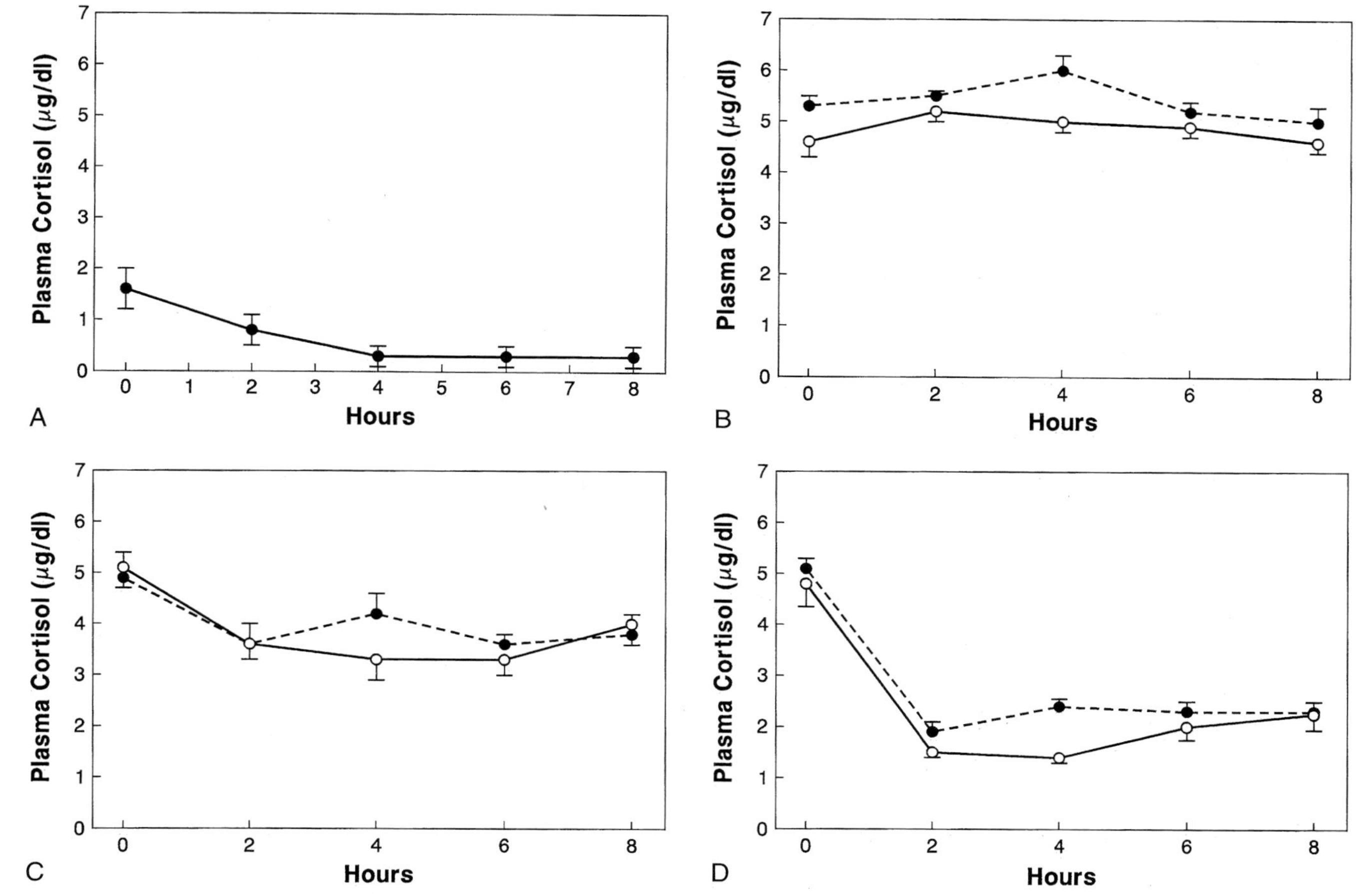

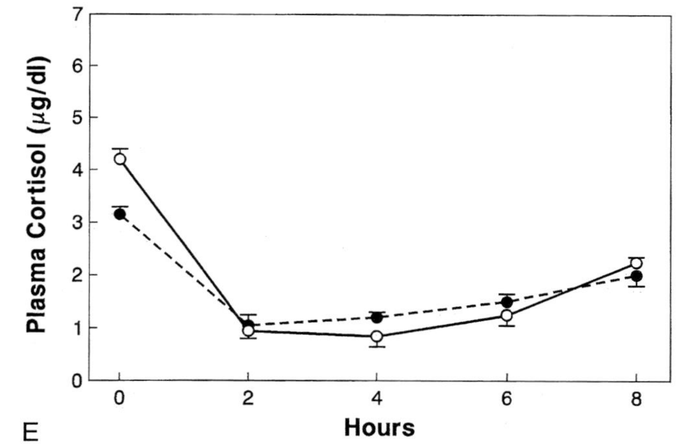

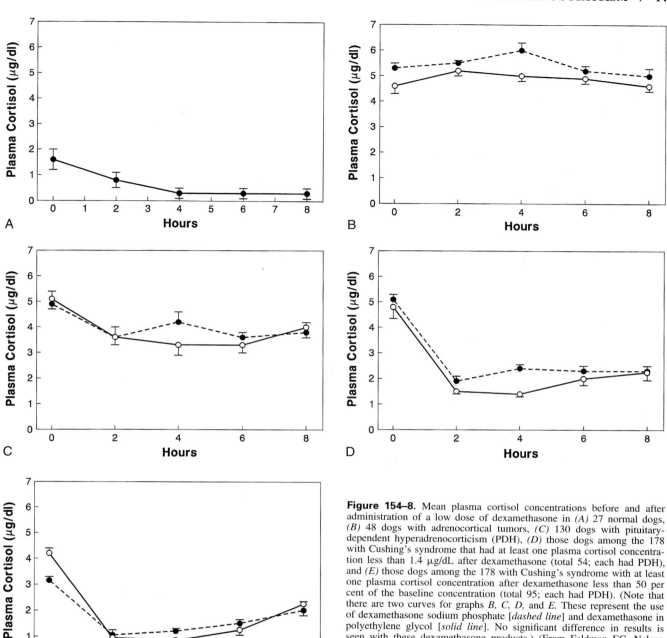

Figure 154–8. Mean plasma cortisol concentrations before and after administration of a low dose of dexamethasone in *(A)* 27 normal dogs, *(B)* 48 dogs with adrenocortical tumors, *(C)* 130 dogs with pituitary-dependent hyperadrenocorticism (PDH), *(D)* those dogs among the 178 with Cushing's syndrome that had at least one plasma cortisol concentration less than 1.4 μg/dL after dexamethasone (total 54; each had PDH), and *(E)* those dogs among the 178 with Cushing's syndrome with at least one plasma cortisol concentration after dexamethasone less than 50 per cent of the baseline concentration (total 95; each had PDH). (Note that there are two curves for graphs *B, C, D,* and *E.* These represent the use of dexamethasone sodium phosphate [*dashed line*] and dexamethasone in polyethylene glycol [*solid line*]. No significant difference in results is seen with these dexamethasone products.) (From Feldman EC, Nelson RW: Canine and Feline Endocrinology and Reproduction, 2nd ed. Philadelphia, WB Saunders, 1996, p 227.)

sion at four and eight hours, respectively.[21] Anticonvulsant medications can cause dogs to have unusual plasma cortisol concentrations. The stress of bathing, hospitalization, illness, and numerous other factors may interfere with test results.

Miscellaneous Screening Tests

Alkaline Phosphatase Isoenzyme. Assay of alkaline phosphatase isoenzymes is not a reliable screening test.[32]

Combined Dexamethasone Suppression and ACTH Stimulation. Combining these screening tests does not yield reliable results and is not recommended.[33, 34]

Liver Biopsy. Abnormal liver enzymes and abnormal liver function tests are common in hyperadrenocorticism. Dogs with naturally occurring hyperadrenocorticism and those given exogenous glucocorticoids usually have histologic evidence of glucocorticoid-induced or steroid hepatopathy. This hepatopathy is histologically characterized by centrilobular vacuolization, perivacuolar glycogen accumulation within hepatocytes, and focal centrilobular necrosis. Steroid hepatopathy is unique to the dog. However, complications of infection or inadequate healing following liver biopsy procedures limit the usefulness of this study, and it is not recommended as a screening test.

Discrimination Tests to Differentiate Between Pituitary-Dependent and Adrenocortical Tumor Hyperadrenocorticism

Low-Dose Dexamethasone Suppression (LDDS) Test

Protocol and Definitions. The four-hour sample can be used as a discrimination test, and the eight-hour sample can be used for both screening and discrimination. The LDDS test can be used to identify dogs with PDH based on three criteria: a four-hour plasma cortisol concentration less than 1.4 μg/dL, a four-hour result less than 50 per cent of the basal level, or an eight-hour result less than 50 per cent of the basal concentration. Any dog with hyperadrenocorticism that has plasma cortisol concentrations that meet one or more of these criteria most likely has PDH.

Results. Approximately 25 per cent of dogs with PDH have a four-hour cortisol concentration less than 1.4 μg/dL, 60 per cent have a four-hour result less than 50 per cent of the baseline value, and 25 per cent have an eight-hour value less than 50 per cent of baseline. Virtually all have an eight-hour plasma cortisol concentration that is consistent with hyperadrenocorticism. Approximately 60 per cent of dogs with PDH demonstrate suppression on the LDDS test as defined by at least one of these criteria.[30] Lack of suppression is considered a nonspecific result, because 40 per cent of PDH dogs and virtually 100 per cent of dogs with adrenocortical tumor do not meet any of these criteria.

High-Dose Dexamethasone Suppression (HDDS) Test

Theory, Protocol, and Interpretation. Regardless of dose, dexamethasone should not suppress plasma cortisol when the source of that cortisol is an adrenocortical tumor. PDH, in contrast, results from chronic oversecretion of ACTH from a tumor that can potentially be suppressed by dexamethasone. Administering larger and larger doses of dexamethasone would eventually suppress pituitary ACTH secretion in most dogs with PDH. The HDDS protocol recommended involves the collection of heparinized blood samples before and four or eight hours after administration of 0.1 mg/kg dexamethasone intravenously. Suppression is defined as a plasma cortisol concentration less than 50 per cent of the baseline concentration four or eight hours after administration or less than 1.4 μg/dL four or eight hours after administration.[30]

Results. Administration of a high dose of dexamethasone does not cause cortisol suppression in dogs with adrenocortical tumor, whereas approximately 75 per cent of dogs with PDH have plasma cortisol concentrations less than 1.4 μg/dL or less than 50 per cent of the baseline concentration at four and/or eight hours. It is not known why some dogs with PDH are extremely resistant to dexamethasone suppression while others suppress in response to high-dose dexamethasone. This variation is not due to pituitary tumor size or location.

Endogenous ACTH Concentrations

Theory and Collection Protocol. Adrenocortical tumors and iatrogenic Cushing's syndrome should suppress pituitary ACTH secretion, and PDH is due to excessive ACTH secretion. Pituitary secretion of ACTH occurs episodically (it is released in bursts), and plasma concentrations fluctuate from minute to minute. In order to diminish the effect of stress or time of day, blood for endogenous ACTH should be obtained between 8 and 9 A.M., after the dog has been hospitalized for a night. Blood obtained for ACTH must be handled quickly, because the disappearance rate of ACTH from fresh whole blood is rapid. Specimens should be centrifuged in plastic and the plasma frozen at −20°C within minutes of collection. Contact with glass must be avoided, because ACTH adheres to glass. Several kits for human ACTH have excellent cross-reactivity in dogs and cats.[35, 36] Any assay must be validated for the species being studied, and test results obtained from control animals must be made available. The baseline plasma ACTH concentration in healthy dogs averages 45 pg/mL, and the reference range is 10 to 110 pg/mL (Fig. 154–9).

Results. Endogenous ACTH concentrations less than 10 pg/mL (undetectable) in dogs with naturally occurring Cushing's are strongly suggestive of a functioning adrenocortical tumor (see Fig. 154–9). Undetectable plasma endogenous ACTH concentrations would also be typical of dogs with iatrogenic Cushing's, but ACTH stimulation test results should reveal the underlying disorder (see Fig. 154–7). Approximately 60 per cent of dogs with adrenocortical tumors have an undetectable ACTH concentration, and the remaining 40 per cent have values of 10 to 40 pg/mL, regardless of whether the tumor is an adenoma or a carcinoma.[6]

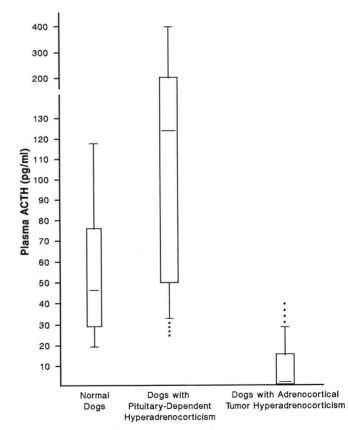

Figure 154–9. Endogenous plasma ACTH concentrations from clinically normal dogs, dogs with functioning adrenocortical carcinomas or adenomas, and dogs with pituitary-dependent hyperadrenocorticism (PDH). Each box represents the interquartile range from the 25th to the 75th percentiles (the middle half of the data). The horizontal bar through the box is the median. The "whiskers" represent the main body of data, which in most cases is equal to the range. Outlying data points are represented by the circles. (From Feldman EC, Nelson RW: Canine and Feline Endocrinology and Reproduction, 2nd ed. Philadelphia, WB Saunders, 1996, p 230.)

ACTH concentrations of 45 pg/mL or greater are consistent with a diagnosis of PDH, and such results are obtained in 85 to 90 per cent of these dogs (see Fig. 154–9). Again, appropriate screening tests must first be used to confirm the diagnosis of Cushing's. Approximately 35 per cent of dogs with PDH have endogenous ACTH concentrations greater than 100 pg/mL, and about 55 per cent have a result between 45 and 100 pg/mL. Only 10 to 15 per cent of PDH dogs have endogenous ACTH concentrations of 10 to 45 pg/mL, values that are considered nondiagnostic.[37]

CT Scans

The use of CT scans has been part of a minor revolution in the high technology of modern veterinary medicine. This sophisticated tool is available primarily at veterinary schools and to some veterinarians working with local human hospitals. CT scans require 30 minutes to two hours of anesthesia to complete. In dogs and cats, CT scans of the abdomen have been successful in identifying normal adrenals versus one large adrenal or bilateral adrenal enlargement.[38] Abdominal radiography is not as sensitive as CT scanning, but ultrasonography is as sensitive as CT in detecting and localizing adrenocortical tumors.[39, 40] Approximately 50 per cent of pituitary tumors are relatively small, contained within the normal pituitary, and can be difficult to discern by CT scanning. About 40 per cent of PDH dogs that have no CNS signs have a visible pituitary tumor on CT. However, those with clinical signs caused by a large pituitary mass would have a visible mass on CT scan.

MRI Scans

Dogs Without CNS Signs. MRI scans can be obtained on dogs heavily sedated with an intravenous mixture of ketamine and diazapam. Sedation is maintained with additional small doses every 10 to 15 minutes throughout the scanning period. Sedation allows intubation, which decreases respiratory movement and improves scan quality. Approximately 50 per cent of dogs with untreated PDH and no signs suggestive of an intracranial mass have easily visualized pituitary tumors on MRI measuring 3 to 13 mm at greatest diameter (Fig. 154–10). Most visible masses extend beyond the dorsal confines of the sella turcica, and most are contrast enhancing. The lateral ventricles were enlarged in several dogs, but this finding was considered an age-related change rather than an indication of obstructive hydrocephalus.[8]

Our experience demonstrates that (1) at least 80 per cent of these tumors are larger one year later, regardless of the success of medical treatment; (2) 15 to 20 per cent of dogs with PDH are at risk for developing neurologic signs due to an enlarging tumor during the first one to two years after diagnosis; (3) o,p'-DDD treatment did not affect tumor growth rate; (4) neurologic signs are associated with tumors 10 mm or greater in diameter; (5) cobalt irradiation should be considered for any PDH dog with a pituitary tumor 8 mm or greater in diameter, and (6) MRI or CT scans of the pituitary in dogs with PDH are helpful in predicting dogs likely to develop problems owing to an enlarging pituitary tumor.[8, 41]

Dogs With PDH and Signs of Intracranial Tumor. We have completed MRI scans in a group of PDH dogs with signs of intracranial tumor. These dogs had a mean age of 9.5 years (younger than the mean for all dogs with PDH) and a mean body weight of 24 kg (larger than the average dog with PDH). MRI scans were definitive in demonstrating the size and nature of the tumor in each dog. All masses were better visualized after administration of the contrast agent (gadolinium DTPA). The masses measured 8 to 24 mm at greatest vertical height (Fig. 154–11). All tumors had expanded dorsally, well beyond the limits of the sella turcica, without causing bone destruction. Some masses elevated the floor of the third ventricle, and some appeared to compress the hypothalamus. Obstructive hydrocephalus was suspected in a few dogs. Tumor-associated necrosis or hemorrhage was not apparent on any scans.[9]

TREATMENT

Approximately 80 to 85 per cent of dogs with naturally occurring hyperadrenocorticism have PDH, and 15 to 20 per cent have functioning adrenal tumors. Therapy may be selected on the basis of the etiology for the Cushing's (pituitary or adrenal), as well as on the veterinarian's experience. Excellent rapport between veterinarian and owner is valuable during the long-term management of a dog or cat that has been diagnosed as having hyperadrenocorticism. The surgical and medical options should be discussed in detail, including what is expected of the owner. One hopes to return such pets to a normal endocrine state, but this is not always possible, and all complications must be discussed. They may have endocrine excesses or deficiencies after treatment, and the prepared owner can better accept these setbacks. Time spent explaining the pathophysiology in lay terms is well worth the effort to improve client understanding.

Surgery

Adrenal Tumor Hyperadrenocorticism

Preoperative Evaluation. Once the diagnosis of Cushing's syndrome and the presence of an adrenal tumor are confirmed, one should attempt to localize the tumor and rule out metastasis. Abdominal ultrasonography is the preferred tool for localizing tumors and identifying abdominal metastasis as well as vessel or organ invasion or compression. Abdominal surgery should not be considered without abdominal ultrasound and thoracic radiographic evaluation. Adrenal tumors that metastasize usually spread to the liver and/or lungs. If metastasis to the liver is suspected, an ultrasound-guided biopsy should be performed to confirm this suspicion. Screening tests, such as radiographs, ultrasound, and CT scans, may also provide valuable information regarding the size of the tumor. Small tumors are much more likely to be benign and easily removed than are tumors as big as or bigger than a normal kidney.

The preoperative evaluation should also be directed at determining whether a particular dog is a reasonable surgical candidate. This assessment should include clinical estimation of health as well as an evaluation of systemic blood pressure, urine protein-creatinine ratio, and serum antithrombin III concentrations. Abnormalities in the latter three may correlate with risk for thromboembolism.[15] Treating a dog at increased risk for anesthetic, surgical, or postsurgical problems for one to three months with ketoconazole or o,p'-DDD may be beneficial in resolving many of the problems associated with Cushing's-related debilitation. This time can also be used to treat any other concurrent problems (e.g., infection) before surgery.

Surgical Approach. The recommended surgical approach is either paracostal or ventral midline laparotomy. A

END

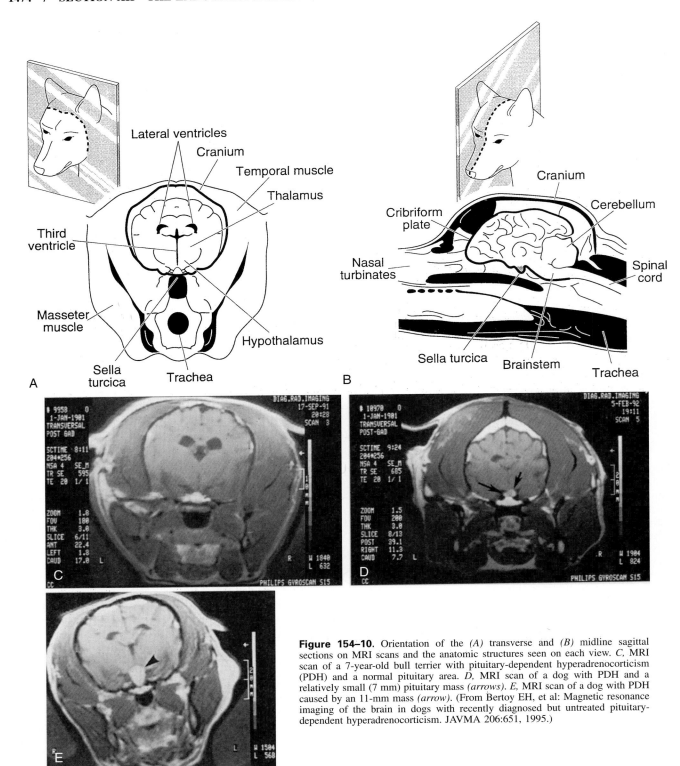

Figure 154–10. Orientation of the (A) transverse and (B) midline sagittal sections on MRI scans and the anatomic structures seen on each view. C, MRI scan of a 7-year-old bull terrier with pituitary-dependent hyperadrenocorticism (PDH) and a normal pituitary area. D, MRI scan of a dog with PDH and a relatively small (7 mm) pituitary mass (arrows). E, MRI scan of a dog with PDH caused by an 11-mm mass (arrow). (From Bertoy EH, et al: Magnetic resonance imaging of the brain in dogs with recently diagnosed but untreated pituitary-dependent hyperadrenocorticism. JAVMA 206:651, 1995.)

ventral midline celiotomy should provide excellent exposure of both adrenal glands and an opportunity to completely evaluate the abdominal contents, especially the liver, for metastasis and/or other problems.[42] However, problems with wound healing are exaggerated by a ventral weight-bearing incision. The paracostal retroperitoneal approach to adrenalectomy also has advantages and disadvantages. Most surgeons prefer ventral midline surgery.

Patient Management During and After Surgery

Glucocorticoid Therapy. The autonomous secretion of cortisol from an adrenocortical tumor causes decreased secretion of pituitary ACTH, resulting in significant atrophy of normal cells within the zona reticularis and zona fasciculata (which synthesize cortisol) of the opposite adrenal. Suppression of endogenous ACTH by the tumor may also cause some atrophy of the zona glomerulosa, which synthesizes aldosterone. Acute hypocortisolism is expected and uniformly occurs after surgery, unless there are functioning metastases. At the time of anesthesia, intravenous fluids (saline or Ringer's solution) should be administered at a maintenance rate. When the adrenal tumor is recognized by the surgeon, dexamethasone should be placed in the intravenous infusion bottle at a dose of 0.1 mg/kg of body weight and infused over a six-hour period. The dose should be repeated two to four time a day subcutaneously. Parenteral medication is usually not continued for more than 48 to 72 hours, because by that time the dog is eating and drinking normally and is not receiving intravenous fluids, so oral medication can be initiated. The dog should receive approximately 0.5 mg/kg of prednisone orally twice a day for two days, then tapered over a period of two to three months. After achieving every-other-day or every-third-day therapy, a trial period with no medication can be undertaken.

Mineralocorticoid Therapy. Postoperatively, the blood pressure, blood urea nitrogen, serum electrolytes, and blood glucose concentrations should be closely monitored. Serum sodium concentrations less than 138 mEq/L and/or serum potassium concentrations greater than 5.5 mEq/L may indicate a need for mineralocorticoid therapy. Mild hyperkalemia and/or hyponatremia have been documented in 40 per cent

of our dogs in the 24- to 48-hour period following surgery. In most, this is a transient problem that resolves within a day or two. Because mineralocorticoid therapy is rather benign, and because it is not possible to determine which dogs will have transient problems and which will have serious mineralocortcoid deficits, treatment with fludrocortisone acetate or desoxycorticosterone pivalate is recommended if these abnormalities persist or worsen.

Prophylaxis Against Thromboembolism. Dogs with hyperadrenocorticism undergoing the prolonged anesthesia and recumbency associated with surgery may be at increased risk for thromboembolism. We currently treat these dogs with plasma (a source of antithrombin III) and heparin during surgery (35 U/kg in the plasma infusion) and 35 U/kg twice subcutaneously after surgery. The subcutaneous heparin dose is then tapered over a period of four days. An infusion of hetastarch is administered intravenously on the fifth postsurgical day (10 mL/kg over a period of six hours). It is thought that the single infusion of hetastarch may decrease the potential for thromboembolism for a period of days.[43]

Pain Control. The abdominal incision and surgery associated with adrenal tumor excision can be painful. However, analgesics that have sedative effects are dangerous, because recumbency increases the risk of thromboembolism. We routinely place fentanyl patches on these dogs 24 hours

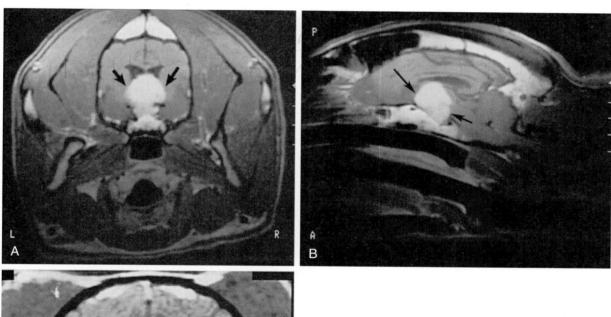

Figure 154–11. *A,* Transverse view of a post-gadolinium MRI scan of a 7-year-old bull terrier with pituitary-dependent hyperadrenocorticism (PDH) caused by a 2.4-cm mass *(arrows)*; the dog developed signs of disorientation and ataxia. *B,* Midline sagittal view of the brain of the same dog (using MRI), showing the densely enhancing mass *(arrows)* arising from the pituitary fossa and causing compression of the floor of the overlying third ventricle. *C,* Post-gadolinium MRI scan of an 8-year-old Boston terrier with PDH and signs of disorientation, ataxia, and circling. (From Feldman EC, Nelson RW: Canine and Feline Endocrinology and Reproduction, 2nd ed. Philadelphia, WB Saunders, 1996, p 237.)

before surgery and have found this to be an excellent and safe method of analgesia while avoiding sedation.

Results (Prognosis). Surgical removal of an adrenocortical tumor can be an extremely difficult soft tissue procedure. In addition, the potential complications (e.g., poor wound healing, immune suppression, thromboembolism) result in a guarded prognosis for any dog undergoing this surgery. In our series, about 80 per cent of dogs have survived the surgery and the first-month recovery period.

Inoperable Mass, Poor Anesthetic Risk, or Obvious Metastasis. Surgery is not recommended for some Cushing's dogs with adrenocortical tumors. The reasons for avoiding surgery include finding a large, obviously inoperable mass on radiographs, ultrasound, or CT scan; finding evidence of metastasis; having an animal that is so debilitated that surgery would likely be terminal; and having an owner who refuses surgery. In these dogs, medical therapy should be considered.

Pituitary-Dependent Hyperadrenocorticism

Hypophysectomy. In humans, surgical removal of the pituitary tumor is the treatment of choice. Although this procedure has been described for dogs, it is not yet commonly performed. Transsphenoidal hypophysectomy will likely become more available, and with increased experience, it may become the treatment of choice.[44, 45]

Adrenalectomy. PDH results in bilateral adrenocortical hyperplasia. Removal of both adrenals results in complete resolution of signs attributed to Cushing's. Because "medical adrenalectomy" is relatively easy to accomplish in dogs using o,p'-DDD, the risk of surgery seems unwarranted, and it is rarely performed.

Medical Management Using o,p'-DDD

Pituitary-Dependent Hyperadrenocorticism

Since the treatment protocol first suggested by Schechter et al. in 1973, chemotherapy with o,p'-DDD has become the most common means of managing dogs with naturally occurring Cushing's. The systemic effects of o,p'-DDD (mitotane, Lysodren), a chemical derived from the insecticide DDT, were first reported in 1949 by Nelson and Woodard. The agent was administered to dogs and was found to be a potent adrenocorticolytic drug, causing progressive necrosis of the zona fasciculata and reticularis. The only other effects are moderate hepatic fatty degeneration, centrolobular atrophy, and congestion.

Dogs with adrenal hyperplasia are more sensitive than dogs with no adrenal disease to the destructive effects of o,p'-DDD. They usually respond after five to nine days of o,p'-DDD therapy and often become ill (hypoadrenal) if medication is not discontinued after the first hint of response. Any dog diagnosed as having PDH and requiring more than 21 consecutive days of o,p'-DDD therapy must be carefully reevaluated. Possible explanations for "resistance" are (1) the dog is not receiving the drug or it is not being absorbed from the gastrointestinal tract, (2) the dog has an adrenocortical tumor, or (3) the diagnosis is incorrect.

Pretreatment Assessments. There are several factors that owners should recognize before initiating o,p'-DDD therapy, including the dog's attitude, activity, daily water intake, and appetite. The most important and the most reliable monitoring tool used in the initial (loading dose) phase of o,p'-DDD therapy is appetite. A small percentage of dogs

respond to the drug in less than 5 days, some take 9 to 21 days, but more than 85 per cent respond in 5 to 9 days. We instruct owners to provide the pet with one third of its normal daily food intake, twice daily. These dogs are usually ravenously hungry, and reducing their daily food allotment further enhances appetite. The owner can then observe the dog for any reduction in appetite. The goal of therapy is to discontinue o,p'-DDD administration before the pet becomes anorexic. In addition to providing the most important monitoring tool, administration of o,p'-DDD to dogs twice a day, with each meal, enhances drug absorption.[46] It would be inappropriate to treat a dog with o,p'-DDD that did not have an excellent to ravenous appetite. Anorexia or poor appetite should cause the veterinarian to question the diagnosis or the advisability of treatment and raise the possibility of concurrent problems.

The Loading Dose Phase. Therapy is begun at home with the owner administering o,p'-DDD at a dosage of 50 mg/kg per day, divided and given twice a day (Fig. 154–12). Glucocorticoids are not advised, but the owner should have a small supply of prednisolone or prednisone tablets in case of emergency. The owner should receive thorough instructions on the actions of o,p'-DDD and should also have specific instructions on when the drug should be discontinued. Administration should be stopped when (1) the dog demonstrates *any* reduction in appetite (this might mean just pausing slightly during meal consumption, stopping to drink some water, or stopping in response to the owner's voice), (2) the polydipsic dog consumes less than 60 mL/kg of water per day; (3) the dog vomits; (4) the dog has diarrhea, or (5) the dog is unusually listless. The first two indications for stopping medication are emphasized, because they are most common.

Because of the potency of o,p'-DDD, the veterinarian is encouraged *not* to rely on the instructions given to the owner. Never provide an owner with more than eight days of o,p'-DDD initially. This drug is highly successful in eliminating the signs of hyperadrenocorticism because of its potency coupled with *close communication between owner and veterinarian.* Either the veterinarian or a technician should call the owner for a verbal report regarding the dog every day beginning with the second day of therapy. In this way, the owner will be impressed with the veterinarian's concern and will observe the animal closely. The dog's appetite should be observed before each administration of o,p'-DDD. If food is rapidly consumed (with or without polydipsia), medication is warranted. The initial loading dose phase is complete when any reduction in appetite is noted or after water intake approaches or falls below 60 mL/kg per day.

Veterinary Monitoring. In addition to making daily phone calls, the veterinarian should see the dog eight to nine days after beginning therapy. At this time a thorough history, physical examination, and ACTH response test should be performed. An evaluation of the blood urea nitrogen, serum sodium, and serum potassium concentrations may also be warranted, although these test results are rarely abnormal. Dogs should have therapy withheld until the ACTH response test results can be evaluated (see Fig. 154–12).

Goals of Therapy. The goals of therapy are to achieve clinical improvement plus an ACTH response test result that is suggestive of hypoadrenocorticism. Successful response is indicated by pre- and post-ACTH plasma cortisol concentrations less than 5 μg/dL. A dog that has a normal or exaggerated response to ACTH before therapy and a normal response to ACTH (post-ACTH cortisol 6 to 15 μg/dL) following the initial phase of therapy is likely to demonstrate

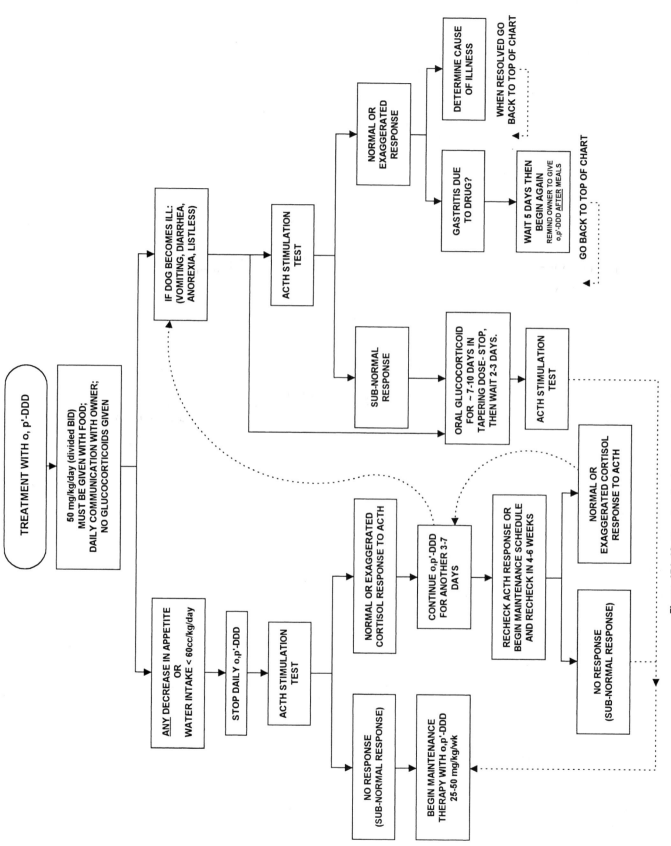

Figure 154-12. Flowchart for the management of hyperadrenocorticism using o,p'-DDD.

END

improvement but continue to have some clinical evidence of Cushing's.

Continuation of o,p'-DDD at the Loading Dose. If a dog with Cushing's has a normal or exaggerated response to ACTH following the initial eight to nine days of therapy, daily medication should be continued for three to seven additional days; the shorter period is used for dogs that have shown a significant (albeit inadequate) response. The ACTH response test should be rechecked every 7 to 10 days until a post-ACTH plasma cortisol concentration less than 5 µg/dL is achieved. Numerous ACTH tests are not usually necessary, because more than 85 per cent of dogs respond during the initial five to nine days of medication, and virtually all respond by the fourteenth day.

Concomitant Glucocorticoids During the Loading Dose Phase. The veterinary literature recommends two distinct protocols for the induction or loading dose phase of o,p'-DDD therapy: concurrent glucocorticoids versus none. Neither method is wrong. There are advantages and disadvantages with each. We do not recommend concurrent glucocorticoids. Rather than the "protection" of glucocorticoids, daily communication with owners is strongly advised. The incidence of o,p'-DDD overdosage is actually lower in dogs that do not receive simultaneous glucocorticoids than in dogs that do. This is true because owners not giving steroids can appreciate mild clinical changes early in therapy and stop the medication before hypocortisolism becomes severe.[47]

Need for Glucocorticoids. If signs of anorexia, vomiting, diarrhea, weakness, or listlessness develop, glucocorticoid therapy is warranted. If the dog has received no glucocorticoids during the initial phase of o,p'-DDD therapy, they should be started. If the dog has been treated with glucocorticoids, the dose needs to be increased. This is also true during the maintenance phase of therapy or if a well-controlled dog undergoes any major stress (illness, trauma, or elective surgery). Prednisone should be given at a dose of 0.5 to 1 mg/kg for two days. If signs develop as a result of o,p'-DDD overdosage, the dog usually shows clinical improvement within one to eight hours of initiating prednisone therapy. If oral therapy is not possible owing to vomiting, parenteral fluids and glucocorticoids are warranted. After a good response is observed, steroids should be tapered over 10 to 14 days. Recurrence of signs demands reinstitution of therapy or raising the dose.

Need for Both Glucocorticoids and Mineralocorticoids. o,p'-DDD is reported to spare the zona glomerulosa and, therefore, mineralocorticoid secretion. Dogs that develop signs of weakness, anorexia, and/or vomiting without electrolyte imbalances require immediate glucocorticoid therapy. Electrolyte disturbances suggestive of deficient mineralocorticoids (increased serum potassium and/or decreased serum sodium concentrations) have resulted from o,p'-DDD administration; these dogs require both glucocorticoid and mineralocorticoid therapy. Severe, inadvertent overdosage of this magnitude is rare (seen in <2 per cent of our closely monitored dogs). Glucocorticoid deficiency is usually transient. Addison's disease (deficiency of both glucocorticoids and mineralocorticoids) in o,p'-DDD-treated dogs can be permanent.

Time Sequence for Improvement in Signs and Biochemical Abnormalities. Dogs with o,p'-DDD-treated PDH usually respond quickly. The most obvious and rapid response is the reduction in appetite, water intake, and urine output seen during the first five to nine days of therapy. Owners often comment that they see an increase in activity during the first or second week of treatment. Other signs

take longer to dissipate. Muscle strength improves within days to weeks, as does reduction in the potbellied appearance. Alopecia, thin skin, acne, calcinosis cutis, and panting often take weeks to months for significant improvement. Dogs with haircoat abnormalities may go through a phase of severe seborrhea associated with a terrible haircoat or worsening alopecia and pruritus that may last one or two months before the haircoat shows significant improvement. Some dogs go through a phase of "puppy haircoat" before the normal adult coat returns (Fig. 154–13). A few dogs have dramatic changes in coat color following successful therapy (Fig. 154–14).

As the external appearance of a dog with Cushing's syndrome improves, internal improvement follows. Improvement in blood pressure and urine protein-creatinine ratio can be detected in three to six months.[15] Urinary tract infections may resolve quickly or linger for prolonged periods owing to pyelonephritis, retention of urine, calculi, and so forth.

Development of Concurrent Problems During Therapy. The anti-inflammatory and immune-suppressive actions of cortisol can mask concurrent problems in dogs with hyperadrenocorticism. Resolution of the hypercortisolism can cause subclinical problems to become obvious. The most common problems masked by hypercortisolism are degenerative arthritis and allergies.

Failure to Respond to o,p'-DDD. It is uncommon for o,p'-DDD to fail to help a dog with PDH. The drug is quite potent, and its effect on destroying the zona fasciculata and zona reticularis is consistent. There can be several reasons for apparent treatment failures: (1) a dog thought to have PDH may have an adrenocortical tumor (adenoma or carcinoma), which is relatively resistant to the cytotoxic effects of o,p'-DDD; (2) the drug itself may not be potent, and replacing the owner's tablets with o,p'-DDD obtained from a new or different bottle may solve an apparent treatment failure; (3) the drug may not have been given with food, and absorption may be adversely affected (crush the tablets and dissolve in 1 to 3 teaspoons of corn oil); (4) a dog may be one of the few that take longer than 14 days to respond; (5) a dog has been diagnosed incorrectly (incorrect diagnoses include any illness that may mimic hyperadrenocorticism, including anticonvulsant therapy); and (6) a dog may have iatrogenic Cushing's syndrome.

Therapy of Concurrent Diabetes Mellitus and Cushing's Syndrome. Approximately 5 to 10 per cent of dogs with Cushing's syndrome also have diabetes mellitus. These dogs should be treated in the same manner as nondiabetic dogs with PDH (o,p'-DDD at 50 mg/kg per day and no glucocorticoids). Because Cushing's syndrome causes insulin antagonism, reduction of circulating cortisol concentrations should reduce the insulin requirement. Failure to plan for this enhanced insulin effectiveness could result in hypoglycemic reactions. The complicated nature of treating this combination of diseases should be carefully explained to the owner. Owners should be asked to obtain a urine sample and check it for glucose at least two or three times daily during the loading dose phase of therapy. Each time the urine is negative for glucose, the subsequent insulin dose should be reduced by 10 to 20 per cent. The hyperadrenocorticism in most of these dogs is controlled in the expected five to nine days.

The ACTH stimulation test should be rechecked within seven days of initiating o,p'-DDD to assess adrenocortical reserve. The recheck protocol for these dogs should proceed as follows: (1) the owner feeds the dog at home; (2) the dog is brought to the veterinary hospital between 7 and 9 AM;

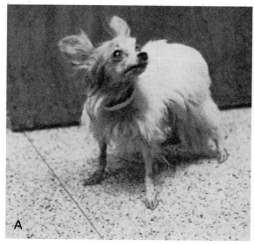

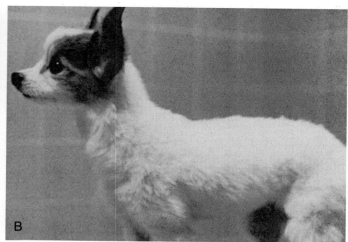

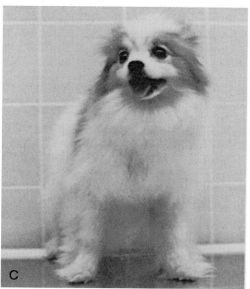

Figure 154–13. Photographs of a Papillon with pituitary-dependent hyperadrenocorticism before therapy *(A)*; six weeks following initial o,p'-DDD therapy, which resulted in the appearance of a new, puppy-like haircoat *(B)*; and 10 weeks later, with a good adult coat *(C)*. (From Feldman EC, Nelson RW: Canine and Feline Endocrinology and Reproduction, 2nd ed. Philadelphia, WB Saunders, 1996, p 248.)

END

(3) the blood glucose is measured, and the owner is observed as insulin is administered; (4) the blood glucose is monitored every one to two hours throughout the day; and (5) one to two hours before the owner picks up the pet in the late afternoon, the ACTH stimulation test is completed. This protocol provides an opportunity to answer two critical questions: What effect has o,p'-DDD therapy had on glycemic control (blood glucose, insulin dosage)? and What effect has o,p'-DDD had on the hyperadrenocorticism?

Approximately 5 to 10 per cent of dogs diagnosed with this combination of diseases require no insulin following successful o,p'-DDD therapy. An additional 70 to 80 per cent require significantly less insulin, and their diabetes mellitus is easier to control. The insulin dose in the remaining dogs is minimally reduced by control of the PDH, but the insulin is more effective in lowering blood glucose concentrations. If none of these three results is observed, the original diagnosis of hyperadrenocorticism should be questioned.

Functioning Adrenocortical Tumors

Background and Protocol. The ideal treatment for a dog with a functioning adrenocortical tumor causing hyper-

adrenocorticism is surgical tumor removal. However, some of these dogs have inoperable tumors or metastases, are too debilitated for major surgery, or have owners who will not allow surgery. The adrenocorticolytic drug o,p'-DDD can be used. Treatment of dogs with adrenocortical tumors with o,p'-DDD is similar to the protocol for those with PDH, using the same initial dose of 50 mg/kg per day. If, after the initial 7 to 10 days of treatment, the ACTH response test demonstrates improvement but not post-ACTH cortisol concentrations in the ideal range (<5 μg/dL), the original 50 mg/kg per day schedule should be continued for an additional 7 to 10 days. Another ACTH stimulation test should be assessed after this second 7 to 10 days. Lack of significant improvement in ACTH response testing after the second 7- to 10-day loading dose phase indicates a need to continue the o,p'-DDD at the same or a higher dosage for an additional 7 to 10 days. Duration of the loading dose phase and dosage requirement are then determined on an individual basis.

Results. Using o,p'-DDD, 43 per cent of 32 dogs with adrenocortical tumors had abnormally exaggerated ACTH response test results after the first 10 to 14 days. Despite concurrent glucocorticoid therapy, 60 per cent suffered adverse effects sometime during treatment as a result of direct drug toxicity or low cortisol concentrations. Over 60 per

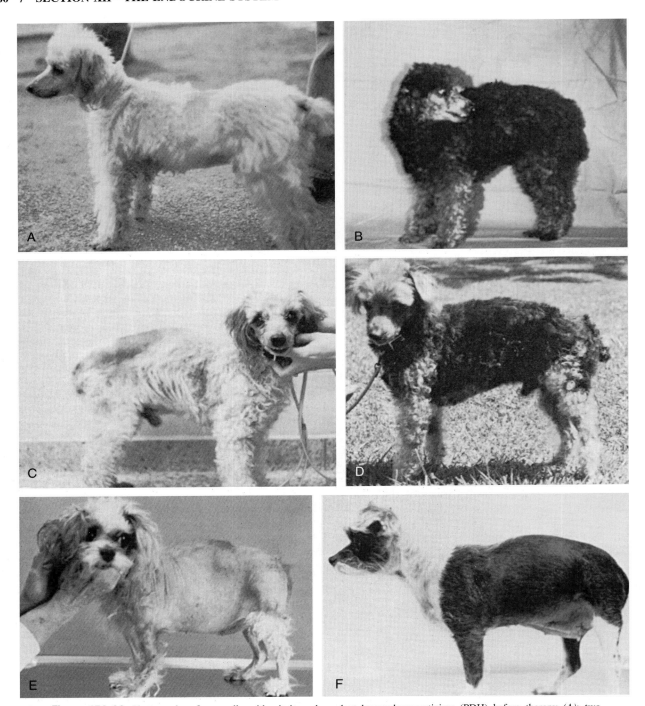

Figure 154–14. Photographs of a poodle with pituitary-dependent hyperadrenocorticism (PDH) before therapy *(A)*; two months following o,p'-DDD therapy *(B)*, showing a dramatic haircoat color change; following a relapse four years later *(C)*; and following reinstitution of o,p'-DDD therapy *(D)*. Photographs of a small mixed breed dog with PDH before therapy *(E)* and two months following o,p'-DDD therapy *(F)*, showing a dramatic haircoat color change. (From Feldman EC, Nelson RW: Canine and Feline Endocrinology and Reproduction, 2nd ed. Philadelphia, WB Saunders, 1996, p 249.)

cent of o,p'-DDD-treated dogs with adrenocortical tumors were considered to have a good to excellent response. Sixty-three per cent of the dogs suffered relapses, and the mean survival period on therapy was only 16 months.[48]

o,p'-DDD Resistance and Histologic Evaluation. The adrenal cortex, specifically the zona fasciculata, of dogs with o,p'-DDD-treated PDH demonstrates acute collapse, necrosis, and hemorrhage. Fibrosis, atrophy, and degenera-

tion were observed in adrenals after chronic therapy. In contrast, reports on dogs with adrenocortical tumors similarly treated with o,p'-DDD usually contain a clear description of tumor histology. The tumor can typically be categorized as an adenoma or a carcinoma.[49] Many of these evaluations contain no mention of destruction or necrosis, lending support to the concept that adrenocortical tumors are more resistant to the lytic effects of the drug.

Maintenance (Long-Term) Therapy With o,p'-DDD

Once the initial daily protocol with o,p'-DDD completes adequate destruction of the adrenal cortex, as determined by clinical signs (reduced appetite and water intake) and ACTH stimulation test results, maintenance therapy should begin. In dogs with PDH, o,p'-DDD does not affect the abnormal pituitary. Therefore, excessive ACTH secretion continues or becomes exaggerated.[35] Failure to continue o,p'-DDD therapy results in regrowth of the adrenal cortices and return of clinical signs. This exacerbation of the disease usually occurs within 2 to 24 months of stopping therapy.

Protocol. Maintenance therapy involves choosing a regimen and altering that regimen as required by the individual dog. Dogs that respond to daily o,p'-DDD therapy within nine days or that have a post-ACTH plasma cortisol concentration of 1 to 4 μg/dL are treated on a maintenance schedule of 25 mg/kg of o,p'-DDD every seven days, divided. Those that initially require more than 10 days of therapy or with a post-ACTH plasma cortisol concentration greater than 4 μg/dL should receive 50 mg/kg every seven days, divided. Whenever possible, dosages should be divided into four to seven treatments per week. For example, a dog requiring 500 mg a week should receive ¼ tablet four times a week. Those dogs with a post-ACTH plasma cortisol less than 1 μg/dL should have medication withheld for two weeks before beginning treatment with 25 mg/kg per week in divided doses.

An ACTH response test should be performed one and three months after beginning the maintenance therapy. If the post-ACTH plasma cortisol concentration begins to rise to or above 4 to 5 μg/dL, the o,p'-DDD dosage should be increased or dissolved in corn oil. Some dogs remain stable for months or years on conservative dosages; others receive o,p'-DDD daily at rather large doses. It is important to tailor the treatment to the needs of each dog. Return of clinical signs suggestive of hyperadrenocorticism should be managed by performing an ACTH stimulation test to confirm disease exacerbation, followed by raising the dose of o,p'-DDD. If the post-ACTH plasma cortisol concentration is above 22 μg/dL, the dog should be treated with daily o,p'-DDD therapy as recommended for the loading dose phase.

Long-Term Monitoring. Many dogs treated with o,p'-DDD remain quite stable on maintenance treatment. It is recommended that these dogs be rechecked with an examination and an ACTH response test every three or four months. Test results allow the veterinarian to adjust maintenance dosages if subclinical problems are occurring. Whenever the post-ACTH plasma cortisol concentration exceeds 5 μg/dL, the dose of o,p'-DDD should be increased. Whenever the post-ACTH plasma cortisol concentration is less than 1 μg/dL, or if the dog exhibits listlessness or anorexia, o,p'-DDD should be transiently discontinued and then the dose reduced.

Stress or Illness. Dogs receiving o,p'-DDD and undergoing any stress (e.g., illness, trauma, elective surgery) should have this drug withheld and be treated with glucocorticoids (usually at a dose of 0.2 mg/kg, adjusted or tapered as needed). The adequately treated dog with PDH has sufficient adrenal reserve for day-to-day living but may not have enough to handle major stress.

o,p'-DDD Overdosage

A minority of dogs (< 2 per cent) develop permanent Addison's disease. Permanent disease is usually associated with hyperkalemia, hyponatremia, and low plasma cortisol concentrations before and following ACTH administration. These dogs often require lifelong mineralocorticoid and glucocorticoid treatment. In the more typical and mild forms of overdosage, the o,p'-DDD-treated dog becomes weak, anorectic, lethargic, or ataxic or develops vomiting and/or diarrhea. Serum chemistry profiles, CBC, and urinalysis from these dogs are often unremarkable. The easiest method of confirming the diagnosis of overdosage is to treat these dogs with 5 to 10 mg of prednisone. Clinical improvement in one to three hours (sometimes it requires 6 to 12 hours) confirms that an overdosage of o,p'-DDD has occurred. Treatment with o,p'-DDD should be transiently discontinued. Prednisone is initially administered to effect (to eliminate all signs), and then the dose is slowly tapered over a period of two to three weeks. As long as the dog needs prednisone, o,p'-DDD is withheld. When the prednisone is discontinued and the dog is stable on no treatment for an additional two to four weeks, o,p'-DDD should again be given, but at a lower dosage.

Prognosis

We have been able to monitor more than 850 o,p'-DDD-treated dogs with PDH. The life expectancy averages 31.4 months. This average includes dogs that lived only days and several that lived longer than 10 years. It appears that good owner observation improves the prognosis. Relapses are common but mild. More than 40 per cent of the dogs had at least one period in which mild to moderate signs of hyperadrenocorticism recurred but responded to an increase in the maintenance dosage. Forty-five per cent of the dogs that died had problems that could have been or were related to the hyperadrenocorticism (thromboembolism, congestive heart failure, infection, diabetic ketoacidosis, or growing pituitary tumor).

Medical Management With Ketoconazole

Ketoconazole (Nizoral), an imidazole derivative, is an orally active broad-spectrum antimycotic drug. The endocrine effects of ketoconazole result from an interaction of the imidazole ring with the cytochrome P-450 component of various mammalian steroidogenic enzyme systems. In vivo, the administration of low doses of ketoconazole leads to a significant reduction in serum androgen concentrations; at higher doses, cortisol secretion is suppressed.[50] This inhibitory effect of ketoconazole on steroid biosynthesis has led to its therapeutic use in the treatment of people with Cushing's syndrome.

Protocol in Canine Cushing's Syndrome

Ketoconazole is administered initially at a dose of 5 mg/kg twice a day for seven days. If no problems with appetite or icterus are noted, the dose should be increased to 10 mg/kg twice a day. After 14 days, an ACTH response test should be completed while the dog remains on the drug. If the condition is not satisfactorily controlled, the dosage should be increased to 15 mg/kg twice a day. The dose requirement should be based on owner opinion, physical examination, blood chemistries, and ACTH stimulation test monitoring. The goals in ACTH stimulation results are pre- and post-ACTH plasma cortisol concentrations less than 5 μg/kg. Clinical remission usually requires 30 mg/kg per day chronically.

Results

We have evaluated the use of this drug in more than 50 dogs with naturally occurring hyperadrenocorticism, including dogs with PDH and dogs with adrenocortical tumors. All underwent treatment with ketoconazole at 30 mg/kg divided into two daily doses. The drug lasts 8 to 16 hours in most dogs and is most effective when administered twice a day. Laboratory data demonstrate that approximately 80 per cent of treated dogs have a rapid reduction in serum cortisol concentration and cortisol responsiveness to ACTH. In dogs treated for more than two months, there was significant improvement in their clinical condition, as evidenced by a reduction in water intake, urine production, appetite, panting, and weight. Regrowth of hair and return of muscle strength were also noted. Signs of toxicity rarely developed. Signs of overdosage were usually those of hypocortisolism.[51]

It appears that 20 to 25 per cent of dogs fail to respond to ketoconazole owing to poor intestinal absorption. Although this is true for many dogs that do not improve, other explanations must be entertained, because some dogs demonstrate an *increase* in pre- and post-ACTH plasma cortisol concentrations when receiving ketoconazole, as compared with levels obtained before treatment. Plasma cortisol concentrations return to pretreatment levels when the drug is discontinued. The major drawbacks to the use of this drug are its expense, the failure of some dogs to respond, and the necessity for twice-a-day administration indefinitely.

Indications

Ketoconazole, with its low incidence of toxicity and negligible effects on mineralocorticoid production, may be an attractive (albeit expensive) alternative in the medical management of canine hyperadrenocorticism. Ketoconazole is readily available through human pharmacies. The effects on enzyme blockage are completely reversible. It may be used as an alternative to o,p'-DDD in the medical management of dogs with malignant, large, or invasive adrenal tumors if surgical intervention is not an option but palliative therapy is desired. Ketoconazole is used most frequently to stabilize dogs before surgery.

Other Medications

L-Deprenyl

L-deprenyl is approved for use in humans with Parkinson's disease and for dogs with hyperadrenocorticism. It acts as an irreversible inhibitor of the enzyme monoamine oxidase type B, thereby promoting normalization of dopamine. Normally, ACTH secretion is controlled, in part, by hypothalamic CRH secretion via positive feedback. It has been hypothesized that ACTH is also controlled via a negative feedback mechanism mediated by dopamine and that PDH may be caused by a lack of this negative suppression of ACTH. This hypothesis was suggested in the 1960s for people with Cushing's syndrome but has never received support, nor has it been proved in dogs. It is now suggested that L-deprenyl, by enhancing dopamine concentrations, may downregulate ACTH and control Cushing's. There has been only one objective report in the veterinary literature on this drug (all others have been sponsored by the manufacturers of L-deprenyl). In that report, no improvement was documented in water intake, urine output, urine concentration, ACTH stimulation test results, low-dose dexamethasone test results, or urine cortisol-creatinine ratios. However, most owners believe that their pets are healthier when receiving the drug.[52] A review of the information supplied to the Food and Drug Administration by the manufacturers of L-deprenyl in order to receive a license to market the drug (obtained through the Freedom of Information Act) found that virtually no supportive data are given. In the first study of 34 dogs (the drug was supplied for free), only five owners still had their pets on the medication at 15 months. Of 52 dogs in the second study, only 19 dogs (36 per cent) were receiving the drug at the ninth month of treatment. In the third study of 39 dogs, 17 (44 per cent) were still on the drug at six months and were thought to have "improved quality of life." Side effects of L-deprenyl include vomiting, diarrhea, restlessness, lethargy, salivation, anorexia, deafness, pruritus, licking, shivering, trembling, and shaking. We do not recommend use of this drug.

Mifepristone (RU486)

RU486 is a 19-norsteroid that has anticortisol activity by virtue of its ability to inhibit cortisol binding competitively at the receptor level. The result is blockage of the feedback effect of cortisol on ACTH secretion, as well as blockage of the systemic effects of cortisol. Thus, people treated with 4 to 6 mg/kg have **increases** in both plasma ACTH and cortisol concentrations, but they are prone to developing signs of cortisol deficiency (weakness, nausea, vomiting). Their serum cortisol concentrations are increased because it is the binding that is inhibited, not hormonal synthesis or secretion. Treatment with mifepristone ameliorates the clinical manifestations of hypercortisolism in more than 50 per cent of people with Cushing's syndrome caused by adrenocortical tumor or in whom the source of ACTH is other than the pituitary (ectopic; not reported in dogs or cats). By contrast, people with pituitary-dependent Cushing's do not respond with any consistency to mifepristone, because their excesses in ACTH and then cortisol overwhelm the receptor blockade.[53]

Trilostane

Trilostane is a competitive inhibitor of 3β-hydroxysteroid dehydrogenase. This causes interference with adrenal steroid biosynthesis. In a trial study on 5 dogs with hyperadrenocorticism weighing 6 to 47 kg, doses of 20 mg once daily to 120 mg twice daily successfully controlled clinical and biochemical changes due to glucocorticoid excess without side effects.[54] This drug has potential as a safe and effective medical therapy for dogs with PDH or with a functioning adrenocortical tumor.

MEDICAL COMPLICATIONS ASSOCIATED WITH HYPERADRENOCORTICISM

Pyelonephritis and Urinary Calculi

Urinary tract infections are common in dogs with Cushing's, and such infections can ascend to the kidneys. Lowered resistance to infection may result from glucocorticoid-induced inhibition of neutrophil and macrophage migration into areas of infection. Dilute urine increases susceptibility to lower urinary tract infection but decreases susceptibility to pyelonephritis.[14]

Approximately 5 to 10 per cent of dogs with Cushing's syndrome have calcium-containing urinary calculi. Glucocorticoids increase calcium excretion, which may result in calculi formation. The increased incidence of infection also contributes to calculi. Dysuria, a sign caused by urolithiasis, may not be obvious, because glucocorticoid excess interferes with inflammatory responses.

Pancreatitis

Dogs with hyperadrenocorticism have been described as being predisposed to pancreatitis. Dogs with Cushing's syndrome commonly eat garbage and have hyperlipidemia, hypercholesterolemia, infection, and so forth. However, pancreatitis is not common.

Diabetes Mellitus

Diabetes mellitus is a straightforward disease to diagnose in dogs and cats. Hyperadrenocorticism is not as easily diagnosed, but the clinical picture of Cushing's is striking, making the diagnosis in most dogs relatively uncomplicated. It is easy to realize when an established Cushing's dog develops diabetes mellitus, because of a sudden increase in thirst, urine output, and glucose in the urine. However, a major dilemma is encountered when attempting to determine whether a dog or cat with established diabetes mellitus has Cushing's. The major clue used by practitioners is the presence of insulin resistance. Resistance, however, is a subjective phenomenon that has myriad differential diagnoses. The clinician would be best served by relying on the clinical presentation of the animal. Does the animal have an appearance consistent with the diagnosis of Cushing's? This question deserves careful consideration, because the clinical signs (polydipsia, polyuria, polyphagia, hepatomegaly), CBC (increase in white blood cell count and "stress" leukogram), serum chemistry profile (increases in cholesterol, alkaline phosphatase, and ALT), and radiography and ultrasonography results of the two diseases are similar. The urine of the diabetic is usually more concentrated than that of the Cushing's diabetic, but both are prone to infection. Various screening tests for Cushing's may be abnormal in diabetics. This is particularly true of the urine cortisol-creatine ratio but may be true of other tests of the pituitary-adrenal axis as well. In addition to being imperfect, endocrine screening tests are expensive, and appropriate usage aids their reliability. Thus, the diagnosis of hyperadrenocorticism in a diabetic dog is more likely if the pet has bilaterally symmetric hair loss, calcinosis cutis, abdominal distention, low blood urea nitrogen and creatinine with a urine specific gravity less than 1.012, and adrenomegaly on abdominal ultrasonography, in addition to unexpectedly high exogenous insulin requirements.

Pulmonary Thromboembolism

Etiology and Clinical Signs. Pulmonary thromboembolism is a potential complication of hyperadrenocorticism as well as of several other disorders (e.g., protein-losing nephropathies, renal failure, pancreatitis, sepsis, diabetes mellitus, immune-mediated hemolytic anemia, cardiac disease, heartworm disease). In Cushing's syndrome, the syndrome is no doubt related to the hypercoagulable state. Venous stasis and injury to the vascular epithelium are known to induce thromboembolic disorders.[55] In Cushing's, embolic tendencies may be related to glomerular protein loss that decreases antithrombin III and/or increases Factors V, VIII, IX, and X, fibrinogen, and plasminogen.[56] Additional predisposing factors include obesity, hypertension, increased hematocrit, sepsis, and prolonged periods of recumbency.[55] Most Cushing's dogs with thromboembolism in our series had recently undergone medical treatment for PDH or surgery to remove an adrenocortical tumor. These dogs usually have acute respiratory distress.

Radiology. Results of thoracic radiology from dogs with pulmonary thromboembolism are not consistent, revealing no abnormalities, hypoperfusion, alveolar infiltrates, or pleural effusion. Alternatively, there may be an increased diameter and blunting of the pulmonary arteries, lack of perfusion of the obstructed pulmonary vasculature, or overperfusion of the unobstructed pulmonary vasculature. Normal thoracic radiographs in a dyspneic dog that lacks large airway obstruction suggest pulmonary thromboembolism.

Blood Gas Analysis. Arterial blood gas results demonstrate decreases in the P_aO_2 (50 to 60 mmHg; normal, 80 to 100 mmHg) and decreases in the P_aCO_2 (17 to 30 mmHg; normal, 35 to 45 mmHg).[57] Initially, there may be respiratory alkalosis, but the effects of hypoxia and the complicated physiology of this syndrome result in lactic acidosis and mild systemic metabolic acidosis.

Diagnosis. Thrombosis may be confirmed with angiography of the lungs or with a radionuclear lung scan. Absence of perfusion defects practically excludes the diagnosis of pulmonary thromboembolism. The presence of significant perfusion defects in lung regions with normal ventilation and no radiographic evidence of pulmonary disease is most diagnostic for pulmonary thromboembolism.[57]

Therapy. Treatment of naturally acquired pulmonary thromboembolism in dogs is not well described. In experimental conditions, thromboemboli begin to dissolve without treatment within hours of their formation, and complete resolution has been documented within days.[57] In naturally occurring disease, persistent prothrombotic tendencies exist, and the fibrinolytic mechanisms in these dogs may be hindered. The goals of therapy are to reverse the prothrombotic state and to alleviate the hemodynamic and pulmonary sequelae responsible for morbidity and mortality.[57] Therapy consists of general support, oxygen, and anticoagulants (heparin 100 to 200 IU/kg intravenously, followed by that same dose subcutaneously every six hours, adjusted to prolong the aPTT by 1.5 to 2 times normal, and/or coumarin [warfarin] 0.2 mg/kg orally, followed by 0.05 to 0.1 mg/kg daily to achieve a prothrombin time of 1.5 to 2 times normal—takes two to seven days to become effective). Warfarin is potentially thrombogenic during the first few days, and this tendency should be counteracted by the anticoagulant effects of heparin. Ideally, antagonizing the coagulation system will prevent the growth of existing thrombi and the formation of new thrombi that may further compromise cardiovascular and respiratory function. Heparin and coumarin do not directly dissolve existing thrombi. Streptokinase and recombinant tissue plasminogen activator rapidly dissolve experimental pulmonary thromboemboli in dogs, but the effectiveness of fibrinolytic agents in treating naturally acquired canine pulmonary thromboembolism has not been critically evaluated. As with anticoagulant therapy, the primary complication of fibrinolytic therapy is life-threatening hemorrhage.[57]

Prognosis. The prognosis for this condition is guarded to grave. Recovery, if it occurs, usually requires at least 7 to 10 days before the dogs can be safely removed from oxygen support. Thus, the treatment can be expensive, and the outcome is usually not promising.

END

Pituitary Macro Tumors and Central Nervous System Signs

Pathophysiology. Occasionally, pituitary tumors in dogs with PDH grow to a size exceeding 1 cm in diameter. Such a mass, whether present at the time of diagnosis or years after beginning treatment, can cause clinical signs due to dorsal expansion and compression of the hypothalamus; invagination of the pituitary stalk, which connects the hypothalamus with the pituitary; or dilatation of the infundibular recess and third ventricle. The clinical signs exhibited by dogs with macro tumors often reflect both the endocrine (Cushing's signs; assuming that therapy has not been initiated) and the space-occupying effects of the tumor.

Predicting which pituitary tumor will cause clinical signs owing to its mass is difficult. We evaluated 21 dogs with untreated and recently diagnosed PDH with no clinical signs suggestive of a large intracranial mass. Each dog underwent brain MRI, and 11 of the 21 dogs had pituitary tumors that ranged in size from 3 to 13 mm at greatest diameter. There were no clinical or endocrine tests that could distinguish dogs with large tumors from those with tumors smaller than 3 mm.[8] In two additional studies of dogs with PDH and clinical signs caused by an enlarging pituitary tumor, each had a mass 1 cm or greater in diameter. Again, no routine clinical pathology or endocrine test result consistently distinguished dogs with small tumors from those with large tumors.[9, 58]

Clinical Signs. When neurologic signs first begin to be recognized, they are almost always subtle—obvious to the owner, but not obvious to the veterinarian. Therefore, knowing the owner and his or her observation skills is quite important. Common initial signs are that the pet seems to be dull and listless and has a poor appetite. These signs may progress to anorexia, restlessness, loss of interest in normal household activities, and brief episodes of disorientation (the differential diagnosis for these signs includes, among many others, o,p'-DDD overdosage). More definitive but late signs exhibited by dogs with macro tumors include altered mentation (obtundation, stupor), ataxia, and aimless pacing (Table 154–6). Some of these dogs may be misdiagnosed as being blind because their mental dullness results in inappropriate responses to visual stimuli (absent menace).

Diagnosis. The specific antemortem diagnosis of a pituitary macro tumor is made with results of CT or MRI scans. Because these studies involve facilities that are not widely available, require anesthesia, and can be expensive, patient selection is of paramount importance. The recognition of typical clinical signs is critical. The untreated PDH dog with a poor appetite but with other signs associated with Cushing's syndrome should be considered a candidate for a large intracranial tumor. A small number of the dogs with macro tumors in our series (20 per cent) were diagnosed before therapy for PDH. Evaluations should confirm the diagnosis of PDH and attempt to identify any cause for the anorexia (e.g., renal failure, pancreatitis, severe hepatopathy). When the anorexia remains unexplained, evaluation of the CNS is warranted.

Signs of anorexia in a treated PDH dog should always be assumed to be caused by hypocortisolism until proved otherwise. Medication (e.g., o,p'-DDD, ketoconazole), should be discontinued, evaluation for unrelated systemic disease (e.g., renal failure, pancreatitis) completed, an ACTH stimulation test performed, and prednisone therapy begun. If all the above information rules out drug overdose and cortisone does not quickly resolve the signs, an intracranial mass should be considered. We have diagnosed this problem within one to six months of beginning treatment in about 30 per cent of dogs with pituitary macro tumors, and about 50 per cent have been diagnosed more than six months after treatment for PDH was started.

Treatment. The macro-tumor syndrome is being recognized with increasing frequency owing to improved diagnostic capabilities (CT and MRI) and an increasing index of suspicion. Conservatively, 15 to 20 per cent of all dogs with PDH develop clinical problems due to a growing pituitary tumor. The primary mode of treating these dogs is photon irradiation. Success, to date, has been limited. Most of the dogs undergoing irradiation have had significant clinical signs and extremely large intracranial masses. Response to treatment will improve as our ability to identify these dogs earlier in the course of their disease improves, so that the radiation is directed at smaller tumors or in dogs less debilitated by the condition.

Modes of Therapy. Modes of therapy are limited. Most dogs with CNS signs have masses much too large for surgical extirpation. Success in resolving some to all of the clinical signs has been achieved with the use of cobalt-60 photon irradiation or with the use of linear accelerator photon irradiation. Treatment usually involves delivery of a predetermined total dose of radiation given in fractions over a period of several weeks. Current doses include 40 to 48 Gy given in 4-Gy doses three times a week for three to four weeks. Alternatively, 3 Gy may be delivered five days a week, with a total dose of 45 to 60 Gy. Irradiation may reduce tumor size and cause a reduction in or elimination of the CNS clinical signs. Reduction of the secretory nature of the pituitary tumor is variable, and secretion may even increase despite a confirmed reduction in tumor size. Therefore, o,p'-DDD or an alternative form of medical therapy may be necessary in addition to pituitary irradiation.[59]

Results. There are few reports in the veterinary literature, and those reports included small numbers of dogs. Response to radiation can be categorized into those dogs failing to respond to or dying during radiation treatment (approximately 33 per cent), dogs that demonstrate some response and that survive for a few months (approximately 33 per cent), and dogs in which a complete resolution of signs and years of survival are noted (approximately 33 per cent). However, if the dogs were first categorized according to tumor size and clinical signs, those with the most subtle signs and the smallest tumors experienced the best responses to treatment, and those with the most worrisome clinical

---

TABLE 154–6. CLINICAL SIGNS CAUSED BY AN ENLARGING PITUITARY TUMOR IN DOGS WITH HYPERADRENOCORTICISM*

Dullness, listlessness	Ataxia
Inappetence (poor appetite)/anorexia (no appetite)	Tetraparesis
	Nystagmus
Restlessness	Circling
Loss of interest in normal activities	Head pressing
Delayed response to various stimuli	Behavior changes
Disorientation/aimless pacing	Blindness
Altered mentation	Seizures
Obtundation	Coma
Stupor	Adipsia
	Loss of temperature regulation
	Erratic heart rate

*Listed in decreasing order of frequency.
From Feldman EC, Nelson RW: Canine and Feline Endocrinology and Reproduction, 2nd ed. Philadelphia, WB Saunders, 1996, p 220.

signs and the largest tumors probably should not have been treated at all.[59]

Success. Treatment success is not dependent on the source of photons (cobalt-60 vs. linear accelerator), the dose per day, or the total dose of radiation delivered to the pituitary tumor. Although these factors are important, the most critical parameter is likely to be the time of diagnosis. A dog with severe clinical signs and a huge tumor (>2 cm in diameter) carries a much poorer prognosis than a dog with subtle signs and a small tumor (0.5 to 1.5 cm in diameter). There is little doubt that brain CT or MRI scanning of all dogs with PDH, with subsequent radiation of dogs with visible pituitary tumors, could be of potential value. This does not seem feasible in the near future. Certainly, we would recommend radiation therapy of any tumor 7 mm or greater in diameter.

The problem lies in identification of dogs most likely to have visible masses. Use of age, sex, breed, and endocrine test results has not been consistent. Clinical signs associated with Cushing's have not proved informative. Clinical signs of a large intracranial tumor are probably observed too late in many dogs.

HYPERADRENOCORTICISM IN CATS

ETIOLOGY

Approximately 75 to 80 per cent of the cats we have diagnosed with Cushing's syndrome had PDH, and 20 to 25 per cent had a functioning adrenocortical tumor. Cats with PDH had pituitary microadenoma, macroadenoma, or adenocarcinoma. Fifty per cent of cats with adrenal tumor had an adenoma, and 50 per cent had a carcinoma.

SIGNALMENT

Cats with Cushing's syndrome are middle-aged or older (average, 10 to 11 years) and are usually of mixed breeding. Approximately 70 per cent of the cats are female, and no breed predilection has been noted.

HISTORY AND PHYSICAL EXAMINATION

The most common clinical signs of diabetes mellitus are polydipsia, polyuria, and polyphagia, and these signs are frequently observed in cats with Cushing's syndrome, because the incidence of diabetes mellitus is extremely high (Table 154–7). In most cats, hyperadrenocorticism is diagnosed following documentation of insulin-resistant diabetes mellitus. Therefore, polyuria and polydipsia develop as a result of hyperglycemia and glycosuria rather than from hypercortisolism. Consistent with this concept is the small incidence of polyuria, polydipsia, and polyphagia in cats receiving exogenous glucocorticoids and the common finding of concentrated urine (>1.020) in most cats with hyperadrenocorticism. Cats with Cushing's that do not have diabetes also do not have polyuria and polydipsia.

Dermatologic signs, most notably extremely fragile, thin, easily bruised skin, constitute the second most common clinical sign in cats with hyperadrenocorticism. These cats may also have an unkempt haircoat, patchy or asymmetric alopecia, muscle wasting, a pot belly (pendulous abdomen), and pigmented skin. Normal feline grooming behavior, or

TABLE 154–7. HISTORY AND PHYSICAL EXAMINATION FINDINGS IN CATS WITH HYPERADRENOCORTICISM

History

Polydipsia/polyuria
Polyphagia
Patchy alopecia
Weight gain/abdominal enlargement
Inactivity/muscle weakness
Poor haircoat/not grooming
Skin infections
Weight loss

Physical Examination

Potbellied appearance
Unkempt (rough) haircoat
Thin, fragile skin (bruises easily)
Muscle wasting
Hepatomegaly
Patchy alopecia
Skin infections

lifting the skin to administer a subcutaneous injection, may result in severe lacerations. These cats have been classified as having the "feline fragile skin syndrome." Dermatologic infections and hepatomegaly are common.

ROUTINE CLINICAL PATHOLOGY

The CBC from cats with hyperadrenocorticism is not contributory to the final diagnosis. Seventy-five to 80 per cent of cats with Cushing's syndrome have randomly obtained urine specific gravities greater than 1.020. However, more than 75 per cent of cats with Cushing's syndrome have diabetes mellitus with hyperglycemia and glycosuria. Proteinuria, pyuria, and bacteriuria are not common in cats with Cushing's. The most frequently observed serum abnormalities are hyperglycemia, hypercholesterolemia, and a mild increase in ALT. These alterations can be attributed to poorly regulated diabetes mellitus.

ESTABLISHING THE DIAGNOSIS

ACTH Stimulation

The ACTH stimulation test in cats is performed by obtaining plasma before and one and two hours after administering 2 U ACTH gel/kg intramuscularly, or before and 30 and 60 minutes after administering 0.125 mg synthetic ACTH/cat intramuscularly. The peak increase in plasma cortisol after ACTH administration occurs more rapidly in cats than in dogs. Two "after" samples are recommended because the peak effect is less consistent in cats, and two values provide better assessment of adrenocortical responsiveness to ACTH. Reference values for cats may be slightly lower than those for dogs. The ACTH stimulation test is not strongly recommended as a diagnostic aid in cats because it is considerably less sensitive than dexamethasone suppression testing. In our laboratory, a post-ACTH cortisol concentration of 16 μg/dL or greater was consistent with hyperadrenocorticism, and one between 13 and 16 μg/dL was borderline.[60] Only 40 to 50 per cent of the cats we have diagnosed with hyperadrenocorticism had abnormally exaggerated test results.

Low-Dose Dexamethasone Suppression Test

Dexamethasone should be given intravenously at a dose of 0.01 to 0.015 mg/kg, with plasma cortisols obtained

END

before and four and eight hours after administration. During the eight-hour test period, the cat should be kept as quiet as possible in its cage. Using the normal values established in one study,[60] post-dexamethasone plasma cortisol concentrations of 1 μg/dL or less at four and eight hours are considered normal. Concentrations of 1.1 to 1.4 μg/dL at four and eight hours are borderline, and concentrations of 1.5 μg/dL or greater at both four and eight hours are consistent with a diagnosis of hyperadrenocorticism. Because 15 to 20 per cent of normal cats fail to demonstrate suppression after this low dose of dexamethasone (or they "escape" transiently from the suppressive effects of dexamethasone), we recommend that cats suspected of having Cushing's syndrome also be tested with a 0.1 mg/kg dose of dexamethasone. Failure to suppress on both these doses is strongly consistent with a diagnosis of hyperadrenocorticism. Approximately 90 per cent of cats with Cushing's syndrome have failed to demonstrate suppression in plasma cortisol concentrations on any of the low-dose dexamethasone test protocols (0.01, 0.015, 0.1 mg/kg).

Urine Cortisol-Creatinine Ratio

The use of urine cortisol-creatinine ratio for feline Cushing's syndrome has gained support. Sensitivity and specificity are similar to those in dogs.[61, 62]

DISCRIMINATION TESTING

The only consistent and reliable therapy to date is surgical removal of one or both adrenals. Therefore, although discrimination testing may be interesting and informative, especially to a surgeon, the management of these cats is often similar, regardless of their underlying disease.

High-Dose Dexamethasone Suppression Tests

Two high-dose dexamethasone tests are recommended. They should be performed on separate days by collecting blood (plasma) samples before and four and eight hours after intravenous dexamethasone administration of 0.1 mg/kg and then 1 mg/kg. Arbitrarily, suppression of post-dexamethasone plasma cortisol concentrations is defined as values less than 50 per cent of baseline. Suppression can also be defined as plasma cortisol concentrations less than 1 μg/dL at four or eight hours. Plasma cortisol concentrations of 1 to 1.5 μg/dL should be considered borderline. If the results are 1.5 μg/dL or greater and less than 50 per cent of baseline, the interpretation would be PDH. Lack of suppression, either on a percentage basis (<50 per cent of baseline) or using absolute values (<1 μg/dL), would be consistent with PDH or with an adrenocortical tumor causing Cushing's syndrome.

Plasma Endogenous ACTH

Using canine and human values, a result greater than 45 pg/mL is consistent with PDH, and one less than 10 pg/mL is consistent with an adrenocortical tumor. However, in cats the normal range is 0 to 110 pg/mL. In 11 of our cats diagnosed with Cushing's syndrome and in 5 from the literature, the results were correct for the final diagnosis. Three cats with adrenal tumor had undetectable to low endogenous plasma ACTH concentration, and 13 cats with PDH had ACTH values that ranged from 9 to more than 1000 pg/mL

(mean, 281 pg/mL). As in dogs and humans, this test can be interpreted reliably only after the diagnosis has been confirmed with acceptable screening test results.

Abdominal Ultrasonography

Ultrasonography is an excellent tool for distinguishing PDH from adrenocortical tumor. Visualizing symmetrically normal or large glands would be suggestive of PDH. If one obviously enlarged, misshapen, and/or compressive adrenal is seen, one should be suspicious of an adrenocortical tumor.

TREATMENT

Hyperadrenocorticism is remarkably debilitating in cats. Although therapy is difficult and the prognosis is guarded, an attempt is usually made to control the disease because of the deteriorating clinical condition of afflicted cats. Adrenalectomy—unilateral in cats with adrenal tumor, or bilateral in cats with PDH—has provided the best results.

Medical Therapy

Transient resolution of hyperadrenocorticism can be extremely beneficial to cats in which surgery is planned. Cats with Cushing's syndrome often have extremely fragile skin, are prone to infection, and heal poorly. Complications from these problems can be catastrophic. These complications can be minimized by presurgical management of the Cushing's. We have had poor responses to o,p'-DDD and to ketoconazole in cats. According to one report, a cat with Cushing's syndrome treated with metyrapone demonstrated transient reduction in baseline and ACTH-stimulated cortisol concentrations and amelioration of clinical signs, and the cat underwent subsequent successful adrenalectomy.[63] The dose at which the best results were described was 65 mg/kg orally twice a day. It is important to point out that this cat was also diabetic and suffered from a severe hypoglycemic reaction after metyrapone treatment was initiated, owing to reduction of cortisol concentrations and decreased insulin antagonism. Unfortunately, metyrapone is not consistently available. At the time of this writing, the drug was available to physicians for investigational use only.

Radiation

Cobalt-60 radiation therapy of several cats with visible pituitary tumors was not successful in resolving hypercortisolism.

Surgical Therapy

In our experience, surgical adrenalectomy (unilateral in cats with adrenocortical tumor; bilateral in cats with PDH) has provided the best response in managing cats with hyperadrenocorticism. The surgery protocol and medical management of cats during and after the procedure are similar to those used in dogs and are only briefly reviewed here.

Pre- and Postsurgical Management. Conservative volumes of intravenous fluids are recommended, plus parenteral antibiotics. Intermediate-acting insulin (Lente) should be administered at 50 per cent of the usual morning dose to those cats with diabetes mellitus. A continuous intravenous infusion of hydrocortisone (625 μg/kg per hour) is recommended from the time of anesthetic induction until 24 to 48 hours after surgery is completed. Oral prednisone (2.5 mg/cat twice a day) should be given to all cats when the hydrocortisone infusion is discontinued. Mineralocorticoid should be administered to those cats undergoing bilateral adrenalectomy or in which hyperkalemia and/or hyponatremia is documented after surgery. Serum electrolyte concentrations should be evaluated twice a day for several days after surgery. Fludrocortisone acetate (0.1 to 0.3 mg/cat) or desoxycorticosterone pivalate (2.2 mg/kg subcutaneously every 25 days) is recommended.

Surgery. Adrenalectomy procedures are well described elsewhere. If discrimination tests are not performed or are not conclusive, the surgeon must be prepared to make decisions during the procedure regarding removal of one or both adrenals. Eight of the cats we have treated were diagnosed as having PDH and had both adrenal glands surgically removed. Two cats had adrenocortical tumors removed (one adenoma and one adenocarcinoma). These two cats were among the three longest living cats following surgery (12 and >30 months, respectively).[64]

Postsurgical Complications. Postoperative complications contributing to death or euthanasia include sepsis, pancreatitis, thromboembolic phenomena, wound dehiscence, and adrenal insufficiency.[64] Sepsis was identified in 50 per cent of our most recently treated cats, causing most of the problems we encountered with morbidity and mortality. Preoperative medical management of the Cushing's syndrome and administration of anticoagulants may be extremely beneficial in preventing many of these complications. Two cats that survived bilateral adrenalectomy, subsequently (2 and 14 months later) developed signs consistent with large intracranial masses. Both were euthanized, and necropsy was allowed in one cat. That cat had a 12-mm pituitary mass that was believed to have caused the clinical signs.

PROGNOSIS

Hyperadrenocorticism must be considered a serious disease with a guarded to grave prognosis in cats. The deleterious effects of chronic hypercortisolism on skin fragility as well as on immune and cardiovascular function are frequently responsible for the death of untreated cats. Medical therapies have had limited success, and surgery has been difficult to perform owing to the debilitated condition of these cats. The longest surviving cats are those that have had an adrenocortical adenoma or carcinoma removed surgically. The most important determinant of long-term prognosis in cats undergoing adrenalectomy is the ability of the owner and the clinician to successfully manage the iatrogenic adrenal insufficiency. Addisonian crises occurred in several of our cats months after surgery and were believed to be responsible for the death of several cats.

REFERENCES

1. Tyrrell JB, et al: Glucocorticoids and adrenal androgens. In Greenspan FS (ed): Basic and Clinical Endocrinology, 3rd ed. Los Altos, CA, Lange Med Publications, 1991, p 323.
2. Halmi NS, et al: Pituitary intermediate lobe in the dog. Two cell types and high bioactive adrenocorticotropin content. Science 211:72, 1981.
3. Peterson ME, et al: Immunocytochemical study of the hypophysis in 25 dogs with pituitary-dependent hyperadrenocorticism. Acta Endocrinol 101:15, 1982.
4. Peterson M: Pathophysiology of canine pituitary-dependent hyperadrenocorticism. Front Hormone Res 17:37, 1987.
5. Leroy J, Feldman EC: Clinical comparison of dogs with pituitary-dependent hyperadrenocorticism of pars distalis versus pars intermedia origin. Proceedings of the Seventh Annual Veterinary Medical Forum, ACVIM, San Diego, 1989, pp 1034.
6. Reusch CE, Feldman EC: Canine hyperadrenocorticism due to adrenocortical neoplasia. J Vet Intern Med 5:3, 1991.
7. Ford SL, et al: Hyperadrenocorticism caused by bilateral adrenocortical neoplasia in dogs: Four cases (1983–1988). JAVMA 202:789, 1993.
8. Bertoy EH, et al: Magnetic resonance imaging of the brain in dogs with recently diagnosed but untreated pituitary-dependent hyperadrenocorticism. JAVMA 206:651, 1995.
9. Duesberg CA, et al: Magnetic resonance imaging for diagnosis of pituitary macrotumors in dogs. JAVMA 206:657, 1995.
10. Findling JW, Tyrrell JB: Anterior pituitary gland. In Greenspan FS (ed): Basic and Clinical Endocrinology, 3rd ed. Los Altos, CA, Lange Medical Publications, 1991, pp 79–132.
11. Mattson A, et al: Clinical features suggesting hyperadrenocorticism associated with sudden acquired retinal degeneration syndrome in a dog. J Am Anim Hosp Assoc 28:199, 1992.
12. Badylak SF, Van Vleet JF: Tissue gamma-glutamyl transpeptidase activity and hepatic ultrastructural alterations in dogs with experimentally induced glucocorticoid hepatopathy. Am J Vet Res 43:649, 1982.
13. Teske E, et al: Corticosteroid-induced alkaline phosphatase isoenzyme in the diagnosis of canine hypercortism. Vet Rec 125:12, 1989.
14. Lulich JP, Osborne CA: Bacterial infections of the urinary tract. In Ettinger SJ, Feldman EC (eds): Textbook of Veterinary Internal Medicine, 4th ed. Philadelphia, WB Saunders, 1995, 1775–1787.
15. Ortega TO, et al: Systemic arterial blood pressure and urine protein/creatinine ratio in dogs with hyperadrenocorticism. JAVMA 209:1724, 1996.
16. Littman MP, et al: Spontaneous systemic hypertension in dogs: Five cases (1981–1983). JAVMA 193:486, 1988.
17. Torres SMF, et al: Effect of oral administration of prednisolone on thyroid function in dogs. Am J Vet Res 52:412, 1991.
18. Penninck DG, et al: Radiologic features of canine hyperadrenocorticism caused by autonomously functioning adrenocortical tumors: 23 cases (1978–1986). JAVMA 192:1604, 1988.
19. Kantrowitz BM, Nyland TG, Feldman EC: Adrenal ultrasonography in the dog. Vet Radiol 27:15, 1986.
20. Barthez PY, et al: Ultrasonographic evaluation of the adrenal glands in dogs. JAVMA 207:1180, 1995.
21. Kaplan AJ, et al: Effects of nonadrenal disease on the results of diagnostic tests for hyperadrenocorticism in dogs. J Vet Intern Med 6:161, 1994.
22. Orth DN: Cushing's syndrome. N Engl J Med 332:791, 1995.
23. Smiley LE, Peterson ME: Evaluation of a urine cortisol:creatinine ratio as a screening test for hyperadrenocorticism in dogs. J Vet Intern Med 7:163, 1993.
24. Feldman EC, Mack RE: Urine cortisol:creatinine ratio as a screening test for hyperadrenocorticism in dogs. JAVMA 200:1637, 1992.
25. Feldman EC, et al: Comparison of aqueous porcine ACTH with synthetic ACTH in adrenal stimulation tests of the female dog. Am J Vet Res 43:522, 1982.
26. Dyer KR, et al: Effects of short- and long-term administration of phenobarbital on endogenous ACTH concentration and results of ACTH stimulation tests in dogs. JAVMA 205:315, 1994.
27. Chauvet AE, et al: Effects of phenobarbital administration on results of serum biochemical analyses and adrenocortical function tests in epileptic dogs. JAVMA 207:1305, 1995.
28. Mack RE, Feldman EC: Comparison of two low dose dexamethasone suppression protocols as screening and discrimination tests in dogs with hyperadrenocorticism. JAVMA 197:1603, 1990.
29. Feldman EC: Comparison of ACTH response and dexamethasone suppression as screening tests in canine hyperadrenocorticism. JAVMA 182:505, 1983.
30. Feldman EC, et al: Use of low- and high-dose dexamethasone tests for distinguishing pituitary-dependent from adrenal tumor hyperadrenocorticism in dogs. JAVMA 209:772, 1996.
31. Toutain PL, et al: Pharmacokinetics of dexamethasone and its effect on adrenal gland function in the dog. Am J Vet Res 44:212, 1983.
32. Wilson SM, Feldman EC: Diagnostic value of the steroid-induced isoenzyme of alkaline phosphatase in the dog. J Am Anim Hosp Assoc 28:245, 1992.
33. Feldman EC: Evaluation of a combined dexamethasone suppression/ACTH stimulation test in dogs with hyperadrenocorticism. JAVMA 187:49, 1985.
34. Feldman EC: Evaluation of a 6-hour combined dexamethasone suppression/ACTH stimulation test in dogs with hyperadrenocorticism. JAVMA 189:1562, 1986.
35. Nelson RW, et al: Effect of o,p'-DDD therapy on endogenous ACTH concentrations in dogs with hypophysis-dependent hyperadrenocorticism. Am J Vet Res 46:1534, 1985.
36. Hegstad RL, et al: Effect of sample handling on adrenocorticotropin concentration measured in canine plasma, using a commercially available radioimmunoassay kit. Am J Vet Res 51:1941, 1990.
37. Feldman EC: The effect of functional adrenocortical tumors on plasma cortisol and corticotropin concentrations in dogs. JAVMA 178:823, 1981.
38. Emms SG, et al: Evaluation of canine hyperadrenocorticism, using computed tomography. JAVMA 189:432, 1986.
39. Voorhout G, et al: Assessment of survey radiography and comparison with x-ray computed tomography for detection of hyperfunctioning adrenocortical tumors in dogs. JAVMA 196:1799, 1990.
40. Voorhout G, et al: Nephrotomography and ultrasonography for the localization of hyperfunctioning adrenocortical tumors in dogs. Am J Vet Res 51:1280, 1990.

END

41. Bertoy EH, et al: One-year follow-up evaluation of magnetic resonance imaging of the brain in dogs with pituitary-dependent hyperadrenocorticism. JAVMA 208:1268, 1996.
42. Scavelli TD, et al: Results of surgical treatment for hyperadrenocorticism caused by adrenocortical neoplasia in the dog: 25 cases (1980–1984). JAVMA 189:1360, 1986.
43. Smiley LE, Garvey MS: The use of hetastarch as adjunct therapy in 26 dogs with hypoalbuminemia: A phase two clinical trial. J Vet Intern Med 8:195, 1994.
44. Meij BP, et al: Transsphenoidal hypophysectomy in beagle dogs: Evaluation of a microsurgical technique. Vet Surg 26:295, 1997.
45. Meij BP, et al: Results of transsphenoidal hypophysectomy in 52 dogs with pituitary-dependent hyperadrenocorticism. Vet Surg 27:246, 1998.
46. Watson ADJ, et al: Systemic availability of o,p'DDD in normal dogs, fasted and fed, and in dogs with hyperadrenocorticism. Res Vet Sci 43:160, 1987.
47. Feldman EC, Nelson RW: Canine and Feline Endocrinology and Reproduction, 2nd ed. Philadelphia, WB Saunders, 1996.
48. Kintzer PP, Peterson ME: Mitotane (o,p'DDD) treatment of dogs with cortisol-secreting adrenocortical neoplasia: 32 cases (1980–1992). JAVMA 205:54, 1994.
49. Feldman EC, et al: Comparison of mitotane treatment for adrenal tumor versus pituitary-dependent hyperadrenocorticism in dogs. JAVMA 200:1642, 1992.
50. Engelhardt D, et al: The influence of ketoconazole on human adrenal steroidogenesis: Incubation studies with tissue slices. Clin Endocrinol 35:163, 1991.
51. Feldman EC, et al: Plasma cortisol response to ketoconazole administration in dogs with hyperadrenocorticism. JAVMA 197:71, 1990.
52. Steffen T, et al: Selegiline HCl (L-deprenyl) for treatment of canine pituitary-dependent hyperadrenocorticism. J Vet Intern Med 11:122, 1997.
53. Spitz IM, Bardin CW: Mifepristone (RU 486)—a modulator of progestin and glucocorticoid action. N Engl J Med 329:404, 1993.
54. Hurley K, et al: The use of trilostane for the treatment of hyperadrenocorticism in dogs. J Vet Intern Med 12:210, 1998.
55. LaRue MJ, Murtaugh P: Pulmonary thromboembolism in dogs: 47 cases (1986–1987). JAVMA 197:1368, 1990.
56. Feldman BF, et al: Hemostatic abnormalities in canine Cushing's syndrome. Res Vet Sci 41:228, 1986.
57. Dennis JS: Clinical features of canine pulmonary thromboembolism. Compend Contin Educ Small Anim Pract 15:1595, 1993.
58. Kipperman BS, et al: Pituitary tumor size, neurologic signs, and relation to endocrine test results in dogs with pituitary-dependent hyperadrenocorticism: 43 cases (1980–1990). JAVMA 201:762, 1992.
59. Théon AP, et al: Megavoltage irradiation of pituitary macrotumors in dogs with neurologic signs. JAVMA (in press).
60. Smith MC, Feldman EC: Plasma endogenous ACTH and plasma cortisol responses to synthetic ACTH and dexamethasone sodium phosphate in healthy cats. Am J Vet Res 48:1719, 1987.
61. Goossens MMC, et al: Urinary excretion of glucocorticoids in the diagnosis of hyperadrenocorticism in cats. Domest Anim Endocrinol 12:355, 1995.
62. Henry CJ, et al: Urine cortisol:creatinine ratio in healthy and sick cats. J Vet Intern Med 10:123, 1996.
63. Daley CA, et al: Use of metyrapone to treat pituitary-dependent hyperadrenocorticism in a cat with large cutaneous wounds. JAVMA 202:956, 1993.
64. Duesberg CA, et al: Adrenalectomy for the treatment of hyperadrenocorticism in 10 cats (1988–1992). JAVMA 207:1066, 1995.

CHAPTER 155

HYPOADRENOCORTICISM

Claudia E. Reusch

HISTORICAL BACKGROUND

In 1855, Thomas Addison published the first report of hypoadrenocorticism in 11 human patients in England. Included in his report were a detailed description of the clinical signs and postmortem findings as well as drawings of the adrenal glands, which at that time were referred to as the suprarenal capsules.[1] Although Addison suspected that these organs were essential for life, it was not until about 1925 that the importance of the adrenal glands became generally accepted. In 1942, Thorn and coworkers[2] described the use of the synthetic crystalline corticosteroid desoxycorticosterone acetate (DOCA), which owing to its extremely weak glucocorticoid activity was not always effective. In the 1950s, cortisol was isolated from blood and was recognized as one of the principal products of the adrenal cortices in humans and in dogs. At that point, the fundamental physiology and control mechanisms of the adrenal cortices were finally understood, adrenal insufficiency was classified into primary and secondary disease, and the three major types of adrenal hormones—i.e., glucocorticoids, mineralocorticoids, and androgens—were recognized. Interestingly, the first cases of canine hypoadrenocorticism were reported shortly after the principles of the disease were understood.[3] The first case of feline hypoadrenocorticism was not published until 30 years later.[4]

ANATOMIC AND MICROSCOPIC FEATURES

The paired adrenal glands are situated in the retroperitoneal space. The left and larger adrenal gland is positioned near the craniomedial border of the left kidney, the right adrenal gland near the hilus of the corresponding kidney. Each adrenal gland consists of two distinct parts, the adrenal medulla and the adrenal cortex, which differ in endocrine function and embryologic origin. The cortex composes approximately 75 per cent of the mass of the adrenal gland and can be divided into three morphologically recognizable zones: the inner zona reticularis, the zona fasciculata, and the outer zona glomerulosa. The zona fasciculata, which is the thickest layer, and the zona reticularis are composed of cells of similar appearance; however, the arrangement of cells in the latter is much looser. Cells of the zona reticularis and the zona fasciculata produce glucocorticoids and androgens. The zona glomerulosa lacks a well-defined structure, and its small cells scattered beneath the capsule produce mineralocorticoids.[5]

ETIOLOGY

Impairment of adrenal function leads to deficient adrenal production of mineralocorticoids and/or glucocorticoids. fAdrenocortical hypofunction is usually due to destruction of the adrenal cortices, referred to as primary adrenocortical insufficiency (Addison's disease) or to deficient pituitary secretion of adrenocorticotropic hormone ACTH, referred to as secondary adrenocortical insufficiency.

PRIMARY ADRENOCORTICAL INSUFFICIENCY (ADDISON'S DISEASE)

Clinical signs of adrenocortical insufficiency do not occur unless approximately 90 per cent of the adrenal cortex is nonfunctional.

Humans. The etiology of Addison's disease has changed over time. Tuberculosis used to be the major cause of adrenocortical insufficiency. However, since the 1950s, autoimmune adrenalitis with resultant adrenal atrophy has accounted for 75 to 80 per cent of cases in developed countries, affecting four times as many women as men. In the active phase of the disease, histologic examination reveals widespread, but variable degrees of, mononuclear cell infiltrates consisting of lymphocytes, plasma cells, and macrophages. In advanced stages, the cortex is replaced by fibrous tissue.[6] Autoimmune Addison's disease is considered synonymous with idiopathic atrophy of the adrenal cortex.[7] Approximately 50 to 60 per cent of patients with autoimmune Addison's disease concurrently suffer from or develop other autoimmune disorders. Two different syndromes have been recognized: autoimmune polyglandular disease (PGD) type I and type II. Type I disease, which probably is an autosomal recessive disorder, usually begins during childhood and is characterized by mucocutaneous candidiasis, hypoparathyroidism, and adrenal cortical failure. The more common PGD type II, also termed Schmidt's syndrome, is characterized by adrenal failure, and autoimmune thyroid disease and/or insulin-dependent diabetes mellitus. The majority of cases are familial; however, the exact mode of inheritance is unknown. Additionally, both syndromes are often associated with other endocrine dysfunctions (e.g., hypogonadism) and nonendocrine disorders (e.g., hypofunction of gastric parietal cells, chronic active hepatitis).

It is now apparent that enzymes involved in steroidogenesis are target autoantigens in autoimmune Addison's disease. Of the three enzymes 17α-hydroxylase, 21α-hydroxylase, and the side-chain cleavage enzyme, 21α-hydroxylase is the major autoantigen in isolated Addison's disease as well as in PGD type I or II.[8, 9] The exact role autoantibodies and T cells play in the destructive process is still unclear. However, since the presence of such autoantibodies strongly indicates an ongoing autoimmune process and their appearance precedes clinical disease, they can be used as a marker for present or developing Addison's disease. Other (however, rare) causes of Addison's disease are bilateral adrenal hemorrhage due to anticoagulant therapy or spontaneous coagulopathy; metastatic malignancy or lymphoma; infectious diseases such as tuberculosis, fungal disease, and acquired immunodeficiency syndrome (AIDS); adrenoleukodystrophy; infiltrative disorders such as amyloidosis and hemochromatosis; familial glucocorticoid deficiency; and drugs such as ketoconazole, metyrapone, and mitotane.

Dogs. Substantially less is known about the etiology of primary hypoadrenocorticism in dogs than in humans, although an autoimmune or idiopathic disturbance is thought to be the most common cause. Several reports describe characteristic bilateral atrophy of the adrenal cortices with mononuclear cell infiltration and fibrosis of the capsule.[10, 11]

Anti-adrenal antibodies were isolated from two dogs with naturally occurring hypoadrenocorticism and from two of six beagles that developed hypoadrenocorticism after inhalation of aerosols of plutonium-238 dioxide.[10, 12] In some breeds, there may be a genetic predisposition and autoimmune PGD, with concurrent Addison's disease and hypothyroidism being the most common combination. Diabetes mellitus, hypoparathyroidism, and hypogonadism may also occur.[13–17] Similar to humans with PGD, nonendocrine disease such as chronic active hepatitis may occur in dogs.[17]

Bleeding disorders and infectious or infiltrative diseases are rare causes of primary hypoadrenocorticism in dogs. Iatrogenic hypoadrenocorticism due to overdoses of o,p'-DDD occurs commonly, although most dogs have only transient signs of glucocorticoid deficiency and less than 2 per cent of these dogs develop permanent, complete Addison's disease. The effect of ketoconazole, which inhibits steroid synthesis by blocking several P-450 enzyme systems, quickly wears off after cessation of the drug.

SECONDARY ADRENOCORTICAL INSUFFICIENCY

Naturally occurring secondary adrenocortical failure due to ACTH deficiency (either direct or due to reduced corticotropin-releasing hormone (CRH) secretion) is rare in humans and not well described in dogs. Destructive lesions in the pituitary or hypothalamus are usually associated with neoplasia, inflammation, or trauma, mostly leading to multiple pituitary hormone deficiencies. In humans, most cases of isolated ACTH deficiency are due to lymphocytic hypophysitis, a disease not yet described in the dog. Iatrogenic secondary adrenocortical insufficiency attributable to long-term glucocorticoid therapy is much more common than the naturally occurring disease. Depending on dose, preparation, duration of treatment, and individual sensitivity, suppression of the hypothalamo-pituitary-adrenocortical axis may persist for weeks or months after cessation of glucocorticoids. Similar long-lasting suppression occurs in dogs and cats treated with progestins.[18, 19] The majority of dogs receiving treatment for any length of time do not develop signs following cessation of therapy. However, a clinical problem may arise if a dog encounters a stressful situation and does not possess sufficient adrenal reserve to meet physiologic demands.

PATHOPHYSIOLOGY

The adrenal cortex consists of two separate functional units: the zona glomerulosa and the inner two zones. These two regions differ with regard to regulation and to secretory products, because of differing enzymatic make-ups (Fig. 155–1).

GLUCOCORTICOIDS

Biologic Effects. The synthesis and release of glucocorticoids (and adrenal androgens) are controlled almost exclusively by ACTH. Secretion of ACTH in turn is controlled by the hypothalamus and higher brain centers via neurotransmitters that regulate the release of CRH and ADH. Almost all tissues in the body are affected by glucocorticoids. One

END

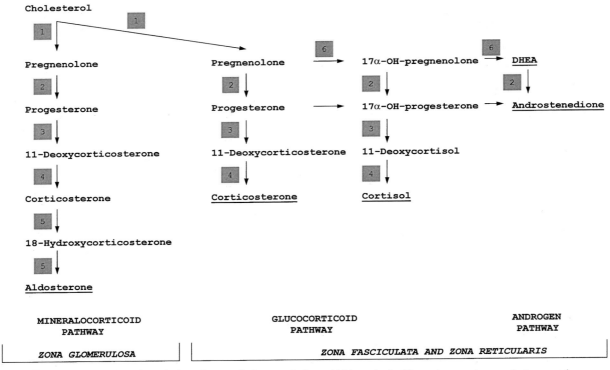

Figure 155–1. Major biosynthetic pathways of adrenocortical steroid biosynthesis. The major secretory products are underlined. 1 = Cholesterol desmolase (side-chain cleavage enzyme, P450scc); 2 = 3β-hydroxysteroid dehydrogenase; 3 = 21β-hydroxylase (P450c21); 4 = 11β-hydroxylase (P450c11); 5 = aldosterone synthase; 6 = 17α-hydroxylase (P450c17). The zona glomerulosa, which produces aldosterone, lacks 17α-hydroxylase and therefore cannot synthesize 17α-hydroxypregnenolone and 17α-hydroxyprogesterone, which are the precursors of cortisol and the adrenal androgens. The zona fasciculata and reticularis produce cortisol, androgens, and small amounts of estrogens. These zones do not contain the aldosterone synthase and therefore cannot convert 11-deoxycorticosterone to aldosterone.

important metabolic effect, particularly during fasting, is the increase in hepatic gluconeogenesis that results from stimulation of gluconeogenic enzymes. Peripheral glucose uptake and metabolism as well as peripheral amino acid uptake and protein synthesis are decreased, and glycerol and free fatty acid release by lipolysis are increased. Glucocorticoids also affect multiple aspects of immunologic and inflammatory reactions and help maintain vascular reactivity and water and electrolyte balance.

Glucocorticoid Deficiency. Regardless of the etiology, glucocorticoid deficiency leads to lethargy, weakness, decreased stress tolerance, and a variety of gastrointestinal symptoms such as anorexia, vomiting, diarrhea, and abdominal pain. Weight loss and fasting hypoglycemia may also occur. Individuals with glucocorticoid deficiency have a decreased glomerular filtration rate and are unable to secrete a water load, probably owing to increased antidiuretic hormone (ADH) secretion. Vascular compensation for hypovolemia is impaired, and vascular collapse is possible.[20]

MINERALOCORTICOIDS

Biologic Effects. Aldosterone is primarily controlled by the renin-angiotensin system. A decrease in the extracellular fluid (ECF) volume leads to an increase in the secretion of renin, which in turn stimulates synthesis of angiotensin II, resulting in increased aldosterone production. Another important direct stimulus for the output of aldosterone is an increase in plasma potassium concentration. Plasma sodium stimulates the production of aldosterone only when the con-

centration is extremely low. Likewise, ACTH plays a minor role in the control of aldosterone secretion, although it can elicit a transient increase. The principal effects of aldosterone are on the maintenance of normal sodium and potassium concentrations and ECF volume. The typical target tissues are the kidneys (primarily collecting ducts), the colon, and the salivary glands, in which sodium is retained in exchange for potassium and hydrogen.

Mineralocorticoid Deficiency. In most dogs with primary adrenocortical insufficiency, all three zones are equally affected and clinical signs reflect both glucocorticoid as well as mineralocorticoid deficiency. Aldosterone deficiency results in loss of sodium, chloride, and water and accumulation of potassium and hydrogen. Hypovolemia stimulates the release of ADH, which enhances the hyponatremia. Cardiac output decreases, resulting in poor tissue perfusion, and decreased glomerular filtration rate (GFR) leads to prerenal azotemia. Despite hypovolemia, urine specific gravity is usually less than 1.030, which is due to an impaired ability of the kidney to concentrate urine (most likely due to renal sodium loss and subsequent medullary washout). Metabolic acidosis is usually mild to moderate and results from decreased tissue perfusion and glomerular filtration rate (GFR) and impaired tubular secretion of hydrogen. The serum concentration of potassium increases, because of the reduced sodium exchange, which is enhanced by impaired glomerular filtration. Hyperkalemia results in generalized muscle weakness, decreased myocardial excitability, increased myocardial refractory period, and slowed conduction. Ventricular fibrillation or cardiac arrest may eventually occur.

CLINICAL FINDINGS

Canine hypoadrenocorticism is a rare disease with an incidence of approximately 0.36 cases per 1000 dogs per year and a prevalence of approximately 1.8 cases per 1000 dogs.[21]

SIGNALMENT

Most dogs with hypoadrenocorticism are between 2 and 7 years of age, although the disease has been reported in dogs 2 months to 14 years of age. Female dogs are more often affected than male dogs, with a ratio of approximately 70:30. This is similar to autoimmune Addison's disease in humans and supports the hypothesis of an immune-mediated pathogenesis in most dogs.[22] It is generally agreed that castrated male dogs have a higher risk of hypoadrenocorticism than intact males. However, the risk in intact versus castrated females is controversial.[16, 21] A genetic predilection to hypoadrenocorticism is suggested by a familial occurrence of the disease in certain breeds such as standard poodles, Leonbergers, and Nova Scotia duck tolling retrievers and some others.[23–26] Several other breeds such the Airedale terrier, basset hound, bearded collie, German shepherd, German shorthaired pointer, Great Dane, Saint Bernard, springer spaniel, and West Highland white terrier[21] seem to be at increased risk, although familial accumulation has not been shown.

HISTORY AND PHYSICAL EXAMINATION

The clinical signs of hypoadrenocorticism are vague and nonspecific, and compatible with other disorders such as primary gastrointestinal, renal, or neuromuscular diseases. The severity of the disease varies markedly. Typically, dogs with hypoadrenocorticism have a waxing-waning course. This can be explained by the slow deterioration of the adrenal cortex, which may still be capable of responding to normal demands but not to a stress situation. However, most owners report on the improvement in the dog's condition after intravenous fluid replacement and glucocorticoid therapy, rather than on the waxing-waning nature of the disease. The majority of dogs with hypoadrenocorticism have chronic progressive problems, which may have been present for up to 1 year. Some dogs are brought to a veterinarian in acute adrenal crisis, which constitutes a medical emergency. However, even in these dogs, a careful history usually suggests that clinical signs of hypoadrenocorticism were present days to months prior to the acute onset of disease.[27] Anorexia, lethargy, vomiting, weight loss, diarrhea, shaking/shivering, and severe muscle weakness are the most common owner concerns (Table 155–1). Hypoglycemic seizures are rare.[28] During physical examination, most dogs appear extremely ill; however, findings are nonspecific. Lethargy, weakness, dehydration, hypothermia, and weak pulse are the principal clinical findings. Bradycardia occurs in less than 30 per cent of affected animals. Normal concentrations of serum glucocorticoids are necessary for function and maintenance of the gastrointestinal mucosa. Thus, a decrease in the concentration of serum glucocorticoids coupled with impaired tissue perfusion may cause gastrointestinal ulceration and hemorrhage. Although hematemesis, hematochezia, and melena are rare, they can be severe.[29] Some dogs develop gastrointestinal hemorrhage only during hospitalization. This

TABLE 155–1. OWNER COMPLAINTS AND PHYSICAL EXAMINATION FINDINGS IN 378 DOGS WITH HYPOADRENOCORTICISM

	% OF DOGS
Owner Complaints	
Anorexia	89
Lethargy	88
Vomiting	72
Weight loss	42
Diarrhea	36
Waxing-waning course of illness	31
Shaking/shivering	23
Polyuria/polydipsia	20
Physical Examination	
Depression	87
Weakness	69
Dehydration	42
Hypothermia[1]	34
Collapse	29
Bradycardia[2]	25
Melena and/or hematochezia	17
Abdominal pain[2]	6

1 = calculation was made from 267 dogs; 2 = calculation was made from 153 dogs.
Data summarized from three different studies.[16, 17, 34]

may be due to increased stress, inadequate fluid replacement, and lack of glucocorticoid therapy. Megaesophagus, which is often reversible, has been described repeatedly; in affected dogs, regurgitation may be seen.[13, 30–33] The cause was originally thought to be altered membrane potential due to abnormal sodium and potassium exchange. However, since the majority of reported cases only suffered from a lack of glucocorticoids, esophageal muscle weakness attributable to glucocorticoid deficiency or to concurrent disease such as hypothyroidism or myasthenia gravis seems more likely.

Since the history and clinical findings are not pathognomonic, a high index of suspicion and a thorough evaluation are necessary to arrive at a correct diagnosis.

CLINICOPATHOLOGIC FINDINGS

HEMOGRAM

In 20 to 30 per cent of dogs with hypoadrenocorticism, there is an initial mild to severe normochromic, normocytic anemia.[16, 17, 33] The most dramatic anemia, with a packed cell volume (PCV) of less than 20, is seen in association with severe gastrointestinal hemorrhage. In many dogs with a low-normal hematocrit, anemia may be apparent only after rehydration. Life-threatening anemia may necessitate blood transfusions. Anemia appears to be caused by a combination of chronic disease and gastrointestinal blood loss. In dogs with glucocorticoid deficiency, one would expect a leukogram opposite to that of the stress leukogram. However, only about 20 per cent of dogs with hypoadrenocorticism have an absolute eosinophilia, and approximately 10 per cent have an absolute lymphocytosis.[16] However, in a dog with severe illness, eosinophil and lymphocyte counts that are normal, rather than decreased, should at least arouse a suspicion of hypoadrenocorticism.

BIOCHEMICAL PROFILE

Sodium and Potassium. Hyperkalemia, hyponatremia, and hypochloremia are typical findings in animals with aldosterone deficiency. Because sodium and potassium concentrations are regulated independently by a variety of mechanisms, these electrolyte changes may occur alone or in combination.

Compilation of the results of three studies showed that although hyperkalemia occurred in 90 per cent and hyponatremia in 83 per cent of dogs diagnosed as having hypoadrenocorticism, hypochloremia was seen in only 46 per cent of dogs. A decrease in the sodium:potassium ratio, which normally ranges from 27:1 to 40:1, occurred in approximately 92 per cent. Electrolyte changes can be mild to severe; the highest reported potassium concentration was 10.8 mEq/L, the lowest sodium 106 mEq/L, and the lowest chloride 68 mEq/L (Table 155–2).[16, 17, 34] Such electrolyte abnormalities in a dog with lethargy, weakness, anorexia, vomiting, and/or diarrhea could indicate hypoadrenocorticism, although they are not specific. Hyperkalemia may occur when potassium is translocated from the intracellular to the extracellular space, when renal excretion is decreased, in cases of pseudohyperkalemia, or, in rare cases, after increased intake (Fig. 155–2). Translocation in turn may occur in acidosis, in acute tumor lysis syndrome, in rhabdomyolysis, or in reperfusion after thromboembolism. However, the most important causes are decreased renal excretion, which occurs in hypoadrenocorticism, oliguric or anuric renal failure, trauma to or rupture of the lower urinary tract, urethral obstruction, dehydration, and decreased sodium intake. A common pathomechanism has been proposed for the latter two causes: increased resorption of sodium and water in the proximal tubules leads to a decrease in fluid volume and thus a decrease in potassium secretion in the distal tubules.[35] This mechanism may be partly responsible for the hyponatremia and hyperkalemia seen in dogs with various gastrointestinal disorders such as trichuriasis and ancylostomiasis[36] and in some dogs with chylothorax.[37] Pseudohyperkalemia is an in vitro phenomenon, which may occur during the blood clotting process in dogs with severe leukocytosis or thrombocytosis, and in Akitas with hemolysis.

Hyponatremia occurs with increased loss through vomiting, diarrhea, hypoadrenocorticism, end-stage renal failure, third-space loss, and osmotic diuresis. In addition, disorders involving hypervolemia such as nephrotic syndrome, congestive heart failure, severe liver disease, psychotic polydipsia, and the syndrome of inappropriate ADH secretion can also cause hyponatremia. Pseudohypernatremia occurs with hyperlipidemia and severe hyperproteinemia. Diagnosis of hypoadrenocorticism is difficult in dogs with normal electrolyte concentrations. However, these cases are uncommon and occur in only 5 to 10 per cent of diagnoses.[21, 32, 33] The reason for this may be that the zona glomerulosa is spared during the gradual destruction of the adrenal cortex in dogs with primary hypoadrenocorticism. These dogs may develop typical electrolyte abnormalities at a later stage. Another reason may be that these dogs have secondary hypoadrenocorticism. Determination of the concentration of endogenous plasma ACTH is necessary to differentiate between primary hypoadrenocorticism without electrolyte abnormalities and secondary hypoadrenocorticism.

Blood Urea Nitrogen, Creatinine, Phosphorus, Urine Specific Gravity. Prerenal azotemia in dogs with hypoadrenocorticism is attributable to hypovolemia and hypotension as a result of decreased renal perfusion and GFR. Blood urea nitrogen (BUN) is increased in a larger percentage of dogs than is creatinine (86 per cent versus 68 per cent; Table 155–2), and the extent of the increase is often larger for BUN than for creatinine. This discrepancy is most likely due to the prerenal origin of the azotemia and to gastrointestinal hemorrhage. Also because of a reduced GFR, anorganic phosphate is increased in approximately 66 per cent of cases. Normally the determination of urine specific gravity is used to differentiate between prerenal and renal azotemia; in prerenal azotemia, it is greater than 1.030. Although dogs with hypoadrenocorticism have prerenal azotemia, 71 per cent of these dogs have a urine specific gravity of less than 1.030.[16, 17] Therefore, these two conditions initially cannot be differentiated. However, in dogs with hypoadrenocorticism, the BUN and creatinine concentrations return to normal within approximately 24 hours after initiation of treatment.

Serum Glucose. Approximately 20 per cent of dogs with hypoadrenocorticism are hypoglycemic (see Table 155–2), although clinical signs of neuroglycopenia such as bizarre behavior, muscle rigidity, stupor, and coma are rarely observed. The role played by hypoglycemia in the genesis of weakness is difficult to assess because other abnormalities, such as electrolyte imbalances or volume depletion, cause weakness in dogs with hypoadrenocorticism. In some cases,

TABLE 155–2. SELECTED BIOCHEMICAL VALUES IN DOGS WITH HYPOADRENOCORTICISM

	NO. OF DOGS	RANGE	% BELOW REFERENCE RANGE	% ABOVE REFERENCE RANGE	REFERENCE RANGES
Sodium mEq/L	371	106–150	83	0	142–155[17] 139–154[16, 34]
Potassium mEq/L	371	3.9–10.8	0	90	4.1–5.5[17] 3.5–5.5[16, 34]
Sodium : potassium ratio	369	11.2–36.2	92	0	27 : 1–40 : 1[17] >27[16, 34]
Chloride mEq/L	260	68–125	46	3	99–117[16, 34]
BUN mg/dL	371	9–311	0.8	86	13–25[17] 8–25[16, 34]
Creatinine mg/dL	371	0.6–20	0	68	0.8–1.9[17] 0.5–1.5[16, 34]
Phosphorus mg/dL	265	2.4–23.4	0.8	66	2.6–6.0[16, 34]
Serum glucose mg/dL	366	4–547	22	11	70–110[17] 60–140[16, 34]
Calcium mg/dL	371	4.6–15.9	8	29	8.9–11.4[17] 8.5–11.5[16, 34]
Urine specific gravity	276	1.004–1.055	71% < 1.030	—	–

Data summarized from three different studies.[16, 17, 34]

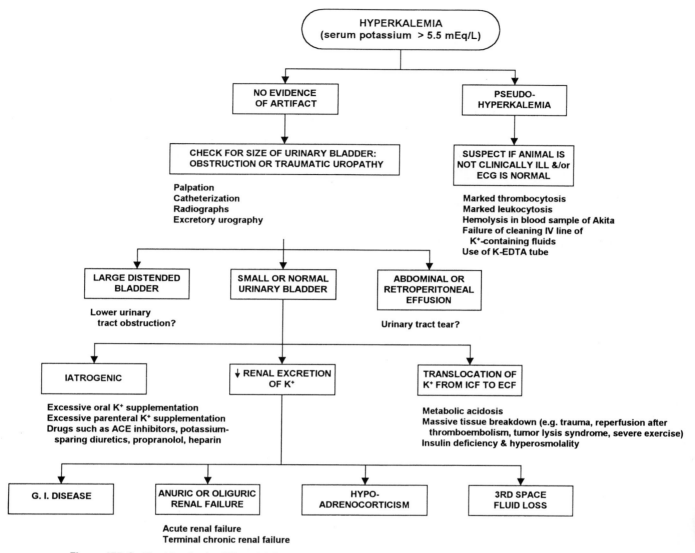

Figure 155–2. Algorithm for the differential diagnosis of hyperkalemia most likely in the presence of other predisposing factors.

hyperglycemia occurs as a result of concomitant diabetes mellitus.

Serum Calcium. Hypercalcemia may occur in hypoadrenocorticism and is detected in about 30 per cent of cases.[16, 38] Dogs with severe hypoadrenocorticism are more likely to develop hypercalcemia than dogs with mild to moderate disease. There appears to be a strong correlation between hyperkalemia and hypercalcemia.[17] In rare cases, hypercalcemia may occur without hyperkalemia. The pathogenesis of hypercalcemia is not fully understood, and more than one factor is probably involved. It is suggested that hemoconcentration is a critical factor.[39] However, since serum calcium concentrations usually decrease rapidly following administration of glucocorticoids, a causal relationship between hypercalcemia and glucocorticoid deficiency is likely. Diminished renal excretion of calcium may be the major cause of hypercalcemia in adrenal insufficiency.[17] The differential diagnoses for combined azotemia, hyperphosphatemia, hyperkalemia, hyponatremia, and hypercalcemia are limited to hypoadrenocorticism, renal failure, and vitamin D toxicosis.

In hypoadrenocorticism, hypercalcemia resolves quickly after initiation of therapy.

Other Clinicopathologic Findings. There appears to be a significant association between hypoadrenocorticism and hypoalbuminemia. One retrospective study demonstrated hypoalbuminemia in 17 of 44 dogs (38.6 per cent) with hypoadrenocorticism, in which albumin levels as low as 1.2 mg/dL were measured. The pathogenesis is speculative; suggested mechanisms include gastrointestinal blood loss, protein-losing enteropathy, malassimilation, and decreased albumin synthesis.[40]

Mild to moderate increases in the activities of alanine aminotransferase and aspartate aminotransferase are reported in approximately 30 to 50 per cent of cases.[16, 34] Possible causes are low cardiac output and poor tissue perfusion. Sometimes, increases in alkaline phosphatase and bilirubin are seen, which may be due to cholestasis associated with glucocorticoid deficiency, although previous glucocorticoid therapy may also account for increased enzyme activities.[16] It has been proposed that in some cases, there may be

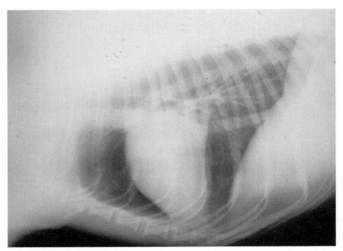

Figure 155–3. Thoracic radiograph of a 4-year old mixed breed dog in acute addisonian crisis. Note the reduced cardiac size, hypolucency of the lung, and reduced diameter of the vascular structures. (From Reusch C, Haehnle B: Endokrine Erkrankungen, Störungen der Drüsen mit innerer Sekretion. *In* Niemand H, Suter PF (eds): Praktikum der Hundeklinik, 9th ed, in preparation, Blackwell Wissenschafts-Verlag GmbH, Berlin.)

primary liver disease attributable to autoimmune processes.[17] Mild to moderate acidosis is often seen.

DIAGNOSTIC IMAGING

Radiographs are usually obtained as part of the routine database in dogs that are chronically or critically ill. Abnormal findings in dogs with hypoadrenocorticism include microcardia, a narrowed caudal vena cava and descending aorta, and hypoperfusion of lung fields (Fig. 155–3). The severity of the radiographic findings usually correlates with the degree of hypovolemia. However, those findings are not specific for hypoadrenocorticism, but reflect volume depletion and decreased tissue perfusion, which may be due to a variety of diseases. Megaesophagus is a rare finding.

It is currently believed that most cases of hypoadrenocorticism result from autoimmune destruction of the adrenal cortices with bilateral atrophy of all three zones. In humans with hypoadrenocorticism, bilateral adrenal gland atrophy has been demonstrated via computed tomography.[41] In a study involving six dogs with hypoadrenocorticism, ultrasonography revealed a significant decrease in length and thickness of the adrenal glands compared with healthy dogs (Fig. 155–4).[42] Thus, it appears that ultrasonographic examination of the adrenal glands represents a useful tool in the diagnosis of hypoadrenocorticism and is suitable as a screening method, especially in emergency cases of acute disease. However, high-quality equipment and expert operator knowledge are required.

BLOOD PRESSURE

Hypotension is present in approximately 90 per cent of humans with primary adrenal insufficiency, whereas in secondary hypoadrenocorticism, it seldom occurs.[6] Little information is available on blood pressure measurements in dogs with hypoadrenocorticism, and hypotension has been reported only occasionally.[17, 43]

ELECTROCARDIOGRAPHY

Hyperkalemia has profound effects on the heart and may cause potentially life-threatening arrhythmias. When clinical examination reveals bradycardia, or when adrenal insufficiency is suspected, an electrocardiogram (ECG) should be performed. In many cases, it can be used to gain an early suspicion of hyperkalemia and immediate therapy can be instituted. As the plasma potassium concentration rises (K^+: 5.5 to 6.5 mEq/L), the first changes in the ECG are the appearance of tall peaked T waves and slowing of the heart rate. With further increase in potassium concentration (K^+: 6.5 to 8.5 mEq/L), typical changes include a decrease in R wave amplitude, widening of the QRS complex, prolongation of the P-R interval, decrease in P wave amplitude, and prolongation of P wave duration. With potassium concentrations greater than 7.5 to 8.5 mEq/L, P waves are no longer visible and there may be a deviation of the ST segment from baseline. Ventricular fibrillation or ventricular asystole may be observed when potassium concentrations increase to greater than 11 mEq/L, although this rarely occurs.[17, 44] The heart rate in dogs with Addison's disease may exceed 120

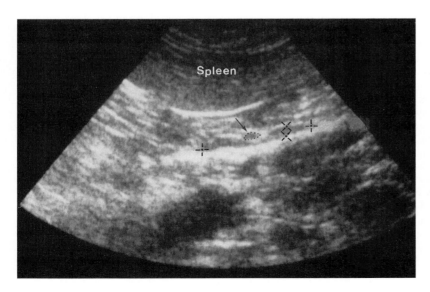

Figure 155–4. Longitudinal sonogram of the left adrenal gland of an 8-year-old West Highland white terrier with Addison's disease imaged in a sagittal plane. Adrenal thickness is indicated by the "x" calipers; the long axis of the adrenal gland is indicated by the "+" calipers; V. phrenicoabdominalis is indicated by "→" caliper. Thickness is 1.5 mm, length 15.2 mm. (This figure has been submitted for publication in the *Journal of the American Animal Hospital Association* and is used with permission. Hoerauf A, Reusch C: Ultrasonographic evaluation of the adrenal glands in 6 dogs with hypoadrenocorticism.)

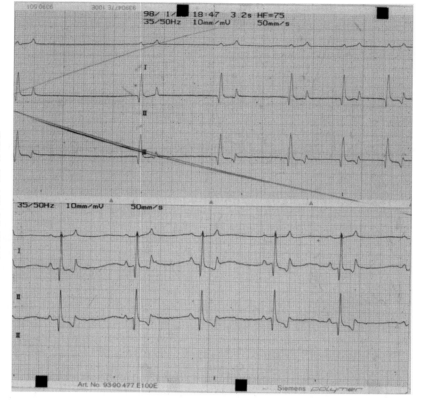

Figure 155–5. Serial ECG segments from an 8-year-old flat-coated retriever with Addison's disease. The upper ECG was taken when the dog was brought to the hospital in acute addisonian crisis. Serum potassium was 10.5 mmol/L (normal range, 4.2–5.1 mmol/L), and serum sodium 134 mmol/L (normal range, 145–156 mmol/L). P waves are absent, QRS is slightly prolonged, heart rate varies between 80 and 100 beats/min. By the time the lower ECG was taken, the dog had recovered and maintenance therapy had been instituted. Serum potassium was 5.6 mmol/L, serum sodium 152 mmol/L. P waves have returned, QRS is of normal duration, and R waves are taller. Heart rate is 80 beats/min and regular. Paper speed is 50 mm/sec, and 1 cm = 1 mv.

beats/minute, and ventricular tachycardia occurs occasionally. It should be kept in mind that the presence and severity of electrocardiographic abnormalities do not always correlate with serum potassium concentrations, because of the concurrent effects of other electrolyte abnormalities, metabolic acidosis, and decreased tissue perfusion. Rarely, severe increases in potassium concentration cause only minimal clinical or electrocardiographic signs (Fig. 155–5).[45]

DIAGNOSTIC PROCEDURES

ACTH STIMULATION TEST

The ACTH stimulation test is the only means of diagnosing hypoadrenocorticism. Sole measurement of basal cortisol concentration or of the urine cortisol:creatinine ratio is inadequate for the assessment of the adrenal reserve, because neither test detects partial adrenocortical insufficiency, and healthy animals as well as those with other diseases may have low basal values. Either synthetic $ACTH_{1-24}$ (Cortrosyn, Organon) or an ACTH gel (if available) can be used. In dogs, blood samples should be obtained before and 1 hour after the intramuscular or intravenous administration of 0.25 mg of synthetic ACTH, or before and 2 hours after the intramuscular administration of 2.2 IU/kg of ACTH gel. The test can be performed either during acute adrenal crisis or after several hours of therapy. In severely dehydrated patients, resorption of ACTH after intramuscular administration may be delayed. In these cases, synthetic ACTH should be administered intravenously or the test should be postponed until the dog or cat is rehydrated.

In comparison with other glucocorticoids, the cross-reactivity of dexamethasone with cortisol in the assay is low. However, prior treatment with dexamethasone can suppress

the hypophyseal-adrenocortical axis and theoretically result in a false-positive ACTH stimulation test result.[46] Thus, because dogs with hypoadrenocorticism respond dramatically to intensive infusion therapy alone, one should initiate treatment by administering intravenous fluids and then perform an ACTH stimulation test, before treatment with corticosteroids. In primary adrenal insufficiency, decreased production of cortisol due to cell destruction results in increased pituitary ACTH secretion. Thus, there will be no further increase in response to exogenous ACTH. In secondary adrenal insufficiency due to a lack of ACTH, the atrophied cells of the zona fasciculata and zona reticularis are unable to respond to an acute stimulation with exogenous ACTH. A post-ACTH cortisol concentration of 2 μg/dL or less confirms the diagnosis of hypoadrenocorticism. Occasionally, in dogs in which the destruction of the adrenal cortex is incomplete, or even in cases with secondary hypoadrenocorticism, the post-ACTH cortisol concentration may be greater than 2 μg/dL. The ACTH stimulation test does not differentiate between primary and secondary hypoadrenocorticism.

ALDOSTERONE

Assessment of the function of the zona glomerulosa usually is not required. In most addisonian dogs, there is complete primary adrenocortical insufficiency and the diagnosis can be based on the results of the ACTH stimulation test and on characteristic electrolyte changes. Theoretically, determination of aldosterone levels would be helpful in dogs with primary hypoadrenocorticism at a stage at which the destruction of the adrenal cortex is limited to the zona glomerulosa, or in hypoadrenal dogs with subclinical changes in mineralocorticoid synthesis. In these animals, the

END

concentration of aldosterone would be decreased after ACTH stimulation but would be normal with secondary hypoadrenocorticism. Determination of aldosterone concentrations should be performed only after ACTH stimulation, because basal values vary greatly.[47] There are a number of assays available, which require serum or heparinized plasma. Samples can be stored at 2 to 8°C for 7 days and at −20°C for 2 months.[17] Data concerning aldosterone concentrations in dogs are limited. In 32 healthy dogs, the basal aldosterone concentration ranged from 2 to 96 pg/mL (mean, 49 pg/mL), and after ACTH stimulation, the concentrations ranged from 146 to 519 pg/mL (mean, 306 pg/mL).[48] In contrast, in 15 dogs with primary hypoadrenocorticism and electrolyte abnormalities, the basal aldosterone concentrations ranged from 0.1 to 1.0 pg/mL (mean, 0.3 pg/mL), and after ACTH stimulation ranged from 0.1 to 91 pg/mL (mean, 13 pg/mL).[17] Further studies involving dogs with partial primary adrenocortical insufficiency or secondary hypoadrenocorticism are required to ascertain whether measurement of aldosterone is a useful diagnostic aid.

ENDOGENOUS ACTH

In dogs with hyperkalemia, hyponatremia, and abnormally decreased cortisol secretion after ACTH stimulation, determination of endogenous ACTH serves only academic interests. However, it is indicated in dogs with abnormally decreased ACTH stimulation test results and normal electrolyte concentrations, because this could indicate partial primary hypoadrenocorticism or secondary hypoadrenocorticism. It should be remembered that hyponatremia also may occur in dogs with secondary hypoadrenocorticism. For determination of endogenous ACTH concentration, blood should be collected before glucocorticoid therapy. Glucocorticoids suppress ACTH concentrations and thus could lead to the erroneous diagnosis of secondary hypoadrenocorticism. Recommendations for handling blood samples for ACTH determination vary. One protocol advises to avoid contact with glass, to pre-cool EDTA tubes, to process samples immediately after collection, and to store the plasma at extremely low temperatures.[17] Another study showed that the stability of the ACTH molecule can be increased by the addition of aprotinin.[49] It was previously recommended to store samples at −70°C; however, storage at −20°C for 1 month appears to be acceptable.[50] Reference values for ACTH vary with the laboratory and usually range from 10 to 110 pg/mL.[16, 17] The assay must be validated for use in the dog. The majority (>90 per cent) of dogs with primary hypoadrenocorticism have marked increases in the concentration of endogenous plasma ACTH, because of the lack of negative feedback. Low or non-measurable plasma concentrations of endogenous ACTH, on the other hand, indicate secondary hypoadrenocorticism. This form of the disease is poorly characterized in dogs, except for iatrogenic cases that occur as a result of glucocorticoid administration. However, because a tumor may be the possible cause, such a diagnosis should be taken seriously.

TREATMENT

EMERGENCY TREATMENT OF ADRENOCORTICAL INSUFFICIENCY

Acute adrenocortical insufficiency, also referred to as addisonian crisis, is a life-threatening situation, which requires immediate treatment. If a tentative diagnosis is made on the basis of clinical, electrocardiographic, or electrolyte abnormalities, appropriate therapy should be initiated. A delay of therapeutic measures until all laboratory results are available may result in death.

Fluid Therapy. Intravenous fluid therapy is the most important component of initial treatment. In an acute addisonian crisis, hypovolemia and shock are usually more life-threatening than hyperkalemia. The fluid of choice is 0.9 per cent (normal) saline solution. The administration of lactated Ringer's solution, as may occur in a case without a clear diagnosis, generally does not constitute a problem, because it only contains 4 mEq/L of potassium, and dilution of serum potassium still occurs. The amount and rate of infusion depend on the degree of dehydration, the extent of ongoing losses through vomiting and diarrhea, and urine output. An initial rate of 60 to 80 mL/kg/hour can be used for the first 1 to 2 hours. After correction of hypovolemia, a rate of 90 to 120 mL/kg/24 hours (1.5 to 2 times the maintenance level) should be used for 36 to 48 hours. In most dogs, clinical signs resolve within this time period and infusion therapy can be slowly discontinued. Fluid therapy results in a marked reduction in serum potassium concentration, restoration of renal perfusion, and correction of acidosis. Monitoring urine output, especially at the start of treatment, aids in the detection of possible oliguric or anuric kidney failure, and to adjust the rate of fluid administration.

Glucocorticoid Therapy. Treatment with glucocorticoids is important. Suitable choices are hydrocortisone hemisuccinate or hydrocortisone phosphate, administered intravenously at 5 mg/kg for the initial treatment and then 1 mg/kg every 6 hours. For animals in shock, a higher dose (50 mg/kg), administered intravenously, may be necessary. Hydrocortisone has glucocorticoid and mineralocorticoid effects, and, therefore, additional mineralocorticoid therapy during the first 24 hours of treatment is usually not necessary.[51] Prednisolone sodium succinate or an equivalent amount of dexamethasone is an alternative choice. To a dog in shock, 15 to 30 mg/kg of prednisolone sodium succinate can be administered intravenously.[52] For less critical situations, 2 to 4 mg/kg, intravenously, may be sufficient. Treatment should be repeated 2 to 6 hours later, as required, and depending on the clinical status of the patient, the prednisolone may be slowly reduced to a maintenance dose of approximately 0.2 mg/kg/day.

Mineralocorticoid Therapy. Intensive fluid and glucocorticoid therapy is usually sufficient to stabilize addisonian dogs and cats. However, in primary hypoadrenocorticism, the administration of mineralocorticoids is required for the maintenance of normal electrolyte balance. When prednisolone (extremely low mineralocorticoid activity) or dexamethasone (no mineralocorticoid activity) is used, desoxycorticosterone pivalate (DOCP, Percorten-V, Novartis) can be administered intramuscularly at a dosage of 2.2 mg/kg every 25 days (see long-term management). In some animals, the initial fluid and glucocorticoid therapy result in such rapid stabilization that parenteral administration can be replaced by oral administration of a mineralocorticoid (fludrocortisone acetate, Florinef, Squibb) at a dose of 0.015 to 0.02 mg/kg/day. In some countries, desoxycorticosterone acetate (DOCA), a rapidly acting steroid, is available and administered intramuscularly at a dose of 0.2 to 0.4 mg/kg, once daily.

Additional Treatment. In rare cases of life-threatening hyperkalemia that cannot be controlled with intravenous isotonic saline solution, the intravenous administration of a

10 per cent glucose solution (4 to 10 mL/kg within 30 to 60 minutes) may be necessary. For myocardial protection, the intravenous infusion of 10 per cent calcium gluconate (0.5 to 1.0 mL/kg over 10 to 20 minutes) under continuous ECG monitoring may be considered. However, in our experience, these additional treatments are not necessary provided that the intravenous therapy is adequate. In dogs with hypoglycemia, glucose solution can be added to isotonic saline so that the final glucose concentration is 2.5 to 5.0 per cent. In dogs with clinical signs of hypoglycemia, repeated boluses of approximately 2 mL/kg of a 25 per cent glucose solution should be given by slow intravenous administration. The degree of metabolic acidosis generally is mild, and bicarbonate required to correct acidosis can be given only when serum concentrations are less than 12 mEq/L. The amount of bicarbonate required to correct acidosis can be calculated from the base deficit obtained from the blood gas analysis; alternatively, the base deficit can also be estimated by subtracting the patients' total venous CO_2 from normal venous CO_2. The number of millieqivalents of bicarbonate needed to correct acidosis is then estimated using the formula: body weight (kg) $\times$ 0.4 $\times$ base deficit. Only about 25 per cent of the calculated amount is administered during the first 6 to 8 hours; further treatment with bicarbonate is usually not necessary.[17]

Monitoring. Monitoring of general attitude and behavior, skin elasticity, capillary refill time, pulse quality, heart rate and rhythm, and urine output should be performed at regular intervals. Determination of electrolyte concentrations and/or an ECG should be carried out every 6 hours. In many cases, the clinical signs and concentrations of BUN, creatinine, and electrolytes return to normal within 24 to 48 hours. Occasionally, this may take longer and other diseases may need to be ruled out.

LONG-TERM MANAGEMENT

PRIMARY HYPOADRENOCORTICISM

Oral treatment is instituted after stabilization of the patient and when it is eating normally and no longer vomiting.

In most dogs, the entire adrenal cortex is affected, which necessitates the administration of both mineralocorticoids and glucocorticoids.

Mineralocorticoids. At present, there are only two mineralocorticoid preparations of importance: fludrocortisone acetate (Florinef; Squibb) and DOCP (Percorten-V, Novartis). The initial dose of fludrocortisone is 0.015 to 0.02 mg/kg per day (1.5 to 2 tablets per 10 kg of body weight), given as a single dose or as divided doses 12 hours apart. Change of dosage should be gradually by 0.05 to 0.1 mg/day (0.5 to 1 tablet). The first re-check should be 1 to 2 weeks after discharge from the clinic. In stable dogs and cats, reevaluation every 1 to 2 months and later once or twice a year is sufficient. Adequate mineralocorticoid replacement is reflected by normal values for the relevant parameters, particularly electrolytes. Mild hyponatremia can usually be corrected by adding salt to the diet without increasing the dose of fludrocortisone. Too high a dose of fludrocortisone can result in hypokalemia, whereas hypernatremia is probably prevented by atrial natriuretic peptide (ANP). In most dogs the required dosage of fludrocortisone increases, particularly during the first 6 to 18 months after initiation of treatment.[17] The reason for this is not clear, but further destruction of the adrenal cortex or a change in the bioavailability of the medication is possible. In a retrospective study involving 190 dogs with hypoadrenocorticism, there was a significant increase in the requirement of fludrocortisone during the course of the study (median, 2.6 years). It rose from an initial median dose of 0.013 mg/kg/day to a final median dose of 0.0226 mg/kg/day.[54] The advantage of fludrocortisone over DOCP is its short half-life, which allows for better control of blood levels. However, a significant disadvantage of fludrocortisone is its glucocorticoid activity. In comparison with hydrocortisone, it has approximately 125 times more mineralocorticoid and approximately 10 times more glucocorticoid potency. Thus, control of mineralocorticoid activity independent of glucocorticoid activity is not possible. A dose that maintains a normal electrolyte balance may therefore result in clinical signs of glucocorticoid excess such as polyuria, polydipsia, polyphagia, and hair loss. In such cases, any salt supplementation of the food should be discontinued and the dosage of any additional glucocorticoids reduced and eventually discontinued. If this does not result in normalization of symptoms, the animal should be treated with DOCP, which has almost exclusive mineralocorticoid activity.

Desoxycorticosterone pivalate is a long-acting insoluble ester of desoxycorticosterone, formulated in a microcrystalline suspension. After its use for many years as an experimental drug, it recently became available to veterinarians as Percorten-V (Novartis). The manufacturer recommends intramuscular administration, but it has been shown that the subcutaneous route is also effective,[53] which means that owners can be taught to inject the drug. The results of a clinical trial by CIBA Animal Health and practicing veterinarians indicated that DOCP was effective in 260 of 262 (99.2 per cent) cases.[21] The recommended dosage is 2.2 mg/kg every 25 days.[17, 53, 55] The actual dosage must be individually tailored for each dog, based on regular reexaminations. Dogs should be reevaluated approximately 12 and 25 days after the initial injection of DOCP. In dogs with hyponatremia and/or hyperkalemia at 12 days post-treatment, the next dose should be increased by 10 per cent. When these abnormalities appear on day 25 but not on day 12 post-treatment, the treatment interval should be shortened by 2 days.[17, 55] In most cases, the recommended dosage of 2.2 mg/kg every 25 days provides excellent control of the condition. Of 60 dogs treated this way, 58 were stable and 2 had symptoms of an addisonian crisis a few days before the next injection, which was subsequently controlled by reducing the treatment interval to 21 days.[55] When the dosage was lower than the one recommended, a shorter treatment interval was required in most animals.[54] When used at the recommended dosage, DOCP does not lead to sodium retention or hypertension[56] and is well tolerated even at 15 times the recommended dose.[57] Side effects such as polydipsia, polyuria, and polyphagia are usually due to concomitant glucocorticoid therapy and disappear by reducing its dosage. In rare cases, DOCP may not be tolerated and a change to fludrocortisone is necessary.

Glucocorticoids. Whether or not glucocorticoids should be administered depends on the dog's clinical status including appetite and general well-being. Only about 50 per cent of dogs on fludrocortisone require additional glucocorticoids.[17] In the majority of cases, it may be prudent to initially administer mineralocorticoids and glucocorticoids together. Later on, the clinician may try to reduce the dosage of the latter and possibly discontinue it altogether. However, should the clinical status worsen, glucocorticoid treatment must be resumed. Glucocorticoids are indicated in conjunction with

END

DOCP. Prednisone or prednisolone is an ideal choice, because of low cost and the fact that blood levels are easily controlled. The recommended dosage is approximately 0.2 mg/kg/day, although a 2- to 10-fold increase in dosage is required in stressful periods such as exertion, illness, trauma, or surgery. The owner should be informed of this and be prepared to administer increased amounts.

SECONDARY HYPOADRENOCORTICISM

Animals with secondary hypoadrenocorticism require glucocorticoid therapy only. A daily dose of approximately 0.2 mg/kg of prednisone or prednisolone is sufficient in most dogs. However, as mentioned previously, the dosage must be increased during stressful periods. If secondary hypoadrenocorticism is suspected based only on the absence of changes in the electrolyte concentrations, but not confirmed by a low concentration of endogenous plasma ACTH, electrolyte profiles should be determined periodically to rule out possible primary hypoadrenocorticism. Iatrogenic secondary hypoadrenocorticism, attributable to abrupt discontinuation of long-term glucocorticoid treatment, is encountered much more frequently than the naturally occurring form of the disease. For its treatment, the administration of glucocorticoids is resumed followed by tapering the dosage until no longer necessary. The time required for the resumption of normal function of the hypothalamic-pituitary-adrenal axis varies, and repeated ACTH stimulation tests may be used for its assessment.[58]

Prognosis. Life-long treatment is necessary. However, with adequate glucocorticoid and/or mineralocorticoid replacement, dogs may lead a normal life of good quality. Even strenuous activities such as hunting and accompanying a jogger are possible. However, it must be emphasized to the owner that uninterrupted administration of medication and an increased dosage of glucocorticoids in stressful situations are critical for the maintenance of the dog's health.

HYPOADRENOCORTICISM IN CATS

Hypoadrenocorticism in cats is rare. The first case was reported in 1983, and since then less than three dozen cases have been described.[4, 17, 59–64] The cause of this disease in cats is not known, although an immune-mediated etiology (leading to primary hypoadrenocorticism) is suspected based on a small number of postmortem findings.[60] Naturally occurring secondary hypoadrenocorticism has not been described in cats. Iatrogenic secondary hypoadrenocorticism may occur after administration of glucocorticoids or progestins, although clinical signs are seldom observed. Cats with hypoadrenocorticism ranged in age from 1.5 to 14 years. There was no sex predisposition, and all affected cats were neutered. All but one belonged to either domestic shorthaired or longhaired breeds. The duration of clinical signs previous to diagnosis varied from several days to 2 to 3 months. Owner complaints were similar to those for dogs, with hypoadrenocorticism and included lethargy, anorexia, weight loss, and, less often, vomiting, polydipsia, and polyuria. The course of the disease can vary. In contrast to dogs, diarrhea has not been reported in any cats with hypoadrenocorticism. The principal findings of a clinical examination are nonspecific and include depression, weakness, dehydration, hypothermia, prolonged capillary refill time, and a weak pulse. Collapse, bradycardia, and painful abdomen occur rarely.[60]

Most cats have characteristic hyponatremia, hyperkalemia, and hypochloremia. Hyperkalemia is less severe than in dogs, and reported values range from 5.4 to 7.6 mEq/L. Hypercalcemia has been reported in only one cat. Mild metabolic acidosis may also occur.[60] Similar to dogs with hypoadrenocorticism, most cats have prerenal azotemia, hyperphosphatemia, and, despite dehydration, a urine specific gravity of less than 1.030. Anemia, lymphocytosis, and eosinophilia are inconsistent features. Because of dehydration, some cats have microcardia and hypoperfusion of the lungs on radiographs. Electrocardiographic abnormalities reported to date are limited to sinus bradycardia in two cats and atrial premature contractions in one.[60] The diagnosis is based on ACTH stimulation testing. Synthetic $ACTH_{1-24}$ (Cortrosyn, Organon, 0.125 mg/cat) or ACTH gel (2.2 mg/kg) may be used. When synthetic ACTH is used, blood samples are collected prior to and 30 and 60 minutes after intramuscular or 60 and 90 minutes after intravenous administration.[65] ACTH gel is administered intramuscularly and blood is collected before and 60 and 120 minutes after injection. A low or an unmeasurable basal cortisol concentration and no or slight increases after ACTH stimulation confirm the diagnosis. The published basal ACTH values of cats with hypoadrenocorticism ranged from 0.1 to 0.8 μg/dL, and the cortisol values after ACTH administration ranged from 0.1 to 1.3 μg/dL.[59, 60, 62] Endogenous plasma ACTH concentrations are used to differentiate between primary and secondary hypoadrenocorticism. The published values for seven cats were markedly increased and ranged from 500 to 800 pg/mL (normal, <10 to 125 pg/mL), which supported a diagnosis of primary hypoadrenocorticism.[60]

The principles of management of cats with hypoadrenocorticism are analogous to those of dogs. For addisonian crisis, initial treatment consists of intravenous infusion of 0.9 per cent saline solution at 40 mL/kg/hour over the first 1 to 4 hours. After correction of dehydration, the rate is reduced to 60 mL/kg/day. Fluid therapy is discontinued when the cat starts to drink and eat and no longer vomits. Glucocorticoids and mineralocorticoids are administered after the ACTH stimulation test. Optimal dosages have not been established. The dosages used in dogs may be used as rough guidelines. Glucocorticoid deficits may be replaced with prednisolone sodium succinate (4 to 20 mg/kg, intravenously) or dexamethasone (0.1 to 2.0 mg/kg, intravenously or intramuscularly).[17] Application should be repeated as required, and dosages should be reduced slowly according to clinical response. Mineralocorticoids can be administered as DOCP (Percorten-V, Novartis) at a dosage of 2.2 mg/kg/q 25 days intramuscularly.[17] Cats do not respond to initial treatment as rapidly as dogs, and apathy, weakness, and anorexia may persist for 3 to 5 days despite adequate treatment.[60] For long-term management, mineralocorticoid treatment such as fludrocortisone acetate (0.05 to 0.1 mg/cat, BID, per os) or DOCP (2.2 mg/kg/q 25 days, intramuscularly) plus glucocorticoid treatment such as prednisolone or prednisone (0.25 to 1.0 mg/cat, BID, per os) are administered.[17] Intramuscular administration of 10 mg of methylprednisolone acetate once a month is an alternative to oral prednisolone or prednisone, if daily pilling is not feasible.[66] The optimal dosages for replacement therapy must be established through periodic reassessment. The long-term prognosis for cats is favorable. As for dogs, owners must be informed of the necessity of correct and uninterrupted periodic administration of medication.

REFERENCES

1. Addison T: On the Constitutional and Local Effects of Disease of the Supra-renal Capsules. London, Highley, 1855.

2. Thorn GW, et al: Addison's disease: Evaluation of synthetic desoxycorticosterone acetate therapy in 158 patients. Ann Intern Med 16:1053, 1942.
3. Hadlow WJ: Adrenal cortical atrophy in the dog. Am J Path 29:353, 1953.
4. Johnssee JS, et al: Primary hypoadrenocorticism in a cat. JAVMA 183:881, 1983.
5. Hullinger RL: The endocrine system. In Evans HE (ed): Miller's Anatomy of the Dog, 3rd ed. Philadelphia, WB Saunders, 1993, p 559.
6. Findling JW, et al: Glucocorticoids and adrenal androgens. In Greenspan FS, Strewler GJ (eds): Basic and Clinical Endocrinology, 5th ed. Stamford, CT, Appleton & Lange, 1997, p 317.
7. Betterle C, Volpato M: Adrenal and ovarian autoimmunity. Soc Eur J Endocrinol 138:16, 1998.
8. Chen S, et al: Autoantibodies to steroidogenic enzymes in autoimmune polyglandular syndrome, Addison's disease, and premature ovarian failure. J Clin Endocrinol Metab 81:1871, 1996.
9. Söderbergh A, et al: Adrenal autoantibodies and organ-specific autoimmunity in patients with Addison's disease. Clin Endocrinol 45:453, 1996.
10. Schaer M, et al: Autoimmunity and Addison's disease in the dog. J Am Anim Hosp Assoc 22:789, 1985.
11. Boujon CE, et al: Pituitary gland changes in canine hypoadrenocorticism: A functional and immunocytochemical study. J Comp Path 111:287, 1994.
12. Weller RE, et al: Hypoadrenocorticism in beagles exposed to aerosols of plutonium-238 dioxide by inhalation. Radiat Res 146:688, 1996.
13. Bowen D, et al: Autoimmune polyglandular syndrome in a dog: A case report. J Am Anim Hosp Assoc 22:649, 1986.
14. Kooistra HS, et al: Polyglandular deficiency syndrome in a boxer dog: Thyroid hormone and glucocorticoid deficiency. Vet Quart 17:59, 1995.
15. Melendez LD, et al: Concurrent hypoadrenocorticism and hypothyroidism in 10 dogs. Proceedings of the 14th ACVIM Forum, San Antonio, TX, 1996 (abstract).
16. Peterson ME, et al: Pretreatment clinical and laboratory findings in dogs with hypoadrenocorticism: 225 cases (1979–1993). JAVMA 208:85, 1996.
17. Feldman EC, Nelson RW (eds): Canine and Feline Endocrinology and Reproduction, 2nd ed. Philadelphia, WB Saunders, 1996.
18. Selman PJ, et al: Progestin treatment in the dog. II. Effects on the hypothalamic-pituitary-adrenocortical axis. Eur J Endocrinol 131:442, 1994.
19. Middleton DJ, et al: Suppression of cortisol responses to exogenous adrenocorticotrophic hormone, and the occurrence of side effects attributable to glucocorticoid excess, in cats during therapy with megastrol acetate and prednisolone. Can J Vet Res 51:60, 1987.
20. Ganong WF: The adrenal medulla and adrenal cortex. In Ganong WF (ed): Review of Medical Physiology, 18th ed. Stamford, CT, Appleton & Lange, 1997, p 334.
21. Kelch WJ: Canine Hypoadrenocorticism (Canine Addison's Disease): History, Contemporary Diagnosis by Practicing Veterinarians, and Epidemiology. Dissertation, The University of Tennessee, Knoxville, 1996.
22. Werner L: Immunological diseases affecting internal organ systems. In Ettinger SJ (ed): Textbook of Veterinary Internal Medicine, 2nd ed. Philadelphia, WB Saunders 1983, p 2158.
23. Shaker E, et al: Hypoadrenocorticism in a family of standard poodles. JAVMA 192:1091, 1988.
24. Smallwood LJ, Barsanti JA: Hypoadrenocorticism in a family of Leonbergers. J Am Anim Hosp Ass 31:301, 1995.
25. Aronson L: Hypoadrenocorticism. J Am Anim Hosp Assoc 32:90, 1996.
26. Burton S, et al: Hypoadrenocorticism in young related Nova Scotia duck tolling retrievers. Can Vet J 38:231, 1997.
27. Kintzer PP, Peterson ME: Primary and secondary canine hypoadrenocorticism. Vet Clin North Am 27:349, 1997.
28. Levy JK: Hypoglycemic seizures attributable to hypoadrenocorticism in a dog. JAVMA 204:526, 1994.
29. Medinger TL, et al: Severe gastrointestinal tract hemorrhage in three dogs with hypoadrenocorticism. JAVMA 202:1869, 1993.
30. Burrows CF: Reversible mega-oesophagus in a dog with hypoadrenocorticism. J Small Anim Pract 28:1073, 1987.
31. Bartges JW, Nielson DL: Reversible megaesophagus associated with atypical primary hypoadrenocorticism in a dog. JAVMA 201:889, 1992.
32. Whitley NT: Megaoesophagus and glucocorticoid-deficient hypoadrenocorticism in a dog. J Small Anim Pract 36:132, 1995.
33. Lifton SJ, et al: Glucocorticoid deficient hypoadrenocorticism in dogs: 18 cases (1986–1995). JAVMA 209:2076, 1996.
34. Melian C, Peterson ME: Diagnosis and treatment of naturally occurring hypoadrenocorticism in 42 dogs. J Small Anim Pract 37:268, 1996.
35. Rose BD: Clinical Physiology of Acid-Base and Electrolyte Disorders, 4th ed. New York, McGraw-Hill, 1994.
36. DiBartola SP, et al: Clinicopathologic findings resembling hypoadrenocorticism in dogs with primary gastrointestinal disease. JAVMA 187:60, 1985.
37. Willard MD, et al: Hyponatremia and hyperkalemia associated with idiopathic or experimentally induced chylothorax in four dogs. JAVMA 199:353, 1991.
38. Peterson ME, Feinman JM: Hypercalcemia associated with hypoadrenocorticism in sixteen dogs. JAVMA 181:802, 1982.
39. Strewler GJ: Paget's disease of bone. West J Med 140:763, 1984.
40. Langlais-Burgess L, et al: Concurrent hypoadrenocorticism and hypoalbuminemia in dogs: A retrospective study. J Am Anim Hosp Assoc 31:307, 1995.
41. Sun ZH, et al: Clinical significance of adrenal computed tomography in Addison's disease. Endocrinol Jpn 39:563, 1992.
42. Hoerauf A, Reusch C: Ultrasonographic evaluation of the adrenal glands in 6 dogs with hypoadrenocorticism. J Am Anim Hosp Assoc 1998 (accepted).
43. Koch J, et al: Duplex Doppler measurements of renal blood flow in a dog with Addison's disease. J Small Anim Pract 38:124, 1997.
44. Tilley LA: Essentials of canine and feline electrocardiography, 3rd ed. Philadelphia, Lea & Febiger, 1992.
45. Willard MD: Disorders of potassium homeostasis. Vet Clin North Am 19:241, 1989.
46. Kemppainen J: Effects of glucocorticoids on endocrine function in the dog. Vet Clin North Am 14:721, 1984.
47. Willard MD, et al: Evaluation of plasma aldosterone concentrations before and after ACTH administration in clinically normal dogs and in dogs with various diseases. Am J Vet Res 48:1713, 1987.
48. Ortega T, et al: Evaluation of fasting serum lipid profiles in dogs with Cushing's syndrome (CS). Lake Buena Vista, FL, Proc 13th ACVIM Forum, 1995 (abstract).
49. Kemppainen RJ, et al: Preservative effect of aprotinin on canine plasma immunoreactive adrenocorticotropin concentrations. Domest Anim Endocrinol 11:355, 1994.
50. Hegstad RL, et al: Effects of sample handling on adrenocorticotropin concentration measured in canine plasma, using a commercially available radioimmunoassay kit. Am J Vet Res 51:1941, 1990.
51. Rijnberk A: Adrenals. In Rijnberk A (ed): Clinical Endocrinology of Dogs and Cats. Dordrecht, Kluwer Academic Publishers, 1996, p 61.
52. Papich MG, Davis LE: Glucocorticoid therapy. In Kirk RW (ed): Current Veterinary Therapy X. Philadelphia, WB Saunders, 1989, p 54.
53. McCabe MD, et al: Subcutaneous adminstration of desoxycorticosterone pivalate for the treatment of canine hypoadrenocorticism. J Am Anim Hosp Assoc 31:151, 1995.
54. Kintzer PP, Peterson ME: Treatment and long-term follow-up of 205 dogs with hypoadrenocorticism. J Vet Int Med 11:43, 1997.
55. Lynn RC, et al: Efficacy of microcrystalline desoxycorticosterone pivalate for treatment of hypoadrenocorticism in dogs. JAVMA 202:392, 1993.
56. Kaplan AJ, Peterson ME: Effects of desoxycorticosterone pivalate administration on blood pressure in dogs with primary hypoadrenocorticism. JAVMA 206:327, 1995.
57. Chow E, et al: Toxicity of desoxycorticosterone pivalate given at high dosages to clinically normal beagles for six months. Am J Vet Res 54:1954, 1993.
58. Behrend EN, Kemppainen RJ: Glucocorticoid therapy. Vet Clin North Am 27:187, 1997.
59. Freudiger U: Literaturübersicht über Nebennierenrinden-Erkrankungen der Katze und Beschreibung eines Falles von primärer Nebennierenrinden-Insuffizienz. Schweiz Arch Tierheilk 128:221, 1986.
60. Peterson ME, et al: Primary hypoadrenocorticism in ten cats. J Vet Int Med 3:55, 1989.
61. Berger SL, Reed J: Traumatically induced hypoadrenocorticism in a cat. J Am Anim Hosp Ass 29:337, 1993.
62. Ballmer-Rusca E: Welche Diagnose stellen Sie? Schweiz Arch Tierheilk 137:65, 1995.
63. Hardy RM: Hypoadrenal gland disease. In Ettinger SJ, Feldman EC (eds): Textbook of Veterinary Internal Medicine, 4th ed, Vol II. Philadelphia, WB Saunders, 1995, p 1579.
64. Berger SL, Reed JR: Traumatically induced hypoadrenocorticism in a cat. J Am Anim Hosp Ass 29:337, 1993.
65. Peterson ME, Kemppainen RJ: Comparison of intravenous and intramuscular routes of administering cosyntropin for corticotropin stimulation testing in cats. Am J Vet Res 53:1392, 1992.
66. Duesberg C, Peterson ME: Adrenal disorders in cats. Vet Clin North Am 27:321, 1997.

END

CHAPTER 156

GASTROINTESTINAL ENDOCRINE DISEASE

Carole A. Zerbe and Robert J. Washabau

GASTROINTESTINAL ENDOCRINOLOGY

ENDOCRINE, NEUROCRINE, AND PARACRINE ACTIVATION

A gastrointestinal hormone is classically defined as a substance that (1) is found in gastrointestinal endocrine cells, (2) is released by physiologic stimuli (e.g., feeding), (3) circulates in blood, (4) binds to a cell receptor at a distant site, and (5) evokes a biologic response.[1, 2] However, the characterization of an event as the physiologic result of a hormonal action may be exceedingly difficult. It is now clear that many substances previously classified as gastrointestinal hormones are neither confined to the gastrointestinal tract nor solely bloodborne. For example, many of the peptides localized in gut endocrine cells (e.g., cholecystokinin, substance P, neurotensin, and somatostatin) also may be found in gut neurons and act as neurocrine substances.[3] As enteric neuropeptides, these substances may evoke similar or different biologic responses. Some of these same peptides (e.g., cholecystokinin, substance P, somatostatin) are also located outside the enteric nervous system in vagal afferent fibers or central nervous system neurons. Thus, some gastrointestinal hormones may also function as enteric or brain neuropeptides. A further complication is that some gut endocrine cells may release peptides into the extracellular fluid from which they diffuse to, and directly act on, neighboring cells. Thus, a gastrointestinal peptide may evoke a biologic response through a paracrine mechanism of activation that operates independently of, or in parallel to, an endocrine mechanism of activation. Finally, some substances (e.g., somatostatin) may evoke biologic responses through endocrine, paracrine, and neurocrine mechanisms—endocrine regulation of gastric acid secretion, paracrine regulation of antral gastrin secretion, and neurocrine regulation of smooth muscle contraction.

Although it is clear that some gastrointestinal peptides evoke biologic responses through an endocrine mechanism, it is equally clear that other gastrointestinal peptides activate cells through a multitude of cellular pathways—endocrine, neurocrine, and paracrine. The endocrine, neurocrine, or paracrine status of each of the well-established gastrointestinal peptides and other bioactive substances is reviewed in this chapter.

GASTROINTESTINAL HORMONES

Gastrin-Cholecystokinin Family

The gastrointestinal hormones[1, 2, 4] and related peptides have been divided into structurally homologous families.

The first family consists of gastrin and cholecystokinin (CCK). Gastrin and CCK share five basic characteristics: (1) partial sequence homology; (2) similar, but not identical, biologic activities; (3) heterogeneity—each hormone exists in different molecular forms; (4) ubiquity—each hormone is synthesized in different cell types; and (5) differential principality—different molecular forms predominate in different tissues and cells.[1, 4, 5]

Gastrin. Gastrin exists in several molecular forms—G-34, G-17, and G-14—gastrin peptides that contain 34, 17, and 14 amino acids, respectively. G-34, also known as big gastrin, is the most abundant form of gastrin in serum. G-17, known as little gastrin, is less abundant than G-34 in serum but is much more potent in stimulating gastric acid secretion. Mini gastrin (G-14) has little biologic effect. Endocrine cells (G cells) in the gastric antrum and duodenum secrete gastrin in response to protein meals and, to a lesser extent, gastric distention.[1, 4, 5] The most important biologic action of gastrin is the stimulation of gastric acid secretion by gastric oxyntic (parietal) cells. A substantial fraction of the gastric acid secretory response to protein meals is, in fact, mediated by gastrin. However, interactions between gastrin, acetylcholine (neurocrine stimulant), and histamine (paracrine stimulant) determine the final gastric acid secretory output.[6] Most evidence suggests that the gastrin effect occurs through the binding of gastrin to gastrin receptors on oxyntic cells, although one study suggests that the gastrin effect might be indirectly mediated through gastrin receptors on gastric mucosal immunocytes.[7] Other important biologic actions of gastrin include stimulation of gastric pepsinogen secretion, gastric mucosal blood flow, antral motility, and pancreatic enzyme secretion and of pancreatic, gastric, and duodenal growth.[1, 4, 5, 8] Pancreatic islet cells (delta cells) are a site of gastrin synthesis and secretion in fetal and neonatal animals.[8] Malignant transformation of these islet cells in adult animals results in functional gastrinomas. All but one of the gastrinomas that have been reported in the dog or cat have been of pancreatic origin (see Gastrinoma).

Cholecystokinin. CCK also exists in several molecular forms: CCK-63, CCK-58, CCK-39, CCK-33, CCK-12, CCK-8, and CCK-5. The predominant forms in serum are CCK-33, CCK-39, and CCK-58 and probably account for most of the gastrointestinal hormone responses.[1, 2, 4] CCK-8 is the predominant form found in neurons and probably accounts for most of the enteric and central nervous system neuropeptide responses. Endocrine cells (I cells) in the duodenum and jejunum secrete CCK in response to intraduodenal fatty acids, amino acids, and hydrogen ion (H^+).[1, 2, 4] As a gastrointestinal hormone, CCK evokes several important biologic responses, most importantly, contraction of the gallbladder and stimulation of pancreatic enzyme secretion. Ivy and Oldberg, in 1928, originally described a humoral mechanism for stimulation of gallbladder contraction and applied the term *cholecystokinin* to this mechanism. Harper and Raper later (1943) described a humoral mechanism for stimulation of pancreatic enzyme secretion and applied the term pancreozymin (PZ). It was not until 1968 that Jorpes and Mutt isolated a single peptide that had both properties. This peptide was subsequently identified as cholecystokinin-pancreozymin (CCK-PZ), or simply CCK. Although CCK receptors have been demonstrated on both gallbladder smooth muscle cells and pancreatic acinar cells, it is now clear that CCK evokes gallbladder contraction and pancreatic enzyme secretion through activation of pre-synaptic cholinergic neurons at both sites.[4, 8]

Other important endocrine actions of CCK include augmentation of pancreatic fluid secretion in the presence of secretin, relaxation of the sphincter of Oddi, inhibition of the gastric emptying of liquids, and stimulation of pancreatic growth.[1, 4] Because of the trophic effects of CCK on pancreatic growth,[8] it has been suggested that canine juvenile pancreatic atrophy might result from CCK deficiency. However, CCK secretory deficiency was not observed in a group of young dogs with exocrine pancreatic insufficiency.[9] CCK has two important biologic actions as an enteric or brain neuropeptide (see Enteric Neuropeptides).

Secretin-Enteroglucagon-Gastric Inhibitory Polypeptide Family

A second structurally homologous gastrointestinal hormone family consists of the gastrointestinal hormones secretin, enteroglucagon, and gastric inhibitory polypeptide (GIP), as well as the enteric neuropeptides vasoactive intestinal polypeptide (VIP) and peptide histidine-isoleucine (PHI). All of these substances share considerable sequence homology.

Secretin. Unlike gastrin and CCK, secretin exists in one form, a 27-amino acid polypeptide. Secretin was the first hormone discovered (Bayliss and Starling, 1902), but the 27 amino acid peptide was not isolated until 1966 by Jorpes and Mutt. Acidification of the duodenum and jejunum by gastric H^+ is the most important stimulus for secretin secretion by endocrine cells (S cells) in the small intestine.[1, 4] Intraduodenal lipid may also stimulate secretin release in some species. The most important biologic action of secretin is stimulating secretion of a bicarbonate-rich pancreatic juice by pancreatic ductal cells.[8] Pancreatic bicarbonate is important in neutralizing gastric acid delivered to the small intestine and in creating an alkaline environment that is close to the pH optimum of pancreatic lipase and co-lipase. Less important biologic actions of secretin are stimulation of secretion of bile bicarbonate and pancreatic enzyme.[1, 8] The latter effect is observed only in the presence of CCK. Secretin has also been identified in brain neurons, but a functional role for secretin in these neurons has not yet been elucidated.

Enteroglucagon. Enteroglucagon and pancreatic glucagon arise from the same gene precursor through post-translational processing. Several molecular forms of enteroglucagon have been characterized, including enteroglucagon or oxyntomodulin, a 37-amino acid peptide; glicentin, a 69-amino acid, C-terminal extended form of oxyntomodulin; glucagon-like peptide (GLP)-1; intervening peptide-2; and GLP-2. Endocrine cells (L cells) in the terminal ileum and colon secrete enteroglucagon(s) in response to intraluminal glucose and lipid. The most important gastrointestinal action of the enteroglucagons is the inhibition of gastric acid secretion.[1, 4] GLP peptides are also involved in the regulation of insulin secretion and glycemic control. GLP-1, for example, is reported to stimulate proinsulin expression, and to delay intestinal glucose absorption through inhibition of gastric emptying.[10] The role of pancreatic glucagon in the regulation of insulin secretion and glycemic control is further discussed in Chapter 153.

Gastric Inhibitory Polypeptide (GIP). GIP is a 54-amino acid peptide that exists in a single molecular form. It is secreted by endocrine cells of the proximal small intestine in response to intraduodenal glucose, fatty acids, and amino acids. Two important biologic actions of GIP are inhibition of gastric acid secretion and stimulation of intestinal fluid secretion. The third, and likely most important, biologic action of GIP is the stimulation of pancreatic insulin release during hyperglycemia. It has been suggested that GIP may function as an "incretin" and may be the substance responsible for increased glucose disposal and enhanced insulin responses during intestinal absorption of glucose.[1, 4]

Somatostatin

Somatostatin, or somatotropin release-inhibiting factor (SRIF), was originally isolated from the hypothalamus and found to inhibit growth hormone and thyrotropin release from the pituitary. A further discussion of these extraintestinal properties of somatostatin may be found in Chapter 147. Somatostatin was subsequently found in gut endocrine cells and gut neurons and shown to have endocrine, neurocrine, and paracrine biologic effects. Two molecular forms of somatostatin have been identified in gut endocrine cells: somatostatin-14 (SS-14) and somatostatin-28 (SS-28). Endocrine cells (D cells) throughout the gastrointestinal tract secrete somatostatin in response to protein, lipid, and bile. As a gastrointestinal hormone, somatostatin inhibits gastric acid and pepsin secretion, pancreatic enzyme and fluid secretion, gallbladder contraction, and intestinal amino acid and glucose absorption.[1, 4] Synthetic forms of somatostatin (Sandostatin) are available for the treatment of gastric acid secretory disorders.[11] In addition to its role as a gastrointestinal hormone, somatostatin also functions as an enteric neuropeptide (e.g., inhibition of intestinal motility) and as a paracrine substance (e.g., inhibition of gastrin secretion).

Motilin

Motilin is a 22-amino acid peptide found in endocrine cells of the proximal small intestine. Motilin secretion is stimulated by H^+ and lipid during the fed state. However, motilin secretion seems to be most important in the interdigestive (fasting) state. During a fast, motilin is episodically released into the serum and initiates phase III of the migrating motility complex (MMC, or interdigestive motility complex).[12] The MMC is a motility pattern that empties the stomach and small intestine of indigestible solids that accumulate during feeding. The cyclic release of motilin from the small intestinal mucosa during fasting is also thought to coordinate gastric, pancreatic, and biliary secretions with phase III of the MMC.[13] It has been shown that microbially ineffective doses of erythromycin (0.5 mg/lb or 1.0 mg/kg) initiate an MMC pattern that is indistinguishable from that induced by motilin. It has thus been suggested that erythromycin and other macrolide-like antibiotics might be useful gastric prokinetic agents.[14]

Neurotensin

Neurotensin is a 13-amino acid peptide, isolated from dog ileal and jejunal mucosal endocrine cells (N cells), for which

END

no definitive endocrine function has been established. Intraluminal lipid stimulates neurotensin release from these endocrine cells. Neurotensin has been shown to inhibit gastric secretion and emptying, stimulate pancreatic secretion, and stimulate gallbladder contraction. One of the most likely potential roles of neurotensin is that of a physiologic enterogastrone that mediates inhibition of acid secretion after fat ingestion.[1, 4]

Pancreatic Polypeptide

Pancreatic polypeptide (PP) is a 36-amino acid peptide that shares sequence homology with the enteric neuropeptide known as neuropeptide Y (NPY). PP is found exclusively in pancreatic islet cells (F cells). PP release is stimulated by protein meals and by cholinergic reflexes. The most important biologic action of PP is the inhibition of pancreatic enzyme and fluid secretion.[1, 4] Islet cell PP secretion likely autoregulates acinar and ductal cell secretions because of the islet-acinar portal venous system. Other possible endocrine functions of PP include relaxation of gallbladder smooth muscle, mild stimulation of gastric acid secretion, and initiation of the MMC along with motilin.[13]

Peptide YY

Peptide YY is a 36-amino acid peptide with structural similarities to PP and to NPY. Peptide YY may function as a physiologic enterogastrone similar to neurotensin in inhibiting pancreatic and gastric secretions.[1, 4]

5-Hydroxytryptamine

5-Hydroxytryptamine (5-HT or serotonin) is found in endocrine cells (i.e., enterochromaffin cells) and enteric neurons throughout the gastrointestinal tract of most animal species.[1, 2, 4] In some species, 5-HT is also found in intestinal mucosal mast cells, pancreatic islet cells, and bronchial endocrine cells. 5-HT secreted by enterochromaffin cells may act through an endocrine or paracrine mechanism to stimulate gastrointestinal smooth muscle contraction and intestinal electrolyte secretion.[2] Tumors of these enterochromaffin cells (i.e., carcinoids) may be associated with hypermotility and secretory diarrhea because of the effects of 5-HT on motility and secretion.

Enteric Neuropeptides

A substance may be defined as an enteric neuropeptide if (1) it can be demonstrated histochemically in enteric neurons, (2) mechanisms for its biosynthesis exist in enteric neurons, (3) it is concentrated in nerve terminals, (4) it is released from nerve terminals by depolarizing stimuli through a calcium-dependent mechanism, and (5) mechanisms for the breakdown, re-uptake, or removal of the substance exist.[3]

The Tachykinins

The tachykinin family is represented by substance P, substance K, neuromedin K, physalaemin, kassinin, and eledoisin. Substance P is probably the most important enteric neuropeptide of this group. Substance P is distributed in enteric neurons throughout the gastrointestinal tract and pancreas, and it is released from these neurons in response to luminal distention or depolarization. Substance P has three important biologic actions as an enteric neuropeptide.[3] First, it causes contraction of gastrointestinal smooth muscle through an indirect effect of mediating cholinergic transmission and a direct effect on smooth muscle during the peristaltic reflex. Second, substance P is located in primary sensory afferent fibers and may be important, along with calcitonin gene–related peptide (CGRP), in pain input to the central nervous system. Finally, substance P neurons stimulate pancreatic enzyme secretion from pancreatic acinar cells.

Vasoactive Intestinal Polypeptide/Peptide Histidine-Isoleucine

The classic enteric neuropeptides VIP and PHI share sequence homology with one another and with the gastrointestinal hormones secretin, enteroglucagon, and GIP. VIP and PHI have many similar biologic activities and are derived from the same biosynthetic precursor. VIP and PHI are released by vagal stimulation and have four important biologic actions[3]: (1) stimulation of pancreatic fluid and bicarbonate secretion, (2) stimulation of salivary and intestinal fluid secretion, (3) increasing intestinal blood flow, and (4) relaxation of gastrointestinal smooth muscle. This last property of VIP/PHI is believed to be important in descending intestinal inhibition (along with somatostatin) and in sphincter relaxation. Functional tumors of VIP-producing cells produce a watery diarrhea syndrome (pancreatic cholera or Verner-Morrison syndrome) in humans. This syndrome has not yet been described in dogs or cats.

Opioids

Opioid neurons are distributed throughout the gastrointestinal tract, spinal cord, brain, and adrenal glands. Methionine-enkephalin, leucine-enkephalin, and dynorphin are the most representative members of the opioid enteric neuropeptide family.[3] At least three different types of binding sites for these opioid peptides can be distinguished in the gut (μ, δ, and κ), but there may be others (ε and σ). The binding sites for these opioids are located on other neurons, smooth muscle cells, and epithelial cells. Opioid binding results in (1) inhibition of contraction of longitudinal smooth muscle through inhibition of acetylcholine release from myenteric plexus neurons, (2) direct stimulation of circular smooth muscle contraction, and (3) inhibition of intestinal water and electrolyte secretion through inhibition of submucosal plexus neurons. These effects account for the potent anti-diarrheal properties of morphine and other opiate alkaloids that have been recognized for centuries.[3]

Bombesins

The bombesins are so named because of their original isolation from the skin of the frog genus *Bombina*. The mammalian bombesins that have been identified as enteric neuropeptides are gastrin-releasing peptide (GRP) and neuromedin B. GRP is released by vagal stimulation, and it stimulates gastrin release from antral G cells. Thus, GRP acts a co-transmitter (along with acetylcholine) to stimulate gastrin release.[3, 5] GRP also stimulates pancreatic acinar cell enzyme secretion.[3, 8]

Somatostatin

In addition to its role as a gastrointestinal hormone, somatostatin (SS-14) has been identified as an enteric neuropeptide in neurons throughout the gastrointestinal tract. Somatostatin inhibits acetylcholine release from myenteric plexus neurons and may be involved in the descending inhibitory reflex of peristalsis.[3] Somatostatin neurons in the submucous plexus have a mucosal projection, suggesting a further role for neuronal somatostatin in the control of mucosal function.

Gastrin-CCK

CCK-8 is an important enteric neuropeptide in the ileum and colon, especially in the cat. Intraluminal distention activates CCK-8–containing neurons, which then stimulate the release of acetylcholine from myenteric plexus neurons. CCK-8 thus acts as an excitatory transmitter in stimulating the peristaltic reflex in ileum and colon.[1, 3] Brain CCK-8 neurons are involved in mediating the satiety response after feeding. Indeed, it has been suggested that humans with bulimia nervosa do not have normal satiety and have an impaired secretion of CCK in response to a meal.[15]

Pancreatic Polypeptides

A 36-amino acid peptide, NPY shares structural similarities with the gastrointestinal hormones PP and peptide YY. Neurons containing NPY decrease acetylcholine release from myenteric plexus neurons, hence inhibit small intestinal smooth muscle contraction.[3]

5-Hydroxytryptamine

In addition to its role as an endocrine/paracrine substance of the gastrointestinal tract, 5-HT is also found in enteric neurons where it is believed to regulate the migrating myoelectrical complex and the intestinal peristaltic reflex.[3]

PARACRINE SUBSTANCES

A substance may be defined as having a paracrine mechanism of activation if (1) the substance is found within an effector cell, (2) receptors for the substance exist on an adjacent paracrine target cell, (3) the effector cell and paracrine target cell are in close proximity, and (4) the substance when applied to the paracrine target cell evokes a biologic response.[1, 2] Histamine, somatostatin, adenosine, and prostaglandins have been shown to satisfy these criteria.

Histamine

Histamine is formed from the decarboxylation of histidine in mast cells found throughout the gastrointestinal tract of the dog. In the dog, gastric mucosal histamine stores appear fully accounted for by mast cells, there being no evidence to indicate histamine is stored in endocrine cells.[6] Histamine released from mast cells diffuses into the interstitial milieu and is believed to bind parietal cell H_2 receptors to stimulate H^+ secretion.[6] A large body of evidence has accumulated in support of this idea, although one study suggests that the histamine effect might be indirectly mediated through histamine receptors on gastric mucosal immunocytes.[7] Regardless, H_2 receptor antagonists have been shown to be potent inhibitors of histamine, acetylcholine, and gastrin-stimulated H^+ secretion. The interaction of these paracrine, neurocrine, and endocrine pathways in the regulation of gastric acid secretion is further discussed in Chapter 136.

Somatostatin

The endocrine and neurocrine roles of somatostatin were discussed earlier in this chapter. As a paracrine substance, somatostatin has an important role in the paracrine inhibition of gastrin release. Somatostatin cells in the gastric antrum have long cytoplasmic processes that terminate adjacent to antral G cells. Paracrine release of somatostatin by these somatostatin cells is postulated to mediate the negative feedback inhibition of H^+ on gastrin release.[16] Somatostatin released from pancreatic islet cells (D cells) may also autoregulate pancreatic insulin and glucagon secretion through a local paracrine mechanism[17] (see also Chapter 153).

Prostaglandins

Prostaglandins are long-chain fatty acids that are distributed throughout the gastrointestinal tract. The role of prostaglandins as paracrine substances is perhaps best understood in the gastric mucosa, where they bind to inhibitory prostanoid receptors on gastric oxyntic cells. These receptors are coupled to inhibitory G proteins and subsequent inhibition of adenylate cyclase and of H^+ secretion.[18] A "cytoprotective effect" of prostaglandins, separate from the direct inhibition of acid secretion, has also been implied. Gastric prostaglandins, for example, stimulate mucosal bicarbonate and glycoprotein secretion, epithelial cell renewal, and mucosal blood flow. These effects are all central to the barrier properties of the gastric mucosa.[19] Synthetic forms of prostaglandins (Cytotec) are now available for the treatment of gastric mucosal barrier disorders.[20, 21] The role of prostaglandins in the maintenance of the gastric mucosal barrier is discussed further in Chapter 136.

DISEASES OF THE GASTROINTESTINAL ENDOCRINE SYSTEM

The major syndromes of gastrointestinal endocrine pathology are diabetes mellitus, islet cell tumors of the pancreas, and carcinoid tumors of the small and large intestine. The syndromes of gastrinoma, pancreatic polypeptidoma, glucagonoma, and carcinoid are discussed separately here.

GASTRINOMA

Islet cell tumors that secrete excessive amounts of gastrin are referred to as gastrinomas. A syndrome of gastric acid hypersecretion, severe peptic ulceration, and islet cell tumors was first described in humans by Zollinger and Ellison in 1955. The eponym Zollinger-Ellison syndrome was soon used to describe this syndrome. These tumors were subsequently found to contain gastrin and are now more appropriately referred to as gastrinomas.

Clinical Features

Gastrinomas are rare, having been reported in only 20 dogs and three cats. They usually develop in female (69 per cent), middle-aged dogs (average, 8.2 years; range, 3.5 to 12 years).[22–34] No breed predilection has been reported. Of the three cats reported, one was 10 and two were 12 years old.[27, 28]

Vomiting and weight loss are the most frequent owner concerns. Depression, lethargy, anorexia, and intermittent diarrhea are also frequently reported complaints. Polydipsia, melena, abdominal pain, hematemesis, hematochezia, and obstipation are reported infrequently. Physical examination is not remarkable in most animals; abdominal pain, fever, and tachycardia were observed in only a small number of animals. One cat affected with gastrinoma had a palpable abdominal mass.

Most of the clinical signs result from gastrin-stimulated gastric acid hypersecretion. Increased gastric acid secretion causes erosive gastritis and duodenitis, gastric mucosal hyperplasia, and eventually gastrointestinal ulceration. Ulceration may be associated with hematochezia, melena, hematemesis, and abdominal pain. Erosive esophagitis and esophageal ulceration associated with gastroesophageal reflux of gastric acid may cause anorexia, regurgitation, and hematemesis. Duodenal acidification causes malabsorption and steatorrhea through inactivation of lipase and bile salts, through direct chemical injury to the intestinal mucosa, and through gastrin inhibition of water and electrolyte absorption.

Laboratory Findings

Regenerative anemia, attributed to gastrointestinal bleeding, was present in 45 per cent of the dogs and cats with gastrinoma. Leukocytosis (50 per cent), neutrophilia (35 per cent), and increased band neutrophils (10 per cent) were also reported. These changes were attributed to gastrointestinal inflammation. The most common biochemical abnormalities of dogs and cats with gastrinoma were increased serum alkaline phosphatase activity, hypoalbuminemia, hyperglycemia, hypokalemia, and hypocalcemia. Other mild to moderate changes were hyponatremia, hypochloremia, alkalosis, acidosis, hypoglycemia, decreased total protein, and increased bilirubin, creatinine, and alanine aminotransferase activity.

The cause of the hyperglycemia was unclear in most cases except in one dog with hyperadrenocorticism and glucocorticoid-induced insulin resistance; extracts of the islet cell tumor in this case yielded adrenocorticotropic hormone in addition to gastrin. The hypoalbuminemia and hypoproteinemia were attributed to loss of serum albumin and other proteins through gastrointestinal erosions and ulcerations. The hypocalcemia was probably artifactual and secondary to decreased serum albumin, although steatorrhea could have contributed through vitamin D malabsorption. The hypokalemia likely resulted from losses in vomitus and diarrhea, as well as from decreased food intake. Frequent vomiting was also associated with hyponatremia, hypochloremia, and metabolic alkalosis in several dogs. Only one dog developed metabolic acidosis. The hypoglycemia observed in two dogs may have resulted from concurrent hyperinsulinemia. The increases in serum alkaline phosphatase, alanine aminotransferase, and bilirubin may have resulted from tumor metastasis to the liver, which was observed in 85 per cent of the cases.

Radiography and Endoscopy

Survey abdominal radiographs were usually normal. Decreased abdominal detail was observed in animals with perforated ulcer and peritonitis. Contrast medium–enhanced studies performed in six dogs revealed plaque-like defects in the fundic or small intestinal mucosa consistent with ulceration, prominent gastric rugal folds, thickened pyloric antrum, complete pyloric obstruction, intestinal thickening, and rapid small bowel transit time. Abdominal ultrasonography in one dog revealed wall thickening of the pylorus and a hyperechoic focus in the liver. Endoscopic examination performed on 10 dogs revealed esophageal inflammation or ulceration (4 dogs), thickened gastric rugae (6 dogs), gastric ulceration or hemorrhage (5 dogs), excessive liquid in the stomach (5 dogs), duodenal ulceration (2 dogs), a hypertrophied pyloric antrum (3 dogs) that impeded passage of the endoscope through the pylorus in one dog, and raised erythematous nodules in the gastric mucosa.

Diagnostic Tests

Diagnostic tests for gastrinoma include evaluation of basal gastric acid secretion and basal serum gastrin concentration, provocative tests such as secretin and calcium stimulation, and somatostatin receptor scintigraphy. Gross and histopathologic findings are also important in the diagnosis of gastrinoma.

Basal Gastric Acid Secretion. Measurement of basal gastric acid secretion is commonly performed in humans as an aid to the diagnosis of gastrinoma. An orogastric aspiration technique for evaluation of pentagastrin-stimulated gastric acid analysis and reference values for volume, pH, H^+ output, and hydrochloric acid output in healthy anesthetized dogs have been reported. However, because of technical difficulties, basal gastric acid secretion has been measured in only four dogs with gastrinoma.

Basal Serum Gastrin Concentration. The best screening test for gastrinoma is measurement of basal serum gastrin concentration. Dogs and cats with gastrinoma have serum gastrin concentrations that vary from 3.2 to 100 times the highest value reported for the normal range. However, hypergastrinemia alone is not diagnostic for gastrinoma and may be increased in dogs in renal failure, gastric outlet obstruction, chronic gastritis, liver disease, and small intestinal resection and during H_2 receptor antagonist therapy. Thus provocative testing is usually necessary to confirm a diagnosis of gastrinoma. Only when serum gastrin concentrations exceed 10 times the normal levels, concurrent with increased gastric acidity, is a diagnosis of gastrinoma considered without provocative testing in humans. Because of the paucity of reported cases, we recommend provocative testing (calcium and secretin challenge) in dogs and cats whenever possible, especially if basal serum gastrin concentrations are increased less than 10-fold. Serum gastrin concentrations have also been measured before and after feeding in normal dogs. However, responses in dogs with gastrinoma have not been evaluated.

Secretin Stimulation. Secretin stimulation is the preferred test in humans with presumed gastrinoma. Secretin stimulates gastrin secretion in humans with gastrinoma but does not stimulate gastrin secretion in healthy humans. Experience with secretin stimulation in small animals with gastrinoma is limited, however. It has been performed in three dogs with gastrinoma and in one dog with a pancreatic polypeptidoma. The test has not been used in cats with gastrinoma. Further limitations of the test are expense, sporadic availability, variable potency, and contaminants that cross-react in the gastrin radioimmunoassay. If the test is to be performed, samples should be collected before and 2, 5, 15, and 30 minutes after an intravenous bolus of secretin administered at a dosage of 2 to 4 U/kg. The 2- and 5-minute blood samples are believed to be most important because the maximum (diagnostic) response is reported to occur at those time points. A diagnostic response in humans is a twofold or greater increase in serum gastrin. Although similar criteria have not been established for the dog, two dogs with gastrinoma had greater than a twofold increase while one dog had a 1.4-fold increase in gastrin within 5 minutes of secretin administration. The reader is referred to the previous edition of this textbook for examples of plasma gastrin response to secretin and calcium challenge.[35]

Calcium Stimulation. Experience with the calcium challenge test in small animals has been limited to two dogs with gastrinoma and one dog with pancreatic polypeptidoma. As with secretin stimulation, calcium infusion stimulates an increase in serum gastrin concentrations in gastrinoma patients but not in nongastrinoma patients. The source of calcium is usually calcium gluconate, which should be administered as a 1-minute intravenous bolus infusion (2 mg/kg) or as an intravenous continuous infusion over several hours (5 mg/kg/h). Serum samples are collected before and at 15, 30, 60, 90, and 120 minutes after administration. Maximum serum gastrin concentrations occurred 60 minutes after calcium bolus infusion in two dogs with gastrinoma. Both dogs had a twofold increase in serum gastrin concentration in response to calcium infusion. In one dog, calcium stimulation, but not secretin stimulation, was diagnostic for gastrinoma. A combined secretin-calcium stimulation test has been shown to be superior to secretin stimulation in the diagnosis of gastrinoma in humans. A 1-minute infusion of 2 mg/kg of calcium gluconate, together with an intravenous bolus of 2 U/kg of secretin, generally causes a twofold increase in gastrin in humans.

Somatostatin Receptor Scintigraphy. Experience with somatostatin receptor scintigraphy is limited to one dog with gastrinoma. This procedure is useful for imaging primary and metastatic gastrinoma, as well as indicating if a patient will be likely to benefit from anti-somatostatin therapy. One affected and two normal dogs were given 2 mCi of ^{111}In pentetreotide, and images were obtained using a gamma counter with a medium energy collimator. Results of scintigraphy were confirmed by finding tumors in the pancreas, duodenum, and multiple sites within the liver. Positive scintigraphic images were consistent with somatostatin binding by tumor cell receptors. This was documented by in vitro autoradiography and a therapeutic response to somatostatin.[25]

Pathology

All but one dog with gastrinoma had an islet cell tumor of the pancreas. In contrast to insulinomas where tumor distribution is nearly equal between lobes of the pancreas, gastrin-secreting tumors occurred most commonly in the right lobe (60 per cent) and body (angle, 40 per cent) of the pancreas with only one report of a tumor in the left lobe of the pancreas (Table 156–1). Tumor location was not given in six other cases. Most dogs and cats had solitary nodules in the pancreas, but multiple masses were found in 3 of 13 animals. In one dog a tumor was missed during surgical exploration. A probable extrapancreatic gastrinoma was described in one dog that had neuroendocrine tumors in the root of the mesentery. However, it could not be determined if these were primary or metastatic foci. At the time of diagnosis the gastrinoma had metastasized in 85 per cent of the cases, with the liver the most common site of metastasis (65 per cent). Metastasis to other sites included lymph nodes, mesentery, spleen, peritoneum, omentum, and serosal surface of the duodenum and jejunum.

Light microscopic appearance of gastrinoma may be consistent with an islet cell tumor but is not specific for gas-

TABLE 156–1. INCIDENCE OF GROSS PATHOLOGY FINDINGS (SURGICAL OR NECROPSY) OF GASTRINOMA IN 20 DOGS AND TWO CATS

PATHOLOGY	NO. OF ANIMALS	%
Tumor location		
Pancreas	20/21	95
Left lobe	1/15*	7*
Body or angle	6/15*	40*
Right lobe	9/15*	60*
Liver	13/20	65
Lymph node	6/20	30
Other (spleen, peritoneum, mesentery)	5/20	25
Gastrointestinal ulceration	21/22	95
Esophagus	4/20	20
Stomach	9/20	45
Duodenum	14/18	78
Jejunum	1/17	6
Perforated ulcers	5/20	25
Miscellaneous		
Gastric hypertrophy	13/18	72
C-cell increase	4/9	44
Adrenocortical hyperplasia	2/9	22
Thyroid follicular cell carcinoma	1/9	11

*One dog had tumor in two limbs of the pancreas.

trinoma. The presence of gastrin in the tumor can be documented by immunocytochemistry or through tissue extraction and radioimmunoassay. Alternatively, ultrastructure of the intracytoplasmic granules can be used to distinguish gastrinomas from other types of islet cell tumors of the dog. Ideally, at the time of surgery (or necropsy) portions of the tumor should be frozen (for immunocytochemistry and hormone extraction), fixed in formalin or Bouin's solution (for routine histopathology and immunocytochemistry), and in glutaraldehyde (for electron microscopy).

Gastrointestinal ulceration was present in 95 per cent of dogs and cats with gastrinoma. Ulceration of the duodenum was the most common occurrence, followed in descending order of frequency by the stomach, esophagus, and jejunum. Perforated duodenal and esophageal ulcers were documented in five dogs. Other pathologic abnormalities included gastric hypertrophy, thyroid C-cell and adrenal hyperplasia, and thyroid follicular cell carcinoma (see Table 156–1). The reader is referred to the previous edition of this textbook for an example of multiple duodenal ulcerations in a dog with gastrinoma.[35]

Therapy

The management of gastrinoma patients should be directed at specific treatment of the primary tumor, control of gastric acid hypersecretion, treatment of gastrointestinal ulceration, and correction of fluid, electrolyte, and acid-base disturbances.

Primary Tumor. Gastrinomas are best treated by surgical resection. Surgery facilitates confirmation of the diagnosis, as well as reduction of tumor mass and gastrin secretory capacity. Because many gastrinomas are quite small, the pancreas should be carefully inspected, both visually and digitally, at the time of surgery. Excessive manipulation should be avoided, however, because of the risk of traumatic pancreatitis. Because most of the tumors are located within the right lobe and body of the pancreas, we recommend that a right lobe pancreatectomy be performed if a specific tumor nodule cannot be located. Indeed, one dog with gastrinoma had a small tumor in the right pancreatic lobe that was not detectable at surgery.

Because metastasis is common at the time of surgery, the liver, lymph nodes, duodenum, mesentery, omentum, and spleen should be carefully examined. If metastasis is considered too extensive for excision, a partial pancreatectomy should be performed with debulking of the primary tumor. Euthanasia is not necessarily recommended because these tumors are slow growing, debulking reduces the gastrin secretory capacity, and medical therapies exist for the treatment of hypergastrinemia and gastric hyperacidity.

Adequate fluid therapy is extremely important in the operative and post-operative periods. This will maintain the pancreatic microcirculation and minimize the development of post-pancreatectomy pancreatitis. Therapies should also be formulated to neutralize gastric acidity and reduce the possibility of gastroesophageal reflux in these patients. Chemotherapy has not yet been used in the treatment of gastrinoma in dogs and cats. However, octreotide (Sandostatin), a somatostatin analogue, has been used successfully for treatment of gastrinoma in two dogs.[25, 29] Somatostatin inhibits both gastrin and hydrogen ion secretion. One animal was successfully treated for more than 10 months with 10 to 20 μg three times daily of octreotide, as well as sucralfate and cimetidine. The other dog was successfully treated with initial doses of 2 μg/kg given twice daily. Dramatic improvement was noted after an increase in dose from two to three times daily. Deterioration in clinical signs led to euthanasia after 14 months at which time octreotide was being given to a final dose of 20 μg/kg three times a day. Necropsy revealed a marked increase in tumor growth and metastasis.

Gastric Hyperacidity. Because of the difficulty in resecting primary and metastatic tumors, gastrinoma patients usually maintain high levels of gastric acid secretion. Specific therapies aimed at controlling gastric acid secretion will usually be necessary. The best therapeutic agents used for reducing gastric acid secretion include the H_2 receptor antagonists, H^+,K^+-ATPase inhibitors (proton pump inhibitors), and somatostatin analogues. Cimetidine (Tagamet), ranitidine (Zantac), famotidine (Pepcid), and nizatidine (Axid) are H_2-receptor antagonists used in small animal practice. They are potent inhibitors of H^+ secretion in dogs and cats. Cimetidine has been effective in controlling clinical signs associated with gastrinoma in several dogs and one cat. The recommended dosage of cimetidine in dogs is 5 to 10 mg/kg orally, subcutaneously, or intravenously every 4 to 6 hours, although gastrinoma patients may require a higher dosage to control gastric acidity. The recommended dosage of ranitidine is 2 mg/kg orally or intravenously every 8 to 12 hours. Famotidine is used at a dose of 0.1 to 0.2 mg/kg orally every 8 hours (Table 156–2).

Omeprazole (Prilosec), an inhibitor of the parietal cell H^+,K^+-ATPase, is a potent inhibitor of gastric acid secretion with a long duration of action in normal dogs.[36, 37] This drug has been successfully used to treat two dogs with gastrinoma. Hematemesis and melena in one dog was unresponsive to treatment with cimetidine and sucralfate but resolved with omeprazole therapy. In this dog, use of omeprazole at 20 mg orally every 24 hours resulted in amelioration of all clinical and laboratory abnormalities. An attempt to lower the dose of omeprazole to 20 mg orally every 2 days was unsuccessful. The dog remained asymptomatic for more than 2 years. In the other dog, omeprazole was discontinued after 7 months because of cost but concurrent treatment with octreotide was continued successfully until euthanasia at 14 months. Based on these limited treatment experiences,

TABLE 156–2. DRUGS USED TO MODIFY GASTROINTESTINAL HORMONES

Histamine (H_2) Receptor Antagonists
Cimetidine (Tagamet), 2–4 mg/lb (5–10 mg/kg) PO, SQ, IV q6h or q8h
Ranitidine (Zantac), 0.5–1.0 mg/lb (1–2 mg/kg) PO, SQ, IV q8h or q12h
Famotidine (Pepcid), 0.1–0.2/mg/kg PO, IV q12h
Nizatidine (Axid), 1.0–3.0 mg/kg SQ, IM, IV q8h
H^+, K^+-ATPase Inhibitors
Omeprazole (Prilosec; Losec) 0.35 mg/lb (0.7 mg/kg) PO q24h
Diffusion Barriers
Sucralfate (Carafate), 1 g q8h for large dogs; 0.5 g q8h for smaller dogs; 0.25 to 0.5 g q8–12h for cats
Synthetic Prostaglandins
Misoprostol (Cytotec), 2–5 μg/kg PO q8h
Somatostatin Analogues
Octreotide (Sandostatin), 10–20 μg PO q8h

omeprazole may be superior to cimetidine as the gastric acid anti-secretory drug of choice for gastrinoma in dogs.

Sandostatin, a somatostatin analogue discussed earlier, directly inhibits gastrin and gastric acid secretion and might be useful in gastrinoma patients. Sandostatin should certainly be considered in a gastrinoma patient when other medical therapies have failed.

Gastrointestinal Ulceration. Gastrointestinal ulceration is common in cats and dogs with gastrinoma. Treatment of ulcers includes surgical resection where appropriate, reduction of gastric acidity as discussed previously, and the use of diffusion barriers and "cytoprotective agents" to promote ulcer healing (see Table 156–2).

Sucralfate (Carafate) is an example of a diffusion barrier used to promote ulcer healing. It is a complex of sulfated sucrose and aluminum hydroxide that when ingested reacts with gastric acid and binds to necrotic tissue proteins. The recommended dosages are 1 g every 8 hours for larger dogs, 0.5 g every 8 hours for smaller dogs, and 0.25 to 0.5 g every 8 to 12 hours for cats.

Misoprostol (Cytotec) is a 16,16-dimethylated synthetic prostaglandin that has cytoprotective properties in addition to its direct acid-inhibitory effect. Synthetic prostaglandins may be useful in restoring the protective properties of the gastric mucosal barrier in ulcer patients. Clinical experience with misoprostol in small animals is still limited. Misoprostol was effective in preventing ulcers in arthritic dogs medicated with acetylsalicylic acid.[20]

Prognosis

Gastrinoma in cats and dogs appears to be highly malignant with gross evidence of metastasis at the time of diagnosis in 85 per cent of the animals. Hence the long-term prognosis is grave. Eleven of 23 animals with gastrinoma died or were euthanized without the benefit of therapy. The prognosis for gastrinoma is likely to improve with heightened degree of suspicion and the increased availability of anti-secretory drugs such as omeprazole and somatostatin analogues.

PANCREATIC POLYPEPTIDOMA

Pancreatic polypeptide is commonly identified by immunocytochemistry within canine pancreatic endocrine tumors secreting gastrin, insulin, or glucagon (75 per cent of 57 dogs).[38] However, elevated plasma PP concentrations have been documented in only one dog with a pancreatic islet cell tumor. In that case the excessive amounts of PP were thought to contribute to the dog's clinical abnormalities.

The clinical syndrome of chronic vomiting, hypertrophic gastritis, duodenal ulceration, pancreatic adenocarcinoma, and fasting hypergastrinemia were highly suggestive of gastrinoma. However, this dog maintained normal serum gastrin concentrations in response to both calcium and secretin, and there was no immunocytochemical staining of gastrin in the pancreatic tumor or its metastases. For these reasons, a gastrin-secreting tumor was thought to be an unlikely cause of the clinical signs in this dog.

Immunocytochemistry revealed intense staining of the pancreatic tumor and its metastases for pancreatic polypeptide. Plasma PP concentrations were also extremely high (637,000 pg/mL; normal dogs < 155 pg/mL). The investigators proposed that high plasma PP concentrations may have contributed to the dog's gastrointestinal ulceration and vomiting because PP decreases pancreatic bicarbonate secretion and mildly increases gastric acid secretion.[1, 2, 4] The tumor also contained insulin, which may have led to the significant hypoglycemia.

GLUCAGONOMA

Glucagonoma is a rare syndrome in humans and dogs. Humans with glucagonoma develop a characteristic rash referred to as necrolytic migratory erythema (NME), diabetes mellitus, venous thromboses, depression, anorexia, weight loss, glossitis or stomatitis, diarrhea, and normocytic normochromic anemia. The rash probably results from hypoaminoacidemia, rather than the hyperglucagonemia, whereas the diabetes mellitus results from the glycogenolytic and gluconeogenic actions of glucagon. The diagnosis of glucagonoma is confirmed by finding elevated plasma glucagon concentrations and a pancreatic islet cell tumor immunoreactive for glucagon.

The authors are aware of five definitive and two presumptive diagnoses of canine glucagoma.[39-44] Affected dog breeds included boxer, standard poodle, fox terrier, Labrador retriever, springer spaniel, Bernese Mountain mixed breed dog, and a mixed breed dog. There were three female and four male dogs with an age range of 5 to 11 years.

Affected dogs had scaling and crusting dermatitis that varied in duration from 3 weeks to 16 months. Footpads were affected in all dogs, followed in descending order of frequency by hocks; ventral abdomen; elbows; perineum; nose; mucocutaneous junctions of the eyes, mouth, anus, and prepuce or vulva; flanks; and distal extremities (Fig. 156-1). Other clinical signs or physical examination findings included depression (57 per cent), peripheral lymphadenopathy (43 per cent), and anorexia (43 per cent).

Laboratory abnormalities included hyperglycemia (86 per cent), glucosuria (43 per cent), increased serum alanine aminotransferase (57 per cent) and alkaline phosphatase (29 per cent), decreased albumin (29 per cent), and anemia in 43 per cent of dogs. Concurrent hyperadrenocorticism was present in one dog. Abdominal radiographs were unremarkable in all dogs. Abdominal ultrasound examination was within normal limits in three dogs, but pancreatic mass (one dog) and hepatic pathologic processes (three dogs) were observed in four other dogs. Ultrasound abnormalities included small liver with increased echogenicity of the portal and hepatic vein walls, diffuse hepatic hyperechogenicity and multiple small hypoechoic foci in the liver, a well-defined hyperechoic area within the liver, and a possible mass in the right lobe of the pancreas.

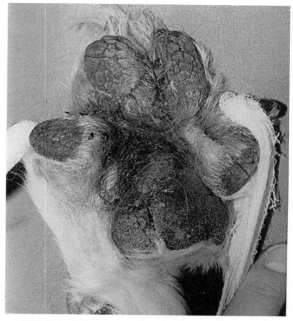

Figure 156-1. Necrolytic migratory erythema of the footpads in a 9-year-old Bernese mountain mixed breed dog with glucagonoma. Note the hyperkeratosis and multiple fissures. (Courtesy of Dr. Karin Allenspach.)

Six of seven dogs had a pancreatic tumor; serial sections of the pancreas failed to reveal neoplasia in one animal. Tumor location within the pancreas involved the right lobe (three dogs), left lobe (one dog), and body (one dog); in another dog the location was undisclosed. Metastasis occurred in 71 per cent of dogs and most frequently involved the liver (57 per cent) and lymph nodes (28 per cent). Pancreatitis was noted in four dogs, three of which occurred postoperatively.

Tumors were positive for glucagon immunocytochemistry in all seven dogs. In four of these dogs the tumors also stained for one or more of the following peptides: insulin, somatostatin, PP, and islet amyloid peptide. Plasma glucagon was increased 2.8 to 7.5 times the upper limit of the normal range in all five dogs tested. Three dogs also had low plasma amino acid concentrations (20 of 24, 4 of 5, and 13 of 18 amino acids tested). Amino acids that were decreased in all three dogs included arginine, histidine, and lysine. Amino acids that were decreased in two dogs included taurine, threonine, serine, glutamine, proline, glycine, alanine, valine, isoleucine, and tyrosine. Phenylalanine was either slightly decreased or within normal limits. Tryptophan was normal or increased, and cystathionine was elevated in tested dogs.

Only one of seven dogs survived its illness. Four dogs were diagnosed with NME associated with diffuse hepatic disease (including neoplasia) and were euthanized days to weeks later when the dog's condition deteriorated. Two other dogs underwent exploratory laparotomy for suspected pancreatic masses. These dogs were euthanized 3 days postoperatively due to pancreatitis. The surviving dog had a tumor of the pancreas and mesenteric lymph node removed at the time of exploratory laparotomy. In that dog plasma glucagon concentrations decreased into the normal range within 1 day. The dermatosis improved within 1 week, and all skin lesions resolved by 45 days after surgery. There was also a remarkable increase in fasting plasma amino acids within 30 days of tumor removal. However, relapse of skin

END

disease occurred 9 months later and the dog was euthanized without necropsy.

NME (also referred to as superficial necrolytic dermatitis) has also been documented in dogs with diabetes mellitus and hepatic disease. Glucagonomas account for only about 10 per cent of dogs with NME. It is important to distinguish these causes, however, because the prognosis for glucagonoma is likely to be better than that for diffuse chronic hepatic disease. Hyperglucagonemia and hypoaminoacidemia may result from significant liver pathology in the absence of functional glucagonoma. Four dogs with glucagonoma were given a poor prognosis with documented or suspected liver disease. Outcome may have differed with altered presumptive diagnosis and/or surgical intervention, although it would appear that dogs are at increased risk for development of post-operative pancreatitis (57 per cent).

Pancreatic glucagonoma was never detected radiographically and was only suspected by abdominal ultrasonography in one dog. Exploratory laparotomy should always be considered if liver function testing is normal and NME is present. As with most islet cell tumors, treatment should be directed at tumor removal or reduction, decreasing excessive hormonal secretion (Sandostatin), and supportive therapy for clinical abnormalities. As clinical awareness and diagnostic testing improves, prognosis for glucagonoma may substantially improve. Suspected dogs should be evaluated for presence of pancreatic mass, liver and lymph node metastasis, plasma glucagon, insulin, and amino acid and fatty acid concentrations. If tumors are located, immunocytochemistry for multiple peptides should be performed on the primary tumor and metastatic sites.

INTESTINAL CARCINOID

Intestinal carcinoid is a rare neoplasm arising from enterochromaffin cells of the gastrointestinal tract. In dogs, carcinoids have been reported in the intestines, liver, and lungs, whereas gastric and intestinal carcinoids have been reported in cats. These tumors most often produce signs of gastrointestinal obstruction or signs associated with metastatic cancer in dogs and cats. A syndrome of facial flushing, bronchoconstriction, abdominal cramping, and diarrhea occurs in some affected humans due to excessive secretion of 5-hydroxytryptamine by the enterochromaffin cells. This carcinoid syndrome has not been very well documented in veterinary species, however. Diarrhea, for example, has been described in only 5 of the 29 cases of carcinoid reported.

Despite the paucity of case reports, it would seem that surgical resection is the treatment of choice for carcinoid. The prognosis is fair because some carcinoids have a rather slow biologic growth rate.

REFERENCES

1. Walsh JH: Gastrointestinal hormones. *In* Johnson LR (ed): Physiology of the Gastrointestinal Tract. New York, Raven Press, 1994, p 1.
2. Merchant JL, et al: Molecular biology of the gut: Model of gastrointestinal hormones. *In* Johnson LR (ed): Physiology of the Gastrointestinal Tract. New York, Raven Press, 1994, p 295.
3. Dockray GJ: Physiology of the enteric neuropeptides. *In* Johnson LR (ed): Physiology of the Gastrointestinal Tract. New York, Raven Press, 1994, p 169.
4. Makhlouf GM: The Handbook of Physiology—The Gastrointestinal System Vol. II. Neural and Endocrine Biology. Washington, DC, American Physiological Society, 1989.
5. Walsh JH: Gastrin. New York, Raven Press, 1993.
6. Soll AH, Berglindh T: Receptors that regulate gastric acid secretory function. *In* Johnson LR (ed): Physiology of the Gastrointestinal Tract. New York, Raven Press, 1994, p 1139.
7. Mezey É, Palkovits M: Localization of targets for anti-ulcer drugs in the cells of the immune system. Science 258:1662, 1992.
8. Chey WY: Hormonal control of pancreatic exocrine secretion. *In* Go VLW (ed): Pancreas, Biology, Pathobiology and Disease. New York, Raven Press, 1993, p 403.
9. Washabau RJ, et al: Cholecystokinin secretion is preserved in canine pancreatic insufficiency. J Vet Intern Med 9:193, 1995.
10. Schirra J, et al: Gastric emptying and release of incretin hormones after glucose ingestion. J Clin Invest 97:92, 1996.
11. Schally AV, et al: Effect of somatostatin analogs on gastric acid secretion in dogs and rats. Int J Pept Prot Res 36:267, 1990.
12. Haga N, et al: Role of endogenous 5-hydroxytryptamine in the regulation of gastric contractions by motilin in dogs. Am J Physiol 270:G20, 1996.
13. Lee KY, et al: A hormonal mechanism for the interdigestive pancreatic secretion in dog. Am J Physiol (Gastrointest Liver Physiol) 14:G759, 1986.
14. Hall JA, Washabau RJ: Gastrointestinal prokinetic therapy: Motilin-like drugs. Compend Contin Ed Pract Vet 19:281, 1997.
15. Geracioti TF, Liddle RA: Impaired cholecystokinin secretion in bulimia nervosa. N Eng J Med 319:683, 1988.
16. Makhlouf GM, Schubert ML: Gastric somatostatin: A paracrine regulator of acid secretion. Metabolism 39:138, 1990.
17. Yamada T: Local regulatory actions of gastrointestinal peptides. *In* Johnson LR (ed): Physiology of the Gastrointestinal Tract. New York, Raven Press, 1987, p 131.
18. Chen MCY, et al: Prostanoid inhibition of canine parietal cells: Mediation by the inhibitory guanosine triphosphate-binding protein of adenylate cyclase. Gastroenterology 94:1121, 1988.
19. Goddard PJ, et al: Luminal surface hydrophobicity of canine gastric mucosa is dependent on a surface mucous gel. Gastroenterology 98:361, 1990.
20. Murtaugh R, et al: Use of a synthetic prostaglandin E₁ (Misoprostol) for prevention of aspirin-induced gastroduodenal ulceration in arthritic dogs. JAVMA 202:251, 1993.
21. Johnston SA, et al: The effect of misoprostol on aspirin-induced gastroduodenal lesions in dogs. J Vet Intern Med 9:32, 1995.
22. Rousseaux CG, et al: Ultrastructure of a canine gastrinoma. J Comp Pathol 97:605, 1987.
23. English RV, et al: Zollinger-Ellison syndrome and myelofibrosis in a dog. JAVMA 192:1430, 1988.
24. Brooks D, et al: Omeprazole in a dog with gastrinoma. J Vet Intern Med 11:379, 1997.
25. Altschul M, et al: Evaluation of somatostatin analogues for the detection and treatment of gastrinoma in a dog. J Small Anim Pract 38:286, 1997.
26. Hayden DW, et al: Gastrin-secreting pancreatic endocrine tumor in a dog (putative Zollinger-Ellison syndrome). J Vet Diagn Invest 9:100, 1997.
27. Van der Gaag I, et al: Zollinger-Ellison syndrome in a cat. Vet Q 10:151, 1988.
28. Eng J, et al: Cat gastrinoma and the sequence of cat gastrins. Reg Pept 37:9, 1992.
29. Lothrop CD, et al: Medical treatment of neuroendocrine tumors of the gastroenteropancreatic system with somatostatin. *In* Kirk RW (ed): Current Veterinary Therapy X. Philadelphia, WB Saunders, 1989, p 1020.
30. Feldman EC, et al: Gastrinoma, glucagonoma, and other APUDomas. *In* Feldman EC, Nelson RW (eds): Canine and Feline Endocrinology and Reproduction, 2nd ed. Philadelphia, WB Saunders, 1996, p 442.
31. Straus E, et al: Canine Zollinger-Ellison syndrome. Gastroenterology 72:380, 1977.
32. Jones BR, et al: Peptic ulceration in a dog associated with an islet cell carcinoma of the pancreas and an elevated plasma gastrin level. J Small Anim Pract 17:593, 1976.
33. Happe RP, et al: Zollinger-Ellison syndrome in three dogs. Vet Pathol 17:177, 1980.
34. Drazner FH: Canine gastrinoma: A condition analogous to the Zollinger-Ellison syndrome in man. Cal Vet 11:6, 1981.
35. Zerbe CA, Washabau RJ: Gastrointestinal endocrine disease. *In* Ettinger SJ, Feldman EC (eds): Textbook of Veterinary Internal Medicine. Philadelphia, WB Saunders, 1995, p 1593.
36. Säfholm C, et al: Effect of 7 years daily oral administration of omeprazole to beagle dogs. Digestion 55:139, 1994.
37. Coruzzi G, et al: Antisecretory activity of omeprazole in the conscious gastric fistula cat: Comparison with famotidine. Pharm Res 21:499, 1989.
38. Zerbe CA, et al: Pancreatic polypeptide and insulin-secreting tumor in a dog with duodenal ulcers and hypertrophic gastritis. J Vet Intern Med 3:178, 1989.
39. Gross TL, et al: Glucagon-producing pancreatic endocrine tumors in two dogs with superficial necrolytic dermatitis. JAVMA 186:1619, 1990.
40. Zerbe CA: Personal communication with Dr. Karin Allenspach, 1998.
41. Miller WH, et al: Necrolytic migratory erythema in a dog with a glucagon-secreting endocrine tumor. Vet Dermatol 2:179, 1991.
42. Torres SMF, et al: Resolution of superficial necrolytic dermatitis following excision of a glucagon-secreting pancreatic neoplasm in a dog. J Am Anim Hosp Assoc 33:313, 1997.
43. Bond R, et al: Metabolic epidermal necrosis in two dogs with different underlying diseases. Vet Rec 136:466, 1995.
44. Torres S, et al: Superficial necrolytic dermatitis and a pancreatic endocrine tumor in a dog. J Small Anim Pract 38:246, 1997.

SECTION XIII

THE REPRODUCTIVE SYSTEM

CHAPTER 157

ESTROUS CYCLE AND BREEDING MANAGEMENT OF THE HEALTHY BITCH

Auke C. Schaefers-Okkens

THE ESTROUS CYCLE

Onset of puberty in the healthy bitch occurs between 6 and 18 months of age. After each estrous cycle, which has a length of about 3 months, an anestrus with a variable duration occurs. The mean interval from onset of one estrous cycle to the next is about 7 months, with a range of 4 to 12 months. The interestrous interval may be regular or variable within individual bitches. After 8 years of age, the duration and frequency of the cycles become less regular and the interestrous interval increases.[1]

The stages of the estrous cycle are proestrus, estrus, and diestrus (metestrus) (Fig. 157–1). The average duration of proestrus is 9 days, with a range of 3 to 17 days. Proestrus is defined as the period when the bitch is sexually attractive while rejecting the male's advances until the first willingness to accept the male. However, early behavioral signs are indistinct. Therefore, it is common to use the onset of sero-sanguineous vaginal discharge and vulvar swelling to mark the first day of proestrus. On average, estrus (the period of mating) has a duration of 9 days, with a range of 3 to 21 days. During estrus the vulva begins to shrink and soften. The vaginal discharge usually persists but generally diminishes. It may remain serosanguineous or turn straw colored. Diestrus begins when the bitch will no longer accept the dog. It has an average duration of about 70 days if we assume that it ends when the plasma progesterone concentration initially declines to a level of less than or equal to 3 nmol/L.

In addition to this behavior-oriented classification of the cycle, it is also possible, and sometimes more appropriate, to concentrate on ovarian function and to classify the follicular phase, the phase of pre-ovulatory luteinization and ovulation, the luteal phase, and the anestrus (see Fig. 157–1).

FOLLICULAR PHASE

As tertiary follicles develop in the ovaries they produce estradiol, leading to peak plasma levels of 180 to 370 pmol/L in late proestrus, 1 to 2 days before the pre-ovulatory luteinizing hormone (LH) surge (Fig. 157–2). On laparoscopic inspection, follicle development is not readily apparent on the ovary because of the ovarian bursa. Furthermore, until mid proestrus, follicular development appears only as clear grayish areas with indistinct boundaries on the ovarian surface. These areas gradually develop into distinct fluid-filled vesicular follicles, which protrude distinctly above the ovarian surface.[2] The external signs of proestrus, such as hyperemia and edema of the vulva and bloody vaginal discharge, are caused by the increased concentrations of estradiol (Fig. 157–3). This also causes lengthening and hyperemia of the uterine horns, enlargement of the cervix (which can be palpated), and thickening of the vaginal wall. The percentage of superficial cells in the vaginal smear increases, and the percentage of parabasal and small intermediate cells decreases. Erythrocytes are numerous, and leukocytes are seen in the early follicular phase but disappear as cornification progresses (Fig. 157–4). Superficial cells dominate as the follicular phase progresses (Fig. 157–5). However, it should be realized that although vaginal cytology provides an indication of the stage of the cycle it is not reliable for timing the pre-ovulatory LH surge or of ovulation.[3] With vaginoscopy it can be observed that the vaginal mucosal folds are swollen, are pale, and have smooth rounded surfaces (balloons) (Fig. 157–6). The increased concentrations of estradiol frequently cause hypertrophy of the floor of the

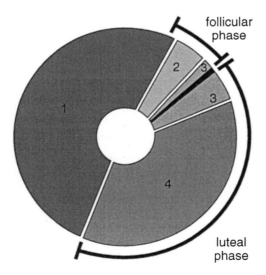

1. anestrus
2. proestrus
3. estrus, ovulation
4. metestrus or diestrus

Figure 157–1. Diagram of the estrous cycle and anestrus in the dog. (From Schaefers-Okkens AC: The ovaries. *In* Rijnberk A [ed]: Clinical Endocrinology of Dogs and Cats. Amsterdam, Kluwer Academic Publishers, 1996. With kind permission from Kluwer Academic Publishers.)

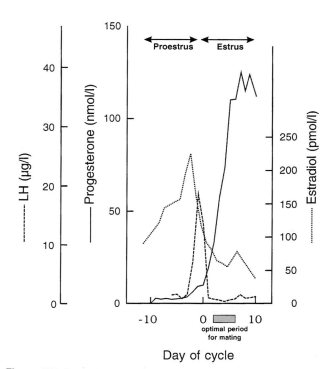

Figure 157–2. Diagram of estradiol, luteinizing hormone, and progesterone concentrations in plasma in relation to commonly observed estrus behavior of the bitch and the optimal period for mating. (From Schaefers-Okkens AC: The ovaries. *In* Rijnberk A [ed]: Clinical Endocrinology of Dogs and Cats. Amsterdam, Kluwer Academic Publishers, 1996. With kind permission from Kluwer Academic Publishers.)

Both LH and follicle-stimulating hormone (FSH) concentrations in plasma are relatively low during the follicular phase. Plasma progesterone levels initially remain low but fluctuate and increase during the second half of the follicular phase, as a result of partial luteinization of the follicles.

PRE-OVULATORY LUTEINIZATION AND OVULATION

The pre-ovulatory surge of LH lasts 24 to 72 hours. It usually starts 1 to 2 days after the estradiol peak and coincides with declining estradiol and rising progesterone concentrations in plasma (see Fig. 157–2). Rapid and extensive luteinization takes place during the pre-ovulatory LH surge. Ovulating follicles, therefore, have many of the characteristics of rapidly developing corpora lutea. Most ova in the dog are ovulated in an immature state as primary oocytes. The process of ovulation can take up to 24 hours. In the first 2 to 3 days after ovulation the oocytes mature; that is, they undergo the first meiotic division and the extrusion of the first polar body, after which fertilization can occur.[4] Plasma progesterone concentrations are 6 to 13 nmol/L at the time of the LH peak and 15 to 25 nmol/L at the time of ovulation, 36 to 48 hours later. Concurrent with the LH peak, a pre-ovulatory surge in FSH occurs that reaches peak concentrations 1 to 2 days after the LH peak. Estrus behavior usually starts synchronously with the pre-ovulatory LH peak (see Fig. 157–2), but some bitches demonstrate estrus behavior days before or after the LH peak.[5] Some bitches, however, exhibit no estrus behavior during the follicular phase, ovulation, and fertilization period. Shrinkage of the vaginal mucosa starts about midway in the follicular phase and continues through the phase of pre-ovulatory luteinization and ovulation, when many longitudinal folds can be observed (Fig. 157–9).

LUTEAL PHASE

Concentrations of progesterone originating from the corpora lutea increase in the peripheral blood during the remainder of the estrus and during the onset of diestrus (metestrus).

posterior vagina, just cranial to the urethral orifice and therefore folding over and covering the urethral orifice (Fig. 157–7). At the end of the follicular phase, that is, during the decline in estradiol and the rise in progesterone concentrations in plasma, shrinkage begins in response to reduced estradiol-dependent water retention. These cyclic changes are most marked in the dorsal median fold and precede those of the mid-vaginal mucosa (Fig. 157–8).

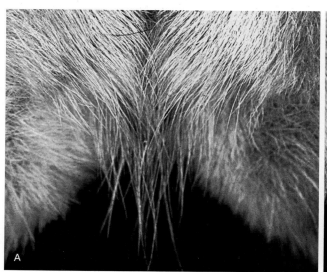
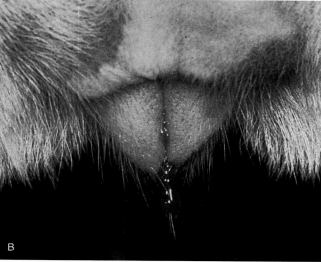

Figure 157–3. The vulva of a beagle bitch during (*A*) anestrus and (*B*) proestrus/estrus. (From Schaefers-Okkens AC: The ovaries. *In* Rijnberk A [ed]: Clinical Endocrinology of Dogs and Cats. Amsterdam, Kluwer Academic Publishers, 1996. With kind permission from Kluwer Academic Publishers.)

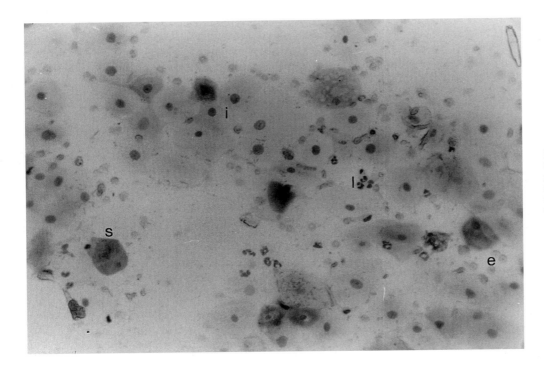

Figure 157–4. Vaginal cytology in the bitch at the onset of the follicular phase, showing primarily intermediate (i) cells, some superficial (s) cells, erythrocytes (e), and leukocytes (l). (May-Grünwald-Giemsa, ×200.)

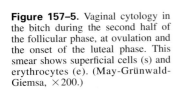

Figure 157–5. Vaginal cytology in the bitch during the second half of the follicular phase, at ovulation and the onset of the luteal phase. This smear shows superficial cells (s) and erythrocytes (e). (May-Grünwald-Giemsa, ×200.)

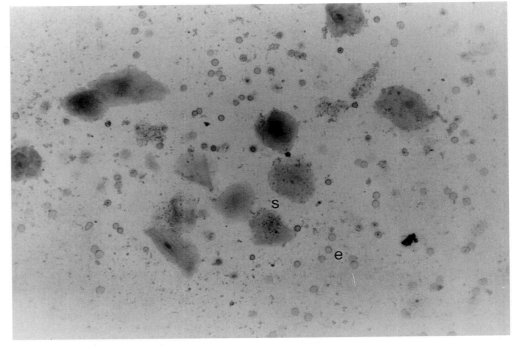

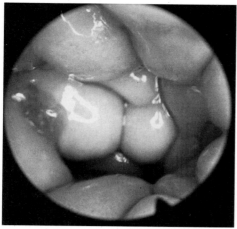

Figure 157–6. Vaginoscopy in the bitch at the onset of the follicular phase. Note the swollen, pale mucosal folds with smooth rounded surfaces (balloons) and the bloody secretion between the folds.

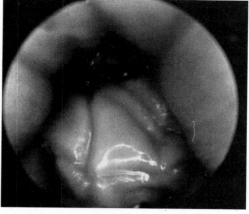

Figure 157–7. A modest vaginal hyperplasia that is observed quite often in the posterior vagina during the follicular phase of the cycle. (From Schaefers-Okkens AC: The ovaries. In Rijnberk A [ed]: Clinical Endocrinology of Dogs and Cats. Amsterdam, Kluwer Academic Publishers, 1996. With kind permission from Kluwer Academic Publishers.)

Estrus behavior is thus seen in the period of a rising plasma progesterone concentration. Increased progesterone concentrations plateau at 10 to 30 days after the LH peak. Thereafter, in non-pregnant bitches, the progesterone secretion declines slowly and reaches a basal level of 3 nmol/L for the first time about 75 days after the start of the luteal phase (Fig. 157–10).

During the initial part of the luteal phase the transition from estrus to diestrus takes place. In this period of time the cytology of the vaginal mucosa changes from primarily superficial cells to chiefly intermediate and parabasal cells and leukocytes (Fig. 157–11). This is an indication that the

fertile period has expired. During the oocyte maturation period, shrinkage of the vaginal mucosa continues and increasing numbers of sharp edged summit profiles appear. In the transition period from estrus to diestrus the mucosa thins and profiles become round. At the start of diestrus a patchwork of red and white areas can be seen (Fig. 157–12).

Prolactin acts as a luteotropic factor in the second half of the luteal phase.[6–8] During the first half of the luteal phase the canine corpus luteum functions independently of pituitary support.[9] Thereafter, inhibition of prolactin secretion causes a sharp decrease in progesterone secretion (Fig. 157–13). Whether or not LH has luteotropic properties in the bitch is

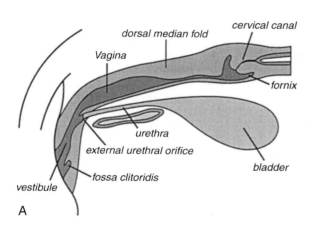

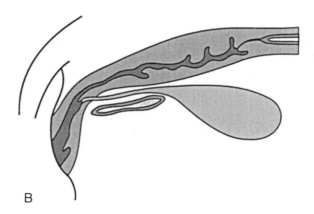

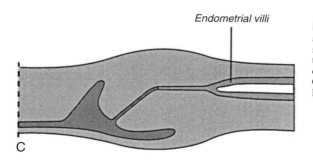

Figure 157–8. A sagittal section through the vestibule, vagina, and cervix of a bitch (A) during anestrus and (B) during the proestrus/estrus period. In this stage the vaginal wall is extremely folded. C, A close-up of the cranial part of the vagina and the cervix during the anestrus period. Note the very short cervical canal. (From Schaefers-Okkens AC: The ovaries. In Rijnberk A [ed]: Clinical Endocrinology of Dogs and Cats. Amsterdam, Kluwer Academic Publishers, 1996. With kind permission from Kluwer Academic Publishers.)

REP

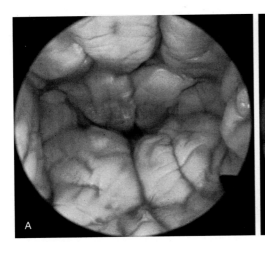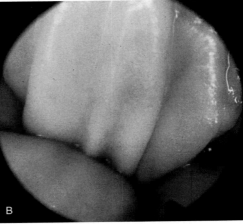

A

B

Figure 157–9. Vaginoscopy at the time of ovulation. The plasma progesterone concentration in this bitch was 22 nmol/L. *A*, The mucosal shrinkage leads to longitudinal folds. *B*, Close-up of the shrinkage of the longitudinal folds of the dorsal median fold of the cranial vagina. (From Schaefers-Okkens AC: The ovaries. *In* Rijnberk A [ed]: Clinical Endocrinology of Dogs and Cats. Amsterdam, Kluwer Academic Publishers, 1996. With kind permission from Kluwer Academic Publishers.)

still unclear. LH levels change little during the luteal phase, with the exception of a slight increase in the second half of the luteal phase (see Fig. 157–10).

The factors that are responsible for initiating the regression of the corpora lutea in the dog are still unknown. Prostaglandin $F_{2\alpha}$ originating from the endometrium is not the causative factor as it is in the cow and sheep. This is demonstrated by the fact that hysterectomy does not influence the length of the luteal phase.[10]

The secretion of prolactin fluctuates. In most non-pregnant bitches the plasma prolactin concentrations vary only slightly during the follicular and luteal phase (around 7 μg/L) (see Fig. 157–10). In the pseudopregnant bitch, however, the plasma prolactin concentration may increase, probably corresponding with the degree of "clinical" pseudopregnancy.

Pseudopregnancy is a syndrome that to one degree or another accompanies the extended luteal phase of all non-pregnant ovarian cycles in the bitch. If the nature of the syndrome is mild it is generally referred to as a physiologic or covert pseudopregnancy. In contrast, overt or clinical pseudopregnancy indicates obvious mammary development and/or behavioral changes that are not distinguishable from the changes of late pregnancy or lactation (see Chapter 158). Generally, in cases of covert pseudopregnancy there may be

slight increases in plasma prolactin concentrations comparing the first half of the luteal phase with the second half of the luteal phase and onset of anestrus.[11, 12] In bitches with overt pseudopregnancy, elevated plasma prolactin levels of around 35 μg/L are found.[13] A rapid decline in progesterone secretion, as occurs for example after ovariectomy during the luteal phase, appears to be an important precipitating factor for pseudopregnancy.

ANESTRUS

The time of the onset of anestrus depends on which criteria are being used to define the end of the luteal phase, such as after 2 to 3 months when mammary development subsides, the first time that the plasma progesterone concentration reaches a level below 3 nmol/L, or the moment that the influence of progesterone on the endometrium is no longer evident. In any case, the transition from the luteal phase into anestrus is gradual and varies considerably among bitches. Although sporadic elevations are observed, plasma estradiol concentrations are usually low and do not begin to rise until before the next proestrus. Plasma FSH concentrations are generally higher than during proestrus.[14] Mean plasma LH concentrations are low. There is an indication that there is a short period of increased LH pulsatility at the end of anestrus. In advanced anestrus the sensitivity of LH responses to various doses of gonadotropin-releasing hormone (GnRH) increases.[15]

The estrous cycle can begin at any time throughout the year and there appears to be little, if any, seasonal influence. Breed differences and strains within breeds can form the basis of variation in mean interestrous intervals. In the collie, for instance, the mean interval is 36 weeks, and in the Alsatian it is 20 to 22 weeks. Some breeds such as the Basenji and Tibetan mastiff, however, have a single annual estrous cycle, which may possibly be influenced by a photoperiod. Environmental factors can also affect the interestrous interval: an anestrous bitch placed in close proximity to a bitch in estrus can show an advance of the onset of proestrus by several weeks. Furthermore, bitches housed together often have synchronous estrous cycles.

It is still not clear which factors influence the transition from anestrus to proestrus. Endogenous opioids may modulate GnRH and LH release by reducing the pulsatility. There is some evidence that factors that decrease opioidergic activity promote LH release and the termination of anestrus.[16]

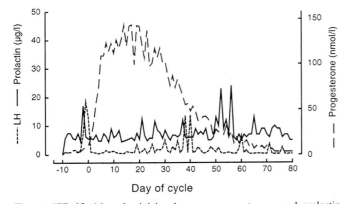

Figure 157–10. Mean luteinizing hormone, progesterone, and prolactin levels in plasma of three dogs during the follicular and luteal phase. The data have been synchronized on day 1, the day after the onset of the follicular phase on which the progesterone concentration in the peripheral blood had reached 16 nmol/L. (From Schaefers-Okkens AC: The ovaries. *In* Rijnberk A [ed]: Clinical Endocrinology of Dogs and Cats. Amsterdam, Kluwer Academic Publishers, 1996. With kind permission from Kluwer Academic Publishers.)

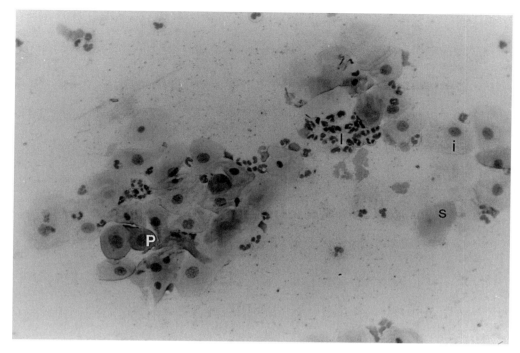

Figure 157–11. Vaginal cytology during diestrus (metestrus), which starts 6 to 10 days after the preovulatory LH peak. This smear shows intermediate cells (i), parabasal cells (p), some superficial cells (s), and leukocytes (l). (May-Grünwald-Giemsa, ×200.)

Pulsatile administration of GnRH has the potential to induce follicle growth and proestrus in dogs. In one study in which GnRH was administered in pulses of 15 to 500 ng/kg every 90 minutes for 7 to 9 days to 36 anestrous bitches, GnRH pulses resulted in proestrus, estrus, ovulation, and pregnancy in 26, 20, 16, and 12 bitches, respectively. Efficacy was dose dependent with high doses of more than 280 ng/kg (n = 12) versus intermediate doses of 85 to 270 ng/kg (n = 12) and low doses of less than 85 ng/kg (n = 12) resulting in a higher incidence of proestrus (100 per cent versus 80 per cent and 33 per cent, respectively), estrus (92 per cent versus 50 per cent and 25 per cent), ovulation (84 per cent versus 42 per cent and 8 per cent), and pregnancy (58 per cent versus 33 per cent and 8 per cent).[17] A fertile estrus could be also induced by administering a timed-release GnRH agonist, followed by a GnRH analogue on the first day of induced estrus. The interestrous interval in 120 and 150 days post-partum bitches was shortened to an average of 191 and

222 days, respectively, compared with an average of 264 days in control bitches. Using this method, three of six bitches for which treatment began at 120 days post partum, six of six at 150 days post partum, and five of six prepubertal (1 year old) bitches became pregnant and produced a litter.[18]

Anestrus can also be terminated by treating bitches with pig LH. In one study, proestrus was induced in all 16 bitches after pig LH was administered three times a day for 7 days; 12 bitches came in estrus, from which 7 ovulated. Bitches

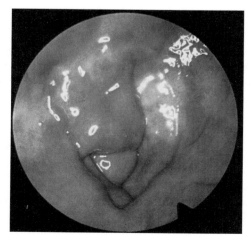

Figure 157–12. Vaginoscopy during diestrus (metestrus). Note the rounded profiles and the patchwork of red and white areas.

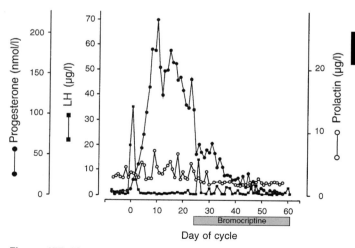

Figure 157–13. Mean progesterone, prolactin, and luteinizing hormone levels in the plasma of four dogs, treated with bromocriptine, 20 μg/kg, twice daily, orally from day 20 to 24 after the onset of the luteal phase until the end of the luteal period (bar). The data have been synchronized on day 1, the day after the onset of the follicular phase on which the progesterone concentration in the peripheral blood had reached 16 nmol/L. Note the shortened luteal phase due to basal prolactin levels caused by bromocriptine treatment. (From Schaefers-Okkens AC: The ovaries. *In* Rijnberk A [ed]: Clinical Endocrinology of Dogs and Cats. Amsterdam, Kluwer Academic Publishers, 1996. With kind permission from Kluwer Academic Publishers.)

REP

in which proestrus but not estrus occurred were all treated in early anestrus.[19] The observed rapid increase of plasma estradiol concentration after LH treatment suggests that increased follicle steroidogenesis is a primary effect of LH. On the other hand, the insufficient reaction to pig LH of bitches in early anestrus may be due to a deficiency of FSH or FSH receptors in this stage of anestrus. Follicular aromatase in rats and most other species studied appears to be primarily under upregulation control by FSH.[20] More research has to be performed concerning basal FSH concentrations and patterns of FSH pulsatility in bitches in different stages of anestrus.

Anestrus can also be shortened considerably by administration of dopamine agonists such as bromocriptine and cabergoline.[6, 16, 21, 22] Both bromocriptine and cabergoline rapidly inhibit prolactin secretion, but the lowering of prolactin secretion does not appear to be the cause of the premature induction of a follicular phase. Treatment with metergoline, in low dosages a serotonin antagonist, also lowers the plasma concentrations of prolactin, but the anestrus period will not be shortened. Therefore, the induction of estrus by dopamine agonists through suppression of prolactin secretion should probably be ruled out. The cause should be sought in other direct or indirect dopaminergic effects.[23] When bromocriptine treatment is started during the luteal phase, the interestrous interval can be shortened from 245 days to 100 days (Fig. 157–14).[6] When started during the anestrus—100 days after the ovulation—the next proestrus can be expected after about 45 days. The fertility of an estrus initiated by bromocriptine treatment appears to be normal.[22]

BREEDING MANAGEMENT OF THE HEALTHY BITCH

Breeding management starts with the determination if the bitch is healthy and if a normal fertility can be expected (Fig. 157–15). For that reason the age and the breeding history of both the bitch and the male dog have to be considered. Thereafter, a complete gynecologic examination of the bitch is needed. Recurring examinations should be performed during the follicular phase, ovulation, and pregnancy. A decrease in fertility may be expected with increasing age. One of the reasons for this diminished fertility may be the development of cystic endometrial hyperplasia (CEH; see Chapter 162).

THE HISTORY CONCERNING THE REPRODUCTION DATA

The reproduction history of the bitch must be considered in the breeding management program. The age of the bitch at her first estrus and the length of the interestrous intervals are important. The bitch that has not experienced an estrus by 18 months of age is considered to have a primary anestrus. One of the major causes of primary anestrus is probably true hermaphroditism or pseudohermaphroditism. If a bitch has experienced estrus, an interval of more than 12 months or an interval that is double the usual interestrous interval for that individual bitch is considered to be a prolonged interestrous interval. One reason for a prolonged anestrus can be hypothyroidism. However, it should be realized that less pronounced cases of hypothyroidism may result in prolonged or abbreviated proestrus or weak estrus symptoms instead of anestrus. Anestrus may also be induced with drugs such as progestagens or glucocorticosteroids. Glucocorticoids probably decrease levels of circulating gonadotropic hormones.[24] In bitches older than 8 years of age, the duration and frequency of the cycles become more irregular and the interestrous interval increases. An apparent prolonged anestrus can be present if the bitch has a silent estrus or if the owner did not observe the estrus properly. Shortened interestrous intervals (intervals of less than 4 months) may be caused by a split heat or are seen in combination with persistent estrus (see Chapter 158).

Attention must also be given to the length of estrous periods. The average length of proestrus and estrus is 9 days each. The bitch is considered to have a persistent estrus if ovulation has not occurred after about 25 days from the onset of proestrus. In that case, the plasma progesterone concentration will be lower than 16 nmol/L and estrus symptoms such as sanguineous discharge, estrus behavior, estradiol influence seen during vaginoscopy, and/or the presence of superficial cells in the vaginal smear are present. Plasma estradiol concentrations are not consistently elevated.[25] Persistent estrus can be caused by ovarian tumors and cysts (see Chapter 158).

Attention should also be given to attempts to mate the bitch and/or the results of matings in previous cycles, previous pregnancies and parturitions, and how many puppies were born. There are a number of problems that can lead to an unsuccessful mating. One problem can be inexperience or behavioral problems from bitch and/or dog. Also anatomic disorders may prevent a normal mating. Strictures, adhesions, septa, and hyperplasia, for example, are common in

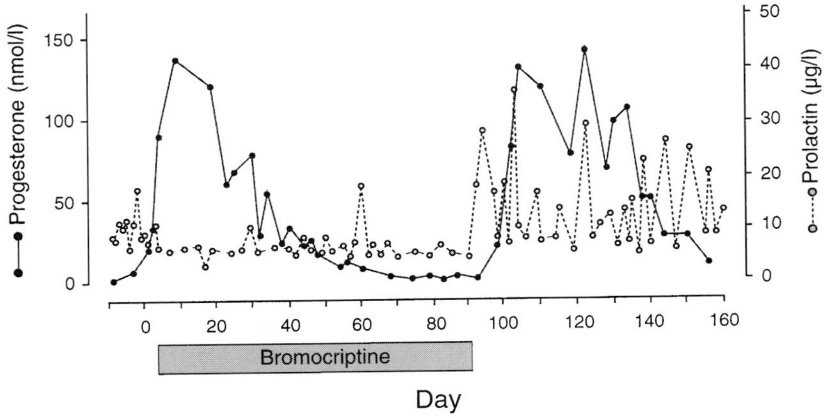

Figure 157–14. Progesterone and prolactin levels in the peripheral blood of one dog, treated with bromocriptine (bar) from ovulation in the first cycle until the onset of the next follicular phase. The luteal phase and especially the anestrus are considerably shortened. (From Schaefers-Okkens AC: The ovaries. In Rijnberk A [ed]: Clinical Endocrinology of Dogs and Cats. Amsterdam, Kluwer Academic Publishers, 1996. With kind permission from Kluwer Academic Publishers.)

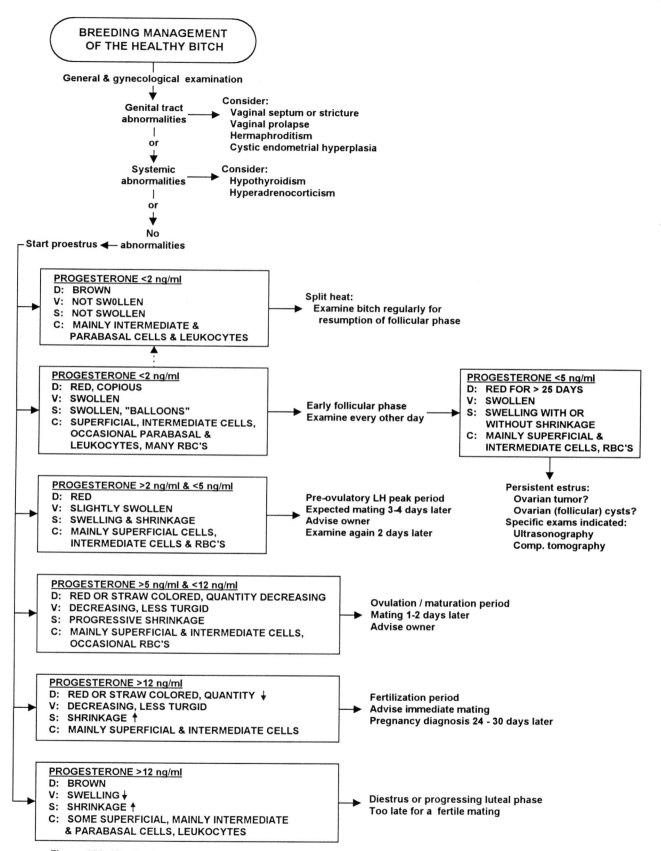

Figure 157–15. Algorithm for the breeding management of the healthy bitch. D = appearance of the vaginal discharge; V = appearance of the vulva; S = appearance of the vaginal mucosa as observed during vaginoscopy; C = vaginal cytology.

bitches.[26] They can be congenital or acquired as a result of local treatment of vaginitis with irritating drugs (see Chapter 163).

Another important reason for a failure to mate or a missed conception is mating at an improper moment. A large number of fertility problems are the result of inappropriate management of the bitch and are avoidable if a proper breeding program is used. Additionally, CEH or CEH-endometritis or infectious diseases such as canine brucellosis or herpesvirus infection may also lead to breeding problems. Infertility due to CEH without endometritis, in which case the bitch does not show signs of a systemic disease, may be diagnosed during an ultrasonographic examination.

Canine brucellosis is a contagious disease for which the clinical manifestations vary greatly. It is characterized in the bitch by generalized lymphadenopathy and by early embryonic death, abortion (mainly between the 45th and 55th days of gestation), and infertility.[27] Canine brucellosis must be considered whenever there is a history of abortion or poor reproductive performance in either sex. The diagnosis can, however, not be established based on clinical signs alone. Serologic tests are necessary to confirm the diagnosis of canine brucellosis. Canine herpesvirus can cause a high percentage of dead puppies in the first weeks after parturition. A marked decrease in fertility has also been described. Infected bitches with antibodies for herpes will probably not suffer permanent infertility.

The Examination of the Bitch

Breeding management starts with a general examination followed by sequential examinations. During the gynecologic portion of the first examination special emphasis should be given to palpation of the uterus and digital evaluation of the vagina. The following items should be examined every other day, starting 5 to 6 days after onset of proestrus: the vulva (size, swelling), vaginal discharge (quantity, color), and vaginoscopic and cytologic findings. Furthermore, the owner should be asked to look for behavioral changes consistent with estrus. Estrus behavior usually occurs synchronously with the pre-ovulatory LH peak (see Fig. 157–2), but this behavior can be observed several days before or after the LH peak or may never be seen. Repeated examinations are carried out to determine if the cycle is progressing normally.

Vaginoscopic and cytologic observations not in agreement with the expected stage of the cycle may be a sign of a fertility disorder, which may or may not be serious. For example, a split heat is not uncommon in both younger and older healthy bitches. In cases of split heat, the follicular phase stops before ovulation and resumes after a few days or weeks. The vaginal discharge changes from red to brown; the smear shows intermediate cells, parabasal cells, and leukocytes; and the swelling of the vaginal mucosal folds diminishes. It is probably caused by prematurely regressing follicles. Ovulation will generally occur if proestrus returns. Treatment is usually not necessary, but close monitoring of the cycle is essential for determining the appropriate mating period.

Sequential examinations should also be carried out to determine the ovulation period. Data concerning vulvar swelling, vaginal discharge, and vaginoscopic and cytologic findings have been described. Because of the variable length of proestrus and estrus, it should be clear that breeding a bitch on pre-set days of the cycle (e.g., 11 to 13 days after onset of proestrus bleeding) will give inconsistent results. Although breeding in accordance with estrus behavior will give better results, some bitches are nevertheless bred too early and others too late. Determination of the ovulation period is, therefore, of value. Several methods have been described to determine the ovulation period and the proper period for mating. The principal methods are measurement of the plasma progesterone concentration and vaginoscopy. Plasma progesterone concentrations should, along with the other examinations, be determined every other day. At the onset of the follicular phase, determined through cytologic and vaginoscopic findings, the time between two determinations of plasma progesterone may be longer than in the progressing follicular phase. Use of an enzyme-linked immunosorbent assay (ELISA) or enzyme immunoassay kit for plasma progesterone determination may be less accurate, especially in medium (progesterone: >3 nnmol/L <16 nnmol/L) plasma progesterone concentrations as compared with a plasma progesterone determination via a radioimmunoassay (RIA).[28, 29] The RIA method is therefore the preferred method for progesterone determination. When frozen or chilled extended semen is being used, and sperm life span is expected to be shorter than in fresh semen, it is especially advisable to determine plasma progesterone concentrations by RIA to ensure accuracy in determining the ovulation day and the fertile period, therefore permitting use of a single insemination. Plasma progesterone concentrations increase slightly at the time of the pre-ovulatory LH peak and rapidly at the onset of ovulation. At this time the plasma progesterone concentration exceeds 16 nmol/L. The onset of the optimal period for mating is 24 hours later and is based on the time needed for maturation of the oocytes, capacitation, and life span of the sperm.[30] With determination of the period for mating using a rapid RIA for the plasma progesterone concentration, it was found that 105 of 112 (94 per cent) bitches with normal fertility became pregnant and 81 of 104 bitches (78 per cent) with suboptimal fertility became pregnant. In the latter group, only 23 per cent of previous matings had been successful.[31]

Determination of the pre-ovulatory LH peak would also provide an excellent parameter for the estimation of the ovulation time. In-hospital ELISA LH kits are available. However, more frequent blood sampling is required than for progesterone because of the risk of missing the pre-ovulatory LH peak. Vaginoscopy can also be used to try to establish the ovulation period. The mucosal changes are, however, a response to hormonal changes and are therefore secondary changes. Additionally, interpretation of the changes is subjective. Vaginoscopy is thus a less reliable method of estimation of the ovulation period than measurement of hormone levels. For experienced veterinarians, it can be a useful tool for monitoring the stage of the cycle, but mating advice based on vaginoscopy should include the recommendation to mate at least twice, with an interval of 48 hours. Vaginal cytology is useful in diagnosing early proestrus, progressing proestrus-estrus, or diestrus. There are, however, no reliable changes in the smear indicative of the pre-ovulatory LH surge or of ovulation. Lastly, ultrasonography is not reliable for ovulation determination.[32]

Additional Examinations

In bitches with previous fertility problems, vaginal culture may be of use. A mixed bacterial flora including *Pasteurella*, beta-hemolytic streptococci, and *Escherichia coli* often inhabits the canine vagina and should not be considered a causative factor for infertility. In an examination of the aerobic bacterial flora of the genital tract of 59 bitches in four breeds during different stages of the cycle and pregnancy—all bitches whelped at least once during this study—culture results were negative in only 5 per cent of the specimens. Although the cultures in general showed a mixed flora, single species were obtained from 18 per cent of the specimens. The aerobic bacterial flora consisted of common opportunistic pathogens.[33] Therefore, bacterial culturing of vaginal swab specimens from bitches without signs of genital disease is of little value. Treatment is indicated in cases of suspected genital inflammation only if there are many bacteria (>100 colonies per culture) or the culture reveals only one species. Treatment may be systemic or local, but locally applied drugs alter the vaginal environment, are often spermicidal, and should therefore not be used shortly before breeding.

Pregnancy diagnosis is important within a breeding management program. Between 26 and 33 days after mating, pregnancy may be diagnosed by abdominal palpation. In some bitches an earlier diagnosis can be made dependent on muscular defense, thickness, breed, and so on. The examination should, however, be repeated in case of a negative finding. In case of a negative or dubious finding, if vesicles of different size and elasticity are palpated, or if only one or two gestational vesicles are found, ultrasonography is indicated. In the last two instances, fetal resorption has frequently been observed, which may warrant further examinations and sequential ultrasonographic examinations during the rest of the pregnancy. Furthermore, in cases of only one or two gestational vesicles the chance and risk of a prolonged pregnancy have to be discussed with the owner.

REFERENCES

1. Anderson AC, Simpson ME: The Ovary and Reproductive Cycle of the Dog (Beagle). Los Altos, CA, Geron-X, 1973.
2. Wildt DE, et al: Relationship of reproductive behavior, serum luteinizing hormone and time of ovulation in the bitch. Biol Reprod 18:561–570, 1978.
3. Concannon PW: Physiology of canine ovarian cycles, pregnancy, parturition and anestrus. In Christiansen IJ (ed): Proceedings of the Symposium on Reproduction in the Dog. Denmark, 1989, pp 32–39.
4. Phemister RD, et al: Time of ovulation in the beagle bitch. Biol Reprod 8:74–82, 1973.
5. Concannon, PW: Canine physiology of reproduction. In Burke TJ (ed): Small Animal Reproduction and Infertility. Philadelphia, Lea & Febiger, 1986, pp 23–42.
6. Okkens AC, et al: Shortening of the interoestrous interval and the lifespan of the corpus luteum of the cyclic dog by bromocriptine treatment. Vet Q 7:173–176, 1985.
7. Okkens AC, et al: Evidence for prolactin as the main luteotrophic factor in the cyclic dog. Vet Q 12:193–201, 1990.
8. Concannon PW, et al: Suppression of luteal function in dogs by bromocriptin. J Reprod Fertil 81:175–180, 1987.
9. Okkens AC, et al: Influence of hypophysectomy on the lifespan of the corpus luteum in the cyclic dog. J Reprod Fertil 77:187–192, 1986.
10. Okkens AC, et al: Evidence for the non-involvement of the uterus in the lifespan of the corpus luteum in the cyclic dog. Vet Q 7:169–173, 1985.
11. Onclin K, Verstegen JP: Secretion patterns of plasma prolactin and progesterone in pregnant compared with nonpregnant beagle bitches. J Reprod Fertil Suppl 51:203–208, 1997.
12. Overgaauw PAM, et al: Incidence of patent Toxocara canis infection in bitches during the oestrous cycle. Vet Q 20:104–107, 1998.
13. Okkens AC, et al: Plasma concentrations of prolactin in overtly pseudopregnant Afghan hounds and the effect of metergoline. J Reprod Fertil Suppl 51:295–301, 1997.
14. Olson PN, et al: Concentrations of reproductive hormones in canine serum throughout late anestrus, proestrus and estrus. Biol Reprod 27:1196–1206, 1982.
15. Van Haaften B, et al: Increasing sensitivity of the pituitary to GnRH from early to late anoestrus in the beagle bitch. J Reprod Fertil 101:221–225, 1994.
16. Concannon PW: Biology of gonadotrophin secretion in adult and prepubertal female dogs. J Reprod Fertil Suppl 47:3–27, 1993.
17. Concannon PW, et al: LH release, induction of oestrus and fertile ovulations in response to pulsatile administration of GnRH to anoestrous dogs. J Reprod Fertil 51:41–54, 1997.
18. Inaba T, et al: Induction of fertile estrus in bitches using a sustained-release formulation of a GnRH agonist (leuprolide acetate). Theriogenology 49:975–982, 1998.
19. Verstegen J, et al: Termination of obligate anoestrus and induction of fertile ovarian cycles in dogs by administration of purified pig LH. J Reprod Fertil 111:35–40, 1997.
20. Gore-Langton RE, Armstrong DT: Follicular steroidogenesis and its control. In Knobil E, Neill JD (eds): The Physiology of Reproduction. New York, Raven Press, 1994.
21. Onclin K, et al: Patterns of circulating prolactin, LH, and FSH during dopamine-agonist induced termination of anestrus in beagle dogs. Biol Reprod Suppl 52:314, 1995.
22. Van Haaften B, et al: Induction of oestrus and ovulation in dogs by treatment with PMSG and/or bromocriptine. J Reprod Fertil Suppl 39:330–331, 1989.
23. Okkens AC, et al: Dopamine agonistic effects as opposed to prolactin concentrations in plasma as the influencing factor on the duration of the anoestrus in the bitch. J Reprod Fertil Suppl 51:55–58, 1997.
24. Kemppainen RJ, et al: Effects of prednisone on thyroid and gonadal endocrine function in dogs. J Endocrinol 96:293–302, 1983.
25. Olson PN, et al: Persistent estrus in the bitch. In Ettinger SJ (ed): Textbook of Veterinary Internal Medicine, 3rd ed. Philadelphia, WB Saunders, 1989, pp 1793–1796.
26. Post K, et al: Vaginal hyperplasia in the bitch: Literature review and commentary. Can Vet J 32:35–37, 1991.
27. Carmichael LE: Canine brucellosis. In Burke TJ (ed): Small Animal Reproduction and Infertility. Philadelphia, Lea & Febiger, 1986, pp 269–275.
28. Manothaiudom K, et al: Evaluation of the Icagen-Target Canine Ovulation Timing Diagnostic Test in detecting canine plasma progesterone concentrations. J Am Anim Hosp Assoc 31:57–64, 1995.
29. Dieleman SJ, Blankenstein DM: Determination of the time of ovulation in the dog by estimation of progesterone in blood: Applicability of an EIA method in comparison to RIA. In: Proceedings of the 11th International Congress on Animal Reproduction and AI, Dublin, Ireland, 1988, pp 21–22.
30. Mahi CA, Yanagimachi R: Maturation and sperm penetration of canine ovaria oocytes in vitro. J Exp Zool 196:189–196, 1976.
31. Van Haaften B, et al: Timing the mating of dogs on the basis of blood progesterone concentration. Vet Rec 125:524–526, 1989.
32. Silva LDM, et al: Assessment of ovarian changes around ovulation in bitches by ultrasonography, laparoscopy and hormonal assays. Vet Radiol Ultrasound 37:313–320, 1996.
33. Bjurström L, Linde-Forsberg C: Long-term study of aerobic bacteria of the genital tract in breeding bitches. Am J Vet Res 53:665–669, 1992.

REP

CHAPTER 158

OVARIAN AND ESTROUS CYCLE ABNORMALITIES

Autumn P. Davidson and Edward C. Feldman

Deviation from anticipated estrous cycle events in a bitch intended for breeding may cause her to be brought to a veterinarian for evaluation. The canine reproductive cycle is divided into four distinct phases, each having characteristic behavioral, physical, and endocrinologic patterns (see Chapter 157). Although considerable variation exists in the normal canine reproductive cycle, breeders often believe that such variations indicate abnormality. The clinician should attempt to differentiate between bitches with normal estrous cycles but unexpected patterns and those with true abnormalities. Detection of individual variations within the normal range of events in a fertile bitch can be crucial to providing effective counseling concerning breeding management. Evaluation of the estrous cycle for actual abnormalities is an important component in assessing an apparently infertile bitch (Fig. 158–1). Variations in normal estrous cycle events can sometimes be traced to specific ovarian disorders.

THE NORMAL CANINE ESTROUS CYCLE

The interestrous interval (from the end of estrus to the beginning of proestrus) normally varies from 4.5 to 10 months in duration, with 7 months being average. The anestrous phase of the interestrous interval is marked by reproductive inactivity, uterine involution, and endometrial repair. The normal bitch is neither attractive nor receptive to male dogs. Minimal mucoid vaginal discharge is present, and the vulva is small. Vaginal cytology is characterized by small parabasal cells with occasional nontoxic neutrophils and small numbers of mixed bacteria. Viewed endoscopically, the vaginal mucosal folds are flat, thin, and pale red. The termination of anestrus (onset of proestrus) follows the pulsatile secretion of gonadotropin-releasing hormone (GnRH) by the hypothalamus, which induces secretion of the pituitary gonadotropins follicle-stimulating hormone (FSH) and luteinizing hormone (LH). Such pulsatile GnRH secretion is a physiologic requirement of gonadotropin release. Following GnRH stimulation during late anestrus, pituitary gonadotrophs release LH in a rapid, transitory pattern and FSH in a slow, sustained pattern. Mean serum concentrations of FSH rise moderately during late anestrus, while episodic surges of LH occur throughout. At the termination of anestrus, the pulsatile release of LH increases, preceding ovarian folliculogenesis of proestrus. Serum estrogen and progesterone concentrations are basal (5 to 10 pg/mL and <1 ng/mL, respectively) in late anestrus. Anestrus normally lasts one to six months.[1, 2]

During proestrus, the bitch attracts male dogs but is not receptive to breeding. She may become more playful or passive concerning the male as proestrus progresses. A serosanguineous-hemorrhagic vaginal discharge of uterine origin is present, and the vulva is mildly enlarged and turgid. The microscopic appearance of exfoliated vaginal epithelial cells shifts over a period of four to seven days from small parabasal cells to small then large intermediate cells, superficial intermediate cells, and finally superficial (cornified) epithelial cells. These changes in exfoliated vaginal cells reflect the degree of estrogen influence on the vaginal mucosa. Red blood cells are usually but not invariably present. Endoscopically, the vaginal mucosal folds appear edematous, pink, and rounded. Serum FSH and LH concentrations are low during most of proestrus, rising during preovulatory surges. Estrogen rises from basal anestrus levels to peak levels (50 to 100 pg/dL during late proestrus), while progesterone remains basal (<1 ng/mL) until rising with the LH surge (2 to 4 ng/mL). The LH surge generally lasts only 12 to 24 hours in the bitch. Proestrus lasts from three days to three weeks, averaging nine days. The follicular phase of the ovarian cycle coincides with proestrus and early estrus.[1, 3]

During estrus, the normal bitch displays receptive or passive behavior with a male dog, enabling breeding. Serosanguineous to hemorrhagic vaginal discharge diminishes to variable degrees. Vulvar enlargement and edema tend to be maximal, but the vulva is soft. Vaginal cytology usually consists of 80 to 100 per cent superficial cells, with no white blood cells. Red blood cells tend to diminish but may persist throughout estrus. Endoscopically, vaginal mucosal folds become progressively wrinkled or crenulated, correlating with ovulation and oocyte maturation. Plasma estrogen progressively declines to basal concentrations. Progesterone concentrations steadily increase (usually 4 to 10 ng/mL at ovulation), marking the onset of the luteal phase of the ovarian cycle. Estrus lasts three days to three weeks, with an average of nine days. The receptive behavior of estrus may precede or shortly follow the LH peak. Duration of receptivity is variable and may not coincide precisely with the fertile period. Receptive behavior reflects decreasing estrogen and increasing progesterone concentrations. Ovulation of infertile primary oocytes begins approximately two days after the LH surge, with oocyte maturation occurring over the following one to three days. The life span of secondary (fertile) oocytes is two to three days.[1–3]

During diestrus, the normal bitch becomes refractory to breeding and gradually less attractive to male dogs. Vaginal discharge diminishes, often becoming mucoid and mildly suppurative before disappearing, and vulvar edema slowly resolves. Vaginal cytology is abruptly altered by the reappearance of parabasal epithelial cells and, frequently, neutrophils. Endoscopically, vaginal mucosal folds appear flattened and flaccid. Plasma estrogen concentrations are low during diestrus, except for a mild rise in the pregnant bitch prior to parturition. Plasma progesterone concentrations steadily increase during the first few weeks of diestrus to a plateau

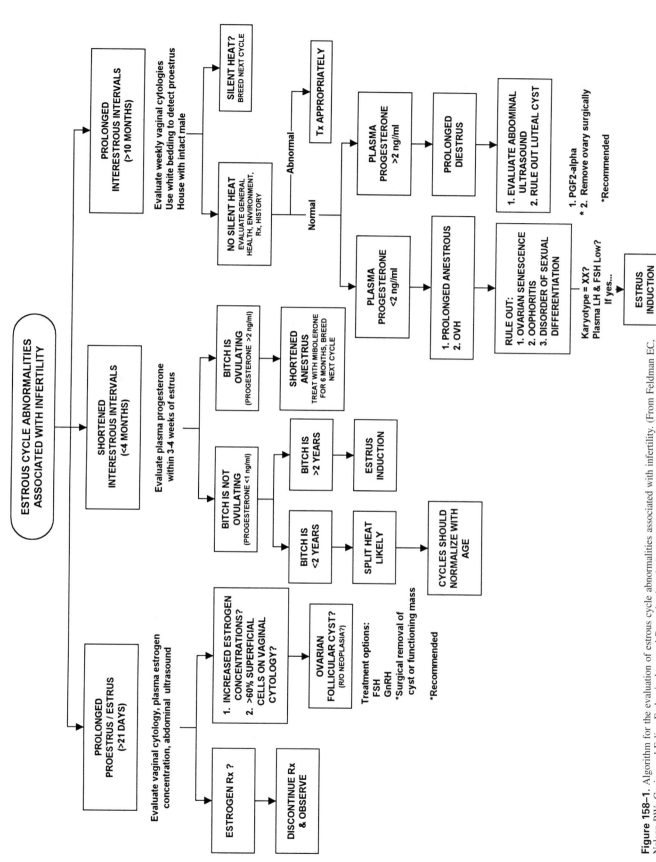

Figure 158–1. Algorithm for the evaluation of estrous cycle abnormalities associated with infertility. (From Feldman EC, Nelson RW: Canine and Feline Endocrinology and Reproduction, 2nd ed. Philadelphia, WB Saunders, 1996, p 630.)

of 15 to 80 ng/mL, before progressively declining in late diestrus. Progesterone secretion is dependent on both pituitary LH and prolactin secretion and causes proliferation of the endometrium and quiescence of the myometrium. Diestrus usually lasts two to three months in the absence of pregnancy. Parturition terminates pregnancy 64 to 66 days after the LH peak, or 56 to 58 days after the onset of diestrus as determined by vaginal cytology. With larger litters, duration of gestation decreases. Prolactin concentrations increase in a reciprocal fashion to declining progesterone concentrations as diestrus terminates. Prolactin concentrations are higher in pregnant bitches. Mammary ductal and glandular tissues increase in response to prolactin.[1-3]

NORMAL VARIATIONS IN THE CANINE ESTROUS CYCLE

When evaluating a bitch for estrous cycle abnormalities, the signalment, medical history, reproductive history, physical examination findings, and results of clinical testing should be considered. Monitoring the bitch over time may be necessary to reach a diagnosis.

DELAYED PUBERTY

The onset of the first estrous cycle occurs after a bitch approaches her adult height and body weight. Small breeds generally begin the first estrous cycle between 6 and 10 months of age, while large breeds may begin as late as 18 to 24 months. Family histories (dam and female siblings) can help predict the onset of reproductive activity. Efforts at differentiating delayed puberty from an actual failure to experience reproductive cycles should be postponed until a bitch is at least 2 years old.

SILENT HEAT CYCLES

The occurrence of a silent heat cycle needs to be ruled out when evaluating a bitch for a reported failure to experience estrous cycles. Fastidious bitches with minimal vulvar swelling or vaginal discharge and few behavioral changes may have estrous cycles that escape detection, especially in the absence of a male dog. Estrous cycles tend to become more apparent as a bitch ages. Performing weekly vaginal cytologies or monthly progesterone assays, housing the bitch near an intact male, or using white bedding can aid in the detection of silent heats. True primary anestrus in a bitch that fails to experience an estrous cycle is most likely due to a disorder of sexual development (see Chapter 165).[3]

SPLIT HEAT CYCLES

Bitches experiencing split heat cycles, in which signs of proestrus or estrus occur without progression to diestrus, may be brought to a veterinarian for evaluation of abnormal, short cycles and/or a lack of sexual receptivity. These cycles typically occur in young bitches and are characterized by periods of bloody vaginal discharge and attractiveness to males, usually without breeding. Much less commonly, such cycles occur in mature bitches with a history of normal past cycles. Waves of folliculogenesis and estrogen secretion without ovulation occur in split heats. Follicular outrace follows, and no luteal phase with progesterone elevation

occurs; thus complete sexual receptivity does not take place. After a period of 2 to 10 weeks, another similar proestrus occurs, which may or may not proceed through diestrus. Eventually, most bitches experiencing split heats progress through a normal estrus to diestrus. The condition is not associated with reproductive pathology, and no treatment is recommended. Cytologies documenting the influence of estrogen on vaginal mucosa early in the cycle, and progesterone assays performed one to two weeks later (≤ 2 ng/mL) documenting folliculogenesis without luteinization, confirm the diagnosis of a split heat.

MANAGEMENT ERRORS

Bitches with a history of failing to permit breeding or failing to conceive after artificial insemination or forced breeding during a perceived fertile period need to be evaluated for kennel management errors. Timing of the receptive and fertile periods during estrus varies significantly among normal bitches. These periods may not correlate with the handler's choice of predetermined breeding dates, typically 10 to 14 days after the onset of vaginal bleeding. Ovulation timing protocols using serial vaginal cytologies, vaginoscopy, and serum progesterone concentrations are useful in identifying the actual fertile period when breeding should occur.[4] Behavioral or physical problems can interfere with a bitch's acceptance of a male for breeding. A dominant bitch exposed to an inexperienced male may not allow breeding even during the appropriate time. Vulvar and vaginal abnormalities such as strictures or septate bands and vaginal hyperplasia may make natural breeding painful and result in a bitch refusing to permit breeding when in estrus (see Chapter 163) (Fig. 158–2).[5] Prebreeding veterinary examination permits early detection of such anatomic problems, enabling correction or adjustment in plans (artificial insemination vs. natural breeding) before the onset of proestrus (see Chapter 157).

PATTERNS OF ABNORMAL ESTROUS CYCLES

Abnormal estrous cycles can be categorized and simplified into several patterns reflecting either prolongation or abbre-

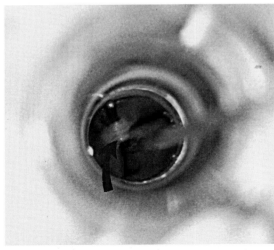

Figure 158–2. Vaginoscopic view of a septate band of tissue in the caudal vagina of an estrous bitch exhibiting pain during breeding efforts. The band is retracted with a spay hook.

viation of a phase of the cycle or an alteration in the normal sequence of events. An owner's interpretation of a bitch's behavior and physical characteristics may not equate with the actual physiologic events, necessitating prospective documentation of the cycle through vaginal cytologies, vaginoscopy, behavioral analysis, and plasma estrogen and progesterone concentrations.

PROLONGED PROESTRUS OR ESTRUS

Prolonged proestrus or estrus occurs when a bitch displays vaginal bleeding (of uterine origin) for more than 21 to 28 consecutive days, accompanied by attractiveness to males. Greater than 80 to 90 per cent superficial cells are seen on vaginal cytologic examination. Such bitches may or may not be receptive to breeding. Prolonged proestrus and/or estrus most likely results from persistent secretion of estrogens, with or without small increases in progesterone secretion. Progesterone enhances sexual receptivity. Endogenous sources of prolonged estrogen and/or progesterone exposure in the bitch include ovarian follicular cysts and secretory neoplasias.[6] Secretory, anovulatory follicular ovarian cysts tend to be solitary, to be lined with granulosa cells, and to exceed normal preovulatory follicles in size, ranging from 1 to 5 cm in diameter (Fig. 158–3). Bilateral follicular cysts may indicate a problem with the hypothalamic-pituitary-ovarian axis. Follicular cysts tend to occur in bitches younger than 3 years of age. Quite uncommonly, ovarian neoplasia capable of producing estrogen occurs, including tumors of epithelial origin (cystadenomas and adenocarcinomas) as well as tumors of gonadal-stromal origin (granulosatheca cell tumors).[7] Ovarian neoplasia tends to occur in bitches older than 5 years of age and can occur unilaterally or, less commonly, bilaterally. Functional ovarian neoplasia and cystic ovarian pathology can occur simultaneously (Fig. 158–4). Cysts in the contralateral ovary, and endometrial hyperplasia accompanying tumor function, occur most frequently with tumors of gonadal-stromal origin.[8]

There are few differential diagnoses for prolonged vaginal bleeding. Vaginal bleeding secondary to infection, inflammation, or neoplasia of the genitourinary tract, a vaginal foreign body, or a coagulopathy should be differentiated from prolonged proestrus or estrus. Excessive exogenous administration of estrogen may be encountered when a bitch is treated for urethral sphincter incompetence with diethylstilbestrol (DES) or when attempts are made to prevent

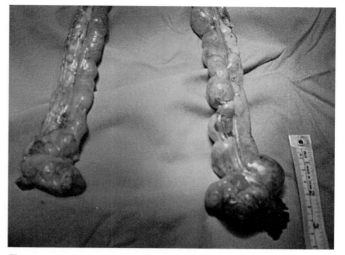

Figure 158–4. Ovarian carcinoma, right ovary *(ruler)*, accompanied by ovarian follicular cysts, left ovary, in a Boxer bitch experiencing estrus for longer than two months.

unwanted pregnancy using DES or estradiol cypionate. Recognized sequelae to chronic estrogen exposure include bone marrow dyscrasias, predisposition to the cystic endometrial gland hyperplasia-pyometra complex, and the development of ovarian cysts.[6–8]

After naturally occurring hyperestrogenism is confirmed through vaginal cytologies and serum estrogen concentrations, abdominal ultrasonography is recommended in an attempt to identify an ovarian follicular cyst or functional neoplasia (Fig. 158–5). Normal preovulatory follicles measure 4 to 9 mm in diameter, making them smaller than follicular cysts and most functional neoplasia.[9] Analysis of the estrogen and progesterone concentrations in fluid from abnormal cystic ovarian structures obtained via ultrasound guidance and histologic analysis of tissues obtained surgically can confirm the diagnosis.

Because follicular cysts may spontaneously undergo atresia or luteinization, not all bitches experiencing prolonged proestrus or estrus require treatment. Progression of the follicular cyst to an atretic follicle or a corpus luteum can be monitored ultrasonographically, via vaginal cytologies, and by serum estrogen and progesterone concentrations.

REP

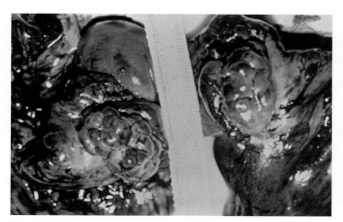

Figure 158–3. Functional, nonovulatory follicular ovarian cysts found in a Mastiff bitch experiencing estrus for longer than three months.

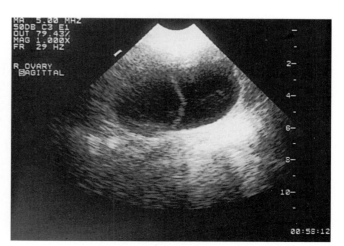

Figure 158–5. Ultrasonographic appearance of a functional, estrogen-secreting, nonovulatory ovarian follicular cyst.

Therapy aimed at terminating prolonged proestrus or estrus becomes necessary if spontaneous regression fails to occur, vaginal bleeding is a continuing nuisance, estrous behavior and the attraction of males are unacceptable, or other complications develop (blood-loss anemia, marrow dyscrasias, vaginal hyperplasia) (Fig. 158–6). Medical and surgical options exist for the treatment of persistent follicular cysts. Medical therapies should not place the reproductive health of the bitch at risk. Progesterone treatment of bitches with functional follicular cysts puts them at increased risk for the development of cystic endometrial hyperplasia-pyometra and is not advised. The use of GnRH (50 to 100 μg/bitch intramuscularly every 24 to 48 hours for up to three doses) or human placental gonadotropin (hCG 11 IU/lb, or 22 IU/kg, intramuscularly every 24 to 48 hours) has been advocated[3, 6] as effective in inducing cyst regression or luteinization, although our success rate with medical treatment has been extremely poor. GnRH does not appear to be antigenic in the bitch and may be the preferred treatment. Successful induction of cyst regression or luteinization is reflected by a reduction in vaginal discharge, diminished attractiveness to males, and normalization of behavior. Serum estrogen concentrations fall, and increased progesterone concentrations support luteinization. Ultrasonographic monitoring of ovarian morphology shows regression of hypoechoic structures. It has been suggested that failure of medical therapies to resolve prolonged proestrus or estrus indicates that ovarian neoplasia is more likely than a follicular cyst,[3, 6] but this has not been our experience. We have found surgical removal of such cysts to be the most expedient means of managing the problem.[3] Removal of the cyst alone is optimal, but resection of the associated ovary is often necessary. Histologic evaluation of the removed tissue usually confirms the diagnosis and permits evaluation for evidence of neoplasia that might warrant additional therapy (Fig. 158–7).[10]

PROLONGED INTERESTROUS INTERVALS

Bitches exhibiting prolonged interestrous intervals may have prolongation of either anestrus or diestrus. Prolonged anestrus occurs when no ovarian activity occurs for longer than 16 to 20 months in a bitch having previously experienced estrous cycles. An actual failure to continue to cycle

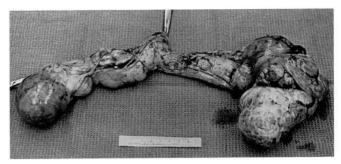

Figure 158–7. Bilateral ovarian neoplasia.

must be differentiated from silent heats. Underlying disease and iatrogenic causes for failure to cycle should be ruled out by a careful history, physical examination, and database.

A bitch presented for evaluation of prolonged intervals between heat cycles may be under the influence of progesterone (≥2 to 5 ng/mL). When progesterone concentrations remain increased for longer than 9 to 10 weeks, prolonged diestrus is probable. The clinical behavior of the bitch cannot be differentiated from that of one experiencing prolonged anestrus. Vaginal cytologies, serial serum progesterone concentrations, and the ultrasonographic appearance of the ovaries and uterus are valuable in establishing a diagnosis.

Prolonged diestrus occurs secondary to the presence of a luteinized, progesterone-secreting ovarian cyst. Progesterone feeds back to the pituitary and hypothalamus, preventing normal ovarian activity. Luteinized cysts can be single or multiple, involving one or both ovaries.[3] Abdominal ultrasonography should identify hypoechoic structures within the affected ovaries (Fig. 158–8). Abdominal radiography rarely provides diagnostic information because the cysts are relatively small. Serum progesterone concentrations of 2 to 5 ng/mL or greater confirm the diagnosis. Treatment with prostaglandin $F_{2\alpha}$ usually causes only a transient decline in serum progesterone levels, indicating partial luteolysis. Surgical removal of the cyst with histologic analysis is the recommended treatment. Separation of the cyst from the affected ovary is optimal but may not be possible.[3] Acquiring a uterine biopsy to evaluate the presence and extent of accompanying cystic endometrial hyperplasia is advisable, as it can provide valuable information concerning the future fertility of the bitch (see Fig. 158–8). Cystic endometrial

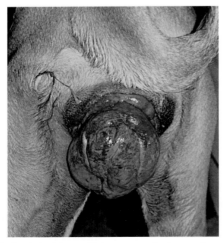

Figure 158–6. Vaginal hyperplasia, present for longer than three months in a Mastiff bitch experiencing prolonged proestrus/estrus secondary to follicular ovarian cysts.

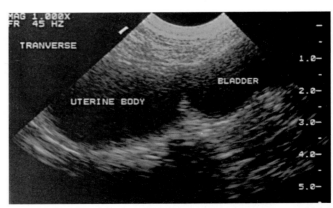

Figure 158–8. Ultrasonographic appearance of cystic endometrial hyperplasia and hydrometra in a Doberman bitch experiencing prolonged interestrous intervals, with elevated plasma progesterone concentrations for longer than four months, due to a luteinized ovarian cyst.

hyperplasia, if present, may resolve after elimination of the cyst.

Nonfunctional ovarian cysts may cause failure to cycle owing to their mass effect. Rete ovarii cysts and subsurface epithelial structure cysts are examples of nonfunctional ovarian cysts. Increases in plasma estrogen or progesterone will not be identified, although these cysts have the potential to produce a wide variety of other steroidal compounds without systemic effect.[3] The diagnosis, initially suspected with abdominal ultrasonography, is confirmed by histologic evaluation of surgically removed tissues.

Premature ovarian failure can result in permanent anestrus. Although the functional longevity of the ovaries of bitches is not known, on average, a decline in function would not be expected before 7 to 10 years of age. Prolonged anestrus owing to premature ovarian failure could be supported by documenting markedly elevated FSH and LH concentrations as occur following ovariohysterectomy. Such increases indicate a lack of negative feedback to the pituitary and hypothalamus, without any other identifiable cause for anestrus.[11] Immune-mediated oophoritis, diagnosed by ovarian histopathology, could result in prolonged anestrus. A mononuclear infiltrate predominated by lymphocytes, plasma cells, and macrophages was reported to occur in both ovaries in a bitch experiencing estrous cycle abnormalities.[12] This is an extremely rare disorder.

Hypothyroidism is a potential cause for failure to cycle, but the diagnosis should be well supported by other clinical signs (lethargy, weight gain, bilaterally symmetric alopecia) and clinical pathologic data (hypercholesterolemia, nonregenerative anemia), as well as by confirmation of subnormal serum thyroid concentrations and increases in serum endogenous thyrotropin (TSH) concentrations. Hypothyroid bitches placed on replacement therapy should begin to cycle within six months of becoming euthyroid.[3, 13, 14] The presence of immune-mediated thyroiditis is thought to have a genetic basis in some breeds. Glucocorticoids can feed back on the pituitary gonadotropins FSH and LH, causing a failure to cycle.[15, 16] Therefore, administration of any steroid medication must be discontinued in a bitch with prolonged anestrus.

SHORTENED INTERESTROUS INTERVALS

Bitches with short (less than 4.5 months) interestrous intervals can fail to conceive owing to incomplete uterine involution and repair, precluding implantation.[3] Classically, bitches experiencing shortened interestrous intervals are normal in other respects. Ovulation and luteinization occur; the secondary oocyte is fertilized but fails to implant successfully. Documentation of this disorder requires evaluation of serial vaginal cytologies during estrus and diestrus and evaluation of serum progesterone concentrations during the luteal phase of at least two consecutive cycles. Currently, there is no reliable, commercially available, consistent preimplantation method of confirming fertilization in the dog. The occurrence of folliculogenesis without ovulation (split heat) and hypoluteiodism (premature luteal failure) should be ruled out by documenting luteal function. Intervention should not take place unless the bitch is older than 3 years, because these abnormalities may resolve naturally with maturity. Therapy consists of inducing anestrus through the use of mibolerone, a potent synthetic androgen causing negative pituitary and hypothalamic feedback and ovarian inactivity, for six months. Mibolerone therapy (follow manufacturer's recommended dosage) should begin six to eight weeks after

an estrus. Potential side effects include clitoral hypertrophy, mucoid vaginal discharge, atrophy of the glandular endothelium, epiphora, and virilized behavior. The bitch should be bred on the first cycle after discontinuation of the drug, which can occur quickly or be delayed six to nine months.[3] Unfortunately, many bitches experience infertility during the first cycle after mibolerone administration.

HYPOLUTEIODISM

The maintenance of canine pregnancy requires serum progesterone concentrations of greater than 1 to 2 ng/mL. Hypoluteiodism, primary luteal failure occurring before term gestation, is a potential but undocumented cause of abortion in dogs.[3, 13, 17] Induction of abortion follows reduction of plasma progesterone concentrations below 2 ng/mL.[3] The diagnosis of abortion caused by premature luteolysis is difficult, requiring documentation of inadequate plasma progesterone concentrations prior to abortion for which no other cause is found. Measurement of precise progesterone concentrations, especially in the critical 1 to 3 ng/mL range, is inaccurate using currently available rapid ELISA kits. Thus, the more time-consuming radioimmunoassays are needed.[18] Progesterone concentrations diminish in response to fetal death; thus documentation of low progesterone concentration after an abortion does not establish the diagnosis of hypoluteiodism as a cause for reproductive failure. Administration of progesterone to maintain pregnancy in bitches with primary fetal abnormalities, placentitis, or intrauterine infection can cause continued fetal growth, with the possibility of dystocia and sepsis. Administration of progesterone to maintain pregnancy in a bitch that does not require therapy can delay parturition, endangering the life of the bitch and her fetuses. Bitches with low progesterone levels and historical late-term loss of pregnancy should be evaluated for premature myometrial activity using uterine monitors (Whelp Wise, Denver, CO). Elaboration of prostaglandins from the endometrium and placenta can result in declining progesterone levels. Pharmacologic intervention to decrease myometrial activity may be indicated. Exogenous progesterone supplementation for bitches with suspected hypoluteiodism can interfere with normal parturition, and oral progesterone supplementation has been complicated by poor lactation, dystocia, and fetal death.[19]

EXAGGERATED PSEUDOCYESIS (PSEUDOPREGNANCY)

Nonpregnant bitches with overt signs of term pregnancy are frequently evaluated because of concerns about parturition. Symptoms exhibited during overt pseudocyesis include weight gain, mammary gland hyperplasia and lactation, mucoid vaginal discharge, inappetence, restlessness, nesting, and mothering of inanimate objects. Abdominal palpation and ultrasonography can establish the presence or absence of fetuses. Alternatively, owners may bring a bitch with overt signs of pseudocyesis to the veterinarian because they find the behavior or physical symptoms objectionable when they know that the bitch is not pregnant.

Pseudocyesis is an exaggeration of the normal physiologic phenomena experienced by any nonpregnant bitch completing the luteal portion of an estrous cycle. These signs are the result of progesterone concentrations declining and prolactin increasing. The clinical expression of pseudocyesis varies

REP

from indiscernible to potentially serious. Clinical signs of pseudocyesis usually are reported from 6 to 12 weeks after estrus. Signs of pseudocyesis are often reported by owners as if its occurrence indicates a reproductive disorder; in fact, pseudocyesis probably establishes that the bitch has a normal pituitary-ovarian axis and estrous cycle.

Bitches exhibiting signs consistent with a diagnosis of pseudocyesis are probably under the influence of prolactin. Similar concentrations can be demonstrated in bitches that have no clinical signs, suggesting that the former may have increased target organ concentrations or heightened peripheral sensitivity to the hormone.[3] The condition is self-limited, usually regressing in one to three weeks, and therapy is not recommended unless the symptoms are unusually prolonged or pronounced. Unusually persistent cases of inappropriate lactation should be evaluated for hypothyroidism, which may result in elevated prolactin concentrations.

Therapy, when recommended, is usually directed at decreasing or eliminating lactation. Therapy is pursued to reduce the likelihood of mastitis occurring secondary to milk stasis or to diminish lactation-induced household soiling. Minimal measures are recommended. Mammary stimulation via licking, mothering behavior, or warm or cold compressing should be discontinued. Simply removing access to water for three or four consecutive nights is often effective, especially if combined with the administration of furosemide (2 mg/kg orally two or three times per day). Dopamine antagonists, of which phenothiazines are a class, enhance prolactin secretion and should *not* be administered. Mild sedation with a non-phenothiazine tranquilizer may be effective.[3]

A variety of hormonal and medical therapies have been employed to reduce or stop lactation in "pseudopregnant" dogs. Side effects, in some cases, outweigh the benefit of these medications. Therapy with gonadal hormones, progesterone, estrogen, or testosterone is not recommended, owing to complications of repetitive cycles of pseudocyesis, symptoms of proestrus or estrus, and virilization behavior, respectively. The androgen mibolerone, administered at 0.008 mg/lb (0.016 mg/kg) orally once daily for five days, has successfully abbreviated the signs of pseudocyesis in approximately 50 per cent of treated cases, although this medication also may cause virilization.[20] Ergot alkaloids are potent prolactin inhibitors (dopaminergic) and can be used to abbreviate exaggerated pseudocyesis. Bromocriptine can be administered at 0.005 to 0.05 mg/lb per day (0.01 to 0.10 mg/kg per day) in divided doses until lactation ceases. Vomiting, depression, and anorexia are reported side effects. Carbergoline, administered at 2.5 μg/lb per day (5 mg/kg per day) once daily for 5 to 10 days, effectively drops prolactin levels and diminishes signs of pseudocyesis with fewer side effects but is not yet available in the United States. Permanent avoidance of clinical pseudocyesis requires ovariohysterectomy.

REFERENCES

1. Shille VM: Reproductive physiology and endocrinology of the female and male. *In* Ettinger SJ (ed): Textbook of Veterinary Internal Medicine. 3rd ed. Philadelphia, WB Saunders, 1989, pp 1777–1790.
2. Davidson AP, Stabenfeldt GH: Reproduction and lactation. *In* Cunningham JG (ed): Textbook of Veterinary Physiology. Philadelphia, WB Saunders, 1997, pp 453–479.
3. Feldman EC, Nelson RW: Canine female reproduction. *In* Feldman EC, Nelson RW (eds): Canine and Feline Endocrinology and Reproduction. 2nd ed. Philadelphia, WB Saunders, 1996, pp 525–671.
4. Goodman MF: Canine ovulation timing. *In* Kay W, et al (eds): Problems in Veterinary Medicine: Canine Reproduction. Philadelphia, JB Lippincott, 1992, pp 433–444.
5. Johnson CA: Vaginal disorders. *In* Ettinger SJ (ed): Textbook of Veterinary Internal Medicine. 3rd ed. Philadelphia, WB Saunders, 1989, pp 1806–1813.
6. Olson PN, et al: Persistent estrus in the bitch. *In* Ettinger SJ (ed): Textbook of Veterinary Internal Medicine. 3rd ed. Philadelphia, WB Saunders, 1989, pp 1792–1796.
7. Poffenbarger EM, Feeney DA: Use of gray-scale ultrasonography in the diagnosis of reproductive disease in the bitch: 18 cases (1981–1984). JAVMA 189:90, 1986.
8. Madewell BR, Theilen GH: Tumors of the genital system. *In* Madewell BR, Theilen GH (eds): Veterinary Cancer Medicine. Philadelphia, Lea & Febiger, 1987, pp 583–600.
9. Yeager AE, et al: Ultrasonographic appearance of the uterus, placenta, fetus, and fetal membranes throughout accurately timed pregnancy in beagles. Am J Vet Res 53:342, 1992.
10. Patnaik AK, Greenlee PG: Canine ovarian neoplasms: A clinicopathologic study of 71 cases, including histology of 12 granulosa cell tumors. Vet Pathol 24:509, 1987.
11. Olson PN, et al: Concentrations of luteinizing hormone and follicle stimulating hormone in the serum of sexually intact and neutered dogs. Am J Vet Res 53:762, 1992.
12. Nickel RF, et al: Oophoritis in a dog with abnormal corpus luteum function. Vet Rec 128:333, 1991.
13. Feldman EC: Infertility. *In* Ettinger SJ (ed): Textbook of Veterinary Internal Medicine. 3rd ed. Philadelphia, WB Saunders, 1989, pp 1838–1858.
14. Scott-Moncrieff JC: Serum canine thyrotropin concentrations in experimental and spontaneous hypothyroidism. *In* Proc Int Symp Canine Hypothyroidism, 1996, pp 47–49.
15. Johnston SD: Canine primary anestrus: Management strategies. *In* Proc Am Anim Hosp Assoc, 1987, pp 187–188.
16. Johnston SD: Clinical approach to infertility in bitches with primary anestrus. Vet Clin North Am Small Anim Pract 21:421, 1991.
17. Concannon PW, et al: Termination of pregnancy and induction of premature luteolysis by the antiprogestagen, mifepristone, in dogs. J Reprod Fertil 88:99, 1990.
18. Hegsted RL, Johnston SD: Use of a rapid, qualitative ELISA technique (Biometallics, Inc) to determine serum progesterone concentrations in the bitch. *In* Proc Soc Theriogenol, 1989, pp 277–287.
19. Scott-Moncrieff JC, et al: Serum disposition of exogenous progesterone after intramuscular administration in bitches. Am J Vet Res 51:893, 1990.
20. Brown JM: Efficacy and dosage titration study of mibolerone for treatment of pseudopregnancy in the bitch. JAVMA 184:146, 1984.

CHAPTER 159

ABNORMALITIES IN PREGNANCY, PARTURITION, AND THE PERIPARTURIENT PERIOD

Catharina Linde-Forsberg and Annelie Eneroth

PREGNANCY

PHYSIOLOGIC CHANGES AND CLINICAL MONITORING

Maternal physiologic alterations during pregnancy are due to increased metabolic demands. Blood volume increases by 40 per cent, which provides an adequate reserve to compensate for the large quantities of blood and fluids lost at parturition. The volume increase is primarily plasma with resulting hemodilution (the hematocrit is around 30 per cent at term). There is an increase in cardiac output caused by enhanced heart rate and stroke volume. The functional residual capacity of the lungs is decreased by anterior displacement of the diaphragm by the gravid uterus, and oxygen consumption during pregnancy increases by 20 per cent. Pregnant animals also have delayed gastric emptying from decreased gastric motility and displacement of the stomach.

It is recommended to examine and maybe also obtain radiographs of bitches at about 45 days of gestation. This allows the veterinarian to answer questions, assess the health of the bitch, and confirm pregnancy as well as count fetuses. Ultrasound is excellent for determining fetal viability and can be performed from day 24 onward.

DURATION OF PREGNANCY

Apparent gestation length in the bitch averages 63 days, with a variation of 56 to 72 days if calculated from the day of the first mating to parturition. This surprisingly large variation is due to the long behavioral estrous period of the bitch. Actual gestation length determined endocrinologically is much more constant, with parturition occurring 65 ± 1 days from the pre-ovulatory luteinizing hormone peak, that is, 63 ± 1 days from the day of ovulation[1] and around 60 days from conception.[2] In one study, a negative correlation was found between length of gestation in the dog and litter size when the litters contained seven or fewer puppies, and a relation between breed and length of gestation was suggested.[3] In another study, no significant variation of mean canine gestation length with litter size was found, although mean gestation length was slightly shorter for nine- and ten-puppy litters.[4]

DISORDERS DURING PREGNANCY

EARLY FETAL LOSS AND ABORTION

The true incidence of early embryonic or fetal death (before 45 days of pregnancy) and spontaneous abortion in the bitch is unknown and may be difficult to determine because pregnancy may pass unnoticed. The bitch may consume aborted fetuses, or resorption of conceptuses may occur until day 45 of pregnancy without noticeable signs. In pigs, the embryonic wastage is reported to be as high as 30 to 50 per cent.[5]

INFECTIOUS AGENTS

Bleeding from the genital tract often precedes an abortion caused by bacterial infections. This is probably due to the effect of bacterial toxins on the placenta and the release of prostaglandin $F_{2\alpha}$, causing the uterus to contract and expel its contents. The underlying cause of bleeding should be diagnosed, and the administration of antibiotics or anti-inflammatory drugs could be used in an attempt to prevent the abortion. A bitch can abort some fetuses and then carry the remainder of the litter to term.

Brucella canis. Abortion caused by *B. canis* usually occurs between 45 and 59 days of gestation and is accompanied by a highly contagious brown to greenish-gray vaginal discharge that lasts for 1 to 6 weeks. Infected bitches may not exhibit other clinical signs. *B. canis* may also cause conception failure, fetal death, and absorption in early stages of gestation, or the birth of weak, infected puppies. The infection is chronic and mostly asymptomatic in adult animals. Infected animals have intermittent bacteremia and shed bacteria through body fluids. Diagnosis is based on serologic testing, bearing in mind that it could take several months after infection before antibody titers rise and that antibiotic treatment may create false-negative test results.

Toxoplasma gondii **and** ***Neospora caninum.*** *T. gondii* and *N. caninum* are both tissue cyst-forming protozoan microorganisms that are vertically transmitted to puppies if a bitch is infected during pregnancy. Infected bitches usually remain clinically normal, but the puppies are severely affected. Toxoplasmosis is known to cause fetal death and is a rare cause of abortion in dogs. Premature birth, stillbirths, and the birth of weak puppies have also been reported due to toxoplasmosis. Neosporosis causes fatal encephalomyelitis and polymyositis in neonatal puppies infected in utero and has experimentally been shown to cause fetal death and resorption.[6]

Canine Herpesvirus. The canine herpesvirus is species specific. In experimental studies it has been demonstrated that the effect of infection is dependent on stage of pregnancy when infection occurs. Infection in early stages causes fetal death and mummification; in midpregnancy it may result in abortion, and in later stages in premature birth. More common in naturally occurring cases is that the puppies are born apparently healthy but become ill during the first 1 or 2 weeks and succumb within days. Often the whole litter is affected; however, sometimes some of the puppies survive but develop kidney malfunction at 7 or 8 months of age. It would appear that some level of immunity is incurred, because bitches that have lost a litter due to herpesvirus infection subsequently may give birth to normal litters. The prevalence of herpesvirus in the dog population is unknown, but it has been suggested to be as high as 48 per cent in breeding kennels in some European countries. Herpesvirus has been isolated from 67 per cent of cases of infertility and abortions in those countries, but it is not clear whether it is the virus itself or a combination of several agents that is the cause.

Hypoluteodism. Inadequate progesterone production by the corpora lutea is a potential cause of fetal death or abortion in some species but has not unequivocally been proven to exist in the dog. A blood sample for progesterone taken at the time of an abortion often will show low concentrations due to the luteolytic effects of the prostaglandin release during fetal expulsion; but, if repeated a week later, normal-for-stage levels of progesterone will be found. Any attempts at treating cases of imminent abortion with progestogens should only be done using the short-acting compounds, because the bitch cannot deliver the litter when under the influence of progesterone.[1]

INSULIN RESISTANCE

The physiologic, increased progesterone concentrations typical of diestrus/pregnancy stimulate growth hormone secretion, which in some individuals may cause downregulation of insulin receptors and inhibition of post-receptor pathways. The condition is typically seen in middle-aged and older bitches. The resulting type II diabetes is transient and in most cases reversible. Once blood progesterone concentration returns to anestrous levels and, thus, the stimulus for growth hormone secretion declines, insulin resistance resolves. Insulin resistance should be suspected in a bitch with supranormal blood insulin concentrations in the presence of normal or increased blood glucose concentration.[7] Treatment should be initiated to prevent permanent damage to the pancreas. There is a poor prognosis for the fetuses, which sometimes become undernourished but sometimes instead grow excessively large (due to the excess in glucose), with a poor survival rate. In the bitch, acromegaly could develop as a result of excessive secretion of growth hormone by the progesterone-stimulated mammary gland. Edema, especially of the head, throat, and legs, is seen in combination with excessive skin and wrinkling and an increase in interdental spaces. In advanced cases, there may be a change in voice, becoming coarse from the edema of the throat. The condition could become life threatening, and it may be necessary to interrupt pregnancy.

HYPOGLYCEMIA

Preparturient hypoglycemia in the bitch is rare. Some dogs may be incorrectly diagnosed as hypocalcemic because they respond to treatment with calcium borogluconate. Affected bitches have been reported to be in late gestation and have a short history of muscle weakness, convulsion, or collapse. Blood testing demonstrates the hypoglycemia.[8–10] The condition improves dramatically after treatment with intravenous glucose solutions and resolves after parturition.

NORMAL PARTURITION

LITTER SIZE

The litter size in dogs varies, ranging from as few as one puppy in the miniature breeds to more than 15 in some of the giant breeds. Litter sizes are smaller in young bitches, increase when 3 to 4 years of age, and decrease as the bitch gets older. A litter size of only one or two puppies predisposes to dystocia because of insufficient uterine stimulation and large puppy size—"the single-puppy syndrome." This can be seen in dog breeds of all sizes. Breeders of the miniature breeds tend to accept small litters but should be encouraged to breed for litter sizes of at least three to four puppies to avoid this complication.

PHYSIOLOGY OF PARTURITION

An understanding of the course and control of normal parturition (eutocia) is necessary for the diagnosis and treatment of abnormal parturition (dystocia). Studies of canine parturition and extrapolations from other species provide information on the physiologic and endocrinologic changes important for normal parturition. Stress produced by the reduction of the nutritional supply by the placenta to the fetus stimulates the fetal hypothalamic-pituitary-adrenal axis, resulting in release of adrenocorticosteroid hormone, and is thought to be the trigger for parturition. An increase in fetal and maternal cortisol is believed to stimulate the release of prostaglandin $F_{2\alpha}$, which is luteolytic, from the fetoplacental tissue, resulting in a decline in plasma progesterone concentration. Withdrawal of the progesterone blockade of pregnancy is a prerequisite for the normal course of canine parturition; bitches given long-acting progesterone during pregnancy fail to deliver.[1] Concurrent with the gradual decrease in plasma progesterone concentration during the last 7 days before whelping there is a progressive qualitative change in uterine electrical activity, and a significant increase in uterine activity occurs during the last 24 hours before parturition with the final fall in plasma progesterone concentration.[11] The change in the estrogen/progesterone ratio is probably a major cause of placental separation and cervical dilation, although, in the dog, estrogens have not been unambiguously shown to increase before parturition as they do in many other species. Estrogens sensitize the myometrium to oxytocin, which in turn initiates strong contractions in the uterus when not under the influence of progesterone. Sensory receptors within the cervix and vagina are stimulated by the distention created by the fetus and the fluid-filled fetal membranes. This afferent stimulation is conveyed to the hypothalamus and results in release of oxytocin. Afferents also participate in a spinal reflex arch with efferent stimulation of the abdominal musculature to produce abdominal straining. Relaxin causes the pelvic soft tissues and genital tract to relax, which facilitates fetal passage. In the pregnant bitch, this hormone is produced by the ovary and the placenta and rises gradually over the last two thirds of pregnancy.[12] Prolactin, the hormone responsible for lactation, starts to rise 3 to 4 weeks after ovulation and surges dramatically with the abrupt decline in serum progesterone just before parturition.

SIGNS OF IMPENDING PARTURITION

Relaxation of the pelvic and abdominal musculature is a consistent but subtle indicator of impending parturition. The most consistent change is the drop in rectal temperature caused by the final abrupt decrease in progesterone concentration. The last week before parturition the rectal temperature of the bitch fluctuates and drops sharply 8 to 24 hours before parturition and 10 to 14 hours after the concentration of progesterone in peripheral plasma has declined to less than 6 nmol/L. This drop in rectal temperature is individual but also may depend on body size. Thus, in miniature breed bitches it can fall to 35°C, in medium-sized bitches it can fall to around 36°C, whereas it seldom falls below 37°C in bitches of the giant breeds. This difference is probably an effect of the surface area/body volume ratio. Several days before parturition the bitch may become restless, seeks seclusion or is excessively attentive, and may refuse all food. She may exhibit nesting behavior 12 to 24 hours before parturition concomitant with increasing frequency and force of uterine contractions. Shivering may be an attempt to increase body temperature. In primiparous bitches, lactation may be established less than 24 hours before parturition, whereas, after several pregnancies, colostrum can be detected as early as 1 week prepartum.

STAGES OF PARTURITION

Parturition is divided into three stages, with the last two stages being repeated for each puppy delivered.

First Stage

The duration of the first stage is 6 to 12 hours. It may last 36 hours, especially in the nervous primiparous animal, but for this to be considered normal the rectal temperature must remain low. Vaginal relaxation and dilation of the cervix occur during this stage. Intermittent uterine contractions, with no signs of abdominal contractions or straining, are present. The bitch may appear uncomfortable, and the restless behavior may become more intense. Panting, tearing up and rearranging of bedding, shivering, and occasional vomiting may be seen. Some bitches show no behavioral evidence of first-stage labor. The inapparent uterine contractions increase both in frequency and intensity toward the end of the first stage.

During pregnancy the orientation of the fetuses within the uterus is 50 per cent heading caudally and 50 per cent cranially, but this changes during first-stage labor as the fetus rotates on its long axis, extending its head, neck, and limbs, resulting in 60 per cent of puppies being born in anterior and 40 per cent in posterior presentation.[13] The fluid-filled fetal membranes are pushed ahead of the fetus by the uterine propulsive efforts and dilate the cervix.

Second Stage

The duration of the second stage is usually 3 to 12 hours and, in rare cases, 24 hours. At the onset of second-stage labor the rectal temperature rises to normal or slightly above normal. The first fetus engages in the pelvic inlet, and the subsequent intense, expulsive uterine contractions are accompanied by abdominal straining. On entering the birth canal the allantochorionic membrane may rupture and a discharge of some clear fluid may be noted. Covered by the amniotic membrane the first fetus is usually delivered within 4 hours after onset of second-stage labor.[14] Normally, the bitch will break the membrane, lick the neonate intensively, and sever the umbilical cord. At times the bitch will need some assistance to open the fetal membranes to allow the newborn to breathe, and sometimes the airways will have to be emptied of fetal fluids. The umbilicus can be clamped with a pair of hemostats and cut with a blunt scissors to minimize hemorrhage from the fetal vessels, leaving about 1 cm of the umbilicus. In case of continuing hemorrhage the umbilicus should be ligated.

Diagnosing Second-Stage Labor. It is of utmost importance that the veterinarian is able to determine whether the bitch is in the second stage or still in the first stage of labor. Inexperienced breeders tend to get nervous during a bitch's first-stage labor, not fully understanding the function of this preparatory stage of parturition during which the recurrence of uterine tones, the softening of the birth canal, and the opening of the cervix take place.

There are three signs that indicate that the bitch has entered into second-stage labor:

- The passing of fetal fluids (first water bag bursts)
- Visible abdominal straining
- The rectal temperature returning to normal level

If one or more of these signs have been observed the bitch is in second-stage labor.

In normal labor the bitch may show weak and infrequent straining for up to 2, and at the most 4, hours before giving birth to the first fetus. If the bitch is showing strong, frequent straining without producing a pup, this indicates the presence of some obstruction and she should not be left for more than 20 to 30 minutes before seeking veterinary advice.

The bitch should be examined if

- She has a greenish discharge but no pup is born within 2 to 4 hours.
- Fetal fluid was passed more than 2 to 3 hours previously but nothing more has happened.
- The bitch has had weak, irregular straining for more than 2 to 4 hours.
- The bitch has had strong, regular straining for more than 20 to 30 minutes.
- More than 2 to 4 hours have passed since the birth of the last puppy and more remain.
- The bitch has been in second-stage labor for more than 12 hours.

Third Stage

The third stage of parturition, expulsion of the placenta and shortening of the uterine horns, usually follows within 15 minutes of the delivery of each fetus. Two or three fetuses may, however, be born before the passage of their placentas occurs. The bitch should be discouraged from eating more than one or two of the placentas because she may develop diarrhea and vomiting may also be induced, with the risk of aspiration pneumonia. Lochia (i.e., the greenish postpartum discharge of fetal fluids and placental remains) will be seen for up to 3 weeks or more, being most profuse during the first week. Uterine involution and vaginal bleeding are normally completed within 12 to 15 weeks.

The bitch should be examined if:

- All placentas have not been passed within 4 to 6 hours (although placental numbers may be difficult to determine because of the bitch eating them).
- The lochia are putrid and/or foul smelling.
- There is continuing severe genital hemorrhage.
- The rectal temperature is higher than 39.5°C.
- The general condition of the bitch is affected.
- The general condition of the puppies is affected.

INTERVAL BETWEEN BIRTHS

Expulsion of the first fetus usually takes the longest. The interval between births in normal uncomplicated parturition is from 5 to 120 minutes.[13] In almost 80 per cent of cases the fetuses are delivered alternately from the two uterine horns. When giving birth to a large litter a bitch may stop straining and rest for more than 2 hours between the delivery of two consecutive fetuses. The second-stage straining will then resume, followed again by the third stage, until all the fetuses are born.

COMPLETION OF PARTURITION

Parturition is usually completed within 6 hours after the onset of second stage labor, but it may last up to 12 hours. It should never be allowed to last for more than 24 hours because of the risks involved both for the bitch and the fetuses.

DYSTOCIA

DEFINITION

Dystocia is defined as difficult birth or the inability to expel the fetus through the birth canal without assistance.

FREQUENCY

Dystocia is a frequent problem in the dog. The true incidence of dystocia in the bitch is probably around 5 per cent overall, but it may amount to almost 100 per cent in some breeds of dogs, especially those of the achondroplastic type and those selected for large heads.

CLINICAL ASSESSMENT

When a case of dystocia is presented, an accurate history and a thorough physical examination of the bitch are important prerequisites for proper management. The three criteria for being in second-stage labor, namely, passage of fetal fluids, visible abdominal straining, and temperature returned to normal, should be assessed. An evaluation of the bitch's general health status should be made and signs of any adverse effects of parturition noted. Observation should be made of the bitch's behavior and the character and frequency

of straining, and the vulva and perineum should be examined noting color and amount of vaginal discharge. Mammary gland development including congestion, distention, size, and presence of milk should be evaluated. Palpation of the abdomen, roughly estimating the number of fetuses and degree of distention of the uterus, should be carried out. Digital examination of the vagina using aseptic technique should be undertaken to detect obstructions and determine the presence and presentation of any fetus in the pelvic canal (Fig. 159–1). In most bitches it is not possible to reach the cervix during first stage, but an assessment of the degree of dilation and tone of the vagina may give some indication of the status of the cervix and the tone of the uterus. Pronounced tone of the anterior vagina may indicate satisfactory muscular activity in the uterus, whereas flaccidity may indicate uterine inertia.[15] The character of the vaginal fluids also will indicate whether the cervix is closed, with the production of a fluid that is scant and sticky creating a certain resistance to the introduction of a finger, or open, when fetal fluids lubricate the vagina, making the exploration easy. When the cervix is closed the vaginal walls also fit quite tightly around the exploring finger, whereas with an open cervix the cranial vagina appears more open.

Radiographic examination is valuable to assess gross abnormalities of the maternal pelvis and number and location of fetuses, to estimate fetal size, and to detect congenital defects or signs of fetal death. In the dead fetus, intrafetal gas will appear 6 hours after death and can be detected radiographically, whereas overlapping of cranial bones and collapse of the spinal column will not be seen until 48 hours have passed after the death of the fetus. Ultrasound examination will determine fetal viability or distress, with normal heart rate being 180 to 240 beats per minute, decreasing in the compromised fetus. Some bitches brought to veterinarians for dystocia have already delivered all fetuses or were never pregnant (i.e., they were pseudo-pregnant). Pseudo-pregnancy is most commonly diagnosed as lactation without pregnancy, but it may include abdominal contractions, nesting behavior, and changes in personality that convince an owner that the pet is pregnant.

DIAGNOSIS

The range of normal variations observed in dogs at parturition makes recognition of dystocia difficult, especially for the inexperienced observer. The following criteria for dystocia may assist in making the diagnosis:

- The rectal temperature has been down and returned to normal with no signs of labor.
- There is a green vulvar discharge but no fetuses have been delivered. (These discharges emanate from the marginal hematoma of the placentas and indicate that at least one placenta is beginning to become separated from the maternal blood supply. They are normal once birth is underway.)
- Fetal fluids were passed 2 to 3 hours earlier but there are no signs of labor.
- Labor is absent for more than 2 hours or is weak and infrequent for more than 2 to 4 hours.
- Strong and persistent non-productive labor occurs for more than 20 to 30 minutes.
- An obvious cause of dystocia is evident (e.g., pelvic fracture or a fetus stuck in the birth canal and partially visible).
- Signs of toxemia (disturbed general condition, general

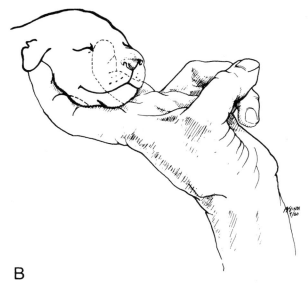

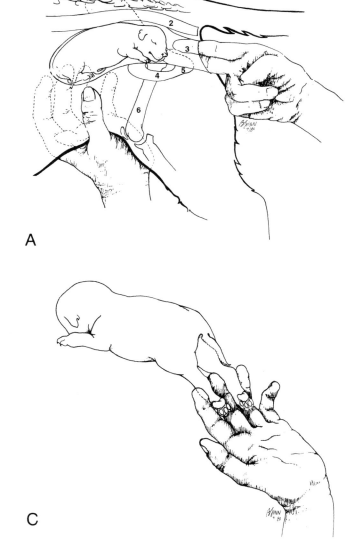

FIGURE 159–1. *A,* Determination of the fetal disposition when the head has entered the vaginal canal. The bitch should be standing for this procedure. 1, Right wing of ilium; 2, rectum; 3, lumen of vaginal vestibule; 4, right half of pubic symphysis; 5, right wing of ischium; 6, right femur. *B,* The index and middle fingers are used to guide the head and to exert moderate traction in a cranial presentation. *C,* Manual traction as applied in a caudal presentation. The fingers should be positioned proximal to the hocks for best results. (From Shille VM: Diagnosis and management of dystocia in the bitch and queen. *In* Bojrab MJ [ed]: Current Techniques in Small Animal Surgery. Philadelphia, Lea & Febiger, 1983, p 338; used with permission.)

REP

edema, shock) are noted when parturition should be occurring.

MATERNAL CAUSES OF DYSTOCIA

Traditionally, dystocia is classified as being of either maternal or of fetal origin, or a combination of both (Table 159–1; Figs. 159–2 and 159–3).

Uterine Inertia

Uterine inertia is by far the most common cause of dystocia in dogs. It is classified into primary and secondary inertia. In primary inertia, the uterus may fail to respond to the fetal signals because there are only one or two puppies and thus insufficient stimulation to initiate labor (the single-puppy syndrome) or because of overstretching of the myometrium by large litters, excessive fetal fluids, or oversized fetuses. Other causes of primary inertia may be an inherited predisposition, nutritional imbalance, fatty infiltration of the myometrium, age-related changes, deficiency in neuroendo-

crine regulation, or systemic disease in the bitch. Primary complete uterine inertia is the failure of the uterus to begin labor at full term. Primary partial uterine inertia occurs when there is enough uterine activity to initiate parturition but it is insufficient to complete a normal birth of all fetuses in the absence of an obstruction. Secondary uterine inertia implies that some fetuses have been delivered and the remainder are in utero due to exhaustion of the uterine myometrium caused by obstruction of the birth canal; this condition should be distinguished from primary inertia.

Management. In cases of primary uterine inertia, the owners should initially be instructed to try to induce straining by actively exercising the bitch—for instance, by running around the house or up the stairs with her. A considerable number of puppies are born in the car on the way to the veterinarian. Most of these would probably have been delivered in the calm and quiet of home had the owners tried to induce straining themselves, thus giving the puppies a better start in life and possibly also resulting in the whole litter being born without further intervention. Another means of induction of straining in the bitch with insufficient labor is by feathering of the dorsal vaginal wall. Feathering is

**TABLE 159–1. CAUSES OF DYSTOCIA IN BITCHES
(182 CASES)**

	FREQUENCY (%)
Maternal Causes	75.3
Primary complete inertia	48.9
Primary partial inertia	23.1
Birth canal too narrow	1.1
Uterine torsion	1.1
Hydrallantois	0.5
Vaginal septum formation	0.5
Fetal Causes	24.7
Malpresentations	15.4
Fetal oversize	6.6
Malformations	1.6
Fetal death	1.1

From Darvelid AW, Linde-Forsberg C: Dystocia in the bitch: A retrospective study of 182 cases. J Small Animal Pract 35:402–407, 1994.

accomplished by inserting two fingers into the vagina and pushing or "walking" with them against the dorsal vaginal wall, thus inducing an episode of straining (the Ferguson reflex). Feathering can also be effective in initiating labor after correction of the position or posture of a fetus.

Nervous voluntary inhibition of labor due to psychologic stress may occur, mainly in the nervous primiparous animal. Reassurance by the owner or administration of a low dose of a tranquilizer may remove the inhibition.[16] Once the first fetus is born, parturition will usually proceed normally.

The bitch with complete primary uterine inertia is usually bright and alert, has a normal rectal temperature, and has no evidence of labor. The cervix is often dilated, and vaginal exploration is easy to perform owing to the presence of fetal fluids, but the fetus may be out of reach because of the flaccid uterus. Before initiation of medical treatment, obstruction of the birth canal must be excluded.

Calcium solutions and oxytocin are the drugs of choice in cases of uterine inertia. Oxytocin has a direct action on the rate of calcium influx into the myometrial cell, which is essential for myometrial contraction. Many do not respond to oxytocin alone but require prior administration of a calcium solution. Therefore, some 10 minutes before the administration of oxytocin, 10 per cent calcium borogluconate, 0.5 to 1.5 mL/kg body weight (2–20 mL), should be given by slow intravenous infusion (1 mL/min) with careful monitoring of the heart rate. Small breed bitches may be prone to hypoglycemia, particularly after prolonged straining. In such cases, a dilute (10 to 20 per cent) glucose solution can be added to the infusion or given intravenously in doses of 5 to 20 mL. The recommended dose of oxytocin for the bitch is 1 to 12 IU given intravenously or 2.5 to 10 IU intramuscularly, which can be repeated at 30-minute intervals. The response to treatment will be reduced with each repeated administration. Higher doses than recommended or too frequent administration may result in prolonged contracture of the myometrium, preventing fetal expulsion and impeding uteroplacental blood flow. The disadvantages of oxytocin include a tendency to cause premature induction of placental separation and cervical closure. If there is no response to treatment after a second administration of oxytocin the puppies should be delivered without further delay, either with the aid of obstetric forceps, if only one or two puppies remain and are within easy reach in the uterine corpus, or by cesarean section.

The long-acting ergotamines should never be used in connection with parturition.

The treatment regimen includes

- The owner runs with the bitch and feathers the vaginal vault.
- A 10 per cent solution of calcium borogluconate is given slowly intravenously while carefully checking the bitch's heart rate.
- The bitch is given 30 minutes to respond to treatment. If straining begins, the treatment can be repeated if necessary or continued with oxytocin.
- If the calcium infusion has no effect within 30 minutes, oxytocin is given intravenously or intramuscularly.
- The bitch again is given 30 minutes to respond to treatment. If straining begins, the treatment can be repeated if necessary, although each additional administration will elicit a weaker response.
- If nothing happens within 30 minutes, it is not likely that further treatment will be successful. The fetuses should be delivered, either by forceps, if only one or two fetuses remain and are within easy reach, or by cesarean section.

Obstruction of the Birth Canal

Obstruction of the birth canal may be of maternal or fetal origin. Some maternal causes for obstruction are listed below:

- *Uterine torsion* and *uterine rupture.* These are acute, life-threatening conditions that can occur during late pregnancy or at the time of parturition. Sometimes a few fetuses are born before parturition stops and the condition of the bitch may quickly deteriorate. Surgery is always required and a quick diagnosis is essential for survival.
- *Uterine malposition* resulting from inguinal herniation usually is detected around week 4 of pregnancy as the fetal uterine enlargements are growing and the contour of the abdomen is markedly disturbed. Sometimes the early stages may be mistaken for mastitis of the rear mammary glands. The condition is corrected by surgery, whereby the uterine horn is repositioned and the herniation sutured. In cases with circulatory disturbance and advanced tissue damage, the uterus will have to be removed.
- *Congenital malformations of the uterus* (e.g., partial or complete aplasia or hypoplasia of one or both uterine horns or of the corpus uteri) or the cervix are rare causes of maternal obstructive dystocia. Symptoms depend on the character and degree of the malformation. In cases of unilateral aplasia of an entire uterine horn, small litter size may be the only presenting sign. Retained fetuses behind partial occlusions require surgery, and the final diagnosis is usually made during the operation.
- *Soft tissue abnormalities* such as neoplasms, vaginal septa, or fibrosis of the birth canal may cause obstructive dystocia. The prepartum relaxation of the vagina often will allow the passage of fetuses. Vaginal septa may consist of remnants from the fetal müllerian duct system. However, they can also occur secondary to vaginal trauma or infection and, if extensive, may prevent the passage of the fetuses. Often, however, they are not so extensive and vaginal relaxation may allow the fetuses to pass. Cervical

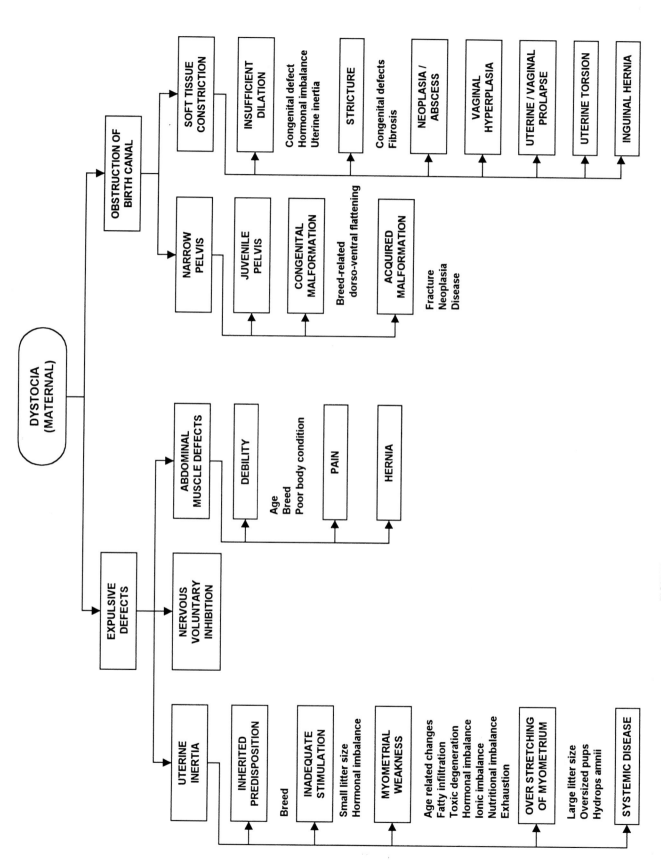

FIGURE 159–2. Algorithm defining the various maternal causes for dystocia.

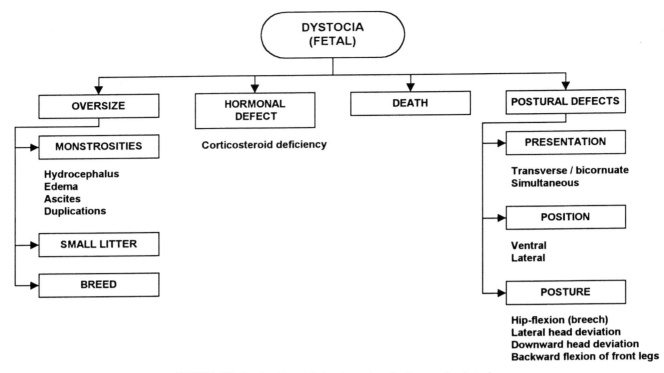

FIGURE 159–3. Algorithm defining the various fetal causes for dystocia.

or vaginal fibrosis usually is secondary to trauma or inflammatory processes and in severe cases will cause dystocia. Surgical intervention may save the puppies. Tumors and septa formations may be removed; but in the cases of fibrosis, surgery is seldom successful because of new scar formation during the healing process.

• *Narrow pelvic canal* causing obstructive dystocia may result from previous pelvic fractures, immaturity, or congenital malformation of the pelvis. The normal pelvis has a vertical diameter greater than the horizontal. Congenitally narrow birth canals exist in some brachycephalic and terrier breeds; in addition, their fetuses have comparatively large heads and wide shoulders. When achondroplasia exists, as in the Scottish terrier, dorsoventral flattening of the pelvis modifies the normal pelvic inlet, which creates an obstruction to the engagement of the fetuses. In a study using indirect pelvimetry, significant differences were found between Scottish terrier bitches whelping normally compared with those with dystocia owing to a too narrow birth canal, confirming the dorsoflattening and also demonstrating a shortening of the pelvis in the bitches with dystocia. The weight of the puppies was the same in both groups.[17] Boston terrier bitches were also studied, and again there was a significantly higher inner pelvic area in the normally whelping bitches, but in this breed also the size of the puppies was of importance because the weight of the pup correlated with the size of the head. In the bulldog, the large, deep chest and pronounced waist causes the gravid uterus to drop down. At parturition, the fetuses are presented at a relatively acute angle to the pelvic inlet. Bulldogs sometimes also have slack abdominal musculature, leading to insufficient uterine contractions and abdominal straining to lift the fetus up into the pelvic cavity.

FETAL CAUSES OF DYSTOCIA

Fetal obstructions may be caused by oversized fetuses, malpresentations/malorientations, or monstrosities, such as hydrocephalus, edema, or various duplications (see Fig. 159–3). Being oversized in itself is a cause for malpresentation. Fetal death may result in dystocia due to malpositioning or inadequate stimulation for parturition to begin. A healthy fetus is active during expulsion, extending its head and limbs, twisting, and rotating to get through. In most breeds the greatest bulk of the fetus lies in its abdominal cavity, whereas the bony parts, the head and the hips, are comparatively small. The limbs are short and flexible and rarely cause serious obstruction to delivery in the normal-sized fetus.

Oversized Fetuses

A puppy weighing 4 to 5 per cent of the weight of the bitch is considered the upper limit for an uncomplicated birth. In the absence of monstrosities, oversized fetuses are often associated with small litter size. In breeds in which miniaturizing exists, great disparity in fetal size within litters may occur with some greatly oversized individuals. In brachycephalic breeds like the Boston terrier, dystocia occurs from the combination of a flattened pelvic inlet and puppies having a large head. In dystocia due to an oversized fetus, sometimes a portion of the fetus may protrude from the vulva. In anterior presentation the head may be born and the shoulders and chest cause obstruction, whereas in posterior presentation the hindlimbs and hips may protrude.

Posterior Presentation

This is considered normal in dogs, occurring in 40 per cent of fetal deliveries. Posterior presentations have, however, been related to a predisposition for dystocia, because mechanical dilation of the cervix may be inadequate, particularly when this involves the first fetus to be delivered. In addition, expulsion is rendered more difficult because the fetus is being delivered against the direction of its hair coat and because the fetal chest instead of being compressed becomes distended by the pressure from the abdominal organs through the diaphragm. Occasionally, the fetus may have the elbows hooked around the pelvic brim, preventing further expulsion. Should the fetus become lodged in the pelvic canal, pressure on the umbilical vessels trapped between the fetal chest wall and maternal pelvic floor may cause hypoxia and reflex inhalation of fetal fluids.

Breech Presentation

Breech presentation (i.e., posterior presentation with hindlegs flexed forward) can be a serious complication, especially in medium- and small-sized breeds. Vaginal exploration will reveal a tail tip and maybe the anus and the bony structure of the pelvis of the fetus.

Lateral or Downward Deviation of the Head

These are two of the most common malpositionings in the dog. Lateral deviation is most common with long-necked breeds such as rough collies, whereas downward deviation is seen in brachycephalic breeds and long-headed breeds such as Sealyham and Scottish terriers. In lateral deviation, vaginal exploration will demonstrate just one front leg, the one contralateral to the direction of the deviation of the head (i.e., when the head is deviated to the left the right front paw will be found and vice versa). When there is a downward deviation of the head, either both front legs and sometimes the nape of the neck of the fetus can be palpated, or both front legs may be flexed backward and only the skull of the fetus be reached.

Backward Flexion of Front Legs

This condition is especially common when the fetus is weak or dead and is sometimes seen in combination with deviation of the head, especially downward. For bitches of the larger or even medium-sized breeds it may be possible to deliver a puppy with one or both front legs flexed.

Transverse or Bicornate Presentation

Sometimes a fetus, instead of progressing from the uterine horn through the cervix to the vagina, will proceed into the contralateral uterine horn, possibly due to some obstruction. Another reason may be that the fetus was implanted close to the corpus uteri (body of the uterus). These cases always require surgery, because there is no possibility for manual correction.

Two Fetuses Presented Simultaneously

Sometimes one fetus from each horn is presented at the same time, jamming the birth canal. When possible, if one is coming backward, this one should be removed first, because it occupies more space.

Management of Fetal Malpresentations

If a fetus is present in the birth canal, manipulation by hand or by obstetric forceps may be attempted. In bitches of the giant breeds it may be possible to insert one hand through the vagina into the uterus and thus extract the puppy. During natural birth the puppy will almost make a full somersault emerging from the loop of the uterine horn, progressing upward to pass through the pelvic canal and then down again through the long vestibulum of the bitch, the vulva being situated some 5 to 15 cm below the level of the pelvic floor. Thus, after the fetus is seized, a gentle traction in posteroventral direction is applied.

Fetal position must be assessed. If the fetus has advanced into and partly through the pelvic canal, it will create a characteristic bulge of the perineal region, below the tail. Easing the vulvar lips upward may reveal the amniotic sac and the position of the fetus. Vaginal exploration and radiographic examination will aid in making a diagnosis in the cases when the fetus has not advanced as far.

The narrowest part of the birth canal is within the rigid pelvic girdle. If external manipulation is to be attempted, the fetus that cannot be easily pulled out may have to be pushed in front of the pelvic girdle, where corrections of position or posture are easier to perform. This should be done between periods of straining of the bitch, never working against the uterine contractions. It should also be remembered that the widest part of the pelvic girdle usually is on the diagonal (see Fig. 159–1); thus, rotating the fetus 45 degrees may create sufficient room for passage. Generous application of obstetric lubricant (liquid paraffin, Vaseline, or a sterile water-soluble lubricant) is helpful, especially if the bitch has been in second-stage labor for some time.

Depending on the position and posture of the fetus a grip should be applied around its head and neck, from above or below, whichever is most convenient, around its pelvis, or around the legs. Care should be taken because the neck and limbs of the fetus are easily torn when pulled. Correction of posture may be obtained by manipulation of the fetus through the abdominal wall with one hand and concurrent transvaginal manipulation with the other. A finger may be introduced into the mouth of the fetus to help correcting a downward deviation of the head. Should it be necessary to change the postures of the limbs, a finger is inserted past the elbow or knee and the limb moved medially in under the fetus and corrected.

A gently applied alternating right-to-left traction of the puppy, gently rocking it back and forth or from side to side and possibly twisting it to a diagonal position within the pelvis, will help free the shoulders or the hips one at a time. A slight pressure applied over the perineal bulge may prevent the fetus from sliding back into the uterus again between strainings.

Obstetric forceps should only be used for assisted traction of a relatively oversized fetus when it is likely the rest of the puppies in the litter are smaller or when just one or two fetuses remain. The forceps is guided with a finger and never introduced farther than to the uterine body because of the risk of getting part of the uterine wall within the grip, thereby causing serious damage. If the head of the fetus can be reached, the grip should be applied around the neck (Pålssons forceps) or across the cheeks. In posterior presentation the grip should be around the fetal pelvis. If the legs can be reached, the grip should be around those, not around the feet.

Outcome of Obstetric Treatment. A study[18] reporting

on treatment outcome shows that digital manipulation including forceps delivery and/or medical treatment for dystocia is successful in only 27.6 per cent of the cases. Around 65 per cent of bitches brought to the clinic because of dystocia thus end up having a cesarean section.

Fetal death increases from 5.8 per cent in bitches brought in within 1 to 4.5 hours after the beginning of second-stage labor to 13.7 per cent in the period between 5 and 24 hours. Overall fetal death was 22.3 per cent. Early diagnosis and prompt treatment is therefore crucial in reducing the puppy death rate in cases of dystocia.

Criteria for Cesarean Section

The indications for cesarean section include the following:

- Complete primary uterine inertia that does not respond to medical treatment
- Partial primary uterine inertia that is refractory to medical management
- Secondary uterine inertia with inadequate resumption of labor
- Abnormalities of the maternal pelvis or soft tissues of the birth canal
- Relative fetal oversize, if considered likely to be repeated in several fetuses
- Absolute oversize, single-puppy syndrome, or fetal monstrosity
- Excess or deficiency of fetal fluids
- Fetal malposition unamenable to manipulation
- Fetal death with putrefaction
- Toxemia of pregnancy and illness of the bitch
- Neglected dystocia
- Prophylactic (history of previous deliveries)

Prophylactic cesarean section should be questioned on ethical grounds if it is performed to assist the propagation of a breed line that cannot reproduce successfully without intervention.

Once a decision has been made to deliver the litter by cesarean section, surgery should be carried out without delay. The bitch has often endured hours of more or less intensive labor and may be suffering from physical exhaustion, dehydration, acid-base disorders, hypotension, hypocalcemia and/or hypoglycemia. The prognosis for both bitch and offspring is good if surgery is performed within 12 hours after the onset of second-stage labor; it continues to be fairly good for the bitch after 12 hours but guarded for the fetuses. If more than 24 hours have passed after the onset of second-stage labor the entire litter is usually dead and further delay compromises the life of the bitch.

POSTPARTURIENT CONDITIONS

It is normal for the bitch to have a slightly elevated rectal temperature, up to 39.2°C, for a couple of days after parturition. It should, however, not exceed 39.5°C. Fever during this period usually emanates from conditions of the uterus or the mammary glands.

PERINATAL LOSS

Based on a number of surveys, puppy losses up to weaning age appear to range between 10 and 30 per cent[19] and average around 12 per cent.[19–21] More than 65 per cent of puppy mortality occurs at parturition and during the first week of life; few puppies die after 3 weeks of age. Inbreeding is said to be associated with a high incidence of fetal and neonatal mortality.

UTERINE DISORDERS

Hemorrhage

Some hemorrhage from the genital tract after parturition is normal, but maternal blood loss should never exceed a scant drip from the vulva. True hemorrhage should be distinguished from normal vaginal postparturient discharge. Excessive hemorrhage after parturition may indicate uterine or vaginal tearing or vessel rupture or may be evidence of a coagulation defect. The hematocrit should be checked, remembering that 30 per cent is normal for the bitch at term. Inspection of the vulva and vagina should be performed in an attempt to locate the source of the bleeding. Oxytocin can be administered to promote uterine involution and contraction of the uterine wall. In more severe cases of uterine hemorrhage an exploratory laparotomy may be necessary. The bitch should be monitored closely for signs of impending shock, and blood transfusion may be required while attempting to determine the cause of hemorrhage.

Retained Placentas/Fetuses

Retained placentas in the bitch may cause severe problems, especially when accompanied by retained fetuses or infection. Clinical signs of retained placenta include a thick dark vaginal discharge. Retained fetuses can be identified by palpation or radiographic or ultrasonographic examination. A retained placenta is often palpable, depending on the size of the bitch and degree of involution of the uterus. Extraction of retained tissue, by careful "milking" of the uterine horn or by using forceps, is sometimes possible. Treatment with 1 to 5 IU oxytocin per dog subcutaneously or intramuscularly two to four times daily for up to 3 days can help expulsion of retained placentas. The long-acting ergot alkaloids should not be used because they may cause closure of the cervix. Antibiotic treatment is advisable if the bitch is showing signs of illness.

Acute Metritis

Acute metritis is an ascending bacterial infection of the uterus in the immediate postpartum period. Dystocia, obstetric manipulation, retained fetuses or placental membranes, or parturition in an unsanitary environment predispose to metritis. Metritis may rarely occur after normal parturition, natural or artificial insemination, or an abortion. Infection usually ascends through an open cervix and is often caused by gram-negative bacteria. Clinical signs include fever, dehydration, depression, anorexia, poor lactation and mothering, and a purulent or sanguinopurulent vaginal discharge. A doughy enlarged uterus may be palpated abdominally. Abdominal radiographic and/or ultrasonographic examination is indicated to evaluate the uterine size and uterine contents. A vaginal culture is recommended. Vaginal cytology will show large numbers of degenerate neutrophils, red blood cells, bacteria, and debris. The complete blood cell count often shows leukocytosis with a left shift. Therapy consists of immediate administration of intravenous fluids and antibiotics and evacuation of uterine contents. The latter may be accomplished by administering oxytocin or prostaglandin $F_{2\alpha}$. There is one high-dose regimen for administration of prostaglandin $F_{2\alpha}$ (0.1–0.25 mg/kg SC once or twice daily for 3–8 days) and one low-dose regimen (0.025–0.05 mg/kg SC six to eight times daily for 2 to 3 days). The high-dose alternative may cause adverse reactions such as abdominal pain, increased pulse and respiratory rate, salivary secretion, and sweating. These reactions appear within 10 minutes of administration and normally disappear again after 30 minutes to 1 hour. It should be remembered, however, that the prostaglandins are not licensed for use in dogs. In more severe cases, ovariohysterectomy is the recommended treatment.

Subinvolution of Placental Sites

In the postparturient period it is normal for the bitch to have a serosanguineous vaginal discharge for 3 to 6 weeks. Normally, the uterine involution is completed within 12 weeks after whelping. Subinvolution of placental sites is suspected if a sanguineous vaginal discharge persists for longer than 6 weeks (Fig. 159–4). The etiology of this condition is unknown, and the bitch often shows no symptoms of illness. Vaginal cytology shows predominantly red blood cells, with syncytial trophoblast–like cells being a useful confirmatory finding. Subinvolution of placental sites almost exclusively affects the young, primiparous animal and, in the majority of cases, resolves spontaneously, with the prognosis for future pregnancy being good. Because of increased risk of anemia, secondary bacterial infection, or rupture of the affected placental sites with subsequent perito-nitis, the bitch should be monitored until the disorder resolves. Ovariohysterectomy is indicated in rare cases of profound permanent bleeding or uterine infection.

Uterine Rupture

Uterine rupture should be considered a possible but uncommon cause of illness in the postparturient period. Uterine rupture can occur when prostaglandin or oxytocin has been administered for treatment of pyometra, metritis, or dystocia. The condition may occur as a result of dystocia or during an apparently normal parturition or may be due to injury occurring in late pregnancy. The clinical signs of uterine rupture include abdominal pain and distention and a rapid deterioration of the condition of the bitch. The diagnosis is confirmed by exploratory laparotomy, and ovariohysterectomy is the usual treatment combined with intravenous fluids and antibiotic therapy.

Uterine Prolapse

Uterine prolapse is an uncommon complication during parturition. It occurs in primiparous as well as multiparous bitches. The prolapse usually occurs immediately or within a few hours after delivery of the last puppy. The prolapse can be complete with both uterine horns protruding from the vulva or may be limited to the uterine body and one horn. Treatments include manual reposition, reposition by means of laparotomy, and amputation. Ovariohysterectomy is usually performed.

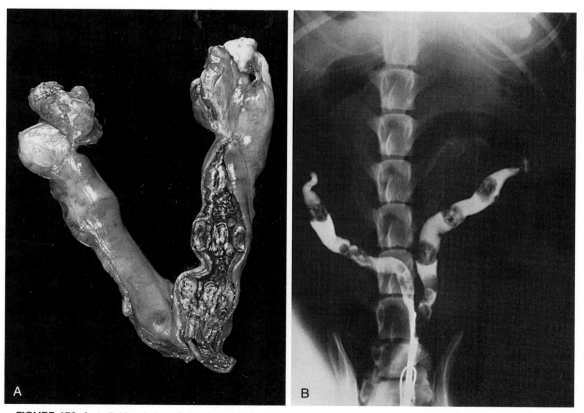

FIGURE 159–4. *A,* Subinvolution of the placental sites. In the unopened left uterine horn the typical oval swellings of the placental areas can be observed. In the opened horn, the placentation zones and the hemorrhage emanating from those areas can be seen. *B,* A hysterographic picture of a bitch with subinvolution of the placental sites, 4 months after whelping. The placentation zones are seen as the darker areas. Normal uterine involution is completed within 12 weeks in the bitch.

REP

Toxic Milk Syndrome

The toxic milk syndrome is poorly documented. Pathologic conditions in the uterus of the bitch may cause toxins to be excreted in the milk. Suckling offspring that are affected by toxic milk syndrome become vocal and uncomfortable. Other signs are diarrhea, salivation, bloating, and a reddened anus. Treatment consists of removing the offspring from the bitch and the administration of fluid therapy and oral glucose until bloating resolves. If the bitch is successfully treated for her uterine condition, the litter can be returned to her after 24 to 48 hours; otherwise, it requires hand rearing.

MAMMARY GLAND DISORDERS

Agalactia

Agalactia, or absence of milk after parturition, may be due to a failure of milk letdown or milk production. True agalactia, failure of milk production, is uncommon but may be observed after premature parturitions/cesarean sections. Failure of milk letdown may occur as a consequence of excessive secretion of epinephrine, resulting from fright or pain, which has a blocking effect on the release of oxytocin. Oxytocin can be administered repeatedly for a few days until milk flow has been established. Primiparous, nervous, or confused bitches may experience temporary agalactia. Reassurance by the owner and administration of low doses of acepromazine orally may help the bitch to settle down, and subsequent suckling by the puppies will enhance milk flow.[14] Other causes of agalactia are physical exhaustion, undernourishment, shock, mastitis, metritis, systemic infection, and endocrine imbalances.

Galactostasis

Milk stasis, galactostasis, causes enlarged and edematous mammary glands, which are firm and warm to the touch. The bitch shows signs of discomfort and pain and fails to let down milk. The condition should be differentiated from mastitis and agalactia. The etiology is unknown in dogs, but it usually involves the two most caudal pairs of mammae in bitches with a high milk production and/or few puppies or in glands with malformed teats, which the offspring avoid to suckle. Another cause can be that nursing comes to an abrupt end owing to death of the litter or sudden weaning. To relieve mammary congestion the owner can apply gentle massage and warm-water compresses to the mammary glands or perform careful milking to relieve some of the pressure. Sometimes it helps to put more aggressively nursing neonates to the bitch. Treatment includes reducing food intake and the administration of a mild diuretic. Neglected galactostasis may lead to mastitis or involution of the mammary gland. Cabergoline (Galastop vet.), a dopamine agonist, at 2.5 to 5 μg/kg/d orally for 4 to 6 days, reduces prolactin secretion and thereby lactation. The use of dopamine agonists should be restricted to bitches that have either lost their litter or have a litter old enough to be weaned.

Acute Mastitis

Acute mastitis in the bitch occurs from hematogenously spread bacterial infections or from bacteria ascending through the teat orifices. Predisposing factors include mammary gland congestion, trauma, and poor sanitary conditions.

The mammary glands become hot, painful, and enlarged; the milk shows increased viscosity and changes in color from yellow to brown depending on the amount of blood and purulent exudate present. Clinical signs include fever, anorexia, and depression in the bitch. The offspring may be restless and crying. Milk cytology reveals the presence of degenerate neutrophils, red blood cells, and bacteria. Culture of the milk often shows growth of *Staphylococcus* species, *Streptococcus* species, or *Escherichia coli*. Treatment consists of adequate antibiotics, application of warm-water compresses, and massage of mammary glands. If abscessation of the glands occurs, surgical débridement and drainage are essential. Untreated acute mastitis may result in gangrenous mastitis and septic shock. Depending on the severity of the condition the litter may stay with the bitch or has to be separated and hand reared.

MISCELLANEOUS DISORDERS

Puerperal Tetany

An acute decrease in extracellular calcium concentration is the cause of puerperal tetany (eclampsia). Eclampsia occurs most commonly in dogs of the small breeds, usually within the first 21 days after whelping but occasionally during late pregnancy or at parturition. Early signs are restlessness, panting, pacing, whining, salivation, tremors, and stiffness. The symptoms aggravate to clonic-tonic muscle spasms, fever, tachycardia, miosis, seizures, and death. Treatment must be instigated immediately and consists of slow intravenous infusion of a 10 per cent calcium borogluconate solution. The dosage required varies from 2 to 20 mL, depending on the degree of hypocalcemia and the size of the bitch. Careful cardiac monitoring for bradycardia and arrhythmias is important. If arrhythmia or vomiting occurs, the infusion must be temporarily halted and then, if necessary, resumed at a slower rate. Because hypoglycemia may follow hypocalcemia, the intravenous administration of a 10 per cent dextrose solution has been recommended. The puppies should be removed from the bitch and hand fed a canine milk replacer for 24 hours. If the litter is 4 weeks old or more, it is advisable to wean them. Oral supplementation of the lactating bitch (having experienced eclampsia) with calcium carbonate at 100 mg/kg body weight per day, divided with meals, and vitamin D is recommended. Prophylactic calcium treatment during the course of pregnancy of bitches expected to develop eclampsia probably is contraindicated, because it may cause a disturbance of the calcium homeostasis.

Disturbances in Maternal Behavior

Good maternal behavior includes nest building, nursing, and protecting, The bitch should spend most of the time with the litter for at least the first 2 weeks. Most bitches have strong maternal instincts, but their behavior depends strongly on their hormonal balance, general health, and the environment. In some breeds there is a higher occurrence of bad mothering, suggesting a heritable factor. Sublimation, close emotional attachment to a human, may cause problems at parturition when the bitch may manifest panic and "regard her offspring with horror and disgust."[16] On the contrary, a bitch may resent human intervention, not accepting assisted-birthing and cesarean-delivered offspring and may sometimes even kill them. Major disturbing factors during and after parturition, mental instability, or pain may cause the mother to kill her neonates. Good health, quiet and familiar surroundings, and, most important of all, presence of her young will promote normal maternal behavior.

REFERENCES

1. Concannon PW, et al: Biology and endocrinology of ovulation, pregnancy and parturition in the dog. J Reprod Fertil 39(Suppl):3–25, 1989.
2. Holst PA, Phemister RD: Onset of diestrus in the beagle bitch: Definition and significance. Am J Vet Res 35:401–406, 1974.
3. Okkens AC, et al: Influence of litter size and breed on variation in length of gestation in the dog. Vet Q 15:160–161, 1993.
4. Johnston SD, et al: Canine pregnancy length from serum progesterone concentrations of 3–32 nmol/L (1 to 10 ng/mL) (abstract). In Concannon PW (ed): Reproduction in Dogs and Other Carnivores. Proceedings of a Satellite Meeting of the 13th International Congress on Animal Reproduction, July 5, 1996, Sydney, p 34.
5. Long S: Abnormal development of the conceptus and its consequences. In Arthur GH, Noakes DE, Pearson H, Parkinson TJ (eds): Veterinary Reproduction and Obstetrics, 7th ed. London, WB Saunders, 1996, p 110.
6. Cole RA, et al: Vertical transmission of Neospora caninum in dogs. J Parasitol 81:208–211, 1995.
7. Ihle SL, Nelson RW: Insulin resistance and diabetes mellitus. Compend Contin Ed Small Anim 13:197–202, 1991.
8. Irvine CHG: Hypoglycemia in the bitch. N Z Vet J 12:140, 1964.
9. Jackson RF, et al: Hypoglycemia-ketonemia in a pregnant bitch. JAVMA 177:1123–1127, 1980.
10. Moore AH, Wotton PR: Preparturient hypoglycemia in two bitches. Vet Rec 133:396, 1993.
11. van der Weyden GC, et al: Physiological aspects of pregnancy and parturition in the bitch. J Reprod Fertil Suppl 39:211–224, 1989.
12. Steinetz BG, et al: Diurnal variation of serum progesterone, but not relaxin, prolactin or oestradiol-17beta in the pregnant bitch. Endocrinology 127:1057–1063, 1990.
13. van der Weyden GC, et al: The intrauterine position of canine fetuses and their sequence of expulsion at birth. J Small Anim Pract 22:503–510, 1981.
14. Wallace MS: Management of parturition and problems of the periparturient period of dogs and cats. Semin Vet Med Surg (Small Anim) 9:28–37, 1994.
15. Jackson PGG: Dystocia in the dog and cat. In Jackson PGG (ed): Handbook of Veterinary Obstetrics. London, WB Saunders, 1995, pp 115–133.
16. Freak MJ: The whelping bitch. Vet Rec 60:295–301, 1948.
17. Eneroth A, et al: A pelvimetric study of bitches with dystocia of the Boston terrier and the Scottish terrier breeds (abstract). In: Proceedings of the Inauguration of the Centre for Reproductive Biology. Uppsala, Sweden, SLU Service/Repro, 1997, p 37.
18. Darvelid AW, Linde-Forsberg C: Dystocia in the bitch: A retrospective study of 182 cases. J Small Anim Pract 35:402–407, 1994.
19. Mosier JE: Introduction to canine pediatrics. Vet Clin North Am Small Anim Pract 8:3–5, 1978.
20. Linde-Forsberg C, Forsberg M: Fertility in dogs in relation to semen quality and the time and site of insemination with fresh and frozen semen. J Reprod Fertil 39(Suppl):299–310, 1989.
21. Linde-Forsberg C, Forsberg M: Results of 527 controlled artificial inseminations in dogs. J Reprod Fertil 47(Suppl):313–323, 1993.

CHAPTER 160

EARLY SPAY AND NEUTER

Margaret V. Root Kustritz and Patricia N. Olson

Early spay and neuter, or prepubertal gonadectomy, refers to the surgical sterilization of sexually immature animals. This topic has received increasing attention, as it has been regarded as a tool to help control pet overpopulation in the United States.[1] Although the United States is reported to have the highest percentage of pet-owning households among the world's 20 major nations,[2] millions of animals are still abandoned and euthanized at humane shelters every year. In 1996, 2.5 million dogs and cats were euthanized at shelters reporting to the National Council on Pet Population Study and Policy.[3] This number is not an accurate reflection of the magnitude of the problem, as it does not include the many nonreporting shelters and veterinary clinics that perform euthanasia, nor does it include animals abandoned to the wild.

In 1992, the American Humane Association (AHA) put forth a resolution supporting further research in early spay and neuter and stated, "the AHA believes that no dog or cat adopted from a shelter should be allowed to reproduce."[4] The following year, the American Veterinary Medical Association stated that it "supports the concept of early (8–16 weeks of age) ovariohysterectomies/gonadectomies in dogs and cats, in an effort to stem the overpopulation problem in these species."[5]

ARGUMENTS FOR EARLY SPAY AND NEUTER

Although most animals that are released from a shelter have a spay/neuter contract, many of those animals are left intact once adopted.[4, 6] Those adopting cats are more likely to comply than are those adopting dogs, with poorest compliance among those adopting male dogs and apparently purebred female dogs.[6] If animals in shelters were neutered before adoption, they would be unable to reproduce and repopulate animal shelters. "Animal from an unwanted litter" was the reason for relinquishment to a shelter in 36.4 per cent of the cases in one study.[6]

No research has been done designating the best age at which to spay or neuter an animal. It is possible that the age of 5 to 7 months, which is the current recommendation in most of the United States, was chosen at a time in history when anesthetics and surgical equipment were less advanced and surgical success was more likely in a larger animal. Prepubertal gonadectomy is commonly performed in noncompanion species, including farm animals (e.g., cattle, sheep, pigs) and laboratory animals (e.g., ferrets, mice).

The "early" spay or neuter surgery is quick, with minimal bleeding and quick recovery. There is less time required of

REP

the surgeon and, subjectively, less stress to the animal. No common, age-related, serious intraoperative or short-term postoperative complications have been reported.[7-9] Ovariohysterectomy and castration are performed routinely. Fine suture material or hemostatic clips may be used for ligation of ovarian or testicular vessels.[8, 9]

ARGUMENTS AGAINST EARLY SPAY AND NEUTER

The underlying cause of pet overpopulation in the United States is not solely excessive reproduction of current dog and cat populations; it is more likely irresponsible pet ownership. A great many of the animals surrendered to humane shelters have been abandoned or surrendered by their owners, who no longer want the responsibility of caring for the animal. Animals that remain as pets in homes are often allowed to reproduce before being gonadectomized; the rate of lifetime litter production did not vary between intact female dogs and cats and animals sterilized pre- or postpubertally in one study.[10] Early spay and neuter surgery does not address these issues and may therefore be limited in its effect on pet overpopulation.

There is conflict in the literature as to whether lower urinary tract disease is more common in neutered than in intact male cats.[11-13] All prospective studies published to date show that urethral diameter does not differ significantly between intact and gonadectomized animals.[14-17] These include two historical studies comparing intact male cats with either males castrated at 5 months of age, with or without subsequent testosterone supplementation,[14] or males castrated or vasectomized at 3 months of age,[15] and two recent studies comparing intact male cats with males gonadectomized at either 7 weeks or 7 months of age.[16, 17] Urethral diameters were evaluated either by direct measurement after dissection[14, 15] or by measurements on lateral projection cystourethrograms at 12 to 22 months of age.[16, 17]

Prepubertal gonadectomy may predispose male cats to an inability to completely extrude the penis at maturity. Dissolution of the balanopreputial fold, the tissue normally joining the penile to the preputial mucosa at birth in cats, is androgen-dependent.[18] Forty per cent of cats neutered at 5 months of age have been reported to have preputial adhesions causing an inability to extrude the penis as adults.[19] Zero to 100 per cent of male cats gonadectomized at 7 weeks of age and 0 to 60 per cent of male cats gonadectomized at 7 months of age have been reported to exhibit an inability to completely extrude the penis at 12 to 22 months of age.[16, 17] The significance of decreased penile extrusion is unknown.

Obesity is a multifactorial problem caused by improper diet, decreased exercise and activity level, breed, age, and sexual status. Obesity is a commonly reported sequela to gonadectomy in the dog and cat, with the problem more common in females than in males. In the dog, retrospective studies demonstrate increased predisposition to obesity in spayed and neutered animals.[20, 21] No prospective study has yet demonstrated this predisposition. One study demonstrated no difference in food intake, weight gain, or back-fat depth in dogs that had been gonadectomized at 7 weeks or 7 months of age or left intact.[22] In the cat, animals gonadectomized at either 7 weeks or 7 months of age have been shown to have greater body weight and larger volumes of falciform fat, measured on lateral abdominal radiographs, than intact controls.[16] In another feline study, animals gonad-

ectomized at 7 weeks or 7 months of age were shown to have higher physical measures of obesity than intact controls; these physical measures included body condition scores and body mass indices (BMI = weight [kg] divided by height [M] times length [M]).[23] In the latter study, all gonadectomized cats were shown to have lower resting metabolic rates than intact cats, as measured by indirect calorimetry.[24] If a physiologic predisposition to obesity due to gonadectomy does exist, there is no evidence that age at the time of gonadectomy would change this effect.

Ovariohysterectomized bitches may be prone to urinary incontinence. Urinary incontinence has been reported to occur in 2.1 to 20.1 per cent of ovariohysterectomized dogs months to years after gonadectomy.[20, 25] Estrogen potentiates the activity of the sympathetic nervous system in maintenance of the closure of the external urethral sphincter. In an estrogen-deficient dog, the sphincter is not maintained in a tightly closed position, and leakage of urine may occur as the dog relaxes. This may exacerbate perivulvar dermatitis, a condition caused by infolding of the vulva secondary to obesity in ovariohysterectomized bitches. Vulvar infolding occurs in bitches spayed prepubertally that maintain an infantile vulva, and in bitches spayed later in life that undergo atrophy of the vulva to a more infantile form. There is no evidence to support a hypothesis that age at gonadectomy would affect onset or progression of estrogen-responsive urinary incontinence and/or perivulvar dermatitis.

An increased incidence of hyperadrenocorticism associated with adrenocortical tumor or nodular hyperplasia has been reported in ferrets, which are commonly gonadectomized prepubertally.[26, 27] One hypothesis is that these abnormalities are due to metaplasia of undifferentiated gonadal cells in the adrenal capsule. However, of 100 cases of proliferative adrenal lesions archived at the Armed Forces Institute of Pathology, almost 30 per cent were in intact females.[28] At present, no increase in adrenal disease has been reported in dogs and cats in areas of the country where early spay and neuter surgeries have been performed for 10 years or more. However, no prospective study has evaluated possible changes in adrenal function after prepubertal gonadectomy.

A common argument against early spay and neuter is that of stunted growth and poor muscle development in prepubertally gonadectomized animals. Gonadal steroids stimulate growth of cartilage and maturation of the physes of the long bones. Prepubertally gonadectomized animals are therefore more likely to show delay in closure of the physes and increased long bone length. This delay in physeal closure and subsequent increase in mature bone length have been demonstrated in dogs and cats gonadectomized at 7 weeks or 7 months of age, compared with intact animals.[16, 22, 29, 30] Whether this predisposes these animals to Salter-type fractures is unknown. Most of the muscle development of male cats is androgen-dependent, and a decrease in muscularity is seen when the animal is castrated, no matter what the age.

Behavioral concerns include retention of juvenile behaviors in prepubertally gonadectomized animals, inability of gonadectomized animals to exhibit behaviors traditionally appropriate to their gender (e.g., increased enthusiasm in intact male hunting dogs), and the impact of surgery during a young animal's fear imprinting period. It has been demonstrated that dogs castrated at 7 weeks or 7 months of age were more active than intact males at 1 year of age.[22] Male and female cats gonadectomized at 7 weeks or 7 months of age have been reported to show less intraspecies aggression and more affection than intact animals.[16] As to ability of gonadectomized animals to function normally for their gender, one study reported that prior sexual experience did not affect retention of male sexual behaviors in dogs.[31] These data may be extrapolated to include hunting and other working behaviors. The significance of performing surgery during the fear imprinting period is unknown. However, one study suggests that animals housed with littermates in a quiet location preoperatively were less likely to resist handling and experience inadequate sedation.[9]

Anesthesia concerns unique to pediatric animals include decreased ability to maintain body temperature owing to lower percentage of body fat and decreased ability to shiver, inadequate metabolization and excretion of drugs owing to immature hepatic enzyme systems, decreased protein binding of drugs and decreased renal function, and predisposition to hypoglycemia with fasting owing to decreased glycogen stores secondary to their smaller liver size and skeletal muscle mass.[32] Pediatric animals should be fasted for no more than 8 to 10 hours before surgery; they should be prepared with minimal clipping and warmed surgical scrub solutions and maintained on a circulating warm water blanket during surgery. Surgery time should be minimized to counter these concerns. Anesthetic regimens that have been shown to provide the smoothest induction and recovery and the best intraoperative analgesia are as follows:

Female puppies: atropine (0.04 mg/kg intramuscularly) and oxymorphone (0.11 mg/kg intramuscularly), followed in 15 minutes by propofol (3.4 mg/kg intravenously) with inhalant isoflurane for maintenance.[33]

Male puppies: atropine (0.04 mg/kg intramuscularly) and oxymorphone (0.22 mg/kg intramuscularly), followed in 15 minutes by propofol (6.5 mg/kg intravenously).[33]

Female kittens: midazolam (0.22 mg/kg intramuscularly) and ketamine hydrochloride (11 mg/kg intramuscularly) with inhalant isoflurane for maintenance.[9]

Male kittens: tiletamine/zolazepam (11 mg/kg intramuscularly).[9]

It is recommended that all female animals be intubated instead of maintained with gas anesthesia by mask, to ensure a patent airway, assist with ventilation if needed, and decrease gas exposure to personnel.[9]

CONCLUSION

Currently available information indicates that early spay and neuter is a safe procedure. Further research and the passage of time are required to allow us to understand any possible long-term effects. At present, only approximately one third of the 27 veterinary schools in North America will perform early spay and neuter surgeries, with the vast majority of those requiring the animal to be at least 4 months of age.[34] Whether the adoption of early spay and neuter programs will significantly impact pet overpopulation remains to be seen, but it is likely that early spay and neuter, coupled with increased enforcement of animal control ordinances, enhanced veterinary and public education, and a change in attitude concerning responsible pet ownership, will successfully help control pet overpopulation.

REFERENCES

1. Lieberman LL: A case for neutering pups and kittens at two months of age. JAVMA 191:518, 1987.
2. Pet Ownership. American Humane Association Fact Sheet. Englewood, CO, 1997.
3. National Shelter Survey: 1996 Results. Presented at the annual meeting of the National Council on Pet Population Study and Policy, Dallas, TX, 1997.
4. Nassar R, Talboy J, Moulton C: Animal Shelter Reporting Study 1990. American Humane Association, Englewood, CO, 1992.
5. Kahler S: Spaying/neutering comes of age. JAVMA 203:591, 1993.
6. Alexander SA, Shane SM: Characteristics of animals adopted from an animal control center whose owners complied with a spaying/neutering program. JAVMA 205:472, 1994.
7. Howe LM: Short-term results and complications of prepubertal gonadectomy in cats and dogs. JAVMA 211:57, 1997.
8. Aronsohn MG, Faggella AM: Surgical techniques for neutering 6- to 14-week-old kittens. JAVMA 202:53, 1993.
9. Faggella AM, Aronsohn MG: Anesthetic techniques for neutering 6- to 14-week-old kittens. JAVMA 202:56, 1993.
10. Manning AM, Rowan AN: Companion animal demographics and sterilization status: Results from a survey in four Massachusetts towns. Anthrozoos 5:192, 1992.
11. Engle GC: A clinical report on 250 cases of feline urologic syndrome. Feline Pract 7:24, 1977.
12. Foster SJ: The ''urolithiasis'' syndrome in male cats: A statistical analysis of the problems, with clinical observations. J Small Anim Pract 8:207, 1967.
13. Duch DS, Chow FC, Hamar DW, et al: The effect of castration and body weight on the occurrence of the feline urological syndrome. Feline Pract 8:35, 1978.
14. Herron MA: The effect of prepubertal castration on the penile urethra of the cat. JAVMA 160:208, 1972.
15. Jackson OF: The treatment and subsequent prevention of struvite urolithiasis in cats. J Small Anim Pract 12:555, 1971.
16. Stubbs WP, Bloomberg MS, Scruggs SL, et al: Effects of prepubertal gonadectomy on physical and behavioral development in cats. JAVMA 209:1864, 1996.
17. Root MV, Johnston SD, Johnston GR, et al: The effect of prepubertal and postpuberal gonadectomy on penile extrusion and urethral diameter in the domestic cat. Vet Radiol Ultrasound 37:363, 1996.
18. Bharadwaj MB, Calhoun ML: Mode of the formation of the preputial cavity in domestic animals. Am J Vet Res 22:764, 1961.
19. Herron MA: A potential consequence of prepubertal feline castration. Feline Pract 1:17, 1971.
20. David G, Rajendran EI: The after-effects of spaying in bitches and cats. Cheiron 9:3, 1980.
21. Sloth C: Practical management of obesity in dogs and cats. J Small Anim Pract 33:178, 1992.
22. Salmeri KR, Bloomberg MS, Scruggs SL, et al: Gonadectomy in immature dogs: Effects of skeletal, physical, and behavioral development. JAVMA 198:1193, 1991.
23. Root MV: Early spay-neuter in the cat: Effect on development of obesity and metabolic rate. Vet Clin Nutr 2:132, 1996.
24. Root MV, Johnston SD, Olson PN: Effect of prepubertal and postpuberal gonadectomy on heat production measured by indirect calorimetry in male and female domestic cats. Am J Vet Res 57:371, 1996.
25. Arnold S, Arnold P, Hubler M, et al: Urinary incontinence in spayed bitches: Prevalence and breed predisposition. Schweiz Arch Tierheilkd 131:259, 1989.
26. Lawrence HJ, Gould WJ, Flanders JA, et al: Unilateral adrenalectomy as a treatment for adrenocortical tumors in ferrets: Five cases (1990–1992). JAVMA 203:267, 1993.
27. Rosenthal KL, Peterson ME, Quesenberry KE, et al: Hyperadrenocorticism associated with adrenocortical tumor or nodular hyperplasia of the adrenal gland in ferrets: 50 cases (1987–1991). JAVMA 203:271, 1993.
28. Olson PN: Early spay and neuter. Proceedings, North American Veterinary Conference, Orlando, FL, 1997, p 25.
29. Root MV, Johnston SD, Olson PN: The effect of prepubertal and postpuberal gonadectomy on radial physeal closure in male and female domestic cats. Vet Radiol Ultrasound 37:363, 1996.
30. Houlton JEF, McGlennon NJ: Castration and physeal closure in the cat. Vet Rec 131:466, 1992.
31. Hart BL: Gonadal androgen and sociosexual behavior of male mammals: A comparative analysis. Psychol Bull 81:383, 1974.
32. Grandy JL, Dunlop CI: Anesthesia of pups and kittens. JAVMA 198:1244, 1991.
33. Faggella AM, Aronsohn MG: Evaluation of anesthetic protocols for neutering 6- to 14-week-old pups. JAVMA 205:308, 1994.
34. Bean B: Veterinary Medical College Survey, 1995. Written correspondence to Dr. Margaret Root Kustritz, June 27, 1995.

REP

CHAPTER 161

CONTRACEPTION AND PREGNANCY TERMINATION

J. Verstegen

Methods for general contraception (including postcoital contraception) and induction of abortion in dogs are necessary to prevent the birth of undesirable litters. There are numerous reasons that justify these protocols: pet overpopulation, preservation of the reproductive potential in animals devoted to breeding, travel, unwanted matings, first estrous matings in young bitches, reproduction management, current health problems or expected problems during labor related to pelvic abnormalities or disproportion between the male and female, and myriad others.

Because of social, cultural, financial, or ethical differences, great variations exist among countries in the management of these problems. In North America, the majority of bitches are surgically sterilized and contraception is rarely used. Furthermore, the products available to control reproduction are few. In the Scandinavian countries, surgical sterilization is ethically controversial and medical contraception is the main technique for population control. Europe appears to fall between these two extreme positions, and a particularly large number of drugs for reproductive purposes are commercially available. Similarly, use of drugs authorized for humans or other species is relatively common.

METHODS OF CONTRACEPTION

SURGICAL CONTRACEPTION

Surgical removal of the gonads in both males and females is the method of choice for preventing reproduction in animals not intended for breeding. This procedure permanently eliminates heat cycles, mating, unwanted pregnancy, and reproductive behavior. These surgeries are safe and inexpensive. Neutering prevents any risk of reproductive failure or disease (e.g., protects against mammary tumors, prostatic diseases, perineal hernia). All animals not dedicated to breeding purposes should be surgically sterilized before puberty. Sterilization prevents the well-known consequences of hormonal impregnation in the bitch: mammary tumors, reproductive tract diseases, or modified behavior during the estrous cycle. It also obviates the need for future possible treatment for abortion induction.

Side effects of surgical sterilization are rare and include direct surgery-related complications (e.g., inflammatory reactions, adhesions, abscesses), the remnant ovarian syndrome (accounting for half the cases of complications described and caused by persistence of ovarian tissue), and obesity. The increased incidence of obesity is probably related to a decreased basal metabolic rate and decreased activity. However, many spayed animals do not experience obesity, and this tendency can be diminished via owner education, increased activity, and restricted feeding. Although primary

incontinence has been described as a "common" complication of sterilization, its incidence is much lower than the incidence of problems associated with dogs and cats that have not been neutered, including the problem of pet overpopulation.

Controversies exist regarding early versus late ovariectomy (see Chapter 160) and also regarding ovariectomy versus ovariohysterectomy (OHE) in young animals.

OVARIECTOMY VERSUS OVARIOHYSTERECTOMY

Spaying has the advantage of significantly reducing the incidence of mammary tumors particularly if performed at a young age, but its protective effects, although controversial, can still be observed in animals committed to surgery as late as 7 to 9 years old (Fig. 161–1). Removal of the uterus and cervix along with the ovaries is supposed to preclude any subsequent development of uterine or cervical disease. However, although most surgery textbooks recommend OHE for routine neutering of young bitches, there is no evidence that conditions such as the cystic endometrial hyperplasia (CEH)–pyometra complex or tumors develop in animals submitted to only an ovariectomy. Published data[1, 2] and our

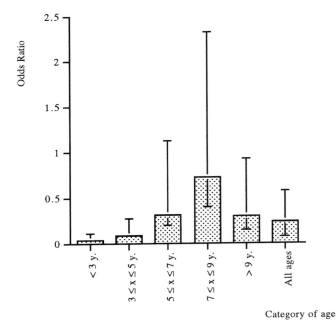

Category of age

Figure 161–1. Odds ratio for the risk of mammary tumor development (all lesions included) related to the age at sterilization with correction for age and progestin treatments.

own experience for more than 20 years with thousands of animals demonstrate that there are no significant differences in the incidence of urogenital problems between ovariectomized and ovariohysterectomized bitches. Ovariectomy performed in young, healthy animals appears to be associated with no significant risk of genital diseases. Indeed, the removal of the ovaries (and consequently of the reproductive steroid hormones) is followed by complete regression and atrophy of the remaining reproductive tract, which is no longer affected by tonic stimuli from the ovaries. The benefit/risk ratio is highly in favor of the ovariectomy for many reasons. The procedure is less invasive (smaller abdominal wall incision, less abdominal trauma), easier to perform, and less time consuming, and there are fewer problems related to anesthesia. Fewer complications are observed than with OHE, as shown by Okkens et al.,[1] who demonstrated that most of the postoperative complications occur at the cervical stump.

Ovariectomy appears to be associated with a lower risk of acquired urinary incontinence than OHE, although this is still controversial and based on preliminary objective controlled studies. Acquired urinary incontinence is a complex entity in which many factors play a role. Among these factors are obesity, breed, and sterilization. The type of surgery performed is also important, OHE being, in our opinion, more often associated with urinary incontinence than ovariectomy. Inflammatory reactions in the pelvic cavity (perhaps secondary to traction exerted on the genital tract during OHE) may lead to diffuse intrapelvic adhesions between the vagina and the urinary tract. These adhesions may cause displacement of the bladder neck in the pelvic cavity while the remaining intrapelvic portion of the genital tract, because of the disappearance of sex hormones, slowly becomes atrophic. Together, these inflammatory reactions and associated fibrosis, adhesions, and atrophic processes, combined with the accumulation of fat in the retroperitoneal "culs-de-sac" often observed in old animals, may cause development of post-sterilization urinary incontinence. When estrogens are used to treat the urinary incontinence, they may act directly on the urethral sphincter competence, as generally proposed. In addition, estrogens probably induce changes in the remaining genital tract, allowing the bladder to descend from the pelvic cavity and move back into the abdomen.

For all the preceding reasons, some demonstrated and some hypothetical, it has been proposed, particularly in European veterinary institutions, that ovariectomy be considered the procedure of choice for all young bitches without evidence of reproductive pathologies (e.g., metrorrhagy, follicular cysts, abortion, cesarean section, CEH, pyometra) or without previous reproductive hormone treatment that could promote uterine diseases. When ovariectomy is used instead of OHE, the quality of the surgery has to be perfect to prevent the in situ ovarian remnant syndrome, which could cause uterine disease.

When possible, surgical castration should be performed in anestrous animals. Sterilization during heat is associated with increased bleeding because of coagulation changes and vascular congestion; sterilization during the luteal phase may be followed by pseudocyesis caused by the rapid decline in serum progesterone concentration and the subsequent increase in prolactin. When sterilization is performed during the luteal phase, adjunctive treatment with an antiprolactin agent must be proposed, particularly for animals that have shown overt pseudopregnancy during the previous cycles. Cabergoline orally administered at 5 μg/kg per day has

proved to be effective in preventing this type of side effect. Bromocryptine can also be used at doses ranging from 10 to 50 μg/kg but given three times a day (short duration of action) for at least 7 days.

MEDICAL TECHNIQUES FOR CONTROLLING REPRODUCTION

CYCLE CONTROL BY STEROID HORMONES

Many different steroid hormones have been used to control reproductive behavior and ovarian cycle activity in the bitch and queen. Steroid hormones are numerous, but the number and type of products available vary greatly from country to country. Among these drugs are the natural steroids progesterone and testosterone and a large variety of synthetic steroids including medroxyprogesterone acetate, chlormadinone acetate, megestrol acetate, delmadinone acetate, melengestrol, proligestone, norethisterone acetate, and mibolerone.[3] Contraceptive steroids that are administered orally have a short duration of action. Those injected have a longer duration of action. However, progesterones used in large dosages and long-acting formulas are known to promote acromegaly, insulin resistance, diabetes mellitus, the development of the CEH-pyometra complex, mammary development, and tumors. Androgen derivatives may induce masculinization of external genitalia. Obesity and increased body weight have also often been described as possible side effects. Therefore, the use of contraceptive steroids is of limited importance and particular attention should be given to the route of administration, dose, duration of treatment, and stage of the cycle at initiation of the treatment.

Data have suggested that many of the adverse side effects attributed to steroid contraceptives may be related to overdosages rather than to the drugs per se. Indeed, for the vast majority of these "old" drugs, no data are available regarding the correct dose, as dose titration studies have not been performed to demonstrate clearly the minimal amount of product needed to prevent the onset of the estrous cycle. These studies are warranted, and results will probably demonstrate that use of these drugs at appropriate dosages may not be associated with significant side effects. Misdorp,[4] in studies of progestogens and mammary tumors in dogs and cats, pointed out a possible dose-related tumorigenic effect of progestins. Moderate doses were associated with a slightly increased risk for benign tumors but no carcinogenic effect, and low doses were associated with a protective effect. It was suggested that the protective effect might result from suppression of ovarian function, leaving the animals at a lower level of exposure to sex steroids than under physiologic conditions. Further studies are needed before condemning the use of progestins as contraceptive agents in dogs. However, it is correct to say that their current use is far from the safest way to control reproduction in dogs and cats.

It is not the author's objective to review all the progestins or testosterone derivatives used for cycle control in dogs and cats as no real discovery has emerged on this topic. The author refers to good reviews published on this subject, particularly in the previous edition of Ettinger and Feldman.[5]

No injectable progestins are available for dogs and cats in the United States. In Europe, medroxyprogesterone acetate, delmadinone acetate, and proligestone are the compounds mostly used. They differ in their relative activity, dose, and duration of action. Injectable progestins should be given to dogs in anestrus, around 3 to 4 months after the previous

REP

heat period, and repeated every 3 to 6 months depending on the drug. Prolonged, continuous treatments are not recommended as they increase the risk of permanent infertility (chemical sterilization), reproductive tract pathology (CEH-pyometra), acromegaly, insulin resistance or diabetes mellitus, or mammary diseases. Care must be taken not to use these drugs in prepubertal animals because irreversible prolonged anestrus is sometimes observed if animals are treated before the first estrous cycle. Because of the potential for adverse effects on fertility and reproductive organs, it is advisable not to use these drugs in animals dedicated to reproduction. The use of progestins during the follicular phase is contraindicated because of the increased risk of uterine pathology.

Administration of progestins during the luteal phase may lead to prolonged pregnancy associated with fetal death, maceration, mummification, and uterine diseases. If a pregnant animal receives an injectable progestagen, one must consider performing a cesarean section. The timing for cesarean section can be determined by a progesterone assay. Indeed, at the end of a normal pregnancy period, a physiologic drop in endogenous progesterone is observed, which can be detected by a specific progesterone assay, but because of the high exogenous plasma progestin content, whelping does not occur. Neonates require commercially available milk, as maternal milk production and lactation are inhibited by the exogenous progestin. Finally, poor involution of placental sites may result. High doses of antibiotics and prostaglandin treatment should be considered.

Oral administration of progestins seems to be better tolerated, but side effects are still sometimes observed. This is particularly true if a high dose or long duration of treatment is used. Diabetes mellitus and mammary lesions are certainly contraindications to such treatments. Administration during pregnancy of orally active progestins is contraindicated because of the risk of fetal feminization. If such treatment is stopped a few days before the supposed date of whelping, whelping and lactation can occur normally. This oral form of short-acting progestin (natural progesterone or megestrol acetate) is of interest in cases of suspected hypoluteoidism (see Chapter 159).

Mibolerone, an androgenic steroid, is approved only in the United States for long-term prevention of estrus in dogs. Because of its toxic effects in cats and worrisome side effects in bitches (e.g., masculinization, fetal androgenization, clitoris enlargement, vaginal discharge), the product has been withdrawn from the European market.

NONSTEROIDAL CONTROL OF CYCLE

Devices

Vaginal devices have been developed. Inflammatory reactions and device expulsion result in unacceptable failure rates.[6] So far, intrauterine devices are not available because of the difficulty of cannulating the canine cervix.

Vaccines

Antifertility vaccines have been studied in dogs and in other species but results have been poor or inconsistent.[6] Immunization against gonadotropin-releasing hormone (GnRH),[7, 8] luteinizing hormone (LH), follicle-stimulating hormone (FSH), or zona pellucida (ZP) proteins is still under investigation and development. ZP immunization appears to be irreversible. The main concerns are related to the immunization process (irritation, skin lesions), vaccine adjuvant, duration of immunity, and efficacy. To date, no contraceptive immunization protocol for dogs has been submitted to large-scale clinical trials. However, this is certainly one route for future development.

Treatments With Gonadotropin-Releasing Hormone Agonists or Antagonists[9, 10]

GnRH antagonists, if available, would be an excellent means of controlling reproduction in dogs. By continuously blocking GnRH receptors at the pituitary level, these antagonists block the synthesis and release of the primary stimulus for LH and FSH secretion. Estrous cycle control is inhibited, whereas modification of the tonic constant release is questionable. However, GnRH antagonists are currently expensive, which is a major block to their development. GnRH antagonists have been associated with side effects, such as mastocyst degranulation and histamine release.

GnRH agonists, when used continuously, are associated, after an initial stimulatory effect on FSH and LH release, with downregulation effects. Gonadotropin receptors are downregulated, and during constant GnRH agonist administration, FSH and LH synthesis and release also seem to be inhibited. Starting the treatment during anestrus unfortunately induces estrus initially, before inducing the downregulation. GnRH agonist implants have been described to prevent estrus for 1 year or longer, but field trials have not been reported.

METHODS OF PREGNANCY TERMINATION

The only information available is that any modification in the estrogen/progesterone ratio or inhibition of progesterone secretion by the corpus luteum interferes with pregnancy. Continuous secretion of progesterone is required during all stages of pregnancy. In dogs, a plasma progesterone level of ± 2 ng/mL appears to be required to maintain pregnancy. No placental or embryonic secretions have been demonstrated to regulate luteal steroidogenesis tonically in dogs. Even if still controversial, both LH and prolactin appear to be luteotropic in dogs. Exogenous prostaglandins as well as endogenous prostaglandins are luteolytic. Prolactin appears to be the main pituitary hormone that sustains the corpus luteum steroidogenesis, and inhibition of its secretion by dopamine agonists or other mechanisms induces the functional arrest of corpora lutea and/or luteolysis. The role of LH is more controversial; some studies have demonstrated that LH can have a stimulating effect on progesterone secretion and that LH inhibition induces luteolysis, whereas other studies have failed to support these conclusions.

Prostaglandin $F_{2\alpha}$ induces luteal arrest by binding to specific receptors. Its administration induces a reduction in corpus luteum blood supply (vasoconstriction) and interferes with luteal steroidogenesis. This is initially associated with a reversible functional arrest characterized by a drop in progesterone secretion if short-acting and low-dose treatment is administered. If prostaglandins are given for a long enough time, irreversible arrest of progesterone production occurs. In bitches, abortion occurs when the plasma progesterone concentration remains below 2 ng/mL for more than 24 to 48 hours. In queens, the progesterone requirement during pregnancy seems to be lower and less well characterized than in bitches. A minimum of 1 ng/mL seems to be required to prevent abortion in this species.

Abortion can be induced in a number of ways:

1. Modification of the estrogen/progesterone ratio. This can apparently be done by either estrogen[11] or corticosteroid[12] injection. Several publications have described the use of estrogen derivatives to induce abortion. They are, however, often associated with side effects and their use is no longer advisable. The use of corticosteroids to induce abortion is controversial. However, they represent an interesting alternative in countries where more sophisticated and expensive drugs are not readily available.[12]

2. Induction of luteal functional arrest or luteolysis. This can be achieved directly using prostaglandins[13, 14] or indirectly using prolactin secretion inhibitors[15] or GnRH antagonists[16] to deplete LH secretion. Prostaglandins have been widely described as inducing abortion by inducing corpora lutea functional arrest and uterine myocontraction. The use of these drugs is, however, associated with numerous non–life-threatening side effects. Dose titration studies have demonstrated that these side effects could be reduced by diminishing the dose (10 to 50 μg/kg versus 250 μg/kg) and, for natural prostaglandins, increasing the number of injections (three to five). Synthetic prostaglandins appear to be associated with fewer side effects and a longer duration of action, allowing alternate-day injections. Full and consistent efficacy of prostaglandins is generally obtained after implantation has occurred. Prolactin secretion inhibitors (and not antagonists) block secretion of prolactin and prevent its essential supportive action on the corpus luteum. They induce abortion indirectly by removing the obligatory corpus luteum support. When they are administered alone, this action occurs with consistency only after day 30 to 40 of pregnancy (pregnancy always being dated from the LH surge, which corresponds approximately to a progesterone serum concentration of 1 to 2 ng/mL [increased from the basal level obtained 1 or 2 days before] or 8 to 9 days before the onset of diestrus; mating cannot be used as a reference as it could occur as early as 2 to 5 days before or 2 to 5 days after the LH surge).

3. Direct inhibition of progesterone secretion by the use of drugs that specifically inhibit steroidogenesis[17] (e.g., epostane). These are not available yet, and many questions remain regarding their actions on the other steroids (mineralocorticoids and glucocorticoids). However, they are an interesting alternative for the future.

4. Inhibition of the action of progesterone at the receptor site by blocking the progesterone receptors using progesterone antagonists that bind to the receptors without inducing any DNA effects. The most extensively studied antiprogestin, mifepristone (RU 486, Roussel-UCLAF, not registered for animal use[18]), has been shown to bind to progesterone receptors with high affinity and to prevent progesterone-induced changes in DNA transcription. These specific drugs are not yet available for use in veterinary medicine except in France, where aglepristone, a specific progesterone antagonist, has been launched. However, for ethical reasons related to the risk of unauthorized use in humans, their future remains questionable. Progesterone antagonists could be used at any time during pregnancy, depriving the embryo and then the uteroplacental unit of its progesterone support. Progesterone antagonists induce embryonic loss without significant clinical signs when given before implantation; fetal death is associated with fetal expulsion (if given after ossification) or no expulsion (if given before ossification). Aglepristone has been administered at a dose of 10 mg/kg twice, at a 24-hour interval, in a study involving 367 bitches. The treatment was effective in 100% of animals not diagnosed as pregnant at the time of treatment and in 94.8% of animals confirmed pregnant on the first day of treatment.[13] No systemic or local side effects were observed except for the development of mammary glands and lactation.

TREATMENTS TO INDUCE ABORTION

TREATMENT OF BITCHES NOT INTENDED FOR BREEDING

For the majority of bitches, the most appropriate technique for preventing the birth of an undesirable litter after unwanted mating or for health reasons is to perform a sterilization by ovariectomy before implantation or by OHE if pregnancy is confirmed.

TREATMENT OF BITCHES INTENDED FOR BREEDING*

Abortion can be induced either before or after implantation. Induction of abortion before implantation is no longer recommended for at least two reasons:

1. It has been clearly shown that less than 50 per cent of bitches are pregnant when only one accidental mating has occurred. This means that at least 50 per cent of animals are unduly treated if pregnancy has not been confirmed.[19]

2. The products available for inducing abortion before implantation are all associated with side effects that can be life-threatening.

It is best and safest for the animal to be treated approximately 25 days after the LH surge, when pregnancy can easily be confirmed. If abortion is then pursued, the safest approach should be used.

Abortion Induction Before Implantation

Two types of treatment can be proposed. The first one prevents implantation by modifying oviductal-uterine motility and secretion, inducing death of the embryo. It is based on the administration of estrogens. The second treatment is based on inhibiting progesterone secretion via the use of prostaglandins. However, the corpus luteum is relatively independent of all hormonal control until at least day 20 to 25 after the LH surge. Therefore, induction of luteal arrest early in diestrus requires using high dosages of prostaglandins associated with many side effects. For this reason, use of prostaglandins to induce abortion before implantation is not recommended.

Large doses of estrogens have been used extensively to prevent implantation. However, their toxic effects make their use dangerous. In clinical practice, diethylstilbestrol (DES), estradiol cypionate (ECP) or benzoate, and mestranol have been widely used to prevent unwanted pregnancies. Numerous protocols are available and reflect the absence of clear, well-constructed studies to define the minimum effective dose of estrogen necessary to induce abortion. Estrogens should never be administered to a bitch intended for breeding. Their side effects (e.g., uterine diseases, hypothalamo-pituitary blockade leading to irreversible sterility, bleeding, medullar aplasia) can irreversibly damage the reproductive function.

The main estrogenic drug used for abortion induction in

REP

---

*Only the available and clinically acceptable treatments are given here.

Europe is estradiol benzoate (Intervet, The Netherlands). In the United States, ECP is used. The ECP is more potent, has a longer duration of action, but is clearly more toxic. DES is no longer available in Europe or the United States as an injectable formulation, and oral DES has been proved to be ineffective for inducing abortion.[20] Neither drug should be used.

Abortion Induction After Implantation

Prostaglandins

Multiple doses of prostaglandins have been demonstrated to prevent pregnancy in bitches by inhibition of progesterone synthesis by corpora lutea. Efficacy is dependent not only dose and frequency but also on the stage of pregnancy. Prostaglandin administration early in diestrus requires higher doses and periods of treatment to achieve results. Early treatment is less efficacious.

Prostaglandins can be used to induce abortion. One mechanism of action is indirect: induction of local vasoconstriction, reducing blood flow to the corpora lutea, and consequently leading to cellular degeneration. Another mechanism of action is direct: binding to specific receptors, interfering with steroidogenesis, and reducing the production of progesterone. Prostaglandins (especially natural prostaglandins) are also known to exert a direct action on the myometrium, inducing contractions. The side effects of natural prostaglandins are related mainly to their stimulant effects on smooth muscles, which appear within minutes after injection and are clearly dose dependent. Adaptation to the side effects seems to occur after repeated treatments, and side effects actually decrease considerably after several injections. Clinical observations include excessive salivation, vomiting, diarrhea, defecation, hyperpnea, ataxia, urination, anxiety, and pupil dilatation followed by constriction.

Prostaglandin analogues may be safer in inducing abortion because they have a greater effect on luteal function and a less intense effect on smooth muscle. Therefore, the adverse effects previously described are not as dramatic. However, in experimental and clinical trials, we have demonstrated that doses of natural prostaglandins of $10 \mu g/kg$ or less and doses of cloprostenol of $1 \mu g/kg$ or less are generally not associated with side effects but retain their biologic action on the corpus luteum. Indeed, cloprostenol at $1 \mu g/kg$ once a day for 5 days is able, after day 25 to 30 of pregnancy, to induce luteal functional arrest characterized by a drop of progesterone secretion below the limit of 2 ng/mL. A dinoprostum dose of 10 $\mu g/kg$ has similar effects, but because of the short half-life of this molecule, it has to be injected at least three to five times a day, making this protocol much more cumbersome in clinical conditions. The author's preference is injection subcutaneously starting at day 30 after mating of 1 to 2 $\mu g/kg$ cloprostenol once a day for 5 to 7 days.

Dopamine Agonist Agents

Prolactin is the main luteotropic hormone in dogs. Inhibition of the synthesis and release of prolactin causes withdrawal of the necessary support for continuing function of corpora lutea. Thus, luteal functional arrest, a drop in progesterone secretion, and (if this treatment is applied during the second part of pregnancy and for a long enough time) luteolysis occur. Prolactin secretion is under tonic inhibitory regulation via hypothalamic dopamine. Centrally, serotonin may also affect prolactin secretion by modifying the dopamine release. Indeed, serotonin acting at the arcuate nucleus of the hypothalamus inhibits dopamine synthesis and release, which, in turn, stimulates prolactin release. Serotonin antagonists increase dopamine release and prolactin inhibition.

Two main classes of prolactin inhibitors exist: direct dopamine agonists and indirect serotonin antagonists. Bromocriptine and cabergoline belong to the first class; they are dopamine D_2 agonists that inhibit prolactin secretion by a direct action on D_2 pituitary receptors. Metergoline belongs essentially to the second class; it is a serotonin antagonist that increases the dopamine inhibiting tone at the hypothalamic level and indirectly inhibits prolactin release.

Bromocriptine (Parlodel, Sandoz, Switzerland; not approved for animal use except in Italy) was the first inhibitor for which an effective dose was established. Its use was not extensive because of the high incidence of emesis observed after use of doses ranging from 50 to 100 $\mu g/kg$ once or twice a day. However, these doses are not consistently effective in inducing abortion and have to be given for at least 5 days and, ideally, to effect, which could take more than 7 days, depending on the period in which the treatment begins. In fact, before day 40 of pregnancy, bromocryptine given orally is far from effective in inducing abortion because of its relatively low potency as an inhibitor of prolactin secretion and its limited duration of action (approximately 8 hours). After day 40, abortion is associated with fetal expulsion and is not recommended. Emesis associated with inappetence can be of considerable concern when bromocriptine is used at the highest dose level.

Cabergoline (Galastop, Vetem Centralvet, Italy; approved in Europe), a more specific dopamine agonist commercially available in Europe but not in the United States, has been developed as an antiprolactin drug; it was used initially in dogs and cats and is now used in humans (for physiologic—postpartum—or pathologic hyperprolactinemia). It is safe and effective, long acting (binding to the dopamine receptors at the pituitary level for more than 48 hours), and available as an easily administered syrup. Vomiting is rarely observed, but when vomiting occurs, it is of short duration and intensity. Oral cabergoline at a dosage of 5 $\mu g/kg/per$ day for 5 days has been demonstrated to induce abortion in 100% of bitches treated orally from 40 days after the LH surge. However, only 25% respond when cabergoline is given from day 30.[21] An injectable formulation administered subcutaneously every other day over 5 days at 1.65 $\mu g/kg$ was more potent (with 100, 66, and 25 per cent of dogs responding when treatments were started at days 40, 30, and 25 after the LH surge, respectively[22]).

Because of its relatively low prolactin-inhibiting activity, short duration of action, and induction of side effects related to its serotoninergic activities (aggressive behavior, excitation, mood changes), metergoline is not used to induce abortion in dogs and cats.

Combination of Low-Dose Prostaglandins and Dopamine Agonists

Encouraging results have been published regarding the simultaneous use of low-dose prostaglandins and a dopamine agonist to induce abortion. The objective of this association is to impair corpus luteum function and, therefore, progesterone release by a double mechanism of action: (1) direct, through the local effects of the prostaglandins on corpus luteum steroidogenesis, and (2) indirect, through withdrawal of the necessary pituitary luteotropic support of prolactin. In this way, an additive if not synergistic effect is obtained, allowing a reduction of the doses and consequently a reduction of the well-known side effects of prostaglandins. This protocol induces abortion in 100% of dogs treated from day 25 after the LH surge (20 to 28 days after first mating). A combination of cloprostenol (1 μg/kg, two subcutaneous injections, 4 days apart) and cabergoline given orally at 5 μg/kg per day for 7 days (see Fig. 161–3) was demonstrated to be experimentally and clinically effective in inducing abortion. Abortion always occurred by resorption 5 to 8 days after the beginning of treatment. No side effects were recorded except, as in all abortive treatment, some vaginal bleeding 5 to 10 days after the beginning of treatment, which matched the sonographic images of resorption.[23] The safety of this type of protocol has been demonstrated both in the short term and in the long term as far as future fertility is concerned. The treatment has to be initiated around day 25, when pregnancy can be confirmed. Before day 25, the corpus luteum is refractory and the confirmation of pregnancy is less reliable. After day 40, as ossification has already occurred, abortion is associated with nonideal fetal expulsion as opposed to what is observed earlier. For these reasons, it is recommended that the treatment be started as soon as the pregnancy diagnosis is made by palpation or sonography.

The use of bromocriptine instead of cabergoline, combined with natural or artificial prostaglandins, has also been described and shown to be effective by the author. In these cases, bromocriptine has to be administered twice a day at 25 μg/kg, compared with daily administration of cabergoline, and if dinoprostum is used instead of cloprostenol, it has to be given three times a day at 10 μg/kg (Figs. 161–2 and 161–3).

This approach to induction of abortion is efficacious. Abortion is induced only when the animal is confirmed to be pregnant, the treatment causes few direct or indirect side effects, and fertility is conserved. This type of treatment is easy to apply, particularly if cloprostenol and cabergoline are used. It ensures the necessary veterinary control related to this important procedure (the animal being seen on the

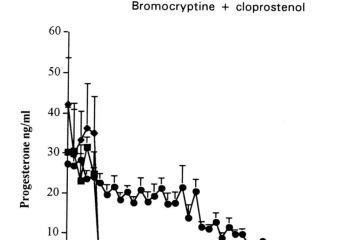

Figure 161–3. Effects on plasma progesterone concentration in a group treated with bromocryptine (20 μg/kg twice a day for 7 days) and cloprostenol (2.5 μg/kg once at day 25 or 1 μg/kg at days 25 and 30) compared with a nontreated control group. A drop below 2 ng is observed in 48 hours. Abortion was always observed.

first and last days of treatment), but at the same time it requires the owner's compliance.

Corticosteroid Treatments

Administration of glucocorticoids was shown to induce abortion in cattle and sheep and several injections terminate pregnancy in dogs when doses of 5 mg/kg are administered intramuscularly every 12 hours for 10 days starting at day 30 or 45 of pregnancy. The ability of oral dexamethasone

Figure 161–2. Effects on plasma progesterone concentration in a group treated with cabergoline (5 μg/kg/d for 7 days) and cloprostenol (2.5 μg/kg once at day 25 or 1 μg/kg at days 25 and 30) compared with a nontreated control group. A drop below 2 ng is observed in 48 hours. Abortion was always observed.

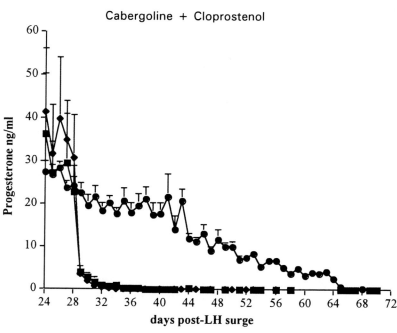
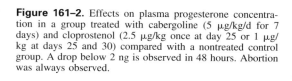

administration to terminate pregnancy has been demonstrated. Dexamethasone was administered orally from day 35 of pregnancy at a dose of 0.2 mg/kg two or three times a day for 5 days, followed by another 3 to 5 days during which the dose was progressively reduced to zero. Abortion was observed in all animals within a few days of the end of the treatment. The exact mode of action is not understood. Dexamethasone may have direct or indirect luteolytic effects. This type of treatment has certainly advantages over the use of estrogens during estrus: the side effects are limited and are unlikely to be life-threatening. The efficacy of this treatment is good, although obvious corticoid-induced side effects (polyphagia, polydipsia, and polyuria) were observed. Additional information is certainly required to determine the exact mode of action, the effects on future fertility, and whether dexamethasone treatment should be recommended as an alternative method of pregnancy termination if other alternatives are not available or if hospitalization or surgery is not possible. Therefore, the use of corticoids to terminate pregnancy cannot be recommended until further information on efficacy and side effects is available.[24]

REFERENCES

1. Okkens AC, Dieleman SJ, Kooistra HS et al: Comparison of long-term effects of ovariectomy versus ovariohysterectomy in bitches. J Reprod Fertil Suppl 51: 227–231, 1997.
2. Janssens LAA, Janssens GHRR: Bilateral flank ovariectomy in the dog—Surgical technique and sequelae in 72 animals. J Small Anim Pract 32:249–252, 1991.
3. England GCW: Pharmacological control of reproduction in the dog and bitch. In Simpson G, England G, Harvey M (eds): Manual of Small Animal Reproduction and Neonatology. London, BSAVA, 1998, pp 197–122.
4. Misdorp W: Progestogens and mammary tumours in dogs and cats. Acta Endocrinol (Copenh) 125:27–31, 1991.
5. Ettinger SJ, Feldman EC: Textbook of Veterinary Internal Medicine, 4th ed. Philadelphia, WB Saunders, 1995, pp 21–46.
6. Concannon PW, Meyers-Wallen V: Current and proposed methods for contraception and termination of pregnancy in dogs and cats. JAVMA 198:1214–1225, 1991.
7. Gonzalez A, Allen AF, Post R, et al: Immunological approaches to contraception in dogs. J Reprod Fertil Suppl 39:189–198, 1989.
8. Singh V: Active immunization of female dogs against LHRH and its effects on ovarian steroids and estrus suppression. Indian J Exp Biol 23:667–675, 1985.
9. Concannon PW: Biology of gonadotropin secretion in adult and prepubertal female dogs. J Reprod Fertil Suppl 47:3–27, 1993.
10. Vickery BH, McRae GI, Goodpasture JC, et al: Use of potent LHRH analogues for chronic contraception and pregnancy termination in dogs. J Reprod Fertil Suppl 39:175–187, 1989.
11. Sutton DJ, Geary MR, Bergman GHE: Prevention of pregnancy in bitches following unwanted mating: A clinical trial using low dose of oestradiol benzoate. J Reprod Fertil Suppl 51:239–243, 1997.
12. Wanke M, Loza ME, Monaschi N, et al: Clinical use of dexamethasone for termination of unwanted pregnancy in dogs. J Reprod Fertil Suppl 51:233–238, 1997.
13. Fieni F, Dumon C, Tainturier D, et al: Clinical protocol for pregnancy termination in bitches using prostaglandine F2alpha. J Reprod Fertil Suppl 51:245–250, 1997.
14. Lange K, Gunzel-Apel AR, Hoppen HO, et al: Effects of low doses of prostaglandin F2alpha during the early luteal phase before and after implantation in beagle bitches. J Reprod Fertil Suppl 51:251–257, 1997.
15. Verstegen J, Onclin K, Donnay I, et al: Luteotropic action of prolactin in dogs and effects of a dopamine agonist cabergoline. J Reprod Fertil Suppl 47:403–409, 1993.
16. Evans JM, Sutton DJ: The use of hormones, especially progestogens to control estrus in bitches. J Reprod Fertil Suppl 39:163–173, 1989.
17. Keister DM, Gutheil RF, Kaiser LD, et al: Efficacy of oral epostane administration to terminate pregnancy in mated laboratory bitches. J Reprod Fertil Suppl 39:241–249, 1989.
18. Concannon PW: Termination of pregnancy and induction of premature luteolysis by the antiprogestagen mefiprestone in dogs. J Reprod Fertil 88:89–96, 1990.
19. Feldman EC, et al: Prostaglandins induction of abortion in pregnant bitches after misalliance. JAVMA 202:1855–1858, 1993.
20. Bowen RA: Efficacy and toxicity of estrogens commonly used to terminate canine pregnancy. JAVMA 186:783–793, 1985.
21. Verstegen J, Ballabio R: Interuption of pregnancy in bitches using cabergoline. Riv Zoot Vet 20:35–43, 1993.
22. Onclin K, Silva L, Verstegen J: Termination of unwanted pregnancy in dogs with the dopamine agonist cabergoline in combination with synthetic analogue of either cloprostenol or alphaprostol. Theriogenology 43:813–822, 1995.
23. Onclin K, Verstegen J: Practical use of a combination of a dopamine agonist and synthetic prostaglandin analogue to terminate unwanted pregnancy in dogs. J Small Anim Pract 37:211–216, 1996.
24. Zone M, Wanke M, Rebuelto M, et al: Termination of pregnancy in dogs by oral administration of dexamethasone Theriogenology 43:487–494, 1995.

CHAPTER 162

THE CYSTIC ENDOMETRIAL HYPERPLASIA/PYOMETRA COMPLEX AND INFERTILITY IN FEMALE DOGS

Edward C. Feldman

THE CYSTIC ENDOMETRIAL HYPERPLASIA/PYOMETRA COMPLEX

PATHOPHYSIOLOGY

Pyometra is a hormonally mediated diestrual disorder. The disease is caused by a bacterial infection within the uterus that results in mild to severe and life-threatening bacteremia and toxemia. Older female dogs commonly develop a condition called cystic endometrial hyperplasia (CEH). This condition is believed to be a result of an exaggerated and abnormal reponse of the endometrium to chronic and repeated exposure to progesterone. CEH predisposes the dog to pyometra. Severe, life-threatening pyometra can occur without cystic endometrial hyperplasia. It is extremely rare, however, for pyometra to occur in a bitch not under the influence of progesterone; that is, pyometra virtually always develops during diestrus (the progesterone-dominated phase of the ovarian cycle). The only exception to this rule occurs when the infection progresses slowly and diestrus has terminated before the diagnosis is confirmed.

Progesterone, Cystic Endometrial Hyperplasia, and Infection

For 9 to 12 weeks after estrus in all normal bitches, the plasma progesterone concentration is increased more than 2 ng/mL. Progesterone supports endometrial growth and glandular secretion while suppressing myometrial activity, allowing accumulation of uterine glandular secretions. These secretions provide an excellent environment for bacterial growth. Bacterial growth is further enhanced by inhibition of leukocyte response within the uterus. Bacterial infections associated with pyometra are caused by normal vaginal bacteria. Therefore, pyometra is the result of combining the ovarian (progesterone) phase of the estrous cycle together with an abnormal endometrium, which allows overgrowth of bacteria normally isolated from this area of the anatomy.

Progesterone-induced CEH typically precedes the development of pyometra in bitches older than 6 years of age. Although pyometra is well recognized and commonly found in bitches younger than 6 years of age, that population is less likely to have CEH. When pathologic hyperplasia becomes progressive and cystic, endometrial thickening is due to an increase in the size and number of endometrial glands. The mucosal epithelial cells have hypertrophic and clear cytoplasm. The stroma becomes edematous, and an inflammatory cell infiltrate is invariably present. Occasionally, the CEH results in an accumulation of fluid within the uterine lumen. A sterile fluid-filled uterus is commonly referred to as hydrometra or mucometra, the thickness of the fluid determining its description. Pyometra is the most common sequela to CEH. Much less frequently, CEH is the cause of infertility and/or chronic endometritis. Confirming the diagnosis of CEH is difficult because it is not usually associated with clinical signs unless the uterine contents become infected and pyometra develops.

Bacteria

Bacterial contamination (not overgrowth) of the uterus appears to be a normal phenomenon during proestrus and estrus. The sources for bacteria are normal vaginal flora. These bacteria ascend through the cervix into the uterus during proestrus and estrus. Significant uterine disease or some other predisposing factor (progesterone or estrogen administration) predisposes bitches to pyometra, because bacteria do contaminate the uterus without pyometra in normal dogs. The bacteria associated with pyometra are *Escherichia coli*. However, staphylococci, streptococci, *Klebsiella*, *Pseudomonas*, *Proteus*, *Hemophilus*, *Pasteurella*, *Serratia*, and other bacteria have been isolated from uteri of bitches with pyometra.[1, 2] All these bacteria, in single or multiple isolates, have been identified in the vaginal tracts of healthy, normal bitches.[3]

Estrogen

The supraphysiologic concentrations of estrogen resulting from exogenous administration (e.g., mismate injections) during estrus or diestrus *dramatically increases risk for developing pyometra*. For this reason, estrogen administration to prevent pregnancy is strongly discouraged.

Two Distinct Pyometra Syndromes

The Older Bitch. The bitch that is older than 7 or 8 years of age is prone to CEH and then pyometra. This appears to be an age-related syndrome.

The Younger Bitch. It is unlikely that CEH is the cause of pyometra in most bitches younger than 6 years of age.

REP

Chronic recurring exposure to progesterone cannot have occurred in these dogs. However, there is a strong correlation between the incidence of pyometra in young dogs and estrogen administration by veterinarians to prevent pregnancy.[2, 4] If the misbred bitch is not of value as a brood bitch, ovariohysterectomy should be recommended. If she is of value, carrying the unwanted pregnancy to term or inducing abortion with prostaglandins is preferable to estrogen administration.

SIGNALMENT AND HISTORY

Traditional Description Versus Clinical Experience

Traditionally, pyometra has been described as a disorder of middle-aged bitches (>6 years of age) after years of repetitive progesterone stimulation of the uterus. However, with the common use of estrogens for mismating in young bitches, pyometra is relatively common in young dogs as well. In our series of more than 160 bitches treated with Prostaglandin $F_{2\alpha}$ ($PGF_{2\alpha}$) for open- and closed-cervix pyometra, the mean age at diagnosis was 2.1 years.

Open-Cervix Pyometra

Owner-reported signs will depend on the patency of the cervix (Table 162–1). An obvious sign in bitches with an open-cervix pyometra is a sanguineous to mucopurulent discharge from the vagina. The discharge is usually first noticed 4 to 8 weeks after the end of estrus. Pyometra has been diagnosed as early as the end of standing heat (estrus) and as late as 12 to 14 weeks later. Other common features include lethargy, depression, inappetence/anorexia, polyuria, polydipsia, vomiting, and diarrhea.[2] Open-cervix pyometra may be recognized quickly by experienced owners.

Closed-Cervix Pyometra

The bitch with closed-cervix pyometra has more worrisome clinical signs at the time of diagnosis when compared with dogs with open-cervix pyometra. This is due to the lack of an easily recognized and early sign of a serious problem, namely, the purulent vaginal discharge seen with open-cervix infection. Instead, owners notice an insidious onset of manifestations that usually include depression, lethargy, inappetence, polydipsia with or without polyuria, and weight loss. These problems, in association with septicemia and toxemia, can result in progressively worsening dehydration, shock, coma, and, eventually, death.

TABLE 162–1. CLINICAL SIGNS COMMONLY SEEN IN BITCHES WITH PYOMETRA

SIGN	PER CENT OF DOGS
Vaginal discharge	85
Lethargy–depression	62
Inappetence/anorexia	42
Polyuria and/or polydipsia	28
Vomiting	15
Nocturia	5
Diarrhea	5
Abdominal enlargement	5

From Feldman EC, Nelson RW: Canine and Feline Endocrinology and Reproduction, 2nd ed. Philadelphia, WB Saunders, 1996, p 607.

PHYSICAL EXAMINATION

Abnormalities on physical examination consistent with pyometra include depression, dehydration, fever, palpable uterine enlargement, and a sanguineous to mucopurulent discharge from the vagina if the cervix is patent ("open"). The rectal temperature can be increased, normal, or decreased. Fever is associated with uterine inflammation and secondary bacterial infection, as well as septicemia or toxemia. With septicemia or toxemia, shock may ensue, with tachycardia, prolonged capillary refill time, weak femoral pulses, and sub-normal rectal temperature.

Uterine enlargement may be obvious; or if much of the purulent material is draining, it may be flaccid to nonpalpable. Furthermore, the size and weight of the dog plus the degree of abdominal relaxation affect the ease of palpating uterine enlargement. Overzealous palpation should be prevented to avoid uterine rupture. A palpable uterus is virtually always considered abnormal in the nonpregnant diestrual bitch. Even if not palpable, illness can be caused by a uterus that is massively inflamed and infected.

CLINICAL PATHOLOGY

White and Red Blood Cells

An absolute neutrophilia (usually exceeding 25,000 cells/mm^3) with variable degrees of cellular immaturity (presence of a left shift, i.e., >300 bands/μL) is common due to infection and septicemia. The infection, if severe and/or chronic, may cause a degenerative left shift with toxic neutrophils. Although increases in total white blood cell counts are common, normal or even decreased counts occur. Some dogs with normal counts do not have evidence of the overwhelming infection seen in closed-cervix pyometra and some are unable to cope with the disease, accounting for the decreased count. Because pyometra is a chronic inflammatory disease, it is not surprising that a mild normocytic, normochromic, non-regenerative anemia (packed cell volume, 28 to 35 per cent) often develops. The septicemia or toxemia associated with the syndrome can be potent suppressors of the bone marrow.

Serum Biochemical Profile

Hyperproteinemia (total protein, 7.5 to 10.0 g/dL) and hyperglobulinemia commonly result from dehydration and/or chronic antigenic stimulation of the immune system. The blood urea nitrogen level may be increased if dehydration and pre-renal uremia are present. Occasionally, serum liver enzyme activities are abnormal as a result of damage caused by septicemia and/or diminished hepatic circulation and cellular hypoxia secondary to dehydration.

Urinalysis and Urine Culture

Isosthenuria (urine specific gravity, 1.008 to 1.015) or hyposthenuria (urine specific gravity <1.008) is common in pyometra. Early in the disease process, the urine specific gravity may be greater than 1.030 simply as a reflection of dehydration and the physiologic response to conserve fluids. With secondary bacterial infection, especially from *Escherichia coli*, toxemia develops that can interfere with the resorption of sodium and chloride in the loop of Henle. This reduces renal medullary hypertonicity, impairing the ability of the renal collecting tubules to resorb free water. Polyuria and compensatory polydipsia result. A reversible renal tubular insensitivity to antidiuretic hormone (ADH; secondary nephrogenic diabetes insipidus), caused by *E. coli* endotoxins, also may account for the loss of concentrating ability. Renal tubular immune complex injury is another proposed mechanism for polydipsia/polyuria.

Urinary tract infections may be suspected if pyuria, hematuria, and/or proteinuria are identified on urinalysis. However, urine obtained by a midstream collection will be contaminated by the vaginal discharge. "Blind" cystocentesis is not recommended on dogs with suspected or known pyometra because of the risk of puncturing the infected uterus. Proteinuria without pyuria or hematuria may be associated with pyometra. Immune complex deposition in the glomeruli can cause a reversible mixed membranoproliferative glomerulonephropathy. The resulting proteinuria gradually resolves with correction of the pyometra.

RADIOLOGY

Pregnancy enhances uterine size and the ability to identify the uterus, which can be visualized radiographically beginning with the third to fourth week of gestation, continuing throughout pregnancy, and for 2 to 4 weeks after whelping. Radiographic visualization of the uterus at other times is abnormal. It is abnormal for a nonpregnant bitch in diestrus to have an easily identified uterus. Abdominal radiographs should be assessed in a bitch with suspected pyometra to confirm the diagnosis and to identify any unexpected problems. With pyometra, a fluid-dense tubular structure, larger than small intestinal loops, is typically seen in the ventral and caudal abdomen (Fig. 162–1A and B).

Two additional problems might be seen radiographically in a dog with pyometra: (1) the presence or absence of peritonitis from uterine rupture and (2) retained fetal tissue from a pregnancy occurring during the present or previous cycle (see Fig. 162–1C and D). Abdominal compression may be of value, using a belly band or wooden spoon to displace intestines from the uterus. Inability to visualize the uterus radiographically does not rule out the presence of a relatively small pyometra with an open cervix.

ULTRASONOGRAPHY

Ultrasound has greatly enhanced the ability to document the presence of pyometra and/or the success of medical treatment. Ultrasound allows determination of the size of the uterus, thickness of the uterine wall, and presence of fluid accumulation within the lumen. In some cases, the character of the fluid within the uterus (serous vs. viscid) can be determined. More importantly, ultrasonography easily identifies fetal remnants or placental tissue, factors that negatively impact potential success with prostaglandin therapy. Endometritis or pyometra can be distinguished from a gravid uterus, and "stump" pyometras can be visualized dorsal and caudal to the bladder.[5]

DIAGNOSIS

Uncomplicated Pyometra

Pyometra should be suspected in any female dog or cat that has not been spayed, especially those with appropriate abnormalities on review of clinical signs, physical examination, laboratory studies, and radiographic or ultrasonographic evaluations. A definitive diagnosis becomes a challenge when the history is vague (especially regarding ovarian cycle activity), when a vulvar discharge is present, yet no uterus is palpable, when no vaginal discharge is observed, when the owner has a primary concern only of polydipsia and polyuria (rare), or when the dog has been previously "spayed" yet clinical signs and clinical pathology suggest pyometra.

A dog could have a copious vaginal discharge without uterine enlargement. The major differential diagnoses for such a situation are vaginal inflammation with or without infection and pyometra that has drained sufficiently to avoid systemic toxemia. In an ovariohysterectomized dog, a "stump pyometra" should also be considered. A carefully obtained history and results of a hemogram, vaginal examination, and, if possible, abdominal ultrasonography should be used to differentiate an open-cervix pyometra from a severe focal vaginal infection. Systemic signs of illness (lethargy, inappetence) may be subtle in a dog with an open-cervix pyometra. However, an isolated vaginal infection rarely causes systemic signs. Likewise, fever, neutrophilic leukocytosis, or hyperproteinemia are suggestive of a uterine problem not a vaginal infection.

Stump Pyometra

Stump pyometra, an uncommon and difficult problem to diagnose, refers to inflammation and bacterial infection of a post-ovariohysterectomy remnant of the uterine body. If the cervix and a portion of the uterine body are left in situ during a "spay" surgery, that area becomes a potential site for future infection. The stump of the uterus is located in an area favoring bacterial growth, and an internal abscess could develop. If remnant ovarian tissue also remains after ovariohysterectomy, ovarian cycles, progesterone secretion, uterine stimulation, and inflammation could occur. These changes would enhance the likelihood for future infection. Stump pyometra due to an ascending infection from the vagina usually occurs without the presence of remnant ovarian tissue because the site is one that becomes infected easily. The diagnosis can be extremely difficult if a vaginal discharge is not present. Clinical signs and laboratory abnormalities are those typically associated with systemic illness, problems rarely encountered with vaginitis. Ultrasonography is the most definitive non-invasive tool for diagnosing this disorder (Fig. 162–2).

SURGICAL TREATMENT

Ovariohysterectomy

Ovariohysterectomy is the preferred treatment for pyometra unless the owner adamantly wants to maintain the reproductive potential of a 6-month-old to 6-year-old dog. Relatively healthy bitches are usually excellent surgical risks, whereas those that are severely ill should be vigorously treated with intravenous administration of fluids and antibiotics effective against *E. coli* (e.g., amoxicillin plus clavulanate [Clavamox], trimethoprim-sulfamethoxazole, cephalosporins) and should undergo proper testing needed to identify abnormalities in serum electrolytes, acid-base status, cardiac rhythm, and fluid status. Complications associated with septicemia, toxemia, and uremia are common. One cannot al-

REP

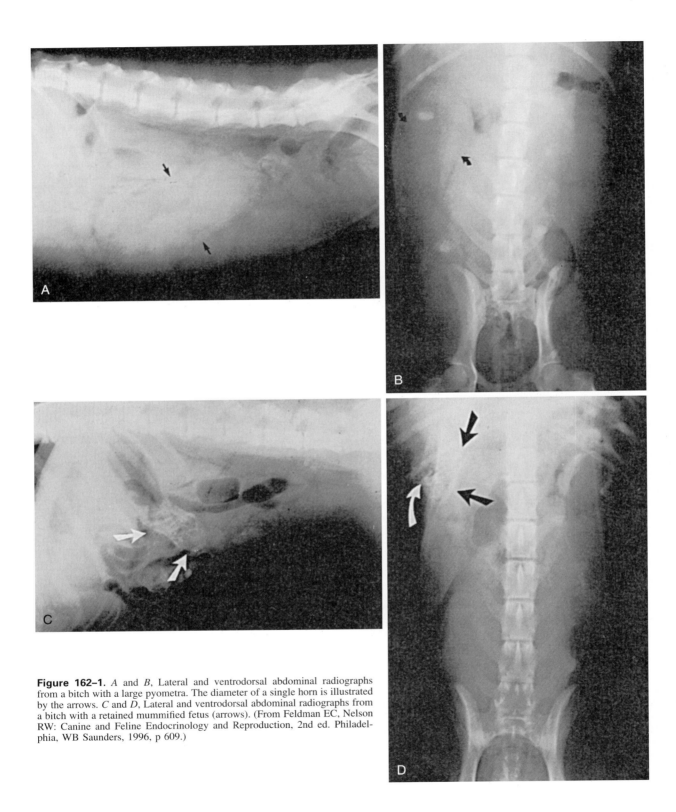

Figure 162–1. *A* and *B*, Lateral and ventrodorsal abdominal radiographs from a bitch with a large pyometra. The diameter of a single horn is illustrated by the arrows. *C* and *D*, Lateral and ventrodorsal abdominal radiographs from a bitch with a retained mummified fetus (arrows). (From Feldman EC, Nelson RW: Canine and Feline Endocrinology and Reproduction, 2nd ed. Philadelphia, WB Saunders, 1996, p 609.)

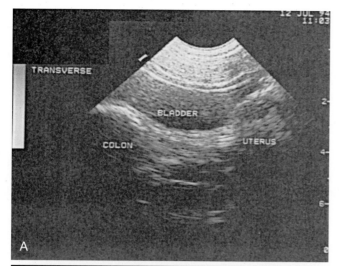

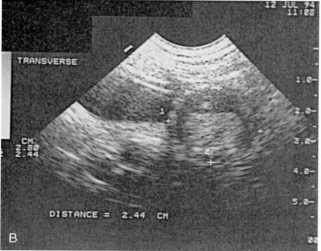

Figure 162–2. Ultrasonography of the abdomen of a bitch demonstrating a stump pyometra that had developed several years after ovariohysterectomy. (From Feldman EC, Nelson RW: Canine and Feline Endocrinology and Reproduction, 2nd ed. Philadelphia, WB Saunders, 1996, p 613.)

ways wait for "stabilization" of the animal before surgery is performed. In some dogs, surgery may not be postponed more than a few hours. Septicemia originating from the diseased uterus is often responsible for the severe illness, and only its surgical removal will allow resolution of the animal's septic state.

Surgical Drainage

Surgical drainage of pyometra is not recommended.

MEDICAL TREATMENT

Prostaglandins

Actions

Prostaglandin $F_{2\alpha}$ has two important physiologic effects. These include contraction of the myometrium (causing expulsion of exudate from the uterus) and inhibiting synthesis of progesterone by the corpora lutea (in contrast to other species, this drug is not likely causing lysis of the corpora

lutea except late in diestrus [Fig. 162–3]). The least consistent effect is relaxation of the cervix.

Clinical Use

Guidelines. Use of $PGF_{2\alpha}$ should be restricted to bitches or queens 6 years of age or younger that are *not* critically ill, that do not have significant concurrent illness, that have an open cervix, and that have an owner who is adamant about saving the animal's reproductive potential. The drug should never be administered to dogs with known cardiac or respiratory disease. Ovariohysterectomy remains the treatment of choice in managing pyometra.

Severely Ill Bitches. Clinical improvement is not usually observed for at least 48 hours, and more often 2 weeks, after beginning $PGF_{2\alpha}$ therapy. Therefore, this drug is *not* for use in severely ill animals that are poor anesthetic risks. It is possible that side effects to $PGF_{2\alpha}$ will cause significant morbidity and/or mortality in critically ill dogs and cats.

Closed-Cervix Pyometra. $PGF_{2\alpha}$ should be used with caution in bitches or queens with a closed-cervix pyometra because of relatively poor therapeutic response and the potential for failure of the cervix to dilate. Lack of cervical dilatation may result in uterine contents being expelled into the peritoneal cavity through the fallopian tubes or through a rupture in the uterine wall.

Drug Licensing. $PGF_{2\alpha}$ is not licensed for use in the bitch, but it is available for use in the cow and mare. However, use of prostaglandins is an established therapy for pyometra in dogs and cats and is within the standard care of these pets.

Initial Evaluation. The bitch to be treated with prostaglandins should first be screened for the presence of fetuses (living or dead) within the uterus, ideally utilizing ultrasonography. Radiography is a relatively poor alternative. The success of $PGF_{2\alpha}$ has been poor in bitches with mummified fetuses and those with fetal skeletal material in utero.

Recommended Agent and Protocol

Choices. Only naturally occurring $PGF_{2\alpha}$ (Lutalyse, Prostin [Upjohn Co, Kalamazoo, MI]) should be used at the

REP

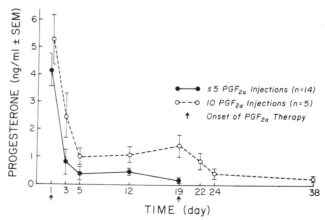

Figure 162–3. Illustration of the dramatic effect prostaglandin $F_{2\alpha}$ has on plasma progesterone concentrations in late diestrus of dogs with pyometra. The solid line reveals the changes seen in bitches requiring one 5-day course of injections. The dashed line reveals progesterone concentrations after onset of prostaglandin therapy earlier in diestrus and having an incomplete result until a second 5-day course of therapy is finished. (From Feldman EC, Nelson RW: Canine and Feline Endocrinology and Reproduction, 2nd ed. Philadelphia, WB Saunders, 1996, p 614.)

TABLE 162–2. PROTOCOL FOR PGF$_{2\alpha}$ THERAPY FOR CANINE OPEN-CERVIX PYOMETRA

1. Establish diagnosis definitively
   a. History and physical examination
   b. Complete blood cell count, other blood tests
   c. Abdominal ultrasonography
   d. Radiography (not as good as ultrasonography)
2. Use natural prostaglandin (Lutalyse)
   a. Day 1: 0.1 mg/kg, SC, once
   b. Day 2: 0.2 mg/kg, SC, once
   c. Days 3–7: 0.25 mg/kg, SC, once daily
3. Antibiotics used during and for 14 days after prostaglandin treatment
4. Re-evaluate
   a. 7 days after completion of PGF$_{2\alpha}$
   b. 14 days after completion of PGF$_{2\alpha}$
5. Re-treat at 14 days if
   a. Purulent vaginal discharge persists
   b. Fever, increased white blood cells, and fluid-filled uterus persist

From Feldman EC, Nelson RW: Canine and Feline Endocrinology and Reproduction, 2nd ed. Philadelphia, WB Saunders, 1996, p 615.

dosages recommended. The LD$_{50}$ for this PGF$_{2\alpha}$ in the bitch is 5.13 mg/kg. Synthetic PGF$_{2\alpha}$ analogues are more potent, and use of these synthetic products at our recommended doses could result in shock and possibly death.

Prostaglandin Therapy and Observation Period. The protocol recommended for use of PGF$_{2\alpha}$ to treat pyometra in dogs involves a progressively increasing dose (Table 162–2); day 1: 0.1 mg/kg SQ once; day 2: 0.2 mg/kg SQ once; days 3 through 7: 0.25 mg/kg SQ once daily. All injections should be administered in the morning to allow observation of the bitch through the day. Seven days after the final day of prostaglandin administration, the bitch should be examined to be certain that her condition has not deteriorated since onset of therapy. If worse, ovariohysterectomy should be recommended. If stable, the bitch should be evaluated an additional 7 days later. Many dogs continue to have a vaginal discharge for the 2-week period after therapy. The discharge typically progresses from purulent to clear, before stopping.[6]

Daily Monitoring. During the initial 7-day course of treatment with PGF$_{2\alpha}$ each bitch should be closely monitored daily with several thorough physical examinations. Rectal temperature, abdominal palpation, hydration status, and any other relevant parameters should be assessed. Side effects to PGF$_{2\alpha}$, especially those witnessed after the first and second injections, can be striking and worrisome (see later). It is strongly recommended that PGF$_{2\alpha}$ be administered in the morning, allowing observation of the animal throughout the day. The first injection *must* be administered in the morning. There is no need for a bitch with an open-cervix pyometra to remain hospitalized. We encourage sending dogs home each night, just as we encourage owners to allow us to keep their bitches for at least 4 hours after each injection. In this way, any unexpected drug-induced side effect can be managed. Bitches with closed-cervix pyometra should be hospitalized throughout the treatment period.

Vaginal Discharge. When treating a dog with closed- or open-cervix pyometra, a prostaglandin-induced discharge from the vulva is not always obvious. It appears that the uterine response to prostaglandins is slow and progressive, occurring over a period of days to weeks, not minutes to hours. As the uterus slowly contracts, the contents are slowly discharged, and most of this material is eaten by the bitch. Close observation of these dogs should allow quick identification and treatment of peritonitis due to uterine rupture or fallopian tube leakage, an extremely rare consequence of treatment. Ultrasonography is the preferred tool for assessing

uterine size, peritonitis, and response to prostaglandins. Of the 162 bitches we haved treated, none has developed peritonitis.

Antibiotics. Fifteen per cent of bitches with pyometra have had positive blood cultures before treatment, supporting the need for antibiotic therapy.[6, 7] Therefore, broad-spectrum antibiotics effective against *E. coli* should be administered.

Side Effects

Bitches should not be fed before PGF$_{2\alpha}$ administration. Several reactions will be observed after administration of PGF$_{2\alpha}$ (Table 162–3). It would be extremely unusual to observe no side effects, especially after the first dose. Within 30 seconds of administration, the bitch may be restless and begin pacing. Hypersalivation and occasional panting then occur, followed by some or all of the following: abdominal pain or cramping, tachycardia, fever, vomiting, and defecation. These reactions disappear within 5 to 60 minutes of the injection. Generally, the side effects due to PGF$_{2\alpha}$ administration last for 20 to 30 minutes. Observance of uterine evacuation after an injection is variable. It is suggested that each PGF$_{2\alpha}$-treated bitch be walked from the time of administration until the side effects completely dissipate. Walking appears to minimize clinical signs. Side effects typically diminish in severity with each dose of PGF$_{2\alpha}$. The bitch exhibiting alarming side effects after the first dose often has no side effects or just a mild reaction after the fifth to seventh dose.

The most worrisome reactions to the administration of PGF$_{2\alpha}$ have included two dogs that had a shock-like syndrome of weakness, pale mucous membranes, and tachycardia with poor pulse quality within seconds of the injection. Each was treated with intravenous administration of fluids and recovered within 45 minutes. Two dogs had ventricular tachycardias within minutes after receiving PGF$_{2\alpha}$. These dogs were managed with an intravenous lidocaine infusion and recovered within 60 minutes. Three of these four dogs completed prostaglandin therapy.

RETREATMENT—PREDICTING THE NEED FOR TWO COURSES OF THERAPY

Bitches with open-cervix pyometra, treated with PGF$_{2\alpha}$, requiring two 7-day courses of medication were compared with those requiring only one course of therapy. Those bitches treated for pyometra less than 5 weeks after the end

TABLE 162–3. INCIDENCE OF REACTIONS IN 62 BITCHES RECEIVING SUBCUTANEOUS PROSTAGLANDIN THERAPY FOR PYOMETRA

REACTION	PER CENT OF DOGS
Restlessness	85
Pacing	85
Hypersalivation	82
Panting	79
Vomiting	73
Abdominal pain or cramping	61
Tachycardia	55
Fever	33
Defecation	30
Uterine evacuation	30

From Feldman EC, Nelson RW: Canine and Feline Endocrinology and Reproduction, 2nd ed. Philadelphia, WB Saunders, 1996, p 616.

of estrus were most likely to require two courses of therapy. Bitches whose previous estrus occurred more than 5 weeks previously usually responded to one course of treatment. Corpora lutea of the bitch appear to become more sensitive to the destructive effects of prostaglandins as diestrus progresses. Therefore, the bitch with pyometra treated more than 5 weeks after the end of estrus is more sensitive to prostaglandins than bitches treated earlier in diestrus.

RESULTS OF TREATMENT

Successful response to $PGF_{2\alpha}$ therapy includes resolution of clinical signs, development of a serous vulvar discharge that then ceases, decrease in the palpable uterine diameter, and a normal leukogram. After a pyometra is surgically extirpated, the peripheral white blood cell count often transiently increases. This is believed to be due to loss of the "sink" into which white blood cells flood, while the bone marrow continues to pour out cells. With medical management of pyometra, the sink remains but the infection clears. Thus, with this form of treatment the white blood cell count should diminish (Fig. 162–4).

Of the more than 160 bitches with open-cervix pyometra we have treated, more than 95 per cent have had complete resolution of pyometra. Approximately 66 per cent of these dogs required one 7-day course of treatment and the remainder have had two courses of treatment. We have not had a dog respond to a third course of medication. Almost 90 per cent of successfully treated dogs have whelped litters, and more than 50 per cent have had more than one litter. Less than 5 per cent re-developed pyometra before or after successfully carrying a litter. Prostaglandin-treated bitches may begin their next estrous cycle early or late. No consistent pattern has been established, and owners should be made aware that an early cycle is possible. We strongly recommend breeding the dog on the cycle immediately after therapy for several reasons: (1) these bitches may have an abnormal uterus, and thus an attempt should be made obtain a litter while it is possible; (2) pregnant dogs may be less susceptible to infection than nonpregnant dogs; and (3) there is no benefit to skipping a cycle. A large number of successfully treated bitches have been spayed after whelping one or more litters. Histologic evaluation of the uteri from these bitches has usually been normal.

The results of prostaglandin therapy in bitches with closed-cervix pyometra have *not* been as positive as with the open-cervix group. There have been fewer dogs treated because the syndrome is less common in our hospital population and because these bitches are often so ill that ovariohysterectomy is recommended with greater conviction. Only 34 per cent of these dogs have responded successfully to $PGF_{2\alpha}$. Treatment failure is due to an inability to evacuate the uterus because of the closed cervix. Should a reliable method develop for dilating the cervix, the ability to help these bitches will improve. Careful monitoring is imperative during prostaglandin therapy for closed-cervix pyometra. Monitoring should consist of abdominal ultrasonography performed before and every 2 or 3 days after beginning therapy. Ultrasonography should reveal decreasing uterine size without evidence of peritonitis. Daily decreases in white blood cell counts should occur as the infection clears. No decrease is expected in the first 2 or 3 days, but a progressive decline toward normal should then follow. Appetite, attitude, and activity should return toward normal. However, the clinical signs in many of these bitches persist for weeks without becoming worse or better. Uterine discharge, as a result of the injections, is not always obvious. Some fastidious bitches keep themselves extremely clean by licking. Thus, constant licking may be the only evidence of an induced open cervix with vaginal discharge.

INFERTILITY OF THE BITCH

DEVELOPING THE PROBLEM LIST

Assessment of the Male

Before embarking on an investigation into the potential causes of infertility in a bitch, the male should be assessed. The primary reason for evaluating the male before the female is that males are so much easier to study. The normal male is continuously fertile (i.e., continuously producing sperm). The female is usually fertile only 1 to 3 weeks per year. The easiest and usually most reliable methods for establishing male fertility are a review of the male's present breeding history, evaluation of his semen, and ensuring that he is *Brucella* negative.

History (Anamnesis)

Definition. Veterinary advice will often be sought after a bitch fails to conceive, if she fails to exhibit "normal" breeding behavior, when her cycles appear to be unusual, or for a myriad of other disturbances. "Infertility," therefore, is a huge category comprising a long list of anatomic, physiologic, behavioral, and husbandry problems.

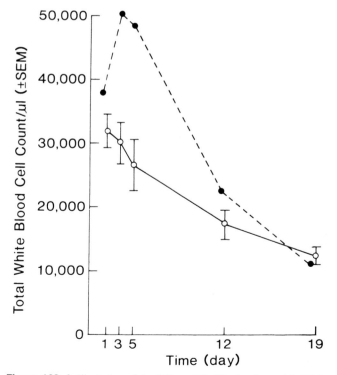

Figure 162–4. Illustration of the falling white blood cell count in bitches with pyometra treated successfully with prostaglandin $F_{2\alpha}$ (solid line) versus the initial increase in total white blood cell count in four dogs with pyometra that were successfully treated by ovariohysterectomy (dashed line). (From Feldman EC, Nelson RW: Canine and Feline Endocrinology and Reproduction, 2nd ed. Philadelphia, WB Saunders, 1996, p 617.)

TABLE 162–4. CLIENT QUESTIONNAIRE—THE INFERTILE BITCH

A. Age _____ Breed _____

B. General medical history (not including reproduction problems)
1. Vaccinations current? _____
2. Previous significant illness requiring hospitalization? If so, please briefly summarize:
   a. _____
   b. _____
3. Does your dog:

	Yes	No
a. Have a vomiting problem?	Yes _____	No _____
b. Have diarrhea?	Yes _____	No _____
c. Drink excessively?	Yes _____	No _____
d. Urinate excessively?	Yes _____	No _____
e. Have normal ability to play and exercise?	Yes _____	No _____
f. Appear to be of normal weight and height?	Yes _____	No _____
g. Have a hair coat problem?	Yes _____	No _____
h. Have any other problem? (If yes, please describe) _____	Yes _____	No _____

4. Has your dog ever had thyroid tests run?   Yes _____ No _____
5. Has your dog received thyroid hormone?
   a. In the past?   No _____ Yes _____ Dose _____
   b. Now?   No _____ Yes _____ Dose _____
6. Is your dog receiving any medication of any type?
   No _____ Yes _____ Drug and dose _____
7. Has your dog ever received or is it now receiving medicine for fleas or scratching?
   No _____ Yes _____ Drug and dose _____
8. Please list all foods and supplements presently being given to your dog:
_____
_____
_____
_____

C. Cycle history
1. Is she cycling?   Yes _____ No _____
2. Time interval between cycles _____
3. Total number of cycles in her life _____
4. How many days is a bloody discharge present (average in last 2 or 3 cycles)? _____
5. How many days does she stand for the male (average in last 2 or 3 cycles)? _____
6. Has a vaginal smear been checked by a veterinarian during a heat? _____
7. Has a series of vaginal smears (several during one heat) ever been checked? _____
8. Have any hormone assays been run?   No _____ Yes _____ Please describe
_____
9. Has your dog received any drug to cause a cycle (no _____ yes _____) or increase fertility? (no _____ yes _____)
   Please explain _____

D. Breeding history
1. Does your bitch allow the male to mount and breed?   No _____ Yes _____
2. How often is your dog bred in a cycle? _____
3. How are breeding dates chosen? _____
4. Has your bitch been bred to a male that has successfully sired litters within the last 6 months?   No _____ Yes _____
   1–2 years?   No _____ Yes _____
5. Have you observed any ties?   No _____ Yes _____
6. Duration of ties (average) _____
7. Inside tie _____? Outside tie _____?
8. Has the bitch been tranquilized prior to breeding or shipping?   No _____ Yes _____
9. Is the bitch bred locally or is she shipped for breeding?

Obtaining a "Complete" History. The initial history should include information regarding how well the owners know the bitch. Is she housed alone, with another bitch(es) that recently completed ovarian cycles, with ovariohysterectomized bitch(es), or with males? Is she normal in height and weight for her breed and for her line? Is she receiving any medication and is she well or ill? To avoid the time-consuming chore of asking all the questions that aid in establishing an answer, a questionnaire is used (Table 162–4).

Age, Breed. Small dogs reach sexual maturity at a younger age than large dogs. Virtually all healthy bitches begin ovarian cycles by 24 to 30 months of age. The first and second cycles may be irregular, unusual, subtle, brief, or long. Infertility evaluations should be delayed in most dogs until 24 to 30 months of age.

Physical Examination

Examine the Problem Area Last. As with any serious problem, the area of concern should be the last to be evaluated, ensuring completion of a thorough physical examination.

Vulva. Examination of the vulva includes checking size, conformation, and presence of any discharge. The small immature vulva or one that is recessed under a fold of tissue owing to body type or obesity may be impediments to normal breeding. A swollen, turgid vulva is suggestive of proestrus. One that is swollen and flaccid can be consistent with estrus (standing heat) or approaching parturition.

Vaginal Discharges. The bitch in anestrus or diestrus usually has no vaginal discharge. A bloody discharge is most suggestive of proestrus, estrus, separation of the placental sites, severe vaginitis, or pyometra. Greenish-black or dark bloody vaginal discharges are associated with placental separation as well as postpartum "lochia." Reddish-brown, yellowish, or grayish thick, creamy, malodorous vaginal discharges are often seen in open-cervix pyometra, metritis, or severe vaginitis. Straw-colored vaginal discharges are sometimes seen when bitches are in estrus. Clear mucus can

TABLE 162–4. CLIENT QUESTIONNAIRE—THE INFERTILE BITCH *Continued*

E. Pregnancy history
   1. Has she had any litters?
      Dates: a. _____   Litter size a. _____
            b. _____   b. _____
            c. _____   c. _____
            d. _____   d. _____
   2. Any abortions? No _____ Yes _____ If so, how do you know she aborted?
   3. Any resorption of puppies?   No _____ Yes _____
      a. If so, how do you know she resorbed puppies?
       _____
      b. How was pregnancy proven? _____
      c. Was pregnancy examined at
         (1) 7 days _____
         (2) 14 days _____
         (3) 21 days _____
         (4) 28 days _____
         (5) 35 days _____
         (6) 45 days _____
   4. Has she ever been treated for mismating? _____
   5. Has she had a *Brucella* titer? _____
      Date of most recent check _____
   6. Has she ever had:
      Pyometra?   Yes _____ No _____
      Vaginitis?   Yes _____ No _____
   7. Has she ever had medication to prevent or delay a heat?
      No _____ Yes_____
      If yes, what drug? _____
         when given? _____
   8. Does she now or has she had an abnormal vaginal discharge?
   _____

F. Kennel history
   Do any other bitches in your kennel have reproductive disorders?
   No _____ Yes _____
G. Pedigree
   Do any other bitches in her line have reproductive disorders?
   No _____ Yes _____

From Feldman EC, Nelson RW: Canine and Feline Endocrinology and Reproduction, 2nd ed. Philadelphia, WB Saunders, 1996, pp 620–621.

precede parturition and is rarely worrisome (see Chapters 23, 157, and 163).

Digital Examination of the Vestibule and Vagina. A digital examination of the vaginal vault should be routinely performed on any bitch evaluated for breeding soundness. If a culture or cytologic study is needed, it should be obtained before the digital examination. The gloved and lubricated index finger should pass easily into the vaginal vault, allowing assessment of the lumen, the urethral opening, and clitoral size and shape. Masses, foreign bodies, strictures, painful vaginitis, or abnormal tissue bands all prevent easy and painless examination.

If digital examination is inconclusive, vaginoscopy provides a more thorough evaluation. The use of an otoscope or a vaginal speculum provides an extremely limited view of the vaginal vault and is of little value. Pediatric proctoscopes are excellent for vaginoscopy (Fig. 162–5), are relatively inexpensive, and can be easily used in all but the

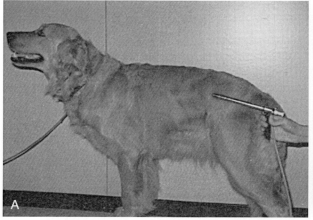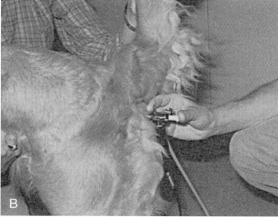

Figure 162–5. *A* and *B*, Vaginoscopy can be performed with a pediatric proctoscope. The instrument is easily passed into the vaginal vault for its thorough inspection. The pediatric proctoscope does not always allow visualization of the cervix despite its length, illustrating the futility of using an otoscope for this procedure. (From Feldman EC, Nelson RW: Canine and Feline Endocrinology and Reproduction, 2nd ed. Philadelphia, WB Saunders, 1996, p 622.)

smallest of miniature breeds because they are available in various diameters and lengths.

Mammary Glands and Ventrum. The mammary glands should be palpated primarily for mammary tumors. They can also be evaluated for lactation, mastitis, inverted teats, or benign nodules. The ventral midline can be checked for evidence of a surgical scar, suggesting previous ovariohysterectomy.

Rectal Examination. A rectal examination ensures that the pelvic canal has been assessed for previous fractures or other unsuspected abnormalities.

OWNER MANAGEMENT PRACTICES

Definition and Common Mistakes. Improper management practices are the cause for a large majority of apparent infertility problems. A bitch that is bred at incorrect times may be normal but fail to conceive as a result of being brought to the male when she is not fertile. Five major errors in breeding management are commonly encountered (assuming that the dog is *Brucella* negative):

1. Many people who own popular male dogs allow only one breeding per cycle. Breeding a female several times helps to eliminate the chance of a poorly timed or mistimed breeding.

2. Many dog owners allow breeding only on certain predetermined days of the cycle—days 11 and 13 (first day of vaginal bleeding is day 1), days 10 and 12, or one day only (such as day 14) may be chosen. Such predetermined dates may not be correct for every dog.

3. Breeding may be timed to begin only after the bloody vaginal discharge of proestrus becomes clear and/or straw colored, a strategy with inconsistent results.

4. The male dog may be allowed to choose the breeding date.

5. The male is assumed to be fertile. Any male can become transiently or permanently infertile. Any time the fertility of the male is questioned, a semen analysis is warranted.

INFERTILITY IN THE *BRUCELLA*-NEGATIVE BITCH THAT HAS NORMAL OVARIAN CYCLES, NORMAL INTERESTROUS INTERVALS, AND ALLOWS BREEDING
(Fig. 162–6)

Initial Approach (see also Chapter 157)

Behavior Observation

The Recommendation. The initial approach to an apparently healthy bitch that fails to conceive is to recommend that an owner adopt a reliable breeding schedule while simultaneously studying ovarian function. In this manner, if the problem is management related, it will be corrected. If the problem is physiologic, it may be identified and treated appropriately. It is important to realize that in the "normal" bitch, proestrus can last 1 to 2 days or as long as 25 days. Correctly identifying day 1 of proestrus is dependent on an owner detecting the first day of vaginal bleeding. Estrus (standing heat) can have a duration of 2 to 20 days. The recommendations, therefore, are to bring the bitch to a dominant male for evaluation of *her* behavior beginning on the second, third, or fourth day of proestrus and continue to do so every other day until *diestrus* is demonstrated by *her* behavior and vaginal cytology. Vaginal smears should be obtained by the owner, once daily, beginning with recognition of proestrus and continuing 2 to 4 days into diestrus. If attempts at mounting are made by the male and the bitch is receptive, breeding should be allowed, regardless of the apparent timing within the ovarian cycle.

Breeding Activity. Once the bitch displays standing heat, she should be bred on that day and every 2 to 4 days thereafter, until she refuses to breed. Breeding is continued on this schedule, regardless of the duration of standing heat, the color of the vaginal discharge, the day of the cycle, or the interpretation of a vaginal cytology smear. This program ensures that live sperm will be present when eggs are available for fertilization (Fig. 162–7).

Male Preference. Some bitches refuse a particular male. The three potential explanations for this frustrating dilemma include (1) the male has been brought to the bitch for mating and she is dominant to him when she is at her home (the bitch will not allow submissive males to breed); (2) the male is submissive regardless of environment;[8] and (3) the bitch is housed with another dominant bitch, interfering with normal behavior.

Ovarian Function: Proestrus and Estrus
(see Chapters 157 and 158)

Review of Shipping Practices

It is not known whether tranquilization or the stress of shipping has an undesirable effect on ovulation or early pregnancy. These are factors that may relate to acquired infertility and are worth avoiding during one cycle to see if the infertility problem can be resolved by keeping the bitch at home and having her locally bred.

Review of Medications

Gonadotropins may have long-term deleterious effects on pituitary function. Progesterone or estrogen administration may result in subclinical CEH, with infertility being the only outward effect that would be seen by the owner or veterinarian.

Hypothyroidism

Hypothyroidism typically causes prolonged interestrous intervals or persistent anestrus. The diagnosis of hypothyroidism should be viewed with suspicion, not because the disease does not exist but simply because most dogs treated for the disease are not so afflicted (see Chapter 151).

Infection

Brucella canis classically causes abortion late in gestation (see Chapter 159). All females in active breeding programs should be evaluated for canine brucellosis before each estrus and all males before breeding each new female.

Virtually all normal bitches harbor aerobic bacteria in the vaginal tract (Table 162–5). Merely isolating bacteria, *Mycoplasma* or *Ureaplasma* from the vagina does not constitute diagnosis of infection; and some organisms, such as *B. canis*, may be difficult to isolate. Thus, a negative culture does not ensure that a bitch is free of serious infection. Pure cultures of one organism were identified from 18 per cent of vaginal swabs from healthy, fertile, bitches, mixed cultures were obtained from 77 per cent, and completely negative results were obtained from only 5 per cent of 826 swabs taken from 59 bitches.[3]

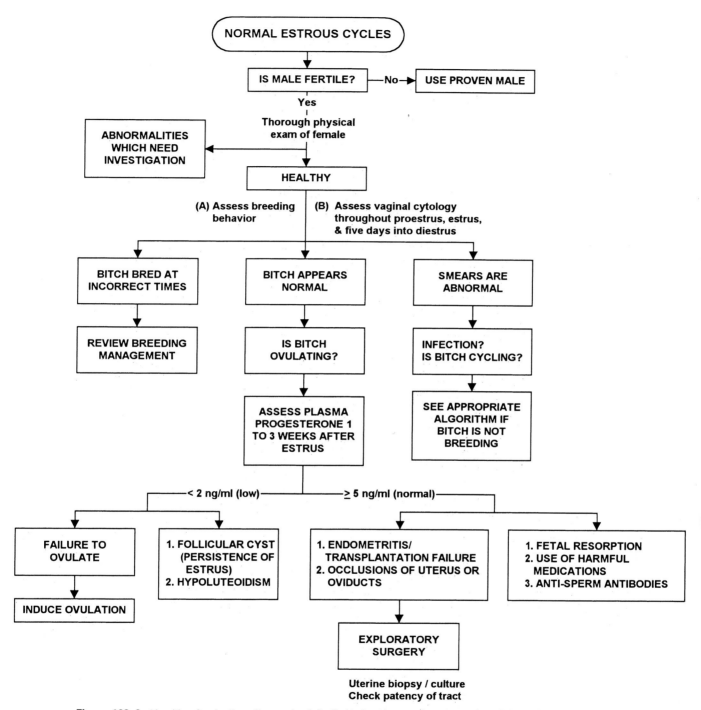

Figure 162–6. Algorithm for the *Brucella*-negative infertile bitch with normal estrous cycle activity and apparent infertility. (Modified from Feldman EC, Nelson RW: Canine and Feline Endocrinology and Reproduction, 2nd ed. Philadelphia, WB Saunders, 1996, p 624.)

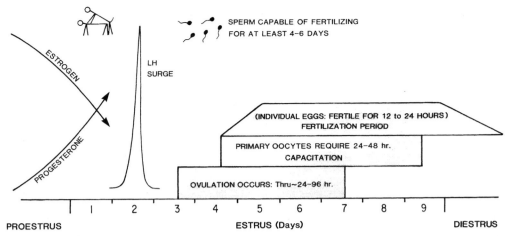

Figure 162–7. An illustration of the hormonal changes and sequence of events concerning the timing of ovulation and fertilization of ova in the average healthy bitch. (From Feldman EC, Nelson RW: Canine and Feline Endocrinology and Reproduction, 2nd ed. Philadelphia, WB Saunders, 1996, p 652.)

Viral infections, specifically herpesvirus, have been isolated in dogs with abortion and stillbirths. However, viral infections as a cause of infertility are not well documented.

Chronic Endometritis—Cystic Endometrial Hyperplasia

The bitch with chronic endometrial disease is likely to be infertile. These dogs could experience normal ovarian cycles, ovulate, have fertilized eggs, but fail to support pregnancy because of the abnormal uterine environment (see earlier).

Fetal Resorption (see Chapter 159)

Hypoluteoidism (see Chapters 158 and 159)

Occlusion of the Uterus or Oviducts

It is impossible to evaluate patency of the uterus and oviducts on a physical examination simply because these structures are too small. Bilateral segmental aplasia or other causes of obstruction of the uterine horns, or occlusion of

both oviducts, rarely results in a bitch that cycles, ovulates, breeds normally, but fails to conceive.[9] Bilateral occlusion prevents the sperm from ever reaching the egg.

THE BITCH WITH SHORTENED INTERESTROUS INTERVALS—LESS THAN 4 1/2 MONTHS
(Fig. 162–8)

Idiopathic Shortened Ovarian Cycles

Physiopathology

The "normal" bitch requires 2 weeks to 1 month for both proestrus and estrus, plus 2 to 2½ months for diestrus and 2 to 5 months for uterine recovery phase (anestrus). This accounts for the 4½- to 8½-month duration of a complete ovarian cycle. A bitch that begins proestrus before completing uterine repair may be infertile. Infertility could be the result of implantation failure caused by an abnormal endometrium that has not recovered from the previous effects of progesterone. Confirmation of these physiopathologic events is difficult. However, the presumptive diagnosis can be made from a careful review of the history.

Owner Management Problems

Before making a diagnosis or instituting therapy, a complete history of the bitch must be obtained and studied. The bitch that cycles at less than 4-month intervals is typically normal in all respects but is infertile as a result of incomplete uterine involution. It is recommended not to treat any bitch for frequent cycles until she is at least 2½ to 3 years of age. In addition, a veterinarian should be allowed to observe and test a bitch through one cycle utilizing physical examination, vaginal cytology, and at least one diestrual plasma progesterone concentration. The presence of "split heats" must be ruled out (see Chapter 158).

Treatment

Treatment for the bitch older than 3 years of age that cycles too frequently is to medically induce a normal anestrus period. This can usually be accomplished by treating the bitch with mibolerone drops (Cheque [Upjohn Co, Kala-

TABLE 162–5. AEROBIC BACTERIA RECOVERED FROM THE VAGINAS OF 59 HEALTHY BREEDING BITCHES

ORGANISM	PER CENT OF BITCHES
Pasteurella multocida	
β-Hemolytic streptococci	98
Escherichia coli	90
Unclassified gram-positive rods	85
Unclassified gram-negative rods	90
Mycoplasma spp.	86
Streptococcus spp.	60
(α-hemolytic, nonhemolytic)	56
Pasteurella spp.	68
Enterococci	44
Proteus mirabilis	25
Staphylococcus intermedius	34
Coryneforms	41
Coagulase-negative staphylococci	22
Pseudomonas spp.	10

All bitches had at least one positive culture; 826 vaginal swab specimens were obtained from these dogs.

Adapted from Bjurstrom L, Linde-Forsberg C: Long-term study of aerobic bacteria of the genital tract in breeding bitches. Am J Vet Res 53:665, 1992.

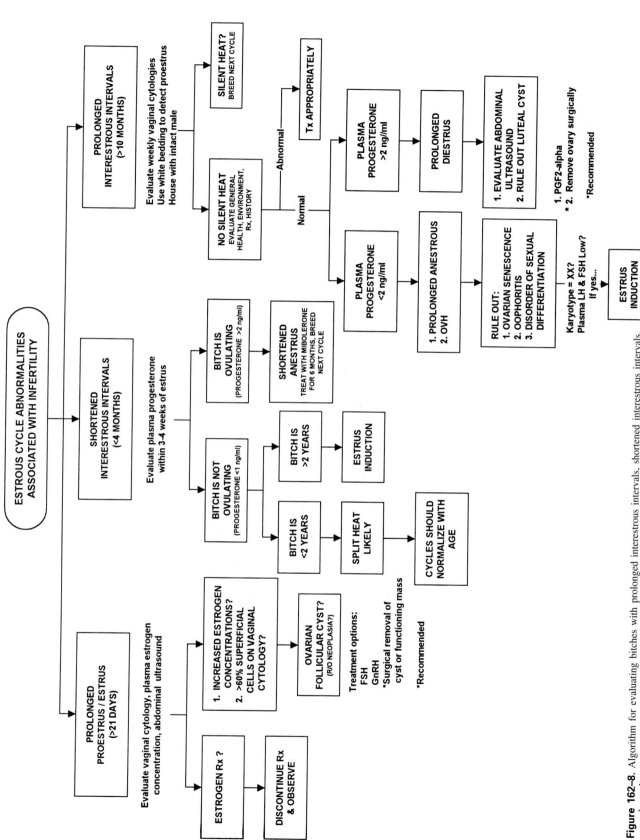

Figure 162–8. Algorithm for evaluating bitches with prolonged interestrous intervals, shortened interestrous intervals, or prolonged proestrus or estrus phases of their estrous cycles. (From Feldman EC, Nelson RW: Canine and Feline Endocrinology and Reproduction, 2nd ed. Philadelphia, WB Saunders, 1996, p 630.)

REP

1561

mazoo, MI]) for a period of 6 months. Medication is started 6 to 8 weeks after the end of the previous standing heat. The drug may induce some virilization. This is reversible and not thought to alter future reproductive performance. The bitch should be bred during the first estrus that follows therapy, which can begin soon or as long as 6 to 9 months later.

Split Heats (see Chapter 158)

Ovulation Failure

Failure to ovulate may result in failure to form corpora lutea and failure to synthesize progesterone. The entire diestrus phase of the ovarian cycle would be skipped, and, therefore, the phase of uterine involution (anestrus) would also be brief.[10] Diagnosis would be based on serial serum progesterone determinations. This diagnosis would be identical to that of *split heats*. In the bitch younger than 3 years of age, no treatment is recommended. In the bitch older than 3 years of age, an attempt to stimulate ovulation can be undertaken with luteinizing hormone or human chorionic gonadotropin (hCG, 500 IU/kg IM) administered the day before or the day after first breeding.[11, 12]

THE BITCH WITH PROLONGED INTERESTROUS INTERVALS—GREATER THAN 10 MONTHS
(see Fig. 162–8)

Idiopathic Prolongation of the Interestrous Interval

Management Practices, History, and Physical Examination

The veterinarian must first determine that the bitch is healthy with a review of the history and physical examination. As a bitch becomes older, the interestrous interval will increase.[13] However, intervals in excess of 8 to 10 months are not typical of the 2- to 6-year-old bitch. Knowing how an owner detects proestrus and estrus ("*heat*") and how closely an owner watches the dog is important. In some instances, a heat may simply be missed by the owner (silent heat; see Chapter 158).

Breed

Certain breeds do experience "long" ovarian cycles. The classic examples are the Basenji and the wolf-hybrid, both of which cycle on a yearly basis.[14] Individuals of any breed may have long interestrous intervals but remain fertile.

In-Hospital Evaluation

General Approach. Prolongation of the interval between ovarian cycles in the bitch can occur secondary to an underlying illness. Any major medical disorder has the potential for delaying the onset of an ovarian cycle. A database (complete blood cell count, serum chemistry profile, urinalysis) is recommended.

Hypothyroidism. See previous discussion and Chapter 151.

Silent Heat (see Chapter 158)

Ovarian Cysts or Neoplasia

Ovarian cysts that secrete progesterone should cause prolonged interestrous intervals. Progesterone provides negative

feedback to the pituitary/hypothalamus, suppressing ovarian activity. This "diestrus" is not usually associated with any clinical signs. The diagnosis is based on demonstrating persistent (>9 to 10 weeks) increases in serum progesterone concentration (>2 to 5 ng/mL) and presence of a cystic structure in one or both ovaries on abdominal ultrasonography (Fig. 162–9). Treatment of this condition is surgical removal of the cyst.

FAILURE TO CYCLE—PRIMARY AND SECONDARY ANESTRUS (Fig. 162–10)

Definition of the Problem

Primary anestrus refers to the bitch that has never had an ovarian cycle, and *secondary anestrus* refers to a bitch that has had one or more ovarian cycles but that subsequently fails to cycle. As with all reproductive disorders, the dog's age, breed, past history, current history, and physical examination should be assessed before any major tests are undertaken. Some large-breed dogs experience the puberal (first) estrus after they reach 2 years of age, whereas small breed dogs may have several silent heat cycles before exhibiting an obvious cycle. Failure to cycle, therefore, is a problem

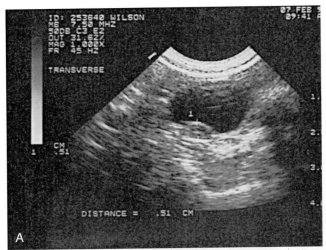

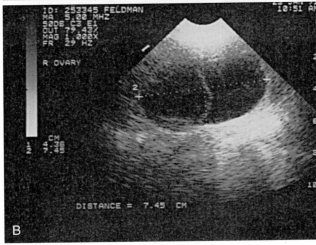

Figure 162–9. Abdominal ultrasonography of two bitches (*A* and *B*) that had ovarian cysts causing prolonged proestrus in each. (From Feldman EC, Nelson RW: Canine and Feline Endocrinology and Reproduction, 2nd ed. Philadelphia, WB Saunders, 1996, p 631.)

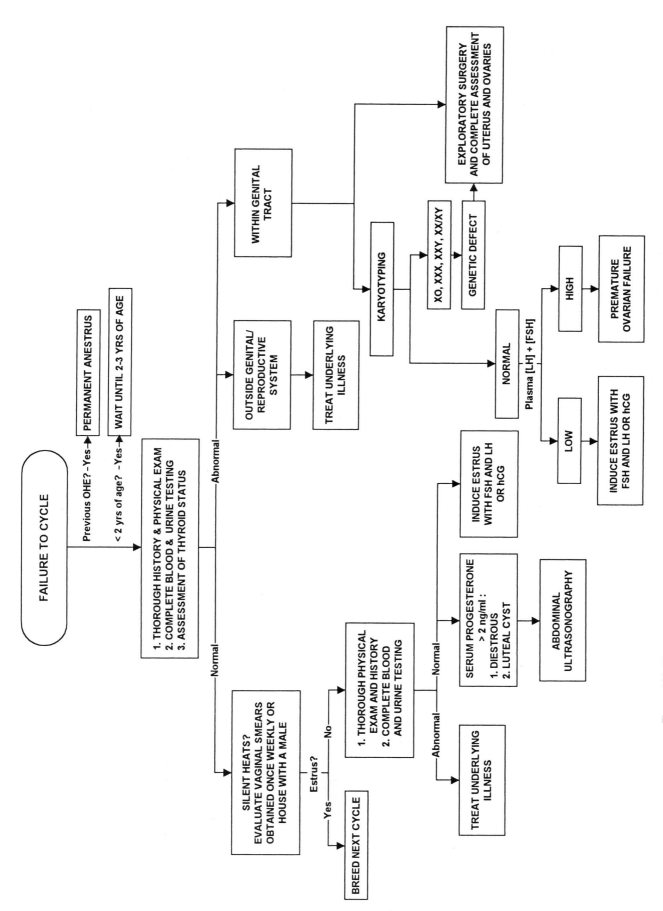

Figure 162–10. Algorithm to aid in the evaluation of a bitch that has an apparent failure to have any estrous cycle activity. (From Feldman EC, Nelson RW: Canine and Feline Endocrinology and Reproduction, 2nd ed. Philadelphia, WB Saunders, 1996, p 634.)

REP

1563

that is usually not pursued until the dog is older than 2 to 3 years of age. Evaluation of dogs with secondary anestrus should include all suggested approaches in the previous section on prolonged interestrous intervals. Secondary anestrus can occur after the onset of thyroid, other endocrine, or non-endocrine disease. If all testing is normal, it would be wise to wait at least 16 to 20 months from the previous cycle, in case one or two heat cycles were silent and, therefore, missed.

Previous Ovariohysterectomy/Premature Ovarian Failure

One cause for failure to cycle is previous ovariohysterectomy. Examination of the ventral midline for an incision scar provides initial evidence for an earlier spay. Premature ovarian failure causes the same biochemical abnormalities as a spay: dramatic increases in serum luteinizing hormone and follicle-stimulating hormone concentrations; assays of these hormones are available.[15]

Silent Heat (see Chapter 158)

Drug-Induced Anestrus

Anestrus may be induced with drugs specifically marketed for that purpose (see Chapter 161) and by drugs that result in anestrus as a side effect. Marketed drugs include androgens that might be used by an owner interested in increasing the strength and/or endurance in an animal without realizing effects on the hypothalamic-pituitary-ovarian axis. Progestagens are used in the treatment of a variety of maladies with prolongation of anestrus (diestrus) as a side effect. Glucocorticoids can have negative feedback effects to the pituitary, suppressing gonadotropin activity and preventing ovarian cycles.

Underlying Disease

Any illness, mild as well as severe (including hypothyroidism), can interfere with ovarian cycle activity in the bitch. Realization of this concept emphasizes the importance of obtaining a thorough history and completing a physical examination. If necessary, a database and other testing may be warranted.

Progesterone-Secreting Ovarian Cyst

This disorder was discussed previously.

Surgical Diagnosis

The diagnostic evaluation of an adult bitch that has never exhibited ovarian cycle activity can be frustrating because it involves use of tests not commonly performed by veterinary practitioners. Many veterinarians view exploratory laparotomy as an expedient means of deriving an answer, bypassing pre-surgical medical testing. During surgery, the abdominal organs should be evaluated for normal versus abnormal appearance and the veterinarian should be prepared to obtain biopsy specimens of ovarian and uterine tissue as well as cultures of the uterine lumen. Although this method is expedient, one may not always be able to distinguish normal from abnormal tissues. Furthermore, the veterinarian may not be able to answer questions raised by an owner or breeder. Surgery, therefore, is tempered with the knowledge that a definitive diagnosis cannot always be made, even after

seeing the organs in question. A thorough medical evaluation should be completed before surgical exploration.

INDUCTION OF ESTRUS

Most studies on induction of estrus have been performed on healthy females, and success has been variable. When similar protocols are utilized on a bitch with a defect in the hypothalamic-pituitary-ovarian axis, one should not expect great results because the explanation for failure includes both a protocol that may not be successful as well as testing an individual that has defects rendering it incapable of responding. The reader is referred to appropriate sources for treatment protocols.

PERSISTENT PROESTRUS AND/OR ESTRUS
(see Fig. 162–8)

Definition and Clinical Signs

Persistent estrus is defined as a bitch willing to breed for longer than 21 to 28 consecutive days in any one ovarian cycle. Alternatively, persistent proestrus/estrus is defined as more than 21 to 28 consecutive days of vaginal bleeding or similar duration of greater than 80 to 90 per cent superficial cells observed on vaginal cytology. These dogs have an enlarged vulva and attract males for prolonged time periods.

Endogenous Estrogen Excess

Young Bitches

Rarely, the young bitch in her first or second ovarian cycle fails to ovulate and may exhibit prolonged proestrus or estrus activity due to continued follicular estrogen secretion. This would appear to be a self-limiting problem owing to inadequate amounts of estrogen to induce the luteinizing hormone surge or for luteinizing hormone to induce ovulation.

Follicular Cysts

Incidence. Most follicular cysts have a granulosa cell lining, are anovulatory, and secrete significant amounts of estrogen. The cysts are usually solitary, occur in bitches younger than 3 years of age, and measure 1 to 1.5 cm in diameter. A few are as large as 5 cm in diameter, and they typically contain a clear, watery fluid.

Clinical Signs and Diagnosis. The clinical signs in bitches with follicular cysts are those typical of estrogen dominance (i.e., the bitch exhibits signs of proestrus and/or estrus). The most common reason for owners to seek veterinary care would be the observation of vaginal bleeding that persists for weeks rather than the expected 7 to 10 days. The diagnosis of follicular cyst is based on observing prolonged vaginal bleeding, persistent estrus behavior, continuous vaginal cytologic changes suggestive of late proestrus or estrus, and chronically increased plasma estrogen concentrations (>20 pg/mL). The finding of a cystic structure in the area of one ovary on abdominal ultrasonography in a female with these problems virtually confirms the diagnosis. Normal preovulatory follicles measure 4 to 9 mm in diameter,[16] and functional cysts are usually larger and, therefore, easier to visualize (see Fig. 162–9).

Treatment. In some bitches treatment is not required because the follicular cyst(s) may spontaneously undergo atresia or they may completely luteinize. This can be moni-

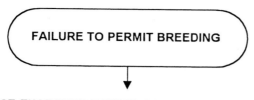

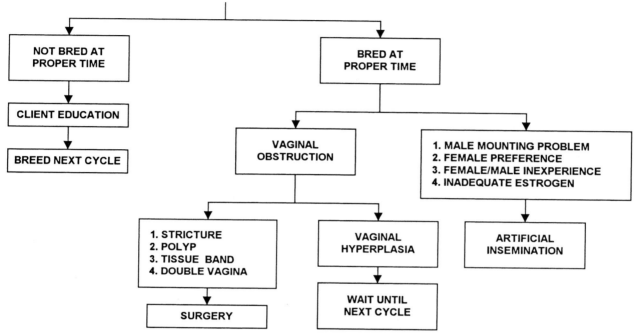

Figure 162–11. Algorithm to aid in the evaluation of a bitch that appears to be healthy but refuses to allow breeding attempts by a male in spite of being in the estrus phase of the ovarian cycle. (From Feldman EC, Nelson RW: Canine and Feline Endocrinology and Reproduction, 2nd ed. Philadelphia, WB Saunders, 1996, p 646.)

tored with abdominal ultrasonography, vaginal cytology, and serum progesterone concentrations. A majority of bitches in our series have not had spontaneous resolution and have been managed surgically. Most often, the associated ovary cannot be separated from the cyst and resection of both structures has been necessary. These bitches have quickly responded to the surgery. The signs of proestrus and/or estrus dissipate within days, and there has not been long-term problems. A large majority of these bitches have remained fertile and have subsequently whelped healthy litters.

FAILURE TO PERMIT BREEDING (Fig. 162–11)

The most common cause for bitches to refuse attempts at mounting by a male is an owner choosing incorrect breeding dates. The other common explanation for this problem is vaginal defects (see Chapter 163).

REFERENCES

1. Stone EA: The uterus. In Slatter DH (ed): Textbook of Small Animal Surgery. Philadelphia, WB Saunders, 1985, pp 1661–1664.
2. Wheaton LG, et al: Results and complications of surgical treatment of pyometra: A review of 80 cases. J Am Anim Hosp Assoc 25:563-568, 1989.
3. Bjurstrom L, Linde-Forsberg C: Long-term study of aerobic bacteria of the genital tract in breeding bitches. Am J Vet Res 53: 665–669, 1992.
4. Bowen RA, et al: Efficacy amd toxicity of estrogens commonly used to terminate canine pregnancy. JAVMA 186:783–788, 1985.
5. Wrigley RH, Finn ST: Ultrasonography of the canine uterus and ovary. In Kirk RW (ed): Current Veterinary Therapy X. Philadelphia, WB Saunders, 1989, pp 1239–1241.
6. Nelson RW, et al: Treatment of canine pyometra and endometritis with prostaglandin F$_{2\alpha}$. JAVMA 181:899–903, 1982.
7. Feldman EC, Nelson RW: Diagnosis and treatment alternatives for pyometra in dogs and cats. In Kirk RW (ed): Current Veterinary Therapy X. Philadelphia, WB Saunders, 1989 pp 1305–1310.
8. Freshman JL: Clinical approach to infertility in the cycling bitch. Vet Clin North Am Small Anim Pract 21:427–435, 1991.
9. Olson PN, et al: Infertility in the bitch. In Kirk RW (ed): Current Veterinary Therapy VIII. Philadelphia, WB Saunders, 1983, pp 925–931.
10. Johnston SD: Noninfectious causes of infertility in the dog and cat. In Laing JA, Morgan WJ, Wagner WC (eds): Fertility and Infertility in Veterinary Practice. London, Balliere Tindall, 1988, pp 160–172.
11. Burke TJ: Causes of infertility. In Burke TJ (ed): Small Animal Reproduction and Infertility: A Clinical Approach to Diagnosis and Treatment. Philadelphia, Lea & Febiger, 1986, pp 227–316.
12. Jones DE, Joshua JO: Infertility. Reproductive Clinical Problems in the Dog, 2nd ed. London, Butterworths, 1988, p 187.
13. Olson PN: Evaluating Reproductive Failure in the Bitch. San Diego, CA, American College of Veterinary Internal Medicine, 1987, pp 103–106.
14. Barton CL: Infertility in the bitch. In Proceedings of the Annual Meeting of the Society for Theriogenology, Austin, Texas, 1987, pp 198–205.
15. Olson PN, et al: Concentrations of luteinizing hormone and follicle-stimulating hormone in the serum of sexually intact and neutered dogs. Am J Vet Res 53:762–766, 1992.
16. Meyers-Wallen VN: Persistent estrus in the bitch. In Kirk RW, Bonagura JD (eds): Current Veterinary Therapy XI. Philadelphia, WB Saunders, 1992, pp 963–966.

REP

CHAPTER 163

VAGINAL DISORDERS

Beverly J. Purswell

ANATOMY

EMBRYOLOGIC ORIGINS OF THE POSTERIOR REPRODUCTIVE TRACT

In normal sexual development of the female dog and cat, the urogenital sinus, genital tubercle, and genital swellings become the vestibule, the clitoris, and the vulva, respectively.[1] The paramesonephric (müllerian) ducts give rise to the uterine tubes (oviducts), uterus, cervix, and vagina.[2] The caudal end of the vaginal canal opens into the vestibule by joining the urogenital sinus at the vaginovestibular junction. Although both the paramesonephric ducts and the urogenital sinus probably contribute to the vaginal epithelium, the vaginal squamous epithelial cells are considered to originate from the urogenital sinus.[2] The urogenital sinus also gives rise to the urinary bladder and the urethra, which enters the vestibule just caudal to the vaginovestibular junction.

ANATOMIC RELATIONSHIP OF THE VAGINA AND VESTIBULE

The vestibule is the common external opening of the urinary and reproductive tracts. Cranially, the vestibule ends at the vagina, where the narrowing of the vaginovestibular junction can be palpated digitally. There is a distinct downward slope to the vestibule starting at the vaginovestibular junction to the ventral commissure of the vulva (Fig. 163–1).

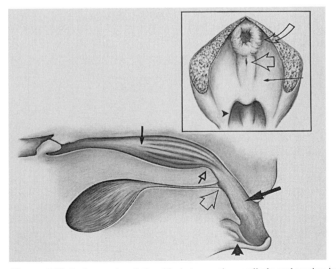

Figure 163–1. Anatomic relationship between the vestibule and vagina in the bitch. The inset shows an annular stricture at the vaginovestibular junction cranial to the urethral opening. Open arrowhead = urethral opening; solid arrowhead = clitoral fossa; open arrow = vaginovestibular junction; solid arrow = vagina; large solid arrow = vestibule.

The urethral opening is located on the ventral floor of the vestibule 0.5 cm distal to the vaginovestibular junction.

The vagina extends from the vaginovestibular junction to the cervix. The bitch has a relatively long vagina, placing the cervix in the abdomen, not the pelvic canal. This length makes examination of the vagina in its entirety difficult without special equipment and impossible with digital palpation. The anterior part of the vagina is quite narrow (5 to 7 mm), making visualization of the cervix and its external os difficult even with endoscopy.[3]

EXAMINATION OF THE VESTIBULE AND VAGINA

VAGINAL CYTOLOGY

Vaginal cytology is the most widely used technique to evaluate the distal reproductive tract of the bitch and is invaluable in interpreting the nature of vulvar discharges. Localization of a disease process may be facilitated by comparing cytology from the vestibule with that of the vagina. Vaginal cytology is indicated any time there is suspected disease of the reproductive tract. Neutrophils in low numbers are normally seen in vaginal cytology at any time except during the peak of the estrogenic phase (mid to late proestrus and the entire estrous phase). Large numbers of neutrophils are seen during early diestrus. This influx is not associated with any disease process and is considered a normal phenomenon. Large numbers of neutrophils during any other stage of the cycle indicate an inflammatory process.

VISUAL AND DIGITAL EXAMINATION

Digital examination of the distal reproductive tract is invaluable in diagnosing a variety of abnormalities. The size of the animal may limit the extent of an examination. Owing to the length of the distal reproductive tract, particularly the length of the vagina, it is impossible to digitally examine the vagina in its entirety. Only the vulva, vestibule, urethral opening, and vaginovestibular junction are adequately evaluated on digital examination. Most abnormalities in this area are best diagnosed with a digital examination and may remain undetected with other forms of inspection.

Vaginoscopy may be performed with an endoscope, proctoscope, or any fiberoptic equipment with sufficient length (15 cm) to inspect the entire vagina. Vaginoscopy can usually be performed on an awake standing bitch, and sedation is not often needed. Rigid equipment such as a proctoscope tends to give better visualization of the vagina owing to the collapsing nature of the vaginal folds. When using flexible fiberoptic endoscopes, insufflation of the vagina with air is necessary for a thorough examination. The outside diameter of the endoscope needs to be 5 mm or less for complete visualization of the anterior vagina and paracervical area.[3] This small diameter may be necessary as well to traverse the narrowing seen at the vaginovestibular junction or when examining small bitches (<20 pounds). Body size does not always correlate with vestibular and vaginal diameter, especially in a prepubertal or ovariectomized bitch. Equipment less than 5 cm in length, such as otoscopes, allow only the vestibule of the vagina to be visualized.

VAGINAL BACTERIAL CULTURES

It has become common practice to request vaginal cultures from bitches prior to breeding. Normal bitches have bacterial flora that may not be distinct from that of bitches with reproductive tract disease.[4,5] The aerobic bacterial flora of the bitch's vagina consists of common opportunistic pathogens whose presence does not influence fertility.[5] Careful interpretation of culture results is mandatory because this area has normal flora, but results obtained during an overt disease process are valuable in choosing appropriate therapy. Isolation of opportunistic aerobic pathogens, anaerobic bacteria, or mycoplasmas in an asymptomatic animal does not constitute evidence of infection.[4] Prophylactic use of antibiotics in apparently healthy breeding bitches may predispose the vagina to colonization by organisms that are known opportunistic pathogens.[6] Vaginal cultures should be obtained only with a guarded swab technique.

VAGINAL ABNORMALITIES

VAGINITIS

By definition, vaginitis describes an inflammatory process that may not be infectious. Inflammation can be identified easily with vaginal cytology and vaginoscopy. The physical signs are irritation evidenced by licking, vulvar discharge, and attraction of male dogs. Vaginal cytology usually demonstrates increased numbers of neutrophils in various stages of degeneration, with or without increased numbers of bacteria. Chronic vaginitis may induce the presence of lymphocytes and macrophages. Vaginoscopy may demonstrate the presence and extent of hyperemia, exudate, and mucosal lesions such as vesicles, ulcers, and lymphoid follicle hyperplasia. An attempt should be made to differentiate other systemic disorders that are associated with similar signs. Urinary tract problems should be ruled out as a cause for vestibular irritation or attraction of male dogs. Dermatologic lesions may cause perineal irritation and excessive licking. Comparing vestibular cytology with vaginal cytology may help localize the problem (Fig. 163–2).

Juvenile (puppy) vaginitis, with its purulent vulvar discharge, is a common malady seen in prepubertal bitches. Juvenile vaginitis may respond to systemic antibacterial therapy or to topical douching, but inevitably the signs return when treatment is discontinued. The condition resolves naturally after the first estrous cycle, if not before. It is advisable to postpone neutering these individuals until after the signs have disappeared on their own or the first estrus has occurred. The vulvar area should be kept clean to avoid secondary skin problems. No other treatment is necessary.

Adult vaginitis can be caused by anatomic abnormalities that lead to accumulation of discharge or urine in the vagina. Accumulation of urine in the vagina may present as urinary incontinence with urine dribbling from the vulva when the bitch changes position. Bacterial or chemical vaginitis is secondary to the predisposing cause. Strictures at the vaginovestibular junction that may cause a problem can be identified by a digital examination. Digital dilatation, surgical dilatation, or vaginectomy may be required to eliminate the problem. Foreign bodies, tumors, or uterine stump granulomas should be ruled out as predisposing causes by vaginoscopy, contrast radiography, or other imaging modalities (Fig. 163–3). Contrast radiography may be helpful in identifying anatomic abnormalities or concurrent urinary tract disease (including acquired ectopic ureters after ovariohysterectomy).[7] Because systemic disease may predispose a bitch to vaginal infections, the general health of the animal should be evaluated. If a predisposing cause is not identified, vaginal cultures should be obtained and appropriate antibacterial therapy instituted. Initial lavage of the vagina may be beneficial to remove the accumulated discharge.

Viral vaginitis has been described in conjunction with canine herpesvirus infections. Genital infections of canine herpesvirus result in diffuse, multifocal, raised vesicular lesions on the vaginal mucosa that characteristically cause no clinical signs in the bitch.[8] No treatment is necessary, but it is advisable to separate the affected animal from any pregnant bitches or neonatal puppies.[9]

ANATOMIC ABNORMALITIES

A variety of congenital abnormalities of the vagina and vestibule exist. Their incidence is unknown, but these abnormalities are not uncommon. Abnormal embryologic development is responsible for the majority of these conditions.

A persistent hymen can occur at the junction of the vagina and vestibule where the paramesonephric duct joins the urogenital sinus. Incomplete perforation of the hymen may present as an annular stricture (see Fig. 163–1 inset) or a vertical annular stricture or a vertical band. Affected bitches may have breeding difficulties, chronic vaginitis, or urinary incontinence unresponsive to conventional therapy due to urine pooling. Digital palpation is the preferred method to diagnose these conditions. Vaginoscopy may bypass the affected area. If these anomalies are incidental findings in an asymptomatic animal, no correction is necessary. A vertical band is usually easily resected, and clinical signs quickly resolve. An annular stricture is more difficult to correct permanently. Digital dilatation can be attempted and may be successful, depending on the extent of the tissue involved. An episiotomy may be required to attain adequate exposure of the vaginovestibular junction for surgical manipulation. The stricture may be excised completely, with the mucosa closed perpendicular to the initial incision in an attempt to enlarge the lumen. Another approach is to make a series of radial incisions perpendicular to the lumen. Both procedures may require frequent and repeated postoperative digital dilatation to prevent recurrence of the stricture. Clinical signs may persist following attempted surgical correction. Vaginectomy is an alternative therapy that alleviates problems associated with the vagina. Bitches with annular strictures may be bred artificially and reevaluated immediately before parturition. Sufficient relaxation usually occurs to allow normal delivery. Surgical intervention at parturition would be necessary in the form of cesarean section or an episiotomy if the relaxation is insufficient to allow whelping.

Vaginal anomalies arise because of problems associated with the paramesonephric duct organogenesis. The external

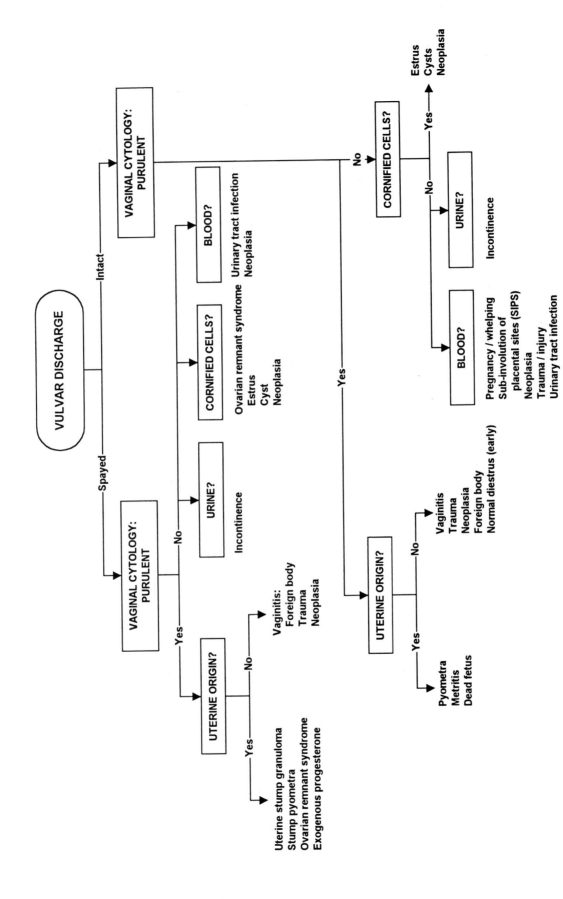

Figure 163–2. Algorithm for the evaluation of vulvar discharge.

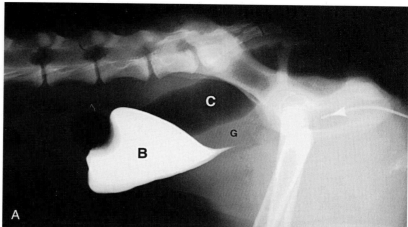

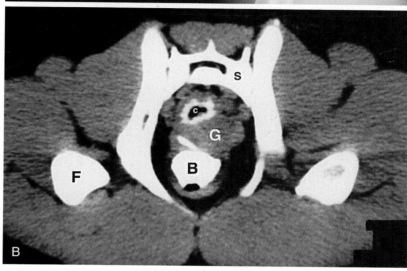

Figure 163–3. Uterine stump granuloma in a 7-month-old spayed bitch presented for urinary incontinence. *A,* Lateral abdominal radiograph obtained after infusion of air into the colon (C) and iodinated contrast medium into the urinary bladder (B). The uterine stump granuloma (G) is evident as a soft tissue mass compressing the neck of the urinary bladder. *B,* Transverse computed tomographic image obtained at the level of the cranial pelvic canal. The granuloma compresses the left ureter at the trigone and indents the left dorsolateral margin of the urinary bladder. S = sacrum; F = femur. (Courtesy of Dr. Jeryl C. Jones.)

genitalia and vestibule are usually normal in these animals, owing to their separate embryologic origin. Incomplete fusion of the paramesonephric ducts results in a vertical septum within the vagina (double vagina). Surgery is indicated if the bitch's intended use is breeding or if clinical signs are present. Concomitant anomalies must be ruled out before attempted correction of any abnormality. Segmental hypoplasia or aplasia of the vagina has been described in the bitch, and surgical correction is not possible. Vaginal diverticula may occur and can fill with debris, causing local inflammation. Surgical removal of the diverticula is indicated to resolve this condition. Contrast radiography and vaginoscopy are helpful in identifying and defining the extent of the various vaginal anomalies. Ovariohysterectomy is indicated when the offending condition is extensive and a total or partial vaginectomy is indicated.

Vulvar anomalies are occasional findings in the bitch with breeding difficulties. Tight bands at the dorsal commissure are a common cause of painful copulation (dyspareunia) and are easily identified with digital palpation. If necessary, the bitch may be bred artificially and reexamined immediately before parturition to assess potential whelping difficulties. Relaxation of the vulva is usually sufficient to allow normal delivery.

Infantile vulvas may be found in prepubertal bitches. The vulva is small and may be inverted to the point of being hidden from view. Vaginitis, perineal irritation, vulvar dis-

charge, or urinary tract disease may be found owing to the infolding of the vulva and distortion of the vestibule and urethral opening. Neutering of these bitches should be postponed until after the first estrus. Eversion of the vulva normally occurs during the first estrus, and the condition is self-correcting.

Faulty urogenital sinus embryogenesis may lead to congenital problems in the vestibule, vulva, and perineum. Open vulvar clefts, perineal dysgenesis, and rectovaginal fistulas have been described and require surgical correction. These distal abnormalities may be associated with other reproductive or urinary tract anomalies and can be acquired or congenital. Clitoral anomalies are usually associated with intersex conditions and take the form of clitoral enlargement with penis-like anatomy. Surgical removal of the clitoris to prevent excoriation is advised whenever the clitoris protrudes from the vulva.

VAGINAL FOLD PROLAPSE, VAGINAL HYPERPLASIA, VAGINAL PROLAPSE

Under the influence of estrogen, some young bitches develop an edematous ventral fold in the distal vaginal mucosa immediately cranial to the urethral opening (Fig. 163–4) that may become large enough to protrude from the vulvar opening. Traditionally, this condition has been referred to as

REP

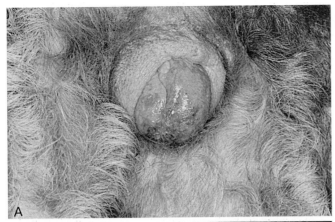
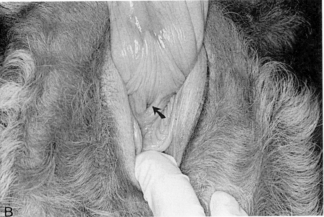

Figure 163–4. Vaginal fold prolapse (vaginal hyperplasia) in a bitch. *A,* Vaginal fold prolapse protruding from the vulva, with excoriation evident. *B,* Vaginal fold prolapse originating anterior to the urethral opening (*arrow*).

vaginal hyperplasia. Histologically, this tissue is no more hyperplastic than the rest of the vagina under the influence of estrogen. Pronounced edema is the major histologic lesion, with fibroplasia resulting from the edema. Prolapse of a vaginal fold occurs almost exclusively when the bitch is under the influence of estrogen. This may occur at the first estrus or become evident during later estrous cycles. Once this condition manifests itself, the tendency is for it to reoccur at each subsequent estrus. The condition is usually self-limited and will resolve once the estrogenic influence is withdrawn at the end of estrus or after ovariohysterectomy. Ovariohysterectomy resolves the condition permanently and is the treatment of choice in a nonbreeding animal. The major worries in affected dogs are infection of this tissue, severe trauma, and urinary tract obstruction. Surgical removal of the prolapsed tissue can be attempted and may resolve the condition permanently in some animals. However, excessive perioperative hemorrhage may be associated with this procedure. Artificial insemination can be performed in affected bitches, with resolution expected with the onset of diestrus. Occasionally, the condition fails to resolve after estrus or recurs at the end of pregnancy when estrogen concentrations increase slightly.[10] The condition is not generally thought to be hereditary, although there is evidence of hereditary predisposition in some family lines and some breeds.

Vaginal prolapse rarely occurs in bitches and queens. It is usually associated with dystocia, tenesmus, or forced extrac-

tion of the male during the genital tie. Uterine prolapse may follow, depending on the cause. Treatment involves replacement of the affected structures. An abdominal approach may be necessary to replace the vagina. An ovariohysterectomy may be performed at the time of correction if so desired.

MISCELLANEOUS VAGINAL DISORDERS

Vaginal lacerations can occur during copulation, obstetric procedures, or vaginoscopy. Hemorrhage from the vulva is the primary sign. A bitch that bleeds from the vulva after breeding should be examined for vaginal tears. The decision must be made whether suturing is necessary or possible. Systemic antibiotics should be administered to prevent infections, particularly dissecting pelvic infections.

Vaginal and vulvar neoplasia represent 2.5 to 3 per cent of all canine tumors.[11] Seventy to 80 per cent of these tumors are benign. These dogs may have perineal enlargement, a mass protruding from the vulva, vulvar discharge, tenesmus, and dysuria (Fig. 163–5). Tumors prolapsing from the vulva must be differentiated from vaginal fold prolapse by evaluating the stage of the estrous cycle and its relationship to the onset of signs, location of the mass, and failure of the mass to regress postestrus. Leiomyomas are the most common benign tumor and are often pedunculated. Leiomyosarcoma is the most common malignant vaginal tumor. Surgical excision is the treatment of choice. Transmissible venereal tumors are more common in younger animals and respond readily to chemotherapy. The prognosis for vaginal and vulvar tumors is good, provided that metastasis has not occurred with the malignant tumors. Ovariohysterectomy is recommended at the time of removal because of the possibility of hormonal influence on the incidence and possible recurrence rate.

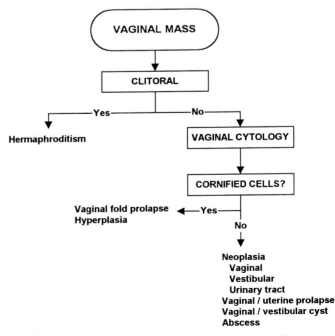

Figure 163–5. Algorithm for the evaluation of a vaginal mass.

REFERENCES

1. Meyers-Wallen VN, Patterson DF: Disorders of sexual development in dogs and cats. *In* Kirk RW (ed): Current Veterinary Therapy X. Philadelphia, WB Saunders, 1989, pp 1261–1269.
2. McEntee K: Reproductive Pathology of Domestic Mammals. San Diego, Academic Press, 1990.
3. Lindsay FEF: Endoscopy of the reproductive tract in the bitch. *In* Kirk RW (ed): Current Veterinary Therapy VIII. Philadelphia, WB Saunders, 1983, pp 912–921.
4. Olson PN, Mather ED: The use and misuse of vaginal cultures in diagnosing reproductive diseases in the bitch. *In* Morrow DA (ed): Current Therapy in Theriogenology. Philadelphia, WB Saunders, 1986, pp 469–475.
5. Bjurstrom L, Linde-Forsberg C: Long-term study of aerobic bacteria of the genital tract in breeding bitches. Am J Vet Res 53:665, 1992.
6. Strom B, Linde-Forsberg C: Effects of ampicillin and trimethoprim-sulfamethoxazole on the vaginal bacterial flora of bitches. Am J Vet Res 54:891, 1993.
7. Holt PE, et al: An evaluation of positive contrast vagino-urethrography as a diagnostic aid in the bitch. J Small Anim Pract 25:531, 1984.
8. Greene CE, Kakuk TJ: Canine herpesvirus infection. *In* Greene CE (ed): Clinical Microbiology and Infectious Diseases of the Dog and Cat. Philadelphia, WB Saunders, 1984, pp 419–429.
9. Evermann JF: Comparative clinical and diagnostic aspects of herpesvirus infections of companion animals with primary emphasis on the dog. Proceedings of the Annual Meeting of the Society for Theriogenology, 1989, pp 335–343.
10. Johnston SD: Vaginal prolapse. *In* Kirk RW (ed): Current Veterinary Therapy X. Philadelphia, WB Saunders, 1989, pp 1302–1305.
11. Withrow SJ, Susaneck SJ: Tumors of the canine female reproductive tract. *In* Morrow DA (ed): Current Therapy in Theriogenology. Philadelphia, WB Saunders, 1986, pp 521–528.

CHAPTER 164

SEMEN EVALUATION, ARTIFICIAL INSEMINATION, AND INFERTILITY IN THE MALE DOG

Gary C. W. England

Major technologic advances have been made in the study of seminal characteristics and spermatozoal function of farm animals and men. However, despite the fact that the collection and evaluation of dog semen has been undertaken since the beginning of this century, information regarding this species is sparse. Interest in canine andrology has recently increased with show dogs being commonly examined before purchase, before use at stud, and when there is concern about infertility. The use of artificial insemination with fresh and preserved semen has also allowed greater examination of semen from fertile stud dogs and has facilitated the establishment of acceptable normal ranges for many seminal characteristics. The aim of this chapter is to review semen collection and evaluation and to consider the application of artificial insemination and the investigation of the infertile male.

SEMEN EVALUATION

The best measure of the fertility of a male is the ability of his spermatozoa to fertilize oocytes and sustain embryogenesis. The principle of semen evaluation relies on the belief that certain characteristics of semen quality are predictive of fertilizing capacity. However, when the range of events that follow ejaculation is considered, it is not surprising that no one test is predictive of absolute fertility.

With the increasing use of artificial insemination, there has been wider access to semen from known fertile dogs, and our knowledge of normal semen quality has improved.

SEMEN COLLECTION

The ejaculate of the dog has three distinct fractions, of which the first and third originate from the prostate. The second fraction is the sperm-rich portion. The method of semen collection may influence the quality of the semen. Collection using an artificial vagina allows mixing of the fractions, and in vitro this may be deleterious to the sperm. Additionally, low spermatozoal motility and sperm immobilization has been reported after collection of dog semen with rubber artificial vaginas. For an accurate assessment of semen quality it has been suggested that separation of the fractions is necessary. To this aim, semen is most commonly collected into plastic centrifuge tubes by means of glass funnels after manipulation of the penis and is facilitated by the presence of a bitch in estrus. During semen collection and assessment it is important to ensure that samples are not temperature shocked. Although dog sperm is less susceptible to this problem than that of other species, warming and insulation of collection equipment should normally be practiced. Many items of equipment are toxic to dog sperm, and all plastic tubes, syringes, and pipettes should be carefully

REP

tested before routine use. Semen may be collected from dogs with poor libido by electrical stimulation; however, this technique requires general anesthesia, the ejaculate volume is usually small, and there is frequently contamination of the ejaculate with urine.

ASSESSMENT OF SEMEN QUALITY

In men, a number of retrospective studies have shown that certain characteristics of the ejaculate are, on average, superior in fertile compared with non-fertile samples, although there is no definitive method of predicting fertility. Table 164–1 contains the mean seminal characteristics from 53 apparently fertile dogs that achieved pregnancy in the 6 months before and 6 months after semen collection. This group of dogs had mated 735 bitches on two occasions during estrus, of which 624 bitches whelped, giving a pregnancy rate of 84.8 per cent. Although all of these dogs are considered to be fertile, these data demonstrate the wide range of seminal characteristics that may be associated with fertility.

SPERMATOZOAL NUMBER

The determination of the total number of spermatozoa per ejaculate is the most accurate measure of sperm production. This is calculated by multiplying the second fraction volume with the spermatozoal concentration, the latter being conventionally measured using a hemocytometer chamber despite the inaccuracies of this method.[1] A relationship has been demonstrated between breed and the number of sperm ejaculated, with larger breeds producing more sperm. For an individual the best assessment of sperm production is the number of sperm produced per day by testicular tissue (the daily sperm production). Although it is not practical to measure this in most animals it can be estimated on the basis of the daily sperm output, following repeated daily sample collection until semen characteristics have stabilized. Five to seven daily collections are required to stabilize the daily sperm output, which is approximately 400×10^6 sperm for most dogs.[2]

The wide normal range of total sperm output for fertile dogs is given in Table 164–1. Interestingly, some of these values are considerably lower than the minimal requirement for fertility suggested by some authors, although Tsutsui and colleagues[3] showed that for optimal fertility a total of only 200×10^6 live spermatozoa were required.

SPERMATOZOAL MORPHOLOGY AND VITAL STAINING

Spermatozoal morphology can be examined in a number of different ways. Frequently, sperm are highlighted using a background stain such as India ink or are specifically stained using, for example, Giemsa. Stains that allow the evaluation of acrosomal morphology (e.g., Spermac) or the assessment of live/dead ratios (such as nigrosin-eosin) are increasingly used. In several species, good relationships have been found between the percentage of live staining spermatozoa and fertility, and this may relate to one of two concepts: (1) the effect of the total number of live spermatozoa on fertility and (2) the interference with fertility by the proportion of dead spermatozoa. In the dog there has been little study of the proportion of dead spermatozoa within the ejaculate; commonly, only the total number of morphologically normal, live-staining spermatozoa are considered.

In other species, techniques for the triple staining of spermatozoa have been investigated, allowing the differentiation of live and dead cells and those that have undergone the acrosome reaction. More recently, the use of fluorescence staining has been studied because this may allow the assessment of the capacitational status of spermatozoa, as well as those that are acrosome-reacted sperm.[4] Such techniques are, however, relatively complicated and not suitable for use in general practice.

SPERMATOZOAL MOTILITY

In dogs, there are no data relating spermatozoal motility to fertility. Considerable attention has however been directed toward the assessment of spermatozoal motility, and both the percentage motile and the character of motility are evaluated. Motility is a temperature-dependent phenomenon, and samples should always be evaluated at a standard temperature on a heated microscope stage. Conventionally, this is 37°C, but 39°C may be more physiologically appropriate.

For subjective assessment of sperm it is worthwhile classifying the character of sperm motility and estimating the percentage of sperm within each category. For example, motility can be considered in five categories:

O—immotile sperm
I—sperm that are motile but not progressive
II—sperm that have sluggish motility and are poorly progressive
III—sperm with reasonable motility and moderate progression
IV—sperm with rapid forward progressive motility.

TABLE 164–1. CHARACTERISTICS OF THE SECOND FRACTION OF THE EJACULATE FROM 53 FERTILE DOGS

CHARACTERISTIC	MEAN	STANDARD DEVIATION	RANGE
Motility (%)	85.2	6.2	42–92
Volume (mL)	1.3	0.4	0.4–3.4
Concentration ($\times 10^6$)	310.5	82	50–560
Total sperm output ($\times 10^6$)	403.4	120	36–620
Hypo-osmotic swelling test (%)	83.1	5.2	62–95
Live normal (%)	75.2	7.9	52–90
Dead normal (%)	10.2	5.4	2–26
Primary abnormal (%)	1.6	2.6	0.12
Secondary abnormal (%)	10.0	5.4	2–24

Only category IV spermatozoa are considered to have normal motility. It is not uncommon for the inexperienced assessor to evaluate the total number of motile sperm (i.e., all those that are not immotile). Only with the use of strict criteria can a relationship with fertility be demonstrated.

In men, some workers have suggested that spermatozoal motility is the best predictor of infertility, although others have questioned this absolute relationship. Holt and associates[5] found that the swimming speed of human sperm correlated well with the results of in vitro fertilization assays and suggested that spermatozoal swimming speeds were one of the most important diagnostic parameters in the prediction of male fertility. In the dog, spermatozoal motility has conventionally been assessed subjectively, although more recently there have been attempts to quantify these measures using computer image analysis techniques. Gunzel-Apel and co-workers[6] evaluated the use of two commercial computerized machines for the assessment of dog sperm motility, but to date there are no data relating these findings to fertility. Further investigations of this technology appear to be warranted, especially considering the useful results obtained in other species.

SEMINAL PLASMA

In addition to the routine assessment of spermatozoal morphology and motility there have been several studies of the composition of dog seminal plasma. Most have found the pH of the first and second fraction to be approximately 6.3 and that of the third fraction to be slightly higher. Others have investigated the electrolyte and carbohydrate concentration and osmolarity of the ejaculate, although overall there have been no substantiated differences identified between fertile and infertile dogs.

More recently, there has been discussion of measurement of seminal plasma alkaline phosphatase and carnitine concentrations for the diagnosis of dogs with obstruction of the tubular genitalia.[7] Because these compounds are thought to originate from the epididymides their absence indicates either obstruction or an incomplete ejaculation. For normal dogs, seminal plasma alkaline phosphatase concentrations are usually greater than 10,000 IU/L.

OTHER CELLS

In men, much importance has been given to the presence of cells other than spermatozoa within the ejaculate. Common hematology stains can be used to facilitate the identification of other cells; however, little attention has been given to them in the dog, with the exception of macrophages[8] and "leukophages."[9] It is common for the presence of inflammatory cells to be noted within the ejaculate, but these frequently originate from the prepuce.

MICROBIOLOGY

There has been considerable debate concerning the role of bacteria within the prostatic fluid and seminal plasma of dogs. Many aerobic and anaerobic organisms are frequently isolated from the prepuce of the dog, and the bacterial flora is usually mixed.[10] It is not surprising that many bacterial species are isolated from the ejaculate. These bacteria, including beta-hemolytic *Streptococcus,* are now considered normal commensal organisms; and although the role of *My-*

coplasma and *Ureaplasma* is less certain,[11] these organisms are frequently isolated in clinically normal fertile dogs.

ASSESSMENT OF SPERMATOZOAL FUNCTION

The functional competence of sperm may be more important than the number of spermatozoa present. The traditional criteria of semen quality are based on descriptive assessments of ejaculate characteristics. However, abnormal spermatozoa have been detected in fertile men, and similarly fertile dogs have been reported with low numbers of normal spermatozoa.[12] These data suggest that it is not simply the number of normal motile gametes that is critical to male infertility but their functional competence.

Recently, the phenomenon of spermatozoal swelling in the presence of hypo-osmotic medium has been used in an attempt to assess the functional capacity of spermatozoal membranes. The ability of spermatozoa to swell in a hypo-osmotic medium was found to be highly correlated with the ability of spermatozoa to penetrate zona-free hamster oocytes. Although some workers have suggested that this test has little practical value, it has been shown to provide a more accurate prediction of the outcome of in vitro fertilization, and in some species pregnancy rates, than conventional semen analysis. The technique has been investigated for use in the dog[13] and found to be reliable and repeatable. It is clear that the hypo-osmotic swelling test may be useful for the assessment of membrane function. However, no data are available relating this to fertility in the dog.

In several species, assessments have been made of sperm-oocyte interactions. The most common test involves evaluation of the number of oocytes penetrated by capacitated sperm, with the aim being to assess the ability of the spermatozoa to hyperactivate and interact with the vitelline membrane and become incorporated into the oocyte. Despite the fact that such techniques do not assess the ability of sperm to ascend the reproductive tract and penetrate the zona, many studies have shown a reasonable correlation with fertility. There have been limited studies of oocyte penetration in the dog, although Hewitt and England[14] showed that such an assay was a viable method for the assessment of semen.

RELATION BETWEEN SEMEN QUALITY AND INFERTILITY

It is often possible to identify those animals with grossly abnormal spermatozoa and those with spermatozoa that are apparently normal. However, frequently the consideration of fertility is not addressed; indeed, the question of whether routine semen analysis serves any useful purpose has been posed. It is, however, this value of detecting major deficiencies in semen quality that is particularly useful, because it may then stimulate further investigation and possible treatment. Invariably, the majority of semen samples lies between the two extremes of excellent or poor quality; and for this reason it is necessary to establish an acceptable normal range. This has been achieved for normal fertile dogs (see Table 164–1). However, because it is unlikely that any one test will provide an accurate prediction of the fertility of a sample, and there is limited information on the evaluation of dog spermatozoal function, the need for further investigation of seminal characteristics in the dog is emphasized. In an attempt to establish a relationship between semen quality

REP

and fertility in dogs, a statistical cut-off was established for morphologically normal sperm at 60 per cent.[15] Above this value, fertility was normal, whereas below this value there was a significant reduction in fertility.

ARTIFICIAL INSEMINATION

Artificial insemination has a number of advantages over natural mating, including that it reduces the requirement to transport animals, overcomes quarantine restrictions, increases the genetic pool available within a country, reduces the risk of disease when unknown animals enter a kennel for mating, may reduce the spread of infectious disease, and may be useful when natural mating is difficult (e.g., bitches that ovulate when they are not in standing estrus, or in males that owing to age, debility, back pain, or premature ejaculation are unable to achieve a natural mating). The greatest area of interest is probably the storage of semen for future use and the international exchange of genetic material. For the latter there are specific requirements when semen is imported into a country, determined by federal agencies. These requirements are aimed at controlling the spread of infectious canine diseases, and many poultry diseases, because semen extenders are often based on egg yolk. Importation regulations vary between countries and should always be checked before transporting semen. In some countries there is limited use of artificial insemination because of the restrictions imposed by the national kennel clubs (in the United States regulations vary between the American Kennel Club and the United Kennel Club) or by breed associations. Artificial insemination of the bitch can be performed with fresh, chilled, or frozen-thawed semen.

METHODS OF SEMEN INSEMINATION

FRESH SEMEN

Fresh semen may be used undiluted, or diluted with an extender solution, to enhance its longevity and control the growth of bacteria by the addition of anti-bacterial agents. Fresh semen artificial insemination may be used when a normal mating is not possible (e.g., an aggressive bitch, unwilling dog, or injury to either dog or bitch). Undiluted semen held at 39°C deteriorates quickly, and for short-term storage until insemination (< 6 hours) it is best to allow the sample to cool to room temperature and preferably to use a semen extender.

CHILLED (COOLED) SEMEN

Semen may be stored for a short period of time by dilution with an extender solution (often based on skim milk) followed by cooling to approximately 5°C. This method allows transportation of semen to the bitch or may be useful when there is short-term unavailability of the dog. When cooled in this way the usable lifespan of the semen is approximately 4 days.

FROZEN SEMEN

Semen may be stored for a long periods of time by dilution with an extender solution (often based on egg yolk, glycerol, and a pH buffer), freezing to −196°C, and subse-

quently thawing. This processing allows semen to be transported over long distances or allows samples to be stored for use in future generations. The lifespan of frozen semen is considered to be several hundred years.

SEMEN PRESERVATION

For the short- or long-term storage of semen the ejaculate is normally diluted with an extender that protects the sperm during cooling/freezing/warming; provides an energy source to sperm; and maintains the pH, osmolarity, and ionic strength. Specific protective agents that may be used include milk proteins, which protect against cold shock, and egg yolk (low-density lipoproteins) and bovine serum albumen, which protect acrosomal and mitochondrial membranes and protect against cold shock. For semen freezing, cryoprotective agents are essential because they prevent ice crystal damage. There are two basic cryoprotectants, those that are penetrating (e.g., glycerol and dimethylsulfoxide) and those that are non-penetrating (e.g., sugars and polyvinylpyrrolidone).

Glucose, fructose, and mannose are glycolyzable sugars that may be included in semen extenders as sources of energy, whereas the larger molecular weight sugars (ribose, arabinose) are often used as non-penetrating cryoprotectants. During storage, hydrogen ions are produced by sperm and therefore the pH decreases. Control of pH is important, and many agents have been used, including phosphate buffer, egg yolk, milk proteins, and zwitterionic buffers (e.g., Tris, Tes, Hepes).

In general, hypotonic extenders are harmful to sperm during freezing because they lead to a gain in intracellular water and redistribution of ions. Hypertonic extenders are less harmful because they lead to loss of water from the sperm and a reduction in the likelihood of intracellular ice crystal formation. Seminal plasma has an osmolarity of 300 mOsm, and therefore most extenders are formulated to approximately 370 mOsm. Frequently antibacterial agents are included in semen extenders to control the proliferation of microorganisms.

PREPARATION OF FRESH DOG SEMEN

Semen is collected as previously described, and the second fraction is evaluated before insemination. The entire second fraction is normally deposited into the vagina close to the cervix using a long inseminating pipette. Uterine insemination (discussed later) increases the chance of conception; however, this is not commonly performed when using fresh semen because pregnancy rates are generally good even with vaginal insemination.

PREPARATION OF CHILLED (COOLED) DOG SEMEN

Semen is collected and evaluated as previously described, and the second fraction of the ejaculate is diluted with an extender solution. A common extender is composed of non-fat dry milk, 2.4 g; glucose, 4.9 g; sodium bicarbonate, 0.15 g; and sufficient deionized water to make the volume up to 100 mL. Antimicrobial agents may then be added, such as penicillin, 150,000 IU, and streptomycin, 150,000 mg. Alternatively, a low-fat pasteurized cow's milk extender can be prepared by heating the milk until it starts to simmer and then allowing it to cool. Extender may be stored frozen and should be warmed to 37°C before use. In each case, before diluting the whole ejaculate, a few drops of semen should be mixed with a small volume of the extender. Provided that the extender has no deleterious effect, the remaining semen can then be diluted with the extender. It is preferable to dilute the semen in a ratio 1:4 (semen:extender), rather than aim to achieve a standard sperm concentration. Once diluted, the extended semen is cooled slowly to 5°C and stored at this temperature. Slow cooling can be achieved by placing the extended semen in a non-toxic insulated vial into a refrigerator. Semen may be transported using a wide-mouthed vacuum flask partially filled with ice cubes. Before insemination the extended semen is normally warmed slowly by placing the vials into a water bath at 37°C. Samples should be allowed to warm for 10 minutes before evaluation. Good-quality semen normally has excellent longevity and remains fertile for up to 4 or 5 days, although frequently the semen is used within 24 hours of collection. In these cases the semen can be treated as if it were fresh and a vaginal insemination performed. When samples have been stored for a prolonged period of time, or when the initial semen quality is poor, it is preferable to perform a uterine insemination.

PREPARATION OF FROZEN-THAWED DOG SEMEN

Before embarking on freezing it is essential to perform an adequate semen evaluation. Sperm are damaged during the cryopreservation process and samples that are initially poor (less than 60 per cent live normal spermatozoal with forward progressive motility) may be unusable after freeze thawing. Although semen freezing extenders and freezing technology is available almost in a "cook book" manner, it should be remembered that the process is intricate and that for optimal post-thaw survival there is a fine balance between the composition of the extender, the cooling rate, equilibration time, freezing rate, and thawing rate. Changing any one of these has consequences for the others, for example, diluting semen with an extender either 1:2 (semen:extender) or 1:5 results in a 25 per cent increase in the final glycerol concentration; this variation may be more damaging to the sperm and will require a different cooling rate, equilibration time, freezing rate, and thawing rate. Many workers do not pay attention to this important aspect of cryopreservation.[16] A common extender contains Tris, 6.06 g; fructose, 2.5 g; citric acid, 3.4 g; and deionized water, 184 mL. To this, glycerol and egg yolk are added to a final concentration of 8 and 20 per cent, respectively. Penicillin and streptomycin are frequently used as described earlier to prevent bacterial growth. Before diluting the whole ejaculate, a test-dilution with a small volume of semen should be performed; and providing that the extender has no deleterious effect, the remaining semen can be diluted with the extender at 37°C. It is preferable to make a volume:volume dilution rather than trying to obtain a standard spermatozoal concentration. To achieve a standard spermatozoal concentration would require the use of several extenders of different composition otherwise the concentration of cryoprotectant (e.g., glycerol, egg yolk) will vary and adversely affect the freeze-thawing process as described earlier. The optimal dilution rate appears to be 1:4 (semen:extender). After dilution the sample is re-evaluated and then placed into insulated vials that are slowly cooled to 5°C.

Spermatozoa requires a pause of several hours during cooling, before freezing, to develop maximal resistance to the effects of freezing. The optimal time taken during the cooling process is related to the glycerol concentration of the extended semen. In some species, the cooling and equilibration time has been shown to influence sample fertility. In the dog, most studies have not fully evaluated cooling rates or equilibration times before freezing and have used arbitrary values, often in the region of 2 to 4 hours.

Once cooled, semen must be packaged before freezing. The pellet method of semen freezing (dropping small volumes of the cooled semen onto a block of dry ice) was adopted in many early studies, although it is now more common to freeze semen in 0.5 or 0.25-mL straws. Although various studies have compared the straw and pellet methods, these have often been flawed because these are not simply alternative packaging methods but they also produce markedly different sample freezing rates. The method chosen, therefore, will be determined by the extender used and the particular cooling rate and equilibration time. Pelleted semen is normally plunged into liquid nitrogen after freezing on the dry ice block. For semen packed in straws, however, a variety of freezing rates have been advocated, generally within the range of −10 to −100°C per minute. It is difficult to express an average rate, because the freezing curve is usually sigmoid in shape and the plateau phase varies in duration depending on the freezing method. For practical freezing, straws are often placed in a wire basket in liquid nitrogen vapor. The height above the liquid nitrogen influences the freezing rate. As discussed previously, this procedure is optimized according to the extender, cooling rate, equilibration time, and size of straw used.

The warming phase of the freeze thaw process is as important to cell survival as the cooling phase. Straws of frozen semen are frequently thawed by immersion in cold or warm water. Rewarming in water at 75°C for a few seconds has been shown to improve motility and acrosome integrity of dog sperm frozen in straws, but the optimal rate will depend on the other freezing conditions. The freeze-thaw process causes a considerable decrease in spermatozoal motility and longevity. For this reason, fertility rates are highest when uterine insemination is performed.

TIMING OF INSEMINATION

The optimal time for insemination may vary according to the type of semen that is to be inseminated; frozen-thawed semen is often of poor quality and must be deposited into the female reproductive tract when fertile oocytes are available. In the bitch, the oocyte is ovulated in an immature state and, unlike other species, cannot be fertilized immediately. Fertilization occurs after maturation of the primary oocyte, extrusion of the polar body, and completion of the first meiotic division. These events are not completed until at least 48 hours after ovulation; however, oocytes remain viable within the reproductive tract for a further 4 to 5 days. The "fertile period" of the bitch is the time during which a mating could result in a conception. It includes the time that oocytes are fertilizable (the 'fertilization period') but precedes this by several days, because sperm can survive within the female reproductive tract "waiting" for ovulation and oocyte maturation. The "fertile period" is, therefore, affected by the longevity of the dog's semen. Poor quality or cryopreserved semen has a short longevity in the female tract; and, therefore, insemination must be performed during the "fertilization period." This is the time when oocytes can be fertilized; it begins 4 days after the pre-ovulatory surge of luteinizing hormone (LH) and terminates 7 days after the pre-ovulatory surge of LH (it therefore extends between 2 to 5 days after ovulation) (Fig. 164–1).

For fresh semen insemination the bitch may be monitored using vaginal endoscopy and vaginal cytology, because these methods can adequately detect the "fertile period." However, for cryopreserved semen, insemination should be performed on the basis of plasma (serum) progesterone (or LH) measurement, because these methods allow the detection of the "fertilization period" (see Chapter 157).

NUMBER OF SPERM INSEMINATED

Successful inseminations with frozen-thawed semen have, in general, used high numbers of spermatozoa and, or, frequent insemination. Success rates of up to 85 per cent have been claimed by inseminating 200 to 800 million frozen-thawed spermatozoa an average of four times per bitch. Such insemination doses are up to four times that required for normal conception with intravaginal insemination of fresh semen.[3]

Intrauterine insemination of spermatozoa requires fewer spermatozoa per insemination than intravaginal insemination, and Farstad and Andersen Berg[17] suggested that 100×10^6 of live spermatozoa gave acceptable conception rates and litter sizes. Commonly, a total of 150 to 200×10^6 motile spermatozoa inseminated on two to three occasions is believed to be adequate, although two insemination doses of 75×10^6 spermatozoa has been successful in the fox.[18] It is likely that the higher the number of spermatozoa per insemination, the higher will be the fertility (up to a threshold value); and the examination of this variable is particularly relevant. Many breeders aim to split ejaculates and sell the maximum number of insemination doses, often at the expense of pregnancy rate and litter size.

TECHNIQUE OF INSEMINATION

Care must be taken during the manipulation of semen before and during an insemination. Certain plastic tubes, syringes (especially those with rubber plungers), and lubricants can have deleterious effects on sperm. All equipment should be tested for toxicity before use in the clinical situation.

Natural mating results in vaginal contractions that propel the ejaculate cranially into the uterus and uterine contractions that propel the ejaculate toward the uterine tube. These contractions are generally absent when a bitch is artificially inseminated, and, therefore, spermatozoal transport is reduced. It is clear that uterine insemination results in a higher pregnancy rate and litter size than vaginal insemination, probably by ensuring that sperm reach the uterotubal junction. Uterine insemination is necessary with frozen-thawed semen to ensure an adequate success.

VAGINAL INSEMINATION

Semen is normally deposited into the vagina close to the cervix using a long inseminating pipette, and the pipette is flushed with warmed physiologic saline. Some workers use the third fraction of the ejaculate to flush the catheter; however, surprisingly in vitro this may have deleterious effects on sperm longevity.[19] The vagina may be stimulated using a finger in an attempt to initiate vaginal and uterine contractions that may propel the ejaculate cranially within the reproductive tract. Additionally, it is common to raise the hindquarters of the bitch to ensure that the semen runs cranially and pools around the cervix. The cervix is normally open during estrus and should allow entry of the ejaculate; however, the cervix appears to close just before the end of the fertilization period.[20]

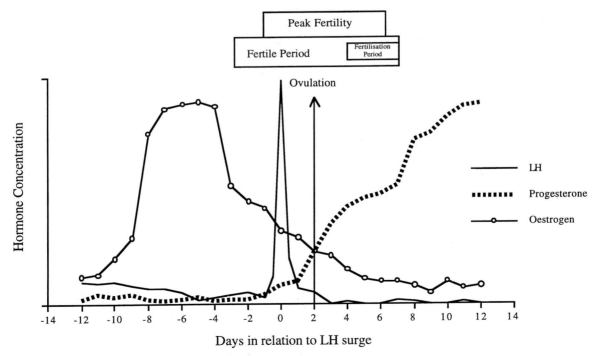

Figure 164–1. Schematic representation of the changes in plasma estrogen, luteinizing hormone, and progesterone in relation to the fertile period and fertilization period of the bitch.

UTERINE INSEMINATION

It is difficult to place a catheter through the cervix because the vagina of the bitch is long and narrow and the cervical opening is small and placed at an angle to the vagina. Several methods have therefore been developed to achieve uterine insemination:

Foley Catheter Technique

An especially designed Foley catheter (manufactured by IMV, Paris, France) may be used to perform an effective uterine insemination. The catheter has two components: an outer sheath with the Foley bulb positioned at its tip and a second catheter with a side exit port that is inserted through the outer sheath. The catheter is inserted into the vagina up to the level of the cervix, and the bulb is inflated so that it forms a seal against the vaginal wall. The inner catheter is then advanced and the semen is deposited, after which the inner catheter is withdrawn inside the Foley catheter, thereby closing the side exit ports. Using this catheter means that semen can only run forward through the cervix and does not drain back along the vagina. The device is left in place for up to 15 minutes to ensure that a pool of semen is located next to the cervix. The Foley bulb may simulate the copulatory tie and result in vaginal contractions. The principle of the technique is excellent, but there is often leakage of semen around, and through, the catheters.

Norwegian Catheter Technique

This device (available from Dr. J. Fougner, Oslo, Norway) consists of an outer plastic sheath and inner metal catheter with rounded bulb-ended tip. The outer plastic catheter is inserted into the vagina to the level of the cervix. The cervix is palpated transabdominally and realigned so that it is continuous with the direction of the vagina. The inner catheter is pushed forward to the cervix and manipulated through the cervix.[18] The technique works well but requires training and considerable practice; however, it may be very difficult to perform in large, obese, or nervous animals that have a tense abdomen.

Endoscopic Technique

This method requires a rigid endoscope, preferably with a mechanism for deflecting a catheter at the endoscope tip.[21] The endoscope is inserted into the vagina and advanced to the level of the cervix. Inflation of the vagina is useful for allowing the identification of the cervical os. The inseminating catheter is inserted through the endoscope, and the deflection device is used to direct the catheter into the cervical os. The technique requires training and practice before catheterization can be achieved reliably. Some bitches need to be sedated, otherwise movement of the bitch makes placement of the catheter difficult.

Surgical Technique

This technique has gained wide acceptance in some countries and is often advocated by veterinarians because, for them, it requires no special training. However, consideration should be given to the ethics of performing a surgical procedure to achieve a pregnancy.

A small caudal ventral midline laparotomy incision is made and the uterine body is lifted into the incision. A 22-gauge over-the-needle intravenous catheter is placed into the lumen of the uterine body, and padded bowel clamps are placed across the cervix. The semen is introduced slowly into the uterus and allowed to run proximally into the uterine horns. After removal of the catheter, pressure is applied to the site to provide hemostasis; usually no sutures are required. The abdominal incision is closed routinely.

SUCCESS WITH ARTIFICIAL INSEMINATION

Owners often have high expectations of artificial insemination. There are, however, a number of factors that influence the subsequent pregnancy rates:

- Initial seminal quality
- Degree of spermatozoal damage (and reduced longevity) caused by preservation
- Spermatozoal damage caused by poor handling techniques
- Number of sperm inseminated
- Timing of insemination
- Site of semen deposition
- Fertility of the bitch

In addition, it may be extremely difficult to preserve the semen from certain dogs. The reason for this phenomenon is not known.

Some workers have reported high success rates with artificial insemination. It is likely that these workers have optimized the parameters that are under their control (e.g., sperm handling, timing of insemination, site of semen deposition). When these factors are not carefully monitored, success rates are low.[22] The "world average" success rates for fertile bitches inseminated at the appropriate time are:

- Fresh semen: 60 to 90 per cent pregnancy rate
- Chilled semen: 50 to 70 per cent pregnancy rate
- Frozen semen: 30 to 60 per cent pregnancy rate

It is clear that there is considerable overlap in the success rates that may be achieved when using artificial insemination. For each of the methods the factors just listed are relevant; however, for chilled semen an additional factor is important—the time between collection and insemination. England and Ponzio[23] demonstrated, in a split-ejaculate experiment, that semen quality of chilled semen deteriorated on a daily basis but that in the first 2 days after collection the quality was always superior to frozen-thawed semen. The mean time taken for the quality of chilled semen to become equal to frozen-thawed semen was approximately 4 days. It may, therefore, be preferable in many cases to used chilled semen, unless the transportation time or other considerations necessitate semen storage for more than 4 days.

PATHOGENS THAT MAY BE TRANSMITTED IN DOG SEMEN

There is little information concerning the transmission of infectious organisms in dog semen. For these reasons, several countries have strict guidelines regarding the health requirements of dogs before the export of semen and the sanitary conditions under which semen is collected and processed. Whereas canine herpesvirus may be transmitted at

REP

coitus, it seems likely that this is by means of direct animal contact rather than transmission within semen. Rabies virus is unlikely to be found in semen except possibly during, or a few days before, overt clinical signs of the disease. Information about other organisms is scant.

INFERTILITY IN THE DOG

A number of abnormalities of the genital tract may result in male infertility, including abnormalities of the penis, sheath, testes, epididymides, vasa deferentia, urethra, and prostate gland. These conditions may result in reduced libido, failure to copulate, or failure of conception after an apparently normal mating. For the present review, consideration is given specifically to infertility associated with abnormal semen quality. When investigating these cases it is imperative to collect a detailed breeding history and to perform a full clinical examination of the reproductive tract.

A number of diagnostic procedures may be performed in addition to semen evaluation. Real-time diagnostic B-mode ultrasound imaging of the testes and epididymides is especially useful because it allows appreciation of the internal architecture, as well as size and shape. Ultrasonography is suitable for the detection of both focal and diffuse lesions that cannot be appreciated by palpation and for the further investigation of lesions that can be palpated. Testicular biopsy specimens may be obtained by incision or needle aspiration,[24] although this may be followed by a marked inflammatory response; incisional biopsies may produce hypospermatogenesis, necrosis, tubular degeneration, fibrosis, and inflammation; and both techniques should be avoided whenever possible. The measurement of circulating plasma hormones may be of value for the confirmation of testicular activity and for the diagnosis of testicular failure. Resting plasma concentrations of testosterone, LH, and follicle-stimulating hormone may be diagnostic; however, concentrations fluctuate markedly, and serial sampling or the response of plasma testosterone to the administration of human chorionic gonadotropin may be of more value.

AZOOSPERMIA

Azoospermia is an apparently normal ejaculate that contains no spermatozoa. This condition is a relatively common finding in clinical practice, and full clinical evaluation including palpation and ultrasonographic examination of the scrotal contents is essential in achieving and accurate diagnosis. There are three main causes of azoospermia, including incomplete ejaculation, obstruction of the outflow tract, and gonadal dysfunction.

INCOMPLETE EJACULATION

Nervous males that are inexperienced may frequently have an incomplete ejaculation. The problem may be unrecognized and incorrectly diagnosed as azoospermia. The likelihood of failing to collect a full sample can be reduced by teasing the dog with a bitch in estrus or a spayed bitch in which methyl-*p*-hydroxybenzoate[25] has been applied to the vulva. Alternatively, vaginal fluid from estrus bitches that has been frozen on cotton swabs can be used. When incomplete ejaculation is suspected, it is most simple to attempt to collect ejaculate from the dog on another occasion. Results of clinical examination of these dogs should be normal.

Carnitine and alkaline phosphatase are present in the canine ejaculate and appear to be of epididymal origin.[7] Absence of these compounds is diagnostic of incomplete ejaculation or obstructive azoospermia. Measurement of alkaline phosphatase is common to many diagnostic laboratories and therefore is a readily available test. Examination of a urine sediment sample after centrifugation can be useful for distinguishing between these two conditions, because dogs with incomplete ejaculation frequently have sperm present within the bladder whereas those with obstruction do not.

OBSTRUCTIVE AZOOSPERMIA

Obstruction of the collecting ducts, epididymides, or ductus deferens may occur in the dog, and there are a number of potential causes, including acute inflammation, spermatocele, sperm granuloma, neoplasia, previous vasectomy, and segmental aplasia.[7] When obstructive azoospermia occurs, there is usually a low concentration of carnitine and alkaline phosphatase and an absence of sperm within the urine as described earlier. In each of these cases there is commonly obvious disease of the scrotum, testes, or epididymides. It is rare for a dog to have obstructive azoospermia without other clinical findings. This emphasizes the need to perform a complete physical examination of the reproductive tract in all cases.

GONADAL DYSFUNCTION

There are a relatively large number of causes of gonadal dysfunction; however, these can most simply be classified as congenital or acquired.

Congenital Gonadal Dysfunction

Phenotypically male dogs with chromosomal abnormalities such as XXY or XX-male syndrome usually have aspermatogenesis. These cases are relatively easy to diagnose because there is usually testicular hypoplasia, which can be readily diagnosed on clinical examination.

Acquired Gonadal Dysfunction

Dogs that were previously normal and fertile and subsequently become azoospermic are interesting to investigate and are the most common problem seen by veterinary practitioners. In an early study, Harrop[26] found that of 200 infertile dogs, 169 had no sperm within the ejaculate and, of these, 158 had previously been proven sires. Cases of functional azoospermia with spermatogenic arrest have been reported in related Shetland collies, Welsh springer spaniels, and Labrador retrievers. Allen and Patel[27] demonstrated the presence of autoantibodies directed against sperm tails in the serum of dogs with azoospermia and concluded that the condition was an autoimmune orchitis. A relationship between focal degenerative orchitis and thyroiditis in a closed colony of beagles has also been identified.[28] An effect of season of the year has been demonstrated in extremely warm climates.[29]

Drugs and toxins are frequently cited as being the cause of azoospermia[7]; however, with the exception of deliberate and prolonged administration of gonadotropin releasing hormone agonists and antagonists, most agents are unable to completely eliminate sperm from the ejaculate, and oligoteratozoospermia rather than azoospermia occurs.

When investigating dogs with acquired azoospermia it is clear that most have normal concentrations of carnitine and alkaline phosphatase within the ejaculate. They may also have normal plasma (serum) values of testosterone and luteinizing hormone, although concentrations of follicle-stimulating hormone may be elevated presumably due to a reduced production of inhibin by the Sertoli cells. Serial measurement of follicle-stimulating hormone may therefore be useful in these cases, as may a testicular biopsy. In reality, however, these tests are somewhat pointless because they simply confirm the diagnosis that can be reached by collection of several ejaculates, and they add nothing to the management of such cases, because the prognosis is hopeless.

OLIGOZOOSPERMIA

Oligozoospermia is the term used to describe low numbers of morphologically normal sperm within the ejaculate. This is rare in dogs but may occur for a variety of reasons:

1. *Incomplete ejaculation.* Incomplete ejaculation may result in a low number of normal sperm within the ejaculate. It can be diagnosed and managed as described previously.

2. *Retrograde ejaculation.* Retrograde ejaculation in dogs is extremely rare. When it occurs there may be a small volume of semen collected despite normal urethral contractions. The majority of the semen is ejaculated in a retrograde manner into the bladder.[30] Lavage of the bladder with physiologic saline and examination of the flushings may be diagnostic. These dogs can be managed by preventing urination before mating or semen collection, although sympathomimetic agents have also been suggested as being useful. Semen may be collected from the bladder after ejaculation and washed free of urine. However, there is often poor motility, and successful insemination requires uterine deposition of the sperm.

3. *"Overuse."* In some, often older dogs, oligozoospermia may occur when there is frequent ejaculation. In these cases it is likely that the daily sperm production is low; but with sexual rest, the extragonadal reserves increase to a suitable value. Careful management of the time of mating is required in these cases.

4. *Recent testicular insult.* It is possible for a particular testicular insult (e.g., pyrexia or toxin) to damage spermatogonia without affecting the spermatocytes. In these cases, oligospermia may be present initially,[31] although later in the course of the pathology abnormal sperm are also present in the ejaculate.

5. *Partial obstruction.* Unilateral obstruction of the collecting ducts, epididymides, or ductus deferens may reduce the number of normal sperm ejaculated. The condition can be diagnosed as described previously.

TERATOZOOSPERMIA

Teratozoospermia is the term used to describe abnormal sperm morphology. A high incidence of morphologically abnormal spermatozoa is often associated with reduced fertility in many animal species. In many cases, morphologic abnormalities result in impaired spermatozoal motility such that teratozoospermia and asthenozoospermia occur concurrently.

Although many authors have reported common dog sperm abnormalities and have suggested minimal values of morphologically normal dog spermatozoa for optimal fertility,

there have been few reports concerning the influence of specific morphologic abnormalities on fertility. One abnormality associated with infertility was first described by Aughey and Renton,[32] when abnormal midpiece droplets were identified in a greyhound. Subsequently, Oettle and Soley[33] noted infertility in a dog in which 80 per cent of spermatozoa had defects of the headbase/midpiece region, manifested by disruption of the midpiece attachment to the head. Defects of the midpiece were also found to be associated with infertility in seven of nine dogs examined by Renton and associates.[34] The most common abnormality in these dogs was swelling of the midpiece region with an incidence ranging from 1 to 96 per cent, although one dog with 94 per cent midpiece defects was apparently fertile.[34] Spermatozoa with midpiece defects and deformed acrosomes have also been found associated with experimental *Brucella canis* infection. In each of these cases the cause of the infertility was not suggested, although Renton and associates[34] noted that there were spermatozoal membrane changes evident electron microscopically. Plummer and colleagues[35] also identified an infertile dog in which 87 per cent of spermatozoa had proximal cytoplasmic droplets. Electron microscopic studies showed that there were axonemal and mitochondrial defects both within these membrane swellings and at other regions of the midpiece. No other specific spermatozoal morphologic abnormalities have been reported to affect fertility in the dog; however, dogs with low numbers of morphologically normal sperm have reduced fertility.[15] Large numbers of primary spermatozoal abnormalities may result from orchitis, congenital defects of spermatogenesis, toxin exposure, administration of hormonal or chemotherapeutic agents, or increased scrotal temperature.[31] Large numbers of secondary spermatozoal abnormalities may occur with epididymal disorders or after the administration of agents (such as reproductive steroids) that have a direct influence on epididymal function.[36] It is also clear that dogs that are azoospermic have previously been oligozoospermic, and serial monitoring may demonstrate a gradual decline in semen quality in these cases.

A relationship between fertility and the percentage of morphologically normal sperm was only found in men with mixed sperm morphologic abnormalities when a strict classification of morphologic normality was used.[37] The use of strict criteria for morphologic assessment should be advocated in the dog.

ASTHENOZOOSPERMIA

Asthenozoospermia refers to normal sperm morphology but a reduction in motility. As previously described, careful assessment of motility is necessary to ensure that these cases are adequately detected. The condition is rare in the dog without concurrent teratozoospermia. There are several recognized causes:

1. *Inappropriate analysis temperature.* Spermatozoal motility should be evaluated at a standard temperature to ensure repeatable and reliable results. Evaluation at temperatures less than 25°C results in an erroneously low value for normal forward progressive motility, whereas spermatozoa rapidly become immotile when temperatures exceed 40°C.

2. *Ejaculate contamination.* Contamination of the ejaculate with toxic compounds (including latex artificial vagina liners, lubricants, certain plastic syringes, urine, water, sterilizing agents) can all reduce motility or produce immotile sperm without producing obvious morphologic changes.

REP

3. *Agglutination of sperm.* In dogs that produce antisperm antibodies, sperm agglutination and poor motility often results. Although the cause of such antibody production is not known in many cases, it has been demonstrated in experimental infection with *Brucella canis.*

4. *Ciliary dyskinesia.* Immotile cilia syndrome is an extremely rare condition in the dog. In the few cases identified there is complete absence of motility. Sperm usually have marked midpiece abnormalities; that is, there is a concurrent teratozoospermia.

NORMOSPERMIA

There are a considerable number of cases when dogs are apparently infertile despite having normal semen quality. In many of these cases there are anatomic, physical, psychological, or management problems that prevent normal courtship, intromission, and ejaculation. Some workers suggest that a positive semen culture, and/or changes in the pH, biochemistry, or cellularity of the prostatic fluid or seminal plasma, can influence fertility. In general, however, a significant alteration from normal for these parameters results in sperm morphologic changes that influence fertility.[38]

CONCLUSION

The development of accurate and repeatable methods for the evaluation of semen, and the establishment of normal acceptable ranges for fertility, has dramatically increased our ability to diagnose and manage dogs with fertility problems and to assist breeders with artificial insemination programs. It is clear, however, that further work in the area is warranted. The development of in vitro techniques to evaluate the functional capacity of spermatozoa and to assess the ability of spermatozoa to interact and survive within the female reproductive tract and associate with and penetrate oocytes will allow us to increase the fecundity of this species.

REFERENCES

1. Mortimer D, et al: A technical note on diluting semen for the haemocytometric determination of sperm concentration. Hum Reprod 4:166, 1989.
2. Olar TT, et al: Relationships among testicular size, daily production and output of spermatozoa, and extragonadal spermatozoal reserves of the dog. Biol Reprod 29:1114, 1983.
3. Tsutsui T, et al: Artificial insemination with fresh semen in beagle bitches. Jpn J Vet Sci 50:193, 1988.
4. Hewitt DA, England GCW: An investigation of capacitation and the acrosome reaction in dog spermatozoa using a dual fluorescent staining technique. Anim Reprod Sci 51:321, 1998.
5. Holt WV, et al: Computer-assisted measurement of sperm swimming speed in human semen: Correlation of results with *in vitro* fertilization assays. Fertil Steril 44:112, 1985.
6. Gunzel-Apel AR, et al: Computer-assisted analysis of motility, velocity and linearity of dog spermatozoa. J Reprod Fertil Suppl 47:271, 1993.
7. Olson PN: Clinical approach for evaluating dogs with azoospermia or aspermia. Vet Clin North Am Small Anim Pract 21:591, 1991.
8. Allen WE: Macrophage cells in the semen of a dog with oligospermia. Vet Rec 109:310, 1981.
9. Hrudka F, Post K: Leukophages in canine semen. Andrologia 15:26, 1983.
10. Allen WE, Dagnall GRJ: Some observations on the aerobic bacterial flora of the genital tract of the dog and bitch. J Small Anim Pract 23:325, 1982.
11. Doig PA: The genital *Mycoplasma* and *Ureaplasma* flora of healthy and diseased dogs. Can J Comp Med 45:233, 1981.
12. England GCW, Allen WE: Seminal characteristics and fertility in dogs. Vet Rec 125:399, 1989.
13. England GCW, Plummer JM: Hypo-osmotic swelling of dog spermatozoa. J Reprod Fertil Suppl 47:261, 1993.
14. Hewitt DA, England GCW: The canine oocyte penetration assay: Its use as an indicator of dog spermatozoal performance in vitro. Anim Reprod Sci 50:123, 1997.
15. Oettle EE: Sperm morphology and fertility in the dog. J Reprod Fertil Suppl 47:257, 1993.
16. England GCW: Cryopreservation of dog semen: A review. J Reprod Fertil Suppl 47:243, 1993.
17. Farstad W, Andersen Berg K: Factors influencing the success rate of artificial insemination with frozen semen in the dog. J Reprod Fertil Suppl 39:289, 1989.
18. Fougner JA: Artificial insemination in fox breeding. J Reprod Fertil Suppl 39:317, 1989.
19. England GCW, Allen WE: Factors affecting the viability of canine spermatozoa: I. Potential influences during processing for artificial insemination. Theriogenology 37:363, 1992.
20. Silva LD, et al: Cervical opening in relation to progesterone and oestradiol during heat in beagle bitches. J Reprod Fertil 104:85, 1995.
21. Wilson MS: Non-surgical intrauterine artificial insemination in bitches using frozen semen. J Reprod Fertil Suppl 47:307, 1993.
22. Goodman MF, Cain JL: Retrospective evaluation of artificial insemination with chilled extended semen in the dog. J Reprod Fertil Suppl 47:554, 1993.
23. England GCW, Ponzio P: Comparison of the quality of frozen-thawed and cooled-rewarmed dog semen. Theriogenology 46:165, 1996.
24. Dahlbom M, et al: Testicular fine needle aspiration cytology as a diagnostic tool in dog infertility. J Small Anim Pract 38:506, 1997.
25. Goodwin M, et al: Sex pheromone in the dog. Science 203:559, 1979.
26. Harrop AE: An aspect of infertility in the dog. Vet Rec 72:362, 1960.
27. Allen WE, Patel JR: Autoimmune orchitis in two related dogs. J Small Anim Pract 23:713, 1982.
28. Fritz TE, et al: Pathology and familial incidence of orchitis and its relation to thyroiditis in a closed beagle colony. Exp Mol Pathol 24:142, 1976.
29. Takeishi M, et al: Studies on reproduction of the dog. Bull Coll Agri Vet Med Nikon 32:224, 1975.
30. Root MV, et al: Concurrent retrograde ejaculation and hypothyroidism in a dog—case report. Theriogenology 41:593, 1994.
31. Myers-Wallen VN: Clinical approach to infertile male dogs with sperm in the ejaculate. Vet Clin North Am Small Anim Pract 21:609, 1991.
32. Aughey E, Renton JP: The ultrastructure of abnormal spermatozoa in a stud dog. J Reprod Fertil 25:303, 1971.
33. Oettle EE, Soley JT: Infertility in a Maltese poodle as a result of a sperm midpiece defect. J South Afr Vet Assoc 56:103, 1985.
34. Renton JP, et al: A spermatozoal abnormality in dogs related to infertility. Vet Rec 118:429, 1986.
35. Plummer JM, et al: A spermatozoal midpiece abnormality associated with infertility in a Lhasa apso dog. J Small Anim Pract 28:743, 1987.
36. England GCW: Effect of progestogens and androgens upon spermatogenesis and steroidogenesis in dogs. J Reprod Fertil Suppl 51:123, 1997.
37. Kruger TF, et al: Sperm morphologic features as a prognostic factor in in vitro fertilization. Fertil Steril 46:1118, 1986.
38. Johnston SD: Performing a complete canine semen evaluation in a small animal hospital. Vet Clin North Am Small Anim Pract 21:545, 1991.

CHAPTER 165

INHERITED AND CONGENITAL DISORDERS OF THE MALE AND FEMALE REPRODUCTIVE SYSTEMS

Mushtaq A. Memon and W. Duane Mickelsen

Veterinarians and dog breeders need to be aware of, and able to recognize, congenital defects that have economic and biomedical consequences. Not only is diagnosis necessary, but also veterinarians should be knowledgeable of methods to reduce, control, or eliminate genetically caused defects. Many genetic conditions in animals are models for human genetic diseases and are valuable as research models. In cases of previously unrecognized conditions, veterinarians should contact veterinary colleges conducting research on genetic diseases.

Genetic problems may spread through a breed or kennel until they are economically disastrous and difficult to control. Many breed associations have programs to monitor and control undesirable genetic traits including genetic defects. Understanding the clinical signs, morphologic or biochemical lesions, and transmission patterns is necessary before advice can be given and control measures instituted.

EMBRYOLOGY OF THE REPRODUCTIVE ORGANS

NORMAL DEVELOPMENT

At fertilization, the sex chromosome constitution of the zygote normally becomes either XX or XY and is then maintained by mitotic division in all cell types, including primary germ cells. In early embryonic life, the gonad is undifferentiated. Normally an ovary develops if the chromosomal sex is XX and testicles develop in the presence of the Y chromosome. In normal embryos (XY), the testes produce two substances necessary for the formation of normal male internal and external structures. Müllerian-inhibiting factor is a glycoprotein produced by the Sertoli cells that causes the müllerian duct system to regress. The second substance is testosterone, a steroid produced by the Leydig cells, which stabilizes the wolffian duct system so that the vas deferens and epididymis are formed.[1]

In the absence of a testis, the indifferent embryo will develop into a phenotypic female. The müllerian duct system persists and forms the oviducts, uterus, and cranial vagina. The wolffian duct system regresses. The urogenital sinus, genital tubercle, and genital swellings form the caudal vagina and vestibule, the clitoris, and the vulva, respectively.[1]

In the female fetus, the paired müllerian ducts join caudally to form the body of the uterus, cervix, and vagina. The vestibule, urethra, and urinary bladder develop from the urogenital sinus. The hymen is formed by the fusion of the müllerian ducts and urogenital sinus. Histologically, the hymen consists of two epithelial linings, with a thin layer of mesoderm in between. The congenital tubercle forms the clitoris, the genital folds contribute to the vestibule, and the genital swellings enlarge to form the vulvar lips.[1]

CAUSES OF CONGENITAL DISORDER

Congenital defects are defined as abnormalities of structure and function present at birth. Purebred dogs are more frequently affected than are crossbreeds.[2, 3]

Genes are chemical entities that control growth and development within environmental limits. They are present in pairs (alleles) located on chromosomes. Dogs have 39 pairs of chromosomes, and cats have 19 pairs. All pairs but one (sex chromosomes) are exactly the same size and shape. Gene pairs are located on the same location (locus) of homologous chromosomes. Such genes on the given locus may be identical and are referred to as homozygous for that locus. A gene has the property to mutate while the other allele remains unchanged.[3]

Recessive Genes. These defects are caused by a related pair of mutant genes, two alleles at a single locus, or one gene inherited from each parent. The defective offspring is homozygous with respect to the mutant gene. Although two defective parents will produce only defective offspring, most defective dogs do not reproduce. Therefore, most defective dogs are born to normal parents. Each normal parent that produces a defective offspring from the two abnormal genes are heterozygotes. If normal homozygotes are mated, they produce only normal offspring. However, when normal dogs that have produced a defective offspring are mated repeatedly, 25 per cent of their offspring will be defective and 75 per cent will be normal.[2] In addition, two thirds of the normal dogs from such parents also carry a hidden abnormal gene (heterozygote) that they can also transmit to their offspring. Therefore, recessive defects can be carried in a breed for several generations by normal carrier animals. Inbreeding is one way of exposing abnormal recessive genes.

Dominant Genes. Dominant inheritance is the reverse of recessive inheritance. In these cases, the dominant genes are passed from one generation to the next and their expressions do not skip generations as recessive genes may do.

They are usually found in parents and offspring. With dominant inheritance, normal, unaffected animals breed true, but defective animals may produce both normal and abnormal offspring.[3] Dominant defects are easily controlled by eliminating all the defective animals.

Incomplete dominance creates three types of animals: normal, slightly defective, and severely deformed. Both the normal and slightly defective breed true, but the severely deformed animals, when mated together, produce one quarter normal, one half slightly defective, and one quarter severely deformed offspring. These defects are easily controlled by eliminating all the defective progeny.

Overdominance is similar to incomplete dominance in that normal, superior, and deformed animals are produced.[3] The normal and deformed breed true, but the superior animals, when mated together, produce one quarter normal, one half superior, and one quarter defective animals. The problem is that the superior animals are usually selected as breeders in preference to normal animals. The cost of mating is a 25 per cent loss of offspring because they are defective.

Chromosomal Defects. A few characteristics are linked with the sex of animals. Chromosomal defects may be introduced by environmental factors, or they may be inherited. Chromosomal aberrations may take different forms such as single and double gaps, breaks, ring chromosomes, and fragmentation.

Ploidy refers to the number of chromosomes within a cell. Haploid (N) is the number in the gamete, whereas diploid (2N) is the normal number in a somatic cell. *Polyploidy* is a condition in which the number of chromosomes in a cell is increased by an exact multiple of the haploid state. *Aneuploidy* is an increase or decrease in the number of one or more chromosomes, but not an entire haploid number.[4] It usually refers to an increase or decrease of one chromosome. One extra chromosome added to a homologous pair is called trisomy; a loss of one from a homologous pair is monosomy.

TYPES OF DISORDERS OF SEXUAL DEVELOPMENT

ABNORMAL CHROMOSOME NUMBERS

XXY Syndrome. In dogs, XXY trisomy results from a female gamete 40,XX and a male gamete 39,XY. This condition can result from nondisjunction during the first or second meiotic division of gametogenesis or from mitotic nondisjunction in the developing zygote.[5] It is referred to as Klinefelter's syndrome and is characterized by wide variation in phenotypic presentation, including testicular hypoplasia and hypoplasia of tubular and accessory reproductive organs, azoospermia, and sterility. Because of this variation in phenotypic presentation of the 79,XXY genotype, cytogenic investigation is necessary to accurately diagnose the condition. A 21-month-old Norwich terrier was reported infertile because of azoospermia resulting from seminiferous tubule dysgenesis.[6] The dysgenesis was attributed to the 79,XXY chromosome complement (Fig. 165–1). Histologically, the testes of this 79,XXY dog consisted of small, spermatogenic seminiferous tubules lined almost exclusively by a one-cell-thick layer of Sertoli cells (Fig. 165–2).

The XXY syndrome has been described in cats as well. These cats may be of any color, but these animals are usually recognized as tricolor (calico) males. Early in female embryonic development, either the paternal or maternal X chromosome is inactivated in a random fashion with each

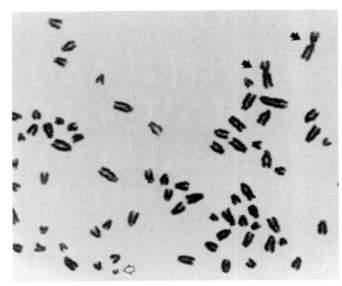

Figure 165–1. Chromosome complement of a 21-month-old male Norwich terrier that was azoospermic. Sex chromosomes are indicated (open arrow, Y chromosome; dark arrows, X chromosomes). (From Nie GJ, Johnston SD, Hayden DW, et al: Azoospermia associated with 79, XXY chromosome complement. Theriogenology Question of the Month. JAVMA 212:1545, 1998.)

cell.[4] Subsequent cell populations bear the same inactivated X chromosome (Barr body). The genes for orange and nonorange coat color are alleles at the X-linked orange locus. The O allele produces orange hair, whereas the O+ allele produces nonorange (black and brown). This calico pattern is seen normally in females heterozygous for these alleles, since only one allele is expressed in each cell population, producing patches of different hair color.[7] Calico males have at least two X chromosomes, each bearing a different allele at the orange locus. Commonly, these aneuploidic cats have an XXY chromosomal picture and are further characterized by testicular hypoplasia.[7] However, other chromosome constitutions are possible (see chimeras and mosiacs later).

XO Syndrome. In humans, this syndrome is called Turner's syndrome, and affected individuals develop as phenotypic females with infantile genitalia and short stature. In dogs that have a normal female phenotype but have not cycled by 24 months of age, the XO syndrome should be considered.

XO syndrome cats are phenotypic females.[4] The XO condition may be recognized by their coat color pattern when family history is known. Matings in which one parent is orange and the other is nonorange should produce female offspring that all have the tortoiseshell pattern. A female that is all orange or all nonorange should be suspected of the XO condition.[7] These kittens have normal ovaries at birth, which apparently become dysgenetic in the adults.[4]

XXX Syndrome. A 79,XXX chromosome constitution was reported in a 4-year-old anestrus bitch.[8] Ovaries without follicles, a small uterus, and a female phenotype were present. Serum gonadotropins were elevated, and serum progesterone levels were low. Although fertile individuals with triple X syndrome have been reported in other species, abnormalities of the estrous cycle and infertility are frequent findings in XXX dogs.[8]

Chimeras and Mosaics. A chimera is an individual composed of two or more cell populations, each population arising from different individuals. A mosaic is also an indi-

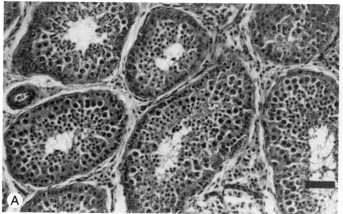
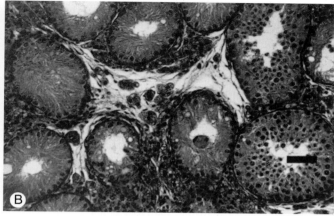

Figure 165–2. Photomicrographs of a hematoxylin and eosin–stained section of testis from a clinically normal dog *(left)* and a trichrome-stained section of testis from a Norwich terrier with a 79,XXY chromosome abnormality *(right)*. Seminiferous tubules in the clinically normal dog consist of Sertoli cells and germ cells in varying stages of maturation as well as small clusters of interstitial cells. In the 79,XXY dog, seminiferous tubules are lined only by Sertoli cells adjacent to a few tubules with germ cell elements. Bar = 50 μm. (From Nie GJ, Johnston SD, Hayden DW, et al: Azoospermia associated with 79,XXY chromosome complement. Theriogenology Question of the Month. JAVMA 212:1545, 1998.)

vidual composed of two or more cell populations having different chromosome constitutions, but the cells originate within the same individual. Whether a chimera or mosaic, the individual is composed of at least two cell populations having different chromosome constitutions.

True hermaphrodites have both ovarian and testicular tissue present in the same individual. One or both gonads may be ovotestes, or one gonad may be an ovary and the other a testis. Most canine true hermaphrodites reported have an XX sex chromosome constitution and will be discussed under the abnormalities of gonadal sex. True hermaphrodite chimeras are rare, and the few reported[9] were XX/XY or XX/XXY with enlarged clitoris (Fig. 165–3) but otherwise female in external appearance. All such dogs have had a history of failure to cycle or chronic vulvar irritation. Internally, testicular and ovarian tissue and a uterus were present. One feline true hermaphrodite cat had an XX/XY chromosomal constitution, a male phenotype externally, a scrotal testis, and an abdominal ovary.[4]

XX/XY chimeras with testes have been reported in dogs

and cats.[9] In the dog, a hypoplastic penis was located in a vulva-like structure. The gonads were located abdominally near the kidneys and contained dysgenic testicular tissue lacking spermatogenesis. The cats were similar, although one cat had small testicles located in the scrotum and spermatozoa present in the epididymis.

XY/XY chimeras with testes have been reported in several fertile male cats with normal male external phenotypes and tortoiseshell coat colors. These cats had normal testicular histology, including spermatogenesis.

ABNORMALITIES OF GONADAL SEX

XX Sex Reversal. A condition in animals in which chromosomal and gonadal sex do not agree is called sex reversal. Only XX sex reversal has been reported in the dog.[10] These dogs have a 78,XX chromosomal constitution with varying amounts of testicular tissue in the gonad. They have at least one ovotestis or testis. Individuals with this condition are XX true hermaphrodites or XX males.

Based upon breeding experiments, anatomic and histologic studies of affected offspring, in the American cocker spaniel, led to the conclusion that XX sex reversal is inherited as an autosomal recessive trait in this breed. Similar conditions have also been observed in families of beagles, English cocker spaniels, Weimaraners, and German shorthaired pointers.[9, 10]

XX True Hermaphrodite. A true hermaphrodite has both ovarian and testicular tissue. It occurs in three forms: unilateral (one gonad is an ovotestis and the other an ovary or testis), bilateral (both gonads are ovotestes), and lateral (a testis and an ovary). The degree of androgen-dependent masculinization of the internal and external genitalia is positively correlated to the proportion of testicular tissue in the gonads.[9] True hermaphroditism comprises only 25 per cent of the reported intersex cases in the dog, with the remainder being male pseudohermaphrodites, female pseudohermaphrodites, and unclassified.

XX Male Syndrome. These dogs have a 78,XX cytogenic constitution and bilateral testes that are usually undescended. The entire wolffian duct system is present bilaterally, and the prostate is present. The prepuce is present but

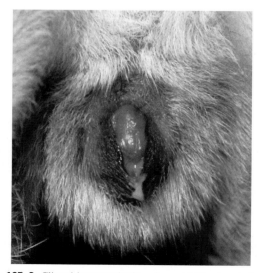

Figure 165–3. Clitoral hypertrophy in a dog exhibiting hermaphroditism.

usually located in an abnormal position such as hypospadia, or abnormal in shape such as hypoplasia or abnormal curvature. These dogs are usually sterile, and spermatogonia are absent even in testes located in the scrotum. Oviducts are absent in these males, but a complete uterus is present. Functionally active müllerian-inhibiting substance (MIS) is produced by the testicular tissue of XX males as well as XX true hermaphrodites.[9] The degree of oviductal regression in each is proportional to MIS production by the ipsilateral gonad.

The male determining histocompatibility antigen (H-Y antigen) likely accounts for the development of testicular tissue in XX hermaphrodites. Theories proposed for the presence of H-Y antigen in the absence of Y chromosome include mutant autosomal genes, mosaicism with an undetected XXY-bearing cell line, undetected XY cells, original XXY zygote with subsequent loss of the Y chromosome, X-Y interchange during meiosis, Y-to-autosomal translocations, and X-chromosome deletions.[11]

ABNORMALITIES OF PHENOTYPIC SEX

In these animals, chromosomal and gonadal sex are in agreement but the genitalia are ambiguous. Affected animals are either male or female pseudohermaphrodites.

Female Pseudohermaphrodites. Female pseudohermaphrodites have an XX chromosome constitution and ovaries, but the internal and external genitalia are masculinized. Those animals exposed to exogenous androgens are 78,XX. The degree of masculinization ranges from mild clitoral enlargement to nearly normal male external genitalia with a prostate internally. The cause is either androgen or progesterone administration during gestation or androgen administration to racing greyhounds. Affected dogs may attract male dogs, have cystic endometrial hyperplasia or pyometra, or have urinary incontinence from urine pooling in the vagina or uterus. Ovariohysterectomy is recommended.

Congenital abnormalities of the canine vagina and vulva include two forms of perforated hymen that have vesical septa or annular strictures, and incomplete fusion of the müllerian ducts that is manifested as elongated vertical septa or double vaginas. Vestibulovaginal strictures are also identified.[12] Bitches with these abnormalities are brought to veterinarians either because of unsuccessful attempts at natural breeding or due to chronic vaginitis in intact or in ovariohysterectomized bitches.[13] Clinical signs most commonly encountered include vaginal discharge, persistent licking, and attracting males. When the defect is corrected surgically, the clinical signs are resolved in most cases.

Premature gonadal failure has been reported[14] in phenotypically female dogs and cats with defective prenatal germ migration (ovarian aplasias), defective prenatal differentiation of the gonadal ridge into ovarian tissue (true hermaphroditism, male pseudohermaphroditism, ovarian dysgenesis in the presence of XO or XXX sex chromosome complements), or defective gamete maturation in the presence of primordial ovarian follicles (lymphocytic oophoritis, thyroid insufficiency). The most common of these is defective gonadal differentiation in animals with true hermaphroditism and failure of gamete maturation in thyroid insufficiency. A common clinical sign of premature gonadal failure in dogs and cats is failure to show a pubertal estrus by 2 years of age.

Male Pseudohermaphrodites. Male pseudohermaphrodites have an XY chromosome constitution and testes, but the internal or external genitalia are to some degree those of a female. Persistent müllerian duct syndrome is a form of inherited male pseudohermaphroditism occurring in miniature schnauzers.[9] Affected dogs are XY with bilateral testes and müllerian duct derivatives: oviducts, uterus, and cranial vagina.

Hypospadias. This is a developmental anomaly that affects both sexes and is characterized by ventral dystopia of the urethral meatus. In the male, the abnormality is noticed in location of the urinary orifice, being ventral and proximal to the normal site in the glans penis (Fig. 165–4). The etiology is thought to be inadequate fetal androgen production. The Boston terrier breed has been suggested to have a familial predisposition for hypospadias. Cryptorchidism is the most common defect found in association with hypospadias.[15]

Cryptorchidism. In dogs, cryptorchidism is the most common disorder of sexual development, occurring in as many as 13 per cent of male dogs. Normally the canine

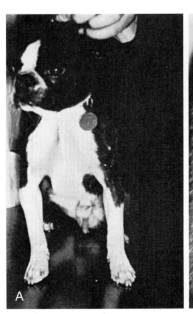
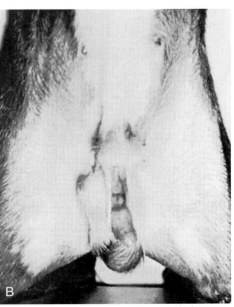

Figure 165–4. Puppy with hypospadias. Note the abnormal locations of the urethral openings. (From Feldman EC, Nelson RW: Canine and Feline Endocrinology and Reproduction, 2nd ed. Philadelphia, WB Saunders, 1996, p 645.)

testes descend to the scrotum by 10 days after birth. Both testicles should be within the scrotum by 8 weeks of age; however, some authors suggest that the diagnosis not be made until 6 months of age. Cryptorchid dogs have been shown to have an increased development of Sertoli cell tumors.[16] Cryptorchidism is seen more commonly in the toy and miniature poodle, Pomeranian, Yorkshire terrier, miniature dachshund, Chihuahua, Maltese, Boxer, Pekingese, English bulldog, miniature schnauzer, and Shetland sheep-dog, and therefore may have a genetic basis.[9] The exact mode of inheritance is not known but is thought to be a sex-limited autosomal recessive. Therefore, both males and females can carry the gene and pass it to their offspring. Treatment of affected individuals is limited to castration. Removal of carrier parents from the breeding population would result in a decrease in frequency of this condition.

DIAGNOSIS, TREATMENT, AND PREVENTION OF SEXUAL DEVELOPMENT DISEASES

A definitive diagnosis of a sexual development disorder is based upon a thorough investigation of each step in sexual development. Karyotype (see Fig. 165–1), gonadal histology (see Fig. 165–2), plasma concentrations of gonadotropins and thyroid hormone, and complete description of the internal and external genitalia are necessary to facilitate the diagnosis.

Differential diagnosis for infertility and irregular estrous cycles in a young bitch should include the possibility of intersexuality. Phenotype and morphologic appearance of external genitalia cannot rule out intersexuality. In cryptorchid phenotypic males, removal of gonads is recommended because cryptorchid testicular tissue has an increased risk of Sertoli cell tumor development. With an enlarged clitoris with the mucosal surfaces exposed to drying or trauma, amputation is indicated. Dogs with hypospadias and malformed penis or prepuce (XX male syndrome) are treated with reconstruction or plastic surgery of the external genitalia.

A complete family history is essential in all cases. Pedigree analysis of the dog and related dogs is extremely helpful in establishing whether the condition is heritable. Genetic counseling and preventative measures for inherited disorders of sexual development depend on knowledge of the mode of inheritance. Various statistical methods are used to analyze such data, and breeding trials may be necessary to confirm inheritance patterns. Many congenital diseases follow simple mendelian inheritance, mostly simple autosomal recessive.[17] Further studies are needed to understand the mode of inheritance of most canine and feline disorders of sexual development.

REFERENCES

1. Meyers-Wallen VN, Patterson DF: Sexual differentiation and inherited disorders of sexual development in the dog. J Reprod Fert Suppl 39:57, 1989.
2. Padgett AB, Bell TG, Patterson WR: Genetic disorders affecting reproduction and parturient care. Vet Clin North Am Sm Anim Pract 16:577, 1986.
3. Leipold HW, Dennis SM: Chromosomal and genetic disorders. In Ettinger SJ (ed): Textbook of Veterinary Internal Medicine, 3rd ed. Philadelphia, WB Saunders, 1989, pp 183–187.
4. Meyers-Wallen VN, Patterson DF: Disorders of sexual development in the dog. In Morrow DA (ed): Current Therapy in Theriogenology, 2nd ed. Philadelphia, WB Saunders, 1986, pp 567–574.
5. Schwartz ID, Root AW: The Klinefelter syndrome of testicular dysgenesis. Endocrinol Metab Clin North Am 20:153, 1991.
6. Nie GJ, Johnston SD, Hayden DW, et al: Azoospermia associated with 79,XXY chromosome complement. Theriogenology Question of the Month. JAVMA 212:1545, 1998.
7. Moran C, Gill CF, Nicholas F: Fertile male tortoiseshell cats. Mosaics due to gene instability. J Hered 75:397, 1984.
8. Johnston SD, Buoen LC, Weber AF, et al: X trisomy in an Airedale bitch with ovarian dysplasia and primary anestrus. Theriogenology 24:597, 1985.
9. Meyers-Wallen VN, Patterson DF: Disorders of sexual development in dogs and cats. In Kirk RW (ed): Current Veterinary Therapy X, Small Animal Practice. Philadelphia, WB Saunders, 1989, pp 1261–1269.
10. Meyers-Wallen VN, Patterson DF: XX sex reversal in American cocker spaniel dogs. Phenotypic expression and inheritance. Human Genetics 80:23, 1988.
11. Thomas TN, Olson PN, Hoopes PJ: Lateral hermaphroditism and seminoma in a dog. JAVMA 189:1596, 1986.
12. Kyles AE, Vaden S, Hardie EM, et al: Vestibulovaginal stenosis in dogs: 18 cases (1987–1995). JAVMA 209:1889, 1996.
13. Archbald LF, Wolfsdorf K: Vaginal constriction, probably a congenital malformation. Theriogenology Question of the Month. JAVMA 208:1651, 1996.
14. Johnston SD: Premature gonadal failure in female dogs and cats. J Reprod Fert Suppl 39:65, 1989.
15. Hayes HM, Wilson GP: Hospital incidence of hypospadias in dogs in North America. Vet Rec 118:605, 1986.
16. Hayes HM, Wilson GP, Pendergrass TW, et al: Canine cryptochidism and subsequent testicular neoplasia: Case control study and epidemiologic update. Teratology 32:51, 1985.
17. Stone DM, Mickelsen WD, Jachy PB, et al: A novel Robertsonian translocation in a family of Walker hounds. Genome 34:677, 1991.

REP

CHAPTER 166

FELINE REPRODUCTION

J. Verstegen

For many years, feline reproduction has been neglected and poorly studied. But over the past decade, new data have been obtained on the ovarian cycle and general reproduction in cats because of the growing interest in cats per se and also because cats serve as models for the preservation of endangered wild feline species.[1, 2] In addition, interest has emerged in relation to the problem of pet overpopulation and birth control.[3] However, many aspects of both female and male feline reproduction remain poorly understood. Indeed, the cat is singular among mammals in many aspects of its reproductive physiology (induced ovulation, pregnancy regulation, high blood testosterone levels).

ANATOMY OF THE GENITAL TRACT

The Queen

The Ovary

The ovary is covered by the peritoneum ("ovarian bursa") presenting a large lateral opening. The ovarian serosa is connected to the uterine serosa by the mesosalpinx and the ovarian ligament. Unlike that in the bitch, the mesosalpinx is relatively free of fat and the ovaries can normally be visualized without any need to open the bursa. The ovary is fixed dorsally to the abdominal wall by the mesovarium and cranially by the suspensory ligament.

The Oviducts

The uterine tubes are not heavily curved and are 4 to 6 cm in length. Their diameter is approximately 1 to 1.5 mm. They curve around the mesovarium and can be observed near the ovary.

The Uterus

The uterus is composed of two uterine horns, 9 to 11 cm in length and 3 to 4 mm in diameter; the uterine body (2 to 3 cm long and 4 to 8 mm in diameter); and the cervix. The size of the horns is relatively similar from one extremity to the other. They present a dorsal concavity and are fixed dorsally by the broad ligament. Palpation of the uterus is normally possible only during estrus or pregnancy. During the other phases of the cycle, the uterus cannot easily be detected except in pathologic conditions.

The Vagina and Vestibule

The vagina (20 to 30 mm) is twice as long as the vestibule (10 to 25 mm). The mucosa is pale with many folds. The ventral part of the cervix is deeply folded. The vestibule is highly muscular. Located on the lateral surfaces are the openings of the two vestibular glands (Bartholin's glands), which are highly developed in this species. The urethra opens ventrally in a small fossa. The vestibule, vagina, and cervix are oriented horizontally in a straight line. The vestibulovaginal junction is narrow, and vaginal examination and obtaining deep vaginal smears are difficult without deep sedation or general anesthesia.[4]

The Vulva and Clitoris

The vulva is pigmented and its external portion is covered by hair. The clitoris is short (2 to 10 mm), located in a small ventral depression, and normally not visible.

The Tomcat

The Testes and Epididymides

The testes of the adult male cat are spherical to ovoid, approximately 1.2 to 2 cm in length and 0.7 to 1.7 cm in diameter. They are oriented craniocaudally in the scrotal sac, which is located close to the body wall just below the anus. The feline testes are usually in the scrotum at birth but may move up and down the inguinal canals in young animals until they finally remain in the scrotum. The epididymides are fixed to the scrotal membrane by the ligament of the tail of the epididymis. The head of the epididymis is located at the cranial dorsomedial aspect of the testis, the body curves around the dorsolateral aspect, and the tail passes medial to the surface of the testis and becomes the ductus deferens. The epididymides are not easily palpated. The ductus deferens is sinuous, follows the testis cranially, and with the rest of the spermatic cord passes through the inguinal ring into the abdominal cavity, penetrating into the dorsal surface of the prostate at its entry site, the colliculus seminalis, into the urethra. The ductus deferens is responsible for the maturation of the spermatozoa; the testes are responsible for their formation. In the cat, unlike some other species, there is no ampulla where the sperm can be stored; thus frequent ejaculation can influence the total amount of sperm ejaculated as there are no reserves.

The Prostate

As in other species, the prostate is an androgen-dependent bilobate organ, approximately 1 cm in length, located 2 to 3 cm from the bladder neck and partially encircling the urethra. The prostate gland is composed of two parts: the pars compacta and the pars disseminata. The latter is disseminated all around the urethra, extending from the bladder neck up to the bulbourethral glands. Few data are available regarding the histologic development, maturation, secretion, and physiology of the prostate in cats. No data exist regarding its role in sperm production and sperm function.

The Bulbourethral Glands

The bulbourethral glands are two tubuloalveolar pea-shaped glands (4 × 3 mm) enclosed in the bulbourethral muscles and located dorsal to the bulb of the penis at the ischial symphysis. They have disseminated ramifications extending cranially to the prostate that are histologically different from the disseminated portion of the prostate gland. Indeed, the secretions of the disseminated glands and the bulbourethral glands are different from that of the prostate. The major products of the bulbourethral glands are sulfated mucopolysaccharides. Their role, other than quantitative, in reproductive physiology has not yet been determined.

The Penis

The penis is located ventral to the scrotum and is composed of two corpora cavernosa penis laterally and the corpus spongiosum penis, which is medial. The glans, which terminates the penis, is a smooth conical structure, 8 to 10 mm long, directed caudally at rest but ventrally during mating. The base of the penis is covered by six to eight circular rows of penile spines leading to approximately 150 to 200 cornified keratinized spines.[5] The presence of these spines is hormone dependent, explaining their total disappearance in castrated males. The exact physiologic role of the spines is still uncertain. Their proposed purposes are to provide sexual stimulation during mating, to prevent female withdrawal, and to increase cervical stimulation. In the fully developed large male, an os penis may be observed.

Semen Characteristics

The volume of semen is difficult to evaluate. Indeed, in this species sperm is generally collected after tranquilization and electroejaculation. Semen collected in this manner may not be representative of that collected from a trained animal used in natural conditions. The volume ranges from 0.02 to 0.3 mL. Feline spermatozoa are generally obtained in higher concentration than in dogs (1.5×10^9 to 2×10^9/mL) but are smaller (26 μm in length compared with 36 μm in dogs). The pH of the ejaculate appears to be higher than in dogs (in the range 7.4 to 8.3). The subjective mobility (optical microscope) is in the range 60 to 95 percent with a mean velocity of 4.5 on a scale of 5. A good ejaculate contains less than 10 percent morphologically abnormal spermatozoa.

PHYSIOLOGY OF FELINE REPRODUCTION

The Queen

Puberty

The average age of puberty in the domestic cat is variable. Cats usually start to show estrus once they have reached a body weight of 2.3 to 2.5 kg, around 6 to 9 months of age, but some animals are observed to enter puberty as early as 3 to 4 months of age or as late as 18 months of age. Breed and line variations demonstrate a certain degree of heredity in sexual maturity. Siamese or Burmese cats appear to be more precocious and reach puberty at a lower body weight than long-haired breeds such as Persians. However, the main factor responsible for both sexual maturity and cyclicity seems to be the amount and duration of sunlight received in relation to day length in outdoor cats or of artificial light in breeding colonies. The onset of puberty usually occurs when the amount of daylight increases at the end of the winter.

Seasonality and Estrous Cycle

In the absence of pregnancy or pseudopregnancy, the cat has repeated estrous cycles every 2 or 3 weeks in spring, summer, and autumn. In breeding colonies with controlled light and in households with evening lighting, cats can become nonseasonal breeders and show estrus during winter. It is believed that photoperiods influence the reproductive processes via the pineal gland and its main hormone melatonin in a manner similar to that in the mare.

Behavioral Cycle

In terms of behavior, the cycle of the queen can be divided into the heat and the nonheat periods.

The heat period can be divided into proestrus and estrus. Together, behavioral proestrus (1 to 4 days) and estrus (2 to 19 days) last an average of 3 to 10 days. Whereas estrus is characterized by male acceptance, proestrus, the first days (from 1 to 4) of behavioral heat, is associated with calling but nonacceptance of the male. Proestrus per se is clinically difficult to detect because some cats express estrous behavior and accept the mating without this preliminary transition period. Follicular growth begins during proestrus, but the plasma estradiol concentration is still low and insufficient to allow full behavioral expression of heat. Estrus begins with the queen allowing the mating and ends with the first refusal. It is characterized by maximal secretion of follicular estrogens.

During heat, the queen rubs against animate and inanimate objects, rolls over, and often becomes extremely affectionate. Such queens may constantly vocalize, with much howling and calling. If touched, especially along the back, the cat

adopts the mating posture: foreend crouched, hindend raised, and tail deflected with paddling movements of the limbs. Male cats are attracted, and when the queen is fully in heat she allows mating. Male thrusting causes the female to vocalize violently the (the coital "scream"), and this is followed immediately by the female forcefully and sometimes aggressively freeing herself from the male neck grip. The queen then shows a temporary disinterest in mating, rolls back and forth, and licks her perineum (the "after-reaction"). This is soon followed by the multiple copulations typically observed throughout estrus. The interval between matings averages approximately 15 to 20 minutes.

Queens as well as males can easily block and hide any reproductive behavior with changes in environmental or social circumstances. It is common for queens to exhibit no signs of estrus when in their home but to exhibit dramatic rollings and callings once released. Males may ignore or attack females in a hostile or unknown environment. On the other hand, some really affectionate queens can have heat signs that are not really different from their usual behavior, making detection of estrus difficult in the absence of a male.

It appears that estrus is shortened by mating, although this is controversial and difficult to assess in conditions other than controlled breeding colonies.

External genitalia show few if any typical changes of estrus. Sometimes there is a little reddening, softening, or edema of the vulva, but no discharge is present. The vulva may become slightly opened in estrus.

Interestrus and Anestrus

In the absence of mating or spontaneous ovulation, heat periods are observed, on average, at intervals of every 10 to 14 days (range 0 to 20 days) throughout the entire reproductive season. The interval without evidence of estrus is called "interestrus." It corresponds to apparent quiescence of the ovaries, which, however, are already preparing for the wave of follicular growth for the next estrus. During the interestrus, the plasma estrogen concentration usually declines to basal values. In some cats, however, sequential follicular growth waves may overlap, estrogen concentrations may not decline, and the queen may appear in constant estrus. This phenomenon is often falsely called "nymphomania" or prolonged estrus.

True ovarian quiescence is only found during "anestrus," which, in contrast to interestrus, is a long period without sexual activity. Anestrus occurs when natural daylight is short (winter) or when the cats are submitted to short artificial lightening periods of 4 to 6 hours a day. Anestrus could be absent in animals submitted to constant long daylight periods, particularly animals that live indoors or in breeding colonies with constant lighting.

Mating and Induced Ovulation

The cat was considered a reflex-mediated induced ovulator; that is, a coital stimulus induces a neural firing reflex that stimulates the mediobasal hypothalamus to synthesize and liberate gonadotropin-releasing hormone (GnRH), which then stimulates the release of pituitary luteinizing hormone (LH), which causes ovulation to take place. However, there is now evidence suggesting that cats may ovulate spontaneously without mating.[6] Nevertheless, the ovulation rate seems to be directly related to the amplitude of the LH surge, which may itself be correlated with the number, interval, and duration of matings. The interval between vaginal stimulation and ovulation is indirectly proportional to the number of matings and to the endocrine status at the time of copulation. Cats that have been in estrus for several days ovulate sooner after mating than cats that have just entered estrus. Although queens may accept males during the second or third day of follicular growth (first or second day of estrus), some cats may not show a sufficient release of LH in response to copulation until the fourth or fifth day. Cats seem to require estrogen impregnation for several days before copulation can induce an LH surge sufficient to cause ovulation. Ovulation can therefore occur as early as 24 hours or as late as 52 hours after the induced LH surge. After ovulation, signs of heat disappear within 24 to 48 hours. An increase in plasma progesterone concentration typically follows ovulation.

If ovulation does not occur, the follicles become atretic and plasma estrogen concentrations decline. Luteinization does not occur, and newly recruited follicles may start to grow after a few days of interestrus.

In the queen, unlike the bitch, events after ovulation depend on whether or not the mating was fertile. Indeed, two situations have been observed.

Ovulation Without Fertilization

When oocytes are not fertilized after ovulation, corpora lutea develop and produce progesterone for a period of about 25 to 45 days. This luteal phase is shorter than that associated with pregnancy and is therefore often called pseudopregnancy. In the cat, pseudopregnancy is not, as in dogs, associated with behavioral changes or lactation. No significant clinical signs are observed other than a prolonged period without signs of estrus. At the end of this short luteal phase of pseudopregnancy, a brief period of interestrus precedes the next estrus, provided that it is still the breeding season. Otherwise, anestrus occurs. For queens living indoors, induction of pseudopregnancy could be a safe way to stop the reproductive behavior for a while. Pseudopregnancy can easily be induced by injection of GnRH or human chorionic gonadotropin (HCG). Mechanical vaginal stimulation has been proposed, but there is no consistent and reliable protocol.

Ovulation and Fertilization

If the queen is mated with a fertile male and successfully inseminated, mature ovulated secondary oocytes are fertilized in the oviducts, where the embryos develop for 4 to 5 days. Embryos then migrate into the uterine horns, where implantation occurs around day 12 to 16 after mating. The biology of pregnancy has not been investigated in cats as thoroughly as it has been in other mammalian species. Pregnancy can be timed accurately when mating has been allowed for only 1 or 2 days and ovulation induced by correctly managed mating. Gestation length is 63 to 68 days in controlled conditions but can range from 62 to 72 days when mating is allowed for several days and the exact day of ovulation is not determined. Ovulation follows efficacious matings by about 30 hours and fertilization of the secondary oocytes that are produced occurs in the oviducts. Blastocysts enter the uterus on day 5 to 6 and migrate from one horn to the other for a few days before attachment (around day 14) and implantation (days 14 to 18). The placenta is of the endotheliochorial type and circumferential-zonary in morphology. Average litter size varies among breeds (from two to five kittens), increases with age (until 5 to 8 years), and

then declines. Spontaneous abortion or resorption is well documented to occur in 5 to 30 percent of pregnancies and can include from one kitten to the entire litter. The litter size is usually smaller in primiparous queens.

Parturition is always associated with a decline in plasma progesterone, but this decline can be observed as early as 5 to 10 days before queening or as late as after parturition. Queens sometimes remain pregnant for days without any significant plasma progesterone concentration, possibly because parturition depends on the local withdrawal of the small amount of progesterone produced by the placenta. The peripartum luteolysis involves the production of prostaglandins, which are well known to induce abortion when administered during pregnancy in queens. The prepartum temperature drop observed in dogs and correlated with the decline in progesterone is not consistently seen cats. Parturition and its phases are similar to those observed in dogs, with a few differences: the placenta is red-brown instead of dark green, and the period of queening can be as short as 1 hour but sometimes as long as 1 or 2 days. Delayed parturition is often observed when environmental stress is present or can be characteristic of some animals. A 12- to 48-hour interruption can be observed without any significant effect on the litter except when placental disruption is present.[7]

At the end of the lactation period, if it is still the breeding season, a brief period of interestrus precedes the next estrus; otherwise, anestrus occurs. In lactating queens, this estrous period usually occurs about 10 to 15 days after weaning. However, in some cases, estrus may be observed in lactating females 10 to 15 days after queening. In this case, if the queen is not mated or if ovulation did not occur, she returns to estrus normally every 10 to 20 days. The first mating after queening is often not fertile because of incomplete uterine involution, but mating during the next estrus may be fertile. It is not rare for a lactating queen to be pregnant again before weaning. Spontaneous or induced follicular growth with estrous behavior and mating has been described during pregnancy, suggesting that the ovaries are responsive to gonadotropins during gestation in this species but confirming the centrally mediated inhibiting effects of progesterone on follicular growth. Because of the multiple matings during the heat period, superfecundation characterized by fertilization of ova with semen from different males and whelping of kittens with different fathers is often observed in natural uncontrolled conditions.

Pregnancy diagnosis can be confirmed by ultrasonography around days 11 to 14, by palpation around days 20 to 25, and by radiography after ossification occurs around days 40 to 45. The techniques are similar to those described for dogs. Some hemographic and biochemical changes similar to those in dogs have been described and are mainly characterized by a normocytic, normochromic anemia. Progesterone assays cannot be used for pregnancy diagnosis before day 40 because they do not distinguish pseudopregnant from pregnant cats. Fetal heartbeats can be detected around days 22 to 25 and can be used to monitor fetal distress. Distress is a concern if heart rates decrease below 200 beats per minute.[8] The growing conceptus of the domestic cat is similar to that of larger mammals with regard to the amount of fluid surrounding the developing fetus. The growth rate is similar to that of the guinea pig and beagle and differs from that of mouse, rat, human, sheep, or cow. Litter size ranges from one to five kittens with an average of 3.7 kittens but with large variations between animals and breeds and with age. Mortality by 8 weeks of age is high and ranges from 15 to 45 percent with an average of about 30 percent.[9, 10]

Endocrine Events During the Reproductive Cycle

Estrogens

Estradiol-17β is produced by the developing follicles from early proestrus to the end of estrus. The estradiol concentration rises over a few days from its basal values at the end of anestrus or interestrus (less than 15 to 20 pg/mL) to more than 40 to 80 pg/mL during estrus. The maximum production is obtained during estrus. The increase in estradiol during follicular development and estrus is essential for estrous behavior and to prepare for the gonadotropin surge associated with mating and ovulation. A difference exists between the follicular phase per se and the behavioral "heat." The follicular phase, as assessed by the estradiol-17β plasma concentration, begins earlier than behavioral heat. If no ovulation occurs, plasma estradiol concentrations return to basal values within a few days. If ovulation does occur, estradiol concentrations decline more dramatically and return to basal values within 2 to 3 days.

During the luteal phase, in pregnant and nonpregnant animals, estradiol concentrations are generally below 20 pg/mL, but they occasionally increase in individual animals, particularly after day 35 to 45 of pregnancy. Indeed, occasional follicular phases with estrous behavior and mating have been observed naturally or after experimental induction[11] in this species. However, superfetation is rare.

Luteinizing Hormone and Follicle-Stimulating Hormone

Dynamic changes in pituitary follicle-stimulating hormone (FSH) secretion at the end of anestrus and interestrus are probably responsible for the induction of follicular growth. However, because of the absence of homologous assay methods, no convincing data are available to confirm this observation.

During proestrus and estrus, before any coital stimulus, plasma LH concentrations are basal. The ovulatory LH surge starts within minutes of vaginal stimulation during mating or, in some instances, spontaneously. These concentrations peak within 2 hours and return to basal concentrations within 12 to 24 hours.[12, 13] The amplitude and duration of the LH surge are highly variable and depend on the intensity, duration, and frequency of the coital stimulus. The LH surge is higher and lasts longer when multiple matings occur than after a single coitus. The optimal LH surge is observed when a maximum of four matings occur within a 2- to 4-hour period. Additional coital stimuli during this time frame or over a longer interval may not significantly increase the LH response. This is apparently due to exhaustion of the pituitary LH content. The amplitude of the peak increases from less than 10 ng/mL before mating to more than 100 ng/mL after maximal stimulation. The duration of the LH surge apparently varies from a few minutes after the coital stimulus to a maximum of 24 hours.

Progesterone

Plasma progesterone is at basal concentrations (<1 ng/mL) in the absence of ovulation. If ovulation does occur, in both pregnant and pseudopregnant cats, plasma progesterone begins to increase within 24 to 50 hours after the LH peak. Concentrations may reach a maximum of 30 to 60 ng/mL around day 20 to 25 after mating.

In pseudopregnant animals, the plasma progesterone concentration begin to decrease around day 25 and reaches basal values around days 30 to 40. The decline in progesterone is slow and progressive, in contrast to that observed at the end of pregnancy, and is similar to that in the nongravid dog. The slow decrease is probably due to lack of the luteolytic factor responsible for the rapid progesterone drop at the end of pregnancy. In pseudopregnant animals, the lifespan of the corpus luteum appears to be preprogrammed to 25 to 35 days because there is no luteotropic support originating from the embryo or placenta to prolong and support progesterone secretion. Hysterectomies performed during the luteal phase in pseudopregnant animals did not change the lifespan of the corpus luteum, demonstrating that the uterus is not involved in luteolysis.

In the pregnant cat, an initial decrease in progesterone occurs around day 25 to 35, but values remain stable at approximately 15 to 30 ng/mL and do not decrease below 1 to 1.5 ng/mL by day 60. In the queen, progesterone is necessary throughout gestation to maintain pregnancy. The queen can still remain pregnant for a few days after a decrease in plasma concentration below 1 ng/mL, which is the apparent minimal progesterone concentration necessary to maintain pregnancy. Corpora lutea remain the main source of progesterone. The placenta either produces a small amount of progesterone insufficient to maintain pregnancy or does not secrete any progesterone at all.[14] Ovariectomy performed during any stage of pregnancy results in a decline in plasma progesterone below 1 ng/mL within 48 hours of surgery. Placental progesterone, if any, is assumed to act locally and not significantly contribute to circulating concentrations.

The cause of the difference in corpus luteum activity between pregnant and pseudopregnant cats is still unknown. Pregnancy may, as in other species, involve some specific luteotropic factors originating from the fetus, the placenta, and/or the pituitary gland. Such a factor may act as a signal to maintain the corpus luteum and prevent its regression. Possible factors involved in sustaining the corpus luteum during pregnancy are prolactin and relaxin. These hormones have been identified as possible luteotropins in other species, such as dogs.

Relaxin

Relaxin is the only hormone specifically associated with pregnancy.[15] Relaxin is secreted primarily by the placenta; the ovaries seem to be a minor source. Plasma relaxin concentrations increase from day 25 to 30 after mating exclusively in pregnant animals. This increase is coincident with or slightly precedes the prolactin increase, which may suggest a possible interplay between the two hormones. They may have a synergistic effect in sustaining progesterone secretion by corpora lutea. Relaxin may act directly on the corpus luteum or may indirectly stimulate prolactin secretion from the pituitary gland. Relaxin may also stimulate still other unknown luteotropic factors.

Prolactin

Prolactin secretion, which is basal during the estrous cycle, increases around day 30 to 35 of gestation in the queen and reaches a maximum a few days before parturition. Prolactin concentrations increase dramatically again during lactation. Prolactin appears to play a major central luteotropic role. The suppression of prolactin by administration of a dopamine agonist such as bromocriptine or cabergoline during pregnancy causes a decline in progesterone secretion in cats that causes abortion when the progesterone concentration drops below 1 ng/mL. Being the main luteotropic hormone in queens, prolactin plays a major role in mammary gland secretion and the maintenance of lactation.

Melatonin

In cats, melatonin secretion is clearly associated with the photoperiod.[16] Plasma melatonin and prolactin concentrations are synchronous and appear to be high during periods of darkness and low during periods of high light intensity. Melatonin and prolactin secretions are likely to play a role in ovarian function in the cat because concentrations of both hormones are lower during periods of ovarian activity (estrus) than during periods of ovarian quiescence (anestrus and interestrus). However, the exact relationship between the secretion of melatonin and prolactin and the follicular growth is not well understood.

Vaginal Cytology

Vaginal cytology in queens is a subtle reflection of hormonal changes associated with the follicular phase, proestrus, and estrus.[17] It allows confirmation of mating by the identification of spermatozoa when performed soon after copulation; however, its value in breeding management is limited. Indeed, the changes observed are less impressive and characteristic than they are in the bitch and great experience is needed to be able to analyze the smear properly.

During the follicular phase, superficial keratinized cells are observed on the smear, reflecting the increased effects of estradiol-17β. A main characteristic of follicular phase vaginal smears is the slight decrease in percentage of nuclear intermediate and basal cells. The most significant indication of estrogen activity is the clearing of the background associated with a reduction in cell debris or mucus[4] (Fig. 166–1). Eosinophilic staining is less consistent and marked than in dogs. Red blood cells are not observed in any stage of the cycle. During interestrus, the majority of cells consist of intermediate and a few basal or parabasal and keratinized nuclear cells. Generally, there is cell debris, which gives the background of the vaginal smear a dirty appearance. During

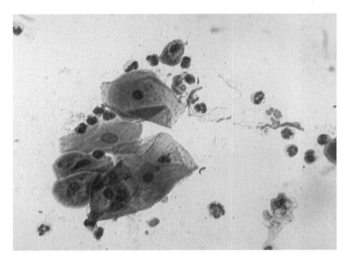

Figure 166–2. Vaginal smear of a pseudopregnant metestrous queen. Many superficial, intermediate, and neutrophilic cells could be observed. (× 250, Hemacolor staining.)

metestrus (luteal phase), the vaginal smear is similar to that of bitches, with superficial, intermediate, and neutrophilic cells decreasing over time. Metestrum cells are not or rarely observed (Fig. 166–2).

During anestrus, cells are rare, mucus is obvious and abundant, and the majority of cells are basal or parabasal with some intermediate cells. Leukocytes can sometimes be observed.

The Male

Puberty, Seasonality, and Reproductive Life

In cats, testicular descent appears to be prenatal. The earliest histologic evidence of spermatogenesis is seen around 20 weeks, and the first spermatozoa appear in the spermatic cord at 30 to 36 weeks of age. In general, spermatozoa are present when the weight of the testes exceeds 1 g and the body weight of the animal reaches about 2.5 to 3.5 kg. Neck biting, mounting, and pelvic movements may occur as early as 4 months, but full reproductive behavior with penile intromission and ejaculation is rarely observed before 8 to 12 months of age. Full sexual activity and maturity are often not observed before 2 years of age in tomcats. Before this age, most males do not fight for hierarchy and seem indifferent to females in estrus. Sexual maturity seems to be associated with changes in appearance of the male's head. The head shape changes dramatically from the typically nonmature appearance to the rounded shape typical of a fully mature tom. Fighting, marking, and mounting behaviors are then observed. The reproductive life of the male cat is supposed to persist as long as 14 years, but it is generally accepted that maximum sexual activity usually lasts 8 to 10 years. Sperm production in cats seems to be seasonally dependent, with maximum numbers during summer months. However, season has no effect on the reproduction of male cats maintained indoors or in controlled catteries under constant artificial lighting.

Endocrine Events During the Reproductive Cycle

Testosterone

A high basal plasma testosterone concentration seems to be characteristic of male cats. Indeed, plasma testosterone is

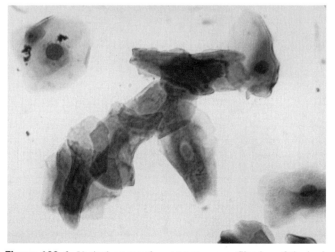

Figure 166–1. Vaginal smear of an estrous queen. Clearing of the background is observed with many superficial and intermediate cells. (× 250, Hemacolor staining.)

elevated in both intact and castrated males as well as in females (4 to 8 ng/mL). Androgen concentrations in the testicular vessels still dramatically exceed those in the peripheral circulation (ratio 1:50). The testosterone production can be stimulated by the injection of HCG or GnRH. Maximum values of 12 to 16 ng/mL are obtained 20 to 24 hours after administration. A portion of the plasma testosterone seems to be of adrenal origin, which can explain the presence of sexual behavior sometimes observed in castrated animals.

REPRODUCTIVE PROBLEMS

The Queen

Anatomic Abnormalities

Congenital defects and intersexuality have been reported but are uncommon in the queen. Among the clinical abnormalities described are the following:

Cystic rete ovarii tubules: dilated ovarian tubules occurring in queens of any age and often observed in cats with the ovarian remnant syndrome.

Uterus unicornis (lack of one uterine horn) or segmental aplasia (lack of development of a portion or portions of the genital tract). These are in general of no clinical significance and are usually detected post mortem or during surgery.

Bartholin's gland abnormalities: mainly cysts. Bartholin's gland in queens appears to be clearly dependent on ovarian steroid hormones, particularly estrogens.[18]

Infertility

Infertility in queens is poorly understood. The causes might be similar to those in bitches, but some species-specific disorders have been described. Knowledge about infertility can be enhanced only by careful and methodic reproductive examinations and good record keeping.[4]

Noninfectious Disorders

Abnormal Mating Behavior. Lack of sexual receptivity has been observed in timid queens, low in social status in a colony. Successful breeding management depends on correct intromission and ejaculation. Indeed, stimulation without intromission could be associated with spontaneous ovulation without fertilization and pseudopregnancy, leading to a false diagnosis of infertility.

Pseudopregnancy and Spontaneous Ovulation. In the past, spontaneous ovulation was considered rare in queens and generally associated with nonfertile matings. However, the concept that cats are primarily copulation-induced ovulators is being reconsidered. There is evidence that spontaneous ovulation is a frequent phenomenon in the presence or absence of males. In colonies, spontaneous ovulation has been described to occur in 30 to 60 per cent of animals and the percentage appears to be higher when a male is present in the same room, even if mating is not allowed. The sexual behavior of queens during heat, which includes rolling, neck rubbing, meowing, licking of their own or another cat's external genitalia, female-female mounting, and neck biting, could induce stimulation of GnRH and LH release, leading to ovulation. A pheromone effect is probably also present, favoring or inducing spontaneous ovulation. Indeed, 67 per cent of females have been

shown to ovulate during the 20 days after the introduction of (but without direct contact with) a male into the room. This suggests a response to some visual or airborne olfactory cues from the male. Every time a queen is suspected of infertility, progesterone has to be checked to ensure that pseudopregnancy has not been spontaneously induced.

Prolonged Heat Behavior. Frequent regular follicular waves may overlap, leading to prolonged periods of estrous behavior and prolonged periods of receptivity. This is most often observed in Siamese queens housed alone without access to males. This prolonged estrous behavior is sometimes called pseudonymphomania, a condition to be differentiated from nymphomania caused by follicular cysts or the centrally mediated nymphomania observed in ovariectomized animals. Mating does not induce ovulation in queens with follicular cysts because the follicles are abnormal, the hypothalamopituitary axis is nonresponsive, or the animal has autoantibodies against its own GnRH, FSH, or LH. The condition frequently recurs in subsequent cycles and is often associated with clinical signs that include weight loss and a sparse, roughened haircoat. Treatment with GnRH or HCG is successful in some cases but sterilization is certainly the treatment of choice.

Persistence of estrous behavior in "neutered" animals can be caused by remnant ovaries. The role of the adrenal cortex, however, cannot be underestimated: excess testosterone can be metabolized to estrogens. This may be responsible for the centrally mediated persistence of estrous behavior. Production of estrogens by the adrenal cortex could also explain the persistent reproductive behavior. Adrenal suppression with short-acting glucocorticoids can result in disappearance of the estrous signs. In cases of centrally mediated persistent estrus, the use of long-acting progestins that block receptors has been successful.

Spontaneous and Iatrogenic Prolonged Anestrus. Prolonged anestrus may be photoperiod related, as variations in daylight exposure have clearly been demonstrated to control the estrous cycle. It can easily be corrected by modifying the duration and intensity of light exposure. Prolonged anestrus can also be socially related, as a stressful position in a hierarchy can induce suppression of estrous behavior and apparent "silent heat." Long-acting progestin injections can also be associated with prolonged anestrus. When progestins are no longer present, estrus can be induced using gonadotropins or antiprolactins.

Mucometra (Also Called Hydrometra). Mucometra (Fig. 166–3) may be a consequence of cystic endometrial hyperplasia, but the exact cause of this pathologic process is not clearly defined and it can be observed in animals without evidence of cystic endometrial hyperplasia. Mucometra may be due to prolonged progestin treatment, but this is not always the case. Endogenous progesterone associated with spontaneous ovulation may be responsible for the occurrence of this asymptomic condition.

Fibroadenomatous Mammary Hyperplasia. This condition is characterized by massive enlargement of the mammary glands. The glands are firm, nonpainful, and not inflammatory but can become infected or necrosed. The stroma is loose and some arborescent glandular structures can be seen (Fig. 166–4). The cats are usually normal and not affected by the often tremendous development of the mammary glands. No milk is observed. This condition is most often observed in young animals after their first ovulation or after progestin treatment to prevent estrus in females or to treat behavioral or skin diseases in both males and females. It is rarely observed soon after pregnancy. The

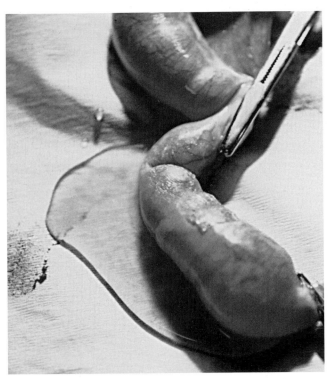

Figure 166–3. A mucometra just after surgical removal. The mucus can be clearly seen leaking from the distended, thin-walled uterus. No clinical symptoms were observed in this animal.

pathology is clearly benign and has to be differentiated from that of mammary tumors, which are usually observed in older animals and are rarely symmetric. The pathology appears hormone dependent and related to oversensibility to progesterone secretion. The influence of progesterone (whether present because of exogenous therapy in the male or female or as an endogenous steroid of ovarian origin) has been demonstrated both directly and indirectly in cats with mammary hypertrophy.[19] Surgery is indicated when the condition is due to spontaneous or induced ovulation. Ovariectomy eliminates the progesterone. In most cases the mammary glands regress in 1 or 2 weeks (Fig. 166–5A and B). Partial or radical mammectomy is not indicated unless large ulcers or skin necrosis is observed. When the disease is related to progestin treatment, the drug should be discontinued. When available, treatment with antiprogestins could be used. Aglepristone has been used at a dose of 10 mg/kg injected three times at 48- to 72-hour intervals.

Infectious Disorders

Cystic Endometrial Hyperplasia–Pyometra Complex. This condition is less common in cats than in dogs. However, its frequency might be underestimated. Clinical signs are few and no significant hematologic (except neutrophilia) or biochemical changes are observed. The etiology is less clear in cats. If a relation between progesterone and pyometra is accepted, high and prolonged plasma progesterone concentrations are observed only when ovulation occurs and not in every cycle as in bitches. The description of a high incidence of pseudopregnancy in cats might corroborate the possible role of repeated and prolonged progesterone impregnation. However, the observation that uterine reactivity to local stimuli (mechanical or biologic) in dogs might

be the first and real inducer of cystic endometrial hyperplasia is also to be taken into account in relation to the feline species.

Pregnancy

Implantation Failure and Abortion

Viral agents are the most commonly reported infectious cause of abortion in queens. Implicated viruses include feline leukemia virus, feline immunodeficiency virus, coronavirus, feline herpesvirus, and feline panleukopenia viruses.

Bacteria reported to cause fetal death and abortion include *Salmonella* sp., *Escherichia coli*, and beta-hemolytic *Streptococcus*. *Toxoplasma gondii* causes abortion after experimental infections, but abortion after natural infections is extremely unusual.

A large variety of bacteria, mycoplasms, or viruses has been detected in infertile cats and cultured from aborted fetuses. In general, infections cause similar clinical signs, and isolation of the causal agent from the placenta or the fetuses is necessary for clear identification of the responsible agent. Among these, feline panleukemia and leukemia viruses and chlamydiae have been proposed as significant pathologic agents.[20] Feline panleukopemia or leukemia infection may result in infertility because of inapparent early embryonic deaths, abortion of mummified or macerated fetuses, or queening of kittens with retinal, cerebellar, or cerebral hypoplasia. In some colonies, abortion has been noted in cats infected with *Chlamydia psittaci*.[21–23] However, queens that have experienced a previous conjunctival or vaginal infection have produced litters identical to those of queens that have been infected conjunctivally before mating or during pregnancy.[24] In breeding colonies, *Chlamydia*, when present, is often thought to be endemic. This is reflected in the prevalence of *Chlamydia* antibodies in 69.4 per cent of sera obtained from feral cats. When *Chlamydia* is endemic in a cat colony, clinical signs may persist in an individual for several weeks and recurrent episodes can occur.

The Tomcat

It is rare to have male cats brought to a veterinarian for infertility or for problems of the internal or external genita-

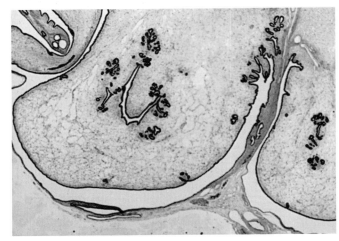

Figure 166–4. Histologic view of the typical aspect of fibroadenomatosis of the mammary gland obtained from a 9-month-old pseudopregnant queen. An intracystic papillary structure with a loose stroma and some glandular structure can be observed.

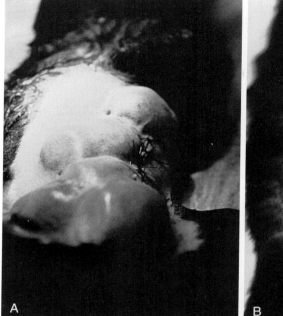
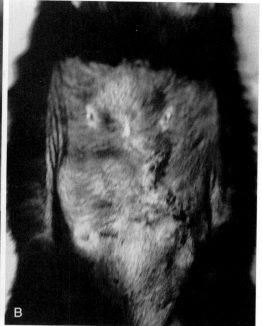

Figure 166–5. Typical mammary development observed in a 9-month-old pseudopregnant queen showing bilateral fibroadenomatosis. *A,* At ovariectomy. *B,* Two weeks after ovariectomy. Quasitotal regression of the dramatic lesions can be observed.

lia. Indeed, most male cats are neutered at a young age, reducing dramatically the incidence of reproductive system problems. Abnormalities of the genitalia other than consequences of fighting or bite wounds are not often reported.

Congenital and Heritable Conditions

Hermaphroditism and Pseudohermaphroditism

True hermaphroditism and abnormalities of gonadal differentiation are rare conditions in cats. Herron and Boehringer[24] reported abnormal testes at the tip of the uterine horns of a 1-year-old phenotypic female blue tabby (male pseudohermaphroditism). The testes contained seminiferous tubules lined with Sertoli cells but no spermatogonia.

Cryptorchidism

The absence of one or both testes in the scrotum is called cryptorchidism. The normal feline testis descends into the scrotum prenatally. However, testes may move freely up and down the inguinal canal before puberty. Therefore, the definitive diagnosis of cryptorchidism should not be made in cats younger than 7 to 8 months of age. Most cats presented for cryptorchidism at 4 months have normal testes at 5 or 6 months. The incidence of cryptorchidism in adult cats ranges from 0.07 to 1.7 per cent, which is much less common than in dogs.[26] Evidence for a hereditary cause of cryptorchidism in cats is not proved, but Persian cats and certain families seem to be predisposed. A simple autosomal recessive sex-linked model has been proposed. Cryptorchidism is more commonly unilateral than bilateral (ratio 3:1). In unilateral cryptorchid animals, both testicles can be equally involved. Cryptorchid cats are most often normal and fertile when the process is unilateral.

Complications (general, behavioral, or pathologic) are rarely observed in cryptorchid cats. The presence or absence of testes in a male can be assessed by the presence of the penile spines, which totally disappear after a male has been castrated. Hormonal evaluation can be undertaken by mea-

suring testosterone concentrations before and after an HCG or GnRH injection. Stimulation tests are required because testosterone concentrations are often close to the minimum detectable value in many normal male cats; therefore, low basal values are not indicative of the absence of testes.

It appears that medical therapies (using GnRH or exogenous gonadotropins) are not successful in correcting abnormal testicular descent. Because this condition may be inherited, cryptorchidism should not be corrected. Such males should be eliminated from breeding programs.

Because testicular neoplasia and testicular cord torsion are uncommon to rare in cats and the heritability of cryptorchidism has not been proved, veterinarians should recommend no treatment or propose castration. Castration should be chosen to eliminate unwanted urination, reproductive behavior, and the problems of male-related odor. If not detected in the abdomen, the cryptorchid testis can often be found in the inguinal ring or under the skin close to the inguinal ring.

Acquired Conditions of the Genitalia

Trauma

Injury to the external genitalia in male cats is often the result of bite wounds, mating, or other accidents. Clinical signs include pain, swelling, and hemorrhage. In all cases of penile wounds, possible urethral damage has to be investigated using techniques such as catheterization and contrast radiography. Superficial penile lesions are usually self-limiting. In cats with more serious lesions, care must to be taken to prevent necrosis and subsequent surgical resection of the penis with perineal urethrostomy is often necessary. For scrotal lesions, general principles of wound management should be followed, including local disinfection, drainage, possibly suturing, and systemic antibiotics if needed. If the animal is not used for breeding, castration with scrotal ablation is the treatment of choice.

Infections

Bacteria are observed within the urethra in more than 90 per cent of normal intact animals. Bacteria include *E. coli,*

REP

Pseudomonas aeruginosa, Proteus mirabilis, Klebsiella oxytoca, Streptococcus spp., *Enteroccocus, Bacillus* spp., and *Staphylococcus* spp. The same organisms can be detected in the semen but are probably contaminants of urethral origin during sperm collection. Bacterial infections of the external genitalia in cats are most often secondary to trauma, bites, or fighting wounds.

Orchitis

Orchitis is rare in the cat but has been described after testicular infection (with tuberculosis, feline infectious peritonitis virus, or aerobic bacteria). Orchitis can be caused by ascending infections from the urinary tract but is most often due to injuries or bite wounds. Tuberculosis has been described in the feline species. One or both testes can be involved. Brucellosis is rare in cats.

Feline infectious peritonitis infections can cause scrotal distention by extension of peritoneal infectious processes through the inguinal ring to the testes. Orchitis caused by bacterial infection is associated with bilateral swelling, fever, lethargy, pain, redness, and anorexia. Furthermore, licking of the lesion may lead to automutilation. Broad-spectrum antibiotics must be administered for at least 2 weeks and, if not successful, must be followed by castration.

Testicular Hypoplasia

This condition is rarely reported in cats because the vast majority are castrated. Testicular hypoplasia can be observed after panleukopenia virus infection in prepubertal cats, with cryptorchidism, and with chromosomal abnormalities. Bilateral hypoplasia may be observed as a sequela of persistent fever, which causes destruction of the germinal layer. Poor libido and variable testicular degeneration leading to azoospermia have also been associated with malnutrition, obesity, hypothyroidism, and hypervitaminosis A.

Neoplasia

Transmissible venereal tumors do not occur in cats. Feline leukemia virus infection was thought to be related to some tumors including testicular and cutaneous tumors overlying the genital region. Sertoli cell tumors are rare and are in general associated with abdominal cryptorchidism. No significant clinical signs are caused by Sertoli cell tumors in cats.

Testicular Torsion

Unilateral torsion of the spermatic cord of both descended and nondescended testes is a rare condition in cats. When it is present, pain is the primary clinical sign.

Penile Hypoplasia and Persistent Penile Frenulum

Penile hypoplasia and failure of separation between the surface of the penis and the preputial mucosa resulting in persistence of the penile frenulum have been described and associated with early castration or genetic conditions. As cats are being neutered at earlier ages, the incidence of these abnormalities and predisposition to urethral obstruction may increase in the future. Urethrostomy is required when penile hypoplasia is associated with urethral obstruction. The persistence of the penile frenulum is often not clinically detectable unless complications of balanoposthitis occur. It might be advisable to check that penile-preputial separation has occurred before castration, particularly in animals younger than 5 months of age.

Phimosis and Paraphimosis

The inability to extrude or to retract the penis from the prepuce may be congenital or acquired after infection or trauma. The preputial hairs of long-haired cats may entangle the orifice, causing clinical signs similar to those of phimosis or paraphimosis. Clipping the hair should resolve the problem. This condition is rare in cats.

Prostatic Diseases

With the rare exception of prostatic neoplasia,[26] prostatic diseases have not been described in cats. Clinical signs of adenocarcinoma are similar to those in dogs and include hematuria, dysuria, pollakiuria, outflow obstruction, anorexia, and weight loss. The condition is usually rapidly progressive and fatal.

Endocrine and Behavioral Conditions

Endocrine Conditions

Plasma testosterone concentrations in the adult intact male cat have been reported to be relatively high. However, large variations exist (ranging from 0 to 23.5 ng/mL). Castration causes a rapid decrease in plasma testosterone concentrations, suggesting that testosterone is primarily of testicular origin. HCG stimulation (250 μg) induces a 3- to 10-fold increase in plasma testosterone concentration after 4 hours and GnRH stimulation (25 μg) a 3- to 15-fold increase after 1 hour.

Behavioral Conditions

Normal breeding behavior of cats is well described. Management of the first mating is important to minimize the risk of acquired behavioral disorders. Acquired behavioral abnormalities of reproduction in the cat include the following.

Lack of Reproductive Behavior and Libido. This may be related to gonadal abnormalities or to immaturity, senility, management conditions, health problems, timing of mating, painful or stressful previous experience, and excessive socialization to humans leading to reduced libido or libido directed toward humans. In certain breeds, particularly Persians and their derivatives (exotic, British), sexual maturity is often observed late (3 years of age and later). In these breeds adult males should not be evaluated for decreased libido until at least 3 years of age.

Inability and/or Refusal to Serve. This may be a consequence of the previously described lack of libido. Refusal to serve is often observed in males that have previously experienced a stressful or painful mating. This could also be related to anatomic or pathologic conditions (inability to extrude the penis [rare], nervous damage to the lumbar and sacral regions of the spinal cord, infections of the genitalia, orchitis and/or epididymides, and other painful or degenerative conditions affecting reproduction).

Infertility in the Tomcat. Possible causes of infertility include poor libido, behavioral disturbances, trauma, and infections. The diagnostic evaluation is similar to that used in dogs. As feline reproduction is a newly developing field, limited information is available.

DRUGS AND TREATMENTS IN FELINE REPRODUCTION

The Queen

Estrus Induction, Infertility, Superovulation

Induction of follicular growth and ovulation can easily be achieved in queens, but a clear indication for estrus induction should be demonstrated before considering such treatment. It is important to know that cats are highly responsive to estrus induction, and overstimulation leading to superovulation or production of numerous anovulatory cystic follicles is common. Such treatment performed inappropriately may cause development of follicular cysts (Fig. 166–6), early embryo resorption caused by an abnormally high plasma estradiol concentration, or infertility. These problems are particularly common in the highly responsive prepubertal or young adult animal. Indications for estrus induction are delayed puberty, prolonged anestrus, and synchronization.

Delayed Puberty

The onset of puberty varies greatly from one animal to another and from one breed to another. For example, it is common for Burmese cats to be 18 to 24 months of age before reaching puberty. Therefore, the veterinarian must know the reproductive tendencies for a particular breed before trying to induce estrus. A clear history must be obtained and a physical examination performed before beginning the treatment.

Prolonged Anestrus

In many cases, the so-called prolonged anestrus is either related to poor estrus detection and management or secondary to progestagen administration.

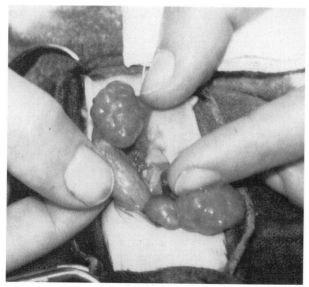

Figure 166–6. Polycystic ovaries observed after estrus induction with PMSG in a 2-year-old queen. The dosage used was too high (100 UI per day for 5 days), and numerous nonovulated follicular cysts could be observed on both ovaries.

Estrus Synchronization

Estrus synchronization may be required for embryo transfer or in association with in vitro procreation techniques. This is particularly true and commonly performed in wild species of felids. These techniques will probably become more efficacious and may be available and useful for small pet animal reproduction problems.

Many treatments have been proposed for inducing estrus in cats, including the use of equine chorionic gonadotropin (ECG) or pregnant mare serum gonadotropin (PMSG), FSH, HCG, and GnRH. Many protocols have been described. Varying doses and protocols have been used. The recommendation here is PMSG (100 to 150 IU) in a single bolus administered to anestral cats, followed 4 to 5 days later by one injection of HCG (50 to 100 IU). This treatment leads to ovulation and pregnancy results comparable to those of natural matings (over 80 per cent). It is important to note that repeated injections of the exogenous gonadotropins (ECG and HCG) may lead to the production of antibodies against FSH and LH, which may cross-react with the endogenous and exogenous hormones and lead to a subsequent decreased response to stimulation or infertility. For this reason, it is recommended that this type of treatment not be repeated and that estrus induction be used only when really needed. In the dog, induction of estrus by the use of buserelin implants or antiprolactinic drugs in bitches with prolonged anestrus has been successful. The use of these drugs in cats has not yet been reported. Data from our laboratory suggest that cabergoline, a dopamine agonist, is efficient at 5 μg/kg per day in inducing a fertile estrus in experimental anestrus-induced cats. However, these results have to be confirmed with a larger number of animals and in clinical situations. GnRH has been recommended at a dosage of 1 μg/kg subcutaneously until signs of estrous behavior are noted or for a maximum of 10 days.

Estrus Prevention or Suppression

Contraception is described in Chapter 161.

Ovulation Induction, Nymphomania, Ovarian Cysts

During estrus, ovulation can be induced mechanically by vaginal stimulation. Exogenous hormones can also be used: GnRH (5 to 25 μg per cat) or HCG (50 to 250 IU per cat) may be administered intramuscularly or intravenously to induce ovulation and therefore terminate estrus. Ovulation generally occurs 24 to 36 hours after the injection and is followed by a 30- to 45-day pseudopregnancy if the animal is not mated or inseminated.

Nymphomania is a complex syndrome in queens. It is usually related to overlapping follicular waves (often observed in Siamese cats) or the presence of ovarian cysts (in old animals or after estrus induction and superovulation), or it may be of central origin (pituitary or hypothalamic). Ovulation induction using GnRH or HCG can temporarily interrupt signs related to ovarian activity. Centrally mediated nymphomania is a rare condition in sterilized animals (particularly Siamese cats), which continuously show estrous behavior despite having been neutered. The exact cause of this condition is still unknown. In centrally mediated nymphomania, administration of progestins may be successful. Ovarian cysts occasionally do not respond to ovulation induction, in which case the treatment of choice is spaying.

REP

Abortion Induction

This is described in Chapter 161.

Pregnancy Maintenance

As in dogs, there is no clear evidence that abortion is caused by hypoluteoidism in cats. However, around day 30 to 45 of pregnancy, significant changes are observed in the function of the corpora lutea. Indeed, around midpregnancy, luteotropic support is required to maintain corpus luteum function. Poor luteal support at this transitional stage, from the period of corpus luteum independence to the corpus luteum hormonally regulated period, can lead to a drop in the plasma progesterone concentration to minimum levels needed to maintain pregnancy (± 1 ng/mL) and can therefore result in abortion. Oral progestins (megestrol acetate, 2.5 mg per cat per day up to day 55 of pregnancy) may be used but should be restricted to cases in which true luteal insufficiency has clearly been diagnosed. Adverse effects on kitten development can result (feminization of male kittens, increased risk of cryptorchidism) and parturition may be impaired (delayed parturition). Injectable progestins should never be used during pregnancy as they prevent the onset of parturition and are associated with mummification or maceration of the fetuses.

Uterine Inertia

Cases of primary or secondary uterine inertia may respond to administration of oxytocin. A dose of 0.5 to 1 IU/kg may be given and repeated a maximum of three times at 20- to 30-minute intervals. The cause of secondary inertia has to be carefully determined before administering oxytocin. Cases of obstructive dystocia are a clear contraindication to use of oxytocin because uterine rupture may result.

Lactation Stimulation or Inhibition

Cats that have undergone cesarean section and some young or stressed queens can experience interference with lactation. Lactation can be stimulated by the administration of dopamine antagonists, which are well known to stimulate prolactin release directly at the pituitary level. Drugs such as metoclopramide (5 mg/kg for 3 to 5 days) can be used safely and successfully. They can be given once or twice daily after parturition or after surgery. Milk production can be enhanced by the postpartum use of oxytocin, assuming that some milk is being produced.

On the other hand, lactation can easily be inhibited by inhibiting prolactin release directly at the pituitary level by giving dopamine agonists (bromocriptine, 10 to 25 μg/kg, or cabergoline, 5 μg/kg, for 5 days) or indirectly by modifying the dopamine release at the hypothalamic level by giving a serotonin antagonist (metergoline). Progestagens, androgens, and androgen-estrogen combinations also have a negative feedback effect and reduce prolactin secretion and lactation. However, they are nonspecific agents associated with other nondesired effects and are not recommended.

Metritis, Pyometra, Placental Retention

Prostaglandins, such as dinoprost, are known to induce luteolysis through a direct luteal cell effect and an indirect blood vessel vasoconstriction reducing corpus luteum blood supply. Prostaglandins also induce smooth muscle contraction, promoting the opening of the cervix and uterine contractions.[27, 28] These effects are the basis for their use in the treatment of pyometra, metritis, or retained placenta. Natural prostaglandins must be used, as their potency in stimulating uterine contractions is significantly higher than that of synthetic prostaglandins. Doses of 20 to 50 μg/kg administered three to five times a day or 200 to 500 μg/kg once or twice a day for 5 to 7 days, plus use of appropriate antibiotics and fluid therapy, are successful treatments. The well-known side effects generally observed when treating dogs with prostaglandins are less significant and much less obvious in cats. Queens clearly tolerate prostaglandins better than bitches and doses up to 200 to 500 μg/kg may be used. However, as in the dog, the advantage of repeated low dosage treatment is certainly best tolerated by the animal. Fertility appears to be conserved after resolution of the condition. However, if reproduction is not necessary, ovariohysterectomy is the preferred treatment. No significant data are available regarding the use of progesterone antagonists such as RU 486 or RU 46534 to treat pyometra in queens.

Placental retention can be treated with oxytocin (1 IU/kg every 20 to 30 minutes with a maximum of three or four injections), particularly if diagnosed early after kittening when uterine sensitivity to oxytocin is most pronounced. To prevent placental retention, injection of oxytocin can be performed routinely.

Postpartum Hemorrhage

Postpartum hemorrhage can be treated using oxytocin and/or ergot derivatives such as ergometrine, which induce uterine contraction and vasoconstriction. However, the cause of the uterine hemorrhage should be clearly identified.

Remnant Ovarian Tissue

Some queens continue to exhibit estrous behavior after sterilization, whereas in others it is unclear whether the queen has been sterilized. Two tests may be used to clarify these situations. An injection of HCG (50 IU, intravenously if possible or intramuscularly, or GnRH, 1 to 5 μg/kg) causes an increase of the plasma estradiol concentration after 1 hour if ovarian tissue is still present. In a sterilized animal, this does not occur. However, as large variations exist in the estradiol assay, the results are not always easy to interpret, particularly with a mild increase. Because of the large intra-assay and individual variations, only a threefold increase should be considered significant. The other way to diagnose the presence of remnant ovarian tissue is to wait for the next period of heat behavior, inject HCG to induce ovulation, and after 1 week take a blood sample to measure the progesterone concentration. If the plasma progesterone concentration is above 1 to 2 ng/mL, a diagnosis of persistence of ovarian tissue can be made. An LH assay could also be proposed, as the LH plasma concentration is always elevated in ovariectomized animals.

The Tomcat

Table 166–1 gives the conditions, dosages, and effects of several agents that may be used in tomcats.

Urine Spraying, Aggressivity and Excitability, Sexual Overt Behavior

In tomcats, urination is used as a communication tool and as a territory marker. This behavior is observed in both

TABLE 166–1. SOME USEFUL DRUGS AND TREATMENTS IN MALE CAT REPRODUCTION

DRUG	INDICATION	DOSAGE	SIDE EFFECTS
Testosterone phenylpropionate or esters	Infertility, reduced libido	0.1–1 mg q 48–72 h, three to five injections IM or SC	High doses can affect fertility, and growth can be blocked by induction of early closure of growth plate. Not indicated for testis descent
Human chorionic gonadotropin (HCG)	Infertility, reduced libido, testis descent, hormonal challenge	50–100 IU repeated if necessary	None are known up to now in male cats. Frequent administration may be associated with antibody production and immunoneutralization of endogenous LH leading to sterility or decreased fertility.
Medroxyprogesterone acetate (MPA)	Hyperexcitability Agressivity, urine marking, male behavior, epilepsy, contraception at high doses Psychogenic alopecia	25–100 mg to be repeated first every 2 weeks then every month or two at half the initial dose SC injection For contraception use more than 50 mg; to be repeated. Urine spraying, 100 mg SC	May affect fertility at high dosage. Mammary development and benign tumors after long-term use, hypoadrenocorticism, diabetus mellitus Growth of white hair or disappearance of hair at injection site
Megestrol acetate (MA)	Same as MPA	2.5 mg per cat every day for 2 weeks, then to effect or once a week. Doses for dermatologic problems are empirical.	Mammary development and benign tumors after long-term use, hypoadrenocorticism, diabetus mellitus
Gonadotropin-releasing hormone (GnRH) agonists	Testis descent, infertility, poor libido	Empirical dosage in this species is 1 µg/kg every 2–3 days.	No significant data available. Might be used to stimulate libido, fertility in a more physiologic way than ECG or testosterone. No side effects expected if low doses are used for short term. Long-term use can lead to downregulation and infertility.
GnRH antagonists	Contraception	No real data are available.	Reversible sterility. Side effects caused by the available drug (mastocyte degranulation).

neutered and intact male cats. Although accepted as normal in feral cats, cat urination in the house is usually considered unacceptable. This behavior may be related to the presence of other cats or animals or possibly to social, environmental, or emotional changes. In intact males, castration decreases plasma testosterone concentrations and can diminish or abolish the behavior and reduce urine odor. The specific male odor is due to both testosterone and retrograde ejaculation, which is normal in the cat. Both are eliminated by castration. Progestagens, such as oral medroxyprogesterone acetate, megestrol acetate, injectable delmadinone acetate, or proligestone, by their central hormonal feedback and central nervous system relaxing effects, can be effective in decreasing these problems. Repeated administration of high dosages is necessary for a significant effect. However, decreasing effectiveness may be observed after repeated administrations. Sedative or psychoactive drugs (diazepam, carbamazepine) can be used to control these behaviors temporarily. Prolonged administration of such agents cannot be recommended because of their metabolic and hormonal side effects at the high dosages needed (diabetes mellitus, Cushing's disease, gain in weight). Behavioral training must always be associated with the medical treatment.

Cryptorchidism

There is no real treatment for stimulating testicular descent in cats and in dogs. Furthermore, such treatments may be considered unethical because the condition is probably inherited. In other species, successful treatment using GnRH, LH, or testosterone has been described, but it is never really clear whether testicular descent occurred as a result of the treatment or would have happened spontaneously. Testosterone or testosterone derivative administration is not recommended because of its general androgenic and anabolic ef-

fects. Testosterone administration to prepubertal animals not only has an irreversible negative feedback on the hypothalamus but also has anabolic effects and interrupts the development of the growth plates. Bilateral castration should be the treatment of choice.

Stimulation of Libido

Poor libido related to gonadal abnormalities, immaturity, or behavioral inhibition can be treated using repeated low doses of testosterone or GnRH or exogenous gonadotropins (HCG). It is important to note that there is no evidence that poor libido is related to low plasma testosterone levels. No dose-titration studies have been performed for these therapies. Doses of 1 to 2 µg of GnRH, 50 to 100 IU of HCG, or 0.1 to 1 mg of methyltestosterone or testosterone propionate per cat every 48 to 72 hours on three to five occasions have been used. As androgens may have negative effects on spermatozoal morphology or continuous negative feedback effects on the hypothalamus, the use of GnRH and HCG is preferred. Reproductive behavior in cats is essentially an acquired trained behavior, and temporary stimulation of libido is usually sufficient to correct the problem permanently.

Other Conditions in Tomcats

Testicular Remnants or Cryptorchidism

As proposed earlier, a GnRH or HCG stimulation test can be performed in animals with male behavior but with no testes in the scrotum. A significant positive increase of testosterone 60 minutes after intravenous injection of GnRH at 1 to 2 µg/kg or HCG at 50 to 100 IU per cat is diagnostic of the presence of testicular tissue. Basal values of testoste-

REP

rone are not reliable. However, a simple, rapid, and easy test is to examine the penis for the presence or absence of keratinized spines, which are clearly hormone dependent. If the spines are not present, it is highly probable that the animal was previously castrated.

Contraception

This is described in Chapter 161.

REFERENCES

1. Wildt DE, Seals US, Rall WF: Genetic resource banks and reproductive technology for wildlife conservation. *In* Cloud JG, Throgaard GH (eds): Genetic Conservation. New York, Plenum, 1993, pp 159–173.
2. Wolfe BA, Wildt DE: Development to blastocysts from in vitro maturation and fertilization of domestic cat oocytes following prolonged cold storage ex situ. J Reprod Fertil 106:135, 1996.
3. Olson P, Moulton C: Pet overpopulation. J Reprod Fertil Suppl 47:433, 1993.
4. Schille VM, Sojka NJ: Feline reproduction. *In* Ettinger SJ, Feldman EC (eds): Textbook of Veterinary Internal Medicine. Philadelphia, WB Saunders, 1995, pp 1690–1698.
5. Aronson LR, Cooper MI: Penile spines of the domestic cat: Their endocrine-behavior relations. Anat Rec 157:71, 1967.
6. Gudermuth DF, Newton L, Daels P, et al: Incidence of spontaneous ovulation in young, group housed cats based on serum and faecal concentrations of progesterone. J Reprod Fertil Suppl 47:177, 1993.
7. Christiansen IJ: Reproduction in the Dog and Cat. London, Baillière Tindall, 1984.
8. Verstegen J, Silva LDM, Onclin K, et al: Echocardiographic study of heart rate in dogs and cats fetuses in utero. J Reprod Fertil Suppl 47:175, 1993.
9. Verstegen J, Onclin K, Silva LDM, et al: Regulation of progesterone during pregnancy in the cat: Studies on the roles of CL, placenta and prolactin secretion. J Reprod Fertil Suppl 47:165, 1993.
10. Root MV, Johnston SD, Olson PN: Estrous length, pregnancy rate, gestation and parturition lengths, litter size and juvenile mortality in the domestic cat. J Am Anim Hosp Assoc 31:429, 1995.
11. Chan SY, Chakraborty PK, Bass EJ, et al: Ovarian-endocrine-behavioural function
12. Concannon P, Hodgson B, Lein D: Reflex LH release in estrous cats following single and multiple copulations Biol Reprod 23:111–117, 1980.
13. Banks DH, Stabenfeldt GH: Luteinizing hormone release in the cat in response to coitus on consecutive days of estrus. Biol Reprod 26:603, 1982.
14. Verstegen J, Onclin K, Potvin N: Morbidity and mortality in neonate kittens: An epidemiological study in Belgium. Proceedings of the Third International Symposium on Reproduction of Dogs, Cats and Exotic Carnivores, Veldhoven, 1996, p 51.
15. Stewart DR, Stabenfeldt GH: Relaxin activity in the pregnant cat. Biol Reprod 32:848, 1983.
16. Leyva H, Madly T, Stabenfeldt GH: Effect of light manipulation on ovarian activity and melatonin and prolactin secretion, in domestic cat. J Reprod Fertil Suppl 39:125, 1989.
17. Shille VM, Lundstrom KE, Stabenfeldt GH: Follicular function in the domestic cat as determined by estradiol 17 beta concentrations in plasma: Relation to estrous behavior and cornification of exfoliated vaginal epithelium. Biol Reprod 21:953, 1979.
18. Hayden DW, Johnston SD, Kiang DT, et al: Feline mammary hypertrophy/fibroadenoma complex: Clinical and hormonal aspects. Am J Vet Res 42:1699, 1981.
19. Wills JM, Gruffydt-Jones TJ, Richmond SJ, et al: Effect of vaccination on feline *Chlamydia psittaci* infection. Infect Immun 55:2653, 1987.
20. Kimura J, Tsukise A, Okano M: Histochemical studies on the dependence of secretory function of the major vestibular gland on ovarian steroid hormones in the cat. J Vet Med Sci 54:1035, 1992.
21. Schwenen PE, Povery RC, Wilson MR: Feline *Chlamydia* infection. Can Vet J 19:289, 1978.
22. Wills JM, Gruffydt-Jones TJ, Richmond SJ, et al: Isolation of feline *Chlamydia psittaci* from cases of conjunctivitis in a colony of cats. Vet Rec 114:344, 1984.
23. Wills JM, Howard J, Gruffydd-Jones TJ, et al: Prevalence of *Chlamydia psittaci* in different cat population in Britain. J Small Anim Pract 29:327, 1988.
24. Herron AA, Boehringer BT: Male pseudohermaphroditism in a cat. Feline Pract 5:30–32, 1975.
25. Millis DL, Hauptman JG, Johnson CA: Cryptorchidism and monorchidism in cats. JAVMA 200:1128, 1992.
26. Hubbard BS, Vulgamott JC, Liska WD: Prostatic adenocarcinoma in a cat. JAVMA 197:1493, 1990.
27. Davidson A, Feldman E, Nelson R: Treatment of feline pyometra in cats using prostaglandins F2 alpha: 21 cases. JAVMA 200:825, 1992.
28. Feldman E, Nelson R: Diagnosis and treatment alternatives for pyometra in dogs and cats. *In* Kirk R (ed): Current Veterinary Therapy X. Philadelphia, WB Saunders, 1989, pp 1305–1328.

SECTION XIV

THE URINARY SYSTEM

CHAPTER 167

CLINICAL APPROACH AND LABORATORY EVALUATION OF RENAL DISEASE

Stephen P. DiBartola

DEFINITIONS

Azotemia is defined as an increased concentration of non-protein nitrogenous compounds in blood, usually urea and creatinine. *Prerenal azotemia* is a consequence of reduced renal perfusion (e.g., severe dehydration, heart failure), and *postrenal azotemia* results from interference with excretion of urine from the body (e.g., obstruction, uroabdomen). *Primary renal azotemia* is caused by parenchymal renal disease. The term *renal failure* refers to the clinical syndrome that occurs when the kidneys are no longer able to maintain their regulatory, excretory, and endocrine functions, resulting in retention of nitrogenous solutes and derangements of fluid, electrolyte, and acid-base balance. Renal failure occurs when 75 per cent of more of the nephron population is non-functional. *Uremia* refers to the constellation of clinical signs and biochemical abnormalities associated with a critical loss of functional nephrons and includes the extrarenal manifestations of renal failure (e.g., uremic gastroenteritis, hyperparathyroidism). The term *renal disease* refers to the presence of morphologic or functional lesions in one or both kidneys, regardless of extent.

CLINICAL APPROACH

The clinician should try to answer the following questions:

1. Is renal disease present?
2. Is the disease glomerular, tubular, interstitial, or a combination of these?
3. What is the extent of the renal disease?
4. Is the disease acute or chronic, reversible or irreversible, progressive or non-progressive?
5. What is the current status of the patient's renal function?
6. Can the disease be treated?
7. What non-urinary complicating factors are present and require treatment (e.g., infection, electrolyte and acid-base disturbances, dehydration, obstruction)?
8. What is the prognosis?

The diagnosis of renal disease begins with a careful evaluation of the history and physical examination findings.

HISTORY

A complete history should be taken, including signalment (age, breed, sex), presenting complaint, husbandry, and review of body systems. The history of the presenting complaint should include information about onset (acute or gradual), progression (improving, unchanging, or worsening), and response to previous therapy. Information about husbandry includes the animal's immediate environment (indoor or outdoor), use (pet, breeding, show, or working animal), geographic origin and travel history, exposure to other animals, vaccination status, diet, and information about previous trauma, illness, or surgery.

Questions relating to the urinary tract include those about changes in water intake and the frequency and volume of urination. The owner should be questioned about pollakiuria, dysuria, or hematuria. Care must be taken to distinguish dysuria and pollakiuria from polyuria and to differentiate polyuria from urinary incontinence. The distinction between pollakiuria and polyuria is important because polyuria may be a sign of upper urinary tract disease whereas pollakiuria and dysuria usually indicate lower urinary tract disease. Occasionally, an owner will complain that the dog is incontinent because it is urinating in the house when in reality it is polyuric but not allowed outdoors frequently enough. Nocturia may be an early sign of polyuria but also can occur as a result of dysuria. Normal urine output ranges from 10 to 20 mL/lb per day in dogs and cats.

Information about the initiation of urination and diameter of the urine stream may be helpful because animals with partial obstruction may experience difficulty initiating urination or may have an abnormal urine stream. If hematuria is present, the owner should be questioned about its timing. Blood at the beginning of urination may indicate a disease process in the urethra or genital tract. Blood at the end of urination or throughout urination may signify a problem in either the bladder or upper urinary tract (kidneys or ureters).

Polydipsia usually is more easily detected by owners than is polyuria. Water intake should not exceed 40 mL/lb per day in dogs and 20 mL/lb per day in cats. It is helpful to describe amounts in quantitative terms familiar to the owner such as cups (approximately 250 mL/cup) or quarts (approximately 1 L/quart). The owner should be questioned about exposure of the animal to nephrotoxins such as ethylene glycol in antifreeze, aminoglycosides (e.g., gentamicin), amphotericin B, thiacetarsamide, and non-steroidal anti-inflammatory drugs (e.g., flunixin meglumine, ibuprofen). Also, one should determine whether the animal has received any drugs that could cause polydipsia and polyuria (e.g., glucocorticoids, diuretics).

PHYSICAL EXAMINATION

A complete physical examination (including fundic and rectal examinations) should be performed. Careful attention

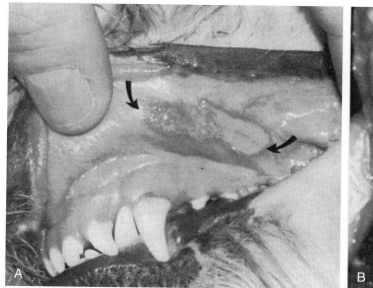 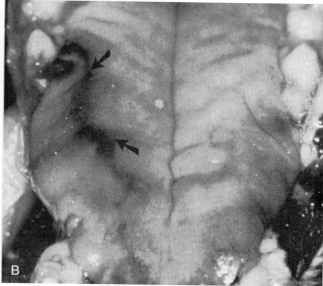

Figure 167–1. *A,* Buccal ulcer. Uremic ulcers often are found in tissue overlying teeth (arrows). Oral ulceration is most commonly observed in dogs with primary (intrinsic) renal azotemia. *B,* Tongue margin necrosis. This lesion may occur in dogs with acute or chronic azotemia.

should be paid to hydration status and to the presence of ascites or subcutaneous edema that may accompany nephrotic disease. The oral cavity is examined for ulcers, tongue tip necrosis, and pallor of the mucous membranes (Fig. 167–1). The presence of retinal edema, detachment, hemorrhage, or vascular tortuosity should be noted on fundic examination. Occasionally, severe hypertension secondary to renal disease will result in acute onset of blindness due to retinal detachment. Young growing animals with renal failure may develop marked fibrous osteodystrophy characterized by enlargement and deformity of the maxilla and mandible (so-called rubber jaw), but this is rare in older dogs with renal failure.

Both kidneys can be palpated in most cats, and the left kidney can be palpated in some dogs. Kidneys should be evaluated for size, shape, consistency, pain, and location. Unless empty, the bladder can be palpated in most dogs and cats. Most chronic renal diseases are associated with normal or small renal size, but several chronic renal diseases of the cat can be associated with renomegaly (e.g., polycystic kidney disease, renal lymphoma, granulomatous nephritis due to feline infectious peritonitis). The bladder should be evaluated for degree of distention, pain, wall thickness, and presence of intramural (e.g., tumors) or intraluminal (e.g., calculi, clots) masses. In the absence of obstruction, a distended bladder in a dehydrated animal suggests abnormal renal function or administration of drugs that impair urinary concentrating ability (e.g., glucocorticoids, diuretics). The prostate gland and pelvic urethra are evaluated by rectal examination. The penis should be exteriorized and examined and the testes palpated. A vaginal examination is performed to evaluate for abnormal discharge, masses, and appearance of the urethral orifice.

LABORATORY EVALUATION OF RENAL FUNCTION

GLOMERULAR FUNCTION

Evaluation of glomerular function is an essential part of the diagnostic approach to patients with suspected renal disease because glomerular filtration rate (GFR) is directly related to functional renal mass. Serum creatinine and blood urea nitrogen (BUN) concentrations are commonly used screening tests, whereas creatinine clearance is useful in patients with suspected renal disease that have normal BUN and serum creatinine concentrations. Clearance of radioisotopes and nuclear imaging are sophisticated techniques that may be used to determine GFR and effective renal plasma flow (ERPF) but do not require urine collection. Evaluation of urinary protein excretion allows assessment of the patient for the presence of primary glomerular disease (e.g., glomerulonephritis, glomerular amyloidosis).

Blood Urea Nitrogen

Urea is synthesized in the liver by means of the ornithine cycle from ammonia derived from amino acid catabolism. The amino acids used in the production of urea arise from the catabolism of exogenous (i.e., dietary) and endogenous proteins. Renal excretion of urea occurs by glomerular filtration, and BUN concentrations are inversely proportional to GFR. Urea is subject to passive reabsorption in the tubules, and this occurs to a greater extent at slower tubular flow rates, which occur during dehydration and volume depletion. Thus, urea clearance is not a reliable estimate of GFR and, in the presence of volume depletion, decreased urea clearance may occur without a decrease in GFR.

The production and excretion of urea do not proceed at a constant rate. Urea production and excretion increase after a high protein meal, and an 8- to 12-hour fast is recommended before measuring BUN concentrations to avoid the effect of feeding on urea production. Gastrointestinal bleeding can increase BUN concentrations because blood represents an endogenous protein load. Clinical conditions characterized by increased catabolism (e.g., starvation, infection, fever) also can increase BUN concentrations. Some drugs may increase BUN concentrations by increasing tissue catabolism (e.g., glucocorticoids, azathioprine) or decreasing protein synthesis (e.g., tetracyclines), but these effects are likely to be minimal. On the other hand, BUN concentrations can be

URO

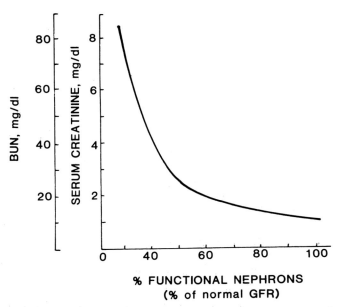

Figure 167–2. Relationship of blood urea nitrogen (BUN) or serum creatinine concentration to percentage of functional nephrons. (From Chew DJ, DiBartola SP: Manual of Small Animal Nephrology and Urology. New York, Churchill Livingstone, 1986.)

decreased by low-protein diets, anabolic steroids, severe hepatic insufficiency, or portosystemic shunting. These non-renal variables limit the usefulness of the BUN concentration as an indicator of GFR. Urea usually is measured by a diacetylmonoxime method, and normal concentrations are 8 to 25 mg/dL in the dog and 15 to 35 mg/dL in the cat.

Serum Creatinine

Creatinine is a non-enzymatic breakdown product of phosphocreatine in muscle, and daily production of creatinine in the body is determined largely by the muscle mass of the individual. Young animals have lower concentrations, whereas males and well-muscled individuals have higher concentrations. Serum creatinine concentration is not affected appreciably by diet. Creatinine is not metabolized and is excreted by the kidneys almost entirely by glomerular filtration. Its rate of excretion is relatively constant in the steady state, and serum creatinine concentration varies inversely with GFR. Thus, *determination of creatinine clearance provides a good estimate of GFR.*

Creatinine is measured by the alkaline picrate reaction, which is not entirely specific for creatinine and measures another group of substances collectively known as non-creatinine chromogens. These substances are found in plasma, where they may constitute up to 50 per cent of the measured creatinine at normal serum concentrations but normally do not appear in urine. As serum creatinine concentration increases due to progression of renal disease and declining GFR, the amount of non-creatinine chromogens is unchanged and contributes progressively less to the total measured serum creatinine concentration. Normal serum creatinine concentrations in the dog and cat are 0.3 to 1.3 mg/dL and 0.8 to 1.8 mg/dL, respectively.

The relationship of BUN or serum creatinine to GFR is a rectangular hyperbola. The slope of the curve is small when GFR is mildly or moderately decreased but large when GFR

is severely reduced (Fig. 167–2). Thus, large changes in GFR early in the course of renal disease cause small increases in BUN or serum creatinine concentrations that may be difficult to appreciate clinically whereas small changes in GFR in advanced renal disease cause large changes in BUN or serum creatinine concentration. The inverse relationship between serum creatinine concentration and GFR is valid only in the steady state.

When non-renal variables have been eliminated from consideration, an increase in BUN or serum creatinine concentration above normal implies that at least 75 per cent of the nephrons are not functioning (see Fig. 167–2). Neither the cause nor the reversibility of this malfunction can be predicted from the magnitude of BUN or serum creatinine concentration. The magnitude of the BUN or serum creatinine concentration cannot be used to predict whether azotemia is prerenal, primary renal, or postrenal in origin and cannot be used to distinguish between acute and chronic, reversible and irreversible, or progressive and nonprogressive processes. The BUN/creatinine ratio in prerenal and postrenal azotemia may be increased owing to increased tubular reabsorption of urea at lower tubular flow rates or easier absorption of urea than creatinine across peritoneal membranes in animals with uroabdomen. A decrease in the BUN/creatinine ratio often follows fluid therapy and reflects decreased tubular reabsorption of urea rather than increased GFR.

Creatinine Clearance

The renal clearance of a substance is that volume of plasma that would have to be filtered by the glomeruli each minute to account for the amount of that substance appearing in the urine each minute. The renal clearance of a substance that is neither reabsorbed nor secreted by the tubules is equal to the GFR. For such a substance in a steady state, the amount filtered equals the amount excreted. Thus,

$$GFR \times P_x = U_x \times V.$$

Dividing both sides of the equation by P_x gives the standard clearance formula (U_xV/P_x), which in this case is equal to the GFR.

Creatinine is produced endogenously and excreted by the body largely by glomerular filtration, and its clearance can be used to estimate GFR in the steady state. Numerous studies in the dog and cat have shown that *endogenous* creatinine clearance in these species is 2 to 5 mL/min per kilogram. Values for glomerular function tests in the dog and cat are presented in Table 167–1.

In chronic progressive renal disease, urinary concentrating

TABLE 167–1. TESTS OF GLOMERULAR FUNCTION IN DOGS AND CATS

TEST	DOG	CAT
Blood urea nitrogen (mg/dL)	8–25	15–35
Serum creatinine (mg/dL)	0.3–1.3	0.8–1.8
Endogenous creatinine clearance (mL/min/kg)	2–5	2–5
Exogenous creatinine clearance (mL/min/kg)	3–5	2–4
^{14}C-inulin clearance (mL/min/kg)	3.3–3.8	3.0–3.5
^{3}H-tetraethylammonium clearance (mL/min/kg)	9–12	7–9
Filtration fraction	0.30–0.38	0.35–0.43
24-hour urine protein excretion (mg/kg/d)	<20	<20
U_{Pr}/U_{Cr}	<0.4	<0.4

ability is impaired after two thirds of the nephron population has become non-functional whereas azotemia does not develop until three fourths of the nephrons have become non-functional. Thus, the main indication for determination of *endogenous* creatinine clearance is the clinical suspicion of renal disease in a patient with polyuria and polydipsia but normal BUN and serum creatinine concentrations. The only requirements for determination of *endogenous* creatinine clearance are an accurately timed collection of urine (usually 12 or 24 hours), determination of the patient's body weight, and serum and urine creatinine concentrations. Failure to collect all urine produced will erroneously reduce the calculated clearance value.

To eliminate the inaccuracy caused by non-creatinine chromogens, some investigators have advocated use of *exogenous* creatinine clearance. In this procedure, creatinine is administered subcutaneously or intravenously to increase serum creatinine concentration approximately 10-fold and reduce the relative effect of non-creatinine chromogens. *Exogenous* creatinine clearance values exceed endogenous creatinine clearance values and closely approximate inulin clearance in the dog. In one study, inulin and *exogenous* creatinine clearances were nearly identical in dogs. The creatinine/inulin clearance ratio was not altered by ablation of 50 to 94 per cent of renal mass and was not affected by gender, dietary protein, or duration of time after renal ablation.[1] *Endogenous* creatinine clearance is a reliable estimate of GFR only when methodology specific for true creatinine is employed.[2] In cats, *exogenous* creatinine clearance may be slightly lower than inulin clearance.

Single-Injection Methods for Estimation of GFR

Single-injection methods using inulin or iohexol have been used in dogs and cats with normal and reduced renal mass to estimate GFR.[3–7] Using these methods, the plasma clearance (mL/min/kg) of a substance that is not bound to plasma proteins and is excreted only by GFR (e.g., inulin, iohexol) is calculated as the quotient of the administered dose divided by the area under the plasma concentration versus the time curve. The plasma clearance of inulin or iohexol then is correlated with exogenous creatinine clearance using linear regression analysis. This technique has the advantage of not requiring collection of urine, but its accuracy depends on the method used to calculate the area under the curve and the number of samples used to make the calculation.

Radioisotopes

Radioisotopes also have been used to determine GFR, ERPF, and filtration fraction (FF) in dogs and cats. The advantages of these procedures are that they do not require collection of urine and are not time consuming. The major disadvantages are the use of radioactive compounds and the need for special equipment and expertise. Published values for radioisotope clearances in dogs and cats are presented in Table 167–1. Values obtained using ^{125}I-iothalamate to measure GFR and ^{131}I-iodohippurate to measure ERPF are slightly higher than values obtained using ^{14}C-inulin and ^{3}H-tetraethylammonium.[8] Also, ERPF values for cats are lower than those observed in dogs and may represent actual species differences in renal blood flow. Thus, FF values were 0.39 in cats and 0.34 in dogs.[8] Quantitative renal scintigraphy[9] and determination of plasma disappearance after single injection[10] using ^{99m}Tc-mercaptoacetyltriglycine also have been used to estimate ERPF in dogs. Nuclear imaging using ^{99m}Tc-diethylenetriaminepentaacetic acid has been used to determine GFR in normal dogs[11] and dogs with renal disease[12] and in normal cats and those with renal dysfunction.[13, 14] This method has the advantage of allowing GFR for individual kidneys to be determined.

Urinary Protein

In animals with persistent proteinuria on routine urinalysis, the severity of proteinuria may be assessed by measuring 24-hour urine protein excretion or performing a urine protein/urine creatinine ratio (U_{Pr}/U_{Cr}). Normal values for 24-hour urine protein excretion in dogs and cats are less than 20 mg/kg per day. Dogs with primary glomerular disease (e.g., glomerulonephritis, glomerular amyloidosis) often have markedly increased 24-hour urine protein excretion values, and those with amyloidosis generally have the highest 24-hour urine protein excretion values.[15, 16]

Determination of U_{Pr}/U_{Cr} eliminates the necessity of a 24-hour urine collection and has been shown to be highly correlated with 24-hour urine protein excretion in dogs[17] and cats.[18] Its value lies in the fact that whereas both urine creatinine and protein concentrations are affected by total urine solute concentration their ratio is not. Normal U_{Pr}/U_{Cr} values in dogs and cats are less than 0.4. In dogs, U_{Pr}/U_{Cr} results are not affected by differences in sex, method of urine collection, fasted versus fed states, or time of day of collection.[19, 20] Pyuria and marked blood contamination of urine samples can result in abnormal U_{Pr}/U_{Cr} ratios in the absence of glomerular disease.[21] Consequently, both the urine protein concentration and U_{Pr}/U_{Cr} ratio must be evaluated in conjunction with urinary sediment findings. Feeding a high-protein diet or induction of renal failure increased 24-hour urine protein and U_{Pr}/U_{Cr} ratios in cats,[22] and administration of prednisone to normal dogs increased U_{Pr}/U_{Cr} ratios from normal to a mean of 1.2 at 30 days and 0.9 at 42 days.[23] Values for 24-hour urine protein excretion and U_{Pr}/U_{Cr} ratio are presented in Table 167–1.

Dogs with proteinuria on screening urinalysis have been shown to have increased U_{Pr}/U_{Cr} values.[15, 17, 20, 24] There is a high degree of overlap between dogs with glomerulonephritis and those with amyloidosis with regard to their 24-hour urine protein excretion and U_{Pr}/U_{Cr} values.[15, 16] Thus, renal biopsy remains the only reliable way to differentiate between these two diseases.

TUBULAR FUNCTION

The kidney is an organ of water conservation. Depending on the needs of the animal, the kidney can produce urine that is highly concentrated or very dilute. Normal urinary concentrating ability is dependent on ability of the hypothalamic osmoreceptors to respond to changes in plasma osmolality, release of antidiuretic hormone (ADH) from the neurohypophysis, and response of the distal nephron to ADH. In addition, medullary hypertonicity must be generated and maintained by the countercurrent multiplier and exchanger systems of the kidney and there must be an adequate number of functional nephrons to generate the appropriate response to ADH. Laboratory tests of tubular function are summarized in Table 167–2.

Urine Specific Gravity and Osmolality

Total urine solute concentration is measured by either urine specific gravity (USG) or urine osmolality (U_{Osm}). The

TABLE 167–2. TESTS OF RENAL TUBULAR FUNCTION IN DOGS AND CATS

TEST	DOG	CAT
Random urine specific gravity	1.001–1.070	1.001–1.080
Urine specific gravity after 5% dehydration	1.050–1.076	1.047–1.087
Urine osmolality after 5% dehydration (mOsm/kg)	1787–2791	1581–2984
Urine-to-plasma osmolality ratio after 5% dehydration	5.7–8.9	NA
Fractional electrolyte clearance (%)		
Sodium	<1	<1
Potassium	<20	<24
Chloride	<1	<1.3
Phosphorus	<39	<73

NA, not available.
Adapted from DiBartola SP: Clinical Evaluation of Renal Function. 16th Annual Waltham/OSU Symposium for the Treatment of Small Animal Diseases. Vernon, CA, Kal Kan Foods, 1992, p 10.

latter is preferable because it depends only on the number of osmotically active particles, regardless of their size. USG is defined as the weight of a solution compared with an equal volume of distilled water. It is dependent on both the number and the molecular weight of the solute particles but has the advantage of requiring only simple, inexpensive equipment for measurement.

Normally, urine is composed of solutes of relatively low molecular weight (e.g., urea, electrolytes) and there is a roughly linear relationship between urine osmolality and specific gravity. The range of urine osmolality corresponding to a given USG value, however, may be relatively wide. If the urine contains appreciable amounts of larger molecular weight solutes such as glucose, mannitol, or radiographic contrast agents, these substances will have a proportionally greater effect on specific gravity than on osmolality.

The term *isosthenuria* (USG 1.007–1.015, U_{Osm} 300 mOsm/kg) refers to urine of the same total solute concentration as unaltered glomerular filtrate. The term *hyposthenuria* refers to urine of lower total solute concentration than glomerular filtrate (USG < 1.007, U_{Osm} < 300 mOsm/kg). Although rarely used clinically, the term *hypersthenuria* (*baruria*) refers to urine of higher total solute concentration than glomerular filtrate (USG > 1.015, U_{Osm} > 300 mOsm/kg). The normal range of total urine solute concentration for dogs and cats is wide (USG 1.001 to 1.080). In a study of normal pet dogs, USG values were found to vary widely (1.006 to >1.050).[25] Samples obtained in the morning had higher USG values than those obtained in the evening, and urine concentration decreased with age but no effect of gender on USG was detected.

Water Deprivation Test

The water deprivation test is a useful test of tubular function and is indicated in evaluation of animals with confirmed polydipsia and polyuria, the cause of which remains undetermined after initial diagnostic evaluation. It usually is performed in animals with hyposthenuria (USG < 1.007) that are suspected to have central or nephrogenic diabetes insipidus or psychogenic polydipsia. An animal that is dehydrated but has dilute urine has already failed the test and should not be subjected to water deprivation. In such an animal, failure to concentrate urine likely is due to structural or functional renal dysfunction or administration of drugs that interfere with urinary concentrating ability (e.g., gluco-

corticoids, diuretics). The water deprivation test is also contraindicated in animals that are azotemic. It should be performed with extreme caution in animals with severe polyuria, because such patients may rapidly become dehydrated during water deprivation if they have defective urinary concentrating ability.

At the beginning of the water deprivation test, the animal's bladder must be emptied and baseline data (body weight, hematocrit, plasma proteins, skin turgor, serum osmolality, urine osmolality, and USG) collected. Water then is withheld, and these parameters are monitored every 2 to 4 hours. Urine and serum osmolalities are the best tests to follow, but osmolality results often are not immediately available to the clinician. Thus, USG and body weight assume the greatest importance for decision making during performance of the test. An increase in total plasma protein concentration is a relatively reliable indicator of progressive dehydration, but increases in hematocrit and changes in skin turgor are not reliable. Serum creatinine and BUN concentrations should not increase during a properly conducted water deprivation test.

Maximal stimulation of ADH release will be present after loss of 5 per cent of body weight. The test is concluded when the patient either demonstrates adequate concentrating ability or becomes dehydrated, as evidenced by loss of 5 per cent or more of its original body weight. It is important when weighing the animal to use the same scale each time and to empty the bladder at each evaluation.

The time required for dehydration to develop during water deprivation varies. Dehydration usually becomes evident within 48 hours in normal dogs and cats but rarely may require a longer period of time. Dogs with diabetes insipidus and psychogenic polydipsia usually become dehydrated after a much shorter period of water deprivation (<12 hours). By the time dehydration is evident, USG usually exceeds 1.045 in normal dogs and cats. Failure to achieve maximal urinary solute concentration does not localize the level of the malfunction, and a structural or functional defect may be present anywhere along the hypothalamic-pituitary-renal axis. Furthermore, animals with medullary solute washout may have impaired concentrating ability regardless of the underlying cause of polyuria and polydipsia.

If there has been less than 5 per cent increase in urine osmolality or less than 10 per cent change in USG for three consecutive determinations or if the animal has lost 5 per cent or more of its original weight, 0.1 to 0.2 U/lb aqueous vasopressin (Pitressin) (up to a total dose of 5 U) or 5 g desmopressin (DDAVP) may be given subcutaneously and parameters of urinary concentrating ability monitored 2 to 4 hours after ADH injection. A further increase in urine osmolality after administration of ADH should not exceed 5 to 10 per cent in normal dogs and cats.

Gradual Water Deprivation

Gradual water deprivation can be performed to eliminate diagnostic confusion caused by medullary solute washout. The owner can be instructed to restrict water consumption to 60 mL/lb per day 72 hours before, 45 mL/lb per day 48 hours before, and 30 mL/lb per day 24 hours before the scheduled water deprivation test. In dogs with psychogenic polydipsia, this will promote endogenous release of ADH, increased permeability of the inner medullary collecting ducts to urea, and restoration of the normal gradient of medullary hypertonicity. An alternate approach is to instruct the owner to reduce water consumption by approximately

10 per cent per day over a 3- to 5-day period (but not < 30 mL/lb/d). This approach should be used only in animals that are otherwise healthy on initial clinical evaluation, and the owner should provide dry food ad libitum and weigh the dog daily to monitor for loss of body weight.

Fractional Clearance of Electrolytes

The extent to which electrolytes appear in the urine is the net result of tubular reabsorption and secretion. The fractional clearance of electrolytes can be used to evaluate tubular function and is defined as the ratio of the clearance of the electrolyte in question to that of creatinine.

$$FC_x = (U_xV/P_x)/(U_{Cr}V/P_{Cr}) = (U_xP_{Cr})/(U_{Cr}P_x)$$

This ratio usually is multiplied by 100 and the fractional clearance value expressed as a percentage. The advantage of this measurement is that a timed urine collection is not necessary. In normal animals, the fractional clearances of all electrolytes are much less than 1.0 (100 per cent), implying net conservation, but values are higher for potassium and phosphorus than for sodium and chloride. Unfortunately, fractional excretion values calculated from "spot" urine samples are highly variable and do not correlate well with values calculated using 72-hour urine samples.[26]

The fractional clearance of sodium may be useful in the differentiation of prerenal and primary renal azotemia. In animals with prerenal azotemia and volume depletion, sodium conservation should be avid and the fractional clearance of sodium very low (≤1 per cent). On the other hand, in animals with azotemia due to primary parenchymal renal disease, the fractional clearance of sodium will be higher than normal (≥1 per cent). Values for fractional electrolyte clearances have been reported for normal dogs,[27] dogs with chronic renal failure,[28] normal cats,[29, 30] and cats with experimentally induced chronic renal failure.[31] Normal values for urinary fractional clearance of electrolytes are summarized in Table 167–2.

ROUTINE URINALYSIS

Urine for urinalysis may be collected by voiding (midstream sample), catheterization, or cystocentesis. Cystocentesis is preferred because it prevents contamination of the sample by the urethra or genital tract, it is simple to perform when the bladder is palpable, there is negligible risk of introducing infection, and it is well tolerated by both dogs and cats. In animals presented for evaluation of hematuria, however, it may be helpful first to evaluate a sample collected by voiding because other methods of urine collection may add red blood cells to the sample as a result of trauma.

When performing the urinalysis, the examiner should use fresh urine whenever possible. Refrigerated urine should be warmed to room temperature before the test. The examiner should note how the sample was collected because this may influence interpretation. Urinalysis is divided into three parts: physical properties, chemical properties, and sediment evaluation.

PHYSICAL PROPERTIES

Appearance

Normal urine is yellow due to the presence of urochrome pigment. Very concentrated urine may be deep amber whereas very dilute urine may be almost colorless. A red or reddish-brown color usually is due to red blood cells, hemoglobin, or myoglobin, whereas a yellow-brown to yellow-green color may be due to bilirubin. Normal urine usually is clear. Cloudy urine often contains increased cellular elements, crystals, or mucus. The most common abnormal odor is ammoniacal and is due to the release of ammonia by urease-producing bacteria.

Specific Gravity

Urine specific gravity is a reflection of the total solute concentration of urine, and the amount of any substance in urine must be interpreted in light of the specific gravity. For example, 4+ protein in 1.010 urine represents more severe proteinuria than 4+ protein in 1.045 urine. USG should be obtained before any treatment because fluids, diuretics, or glucocorticoids may alter specific gravity.

CHEMICAL PROPERTIES

pH

Urine pH varies with diet and acid-base balance. Normal urine pH for dogs and cats is 5.0 to 7.5. Causes of acidic urine pH include meat diet, administration of acidifying agents, metabolic acidosis, respiratory acidosis, paradoxical aciduria in metabolic alkalosis, and protein catabolic states. Causes of alkaline urine pH include urinary tract infection by a urease-positive organism, cereal diet, urine allowed to stand exposed to air at room temperature, post-prandial alkaline tide, administration of alkalinizing agents, metabolic alkalosis, respiratory alkalosis, and distal renal tubular acidosis.

Protein

Random urine samples from normal dogs contain small amounts of protein (up to 50 mg/dL). Commonly used dipstick methods for protein determination are much more sensitive to albumin than globulin. In evaluation of proteinuria, it is critical to localize the origin of the protein loss. This is done by history, physical examination, and a critical evaluation of the urine sediment. Persistent, moderate to heavy proteinuria in the absence of urine sediment abnormalities is highly suggestive of glomerular disease (glomerulonephritis or glomerular amyloidosis). If the sediment is active and proteinuria is mild to moderate, inflammatory renal disease or disease of the lower urinary or genital tract should be considered.

Glucose

Glucose in the glomerular filtrate is almost completely reabsorbed in the proximal tubules and is not normally present in the urine of dogs and cats. If blood glucose concentration exceeds the renal threshold (approximately 180 mg/dL in the dog and 300 mg/dL in the cat), glucose will appear in the urine (glucosuria). Most dipstick tests utilize a colorimetric test based on an enzymatic reaction (glucose oxidase) specific for glucose. Causes of glucosuria include diabetes mellitus, stress or excitement in cats, administration of glucose-containing fluids, and renal tubular diseases such as primary renal glucosuria and Fanconi's syndrome. Glucosuria also may be observed occasionally in

URO

dogs and cats with chronic renal disease, in those with tubular injury caused by nephrotoxins, and in some dogs with familial renal disease.

Ketones

Beta-hydroxybutyrate, acetoacetate, and acetone are ketones, the products of exaggerated and incomplete oxidation of fatty acids. They are not normally present in the urine of dogs and cats. The nitroprusside reagent present in dipstick tests reacts with acetone and acetoacetate, but it is much more reactive with acetoacetate. It does not react with beta-hydroxybutyrate. Causes of ketonuria include diabetic ketoacidosis, starvation or prolonged fasting, glycogen storage disease, low carbohydrate diet, persistent fever, and persistent hypoglycemia. Ketonuria occurs more readily in young animals, and, of the causes just listed, diabetic ketoacidosis is the most important cause in adult dogs and cats.

Occult Blood

Dipstick tests are very sensitive but do not differentiate among erythrocytes, hemoglobin, and myoglobin. The test is more sensitive to hemoglobin than to intact erythrocytes, and the former causes a diffuse color change whereas the latter cause spotting of the reagent pad. A positive test must be interpreted in light of the urine sediment findings (i.e., presence or absence of red blood cells). Free hemoglobin (secondary to hemolysis) is the most common abnormal pigment found in urine. Potential causes of hemolysis include transfusion reaction, autoimmune hemolytic anemia, disseminated intravascular coagulation, postcaval syndrome of dirofilariasis, splenic torsion, and heat stroke. Myoglobinuria is less common but may occur if there is severe rhabdomyolysis (e.g., status epilepticus, crushing injury). For proper interpretation, the occult blood reaction must be considered together with the urine sediment findings (e.g., hematuria).

Bilirubin

Bilirubin is derived from the breakdown of heme by the reticuloendothelial system. It is transported to the liver where it is conjugated with glucuronide and excreted in the bile. Only direct-reacting or conjugated bilirubin appears in the urine. The canine kidney can degrade hemoglobin to bilirubin, and the renal threshold for bilirubin is low in dogs. Thus, in dogs with liver disease, bilirubin may be detected in the urine before its serum concentration is increased. It is not unusual to find small amounts of bilirubin in concentrated urine samples from normal dogs, especially males. Bilirubin is absent from normal feline urine. The causes of bilirubinuria are hemolysis (e.g., autoimmune hemolytic anemia), liver disease, extrahepatic biliary obstruction, fever, and starvation.

Leukocyte Esterase Reaction

Indoxyl released by esterases from intact or lysed leukocytes reacts with a diazonium salt and is detected as a blue color reaction after oxidation by atmospheric oxygen. This test is specific for pyuria in canine urine samples but has low sensitivity (many false-negative results).[32] In cats, the leukocyte esterase test was found to be moderately sensitive but highly nonspecific (many false-positive results) for detection of pyuria.[33]

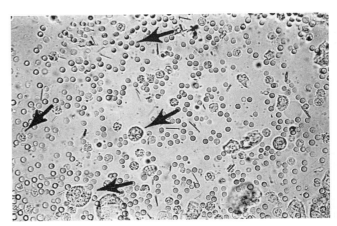

Figure 167–3. Photomicrograph of an abnormal urine sample. Arrow at top indicates red blood cells (RBCs), arrow at left indicates a white blood cell (WBC), whereas central and bottom arrows indicate two different sizes of transitional epithelial cells. RBCs in urine may resemble those in blood or may shrink or swell in response to variations in urine osmolality.

URINARY SEDIMENT EXAMINATION

Depending on the criteria used for data analysis, as few as 3 per cent or as many as 16 per cent of dogs and cats with normal findings on physical and chemical evaluation of urine may have important urinary sediment abnormalities (e.g., pyuria, bacteriuria, microscopic hematuria).[34] The sediment examination should be performed on fresh urine samples because casts and cellular elements degenerate rapidly at room temperature. Urine should be centrifuged at 1000 to 1500 rpm for 5 minutes and the sediment stained with Sedi-Stain (Becton Dickinson, Franklin Lakes, NJ) or examined unstained depending on individual preference. When evaluating the urine sediment, the examiner should keep in mind the method of urine collection because it will influence

TABLE 167–3. CAUSES OF HEMATURIA IN DOGS AND CATS

Urinary Tract Origin (Kidneys, Ureters, Bladder, Urethra)

Trauma
    Traumatic collection (e.g., catheter, cystocentesis)
    Renal biopsy
    Blunt trauma (e.g., automobile accident)
Urolithiasis
Neoplasia
Inflammatory disease
    Urinary tract infection
    Feline urologic syndrome (idiopathic feline lower urinary tract disease)
    Chemically induced inflammation (e.g., cyclophosphamide-induced cystitis)
Parasites
    Dioctophyma renale
    Capillaria plica
Coagulopathy
    Warfarin intoxication
    Disseminated intravascular coagulation
    Thrombocytopenia
Renal infarction
Renal pelvic hematoma
Vascular malformation
    Renal telangiectasia (Welsh corgi)
    Idiopathic renal hematuria

Genital Tract Contamination (Prostate, Prepuce, Vagina)

Estrus
Inflammatory, neoplastic, and traumatic lesions of the genital tract

TABLE 167-4. CAUSES OF PYURIA

Urinary Tract Origin (Kidneys, Ureters, Bladder, Urethra)

Infectious
    Urinary tract infection (e.g., pyelonephritis, cystitis, urethritis)
Noninfectious
    Urolithiasis
    Neoplasia
    Trauma
    Chemically induced (e.g., cyclophosphamide)

Genital Tract Contamination (Prostate, Prepuce, Vagina)

interpretation. Also, the USG should be considered because this will influence the relative numbers of formed elements. The number of casts is recorded per low-power field (lpf), whereas numbers of red blood cells, white blood cells, and epithelial cells are recorded per high-power field (hpf).

Red Blood Cells

Occasional red blood cells are considered normal in the urine sediment. Normal values are voided sample, 0 to 8/hpf; catheterized sample, 0 to 5/hpf; and cystocentesis sample, 0 to 3/hpf. Excessive numbers of red blood cells in urine is called *hematuria* (Fig. 167–3). It may be microscopic or macroscopic. The causes of hematuria are summarized in Table 167–3.

White Blood Cells

Occasional white cells are considered normal in the urine sediment. Normal values are voided sample, 0 to 8/hpf; catheterized sample, 0 to 5/hpf; and cystocentesis sample, 0 to 3/hpf. An increased number of white cells in the urine sediment is called *pyuria* (Fig. 167–4) and, in an appropriately collected urine sample, is indicative of inflammation somewhere in the urinary tract. The presence of white cells does not help localize the lesion unless there are white cell

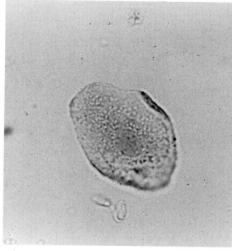

Figure 167–5. Photomicrograph of a squamous epithelial cell in the urine. Note the small nucleus, irregular cell shape, and folding of cytoplasmic margins in some areas.

casts indicating renal origin. Urinary tract infection is the most common cause of pyuria, but genital tract contamination also may cause pyuria in voided or catheterized samples (Table 167–4).

Epithelial Cells

Both squamous and transitional epithelial cells may be found in the urine sediment, but they are often of little diagnostic significance. Squamous cells are large, polygonal cells with small round nuclei (Fig. 167–5). They are common in voided or catheterized samples owing to urethral or vaginal contamination. Occasional squamous cells are normal, and increased numbers may be present during estrus.

Transitional epithelial cells are variable-sized cells derived from the urothelium from the renal pelvis to the urethra (Fig. 167–6). Although their size generally increases from renal pelvis to urethra, the finding of small transitional cells in the urine sediment does not have localizing value. Caudate cells are transitional cells with tapered ends thought to originate from the renal pelvis (Fig. 167–7). Occasional transitional

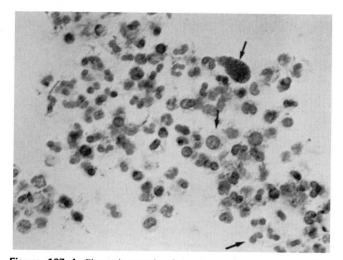

Figure 167–4. Photomicrograph of an abnormal urine sample. White blood cells (WBCs) in urine are subject to degenerative changes that may complicate their identification. They may shrink in concentrated urine or swell in dilute urine. WBCs usually are one and one-half to two times the size of red blood cells. Clumps of WBCs often are associated with infection. Occasional transitional epithelial cells also are present in this field. Arrow, bottom right, denotes neutrophil with swollen cytoplasm and easily identifiable polymorphonuclear nucleus. Occasional transitional epithelial cells also are present (top arrows).

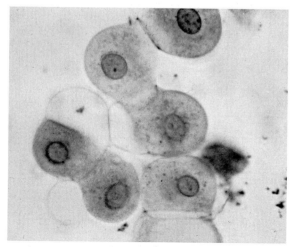

Figure 167–6. Photomicrograph of a raft of transitional epithelial cells in the urine.

URO

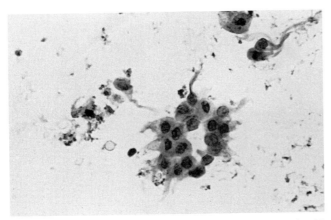

Figure 167–7. Photomicrograph of caudate epithelial cells in urine. The tails on these small epithelial cells suggest their origin from the renal pelvis.

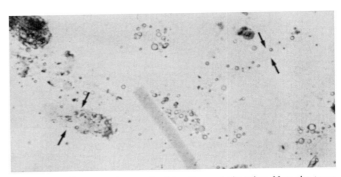

Figure 167–8. Photomicrograph of hyaline casts in urine. Note the transparent nature of these casts (between arrows). It is easy to miss these casts, because their optical density is very low, necessitating low illumination for optimal visualization. The darker cast in the center of the field is a waxy cast. There are many lipid droplets in the background.

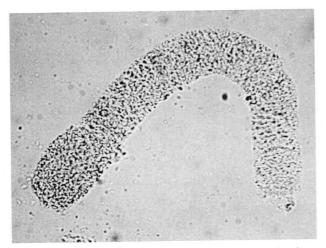

Figure 167–9. Photomicrograph of a finely granular cast in urine.

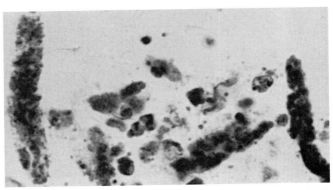

Figure 167–10. Photomicrograph of coarsely granular casts in urine. A "shower" of casts is seen in this field. The cast at the left contains coarse granules, whereas the one on the far right is a cellular cast undergoing degeneration.

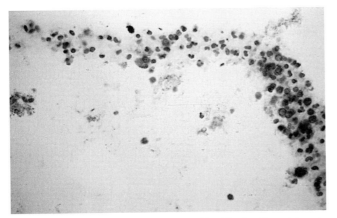

Figure 167–11. Photomicrograph of a white blood cell cast in urine. Neutrophils can be seen within this cast. Their presence suggests renal bacterial infection (i.e., pyelonephritis).

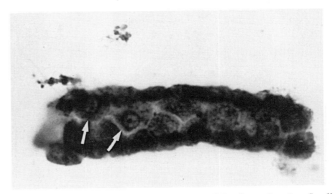

Figure 167–12. Photomicrograph of an epithelial cell cast in urine. Small renal epithelial cells can be identified in this cast (white arrows). (Courtesy of Nancy Facklam.)

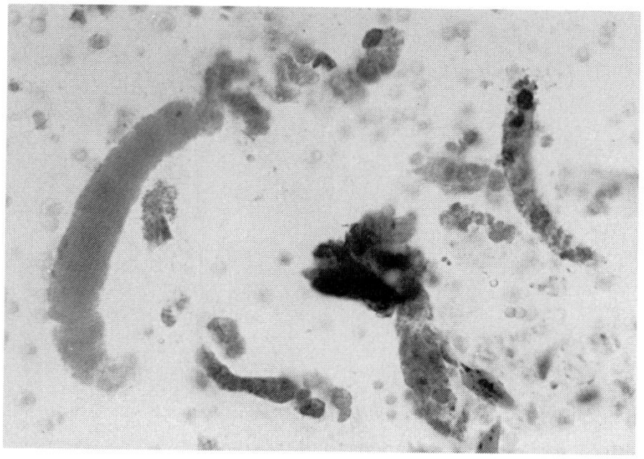

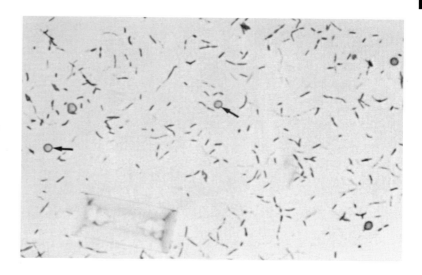

Figure 167–13. Photomicrograph of a urine sample containing waxy and granular casts. The cast at the left is waxy, whereas the others are granular. Notice that the waxy cast is translucent compared with the transparent nature of hyaline casts. Waxy casts are brittle and often have cracks or sharply broken ends.

cells are normal, and increased numbers may be present if there is infection, irritation, or neoplasia of the urinary tract. Renal cells are small epithelial cells from the renal tubules, and their renal origin can only be determined if they are observed in cellular casts. Neoplastic epithelial cells are best identified using conventional blood cell stains (e.g., Wright-Giemsa).

Casts

Casts are cylindric molds of the renal tubules composed of aggregated proteins or cells. They form in the ascending limb of Henle's loop and distal tubule because of maximal acidity, highest solute concentration, and lowest flow rate in this area. The presence of casts in the urinary sediment indicates activity in the kidney itself and thus is of localizing value. Occasional hyaline (Fig. 167–8) and granular (Fig. 167–9) casts per low-power field are considered normal. No cellular casts should be observed in sediment from normal urine. Excretion of abnormal numbers of casts in the urine is called *cylindruria*. The types of casts observed in the urine sediment are hyaline, granular, cellular, and waxy. Hyaline casts are pure protein precipitates (Tamm-Horsfall mucoprotein and albumin). They are difficult to see and

dissolve rapidly in dilute or alkaline urine. Small numbers of hyaline casts may be noted with fever or exercise. They are commonly found in renal diseases associated with proteinuria (glomerulonephritis and glomerular amyloidosis). Coarsely (Fig. 167–10) and finely (see Fig. 167–9) granular casts represent the degeneration of cells in other casts or precipitation of filtered plasma proteins and are suggestive of ischemic or nephrotoxic renal tubular injury. Fatty casts are a type of coarsely granular cast containing lipid granules and may be found in nephrotic syndrome or diabetes mellitus. Cellular casts include white cell or pus casts (suggestive of pyelonephritis) (Fig. 167–11), red cell casts (fragile and rarely observed in dogs and cats), and renal epithelial cell casts (Fig. 167–12) (suggestive of acute tubular necrosis or pyelonephritis). Waxy casts represent the final stage of degeneration of granular casts, are relatively stable, and suggest intrarenal stasis (Fig. 167–13). They often are very convoluted with cracks and blunt ends.

Organisms

Normal bladder urine is sterile. The distal urethra and genital tract harbor bacteria, and voided or catheterized urine samples may be contaminated with bacteria from the distal urethra, genital tract, or skin. Contamination from the urethra in voided or catheterized specimens usually does not result in large enough numbers of bacteria to be visualized microscopically in the urine sediment. If allowed to incubate at room temperature, however, these contaminants may proliferate. To be readily apparent microscopically, there must be more than 10^4 rods/mL urine or more than 10^5 cocci/mL urine. The presence of large numbers of bacteria in urine collected by catheterization or cystocentesis suggests the presence of urinary tract infection (Fig. 167–14). Usually, there is accompanying pyuria. Particulate debris in the sediment may be confused with bacteria and cause false-positive results. Also, the bottle of stain may be contaminated with bacteria. The microscopic absence of bacteria in the sediment does not rule out urinary tract infection. Yeast and fungal hyphae in the sediment usually are contaminants.

Crystals

The solubility of crystals is dependent on urine pH, temperature, and specific gravity. Crystals commonly are present in urine of dogs and cats and often are of little diagnostic

URO

Figure 167–14. Photomicrograph of a urine sample containing bacteria. Chains of bacterial rods are present in this field. Also present are red blood cells (arrows) and a large struvite crystal. Bacteria are most readily identified in urine when they are rods and often are observed in association with clumped white blood cells or within white blood cells.

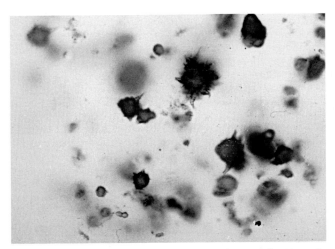

Figure 167–15. Photomicrograph of a urine sample containing ammonium biurate crystals. These crystals may be observed in normal Dalmatian dogs as well as in dogs with liver disease or portosystemic shunts.

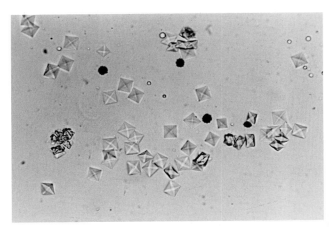

Figure 167–17. Photomicrograph of a urine sample containing calcium oxalate dihydrate crystals. These crystals may be observed in the urine of normal dogs as well as in those with calcium oxalate urolithiasis or acute renal failure due to ethylene glycol ingestion. Note the typical "Maltese cross" appearance within a rhomboidal structure. These crystals can vary markedly in size.

significance. Struvite, amorphous phosphates, and oxalates are examples of crystals that may be found in normal urine samples. Uric acid, calcium oxalate, and cystine typically are found in acidic urine, whereas struvite ($MgNH_4PO_4 \cdot 6H_2O$ or so-called triple phosphate), calcium phosphate, calcium carbonate, amorphous phosphate, and ammonium biurate typically are found in alkaline urine. Characteristic crystals also may be found in the urine sediment of animals receiving specific drugs, especially sulfonamides. Bilirubin crystals may be found in concentrated samples of normal dog urine. Urates are commonly observed in the urine of Dalmatian dogs and may be seen in the urine of animals with liver disease or portosystemic shunts (Fig. 167–15). Struvite crystals may be observed in the urine of cats with feline urologic syndrome, in dogs and cats with struvite urolithiasis, or in the urine of normal animals (Fig. 167–16). In oliguric acute renal failure, the presence of calcium oxalate crystals (Figs. 167–17 and 167–18) is highly suggestive of ethylene glycol intoxication. The presence of cystine crystals in urine of dogs and cats is abnormal and suggestive of cystinuria (Fig. 167–19).

Miscellaneous

Sperm commonly are found in urine samples from normal intact male dogs. Rarely, parasite ova of *Dioctophyma renale*

or *Capillaria plica* or microfilaria of *Dirofilaria immitis* may be observed in the urine sediment. Refractile lipid droplets may occur in diabetes mellitus or nephrotic syndrome. They also may be observed in cats due to degeneration of lipid-laden tubular cells.

MICROBIOLOGY

Clinical signs and urinalysis findings provide supportive evidence, but microbiology is required to conclusively diagnose urinary tract infection (UTI). The kidneys, ureters, bladder, and proximal urethra of normal dogs and cats are sterile, whereas a resident bacterial flora populates the distal urethra, prepuce, and vagina. Urinary tract infection occurs when bacteria colonize areas of the urinary tract that normally are sterile. Aerobic gram-negative bacteria account for the majority of UTI in dogs and cats, and the remainder are caused by gram-positive organisms. *Escherichia coli* is the most common organism implicated in UTI of dogs and cats. Other organisms isolated include *Proteus* spp., coagulase-positive staphylococci, and streptococci. *Pasteurella multo-*

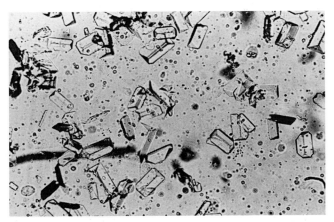

Figure 167–16. Photomicrograph of a urine sample containing struvite crystals. These crystals may be observed in the urine of normal dogs and cats and are more common in alkaline urine.

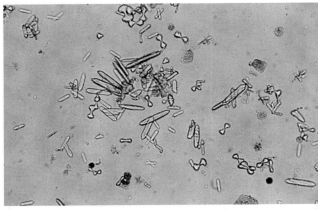

Figure 167–18. Photomicrograph of a urine sample containing calcium oxalate monohydrate crystals. Previously misnamed hippurate, these "picket fence"- and "dumbbell"-shaped crystals may be found in the urine of dogs with acute renal failure due to ethylene glycol ingestion.

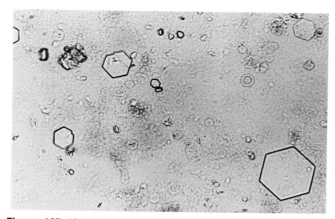

Figure 167–19. Photomicrograph of a urine sample containing cystine crystals. These crystals usually are found in acidic urine and are not found in normal animals. Their presence suggests cystinuria with or without cystine urolithiasis.

cida occasionally is isolated from cats with UTI. *Enterobacter* spp., *Klebsiella* spp., and *Pseudomonas aeruginosa* are observed less commonly in dogs and rarely in cats.

Results obtained by bacterial culture of urine are dependent on the method of urine collection. Voided urine has the greatest potential for bacterial contamination. Catheterization may inoculate the bladder with bacteria from the distal urethra, but urine collected by cystocentesis should be sterile in normal animals. Quantitative bacterial culture of urine allows determination of the number of bacterial colonies (colony-forming units [cfu]) that grow from 1 mL of urine (cfu/mL). Ideally, urine should be submitted for culture within 30 minutes of collection. If this is not possible, the sample may be refrigerated for up to 6 hours without significant loss of bacterial growth. Chemical preservation using a solution of boric acid, glycerol, and sodium formate in combination with refrigeration has been effective in maintaining bacterial viability in canine urine samples for up to 72 hours.[35]

Bacterial culture of midstream-voided urine samples from normal dogs and cats often results in growth of less than 10^3 to greater than or equal to 10^5 cfu/mL. Therefore, culture of voided urine is not recommended in evaluation of patients for UTI. If, however, no growth is obtained from a voided urine sample, UTI can be excluded as a diagnosis. Bacterial growth of greater than or equal to 10^5 cfu/mL may result from culture of urine obtained from catheterization in 20 per cent of normal female dogs. Thus, using 10^5 cfu/mL as indication of UTI in female dogs will result in a substantial number of false-positive results. Also, the procedure of urethral catheterization itself may cause UTI in 20 per cent of normal female dogs. Consequently, collection of urine by cystocentesis is recommended for establishing a diagnosis of UTI in female dogs. Isolation of bacteria from urine collected by catheterization of male dogs is uncommon, and more than 10^3 cfu/mL is recommended for establishing a diagnosis of UTI in urine samples collected by catheterization from male dogs. In both male and female cats, growth of more than 10^3 cfu/mL in samples collected by catheterization is considered compatible with UTI. Urine samples obtained by cystocentesis from normal dogs and cats should yield no growth because this procedure bypasses the normal bacterial flora of the urethra and genital tract. Consequently, results obtained by cystocentesis are the standard against which results obtained using voided or catheterized samples

are compared. Small numbers of organisms from the skin or environment occasionally contaminate samples obtained by cystocentesis, and growth of less than 10^3 cfu/mL may be considered suggestive of contamination. Isolation of bacteria from urinary tissues obtained during surgery indicates UTI regardless of number. Colony counts used to establish a diagnosis of UTI for different methods of urine collection are summarized in Table 167–5.

Microscopic examination of Gram-stained smears of urine also may be helpful in diagnosis of UTI. In one study, one drop of uncentrifuged urine was allowed to dry, Gram stained, and examined under oil immersion. The presence of two or more organisms per field was correlated with bacterial counts of greater than or equal to 10^3 cfu/mL, whereas no organisms were visible in specimens with less than 10^3 cfu/mL.[35]

RADIOLOGY

Radiography provides precise information about renal size that frequently cannot be obtained from physical examination. To correct for variation in patient size and radiographic magnification, renal size is evaluated in reference to surrounding anatomic landmarks, usually the second lumbar vertebra (L2) on the ventrodorsal view. The left kidney normally is well visualized in the dog, but the right kidney often cannot be seen as well, especially its cranial pole. In the dog, the left kidney (near vertebra L2 to L5) is located caudad to the right kidney (near vertebra T13 to L3). In the cat, the kidneys lie near vertebra L3 with the right kidney positioned slightly craniad to the left. Renal size in dogs and cats can be assessed radiographically and compared with the length of vertebra L2. On the ventrodorsal view, the kidney-to-L2 ratio is 2.5 to 3.5 in dogs and 2.4 to 3.0 in cats.

Excretory urography is performed by taking sequential abdominal radiographs after intravenous administration of

TABLE 167–5. ASSESSMENT OF QUANTITATIVE URINE CULTURE RESULTS IN DOGS AND CATS

METHOD OF COLLECTION	SPECIES	SEX	COLONY COUNT INDICATIVE OF URINARY TRACT INFECTION (UTI)
Cystocentesis*	Dog	Male	$>10^2$ cfu/mL
		Female	$>10^2$ cfu/mL
	Cat	Male	$>10^2$ cfu/mL
		Female	$>10^2$ cfu/mL
Catheterization	Dog	Male	$>10^3$ cfu/mL
		Female	$>10^5$ cfu/mL†
	Cat	Male	$>10^3$ cfu/mL
		Female	$>10^3$ cfu/mL
Midstream voided	Dog	Male	Unreliable‡
		Female	Unreliable‡
	Cat	Male	Unreliable‡
		Female	Unreliable‡

*Growth of small numbers of a single organism ($\leq 10^2$ cfu/mL) from urine samples collected by cystocentesis is suggestive of skin contamination during collection. Growth of large numbers ($>10^3$ cfu/mL) of multiple organisms from urine samples collected by cystocentesis is suggestive of needle puncture of bowel and contamination by intestinal flora.

†This guideline may result in erroneous diagnosis of UTI because $>10^5$ cfu/mL may be obtained from urine samples collected by catheterization in 20 per cent of normal female dogs. Also, the procedure of urethral catheterization itself may cause UTI in 20 per cent of normal female dogs. Collection of urine by cystocentesis is recommended for establishing diagnosis of UTI in female dogs.

‡Culture of midstream-voided urine samples from normal dogs and cats may result in growth of $\geq 10^5$ cfu/mL. In the absence of prior antimicrobial therapy, a negative result on a voided sample excludes a diagnosis of UTI.

URO

an iodinated organic compound. The contrast medium is filtered and excreted by the kidneys, and the quality of the study is partially dependent on the patient's GFR. Radiographs should be taken at appropriate intervals (e.g., < 1 min, 5 min, 20 min, 40 min) to obtain maximal information about the renal parenchyma and collecting system. Excretory urography is useful in evaluation of abnormalities in renal size, shape, or location; filling defects in the renal pelvis or ureters; certain congenital defects (e.g., unilateral agenesis); renomegaly; acute pyelonephritis; and rupture of the upper urinary tract. Excretory urography should not be performed in dehydrated patients or in those with known hypersensitivity to contrast media. Although excretory urography normally is a safe procedure, decreased GFR may persist for several days after intravenous administration of contrast agents to normal dogs, and acute renal failure has been reported in a dog after excretory urography.[36] The general technique and interpretation of excretory urography in dogs and cats have been reviewed elsewhere.[37] Ultrasound-guided percutaneous antegrade pyelography has been used to localize ureteral obstruction in dogs and cats.[38]

ULTRASONOGRAPHY

Renal ultrasonography is a non-invasive imaging technique that does not depend on renal function, has no known adverse effects on the patient, and allows characterization of internal renal architecture. The major advantage of ultrasonography is its ability to discriminate among renal capsule, cortex, medulla, pelvic diverticula, and renal sinus.[39–42] Normally, the kidney is less echogenic than the liver or spleen. Collagen and fat provide highly reflective acoustic interfaces and account for the observation that the renal capsule, diverticula, and sinus are the most echogenic structures in the kidney. The renal medulla normally is less echogenic than the renal cortex because of its higher water content and fewer acoustic interfaces.[41] The hyperechogenicity of renal cortex relative to medulla varies among normal cats and has been attributed to variations in the amount of fat present in proximal tubular cells.[43]

Renal length and volume as determined by ultrasonography are linearly related to body weight in dogs.[44, 45] In cats, renal length as determined by ultrasonography ranged between 3.0 and 4.3 cm.[46] Measurements of renal size determined by excretory urography exceed those obtained by ultrasonography.[39, 46] This difference is due to osmotic diuresis and radiographic magnification effects during excretory urography and to indistinct renal margins and inaccurate choice of scanning planes during ultrasonography.[44, 46]

Renal ultrasonography is useful for differentiating solid from fluid-filled lesions and for determining the distribution of lesions within the kidney (i.e., focal, multifocal, diffuse).[47] A pattern of multiple anechoic cavitations is highly suggestive of polycystic kidney disease.[48, 49] Cysts are smooth, sharply demarcated, anechoic lesions that demonstrate through-transmission.[40] The renal pelvis is dilated with anechoic fluid in hydronephrosis, and the kidney is surrounded by an accumulation of anechoic fluid in cats with perinephric pseudocysts. Organized hematomas, abscesses, and necrotic nodules result in a pattern of mixed echogenicity. Focal or diffuse lesions of mixed echogenicity that disrupt normal anatomy often are tumors.[47] Poorly vascularized tumors of homogenous cell type (e.g., lymphosarcoma) may produce hypoechoic lesions that occasionally may be misinterpreted as cysts.[47, 48] Diffuse parenchymal renal diseases character-

ized by cellular infiltration with preservation of normal renal architecture (e.g., chronic tubulointerstitial nephritis) may produce diffuse hyperechogenicity but occasionally are characterized by a normal ultrasonographic appearance. Consequently, normal renal ultrasonography does not eliminate the possibility of renal disease.

Ethylene glycol intoxication also causes renal hyperechogenicity. Within 4 hours of ethylene glycol ingestion, renal cortical echogenicity exceeded that of liver and approached that of spleen.[50, 51] Medullary echogenicity was increased to a lesser extent. Increased cortical and medullary echogenicity with relative hypoechogenicity of the corticomedullary junction and inner medulla resulted in a "halo" sign that correlated with the onset of anuria. Renal hyperechogenicity in ethylene glycol intoxication is attributed to deposition of calcium oxalate crystals in the kidneys.

An echogenic line in the outer zone of the medulla and paralleling the corticomedullary junction (so-called medullary rim sign) has been observed in ethylene glycol intoxication but also in acute tubular necrosis, hypercalcemic nephropathy, granulomatous nephritis due to feline infectious peritonitis, and chronic tubulointerstitial nephritis.[52, 53] This lesion also has been observed in normal cats[43] and is attributed to mineralization of tubular basement membranes.

Intrarenal resistance to blood flow may be assessed during duplex Doppler ultrasonography and evaluated by calculation of the resistive index. Normal values for renal resistive index in normal, non-sedated dogs are approximately 0.6.[54] Somewhat lower values have been reported in normal, sedated dogs (0.32–0.57)[55] and cats (0.52–0.63).[56] Higher than normal values for resistive index have been reported in some renal diseases of dogs and cats[57] but not in experimentally induced aminoglycoside nephrotoxicosis.[58]

RENAL BIOPSY

Renal biopsy allows the clinician to establish a histologic diagnosis and should be considered when the information obtained is likely to alter patient management. Examples of such situations include differentiation of protein-losing glomerular diseases, differentiation of acute renal failure from chronic renal failure, determination of the status of tubular basement membranes in acute renal failure, and establishing the response of the patient to therapy or the progression of previously documented renal disease. A renal biopsy should not be performed until thorough clinical evaluation of the patient has been completed.

Several techniques for renal biopsy are available and include blind percutaneous, laparoscopic, keyhole, open, and ultrasound-guided approaches. The choice of technique is dependent largely on the experience and technical skill of the operator, the species to be sampled, and the size of sample required. The blind percutaneous technique works well in cats because their kidneys can be readily palpated and immobilized. Laparoscopy allows direct visualization of the kidney and detection of hemorrhage but requires special equipment and expertise. The keyhole approach is occasionally employed in dogs but is useful only if the operator is experienced with the technique. In one study of renal biopsy techniques in dogs, modifications of the keyhole technique and use of laparoscopy did not improve the quality of the biopsy specimen obtained or reduce the complication rate.[59] If the operator is relatively inexperienced with renal biopsy or a larger sample is required, wedge biopsy by laparotomy is recommended. Advantages of this procedure include the

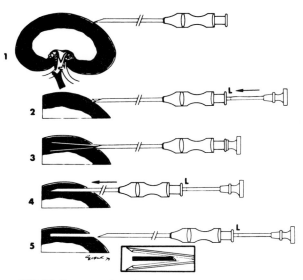

Figure 167–20. Demonstration of renal biopsy technique using a Franklin-modified Vim-Silverman needle. (1) The tip of the outer cannula with stylet is in contact with the renal capsule. (2) The stylet is replaced by the cutting prong. (3) The cutting prongs are advanced into the renal cortex. (4) The outer cutting cannula is advanced over the cutting prongs. (5) The outer cannula and cutting prongs are removed from the kidney. (From Osborne CA: Kidney biopsy. Vet Clin North Am 4[2]:351, 1974.)

ability to visually inspect the kidneys and other abdominal organs, to choose the specific biopsy site, to take an adequately sized sample, and to observe the kidney for hemorrhage. Most techniques necessitate general anesthesia to provide adequate patient restraint and analgesia. At our hospital, renal biopsy in dogs is performed under ultrasound guidance using the Bard Biopty biopsy instrument (C. R. Bard, Inc, Covington, GA) with the animal under ketamine and diazepam anesthesia. Occasionally, tissue architecture is less important (e.g., renal lymphosarcoma, feline infectious peritonitis), and aspiration of the kidney using a 23- or 25-gauge needle may provide useful material for cytology.

Before renal biopsy, an intravenous catheter should be placed and clotting ability evaluated by buccal mucosal bleeding time and estimation of platelet numbers. The patient's hematocrit and plasma proteins should be determined before biopsy but after adequate rehydration with parenteral fluids. Hematocrit and plasma proteins may then be monitored after biopsy to detect hemorrhage.

The most commonly employed biopsy instruments are the Franklin-modified Vim-Silverman needle and the Tru-Cut biopsy needle. Excessive penetration of the kidney with the outer cannula of the Franklin-modified Vim-Silverman instrument should be avoided to prevent retrieval of an insufficient amount of renal cortex. Care should be taken when directing the angle of the biopsy instrument so as to avoid the renal hilus and major vessels. Samples containing large amounts of medulla are more likely to contain large vessels and lead to infarction of renal tissue. Therefore, it is recommended that the biopsy needle be directed along the long axis of the kidney, solely through cortical tissue (Fig. 167–20). Because of the small size of feline kidneys, it is common to obtain relatively large amounts of medullary tissue and this has been associated with infarction and fibrosis.

After biopsy using the open approach or keyhole technique, the kidney should be digitally compressed for 5 minutes and, after release, the abdomen inspected for hemor-

rhage. The biopsy sample may be dislodged from the biopsy instrument using a stream of sterile saline from a syringe or, alternatively, the biopsy instrument may be immersed directly in fixative. For routine histopathology, the sample should be fixed in buffered 10 per cent formalin for at least 3 to 4 hours. For immunofluorescence studies, the sample can be preserved in Michel's transport medium. Immunopathology studies also may be performed by a peroxidase-antiperoxidase method using formalin-fixed samples without need for special preservation of the sample.[60]

After renal biopsy, a brisk fluid diuresis should be initiated to prevent potential clot formation in the renal pelvis. The patient's hematocrit and plasma proteins should be monitored at appropriate intervals over the next 12 to 24 hours to detect serious hemorrhage.

The most common complication of renal biopsy is hemorrhage. Subcapsular hemorrhage commonly occurs at the site of biopsy, and many patients experience microscopic hematuria during the first 48 hours after biopsy. Macroscopic hematuria is less common. Severe hemorrhage into the peritoneal cavity is rare and usually is associated with improper technique. Such hemorrhage must be treated aggressively by compression bandage of the abdomen, fresh whole blood transfusion, and exploratory surgery if necessary.

Linear infarcts in the path of the biopsy needle are observed commonly after renal biopsy in both dogs and cats. These are small and superficial when the biopsy is limited to renal cortex. If, however, an arcuate artery is damaged by passage of the biopsy needle through the corticomedullary junction, a wedge-shaped infarct may occur. This is more common in the cat because of the small size of the kidneys in relation to the length of the biopsy needle.

Hydronephrosis occasionally complicates renal biopsy. If penetrated by the biopsy needle, bleeding into the renal pelvis and clot formation can occur, leading to obstruction and hydronephrosis. This complication should be considered if the biopsy report indicates the presence of transitional epithelium at one end of the biopsy or if progressive renal enlargement is detected after renal biopsy. The risk of this complication is minimized by limiting the biopsy site to the renal cortex and instituting a fluid diuresis afterward.

REFERENCES

1. Finco DR, Brown SA, Crowell WA, et al: Exogenous creatinine clearance as a measure of glomerular filtration rate in dogs with reduced renal mass. Am J Vet Res 52:1029–1032, 1991.
2. Finco DR, Tabaru H, Brown SA, et al: Endogenous creatinine clearance measurement of glomerular filtration rate in dogs. Am J Vet Res 54:1575–1578, 1993.
3. Brown SA: Evaluation of a single-injection method for estimating glomerular filtration rate in dogs with reduced renal function. Am J Vet Res 55:1470–1474, 1994.
4. Brown SA, Haberman C, Finco DR: Use of plasma clearance of insulin for estimating glomerular filtration rate in cats. Am J Vet Res 57:1702–1705, 1996.
5. Brown SA, Finco DR, Boudinot D, et al: Evaluation of a single injection method using iohexol for estimating glomerular filtration rate in cats and dogs. Am J Vet Res 57:105–110, 1996.
6. Miyamoto K: Evaluation of single injection method of inulin and creatinine as a renal function test in normal cats. J Vet Med Sci 60:327–332, 1998.
7. Haller M, Muller W, Binder H, et al: Single injection inulin clearance: A simple method for measuring glomerular filtration rate in dogs. Res Vet Sci 64:151–156, 1998.
8. Fettman MJ, Allen TA, Wilke WL, et al: Single-injection method for evaluation of renal function with ^{14}C-inulin and ^{3}H-tetraethylammonium bromide in dogs and cats. Am J Vet Res 46:482–485, 1985.
9. Itkin RJ, Krawiec DR, Twardock AR, et al: Quantitative renal scintigraphic determination of effective renal plasma flow in dogs with normal and abnormal renal function using ^{99m}Tc-mercaptoacetylglycine. Am J Vet Res 55:1660–1665, 1994.
10. Itkin RJ, Krawiec DR, Twardock AR, et al: Evaluation of the single-injection plasma disappearance of technetium-99m mercaptoacetyltriglycine method for

determination of effective renal plasma flow in dogs with normal or abnormal renal function. Am J Vet Res 55:1652–1659, 1994.

11. Krawiec DR, Badertscher RR, Twardock AR, et al: Evaluation of ^{99m}Tc-diethylene-triaminepentaacetic acid nuclear imaging for quantitative determination of glomerular filtration rate of dogs. Am J Vet Res 47:2175–2179, 1986.

12. Krawiec DR, Twardock AR, Badertscher RR, et al: Use of 99mTc diethylenetriaminepentaacetic acid for assessment of renal function in dogs with suspected renal disease. JAVMA 192:1077–1080, 1988.

13. Rogers KS, Komkow A, Brown SA, et al: Comparison of four methods of estimating glomerular filtration rate in cats. Am J Vet Res 52:961–964, 1991.

14. Uribe D, Krawiec DR, Twardock AR, et al: Quantitative renal scintigraphic determination of the glomerular filtration rate in cats with normal and abnormal kidney function, using ^{99m}Tc-diethylenetriaminepentaacetic acid. Am J Vet Res 53:1101–1107, 1992.

15. Center SA, Wilkinson E, Smith CA, et al: 24-hour urine protein/creatinine ratio in dogs with protein-losing nephropathies. JAVMA 187:820–824, 1985.

16. DiBartola SP, Tarr MJ, Parker AT, et al: Clinicopathologic findings in dogs with renal amyloidosis: 59 cases (1976–1986). JAVMA 195:358–364, 1989.

17. White JV, Olivier NB, Reimann K, et al: Use of protein-to-creatinine ratio in a single urine specimen for quantitative estimation of canine proteinuria. JAVMA 185:882–885, 1984.

18. Monroe WE, Davenport DJ, Saunders GK: Twenty-four hour urinary protein loss in healthy cats and the urinary protein-creatinine ratio as an estimate. Am J Vet Res 50:1906–1909, 1989.

19. Jergens AE, McCaw DL, Hewett JE: Effects of collection time and food consumption on the urine protein/creatinine ratio in the dog. Am J Vet Res 48:1106–1109, 1987.

20. McCaw DL, Knapp DW, Hewett JE: Effect of collection time and exercise restriction on the prediction of urine protein excretion using urine protein/creatinine ratio in dogs. Am J Vet Res 46:1665–1669, 1985.

21. Bagley RS, Center SA, Lewis RM, et al: The effect of experimental cystitis and iatrogenic blood contamination on the urine protein/creatinine ratio in the dog. J Vet Int Med 5:66–70, 1991.

22. Adams LG, Polzin DJ, Osborne CA, et al: Correlation of urine protein/creatinine ratio and twenty-four-hour urinary protein excretion in normal cats and cats with surgically induced chronic renal failure. J Vet Int Med 6:36–40, 1992.

23. Waters CB, Adams LG, Scott-Moncrieff JC, et al: Effects of glucocorticoid therapy on urine protein-to-creatinine ratios and renal morphology in dogs. J Vet Int Med 11:172–177, 1997.

24. Grauer GF, Thomas CB, Eicker SW: Estimation of quantitative proteinuria in the dog using the urine protein-to-creatinine ratio from a random voided sample. Am J Vet Res 46:2116–2119, 1985.

25. van Vonderen IK, Kooistra HS, Rijnberk A: Intra- and interindividual variation in urine osmolality and urine specific gravity in healthy pet dogs of various ages. J Vet Int Med 11:30–35, 1997.

26. Finco DR, Brown SA, Barsanti JA, et al: Reliability of using random urine samples for spot determination of fractional excretion of electrolytes in cats. Am J Vet Res 58:1184–1187, 1997.

27. Lulich JP, Osborne CA, Polzin DJ, et al: Urine metabolite values in fed and nonfed clinically normal beagles. Am J Vet Res 52:1573–1578, 1991.

28. Hansen B, DiBartola SP, Chew DJ, et al: Clinical and metabolic findings in dogs with chronic renal failure fed two diets. Am J Vet Res 53:326–334, 1992.

29. Russo EA, Lees GE, Hightower D: Evaluation of renal function in cats using quantitative urinalysis. Am J Vet Res 47:1308–1312, 1986.

30. Hoskins JD, Turnwald GH, Kearney MT, et al: Quantitative urinalysis in kittens from four to thirty weeks after birth. Am J Vet Res 52:1295–1299, 1991.

31. Adams LG, Polzin DG, Osborne CA, et al: Comparison of fractional excretion and 24-hour urinary excretion of sodium and potassium in clinically normal cats and cats with induced chronic renal failure. Am J Vet Res 52:718–722, 1991.

32. Vail DM, Allen TA, Weiser G: Applicability of leukocyte esterase test strip in detection of canine pyuria. JAMVA 189:1451–1453, 1986.

33. Holan KM, Kruger JM, Gibbons SN, et al: Clinical evaluation of a leukocyte esterase test-strip for detection of feline pyuria. Vet Clin Pathol 26:126–131, 1997.

34. Fettman MJ: Evaluation of the usefulness of routine microscopy in canine urinalysis. JAVMA 190:892–896, 1987.

35. Allen TA, Jones RL, Purvance J: Microbiologic evaluation of canine urine: Direct microscopic examination and preservation of specimen quality for culture. JAVMA 190:1289–1291, 1987.

36. Ihle SL, Kostolich M: Acute renal failure associated with contrast medium administration in a dog. JAVMA 199:899–901, 1991.

37. Johnston GR, Walter PA, Feeney DA: Diagnostic imaging of the urinary tract. *In* Osborne CA, Finco DR (eds): Canine and Feline Nephrology and Urology. Baltimore, Williams & Wilkins, 1995, pp 230–276.

38. Rivers BJ, Walter PA, Polzin DJ: Ultrasonographic-guided, percutaneous antegrade pyelography: Technique and clinical application in the dog and cat. J Am Anim Hosp Assoc 33:61–68, 1997.

39. Konde LJ, Wrigley RH, Park RD, et al: Ultrasonographic anatomy of the normal canine kidney. Vet Radiol 25:173–178, 1984.

40. Konde LJ, Park RD, Wrigley RH, et al: Comparison of radiography and ultrasonography in the evaluation of renal lesions in the dog. JAVMA 188:1420–1425, 1986.

41. Wood AKW, McCarthy PH: Ultrasonographic-anatomic correlation and an imaging protocol of the normal canine kidney. Am J Vet Res 51:103–108, 1990.

42. Walter PA, Johnston GR, Feeney DA, et al: Renal ultrasonography in healthy cats. Am J Vet Res 48:600–607, 1987.

43. Yeager AE, Anderson WI: Study of association between histologic features and echogenicity of architecturally normal cat kidneys. Am J Vet Res 50:860–863, 1989.

44. Barr FJ: Evaluation of ultrasound as a method of assessing renal size in the dog. J Small Anim Pract 31:174–179, 1990.

45. Barr FJ, Holt PE, Gibbs C: Ultrasonographic measurement of normal renal parameters. J Small Anim Pract 31:180–184, 1990.

46. Walter PA, Feeney DA, Johnston GR, et al: Feline renal ultrasonography: Quantitative analyses of imaged anatomy. Am J Vet Res 48:596–599, 1987.

47. Walter PA, Feeney DA, Johnston GR, et al: Ultrasonographic evaluation of renal parenchymal diseases in dogs: 32 cases (1981–1986). JAVMA 191:999–1007, 1987.

48. Walter PA, Johnston GR, Feeney DA, et al: Applications of ultrasonography in the diagnosis of parenchymal kidney disease in cats: 24 cases (1981–1986). JAVMA 192:92–98, 1988.

49. Biller DS, Chew DJ, DiBartola SP: Polycystic kidney disease in a family of Persian cats. JAVMA 196:1288–1290, 1990.

50. Adams WH, Toal RL, Walker MA, et al: Early renal ultrasonographic findings in dogs with experimentally induced ethylene glycol nephrosis. Am J Vet Res 50:1370–1375, 1989.

51. Adams WH, Toal RL, Breider MA: Ultrasonographic findings in dogs and cats with oxalate nephrosis attributed to ethylene glycol intoxication: 15 cases (1984–1988). JAVMA 199:492–496, 1991.

52. Barr FJ, Patteson MW, Lucke VM: Hypercalcemic nephropathy in three dogs: Sonographic appearance. Vet Radiol 30:169–173, 1987.

53. Biller DS, Bradley GA, Partington BP: Renal medullary rim sign: Ultrasonographic evidence of renal disease. Vet Radiol 33:286–290, 1992.

54. Nyland TG, Fisher PE, Doverspike M, et al: Diagnosis of urinary tract obstruction in dogs using duplex Doppler ultrasonography. Vet Radiol Ultrasound 34:348–352, 1993.

55. Rivers BJ, Walter PA, Letourneau JG, et al: Duplex Doppler estimation of resistive index in arcuate arteries of sedated, normal female dogs: Implications for use in the diagnosis of renal failure. J Am Anim Hosp Assoc 33:69–76, 1997.

56. Rivers BJ, Walter PA, O'Brien TD, et al: Duplex Doppler estimation of Pourcelot resistive index in arcuate arteries of sedated normal cats. J Vet Intern Med 10:28–33, 1996.

57. Rivers BJ, Walter PA, Polzin DJ, et al: Duplex Doppler estimation of intrarenal Pourcelot resistive index in dogs and cats with renal disease. J Vet Intern Med 11:250–260, 1997.

58. Rivers BJ, Walter PA, Letourneau JG, et al: Estimation of arcuate artery resistive index as a diagnostic tool for aminoglycoside-induced nephrotoxicosis. Am J Vet Res 57:1546–1544, 1996.

59. Wise LA, Allen TA, Cartwright M: Comparison of renal biopsy techniques in dogs. JAVMA 195:935–939, 1989.

60. Arthur JE, Lucke VM: An immunohistological study of feline glomerulonephritis using the peroxidase-antiperoxidase method. Res Vet Sci 37:12, 1984.

CHAPTER 168

ACUTE RENAL FAILURE

Larry D. Cowgill and Denise A. Elliott

Acute renal failure (ARF) is a clinical syndrome characterized by the sudden onset of hemodynamic, filtration, and excretory failure of the kidneys with subsequent accumulation of metabolic (uremia) toxins and dysregulation of fluid, electrolyte, and acid-base balance. ARF must be distinguished from other presentations of acute uremia, which include combinations of prerenal azotemia, postrenal azotemia, and at times chronic renal failure. Oliguria and anuria characterize severe forms of ARF, but this classical feature of the syndrome is unpredictable. Nonoliguric forms of ARF are common and must be differentiated from the polyuria associated with chronic renal failure. Excretory failure promotes a rapid (hours to days) and progressive increase in blood urea nitrogen (BUN), serum creatinine, and phosphate and variable degrees of hyperkalemia and metabolic acidosis. In contrast to chronic renal failure, ARF is potentially reversible if diagnosed early after onset and the animal is supported while the renal injury is repaired. Delays or failure to initiate therapy may result in irreversible renal damage and death of the animal.

The clinical presentations of acute and chronic renal failure may be quite similar and clinicians must distinguish between these conditions to administer appropriate therapy and render an accurate prognosis. ARF may complicate other surgical or medical conditions. ARF has been identified as a bystander of generalized systemic inflammatory response causing multiple-organ dysfunction.[1]

ETIOLOGY OF ACUTE UREMIA

The etiology of ARF is multifactorial but classified as prerenal, intrinsic renal parenchymal, and postrenal according to the functional origin, extent, and duration of the conditions inciting the syndrome.

PRERENAL ACUTE RENAL FAILURE

Prerenal failure (azotemia) is a functional decline in glomerular filtration resulting from deficiencies in renal blood flow or perfusion pressure or excessive vasoconstriction. Prerenal azotemia is a common cause of mild azotemia (serum creatinine concentrations less than 4 mg/dL and BUN concentrations less than 80 mg/dL), but it can coexist with other causes of acute excretory failure and severe azotemia. Prerenal failure is not associated with morphologic damage to the kidney and is entirely reversible with timely correction of the underlying hemodynamic deficiencies. It develops as a coordinated neural and humoral response to hemodynamic deficiencies, hypotension, and hypovolemia to preserve perfusion to vital organs such as the heart and brain. The onset of these hemodynamic deficiencies increases renal salt and water conservation and urine concentration through activation of the sympathetic nervous system, the renin-angioten-

sin-aldosterone system, and the release of antidiuretic hormone.

At mean systemic blood pressures exceeding 80 mmHg, glomerular filtration is autoregulated. Severe or persisting hemodynamic deficiencies (systemic blood pressure less than 80 mmHg) exceed the autoregulatory capacity of the glomerulus and filtration failure ensues.[2, 3] Azotemia and increased urine specific gravity are hallmarks of prerenal azotemia but may be masked by underlying conditions (chronic renal failure, adrenal insufficiency, hepatic insufficiency) that impair renal concentrating ability. Prerenal azotemia may develop during mild hemodynamic deficiencies in animals with preexisting heart failure or compensated chronic renal failure that depend on activated autoregulatory mechanisms to preserve basal filtration pressure. Similarly, nonsteroidal anti-inflammatory drugs (NSAIDs) and angiotensin-converting enzyme (ACE) inhibitors may independently exacerbate prerenal azotemia by decompensating glomerular function in animals whose filtration is dependent on prostaglandin- and angiotensin II–mediated compensation of glomerular hemodynamics.

RENAL PARENCHYMAL ACUTE RENAL FAILURE

Renal parenchymal ARF is produced by intrinsic damage to the vasculature, glomeruli, tubular epithelium, or interstitium of the kidney. It can develop as a continuation of prerenal hemodynamic deficiencies or ischemic events, exogenous toxins that directly target the kidneys, intrinsic renal diseases, or systemic diseases with renal manifestations (Tables 168–1 and 168–2). The causes of hemodynamically mediated ARF are identical to those promoting prerenal azotemia, but the events have progressed in time or severity to generate morphologic damage that cannot be reversed readily.

Glomerular filtration is dependent on the delivery of blood to the glomerulus. Hypotension, hypovolemia, circulatory collapse, excessive renal vasoconstriction, and ischemia predispose to filtration failure and acute uremia (see Table 168–1).[1, 4] Renal ischemia may also develop from renal arterial thrombosis, disseminated intravascular coagulation, incompatible blood transfusions, or septic thrombi. Vasculitis, pancreatitis, hypoproteinemia, heat stroke, and gastric torsion pose a high risk for ischemic acute uremia.[3, 4] Clinicians must be vigilant to conditions associated with these hemodynamic events and their potential to induce ARF. Age and preexisting renal disease may impose additional risks of ARF.

Renal parenchymal ARF results from exogenous or endogenous nephrotoxins, intrinsic renal diseases, or systemic diseases with secondary renal manifestations. Nephrotoxins are chemicals or drugs that produce direct epithelial injury resulting in sublethal cell damage or cell death.[5] Alternatively, they may decrease renal blood flow, initiating hy-

TABLE 168–1. ETIOLOGY OF ACUTE UREMIA

HEMODYNAMIC

Shock/ Hypovolemia	Systemic Disease	Ischemia
Hemorrhage	Pancreatitis	Thromboembolic occlusion
Hypotensive shock	Peritonitis	
Septic shock	Hepatic failure (hepatorenal)	Malignant hypertension
Cardiogenic shock	Disseminated intravascular coagulation	
Prolonged or deep anesthesia	Adrenal insufficiency	
Hypovolemia	Vasculitis	
Heat stroke		
Trauma		
Burns		
Diuretic abuse		

INTRINSIC RENAL PARENCHYMAL

Infectious	Systemic-Renal Disease	Miscellaneous
Leptospirosis	Multiple organ failure	Nephrotoxins (see Table 168–2)
Pyelonephritis	Glomerulonephritis	
Feline infectious peritonitis	Systemic lupus erythematosus	Neoplasia (lymphoma)
Borreliosis	Renal artery thrombosis	Hypercalcemia
Leishmaniasis	Renal vein thrombosis	Trauma (avulsion)
Babesiosis	Urinary outflow obstruction	Malignant hypertension
Septicemia (septic emboli)	Hemolytic-uremic	Oxalate nephrosis
	Hemepigmenturia—crush syndrome	
	Polycythemia	

poxia-induced cell injury and death. Nephrotoxins react directly with apical, basolateral, or subcellular membranes of tubular cells to alter their permeability, disrupt their protein makeup, or activate phospholipases. They may promote free radical generation, interfere with lysosome function, activate cellular endonucleases and proteinases, interfere with oxidative phosphorylation, and shut down energy-dependent cellular processes.[5, 6] Nephrotoxins are diverse but animals are usually exposed to organic compounds and solvents, antimicrobials, vasoactive drugs, and miscellaneous therapeutics.[7]

Ethylene glycol intoxication is one of the most common causes of ARF and the second most common intoxication recognized in companion animals.[8] Automobile antifreeze is the usual source of exposure, but ethylene glycol is used commonly in a variety of household products including cleaning supplies, lacquers, cosmetics, and flavoring extracts. Ethylene glycol per se is not directly nephrotoxic; its metabolites (glycoaldehyde, glyoxylic acid, glycolate, and oxalic acid) mediate the renal injury. Deposition of calcium oxalate crystals in the tubular lumen contributes to tubular obstruction and back leak, but crystallization is a minor contributor to its overall nephrotoxicity.[9]

Aminoglycoside antimicrobials (neomycin, gentamicin, tobramycin, amikacin, and netilmicin) are polycations with low protein binding capabilities and thus are freely filtered by the glomerulus. Aminoglycosides interact with the negatively charged phospholipids on the brush border membrane of the proximal tubule and accumulate in the proximal epithelium by pinocytosis.[10] Once internalized, they bind to subcellular organelles and disrupt lysosomal function and the structure of cellular membranes. Aminoglycosides also increase production of free radicals and alter the ultrafiltration coefficient of glomerular capillaries. The nephrotoxicity of aminoglycosides is enhanced by concentrative uptake in the proximal tubule, high or repeated daily dosing, preex-

isting renal insufficiency, advanced age, volume depletion, renal ischemia, or concurrent exposure to other nephrotoxins such as NSAIDs. Extracellular fluid (ECF) volume expansion before aminoglycoside administration reduces their accumulation in the renal cortex and decreases their nephrotoxicity.

Amphotericin B is a polyene antibiotic that complexes with sterol moieties of cell membranes, forming pores that disrupt their integrity and increase their permeability. Renal blood flow and glomerular filtration rate (GFR) decrease because of an acute increase in renal vascular resistance after administration. Its toxicity is lessened by sodium loading to ensure that the ECF volume is replete before drug administration or administration of liposome-encapsulated amphotericin B.[11]

Cisplatin is an alkylating antineoplastic agent concentrated within and excreted primarily by the kidney. Its toxic-

TABLE 168–2. NEPHROTOXIC CAUSES OF ACUTE RENAL FAILURE

THERAPEUTIC AGENTS	NONTHERAPEUTIC AGENTS
Antimicrobial agents	**Heavy metals**
Aminoglycosides	Mercury
Penicillins	Uranium
Nafcillin	Lead
Cephalosporins	Bismuth salts
Sulfonamides	Chromium
Quinolones	Arsenic
Carbapenems	Gold
Rifampin	Cadmium
Tetracyclines	Thallium
Vancomycin	Copper
Aztreonam	Silver
Antifungal agents	Nickel
Amphotericin B	Antimony
Antiviral agents	**Organic compounds**
Acyclovir	Ethylene glycol
Foscarnet	Carbon tetrachloride
Antiprotozoal agents	Chloroform
Pentamidine	Pesticides
Sulfadiazine	Herbicides
Trimethoprim-sulfamethoxazole	Solvents
Dapsone	**Miscellaneous agents**
Thiacetarsamide	Gallium nitrate
Cancer chemotherapy agents	Diphosphonates
Cisplatin and carboplatin	Mushrooms
Methotrexate	Calcium antagonists
Doxorubicin (Adriamycin)	Snake venom
Azathioprine (Imuran)	Bee venom
Radiocontrast agents	Myoglobin
Nonsteroidal anti-inflammatory agents	Hemoglobin
Diuretics	Illicit drugs
Angiotensin-converting enzyme inhibitors	
Immunosuppressive agents	
Cyclosporine	
FK-506	
Interleukin-2	
Miscellaneous therapeutic agents	
Allopurinol	
Cimetidine	
Apomorphine	
Deferoxamine	
Streptokinase	
ε-Aminocaproic acid	
Dextran 40	
Lipid-lowering agents	
Methoxyflurane	
Penicillamine	
Acetaminophen	
Tricyclic antidepressants	

ity is dose related, progressive, irreversible and thought to be caused by activation to a positively charged and highly reactive electrophilic compound that forms intra- and interstrand cross-links with DNA. A solute diuresis induced before drug administration reduces its toxicity.[12] Carboplatin, an analogue of cisplatin, has less nephrotoxicity and can be used as an alternative to cisplatin.[12]

NSAIDs inhibit prostaglandin metabolism, which maintains renal blood flow during states of hypoperfusion.[6] Prostaglandin synthesis is stimulated when systemic circulation is compromised and renal sodium reabsorption, renin secretion, and water reabsorption are increased by angiotensin II, vasopressin, and catecholamine-mediated events. Regionally generated prostaglandins PGE_2 and PGI_2 have counterbalancing vasodilator effects on the renal vasculature to preserve renal blood flow and glomerular filtration during these hemodynamically propagated vasoconstrictive stresses.[13] By disrupting these effects, NSAID administration shifts the circulatory balance predisposing to unopposed vasoconstriction and renal ischemia during circulatory distress. The nephrotoxicity of NSAIDs may be exacerbated in animals with congestive heart failure, nephrotic syndrome, renal insufficiency, diabetes mellitus, hypertension, cirrhosis, and anesthesia in which blood volume is compromised and the predisposition for increased renal vascular tone is heightened.[13]

ACE inhibitors blunt angiotensin II–mediated vasoconstriction of the efferent arteriole, resulting in decreased efferent arteriolar resistance, glomerular capillary pressure, and GFR.[13] ARF can be manifest after administration of ACE inhibitors in animals with sodium depletion, diuretic abuse, congestive heart failure, and chronic renal insufficiency when the maintenance of basal GFR is dependent on angiotensin II effects.

INTRINSIC RENAL DISEASE

Intrinsic renal diseases are acquired infectious, immune-mediated, neoplastic, or degenerative diseases expressed primarily in the kidney (see Table 168–1). If fulminating and extensive, intrinsic renal disease produces an acute uremic crisis that must be differentiated from ischemic or nephrotoxic etiologies. Acute pyelonephritis develops from reflux of bacteria in the urine of animals with lower urinary tract infection and is an important cause of acute uremia in both dogs and cats. The azotemia may be moderate or severe and associated with variable degrees of urine formation. Suppurative nephritis is a less common infection resulting from hematogenous deposition or septic embolization of the kidneys in animals with bacteremia or septicemia.

Leptospirosis is a specific infectious zoonosis of dogs with predominantly hepatonephric manifestations. It has been recognized regionally with increasing frequency in the past 10 years. Leptospirosis was a well-characterized infection in dogs caused by two organisms, *Leptospira interrogans* serovars *canicola* and *icterohaemorrhagiae*. These serovars produced syndromes consisting of acute hemorrhagic diathesis, subacute icterus, or subacute uremia. Widespread use of a bivalent vaccine against *L. canicola* and *L. icterohaemorrhagiae* led to near extinction of leptospirosis in the canine population. However, retrospective studies of dog populations in the eastern United States and our own retrospective analysis in northern California have documented a reappearance of the disease and change in its epidemiology, with *Leptospira pomona, L. bratislava,* and *L. grippotyphosa* emerging as the most commonly identified serovars.[14, 15] The available bivalent vaccine does not provide immunity to these emerging serovars, leaving the canine population unprotected and at risk for infection. The change in etiologic serovars has been accompanied by a corresponding change in the clinical syndrome to one of ARF rather than one with hepatorenal or coagulation manifestations.[14, 15] Leptospirosis should be included routinely in the differential diagnosis of all dogs with acute parenchymal failure.

POSTRENAL ACUTE RENAL FAILURE

Postrenal ARF denotes obstruction or diversion of urine outflow and consequent accumulation of excretory products within the body. With early recognition and correction of underlying disorders, the azotemia resolves quickly without permanent morphologic damage to the kidneys. If treatment is delayed, the animal may die from the consequences of acute uremia or develop secondary structural damage to the kidneys. The most common causes of postrenal ARF include partial or complete obstruction of the urethra or bladder by discrete uroliths, mucous plugs, blood clots, or intra- or extraluminal mass lesions. Bilateral ureteral obstruction or unilateral obstruction in a solitary functional kidney by calcium oxalate uroliths is being recognized with increased frequency as a cause of postrenal azotemia in cats. Rupture of the urinary tract diverts urine into the retroperitoneal space (ureteral), peritoneal cavity (ureteral, bladder), or pelvic interstitium (urethra) and causes oligoanuria and uremia.

PATHOPHYSIOLOGY OF ACUTE RENAL FAILURE

"Acute tubular necrosis" (or nephrosis) designates acute uremia resulting from ischemic or toxic injury to the kidney. Histopathologically, degenerative or (less commonly) necrotic foci of renal tubules are distributed heterogeneously throughout the kidney with minimal interstitial inflammatory infiltrates. In both toxic and ischemic forms of ARF, the straight portion of the proximal tubule (S3 segment) is the most severely affected, and the convoluted tubular segments (S1 and S2 segments) are often spared.

PHASES OF ACUTE RENAL FAILURE

ARF classically proceeds through three clinical phases—initiation, maintenance, and recovery (Fig. 168–1).[16] The initiation phase is the period in which the animal is subjected to the renal insult, parenchymal injury evolves, and the tubular epithelium undergoes sublethal injury.[16] If the insult is sustained, cell death is the result of apoptosis or necrosis. At this stage a progressive decline in the GFR, loss of urine concentrating ability, and development of oliguria or polyuria and azotemia are seen. Renal tubular cells and casts may be observed in increased numbers in the urine sediment, and glucose, protein, and renal tubular enzymes may be detected in the supernatant. The initiation phase may last from hours to days but is unrecognized because the changes in GFR and urine specific gravity are not clinically apparent. Intervention during this stage often prevents progression to more severe injury.

The initiation phase becomes the maintenance phase as a critical amount of irreversible epithelial damage is established. GFR and renal blood flow are decreased, urine output

URO

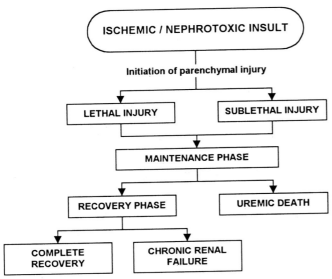

Figure 168–1. Clinical phases of acute renal failure. In the initiation phase, renal damage and sublethal cellular injury evolve but renal failure is not evident. In the maintenance phase, the inciting events have ceased, cellular damage is established, and signs of uremia become apparent. The recovery phase involves tubular regeneration and repair and partial or complete return of renal function.

is generally diminished, and the complications of uremia develop. Elimination of inciting factors at this stage does not alter the existing damage or the rate of recovery.[17] The maintenance phase may last from days to several weeks. A prolonged maintenance phase with severe oliguria increases the likelihood of a slower rate of recovery and permanent renal dysfunction.

The recovery phase is the period of repair and regenera-tion of renal tissue and restoration of renal function. Urine output increases and there is progressive resolution of the azotemia; however, molecular evidence of regeneration may be detected at much earlier stages of the disease. The in-creased urine production may not correspond with improve-ments in GFR, causing changes in the azotemia to lag behind. The polyuria characteristic of this phase is a physio-logic response to the accumulated water, salt, and osmoti-cally active solutes or a pharmacologic response to diuretic administration. Recovery depends on restoration of suble-thally injured cells, removal of intratubular debris, and re-population of the necrotic epithelium by replication of viable renal cells in the areas of cell loss. After ischemic or toxic injury, induced growth factors alter gene expression, en-abling the normally quiescent surviving epithelium to reenter the cell cycle, replicate, and repopulate the necrotic epithe-lium.[18, 19] The recovery phase may last from weeks to months. Many animals recover adequate or even normal renal function after weeks of anuria during the 6 to 12 months after ethylene glycol intoxication.

PATHOGENESIS OF ACUTE RENAL FAILURE

Four functional and pathologic alterations have been shown to participate to variable degrees in the initiation and maintenance phases of ARF on the basis of animal models of ARF (Fig. 168–2): (1) reduction of the glomerular capillary ultrafiltration coefficient (K_f) and permeability, (2) intratubu-lar obstruction, (3) back leak of filtrate across disrupted tubular epithelium, and (4) intrarenal vasoconstriction and renal medullary hypoxia.[16, 18]

Decreased ultrafiltration coefficient (K_f) reduces GFR through a decrease in either effective surface area or hydrau-lic conductivity of glomerular capillaries. Transmission and scanning electron microscopy in animal models of ARF

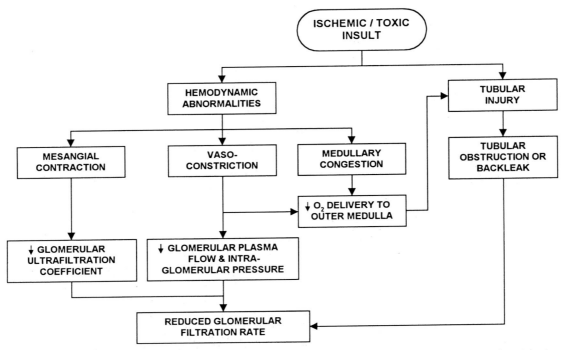

Figure 168–2. Diagrammatic schema showing the pathogenesis of acute renal failure and illustrating the central participation of decreases in glomerular ultrafiltration coefficient, intratubular obstruction, tubular back leak, and arterial vasoconstriction and medullary congestion to the development of filtration failure.

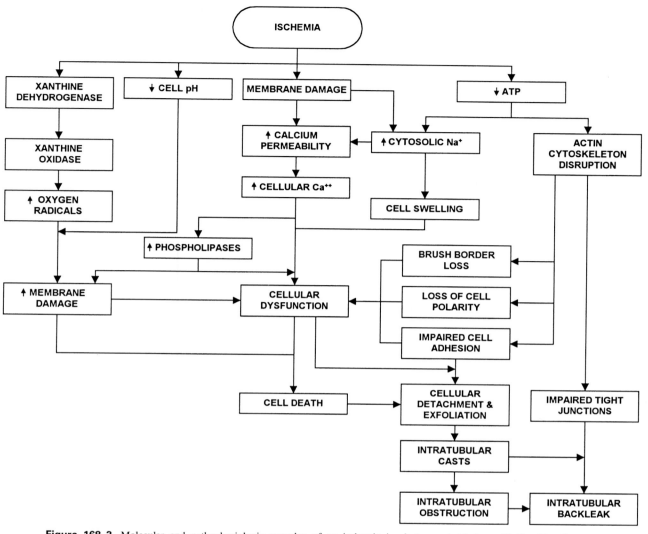

Figure 168–3. Molecular and pathophysiologic sequelae of an ischemic insult to renal tubular epithelia. The diagram illustrates the multifactorial events that result ultimately in sublethal cellular dysfunction or cell death.

demonstrated both loss and fusion of normal foot processes and marked disruption of podocyte architecture. Vasoconstriction initiated by angiotensin II and other vasoactive agents or contraction of the mesangium by ischemia, toxins, thromboxane A_2, endothelin, and platelet-activating factor in the induction phase of ARF reduces effective glomerular surface area and K_f. It is likely that both alterations participate in ischemic and toxic forms of ARF.[19, 20]

Intratubular obstruction develops from tubular cast formation produced by desquamated epithelial cells or cellular debris such as brush border membranes and intracellular organelles combined with intratubular proteins. Tubular obstruction can also occur by precipitation of heme pigments during hemolytic events or calcium oxalate crystals after antifreeze poisoning or by extratubular compression secondary to interstitial edema and inflammation. Tubular obstruction impedes the flow of tubular fluid, increases the intratubular hydrostatic pressure, decreases net ultrafiltration pressure, and halts single-nephron glomerular filtration.

Back leak of tubular fluid across the disrupted epithelium into the interstitium has been demonstrated in both animal models and human forms of ARF. Back leak is facilitated by tubular obstruction and increased intratubular pressure. It

may account for loss of as much as 50 per cent of glomerular filtrate and is greater in oliguric than in nonoliguric renal failure.

Intrarenal vasoconstriction may decrease renal blood flow by 50 percent or more after exposure to a renal insult in both experimental and natural forms of ARF. Renal blood flow is mostly directed to the cortex to optimize GFR and solute reabsorption. The reduced renal blood flow seen in the initial stages of ARF contributes to the early filtration failure, but changes in the intrarenal distribution of blood flow, particularly the outer medulla, appear more significant for the development and maintenance of ARF.[21]

CELLULAR BIOLOGY OF RENAL ISCHEMIA

Global or regional renal ischemia impairs the supply of oxygen to the tubular epithelium with consequent decreases in cellular energy stores, depletes ATP reserves, and initiates biochemical events responsible for cellular dysfunction, sublethal injury, and cell death (Fig. 168–3).[22, 23] Susceptibility of segmental tubular epithelia to ischemia depends on their respective glycolytic capacity, ATP requirements, and bal-

URO

ance between energy supply and demand. Poor medullary perfusion, hypoxia, and the high metabolic requirements of the pars recta (S3 segment) are responsible for the heightened susceptibility of this tubular region to ischemic damage. With sustained hypoxia complex metabolic processes result in intercellular accumulation of sodium and chloride, cellular swelling, increased cytosolic calcium, activation of calcium-dependent proteases and lipases, disruption of cytoskeletal microfilaments, and generation of oxygen free radicals.[22-24] Oxygen free radicals cause direct cellular damage via several mechanisms leading to disruption of vital cytoskeletal functions. This causes loss of epithelial transport orientation and tight junction integrity, back leak of glomerular filtrate, cellular detachment and sloughing, intratubular cast formation, and disruption of the architecture and shedding of microvilli characteristic of ARF.[22-25]

CELLULAR BIOLOGY OF NEPHROTOXIC ACUTE RENAL FAILURE

The kidney is predisposed to nephrotoxic damage because its rich blood supply enhances delivery of toxins for filtration and exposure to the tubular epithelium. Urinary concentrating and countercurrent mechanisms concentrate toxins within the tubular lumen and interstitium. After cellular uptake, the intracellular metabolism of toxins may generate reactive intermediates and toxic metabolites capable of injuring epithelial cells directly. The proximal tubule is the primary target of nephrotoxic injury; however, vulnerability of discrete nephron segments depends on differences in delivery, transport, uptake, and biotransformation of specific toxins at each site. Volume depletion and preexisting renal insufficiency exacerbate the toxicity of most substances.[6]

CELLULAR REPAIR AND REGENERATION

Recovery of renal function after an ischemic or toxic insult is dependent on repair of sublethally injured cells, removal of necrotic cells and intratubular debris, and replication and repopulation of a contiguous renal tubular epithelium. Structural and morphologic recovery must occur despite functional failure and the attendant uremia. Cellular recovery is fostered by hormones and growth factors including thyroid hormone, epidermal growth factor, transforming growth factor alpha, insulin-like growth factor, and adenine nucleotides whose activities are promoted by the cellular damage.

DIAGNOSIS OF ACUTE UREMIA

The clinical presentation of acute uremia depends on its cause and severity, previous therapy, and concurrent diseases. It may be valuable to differentiate quickly and accurately the following presentations of an acute uremic crisis: (1) prerenal azotemia, (2) prerenal azotemia complicating chronic renal failure, (3) acute (parenchymal) renal failure (ARF), (4) prerenal azotemia complicating ARF, (5) chronic end-stage renal failure, and (6) postrenal azotemia. These conditions may appear similar. The diagnosis is established from a comprehensive database that includes history, physical examination, laboratory testing, diagnostic imaging, histopathology, and special diagnostic testing.

HISTORY

The history should document a sudden onset of illness of less than a week's duration; however, animals with acute uremia secondary to underlying systemic or urinary disease may have a longer duration of illness. Historical signs consistent with acute uremia may be nonspecific and include listlessness, depression, weakness, anorexia, vomiting, and diarrhea. Less commonly, seizures, syncope, ataxia, and dyspnea may be reported. Exposure to nephrotoxic chemicals or plants, new environmental conditions, ill animals, or trauma should be ascertained. Recent surgery, diagnostic testing, drugs, and blood loss increase risk for renal injury. Historical oliguria or anuria is consistent with acute uremia, but a history of normal or increased urine production does not exclude the diagnosis. Historical weight loss, polyuria, polydipsia, nocturia or isosthenuria, and laboratory evidence of preexisting renal insufficiency suggest underlying chronic renal insufficiency. Animals with asymptomatic chronic renal insufficiency may become decompensated for any of a variety of reasons, precipitating a seemingly acute uremic crisis.

PHYSICAL EXAMINATION

Animals with ARF are generally depressed but responsive and have normal weight and haircoat. They are variably dehydrated on initial examination. Hypothermia, oral ulceration, "uremic breath," bile-stained fur, scleral injection, cutaneous bruising, discoloration or necrosis of the tongue, tachycardia or bradycardia, tachypnea, abdominal pain, muscle fasciculations, seizures, and palpably enlarged kidneys are consistent features of moderate to severe ARF. In the absence of hemorrhage or hemolysis, mucous membranes are pink. Lameness, icterus, fever, discolored urine, back or flank pain, and dysuria are associated with some etiologies of ARF. ARF is frequently concurrent with other diseases or even chronic renal failure whose physical manifestations may dominate the clinical presentation and mask its characteristic features. Uremic animals are typically hypothermic, and the presence of a normal or slightly elevated body temperature suggests the presence of fever and an underlying infectious or inflammatory etiology.

LABORATORY ASSESSMENT

General—Blood

The initial laboratory evaluation should include a complete blood count, comprehensive biochemical profile (serum creatinine, urea, phosphate, calcium, bicarbonate, sodium, potassium, chloride, glucose, albumin, globulin, hepatic transaminases, and bilirubin), urinalysis with sediment examination, and urine culture. Serum lipase may be included if an animal is suspected of having pancreatitis. The complete blood count is nonspecific for acute uremia but may reflect primary or secondary complications of diagnostic relevance. Nonregenerative anemia is characteristic of chronic renal failure, whereas a normal or increased red blood cell count, hematocrit, and hemoglobin concentration are consistent with prerenal azotemia or ARF. The hemogram should be interpreted carefully to prevent overestimation of actual red blood cell mass in animals with dehydration and underestimation of actual red cell mass in overhydrated animals.

For comparable azotemia, animals with ARF have more

profound disturbances of serum mineral, electrolyte, and bicarbonate concentrations than animals with prerenal azotemia or chronic renal failure. In ARF, serum phosphate concentration generally exceeds that of creatinine and may be associated with mild to moderate hypocalcemia. Serum calcium concentration may be less than 7.0 mg/dL in animals with acute ethylene glycol intoxication. In contrast, serum calcium is usually normal or moderately elevated in proportion to serum creatinine and phosphate in animals with chronic renal failure.[26] Serum potassium concentration varies considerably depending on the extent of vomiting and diuretic administration. Typically, it is increased (between 5.5 and 9.0 mEq/L) in proportion to the degree of azotemia. Serum bicarbonate concentration decreases with the severity of the renal failure such that bicarbonate deficits of 5, 10, and 15 mEq/L are associated with mild, moderate, and severe degrees of acute uremia, respectively.

Serum lipase, osmolality, oncotic pressure, lactate, and blood gas analysis may be indicated for specific diagnostic, therapeutic, or monitoring purposes. The intratubular enzymes gamma-glutamyltranspeptidase (GGT) and N-acetyl-β-D-glucosaminidase (NAG) can be measured in the urine as an index of cellular leakage and early predictor of acute tubular injury or necrosis, but they have not been adopted widely in veterinary diagnostics. Carbamylated hemoglobin is the nonenzymatic and nonreversible reaction product of cyanate, a urea metabolite, with hemoglobin. The blood concentration of carbamylated hemoglobin reflects time of exposure of blood to the azotemia and has been shown to differentiate dogs with acute azotemia from those with normal renal function or chronic renal failure.[27]

General—Urine

Urinalysis is fundamental to the evaluation of renal disease and the differentiation of azotemia. Both renal concentrating and diluting abilities become impaired in the early stages of acute parenchymal renal failure resulting in a urine specific gravity that is relatively fixed in the range 1.008 to 1.018. A urine specific gravity greater than 1.030 for dogs or greater than 1.035 for cats in the presence of azotemia indicates prerenal filtration failure.[28] A urine specific gravity between 1.012 and 1.029 (dogs) or 1.012 and 1.034 (cats) associated with azotemia suggests a prerenal component superimposed on intrinsic renal insufficiency ("prerenal-on-acute" or "prerenal-on-chronic" disease) or an underlying urine concentrating defect. Glucosuria in the absence of hyperglycemia indicates abnormal proximal tubular function and suggests ongoing tubular necrosis. It is a useful discriminator between acute parenchymal renal failure and other types of acute uremia but is recognized inconsistently.[7] Qualitative (dipstick) proteinuria is detected in most uremic animals but has little discriminatory importance. The urine sediment examination may reveal variable red blood cells, white blood cells, casts, crystals, yeast, fungi, or bacteria that aid the differential diagnosis and etiology of the uremia and should be performed routinely on freshly obtained urine. The presence of granular and hyaline casts reflects active renal pathology with epithelial shedding or necrosis. Casts are detected in approximately 30 per cent of dogs with ARF, but their absence does not exclude the diagnosis of acute parenchymal injury.[7] Calcium oxalate crystalluria is indicative of hyperoxaluria associated with ethylene glycol intoxication, lily toxicity, or oxalate nephrosis in cats.[8, 28, 29]

Diagnostic Imaging

Diagnostic imaging including survey radiography and ultrasonography is indicated in the evaluation of uremic animals. Ultrasonography is complementary to diagnostic radiography and is a preferred screening method for urinary imaging in acutely uremic animals.[30] Ultrasonography is rapid, noninvasive, and provides greater delineation of renal geometry, intrarenal architecture, parenchymal consistency, and outflow integrity than survey radiography.[30] It provides a more definitive assessment of renal and abdominal pathology, including nephritis, pyelonephritis, nephrolithiasis, hydronephrosis, pancreatitis, abdominal neoplasia, prostatitis, and ascites. Ultrasonic imaging facilitates collection of diagnostic specimens by guided percutaneous fine-needle aspiration or biopsy techniques for cytology, culture, and histopathology. Color flow Doppler sonography can be used to document intraparenchymal blood flow in the kidney and is useful in the assessment of renal ischemia. The ultrasonographic appearance of kidneys with oxalate nephrosis is characterized by mild to marked increases in cortical echogenicity with variable degrees of lesser echo intensity at the cortical medullary junction (halo sign) and supports a presumptive diagnosis of ethylene glycol intoxication (Fig. 168–4).[31] Excretory urography, renal scintigraphy, computed tomography, and magnetic resonance imaging may be indicated in selected patients.

Histology

Few diagnostic procedures surpass the interpretive value of renal histology for evaluation of acute uremia. The pathologic (and etiologic) basis for the disease, its potential reversibility, and its duration can often be obtained from a percutaneous renal biopsy. Details of the techniques, indications,

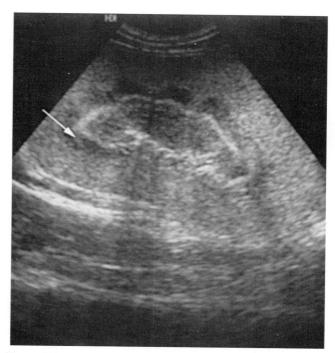

Figure 168–4. Ultrasonographic image of the kidney from a dog acutely poisoned with antifreeze within 24 hours of presentation. The marked increase in cortical and medullary echogenicity with variable echo intensity (arrow) at the cortical medullary junction (halo sign) is a consistent finding with ethylene glycol intoxication.

URO

and contraindications for renal biopsy have been described.[32] Percutaneous needle techniques can be performed in both dogs and cats with a minimum of sedation or anesthesia and obviate the need for surgery. Renal biopsy should not be performed if the animal is likely to undergo hemodialysis. The heparinization required during hemodialysis places the biopsy site at risk for hemorrhage. If indicated, the biopsy can be obtained subsequently on an interdialysis day.

Serology

Serology for leptospirosis should be performed on all dogs from endemic regions with acute uremia. The evaluation should include titers to *L. pomona*, *L. bratislava*, and *L. grippotyphosa* in addition to *L. canicola* and *L. icterohaemorrhagiae*. Strict criteria for serologic conformation of an active leptospiral infection have not been established and laboratory variation makes standardization difficult. A microscopic agglutination titer above 1:100 indicates positive serology, and a rise between paired titers suggests active infection.[33] Ambiguity in the diagnosis arises when only a single titer is available for analysis. Previous retrospective studies arbitrarily established single titers of above 1:800 and above 1:3200 to nonvaccinal serovars as criteria for a positive diagnosis of leptospirosis in dogs.[14, 15] However, laboratory variation and differences in humoral responses produced by each serovar make a strict serologic criterion difficult to assign. Vaccination can produce titers as high as 1:1250 to serovars *icterohemorrhagiae* and *canicola* in dogs. However, vaccination should not produce titers to nonvaccinal serovars that exceed those of vaccinal agents.[33] For diagnostic purposes, a single elevated titer to a nonvaccinal serovar accompanied by clinical signs of leptopsirosis must be considered highly suggestive of active infection. A single microscopic agglutination titer of 1:800 or more for nonvaccinal serovars, evidence of seroconversion between paired acute and convalescent titers, presence of typical clinical signs of leptospirosis, and response to antimicrobial therapy are sufficient to substantiate the diagnosis.

Ethylene Glycol

Laboratory diagnosis of ethylene glycol intoxication can be made presumptively by the presence of increased serum osmolality, osmolal gap, profound metabolic acidosis, increased anion gap, and the presence of calcium oxalate crystalluria.[8, 29] Confirmation of the diagnosis and documentation of the degree of intoxication and response to therapy are best achieved by chemical analysis for ethylene glycol or its toxic metabolites in blood or urine by commercial laboratories (Fig. 168–5). Despite suggestions that ethylene glycol is usually undetectable in the serum or urine by 48 to 72 hours after ingestion, we consistently document concentrations of both ethylene glycol and glycolic acid between several hundred and several thousand ppm in the blood of anuric dogs and cats up to and beyond this time frame.[8, 29, 34, 35] These observations indicate a continued need to initiate antidotal therapy or dialysis to prevent ongoing nephrotoxicity even at late stages of presentation.

CLINICAL CONSEQUENCES OF ACUTE RENAL FAILURE

The clinical consequences of ARF can be attributed to failure of the excretory, metabolic, and endocrine functions

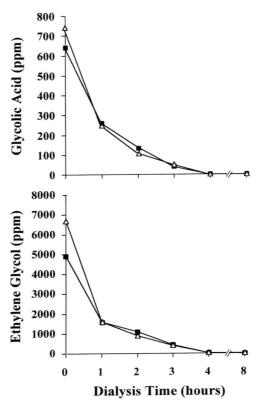

Figure 168–5. Changes in serum glycolic acid (upper panel) and ethylene glycol (lower panel) concentrations in two dogs treated with hemodialysis after simultaneous exposure to antifreeze 4 to 6 hours before presentation. Despite the extremely high initial concentrations of these toxicants, both dogs recovered uneventfully with no evident renal injury after a single dialysis treatment.

of the kidney, predisposing and concurrent diseases, and iatrogenic complications and interventional therapy. The diagnostic evaluation should document foreseeable complications of ARF, and the therapeutic approach must be sufficiently comprehensive to ameliorate the morbid manifestations of each clinical disorder without predisposing the animal to therapeutic risks that might be life threatening.

ALTERATIONS IN BODY FLUID VOLUME—HYPOVOLEMIA AND HYPERVOLEMIA

Disorders of fluid balance constitute some of the most common and clinically significant abnormalities of ARF yet underlie its therapeutic foundations. The fluid status of the animal must be estimated and reassessed at regular intervals in response to therapy (Table 168–3). Most animals with ARF are hypovolemic at *initial* presentation because of inadequate fluid intake and excessive fluid losses associated with vomiting, diarrhea, fever, polyuria, and hemorrhage.[4] Dehydration and hypovolemia exacerbate the azotemia by superimposed prerenal contributions to the underlying uremia and predispose the kidneys to additional ischemic injury. Overhydration and hypervolemia are predictable consequences of hospitalization and fluid management. Hypervolemia imposes risks of pulmonary and peripheral edema, pleural effusion, systemic hypertension, and congestive heart failure (Fig. 168–6). Once administered, an excessive fluid load may be difficult or impossible to correct in oliguric animals.

TABLE 168–3. ASSESSMENT OF BODY FLUID VOLUME

Hypovolemia
    Clinical signs
        Decrease in historical weight
        Loss of skin turgor
        Dry or tacky mucous membranes
        Prolonged capillary refill time
        Sunken eyes
        Poor pulse quality
        Vascular collapse (jugular and peripheral veins, vena cava)
        Low central venous pressure
        Tachycardia
        Systemic hypotension
        Microcardia
        Cool extremities
        Oliguria
    Laboratory:
        Increased hematocrit and plasma protein concentration
        Increased urine specific gravity (prerenal azotemia)
Hypervolemia
    Clinical Signs
        Increase in historical weight
        Increased skin turgor
        Chemosis
        Serous nasal discharge
        Edema, ascites, pleural effusion
        Strong pulses
        Venous engorgement, jugular pulses
        Elevated central venous pressure
        Tachycardia
        Tachypnea
        Increased breath sounds, crackles, or wheezes on thoracic
          auscultation
        Systemic hypotension
    Laboratory
        Hemodilution (decreased hematocrit and plasma proteins)

INADEQUATE URINE PRODUCTION

Oliguria or anuria is a hallmark and life-threatening feature of ARF. Oliguria is defined as urine production of less than 0.27 mL/kg/hour (6.5 mL/kg/day), whereas anuria means essentially no urine formation. It is important to determine whether the oliguria is a functional result of prerenal disorders or is secondary to postrenal diseases. After restoration of systemic blood pressure and ECF volume, bladder size and urethral patency must be assessed. Approximately 50 percent of animals with parenchymal ARF have oliguria and the other half have either normal or increased urine production. The causes and pathophysiologic basis for the oliguria or anuria are multifactorial and vary during the course of the disease (see Pathophysiology of Acute Renal Failure).

Solute retention, overhydration, hyperkalemia, and metabolic acidosis become life threatening if the oliguria or anuria is not responsive to initial therapy. Administration of all enteral and parenteral supplements, blood products, and maintenance solutions becomes problematic or contraindicated in oliguric or anuric animals despite their ongoing needs. Fluid overload and pulmonary edema develop consistently in aggressively managed oliguric animals. The conversion from an oliguric to a nonoliguric state facilitates use of these essential therapies but may not correspond with improvement in GFR or the prognosis for recovery.

CARDIOVASCULAR COMPLICATIONS

Cardiovascular disorders may develop from the underlying cause of the ARF, the uremia per se, or the imposed therapy. Volume overload, cardiac arrhythmias, biventricular dilatation, heart failure, hypertension, pericarditis, and pericardial effusion and tamponade are possible consequences. Abnormalities in myocardial contractility and excitability may be triggered or worsened by hypervolemia, acidosis, hyperkalemia, and other uremia toxins. It is rarely possible or necessary to define the exact cause of the cardiovascular signs, which are managed supportively while the underlying disease and uremia are resolved. Bradycardia (hyperkalemia), supraventricular or ventricular premature contractions, and paroxysmal ventricular tachycardia are consistent electrocardiographic abnormalities. Congestive heart failure may precede the onset of ARF but becomes exacerbated by the metabolic, acid-base, and electrolyte disturbances associated with the uremia or its attending fluid therapy. Signs that mimic congestive heart failure may be attributed to fluid overload caused by attempts to rehydrate and diurese oliguric animals. Most animals with acute uremia we have examined before hemodialysis have moderate to severe hypertension and are overhydrated because of previous fluid therapies. The kidneys, heart, eyes, and brain are targets of systemic hypertension. Manifestations include acute blindness resulting from retinal detachment, hyphema, retinal hemorrhage, left ventricular hypertrophy, myocardial ischemia, hypertensive encephalopathy (intermittent confusion, depression, and collapse), dementia, and cerebrovascular hemorrhage causing seizures, coma, and death.[36]

Cardiac arrest may result from severe hyperkalemia or the collective metabolic, acid-base, and electrolyte disturbances of acute uremia. We frequently observe a "vomit and die syndrome" in animals with acute uremia, severe gastroenteritis, and protracted vomiting. The "syndrome" is characterized by bradycardia (heart rates less than 80 beats per minute) and vomiting. Because many animals are normokalemic, it is presumed that the bradycardia is secondary to increased vagal tone associated with the gastroenteritis. An acute episode of vomiting promotes further vagal stimulation, progressive bradycardia, and cardiac arrest. The condition may be prevented with anticholinergic drugs, which should be given prophylactically to vomiting animals with bradycardia.

PULMONARY COMPLICATIONS

Respiratory complications of acute uremia include pulmonary edema, pneumonia, uremic pneumonitis, pleural effu-

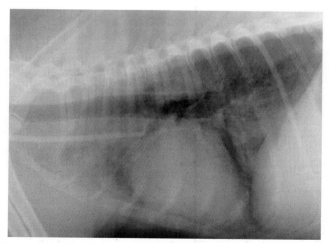

Figure 168–6. Lateral thoracic radiograph of a dog with acute renal failure illustrating severe pulmonary edema and pleural effusion secondary to excessive fluid administration.

sion, and pulmonary artery thromboembolism. Respiratory disease is common in severely uremic animals, frequently life threatening, and often refractory to therapy. The incidence of pulmonary complications has not been defined in uremic animals, but they represent a significant cause of morbidity in as many as 50 percent of human patients with ARF and a significant risk factor for death.[37] These observations are entirely consistent with our experience in dogs and cats. Interstitial or alveolar edema and pleural effusion resulting from excessive fluid administration and volume overload are arguably the most prevalent pulmonary disorders. Some degree of pulmonary congestion is predictable in virtually every animal treated with aggressive fluid therapy. Fluid intolerance is exacerbated in animals with preexisting heart disease, and the signs of fluid overload must be distinguished from those of congestive heart failure to provide appropriate therapy. Other causes of respiratory compromise include aspiration pneumonia in animals with protracted vomiting, uremic pneumonitis (adult respiratory distress syndrome), and pulmonary artery thromboembolism. Respiratory failure requiring ventilatory support is associated with a grave prognosis for recovery. Respiratory arrest is a frequent complication of respiratory distress in uremic patients.[38]

NEUROMUSCULAR DISORDERS

Neurologic manifestations of acute uremia reflect diffuse and nonspecific alterations of cerebral cortical and peripheral neuromuscular functions broadly termed *uremic encephalopathy*. The severity and progression of the neurologic signs generally correlate with the magnitude and progression of the azotemia. Typical signs include dullness, lethargy, impaired mentation, altered behavior, confusion, stupor, tremors, seizures, coma, muscular cramps, myoclonus, hypotonic peripheral reflexes, fatigue, muscle weakness, and peripheral neuropathies that are caused by the uremia per se or are a manifestation of the underlying etiology (e.g., ethylene glycol intoxication). Uremic encephalopathy improves with resolution of the azotemia, but no singular uremic toxin or pathogenesis has been identified for these diverse disorders. An increased brain calcium content secondary to hyperparathyroidism has been implicated for some of the central nervous system (CNS) manifestations.[39] Drugs including H_2-receptor blockers (cimetidine, ranitidine, famotidine) and metoclopramide may induce CNS dysfunction in uremic animals when given at conventional doses. These findings reinforce the need to modify the dosage or frequency of administration of medications that undergo renal excretion. Cerebrovascular hemorrhage, electrolyte disorders, and hypertensive encephalopathy also contribute CNS signs observed in uremia.

ELECTROLYTE AND ACID-BASE DISTURBANCES

Electrolyte imbalances are frequently the most life-threatening complications of acute uremia. Hyperkalemia in particular causes early morbidity and mortality and must be quickly identified and corrected. Hyperkalemia is caused by inadequate potassium excretion related to decreased filtration, decreased delivery of sodium to the cortical collecting duct, injury to potassium secretory sites along the nephron, and inability to augment renal potassium secretion.[40] Hyperkalemia may be further aggravated by cell lysis and release of potassium from intracellular stores (crush injuries, tumor lysis, myositis), cellular shifts of potassium associated with systemic acidosis, increased potassium load related to the diet or potassium-containing enteral or parenteral solutions, and drugs that interfere with renal potassium homeostasis (beta-adrenergic blockers, ACE inhibitors).[41] The adverse effects of hyperkalemia stem from reduction of the transmembrane potassium gradient and changes in cell membrane excitability, increased resting membrane potential, and persistent depolarization of resting membrane potential.[37] Peripheral conducting and contractile cells are most significantly affected by these changes, producing generalized muscular weakness, reduced cardiac contractility, disturbed cardiac conduction, cardiac arrhythmias, and neurologic abnormalities. The electrocardiographic abnormalities of the hyperkalemia commence at serum potassium concentrations greater than 6.5 or 7.0 mEq/L, are also influenced by the rate of rise, and are discussed further in Chapters 62 and 155.

In acute uremia metabolic acidosis invariably develops from ongoing or excessive production of nonvolatile metabolic acids, impaired filtration of the acid load, and decreased reabsorption of bicarbonate and generation of ammonia to facilitate net acid excretion. The severity of the acidosis may be exacerbated by concurrent diabetic ketoacidosis, lactic acidosis, or ethylene glycol or salicylate intoxication.[34] Severe metabolic acidosis produces tachypnea and increased tidal respiration (Kussmaul's respiration), decreased cardiac contractility, cardiac arrhythmias, peripheral arterial vasodilatation, and central vasoconstriction that can aggravate pulmonary edema.[42] Depression, lethargy, stupor, and coma are predictable neurologic sequelae. Metabolic acidosis also promotes breakdown of skeletal proteins contributing to the azotemia and loss of lean body mass.

Metabolic alkalosis may be the predominant acid-base disorder in animals with ECF volume contraction or intractable vomiting or those receiving sodium bicarbonate. Mixed acid-base disturbances (metabolic acidosis–respiratory acidosis or metabolic acidosis–respiratory alkalosis) are commonly diagnosed in animals with concurrent pulmonary edema or hemorrhage, pleural effusion, pneumonia, aspiration pneumonia, hyperventilation, or pulmonary thromboemboli. The respiratory component of these disturbances is evident only on blood gas analysis and must be managed with ventilatory support.

Abnormalities in serum sodium concentration are less common and generally represent disturbances in water metabolism. Hyponatremia results from iatrogenic administration of fluids low in sodium for volume restoration or maintenance requirements. Hyponatremia may be induced by conditions that contribute to the acute uremia such as pancreatitis, adrenal insufficiency, or diuretic administration, which cause excessive losses of sodium in vomitus, stool, or urine. Transient hyponatremia may follow the administration of mannitol or synthetic colloid solutions as a result of free water shifts from the cellular to the extracellular space. Excessive free water loads can also be supplied with enteral administration of nutritional supplements to animals with limited excretory capacity. Hypernatremia occurs in animals with excessive free water losses resulting from heat prostration or diabetes insipidus. More commonly, hypernatremia is an iatrogenic complication of excessive administration of sodium bicarbonate or hypertonic saline in the initial management of acute uremia or failure to provide for insensible water requirements with parenteral fluids used for diuresis.

UREMIC INTOXICATIONS

A myriad of ill-defined "uremia toxins" of diverse molecular size and chemical classification accumulate in animals with excretory failure of the kidneys or altered metabolism. Collectively, uremia toxins contribute to many of the classical complications of acute uremia in direct proportion to the severity of the azotemia. Gastrointestinal disorders include anorexia, nausea, vomiting, fetid breath, stomatitis, oral ulcerations, necrosis of the tip and lateral margins of the tongue, gastritis, gastrointestinal ulcers, hematemesis, gastrointestinal bleeding, enterocolitis, diarrhea, intussusception, and ileus.[43] Conversion of secretory urea to ammonia by urease-producing bacteria in the oral cavity and gastrointestinal tract is considered partly responsible for development of uremic lesions in the oral cavity, stomach, and bowel. Gastritis and gastric ulceration exacerbate the anorexia, nausea, and vomiting associated with acute uremia. Gastric lesions are often associated with hypergastrinemia as a result of increased secretion or reduced renal clearance of gastrin. Hypersecretion of gastric acid and direct damage to the gastric mucosa, submucosa, and vasculature by uremia toxins contribute further to the gastritis.[44] Reduced protection by the gastric mucous barrier and increased diffusion of acid into the gastric wall induce inflammation, ulceration, hemorrhage, and perpetuation of the gastric injury (see Chapter 169). Vomiting is also induced by direct effects of uremia toxins on the D_2-dopaminergic receptors in the chemoreceptor trigger zone.[45] Reflux esophagitis may develop after severe and persistent vomiting.

Uremic bleeding is manifest as purpura, petechia, ecchymosis, bruising, bleeding from gum margins and venipuncture sites, epistaxis, and gastrointestinal blood loss. The gastrointestinal blood loss can be occult or overt and contribute to anemia. Impaired platelet–vessel wall interaction induced by uremia toxins causes uremic bleeding, but the initiating renal insult, concomitant hepatic dysfunction, and therapeutic interventions may contribute to bleeding tendencies. In addition, uremia toxins cause or contribute to the hypothermia, uremic pneumonitis, and carbohydrate intolerance sometimes seen. Hypothermia is most pronounced in animals with severe uremia and body temperature may approach 96°F or lower. Hypothermia resolves with correction of azotemia by dialysis, indicating that the cause is a low-molecular-weight solute. A normal temperature in animals with moderate azotemia (BUN greater than 100 mg/dL) suggests the presence of fever and an underlying infectious or inflammatory process. Carbohydrate intolerance is a laboratory curiosity in azotemic animals characterized by moderate hyperglycemia. Fasting serum glucose concentrations may approach 150 mg/dL but can increase significantly in animals receiving hypertonic glucose solutions or parenteral nutrition.

CONSERVATIVE MEDICAL MANAGEMENT OF ACUTE RENAL FAILURE

Recommendations for the medical management of ARF in animals have changed little over the past 25 years and remain largely anecdotal and based on personal preferences. Conventional recommendations are directed at preventing ARF in animals highly predisposed to renal injury, eliminating ongoing renal insults, and providing supportive management of identified biochemical, metabolic, and clinical consequences of established ARF. The mechanisms underlying

the impaired glomerular hemodynamics, tubular disruption, and intratubular obstruction that mediate ARF have been characterized. Cellular energetics, cytosolic calcium, oxidant stress, necrosis, apoptosis, nitric oxide, epithelial cytoskeleton, and growth promoters are but a few of the participants in the pathogenesis of ARF (see Pathophysiology of Acute Renal Failure). "Designer therapies" have evolved to counteract specific pathophysiologic events in discrete and carefully contrived experimental models of ARF. Despite the pharmacologic promise of these therapies to prevent or ameliorate development of experimental ARF or to accelerate renal regeneration and repair in the models, none have become established. It would be naive to extend the same expectations to a clinical venue in which patients have heterogeneous risks and predispositions for ARF of diverse etiology, severity, duration, and multisystemic expression. Conventional approaches to the management of ARF thus remain supportive and targeted to the predicted and documented clinical consequences of acute uremia. Therapeutic strategies for the management of acute uremia are stratified into prevention, conservative therapy, and dialysis to accommodate the therapeutic requirements of the patient.

PREVENTION OF ACUTE RENAL INJURY

The greatest priorities in the management of acute uremia are to anticipate clinical settings and recognize high-risk patients predisposed to a uremic crisis and to **prevent** its development. Judicious intervention may prevent the development of ARF or correct a functional insufficiency before the onset of intrinsic renal injury. Animals with preexisting renal disease, advanced age, dehydration, hypovolemia, hypotension, sepsis, fever, electrolyte and acid-base imbalances, systemic diseases, or multiple organ failure are at increased risk for ARF and warrant extra precautions and surveillance. "Red flag" clinical settings include prolonged anesthesia and surgery; trauma; concurrent use of vasoactive drugs, NSAIDs, or nephrotoxic drugs (aminoglycosides, cisplatin); and high environmental temperatures. Risk factors for acute uremia are cumulative and result in an additive potential for renal injury. Table 168–4 illustrates these points in the therapeutic approach to acute antifreeze poisoning.

The most consistent renal protectant is correction of existing fluid deficits and mild ECF volume expansion (3 to 5 per cent). Mild volume expansion is especially beneficial before administration of known nephrotoxic drugs (aminoglycosides, cisplatin, amphotericin B) or surgical intervention. Mannitol administered before exposure to hemodynamic or nephrotoxic insults has been shown to prevent or moderate the severity of experimental renal injury and exposure to selected nephrotoxins.[46] Mannitol increases intravascular volume and renal perfusion, decreases renal vascular resistance, enhances tubular fluid flow, promotes renal solute excretion, and protects against oxidative free radical damage.[46] Mannitol (10 to 25 per cent solution) should be administered only to fluid-replete animals as an initial bolus of 0.5 to 1.0 g/kg intravenously over 15 to 30 minutes followed by a continuous-rate infusion at 1.0 to 2.0 mg/kg/min intravenously for the duration of potential ischemic or nephrotoxic insult.

CONVENTIONAL (CONSERVATIVE) MANAGEMENT OF ESTABLISHED ACUTE RENAL FAILURE

The conventional strategy for the management of existing ARF involves elimination of known causes of the renal

URO

TABLE 168–4. THERAPEUTIC APPROACH TO ACUTE ANTIFREEZE POISONING

Therapeutic Plan	Therapeutic Options	
Prevent ongoing exposure (<2 hours)	1. Induce vomiting 2. Perform gastric lavage 3. Administer activated charcoal	
Correct ECF deficits, correct dehydration	1. Correct ECF volume deficits (saline, lactated Ringer's solution) 2. Correct hypocalcemia (if present) 3. Correct metabolic acidosis (if present) 4. Initiate maintenance fluids/replace ongoing losses	
Document urine production promote diuresis	1. Establish urinary catheter, monitor urine output 2. Administer mannitol and/or furosemide and/or dopamine	
Administer antidote	1. Ethanol (20%): (dogs, cats)	5.5 mL/kg IV q4h five times *then* 5.5 mL/kg IV q6h four times
or	2. Ethanol (30%): (dogs, cats)	1.3 mL/kg IV bolus, *then* 0.42 mL/kg/h IV for 48 hours
Eliminate toxin and/or metabolites	3. 4-Methyl-pyrazole: (dogs)	20 mg/kg IV, *then* 15 mg/kg IV at 12 and 24 hours, *then* 5 mg/kg IV at 36 hours
	4. Hemodialysis (dogs, cats)	
Manage ARF or oliguria	1. Conventional medical therapy 2. Hemodialysis	

ARF = acute renal failure; ECF = extracellular fluid.

injury and supportive therapy directed to the life-threatening consequences of acute uremia. In many cases the inciting insult has passed or cannot be identified. In circumstances in which the etiology is ongoing, every effort should be made to eliminate further exposure. Administration of nephrotoxic drugs should be discontinued or their dosage modified to a nontoxic level. Systemic infections such as *Leptospirosis* infections should be aggressively treated with appropriate antimicrobial therapy, and hemodynamic catastrophes must be resolved rapidly to promote euvolemia and normotension. The goals of conventional medical therapy are to correct the existing and ongoing hemodynamic deficiencies, alleviate fluid volume and biochemical abnormalities, and eliminate uremic toxicities until the existing renal damage is repaired or compensatory adaptations occur. Animals with mild renal damage may regain adequate function within 3 to 5 days. Animals with moderate or severe renal damage may require many weeks for renal repair, yet most die from uremia within 5 to 10 days. The disparity between the window of effective medical therapy and the reestablishment of renal function underlies the poor prognosis associated with ARF.

ALTERATIONS IN RENAL HEMODYNAMICS AND EXTRACELLULAR FLUID VOLUME

Fluid therapy remains the foundation of the medical therapy for ARF in animals. The therapeutic objectives are to normalize fluid balance, resolve hemodynamic inadequacies, and promote urine formation. The replacement fluid should mimic as closely as possible the type of fluid lost from the body and effectively restore intravascular volume. Estimated volume deficits should be corrected intravenously with isotonic saline or balanced (isonatric) polyionic solutions within the first 2 to 4 hours of therapy (see Chapter 78). These solutions provide the greatest restoration of ECF volume and blood pressure. There is no indication for subcutaneous replacement of the fluid deficits. Half-strength saline (0.45 per cent) and 2.5 per cent glucose solutions may be use as replacement solutions for animals with mild hypernatremia and excessive free water losses or hypotonic losses associated with vomiting or diarrhea. In general, half-strength saline is inappropriate as the first-choice solution for volume restoration (see Chapter 78). Severe blood losses should be replaced with compatible whole blood or packed red blood cells in saline or colloidal solutions such as plasma, hetastarch, or dextran to restore intravascular volume and oxygen carrying capacity. Glucose in water (5.0 per cent) or hyponatric "maintenance" solutions are distributed widely throughout total body water and are inappropriate replacement solutions for animals with hypovolemia and contraction of extracellular volume. These solutions should be reserved for insensible or maintenance losses later in the course of treatment. The initial use of these fluids predisposes oliguric or anuric animals to overhydration and hyponatremia without effective restoration of ECF volume and renal hemodynamics. The initial replacement volume (mL) is calculated from clinical estimates of dehydration according to the formula Volume replacement (mL) = [body weight (kg)] × [estimated deficit (per cent)] × 1000.

The estimated volume deficit is replaced intravenously over 2 to 4 hours in most animals to restore renal perfusion and promote urine production in a timely interval. Fluid deficits should be replaced rapidly (up to 90 mL/kg/hour) in animals with profound hypovolemia and hypotension to prevent prolonged ischemia of peripheral tissues and further progression or exacerbation of the ARF. The rate of fluid replacement must be tempered in animals with a past history of or current cardiovascular disease to prevent circulatory congestion. Sequential monitoring of central venous pressure (CVP) facilitates safe and efficient fluid administration to these animals. An increase in CVP of 5 to 7 cm H_2O above baseline or an absolute CVP greater than 10 cm H_2O predicts an excessive rate or volume of fluid administration and warrants slowing or discontinuing further fluid administration.

A brisk diuresis (urine production greater than 1 mL/kg/ hour) and improvement in the azotemia after restoration of fluid deficits indicate significant prerenal contributions to the ARF. If the estimated volume replacement fails to promote a diuresis, the hydration status of the animal should be reassessed to ensure that the deficits are replete. Additional saline or balanced electrolyte solution can be administered to produce mild (3 to 5 per cent of body weight) volume expansion to help stimulate urine production. Maintenance fluid requirements including insensible free water requirements (20 to 25 mL/kg/day) and ongoing urinary and gastrointestinal losses (measured or estimated) must be provided after fluid deficits are restored to maintain fluid balance. Free water losses are best provided intravenously as 5 per cent glucose solutions if the animal is vomiting or by mouth after oral intake is tolerated. Urinary and gastrointestinal fluid losses can be replaced with equivalent volumes of lactated Ringer's or balanced replacement solutions. Alternatively, maintenance fluid requirements can be satisfied with half-strength saline (0.45 per cent) or lactated Ringer's and 2.5 per cent glucose solutions or formulated maintenance solutions. Exclusive use of normal saline or balanced replacement solutions in animals with restricted water intake causes hypernatremia after 3 to 5 days of fluid administration resulting from failure to replace ongoing insensible water losses (see Table 168–3).

Hypervolemia is a common complication of overzealous fluid administration or failure to monitor fluid balance. When overhydration is recognized, further fluid administration is contraindicated and diuretics or dialysis may be required to resolve the fluid burden.

INADEQUATE URINE PRODUCTION

Conversion from an oliguric or anuric to a nonoliguric state facilitates management of ARF. For these reasons, induction of an effective diuresis is given a high therapeutic priority, supporting the empirical use of diuretics (mannitol and furosemide) and vasodilators (dopamine). Despite incontrovertible evidence that prophylactic administration of diuretics and vasoactive drugs promotes urine formation in experimental ARF, their efficacy in established ARF remains controversial and unsubstantiated.[18, 46, 47] If delayed beyond a few hours from the initiation phase of ARF, their efficacy in altering the course, morphology, or outcome of the disease becomes negligible. The increased production of urine induced by diuretics offers reassurance to clinicians but may not equate with improving renal function. Diuretics are generally advocated for acute oliguric renal failure because risks and contraindications for their use are few and there are no alternatives. The use of diuretic drugs should never supplant judicious fluid and hemodynamic support. For established ARF, potential benefits of diuretics include (1) induction of a diuresis and conversion from an oliguric or anuric to a nonoliguric state, (2) potential for a more benign course, (3) disclosure of less severe renal injury, (4) better regulation of fluid and electrolyte balance, and (5) opportunity to provide parenteral nutrition.

Hypertonic mannitol is proposed to decrease renal vascular resistance; increase renal blood flow; reverse cellular swelling; increase solute excretion and osmotic tubular fluid flow; disperse tubular debris, casts, and obstructions; and scavenge toxic free radicals.[46, 48] Despite the extensive literature on the benefits of hypertonic mannitol in experimental forms of ARF, reports of its efficacy in the treatment of clinical forms of ARF in dogs or cats are not available. Mannitol should be given in preference to loop diuretics for initial treatment except in animals with severe fluid overload, pulmonary edema, or congestive heart failure. Mannitol (10 to 25 per cent solution) is administered to fluid replete animals as a slow intravenous bolus at 0.25 to 1.0 g/kg. If a significant diuresis is established within 30 to 60 minutes, the mannitol can be continued as a constant-rate intravenous infusion at 1 to 2 mg/kg/min or as intermittent intravenous boluses of 0.25 to 0.5 g/kg every 4 to 6 hours during the subsequent 24 to 48 hours. If an adequate diuresis is not established by 60 minutes, an additional 0.25 to 0.5 g/kg intravenous bolus may be repeated cautiously, but further administration is contraindicated because of the risks of ECF volume expansion, hypervolemia, mannitol intoxication, and potential nephrotoxicity.[4, 49] The more established the onset of uremia, the lower the expectation that mannitol will promote a diuresis or influence the course of the disease.

Furosemide (a loop diuretic) is a potent natriuretic agent that can be used alone or in combination with mannitol or dopamine to promote urine formation. In general, furosemide is less effective than mannitol at improving renal function.[46]

The mechanisms of furosemide's actions are not known with certainty but are considered similar to those of mannitol. In experimental models of ARF, its renal protection is correlated with the induction of a solute diuresis, enhanced osmolar clearance and tubular fluid flow, and relief of intratubular obstruction. Furosemide also has vasodilatation effects that may partially contribute to its actions.

The diuresis induced by furosemide may not correlate with changes in GFR, renal morphology, or the clinical course of ARF. In early stages of ARF, furosemide may unmask incipient or less severe ARF, promote formation of urine, and facilitate management of overhydration and hyperkalemia. Because of the limited risk associated with a short course of therapy, furosemide has been advocated routinely for humans and animals when fluid replacement alone fails to promote a diuresis. Furosemide is given initially at 2 to 6 mg/kg intravenously only after existing fluid deficits have been corrected. If an adequate diuresis of greater than 1 ml/kg/hour is not confirmed within 30 minutes, the initial dose or a higher dose can be repeated or it can be combined with dopamine. If a diuresis is achieved, the dosage can be repeated every 6 to 8 hours or provided as a constant-rate infusion at 0.25 to 1.0 mg/kg/hour to extend the diuresis for 24 to 48 hours. Fluid balance must be monitored carefully to prevent volume contraction. There is little indication for use of furosemide in animals with nonoliguric ARF except to eliminate excessive fluid loads or to increase potassium excretion in animals with hyperkalemia. Diuretics should be administered cautiously to nonoliguric animals. If improperly monitored, diuretics may deplete circulating volume, precipitating a prerenal insult on established renal injury.

Dopamine is a catecholamine and renal vasodilating agent with the potential to increase renal blood flow, glomerular filtration, and renal sodium excretion. In dogs, doses between 0.5 to 1 $\mu g/kg/min$ primarily activate dopamine-specific D_1- and D_2-receptors on vascular smooth muscle cells and postganglionic sympathetic nerves to induce vasodilation. Doses between 2 and 3 $\mu g/kg/min$ activate beta$_1$-receptors to increase cardiac output, whereas higher doses stimulate alpha$_2$-receptor activation, causing undesired vasoconstriction. Dopamine has additional direct and indirect diuretic and natriuretic potential. Overall, the effects of dopamine support maintenance of systemic arterial pressure and renal perfusion. At doses between 0.5 and 3 $\mu g/kg/min$, dopamine may increase urine formation and facilitate the conversion from an oliguric to a nonoliguric state. Higher doses may cause renal vasoconstriction, tachycardia, and cardiac arrhythmias and are contraindicated in ARF. Dopamine and furosemide are often synergistic in their effects to increase urine production.[50] Once a diuresis is established, the combined therapy should be continued until renal function improves and fluid and electrolyte balance can be maintained without drug therapy. If a diuretic response is not induced with aggressive therapy during the initial hours of oliguria, there is little likelihood that continued efforts will be effective. Fluid administration must be curtailed to prevent overhydration, and alternative therapy, including dialysis, should be initiated.

Studies in anesthetized cats document a different spectrum of dopaminergic effects that suggest a lack of dopamine-specific receptor activity in the kidneys of this species. Low-dose dopamine infusion (1 to 3 $\mu g/kg/min$) caused no significant changes in mean arterial blood pressure, heart rate, urine output, or sodium excretion.[51] Only at doses greater than 10 $\mu g/kg/min$ did dopamine infusion result in dose-dependent increases in urine output and sodium excre-

URO

tion. However, the diuretic response was associated with variable decreases in GFR, renal vasoconstriction, and inconsistent changes in mean arterial blood pressure and renal blood flow. These findings are most consistent with effects induced by stimulation of alpha-adrenoreceptors by the higher dopamine doses. The use of dopamine to stimulate a diuresis and natriuresis in cats with acute oliguria is conceptually inappropriate.

MANAGEMENT OF ELECTROLYTE AND ACID BASE DISORDERS

Hyperkalemia is the most common electrolyte disorder threatening animals with acute uremia. Its management is determined by the severity of the hyperkalemia and concurrent cardiac, electrocardiographic, and neuromuscular disturbances. Management strategies include antagonism of the membrane effects of hyperkalemia, redistribution of potassium from the extracellular to the intracellular fluid compartments, or removal of potassium from the body (Table 168–5).

Severe hyperkalemia (potassium greater than 8 mEq/L) is generally associated with extreme electrocardiographic disturbances and is imminently life threatening (see Chapter 155). For severe hyperkalemia, calcium gluconate (10 per cent solution) is administered at 0.5 to 1.0 mL/kg as a slow intravenous bolus over 10 to 15 minutes as a specific antagonist to the cardiotoxicity as required to correct electrocardiographic abnormalities (see Table 168–5). The use of calcium chloride is not recommended because of its potency, acidifying tendency, and caustic irritation if injected extravascularly. Rapid injection of calcium solutions may cause hypotension and cardiac arrhythmias; therefore, arterial blood pressure and an electrocardiogram should be monitored during calcium administration. The infusion should be halted temporarily if S-T segment elevation, Q-T interval shortening, progressive bradycardia, or hypotension is observed. The effects of calcium infusion on the electrocardiogram are rapid in onset but short lived (approximately 25 to 35 minutes) and there is no effect to lower the serum potassium. Calcium infusion should be regarded as a "stop-gap" therapy to correct the immediate, life-threatening cardiotoxic effects of the hyperkalemia until longer lasting controls are initiated. After calcium administration, temporary reduction of serum potassium can be achieved by promoting its translocation from the extracellular to the intracellular fluid space with sodium bicarbonate or insulin and glucose administration (see Table 168–5). During these reprieves, therapy must be instituted to provide long-term regulation of serum potassium.

Moderate hyperkalemia (6.0 to 8.0 mEq/L) may resolve with adequate diuresis and administration of furosemide to promote kaluresis. If a significant diuresis is not established or serum potassium is not controlled with diuretic therapy, potassium-containing fluids should be stopped and sodium bicarbonate should be given to correct the existing bicarbonate deficit. Sodium bicarbonate can be administered at 1 to 2 mEq/kg intravenously over 20 minutes in the absence of measured serum bicarbonate concentrations (see Table 168–5). Beneficial effects usually begin within 10 minutes and may persist for 1 to 2 hours. Bicarbonate administration increases extracellular pH, which translocates potassium into cells in exchange for hydrogen ions. Administration of bicarbonate is contraindicated in animals with metabolic alkalosis and must be used judiciously in volume-overloaded animals. Sodium bicarbonate administration may lower serum calcium concentrations and precipitate a hypocalcemic crisis in animals with preexisting hypocalcemia.

If sodium bicarbonate administration is inappropriate or not effective, 20 per cent glucose may be administered at 1.5 g/kg intravenously as an option. Glucose stimulates insulin release and promotes the transcellular uptake of potassium. Alternatively, regular insulin can be given intravenously at 0.1 to 0.25 units/kg in combination with glucose at 1 to 2 g per unit of administered insulin.

Mild hyperkalemia (potassium 6.0 mEq/L or less) is rarely problematic but should be monitored at regular intervals. In most circumstances, mild hyperkalemia resolves with the initial (potassium-free) fluid replacement. For long-term control in refractory cases, sodium polystyrene sulfonate resin may be given orally with sorbital (30 g slurry with 70 per cent sorbitol every 2 hours). This resin exchanges sodium for potassium across intestinal epithelium and increases the gastrointestinal removal of potassium. Although effective for control of low-grade hyperkalemia, exchange resins have no role in the management of life-threatening hyperkalemia. The acceptability of these preparations is low because of persistent side effects including nausea, constipation, gastrointestinal ulceration, and necrosis. If conventional therapy fails to provide an immediate or lasting resolution of the hyperkalemia, peritoneal dialysis or hemodialysis is indicated.

HYPOKALEMIA

Hypokalemia may develop during the diuretic stage of ARF if renal potassium losses exceed inputs. The use of diuretics, inadequate dietary potassium intake, vomiting, and diarrhea may contribute to the development of hypokalemia. Hypokalemia is usually a laboratory abnormality but clinical signs (muscle weakness, fatigue, vomiting, anorexia, gastrointestinal ileus, and cardiac arrhythmias) may be noted if the serum potassium concentration is less than 2.5 mEq/L. Ventroflexion of the neck may be observed in cats. Potassium depletion has also been associated with the develop-

TABLE 168–5. MANAGEMENT OF HYPERKALEMIA IN ACUTE RENAL FAILURE

THERAPY	MECHANISM OF ACTION
Mild hyperkalemia ($\leq$6.0 mEq/L) IV fluids (0.9% saline, lactated Ringer's solution)	Plasma volume expansion, dilutes K^+, and increases GFR and renal potassium excretion
Moderate hyperkalemia (6.0 to 8.0 mEq/L) Sodium bicarbonate (1–2 mEq/kg IV slowly over 20 minutes)	Translocates K^+ to intracellular space in exchange for H^+
Dextrose (20–50%) (1.5 g/kg IV bolus)	Dextrose stimulates insulin release which promotes transcellular entry of K^+ into cells
Regular insulin and dextrose (20–50%) (insulin at 0.1–0.25 U/kg plus dextrose at 1–2 g/U IV)	Insulin promotes transcellular entry of K^+ into cells
Severe hyperkalemia ($\geq$8.0 mEq/L) Calcium gluconate (10%) (0.5–1.0 mL/kg over 10–15 minutes; monitor the ECG during administration)	Specific antagonist of the cardiotoxic effects of K^+

ECG = electrocardiogram; GFR = glomerular filtration rate.

ment of progressive renal disease and azotemia in cats (see Chapters 61 and 169).

Oral potassium supplementation at 1 to 3 mEq K^+/kg/day is usually beneficial to animals able to eat. Guidelines for parenteral potassium supplementation (via intravenous fluids) are based on the serum potassium concentrations. Serum potassium is rarely less than 2.0 mEq/L in animals with acute uremia, and an increase in potassium content of fluid solutions to 20 to 30 mEq/L is usually sufficient to restore normokalemia. Potassium supplementation should be performed cautiously in uremic animals and serum potassium should be evaluated frequently.

ACID-BASE IMBALANCES

Treatment of prevailing acid-base disorders requires assessment of serum bicarbonate or blood gas analysis. Mild to moderate metabolic acidosis (serum bicarbonate above 16 mEq/L) often resolves after fluid replacement and the onset of a diuresis. Metabolic acidosis should be treated with intravenous sodium bicarbonate if the serum bicarbonate is less than 16 mEq/L. The goal of bicarbonate replacement is to ameliorate, not necessarily normalize, the metabolic acidosis. Serum pH should be corrected to approximately 7.2 to stabilize cardiac conduction and contractility. The initial bicarbonate replacement dose (mEq) = [body weight (kg) × 0.3 × bicarbonate deficit (desired bicarbonate − measured bicarbonate)]. One half of the calculated replacement is administered intravenously over 20 to 30 minutes, and the remainder is provided with intravenous fluids during the following 2 to 4 hours.

Equilibration of the initial bicarbonate dose requires 2 to 4 hours, but most uremic animals have an ongoing requirement for sodium bicarbonate of approximately 80 to 90 mEq/kg/day to offset production of metabolic acids. Serum bicarbonate (blood gases and electrolytes) should be reassessed after the initial replacement and at least daily to determine whether the deficit is replete or additional therapy is required. Excessive sodium bicarbonate administration can promote metabolic alkalosis, ECF volume overload, pulmonary edema, and hypertension. Serum potassium and ionized calcium concentrations may decline precipitously with overcorrection of the acidemia, causing secondary hypoventilation, hypercapnia, shift in oxyhemoglobin dissociation, reduced tissue oxygen delivery, and paradoxical cerebral acidosis with rapid increases in serum pH. Alternative alkalizing agents, including sodium acetate, sodium lactate, sodium or potassium citrate, and calcium carbonate, require hepatic metabolism to generate bicarbonate and have shown no clear advantage over sodium bicarbonate therapy (see Chapter 78).

Mild to moderate metabolic alkalosis (serum bicarbonate 28 to 35 mEq/L) usually resolves with administration of normal saline or balanced electrolyte solutions to correct ECF volume and chloride deficits. Persistent vomiting must be controlled with antiemetics to prevent persisting metabolic alkalosis. Respiratory acid-base disorders may predominate or contribute to the acid-base profile of animals with concurrent pulmonary complications. Management of the respiratory components of the acid-base disorders requires correction of any underlying pulmonary disease.

UREMIA INTOXICATIONS

"Uremia toxins" must be removed from the body by restoration of excretory function, intensive fluid diuresis, or dialysis to resolve the signs attributable to the azotemia. Immediate recovery of excretory function is rarely possible, and symptomatic therapies must be instituted to ameliorate the uremic intoxications (Table 168–6).

Oral and Gastrointestinal Oral hygiene, stomatitis, and oral ulcerations can be improved dramatically by rinsing the oral cavity every 6 to 8 hours with solutions containing 0.1 to 0.2 per cent chlorhexidine. This therapy reduces bacterial contamination, helps to prevent and heal oral ulcers, and relieves discomfort. Pain caused by lingual necrosis or severe ulceration can be managed further with topical lidocaine preparations.

Antiemetic therapy is necessary to manage fluid and electrolyte balance and to support nutritional requirements. All oral fluids and food should be discontinued until vomiting has been controlled for 12 to 24 hours. H_2-receptor antagonists such as cimetidine, ranitidine, and famotidine have become mainstays for the pharmacologic management of gastritis, vomiting, and gastric ulceration (see Table 168–6) (see Chapter 136). H_2-receptor antagonists undergo 50 to 70 per cent renal elimination, and their dose should be reduced in proportion to the degree of excretory failure to prevent CNS-mediated side effects. Omeprazole is the most potent inhibitor of gastric acid secretion currently available. Its metabolite inactivates H^+, K^+-adenosinetriphosphatase (H^+, K^+-ATPase) activity irreversibly, preventing secretion of hydrogen ions into the stomach. Acid secretion resumes only after synthesis of new H^+, K^+-ATPase antiporters by the parietal cells (see Chapter 136).

Oral antacids are also used to neutralize gastric acidity but require frequent administration to ensure continuous efficacy. Their usefulness is limited further in animals with protracted vomiting who cannot tolerate oral medications. Sucralfate and prostaglandin analogues may be indicated and be useful for managing gastric ulceration (see Chapter 136).

Centrally acting antiemetics should be added to the therapeutic scheme if vomiting cannot be controlled by restricted oral intake and treatment of the gastritis (see Table 168–6). Metoclopramide is a D_2-dopaminergic antagonist that directly suppresses the chemoreceptor trigger zone. It also has prokinetic effects on the stomach to promote gastric emptying, which is often delayed in uremic animals. Metoclopramide can be provided by either the oral or the parenteral route and is most effective when administered as a constant intravenous infusion (see Table 168–6). Metoclopramide is excreted by the kidneys and the dosage needs modification in animals with severe uremia. Phenothiazine derivative antiemetics (chlorpromazine, prochlorperazine, acepromazine) suppress vomiting at the chemoreceptor trigger zone and/or the emetic center. They are effective antiemetics in uremic animals but are used infrequently because of the hypotensive and sedative side effects characteristic of this class of drugs. Phenothiazine derivative antiemetics (especially acepromazine) should be considered for animals with intractable vomiting who remain unresponsive to other therapeutics if the adverse effects can be accepted. Domperidone and cisapride are additional prokinetic agents used to treated delayed gastric emptying and uremic gastritis (see Chapter 136).

Uremic bleeding is rarely life threatening but it can be extensive and may lead to anemia. Uremic bleeding improves with resolution of the azotemia. Transfusion of packed red blood cells is indicated for animals with severe anemia or active bleeding. Transfusion of platelet-rich plasma does not improve platelet function or reduce bleeding time as the platelet's function becomes abnormal upon exposure to uremic plasma.[52] Administration of recombinant hu-

URO

TABLE 168–6. THERAPEUTIC AGENTS USED IN THE MANAGEMENT OF GASTROINTESTINAL UREMIC INTOXICATIONS*

AGENT	INDICATION, MECHANISM	CONVENTIONAL DOSAGE
Chlorhexidine (CHX-Guard)	Stomatitis, oral ulceration Bactericidal agent	0.1–0.2% sol topical q6–8h
Cimetidine† (Tagamet, Smith Kline French)	Esophagitis, gastritis, gastric ulceration or hemorrhage H_2-receptor antagonist	5–10 mg/kg PO, IM, IV q4–6h (dog) 5–10 mg/kg PO, IM, IV q6–8h (cat)
Ranitidine† (Zantac, Glaxo)	Esophagitis, gastritis, gastric ulceration or hemorrhage H_2-receptor antagonist	0.5–2.0 mg/kg PO, IV q8–12h
Famotidine† (Pepcid, Merck Sharp Dohme)	Esophagitis, gastritis, gastric ulceration or hemorrhage H_2-receptor antagonist	0.5–1.0 mg/kg PO, IM, IV q12–24h
Omeprazole (Prilosec, Merck Sharp Dohme)	Esophagitis, gastritis, gastric ulceration or hemorrhage H^+, K^+-ATPase proton pump blocker	0.5–1.0 mg/kg PO q24h
Sucralfate (Carafate, Marion)	Esophagitis, gastritis, gastric ulceration or hemorrhage Cytoprotective agent	0.5–1.0 g PO q6–8h (dog) 0.25–0.5 g PO q8–12h (cat)
Misoprostol (Cytotec, Searle)	Esophagitis, gastritis, gastric ulceration or hemorrhage Cytoprotective agent—PGE_1 analogue	1–5 μg/kg PO q6–12h
Metoclopramide† (Reglan, Robins)	CRTZ antiemetic, prokinetic agent D_2-dopaminergic antagonist, $5HT_3$-serotoninergic antagonist	0.1–0.5 mg/kg PO, IM, SQ q6–8h 0.01–0.02 mg/kg/h CRI
Chlorpromazine (Thorazine, Smith Kline French)	CRTZ, emetic center antiemetic Alpha$_2$-adrenergic, D_2-dopaminergic, H_1-histaminergic, M_1-cholinergic antagonists	0.2–0.5 mg/kg IM, SQ q6–8h
Prochlorperazine (Compazine, Smith Kline French)	CRTZ, emetic center antiemetic Alpha$_2$-adrenergic, D_2-dopaminergic, H_1-histaminergic, M_1-cholinergic antagonists	0.1–0.5 mg/kg IM, SQ q8–12h
Acepromazine (PromAce, Fort Dodge)	CRTZ, emetic center antiemetic Alpha$_2$-adrenergic, D_1-dopaminergic, H_1-histaminergic, M_1-cholinergic antagonists	0.01–0.05 mg/kg IM, SQ q8–12h
Cisapride (Propulsid, Janssen Pharmaceutica)	Prokinetic agent $5\text{-}HT_4$ receptor agonist, $5\text{-}HT_1$, $5\text{-}HT_3$ receptor antagonist	0.1–0.5 mg/kg PO q8–12h

*Most of these drugs have not been approved for use in the dog or cat.
†Agent undergoes renal excretion and the dosage must be adjusted accordingly to prevent toxicity.
ATPase = adenosinetriphosphatase; CRI = constant-rate infusion; CRTZ = chemoreceptor trigger zone; 5-HT = 5-hydroxytryptamine; PGE_1 = prostaglandin E_1.

man erythropoietin should be considered for animals receiving dialysis or prolonged supportive management after the uremic crisis.

Uremic animals have increased susceptibility to infection because of impaired immunity and cellular host defenses. The deficiencies are compounded by widespread breaches of mucosal integrity by gastrointestinal ulceration, intravenous and bladder catheterization, parenteral medications and nutrition, and intervention with hemodialysis, peritoneal dialysis, and immunosuppressive drugs.[53] Infection may be difficult to identify as uremia dampens the febrile response. Strict asepsis during catheter placement and meticulous catheter site care are mandatory. If infection is suspected, blood, urine, and catheter tip cultures should be obtained and broad-spectrum antibiotic therapy instituted while awaiting organism identification. Prophylactic use of antibiotics may foster the development of bacterial resistance and superinfections.

Respiratory complications arise from overhydration. Treat by discontinuing fluid administration and by giving diuretics to achieve an appropriate dry weight. Animals with severe pulmonary edema and oliguria may require peritoneal dialysis or hemodialysis with ultrafiltration to alleviate the fluid burden. Aspiration pneumonia should be treated with aggressive antiemetic therapy, parenteral broad-spectrum antibiotics, and supplemental oxygen or ventilatory support. Uremic pneumonitis is a complication of severe azotemia resulting in the respiratory distress syndrome, noncardiogenic pulmonary edema, respiratory compromise, or failure.[38] Uremic pneu-monitis is treated supportively with supplemental oxygenation or mechanical ventilation. Uremic pneumonitis improves with resolution of the azotemia and is an indication for dialysis.

NUTRITIONAL MANAGEMENT OF ACUTE RENAL FAILURE

Protein-calorie malnutrition contributes to many aspects of the uremic syndrome including impaired immune function, increased susceptibility to infection, delayed wound healing, decreased strength, and poor quality of life. The imposed catabolism exacerbates hyperkalemia, hyperphosphatemia, acidosis, and azotemia; increases morbidity and mortality; and influences the outcome of ARF. Anorexia, nausea and vomiting, coexisting catabolic illnesses, uremia toxins, and endocrine abnormalities including insulin resistance and hyperparathyroidism contribute to the nutritional inadequacies. Metabolic acidosis is a major stimulus for breakdown of muscle protein in acute uremia and a contributor to the catabolism.[54]

Accurate assessment of the nutritional status of uremic animals is necessary to guide nutritional therapy. Change in body weight is the simplest parameter for assessing nutritional status but is flawed by alterations in hydration that mask significant losses of lean body mass or fat stores. Body condition scoring is a useful index for sequentially assessing body composition but is qualitative and subject to hydration and experience of the evaluator. Bioelectrical impedance analysis is a new, safe, noninvasive, and reproducible method for precisely quantitating changes in total body water, ECF volume, body cell mass, and fat-free mass with potential application to uremic animals.[55]

Goals of nutritional therapy are to meet the energy and nutrient requirements of the animal; alleviate the azotemia; minimize disturbances in fluid, electrolyte, vitamin, mineral, and acid-base balance; and aid renal regeneration and repair. The optimal nutritional regime for dogs and cats with ARF has not been defined, but a formulation providing high energy and moderated protein, potassium, and phosphate as prescribed for chronic renal failure is logical. Energy supplied must be sufficient to prevent catabolism of endogenous protein to spare lean body mass and to minimize the azotemia. The *illness energy requirement* for animals with acute uremia can be determined from the *resting energy requirement* [RER (kcal/day) = $70(Wt_{kg})^{0.75}$ or RER (kcal/day) = $70 + (30 \times Wt_{kg})$], where Wt_{kg} is the body weight in kilograms times a stress factor (1.2 to 1.4 for uremic dogs and 1.2 for uremic cats) (see Chapters 70 and 71). Carbohydrate and fat provide the nonprotein sources of energy required in the diet. Diets, liquid enteral formulations, or parenteral solutions designed for the management of renal failure may be used. They have a relatively high fat content, because fat provides approximately twice as much energy per gram as carbohydrate and increases the energy density of the formulation (see Chapter 71).

Controlled reduction of nonessential protein in the nutritional formulation is required to minimize urea generation while avoiding protein malnutrition. The optimal protein requirements for animals with ARF are not known and are probably influenced by underlying and coexistent clinical conditions. Consequently, the minimum protein requirements for normal dogs (1.25 to 1.75 g/kg/day; 8 to 10 per cent protein on a metabolizable energy basis) and cats (3.8 to 4.4 g/kg/day; 20 to 25 percent protein on a metabolizable energy basis) are generally adopted for uremic animals. This degree of restriction may not be necessary or desired for animals with mild or moderate azotemia. More liberal protein prescriptions can be provided. Phosphorus, sodium, potassium, and magnesium intake should be restricted to prevent accumulation of these minerals, but intakes must be modified according to the clinical and biochemical dictates of the animal.

Delivery of nutritional therapy is constrained by inappetence of the animal and the gastrointestinal manifestations of the uremia. Oral or enteral feeding may not be possible or recommended in the initial stages of ARF because of gastritis, pancreatitis, or uncontrolled vomiting. Peripheral parenteral nutrition or total parenteral nutrition is indicated for these animals to provide interim nutritional support. Peripheral parenteral nutrition is formulated with isotonic solutions administered through a peripheral vein. However, complete nutritional requirements cannot be met by this technique, and it should be used only as an adjunct to oral intake or to supply partial nutritional support not in excess of 5 days. Total parenteral nutrition is formulated to provide all essential nutrients for indefinite periods but requires central venous administration because of the hypertonicity of the nutrient solutions. (see Chapter 71). Appetite stimulants including benzodiazepine derivatives, serotonin antagonists, or anabolic steroids may be effective in inappetent animals who can tolerate oral feeding.[56] Oral or enteral tube feeding is recommended in animals that are not vomiting but that refuse to eat sufficiently to achieve caloric adequacy. The indications, complications, and technical aspects of enteral feeding have been reviewed (see Chapter 71). Percutaneous gastrostomy tubes are invaluable aids for the long-term nutritional support of animals with prolonged recovery times. Caloric and protein requirements can be met readily by intermittent or continuous administration of blended therapeutic diets or liquid enteral preparations formulated for the management of renal insufficiency. The clinical benefits of enteral or parenteral nutritional support cannot be overemphasized, but it may not be possible to supply the volume load required for nutritional adequacy in oliguric animals without dialysis to alleviate the attending overhydration.

RENAL REPLACEMENT THERAPY (DIALYSIS)

ARF is the most common indication for dialytic intervention in dogs and cats.[35] Without dialysis, animals with severe renal failure generally die with complications of uremia before renal repair can be achieved. Dialysis extends the life expectancy of these animals, allowing potential recovery. The limited number of regional facilities providing dialytic services make their availability problematic but not impossible. Once indicated, the initiation of dialysis cannot be delayed. General guidelines for selection of patients and indications for dialytic therapy are outlined in Table 168–7. Selection of patients is based on subjective criteria predicting the likelihood for return of adequate renal function. Three to 4 weeks of supportive care has been a historical benchmark for distinguishing reversible from irreversible renal failure. However, these criteria are now inadequate and must be redefined for patients receiving dialytic care. With dialytic support, some animals with seemingly irreversible disease can recover sufficient renal function (or normal function) with 4 to 6 months of treatment.

Animals with severe oliguria or anuria in whom an effective diuresis cannot be initiated or maintained with replacement fluids, osmotic or chemical diuretics, and renal vasodilators should be transferred immediately to a referral center where dialysis can be performed. Further attempts with conservative therapies are nonproductive, cause deterioration of the animal's condition, delay the start of dialysis, and predispose the animal to life-threatening hypervolemia. Dialysis is also uniquely suited for the management of acute poisoning when the toxin is dialyzable. Toxins and their metabolites can be removed rapidly and completely from the body with dialysis. Hemodialysis is particularly effective for ethylene glycol intoxication and superior to treatment with either

URO

TABLE 168–7. INDICATIONS FOR DIALYTIC THERAPY IN ANIMALS

Acute uremia
1. Failure of fluid administration, diuretics, or vasodilator therapy to initiate an adequate diuresis
2. Failure of conventional therapy to control the biochemical and clinical manifestations of acute uremia
3. Life-threatening fluid overload
4. Life-threatening electrolyte or acid base disturbances
5. BUN ≥ 100 mg/dL; serum creatinine ≥ 10 mg/dL
6. Clinical course refractory to conservative therapy for more than 24 hours

Miscellaneous
1. Severe overhydration, pulmonary edema, congestive heart failure
2. Acute poisoning, drug overdose

BUN = blood urea nitrogen.

alcohol or 4-methylpyrazole, which merely delays its metabolism without facilitating its removal from the body. Timely and aggressive hemodialysis can eliminate ethylene glycol and its glycolic metabolites within hours, preventing development of renal injury (see Fig. 168–5). Animals with impaired urine production have a limited ability to excrete the toxin, which may persist as long as 7 days despite administration of alcohol or 4-methylpyrazole. Institution of hemodialysis eliminates the residual toxins and precludes ongoing renal injury. Dialysis is the most effective therapy for managing animals with iatrogenic overhydration, life-threatening pulmonary edema, or therapies requiring delivery of large volumes of fluid in animals with limited excretory capacity.[35]

Peritoneal dialysis is a seemingly straightforward procedure in which dialysate is instilled into the abdominal cavity and, by diffusive and convective transport, uremic wastes and excess fluid transfer from plasma to equilibrate with the dialysate across the limiting barrier of the peritoneal lining. The peritoneal limiting membrane is more complex than the artificial barriers of hemodialyzers. It is composed of the capillary endothelium and basement membrane, loose connective tissue, and the mesothelial surface of the peritoneum.[35] The technical simplicity of peritoneal dialysis makes it an enticing therapy ostensibly within the scope of modern veterinary practice. However, technical and medical complications associated with peritoneal access and peritoneal exchange and the personnel demands of the procedure usually prove formidable to the clinician and fatal for the patient.

Hemodialysis is similar conceptually to peritoneal dialysis except that an artificial membrane replaces the peritoneal lining as an exchange surface. Blood is interposed directly with the dialysate across the membrane, and the dialytic process occurs outside the animal's body. Solutes and water transfer across the artificial membrane along diffusive and hydrostatic gradients between plasma water and the dialysate in a hemodialyzer. During dialysis, waste solutes and excessive water loads are removed from the animal in a manner analogous to their excretion by healthy kidneys. Hemodialysis is technically feasible, safe, efficacious, and indispensable for both dogs and cats with life-threatening uremia.[35, 57] Awareness and acceptance of hemodialysis by primary care veterinarians are growing, and there is increased demand by pet owners for this level of service.

Transplantation of renal allografts from unrelated dogs and cats has become more successful in the past 10 years and provides an alternative for animals who sustain irrevocable renal injury.[58, 59] Many of these animals require an interim course of hemodialysis to correct current uremia and to provide preoperative stabilization while the donor is sought and evaluated. Transplantation early in the course of disease for severe conditions such as antifreeze poisoning may also prove more cost effective than a protracted course of hemodialysis with unpredictable recovery.

OUTCOME AND PROGNOSIS

The prognosis for recovery from ARF depends on the nature and extent of the underlying renal injury, the presence of comorbid diseases, the extent and severity of multiple organ involvement, and the availability of diagnostic and therapeutic services. There is little basis in the veterinary literature for accurately predicting the importance of these independent variables. A review of 99 cases of ARF in dogs caused by the usual etiologies documented a mortality of nearly 60 per cent from death or euthanasia.[7] Nearly 60 per cent of the surviving dogs subsequently developed chronic renal failure and only 44 percent recovered normal renal function. The severity of the azotemia; presence of hypocalcemia, anemia, and proteinuria; specific etiology (ethylene glycol intoxication); and comorbid systemic disease (disseminated intravascular coagulation) were associated with failure to survive. In this series, 92 per cent of dogs with a history of ethylene glycol ingestion died or were euthanized because of the poor prognosis. In a another series of cases, 100 per cent of dogs with confirmed ethylene glycol poisoning and concurrent azotemia died or were euthanized despite medical therapy.[60] Survival of dogs with hospital-acquired ARF was reported to be only 38 percent; age and initial urine production were significant contributors to the mortality.[61] In contrast to these outcomes, 9 of 15 cats (60 per cent) with severe ARF secondary to pyelonephritis and ethylene glycol intoxication who were refractory to conventional therapy and managed with hemodialysis recovered sufficient or nearly normal renal function to survive without dialysis. Forty-four per cent of the cats with ethylene glycol intoxication with severe azotemia warranting hemodialysis survived despite being oliguric or anuric at presentation. One hundred per cent of cats with acute pyelonephritis survived.[57] In these animals, as in other series, the magnitude of the azotemia at presentation did not predict survivability.[57, 61] Similarly, approximately 60 per cent of all dogs treated for ARF and approximately 60 per cent of dogs treated for ethylene glycol intoxication with hemodialysis at the University of California survive and are not dialysis dependent. However, in many instances, recovery requires months of dialytic support.

The outcome for dogs with acute leptospirosis is more favorable. In one series, 86 per cent of 14 dogs presenting with severe azotemia (serum creatinine, 11.2 ± 4.5 mg/dL; BUN, 171 ± 66 mg/dL) requiring hemodialysis survived. Similarly, 82 per cent of 22 dogs with moderate azotemia (serum creatinine, 5.1 ± 2.9 mg/dL; BUN, 87 ± 52 mg/dL) who were managed with conventional medical therapy survived. Both groups of dogs recovered with comparable and essentially normal renal function.

ARF is a serious and frequently fatal disease in both dogs and cats. Recovery is best for animals with infectious etiologies and worst for animals with nephrotoxic causes or multiple organ failure. Early recognition, aggressive and appropriate fluid therapy, and supportive therapy with dialysis offer the greatest opportunity for a favorable outcome.

REFERENCES

1. Kierdorf HP, Seelinger S: Acute renal failure in multiple organ dysfunction syndrome. Kidney Blood Press Res 20:164–166, 1997.
2. Kon V, et al: Role of renal sympathetic nerves in mediating hypoperfusion of renal cortical microcirculation in experimental congestive heart failure and acute extracellular fluid volume depletion. J Clin Invest 76:1913–1920, 1985.
3. Badr KF, Ichikawa I: Prerenal failure: A deleterious shift from renal compensation to decompensation. N Engl J Med 319:623–629, 1988.
4. Grauer GF: Fluid therapy in acute and chronic renal failure. Vet Clin North Am 28:609–602, 1998.
5. Schnellmann R: Pathophysiology of nephrotoxic cell injury. *In* Schrier R, Gottschalk C (eds): Diseases of the Kidney, 6th ed. Boston, Little, Brown, 1997, pp 1049–1067.
6. Swan S, Bennet W: Nephrotoxic acute renal failure. *In* Lazarus J, Brenner BM (eds): Acute Renal Failure, 3rd ed. New York, Churchill Livingstone, 1993, pp 357–392.
7. Vaden SL, et al: A retrospective case-control of acute renal failure in 99 dogs. J Vet Intern Med 11:58–64, 1997.
8. Thrall MA, et al: Advances in therapy for antifreeze poisoning. Calif Vet 52:18, 1998.
9. Don B, et al: Acute renal failure associated with pigmenturia or crystal deposits.

In Schrier R, Gottschalk C (eds): Diseases of the Kidney, 6th ed. Boston, Little, Brown, 1997, pp 1273–1299.

10. Molitoris B, et al: Mechanism of ischemia-enhanced aminoglycoside binding and uptake by proximal tubule cells. Am J Physiol 264:F907–F916, 1993.

11. Moreau P, et al: Reduced renal toxicity and improved clinical tolerance of amphotericin B mixed with intralipid compared with conventional amphotericin B in neutropenic patients. J Antimicrob Chemother 30:535–541, 1992.

12. Safirstein R: Renal diseases induced by antineoplastic agents. *In* Schrier R, Gottschalk C (eds): Diseases of the Kidney, 6th ed. Boston, Little Brown, 1997, pp 1153–1165.

13. Palmer B, Henrich W: Nephrotoxicity of nonsteroidal anti-inflammatory agents, analgesics, and angiotensin-converting enzyme inhibitors. *In* Schrier R, Gottschalk C (eds): Diseases of the Kidney, 6th ed. Boston, Little, Brown, 1997, pp 1167–1188.

14. Harkin KR, Gartrell CL: Canine leptospirosis in New Jersey and Michigan: 17 cases (1990–1995). J Am Anim Hosp Assoc 32:495–501, 1996.

15. Birnnaum N, et al: Naturally acquired leptospirosis in 36 dogs: Serological and clinicopathological features. J Small Anim Pract 39:231–236, 1998.

16. Bock HA: Pathogenesis of acute renal failure: New aspects. Nephron 76:130–142, 1997.

17. Myers B, Moran S: Hemodynamically medicated acute renal failure. N Engl J Med 314:97–104, 1986.

18. Thadhani R, et al: Acute renal failure. N Engl J Med 334:1448–1460, 1996.

19. Schena FP: Role of growth factors in acute renal failure. Kidney Int 53:S11–S15, 1998.

20. Nissenson AR: Acute renal failure: Definition and pathogenesis. Kidney Int 53:S7–S10, 1998.

21. Brezis M, Rosen S: Hypoxia of the renal medulla—Its implications for disease. N Engl J Med 332:647–655, 1995.

22. Weinberg J: The cell biology of ischemic renal injury. Kidney Int 39:476–500, 1991.

23. Bonventre J: Mechanisms of ischemic acute renal failure. Kidney Int 43:1160–1178, 1993.

24. Molitoris B: Na/K ATPase that redistributes to apical membrane during ATP depletion remains functional. Am J Physiol 265:F693–F697, 1993.

25. Goligorsky M, DiBona G: Pathogenetic role of Arg-Gly-Asp recognizing integrins in acute renal failure. Proc Natl Acad Sci U S A 90:5700–5704, 1993.

26. Kruger JM, et al: Hypercalcemia and renal failure. Etiology, pathophysiology, diagnosis, and treatment. Vet Clin North Am 26:1417–1445, 1996.

27. Vaden SL, et al: Use of carbamylated hemoglobin concentration to differentiate acute from chronic renal failure in dogs. Am J Vet Res 58:1193–1196, 1997.

28. Osborne CA, et al: A clinician's analysis of urinalysis. *In* Osborne CA, Finco DR (eds): Canine and Feline Nephrology and Urology. Baltimore, Williams & Wilkins, 1995, pp 136–205.

29. Grauer GF, et al: Early clinicopathologic findings in dogs ingesting ethylene glycol. Am J Vet Res 45:2299–2303, 1984.

30. Rivers BJ, Johnston GR: Diagnostic imaging, strategies in small animal nephrology. Vet Clin North Am 26:1505–1517, 1996.

31. Adams WH, et al: Ultrasonographic findings in dogs and cats with oxalate nephrosis attributed to ethylene glycol intoxication: 15 cases (1984–1988). JAVMA 199:492–496, 1991.

32. Osborne CA, et al: Percutaneous needle biopsy of the kidney. Indications, applications, technique, and complications. Vet Clin North Am 26:1461–1504, 1996.

33. Heath SE, Johnson R: Leptospirosis. JAVMA 205:1518–1523, 1994.

34. Dial SM, et al: Efficacy of 4-methylpyrazole for treatment of ethylene glycol intoxication in dogs. Am J Vet Res 12:1762–1770, 1994.

35. Cowgill LD, Langston CE: Role of hemodialysis in the management of dogs and cats with renal failure. Vet Clin North Am 29:1347–1378, 1996.

36. Bartges JW, et al: Hypertension and renal disease. Vet Clin North Am 26:1331–1345, 1996.

37. Bullock ML, et al: The assessment of risk factors in 492 patients with acute renal failure. Am J Kidney Dis 5:97–103, 1985.

38. Grassi V, et al: Uremic lung. Contrib Nephrol 106:36–42, 1994.

39. Fraser CL, Arieff AI: Metabolic encephalopathy as a complication of renal failure: Mechanisms and mediators. New Horiz 2:518–526, 1994.

40. Giebisch G, et al: Control of renal potassium excretion. *In* Brenner BM (ed): The Kidney, 5th ed. Philadelphia, WB Saunders, 1996, pp 371–407.

41. Rastegar A, DeFronzo R: Disorders of potassium and acid-base metabolism in association with renal disease. *In* Schrier R, Gottschalk C (eds): Diseases of the Kidney, 6th ed. Boston, Little, Brown, 1997, pp 2451–2475.

42. Shapiro J: Pathogenesis of cardiac dysfunction during metabolic acidosis: Therapeutic implications. Kidney Int 51:S47–S51, 1997.

43. Krawiec D: Managing gastrointestinal complications of uremia. Vet Clin North Am 26:1287–1292, 1996.

44. Goldstein RE, et al: Gastrin concentrations in plasma of cats with chronic renal failure. JAVMA 213:826–828, 1998.

45. Washabau RJ, Elie MS: Antiemetic therapy. *In* Bonagura JD, Kirk RW (eds): Kirk's Current Veterinary Therapy XII. Philadelphia, WB Saunders, 1995, pp 679–684.

46. Levinsky NG, Bernard DB: Mannitol and loop diuretics in acute renal failure. *In* Brenner BM, Lazarus JM (eds): Acute Renal Failure. New York, Churchill Livingstone, 1988, pp 841–856.

47. Kellum JA: Use of diuretics in the acute care setting. Kidney Int 53:S67–S70, 1998.

48. Better OS, et al: Mannitol therapy revisited (1940–1997). Kidney Int 51:886–894, 1997.

49. Visweswaran P, et al: Mannitol-induced acute renal failure. J Am Soc Nephrol 8:1028–1033, 1997.

50. Graziani G, et al: Dopamine and furosemide in oliguric acute renal failure. Nephron 37:39–42, 1984.

51. Clark KL, et al: Do renal tubular dopamine receptors mediate dopamine-induced diuresis in the anesthetized cat? J Cardiovasc Pharmacol 17:267–276, 1991.

52. Livio M, et al: Uraemic bleeding: Role of anemia and beneficial effect of red cell transfusions. Lancet 2:1013–1015, 1982.

53. Haag-Weber M, Horl, WH: Uremia and infection: Mechanisms of impaired cellular host defense. Nephron 63:125–131, 1993.

54. Mitch WE, et al: Protein and amino acid metabolism in uremia: Influence of metabolic acidosis. Kidney Int 27:S205–S207, 1989.

55. Bioelectrical impedance analysis in body composition measurement: National Institutes of Health Technology Assessment Conference Statement. Am J Clin Nutr, 64:524S–532S, 1996.

56. Cowan LS, et al: Effect of stanozolol on body composition, nitrogen balance, and food consumption in castrated dogs with chronic renal failure. JAVMA 211:719–722, 1997.

57. Langston CE, et al: Applications and outcome of hemodialysis in cats: A review of 29 cases. J Vet Intern Med 11:348–355, 1997.

58. Mathews KG, Gregory CR: Renal transplants in cats: 66 cases (1987–1996). JAVMA 211:1432–1436, 1997.

59. Gregory CR: Clinical renal transplantation. *In* Osborne CA, Finco DR (eds): Canine and Feline Nephrology and Urology. Baltimore, Williams & Wilkins, 1995, pp 597–600.

60. Connally HE, et al: Safety and efficacy of 4-methylpyrazole as treatment for suspected or confirmed ethylene glycol intoxication in dogs. 107 cases (1983–1995). JAVMA 209:1880–1883, 1996.

61. Behrend EN, et al: Hospital-acquired acute renal failure in dogs: 29 cases (1983–1992). JAVMA 208:537–541, 1996.

URO

CHAPTER 169

CHRONIC RENAL FAILURE

David J. Polzin, Carl A. Osborne, Frédéric Jacob, and Sheri Ross

OVERVIEW OF CHRONIC RENAL FAILURE

Chronic renal failure (CRF) is the most common renal disease in dogs and cats. It is defined as primary renal failure that has persisted for an extended period, usually months to years. Regardless of the cause(s) of nephron loss, irreversible renal structural lesions characterize CRF.[1] After correcting reversible primary diseases and/or prerenal or postrenal components of renal dysfunction, further improvement in renal function should not be expected in patients with CRF, because compensatory and adaptive changes designed to sustain renal function have largely already occurred. Likewise, unless additional renal injury occurs, rapid deterioration of intrinsic renal function is unusual. Therefore, renal function typically remains stable for weeks to months. Nonetheless, in some dogs and cats with CRF, renal function progressively declines over months to years.[2-4] Surprisingly, it may not be necessary for the disease process responsible for the initial renal injury to persist for progressive dysfunction to occur. Irrespective of underlying causes, CRF is often described as an irreversible and progressive disease.

In spite of the poor long-term prognosis, patients with CRF often survive for many months to years with a good quality of life. Although no treatment can correct existing irreversible renal lesions of CRF, the clinical and biochemical consequences of reduced renal function can often be ameliorated by symptomatic and supportive therapy. Advances in understanding the spontaneously progressive nature of CRF have provided clues to how this self-perpetuating deterioration of renal function might be deterred.[2] In addition, hemodialysis and renal transplantation, the mainstays of treatment for CRF in humans, are becoming viable therapeutic options for some dogs and cats with renal failure.

AFFECTED POPULATION

Although frequently considered a disease of older animals, CRF occurs with varying frequency in dogs and cats of all ages. In a survey of 170 canine and 36 feline patients with CRF, the mean age of diagnosis was 7.0 years for dogs and 7.4 years for cats.[5] In another study of 119 dogs with CRF, the mean age of diagnosis was 6.5 years.[5] In a review of renal failure in cats, 53 per cent of affected cats were older than 7 years, but animals ranged in age from 9 months to 22 years.[6]

In a study of the age distribution of renal failure in cats, 37 per cent of cats were younger than 10 years, 31 per cent were between 10 and 15, and 32 per cent were older than 15 years.[7] In a study of 80 cats with CRF the mean age was 12.6 years.[4] Renal failure was recognized with increased frequency in Maine coon, Abyssinian, Siamese, Russian blue, and Burmese cats.

Although renal failure occurs less commonly in dogs than in cats, its incidence increases similarly with age. Eighteen per cent of dogs with renal failure were younger than 4 years, 17 per cent between 4 and 7, 20 per cent between 7 and 10, and 45 per cent older than 10 years.

CAUSES OF CHRONIC RENAL FAILURE

CRF may be congenital, familial, or acquired in origin. Congenital and familial causes of CRF can often be suspected on the basis of breed and family history, age of onset of renal disease or failure, or radiographic and ultrasonographic findings (e.g., polycystic kidney disease).[8] Acquired CRF may result from any disease process that injures renal glomeruli, tubules, interstitium, and/or vasculature and causes sufficient irreversible loss of functional nephrons to result in primary renal failure. In a study of biopsy findings in 36 dogs and 47 cats with primary renal azotemia, chronic tubulointerstitial nephritis was the most common finding with a prevalence of 58.3 per cent in dogs and 70.4% in cats,[9] and the prevalence of glomerulonephritis was 27.8 per cent in dogs and 14.8 per cent in cats; Other lesions identified in dogs included amyloidosis (5.6 per cent) and renal dysplasia and in cats included lymphoma (10.6 per cent), amyloidosis (2.1 per cent), and tubulonephrosis (2.1 per cent).

Regardless of the pathologic diagnosis, initiating factors responsible for CRF remain unclear in the majority of dogs and cats. Glomerulopathies have been linked to a variety of neoplastic, metabolic, infectious, and noninfectious inflammatory processes.[10] Causes of tubulointerstitial lesions in dogs and cats are rarely established. Pyelonephritis can cause tubulointerstitial lesions but is not thought to be a major cause of CRF in dogs and cats. Periodontal disease has been linked to renal histologic changes in dogs,[11] but the clinical significance of this association is far from clear. Feline immunodeficiency virus (FIV) infection has been linked to renal disease in cats, although few cats with CRF are FIV positive.[12, 13]

Inability to identify the inciting cause of renal failure derives from three phenomena related to the evolution of progressive renal diseases: (1) the various components of nephrons (glomeruli, tubules, peritubular capillaries, and interstitial tissue) are functionally interdependent; (2) morphologic and functional abnormalities of the kidneys can be manifested clinically in only a limited number of ways, irrespective of underlying cause; and (3) after maturation, new nephrons cannot be formed to replace others irreversibly destroyed by disease. Progressive irreversible lesions initially localized to one portion of the nephron are eventually responsible for development of lesions in the remaining but initially unaffected portions of nephrons. For example, progressive lesions confined initially to glomeruli decrease peritubular capillary perfusion of tubules and thus induce tubule cell atrophy, degeneration, and necrosis. Ultimately, nephron destruction initiated by progressive glomerular disease stimulates repair by fibrosis. Likewise, generalized progressive pyelonephritis damages or destroys tubules and glomeruli and stimulates repair by fibrosis. If the majority of nephrons have been destroyed, these events are associated with reduction in renal size, capsular adhesions, and generalized pitting of the capsular surface of the cortex.

Because of the structural and functional interdependence of various components of nephrons, differentiation of various generalized, progressive renal diseases that have reached an advanced stage may be difficult. Functional and structural changes prominent during earlier phases of progressive generalized renal diseases may permit identification of a specific cause and/or localization of the initial lesion to one or more components of the nephrons. With time, however, destructive changes of varying severity (atrophy, inflammation, fibrosis, and mineralization of diseased nephrons), superimposed on compensatory and adaptive changes (hypertrophy and hyperplasia) of partially and totally viable nephrons, provide a gross and microscopic similarity to the findings in these diseases. The important point is that primary irreversible progressive diseases of glomeruli, tubules, vessels, and interstitial tissue may lead to chronic generalized nephropathy.

At one time, poor understanding of renal response to injury and lack of laboratory and biopsy techniques with which to detect antemortem lesions at an early stage of development led to the widespread but erroneous assumption that the vast majority of "chronic generalized nephropathy" was caused by a specific disease entity called "chronic interstitial nephritis" (so-called CIN). Indeed, primary irreversible progressive diseases of the renal interstitium (chronic interstitial nephritis) can cause chronic generalized nephropathy characterized by reduction in renal size, and interstitial nephritis, whether it be acute or chronic, is a valid descriptive term. When used as a morphologic diagnosis, however, it suggests that the underlying disorder is characterized by morphologic and functional abnormalities of interstitial tissue, which, if progressive, may induce changes in the renal tubules, glomeruli, and vessels. True interstitial nephritis is distinguished from other types of primary renal disease by changes that initially and predominantly affect interstitial tissue. Unfortunately, many chronic generalized diseases of the kidneys that originate in vessels, glomeruli, or tubules are associated with a marked degree of interstitial inflammation and fibrosis.

The term end-stage kidney disease implies the presence of renal diseases that are generalized, progressive, irreversible, and at an extremely advanced or "end" stage of development. End-stage kidneys are one step beyond chronic generalized nephropathy. The histopathologic appearance of such kidneys is consistently characterized by sclerotic glomeruli, abundant mononuclear tubulointerstitial infiltrate, dilated tubules, and simplified tubular epithelium.

Despite the generalized nature of irreversible renal lesions, active renal disease may be present and contribute to progression of CRF. It is particularly important that active renal diseases that may be amenable to treatment not be overlooked. Renal diseases potentially amenable to specific therapy include bacterial pyelonephritis, chronic urinary obstruction, nephrolithiasis, renal lymphoma (particularly in cats), and some immune-mediated renal diseases.

CLINICAL CONSEQUENCES OF CHRONIC RENAL FAILURE

UREMIA

The onset and spectrum of clinical and biochemical events in patients with CRF may vary depending on the nature,

severity, duration, and rate of progression of the underlying disease; presence of coexistent but unrelated disease(s); age and species of the patient; and administration of therapeutic agents. In most instances, however, uremia is the clinical state toward which all progressive, generalized renal diseases ultimately converge, and associated signs are more similar than dissimilar. Diverse clinical and laboratory findings characterize uremia and emphasize the polysystemic nature of CRF (Table 169–1).

Uremia is the pathophysiologic clinical syndrome that accompanies renal failure. It results from retention of substances normally removed by healthy kidneys (Table 169–2). Intake of precursors of some of these substances as food also contributes to signs of uremia, as do derangements in hormonal and enzymatic homeostasis (Table 169–2). The unsuccessful search for "the" uremic toxin has been overemphasized; this approach fails to take into account the cumulative result of retention of innumerable compounds and deficiencies of others.[14]

GASTROINTESTINAL CONSEQUENCES

Gastrointestinal complications are among the most common and prominent clinical signs of uremia. Anorexia and weight loss are common, nonspecific findings which may precede other signs of uremia in dogs and cats. Anorexia appears to be multifactorial in origin (Table 169–3). The patient's appetite may be selective for certain foods, and it may wax and wane throughout the day. Factors promoting weight loss and malnutrition include anorexia, nausea, vomiting and the subsequent reduction in nutrient intake, hormonal and metabolic derangements, and catabolic factors related to uremia, particularly acidosis.

TABLE 169–1. CLINICAL FEATURES OF CHRONIC RENAL FAILURE

Historical and physical findings:
  General: depression, fatigue, weakness, polydipsia, dehydration, weight loss, and malnutrition
  Gastrointestinal: anorexia, nausea, vomiting, diarrhea, gastrointestinal ulcers, uremic stomatitis, xerostomia, uriniferous breath, and constipation
  Urinary system: polyuria, nocturia, palpation reveals small, often irregular kidneys
  Cardiopulmonary: arterial hypertension, heart murmurs, cardiomegaly, cardiac rhythm disturbances, dyspnea, pericarditis, and edema
  Neuromuscular: dullness, drowsiness, lethargy, irritability, tremors, gait imbalance, flaccid muscle weakness, myoclonus, behavioral changes, dementia, isolated cranial nerve deficits, seizures, stupor, and coma
  Eyes: scleral and conjunctival injection, retinopathy, acute-onset blindness
  Skin and hair coat: pallor (anemia), bruising (coagulopathy), increased shedding, unkempt appearance and loss of normal sheen of coat
Laboratory findings:
  Acidosis
  Anemia: usually normochromic, normocytic
  Azotemia
  Hyperamylasemia, hyperlipasemia
  Hypercalcemia or hypocalcemia
  Hypermagnesemia
  Hyperparathyroidism: renal secondary
  Hyperphosphatemia
  Hypokalemia
  Proteinuria
  Radiology: reduced renal size, irregular renal contours, renal mineralization, evidence of osteomalacia or osteitis fibrosa
  Reduced urine concentrating ability
  Renal isotope scan: reduced renal size and function
  Ultrasonography: reduced renal size, increased echogenicity

URO

TABLE 169–2. FACTORS CONTRIBUTING TO THE UREMIC SYNDROME

A. Some currently recognized uremic solutes

Nitric oxide	Guanidinoacetate
Urea	Hippurate
Methylguanidine	*myo*-Inositol
Phenol	ADMA or SDMA
Phosphate	Dimethylarginine
p-Cresol	Spermine
Creatinine	CMPF
Hypoxanthine	Pseudouridine
Spermidine	Indoxyl sulfate
Xanthine	Phenylacetylglutamine
Urate	β-Endorphin
Guanidinosuccinic acid	Parathormone
Indole acetate	β$_2$-Microglobulin

B. Hormonal disturbances that may occur in uremia
   Impaired production of erythropoietin
   Renal secondary hyperparathyroidism
   Abnormal carbohydrate metabolism (altered glucose metabolism, pancreatic glucose–induced insulin secretion, and target organ sensitivity to insulin)
   Low-normal or depressed levels of thyroxine and triiodothyronine associated with abnormal pituitary responsiveness
   Elevated basal levels of growth hormone
C. Enzymatic and metabolic systems that may be depressed in uremia
   Gluconeogenesis
   Lactate dehydrogenase activity
   Mitochondrial storage of calcium and oxygen consumption
   Alkaline phosphatase isoenzyme activity
   Insulin degradation
   Na$^+$,K$^+$-ATPase activity
   Tubular anion transport
   Production and metabolic clearance of calcitriol
   DNA repair ability

ADMA = asymmetric demethylarginine; SDMA = symmetric dimethylarginine; CMPF = carboxymethylpropylfuranpropionic acid; ATPase = adenosinetriphosphatase.

From Vanholder R: The uremic syndrome. *In* Greenberg A (ed.): Primer on Kidney Diseases, 2nd ed. San Diego, Academic Press, 1998, pp 403–407.

Vomiting is a frequent but inconsistent finding in uremia. It results from the effects of as yet unidentified uremic toxins on the medullary emetic chemoreceptor trigger zone and from uremic gastroenteritis. The severity of vomiting correlates crudely with the magnitude of azotemia. Because uremic gastritis may be ulcerative, hematemesis may occur. Vomiting may be a more frequent complaint in uremic dogs than cats. Nonetheless, vomiting is reportedly found in one quarter to one third of cats with clinical signs of uremia.[4]

Uremic gastropathy is characterized microscopically by glandular atrophy, edema of the lamina propria, mast cell infiltration, fibroplasia, mineralization, and submucosal arteritis.[15] Elevated gastrin levels have been implicated in the development of uremic gastropathy. Gastrin induces gastric acid secretion directly by stimulating receptors located on gastric parietal cells as well as by increasing histamine release from mast cells in the gastric mucosa. Enhanced histamine release may also promote gastrointestinal ulceration and ischemic necrosis of the mucosa through a vascular mechanism characterized by small venule and capillary dilatation, increased endothelial permeability, and intravascular thrombosis.[16] Because up to 40 per cent of the circulating gastrin is metabolized by the kidneys, reduced renal function may promote hypergastrinemia. Indeed, elevated gastrin levels have been documented in cats with spontaneous CRF.[17]

Gastrin-induced gastric hyperacidity may lead to uremic gastritis, gastrointestinal hemorrhage, and nausea and vomiting. Back-diffusion of hydrochloric acid and pepsin into the stomach wall may lead to hemorrhage, inflammation, and release of histamine from mast cells. Thus, the cycle may be perpetuated as mast cell–derived histamine causes further stimulation of parietal cells to produce hydrogen ions. However, gastric hyperacidity is not universally found. Hypergastrinemia may not be the primary reason for uremic gastritis. Other factors implicated in the genesis of uremic gastropathy include psychologic stress related to illness, an increase in proton back-diffusion caused by high urea levels, erosions caused by ammonia liberated by bacterial urease acting on urea, ischemia caused by vascular lesions, decreased concentration and turnover of gastric mucous, and biliary reflux related to pyloric incompetence (which may be an indirect consequence of elevated gastrin levels).

Dysphagia and oral discomfort occurred in 7.7 per cent of uremic cats and 38.5 per cent of 80 cats with end-stage renal failure.[4] Periodontal disease was observed in 30.8 per cent of uremic cats and 34.6 per cent of cats with end-stage CRF. Halitosis was reported in 7.7 per cent of cats in both groups. Moderate to severe CRF may result in uremic stomatitis characterized by oral ulcerations (particularly located on the buccal mucosa and tongue), brownish discoloration of the

TABLE 169–3. EXAMPLES OF SOME METABOLIC DEFICITS AND EXCESSES CONTRIBUTING TO ANOREXIA, NAUSEA, AND VOMITING IN PATIENTS WITH RENAL FAILURE

METABOLIC ABNORMALITY	CAUSE	SEQUELA
Polyuria associated with impaired polydipsia	Impaired tubular reabsorption of water, nausea, vomiting	Dehydration, anorexia; others
Hypokalemia	Impaired tubular reabsorption of potassium (?), inadequate intake of potassium	Anorexia, muscle weakness, chronic vomiting, nephropathy, others
Metabolic acidosis	Impaired glomerular filtration of acid catabolites, impaired tubular secretion of hydrogen ion, impaired tubular reabsorption of bicarbonate	Anorexia, nausea, vomiting, hypokalemia, bone demineralization, others
Nonregenerative anemia	Impaired renal production of erythropoietin	Anorexia, weakness, cold intolerance
Hypergastrinemia	Impaired renal clearance of gastrin from blood	Anorexia, nausea, and vomiting related to gastric hyperacidity
Hyperparathormonemia	Renal secondary hyperparathyroidism causing parathyroid hormone–mediated interference of insulin release	Mild hyperglycemia leading to inappetence
Retention of catabolic wastes such as guanidine	Stimulation of medullary emetic chemoreceptor trigger zone	Anorexia, nausea, and vomiting
Retention of urea	Impaired glomerular filtration, degradation of urea to ammonia by urease-producing bacteria in the mouth (especially in tartar)	Caustic stomatitis

dorsal surface of the tongue, necrosis and sloughing of the anterior portion of the tongue (associated with fibrinoid necrosis and arteritis), and uriniferous breath. The mucous membranes may also become dry (xerostomia). Degradation of urea to ammonia by bacterial urease may contribute to many of these signs.

Uremic enterocolitis, manifested as diarrhea, may occur in dogs and cats with severe uremia, but it is typically less dramatic and less common than uremic gastritis. Owners of 80 cats with spontaneous CRF did not report diarrhea.[4] However, when present, uremic enterocolitis is often hemorrhagic. Considerable gastrointestinal hemorrhage may initially escape clinical detection. Intussusception may occasionally complicate uremic enterocolitis. Constipation is a relatively common complication of CRF, particularly in cats. It appears to be primarily a manifestation of dehydration.

IMPAIRED URINE CONCENTRATING ABILITY, POLYURIA, POLYDIPSIA, AND NOCTURIA

Among the earliest and most common clinical manifestations of CRF is onset of polyuria, polydipsia, and sometimes nocturia related to reduced urine concentrating ability. Polydipsia was the single most commonly reported clinical sign in a study of 80 cats with CRF.[4] Cat owners recognized polydipsia more than twice as often as polyuria. Urine specific gravity values were usually below 1.030, typically below 1.020.

Decreased urine concentrating ability results from several factors, including increased solute load per surviving nephron (solute diuresis), disruption of the renal medullary architecture and countercurrent multiplier system by disease, and primary impairment of renal responsiveness to antidiuretic hormone (ADH). Loss of renal responsiveness to ADH may result from an increase in distal renal tubular flow rate, which limits equilibration of tubular fluid with the hypertonic medullary interstitium. In addition, ADH-stimulated adenylate cyclase activity and water permeability in the distal nephron may be impaired in uremia.[18] Polydipsia is, of course, compensatory for polyuria. If fluid intake fails to keep pace with urinary fluid losses, dehydration ensues because of the inability to conserve water by concentrating urine. Dehydration subsequent to inadequate fluid intake appears to be a common problem in cats with CRF.

ARTERIAL HYPERTENSION

Arterial hypertension is purported to be among the most common complications of CRF. It reportedly occurs in approximately two thirds of cats with CRF[19] and from 50 to 93 per cent of dogs with renal failure.[20] Dogs with glomerular diseases may be at particular risk for hypertension. In contrast, a recent study from England suggested that hypertension may be unusual in dogs with CRF.[21, 22] The prevalence and clinical importance of hypertension in dogs and cats remain to be more clearly established. There appears to be a consensus among veterinary nephrologists that systolic blood pressures exceeding 200 mmHg may lead to end-organ injury in dogs and cats with CRF and therefore warrant detection and treatment.

By definition, hypertension is present when there is persistent elevation of either systolic or diastolic blood pressure or when a patient is taking antihypertensive medication (regardless of the blood pressure level).[23] It is generally accepted that the systolic blood pressure in awake, nonanxious cats should not exceed 160 to 170 mmHg.[24–27] Hypertension in cats should probably be defined as systolic pressures in excess of 170 mmHg. Diastolic pressures should probably not exceed 100 mmHg, although our normal range for diastolic pressures established in 103 normal cats (using an oscillometric method) extends up to 124 mmHg. However, using Doppler methods of measuring blood pressure, it is often difficult to obtain reliable diastolic blood pressures. Fortuitously, the preponderance of epidemiologic data in humans suggests that systolic, not diastolic, blood pressure is the primary determinant of pressure-related risk.[23] In addition, isolated diastolic hypertension is believed to be rare in cats.

In dogs, systolic blood pressure should not exceed 180mm Hg.[25, 26] Diastolic pressures should not exceed 100mm Hg, although our normal range for diastolic pressures established in 113 normal dogs extends up to 130 mmHg. Age and breed were shown to have important effects on normal blood pressure values in an extensive study of normal blood pressures in dogs.[21] In this study, blood pressure increased with age and sight hounds had particularly greater mean pressures than other breeds.

Diagnosis of hypertension should be based on a series of blood pressure determinations performed during at least three different hospital visits. Except when systolic pressures are above 200 mmHg and/or clear evidence of end-organ injury is present, rapid diagnosis and pharmacologic intervention are unnecessary and unwise.

Hypertension reflects an imbalance between cardiac output and systemic vascular resistance, the two determinants of systemic blood pressure. Regardless of the cause of hypertension, some form of renal dysfunction is probably essential for development and maintenance of hypertension.[28] The kidneys play a dominant role in long-term control of blood pressure. Normally, an elevation in renal arterial perfusion pressure results in excretion of sodium and water, a phenomenon known as pressure natriuresis. In theory, whenever arterial pressure is elevated, activation of pressure natriuresis promotes excretion of sodium and water until blood volume is reduced sufficiently to restore normal blood pressure. It is predicted that the kidney, as a servocontroller of arterial pressure, exhibits infinite negative feedback gain for long-term control of blood pressure by adjusting blood volume. The logical consequence of this predicted role of the kidneys is that hypertension can occur only when there is an impairment in sodium and water excretion. Specifically, the renal pressure-natriuresis relationship must be reset for hypertension to occur. This line of reasoning provides a plausible explanation for hypertension in the setting of CRF (Fig. 169–1A). However, blood volume alone does not directly determine blood pressure, because large portions of blood are contained within capillary networks, venous beds, and the spleen, which are distensible capacitance compartments.[29] These are not in direct equilibrium with the arterial circuit. Hypertension develops only when the increase in extracellular fluid volume influences the primary determinants of blood pressure, cardiac output and peripheral resistance (Fig. 169–1B).

Although hypertension has long been considered an asymptomatic condition, it is now recognized that human patients do experience a constellation of symptoms that correlate with the blood pressure level, including headache, fatigue or weakness, lack of stamina, exercise intolerance, cardiac "awareness," dizziness, nervousness, sleep disturbances, and chest pain.[23] It is unclear whether hypertension

URO

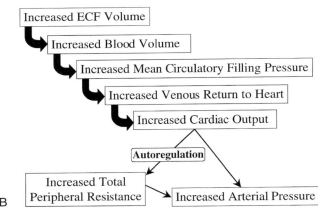

A

B

Figure 169–1. *A,* Schematic representation of one view of the relationship between renal disease or renal failure and the development of arterial hypertension. *B,* Sequence of events through which increased extracellular fluid (ECF) volume occurring as a consequence of renal retention of salt and water leads to increased arterial pressure.

is associated with clinically detectable constitutional signs in dogs and cats.

Hypertension appears to induce pathologic effects largely through vascular injury. Sustained arterial hypertension may result in muscular hypertrophy and hyperplasia, fibrinoid necrosis, loss or fragmentation of the internal elastic lamina, hyalinization, myoarteritis, and capillary occlusion of small arteries and arterioles.[20, 30] Ischemia, decreased tissue perfusion, and hemorrhage subsequent to hypertension-induced vascular lesions result in organ damage. Organs especially prone to hypertensive injury include the eyes, brain, kidneys, and cardiovascular system (see Chapter 50).

Neurologic complications appear to be relatively common among hypertensive CRF cats with active hypertensive retinopathy.[24] Neurologic signs reported in these cats included seizures, sudden collapse or death, intermittent dragging of one or both hindlegs, nystagmus, and decorticate posturing of one or both forelegs.[24]

Cardiovascular complications of arterial hypertension appear to be common although seemingly of little clinical consequence in most cats and dogs. Systolic heart murmurs are a common sign of hypertension in cats, occurring in 42 per cent of affected cats in one study.[24] Murmurs are likewise common in dogs with CRF, but the incidence of valvular murmurs in older dogs is sufficiently great to confound any obvious association with hypertension. Cardiac changes observed on thoracic radiographs in hypertensive cats in-

cluded cardiomegaly; an undulating, tortuous thoracic aorta; and prominent aortic arch. Other cardiac findings included left ventricular hypertrophy shown by echocardiography and atrial or ventricular premature beats. Although cardiac failure may result from sustained hypertension, hypertension appears unlikely to induce cardiac failure in a previously normal heart.

It is generally accepted, although unproved, that hypertension generally results from, rather than causes, CRF in dogs and cats. Occasionally patients are presented with marked elevations in blood pressure (greater than 220 mmHg) and rapidly deteriorating renal function. It appears likely that accelerated hypertension is contributing to deterioration of renal function in these patients, and efforts to reduce blood pressure rapidly and aggressively appear warranted.

NEUROMUSCULAR CONSEQUENCES

Encephalopathies and Neuropathies

Metabolic encephalopathies and, rarely, peripheral neuropathies may occur in dogs and cats with uremia (Table 169–4).[31, 32] It is reported that as many as 65 per cent of dogs and cats with primary renal failure have neurologic manifestations. In patients with neurologic signs, altered consciousness (31 per cent of patients) and seizures (29 per cent of patients) were the most common signs.[32] In our experience, acute onset of altered mentation is an important neurologic finding that typically heralds a poor short-term prognosis in dogs and cats with CRF. Other common signs include limb weakness, ataxia, and tremors. Patients may present with what has been described as the "twitch-convulsive" state, characterized by simultaneous tremor, myoclonus, and seizures. Neurologic signs may be cyclic and episodic.

Clinical signs of neurologic dysfunction are atypical in humans until the glomerular filtration rate (GFR) has declined below 10 per cent of normal.[31] There does not appear to be a correlation between the severity of clinical signs and the severity of renal dysfunction. The severity and rate of progression of neurologic signs appear to vary directly with the rapidity with which renal failure develops.[31]

TABLE 169–4. NEUROLOGIC SIGNS THAT MAY BE ATTRIBUTABLE TO UREMIA

Altered consciousness:	
Confusion	Delirium
Agitation	Restlessness
Dementia	Dullness
Drowsiness	Lethargy
Weakness	Stupor
Coma	Seizures
Abnormal motor responses:	
Abnormal motor tone	Spasms of rigidity
Tremors	Gait imbalance
Myoclonus	Muscle fasciculations
Twitching	Paratonia
Flaccidity	Focal seizures
Peripheral nerve signs:	
Cranial nerve signs	Facial asymmetry
Miosis	Nystagmus
Vestibular dysfunction	Deafness
Hyperreflexia	Autonomic dysfunction
Asymmetric variations in deep tendon reflexes	

From Frasier C: Neurological manifestations of renal failure. In Greenberg A (ed): Primer on Kidney Diseases. San Diego, Academic Press, 1998, pp. 459–464; Fenner W: Uremic encephalopathy. In Bonagura RW (ed): Current Veterinary Therapy XII. Philadelphia, WB Saunders, 1995, pp 1158–1161.

The pathogenesis of uremic neurologic signs remains unclear, but important roles for parathyroid hormone (PTH) and the uremic environment are suspected.[31, 33] Both the sodium-potassium adenosine triphosphate pump and several of the calcium pumps are altered in uremia. Alterations in the calcium pumps have been thought to be due at least in part to PTH acting through monophosphate-independent pathways.[31] Calcium pumps are particularly suspected of playing a role in uremic encephalopathy because they mediate neurotransmitter release and information transfer at nerve terminals. Tremors, myoclonus, and tetany may develop as a result of hypocalcemia. Arterial hypertension may also lead to neurologic signs in patients with otherwise well-controlled renal failure. Hypertensive encephalopathy associated with an acute severe increase in blood pressure and cerebrovascular hemorrhage has been described in humans. Hypertension may also cause brain ischemia related to local vascular autoregulation. Clinical signs are acute in onset and may include seizures, behavioral changes, dementia, isolated cranial nerve deficits, and death.[34] Many of the patients in which we have recognized acute-onset neurologic signs have had hypertension.

Myopathies

Hypokalemic polymyopathy is occasionally observed in association with CRF, primarily in cats. Because of the impact of potassium on resting cell membrane potentials, potassium imbalances are typically manifest clinically as neuromuscular dysfunction. Hypokalemia increases the magnitude (i.e., increases electronegativity) of the resting potential, thereby hyperpolarizing the cell membrane and making it less sensitive to exciting stimuli. The cardinal and most dramatic sign of hypokalemia, regardless of cause, is generalized muscle weakness. Muscle weakness and pain associated with hypokalemic polymyopathy commonly present clinically as cervical ventriflexion and a stiff, stilted gait.[35, 36] Mild cardiac rhythm disturbances may also occur. Serum creatinine kinase and other muscle enzyme activities may be elevated with hypokalemic polymyopathy. In severe instances, rhabdomyolysis may occur. Diets designed for cats with CRF are typically supplemented with potassium; this appears to have reduced the incidence of hypokalemic polymyopathy.

OCULAR CONSEQUENCES

Scleral and conjunctival injections are common manifestations of advanced uremia. Ocular complications are among the more easily detected clinical consequences of arterial hypertension in dogs and cats with CRF. In the absence of hyphema or retinal detachment, slow pupillary light responses may be recognized. Ophthalmoscopy findings may include retinal arterial tortuosity, perivasculitis, papilledema, retinal edema and detachment, and retinal and vitreal hemorrhage.[26, 38] Hyperreflective scars may be seen in cats with previous hypertension injury. Extensive retinal or vitreal hemorrhage or retinal detachment may result in apparent acute onset of blindness. Hyphema with secondary development of glaucoma is an additional potential cause of blindness. In one study, over 50 per cent of cats with CRF and arterial hypertension had retinal lesions develop at some time during the course of their disease.[38] Only 2 of 23 cats with CRF examined in this study were blind. Retinal lesions are typically bilateral.[24] Another study found that acute onset

of blindness was the initial presenting clinical sign in only 1 of 80 cats with CRF, and only one additional episode of blindness was reported during follow-up evaluations of these cats.[4] These researchers concluded that blindness is not a common complication of CRF in cats. Because hypertension may otherwise be clinically silent, fundic examination should be performed in all dogs and cats diagnosed with CRF. Dogs or cats presenting with acute blindness and hyphema should be evaluated for arterial hypertension and renal failure.

Although retinas reattach and hemorrhage clears, the prognosis for sight after retinal detachment and retinal hemorrhage secondary to hypertensive retinopathy appears to be poor. Vision failed to return in 25 of 26 blind cats in a compilation of three studies.[24, 39, 40] Nonetheless, blind cats did not necessarily have a poor prognosis for long-term survival.

The mechanisms of hypertensive retinopathy is related to the effect of long-standing elevations in blood pressure on the retinal vasculature. Chronic hypertension leads to sustained retinal arteriolar vasoconstriction in an attempt to autoregulate local blood flow. Occlusion of precapillary arterioles can lead to ischemia and retinal degeneration. Ultimately, as the integrity of vascular smooth muscle cells and endothelial cells is lost, plasma and/or cellular constituents of blood leak into the surrounding tissues.

HEMORRHAGIC CONSEQUENCES OF UREMIA

Uremia may also be characterized by a hemorrhagic diathesis that typically presents as bruising, gastrointestinal hemorrhage with hematemesis or melena, bleeding from the gums, or hemorrhage subsequent to venipuncture. Gastrointestinal hemorrhage can be an important route of blood loss leading to anemia and exacerbating azotemia and uremia. Bleeding in patients with renal failure results from an acquired qualitative platelet defect and abnormalities in the interaction of platelets and the vessel wall.[41, 42] Platelet numbers and clotting factors are generally normal in renal failure. Clinical bleeding and defective platelet function correlate best with a prolonged bleeding time.

Uremic platelet dysfunction appears to be multifactorial in origin. Abnormal platelet aggregability, diminished thromboxane A[2] production, abnormal intracellular calcium mobilization, and increased intracellular cyclic adenosine monophosphate (cyclic AMP) have been described in uremic platelets.[42] Abnormal glycoprotein function may impair platelet adhesiveness to the subendothelium. In addition, uremia may be associated with increased release of prostacyclin and nitric oxide, which may also impair adhesion of platelets to the endothelium. Uremic toxins have also been implicated in impairing platelet function.

Administration of desmopressin (1-deamino[8-D-arginine] vasopressin, DDAVP) has been shown to shorten bleeding times and improve clinical bleeding in uremic humans.[42] DDAVP is thought to stimulate release of large multimeric von Willebrand's factor complexes from endothelial cells and platelets. Unfortunately, development of tachyphylaxis often limits the usefulness of DDAVP after two or three doses. Alternative therapies have included administration of cryoprecipitates or conjugated estrogens, which may have similar effects. Increasing hematocrit values to above 30 vol% by transfusion or administration of erythropoietin has also been shown to improve bleeding times in humans. Increasing hematocrit may improve bleeding times by a

URO

rheologic effect or by increasing hemoglobin concentrations, which may in turn inactivate the platelet-inhibiting effects of nitric oxide.

LABORATORY FINDINGS

Acidosis

Metabolic acidosis is a well-recognized component of CRF. It results primarily from the limited ability of failing kidneys to excrete hydrogen ions, secondary to disordered ammoniagenesis, decreased filtration of phosphate and sulfate compounds, and decreased maximal renal tubular proton secretion.[43] Bicarbonate wasting may also contribute. Bicarbonate wasting and chloride retention result in hyperchloremic (normal anion gap) acidosis. When phosphate and organic acid (uric acid, hippuric acid, lactic acid) retention is sufficient, high-anion-gap acidosis results.

A combination of tubular reabsorption of filtered bicarbonate and excretion of hydrogen ions with ammonia and urinary buffers, primarily phosphate, maintains normal acid-base balance. As renal mass declines, hydrogen ion excretion is maintained largely by increasing the quantity of ammonium excreted by surviving nephrons. However, at some level of renal dysfunction, the capacity to increase renal ammoniagenesis further is lost and metabolic acidosis ensues. Decreased medullary recycling of ammonia caused by structural renal damage may also contribute to impaired ammonium excretion.

In retrospective case series, 63 per cent and 80 per cent of cats with CRF had metabolic acidosis.[6, 7] However, the prevalence of metabolic acidosis in a prospective study was zero among nonuremic CRF cats, 8 per cent among "uremic" cats, and 50 per cent among cats with end-stage CRF.[4] There is some evidence that feline kidneys may respond differently to metabolic acidosis compared with kidneys of other mammalian species. Apparently, acidosis fails to increase the rate of production of ammonia in cultured feline proximal tubular cells.[44] Whether this characteristic causes cats to be at increased risk for developing metabolic acidosis is unknown, but the unexpectedly high incidence of acidosis in cats with CRF would be consistent with this suggestion. Species-related differences in renal acid excretion aside, it is likely that the high incidence of uremic acidosis in cats is related, at least in part, to the acidifying nature of many cat foods.

Chronic metabolic acidosis promotes a variety of adverse clinical effects including anorexia, nausea, vomiting, lethargy, weakness, muscle wasting, weight loss, and malnutrition. Alkalization therapy appears to be of value in reversing these signs. In addition, chronic mineral acid feeding to dogs has been shown to increase urinary calcium excretion and progressive bone demineralization, the magnitude of which depends on age and dietary calcium levels. Studies of the effects of dietary acidification in cats have revealed that chronic metabolic acidosis can cause negative calcium balance and bone demineralization or negative potassium balance, which may in turn promote hypokalemia, renal dysfunction, and taurine depletion.[45]

Severe acidemia may result in decreased cardiac output, arterial pressure, and hepatic and renal blood flows and centralization of blood volume.[46] Centralization of blood volume results from peripheral arterial vasodilatation and central venoconstriction. Decreases in central and pulmonary vascular compliance may predispose patients to pulmonary edema during fluid administration, an effect that may be particularly important in patients with acute uremic crises requiring intensive fluid therapy. Acidemia also promotes reentrant arrhythmias and a reduction in the threshold for ventricular fibrillation. Severe acidosis may also influence carbohydrate and protein metabolism, serum potassium concentrations, and brain metabolism.[46]

Metabolic acidosis has been theorized to enhance progression of renal failure by promoting renal ammoniagenesis and activation of the alternative complement pathway.[47, 48] Reducing renal ammoniagenesis and renal tubular peptide catabolism was accompanied either by reduced renal tubular injury or by tubular hyperfunction in human patients with CRF. It has been concluded that metabolic acidosis neither causes nor exacerbates chronic renal injury. Furthermore, treatment of uremic acidosis was deemed unlikely to influence disease progression in patients with CRF. Studies performed in our laboratory in cats with induced CRF have likewise failed to identify an adverse effect of chronic acidosis on renal structure or function. (James K, Polzin DJ, Osborne CA: Unpublished observations).

Of great clinical importance is the observation that chronic acidosis may promote protein malnutrition in patients with CRF. Protein catabolism is increased in patients with acidosis to provide a source of nitrogen for hepatic glutamine synthesis, glutamine being the substrate for renal ammoniagenesis.[50, 51] Evidence from studies of rat muscle suggests that uremia directly impairs insulin-stimulated protein synthesis independent of metabolic acidosis. On the other hand, protein degradation is stimulated by metabolic acidosis, even in nonuremic states. The combined effects of reduced protein synthesis related to uremia and accelerated proteolysis related to acidosis promote elevations in blood urea nitrogen (BUN), increased nitrogen excretion, and negative nitrogen balance typical of uremic acidosis. Altered branched-chain amino acid metabolism appears to be involved. Chronic metabolic acidosis increases the activity of muscle branched-chain keto acid dehydrogenase, the rate-limiting enzyme in branched-chain amino acid catabolism. This is important in that branched-chain amino acids are rate limiting in protein synthesis and play a role in regulation of protein turnover. Alkalization therapy effectively reverses acidosis-associated protein breakdown. Although glucocorticoids appear to be essential for acidosis-induced protein catabolism, this response can be blocked in uremic animals by correcting acidosis despite persistent increases in glucocorticoid levels. Excessive protein catabolism may lead to protein malnutrition despite adequate dietary intake. This process may then accelerate breakdown of endogenous cationic and sulfur-containing amino acids, promoting further acidosis.

Acidosis poses a particularly vexing problem for patients with CRF consuming protein-restricted diets. Dietary protein requirements appear to be similar for normal humans and humans with CRF unless uremic acidosis is present. When acid-base status is normal, adaptive reductions in skeletal muscle protein degradation protect patients consuming low-protein diets from losses in lean body mass. Metabolic acidosis blocks the metabolic responses to dietary protein restriction in two ways: it stimulates irreversible degradation of the essential, branched-chain amino acids and stimulates degradation of protein in muscle.[51] Thus, acidosis may limit the ability of humans to adapt to dietary protein restriction. Metabolic acidosis also suppresses albumin synthesis in humans and may reduce the concentration of serum albumin.

Anemia

A progressive hypoproliferative anemia is characteristic of dogs and cats with moderate to advanced CRF. Although affected by the patient's age, species, specific renal diagnosis, and concurrent diseases, the severity and progression of the anemia and clinical signs correlate with the degree of renal failure and worsen with progressive renal failure in both dogs and cats.[53]

Anemia in patients with CRF is multifactorial and may be exacerbated by concurrent illness. Although experimental and clinical evidence exists for the supporting roles of shortened red cell life span, nutritional abnormalities, erythropoietic inhibitor substances in uremic plasma, blood loss, and myelofibrosis, erythropoietin deficiency has clearly emerged as the principal cause of anemia in humans and animals with CRF.[53, 54] The renal peritubular capillary endothelial cells are the major source of erythropoietin synthesis. It may also be produced by renal interstitial fibroblasts. The kidneys synthesize erythropoietin on demand in response to intrarenal tissue hypoxia caused by either decreased oxygen carrying capacity (anemia) or decreased oxygen content (hypoxia).[55] Many CRF patients have a relative, rather than absolute, erythropoietin deficiency in that plasma levels exceed the normal range.[56, 57] However, erythropoietin levels are lower than those in equivalently anemic but nonuremic patients. Anemic cats with CRF have been reported to have erythropoietin levels similar to those of normal cats.[58] Several hypotheses have been proposed to account for the erythropoietin deficiency of CRF: (1) decreased renal mass resulting in an insufficient cellular capacity for new hormone synthesis, (2) lowered set point for response to the hypoxic stimulus, and (3) increased plasma proteolytic activity resulting in accelerated erythropoietin degradation.[57, 59]

Other clinically important causes of anemia in dogs and cats with CRF are iron deficiency and chronic gastrointestinal blood loss. In most patients, iron deficiency can be detected only by measuring serum iron, staining bone marrow biopsy samples for iron content, or observing the response to iron supplementation. Chronic gastrointestinal hemorrhage may or may not be evident on the basis of stool color. It can be suspected on the basis of (1) a hematocrit level that is unexpectedly low relative to the magnitude of renal dysfunction and (2) an elevation in the serum urea nitrogen to serum creatinine ratio.

Azotemia

Azotemia is defined as an excess of urea or other nitrogenous compounds in the blood. Loss of renal function leads to accumulation of a wide variety of nitrogen-containing compounds, including urea and creatinine. Many waste products of protein catabolism are excreted primarily by glomerular filtration. Thus, patients with primary renal failure have an impaired ability to excrete proteinaceous catabolites because of a marked reduction in GFR. Retention of metabolic waste may be further aggravated by impaired tubular secretion and by extrarenal factors that promote renal hypoperfusion and increased catabolism of body tissues. Although accumulation of proteinaceous wastes is largely the result of decreased renal excretion or increased protein catabolism, production of some compounds may also be increased (e.g., guanidine). Because these compounds are derived almost entirely from protein degradation, their production increases when dietary protein increases. A direct cause-and-effect relationship has not been proved in many instances, but it is generally believed that retained protein catabolites contribute significantly to production of uremic signs and many of the laboratory abnormalities found in patients with renal failure.

In human patients with renal failure, maintaining average BUN concentrations close to 50 mg/dL has been shown to be associated with fewer complications than maintaining the average BUN at approximately 90 mg/dL by less intensive dialysis.[60] Likewise, adding a sufficient quantity of urea to the dialysis bath of otherwise "well-dialyzed" patients to raise the BUN to about 140 mg/dL for more than 1 week reproduced uremic signs. On the other hand, moderate increases in BUN do not seem to be associated with uremic symptoms when renal function is otherwise normal.[60] Urea is synthesized using nitrogen derived from amino acid catabolism. Urea may be excreted by the kidneys, retained in body water, or metabolized to ammonia plus carbon dioxide by bacteria in the gastrointestinal tract. Ammonia produced in the gastrointestinal tract is recycled to urea in the liver, yielding no net loss of nitrogen or urea. Regardless of whether urea per se is toxic, BUN concentrations are typically directly related to the protein content of the diet. Furthermore, in patients with renal failure, BUN concentrations tend to correlate reasonably well with clinical signs of uremia. For practical purposes, BUN may thus be viewed as a measure of retained "uremic toxins."

In addition to increasing protein intake and declining renal function, BUN concentrations may also be increased by gastrointestinal hemorrhage, enhanced protein catabolism (e.g., in sepsis, pyrexia, burns, or starvation), decreasing urine volumes (caused by prerenal factors such as dehydration), and certain drugs (glucocorticoids and azathioprine by increasing protein catabolism; tetracyclines by decreasing protein synthesis). Urea nitrogen concentrations may decline with portosystemic shunts, hepatic failure, and low-protein diets. Reduced BUN concentration may also indicate malnutrition.

Because so many extrarenal factors influence BUN concentration, it is not a particularly useful measure of glomerular filtration rate in patients with CRF. Serum creatinine measurements more accurately reflect changes in renal function. Although clearance techniques are more accurate, the serum creatinine concentration remains the most commonly used measure of renal function. Creatinine, a nonenzymatic breakdown product of muscle phosphocreatine, is excreted almost exclusively by glomerular filtration. Daily creatinine production is largely determined by muscle mass. Serum creatinine concentrations may underestimate renal function in exceptionally well-muscled individuals and overestimate renal function in patients with reduced muscle mass.

BUN concentrations should be interpreted with knowledge of simultaneously obtained serum creatinine values, particularly in patients consuming reduced-protein diets. The ratio of BUN to serum creatinine concentration should decline when dietary protein intake is reduced. In patients consuming reduced-protein diets, an increase in the ratio of BUN to serum creatinine concentrations may suggest poor dietary compliance, enhanced protein catabolism, gastrointestinal hemorrhage, dehydration, or declining muscle mass.

Hyperphosphatemia

The kidneys play a pivotal role in regulating phosphorus balance. The kidneys are the primary route of phosphorus excretion. Renal phosphorus excretion is the net of glomerular filtration less tubular reabsorption of phosphorus. If dietary phosphorus intake remains constant, a decline in GFR leads to phosphorus retention and ultimately hyperphosphatemia. However, during the early stages of renal failure, serum phosphorus concentrations typically remain within the normal range because of a compensatory decrease in

URO

phosphate reabsorption in the surviving nephrons. This renal tubular adaptation is largely an effect of renal secondary hyperparathyroidism (see later). Increased PTH levels promote renal excretion of phosphate by reducing the tubular transport maximum for phosphate reabsorption in the proximal tubule via the adenylate cyclase system. When GFR declines below about 20 per cent of normal, this adaptive effect is maximized and hyperphosphatemia ensues.

In dogs and cats with CRF, serum phosphorus concentrations typically parallel serum urea nitrogen concentrations. Thus, hyperphosphatemia is common in azotemic patients but unexpected in patients with nonazotemic renal disease. The primary consequence of hyperphosphatemia is development and progression of secondary hyperparathyroidism. Increases in serum PTH activities in dogs and humans with CRF are closely associated with the degree of hyperphosphatemia (Fig. 169–2),[61, 62] and hyperphosphatemia was found to be 72 per cent efficient in predicting hyperparathyroidism in cats with CRF.[63] An additional consequence of hyperphosphatemia is a predisposition to metastatic calcification when the Ca × PO$_4$ product is elevated. A Ca × PO$_4$ product of 42 to 52 is considered desirable for humans with renal failure.[64] The likelihood of soft tissue calcification increases greatly when the Ca × PO$_4$ product exceeds 60. Calcification is especially prominent in proton-secreting organs, such as the stomach and kidneys, in which basolateral bicarbonate secretion results in an increase in pH that promotes calcium hydrogen phosphate (brushite) precipitation.[65] However, myocardium, lung, and liver are also commonly mineralized in patients with CRF.

Hyperphosphatemia does not appear to induce clinical signs directly. However, hyperparathyroidism and soft tissue calcification may contribute to morbidity and mortality in CRF.[66] Secondary hyperparathyroidism causes renal osteodystrophy and PTH is a purported uremic toxin that may contribute to many signs of uremia.[67, 68]

Hyperphosphatemia has been directly linked to increased mortality in humans and dogs with CRF.[66, 69, 70] In humans with CRF receiving hemodialysis therapy, the adjusted relative risk of mortality was stable in patients with serum phosphate concentrations below 6.5 mg/dL but increased significantly above this level. The overall mortality risk associated with hyperphosphatemia was 1.06 per 1 mg/dL increase in serum phosphorus. The calcium × phosphate product showed a mortality risk trend similar to that seen for phosphate, with patients with Ca × PO$_4$ products greater than 72 having a relative mortality risk of 1.34 compared with that associated with products between 42 and 52 mg^2/dL^2.[66] Analysis of calcium revealed no correlation with relative risk of death.

Interestingly, in humans receiving dialysis, markers traditionally associated with improved nutritional status were significantly associated with higher serum phosphorus levels.[66] Presumably, improved nutrition was associated with increased consumption of foods containing phosphorus. There appeared to be a competing risk and benefit of having higher serum phosphorus levels and improved nutrition.

Renal Secondary Hyperparathyroidism

Incidence. In a study of cats with spontaneous CRF, the overall prevalence of renal secondary hyperparathyroidism was 84 per cent.[63] Hyperparathyroidism occurred in 100 per cent of cats with end-stage CRF and 47 per cent of clinically normal cats with only biochemical evidence of CRF. Hyperparathyroidism was even detected in some cats with normal serum calcium and phosphate concentrations.

Pathophysiology. The pathogenesis of hyperparathyroidism in CRF is controversial. Renal secondary hyperparathyroidism occurs in association with hyperphosphatemia, low circulating 1,25-dihydroxycholecalciferol (calcitriol) levels, reduced blood ionized calcium concentration, and skeletal resistance to the calcemic action of PTH. However, in early to moderate renal failure, it is difficult to dissect out the specific factors responsible for hyperparathyroidism because the increase in PTH serves to prevent hypocalcemia, hyperphosphatemia, and the decrease in calcitriol.[71] At least in human patients, hyperparathyroidism develops early in CRF while serum calcium and phosphorus concentrations remain within normal limits.[72]

Relative or absolute deficiency of calcitriol has been hypothesized to play a pivotal role in the development of renal secondary hyperparathyroidism.[73] Calcitriol, the most active form of vitamin D, is formed by 1-α-hydroxylation of 25-hydroxycholecalciferol in renal tubular cells. PTH promotes renal 1-α-hydroxylase activity and formation of calcitriol. In turn, calcitriol limits PTH synthesis by feedback inhibition. Early in the course of CRF, the inhibitory effects of phos-

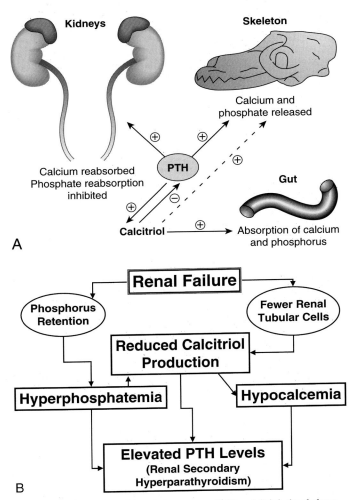

Figure 169–2. *A,* Normal interactions among PTH, calcitriol, the skeleton, kidneys, and gastrointestinal tract. The (+) indicates enhancement; (−) indicates suppression. The dotted line between calcitriol and the skeleton indicates a permissive effect. *B,* Sequential pathogenesis of renal secondary hyperparathyroidism.

phate retention on renal tubular 1-α-hydroxylase activity limit calcitriol production.

In more advanced renal failure, only serum calcium was found to correlate with serum PTH activity.[62] Impaired intestinal absorption of calcium related to low serum calcitriol levels probably plays an important role in hyperparathyroidism in these patients with advanced renal failure. Blood ionized calcium concentrations are often reduced in cats with spontaneous CRF; in one study, over 50 per cent of cats with advanced end-stage CRF were hypocalcemic.[63]

Clinical Consequences. Although renal secondary hyperparathyroidism and renal osteodystrophy are well-documented effects of CRF, clinically important renal osteodystrophy is rare in dogs and cats.[63, 68] In dogs, it most often occurs in immature patients, presumably because metabolically active growing bone is more susceptible to the adverse effects of hyperparathyroidism. For unexplained reasons, bones of the skull and mandible may be the most severely affected and may become so demineralized that the teeth become movable and the jaw can be bent or twisted without fracturing ("rubber jaw" syndrome). Marked proliferation of connective tissue associated with the maxilla may cause distortion of the face. The skull and mandible do not appear to be predisposed to renal osteodystrophy in cats.[63] Pathologic fractures are seemingly uncommon in dogs and cats with CRF. Other possible but uncommon clinical manifestations of severe renal osteodystrophy include skeletal decalcification, cystic bone lesions, bone pain, and growth retardation.

Although bone and kidneys are the classical target organs for PTH, studies have shown that in renal failure PTH may also affect function of nonclassical organs and tissues, including brain, heart, smooth muscles, lungs, erythrocytes, lymphocytes, pancreas, adrenal glands, and testes.[78] Toxicity of PTH appears to be mediated through enhanced entry of calcium into cells with PTH or PTH2 membrane receptors.[74, 78] Sustained PTH-mediated calcium entry leads to inhibition of mitochondrial oxidation and production of ATP. Extrusion of calcium from cells is reduced because of the impairment of ATP production and disruption of the sodium-calcium exchanger. Persistently increased basal cytosolic calcium levels promote cellular dysfunction and death.[61]

Hyperparathyroid-induced cellular dysfunction may lead to carbohydrate intolerance, platelet dysfunction, impaired cardiac and skeletal muscle function (because of impaired mitochondrial energy metabolism and myofiber mineralization), inhibition of erythropoiesis, altered red cell osmotic resistance, altered B-cell proliferation, synaptosome and T-cell dysfunction, and defects in fatty acid metabolism.[14, 74] Potential nonskeletal clinical consequences of hyperparathyroidism include mental dullness and lethargy, weakness, inappetence, and an increased incidence of infections because of immunodeficiency.[74] Excess PTH levels may also promote nephrocalcinosis and consequent progressive loss of renal function.[74] PTH has thus been hypothesized to function as a uremic toxin, although the precise contribution of hyperparathyroidism to the uremic syndrome remains unresolved.

Renal secondary hyperparathyroidism may be associated with substantial enlargement of the parathyroid glands. This finding may be of clinical importance in cats because of frequent coincident hyperthyroidism, which may be suggested by the presence of a thyroid nodule palpable in the cervical region. Hyperplastic parathyroid glands were palpable as paratracheal masses in 11 of 80 cats with spontaneous CRF.[63] Care should be taken to differentiate parathyroid hyperplasia from hyperthyroidism in cats with paratracheal masses.

Quantifying Parathyroid Hormone in Uremia. For patients with renal failure, PTH levels should be determined by methods that measure intact PTH using a two-site immunoradiometric or immunochemiluminometric assay.[79] The two-site method utilizes antibodies directed against two different regions of the intact PTH molecule. A commercially available two-site immunoradiometric assay (Allegro Intact PTH) has been validated for use in dogs and cats.[80, 81] This assay utilizes antiserum to the midregion-carboxyl terminal (residues 39 to 84) absorbed onto polystyrene beads. Only intact PTH is recognized because it is the only form of the peptide to have both determinants. More traditional midregion PTH assays typically detect the species of hormone containing amino acids 43 to 68 of the PTH molecule. However, because renal failure results in reduced renal clearance of midregion PTH fragments, these methods do not accurately reflect parathyroid glandular secretion. Thus, renal secondary hyperparathyroidism is best monitored by use of a two-site assay for intact hormone.[79]

Hypercalcemia, Hypocalcemia, and Hypermagnesemia

As would be predicted in patients with hyperphosphatemia and reduced calcitriol levels, hypocalcemia is the most common disorder of calcium found in patients with renal failure. Ionized hypercalcemia was detected in 6 per cent and ionized hypocalcemia in 26 per cent of 80 cats with spontaneous CRF.[63] Furthermore, the mean blood ionized calcium concentration was significantly lower in cats with CRF in this study than in normal control cats, and over half of the cats with advanced end-stage CRF were hypocalcemic. However, when the same 80 cats were evaluated using total serum calcium concentrations, hypercalcemia was found in 21 per cent of the cats and hypocalcemia was detected in only 8 per cent. Clearly, serum total calcium concentrations do not reliably reflect ionized calcium concentrations in cats with CRF. Similar discrepancies have been observed in dogs with CRF.[82] The mechanism of serum total hypercalcemia in the presence of normal to reduced blood ionized calcium concentrations is unclear but may be related to increased concentrations of calcium complexed to retained organic and inorganic anions such as citrate, phosphate, or sulfate.

In patients with hypercalcemia, it is important to ascertain whether hypercalcemia is the cause rather than the result of CRF.[82] Hypercalcemia caused by malignancy or hypervitaminosis D is most likely to induce renal failure. One way to discriminate the cause-effect relationship between hypercalcemia and renal failure is to determine the patient's blood ionized calcium concentration. Only ionized hypercalcemia promotes renal failure. However, true ionized hypercalcemia may occur in patients with CRF as a consequence of excessive dosages of calcitriol or calcium-containing intestinal phosphate-binding agents or in patients with severe renal secondary hyperparathyroidism with marked hyperplasia of the parathyroid glands. We have also seen small increases in ionized calcium concentrations in dogs with early to moderate CRF that are not receiving calcitriol or calcium therapy and do not have advanced hyperparathyroidism. The mechanism of ionized hypercalcemia in these dogs is unclear.

Hypermagnesemia is common in CRF because the kidneys are primarily responsible for magnesium excretion.[63] For this reason, magnesium-containing drugs (e.g., antacids and laxatives) should be avoided in patients with CRF.

URO

Hypokalemia

An association between polyuric renal failure and hypokalemia has been recognized in cats by several investigators.[7, 83, 84] In contrast, hypokalemia appears to be an uncommon finding at presentation in dogs with CRF, occurring primarily as an iatrogenic complication of fluid therapy in this species. A particularly intriguing concept is that hypokalemia may be a cause of CRF in cats rather than simply a consequence of it. In an uncontrolled study of the long-term effects of feeding a potassium-restricted, acidifying diet, evidence of renal dysfunction developed in three of nine cats and renal lesions consisting of lymphoplasmacytic interstitial nephritis and interstitial fibrosis were observed in five of the nine cats.[85] However, it is not clear whether potassium depletion or hypokalemia precedes the onset of renal failure. In another study, four of seven cats with induced CRF fed a diet containing 0.3 per cent potassium developed hypokalemia but four cats with normal renal function fed the same diet did not develop hypokalemia.[86] Interestingly, muscle potassium content has been shown to be decreased in normokalemic cats with spontaneous CRF, indicating that a total body deficit of potassium may develop well before the onset of hypokalemia.[87] The latter findings support the concept that reduced renal function precedes the development of hypokalemia.

The mechanism of hypokalemia in cats with CRF has remained elusive, but inadequate intake, dietary factors, and increased renal losses appear to be likely candidates. Inadequate intake of potassium could reflect decreased appetite or insufficient dietary potassium content. Dietary risk factors for hypokalemia include acidifying diets, reduced magnesium content, and high protein content. It has yet to be proved that renal potassium wasting occurs in cats with CRF.

Potassium is normally regulated closely by the kidneys. It is excreted primarily via renal tubular secretion, and small quantities are lost in feces and sweat. Although large quantities of K^+ appear in glomerular filtrate, essentially all is reabsorbed before reaching the distal tubules. The majority of potassium appears in urine as a result of potassium secretion from tubular cells into the lumen in the distal nephron. Potassium excretion in these segments of the nephron is quite sensitive to tubular flow rates; rapid urine formation promotes potassium secretion, and slow urine formation limits potassium secretion. Distal potassium secretion is modulated by potassium reabsorption by the intercalated cells in the cortical and outer medullary collecting tubules. Thus, in potassium depletion, net potassium absorption rather than secretion may occur in the distal nephron.

In patients with CRF, the residual nephrons maintain potassium balance by increasing distal tubular secretion of potassium. Gastrointestinal secretion of potassium (primarily in the colon) also appears to increase in CRF and may play an important role in modulating potassium balance. Because of these adaptations, most dogs and cats with CRF are able to tolerate normal dietary potassium intake (about 0.6 per cent dry matter) until renal dysfunction is severe. However, the ability to excrete a potassium load rapidly may be impaired in CRF, resulting in transient hyperkalemia.

Although hypokalemia continues to be detected with some regularity in cats with CRF, its neuromuscular manifestations are becoming increasingly uncommon. Presumably this change is the result of the increase in the potassium content of feline diets that has occurred over the past decade in response to the problem of hypokalemia in cats with CRF. Although generalized muscle weakness has been described as the cardinal sign of hypokalemia, decreased renal function and anorexia are probably more common manifestations of hypokalemia in cats with CRF. In many cats with CRF and hypokalemia, renal function improves after potassium supplementation and restoration of normokalemia, suggesting that hypokalemia may induce a reversible, functional decline in GFR. Renal function was shown to be adversely affected in normal cats when an acidified, potassium-restricted diet was fed.[88] Potassium depletion and acidosis appeared to have additive effects in impairing renal function in this study. These researchers hypothesized that in cats with CRF, a self-perpetuating cycle of excessive urinary potassium losses and whole body potassium depletion may develop that is likely to decrease renal function further. Feeding acidified diets or dietary acidifiers to cats with CRF was suggested to exacerbate their tendency to develop potassium depletion.

By influencing cell metabolism, potassium imbalances may disrupt a variety of cell functions. Hypokalemia-impaired protein synthesis has been hypothesized to promote weight loss and a poor haircoat.[89] Marked potassium depletion has also been linked to polyuria resulting from decreased renal responsiveness to ADH. This antagonism to ADH appears to be due to interference with the generation and action of cyclic AMP and to impairment of the countercurrent mechanism. Locally generated prostaglandins may mediate at least part of this effect.

Proteinuria

Urinary protein excretion is typically mildly increased in dogs and cats with CRF. The magnitude of proteinuria is often as much as 1.5- to 2-fold normal. As a rule, proteinuria is considered a hallmark of glomerular injury and dysfunction. However, the observation that the magnitude of proteinuria may change rapidly when dietary protein intake is increased or decreased has led some researchers to propose that proteinuria in CRF may be related, at least in part, to hemodynamic and physiologic alterations rather than glomerular injury.[90, 91] Disturbances in intraglomerular hemodynamics can induce proteinuria even in the absence of detectable structural abnormalities in the filtration barrier.[90] Presumably, reducing dietary protein intake reduces proteinuria in patients with CRF by reducing intraglomerular hypertension. However, acute and chronic effects of a high dietary protein intake on proteinuria are probably different. Although acute increases in proteinuria associated with high-protein feeding may be of hemodynamic and physiologic origin, the magnitude of this proteinuria typically remains stable. Progressive increases in proteinuria that occur with chronic high-protein feeding are more likely to represent development of glomerular structural lesions. Studies in our laboratory have indicated that in dogs with induced CRF, onset of an increasing magnitude of proteinuria may precede a decline in renal function. Increasing proteinuria has been shown to be an adverse prognostic factor in humans with CRF.[92, 93] There is evidence that this may also hold for dogs.[94]

DIAGNOSTIC EVALUATION OF PATIENTS WITH CHRONIC RENAL FAILURE

See Table 169–5.

TABLE 169–5. DIAGNOSTIC DATABASE FOR PATIENTS WITH CHRONIC RENAL FAILURE

1. Medical history and physical examination
2. Urinalysis
3. Urine culture
4. Complete blood count
5. Serum urea nitrogen concentration
6. Serum creatinine concentration
7. Serum (or plasma) electrolyte and acid-base profile including
   a. Sodium, potassium, and chloride concentrations
   b. Bicarbonate or total CO_2 concentrations
   c. Calcium and phosphorus concentrations
8. Arterial blood pressure (rule out systemic hypertension)
9. Kidney-bladder-urethra survey radiographs
   a. Kidneys—size, shape, location, number
   b. Uroliths or masses affecting kidneys, ureters, or urethra
   c. Urinary bladder—size, shape, location, uroliths
10. Consider
    a. Freezing aliquots of serum (or plasma) and urine for additional diagnostic determinations that may be desired later
    b. Renal ultrasonography (rule out urinary obstruction, renal uroliths, pyelonephritis, renal cystic disease, and renal neoplasia)
    c. Intravenous urography (rule out urinary obstruction, renal uroliths, pyelonephritis, renal cystic disease, and renal neoplasia)
    d. Determining glomerular filtration rate (for cats with hyperthyroidism and early renal failure, for patients with marginal renal dysfunction, or when precise drug dosing regimens are necessary; may also be used to "track" progression of renal failure)[116]
    e. Determining concentration of carbamylated hemoglobin when differentiation of acute from chronic renal failure is unclear from the clinical and other laboratory findings[153]
    f. Renal biopsy (may provide etiologic diagnosis; indicated primarily when kidneys are normal in size or enlarged)

DETERMINING PROGNOSIS FOR CHRONIC RENAL FAILURE

The prognosis for patients with CRF is usually subcategorized according to the probability of immediate survival (short-term prognosis) and survival over the subsequent months to years (long-term prognosis). A guarded prognosis indicates that the chances for recovery are unpredictable. Fair, good, or excellent prognoses indicate varying degrees of probable recovery; poor or grave prognoses indicate that recovery is improbable or hopeless. Loss of renal function is permanent in patients with CRF; recovery refers to improvement of biochemical deficits and excesses and amelioration of clinical signs rather than recovery of renal function.

Factors to be considered in establishing meaningful prognoses for patients with CRF include (1) severity of clinical signs and complications of uremia, (2) probability of improving renal function (reversibility, primarily of prerenal, postrenal, and newly acquired primary renal conditions), (3) severity of intrinsic renal functional impairment, (4) rate of progression of renal dysfunction with or without therapy, (5) primary renal disease, and (6) age of the patient.

Severity of uremic signs is often a relatively good predictor of short-term prognosis. Patients with stable CRF without clinical signs of uremia usually have a good short-term prognosis. Patients with severe clinical signs of uremia typically have a guarded to poor short-term prognosis without therapy. However, it is best to determine whether renal function and clinical signs can be therapeutically improved in such cases before establishing the short-term prognosis. A uremic crisis often occurs in patients with CRF as a consequence of superimposed acute renal failure or prerenal or postrenal conditions. Although CRF is an irreversible condition, improvement of renal function is potentially pos-

sible when uremia results from the sum effects of CRF and a potentially reversible cause of azotemia. If treatment improves renal function and ameliorates clinical signs of uremia, the short-term prognosis may become guarded to good.

Severity of renal dysfunction as determined by serum creatinine concentration or endogenous creatinine clearance provides a less accurate means of assessing short-term prognosis than does the clinical condition of the patient. Short-term prognosis should not be established on the basis of a single measurement of the severity of renal dysfunction. The relationship between magnitude of renal dysfunction and clinical signs of uremia is often unpredictable. In addition, a single determination of renal function is unable to assess the potential for improvement in renal function.

Severity of renal dysfunction is typically more useful in establishing long-term prognoses. In general, severe renal dysfunction is associated with shorter long-term survival and, often, a lower quality of life. This generalization is supported by findings of a study of cats with spontaneous CRF.[4] Mean plasma creatinine concentration and mean survival were 2.6 mg/dL and 397 days for compensated CRF cats, 3.6 mg/dL and 313 days for uremic cats, and 10.3 mg/dL and less than 3 days for cats with end-stage renal failure. Similarly, our experience has been that the long-term prognosis for cats with serum creatinine concentrations less than about 4.5 mg/dL and dogs with serum creatinine concentrations below about 3 mg/dL is typically good. However, the prognosis should be established in light of the clinical condition of the patient, rate of progression of renal dysfunction, response to therapy, cause of the underlying renal disease (if known), and other complicating factors (e.g., urinary tract infection, nephrotic syndrome). Although notable individual exceptions exist, glomerulopathies reportedly have particularly poor long-term prognoses in dogs. In a study of 137 dogs with protein-losing glomerulopathies, median survival time was only 28 days.[10] In contrast, it has been reported that many cats with membranous glomerulonephropathy may have long-term survival or even recoveries.[95]

CONSERVATIVE MEDICAL MANAGEMENT OF CHRONIC RENAL FAILURE

OVERVIEW OF TREATMENT

The clinical and laboratory effects of CRF result from loss of renal excretory, regulatory, and biosynthetic functions. Renal excretory function entails the elimination of waste products of metabolism, toxins, and drugs. Regulatory function refers to the role the kidneys play in maintaining fluid and electrolyte balance. The biosynthetic functions of the kidneys include the formation of a variety of regulatory autacoids and hormones that have important local and systemic functions. This overview provides a somewhat oversimplified version of the link between loss of renal functions and clinical and laboratory findings in renal failure, but it nonetheless provides a framework for describing the conservative medical management of CRF (Table 169–6).

Conservative medical management of CRF consists of supportive and symptomatic therapy designed to correct deficits and excesses in fluid, electrolyte, acid-base, endocrine, and nutritional balance and thereby minimize the clinical and pathophysiologic consequences of reduced renal function. It should not be expected to halt, reverse, or eliminate renal lesions responsible for CRF. Therefore, conserva-

URO

TABLE 169–6. CONSERVATIVE MEDICAL MANAGEMENT OF CHRONIC RENAL FAILURE

Ameliorating clinical consequences of excretory failure
    Dietary management of renal failure
    Modification of drug dosages in renal failure
Ameliorating clinical consequences of regulatory failure
    Minimizing hyperphosphatemia
    Minimizing hypokalemia
    Minimizing metabolic acidosis
    Correcting and preventing dehydration
    Minimizing arterial hypertension
Ameliorating clinical consequences of biosynthetic failure
    Treatment of anemia of chronic renal failure
    Treatment of calcitriol deficit

tive medical management is most beneficial when combined with specific therapy directed at correcting the primary cause of renal disease. Over the past decade, conservative medical management has come to include therapy designed to limit the progressive loss of renal function that may result from adaptive and compensatory events that develop in CRF.

Specific therapy of renal disease consists of therapy designed to slow or stop development of primary renal lesions by influencing the etiopathogenic (disease-specific) processes responsible for the lesions. Examples of specific treatment include correction of hypercalcemia that has caused calcium nephropathy, administration of antibiotics to eliminate bacterial infections, administration of antimycotic agents to eliminate mycotic infections, removal of lesions causing obstructive uropathy (e.g., tumors or uroliths), and correction of abnormal renal perfusion that has caused ischemic renal lesions. Although determining the initiating disease process in dogs and cats with CRF is frequently difficult or impossible, the value of formulating specific therapy on the basis of an etiologic-pathologic diagnosis should not be overlooked. Because renal lesions responsible for CRF are irreversible, they cannot be completely reversed or eliminated by specific therapy. Progression of renal lesions and thus failure may be slowed or stopped by therapy designed to eliminate active renal diseases. Therefore, diagnostic efforts directed especially at detecting treatable renal diseases should be made before formulating plans for conservative medical management. In addition, nonrenal conditions that may aggravate or precipitate uremic crisis (i.e., prerenal and postrenal causes) should be sought and corrected.

Hemodialysis, chronic ambulatory peritoneal dialysis, and renal transplantation are the mainstays of treatment of advanced CRF in humans. These methods have been used for treatment of renal failure in dogs and cats, but their routine application has been severely limited by their expense, technical difficulties, and limited experience on the part of most veterinarians. The current status of these treatment methods in dogs and cats has been reviewed.[96–99]

Conservative medical management is intended for patients with compensated CRF; it is not intended for patients unable to eat or accept oral medications because of severe uremia. Clinical signs and complications of uremia should be managed as described in the section on acute renal failure before attempting conservative medical management.

The goals of conservative medical management of patients with chronic primary renal failure are to (1) ameliorate clinical signs of uremia; (2) minimize disturbances associated with excesses or losses of electrolytes, vitamins, and minerals; (3) support adequate nutrition by supplying daily protein, calorie, and mineral requirements; and (4) modify progression of renal failure. These goals are best achieved when recommendations regarding conservative medical management are individualized to the patient's needs on the basis of clinical and laboratory findings. Because CRF is progressive and dynamic, serial clinical and laboratory assessment of the patient and modification of the therapy in response to changes in the patient's condition are an integral part of conservative medical management.

AMELIORATING CLINICAL CONSEQUENCES OF EXCRETORY FAILURE

Dietary Therapy

Dietary Modifications in Renal Failure. In the past, the emphasis in dietary therapy of CRF has been on reducing protein content.[100, 101] Although protein content continues to play an important role in diet formulation, other dietary modifications are also important in managing patients with renal failure (Table 169–7). Diets recommended for dogs and cats with renal failure are modified from typical maintenance diets in several ways, including reduced protein, phosphorus, and sodium content; increased B-vitamin content and caloric density; and a neutral effect on acid-base balance. Feline renal failure diets are typically supplemented with additional potassium. Canine renal failure diets may have an increased ratio of ω-3 to ω-6 polyunsaturated fatty acids (PUFAs).[94]

Evidence from a randomized controlled clinical trial on the effectiveness of dietary protein restriction in ameliorating clinical signs of uremia in cats with spontaneous CRF supports the efficacy of such therapy in cats.[102] In this study, cats with CRF were randomly assigned to be fed either a diet containing 15.1 g protein and 0.23 g phosphorus per MJ metabolizable energy (25 cats) or a diet containing 23.6 g protein and 0.48 g phosphorus per MJ metabolizable energy (10 cats). Cats were studied for 24 weeks after diet assignment. Body weight, packed cell volume, serum albumin, and total protein values declined in cats fed the 23.6 g protein diet. In contrast, these values increased in cats fed the 15.1 g protein diet. Over the 24 weeks of study, clinical deterioration was reported for cats in both groups with respect to halitosis, gingivitis, appetite, and body condition. However, deterioration was subjectively judged to be less apparent in cats fed the 15.1 g protein diet. Unfortunately, the method for assessing these clinical observations was not reported. Mean BUN and serum creatinine concentration values progressively declined during the study in cats fed the 15.1% g protein diet but progressively increased in cats fed the 23.6 g protein diet. Likewise, serum phosphorus concentrations increased in the 23.6 g protein group and declined in the 15.1 g protein group. The authors concluded that the protein- and phosphorus-restricted diet was beneficial in slowing the rate of clinical deterioration in cats with CRF as assessed by both owners and clinicians. The apparent benefit of dietary protein and phosphorus restriction on slowing progression of CRF and enhancing survival has been further supported by preliminary results of another prospective study of cats with spontaneous renal failure.[103]

Most studies of dietary therapy of canine CRF have been performed using induced models of CRF rather than clinic patients. Although protein restriction is generally accepted as beneficial in ameliorating clinical signs of uremia, data on its effects in dogs with CRF are limited.[100, 104–106] Dietary phosphorus restriction has been linked to prolonged survival and a slower decline in renal function in dogs with induced

TABLE 169–7. CHARACTERISTICS OF TYPICAL RENAL FAILURE DIETS

DIET MODIFICATION	PURPOSE
Decreased protein	Reducing dietary protein intake limits production and subsequent retention of proteinaceous catabolites that contribute to malnutrition and uremic signs. Clinical signs of uremia are crudely related to blood urea nitrogen concentrations, a clinical marker of retained proteinaceous catabolites. Current evidence suggests that protein restriction probably has only a minimal effect, if any, on progression of renal failure.[69, 102, 103, 149, 154, 159]
Decreased phosphorus	The rationale underlying reduced dietary phosphorus content is to minimize hyperphosphatemia and its attendant consequences including renal secondary hyperparathyroidism, soft tissue calcification, progression of renal failure, and enhanced mortality.[61, 62, 70, 107] Dietary phosphorus restriction has been shown to increase survival and slow progression of renal failure in dogs with induced CRF, but similar data are lacking for cats.[69, 70, 107] In concert with protein restriction, phosphorus restriction appears to enhance survival and limit progressive renal failure in cats.[102, 103] Because protein is a major dietary source of phosphorus, diets are usually reduced in both protein and phosphorus.
Decreased sodium	Sodium restriction is designed to limit arterial hypertension. However, data on the effectiveness of salt restriction in ameliorating hypertension in dogs and cats with CRF are scant.[20] Nonetheless, reduced sodium diets may be justified because the effectiveness of some antihypertensive regimes may be impaired unless sodium retention is limited. In addition, dietary "salt" restriction appears to slow progression of renal failure in humans with CRF.[155] In the past, adding salt to the diet had been recommended to enhance renal function; however, later studies suggest that dietary salt consumption does not have a major impact on renal function in dogs.[156]
Increased B vitamins	Water-soluble B vitamins, particularly vitamin B_6, may be lost in increased quantities with polyuria, and reduced food intake typical of many patients with renal failure may limit B vitamin intake. As a consequence, renal failure diets often contain increased quantities of B vitamins.[157]
Increased caloric density	Because of altered taste sensation (known to occur in humans; hard to confirm in dogs and cats), decreased palatability of renal failure diets, nausea, vomiting, and poor appetite, food intake may be reduced in patients with renal failure. Increased caloric density, usually in the form of a high fat content, partially compensates for this effect.
Neutral acid-base balance	Patients with CRF have reduced ability to excrete acid. Avoiding excess ingestion of acidifying compounds limits the extent of metabolic acidosis in patients with CRF. Metabolic acidosis has been shown to promote malnutrition and impair adaptation to reduced protein diets in humans. In addition, acidosis can promote clinical signs similar to those seen in uremic patients (nausea, vomiting, and lethargy).
Increased potassium	*Cats:* For reasons that remain unclear, cats with CRF are predisposed to hypokalemia. Subjectively, increased dietary potassium content appears to reduce the incidence of hypokalemia. However, a study suggested that potassium supplementation of cats with CRF fails to restore muscle potassium stores.[87]
Increased ratio of ω-3 to ω-6 PUFAs	*Dogs:* In dogs with induced CRF, supplementing diets with ω-6 PUFA has been shown to enhance renal injury, whereas ω-3 PUFA supplementation appears renoprotective.[94] Dogs with induced CRF fed ω-3 PUFA had preservation of renal structure and function and minimal proteinuria and were protected from progression to end-stage CRF compared with dogs with CRF fed ω-6 PUFA or saturated fatty acid–supplemented diets.

CRF = chronic renal failure; PUFA = polyunsaturated fatty acid.

renal failure.[69, 70, 107] It has been shown that dietary supplementation with ω-3 PUFAs may be renoprotective in dogs with CRF by preserving renal structure and function, minimizing proteinuria, and preventing progression to end-stage renal failure.[94] All of these findings need to be confirmed by randomized controlled clinical trials in dogs with spontaneous CRF.[108]

A newer area of dietary therapy of CRF under investigation is the possibility of enhancing gastrointestinal excretion of nitrogenous wastes by using dietary fiber.[109–111] It appears from preliminary studies that a varying percentage of nitrogenous waste excretion can be diverted from renal to gastrointestinal excretion. This approach may allow diets with greater protein content to be fed to dogs with CRF or, alternatively, allow greater efficacy in ameliorating clinical signs of uremia. To date, it has been shown only that urea nitrogen levels may be modestly reduced using this approach. However, urea is not recognized as a major toxin of the uremic syndrome. Whether intestinal nitrogen "trapping" would result in improved quality of life needs to be established.

Indications for Diet Therapy. There are no studies of dogs or cats with CRF that indicate clearly criteria for initiation of dietary therapy. In the past, an often-cited guideline has been to initiate therapy when serum creatinine exceeds 2.5 mg/dL or the BUN concentration exceeds 60 to 80 mg/dL. Another guideline is to initiate dietary therapy when clinical signs likely to be attributable to excessive protein intake are apparent. Both of these guidelines suffer

from being inexorably linked to diet protein content as the primary justification for dietary intervention.

We currently recommend dietary therapy at the time of diagnosis of CRF, regardless of the severity of disease. Several lines of reasoning provide a rational basis for this recommendation. From a practical standpoint, the patient may have less resistance to diet change earlier in the course of disease simply because the gastrointestinal consequences of CRF are less prominent and there is less pressure to change the diet rapidly. Hyperparathyroidism typically develops early in the course of CRF and can be effectively managed using dietary therapy at this stage of disease. However, the adverse clinical consequences of renal hyperparathyroidism are poorly documented in dogs and cats, particularly early in the course of disease. It is unclear what impact, if any, early intervention with phosphorus and/or protein restriction or ω-3 PUFA supplementation (in dogs) would have on limiting progression of CRF. However, there is no convincing evidence that early intervention would be harmful if the guidelines provided here are followed (Fig. 169–3). In patients with progressive disease, it is logical that dietary protein restriction would forestall the time at which uremic signs may develop. It may also provide a "buffer" against development of uremic signs should CRF be complicated by events that may promote mild additional prerenal azotemia (e.g., mild dehydration caused by vomiting associated with dietary indiscretion).

In cats, the need to avoid acidifying diets and the need to provide adequate dietary potassium are additional reasons

URO

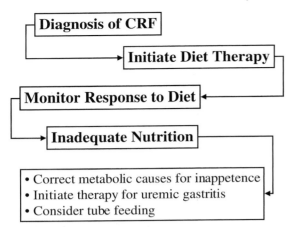

Figure 169–3. Schematic representation of the approach to dietary management of patients with renal failure.

for early intervention with dietary therapy for CRF. Many feline maintenance diets are acidified in order to minimize the risk that struvite-containing uroliths or urethral plugs will form. These conditions are usually not of concern in cats with CRF, and acidifying diets should generally be viewed as contraindicated in cats with CRF.

Monitoring Dietary Therapy. The clinical response to diet modification should be monitored to ensure that unanticipated consequences or malnutrition does not occur. We do not recommend dietary therapy unless the response to treatment is monitored. Evaluation of a routine urinalysis for signs of active renal disease or urinary tract infection is also desirable. The frequency of monitoring depends on the severity of renal dysfunction, complications present, and other therapies employed in managing the patient. We recommend evaluating patients that have not yet developed overt clinical signs at least every 4 months.

Malnutrition. Malnutrition is usually detected clinically as weight loss, declining values for serum albumin concentration (or total plasma protein), anemia, and subjective evidence of decreased muscle mass. Reduced values for serum urea nitrogen may also indicate inappetence and malnutrition. The perfect method for evaluating nutritional status has not yet been devised, and the methods suggested here are relatively insensitive for detecting early malnutrition.

Malnutrition in patients with CRF usually results from inadequate food intake rather than deficiencies in diet formulation, although diets exceptionally restricted in protein content have been reported to promote protein malnutrition.[112] Most commercially available diets designed for patients with renal failure appear to contain sufficient protein to sustain adequate nutrition when consumed in appropriate quantities.

When malnutrition is evident, we recommend a stepwise approach designed to facilitate adequate food intake (see Fig. 169–3). The first step is to ensure that metabolic causes of decreased appetite have been corrected (see Table 169–3). Common metabolic derangements that may promote anorexia include prerenal azotemia caused by dehydration, dietary indiscretion, or gastrointestinal hemorrhage; acidosis; hypokalemia; anemia; and drug-associated anorexia. Some antibiotics and enalapril are particularly prone to induce anorexia, but increased levels of any drug normally excreted by the kidneys should be suspected of potentially promoting anorexia in patients with CRF. Inappetence also appears to be an occasional complication of urinary tract infection.

When metabolic causes of anorexia have been excluded

or corrected, therapy for uremic gastroenteritis should be initiated. This recommendation assumes that nausea and gastrointestinal distress may be the cause of anorexia even in patients that are not vomiting. Therapy for uremic gastroenteritis includes administration of an H_2 antagonist, often combined with an antiemetic. Oral H_2 antagonists ranitidine at a dosage of 0.5 to 1 mg/lb and famotidine at 0.25 to 0.5 mg/lb are used every 12 to 24 hours. They are partially excreted by the kidneys and dosage adjustments of 50 to 75% (ranitidine) and 10 to 25% (famotidine) may be necessary with marked reduction in renal function.[113] Ranitidine may cause false-positive urine protein readings on Multistix.

The antiemetic most commonly recommended for patients with CRF is metoclopramide. It is administered orally or subcutaneously at a dose of 0.05 to 0.2 mg/lb every 8 hours. The kidneys excrete metoclopramide, and the dosage should be reduced by 50 per cent in advanced renal failure.[113] Phenothiazine-derived antiemetics are likely to be effective in patients with CRF, but their sedative and hypotensive effects limit their usefulness.

If therapy with histamine blocking agents and antiemetics fails to restore normal appetite, tube feeding should be considered. Nasogastric feeding with liquid diets may be used in the short term to support nutrition and restore appetite; however, for long-term nutritional support, the clinician should consider placing a percutaneous gastrostomy (PEG) tube. Long-term PEG tube feeding is useful for maintaining nutrition as well as hydration. In our hands, patients with PEG tubes have had extended periods of good quality of life.

Modification of Drug Dosages in Renal Failure

Because the kidneys are responsible for elimination of many drugs from the body, renal drug clearance is reduced in renal failure, causing the half-life of the drug to be prolonged. In addition, distribution, protein binding, and hepatic biotransformation of drugs may be altered in renal failure. For example, two protein binding defects are seen in renal failure.[14] One group of primarily acidic drugs shows decreased binding leading to increases in free, active drug fractions in plasma (e.g., theophylline, methotrexate, diazepam, digoxin, and salicylate). The effect of this change in binding is that lower doses of drugs are required to achieve therapeutic levels and conventional doses may result in toxic levels. Basic drugs, such as propranolol or cimetidine, have increased binding, leading to a decrease in free drug levels and thus diminishing the therapeutic effect. Increased total drug levels may be required to achieve the desired therapeutic effect with these drugs. However, these effects may be complicated by decreased renal clearance of the drugs. Furthermore, accumulation of active drug metabolites may augment drug potency or toxicity.[14]

The sum effect of these changes is that for many drugs normally excreted by the kidneys, there is a tendency for drug to accumulate in patients with renal failure. Excessive drug accumulation promotes an increased rate of adverse drug reactions and nephrotoxicity. Patients with preexisting renal disease and renal failure may also be predisposed to nephrotoxicity. For these reasons, nephrotoxic drugs and drugs requiring renal excretion should generally be avoided in patients with renal failure. If drugs requiring renal excretion must be administered to patients with renal failure, dosage regimens should be adjusted to compensate for decreased organ function.

Because drug accumulation in patients with CRF is primarily a result of reduced renal drug clearance, dosage adjustments should be made according to changes in drug clearance.[114] Changes in renal drug clearance are usually assumed to parallel changes in GFR. Therefore, drug clearance may be estimated by measuring creatinine clearance (C_{cr}). Drug dosage may then be adjusted according to the percentage reduction in C_{cr} (i.e., the ratio of the patients C_{cr} to normal C_{cr}), also known as the dose fraction (K_f)[114]: K_f = (patients C_{cr}/normal C_{cr}). Dosage regimens can be adjusted by decreasing the normal dose or increasing the normal dosage interval in direct proportion to K_f. For drugs excreted 100 per cent unchanged by the kidneys, a precise increase in dosage interval may be calculated by dividing the normal dosing interval by K_f: modified dose interval = (normal dose interval/K_f).

Dosages of antimicrobial drugs may be modified according to three general patterns, depending on the fraction of the drug eliminated by the kidneys (Table 169–8): (1) doubling the dosing interval or halving the drug dosage in patients with severe reduction in renal function, (2) increasing the dosage interval according to ranges of creatinine clearance values, and (3) precise dosage modification as described earlier.[114] Drugs in the first category are relatively nontoxic. Drugs requiring dosage modification according to C_{cr} values are more likely to be toxic. For drugs in this class, the dosing interval is increased twofold when C_{cr} is between 1.0 and 0.5 mL/min/kg, threefold when C_{cr} is between 0.5 and 0.3 mL/min/kg, and fourfold when C_{cr} is less than 0.3 mL/min/kg. Some relatively toxic antimicrobial drugs that are excreted solely by glomerular filtration (particularly aminoglycoside antibiotics) require precise dosage modification according to K_f. For these drugs, increased interval, fixed dosage regimens appear to result in less nephrotoxicity than reduced dosage, fixed interval methods. A combination of dosage reduction and interval extension has been recommended for animals with severe renal dysfunction (C_{cr} less than 0.7 mL/min/kg). A nomogram is available for calculating dosages and dosage intervals for these patients.[114]

As already described, C_{cr} is the preferred measure of renal dysfunction for modifying drug therapy in CRF. However, serum creatinine concentration is a more universally available measure of renal dysfunction than C_{cr}. A regression equation relating serum creatinine concentration to GFR in dogs has been established.[115] The authors of this study cautioned that, because the derived equation did not differ from the theoretic inverse relationship between GFR and serum creatinine concentration, the advantages of this method of estimating GFR in the dog need to be established.

Although the relationship between serum creatinine concentration and C_{cr} is not linear, the reciprocal of serum creatinine concentration may be used to approximate C_{cr} when the serum creatinine concentration is less than 4 mg/dL. This rule of thumb overestimates C_{cr} when the serum creatinine concentration exceeds 4 mg/dL. The serum urea nitrogen concentration is influenced by many extrarenal factors and does not provide an accurate basis for modifying drug dosage regimens. Despite the increased expense and effort involved, it is recommend that C_{cr} be used as the basis for modifying drug dosage schedules whenever possible. This recommendation is particularly relevant when a potentially nephrotoxic drug must be administered. Newer single-injection methods of establishing GFR provide a simpler method for estimating GFR.[116]

Another means of adjusting drug dosage in patients with CRF is to monitor plasma drug concentrations. On the basis of knowledge of specific therapeutic ranges and toxic levels of the drug, dosage may be adjusted according to measured plasma drug concentrations.[117] Use of therapeutic drug concentrations for monitoring therapy is particularly advisable when toxic drugs such as aminoglycosides must be administered to patients with CRF.

TABLE 169–8. DRUG DOSAGE MODIFICATIONS FOR PATIENTS WITH RENAL FAILURE

DRUG	ROUTE(S) OF EXCRETION*	NEPHROTOXIC?	DOSAGE ADJUSTMENT IN RENAL FAILURE†
Amikacin	R	Yes	Pr
Amoxicillin	R	No	D/I
Amphotericin B	O	Yes	Pr
Ampicillin	R,(H)	No	D/I
Cephalexin	R	No	C_{cr}
Cephalothin	R,(H)	No(?)	C_{cr} or D/I
Clindamycin	H,(R)	No	N
Chloramphenicol	H,(R)	No	N,A
Cyclophosphamide	H,(R)	No	N
Corticosteroids	H	No	N
Dicloxacillin	R,(H)	No	N
Digoxin	R,(O)	No	Pr
Doxycycline	GI,(R)	?	N
Furosemide	R	No(?)	N
Gentamicin	R	Yes	Pr
Heparin	O	No	N
Kanamycin	R	Yes	Pr
Neomycin	R	Yes	C/I
Nitrofurantoin	R	No	C/I
Penicillin	R,(H)	No	D/I
Propranolol	H	No	N
Streptomycin	R	Yes	C_{cr}
Sulfisoxazole	R	Yes	C_{cr}
Tetracycline	R,(H)	Yes	C/I
Tobramycin	R	Yes	Pr
Trimethoprim-sulfamethoxazole	R	Yes	C_{cr},A

* Routes of excretion: R = renal; H = hepatic; GI = gastrointestinal; O = other (minor route in parentheses).
† Dosage modification: N = normal; D/I = half-dose or double dosage interval (in severe renal dysfunction); C_{cr} = adjust according to creatinine clearance (see text); Pr = precise dosage modification (see text—adjust according to K_f); C/I = contraindicated; A = avoid in advanced renal failure.

URO

The potential risks and benefits associated with use of nephrotoxic drugs and drugs requiring renal excretion should always be considered before initiating therapy with such drugs in patients with CRF. Careful clinical and laboratory monitoring for toxicosis and pharmacologic effect (i.e., is the drug producing the desired effect?) is essential.

AMELIORATING CLINICAL CONSEQUENCES OF REGULATORY FAILURE

Hyperphosphatemia

Hyperphosphatemia per se rarely causes clinical signs in dogs and cats with CRF. Nonetheless, minimizing phosphorus retention and hyperphosphatemia is an important therapeutic goal in patients with CRF because it appears to prolong survival and limit renal secondary hyperparathyroidism, renal osteodystrophy, and soft issue calcification.[66, 68–70, 107, 118] Hyperphosphoremia is managed by restriction of dietary phosphorus intake, oral administration of intestinal phosphorus binding agents, or a combination of these methods. Optimal control of hyperphosphoremia may be achieved by reducing dietary phosphorus intake "in proportion" to the decrease in GFR.

Although dietary phosphorus restriction has been shown to prolong survival in dogs with CRF, phosphorus restriction alone may not normalize serum PTH levels.[61, 69] Studies of human patients with CRF suggest that, in addition to phosphorus restriction, dietary calcium supplementation may be required to normalize PTH levels.[72] Normalization of PTH in dogs and cats with CRF may be achieved through administration of calcitriol (see later).[68] Nagode and colleagues[68] suggested that normalization of PTH levels using calcitriol therapy may provide clinical benefits that cannot be achieved by phosphorus restriction alone, including amelioration of many clinical signs associated with CRF. However, clinical trials of long-term calcitriol therapy are needed to establish the role of this therapy in dogs and cats with CRF.

Dietary Phosphorus Restriction. Dietary phosphorus restriction is an important and effective first step toward normalizing phosphorus balance. It may normalize serum phosphorus concentrations in mild to moderate CRF and reduce the quantity of phosphorus that must be bound by intestinal phosphorus binding agents in patients with more severe hyperphosphatemia. Dietary phosphorus restriction is usually initiated when hyperphosphatemia is recognized. However, because hyperparathyroidism may occur before serum phosphorus concentrations exceed normal limits and fasting serum phosphorus may not accurately reflect overall phosphorus metabolism, phosphorus restriction may be indicated before the onset of overt hyperphosphatemia.[72]

Because proteinaceous foods are the major dietary phosphorus sources, protein-restricted diets are usually lower in phosphorus content. Typical commercial dog foods contain approximately 1 to 2 per cent phosphorus on a dry matter basis and provide about 2.7 mg/kcal or more phosphorus. Modified protein diets designed for dogs with renal failure may contain as little as 0.13 to 0.28 per cent phosphorus on a dry matter basis and provide about 0.3 to 0.5 mg/kcal phosphorus. Typical commercial cat foods contain from 1 to 4 per cent phosphorus on a dry matter basis and provide about 2.9 mg/kcal or more phosphorus. Modified protein diets designed for cats with renal failure may contain as little as 0.5 per cent phosphorus on a dry matter basis and provide about 0.9 mg/kcal phosphorus.

Phosphorus retention in CRF appears to occur in multiple compartments. As dietary phosphorus restriction reduces serum phosphorus levels, phosphorus leaches out of tissues, delaying the overall reduction in serum phosphorus concentration. Thus, serum phosphorus concentrations should be determined after the patient has been consuming the phosphorus-restricted diet for about 2 to 4 weeks. Samples obtained for determinations of serum phosphorus concentration should be collected after a 12-hour fast to avoid postprandial effects. Sample hemolysis should be avoided because red blood cells contain substantial quantities of phosphorus.

The minimum goal of therapy is to bring serum phosphorus concentration to within the normal range. It is unclear whether further reducing the serum phosphorus concentration within the normal range is of any clinical benefit. Unfortunately, as renal failure becomes more advanced, dietary phosphorus restriction alone often fails to prevent hyperphosphatemia. When hyperphosphoremia persists despite dietary phosphorus restriction, administration of intestinal phosphorus binding agents should be considered.

Intestinal Phosphorus Binding Agents. Phosphorus binding agents should be used in conjunction with dietary phosphorus restriction when dietary therapy alone fails to reduce serum phosphorus concentrations to within the normal range. Intestinal phosphorus binding agents render ingested phosphorus and the phosphorus contained in saliva, bile, and intestinal juices unabsorbable. Because the primary goal is limiting absorption of phosphorus contained in the diet, administration of phosphorus binding agents should be timed to coincide with feeding. These agents are best administered with or mixed into the food or given just before each meal. It is desirable to reduce dietary phosphorus intake before initiating therapy with intestinal phosphorus binding agents in order to reduce the quantity of phosphorus that must be bound. High dietary phosphorus content may greatly limit the effectiveness of phosphorus binding agents or substantially increase the dosage required to achieve the desired therapeutic effect. Administration of 1500 to 2500 mg of aluminum carbonate to dogs with moderate CRF failed to correct hyperphosphoremia consistently when dogs were fed diets containing more than 1.0 per cent phosphorus on a dry matter basis.[119] Phosphorus binding agents appear to be ineffective in controlling hyperphosphoremia when dietary phosphorus intake exceeds 2.0 g/day in humans.[120]

Currently available phosphorus binding agents include aluminum-based and calcium-based compounds. Aluminum-containing intestinal phosphorus binding agents include aluminum hydroxide, aluminum carbonate, and aluminum oxide. Initial doses of 15 to 40 mg/lb/day have been recommended for these aluminum-based phosphorus binding agents. They are available over the counter from most pharmacies as antacid preparations and are available as liquids, tablets, or capsules. In humans, capsules are less effective than liquids, but the patient's compliance may be better with tablets or capsules.[121] Sucralfate, a complex polyaluminum hydroxide salt of sulfate used primarily for treatment of gastrointestinal ulcerations, may also be effective in binding phosphorus in the intestine.[122] Although they are quite effective for binding phosphorus, an important disadvantage of long-term use of aluminum-containing antacids in humans with CRF has been development of aluminum toxicity. Encephalopathies, microcytic anemia, and bone disease (particularly osteomalacia) related to aluminum toxicity have been extensively reported in human patients treated with these drugs. The potential for toxicity of aluminum salts in dogs and cats has been confirmed, but clinical evidence of toxic accumulation of aluminum has not been reported in these species.

Calcium-based phosphorus binding agents such as calcium acetate, calcium carbonate, or calcium citrate may be more effective than aluminum-based phosphorus binding agents.[121] In addition, calcium-based phosphorus binding agents do not entail the risk of aluminum toxicity that accompanies use of aluminum-based phosphorus binding agents. Unfortunately, calcium-based products may promote clinically significant hypercalcemia; therefore, it is necessary to monitor serum calcium concentrations intermittently when using these drugs. On the other hand, they may be used between meals as a source of additional dietary calcium. In humans with CRF, calcium supplementation increased the efficacy of phosphorus restriction in normalizing renal secondary hyperparathyroidism.[72]

Calcium carbonate and calcium acetate may be used alone or concurrently with aluminum-based binding agents to limit risks of hypercalcemia and aluminum toxicity. Calcium citrate may promote absorption of aluminum and should therefore not be used in concert with aluminum-based binding agents. Calcium acetate is the most effective calcium-based phosphorus binding agent as well as the agent least likely to induce hypercalcemia because it releases the least amount of calcium compared with the amount of phosphorus it binds. Initial doses of 30 to 45 mg/lb/day have been recommended for calcium acetate and 45 to 75 mg/lb/day for calcium carbonate. It is particularly important that calcium-based phosphorus binding agents be administered with meals both to enhance the effectiveness of phosphorus binding and to minimize absorption of calcium and the risk of hypercalcemia. Some calcium carbonate preparations may not be effective because they fail to dissolve well in the gastrointestinal tract; this may be investigated by examining the stool or obtaining radiographs of the abdomen for evidence of tablets failing to dissolve.

The dosage of phosphorus binding agents should be individualized to achieve the desired serum phosphorus concentration. The effectiveness of therapy should be assessed by serial evaluation of serum phosphorus concentrations at about 2- to 4-week intervals. Dosages of calcium-based phosphorus binding agents should be decreased if serum calcium concentrations exceed normal limits; additional aluminum-based agents should be used in these patients if hyperphosphoremia persists. A nonabsorbable calcium- and aluminum-free phosphate binder, sevelamer hydrochloride (RenaGel) has recently become available.[123]

Hypokalemia

Potassium replacement therapy is indicated for cats with hypokalemia (serum potassium concentrations less than 4.0 mEq/L) even in absence of overt clinical signs of hypokalemia. Oral administration is the safest and preferred route of administration. Parenteral therapy is generally reserved for patients requiring emergency reversal of hypokalemia or for patients that cannot or do not accept oral therapy. Acidosis is a major risk factor for hypokalemia and should be rectified early in the management of hypokalemia.

Potassium may be supplemented as the gluconate or citrate salt. Potassium chloride is not recommended because of its acidifying nature. Potassium gluconate may be administered orally as tablets, flavored gel, or in a palatable powder form (Tumil-K). Potassium citrate solution (Polycitra-K Syrup) is an excellent alternative that has the advantage of providing simultaneous alkalinization therapy. Depending on the size of the cat and severity of hypokalemia, potassium gluconate is given initially at a dose of 2 to 6 mEq per cat per day. Potassium citrate is initially given at a dose of 20 to 30 mg/lb/day divided into two or three doses. If muscle weakness is present, it usually resolves within 1 to 5 days after initiating parenteral or oral potassium supplements. Potassium dosage should thereafter be adjusted on the basis of the clinical response of the patient and serum potassium determinations performed during the initial phase of therapy. In patients with hypokalemic polymyopathy, it may be necessary to monitor serum potassium concentrations every 24 to 48 hours during the initial phase of therapy. The final maintenance dosage is established by monitoring serum potassium concentrations every 7 to 14 days and adjusting the dosage accordingly. It is unclear whether all cats require long-term potassium supplementation, but preliminary evidence suggests that such therapy is likely to be required by many older cats with CRF.[83]

Routine supplementation of low oral doses of potassium (2 mEq/day) has been recommended for all cats with chronic renal disease.[83] This recommendation appears to be based on the as yet unproved hypothesis that in some cats with CRF, hypokalemia and potassium depletion might promote a self-perpetuating cycle of declining renal function, metabolic acidosis, and continuing potassium losses. It is proposed that supplementation may stabilize renal function before potassium depletion exacerbates the disease. Although the safety and efficacy of this approach have not been evaluated, we have routinely provided oral potassium supplementation to cats with CRF having serum potassium concentrations less than 4.5 mEq/L with no obvious adverse effects. The authors report that they have observed positive responses in several normokalemic cats that had CRF and were treated with potassium supplementation. However, results of a clinical trial suggested that daily supplementation for 6 months with 4 mEq of potassium gluconate was not demonstrably superior to providing sodium gluconate in restoring muscle potassium stores in cats with CRF that initially had normal serum potassium concentrations.[87] The small number of cats enrolled limited interpretation of this clinical trial. In addition, the median muscle potassium content increased in the potassium-supplemented cats from 328 to 402 mEq/kg, a value close to the value of 424 mEq/L established for normal cat muscle. Thus, although the value of providing supplemental potassium to cats with CRF with normal serum potassium concentrations has not been established, it is clear that muscle potassium and probably total body potassium stores are likely to be reduced in cats with CRF, presumably putting them at risk for developing hypokalemia. Furthermore, there is evidence from this study that chronic potassium supplementation of 2 to 4 mEq/day is unlikely to be associated with significant adverse events.

Diets that are acidifying and restricted in magnesium content may promote hypokalemia and should therefore generally be avoided for cats with CRF. Intensive fluid therapy during uremic crises, particularly with potassium-deficient fluids, may promote hypokalemia even in cats or dogs that were not previously hypokalemic. Serum potassium concentrations should be monitored during fluid therapy and maintenance fluids should be supplemented with potassium chloride to prevent induction of hypokalemia (concentrations of 13 to 20 mEq/L are appropriate for maintenance fluids). Care should be taken to ensure that fluids are administered so that potassium is delivered intravenously at a rate not to exceed 0.5 mEq/kg/hour.

URO

Metabolic Acidosis

Alkalinization therapy designed to correct metabolic acidosis is an important part of the overall management of patients with CRF. Potential benefits of alkalinization therapy in patients with chronic renal failure include (1) improving signs of anorexia, lethargy, nausea, vomiting, muscle weakness, and weight loss that may be caused by uremic acidosis[124]; (2) preventing the catabolic effects of metabolic acidosis on protein metabolism in patients with CRF, thereby promoting adaptation to dietary protein restriction[51]; (3) enhancing the patient's capacity to adapt to additional acid stress resulting from such factors as diarrhea, dehydration, or respiratory acidosis; (4) limiting skeletal damage (demineralization and inhibited skeletal growth) resulting from bone buffering; and (5) rectifying the adverse effects of severe acidosis on the cardiovascular system (impaired myocardial contractility and enhanced venoconstriction).[46]

Because even mildly reduced plasma bicarbonate concentrations may promote some of the adverse effects of chronic metabolic acidosis, oral alkalinization therapy is indicated when the serum bicarbonate concentration declines to 17 mEq/L or below (total CO_2 concentrations of 18 mEq/L or below). A word of caution is necessary regarding the use of serum total CO_2 concentrations determined with chemical autoanalyzers to monitor metabolic acidosis and therapy. When blood collection tubes are not fully filled or left exposed to air while awaiting analysis, the vacuum or air above the tube can draw CO_2 out of the serum, falsely lowering CO_2 concentrations. This may result in a falsely low total CO_2 reading and an incorrect conclusion that the patient has metabolic acidosis.[125] In addition, there may be a substantial systematic difference between blood bicarbonate concentrations determined by blood gas analysis and serum total CO_2 concentrations determined with autoanalyzers because of inherent differences in the analytic methods. Appropriate reference ranges are equipment and method specific; therefore, published ranges for therapeutic goals must be extrapolated with caution. It is possible that problems associated with clinical determination of acid-base status may have resulted in artifactually expanded reference ranges and clinician mistrust of the accuracy of total CO_2 determinations, resulting in underappreciation of the true prevalence of metabolic acidosis in CRF.

Oral sodium bicarbonate is the alkalinizing agent most commonly used for patients with metabolic acidosis of CRF. Because the effects of gastric acid on oral sodium bicarbonate are unpredictable, the dosage should be individualized for each patient. The suggested initial dose of sodium bicarbonate is 3 to 5 mg/lb body weight given every 8 to 12 hours. Unfortunately, many dogs and cats find sodium bicarbonate distasteful unless given as tablets.

Potassium citrate is a particularly attractive alternative alkalinization agent. Potassium citrate may offer the advantage, at least in cats, of allowing the simultaneous treatment of both hypokalemia and acidosis with a single drug. Metabolic acidosis when accompanied by potassium depletion or magnesium depletion may respond poorly to alkali therapy alone. There is a risk of overalkalinization, however, in that potassium doses required for adequate correction of hypokalemia may exceed the citrate dose required to correct acidosis. Starting doses of 18 to 35 mg/lb every 8 to 12 hours are recommended.

Regardless of the alkalinizing agent chosen, administration of several smaller doses is preferred to a single large dose in order to minimize fluctuations in blood pH. The patient's response to bicarbonate therapy should be determined by measuring blood bicarbonate or serum (plasma) total CO_2 concentrations 10 to 14 days after initiating therapy. Ideally, blood should be collected just before administration of the drug. The goal of therapy is to maintain blood bicarbonate (or serum total CO_2) concentrations within the normal range. Dosage should be adjusted according to changes in blood bicarbonate (or serum total CO_2) concentrations. Urine pH is often insensitive as a means of assessing the need for or response to treatment and is not routinely recommended for these purposes.

Dehydration

Fluid balance in patients with polyuric renal failure is maintained by compensatory polydipsia. If water consumption is insufficient to balance excessive water loss associated with polyuria, dehydration and renal hypoperfusion may precipitate uremic crisis. If dehydration and decreased renal blood flow persist, additional renal damage may occur. For these reasons, fresh, clean, unadulterated water should be available in adequate quantities at all times.

Cats and some dogs with CRF may fail to consume sufficient water to prevent volume depletion. We have had some success using various flavored liquids (e.g., clam juice, tuna broth) to promote additional fluid consumption. Such fluids should generally be used to supplement fluid consumption, not as a substitute for water consumption. The impact of the mineral and electrolyte content of such supplemental fluids should be considered. For example, milk provides large quantities of phosphate, and broth may contain large quantities of sodium.

For patients whose voluntary fluid intake is inadequate to prevent dehydration, supplemental fluids may be administered subcutaneously at home by the owner. Ideally, fluids selected for chronic parenteral administration should provide free water as well as electrolytes for maintenance (so-called maintenance fluids composed of approximately two thirds dextrose 5 per cent in water and one third balanced electrolyte solution such as lactated Ringer's solution, supplemented with potassium chloride). Unfortunately, fluids containing dextrose may be irritating when administered subcutaneously. Chronic administration of lactated Ringer's solution or normal saline as the principal maintenance fluid source may cause hypernatremia because they fail to provide sufficient electrolyte-free water. Nonetheless, we most often use balanced electrolyte solutions for maintaining hydration. A typical cat or small dog receives 75 to 150 mL of fluids given daily or as needed. Most often, the pet owner gives the subcutaneous injection at home. Chronic subcutaneous fluid therapy can result in fluid overload in some patients, particularly when fluid volumes in excess of those recommended here are used. We have seen several cats given large quantities of fluid (200 to 400 mL/day) present with severe dyspnea caused by pleural effusion. This condition can usually be avoided by reducing the volume of fluids administered.

In our experience, polyuric dogs with renal failure frequently consume inadequate quantities of fluid during periods of hospitalization. If insufficient thirst leads to negative body water balance characterized by rapid loss of body weight, loss of skin pliability, and/or hemoconcentration, supplemental fluids should be given orally or parenterally. In selected patients, prophylactic fluid therapy during periods of hospitalization may be prudent.

Arterial Hypertension

Rationale for Treatment. In humans, pharmacologic reduction of blood pressure reduces the risk of premature cardiovascular morbid and fatal events as well as all-cause mortality.[23] It is unclear whether similar benefits accrue in dogs or cats with arterial hypertension of any origin. Although pharmacologic control of hypertension reportedly failed to increase survival time in cats with CRF, the finding that treatment appeared to prevent additional episodes of neurologic signs provides a modicum of justification for therapeutic intervention.[24] The long- and short-term prognosis for cats with neurologic signs is generally poor. Although it is clear that similar adverse ocular and neurologic events occur in dogs, less is known of their incidence and prognostic implications than for cats. There is little convincing evidence that hypertension leads to cardiac or renal failure in dogs or cats. Epidemiologic studies of the effects of hypertension and its treatment in dogs and cats are greatly needed.

Indications for Treatment. Before initiating therapy for arterial hypertension, the diagnosis must be firmly established by documenting elevated arterial blood pressures during a minimum of three separate blood pressure determinations. Systolic blood pressure values persistently exceeding 180 mmHg for dogs and 170 mmHg for cats are evidence of arterial hypertension, regardless of diastolic pressure values. Diastolic pressure values should probably not exceed 100 mmHg in either species.

In human medicine, the term *hypertensive urgency* is defined as a blood pressure elevation in the absence of ongoing pressure-related symptoms that is high enough to engender concerns regarding development of pressure-related target organ damage.[23] The terms *accelerated hypertension* and *malignant hypertension* are used in human medicine to describe severe hypertension with evidence of end-organ injury. Blood pressures in humans with these conditions typically exceed 200/130 and, by definition, retinal lesions of hypertension are present. Hypertension-associated neurologic signs, heart failure, or renal failure may be present in addition to the ocular lesions. Malignant hypertension is discriminated from accelerated hypertension by the presence of papilledema. Hypertensive humans with pressure-related target organ damage have a severalfold higher risk for pressure-related clinical complications at a given blood pressure level than hypertensives with similar levels of pressure without target organ damage.[23] On this basis, immediate initiation of therapy may be warranted in dogs and cats with clinical signs consistent with pressure-related end-organ injury (e.g., hypertensive retinopathy with retinal detachment, acute-onset neurologic signs) and/or blood pressure values exceeding 200 mmHg.[25]

General Goals and Guidelines for Treatment. Treatment for arterial hypertension should be initiated cautiously with the goal being to reduce systolic blood pressure below 180 mmHg in dogs and 170 mmHg in cats. In humans, a reasonable time frame for attainment of normal blood pressure is measured in months, not days or weeks.[23] In most instances, there is little to be gained by rapid reduction of blood pressure. Thus, it is rational to initiate therapy using a single, orally administered antihypertensive medication. The exceptions to this rule are patients with characteristics of accelerated or malignant hypertension. These patients require rapid reduction of blood pressure, usually through intravenous therapy with sodium nitroprusside.

In general, antihypertensive therapy should be initiated using a single drug (monotherapy) at the lowest effective dose. The dose should then be titrated according to blood pressure response. Response to therapy should be determined after 2 to 4 weeks by again measuring blood pressure. Hypotension is usually the first sign that drug dosage needs to be reduced, and it may be apparent clinically as weakness, lethargy, or anorexia. Serum urea nitrogen and creatinine concentrations should be monitored during antihypertensive therapy because hypotension promotes prerenal azotemia and may precipitate uremic crises.

If therapy has not reduced blood pressure to the target range within 2 to 4 weeks, (1) the drug dosage may be increased to a higher but nontoxic level, (2) the drug may be changed to another class of antihypertensive drug, or (3) a second drug may be added to the treatment regimen. When a partial but inadequate response to therapy is seen after 2 to 4 weeks of treatment, consider attempting to improve the response by increasing the drug dosage. In humans, the probability of normalizing blood pressure with monotherapy is significantly influenced by the magnitude of the pretreatment pressure elevation. Whether this is true in dogs and cats remains unclear, but it seems prudent to consider adding a second drug in preference to switching the class of drugs in patients that remain markedly hypertensive after monotherapy.

Although specific guidelines for treatment of arterial hypertension have not been established for dogs and cats, studies have provided information on the effectiveness of some antihypertensive medications in cats.[24, 25, 126, 127] Currently, the dihydropyridine calcium antagonist amlodipine besylate is the drug of choice for hypertension in cats with CRF. Amlodipine is an intrinsically long-acting, vasoselective calcium antagonist structurally related to nifedipine, but with unique binding and pharmacologic properties that distinguish it from other agents of its class. It does not significantly depress heart rate, nor does it produce significant negative inotropic effects or electrophysiologic disturbances. Studies indicate that amlodipine is a potent antihypertensive agent with natriuretic and diuretic properties that may enhance its ability to reduce blood pressure without attendant fluid retention. It appears to be successful as antihypertensive monotherapy in a majority of cats.

If amlodipine alone is unsuccessful, a second drug should be added. However, the optimal drug to add in this situation is less clear. In cats in which the renin-angiotensin system is activated, an angiotensin-converting enzyme (ACE)–inhibiting drug such as enalapril would be a logical choice.[126] Alternatively, beta-antagonists such as propranolol or atenolol may be suitable, as in one study they were effective alone or in combination therapy in 8 of 20 cats.[24] However, they were reportedly ineffective as long-term monotherapy in six cats in another study.[126] As a rule, diuretics are not recommended as antihypertensives in cats with CRF because of their tendencies to promote dehydration and hypokalemia.

Pharmacologic management of canine hypertension has been less well described. ACE inhibitors have been used extensively to manage hypertension in dogs with CRF. The rationale underlying their use is related to their seemingly beneficial and potentially renoprotective effects in lowering intraglomerular pressures and reducing proteinuria.[128] However, there are no reliable clinical data on the effectiveness of ACE inhibitors for reducing blood pressure or preventing end-organ injury in dogs with hypertension and CRF. Nonetheless, an ACE inhibitor, usually enalapril, or amlodipine besylate is probably the first-choice drug for monotherapy

URO

of hypertension in dogs with CRF. In dogs with anorexia or other gastrointestinal signs, amlodipine may be a better choice because anorexia is a common side effect of enalapril. If the selected drug fails to restore normal blood pressures within 2 to 4 weeks, it is appropriate to switch to dual drug therapy by adding an agent from the other drug class (i.e., start with amlodipine and add an ACE inhibitor if necessary, or start with an ACE inhibitor and add amlodipine if necessary).

ACE inhibitors have generally been safe antihypertensive agents for dogs with CRF. However, captopril appears to be associated with a higher rate of renal injury than other ACE inhibitors; it should generally be avoided in patients with CRF. Similarly, patients with congestive heart failure are at increased risk of adverse renal functional compromise with use of ACE inhibitors. In these patients, it may be desirable to begin therapy with amlodipine in preference to an ACE inhibitor.

Managing Accelerated or Malignant Hypertension. Patients with clinical presentations consistent with accelerated or malignant hypertension should be hospitalized and treatment initiated with constant-rate intravenous infusion of sodium nitroprusside. Such therapy requires continuous monitoring of blood pressure. The goal of treatment is not normalization of blood pressure but a gradual reduction in mean arterial pressure of no more than 15 to 20 per cent.[23] Overzealous reduction of pressure may induce iatrogenic target organ ischemia as a consequence of tissue hypoperfusion.

An alternative therapy that may be considered when intensive management of such patients is not feasible is a combination of hydralazine with furosemide (1 to 2 mg/lb every 8 hours). A beta-antagonist may be added to this regimen if an adequate therapeutic response has not been detected within 12 hours. In some cats, oral therapy with amlodipine may effectively reduce pressures within 12 to 24 hours.

Patients presenting with accelerated or malignant hypertension should probably be evaluated for complicating factors contributing to their hypertension, including glomerulonephritis, hyperthyroidism, hyperadrenocorticism, or pheochromocytoma.[23]

AMELIORATING CLINICAL CONSEQUENCES OF BIOSYNTHETIC FAILURE

Treatment of Anemia of Chronic Renal Failure

General Guidelines for Minimizing Anemia. An obvious but often overlooked consideration is minimizing iatrogenic blood loss. Such loss is especially likely to be a problem in hospitalized cats and small dogs undergoing repeated sampling for diagnostic tests and monitoring. The quantities of blood collected from these patients should be recorded and monitored.

Chronic low-grade gastrointestinal blood loss can also result in moderate to severe anemia in CRF patients that would otherwise have sufficient endogenous erythropoietin production to maintain their hematocrit values in the low-normal range. Many of these patients lack overt gastrointestinal signs. Elevation of the BUN/creatinine ratio above what is expected for the patient's diet and iron deficiency may provide indirect evidence of occult gastrointestinal blood loss. Because of difficulty in confirming gastrointestinal hemorrhage, therapeutic trials with histamine H_2-receptor antagonists may be necessary to support the clinical diagnosis. Improvements in hematocrit and/or appetite indicate a positive response.

Iron deficiency is a relatively common problem in dogs and cats with CRF. In one study, three of six dogs and three of seven cats with CRF had serum iron concentrations below the reference range and transferrin saturations less than 20 per cent.[129] Whether this is related primarily to inadequate intake and absorption or increased losses related to gastrointestinal blood loss is unclear. Unfortunately, iron status can be difficult to assess in dogs and cats. Serum iron levels can be used to screen for both iron deficiency and anemia of chronic inflammatory disease as contributing factors in the diagnostic evaluation of anemia in CRF patients. However, when studied in dogs, serum iron levels did not always reflect the body iron stores; that is, normal values can be seen in patients with iron deficiency.[130] Unfortunately, serum ferritin levels, which are used routinely in humans for diagnosis of iron deficiency, are not available commercially for dogs and cats. Determining the stainable iron content in bone marrow is helpful in assessing body iron stores and may detect problems not identified by serum iron levels or transferrin saturation.[131] Transferrin saturation (estimated by dividing serum iron by total iron binding capacity) appears to be valuable in assessing the ability of the mobilizable iron stores (perhaps independent of total tissue iron stores) to meet the demands of erythropoiesis and, thus, is particularly useful in evaluating patients during periods of increased erythropoiesis such as during recombinant human erythropoietin (rHuEPO) therapy.[132]

Oral supplementation with iron sulfate is the preferred therapy for iron deficiency anemia and for prevention of iron-deficient erythropoiesis in patients starting erythropoietin replacement therapy. Iron dextrans should be reserved for patients intolerant of oral therapy because of the risk of anaphylaxis, shunting of iron to reticuloendothelial storage, and risk of iron overload.[133] Although serum iron levels and transferrin saturation should be monitored to adjust therapy, starting doses of iron sulfate of 50 to 100 mg/day for cats and 100 to 300 mg/day for dogs have been recommended. Iron supplements may be associated with gastrointestinal upset and diarrhea, so small divided doses may be preferable.

Other nutritional abnormalities, in addition to iron deficiency, may contribute to anemia in patients with CRF. Protein malnutrition, with its attendant changes in plasma amino acid and hormone concentrations, is known to cause suboptimal erythropoiesis and anemia. Similar changes occur in human patients with CRF and may reflect mild protein-calorie malnutrition commonly present in advanced CRF. Changes in vitamin and mineral metabolism in patients with CRF are not well understood. Although they have not been examined in dogs and cats, deficiencies that might theoretically induce nutritional anemia include riboflavin (vitamin B_2), cobalamin (vitamin B_{12}), folate, niacin and pyridoxine (vitamin B_6) deficiencies. Vitamin status cannot be easily determined in dogs and cats; however, deficiencies should be suspected in patients with protein-calorie malnutrition or gastrointestinal malabsorption.

Risk of nutritional deficiencies can be minimized through early institution of proper diet and supplements. Preventing protein-calorie malnutrition has far-reaching benefits in reducing morbidity that extend beyond its role in renal anemia. B vitamins, folate, and niacin can be provided as an oral supplement often with iron.[53] Care must be taken with multivitamins not to oversupplement the fat-soluble vitamins A and D.

Red blood cells in uremic plasma have a decreased life

span. Proposed mechanisms for this mild hemolytic tendency include a malfunctioning of the membrane Na^+, K^+-adenosinetriphosphatase pump and impaired regeneration of reduced glutathione needed to prevent hemoglobin oxidation.[57] Cat hemoglobin is especially prone to oxidative stress; a retrospective survey showed that a higher percentage of cats with CRF than normal cats had Heinz's bodies.[134] They also showed that in cats with CRF, those that had Heinz's bodies were more anemic than those that did not. Drugs and foods (e.g., onions, propylene glycol, methylene blue, sulfonamides) that promote the formation of Heinz's bodies should be avoided in uremic pets whenever possible.

PTH has been postulated for many years to play a role in the pathogenesis of anemia of CRF. It has been shown to inhibit the growth of all bone marrow cell lines in vitro, not specifically the erythroid line. Leukopenia and thrombocytopenia are not characteristic of CRF, which argues against an important role for PTH-induced bone marrow suppression.[54] In a clinical series of canine CRF patients with anemia, the authors found no correlation between PTH levels and the degree of anemia.[56] A relationship between serum phosphorus and anemia had been found in earlier studies.[135] It has been postulated that increased serum phosphorus leads to increased intracellular red cell phosphorus. This in turn increases red cell 2,3-diphosphoglycerate (2,3-DPG) levels, a noteworthy finding in anemic CRF patients.[56] Increased 2,3-DPG levels are thought to exacerbate renal anemia by causing a rightward shift in the oxyhemoglobin dissociation curve, which improves tissue oxygenation and decreases the stimulus for erythropoietin synthesis. Although the determination of the clinical importance of PTH and serum phosphorus awaits further study, their proven impact on mineral metabolism and progression of CRF warrants their evaluation and treatment in any case.

Anabolic Steroids. Anabolic steroids were at one time the mainstay of therapy for anemia in CRF. Although controlled safety and efficacy studies in dogs and cats are lacking, the clinical impression is that therapy with anabolic steroids has been disappointing. With the advent of rHuEPO therapy, androgens have largely fallen out of favor for treatment of renal anemia in human and veterinary medicine. In studies of human patients and clinical experience with veterinary patients, androgens appear to work in only a small percentage of patients (usually those mildly affected), have a long delay to onset of action, and may be associated with undesirable side effects.

Blood Transfusion. Transfusions of packed red blood cells or whole blood may be indicated for anemic CRF patients who need rapid correction of their anemia, as in preparation for surgery. For some patients, repeated transfusions can be used for long-term maintenance of hematocrit. However, several drawbacks have limited the use of this therapy in dogs and cats, including lack of availability and expense of blood products, increasing risk of transfusion reactions with multiple transfusions, risk of transfer of infectious agents, and decreased life span of transfused cells in uremic patients. Even for the first transfusion, only compatible blood products (as determined by cross-matching) should be used in both dogs and cats. The post-transfusion target hematocrit should be the low end of the normal range. This is adequate to reverse the anorexia and fatigue associated with the anemia while minimizing the complications of too rapid an increase in blood volume and viscosity such as circulatory overload, hypertension, and seizures.

Hormone Replacement Therapy. Hormone replacement therapy using rHuEPO has become the treatment of choice for anemia of CRF in cats and dogs when hematocrit values decline below about 20 per cent and clinical signs are attributable to the anemia.[136] Administration of rHuEPO causes a dose-dependent increase in hematocrit.[129] Correction of hematocrit to low normal takes approximately 2 to 8 weeks, depending on the starting hematocrit and dose given. As the anemia is corrected, most clients report that their pets show increases in appetite, body weight, energy level, and sociability.

Initially, epoetin usually is administered at a dosage of 22 to 66 units/lb subcutaneously three times weekly. Most dogs and cats should be started at 44 units/lb administered three times weekly. Hematocrit is monitored weekly until a target hematocrit of approximately 30 to 40 per cent for cats and 37 to 45 per cent for dogs is achieved.[129] When anemia is severe (hematocrit less than 14 per cent) but does not require transfusion, daily therapy with 66 units/lb may be preferred for the first week. In the presence of hypertension or when anemia is not severe, a dosage of 22 units/lb three times per week may help to prevent increases in blood pressure and iron-deficient erythropoiesis. When a hematocrit at the low end of the target range is reached, the dosing interval should be decreased to twice weekly. Most animals require 22 to 44 units/lb two to three times weekly to maintain their hematocrit in the target range; however, the dose and dosing interval required to maintain patients in the normal range can be highly variable. Ongoing monitoring of hematocrit is necessary to allow adjustments in dose and dosing interval. Animals requiring more than 66 units/lb three times weekly should be evaluated for erythropoietin resistance. Because of the lag time between the dosage adjustment and effect on hematocrit, patience must be exercised so as not to adjust the dose too frequently, resulting in rapid, unpredictable changes in hematocrit and inability to find a stable dosing regimen. Avoiding iatrogenic polycythemia is especially important.

The basis for individual differences in response to rHuEPO is incompletely understood. Several causes of blunted response or failure to resolve renal anemia with rHuEPO therapy have been identified: functional or absolute iron deficiency, anti-rHuEPO antibody formation, ongoing gastrointestinal blood loss or hemolysis, concurrent inflammatory or malignant disease, and aluminum overload (not documented in veterinary patients). Owner errors related to drug storage, handling, or administration may account for some instances of poor response to rHuEPO therapy.

The demand for iron associated with stimulated erythropoiesis is high, and human patients without preexisting iron overload exhaust iron storage during therapy. Although it is more difficult to assess, the same appears true of dogs and cats. Oral iron supplements are therefore recommended for all patients receiving rHuEPO therapy.

Seizures have been observed in human, canine, and feline CRF patients being treated with rHuEPO who have no prior history of a seizure disorder.[129, 136] Hypertensive and uremic encephalopathies are the most likely potential explanations as, at least in veterinary medicine, they appear to occur more frequently in animals with advanced disease. Allergic reactions including cutaneous or mucocutaneous reactions or cellulitis, sometimes with fever and arthralgia, were uncommonly observed in both dogs and cats early in the course of rHuEPO therapy. Lesions generally resolve within a few days and some had not recurred when therapy was reinstated. Abnormalities in serum chemistries beyond preexisting ones related to CRF have not been noted, although declines in serum iron and transferrin saturation are common. There is no evidence in clinical patients (humans, dogs, or cats) that correction of anemia or rHuEPO therapy itself promotes progression of renal insufficiency.

The most important complication associated with use of rHuEPO is the problem of refractory anemia related to development of neutralizing anti-rHuEPO antibodies.[129] The rHuEPO protein appears to be immunogenic in many, but not all, dogs and cats, with antibody titers developing at variable times (4 weeks to several months) after the onset of therapy. Antibody titers decline after cessation of therapy, and limited attempts at immunosuppressive therapy have thus far not been successful in abrogating the response. In the absence of a widely available anti-erythropoietin antibody assay, bone marrow myeloid/erythroid ratios provide the best method to ascertain whether rHuEPO resistance is due to antibody formation. After therapy is stopped and antibody titers decline, suppressed erythropoiesis is reversible and pretreatment levels of erythropoiesis are attained.[129]

The relatively high prevalence of anti-rHuEPO production prompts the question of when to initiate rHuEPO therapy. When hematocrit values are below 20 per cent anemia probably contributes to adverse clinical signs characteristic of uremia. Generally, these hematocrit guidelines can be used to judge the severity of anemia. In addition, degree of azotemia, expected rate of progression of CRF, appetite and willingness to eat therapeutic diets, and rate of progression of anemia must all be considered in the risk-benefit analysis of when to start therapy. Many cat owners consider quality of life to be as important as or more important than quantity of life, and the advantages and disadvantages of rHuEPO therapy should be discussed with the owners when anemia appears to be contributing to the patient's deteriorating quality of life. Premature initiation of epoetin therapy with subsequent development of anti-erythropoietin antibodies may deprive the patient of the clinical benefits of this therapy when clinical signs of anemia eventually do develop and rHuEPO can be of greatest clinical benefit.

Calcitriol Therapy

Rationale for Calcitriol Therapy. An important consequence of reduced calcitriol production in CRF is renal secondary hyperparathyroidism. Presumably, extraskeletal clinical benefits that may accrue from calcitriol therapy are mediated through reducing PTH levels. The effectiveness of calcitriol therapy in reducing PTH levels in dogs and cats with CRF is well recognized, PTH secretion being modulated by calcitriol at the transcriptional level. Although PTH has been proposed as a potential uremic toxin responsible for many constitutional signs of uremia, the clinical benefits of reducing PTH levels remain controversial. Finco and colleagues,[137, 138] using parathyroidectomy combined with an experimental model of renal failure, concluded that increased PTH levels do not contribute in an important way to clinical signs of uremia in dogs. However, these studies did not directly address the issue of effectiveness of calcitriol therapy in managing clinical signs of dogs and cats with CRF.

Nagode and colleagues[68] have published results of a survey of veterinarians who use calcitriol in management of dogs and cats with CRF. Results of this survey indicate a high level of enthusiasm for calcitriol among veterinarians using the drug. Clinical impressions concerning use of calcitriol in dogs and cats suggest that patients seem (1) brighter and more alert and interactive with owners, (2) to have an improvement in appetite, (3) to be more physically active than before treatment, and (4) to have longer life spans. Furthermore, these authors provided pathophysiologic support for the purported benefits of calcitriol therapy through referenced studies of multiple species.

Despite reported favorable impressions concerning the use of calcitriol, its role in managing dogs and cats with CRF requires confirmation by randomized, controlled clinical trials. It is important to recognize that nonexperimental evidence from the recalled experiences of clinicians and other experts tends to overestimate the efficacy of therapy for several reasons.[139] Clinicians are more likely to recognize and remember favorable outcomes when management recommendations are followed and follow-up appointments are kept. Because high compliance is a marker for better outcomes, even when treatment is useless, uncontrolled clinical experiences may cause clinicians to conclude that compliant patients must have been receiving efficacious therapy. Routine clinical practice is never "blind," and both patients and owners know when active treatment is being received. Again, the desire of pet owners and clinicians for success and the placebo effect can cause both parties to overestimate efficacy.

Guidelines for Using Calcitriol. Although potentially beneficial in CRF patients, calcitriol therapy must be undertaken with caution because hypercalcemia is a potentially serious complication of calcitriol therapy. Calcitriol therapy does not directly impair renal function, but sustained calcitriol-induced hypercalcemia can result in a reversible or irreversible reduction in GFR. Although hypercalcemia reportedly occurs in 30 to 57 per cent of humans treated with calcitriol, Chew and Nagode[73] reported that hypercalcemia was an uncommon side effect in dogs with CRF when calcitriol was administered at low dosages. Hypercalcemia was reported to be most likely to occur when calcitriol therapy was combined with calcium-containing phosphate binding agents, particularly with calcium carbonate.[140] It resolved when oral calcium carbonate therapy was terminated.

Serum phosphate concentration must be normalized before initiating calcitriol therapy because hyperphosphatemia enhances the tendency for calcitriol to promote renal mineralization and injury. In addition, combining phosphorus restriction with calcitriol therapy appears beneficial, with an additive effect in reducing plasma PTH activities.[141] Treatment of hyperparathyroidism with supplemental calcitriol may, however, promote hyperphosphatemia through increased intestinal phosphate absorption.[66] Thus, serum calcium and phosphorus concentrations should be carefully monitored in patients receiving calcitriol. Synthetic vitamin D analogues that suppress PTH but do not stimulate intestinal vitamin D receptors are currently under investigation.

Calcitriol (Rocaltrol capsules) rapidly and effectively suppresses renal secondary hyperparathyroidism. An important advantage of calcitriol over other forms of vitamin D therapy in CRF is that calcitriol does not require renal activation for maximum efficacy. Nagode and Chew[142] have recommended a dosage 0.75 to 1.65 ng/lb body weight per day given orally to dogs with CRF. Similar doses may be effective in cats with CRF as well. Because it enhances intestinal absorption of calcium and phosphorus, calcitriol should not be given with meals. Custom-made capsules containing appropriate doses of calcitriol for use in dogs and cats are available upon prescription from compounding pharmacies. The optimal maintenance dosage for calcitriol must be determined for each patient on the basis of serial evaluation of serum calcium and phosphate concentrations and plasma PTH activities. The recommended end point of calcitriol therapy is normalization of PTH activity in the absence of hypercalcemia.

Because the onset of hypercalcemia after initiation of vitamin D therapy is unpredictable and may occur after days to months of treatment, continued monitoring of serum calcium, phosphate, and creatinine concentrations is necessary to detect hypercalcemia, hyperphosphatemia, or deteriorating renal function before irreversible renal damage ensues. Serum calcium, phosphorus, urea nitrogen, and creatinine concentrations should be monitored 1 week and 1 month after initiating calcitriol therapy and monthly thereafter.[140] The product of serum calcium and phosphorus concentrations should not exceed 60, although values between 42 and 52 may be ideal.[62] Calcitriol's rapid onset (about 1 day) and short duration of action (half-life less than 1 day) permit rapid control of unwanted hypercalcemia, but early detection of hypercalcemia is indicated to limit the extent of renal injury. If hypercalcemia develops, it is advisable to stop treatment completely rather than reduce the dose. Therapy may be reinstituted with a reduced dosage after serum calcium concentration returns to normal.

MINIMIZING PROGRESSION OF RENAL FAILURE

THE PROGRESSIVE NATURE OF CHRONIC RENAL FAILURE

CRF has long been recognized as a progressive disease. It was generally assumed that progression of renal failure resulted from continuing renal damage induced by whatever disease process was responsible for the onset of CRF. However, it was observed in rodents that loss of a critical mass of functional renal tissue invariably led to failure of the remaining nephrons, suggesting that renal insufficiency may progress to end-stage renal failure through mechanisms that are independent of the initiating insult (Fig. 169–4). For example, removal of approximately three quarters or more of the functional renal mass in rats by surgical resection, infarction, or a combination of these techniques resulted in a syndrome of progressive azotemia, proteinuria, arterial hypertension, and, eventually, death caused by uremia.[143] Progression occurred in this rodent model of renal failure despite the fact that remaining renal tissue was initially normal, albeit reduced in quantity. Although the initiating cause of CRF is probably a primary cause of progression of CRF in many patients, spontaneous progression of renal failure probably contributes to the genesis of end-stage renal failure in many patients.

In contrast to findings in rats, spontaneous progression of induced renal failure in dogs and cats has been more difficult to confirm. Numerous studies have been performed in an attempt to determine whether findings in rodents are relevant to dogs. These studies showed that reducing renal mass in dogs led to mild proteinuria, glomerulopathy, and tubulointerstitial renal lesions. These findings are consistent with observations in rats. In general, however, reducing renal mass by 7/8 or less is not consistently associated with a progressive decline in GFR. In a 2 year study, we observed a pattern of declining GFR values in 4 of 15 dogs with 11/12 reduction in renal mass. Renal function had remained stable or improved during the first year of study in these four dogs. The initial sign of progressive renal injury in these dogs was increasing proteinuria. In studies performed at the University of Georgia, a progressive decline in GFR was detected in dogs in which renal mass had been reduced by 15/16.[69] These findings suggest that a progressive decline in renal function develops in dogs with a marked reduction in renal mass. The findings are not inconsistent with the observation that detectable progressive deterioration of GFR in humans may not become obligatory until serum creatinine concentrations exceed 4 mg/dL.[144]

Studies of induced kidney failure have thus far failed to demonstrate clear evidence of spontaneous progression of renal failure in cats, although proteinuria, glomerulopathy, and tubulointerstitial lesions do develop in cats after ablation of substantial quantities of renal tissue.[145–147] In contrast, it is apparent that many cats with spontaneous CRF have progressive renal failure.[4] It is apparent that experimental models of kidney failure may be limited in their ability to replicate spontaneous disease.

The typical courses of spontaneous CRF in dogs and cats and risk factors that may promote progression have not been established. Risk factors that are associated with accelerated

URO

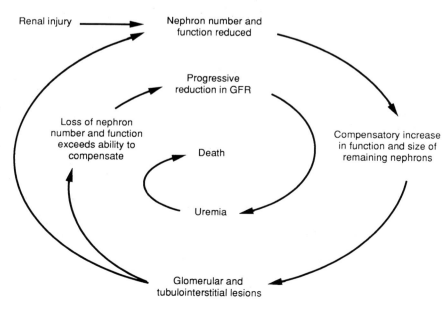

Figure 169–4. Relation between renal injury, loss of nephrons, renal compensatory adaptations, and the ultimate progression of renal failure. To initiate the central spiral, a critical loss of nephron mass must occur. The quantity of renal tissue that must be lost to initiate this process appears to vary from species to species. (From Churchill JA, et al.: The influence of dietary protein intake on progression of chronic renal failure in dogs. Semin Vet Med Surg 7:246, 1992.)

progression of renal failure in humans include arterial hypertension, proteinuria, and a higher level of serum creatinine at the time of diagnosis. In human patients with CRF, the rate of decline in GFR varies between patients and is influenced to some degree by the underlying renal disease, with glomerular diseases, diabetic glomerulopathy, and hypertension tending to progress more rapidly than tubulointerstitial diseases.[148]

PROGRESSION OF RENAL FAILURE—PATHOPHYSIOLOGIC MECHANISMS

Current understanding of mechanisms of progression and how they may relate to management of canine and feline CRF has been reviewed.[2] A summary of pathophysiologic mechanisms that have been proposed to influence progression of renal failure is presented in Table 169–9.

Mechanisms responsible for spontaneous self-perpetuation of CRF have not been fully elucidated but are thought to be related in part to adverse consequences of compensatory adaptations that follow reduction in nephron numbers. Although compensatory adaptations, broadly termed compensatory hypertrophy and hyperfunction, may be initially beneficial in facilitating fluid and solute homeostasis and enhancing waste excretion, some may eventually prove injurious to surviving nephrons. Increased GFR in surviving nephrons, termed hyperfiltration, is driven largely by vasodilation of the arterioles supplying these nephrons with increases in their plasma flow and glomerular capillary pressures. Arterial hypertension may accelerate the effects of arteriolar vasodilatation by transmission of systemic hypertension to the glomerulus. The cellular mechanism whereby increased glomerular capillary pressure leads to scarring and eventual occlusion of these vessels is uncertain but probably involves pressure- or tension-induced increased synthesis of mesangial matrix as well as mechanical disruption of the capillary walls leading to proteinuria.[148]

Proteinuria may promote progressive renal injury in many ways. Excessive proteinuria may injure renal tubules via a toxic or receptor-mediated pathway or via overload of lysosomal degradative mechanisms.[1] Resorption of excessive quantities of filtered plasma proteins by proximal tubular cells liberates various small molecules and substances bound to the proteins. In particular, removal of iron from transferrin may promote local synthesis of reactive oxygen species.[148]

TABLE 169–9. FACTORS THAT MAY INFLUENCE PROGRESSION OF CHRONIC RENAL FAILURE

Compensatory functional adaptations
  Glomerular capillary vasodilation
  Glomerular hyperperfusion and hyperfiltration
  Glomerular capillary hypertension
Compensatory renal hypertrophy
Proteinuria
Arterial hypertension
Metabolic adaptations
  Renal tubular hyperfunction with increased oxygen consumption and generation of reactive oxygen species
  Increased renal ammoniagenesis
Disordered divalent iron metabolism
  Excessive dietary phosphorus intake and hyperphosphatemia
  Elevated calcium-phosphorus product
  Renal secondary hyperparathyroidism
Disordered lipid metabolism
Nephrotoxicity of protein metabolites

From Brown et al,[2] Hostetter,[148] and Polzin.[160]

Small lipids bound to filtered proteins may also be liberated during resorption. Inflammatory or chemotactic properties of these lipids may promote tubulointerstitial disease. Finally, inspissation of filtered proteins related to water extraction in the distal nephron may lead to cast formation and intrarenal obstruction.

The cardinal feature of progressive renal disease is tubulointerstitial fibrosis. Thus, although glomerular structural and functional adaptations may play a role in initiating self-perpetuating renal disease, tubulointerstitial disease plays a crucial role in the ultimate outcome of the process.[1] Two possible explanations for the link between glomerular and tubulointerstitial injuries have been proposed. As described before, proteinuria, the hallmark of glomerular injury, may lead to tubular injury. Alternatively, changes in the glomerular capillaries may be transmitted to the interstitial capillaries, leading to microvascular endothelial injury. Renal interstitial microvascular injury, perhaps complicated by tubular injury, may promote interstitial fibrosis, at least in part through ischemia.

MODIFYING PROGRESSION OF CHRONIC RENAL FAILURE—THERAPEUTIC IMPLICATIONS

Although dietary protein restriction had been proposed as a means of slowing progression of CRF, studies have failed to confirm a role for dietary protein restriction in limiting progression of renal failure in dogs. A meta-analysis of studies of the impact of protein restriction on progression of renal failure in humans led to the conclusion that protein restriction probably does slow the decline of renal function in humans with CRF but that the effect is small and perhaps of little practical clinical importance.[149, 150] Because of the small number of dogs that have been studied, a small beneficial effect of protein restriction in limiting progression of renal failure cannot be ruled out. However, limiting dietary phosphorus intake and increasing the ratio of ω-3 to ω-6 PUFA's in the diet do appear to slow progression of renal failure in dogs with induced CRF.[70, 94] The effectiveness of these "renoprotective" interventions needs to be established in naturally occurring canine CRF. To date, no therapeutic interventions have been shown to influence the progression of feline CRF.

HEMODIALYSIS

Hemodialysis is being used successfully to manage renal failure in dogs and cats.[96, 97] An excellent review of the status and application of hemodialysis in dogs and cats has been published.[97] Although the most obvious application of hemodialysis is in managing patients with acute renal failure, there may be patients with CRF for which hemodialysis may be considered a suitable adjunct to conservative medical management. Hemodialysis is most likely to be beneficial when the serum urea nitrogen concentration exceeds 90 mg/dL and the serum creatinine concentration exceeds 8 mg/dL.[97] These patients are likely be at or to exceed the effective limits of conservative medical management. Intermittent hemodialysis may provide the additional excretory "boost" necessary to provide an adequate quality of life.[97] Dogs with serum creatinine concentrations between 8 and 10 mg/dL need a twice-weekly dialysis schedule, and those with serum creatinine concentrations in excess of 10 mg/dL require dialysis three times weekly. However, in a report on hemodialysis in cats, it was suggested that technical complications and chronic debility appear to limit the success of hemodialysis for cats with CRF.[96] Although 9 of 15 (60%) of cats with a diagnosis of acute renal failure survived in this study, none of 6 cats with CRF and only 1 of 8 cats with acute exacerbation of CRF survived.

Hemodialysis may also play an important role in a renal transplant program. It is useful for preoperative support and conditioning of patients awaiting renal transplantation. After transplantation, hemodialysis can be used to support the patient during episodes of acute transplant rejection.

RENAL TRANSPLANTATION

The first successful long-term renal transplant in a clinical feline patient was performed in 1984. Since then, renal transplantation has become a viable therapeutic option for cats in which conservative medical management has been or is becoming unsuccessful. Long-term immunosuppression with a combination of oral prednisolone and cyclosporin has proved to be quite successful, although regular monitoring of cyclosporin levels is required. The cat's quality of life after discharge from the hospital and during immunosuppressive therapy is reportedly good. In a report on 66 cats undergoing renal transplantation at the University of California College of Veterinary Medicine, 47 cats (71 per cent) survived until discharge and 19 (29 per cent) died during the perioperative period.[98] With experience and improved surgical technique, the authors reported that the postoperative survival rate had increased to 79 per cent during the second half of this study. Of 46 surviving cats available for follow-up evaluation, 18 were still alive with mean survival time of 26 months (range 7 to 81 months). Mean survival time of the 28 cats that had died was 15 months (range 1 to 74 months). Causes of death among the nonsurvivors included renal failure and renal failure–related complications, immunosuppressive-related diseases, and cardiac disease. Five of nine renal-related deaths were associated with renal

rejection. Twelve cats had 19 episodes of allograft rejection. During 11 of the 19 rejection episodes, cats responded favorably to antirejection treatment.

Canine renal transplantation has proved to be a much greater challenge, apparently because of inherent difficulty in inducing suppression of the canine immune system. However, studies at the Ontario Veterinary College using rabbit anti–dog thymocyte serum to modulate the canine immune response to allograft transplantation, have yielded promising results.[151, 152] This therapy has been combined with prednisolone, cyclosporin, and azathioprine to yield periods of successful renal allograft survival extending to 2 years. Routine immunosuppression schedules did not yield such promising results for canine renal transplantation.

Recommended criteria for selection of a feline transplant recipient include (1) early decompensated renal failure (conservative management is no longer effective), (2) moderate weight loss (loss no greater than 20 per cent of healthy body weight), (3) no evidence of cardiac dysfunction, (4) no history of bacterial urinary tract infections, (5) no secondary medical conditions (e.g., inflammatory bowel disease, oxaluria), and (6) negative tests for feline leukemia virus (FeLV) and FIV.[99] Renal transplant donors must be healthy adult cats that are similar to or larger in size than the transplant recipient. They must also have normal urinary tract health and anatomy, be FeLV and FIV negative, and have blood cross-matching compatible with the recipient. Most centers performing renal transplantation require that the owner of the transplant recipient adopt the donor cat.

There are also owner-related criteria that should be considered when referring a cat for transplantation. The ideal pet owner for renal transplant recipients is intelligent, emotionally stable, cooperative, and not demanding and has reasonable expectations and the support of friends and family. Owners must also fully understand the commitment that they are making. Immediate and long-term expenses related to the transplantation cannot be an issue for owners. They should expect to pay upward of $3000 to $7000 in surgery-related expenses and up to several hundred dollars per month

TABLE 169–10. GUIDELINES FOR MONITORING PATIENTS WITH CHRONIC RENAL FAILURE

TEST	PURPOSE
History	To assess response to therapy; to ascertain compliance with recommendations and owner-perceived problems with therapy; to detect communication problems with the client; to detect new problems or complications; to encourage client compliance
Physical examination	To detect new problems or complications; to assess hydration; to assess nutritional status and well-being of the animal
Body weight	To assess nutritional and hydration status
Serum creatinine concentration	To assess severity and progression of renal dysfunction; to detect concomitant prerenal and postrenal azotemia
BUN concentration	To assess compliance with dietary recommendations; to detect concomitant prerenal and postrenal azotemia
Urinalysis	To detect urinary tract infection; to detect changes in urine sediment or urine chemistries that may suggest active or changing renal lesions that may warrant specific therapy or changes in therapy; to monitor proteinuria
Serum phosphorus concentration	To determine success of dietary phosphorus restriction and to adjust dosages of intestinal phosphate binders
Serum calcium concentration	To assess need for and to adjust dosage of calcium supplements and vitamin D
Serum albumin concentration	To assess nutritional status; important for monitoring impact of urinary protein loss in patients with glomerulopathies; necessary for interpretation of serum calcium values and assessing influence on protein-bound drugs
Total CO_2 concentration	To assess need for alkalinization therapy; necessary for adjusting dosage of alkalinization therapy
PCV or CBC	To assess response to therapy for anemia; may also be useful for assessing nutritional status
Urine culture	Indicated (1) if urinalysis supports possible UTI, (2) to confirm that previously detected and treated UTIs have been successfully eradicated, (3) as routine part of follow-up studies in patients with recurrent UTI and CRF

BUN = blood urea nitrogen; CBC = complete blood count; CRF = chronic renal failure; PCV = packed cell volume; UTI = urinary tract infection.

in drug and monitoring expenses for the remainder of the cat's life. Medication must be given according to the prescribed dosing schedule (typically every 12 hours) or transplant rejection may occur. In addition, owners need full-time access to a veterinarian familiar with managing transplant recipients should complications arise. Table 169–10 outlines Minimum requirements for study after transplantation.

REFERENCES

1. Fine LG, Orphanides C, Norman JT: Progressive renal disease: The chronic hypoxia hypothesis. Kidney Int 53(Suppl 65):S-74–S-78, 1998.
2. Brown SA, Crowell WA, Brown CA, et al: Pathophysiology and management of progressive renal disease. Vet J 154:93–109, 1997.
3. Brown S, Finco D: The chronic course of renal function following 15/16 nephrectomy in dogs. J Vet Intern Med 4:125A, 1990.
4. Elliot J, Barber PJ: Feline chronic renal failure: Clinical findings in 80 cases diagnosed between 1992 and 1995. J Small Anim Pract 39:78–85, 1998.
5. Polzin DJ, Osborne CA, O'Brien TD: Diseases of the kidneys and ureters. In Ettinger SJ (ed): Textbook of Veterinary Internal Medicine, 3rd ed. Philadelphia, WB Saunders, 1989, pp 1963–2046.
6. DiBartola SP, Rutgers HC, Zack PM, et al: Clinicopathologic findings associated with chronic renal disease in cats: 74 cases (1973–1984). JAVMA 190:1196–1202, 1987.
7. Lulich J, Osborne C, O'Brien T, et al: Feline renal failure: Questions, answers, questions. Compend Contin Educ Pract Vet 14:127–152, 1992.
8. Lees G: Congenital renal diseases. Vet Clin North Am 26:1379–1399, 1996.
9. Minkus G, RC, Horauf A, et al: Evaluation of renal biopsies in cats and dogs—Histopathology in comparison with clinical data. J Small Anim Pract 35:465–472, 1994.
10. Cook AK, Cowgill LD: Clinical and pathological features of protein-losing glomerular disease in the dog: A review of 137 cases (1985–1992). J Am Anim Hosp Assoc 32:313–322, 1996.
11. DeBowes LJ Mosier D, Logan E, et al: Association of periodontal disease and histologic lesions in multiple organs from 45 dogs. J Vet Dent 13:57–60, 1996.
12. Thomas JB, Robinson WF, Chadwick BJ, et al: Association of renal disease indicators with feline immunodeficiency virus infection. J Am Anim Hosp Assoc 29:320–326, 1993.
13. Poli A, Abramo F, Matteucci D, et al: Renal involvement in feline immunodeficiency virus infection: p24 antigen detection, virus isolation and PCR analysis. Vet Immunol Immunopathol 46:13–20, 1995.
14. Vanholder R: The uremic syndrome. In Greenberg A (ed): Primer on Kidney Diseases, 2nd ed. San Diego, Academic Press, 1998, pp 403–407.
15. Chew D, DiBartola S: Diagnosis and pathophysiology of renal disease. In Ettinger, SJ (ed): Textbook of Veterinary Internal Medicine, 3rd, ed. Philadelphia: WB Saunders, 1989, pp 1893–1961.
16. Lemarié RJ, Lemarié SL, Hedlund CS: Mast cell tumors: Clinical management. Compend Contin Educ 17:1085–1101, 1995.
17. Goldstein RE, Marks SL, Kass PH, et al: Gastrin concentrations in plasma of cats with chronic renal failure. JAVMA 213:826–828, 1998.
18. Meyer T, Scholey J, Brenner B: Nephron adaptation to renal injury. In Brenner B, Rector F (eds): The Kidney, 4th ed. Philadelphia, WB Saunders, 1991, pp 1871–1908.
19. Kobayashi D, Peterson M, Graves T, et al: Hypertension in cats with chronic renal failure or hyperthyroidism. J Vet Intern Med 4:58–62, 1990.
20. Cowgill L, Kallet A: Systemic hypertension. In Kirk, R. (ed): Current Veterinary Therapy IX. Philadelphia, WB Saunders, 1986, pp 360–364.
21. Bodey AR, Michell AR: An epidemiologic study of blood pressure in domestic dogs. J Small Anim Pract 37:116–125, 1996.
22. Michell AR, Bodey AR, Gleodhill A: Absence of hypertension in dogs with renal insufficiency. Ren Fail 19:61–68, 1997.
23. Flack J: Therapy of hypertension. In Greenberg, A (ed): Primer on Kidney Diseases, 2nd ed. San Diego, Academic Press, 1998, pp 506–516.
24. Littman M: Spontaneous systemic hypertension in 24 cats. J Vet Intern Med 8:79–86, 1994.
25. Henik R: Systemic hypertension and its management. Vet Clin North Am 27:1355–1372, 1997.
26. Bartges JW, Willis AM, Polzin DJ: Hypertension and renal disease. Vet Clin North Am 26:1331–1345, 1996.
27. Stiles J, Bistner S, Polzin D: The incidence of retinopathy in hypertensive cats. San Diego, American College of Veterinary Ophthalmologists, 1992, p 476.
28. Cowley AW Jr, Roman RJ: The role of the kidney in hypertension. JAMA 275:1581–1589, 1996.
29. Textor S: Pathogenesis of hypertension. In Greenberg A (ed): Primer on Kidney Diseases, 2nd ed. San Diego, Academic Press, 1998, pp 491–495.
30. Weber MA, Smith DHG, Neutel JM, et al: Cardiovascular and metabolic characteristics of hypertension. Am J Med 91(Suppl 1A):4S–10S, 1991.
31. Frasier C: Neurological manifestations of renal failure. In Greenberg A (ed): Primer on Kidney Diseases. San Diego, Academic Press, 1998, pp 459–464.
32. Fenner W: Uremic encephalopathy. In Bonagura RW (ed): Current Veterinary Therapy XII. Philadelphia, WB Saunders, 1995, pp 1158–1161.
33. Lazarus J, Hakim R: Medical aspects of hemodialysis. In Brenner B, Rector F (eds): The Kidney, 4th ed. Philadelphia, WB Saunders, 1991, pp 2223–2298.
34. Littman M: Update: Treatment of hypertension in dogs and cats. In Kirk R, Bonagura J (eds): Current Veterinary Therapy XI. Philadelphia, WB Saunders, 1992, pp 838–841.
35. Grevel V, Opitz M, Stteb C, et al: Myopathy due to potassium deficiency in eight cats and a dog. Berl Munch Tierarztl Wochenschr 106:20–26, 1993.
36. Dow SW, LeCouteur RA, Fettman MJ, et al: Potassium depletion in cats: Hypokalemic polymyopathy. JAVMA 191:1563–1568, 1987.
37. Cotton J, Knochel J: Correction of a uremic cellular injury with a protein-restricted, amino acid supplemented diet. Am J Kidney Dis 5:233, 1983.
38. Stiles J, Polzin D, Bistner S: The prevalence of retinopathy in cats with systemic hypertension and chronic renal failure or hyperthyroidism. J Am Anim Hosp Assoc 30:564–572, 1994.
39. Littman M: Spontaneous systemic hypertension in cats. J Vet Intern Med 4:126A, 1990.
40. Morgan RV: Systemic hypertension in four cats: Ocular and medical findings. J Am Anim Hosp Assoc 22:615–621, 1986.
41. Eschbach J, Adamson J: Hematologic consequences of renal failure. In Brenner B, Rector F (eds): The Kidney, 4th ed. Philadelphia, WB Saunders, 1991, pp 2019–2035.
42. Himmelfarb J: Hematological manifestations of renal failure. In Greenberg A (ed): Primer on Kidney Diseases. San Diego, Academic Press, 1998, pp 465–471.
43. Kimmel P: Management of the patient with chronic renal disease. In Greenberg A (ed): Primer on Kidney Diseases. San Diego, Academic Press, 1998, pp 433–440.
44. Lemieux J, Lemieux C, Duplessis S, Berkofsky J: Metabolic characteristics of the cat kidney: Failure to adapt to metabolic acidosis. Am J Physiol 259:R277–R281, 1990.
45. Fettman M, Coble J, Hamar D, et al: Effect of dietary phosphoric acid supplementation on acid-base balance and mineral and bone metabolism in adult cats. Am J Vet Res 53:2125–2135, 1992.
46. Adrogué HJ, Madias NE: Management of life-threatening acid-base disorders. N Engl J Med 338:26–34, 1998.
47. Nath KA, Hostetter MK, Hostetter TH: Pathophysiology of chronic tubulointerstitial disease in rats: Interactions of dietary acid load, ammonia, and complement component C3. J Clin Invest 76:667–675, 1985.
48. Nath KA, Hostetter MK, Hostetter TH: Ammonia-complement interaction in the pathogenesis of progressive renal injury. Kidney Int 36:S-52–S-54, 1989.
49. Throssell D, Brown J, Harris KPG, Walls J: Metabolic acidosis does not contribute to chronic renal injury in the rat. Clin Sci 89:643–650, 1995.
50. Mitch W, Jurkovitz C, England B: Mechanisms that cause protein and amino acid catabolism in uremia. Am J Kidney Dis 21:91–95, 1993.
51. Mitch W: Mechanisms causing loss of lean body mass in kidney disease. Am J Clin Nutr 67:359–366, 1997.
52. Stein A, Moorhouse J, Iles-Smith H, et al: Role of improvement in acid-base status and nutrition in CAPD patients. Kidney Int 52:1089–1095, 1997.
53. Cowgill LD: Pathophysiology and management of chronic progressive renal failure. Semin Vet Med Surg (Small Anim) 7:175–182, 1992.
54. Eschbach J, Haley N, Adamson J: The anemia of chronic renal failure: Pathophysiology and effects of recombinant erythropoietin. Contrib Nephrol 78:24–37, 1990.
55. Nissenson A, Nimer S, Wolcott D: Recombinant human erythropoietin and renal anemia: Molecular biology, clinical efficacy, and nervous system effects. Ann Intern Med 114:402–416, 1991.
56. King LG, Giger U, Diserens D, et al: Anemia of chronic renal failure in dogs. J Vet Intern Med 6:264–270, 1992.
57. Hocking W: Hematologic abnormalities in patients with renal diseases. Hematol Oncol Clin North Am 1987:229–260, 1987.
58. Cook SM, Lothrop CD Jr: Serum erythropoietin concentrations measured by radioimmunoassay in normal, polycythemic, and anemic dogs and cats. J Vet Intern Med 8:18–25, 1994.
59. Chandra M, Clemons G, McVicar M: Relation of serum erythropoietin levels to renal excretory function: Evidence for lowered set point for erythropoietin production in chronic renal failure. J Pediatr 113:1015–1021, 1988.
60. Mitch W, Walser M: Nutritional therapy of the uremic patient. In Brenner B, Rector F (eds): The Kidney, 4th ed. Philadelphia, WB Saunders, 1991, pp 2186–2222.
61. Nagode LA, Chew DJ: Nephrocalcinosis caused by hyperparathyroidism in progression of renal failure: Treatment with calcitriol. Semin Vet Med Surg (Small Anim) 7:202–220, 1992.
62. Kates DM, Sherrard DJ, Andress DL: Evidence that serum phosphate is independently associated with serum PTH in patients with chronic renal failure. Am J Kidney Dis 30:809–813, 1997.
63. Barber PJ, Elliott J: Feline chronic renal failure: Calcium homeostasis in 80 cases diagnosed between 1992 and 1995. J Small Anim Pract 39:108–116, 1998.
64. Kates DMA: Control of hyperphosphatemia in renal failure: Role of aluminum. Semin Dial 9:310–315, 1996.
65. Brushinsky D: Disorders of calcium and phosphorus homeostasis. In Greenberg A (ed): Primer on Kidney Diseases, 2nd ed. San Diego, Academic Press, 1998, pp 106–113.
66. Block GA, Hulbert-Shearon TE, Levin NW, Port FK: Association of serum phosphorus and calcium × phosphate product with mortality risk in chronic hemodialysis patients: A national study. Am J Kidney Dis 31:607–617, 1998.
67. Massry SG, Smogorzewski M: Mechanisms through which parathyroid hormone mediates its deleterious effects on organ function in uremia. Semin Nephrol 14:219–231, 1994.
68. Nagode LA, Chew DJ, Podell M: Benefits of calcitriol therapy and serum

phosphorus control in dogs and cats with chronic renal failure. Vet Clin North Am 26:1293–1330, 1996.

69. Finco D, Brown S, Crowell W, et al: Effects of dietary phosphorus and protein in dogs with chronic renal failure. Am J Vet Res 53:2264–2271, 1992.

70. Brown SA, Crowell WA, Barsanti JA, et al: Beneficial effects of dietary mineral restriction in dogs with marked reduction of functional renal mass. J Am Soc Nephrol 1:1169–1179, 1991.

71. Felsenfeld A: Considerations for the treatment of secondary hyperparathyroidism in renal failure. J Am Soc Nephrol 8:993–1004, 1997.

72. Martinez I, Saracho R, Montenegro J, Llack F: The importance of dietary calcium and phosphorus in the secondary hyperparathyroidism of patients with early renal failure. Am J Kidney Dis 29:496–502, 1997.

73. Chew D, Nagode L: Calcitriol in treatment of chronic renal failure. In Kirk R, Bonagura J (eds): Current Veterinary Therapy XI. Philadelphia, WB Saunders, 1992, pp 857–860.

74. Nagode L, Chew D, Steinmeyer C, et al: Renal secondary hyperparathyroidism: Toxic aspects, mechanisms of development, and control by oral calcitriol treatment. Washington, DC, 11th Annual Veterinary Medical Forum, 1993, pp 154–157.

75. Almaden Y, Canalejo A, Hernandez A, et al: Direct effect of phosphorus on PTH secretion from whole rat parathyroid glands in vitro. J Bone Miner Res 11:970–976, 1996.

76. Lopez-Hilker S, Dusso A, Rapp N, et al: Phosphorus restriction reverses hyperparathyroidism in uremia independent of changes in calcium and calcitriol. Am J Physiol 259:F432–F437, 1990.

77. Combe C, Aparicio M: Phosphorus and protein restriction and parathyroid function in chronic renal failure. Kidney Int 46:1381–1386, 1994.

78. Bro S, Olgaard K: Effects of excess PTH on nonclassical target organs. Am J Kidney Dis 30:606–620, 1997.

79. McPhee SJ, Lingappa VR, Ganong WF, Lange JD: Pathophysiology of Disease, 2nd ed. Stamford, CT, Appleton & Lange, 1997.

80. Barber PJ, Elliot J, Torrance AG: Measurement of feline intact parathyroid hormone: Assay validation and sample handling. J Small Anim Pract 34:614–620, 1993.

81. Torrance AG, Nachreiner R: Human-parathormone assay for use in dogs: Validation, sample handling studies, and parathyroid function testing. Am J Vet Res 50:1123–1127, 1989.

82. Kruger JM, Osborne CA, Nachreiner RF, Refsal KR: Hypercalcemia and renal failure. Vet Clin North Am Small Anim Pract 26:1417–1445, 1996.

83. Dow S, Fettman M: Renal disease in cats: The potassium connection. In Kirk R, Bonagura J (eds): Current Veterinary Therapy XI. Philadelphia, WB Saunders, 1992, pp 820–822.

84. DiBartola S: Hypokalemic nephropathy. In August J (ed): Consultations in Feline Internal Medicine 2. Philadelphia, WB Saunders, 1994, pp 319–324.

85. DiBartola S, Buffington C, Chew D, et al: Development of chronic renal disease in cats fed a commercial diet. JAVMA 202:744–751, 1993.

86. Adams LG, Polzin DJ, Osborne CA, et al: Effects of dietary protein and calorie restriction in clinically normal cats and in cats with surgically induced chronic renal failure. Am J Vet Res 54:1653–1662, 1993.

87. Theisen SK, DiBartola SP, Radin MJ, et al: Muscle potassium content and potassium gluconate supplementation in normokalemic cats with naturally occurring chronic renal failure. J Vet Intern Med 11:212–217, 1997.

88. Dow SW, Fettman MJ, Smith KR, et al: Effects of dietary acidification and potassium depletion on acid-base balance, mineral metabolism and renal function in adult cats. J Nutr 120:569–578, 1990.

89. Dow SW, Fettman MJ, LeCouteur RA, et al: Potassium depletion in cats: Renal and dietary influences. JAVMA 191:1569–1575, 1987.

90. Kanwar Y, Liu Z, Kashihara N, et al: Current status of the structural and functional basis of glomerular filtration and proteinuria. Semin Nephrol 11:390–413, 1991.

91. Neugarten J, Kozin A, Gayner R, et al: Dietary protein restriction and glomerular permselectivity in nephrotoxic serum nephritis. Kidney Int 40:57–61, 1991.

92. Stenvinkel P, Alvestrand A, Bergstrom J: Factors influencing progression in patients with chronic renal failure. J Intern Med 226:183–188, 1989.

93. Wright J, Salzano S, Brown C, et al: Natural history of chronic renal failure: A reappraisal. Nephrol Dial Transplant 7:379–383, 1992.

94. Brown SA, Brown CA, Crowell WA, et al: Beneficial effects of chronic administration of dietary ω-3 polyunsaturated fatty acids in dogs with renal insufficiency. J Lab Clin Med 131:447–455, 1998.

95. Arthur JE, Lucke VM, Newby TJ, Bourne FJ: The long-term prognosis of feline idiopathic membranous glomerulonephropathy. J Am Anim Hosp Assoc 22:731–737, 1986.

96. Langston CE, Cogwill LD, Spano JA: Applications and outcome of hemodialysis in cats: A review of 29 cases. J Vet Intern Med 11:348–355, 1997.

97. Cowgill LD, Langston CE: Role of hemodialysis in management of dogs and cats with renal failure. Vet Clin North Am 26:1347–1378, 1996.

98. Mathews KG, Gregory CR: Renal transplants in cats: 66 cases (1987–1996). JAVMA 211:1432–1436, 1997.

99. Gregory C: Renal transplantation in cats. Compend Contin Educ 15:1325–1338, 1993.

100. Devaux C, Polzin DJ, Osborne CA: What role does dietary protein restriction play in the management of chronic renal failure in dogs. Vet Clin North Am 26:1247–1267, 1996.

101. Polzin DJ, Osborne CA, Lulich JP: Diet therapy guidelines for cats with chronic renal failure. Vet Clin North Am 26:1269–1275, 1996.

102. Harte J, Markwell PJ, Moraillon RM, et al: Dietary management of naturally occurring chronic renal failure in cats. J Nutr 124:2660S–2662S, 1994.

103. Elliot J, Barber PJ, Rawlings JM, Markwell PJ: Effect of phosphate and protein restriction on progression of chronic renal failure in cats. J Vet Intern Med 12:221A, 1998.

104. Polzin DJ, Osborne CA, Hayden DW, et al: Influence of reduced protein diets on morbidity, mortality, and renal function in dogs with induced chronic renal failure. Am J Vet Res 45:506–517, 1984.

105. Polzin DJ, Osborne CA, Hayden DW, Stevens JB: Experimental evaluation of reduced protein diets in the management of primary polyuric renal failure: Preliminary findings and their significance. Minn Vet 21:16–29, 1981.

106. Barsanti J, Finco D: Dietary management of chronic renal failure in dogs. J Am Anim Hosp Assoc 21:371–376, 1985.

107. Finco D, Brown S, Crowell W, et al: Effects of phosphorus/calcium-restricted and phosphorus/calcium-replete 32% protein diets in dogs with chronic renal failure. Am J Vet Res 53:157–163, 1992.

108. Polzin D: Importance of clinical trials in evaluating therapy of renal diseases. Vet Clin North Am 26:1519–1525, 1996.

109. Bliss DZ ST, Schleifer CR, Settle RG: Supplementation with gum arabic fiber increases fecal nitrogen excretion and lowers serum urea nitrogen concentration in chronic renal failure patients consuming a low-protein diet. Am J Clin Nutr 63:392–398, 1996.

110. Tetens I, Livesey G, Eggum BO: Effects of the type and level of dietary fibre supplements on nitrogen retention and excretion patterns. Br J Nutr 75:461–469, 1996.

111. Tetrick MA, Sunrold GD, Reinhart GA: Clinical experience with canine renal failure patients fed a diet containing a fermentable fiber blend. In Reinhart GCD (ed): Recent Advances in Canine and Feline Nutrition. Wilmington, OH: Orange Frazer Press, 1998, pp 425–432.

112. Polzin D, Osborne C, Stevens J, et al: Influence of modified protein diets on nutritional status of dogs with experimental chronic renal failure. Am J Vet Res 44:1694–1702, 1983.

113. Bennett WM, Aronoff GR, Golper TA, Morrison G, et al: Drug Prescribing in Renal Failure, 2nd ed. Philadelphia, American College of Physicians, 1991.

114. Riviere J: Calculation of dosage regimes of antimicrobial drugs in animals with renal and hepatic dysfunction. JAVMA 185:1094–1097, 1984.

115. Finco DR, Brown SA, Vaden SL, Fergusson DC: Relationship between plasma creatinine concentration and glomerular filtration rate in dogs. J Vet Pharmacol Ther 18:418–421, 1995.

116. Brown SA, Finco DR, Boudinot FD, et al: Evaluation of a single injection method, using iohexol, for determining glomerular filtration rate in cats and dogs. Am J Vet Res 57:105–110, 1996.

117. Neff-Davis C. Clinical monitoring of drug concentrations. In Davis L (ed): Manual of Therapeutics in Small Animal Practice. New York, Churchill Livingstone, 1985, pp 633–655.

118. Chew D, DiBartola S, Nagode L, et al: Phosphorus restriction in the treatment of chronic renal failure In Kirk R, Bonagura J (eds): Current Veterinary Therapy XI. Philadelphia, WB Saunders, 1992, pp 853–857.

119. Finco DR, Crowell WA, Barsanti JA: Effects of three diets on dogs with induced chronic renal failure. Am J Vet Res 46:646–653, 1985.

120. Massry S: Prevention and treatment in divalent ion metabolism in renal failure. Semin Nephrol 6:114–121, 1986.

121. Coburn J, Slatopolsky E: Vitamin D, parathyroid hormone, and the renal osteodystrophies. In Brenner B, Rector F (eds): The Kidney, 4th ed. Philadelphia, WB Saunders, 1991, pp 2036–2120.

122. Mikiciuk MG, Thornhill JA: Control of parathyroid hormone in chronic renal failure. Compend Contin Educ (Small Anim) 11:831–836, 1989.

123. Chertow GM, Burke SK, Lazarus JM, et al: Poly[allylamine hydrochloride] (RenaGel): A noncalcemic phosphate binder for treatment of hyperphosphatemia in chronic renal failure. Am J Kidney Dis 29:66–71, 1997.

124. Rose B: Clinical Physiology of Acid-Base and Electrolyte Disorders, 4th ed. New York, McGraw-Hill, 1994.

125. James KM, Polzin DJ, Osborne CA: Serum total carbon dioxide concentrations in canine and feline blood: The effect of underfilling blood tubes and comparison with blood gas analysis as an estimate of plasma bicarbonate. Am J Vet Res 58:343–347, 1997.

126. Jensen J, Henik RA, Brownfield M, Armstrong J: Plasma renin activity and angiotensin I and aldosterone concentrations in cats with hypertension associated with chronic renal disease. Am J Vet Res 58:535–540, 1997.

127. Snyder P: Amlodipine: A randomized, blinded clinical trial in 9 cats with systemic hypertension. J Vet Intern Med 12:157–162, 1998.

128. Brown SA, Walton CL, Crawford P, Bakris GL: Long-term effects of antihypertensive regimens on renal hemodynamics and proteinuria. Kidney Int 43:1210–1218, 1993.

129. Cowgill LD, James KJ, Levy JK, et al: Use of recombinant human erythropoietin for management of anemia in dogs and cats with renal failure. JAVMA 212:521–528, 1998.

130. Weeks B: Development and application of an immunoassay for canine serum ferritin as a means of estimation of iron stores and evaluating dietary iron adequacy in dogs. Kansas State University, 1988.

131. Burns E, Goldberg S, Lawrence C, et al: Clinical utility of serum tests for iron deficiency in hospitalized patients. Am J Clin Pathol 93:240–253, 1990.

132. Kooistra M, van Es A, Struyvenberg A, et al: Iron metabolism in patients with the anaemia of end-stage renal disease during treatment with recombinant human erythropoietin. Br J Haematol 79:634–639, 1991.

133. Hutchins L, Lipschitz D. Iron and folate metabolism in renal failure. Semin Nephrol 5:142–146, 1985.

134. Christopher M: Relation of endogenous Heinz bodies to disease and anemia in cats; 120 cases (1978–1987). JAVMA 194:1089–1095, 1989.

URO

135. Connelly T, Caro J, Erslev A, et al: The effect of a low-phosphate diet on hematocrit and oxgen transport in uremic rats. Am J Hematol 12:55–61, 1982.

136. Cowgill L: Medical management of the anemia of chronic renal failure, *In* Osborne CA (ed): Canine and Feline Nephrology and Urology. Baltimore, Williams & Wilkins, 1995, pp 539–554.

137. Finco DR, Brown SA, Cooper T, et al: Effects of parathyroid hormone depletion in dogs with induced renal failure. Am J Vet Res 55:867–873, 1994.

138. Finco DR, Brown SA, Crowell WA, et al: Effects of parathyroidectomy on induced renal failure in dogs. Am J Vet Res 58:188–195, 1997.

139. Sackett D: Rules of evidence and clinical recommendations. Can J Cardiol 9:487–489, 1993.

140. Chew D, Nagode L, Carothers M, et al: Calcitriol treatment of renal secondary hyperparathyroidism in dogs and cats. Washington, DC, 11th Annual Veterinary Medical Forum, 1993, pp 164–167.

141. Brown S, Finco D: Efficacy of calcitriol in suppressing plasma parathyroid hormone (PTH) in dogs with renal disease. Washington, DC, 11th Annual Veterinary Medical Forum, 1993, pp 158–160.

142. Nagode L, Chew D: The use of calcitriol in treatment of renal disease of the dog and cat. Purina International Nutrition Symposium, 1991, pp 39–49.

143. Hostetter T: The hyperfiltering glomerulus. Med Clin North Am 62:387–398, 1984.

144. Dezie C, Renda S, Bichet D, et al: The evolution of chronic renal failure. Kidney Int 29:317A, 1986.

145. Adams L, Polzin D, Osborne C, et al: Influence of dietary protein/calorie intake on renal morphology and function in cats with 5/6 nephrectomy. Lab Invest 70:347–357, 1994.

146. Ross LA, Finco DR, Crowell WA: Effect of dietary phosphorus restriction on the kidneys of cats with reduced renal mass. Am J Vet Res 43:1023–1026, 1982.

147. Finco DR, Brown SA, Brown CA, et al: Protein and calorie effects on progression of induced chronic renal failure in cats. Am J Vet Res 59:575–582, 1998.

148. Hostetter T: Progression of renal disease. *In* Greenberg A (ed): Primer on Renal Diseases. San Diego, Academic Press, 1998, pp 429–432.

149. Kasiske BL, Lakatua JD, Ma JZ, Louis TA: A meta-analysis of the effects of dietary protein restriction on the rate of decline in renal function. Am J Kidney Dis 31:954–961, 1998.

150. Martinez-Maldonado M, Sattin RW: Rate of progression of renal disease and low-protein diet. Am J Kidney Dis 31:1048–1049, 1998.

151. Mathews KA, Holmberg DL, Johnson K, et al: Renal allograft survival in outbred mongrel dogs using anti–dog thymocyte serum in combination with immunosuppressive drug therapy with or without blood donor bone marrow. Vet Surg 23:347–357, 1994.

152. Mathews KA, GG, Mallard BA: Clinical, biochemical, and hematological evaluation of normal dogs after administration of rabbit anti-dog thymocyte serum. Vet Surg 22:213–230, 1990.

153. Vaden SL, Gookin J, Trogdon M, et al: Use of carbamylated hemoglobin concentration to differentiate acute from chronic renal failure in dogs. Am J Vet Res 58:1193–1196, 1997.

154. Polzin DJ, OC, O'Brien TD, Hostetter TH: Effects of protein intake on progression of canine chronic renal failure. J Vet Intern Med 7:125A, 1993.

155. Cianciaruso B, Bellizzi V, Minutolo R, et al: Salt intake and renal outcome in patients with progressive renal disease. Miner Electrolyte Metab 24:296–301, 1998.

156. Greco D, Lees G, Dzendzel G, et al: Effect of dietary sodium intake on glomerular filtration rate in partially nephrectomized dogs. Am J Vet Res 55:152–159, 1994.

157. Stein G SS, Sperschneider H, Richter R, et al: Vitamin status in patients with chronic renal failure. Contrib Nephrol 65:33–42, 1988.

158. Henik R: Diagnosis and treatment of feline systemic hypertension. Compend Contin Educ 19:163–179, 1997.

159. Ross LA: Hypertension and chronic renal failure. Semin Vet Med Surg (Small Anim) 7:221–226, 1992.

160. Polzin D, Osborne CA: Pathophysiology of renal failure and uremia. *In* Osborne CA, Finco DR (eds): Canine and Feline Nephrology and Urology. Baltimore, Williams & Wilkins, 1995, pp 335–367.

CHAPTER 170

GLOMERULAR DISEASE

Gregory F. Grauer and Stephen P. DiBartola

The two major glomerular diseases of dogs and cats are immune complex glomerulonephritis and amyloidosis. Both diseases may cause massive proteinuria and lead to progressive loss of functional renal mass. Classically, the nephrotic syndrome has been considered to include proteinuria, hypoalbuminemia, hypercholesterolemia, and ascites or subcutaneous edema. Proteinuria without inflammatory urinary sediment findings is the hallmark of glomerular disease.

As the number of renal biopsies performed in veterinary medicine has increased in recent years it has become apparent that glomerular disease is not only common in dogs but also a leading cause of chronic renal insufficiency and failure. Glomerulonephritis usually is caused by the presence of immune complexes in glomerular capillary walls. These immune complexes initiate a series of events that can result in glomerular cell proliferation and thickening of capillary walls and ultimately may lead to glomerular hyalinization and sclerosis. Irreversible damage to the glomerulus renders the entire nephron non-functional; and if the disease is progressive, glomerular filtration decreases, resulting in azotemia and renal failure. In dogs with amyloidosis, amyloid fibrils are deposited in the mesangium and glomerular capillary walls and interfere with normal glomerular function by their physical presence. Use of the urine protein/creatinine ratio to quantitate urinary protein loss has facilitated the diagnosis of glomerular disease in dogs and cats. Ultimately, however, differentiation of glomerulonephritis from glomerular amyloidosis requires histologic examination of renal biopsy specimens.

NORMAL GLOMERULAR STRUCTURE AND FUNCTION

The glomeruli function as filters across which an ultrafiltrate of plasma is created by the force of cardiac contraction. The filtration barrier is composed of three major components: the fenestrated endothelium of the glomerular capillary, the glomerular basement membrane, and the visceral epithelial cells (podocytes) (Figs. 70–1 and 170–2). The interdigitating foot processes of the podocytes and the slit diaphragms between them are negatively charged owing to the presence of acidic glycoproteins. The basement membrane and endothelium also contain negatively charged glycoproteins.

The normal glomerulus functions both as a size- and a charge-selective filter. Its size-selective properties are

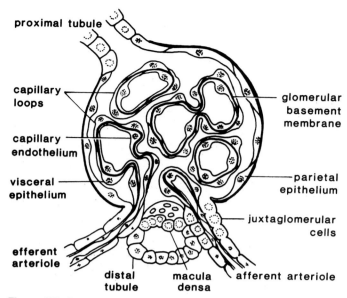

Figure 170–1. Normal glomerular morphology. (Adapted from Ham AW, Cormack DH: Histology, 8th ed. Philadelphia, JB Lippincott, 1979.)

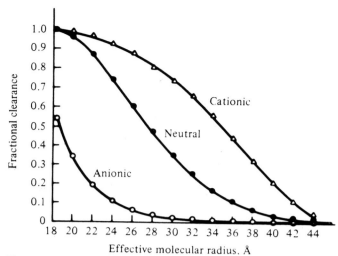

Figure 170–3. Charge selectivity of the glomerulus demonstrated by fractional clearance of anionic, neutral, and cationic dextrans. Fractional clearances (the ratio of the filtration of a substance to that of inulin, which is freely filtered) of anionic, neutral, and cationic dextrans as a function of effective molecular radius. Both molecular size and charge are important, because smaller or cationic molecules are more easily filtered. As a reference, the effective molecular radius of albumin is about 36 Å. (From Rose BD: Pathophysiology of Renal Disease. New York, McGraw-Hill, 1987, p 13.)

thought to reside primarily in the basement membrane and are such that circulating macromolecules greater than 34 nm in diameter are excluded from filtration. Serum albumin with a molecular weight of 69,000 daltons and effective molecular diameter of 36 nm is normally excluded from filtration. The negatively charged glomerular capillary wall restricts filtration of circulating negatively charged macromolecules so that the fractional clearance of particles of similar size differs substantially, depending on their charge (Fig. 170–3).

PATHOGENESIS OF GLOMERULONEPHRITIS

Soluble circulating antigen-antibody complexes may be deposited or trapped in the glomerulus when a mild antigen excess exists or when antigen and antibody molecules are present in approximately equal numbers in the plasma (Fig.

170–4). If a large antibody excess exists, complexes tend to be large and insoluble and are rapidly removed from the circulation by phagocytic cells. If a large antigen excess exists, the immune complexes do not readily bind complement and have a reduced capacity to produce immunologic injury. Glomerular deposition of pre-formed immune complexes usually results in a lumpy-bumpy or granular immunofluorescence pattern with mesangial and subendothelial location of the antigen-antibody complexes (Fig. 170–5).

In contrast to the glomerular deposition of pre-formed complexes, in situ formation of immune complexes can occur within the glomerular capillary wall when circulating antibodies react with endogenous glomerular antigens or "planted" non-glomerular antigens in the glomerular capillary wall (see Fig. 170–4). True autoimmune glomerulonephritis with antibodies directed against endogenous glomerular basement membrane material has not been recognized in dogs and cats with naturally occurring glomerulonephritis. Non-glomerular antigens, however, may localize in the glomerular capillary wall due to electrical charge interaction or biochemical affinity with the glomerular basement membrane. When antibodies present in plasma react with antigens in situ, either a smooth linear or granular lumpy-bumpy pattern of immunofluorescence may result (see Fig. 170–5). In this instance, the location of the complexes usually is subepithelial. The glomerulonephritis in dogs associated with heartworm disease occurs in part due to in situ immune complex formation.[1]

The glomerulus provides a unique environment for injurious factors (i.e., immune complexes) to stimulate production of bioactive mediators (e.g., eicosanoids, cytokines, growth factors, nitric oxide). These mediators may be produced by endogenous glomerular cells or by recruited blood cells (e.g., neutrophils, platelets). T lymphocytes are thought to be involved in immune-mediated glomerular injury associated with the recognition of antigen and their subsequent activation. Mesangial cells can also activate T lymphocytes,

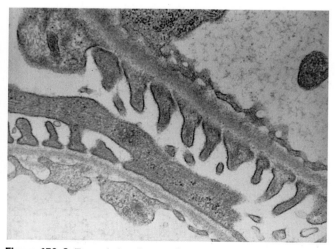

Figure 170–2. Transmission electron photomicrograph of a canine glomerular capillary wall demonstrating the endothelial surface, the glomerular basement membrane, and the epithelial cell (podocyte) foot processes.

URO

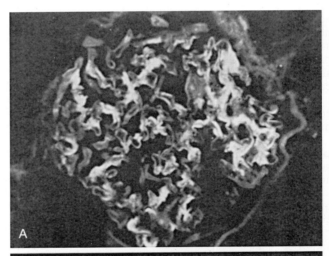

> antibody
• antigen
△ complement
⌗ damaged GBM
∴ lysosomal enzymes

▲ planted Ags
• intrinsic glomerular antigens

Figure 170–4. Immunologic mechanisms of glomerular injury. Schematic representation of the two major types of immunologically mediated glomerular injury. Circulating soluble immune complexes have become trapped in the glomerular filter and have fixed complement. Chemotactic complement components have attracted neutrophils to the area. The release of free oxygen radicals and lysosomal enzymes from the neutrophils has resulted in damage to the glomerulus *(top)*. GBM = glomerular basement membrane. Damage may also result from attachment of autoantibodies directed against fixed intrinsic glomerular antigens *(bottom, left)*. Finally, damage may result from attachment of antibodies directed against planted non-glomerular antigens *(bottom, right)*. Ags = antigens. (From Chew DJ, DiBartola SP: Manual of Small Animal Nephrology and Urology. New York, Churchill Livingstone, 1986, p 232.)

which, in turn, activate and stimulate other mononuclear cells.[2]

Eicosanoids are cyclooxygenase and lipoxygenase products of arachidonic acid metabolism. Prostaglandins and thromboxanes are produced by the action of cyclooxygenase, whereas leukotrienes are lipoxygenase products. Thromboxanes induce platelet aggregation, are chemotactic for neutrophils, and cause both vasoconstriction and mesangial cell contraction, which may result in decreased glomerular filtration. Thromboxane also interferes with the mesangial phagocytosis and disposal of aggregated proteins and immune complexes.[3] Conversely, prostaglandins inhibit platelet aggregation and tend to have anti-inflammatory, vasodilatory effects within the kidney. Like thromboxanes, leukotrienes decrease glomerular filtration by vasoconstriction and mesangial cell contraction.[4, 5] In addition, leukotrienes attract neutrophils and promote leukocyte adhesion and activation as well as mesangial cell proliferation and production of extracellular matrix proteins.[6] Increased urinary excretion of thromboxane is thought to be a general marker of glomerular inflammation, whereas increased urinary excretion of leukotrienes is more specific for acute inflammation.[7]

Cytokines and growth factors are produced by inflammatory cells and resident glomerular cells during glomerular injury. Tumor necrosis factor, interleukins, platelet-derived growth factor, transforming growth factor-beta, epidermal growth factor, and fibroblast growth factor contribute to

mesangial cell proliferation, mesangial matrix production, inflammatory cell adhesion, increased vascular permeability, intraglomerular coagulation and fibrin deposition, and glomerulosclerosis.[8–10] These peptides are thought to have paracrine and autocrine actions and can act synergistically. Platelet-activating factor is a potent lipid-derived autacoid that contributes to glomerular inflammation by promoting neutrophil infiltration, eicosanoid production, and increased vascular permeability.[11] Platelet-activating factor can be produced by neutrophils, macrophages, platelets, and glomerular endothelial and mesangial cells, and the effects of platelet-activating factor are often exerted through the release of thromboxane.[8] Platelet-activating factor is also a positively charged molecule that can neutralize the negative charges of the heparan sulfates and proteoglycans of the glomerular capillary walls and therefore enhance albuminuria.

After formation or deposition of immune complexes in the glomerular capillary wall, several factors, including activation of the complement system, infiltration of neutrophils and macrophages, platelet aggregation, activation of the coagulation system, and fibrin deposition, contribute to glomerular inflammation (Fig. 170–6). The location of the immune complexes within the glomerular capillary wall may influence the immune response. For example, subepithelial im-

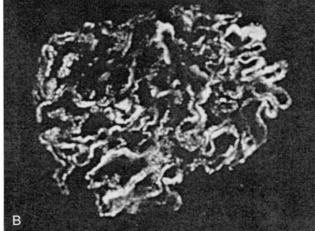

Figure 170–5. Immunofluorescent patterns of glomerular disease. *A,* Linear continuous immunofluorescence suggestive of in situ formation of immune complexes. *B,* Lumpy-bumpy discontinuous pattern of immunofluorescence characteristic of immune-complex deposition glomerulonephritis. (Courtesy of RM Lewis and CA Smith.)

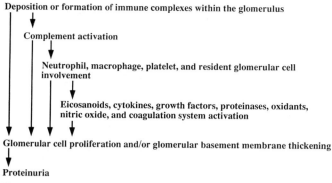

Deposition or formation of immune complexes within the glomerulus

↓

Complement activation

↓

Neutrophil, macrophage, platelet, and resident glomerular cell involvement

↓

Eicosanoids, cytokines, growth factors, proteinases, oxidants, nitric oxide, and coagulation system activation

↓

Glomerular cell proliferation and/or glomerular basement membrane thickening

↓

Proteinuria

Figure 170–6. Summary of immunologic mechanisms of glomerulonephritis and proteinuria.

mune complexes activate complement and result in proteinuria, but an inflammatory response involving neutrophils and macrophages usually is lacking. Local subepithelial activation of complement causes the membrane attack complex (C5b-9) to be assembled and inserted into the lipid bilayer of cell membranes, increasing glomerular permeability.[12] This complex also induces activation of phospholipase A_2, which results in increased eicosanoid production.[13] Complement activation also produces chemotactic fragments that attract neutrophils and macrophages, but the basement membrane separates the immune deposits from the circulation and may prevent adherence of inflammatory cells. Furthermore, diffusion of complement-derived chemotactic factors toward the capillary lumen where neutrophil adherence could occur usually is prevented by filtration forces. Consequently, subepithelial immune complexes may increase glomerular permeability in the absence of inflammatory cells.

If immune complexes form or are deposited closer to the capillary lumen (i.e., in subendothelial locations), there often is more histologic evidence of inflammation. Neutrophils and macrophages localize in the glomerulus in response to several soluble mediators, including complement (C5a), platelet activating factor, platelet-derived growth factor, and eicosanoids.[14] Neutrophils attach to complement (C3b) or the Fc portion of immunoglobulins within the glomerulus and attempt to phagocytose immune complex material, resulting in release of oxidants and proteinases. The principal oxidant involved in neutrophil-mediated injury is H_2O_2.[15] Hydrogen peroxide combines with Fe^{2+} to form toxic hydroxyl radicals and can react with halides in the presence of neutrophil-derived myeloperoxidase to form toxic hypohalous acids. Reactive oxygen species can also be generated by mesangial cells in response to cytokines and immunoglobulins. Oxidants activate proteinases and thereby potentiate their action. Elastase and cathepsin G are neutrophil proteinases that have been detected in the urine of animals with glomerulonephritis, and these proteinases degrade glomerular basement membranes in vitro.[16]

Macrophages attracted to the glomerulus associated with immune complex deposition or formation can produce proteinases and oxidants in addition to several other potential inflammatory mediators, including eicosanoids, growth factors, cytokines, complement fragments, and coagulation factors. Platelet activation and aggregation occur secondary to endothelial damage or antigen-antibody interaction and exacerbate glomerular damage by release of eicosanoids and facilitation of the coagulation cascade. Nitric oxide produced by platelets, neutrophils, macrophages, and endothelial cells

within inflamed glomeruli can induce cytotoxicity by forming an iron-nitrosyl-sulfur complex that inhibits iron-dependent enzymes and causes cessation of DNA replication.[17]

The glomerulus responds to these insults by cellular proliferation, thickening of the glomerular basement membrane, and, if the injury persists, hyalinization and sclerosis (Fig. 170–7 and Table 170–1). Mesangial cell proliferation and mesangial matrix expansion are considered to be precursors of glomerulosclerosis. Regulation of excessive mesangial matrix production and glomerular cell proliferation may prevent irreversible glomerular damage. Matrix metalloproteinases are enzymes that degrade glomerular mesangial matrix and therefore have a role in preventing mesangial matrix expansion. Similarly, programmed cell death (apoptosis) triggered by cytokines and lymphocytes may be critical for successful remodeling of the glomerulus subsequent to inflammation injury. Altered regulation of apoptotic cell death and glomerular metalloproteinase activity is thought to contribute to the development of glomerulosclerosis.[18, 19]

On histologic evaluation of renal biopsy specimens from patients with primary glomerular disease, tubulointerstitial injury is frequently observed. Several mediators of this injury have been proposed, including antibodies, lysosomal enzymes, reactive oxygen species, and complement. Tubular obstruction by casts or cellular debris may also cause tubular damage. In rats with mesangioproliferative glomerulonephritis and proteinuria, the development of tubulointerstitial lesions is associated with activation of serum complement at the level of the tubular brush border.[20] In proteinuric glomerular disease, antibodies also may be filtered into the urinary space where they may react with tubular antigens present on the apical surface.[21] Proteinuria itself may contribute to tubular damage by increasing the amount of tubular protein reabsorption and lysosomal processing. This protein reabsorption may result in lysosomal swelling and rupture, with subsequent tubulointerstitial injury. Finally, filtration of transferrin in protein-losing glomerular disease can be associated with hydroxyl-radical formation and tubular damage.[22]

Once a glomerulus or tubule has been irreversibly damaged, the entire nephron becomes non-functional. Fibrosis

URO

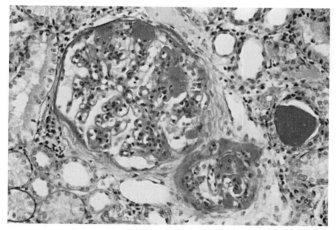

Figure 170–7. Advanced membranoproliferative glomerulonephritis. The large glomerulus shows hypercellularity with prominent focal accumulations of mesangial matrix material and thickened glomerular capillary walls. Adhesions to Bowman's capsule and periglomerular fibrosis are also present. The small glomerulus is irreversibly damaged and obsolescent. A hyaline cast is present in a tubule *(right;* PAS stain, original magnification × 200). (Reprinted with permission from Grauer GF: Glomerular disease and proteinuria. *In* Allen DG [ed]: Small Animal Medicine. Philadelphia, JB Lippincott, 1991, pp 615–623.)

TABLE 170–1. PATHOLOGIC FINDINGS IN DOGS WITH GLOMERULONEPHRITIS

REFERENCE	LIGHT MICROSCOPY	IMMUNOFLUORESCENCE	ELECTRON MICROSCOPY
Murray 1971 (n = 1)	Mesangioproliferative	ND	Subepithelial deposits, foot process fusion
Osborne 1973 (n = 1)	Membranous	Discontinuous Igs; C	Subepithelial, subendothelial, and mesangial deposits; foot process fusion
Lewis 1976 (n = 50)	Proliferative, membranous	ND	ND
Rouse & Lewis 1975 (n = 15)	Proliferative, membranous	Discontinuous IgG; C*	ND
Kurtz 1972 (n = 8)	Mesangioproliferative	Discontinuous IgG; C	Mesangial and subendothelial deposits; foot process fusion†
Murray 1974 (n = 42)	Proliferative, membranous	IgG; C3	Subepithelial and membranous deposits
Muller-Peddinghaus 1977 (n = 94)	Membranous, membranoproliferative, mesangioproliferative, mesangiosclerosing	Discontinuous IgG; C3	Subepithelial, subendothelial, and mesangial deposits
Jaenke 1986 (n = 14)	Membranous	IgG, IgA	Subepithelial‡
MacDougall 1986 (n = 40)	Focal, mesangioproliferative, endocapillary, mesangiocapillary, crescentic, sclerosing	IgG, IgM; C3	Mesangial, subepithelial, intramembranous, and subendothelial deposits§
Wright 1981 (n = 5)	Membranous	IgG; C3	Subepithelial, intramembranous, and mesangial deposits; foot process fusion‖
DiBartola 1980 (n = 11)	Membranous, membranoproliferative Mesangioproliferative	Linear and discontinuous IgG, IgA, IgM	ND
Stuart 1975 (n = 18)	Mesangioproliferative	Discontinuous IgG	Mesangial and subendothelial deposits
Biewenga 1986 (n = 44)	Membranous, membranoproliferative, mesangioproliferative	C_3; IgG, IgA, IgM	ND
Center 1987 (n = 41)	Membranous, membranoproliferative, mesangioproliferative	Discontinuous and linear C_3; IgG, IgA, IgM	ND
Cook 1996 (n = 106)	Membranous, membranoproliferative, glomerulosclerosis	IgM, IgG, IgA; C3	ND
Dambach 1997 (n = 49)	Mesangioproliferative, membranous	Irregular C3; IgG, IgM	Subendothelial deposits

ND = not determined.
*Negative elution studies.
†Subepithelial deposits not observed.
‡Recovered or developed glomerular sclerosis.
§No membranous nephropathy and no minimal change disease observed.
‖All cases were idiopathic.

and cellular infiltration of irreversibly damaged nephrons may result in a diagnosis of chronic interstitial disease. For many years, primary chronic interstitial nephritis was thought to be the major cause of chronic renal failure in dogs; however, much end-stage renal disease in dogs actually represents primary, progressive glomerular disease. As more nephrons become injured, glomerular filtration decreases. Remaining viable nephrons compensate for the decrease in nephron numbers with increased single-nephron glomerular filtration rates (Fig. 170–8). This "hyperfiltration" within remnant nephrons may exacerbate proteinuria and enhance glomerular hyalinization and sclerosis. Increased glomerular

capillary pressure and flow damages glomerular cells, causing release of cytokines and growth factors that contribute to extracellular matrix expansion. Damage to glomerular capillary endothelial cells also exposes the extracellular matrix. Platelets can adhere to this matrix, initiating coagulation and eventually fibrin deposition, which often is an irreversible lesion. Hyperfiltration in remnant nephrons has been documented in dogs,[23] but a causal relationship between glomerular hyperfiltration and glomerulosclerosis or glomerular fibrin deposition has not been established.

Several infectious and inflammatory diseases have been associated with glomerular deposition or in situ formation of immune complexes in dogs and cats (Table 170–2). In many cases, however, the antigen source or underlying disease process is not identified and the glomerular disease is referred to as idiopathic. Endogenous immunoglobulins or complement may be detected within glomeruli using various immunologic techniques, but the offending antigen rarely is identified. It is interesting to note that *Helicobacter pylori* antigen has been discovered in glomeruli from humans with membranous glomerulonephritis and therefore may be involved in the pathogenesis of this nephropathy.[24] There also is increasing evidence in humans that genetic and immunogenetic factors have a role not only in initiating glomerulonephritis but also in determining its severity.

Glomerulonephritis usually is categorized according to histopathologic findings because the underlying cause of the lesion often is unknown. Glomerular basement membrane thickening is referred to as membranous glomerulonephritis,

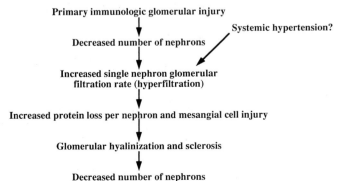

Figure 170–8. Proposed pathogenesis of progressive loss of nephrons secondary to primary immunologic glomerular injury.

whereas increased cellularity is referred to as proliferative glomerulonephritis. A combination of basement membrane thickening and increased cellularity is referred to as membranoproliferative glomerulonephritis. Glomerular scarring associated with increased mesangial matrix is referred to as glomerulosclerosis.

PATHOGENESIS OF AMYLOIDOSIS

Amyloidosis refers to a diverse group of diseases characterized by extracellular deposition of fibrils formed by polymerization of protein subunits with a specific biophysical conformation called the beta-pleated sheet.[25–29] This specific biophysical conformation is responsible for the unique optical and tinctorial properties of amyloid deposits as well as their insolubility and resistance to proteolysis in vivo. Amyloid deposits have a homogeneous, eosinophilic appearance when stained by hematoxylin and eosin and viewed by conventional light microscopy. They demonstrate green birefringence after Congo red staining when viewed under polarized light. The clinical diagnosis of amyloidosis is based on these pathologic findings. Amyloid fibrils are variable in length, non-branching, and 7 to 10 nm in width when viewed by transmission electron microscopy. Congo red–stained amyloid deposits from animals with reactive (secondary) amyloidosis lose their affinity for Congo red after permanganate oxidation. This feature is useful in the preliminary differentiation of reactive from other types of amyloidosis. A notable exception is beta$_2$-microglobulin, which also is permanganate sensitive. Beta$_2$-microglobulin–associated amyloidosis occurs in humans after long-term hemodialysis and has not been observed in domestic animals.

Amyloid syndromes are classified by the distribution of

TABLE 170–2. DISEASES ASSOCIATED WITH GLOMERULONEPHRITIS IN DOGS AND CATS

DOGS	CATS
Infectious	Infectious
Infectious canine hepatitis	Feline leukemia virus
Bacterial endocarditis	Feline infectious peritonitis
Brucellosis	Mycoplasmal polyarthritis
Dirofilariasis	
Ehrlichiosis	
Leishmaniasis	
Pyometra	
Borelliosis	
Chronic bacterial infections	
Rocky Mountain spotted fever	
Trypanosomiasis	
Septicemia	
Helicobacter infection?	
Neoplasia	Neoplasia
Inflammatory	Inflammatory
Pancreatitis	Pancreatitis
Systemic lupus erythematosus	Systemic lupus erythematosus
Polyarthritis	Other immune-mediated diseases
Prostatitis	Chronic skin disease
Hepatitis	
Inflammatory bowel disease	
Immune-mediated hemolytic anemia	
Other	Other
Hyperadrenocorticism and long-term high-dose corticosteroids?	Idiopathic
Idiopathic	Familial
Familial	Non-immunologic—hyperfiltration?
Non-immunologic—hyperfiltration?	Diabetes mellitus?
Diabetes mellitus?	

the deposits (i.e., systemic or localized) and by the nature of the responsible fibril protein and its precursor (Table 170–3). Localized syndromes usually affect one organ and are uncommon in domestic animals. Examples of localized amyloidosis in domestic animals include immunoglobulin-associated amyloidosis of the nasal cavity in horses[30, 31] and pancreatic islet cell amyloid in domestic cats characterized by the presence of a polypeptide hormone called islet amyloid polypeptide.[32] Localized amyloid deposits also have been observed in the brain and lung of aged dogs. The amyloid protein in the cerebral vessels of aged dogs was related immunohistochemically to beta protein found in elderly humans with Alzheimer's disease,[33] and the protein found in the pulmonary vasculature of dogs was determined to be apolipoprotein A-I.[34, 35]

Systemic syndromes affect more than one organ and include reactive, immunoglobulin-associated, and heredofamilial syndromes. Reactive (secondary) amyloidosis is a systemic syndrome characterized by tissue deposition of amyloid A (AA) protein. Naturally occurring systemic amyloidosis in domestic animals is an example of reactive amyloidosis. Familial amyloidosis in the Abyssinian cat and Shar Pei dog also are examples of reactive systemic amyloidosis.[36, 37] Immunoglobulin-associated (primary) amyloidosis is characterized by tissue deposition of amino terminal fragments of immunoglobulin light chains (AL amyloid). In humans, immunoglobulin-associated amyloidosis usually is systemic (e.g., amyloidosis complicating plasma cell dyscrasias) but also can be localized (e.g., solitary amyloid nodules in the skin, respiratory tract, and urogenital tract). Immunoglobulin-associated amyloidosis has been documented in domestic animals.[30, 38–40] In humans, amyloidosis associated with genetic variants of transthyretin may be systemic (e.g., familial neuropathic syndromes) or localized (e.g., senile cardiopathic syndromes). This type of amyloid has not been recognized in veterinary medicine. Proteins that have been associated with amyloidosis in humans and domestic animals are summarized in Table 170–3.

Tissue deposits from animals with reactive systemic amyloidosis contain AA protein, which is an amino-terminal fragment of an acute-phase reactant called serum amyloid A (SAA) protein. AA protein has been characterized in several species of domestic animals.[36, 41–43] In all species studied, the amino acids at positions 33 to 45 are the same, suggesting an important functional role for this portion of the molecule.

SAA protein is the product of two genes (SAA1 and SAA2) located on the short arm of chromosome 11 in humans. In humans, six polymorphic forms of SAA protein have been identified corresponding to five alleles for SAA1 and two alleles for SAA2. In mice, there is one form each of SAA protein from the SAA1 and SAA2 genes. Five forms of SAA protein have been identified in the dog,[44] and three of these have been demonstrated in AA deposits.[37] The distribution of SAA polymorphs in plasma does not seem to be influenced by the inflammatory stimulus or the presence or absence of amyloidosis.[45] In mice, only SAA2 appears to be amyloidogenic, but specific amyloidogenic forms of SAA have not been recognized in humans and dogs.[37]

SAA protein is one of several acute-phase reactants synthesized by the liver in response to tissue injury. Cytokines (e.g., interleukin-1, interleukin-6, tumor necrosis factor) released from macrophages after tissue injury stimulate hepatocytes to synthesize and release SAA protein. SAA protein released from hepatocytes binds to high-density lipoproteins (HDL), where it displaces other apolipoproteins. The normal serum concentration of SAA protein is approximately 1 mg/

URO

TABLE 170–3. PROTEINS ASSOCIATED WITH AMYLOID SYNDROMES IN HUMANS AND DOMESTIC ANIMALS

PROTEIN	DISTRIBUTION	MAJOR ORGANS AFFECTED	DISEASE ASSOCIATION	SPECIES
Serum amyloid A	Systemic	Various	Reactive systemic amyloidosis	Various
Immunoglobulin light chains	Systemic	Various	Plasma cell dyscrasias	Human, dog
	Localized	Lung, skin, urinary tract	Local nodular lesions	Human
	Localized	Nasal cavity	Nasal hemorrhage	Horse
	Localized	Skin	Plasmacytoma	Cat
Transthyretin (prealbumin)	Systemic	Various	Peripheral neuropathy	Human
	Localized	Heart	Cardiomyopathy	Human
			Senescence	Human
Apolipoprotein A-I	Systemic	Various	Peripheral neuropathy	Human
	Localized	Lung	Senescence	Dog
Apolipoprotein A-II	Systemic	Various	Accelerated senescence	Mouse
Gelosin	Systemic	Various	Cranial neuropathy	Human
			Corneal lattice dystrophy	
Islet amyloid polypeptide	Localized	Pancreas	Diabetes mellitus, insulinoma?	Human
				Cat
Calcitonin	Localized	Thyroid	Thyroid medullary carcinoma	Human
Atrial natriuretic peptide	Localized	Heart	Senescence	Human
Beta-microglobulin	Localized	Joints	Chronic hemodialysis	Human
Beta-protein	Localized	Brain	Alzheimer's disease	Human
			Down syndrome	
		Brain	Senescence	Dog
Cystatin C	Localized	Brain	Cerebral hemorrhage	Human
Prion protein	Localized	Brain	Encephalopathy	Human
		Brain	Encephalopathy (scrapie)	Sheep
		Brain	Encephalopathy	Cattle
Keratin	Localized	Skin	Macular and lichen amyloid	Human
Fibrinogen Aα	Systemic	Kidneys	Renal disease, hypertension	Human
Lysozyme	Systemic	Kidneys, liver	Renal disease, hepatomegaly	Human

L, but its concentration increases 100 to 1000-fold after tissue injury (e.g., inflammation, neoplasia, trauma, infarction). The serum concentration of SAA protein begins to increase 2 to 4 hours after an inflammatory stimulus, peaks at 12 to 18 hours, and decreases to baseline by 36 to 48 hours if the inflammatory stimulus is removed. If inflammation persists, SAA protein concentration remains increased.

SAA protein presumably has a critical role in the body's response to tissue injury, but its actual biologic function remains a mystery. The fact that endotoxins bind to HDL has led to speculation that one function of SAA protein may be to confer a rapid clearance rate on HDL and thus enhance the elimination of endotoxin or products of tissue injury from the body. Other suggested roles include an immunosuppressive effect, inhibition of platelet aggregation, regulation of the oxidative burst in neutrophils, and stimulation of collagenase production by fibroblasts. SAA protein may increase the affinity of HDL for macrophages and other reticuloendothelial cells, thus directing SAA to sites of inflammation and macrophage accumulation.[46] These sites include the splenic perifollicular zone, hepatic sinusoids, and glomerular mesangium, all of which also are sites where amyloid deposition first is recognized.

SAA protein serves as the precursor of AA protein in tissues. This was demonstrated by administering human SAA protein intravenously to mice previously stimulated to develop amyloidosis by casein administration. Human A protein subsequently was identified immunohistochemically in the amyloid deposits of the affected mice.[47] It is not clear whether SAA protein is partially degraded to AA protein in plasma and then deposited in tissues or whether SAA protein is deposited in tissues and then partially cleaved to AA protein to initiate fibril formation.

The concentration of SAA protein is increased in plasma before amyloid deposits are observed in tissues. Colchicine administered during this phase may prevent the formation of amyloid-enhancing factor.[48] Amyloid-enhancing factor is a glycoprotein that rapidly accelerates the formation of amyloid fibrils, possibly by acting as a nidus for amyloid fibril crystallization and growth. In the rapid deposition phase, the amount of amyloid in deposits increases. Colchicine given during this phase will delay but not prevent tissue deposition of amyloid and will decrease SAA protein concentration. Colchicine impairs secretion of SAA protein from hepatocytes by binding to microtubules and preventing its release. Colchicine can prevent development of reactive amyloidosis when given prophylactically to a patient population with a known high risk of reactive amyloidosis (i.e., humans with familial Mediterranean fever).[49] Dimethylsulfoxide given during the rapid deposition phase will cause resolution of amyloid deposits and decrease SAA protein concentration.

Amyloid P component, a glycoprotein related in structure to C-reactive protein, and glycosaminoglycans (e.g., heparan sulfate, dermatan sulfate) commonly are found in amyloid deposits regardless of their chemical composition. It is unclear whether these substances have specific roles in the pathogenesis of amyloid deposition or are bound non-specifically to the deposits. Their carbohydrate content, however, probably accounts for the staining of amyloid by periodic acid–Schiff and Lugol's iodine. Scintigraphy using iodine-123 (^{123}I)–labeled serum amyloid P (SAP) has been used to quantify total-body burden of amyloid deposits in humans with amyloidosis and to monitor the response of these patients to treatment.[27] This technique is very sensitive and specific, and it is not dependent on the type of amyloid deposits present (e.g., AA, AL) because SAP is found in all amyloid deposits regardless of type. These studies show that amyloid deposits are not static but change over time and in some instances do respond to therapy. In humans, studies with SAP scintigraphy using ^{123}I-labeled and, more recently, technetium-99m–labeled SAP have shown stabilization (50 per cent of patients) or substantial regression (50 per cent of patients) of amyloid deposits over a 2- to 3-year period if the underlying acute-phase response remits or is effectively treated.[50] There is poor correlation, however, between the quantity of visceral amyloid detected by SAP scintigraphy and organ function as assessed by routine clinical tests. In one study, ^{123}I-labeled SAP scintigraphy was used to evaluate amyloid deposits in Oriental shorthair cats with amyloidosis.[51]

Chronic inflammation and a prolonged increase in SAA protein concentration are necessary prerequisites for development of reactive amyloidosis. Despite this, only a small percentage (5–15 per cent) of animals with chronic inflammatory disease develop amyloidosis. Thus, other factors must also be important in development of amyloidosis. Genetic factors probably are involved. Proteases initially degrade SAA to AA-like intermediates and then to soluble peptides. In mice with casein-induced amyloidosis, Kupffer cells degrade SAA to an AA-like intermediate whereas Kupffer cells from control mice degrade this intermediate further.[52] The second stage of the degradative process may be defective in some individuals and may be a predisposing constitutional factor to amyloidosis.

Normal serum has AA-degrading activity, which may be decreased in serum from patients with chronic inflammatory disease and in those with amyloidosis.[53] This activity is correlated with serum albumin concentration, and hypoalbuminemia in amyloidosis may contribute to decreased AA-degrading activity. Chronic inflammation may contribute to amyloidosis by increasing the concentration of other acute-phase proteins that are protease inhibitors (e.g., anti-trypsin, anti-chymotrypsin). Chronic inflammation also results in a persistent increase in SAA protein concentration, which may then act as a substrate for the formation of AA deposits.

Among the domestic animals, reactive amyloidosis is most common in the dog.[54] It is relatively uncommon in domestic cats, with the exception of the Abyssinian, Siamese, and Oriental shorthair breeds. Diseases that have been observed in association with reactive systemic amyloidosis in the dog include chronic infectious or non-infectious inflammatory diseases and neoplasms, but there is no discernible associated inflammatory or neoplastic disease in the majority of dogs and cats presented with reactive systemic amyloidosis.[55] Amyloidosis has been reported in grey collie dogs with cyclic hematopoiesis and in dogs with ciliary dyskinesia and recurrent respiratory infections.[56]

The cause of the specific tissue tropisms of different amyloid proteins is poorly understood. Transthyretin has a predilection for the peripheral nervous system and heart. AA protein has a predilection for kidney, spleen, and liver. AL amyloid has a predilection for the kidney, spleen, liver, tongue, heart, and musculoskeletal system. The cause of species differences in the tissue tropisms of reactive amyloid deposits also is unknown. In the dog, AA deposits are most common in the kidney and clinical signs are due to renal failure and uremia. The spleen, liver, adrenal glands, and gastrointestinal tract also may be involved, but associated clinical signs are rare. In Shar Pei dogs with amyloidosis, liver involvement may lead to clinical signs in some dogs.[57, 58] In the Abyssinian cat, there is widespread deposition of amyloid deposits[59] but clinical signs are due to renal failure and uremia. In Siamese and Oriental shorthair cats there is a predilection for deposition of amyloid in the liver, leading to hepatic rupture and hemorrhage.[60–62]

CLINICAL FINDINGS IN GLOMERULAR DISEASE

SIGNALMENT

Dogs with immune complex glomerulonephritis range in age from young to old. In one study, the mean age was 7 years.[63] There does not appear to be a sex predilection in dogs with glomerulonephritis; however, in two studies Labrador and golden retrievers were represented most frequently.[64, 65] The mean age of cats with glomerulonephritis is 4 years (range, <1 to 12 years), 75 per cent are males, and there appears to be no breed predilection.[66] Familial glomerulopathies have been described in Doberman pinschers, Samoyeds, rottweilers, greyhounds, Bernese mountain dogs, English cocker spaniels, and soft-coated wheaten terriers.[67–73]

Most dogs and cats with renal amyloidosis are older than 5 years of age at the time of diagnosis. Beagles, collies, and Walker hounds were at increased risk and German shepherd and mixed breed dogs were at decreased risk for renal amyloidosis in one study,[55] and glomerular amyloidosis has been reported in a family of older beagles.[74] Systemic reactive amyloidosis occurs as a familial disease in Abyssinian,[75] Siamese, and Oriental shorthair cats[60–62] and in Chinese Shar Pei dogs.[37, 76–78] Renal amyloidosis has been reported in older beagles[74] and in a group of English foxhounds 4 to 8 years of age.[79] Abyssinian cats and Shar Pei dogs with familial amyloidosis usually are younger than 6 years of age when examined for clinical signs of renal failure.

HISTORY

The presenting complaint in dogs and cats with glomerulonephritis is variable and depends on the severity and duration of urine protein loss as well as the presence or absence of renal failure and complications (e.g., thromboembolism, hypertension). There may be no clinical signs associated with mild to moderate urinary protein loss, or the signs are non-specific (e.g., weight loss and lethargy). If protein loss is severe (serum albumin concentration <1.0–1.5 g/dL), edema or ascites may occur, but this is relatively uncommon (Table 170–4). If the glomerular disease has caused destruction of 75 per cent or more of the nephrons, clinical signs

URO

TABLE 170–4. SIGNS ASSOCIATED WITH DIFFERENT MANIFESTATIONS OF GLOMERULAR DISEASE

STAGE OF DISEASE	CLINICAL SIGNS	LABORATORY FINDINGS
Mild to moderate proteinuria	Lethargy, mild weight loss, decreased muscle mass	Serum albumin <3.0 mg/dL but >1.5 mg/dL
Marked proteinuria (>3.5 g/d)	Severe muscle wasting; weight gain may occur, however, due to edema or ascites	Serum albumin <1.5 mg/dL Hypercholesterolemia/hyperlipidemia
Renal insufficiency/failure	Depression, anorexia, nausea, vomiting, weight loss, polyuria-polydipsia	Azotemia, isosthenuria or minimally concentrated urine, hyperphosphatemia, non-regenerative anemia
Pulmonary thromboembolism	Acute dyspnea or severe panting and minimal radiographic findings	Hypoxia, normal or low P_{CO_2}, fibrinogen >300 mg/dL, antithrombin III <70% of normal

of acute or chronic renal failure may develop. These include polyuria, polydipsia, anorexia, and vomiting. Occasionally, signs associated with an underlying infectious, inflammatory, or neoplastic disease may be the reason the owner seeks veterinary care. Rarely, dogs may have acute dyspnea or severe panting owing to pulmonary thromboembolism, or emboli may occur in other vessels (e.g., femoral arteries with caudal paresis). This complication has not been reported in cats with glomerular disease. Acute blindness due to retinal detachment may occur secondary to systemic hypertension. In many cases, however, asymptomatic proteinuria is detected on urinalysis during an annual examination or clinical evaluation of another medical problem.

A unique, rapidly progressive form of immune complex glomerulonephritis associated with *Borrelia burgdorferi* infection has been described in dogs.[65, 80] In this syndrome, membranoproliferative glomerulonephritis is accompanied by diffuse tubular necrosis and interstitial inflammation that results in renal failure and death. Affected dogs were younger (5.6 years) compared with dogs with other forms of glomerulonephritis, and Labrador and golden retrievers were 6.4 and 4.9 times more likely, respectively, to develop this lesion.[65]

Clinical findings in amyloidosis depend on the organs affected, the amount of amyloid present, and the reaction of affected organs to the presence of amyloid deposits. In dogs and cats, renal amyloid deposits lead to progressive disease and the observed clinical signs usually are those of chronic renal failure and uremia. Amyloid deposits in other tissues frequently cause no clinical signs. Hepatic involvement may be severe and lead to spontaneous hepatic rupture and peritoneal hemorrhage in Shar Pei dogs[57, 58] and in Oriental and Siamese cats with familial amyloidosis.[60–62]

PHYSICAL FINDINGS

Physical examination findings in dogs and cats with glomerular disease are variable and when present usually are related to chronic renal failure. Weight loss, dehydration, poor haircoat, and oral ulceration may be observed. The kidneys often are small, firm, and irregular in animals with chronic renal failure due to glomerular disease, but they can be normal-sized in non-azotemic, proteinuric animals. Other physical findings may be related to the presence of primary inflammatory or neoplastic diseases. Many affected Shar Pei dogs have a previous history of episodic joint swelling (usually the tibiotarsal joints) and high fever that resolve within a few days, regardless of treatment.[76, 77, 81] This tibiotarsal joint swelling with fever syndrome also has been observed in Shar Pei dogs without documented amyloidosis and resembles familial Mediterranean fever (FMF) in humans.[77, 81] Recently, the gene responsible for FMF in humans has been located on chromosome 16.[82] The gene product is a novel protein named pyrin or marenostrin, is expressed exclusively in granulocytes, and appears to be involved in the downregulation of mediators of inflammation.[83, 84]

DIAGNOSIS OF GLOMERULAR DISEASE

The diagnosis of glomerular disease often is a challenge because the clinical signs can be quite varied. Different glomerular diseases can manifest the same clinical signs, and a specific glomerular disease can manifest different clinical signs in different animals or even different clinical signs in the same individual at different times. Proteinuria is the hallmark clinicopathologic abnormality of glomerular disease, but proteinuria can also be caused by physiologic or pathologic non-renal conditions (Fig. 170–9). Non-glomerular proteinuria usually can be differentiated from glomerular proteinuria on the basis of history, physical examination, and urine sediment analysis. Urinary protein excretion should be quantitated whenever the dipstick method or sulfosalicylic acid test for proteinuria is repeatedly positive and the urine sediment examination is normal or contains hyaline or granular casts.

Calculation of the urine protein/creatinine ratio in dogs and cats using the trichloroacetic acid–Ponceau S or Coomassie brilliant blue tests has been shown to accurately reflect the quantity of protein excreted in the urine over a 24-hour period. This test has greatly facilitated the diagnosis of glomerular disease. Furthermore, the magnitude of proteinuria is roughly correlated with the severity of the underlying glomerular lesion, making the urine protein/creatinine ratio a useful parameter to assess progression of disease or response to therapy.

Daily urinary protein excretion in normal dogs is less than 20 mg/kg. Linear regression studies have demonstrated that multiplying the urine protein/creatinine ratio by 20 (Coomassie brilliant blue method) or 30 (trichloroacetic acid–Ponceau S method) will yield an approximation of the 24-hour urinary protein excretion in milligrams per kilogram per day.[85] A urine protein/creatinine ratio less than 1.0 is considered normal in dogs and cats. Significant proteinuria is usually associated with a urine protein/creatinine ratio of greater than 3.0. A complete urinalysis should be obtained at the time a urine protein/creatinine ratio is evaluated because hematuria or pyuria may result in clinically significant non-glomerular proteinuria. The urine protein/creatinine ratio cannot be used to distinguish pathologic renal proteinuria from post-renal proteinuria caused by infection or hemorrhage.[86, 87]

There does not appear to be a relationship between urinary protein excretion and glomerular filtration rate in dogs with renal disease, but the magnitude of proteinuria is correlated with the nature of the glomerular lesion. Urine protein excretion in dogs with glomerulonephritis usually is greater than in dogs with glomerular atrophy or interstitial nephritis and lower than in dogs with amyloidosis.[64] A mean urine protein/creatinine ratio of 20.4 was observed in 31 dogs with amyloidosis as compared with 11.1 in 106 dogs with glomerulonephritis.[64] In one study, however, dogs with membranous

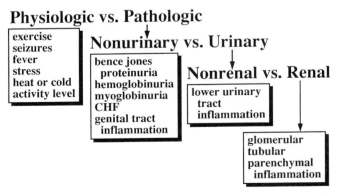

Figure 170–9. Classification scheme for various types of proteinuria. Localization of proteinuria usually can be accomplished by assessing information gained from the history, physical examination, and urine sediment examination.

glomerulonephritis had more severe proteinuria than dogs with amyloidosis,[88] and therefore the urine protein/creatinine ratio cannot be relied on for diagnosis. Moderate to marked proteinuria is common in dogs with amyloidosis because of the predominant glomerular location of the deposits.[55] Proteinuria is mild or absent in animals with medullary amyloidosis without concurrent glomerular involvement. Thus, absence of proteinuria does not rule out a diagnosis of amyloidosis, especially in cats and Shar Pei dogs. Also, if the glomerular disease results in loss of at least three fourths of the nephrons, the accompanying decrease in glomerular filtration rate may decrease the magnitude of the proteinuria.[89]

Hypoalbuminemia occurs in many dogs and cats with glomerular disease. In a recent study of 106 dogs with glomerulonephritis, the average serum albumin concentration was 2.1 g/dL.[64] More severe hypoalbuminemia (<2.1 g/dL) was found in 70 per cent of dogs with amyloidosis.[55] In dogs with amyloidosis, loss of protein by means of the glomeruli probably is the most important factor responsible for hypoalbuminemia. The mechanism presumably is different in cats with renal medullary amyloidosis, because affected cats do not have marked proteinuria.

Other laboratory findings in dogs and cats with renal failure due to glomerular disease include non-regenerative anemia, lymphopenia, azotemia, hyperphosphatemia, hypercholesterolemia, mild hypocalcemia secondary to hypoalbuminemia, mild hyperglycemia due to insulin resistance, and metabolic acidosis. Azotemia may be absent or mild at presentation in approximately 50 per cent of dogs with glomerulonephritis or renal amyloidosis[55, 64] but is commonly observed at presentation in cats and Shar Pei dogs with amyloidosis. When present, azotemia can reflect prerenal (i.e., dehydration) and renal (i.e., >75 per cent loss of nephrons) factors. Isosthenuria is observed in most dogs and cats with chronic renal failure due to glomerular disease. Severe medullary interstitial amyloid deposits, however, may also contribute to defective concentrating ability by their physical presence and lead to interference with urinary concentrating ability before the onset of azotemia. Isosthenuria without proteinuria is common in cats with renal medullary amyloidosis. Hyaline and granular casts are observed commonly in the urine sediment of dogs and cats with glomerular disease.[55, 64]

If persistent proteinuria of renal origin is identified, a renal biopsy is indicated to differentiate glomerular amyloidosis from glomerulonephritis. This distinction is important because glomerulonephritis in dogs and cats may have a variable course characterized by clinical remission or stable renal function for an extended period of time whereas amyloidosis generally is a progressive, fatal disease. Renal biopsy should be considered only after less invasive tests (e.g., complete blood cell count, serum biochemistry profile, urinalysis, urine protein/creatinine ratio, blood pressure measurement, abdominal radiographs, renal ultrasonography) have been performed and an assessment of clotting ability (e.g., buccal mucosal bleeding time, platelet count) has been completed.

The renal cortex should be sampled to obtain an adequate number of glomeruli and to avoid major vessels and nerves in the region of the renal pelvis. Care must be taken in handling and fixation of the renal biopsy specimen to avoid artifactual changes. A Congo red stain should be requested in addition to routine periodic acid–Schiff because small deposits of amyloid can be missed. Regardless of their chemical type, amyloid deposits appear green and birefrin-gent when stained with Congo red and viewed under polarized light (Fig. 170–10). Whenever possible, immunofluorescence or immunoperoxidase staining and electron microscopy should be employed to maximize the information gained from the biopsy specimen. These tests allow for more complete characterization of glomerulonephritis. Biopsy information is also important in establishing a prognosis and formulating a treatment plan. Empirical approaches to treatment without biopsy will add little to our knowledge base about glomerular diseases in dogs and cats.

The renal biopsy not only confirms the diagnosis but also aids in prognostication. In children with lupus nephritis, the initial histologic classification of the biopsy is the most reliable prognostic factor for disease progression.[90] In general, glomerulosclerosis and tubulointerstitial lesions warrant a guarded to poor prognosis. In people with glomerular disease, the degree of glomerular hypertrophy and tubulointerstitial changes are independent risk factors for a poor outcome.[91]

Renal biopsy specimens may be obtained percutaneously using the keyhole technique or by ultrasonographic or laparoscopic guidance. Frequently, however, the best way to obtain a cortical renal biopsy is at laparotomy, when both kidneys can be adequately assessed and treated. A surgical wedge biopsy (2 mm wide by 0.75 to 1 cm long by 3 to 4 mm deep) will include plenty of glomeruli for diagnosis and adequate tissue for immunofluorescent/immunocytochemical techniques as well as electron microscopy. These latter tests should be performed whenever possible to maximize the information gained from the biopsy specimen. It is important to consult with the histopathology laboratory before the biopsy procedure to ensure the proper fixatives are used if specialized microscopy tests are to be performed.

Hemorrhage is the major complication of renal biopsy. Most animals will have microscopic hematuria for 1 to 3 days after the biopsy, and overt hematuria is not uncommon. Severe hemorrhage occurs less than 3 per cent of the time and is almost always associated with faulty biopsy technique. Assessment of blood clotting and a platelet count should always be performed before the biopsy. Contraindications to renal biopsy include a solitary kidney, a coagulopathy, severe systemic hypertension, and renal lesions associated with fluid accumulation (e.g., hydronephrosis renal cysts and abscesses). In addition, a renal biopsy should not be performed by inexperienced clinicians or in animals that are not adequately restrained.

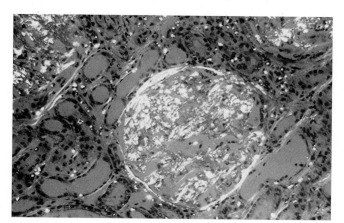

Figure 170–10. Congo red-stained section showing typical birefringence of glomerular amyloid deposits.

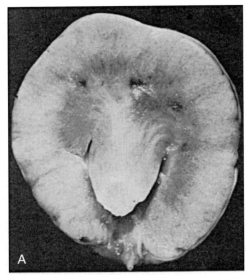

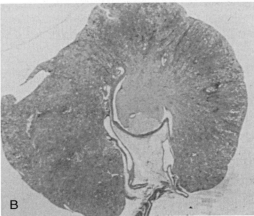

Figure 170–11. Medullary amyloid deposition in a cat leading to papillary necrosis (*A*, gross specimen; *B*, low-power microscopic view).

In dogs other than Shar Pei dogs, amyloidosis is primarily a glomerular disease and can be diagnosed by renal cortical biopsy. In cats, medullary amyloidosis may occur without glomerular involvement and renal cortical biopsies will be negative for amyloidosis. Medullary amyloidosis without discernible glomerular involvement occurs in many cats with amyloidosis, including at least 25 per cent of Abyssinian cats with familial amyloidosis. Medullary amyloidosis without glomerular involvement also occurs in many Shar Pei dogs with familial amyloidosis.[76, 77] In these cases, amyloidosis can be difficult to document clinically unless sufficient medullary tissue is obtained at the time of renal biopsy.

Renal papillary necrosis may occur in cats and Shar Pei dogs with medullary amyloidosis.[75, 76] This lesion is thought to be due to direct interference with blood flow to the inner medulla through the vasa recta by medullary amyloid deposits. It can be observed grossly and in transverse histologic sections of affected kidney (Fig. 170–11). Papillary necrosis was thought to be associated with acute renal failure due to amyloidosis in English foxhounds.[79] Chronic tubulointerstitial lesions (e.g., interstitial fibrosis, lymphoplasmacytic inflammation, tubular atrophy, and dilatation) indicative of end-stage renal disease and of varying severity may be observed in dogs and cats with glomerular disease. Renal involvement predominates in most dogs with amyloidosis,

but small amounts of amyloid may be observed in spleen or liver and occasionally in the gastrointestinal tract, adrenal glands, and pancreas. The extrarenal distribution of amyloid deposits in Abyssinian cats[59] and Shar Pei dogs[76] with familial amyloidosis includes adrenal glands, thyroid glands, spleen, liver, myocardium, gastrointestinal tract, lymph nodes, and pancreas. Tissue deposits in these extrarenal locations usually are clinically silent and cause no readily apparent problems for the affected animal. An important exception to this observation is hepatic amyloid deposition leading to hepatic hemorrhage in Chinese Shar Pei dogs[57, 58] and in Siamese and Oriental shorthair cats.[60–62]

TREATMENT OF GLOMERULAR DISEASE

GLOMERULONEPHRITIS

Ideally, elimination of the source of antigenic stimulation is the primary goal of therapy for glomerulonephritis because the disease is mediated by immunopathogenic mechanisms (Table 170–5). For example, proteinuria associated with dirofilariasis in dogs often improves or resolves after successful treatment of parasitic infection. Unfortunately, elimination of the antigen source often is not possible because the antigen source or underlying disease may not be identified or may be impossible to eliminate (e.g., neoplasia).

Based on results in humans, immunosuppressive drugs have been recommended in dogs and cats with glomerulonephritis. Corticosteroids, azathioprine, chlorambucil, cyclophosphamide, and cyclosporine have been used clinically or experimentally to prevent immunoglobulin production by B cells or to alter the function of T helper or T suppressor cells. Despite widespread use of immunosuppressive agents, there has been only one controlled clinical trial in veterinary medicine assessing the effects of immunosuppressive treatment. In this study, cyclosporine treatment was found to be of no benefit in reducing proteinuria associated with idiopathic glomerulonephritis in dogs.[92] A major factor confounding interpretation of studies designed to assess the efficacy of immunosuppressive drugs in treatment of glomerulonephritis is the variable biologic behavior of different types of glomerulonephritis. In humans, for example, proliferative and membranoproliferative types of glomerulonephri-

TABLE 170–5. TREATMENT GUIDELINES FOR GLOMERULONEPHRITIS

1. Identify and correct any underlying disease processes
2. Immunosuppressive treatment?
   a. Cyclophosphamide, 2.2 mg/kg q24h for 3 or 4 days, and then discontinue for 4 or 3 days, respectively
   b. Azathioprine, 2 mg/kg q24h (dogs only)
   c. Cyclosporine 15 mg/kg q24h (dogs only)
3. Anti-inflammatory—hypercoagulability treatment
   a. Aspirin, 0.5 mg/kg q12–24h
   b. Thromboxane synthetase inhibitors or thromboxane receptor antagonists
   c. Warfarin—titrate dose based on prothrombin time; see text
4. Supportive care
   a. Dietary: sodium restriction, high-quality/low-quantity protein
   b. Hypertension: dietary sodium restriction
      Enalapril, 0.5 mg/kg q12–24h
   c. Edema/ascites: dietary sodium restriction
      Cage rest
      Furosemide, 1–2 mg/kg as needed if necessary—caution: volume contraction and reduced glomerular filtration rate may result
      Paracentesis for patients with tense ascites and/or respiratory distress
      Plasma transfusions?

tis have a poor prognosis as compared with the membranous type.[93, 94]

The association between hyperadrenocorticism or long-term exogenous corticosteroid administration and glomerulonephritis and thromboembolism in the dog, as well as the lack of consistent therapeutic response to corticosteroids, raises questions about use of corticosteroids in dogs with glomerulonephritis. In a retrospective study of dogs with naturally occurring glomerulonephritis, treatment with corticosteroids appeared to be detrimental, leading to azotemia and worsening of proteinuria.[63] Consequently, routine use of corticosteroids to treat glomerulonephritis in dogs is not recommended. Treatment with corticosteroids is indicated, however, if the underlying disease process is known to be steroid responsive (e.g., systemic lupus erythematosus).

Alternatively, or in combination with immunosuppressive drugs, treatment may be aimed at decreasing glomerular inflammation caused by the presence of immune complexes. Increased urinary excretion of thromboxane has been detected in dogs with experimentally induced and spontaneous glomerulonephritis.[95–97] Thromboxane is thought to arise primarily from platelets that are attracted to the glomerulus in immune complex disease. Furthermore, platelet survival is decreased in several types of glomerulonephritis in humans, and platelet depletion attenuates glomerulonephritis.[98] These findings suggest that platelets and thromboxane have an important role in the pathogenesis of glomerulonephritis. Thromboxane synthetase inhibitors decreased proteinuria, glomerular cell proliferation, neutrophil infiltration, and fibrin deposition in dogs with experimental and naturally occurring glomerulonephritis.[95–97]

Dipyridamole, a vasodilator and antiplatelet drug, has also been used successfully in rats and humans to decrease the role of platelets in glomerulonephritis.[99, 100] Aspirin, dipyridamole, and ticlopidine have been used to decrease platelet aggregation in dogs with heartworm disease,[101, 102] but controlled studies assessing the efficacy of these drugs for canine and feline glomerulonephritis are lacking. Appropriate dosage is probably important if nonspecific cyclooxygenase inhibitors such as aspirin are used to decrease glomerular inflammation and platelet aggregation. An extremely low dosage of aspirin (0.25 mg/lb orally once or twice a day) may selectively inhibit platelet cyclooxygenase without preventing the beneficial effects of prostacyclin formation (e.g., vasodilatation, inhibition of platelet aggregation). Treatment of experimentally induced glomerulonephritis in laboratory animals with prostaglandin analogues, leukotriene antagonists, and omega-3 fatty acids to enhance prostaglandin activity also has been successful.[103, 104] Protein-losing glomerular disease in the dog frequently is complicated by systemic hypertension, hypercholesterolemia, and increased platelet aggregation and hypercoagulability. All of these abnormalities could contribute to the development of glomerulosclerosis and a progressive decline in renal function. Omega-3 fatty acid supplementation has been shown to decrease hypertension, serum triglyceride and cholesterol concentrations, and platelet aggregation in humans with nephrotic syndrome.[105, 106]

There is a growing body of evidence indicating that angiotensin-converting enzyme (ACE) inhibitors reduce protein excretion in humans and animals with glomerulonephritis. In dogs with unilateral nephrectomies and experimentally induced diabetes mellitus, ACE inhibitor administration reduced glomerular transcapillary hydraulic pressure and glomerular cell hypertrophy as well as proteinuria.[107] In another study, ACE inhibitor treatment of Samoyed dogs with X-linked hereditary nephritis decreased proteinuria, improved renal excretory function, decreased glomerular basement membrane splitting, and prolonged survival compared with findings in control dogs.[108] In addition, in clinical trials involving humans with glomerulonephritis or chronic renal failure, administration of ACE inhibitors slowed the decline in glomerular filtration rate whether they received placebo or conventional antihypertensive treatment.[109, 110] In one 2-year double-blind prospective study involving 29 non-diabetic proteinuric humans, the short-term antiproteinuric effects of enalapril correlated inversely with the slope of renal functional decline.[111] This observation was confirmed in another long-term study of proteinuric, non-diabetic renal disease in humans[112] and may be important in the identification of patients that will have long-term protection of renal function associated with ACE inhibitor treatment.

Treatment with ACE inhibitors probably decreases proteinuria and preserves renal function associated with glomerular disease by several mechanisms. In dogs, administration of lisinopril decreases efferent glomerular arteriolar resistance, which results in decreased glomerular transcapillary hydraulic pressure and decreased proteinuria.[107] In rats, administration of enalapril prevents the loss of glomerular heparan sulfate that can occur with glomerular disease.[113] Administration of ACE inhibitors also is thought to attenuate proteinuria by decreasing the size of glomerular capillary endothelial cell pores in humans.[114] In addition, the antiproteinuric and renal protective effects of ACE inhibitors may be associated with improved lipoprotein metabolism. Lipid deposition in the glomerular mesangium can contribute to proteinuria and glomerulosclerosis. In humans with nephrotic range proteinuria, administration of ACE inhibitors not only decreases proteinuria but also reduces plasma concentrations of low-density lipoprotein cholesterol and triglycerides.[106, 115] Finally, administration of ACE inhibitors in dogs slows glomerular mesangial cell growth and proliferation that can alter the permeability of the glomerular capillary wall and lead to glomerulosclerosis.[107] Additional controlled trials to assess the efficacy and safety of various treatments for canine and feline glomerulonephritis are needed. Until results of such trials become available, immunosuppressive and anti-inflammatory drugs should be used only after the owner has been informed of the potential risks and lack of proven efficacy of such treatment. If immunosuppressive or anti-inflammatory drugs are used, proteinuria and serum creatinine concentration should be monitored to assess the effect of treatment. In some instances, treatment can exacerbate glomerular lesions and proteinuria.

Supportive therapy should be aimed at alleviating systemic hypertension, decreasing edema or ascites, and reducing the risk of thromboembolism. Sodium-restricted diets (< 0.3 per cent of dry matter) should be employed due to the high frequency of systemic hypertension in animals with glomerular disease. If systemic hypertension is not controlled by dietary sodium restriction, vasodilator therapy should be considered. Angiotensin-converting enzyme inhibitors (e.g., enalapril) usually are recommended as the drugs of choice.

Dogs and cats with edema or ascites should be treated with cage rest and dietary sodium restriction. Paracentesis and diuretics are reserved for animals experiencing respiratory distress and abdominal discomfort. Overzealous use of diuretics may cause dehydration and acute renal decompensation. Plasma transfusions provide only temporary benefit. In the past, dietary protein supplementation was recommended to offset the effects of proteinuria and reduce edema

URO

and ascites. There is concern, however, that normal or high levels of dietary protein may contribute to the progression of renal disease by causing glomerular hyperfiltration, increased proteinuria, and, ultimately, glomerulosclerosis. When humans with glomerulonephritis were fed high-protein diets, albumin synthesis increased, but proteinuria also increased and serum albumin concentration actually decreased.[116] Conversely, restriction of dietary protein in rats with experimentally induced glomerulonephritis resulted in weight loss, but renal function was markedly improved and histologic abnormalities were attenuated. The renin-angiotensin-aldosterone system is modulated by dietary protein, and angiotensin II may be responsible for the increased glomerular permselectivity mediated by dietary protein.[116] Therefore, mild to moderate dietary protein reduction using high-quality protein is recommended (e.g., mildly reduced protein diets used in early chronic renal failure).

Prophylactic therapy with anticoagulants may be beneficial in animals with severe proteinuria, and measurement of antithrombin III and fibrinogen concentrations may identify those at greatest risk of thromboembolism. Dogs with antithrombin III concentrations less than 70 per cent of normal and fibrinogen concentrations greater than 300 mg/dL likely have increased risk for thromboembolism and are candidates for anticoagulation. Coumadins and aspirin have been employed for anticoagulant therapy in proteinuric dogs. Anticoagulant treatment may serve a dual purpose because fibrin accumulation within glomeruli is a frequent and often irreversible consequence of glomerulonephritis.

Warfarin is highly protein bound, and its dosage must be individualized. An initial dosage of 0.1 mg/lb orally once daily has been recommended for dogs.[117] Prothrombin time should be monitored and the dosage of warfarin adjusted so that prothrombin time is maintained at one and one-half times baseline.[117] Prothrombin time should be re-evaluated if marked changes occur in serum albumin concentration or drugs are added to the treatment regimen. This is especially important for drugs that are highly protein bound (e.g., aspirin).

Low-dose aspirin therapy is easily administered on an outpatient basis and does not require extensive monitoring. Quite low doses of aspirin (0.25 mg/lb orally twice daily) have been reported to inhibit platelet aggregation in dogs more effectively than 5 mg/lb orally once daily.[118] It is unclear whether anti-platelet therapy is necessary in cats with glomerular disease, because thromboembolism as a consequence of nephrotic syndrome is rare in this species.

AMYLOIDOSIS

Underlying inflammatory or neoplastic disease processes should be diagnosed and treated if possible. Unfortunately, such treatment is unlikely to alter the course of the disease in animals with established chronic renal failure and uremia. Dehydration should be corrected by appropriate fluid therapy. Renal failure is managed according to the principles of conservative medical treatment (see Chapters 168 and 169). Aggressive cytotoxic therapy using drugs such as chlorambucil, cyclophosphamide, or azathioprine has been beneficial in some humans with reactive amyloidosis, especially those with juvenile rheumatoid arthritis.[50]

Mechanisms by which dimethylsulfoxide (DMSO) may benefit animals with amyloidosis include solubilization of amyloid fibrils, reduction in the serum concentration of the precursor protein SAA, and reduction of interstitial inflammation and fibrosis in the affected kidneys. Solubilization of fibrils probably does not occur to any clinically significant extent because the amount of amyloid in the kidneys of humans who improve clinically after DMSO therapy is unchanged. Reduction of renal interstitial inflammation and fibrosis may result in improvement of renal function and reduction in proteinuria. The side effects of DMSO therapy must be considered before making a treatment decision. Administration of DMSO results in nausea (in humans) and an unpleasant garlic-like odor, which is thought to be due to the metabolite, dimethyl sulfite. These factors may lead to failure of owner compliance and anorexia with decreased water consumption in the affected animal, thus worsening pre-renal azotemia. Peri-vascular inflammation and local thrombosis may occur if undiluted DMSO is administered intravenously.[119] Subcutaneous administration of undiluted DMSO may cause pain. The author has diluted 90 per cent DMSO 1:4 with sterile water before administering it subcutaneously at a dosage of 40 mg/lb three times per week. Whether or not DMSO is beneficial in treatment of renal amyloidosis in dogs remains controversial.

Colchicine impairs the release of SAA from hepatocytes by binding to microtubules and preventing secretion. Colchicine prevents development of amyloidosis in patients with FMF and promotes stabilization of renal function in those with nephrotic syndrome but without overt renal failure.[49, 50, 120, 121] There is no evidence, however, that it is beneficial once amyloidosis has resulted in renal failure. Colchicine is somewhat toxic in humans, and its side effects include vomiting, diarrhea, and nausea.[122] There has been no reported experience with this drug in treatment of dogs and cats with established renal failure due to amyloidosis, although it has been used in some Shar Pei dogs with recurrent fever of unknown origin and hepatic amyloidosis.[57] It is interesting to speculate whether administration of colchicine to Shar Pei dogs with recurrent fever and tibiotarsal joint swelling could prevent development of renal amyloidosis as it does in humans with FMF. It may be reasonable to consider daily treatment with 0.01 to 0.02 mg/lb. This dosage was used safely in a dog with hepatic fibrosis.[123] In humans with FMF, treatment prevents febrile attacks in 65 per cent of patients, partially resolves attacks in 30 per cent, and is ineffective in 5 per cent.[50] Interestingly, colchicine prevents development of amyloidosis even in those patients whose recurrent febrile episodes fail to respond. The dosage of colchicine required in humans may be as high as 1.5 to 2.0 mg/d.[50] Even after the appearance of amyloid deposits, colchicine can cause remission of proteinuria and nephrotic syndrome provided that renal failure has not developed.

Other experimental treatments for amyloidosis include terbutaline and aminophylline to increase cyclic adenosine monophosphate and inhibit amyloid deposition[124] and 4'-iodo-4'-deoxydoxorubicin to inhibit amyloid fibril formation and promote resorption of AL amyloid deposits.[125, 126] These treatments have not been applied to dogs or cats, clinically.

COMPLICATIONS OF GLOMERULAR DISEASE

Consequences of severe urinary protein loss include sodium retention and edema or ascites, hypercholesterolemia, hypertension, hypercoagulability, muscle wasting, and weight loss.

Sodium Retention. The classic explanation for edema or ascites involves activation of the renin-angiotensin-aldosterone system. Decreased plasma oncotic pressure due to hypoalbuminemia allows fluid to escape from the vascular compartment into the interstitial space. This initiates the formation of edema, and the resultant decreased plasma volume and cardiac output stimulate increased renin-angiotensin-aldosterone activity, causing retention of water and salt and further edema formation. Aldosterone concentrations, however, frequently are normal or low in humans with nephrotic syndrome, and treatment with angiotensin-converting enzyme inhibitors does not always prevent sodium retention. It has been hypothesized, therefore, that intrarenal mechanisms, independent of aldosterone, may contribute to sodium retention in patients with glomerular disease (Fig. 170–12). The mechanism of this aldosterone-independent renal sodium retention has been proposed to be either increased sodium reabsorption at the level of the distal nephron or a defect in glomerular filtration of sodium and water.

Hyperlipidemia. Hypercholesterolemia (mean, 312 mg/dL) has been observed in dogs with glomerulonephritis.[64] It has also been observed in 86 per cent of dogs with glomerular amyloidosis.[55] The hypercholesterolemia and hyperlipidemia associated with nephrotic syndrome probably occur due to a combination of increased hepatic synthesis and decreased catabolism of proteins and lipoproteins.[127] Large molecular weight, cholesterol-rich lipoproteins that are not easily lost through the damaged glomerular capillary wall accumulate, whereas smaller molecular weight proteins such as albumin and antithrombin III are lost in the urine. In nephrotic patients, plasma albumin concentrations are inversely correlated with plasma cholesterol concentrations[128] and cholesterol and lipid concentrations tend to increase as albumin concentration decreases. Decreased plasma albumin concentration is thought to stimulate hepatic synthesis of very low density lipoproteins.[129] At the same time, there is decreased hepatic catabolism of lipoproteins associated with abnormal lipoprotein lipase function.

Normal lipoprotein lipase function requires heparin sulfate as a cofactor, and concentrations of heparin sulfate frequently are decreased in nephrotic patients. The decrease in heparin sulfate has been linked to increased urinary loss of another glycoprotein, orosomucoid.[130] Additionally, diversion of necessary sugar intermediates as the liver replaces the lost orosomucoid causes decreased production of heparin sulfate.[131] Orosomucoid has an important role in maintaining glomerular permselectivity by interacting with the capillary charge barrier.[132] Consequently, urinary loss of orosomucoid not only contributes to the hyperlipidemia of the nephrotic syndrome but also exacerbates proteinuria. Renal deposition of lipid is a feature of chronic glomerular disease, and hypercholesterolemia and hyperlipidemia may contribute to further glomerular damage.[127] Mesangial cells that accumulate lipids resemble foam cells observed in atheromatous plaques,[127] and hypercholesterolemia in conjunction with hypertension exacerbates proteinuria and glomerulosclerosis in rats.[133]

Hypertension. Systemic hypertension may occur in dogs and cats with glomerular disease owing to some combination of sodium retention, glomerular vascular fibrosis, impaired release of renal vasodilators, exaggerated responsiveness to normal pressor mechanisms, and activation of the renin-angiotensin system. Systemic hypertension has been associated with immune-mediated glomerulonephritis, glomerulosclerosis, and amyloidosis and may occur in up to 84 per cent of dogs with glomerular disease.[134] Retinal hemorrhage, detachment, and papilledema may result from systemic hypertension and blindness may be the presenting complaint in hypertensive dogs and cats. Blood pressure measurements should be obtained in all animals with suspected glomerular disease because control of systemic hypertension may slow progression of the glomerular disease.

Hypercoagulability. Hypercoagulability and thromboembolism associated with the nephrotic syndrome occur secondary to several abnormalities in the coagulation system. In addition to the mild thrombocytosis often observed in nephrotic patients, platelet hypersensitivity occurs in association with hypoalbuminemia and results in increased platelet adhesion and aggregation. Plasma arachidonic acid normally is protein bound, but more arachidonic acid is free to bind to platelets in the presence of hypoalbuminemia. This may result in increased thromboxane production by platelets and increased platelet aggregation. Platelets from humans with glomerular disease have increased capacity to generate thromboxane. Hypercholesterolemia also may contribute to platelet hyperaggregability by altering platelet membrane composition or affecting platelet adenylate cyclase response to prostaglandins. Loss of antithrombin III (molecular weight, 65,000 daltons) in urine also results in hypercoagulability. Antithrombin III acts in concert with heparin to inhibit serine proteases (clotting factors II, IX, X, XI, and XII) and normally has a vital role in modulating thrombin and fibrin production. Finally, altered fibrinolysis and increases in the concentration of large molecular weight coagulation factors (factors II, V, VII, VIII, and X) may lead to a relative increase in coagulation factors as compared with regulatory proteins.

The pulmonary arteries are the most common site for thromboembolism (Fig. 170–13), but emboli also may lodge in mesenteric, renal, iliac, coronary, and brachial arteries, as well as in the portal vein. Dogs with pulmonary thromboembolism are usually dyspneic and hypoxic with minimal pulmonary parenchymal radiographic abnormalities. Treatment of pulmonary thromboembolism is difficult, expensive, and frequently unrewarding; therefore, early prophylactic treatment is important.

PROGNOSIS FOR GLOMERULONEPHRITIS

The prognosis for dogs and cats with glomerulonephritis is variable and is best based on a combination of factors,

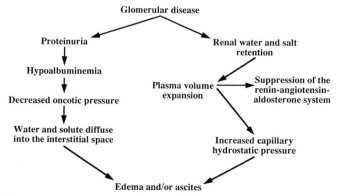

Figure 170–12. Theory of edema formation in nephrotic patients. This theory involves suppression of the renin-angiotensin-aldosterone system.

URO

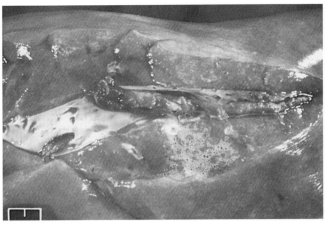

Figure 170–13. Thrombus in the main pulmonary artery of a dog with glomerulonephritis and nephrotic syndrome.

including severity of renal dysfunction (e.g., magnitude of proteinuria, presence or absence of azotemia), assessment of renal histology, and response to therapy. Clinical experience suggests that glomerulonephritis is progressive in many instances. In cats with membranous glomerulonephritis, there may be slow or rapid progression of renal disease, prolonged remissions, or complete recovery.[135] Except for uremia, clinical signs in cats were not helpful prognostic indicators, but intramembranous and subepithelial immune complexes containing IgA or IgM were associated with a less favorable long-term prognosis.[135] In a retrospective study of dogs with glomerulonephritis, mean survival time was 87 days, regardless of treatment.[64] In humans, histologic evidence of proliferative or membranoproliferative glomerulonephritis as well as azotemia, anemia, and hypertension are findings associated with a less favorable prognosis.[93, 94, 136, 137] The prognosis for dogs and cats with renal amyloidosis is uniformly poor. It is a progressive disease leading to chronic renal failure and uremia. In one study of dogs with renal amyloidosis, survival times were available for 12 animals and ranged from 2 to 20 months,[55] whereas in another study survival time for 25 dogs averaged only 49 days.[64]

REFERENCES

1. Grauer GF, et al: Experimental *Dirofilaria immitis*–associated glomerulonephritis induced in part by *in situ* formation of immune complexes in the glomerular capillary wall. J Parasitol 75:585, 1989.
2. Merkel F, et al: T cell involvement in glomerular injury. Kidney Blood Press Res 19:298, 1996.
3. Nagamatsu T, et al: Thromboxane A2 interferes with disposal process of aggregated protein in glomeruli. Jpn J Pharmacol 75:381, 1997.
4. Katoh T, et al: Leukotriene D₄ is a mediator of proteinuria and glomerular hemodynamic abnormalities in passive Heymann nephritis. J Clin Invest 91:1507, 1993.
5. Badr KF: Five-lipooxygenase products in glomerular injury. J Am Soc Nephrol 3:907, 1992.
6. Spurney RF, et al: Enhanced renal leukotriene production in murine lupus: Role of lipoxygenase metabolites. Kidney Int 39:95, 1991.
7. Lefkowith JB, et al: Urinary eicosanoids and the assessment of glomerular inflammation. J Am Soc Nephrol 2:1560, 1992.
8. Wardle EN: Advances in pharmacology and therapy of nephritides. Nephron 66:129, 1994.
9. Ostendorf T, et al: Cytokines and glomerular injury. Kidney Blood Press Res 19:281, 1996.
10. Taniguchi Y, et al: Role of transforming growth factor beta-1 in glomerulonephritis. J Int Med Res 25:71, 1997.
11. Ortiz A, et al: The role of platelet-activating factor (PAF) in experimental glomerular injury. Lipids 26:1310, 1991.
12. Feucht HE: Role of complement in glomerular injury. Kidney Blood Press Res 19:290, 1996.
13. Cybulsky AV: Release of arachidonic acid by complement C5b-9 complex in glomerular epithelial cells. Am J Physiol 261:F427, 1991.
14. Couser WG: Mediation of immune glomerular injury. Am J Nephrol 1:13, 1991.
15. Rohrmoser MM, Mayer G: Reactive oxygen species and glomerular injury. Kidney Blood Press Res 19:263, 1996.
16. Johnson RJ, et al: Oxidants in glomerular injury. *In* Wilson CB, Brenner BM, Stein J (eds): Contemporary Issues in Nephrology, vol 18. New York, Churchill Livingstone, 1988, p 87.
17. Cook HT, Sullivan R: Glomerular nitrite synthesis in *in situ* immune complex glomerulonephritis in the rat. Am J Pathol 139:1047, 1991.
18. Wagrowska-Danilewicz M, Danilewicz M: A study of apoptosis in human glomerulonephritis as determined by in situ non-radioactive labelling of DNA strand breaks. Acta Histochemica 99:257, 1997.
19. Sagar S, et al: Glomerular metalloprotease activity modulates the development of focal segmental glomerulosclerosis. Clin Nephrol 44:356, 1995.
20. Morita Y, et al: The role of complement in the pathogenesis of tubulointerstitial lesions in rat mesangial proliferative glomerulonephritis. J Am Soc Nephrol 8:1363, 1997.
21. Eddy AA: Experimental insights into the tubulointerstitial disease accompanying primary glomerular lesions. J Am Soc Nephrol 5:1273, 1994.
22. Alfrey AC, et al: Role of iron in tubulointerstitial injury in nephrotoxic serum nephritis. Kidney Int 36:753, 1989.
23. Brown SA, et al: Dietary protein intake and the glomerular adaptations to partial nephrectomy in dogs. J Nutr 121:S125, 1991.
24. Nagashima R, et al: *Helicobacter pylori* antigen in the glomeruli of patients with membranous nephropathy. Virchows Arch 431:235, 1997.
25. Sipe JD: Amyloidosis. Annu Rev Biochem 61:947, 1992.
26. Husby G: Amyloidosis. Semin Arthritis Rheum 22:67, 1992.
27. Hawkins PN: Amyloidosis. Blood Rev 9:135, 1995.
28. Bellotti V, Merlini G: Current concepts on the pathogenesis of systemic amyloidosis. Nephrol Dial Transplant 11:53, 1996.
29. Falk RH, et al: The systemic amyloidoses. N Engl J Med 337:898, 1997.
30. van Andel ACJ, et al: Amyloid in the horse: A report of nine cases. Equine Vet J 20:277, 1988.
31. Shaw DP, et al: Nasal amyloidosis in four horses. Vet Pathol 24:183, 1987.
32. Johnson KH, et al: Islet amyloid, islet amyloid polypeptide and diabetes mellitus. N Engl J Med 321:513, 1989.
33. Ishihara T, et al: Immunohistochemical and immunoelectron microscopical characterization of cerebrovascular and senile plaque amyloid in aged dogs' brains. Brain Res 548:196, 1991.
34. Johnson KH, et al: Pulmonary vascular amyloidosis in aged dogs: A new form of spontaneously-occurring amyloidosis derived from apolipoprotein AI. Am J Pathol 141:1013, 1992.
35. Roertgen KE, et al: Apolipoprotein AI–derived pulmonary vascular amyloid in aged dogs. Am J Pathol 147:1311, 1995.
36. DiBartola SP, et al: Isolation and characterization of amyloid protein AA in the Abyssinian cat. Lab Invest 52:485, 1985.
37. Johnson KH, et al: AA amyloidosis in Chinese Shar-Pei dogs: Immunohistochemical and amino acid sequence analysis: Amyloid. Int J Exp Clin Invest 2:92, 1995.
38. Carothers MA, et al: Extramedullary plasmacytoma and immunoglobulin-associated amyloidosis in a cat. JAVMA 195:1593, 1989.
39. Giesel O, et al: Myeloma associated with immunoglobulin lambda-light chain derived amyloid in a dog. Vet Pathol 27:374, 1990.
40. Schwartzman RM: Cutaneous amyloidosis associated with a monoclonal gammopathy in a dog. JAVMA 185:102, 1984.
41. Benson MD, et al: A unique insertion in the primary structure of bovine amyloid AA protein. J Lab Clin Med 113:67, 1989.
42. Benson MD, et al: Identification and characterization of amyloid protein AA in spontaneous canine amyloidosis. Lab Invest 52:448, 1985.
43. Sletten K, et al: The amino acid sequence of an amyloid fibril protein AA isolated from the horse. Scand J Immunol 26:79, 1987.
44. Sellar GC, et al: Dog serum amyloid A protein: Identification of multiple isoforms defined by cDNA and protein analyses. J Biol Chem 266:3505, 1991.
45. Maury CPJ, et al: Serum amyloid A protein (SAA) subtypes in acute and chronic inflammation. Ann Rheum Dis 44:711, 1985.
46. Kisilevsky R, Young ID: Pathogenesis of amyloidosis. Baillieres Clin Rheumatol 8:613, 1994.
47. Husebekk A, et al: Transformation of amyloid precursor SAA to protein AA and incorporation in amyloid fibrils *in vivo*. Scand J Immunol 21:283, 1985.
48. Brandewein SR, et al: Effect of colchicine on experimental amyloidosis in two CBA/J mouse models. Lab Invest 52:319, 1985.
49. Zemer D, et al: Colchicine in the prevention and treatment of amyloidosis of familial Mediterranean fever. N Engl J Med 314:1001, 1986.
50. Tan SY, et al: Treatment of amyloidosis. Am J Kidney Dis 26:267, 1995.
51. Piirsalu K, et al: Role of I-123 serum amyloid protein in the detection of familial amyloidosis in Oriental cats. J Small Anim Pract 35:581, 1994.
52. Fuks A, Zucker-Franklin D: Impaired Kupffer cell function precedes development of secondary amyloidosis. J Exp Med 161:1013, 1985.
53. Bausserman LL, Herbert PN: Degradation of serum amyloid A and apolipoproteins by serum proteases. Biochemistry 23:2241, 1984.
54. DiBartola SP, Benson MD: Review: The pathogenesis of reactive systemic amyloidosis. J Vet Intern Med 3:31, 1989.

55. DiBartola SP, et al: Clinicopathologic findings in dogs with renal amyloidosis: 59 cases (1976–1986). JAVMA 195:358, 1989.
56. Edwards DF, et al: Primary ciliary dyskinesia in the dog. Probl Vet Med 4:291, 1992.
57. Loeven K: Hepatic amyloidosis in two Chinese Shar Pei dogs. JAVMA 204:1212, 1993.
58. Loeven KO: Spontaneous hepatic rupture secondary to amyloidosis in a Chinese Shar pei. J Am Anim Hosp Assoc 30:577, 1994.
59. DiBartola SP, et al: Tissue distribution of amyloid deposits in Abyssinian cats with familial amyloidosis. J Comp Pathol 96:387, 1986.
60. Blunden AS, Smith KC: Generalized amyloidosis and acute liver hemorrhage in four cats. J Small Anim Pract 33:566, 1992.
61. Zuber RM: Systemic amyloidosis in Oriental and Siamese cats. Aust Vet Pract 23:66, 1993.
62. van der Linde-Sipman JS, et al: Generalized AA-amyloidosis in Siamese and Oriental cats. Vet Immunol Immunopathol 56:1, 1997.
63. Center SA, et al: Clinicopathologic, renal immunofluorescent, and light microscopic features of glomerulonephritis in the dog: 41 cases. JAVMA 190:81, 1987.
64. Cook AK, Cowgill LD: Clinical and pathological features of protein-losing glomerular disease in the dog—a review of 137 cases (1985–1992). J Am Anim Hosp Assoc 32:313, 1996.
65. Dambach DM, et al: Morphologic, immunohistochemical, and ultrastructural characterization of a distinctive renal lesion in dogs putatively associated with Borrelia burgdorferi infection: 49 cases (1987–1992). Vet Pathol 34:85, 1997.
66. DiBartola SP, Rutgers HC: Diseases of the kidney. In Sherding RG (ed): The Cat: Diseases and Clinical Management, 2nd ed. New York, Churchill Livingstone, 1994.
67. Picut CA, Lewis RM: Juvenile renal disease in the Doberman pinscher: Ultrastructural changes of the glomerular basement membrane. J Comp Pathol 97:587, 1987.
68. Cook SM, et al: Renal failure attributable to atrophic glomerulopathy in four related Rottweilers. JAVMA 202:107, 1993.
69. Carpenter JL, et al: Idiopathic cutaneous and renal glomerular vasculopathy of greyhounds. Vet Pathol 25:401, 1988.
70. Reusch C, et al: A new familial glomerulonephropathy in Bernese mountain dogs. Vet Rec 134:411, 1994.
71. Littman MP, Giger U: Familial protein-losing enteropathy (PLE) and/or protein-losing nephropathy (PLN) in soft-coated Wheaten terriers. In Proceedings of the 8th ACVIM Forum, Washington, DC, 1990, p 1135.
72. Ross LA: Feline renal failure. In Breitschwerdt EB (ed): Contemporary Issues in Small Animal Practice: Nephrology and Urology. New York, Churchill Livingstone, 1986, p 109.
73. Lees GE, et al: Glomerular ultrastructural findings similar to hereditary nephritis in 4 English Cocker Spaniels. J Vet Intern Med 11:80, 1997.
74. Bowles MH, Mosier DA: Renal amyloidosis in a family of beagles. JAVMA 201:569, 1992.
75. Boyce JT, et al: Familial renal amyloidosis in Abyssinian cats. Vet Pathol 21:33, 1984.
76. DiBartola SP, et al: Familial renal amyloidosis in Chinese Shar pei dogs. JAVMA 197:483, 1990.
77. Rivas AL, et al: A canine febrile disorder associated with elevated interleukin-6. Clin Immunol Immunopathol 64:36, 1992.
78. Rivas AL, et al: Inheritance of renal amyloidosis in Chinese Shar pei dogs. J Hered 84:438, 1993.
79. Mason NJ, Day MJ: Renal amyloidosis in related English foxhounds. J Small Anim Pract 37:255, 1996.
80. Grauer GF, et al: Renal lesions associated with Lyme borreliosis in a dog. JAVMA 193:237, 1988.
81. May C, et al: Chinese Shar pei fever syndrome: A preliminary report. Vet Rec 131:586, 1992.
82. Babior BM, Matzner Y: The familial Mediterranean fever gene-cloned at last. N Engl J Med 337:1548, 1997.
83. Ben-Chetrit E, Levy M: Familial Mediterranean fever. Lancet 351:659, 1998.
84. Pras M: Familial Mediterranean fever: From the clinical syndrome to the cloning of the pyrin gene. Scand J Rheumatol 27:92, 1998.
85. Lulich JP, Osborne CA: Interpretation of urine protein-creatinine ratios in dogs with glomerular and non-glomerular disorders. Compend Contin Ed Pract Vet 12:59, 1990.
86. Bagley RS, et al: The effect of experimental cystitis and iatrogenic blood contamination on the urine protein/creatinine ratio in the dog. J Vet Intern Med 5:66, 1991.
87. Myers NC, et al: The influence of naturally-occurring urinary tract infections on the urine protein/creatinine ratio in dogs (abstract). J Vet Intern Med 7:126, 1993.
88. Biewenga WJ: Proteinuria in the dog: A clinicopathological study in 51 proteinuric dogs. Res Vet Sci 41:257, 1986.
89. Jaenke RS, Allen TA: Membranous nephropathy in the dog. Vet Pathol 23:718, 1986.
90. Baqi N, et al: Lupus nephritis in children: A longitudinal study of prognostic factors and therapy. J Am Soc Nephrol 6:924, 1996.
91. Shiiki H, et al: Clinical and morphological predictors of renal outcome in adult patients with focal and segmental glomerulosclerosis. Clin Nephrol 46:362, 1996.

92. Vaden SL, et al: The effects of cyclosporin versus standard care in dogs with naturally occurring glomerulonephritis. J Vet Intern Med 9:259, 1995.
93. Bohle A, et al: The long-term prognosis of the primary glomerulonephritides. Pathol Res Pract 188:908, 1992.
94. McCurdy DK, et al: Lupus nephritis: Prognostic factors in children. Pediatrics 89:240, 1992.
95. Longhofer SL, et al: Effects of thromboxane synthetase inhibition on immune complex glomerulonephritis. Am J Vet Res 52:480, 1991.
96. Grauer GF, et al: Effects of a thromboxane synthetase inhibitor on established immune complex glomerulonephritis in dogs. Am J Vet Res 53:808, 1992.
97. Grauer GF, et al: Treatment of membranoproliferative glomerulonephritis and nephrotic syndrome in a dog with a thromboxane synthetase inhibitor. J Vet Intern Med 6:77, 1992.
98. Johnson RJ, et al: Platelets mediate neutrophil-dependent immune complex nephritis in the rat. J Clin Invest 82:1225, 1988.
99. Camara S, et al: Effects of dipyridamole on the short term evolution of glomerulonephritis. Nephron 58:13, 1991.
100. De La Cruz JP, et al: Effect of dipyridamole with or without aspirin on urine protein excretion in patients with membranous glomerulonephritis. Eur J Clin Pharmacol 43:307, 1992.
101. Boudreaux MK, et al: Effects of treatment with aspirin or aspirin/dipyridamole combination in heartworm-negative, heartworm-infected, and embolized heartworm-infected dogs. Am J Vet Res 52:1992, 1991.
102. Boudreaux MK, et al: Effects of treatment with ticlopidine in heartworm-negative, heartworm-infected, and embolized heartworm-infected dogs. Am J Vet Res 52:2000, 1991.
103. Donaidio JV, et al: Omega-3 polyunsaturated fatty acids: A potential new treatment of immune renal disease. Mayo Clin Proc 66:1018, 1991.
104. Badr KF: 15-Lipoxygenase products as leukotriene antagonists: Therapeutic potential in glomerulonephritis. Kidney Int 42(Suppl 38):101, 1992.
105. Hall AV, et al: Omega-3 fatty acid supplementation in primary nephrotic syndrome: Effects on plasma lipids and coagulopathy. J Am Soc Nephrol 3:1321, 1992.
106. Appel LJ, et al: Does supplementation of diet with fish oil reduce blood pressure? A meta-analysis of controlled clinical trials. Arch Intern Med 153:1429, 1993.
107. Brown SA, et al: Long-term effects of antihypertensive regimens on renal hemodynamics and proteinuria. Kidney Int 43:1210, 1993.
108. Grodecki KM, et al: Treatment of X-linked hereditary nephritis in Samoyed dogs with angiotensin converting enzyme (ACE) inhibitor. J Comp Pathol 117:209, 1997.
109. Ihle B, et al: The effect of converting enzyme inhibition (ACEI) on progression chronic renal insufficiency. J Am Soc Nephrol 33:284, 1992.
110. Kamper A, et al: Effect of enalapril on the progression of chronic renal failure: A randomized controlled trial. Am J Hypertension 5:423, 1992.
111. Apperloo AJ, et al: Short-term antiproteinuric response to antihypertensive treatment predicts long-term GFR decline in patients with non-diabetic renal disease. Kidney Int 45:S174, 1994.
112. Gansevoort RT, et al: Long-term benefits of the antiproteinuric effect of angiotensin-converting enzyme inhibition in nondiabetic renal disease. Am J Kidney Dis 22:202, 1993.
113. Erhley CM, et al: Renal hemodynamics and reduction of proteinuria by a vasodilating beta blocker versus an ACE inhibitor. Kidney Int 41:1297, 1992.
114. Morelli E, et al: Effects of converting-enzyme inhibition on barrier function in diabetic glomerulonephropathy. Diabetes 39:76, 1990.
115. Keilani T, et al: Improvement of lipid abnormalities associated with proteinuria using fosinopril and angiotensin-converting enzyme inhibitor. Ann Intern Med 118:246, 1993.
116. Kaysen GA: Albumin metabolism in nephrotic syndrome: The effect of dietary protein intake. Am J Kidney Dis 12:461, 1988.
117. Loughman C, et al: Warfarin therapy in dogs and comparison of coagulation parameters for monitoring therapy (abstract). J Vet Intern Med 7:129, 1993.
118. Rackear DG, et al: The effect of three different dosages of acetylsalicylic acid on canine platelet aggregation. J Am Anim Hosp Assoc 24:23, 1988.
119. Spyridakis L, et al: Amyloidosis in a dog: Treatment with dimethylsulfoxide. JAVMA 189:000, 1986.
120. Majeed HA, Barakat M: Familial Mediterranean fever (recurrent hereditary polyserositis) in children: Analysis of 88 cases. Eur J Pediatr 148:636, 1989.
121. Famaey JP: Colchicine in therapy: State of the art and new perspectives for an old drug. Clin Exp Rheumatol 6:303, 1988.
122. Levy M, et al: Colchicine: A state-of-the-art review. Pharmacotherapy 11:196, 1991.
123. Boer HH, Nelson RW: Colchicine therapy for hepatic fibrosis in a dog. JAVMA 185:303, 1984.
124. Brandwein S, et al: Combined treatment with terbutaline and aminophylline inhibits experimental amyloidosis in mice. Arthritis Rheum 37:1757, 1994.
125. Gianni L, et al: New drug therapy of amyloidoses: Resorption of AL-type deposits with 4'-iodo-4'-deoxydoxorubicin. Blood 86:855, 1995.
126. Merlini G, et al: Interaction of the anthracycline 4'-iodo-4'-deoxydoxorubicin with amyloid fibrils: Inhibition of amyloidogenesis. In Proceedings of the National Academy of Sciences U S A 92:2959, 1995.
127. Wheeler DC, et al: Hyperlipidemia in nephrotic syndrome. Am J Nephrol 9(Suppl):78, 1989.

URO

128. Ballmer PE, et al: Elevation of albumin synthesis rates in nephrotic patients measured with [l-^{13}C] leucine. Kidney Int 41:132, 1992.
129. Appel GB, et al: The hyperlipidemia of the nephrotic syndrome: Relation to plasma albumin concentration, oncotic pressure, and viscosity. N Engl J Med 312:1544, 1985.
130. Kaysen GA: Hyperlipidemia in the nephrotic syndrome. Am J Kidney Dis 12:548, 1988.
131. Kaysen GA, et al: Mechanisms and consequences of proteinuria. Lab Invest 54:479, 1986.
132. Haraldsson BS, et al: Glomerular permselectivity is dependent on adequate serum concentrations of orosomucoid. Kidney Int 41:310, 1992.
133. Tolins JP, et al: Interactions of hypercholesterolemia and hypertension in initiation of glomerular injury. Kidney Int 41:1254, 1992.
134. Cowgill LD: Clinical significance, diagnosis and management of systemic hypertension in dogs and cats: Managing Renal Disease and Hypertension. Topeka, Hill's Pet Products and Harmon Smith, 1991, p 35.
135. Arthur JE, et al: The long-term prognosis of feline idiopathic membranous glomerulonephropathy. J Am Anim Hosp Assoc 1986:731, 1986.
136. Widstam-Attrops U, et al: Proteinuria and renal function in relation to renal morphology. Clin Nephrol 38:245, 1992.
137. Levey AS, et al: Progression and remission of renal disease in the lupus nephritis collaborative study. Ann Intern Med 116:114, 1992.

CHAPTER 171

BACTERIAL INFECTIONS OF THE URINARY TRACT

Gerald V. Ling

By definition, urinary tract infection (UTI) is present when bacteria can be demonstrated in renal, ureteral, or bladder urine, because urine that is stored in the bladder, and urine that is presented to it from the kidneys, is bacteriologically sterile in normal animals. Use of the term UTI is more appropriate than use of more specific terms (cystitis, pyelonephritis) and connotes the lack of successful attempts to localize the infection within the tract to the level of the bladder or the kidneys. Localization of UTI is a time-consuming and often difficult process in dogs, but it can be accomplished in this species by means of percutaneous nephropyelocentesis[1] and culture of the specimen, by urinary bladder washout studies,[2, 3] or by measurement of certain enzymes that are elaborated into the urine when the kidneys have sustained cellular damage from infection, trauma, ischemia, or toxic insult.[4, 5] There is no clinical reason to attempt localization, however, because knowledge of the location of the infection within the tract does not alter the selection of the antimicrobial agent, the dose used, the duration of therapy (usually), or the follow-up regimen. Exceptions to this generalization occur in intact male dogs with UTI in which the infection has extended to the prostate and in dogs of either gender that have unilateral renal abscess.

In human beings, UTI usually is accompanied by signs and symptoms that indicate the presence of infection (e.g., a feeling of malaise accompanied by urgency to void, hematuria, increased frequency of voiding), fever, and localized flank (renal) pain when pyelonephritis is present. Some dogs with UTI have signs of pollakiuria, hematuria, or foul-smelling urine, but rarely do they have fever or evidence of renal pain during abdominal palpation, nor do they act depressed. Unfortunately, approximately 80 per cent of dogs and an undetermined percentage of cats have no clinically observable signs whatsoever when they have UTI. Therefore, the diagnosis of UTI in dogs and cats must be made in the laboratory from results of careful microscopic examination of the urine sediment followed by results of bacterial culture of the urine.

It has been inferred that UTI in dogs and cats may have no clinical significance unless there is evidence of response to the infection by increased numbers of white blood cells (WBCs) in the urine sediment, and unless clinical signs are present. However, it must be remembered that the host-parasite interactions in UTI are influenced by many factors that affect the response of the animal to the infection. Some animals that have diseases such as diabetes mellitus or hyperadrenocorticism, or that are receiving corticosteroids or antineoplastic drugs, are not able to mount a consistent urinary WBC response to UTI. Moreover, certain bacteria (e.g., *Pseudomonas* spp. in males, *Streptococcus* spp. in females) do not invoke a urinary WBC response in all dogs and cats. A urinary WBC response may be inapparent in animals that produce quite dilute urine, because the number of urine WBCs may be reduced to nonsignificance by dilution. The magnitude of a urinary WBC response to UTI also seems to be variable at different times within the same animal. If several urine specimens are examined from a single animal with UTI, sometimes there will be excessive WBCs in the sediment, and sometimes the number of WBCs will be within the accepted normal range.

Urinary infections, whether they occur as single episodes, recurrent episodes, or persistent infections, can be associated with significant sequelae regardless of whether clinical signs are present or absent. The sequelae in both dogs and cats include struvite ($MgNH_4PO_4 \cdot 6H_2O$) urolithiasis in cases of UTI that are caused by *Staphylococcus intermedius*. In intact male dogs, UTI can extend to the prostate and is thought to be the most common source of bacteria in prostatitis. Pyelonephritis with progressive renal scarring and eventual renal failure may be a sequel to long-standing UTI that has been clinically inapparent until signs of renal failure are observed. UTIs can extend to the spermatic cords and testicles of male dogs and may be a cause of infertility in both males and females. Septicemia and death can result when large doses of immune-suppressive agents are given to dogs with clinically inapparent UTI. In one study, 39 per cent of dogs that received long-term corticosteroid therapy for chronic skin diseases developed UTI as a complication during treatment.[6] Lumbosacral discospondylitis is thought to be secondary to UTI in some instances.

At the current state of our knowledge, it is not possible to say that UTI caused by organism "A" should be treated, whereas infection caused by organism "B" may be ignored. Also, clinical signs of UTI or the lack thereof is not an adequate predictor of morbidity and cannot be used with confidence in decisions regarding whether to treat. Early recognition, proper treatment, and vigorous follow-up of all UTIs in dogs and cats regardless of the species of the infecting bacteria, the presence or absence of clinical signs, or the number of WBCs in the urine sediment are, therefore, strongly recommended. The serious consequences of UTI are nearly always preventable if the infection is recognized early and is treated properly. Therefore, it is important to conduct a complete urinalysis, including a careful urine sediment examination, as part of any routine or baseline laboratory studies and to collect the urine in such a way as to virtually eliminate the possibility of contamination of the specimen with WBCs and bacteria from the urethra or from outside the urinary tract (e.g., vagina or prepuce) so that an accurate assessment of the presence or absence of UTI can be made.

UTI is thought to be the most common infectious disease in dogs. It has been estimated that as many as 10 per cent of all canine patients that are seen by veterinarians for any reason have UTI in addition to the problems for which they are presented.[7] In one study, female dogs had about 57 per cent of the episodes of UTI and males about 43 per cent.[8] Nine bacterial genera accounted for 95.3 per cent of the urinary infections: *Escherichia coli* (44.1 per cent), *Staphylococcus* spp. (11.6 per cent), *Proteus* spp. (9.3 per cent), *Klebsiella* spp. (9.1 per cent), *Enterococcus* spp. (8 per cent), *Streptococcus* spp. (5.4 per cent), *Pseudomonas* spp. (3 per cent), *Mycoplasma* spp. (2.5 per cent), and *Enterobacter* spp. (2.3 per cent). Females predominated in infections with all these genera except for *Klebsiella* spp., *Mycoplasma* spp., and *Enterobacter* spp., in which males predominated. Age at diagnosis of UTI tended to be similar between genders. Infection with a single bacterial species was responsible for more than 72 per cent of UTI in both genders; two or three bacterial isolates were present in about 28 per cent. Differences appeared to exist with regard to the prevalence of the various bacterial species among breeds of dogs, among ages within individual breeds, and between genders within individual breeds.[8]

Bacterial infection of the urinary tract occurs occasionally in cats. The prevalence of UTI in the feline population is not known but has been estimated to be in the range of 0.1 to 1 per cent,[7] at least 10 times less than the estimated prevalence of UTI in dogs. As in dogs, cats often do not have clinical signs when UTI is present. Cats with dysuria, pollakiuria, and hematuria—signs that have been characterized as feline urologic syndrome (FUS)—usually, but not always, have bacteriologically sterile bladder urine. The consequences of UTI in cats are similar to those in dogs, except that prostatitis, orchitis, septicemia, and discospondylitis are not recognized sequelae of UTI in cats.

Bacteria belonging to nine different genera cause nearly 99 per cent of bacterial UTI in cats.[9] *Escherichia coli*, the most prevalent species, accounts for about 52 per cent of the infections. Following in descending order of prevalence are *Staphylococcus* spp. (19 per cent), *Streptococcus/Enterococcus* spp. (12.5 per cent), *Klebsiella* spp. (5 per cent), *Proteus* spp. (4 per cent), *Mycoplasma* spp. and *Pasteurella* spp. (2 per cent each), and *Pseudomonas* spp. and *Enterobacter* spp. (1 per cent each). Fifty-five per cent of the cats in one study were males, and 45 per cent were females. Male cats probably have more UTIs than do females, partially as a result of passage of urethral catheters in males that have blocked or partially blocked urethras secondary to FUS. Also, there seems to be an increased prevalence of UTI in male cats that have undergone perineal urethrostomy.[10]

PATHOGENESIS

The prepuce and vagina are thought to be the primary portals of entry of uropathogenic bacteria in dogs and cats. Urinary bacterial pathogens, usually of fecal origin, are thought to attach themselves to epithelial cells at these sites, colonize there, and ascend the urethra from that point. These bacteria have special properties, called virulence factors, that enable them to adhere to and colonize the urinary tract.[11] The virulence factors include (1) special attachment (adherence) structures that protrude from the surface of certain bacteria, which enable them to attach to specific molecular sequences on the surface of uroepithelial cells; (2) secretion by certain bacteria of a compound called aerobactin, which extracts essential iron for use in bacterial metabolism from host iron-binding proteins; (3) hemolysin, a substance secreted by certain bacteria that causes injury to host cells, increases inflammation, and impairs certain host defenses; and (4) secretion of a bacterial polysaccharide capsular material that inhibits phagocytosis of the bacteria by host cells. These and other virulence factors have been most extensively studied in *E. coli* and were the subject of an in-depth review.[12]

Host defense mechanisms that protect the external urethral orifice from bacterial invasion have been of great interest to urologists for many years. Passage of a normal stream of urine (i.e., passive washout), the secretion of vaginal and preputial mucus, and the local secretion of immunoglobulin A (IgA) all seem to play a role in prevention of bacterial invasion of the urinary tract in human beings. It may be assumed that they play a similar role in dogs and cats, although conclusive evidence of this has not been gathered in these species. Several species of bacteria inhabit the prepuce, vagina, and distal urethra of dogs and cats.[13–15] The presence of these normal flora also may play a protective role in preventing uropathogenic bacteria from colonizing these sites, but this is somewhat speculative. Instrumentation of the tract with urinary catheters and endoscopic apparatus plays a large role in introducing bacteria into the bladder. The mere fact of passing a catheter is associated with risk of UTI (especially in female dogs) because of the passive transport of organisms past the protective barrier at the external urethral orifice.[16]

DIAGNOSTIC METHODS

Specimen Collection and Handling Methods. Complete urinalysis, including microscopic examination of the urine sediment, is an inexpensive, rapid, and relatively accurate method of ascertaining the presence or absence of UTI.[17] However, one simple but often overlooked aspect of speci-

URO

men collection is of the utmost importance in accurately diagnosing UTI in dogs and cats. In order to achieve acceptable accuracy, the urine specimen must be obtained in a manner that virtually eliminates the possibility of contamination of the specimen with WBCs or bacteria from the urethra, vagina, or prepuce. Both resident and transient bacteria may act as contaminants when urine specimens are collected by catheterization of the bladder or by sampling of the urine during voiding. The concept of "significant bacteriuria" (UTI) versus "insignificant bacteriuria" (contamination) originated in an attempt to solve problems of interpretation caused by bacterial contamination of urine specimens from human beings.[18] In dogs, cultures of urine specimens obtained by catheterization are said to be indicative of UTI (i.e., significant bacteriuria) if the number of bacteria is 10,000 colonies/mL or greater in males and 100,000 colonies/mL or greater in females. Significant bacteriuria in both genders is 100,000 colonies/mL or greater in urine that is obtained by sampling of voided urine. In cats, significant bacteriuria is 1000 colonies/mL or greater for catheterization specimens and 10,000 colonies/mL or greater for voided specimens, although it has been reported that a few voided specimens from cats contained as many as 100,000 contaminant colonies/mL.[19] Significant bacteriuria is considered to be any bacterial growth in specimens that have been collected by antepubic cystocentesis from either dogs or cats. Growth within an individual urine specimen of more than three bacterial species should be considered evidence of contamination of the specimen, regardless of the collection method.

Increased numbers of urine WBCs and the presence of bacteria in the urine sediment are the two most reliable indicators of UTI. In fact, they were associated with bacterial growth on culture (i.e., UTI) in more than 92 per cent of samples that were collected by antepubic cystocentesis.[17] Cystocentesis is the only method of urine sampling that results in an uncontaminated specimen. It is safe, rapid, and simple to perform and is not traumatic or painful to dogs and cats if it is done properly using a few simple guidelines.[7, 20] This method of urine collection has been used routinely by faculty, students, and technical staff at the University of California Veterinary Medical Teaching Hospital for more than 20 years in more than 60,000 samplings with virtually no adverse effects.

A newer method of obtaining a urine sample by cystocentesis involves the use of a diagnostic ultrasound unit. After the animal is placed in dorsal recumbency in a padded V-shaped table, the ultrasound scan head is placed on the abdomen such that the urinary bladder is visualized on a television screen. A needle can be passed down the ultrasound beam and into the bladder quite easily with minimal practice, and a sample can be obtained from animals even when only a small amount of urine is present. If the needle fails to enter the urinary bladder (i.e., no urine can be withdrawn into the syringe after needle placement), the needle should be removed from the abdomen and both needle and syringe replaced before repeating the procedure. This is necessary because the needle and syringe have likely been contaminated with bacteria from the skin or from intestinal contents because of inadvertent passage of the needle through a loop of bowel.

Catheterization of male dogs and cats to obtain a specimen for sediment examination or bacterial culture is acceptable but is recommended only if cystocentesis cannot be conducted. The specimen usually will be contaminated with WBCs and bacteria from the urethra. The magnitude of this contamination is variable in males. Catheterization of female dogs and cats to obtain a specimen for urine sediment examination or bacterial culture is not recommended, because the specimen will nearly always be grossly contaminated with WBCs and bacteria from the vagina and/or urethra. The presence of these cells may result in a false impression of UTI, either because the urine sediment contains excessive WBCs and/or bacteria from the vagina or urethra, or because the urine culture is positive for growth as a result of contamination of the urine specimen by bacteria from the urethra or vagina.[21] Contamination of urine specimens obtained by catheterization may be reduced somewhat by discarding the first few milliliters of urine that flows from or is withdrawn from the catheter.

Catheterization of female dogs and cats to obtain a urine specimen is not a sterile procedure. Even though care can be taken to cleanse the vulva before insertion of the catheter, there is no practical way to eliminate bacteria that normally adhere to the vaginal and urethral mucosa. Regardless of how carefully the catheterization is conducted, bacteria are nearly always introduced into the bladder as a result of contact of the catheter tip with the vaginal and urethral mucosa. It has been reported that 20 per cent of normal female dogs developed UTI following catheterization for urine sampling,[16] and the percentage is likely to be higher in animals that are systemically ill, are immune suppressed, or have an abnormal urinary tract. Although similar studies have not been reported in cats, the prevalence of catheter-induced UTI in this species is likely to be similar to that reported in dogs. Indwelling catheters (i.e., in place >24 hours) were associated with development of UTI in 20 of 36 (56 per cent) normal male cats[22] and in 11 of 20 (55 per cent) dogs.[23]

Collection of a sample of voided urine for urine sediment examination or for bacterial culture is not acceptable practice because it is not possible to prevent contamination of the specimen with WBCs and bacteria from the urethra, vagina, or prepuce. The results of urine sediment WBC counts, bacterial counts, and bacterial cultures from specimens of voided urine are nearly always inaccurate. In one study of the magnitude of contamination in samples of voided urine, in dogs that had bacteriologically sterile urine when samples were collected by cystocentesis, there was bacterial growth in 85 per cent of the samples that were collected by voided midstream sampling.[21] Voided urine samples that have no WBCs or bacteria in the sediment are as good as specimens collected by cystocentesis for determining that UTI is not present. Thus, it is possible to establish the absence, but not the presence, of UTI with urine collected by this method.

Urine specimens should be refrigerated within minutes after collection if urinalysis or urine culture cannot be conducted within 15 minutes. Gram-negative enteric bacteria (e.g., E. coli) are capable of doubling their number every 30 minutes in urine specimens held at room temperature. If an enteric species and a nonenteric species that has a longer doubling time (e.g., staphylococci) are present in such a specimen, the enteric species can overgrow the nonenteric species. Also, false-negative results (i.e., failure of bacteria to grow on culture) can occur when a urine specimen is refrigerated for an extended period (12 to 24 hours, depending on the bacterial species present) or if the specimen is allowed to freeze. It should be a priority to process all urine specimens as soon as possible after collection to avoid potential handling problems.

Urinalysis and Urine Sediment Examination. The only test conducted during the macroscopic portion of the urinalysis that is of direct assistance in assessing the presence or absence of UTI is the urine specific gravity. For acceptable accuracy, this parameter should be measured directly with a refractometer. Some urine dipsticks have a test pad for specific gravity, but the results do not correlate well with those obtained by refractometer.[24] Knowledge of urine specific gravity is useful, in that a specific gravity greater than 1.013, when associated with normal numbers of WBCs and no visible bacteria on the urine sediment examination, is highly suggestive of the absence of UTI. However, a specific gravity less than 1.013 can mask the presence of UTI by diluting urine WBCs and bacteria to below the limit of determination. This may give a false impression of the absence of UTI.

Tests for protein and blood are often positive in cases of UTI, but their specificity is low because such results can also be caused by diseases or disorders not related to UTI. The urine pH value, by itself, is not a reliable indicator of the presence of UTI, even though UTI caused by *Proteus* spp. is often associated with basic urine pH. Diet, specimen handling, and postprandial state are variables that most often influence the urine pH. Urine dipsticks also have a test pad for nitrite that is supposed to test for nitrate-reducing urine bacteria. False-negatives are a significant problem in canine and feline urine; therefore, the test cannot be used reliably to detect UTI in dogs and cats.[24]

After completion of the macroscopic portion of the urinalysis, a standard volume (e.g., 5 mL) of remaining urine should be placed into a tube and centrifuged at $100 \times G$ for three to five minutes in order to concentrate the formed elements of the specimen. The supernatant is then decanted and the material remaining in the bottom of the tube used for the microscopic portion of the analysis. One well-mixed drop of this material can be placed on a clean, dry microscope slide and covered with a coverslip. New methylene blue stain may be used to enhance the visualization of certain formed elements in the preparation. The preparation should be scanned using the low-power ($10\times$) objective of the microscope and more closely for cellular detail and the presence of bacteria using the high-power ($40\times$) objective. WBCs, red blood cells, and epithelial cells are reported in numbers per high-power field (hpf); bacteria are noted to be present or absent, their morphologic characteristics (cocci, rods) are noted, and their numbers are reported as 1 to $4+$/hpf. Other formed elements (e.g., casts, parasite ova) are noted. For a complete examination, approximately 100 high-power microscopic fields should be scanned during the sediment examination.[17]

Bacterial Culture. If increased numbers of WBCs are found or bacteria are seen during microscopic examination of the urine sediment, a portion of the urine specimen should be cultured so that the species of the infecting bacteria can be identified. Inoculation of urine onto blood agar and MacConkey agar plates and incubation of the plates at the veterinary clinic is much cheaper than if the specimen is sent to a commercial diagnostic laboratory for the same service. The techniques of culturing and tentative species identification are easy to master by either a veterinarian or a member of the technical staff of a veterinary hospital.

All but one of the species of bacteria that are commonly associated with canine and feline UTI grow rapidly on culture media so that recognizable colonies are present following overnight incubation at 37°C. The exception is *Mycoplasma* spp., which take two to five days to appear. Moreover, the colonies are quite distinctive for most of the bacterial species that cause UTI, so that following incuba-

tion, the plates can be examined at the veterinary clinic and a tentative species identification made that is based on visual colony morphology and in vitro growth characteristics. This capability often allows the selection of an appropriate antimicrobial agent sooner than if the specimen is sent to a commercial laboratory.[25]

Antibacterial Susceptibility Testing. The terms "sensitive or susceptible" and "resistant" are often used in discussions of antimicrobial therapy of bacterial pathogens. An understanding of what the terms mean is basic to the successful use of antibiotics in the treatment of infectious diseases. The terms may be defined as the ability (resistant) or the lack of ability (sensitive or susceptible) of a specific species or strain of bacteria to grow and reproduce in the presence of a specific concentration of a specific antimicrobial agent. The terms are relative to certain inherent and/or acquired characteristics within the infecting bacterial population (e.g., penicillinase enzyme production, resistance acquired from plasmids) and to the concentration of each antimicrobial agent that is attainable at the site of the infection.

Antibacterial susceptibility tests are used to predict the outcome of therapy in human and animal patients with infectious diseases and are best conducted at a commercial diagnostic laboratory. Conducting susceptibility testing in a veterinary clinic is not acceptable practice, primarily because the level of accuracy achievable is usually very low, and quality control, an essential ingredient of accurate testing, is usually absent.

Antibacterial susceptibility testing techniques are usually used to determine the minimal inhibitory concentration (MIC), which is defined as the least amount of an antibiotic that inhibits growth of the test species or strain of bacteria in a defined and reproducible set of in vitro conditions. All the standard methods of susceptibility testing used in veterinary medicine determine MIC values whether they are reported as such or not.

The standard agar-disk diffusion method used by many commercial laboratories is the Kirby-Bauer method. It is based on attainable concentrations of antimicrobics in human plasma but has been used to test bacterial isolates from animals on the assumption (not always correct) that plasma levels of antimicrobial agents are similar in all species. Susceptibilities of urinary bacterial isolates cannot be measured with accuracy by this method because attainable antimicrobial concentrations in urine are much higher than those in plasma. Thus, MIC values that are within the range of serum concentrations may be accurately determined, but those that are higher than attainable serum concentrations cannot be measured with this test. A modification of the agar-disk diffusion method may be used for testing bacterial isolates from urine.[26]

The broth or agar dilution method involves direct measurement of the MIC from a series of dilutions of each antimicrobial agent (usually serial twofold dilutions) in broth or agar. A standard number of organisms of the test bacterial species (the one causing UTI in the animal) are grown in media in the laboratory and inoculated into each dilution. After incubation, the MIC is recorded as the test tube, well, or agar plate containing the least amount of the antimicrobial agent that prevented growth of the test bacteria. Recent developments in this method include machinery that dilutes and inoculates broth automatically in disposable plastic trays containing 96 tiny wells aligned in rows. Serial dilutions of each of 8 or 12 antimicrobics can be carried out automatically in many trays, which are then stored frozen at −60°C

URO

or are lyophilized and stored at room temperature until they are used. Each test bacterium is grown in broth to a predetermined organism density, and an entire tray is inoculated in a single rapid operation. After incubation, a magnification system or computer-aided automatic reading device is used to visualize the wells to determine the MIC of each antimicrobial for the test bacteria. The MIC is read as the clear well in each row that contains the least amount of each antimicrobial agent.

Because of automated advances in microdilution hardware and techniques, this method of susceptibility testing is now the method of choice in many commercial diagnostic laboratories and in most veterinary teaching hospitals. The ability to conduct many tests quickly and accurately makes this method highly suitable to commercial ventures.

Predicting Antibacterial Susceptibility Without Susceptibility Testing. It is not necessary to conduct susceptibility testing on all urinary bacterial isolates. In cases of canine UTI involving members of several common urinary bacterial species, data are available that can be used to select an appropriate antimicrobial agent with at least a 90 per cent confidence level without the need for susceptibility testing. These several species are said to be predictable with regard to their susceptibility to certain antimicrobial agents. Susceptibility testing is mandatory in cases of UTI in which two or more bacterial species are isolated simultaneously from the urine, when the bacteria causing the UTI are uncommon or unusual species (e.g., *Acinetobacter* sp.), or when the bacteria are less than 90 per cent predictable with regard to their antimicrobial susceptibility (e.g., *Enterobacter* spp.).

Members of *Staphylococcus* spp., *Streptococcus* spp., *Enterococcus* spp., *Proteus mirabilis*, and *Pseudomonas* spp. are able to alter their susceptibility to many antimicrobials by only small increments from bacterial generation to generation. They are generally not capable of changing from susceptible to resistant, at least in terms of urinary antimicrobial concentrations, within a single generation or even within several generations. Thus, each of these species is predictable with regard to its spectrum of antimicrobial susceptibility in the urinary tract. Staphylococci, streptococci, enterococci, and *Proteus mirabilis* are predictably susceptible (>90 per cent confidence) to a simple penicillin (ampicillin, amoxicillin). *Pseudomonas* spp. are predictably susceptible to a tetracycline.

Some members of the enteric group of bacteria that commonly infect the urinary tract, specifically *E. coli*, *Klebsiella* spp., and *Enterobacter* spp., are capable of major changes in their susceptibility to several classes of antibiotics within a single bacterial generation. They accomplish this by exchanging small pieces of extrachromosomal DNA, called plasmids, among themselves. Some of the plasmids contain genetic information that, when incorporated into the bacterial DNA, acts to code for changes in the metabolism of the bacteria that result in production of chemicals (e.g., enzymes such as penicillinase) that destroy or modify antimicrobial molecules, cause alterations in cell membrane permeability to antimicrobials, or in other ways protect the bacteria from the harmful effects of antimicrobials. These bacteria are said to be unpredictable (<90 per cent confidence level) with regard to their susceptibility to most antibiotics because of this unique capability for rapid self-protective genomic manipulation. Therefore, susceptibility testing of these bacteria is mandatory.

SELECTION OF AN ANTIBACTERIAL AGENT

The basic goal of all antibacterial therapy is to provide antibacterial activity at the site of infection that is in excess of that needed to inhibit growth of the infecting bacteria or to kill them outright (i.e., bacteriostatic or bactericidal activity). Although achieving this goal in actual disease situations in animals is sometimes difficult in some organs and tissues of the body, even with modern antibacterial agents, this is not the case in the urinary tract. All the common antibacterials that are recommended for use in UTI in animals develop high urine concentrations following administration of standard oral or injected doses. It has been determined that in order to have optimal therapeutic effectiveness, the urinary concentration of an antibiotic must exceed its growth-inhibiting concentration (MIC) for the infecting bacteria by at least fourfold.[27, 28] If the average urine concentration of an antibiotic is equal to or greater than that of the MIC value multiplied by four, the drug will be at least 90 per cent effective. If it is less than the MIC × 4, the drug will be minimally effective.[27]

When planning treatment of UTI, one should choose an antibiotic that (1) will result in urine concentrations that exceed the MIC for the infecting species of bacteria at least fourfold, (2) is in a form that is easy for the client to administer (thus improving client compliance), (3) has few (if any) undesirable or toxic side effects, and (4) is relatively inexpensive. The drug should be administered often enough to maintain inhibitory urine concentrations and long enough to rid the urinary tract of the infecting agent.

The optimal duration of antibacterial therapy for canine and feline UTI is unknown. At various times, there have been advocates of single-dose therapy and of therapy lasting three days, one week, two weeks, and three weeks. Similar therapeutic regimens have been proposed for use in human beings with UTI. However, there is good evidence that two weeks is close to the optimal duration for treatment of most UTI in dogs and cats. My colleagues and I have used this duration of treatment for more than 20 years and have published the cure rates obtained with therapy lasting two weeks for a variety of antibacterial agents in a variety of bacterial species.[28–33]

Even though bacteria that cause UTI invade the wall of the urinary tract and are not limited to the urine, urine concentrations of antimicrobial agents are thought to be more important than plasma concentrations in the successful treatment of UTI.[27, 34, 35] Each of the antimicrobials commonly used in the treatment of UTI is eliminated in large quantities in the urine, quantities that may attain as much as 50 times peak plasma concentrations. To aid in the success of therapy, the amount of antimicrobial agent in the animal's urine should be maintained at a high concentration during most of each treatment interval (dosing interval), which is the elapsed time between doses. Most antibacterial agents that are used in the treatment of UTI have short therapeutic half-lives (i.e., rapid absorption and rapid excretion of the active compound and its metabolites into the urine). Because of short therapeutic half-lives and the frequent voiding patterns of most animals, it is desirable to administer most antimicrobial agents three times a day to animals with UTI. Most household dogs are able to retain urine without voiding for at least eight hours, so the owner of a dog with UTI should be instructed to restrict the pet's freedom to urinate to a short time just before the pet is due to receive the next dose of medication. Implementation of this restriction is not always possible, but it is a simple strategy that results in significant antimicrobial levels in the urine for much longer periods than would be the case if the pet were allowed to urinate at will.

It may be tempting to initiate treatment on the basis of an animal's clinical signs alone, or on the basis of signs and the results of a urinalysis. This approach is not acceptable in canine and feline medicine for three reasons: (1) because representatives of nine bacterial genera commonly cause UTI in dogs and cats, it is not possible to predict with accuracy which bacterial species is present or to which antimicrobial it might be susceptible; (2) diagnosis is difficult because most dogs and cats do not manifest clinical signs of UTI; and (3) bacterial isolates from the urine of dogs and cats, especially *E. coli*, *Klebsiella* spp., and *Enterobacter* spp., may have acquired resistance to one or more of the commonly used antimicrobials because animals are more frequently exposed to antimicrobials and/or to antimicrobial residues.[36] Therefore, to initiate proper management of UTI, the bacterial species causing the infection must be identified by culture of the urine. When the species of bacteria is known, selection of an appropriate antibiotic may be made with great accuracy, often without the need for susceptibility testing, because many urinary pathogens have predictable susceptibilities to one or more antibiotics.

Greater than 72 per cent of canine UTIs are caused by a single bacterial species. In addition, two bacterial species or two morphologically different strains of the same species are found in about 20 per cent of UTIs in both genders. Three bacterial species or strains can be found in an additional 6 to 8 per cent in each gender.[8] Mixed bacterial infections (two or three organisms) nearly always require susceptibility testing for proper management. Selection of an antimicrobial agent depends on the species of the bacteria encountered and on their combined susceptibilities.

Bacterial culture, instead of urine sediment examination, is strongly recommended for all follow-ups in dogs and cats with UTI. Examination of urine sediment for WBCs and bacteria is not reliable for assessment of the success or failure of antibacterial therapy in UTI. The range of variation of bacterial numbers in infected urine is from less than 1000 colonies/mL to greater than 1 million colonies/mL. If the numbers of infecting bacteria in the follow-up urine specimen are less than 10,000/mL, a false impression of cure may result, because bacteria usually cannot be demonstrated during microscopic examination of the urine sediment if their numbers are below this figure. Also, for unknown reasons, the number of urine WBCs may unpredictably decrease to within the normal range during the treatment of UTI, even when infection is still present and the antibiotic used has been ineffective in eradicating the infecting bacterial species.

THERAPEUTIC STRATEGIES

Single, Uncomplicated Episodes of UTI. Nearly 75 per cent of UTIs in dogs,[7] and approximately 85 per cent of UTIs in cats,[9] regardless of gender, occur as single episodes and seemingly do not recur. After the infecting bacteria have been identified and the antimicrobial susceptibility established by consulting a predictability table or by susceptibility testing of the bacteria, treatment is initiated with an appropriate antimicrobial agent at full dosage and recommended dosing interval (Fig. 171–1). A urine specimen for follow-up bacterial culture should be taken between the seventh and tenth days of treatment to ascertain the actual (in vivo) effectiveness of the therapy. If growth of bacteria is not observed, the treatment is successful and should be continued for the remainder of the two-week period. A follow-up urine culture should be conducted on a urine specimen obtained one to two weeks after completion of the therapeutic course. The results of this culture indicate whether the UTI has recurred following completion of the therapy. If this culture is negative, no further testing or treatment is needed.

If growth of the same or a different species of bacteria is observed in the urine specimen taken between the seventh and tenth days of therapy, the treatment has failed and another antimicrobial agent must be substituted, using a new susceptibility test as a guideline for drug selection. Culture of the urine should be conducted 7 to 10 days after beginning the substitute antimicrobial and one to two weeks after completion of the new course of therapy (see Fig. 171–1).

Persistent UTI. In persistent UTI, bacteriuria continues in spite of treatment with one or more seemingly appropriate antimicrobial agents. The usual definition of persistent UTI is more than three positive cultures in succession with no periods of sterile urine in between, with an elapsed time of not less than one week or more than eight weeks between each culture. Usually the same bacterial species is isolated from all the cultures, but occasionally in dogs, a series of positive cultures may include two or even three different species. Fortunately, persistent UTI is rare in both dogs and cats.[3, 9]

Persistent UTI usually is caused by gram-negative enteric species (e.g., *E. coli*, *Klebsiella* spp., or *Enterobacter* spp.) that are able to adapt their antimicrobial resistance to meet the challenge of the presence of antibiotics, by the presence of a nidus of infection within the tract (e.g., calculi, foreign bodies), or by the presence of prostatitis or unilateral pyelonephritis. Less commonly, it is the result of lack of owner compliance with the prescribed dosage or dosing interval or of interaction of the antibiotic with another drug or with some portion of the animal's diet. Urachal remnants that remain patent through part of their length may trap infected urine and have been suggested as a cause of persistent UTI. The presence of a patent urachus may be determined by the use of positive-contrast cystography. Surgical removal of these remnants may resolve persistent UTI in some cases. This surgery is sometimes performed in lieu of proper medical management, but surgical removal should be considered only if proper medical management has failed to resolve the infection.

Urine culture and susceptibility testing in animals with persistent UTI should be conducted *on a weekly basis* in order to be able to quickly and accurately respond to changes in the antibacterial resistance pattern of the isolates.

Recurrent UTI. In recurrent UTI, bacteriologic cure is only temporary; infection returns in days or weeks following cure of the previous episode. The usual definition of recurrence is more than three successfully treated episodes of UTI in a dog or cat within a single year in which each episode is followed by a period of bacteriologically sterile urine. Recurrent UTI is uncommon in dogs and rare in cats. Experience indicates that recurrence of UTI is almost always caused by bacterial reinfection with a different strain or species rather than by bacterial relapse (infection with the same strain or species).[3, 9]

URO

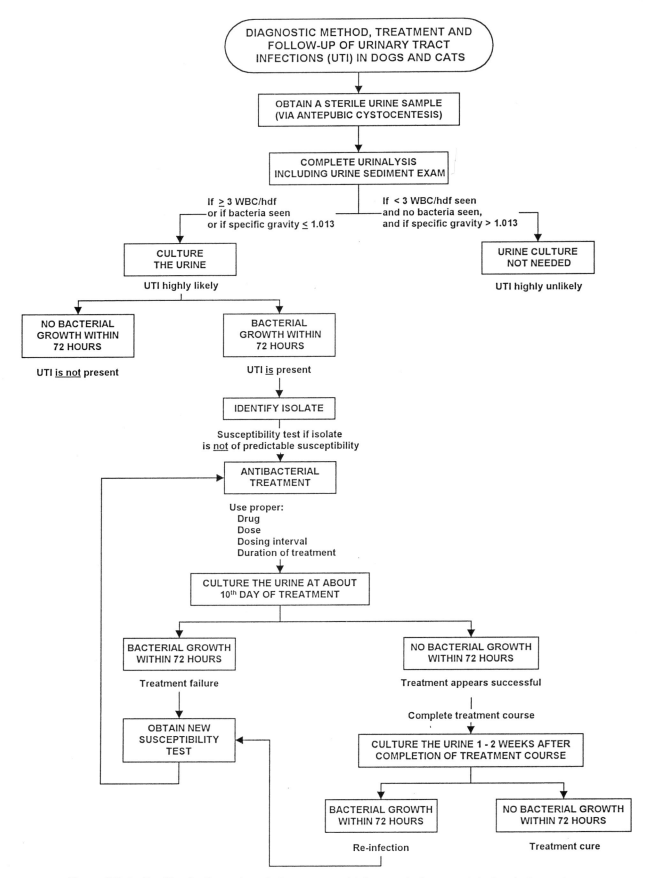

Figure 171–1. Algorithm for diagnostic method, treatment, and follow-up of urinary tract infections in dogs and cats.

When episodes of UTI occur only once or twice each year, administration of the appropriate oral antimicrobial agent at full dose for two weeks, as previously described, is the preferred approach to successful management. However, when UTIs occur more than three times in a single year, administration of an appropriate antimicrobial at full dose to treat a specific infection should be followed by long-term, once-daily preventive antimicrobial administration (Table 171–1). The goal of preventive therapy is to lengthen the intervals between episodes of UTI and to prevent reinfection.

PREVENTION OF ADDITIONAL EPISODES OF UTI

Physicians have advocated the use of once-daily, long-term preventive antibiotic therapy for recurrent UTI in women since 1974.[37] This regimen results in a reduction of the rate of reinfection to about one tenth the rate in untreated patients. Development of resistant bowel flora during use of long-term preventive therapy seemingly has not been a problem.[38–40] We have used this regimen for nearly 20 years with similar results in dogs of either gender that have had multiple episodes of UTI. When the urine is culture-negative, long-term preventive therapy is administered, one dose daily, using the antibiotic that resulted in bacteriologic cure of the latest episode. Therapy is continued daily for six months if the urine remains culture-negative. Because most canine UTIs are asymptomatic, urine cultures must be conducted at frequent intervals (about every four weeks if the most recent UTI was gram-negative; about every 12 weeks if the most recent UTI was gram-positive) during preventive therapy to reassess the status of the urinary tract with regard to reinfection. If reinfection occurs during the preventive regimen, an appropriate antimicrobial (based on a new susceptibility test) should be substituted at full dose and recommended dosing interval for two weeks. Preventive therapy, using the substitute antimicrobial, should be reinstituted following successful completion of full-dose therapy when the urine is once again culture-negative.

If the multiple episodes of UTI are caused by *Staphylococcus* spp., *Streptococcus* spp., *Enterococcus* spp., or *Proteus mirabilis*, a simple penicillin (e.g., ampicillin, amoxicillin) should be used as both the full-dose and the preventive therapeutic agent. If the episodes of UTI are caused by *Pseudomonas* spp., a tetracycline should be used as both the full-dose and the preventive agent. If the episodes of UTI are caused by *E. coli*, *Klebsiella* spp., or *Enterobacter* spp., cephalexin, cefadroxil, trimethoprim/sulfa, enrofloxacin, or amoxicillin/clavulanic acid are among the drugs that may be used as both the full-dose and the low-dose preventive agent. However, in the latter case, final selection of one of these drugs should always be based on results of susceptibility testing of the latest isolate, because these bacteria are not predictable with regard to their antimicrobial susceptibility.

Follow-up urine specimens taken from dogs and cats with multiple episodes of UTI should be collected only by cystocentesis. The urinary tracts of these animals are more susceptible to bacterial infection than are urinary tracts of normal animals. Introduction of a urinary catheter, regardless of how carefully and aseptically the procedure is conducted, always introduces bacteria as a result of passage of the catheter. Bacteria seem to have an increased chance of colonizing the urinary tract and initiating an iatrogenic episode of UTI in these animals.

Following completion of the six-month preventive regimen, a surveillance procedure is recommended that includes reculture of a urine specimen from the dog or cat once every two to three months for the next two years. A two-week course of appropriate antimicrobial therapy must be administered, and follow-up urine cultures conducted, if UTI is discovered during the surveillance period.

CAUSES OF THERAPEUTIC FAILURE IN UTI

Causes of failure to cure an episode of bacterial UTI in any species can be grouped into two broad categories: failure of the antibiotic to come into contact with the infecting bacteria, or failure of the antibiotic to inhibit growth of or to kill the infecting bacteria even though the two are in direct contact.

Therapeutic failure resulting from lack of direct contact between the antimicrobial drug and the infecting bacteria is usually caused by failure of intestinal absorption of the drug. This may be due to improper administration of the drug by the owner, such that the animal rejects the pill or capsule (i.e., spits it out or vomits it), or administration of the drug inside a large piece of meat or other food item that acts as a protective coating around the drug and prevents its absorption. Interaction of the drug in the intestinal tract with food substances or with another drug, leading to inactivation of the drug before it can be absorbed, also may occur. The presence of a nidus or reservoir of infection within the urinary tract (e.g., urinary calculi, infection of the prostate) may provide a haven for bacteria that is completely isolated from exposure to certain antibiotics.

Causes of therapeutic failure in cases in which the antibiotic is present in the urine include development of acquired resistance by bacterial species such as *E. coli*, *Klebsiella* spp., and *Enterobacter* spp. The presence of a nidus or reservoir of infection within the urinary tract (e.g., urinary calculi, pyelonephritis with renal scarring, patent urachus

---

TABLE 171–1. SUMMARY OF RECOMMENDATIONS FOR PREVENTIVE THERAPY FOR RECURRENT URINARY TRACT INFECTIONS

1. If the infections have been caused by gram-positive bacteria (i.e., staphylococci, streptococci, enterococci) or by *Proteus mirabilis,* give one third to one fourth of the total daily dosage of ampicillin or amoxicillin once daily. This therapy should be continued for six months. Urine cultures should be performed once every three months (collect the samples only by cystocentesis).
2. If the infections have been caused by gram-negative bacteria (i.e., *Escherichia coli, Klebsiella* spp., *Enterobacter* spp.) or have been mixtures of gram-positive and gram-negative bacteria, give one third of the total daily dosage of amoxicillin/clavulanic acid, cephalexin, or cefadroxil once daily, or one half of the total daily dosage of trimethoprim/sulfa or enrofloxacin once daily. Selection of a drug from among those listed should be based on susceptibility test results of the latest isolate and in vivo results of the latest therapy. The rule is to use the drug for long-term preventive therapy that resulted in cure of the latest episode of infection. This therapy should be continued for six months. Urine cultures should be performed once a month (collect the samples only by cystocentesis).
3. If infection occurs during long-term preventive therapy, treat it with an appropriate antibiotic (as for single, uncomplicated urinary tract infection), selection of which must be based on susceptibilty test results of the isolate. Resume long-term preventive therapy as per the recommendations in this table after the "breakthrough infection" has been cured.

Note: Long-term preventive therapy should be used only when the animal's urinary tract is bacteriologically sterile. The goal of this strategy is to prevent additional episodes of urinary tract infection.

URO

that traps infected urine, urinary neoplasm, or infection of the prostate) may provide a haven for bacteria that is isolated from exposure to bacteriostatic or bactericidal concentrations of antimicrobials. Failure on the part of the owner to give the drug as directed (i.e., lack of compliance) may take the form of infrequent administration of the drug or administration of incorrectly low doses of the drug, resulting in ineffective concentrations of drug in the urine. Failure to attain proper concentration of the drug in the urine because of concurrent disease (e.g., polyuria from any cause) may play a role in certain animals. Failure to mount a response to the presence of bacteria occurs occasionally in immune-suppressed animals and may be a cause of persistence of bacteriuria.

The most common cause of therapeutic failure in UTI is acquired drug resistance on the part of the infecting agent. Existence of this problem may be ascertained by review of susceptibility results of the latest isolates. If therapeutic failure is a result of acquired resistance, a new antimicrobial agent must be selected. The selection must always be based on results of susceptibility testing of the latest isolate.

REFERENCES

1. Ling GV, et al: Percutaneous nephropyelocentesis and nephropyelostomy in the dog: A description of the technique. Am J Vet Res 40:1605, 1979.
2. Finco DR, et al: Evaluation of methods for localization of urinary tract infection in the female dog. Am J Vet Res 40:707, 1979.
3. Ling GV: Unpublished data.
4. Adelman RD, et al: Furosemide enhancement of experimental gentamicin nephrotoxicity: Comparison of functional and morphological changes with activities of urinary enzymes. J Infect Dis 140:342, 1979.
5. Adelman RD: Personal communication.
6. Ihrke PJ, et al: Urinary tract infection associated with long-term corticosteroid administration in dogs with chronic skin diseases. JAVMA 186:43, 1985.
7. Ling GV: Urinary tract infections. In Lower Urinary Tract Diseases of Dogs and Cats. Philadelphia, Mosby Year Book, 1995, pp 115–128.
8. Ling GV, et al: Urinary tract infection in dogs. I: Method of specimen collection and interrelations of organism prevalence and host age, and gender among 8,354 infections (1969–1995). Am J Vet Res, in press.
9. Davidson AP, et al: Urinary tract infections in cats: A retrospective study, 1977–1989. Calif Vet 46(4):32, 1992.
10. Griffin DW, et al: Prevalence of bacterial urinary tract infection after perineal urethrostomy in cats. JAVMA 200:681, 1992.
11. Senior DF: Bacterial urinary tract infections: Invasion, host defenses, and new approaches to prevention. Compend Contin Educ 7:334, 1985.
12. Johnson JR: Virulence factors in Escherichia coli urinary tract infection. Clin Microbiol Rev 4:80, 1991.
13. Hirsh DC, et al: The bacterial flora of the normal canine vagina: Comparison with the bacterial flora of vaginal exudates. J Small Anim Pract 18:25, 1971.
14. Ling GV, et al: Aerobic bacterial flora of the prepuce, urethra and vagina of normal adult dogs. JAVMA 172:914, 1977.
15. Platt AM, et al: Bacterial flora of the canine vagina. Southwest Vet 27:76, 1964.
16. Biertuempfel PH, et al: Urinary tract infection resulting from catheterization of healthy adult dogs. JAVMA 178:989, 1981.
17. Ling GV, et al: Microscopic examination of canine urine sediment. Calif Vet 30:14, 1976.
18. Kass EH: Bacteriuria and the diagnosis of infections of the urinary tract. Arch Intern Med 100:709, 1957.
19. Lees GE, et al: Results of analyses and bacterial cultures of urine specimens obtained from clinically normal cats by three methods. JAVMA 184:449, 1984.
20. Ling GV: Antepubic cystocentesis in the dog: An aseptic technique for routine collection of urine. Calif Vet 30(8):50, 1976.
21. Comer KM, et al: Results of urinalysis and bacterial culture of canine urine obtained by antepubic cystocentesis, catheterization, and midstream voided methods. JAVMA 179:891, 1981.
22. Lees GE, et al: Adverse effects caused by polypropylene and polyvinyl feline urinary catheters. Am J Vet Res 41:1836, 1980.
23. Barsanti JA, et al: Urinary tract infection due to indwelling bladder catheters in dogs and cats. JAVMA 187:384, 1985.
24. Lees GE, et al: Urinary disorders. In Willard MD, et al (eds): Small Animal Clinical Diagnosis by Laboratory Methods, 2nd ed. Philadelphia, WB Saunders, 1994, pp 115–146.
25. Ling GV: Urine culture techniques and identification of bacteria. In Lower Urinary Tract Diseases of Dogs and Cats. Philadelphia, Mosby Year Book, 1995, pp 37–42.
26. Ericsson HM, et al: Antibiotic sensitivity testing. Acta Path Microbiol Scand, sec B, suppl 217, 1971.
27. Klastersky J, et al: Antibacterial activity in serum and urine as a therapeutic guide in bacterial infections. J Infect Dis 129:187, 1974.
28. Ling GV, et al: Canine urinary tract infections: A comparison of in vitro antimicrobial susceptibility test results and response to oral therapy with ampicillin or with trimethoprim-sulfa. JAVMA 185:277, 1984.
29. Ling GV, et al: Penicillin-G or ampicillin for oral treatment of canine urinary tract infections. JAVMA 171:358, 1977.
30. Ling GV, et al: Chloramphenicol for oral treatment of canine urinary tract infections. JAVMA 172:914, 1978.
31. Ling GV, et al: Trimethoprim in combination with a sulfonamide for oral treatment of canine urinary tract infections. JAVMA 174:1003, 1979.
32. Ling GV, et al: Tetracycline for oral treatment of canine urinary tract infection caused by Pseudomonas aeruginosa. JAVMA 179:578, 1981.
33. Ling GV, et al: Cephalexin for oral treatment of canine urinary tract infection caused by Klebsiella pneumoniae. JAVMA 182:1346, 1983.
34. Stamey TA, et al: The localization and treatment of urinary tract infections: The role of bactericidal urine levels as opposed to serum levels. Medicine 44:1, 1965.
35. Stamey TA, et al: Serum versus urinary antimicrobial concentrations in cure of urinary-tract infections. N Engl J Med 291:1159, 1974.
36. Hirsh DC, et al: Incidence of R-plasmids in fecal flora of healthy household dogs. Antimicrob Agents Chemother 17:313, 1980.
37. Harding GKM, et al: A controlled study of antimicrobial prophylaxis of recurrent urinary infection in women. N Engl J Med 291:597, 1974.
38. Knothe H: The effect of a combined preparation of trimethoprim and sulphamethoxazole following short-term and long-term administration on the flora of the human gut. Chemotherapy 18:285, 1973.
39. Martinez FC, et al: Effect of prophylactic, low dose cephalexin on fecal and vaginal flora. J Urol 133:994, 1985.
40. Stamey TA, et al: Prophylactic efficacy of nitrofurantoin macrocrystals and trimethoprim-sulfamethoxazole in urinary infections. Biologic effects on the vaginal and rectal flora. N Engl J Med 296:780,1977.

CHAPTER 172

PROSTATIC DISEASES

Margaret V. Root Kustritz and Jeffrey S. Klausner

ANATOMY AND PHYSIOLOGY

The prostate, the only accessory sex gland of the male dog, is a retroperitoneal organ with only the craniodorsal surface covered by peritoneum.[1] It is bounded by the rectum dorsally and the symphysis pubis ventrally (Fig. 172–1) and completely encircles the urethra at the bladder neck. It is surrounded by a fibromuscular capsule and is divided into two lobes by a median raphe, which is palpable on the dorsal surface per rectum.[1–3] Its position is abdominal until the urachal remnant breaks down at about 2 months of age; it then is pelvic until it becomes enlarged with advancing age or disease, at which time it may pull the bladder cranially and be palpable abdominally.[1, 4, 5]

Histologically, the glandular epithelial cell population differs with distance from the urethra from low cuboidal to tall columnar.[6] These glandular cells are divided into indistinct lobules by bands of smooth muscle.[2, 4] Blood is supplied by branches of the prostatic artery and drained by the prostatic and urethral veins.[1] Lymph drainage is to the iliac lymph nodes.[1] The hypogastric and pelvic nerves provide sympathetic and parasympathetic innervation.[7]

Prostate growth and secretion are androgen dependent.[3] Castration leads to decreased prostate volume, atrophy of glandular and stromal elements, and decreased ability to take up and metabolize androgens.[3, 8, 9] The principal androgen regulating prostatic growth is 5α-dihydrotestosterone (5α-DHT), which is formed from testosterone by the enzyme 5α-reductase.[8] Although 5α-DHT and testosterone share the same intracellular androgen receptor, 5α-DHT exerts a greater effect because it binds to the receptor with an affinity two times greater than that of testosterone and has a fivefold slower dissociation rate than testosterone.[10] Locally produced growth factors, such as transforming growth factor-β secreted from myofibroblasts, may also act as modulators of epithelial cell growth and function.[6, 11]

The prostate gland secretes seminal plasma through hormonal and nervous system control.[7] Expulsion of prostatic fluid into the urethra is stimulated by the sympathetic nervous system.[7, 12, 13] Prostatic fluid makes up the first and third fractions of the canine ejaculate and acts to thin and increase the volume of the ejaculate and, possibly, aids in sperm transport.[3, 14] Prostatic fluid is secreted constitutively and is normally expelled into the prostatic urethra, from where it drains into the urinary bladder and penile urethra.

HISTORY, PHYSICAL EXAMINATION FINDINGS, AND DIAGNOSTIC TESTS

HISTORY

Urethral discharge, hematuria, and rectal tenesmus are the most frequent signs in dogs with prostatic disease.[15] These

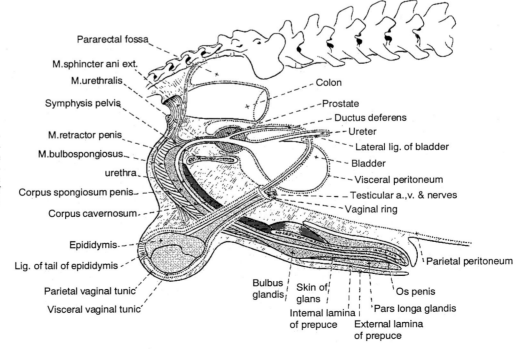

Figure 172–1. Diagram of relationship of the prostate to other structures in the caudal abdomen of the male dog. (From Evans H, Christensen G: The urogenital system. *In* Evans H [ed]: Miller's Anatomy of the Dog, 3rd ed. Philadelphia, WB Saunders, 1993, p 494.)

Pararectal fossa
M.sphincter ani ext.
M.urethralis
Symphysis pelvis
M.retractor penis
M.bulbospongiosus
urethra
Corpus spongiosum penis
Corpus cavernosum
Epididymis
Lig. of tail of epididymis
Parietal vaginal tunic
Visceral vaginal tunic

Colon
Prostate
Ductus deferens
Ureter
Lateral lig. of bladder
Bladder
Visceral peritoneum
Testicular a.,v. & nerves
Vaginal ring
Parietal peritoneum
Os penis
Pars longa glandis
External lamina of prepuce
Internal lamina of prepuce
Skin of glans
Bulbus glandis

URO

signs can also occur in dogs with lower urinary tract and intestinal disease. Physical examination and diagnostic tests are required to localize the disease to the prostate. Signs of prostatic disease vary with the type of disorder that is present (Table 172–1). Dogs with benign prostatic hyperplasia (BPH) are often asymptomatic, although they may demonstrate rectal tenesmus, bloody urethral discharge, or hematuria. Dogs with acute bacterial prostatitis may have depression, anorexia, vomiting, and bloody urethral discharge. Straining to urinate, urethral discharge, anorexia, and depression are seen in dogs with prostatic abscesses. Recurring urinary tract infection is often a clue to the presence of chronic bacterial prostatitis. Dogs with prostatic cysts may be asymptomatic or may demonstrate dysuria and urethral discharge. Dogs with prostatic neoplasia may have decreased appetite, weight loss, urethral discharge, dysuria, and/or rear limb weakness. Prostatic disease may be associated with hypospermia and infertility.[16]

PHYSICAL EXAMINATION

Dogs suspected of having prostatic disease should receive a thorough physical examination and complete examination of the prostate. The prostate is best examined by digital rectal examination. It is often helpful to use a second hand to palpate the prostate per abdomen and to push the prostate toward the pelvic canal.[17] This aids in palpating the caudal surface of the prostate. In large dogs, elevating the forequarters may facilitate examination of the prostate. The prostate should be evaluated for size, symmetry, shape, pain, and movability in the pelvic canal. The normal prostate is smooth and symmetric, non-painful, and freely movable. The median dorsal groove of the prostate is easily palpated. Prostatic size varies with breed, body weight, and age. Scottish terriers are reported to have prostate glands that are larger than the prostate glands of other breeds of similar weight and age.[18]

EVALUATION OF PROSTATIC FLUID

Evaluating prostatic fluid cytology and culturing prostatic fluid are useful means of differentiating between BPH, bacte-

TABLE 172–1. CLINICAL SIGNS OF PROSTATIC DISORDERS

DISORDER	CLINICAL SIGNS
Benign prostatic hypertrophy	Asymptomatic
	Urethral discharge
	Rectal tenesmus
	Hematuria
Acute bacterial prostatitis	Fever, anorexia, depression
	Vomiting
	Urethral discharge
	Rear limb weakness
Prostatic abscess	Fever, anorexia, depression
	Urethral discharge
	Dysuria
	Rectal tenesmus
Chronic bacterial prostatitis	Recurrent urinary tract infection
Prostatic retention cyst	Dysuria
	Hematuria
	Urethral discharge
	Rectal tenesmus
Prostatic neoplasia	Anorexia, weight loss, depression
	Rear limb weakness
	Urethral discharge
	Dysuria

rial prostatitis, and prostatic neoplasia. Samples for cytologic analysis and culture can be obtained from the urethral discharge or by ejaculation, prostatic massage, or aspiration biopsy of the prostate. Prostatic fluid can reflux into the bladder, resulting in abnormalities in the urinalysis.

Urethral Discharge. Urethral discharge is a frequent finding in dogs with prostatic disease.[15] Urethral discharges can result from preputial disease, urinary incontinence, urethral disease, or prostatic disease. Preputial disease is ruled out by careful physical examination. Comparing cytology, pH, and specific gravity of the discharge with urine collected by cystocentesis is helpful in eliminating urinary incontinence as a cause of the discharge.[17] Urethral disease is often associated with straining to urinate, a clinical sign that is infrequent with prostatic disease other than prostatic cancer.

Urethral discharge can be collected for cytologic examination by retracting the prepuce and allowing a few drops of discharge to drip on a glass slide. Because of the resident urethral flora, culture of urethral discharges may be of little value in identifying a primary bacterial pathogen. If the urethral discharge is cultured, it is helpful to perform a quantitative bacterial culture. When a single organism is isolated in large numbers (>100,000/mL) it is more likely to be a pathogen than a urethral contaminant, especially if the cytology of the fluid is consistent with infection.[17]

Semen Evaluation. Prostatic fluid is the third (and some of the first[14]) portion of the ejaculate. It follows the sperm-rich fraction and makes up approximately 95 per cent of the volume of the ejaculate.[19] Prostatic fluid, which is normally clear and is relatively acellular, can be analyzed cytologically and can be cultured. A few red and white blood cells and occasional squamous epithelial cells may be noted in normal prostatic fluid.[20] As with urethral discharges, it is best to perform quantitative culture of prostatic fluid to aid in differentiating bacterial pathogens from urethral contaminants. The technique of obtaining an ejaculate sample has been well described.[16, 17, 21]

Prostatic Massage. Small quantities of prostatic fluid can be obtained by prostatic massage. This technique is especially useful if the dog is in pain during palpation of the prostate, which often makes obtaining ejaculates impossible. Prostatic massage is performed by removing urine from the urinary bladder, placing the tip of a urinary catheter in the prostatic urethra using rectal palpation as a guide, gently massaging the prostate per rectum for 1 to 2 minutes, and aspirating material into the catheter. The collected material can be analyzed cytologically and cultured. A small amount of clear, acellular fluid can be collected from a normal dog. Flushing 5 mL of sterile saline through the catheter before and after massage may facilitate collection of prostatic fluid.[22]

RADIOLOGY

Survey abdominal radiographs are useful in determining size, shape, and location of the prostate. The normal prostate gland is symmetric, has a smooth border, and is located just cranial to the pelvis and caudal to the urinary bladder. On the lateral radiograph, there may be a triangular fat pad between the ventral caudal aspect of the urinary bladder, the cranial ventral portion of the prostate gland, and the caudal ventral abdominal wall.[23] The normal size of the prostate varies in different breeds and sizes of dogs. Prostatomegaly is a frequent sign of prostatic disease (Table 172–2). An enlarged prostate may displace the colon dorsally and the

TABLE 172–2. RADIOGRAPHIC AND ULTRASONOGRAPHIC LESIONS IN DOGS WITH PROSTATIC DISORDERS

DISORDER	RADIOGRAPHIC LESIONS	ULTRASONOGRAPHIC LESIONS
Benign prostatic hypertrophy	Mild to moderate prostatomegaly	Normal to slightly hyperechoic with or without multiple hypoechoic areas
Acute bacterial prostatitis	Mild to moderate prostatomegaly; loss of prostatic detail	Focal or diffusely hyperechoic
Prostatic abscess	Mild to moderate prostatomegaly	Focal or diffusely hyperechoic; focal hypoechoic/anechoic areas
Chronic bacterial prostatitis	Normal; infrequent prostatic mineralization	Focal or diffusely hyperechoic
Prostatic retention cyst	Prostatomegaly; abdominal mass	Large hypoechoic or anechoic mass
Prostatic neoplasia	Mild to severe prostatomegaly; mineralization	Focal or diffusely hyperechoic

Adapted from Barsanti JA, Finco DR: Prostatic diseases. *In* Ettinger S, Feldman E (eds): Textbook of Veterinary Internal Medicine, 4th ed. Philadelphia, WB Saunders, 1995, p 1662.

bladder cranially. Prostatomegaly has been defined as a dorsal ventral prostatic dimension greater than 70 per cent of the distance between the sacral promontory and the pubis on the lateral radiograph.[24] The normal prostatic silhouette may become indistinct with retroperitoneal extension of prostatitis or cancer. Radiopaque densities within the prostate may be caused by calculi within the prostatic urethra or by mineralization of the parenchyma.

Positive contrast retrograde urethrocystography is useful for evaluating the prostatic urethra (Fig. 172–2).[23] When the prostatic urethra is maximally distended, it has smooth margins and a larger diameter than the membranous or penile urethra.[25] A small amount of urethroprostatic reflux (less than one prostatic urethral diameter into the prostatic parenchyma) is normal. Contrast urethrograms may reveal narrowing of the prostatic urethra, an irregular pattern to the mucosal margin, or abnormal urethroprostatic reflux. These lesions are often identified in dogs with prostatic neoplasia.[26]

ULTRASONOGRAPHY

Ultrasonography is more sensitive than survey radiography for detecting intraparenchymal prostatic disease and is especially useful for guiding a biopsy needle into parenchymal lesions. The prostate can be evaluated for shape, size, symmetry, echogenicity, and cavitations. The normal prostatic sonogram has a uniform, homogeneous background echogenicity.[23] The coarsely hyperechoic echotexture is distributed uniformly throughout the parenchyma (Fig. 172–3). The urethra can be traced throughout the prostate. The normal prostate appears symmetric with smooth borders. Abnormal findings include the presence of cavitations; focal, multifocal or diffuse echotexture changes; change in prostatic size; and an irregular margin (see Table 172–2).

PROSTATIC ASPIRATION

Aspiration biopsy provides an excellent means for establishing a diagnosis in animals with signs of prostatic disease. Cytologic evaluation of prostatic aspiration samples correctly predicted the diagnosis in 96 per cent of dogs with various prostatic disorders.[27] Aspiration should be avoided if one suspects a prostatic abscess because aspiration may increase the risk of peritonitis.[21] The presence of fever, anorexia, leukocytosis, and cavitary lesions on ultrasonograms increases the likelihood of an abscess within the prostatic parenchyma.

Aspiration can be performed by rectal, perirectal, or transabdominal techniques. Transrectal aspiration can be performed without sedation or prior bowel preparation, and complications are rare.[26] Bleeding postbiopsy occurs occasionally but virtually always resolves without need for specific therapy. Transrectal biopsy is best done using the Franzen needle guide (Percision Dynamics Corp, Burbank, CA)

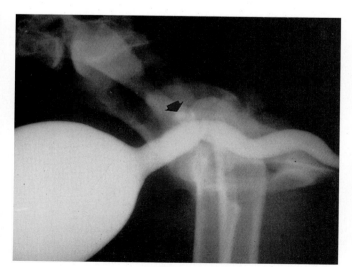

Figure 172–2. Positive contrast urethrogram of a normal dog. Note the small quantity of urethroprostatic reflux (arrow).

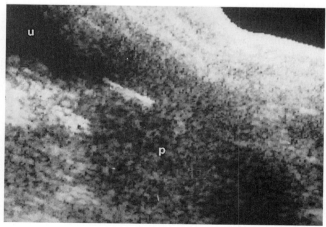

Figure 172–3. Prostatic sonogram of a normal dog. Note the uniform, homogeneous background of the prostate (p) and the location of the urinary bladder (u).

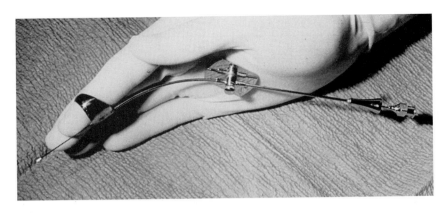

Figure 172–4. Transrectal biopsy of the prostate is performed using a Franzen needle guide.

(Fig. 172–4). Surgical gloves are worn under and over the needle guide. The prostate is palpated per rectum with the index finger placed through the needle guide. The prostate is stabilized with the index finger and by abdominal palpation using the other hand. The needle guide is held against the prostate, and an assistant rapidly advances the aspiration needle through the rectal wall into the prostate. After placement of the needle in the prostate, vigorous aspiration results in a small quantity of material that can be spread on a microscopic slide for cytologic evaluation (Fig. 172–5). Normal prostatic epithelial cells are cuboidal to columnar and uniform in size (10–15 μm in diameter) with a central to basilar nucleus and finely granular basophilic cytoplasm (Fig. 172–6).[27]

Perirectal prostatic aspiration is performed using a long needle such as a spinal needle. With the dog positioned in lateral recumbency, the needle is inserted lateral to the anus and passed into the prostate and an aspirate is obtained. A finger inserted into the rectum aids in guiding the needle into the prostate. It may be helpful to push the prostate caudally toward the pelvic canal.[3, 21]

Transabdominal aspiration is performed by guiding a long needle into the prostate either by palpation or using ultrasound guidance.[28] Ultrasound-guided aspiration allows sonographic visualization of the area to be sampled and may increase the likelihood of obtaining a diagnostic aspiration. Only mild sedation is required in most dogs. Some specialists routinely aspirate prostatic cysts using ultrasound guidance with 22-gauge needles, *especially* if it is suspected that

the cyst is in fact an abscess. The determination on whether to aspirate depends on location and cyst wall thickness. In general, intraprostatic cysts are thick walled and are routinely aspirated under ultrasound guidance. Paraprostatic cysts tend to be thin walled and are not usually considered safe for aspiration. Aspirated material can be evaluated cytologically as well as with culture. The culture results determine whether a cyst is, in fact, an abscess.

PROSTATIC BIOPSY

Biopsy of the prostate, which can provide material for histopathologic evaluation and culture, is the most accurate method to distinguish prostatic disorders. A prostatic biopsy can be obtained percutaneously or surgically. As with aspiration, percutaneous biopsy of the prostate is contraindicated if one suspects a prostatic abscess. Percutaneous biopsy is performed either transabdominally or perirectally[20, 29] using a Tru-Cut biopsy needle (Travenol Laboratories, Inc, Deerfield, IL). Transabdominal biopsy is simple in dogs where the prostatic mass is easily palpated abdominally and can be immobilized through the skin during the procedure. After sedation or general anesthesia, the dog's skin is shaved and surgically prepared and a small stab incision is made with a Number 11 scalpel blade to permit passage of the biopsy instrument. Ultrasound-guided biopsy enhances the accuracy of the needle core biopsy, can specifically avoid certain areas, increases the likelihood of a diagnostic procedure,

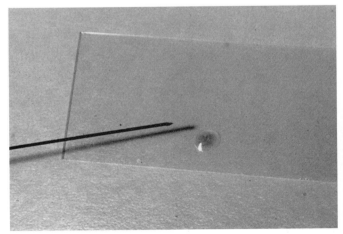

Figure 172–5. Needle aspiration biopsy of the prostate results in a small quantity of material that can be spread on a microscopic slide for microscopic evaluation.

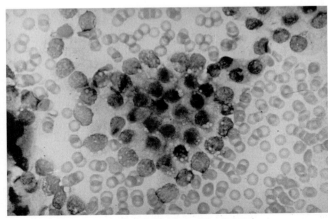

Figure 172–6. Photomicrograph of a group of normal prostatic epithelial cells from a dog with benign prostatic hypertrophy obtained by aspiration biopsy.

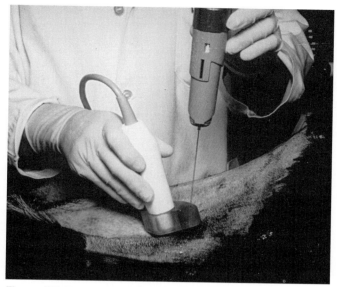

Figure 172–7. Ultrasound-guided biopsy enhances the accuracy of prostatic biopsy.

and minimizes the risk of post-biopsy complications (Fig. 172–7).[30] Perirectal biopsy is performed by passing the biopsy needle along the side of the rectum using rectal palpation to guide the needle into the prostate.[29] Transient hematuria, orchitis, and scrotal edema are occasional complications of needle biopsy.[29, 30]

PROSTATIC DISEASES

The prevalence of canine prostatic disease is reported to be 2.5 per cent.[15] The normal prostate gland increases in volume until the dog reaches 4 to 6 years of age, at which time growth plateaus and prostatic function, as assessed by ejaculate volume and total protein content of the ejaculate, peaks before abruptly declining.[31, 32] Prevalence of all types of prostatic disease increases with age, with a mean reported age of 8.9 years for onset of clinical signs.[15] Doberman pinschers are reported to have a high prevalence of prostatic disease.[15] Sexually intact dogs are most likely to have prostatic disease, although prostatic adenocarcinoma occurs in both intact and castrated dogs.[15, 26] Canine prostatic diseases include BPH, squamous metaplasia, acute and chronic bacterial prostatitis, prostatic abscesses, prostatic retention (true) cysts and paraprostatic cysts, prostatic neoplasia, and prostatic calculi.

BENIGN PROSTATIC HYPERTROPHY/HYPERPLASIA

BPH is commonly seen in older men and dogs. The dog is the only domestic species known to exhibit this disorder.[2] In men, it is characterized by hyperplasia of stromal cells within periurethral tissues.[4] In the dog, both hypertrophy (increased cell size) and hyperplasia (increased cell number) occur with diffuse glandular proliferation and an overall increase in volume and weight of the prostate.[4]

BPH is a natural consequence of aging; 16 per cent of dogs have histologic evidence of BPH by 2 years of age, whereas 50 per cent of dogs have histologic evidence of BPH by 4 to 5 years of age.[33] Both estrogens and androgens must be present for significant hypertrophy/hyperplasia to

occur.[3, 4, 31, 34–40] Aged dogs with BPH have been demonstrated to secrete 40 per cent less testosterone, 15 per cent less 5α-DHT, and 60 per cent more estradiol than normal dogs.[34] This altered estrogen:androgen ratio sensitizes the prostate to 5α-DHT by means of estrogen priming.[3, 41, 42] Estrogens may increase the number of androgen receptors in prostatic tissue and may form metabolites with free radical activity that damage the prostate, altering its response to 5α-DHT.[4, 38, 42, 43] In addition, prostates with BPH have an increased ability to metabolize androgens; a high correlation exists between size of the prostate and ability to form 5α-DHT from testosterone.[38, 39] Local growth factors and catecholamines may also have a role in mediating growth and contractility of the gland.[6, 12, 13] Small intraparenchymal cysts containing bloody or serosanguineous fluid may form; and as the gland develops increased vascularity, there is an increased tendency for prostatic bleeding.[4, 43, 44]

Clinical Signs. In man, pollakiuria is the most common presenting sign of BPH, presumably due to the periurethral location of hyperplasia and increased contractility of the gland.[4, 12, 13] In the dog, signs are referable to increased size of the gland and subsequent pressure on the rectum and surrounding structures. Bloody to serosanguineous urethral discharge unrelated to urination, hematuria, rectal tenesmus, hemospermia, and infertility may occur.[3, 15, 45] Systemic signs of disease are uncommon. BPH is only seen in intact animals. The hypertrophied/hyperplastic prostate will be symmetrically enlarged and non-painful when palpated per rectum.[15]

Diagnosis. Radiographically, the gland will be enlarged and may displace the bladder cranially and the rectum dorsally.[46] Mean normal area will not be as large nor the gland as asymmetric as in neoplasia or cystic prostatic disease.[3] The prostate is enlarged if it encompasses 70 per cent or more of the distance from the cranial aspect of the pubic bone to the sacral promontory on a lateral projection radiograph.[46] Ultrasonographically, the homogeneous parenchyma will be normal to slightly hyperechoic and single to multiple, small, fluid-filled parenchymal cysts may be noted.[24] Prostatic fluid, collected by ejaculation or prostatic massage, will vary in color from clear (normal) to red-brown. Prostatic fluid cytology may reveal increased numbers of red blood cells, and bacterial cultures will be non-significant (less than 100,000 bacteria/mL). Prostatic biopsy is rarely necessary to confirm the diagnosis.

Treatment. Bilateral orchiectomy is the treatment of choice. No medical therapy has yet been shown to be as effective as castration in decreasing prostatic size and causing long-term resolution of clinical signs.[8] Involution of the gland begins within days of surgery.[44] Decrease in prostatic size of 50 per cent is demonstrable in 3 weeks, with a decrease of 70 per cent by 9 weeks after castration.[44] However, castration causes permanent infertility and may be inappropriate as a first-choice treatment in valuable breeding animals.

Oral (diethylstilbestrol, 0.2–1.0 mg/d PO for 5 days) and injectable (estradiol cypionate, 0.1 mg/kg to a maximum total dosage of 2 mg) estrogen preparations have been shown to decrease prostatic size and signs of BPH.[4, 43, 47] Estrogens inhibit pituitary luteinizing hormone release by negative feedback with subsequent decline in serum testosterone concentration.[3, 4, 48] However, estrogens also induce squamous metaplasia of the gland and secretory stasis, which predispose the gland to ascending infection.[3, 4, 43, 48–50] In addition, estrogens may cause fatal bone marrow suppression in susceptible animals.[4] Because of their side effects, estrogens

URO

cannot be recommended as a routine treatment for BPH. An anti-estrogen compound, tamoxifen, has been shown to have some effect on decreasing prostatic size in BPH but does not inhibit androgen-induced stromal proliferation.[50]

Megestrol acetate (Ovaban, 0.5 mg/kg/d PO for 4–8 weeks) and medroxyprogesterone acetate (3–4 mg/kg SQ) have been shown to decrease serum testosterone concentration, to inhibit 5α-reductase activity, to decrease prostatic androgen receptor numbers, and, possibly, to competitively inhibit binding of 5α-DHT to intracellular receptors.[4, 15, 16, 43, 48, 51, 52] Prostate size is decreased and clinical signs resolve after 4 to 7 weeks of therapy.[16, 51, 52] No changes are noted in total sperm number, libido, or testicular size and consistency after treatment.[51, 52] Signs typically recur 10 to 24 months after treatment following a single dose of medroxyprogesterone acetate.[52] Diabetes mellitus has been reported after treatment with medroxyprogesterone acetate in one dog.[44] Progestins are not approved for use in male dogs in the United States.

5-Alpha-reductase inhibitors are effective in BPH by suppressing conversion of testosterone to 5α-DHT. Chlormadinone acetate decreases prostatic size and resolves clinical signs but may cause reduced fertility.[53–57] Finasteride (Proscar) appears to be the most effective drug in this class for treating canine BPH.[8, 58–63] At doses of 1 to 5 mg/kg per day, finasteride causes atrophy of glandular and stromal compartments of the prostate and a decrease in prostatic weight and volume.[8, 58, 61–63] Prostatic size decreases significantly after 4 weeks of treatment; maximum atrophy is noted after 6 to 9 weeks of therapy.[8, 59, 62, 63] Although intraprostatic 5α-DHT concentration will decrease with treatment, serum 5α-DHT concentration may remain unchanged.[8, 62, 64] Decrease in prostatic size is positively correlated with dose and duration of treatment.[61] However, treatment with a lower dose of finasteride (0.1–0.5 mg/kg/d) is being investigated and appears to be effective (Kamolpatana K, personal communication, 12/5/98). The prostate returns to pre-treatment size 7 weeks after cessation of therapy.[63]

Treatment with finasteride has not been demonstrated to cause changes in testicular weight, testicular histomorphology, or daily sperm production.[57, 65] As prostatic size decreases, a significant decrease in prostatic fluid volume ejaculated occurs.[63] This does not appear to alter fertility. In one study, all bitches bred to males that had been treated with finasteride at a dose of 1.0 mg/kg per given day orally for 21 days became pregnant.[63] It is not recommended that men attempt to father children while on the drug. Finasteride has not been evaluated for teratogenicity in the dog, but normal puppies have been born after its use.[63] Side effects have not been associated with administration of finasteride.[63] The drug is not approved for use in male dogs in the United States.

Flutamide and hydroxyflutamide are androgen receptor antagonists that act by competitively binding to the intracellular testosterone and 5α-DHT receptors in prostatic epithelial cells. At oral doses of 2.5 to 5.0 mg/kg per day, these drugs have been demonstrated to significantly decrease prostatic size within 6 to 7 weeks.[43, 66] The prostate undergoes glandular epithelial atrophy and a decrease in the number of intracellular secretory granules.[65] No change in libido, overall sperm production, or fertility has been noted.[43] Flutamide and hydroxyflutamide are not approved for use in the United States.

Miscellaneous treatments reported for canine BPH include ketoconazole,[15, 22] nutritional supplements, smooth muscle relaxants (doxazosin mesylate [Cardura, Roerig, New York]), catecholamine receptor blockers,[67] gossypol,[68] electrovapori-zation,[69, 70] transurethral collagenase injection,[71] transurethral light treatment after photosensitization,[72] transurethral high-intensity focused ultrasound,[73, 74] and rotoresect mechanical ablation plus high-frequency tissue coagulation.[75]

SQUAMOUS METAPLASIA

Squamous metaplasia is a morphologic change from normal cuboidal or columnar epithelium to squamous epithelium within the prostate. Secretory stasis accompanies this morphologic change.[41] Squamous metaplasia is induced by increased serum estrogen concentration, either from exogenous administration of estrogen or from the relative increase in serum estrogen concentration that occurs in normal aged dogs as androgen secretion declines.[4, 42, 76] Consequences of squamous metaplasia are not well defined, but it may predispose to prostatitis, retention (true) cysts, and prostatic neoplasia.[3, 44]

PROSTATITIS/PROSTATIC ABSCESS

Prostatitis (bacterial infection of the prostate) usually results from ascending infection from the normal urethral flora.[77] Prostatitis is often secondary to a primary disorder. BPH, squamous metaplasia, and prostatic neoplasia predispose the gland to infection by altering normal defense mechanisms that prevent retrograde movement of bacteria. These defense mechanisms include normal urine flow during micturition, the urethral high-pressure zone, bactericidal effects of prostatic fluid, and local IgA production.[44, 78] Organisms most commonly isolated include *Escherichia coli, Mycoplasma* sp., *Staphylococcus* sp., *Streptococcus* sp., *Klebsiella, Proteus,* and *Pseudomonas.*[3, 4, 19, 41, 44] *Brucella canis* has also been identified in canine prostatitis cases.[4] In 70 per cent of cases, a single organism will be isolated.[78] Granulomatous prostatitis resulting from systemic fungal infection such as blastomycosis and cryptococcosis has been described but is rare.[44]

Clinical Signs. Presenting signs vary with the course of the disease. Dogs with acute prostatitis may demonstrate prostatic pain, fever, lethargy, weakness, hematuria, urethral discharge, infertility, and unwillingness to breed.[15, 41] In chronically infected dogs, fewer systemic signs will be seen.[15] Dogs with a prostatic abscess may be asymptomatic or have signs of sepsis due to fulminating infection and peritonitis.[4] All dogs with prostatitis are likely to show evidence of urinary tract infection; all intact male dogs with recurrent urinary tract infection should be assumed to have prostatic involvement.[41, 43, 78] Prostatitis is more likely to be noted in intact than in neutered dogs but may occasionally be seen in castrated dogs with infection secondary to prostatic neoplasia.[79] The infected prostate gland may or may not be enlarged. Asymmetric prostatomegaly may be severe if a prostatic abscess is present.

Diagnosis. Radiographically, prostatomegaly and prostatic mineralization may be evident (see Table 172–2).[46] In chronic prostatitis, ultrasonography reveals a diffuse increase in prostatic parenchymal echogenicity (Fig. 172–8).[24] Abscesses are visible as hypoechoic to anechoic lesions with distant enhancement and cannot be differentiated from cysts or hematomas.[24]

Prostatic fluid, collected by ejaculation or prostatic massage, typically reveals an increased number of red and white blood cells. Bacteria may be seen within neutrophils.[15, 78]

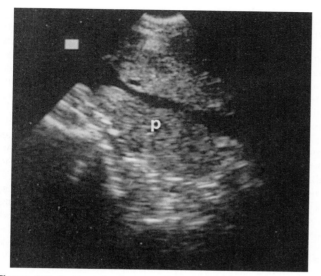

Figure 172–8. Prostatic sonogram from a dog with chronic bacterial prostatitis. Note the diffuse increase in prostatic echogenicity (p).

Culture of prostatic fluid typically reveals large numbers of a single bacterial species. Inflammatory cytology and pure growth of greater than 100,000 bacteria/mL of a single organism have been shown to correlate with a histopathologic diagnosis of infection in 80 to 90 per cent of cases.[43, 80] Comparing urine and urethral cytology and culture results with results obtained from prostatic fluid analysis may increase the accuracy of prostatic fluid evaluation in the diagnosis of bacterial prostatitis.[80] Changes in blood leukocyte counts and prostatic fluid pH do not appear to be helpful in the diagnosis of prostatitis.[43, 81]

Aspiration or needle prostatic biopsy can be useful in the diagnosis of prostatitis but may lead to seeding of bacteria along the needle tract with subsequent peritonitis.[3, 82] Biopsy should not be performed if one suspects a prostatic abscess.

Treatment. Infection is more readily cleared from the prostate of castrated dogs than intact dogs.[79] Castration may promote resolution of disorders predisposing to prostatitis such as BPH. Similarly, treatment with agents that reduce prostatic size such as the 5α-reductase inhibitor finasteride may hasten resolution of prostatitis.

When possible, antibiotic choice should be based on culture and sensitivity. In acute prostatitis, the blood-prostate barrier is disrupted, allowing most antibiotics to readily diffuse into prostatic tissue.[4] In chronic prostatitis or abscess formation, antibiotics that can penetrate the intact blood-prostate barrier or capsule of the abscess must be used. Characteristics of a suitable antibiotic include high lipid solubility, low protein binding, and a pKa complementary to the pH of the prostatic fluid. The pKa should allow antibiotic ionization and trapping within the prostate.[4, 15, 78] Acidic prostatic fluid (pH less than 7.2) will ionize antibiotics with a high pKa, and basic prostatic fluid (pH greater than 7.4) will ionize antibiotics with a low pKa.[4, 78] Examples of antibiotics with poor movement into prostatic tissue due to low lipid solubility include tetracyclines, aminoglycosides, cephalosporins, and ampicillin.[4, 78] Examples of antibiotics that readily penetrate the prostatic capsule include chloramphenicol, trimethoprim-sulfamethoxazole, and enrofloxacin.[15] Chloramphenicol has high protein binding and must be used at the high end of the dose range.[4] Owners should be cautioned of the human health hazards of this drug.

Trimethoprim-sulfamethoxazole may cause anemia and keratoconjunctivitis sicca if given long term. Concurrent administration of 5/mg/d of folic acid may ameliorate these problems.[83] Enrofloxacin (Baytril) has a low molecular weight favoring tissue penetration, is a zwitterion with 2 pKas, and is highly lipid soluble.[84] It achieves serum and intraprostatic concentrations well above the minimum inhibitory concentration of most pathogens when administered at a dose of 5 mg/kg twice a day.[84] Ciprofloxacin does not penetrate the prostate as well as enrofloxacin.[84] In general, prostatic infections caused by gram-positive organisms are most successfully treated with erythromycin, clindamycin, chloramphenicol, or trimethoprim, whereas gram-negative infections are best treated with chloramphenicol, enrofloxacin, or trimethoprim.[44]

Antibiotic therapy should be continued for at least 3 to 6 weeks.[15, 44] Prostatic fluid and urine should be cultured 1 to 2 weeks after completion of treatment and again 2 to 4 weeks later to ensure clearance of infection.[15, 44, 79] If infection recurs, appropriate antibiotic therapy should be instituted for 3 months. Chronically infected dogs may benefit from castration or long-term treatment with a 50 per cent–reduced dose of antibiotic given once daily.[78, 79]

Treatment of prostatic abscesses is problematic; a 1-year survival rate of 50 per cent after therapy has been reported.[44] Antibiotic therapy should be instituted as described earlier. Safely obtaining a sample for culture and sensitivity may be difficult with a large, solitary abscess. Empirical treatment with a highly diffusible antibiotic, such as enrofloxacin, may be required. Therapy with finasteride or castration may facilitate abscess resolution, but pockets of abscessation may persist despite decrease in prostatic size. The prostate should be monitored with ultrasonography to ensure resolution of the abscess.[44] In many cases, marsupialization or placement of Penrose drains will be necessary to obtain adequate drainage of the abscess cavity, but morbidity is high.[84] Reported complications include incontinence, chronic draining stomas, peritonitis, septic shock, and death.[4, 78] Newer surgical techniques appear to decrease morbidity.[85, 86]

PROSTATIC RETENTION (TRUE) CYSTS/ PARAPROSTATIC CYSTS

Numerous small prostatic cysts may occur with BPH and are treated as noted earlier for BPH.[3, 15] Retention (true) cysts are thin-walled structures within the prostatic parenchyma containing non-purulent fluid. The etiology of prostatic retention cysts is unknown. They may result from prostatic ducts that have become obstructed and dilated secondary to squamous metaplasia from exposure to endogenous or exogenous estrogens.[3, 15] Paraprostatic cysts are most commonly seen craniolateral or caudal to the bladder and prostate in older, large-breed dogs.[15, 87] They are thin-walled structures outside the prostatic parenchyma that often contain malodorous fluid containing fibronecrotic debris.[87–89] The etiology is unknown but these may be vestiges of the müllerian ducts.[3]

Clinical Signs and Diagnosis. With either retention cysts or paraprostatic cysts, dogs may have anorexia, weakness, abdominal distention, hematuria, or dysuria.[41, 87–89] Radiographically, the prostate will appear to be enlarged.[46] Contrast radiography may be required to differentiate a paraprostatic cyst from true prostatomegaly. Mineralization may be present in the wall of paraprostatic cysts.[87] Ultrasonography is useful in differentiating retention cysts from parapros-

URO

tatic cysts. Infusion of saline into the urinary bladder through a urethral catheter may be helpful in defining structures.[87]

Treatment. Both retention cysts and paraprostatic cysts are best treated by surgical removal, with or without concurrent subtotal prostatectomy.[15, 90] Surgical drainage may be attempted, but infection is a common complication.[15] Castration may aid in resolution of retention cysts. Effect of castration on resolution of paraprostatic cysts is unknown.

PROSTATIC NEOPLASIA

Prostatic neoplasia is an uncommon, insidious disease of older dogs and cats.[26, 91–100] Less than 1 per cent, of dogs in necropsy studies have been documented to have prostatic neoplasia, although the disease may be slightly more prevalent because of the lack of clinical signs referable to the prostate in some dogs.[97] Prostatic neoplasia is less common than bacterial prostatitis or BPH, occurring in approximately 7 per cent of dogs with signs of prostatic disease.[15] The disorder has been rarely documented in cats.[101, 102]

Adenocarcinomas are the most frequent prostatic cancer, although undifferentiated carcinoma, transitional cell carcinoma, leiomyosarcoma and hemangiosarcoma have also been noted.[103–106] Transitional cell carcinomas may extend into the prostate from the bladder or urethra or arise from prostatic periurethral ductal cells.[107] Benign prostatic tumors have not been reported.

Carcinomatous prostates are usually large, are irregular, and may be cystic.[104] There is no specific anatomic region that is involved most frequently. Tumors are usually diffuse throughout the prostate and may extend into the neck of the bladder, resulting in obstruction to bladder outflow or ureteral obstruction. They may also extend into the urethra and pelvic and colonic musculature.

Leav and Ling identified three histologic types of adenocarcinomas: intra-alveolar proliferative, small acinar, and undifferentiated.[104] The intra-alveolar proliferative type is most often seen and is composed of variably sized and shaped alveoli lined by multiple layers of epithelial cells. Cells are irregularly arranged and not bordered by a basement membrane. The small acinar type is characterized by cells arranged in small acini surrounded by fibrous connective tissue. The undifferentiated type is composed of sheets of pleomorphic epithelial cells. In addition to neoplasia, cancerous prostates may have inflammatory changes, necrosis, BPH, hemorrhage, and fibrous connective tissue proliferation. BPH has been noted in intact, but not in castrated, dogs.[26]

A precancerous lesion (high-grade prostatic intraepithelial neoplasia) has been described in canine prostates.[108, 109] The lesion is present in 55 per cent of normal 7- to 17-year-old sexually intact dogs, 9 per cent of 7- to 17-year-old castrated dogs, and 8 per cent of 1- to 4-year-old sexually intact dogs. The lesion is similar to lesions of prostatic intraepithelial neoplasia that have been described in humans.

Prostatic adenocarcinoma occurs most commonly in medium- to large-breed dogs.[97] The average age at presentation is 8 to 10 years.[26, 110] Prostatic carcinoma has been identified in both intact and castrated male dogs.[26, 98, 111] In two case series, the prevalence of castrated dogs with prostatic carcinoma ranged from 32 to 43 per cent.[26, 98] The risk of prostatic carcinoma in a castrated male dog is approximately two times greater than the risk in an intact male dog, and the risk appears to increase with the time that the dog has been castrated.[26] A dog that has been castrated for at least 10 years has four times the risk of developing a carcinoma as an intact dog.

The cause of canine prostatic carcinoma is unknown, although castration and increasing age appear to increase risk.[26, 112] In a man, endocrine dependence of the normal prostate and the ability to effect prostate cancer growth rates through hormonal manipulation suggest a possible hormonal etiology for prostatic cancer. The role of testosterone in inducing or promoting prostate cancer is unclear. Prostate cancer has been experimentally induced in rats by prolonged testosterone administration,[113, 114] and high levels of circulating testosterone have been identified in some,[115] but not in all, studies of human patients with prostate carcinoma.[116, 117] On the other hand, prostatic cancer is rare in eunuchs and in prisoners castrated for sexual offenses. In both humans and dogs, the adrenal gland may provide a source of androgens and estrogens after castration.[118, 119]

Metastatic disease is often present at the time of diagnosis of prostatic carcinoma. Spread to bones, especially the lumbar vertebrae and pelvis, has been noted in 23 to 42 per cent of cases (Waters D et al, unpublished data).[104, 120, 121] Bone scintigraphy may increase the likelihood of detecting bony metastases.[122] Eighty per cent of dogs with bone metastasis have concurrent visceral metastasis (Waters D et al, unpublished data). Other frequent metastatic sites include lung, iliac lymph nodes, colon, rectum, and bladder.[26, 97, 99, 104, 121]

Clinical Signs. Clinical signs in dogs with prostatic carcinoma include rectal tenesmus, constipation, dyschezia, anorexia, weight loss, straining to urinate, hematuria, hemorrhagic urethral discharge, and rear limb weakness. Defecation abnormalities (e.g., constipation, frequent bowel movements, ribbon-like stools) occur in 45 per cent of dogs, anorexia and weight loss in 35 per cent, and signs related to the urinary tract (e.g., hematuria, incontinence, dysuria) in approximately 40 per cent.[26] Signs of urinary tract dysfunction without signs of gastrointestinal dysfunction develop more commonly in neutered than intact dogs. Gastrointestinal abnormalities are more frequent in intact than in neutered dogs. Dogs with metastases to bones are more likely to demonstrate weight loss and lumbar pain.[121] Hematuria and urethral obstruction have been noted in cats with prostatic carcinomas.[100, 123]

Physical examination typically reveals prostatomegaly. Enlargement may be asymmetric or symmetric, and the prostate may be adhered to the pelvic floor. As would be expected, prostatomegaly is noted more often in intact than in castrated dogs.[26] Identification of an enlarged prostate in a castrated dog should raise the index of suspicion of neoplastic disease. Other frequently identified abnormalities include depression, abdominal pain, pain in response to rectal palpation, presence of a caudal abdominal mass, lumbar pain, hematuria, lameness, and enlargement of the sublumbar lymph nodes.[26, 104, 110] If urine outflow is obstructed, the urinary bladder may be enlarged and painful.

Diagnosis. The diagnosis of prostatic carcinoma can be established by identifying neoplastic cells in prostatic massage samples, needle aspirates, needle core biopsy specimens, or incisional prostatic biopsy specimens (Fig. 172–9).[27, 124] Because dogs with prostatic carcinoma typically have prostatic pain, semen samples are difficult to collect. Cytologic evaluation of prostatic carcinomas typically reveals large, pleomorphic cells with prominent nucleoli and vacuolated cytoplasm. The cells are usually in small to large clusters, clumps, or sheets.[3, 27] Complete blood cell counts reveal leukocytosis and neutrophilia in approximately half the dogs with prostatic carcinoma.[26] Regenerative or non-

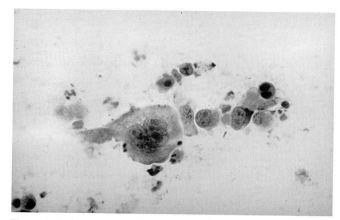

Figure 172–9. Needle aspiration biopsy sample of the prostate from a dog with prostatic adenocarcinoma.

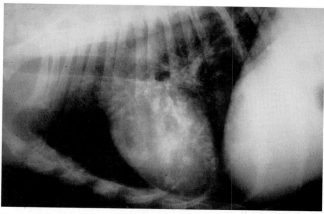

Figure 172–11. Lateral chest radiograph from a dog with prostatic adenocarcinoma and pulmonary metastasis. Note the multiple nodular densities within the pulmonary parenchyma.

regenerative anemia is present in approximately 25 per cent of cases. Neoplastic cells were noted in the blood from one dog.[92]

Urinalyses usually reveal hematuria, although urinary tract inflammation (hematuria, pyuria, proteinuria) with or without bacterial infection may be noted.[22, 26, 110] Bacterial urinary tract infection has been identified in 36 per cent of dogs with prostatic carcinoma.[26] Atypical cells are occasionally noted in the urine, but because the urine environment can cause cellular atypia, morphologic changes must be evaluated with caution.[22, 27]

On biochemistry profiles, serum alkaline phosphatase is increased in 70 per cent of dogs with prostatic carcinoma.[26] Although the cause of the increase is not always known, bone metastases, hepatic metastases, and corticosteroid therapy may play a role. Other biochemical abnormalities identified in dogs with prostatic carcinoma include hypocalcemia (35 per cent), hypercalcemia (5 per cent), and hypoalbuminemia (25 per cent).[26] Azotemia may be noted if bilateral urethral or ureteral obstruction is present.

In man, evaluation of serum biochemical markers (acid phosphatase and prostate-specific antigen) has been useful in detecting prostatic carcinoma cases. Acid phosphatase levels were useful in the detection of prostatic carcinoma in one canine study,[125] but increased serum levels could not be detected in another.[126] Prostate-specific antigen cannot be detected in canine serum, but canine prostatic secretory esterase (CPSE), a similar protein, is increased in dogs with prostatic disease. Unfortunately, highest elevations of CPSE are found in BPH, not carcinoma.[126] Immunohistochemical staining of canine prostatic carcinomas reveals low levels of acid phosphatase, prostate-specific antigen and CPSE.[126, 127]

Prostatomegaly and prostatic mineralization are the most common radiographic findings in dogs with prostatic carcinoma (Fig. 172–10).[26, 46] An enlarged prostate typically displaces the colon dorsally and the bladder cranially. The prostatic border may be smooth, irregular, or indistinct. Sublumbar lymph nodes may be enlarged. Lumbar vertebra and the pelvis should be examined carefully for the presence of lysis or bony proliferation suggestive of metastatic disease. Thoracic radiographs should be obtained to check for pulmonary metastases. Metastatic lesions appear as single or multiple nodular densities or a diffuse increase in unstructured interstitial density (Fig. 172–11). Pulmonary metastasis

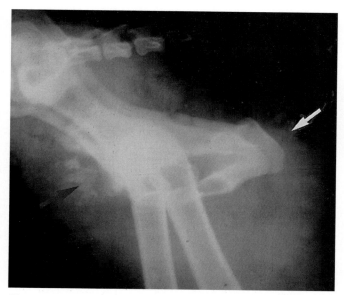

Figure 172–10. Lateral abdominal radiograph from a dog with a prostatic adenocarcinoma and metastasis to the perineum. Note the intraprostatic mineralization (black arrow) and mineralization of the perineal metastasis (white arrow).

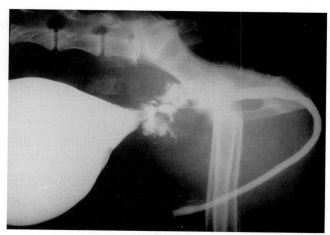

Figure 172–12. Positive contrast urethrogram from a dog with prostatic adenocarcinoma. Note the prostatomegaly and intraprostatic reflux of contrast agent.

URO

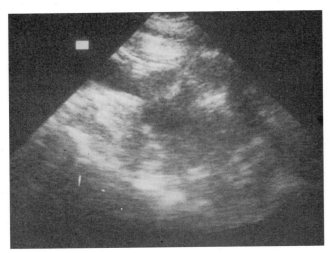

Figure 172–13. Prostatic sonogram from a dog with prostatic adenocarcinoma. Note the hyperechoic and hypoechoic areas and the irregular prostatic margin.

is present at the time of initial diagnosis in greater than 40 per cent of dogs with prostatic adenocarcinomas.[26]

A positive contrast urethrogram often reveals abnormal prostatic reflux and an irregular contour and narrowing of the prostatic urethra (Fig. 172–12).[46, 128] Ultrasonographic findings include coalescing areas of focal to multifocal increased echogenicity and prostatomegaly in approximately 70 per cent of cases; mineralization and cavitary lesions also may be noted (Fig. 172–13).[26, 129] Lesions may be difficult to distinguish from those associated with chronic bacterial prostatitis. Sub-lumbar lymph nodes may be enlarged.

Treatment. Treatment of dogs with prostatic carcinoma has not been rewarding. Most dogs have extensive local and metastatic disease at the time of diagnosis.[26] A thorough staging evaluation including abdominal and thoracic radiographs will be useful in guiding therapeutic decisions. External-beam radiation therapy may provide short-term benefits in dogs without extensive metastatic disease.[26, 130] Median survival time in ten dogs treated with radiation therapy was 114 days.[130] Prostatectomy can be attempted, but urinary incontinence is a frequent complication, and 9 months is the longest reported postoperative survival.[131, 132] No response has been noted to orchiectomy, estrogen, or ketoconazole therapy.[26] Chemotherapy with cisplatin and doxorubicin has been attempted, but results to date have not been encouraging. A retained urethral catheter may provide symptomatic relief in dogs with prostatic cancer and urethral obstruction.[133]

Prognosis. The prognosis in dogs with prostatic carcinoma is poor. Survival is typically 1 to 2 months after diagnosis, although one dog survived 19 months without therapy.[26] External-beam radiation therapy may provide palliative relief in dogs without extensive metastatic disease.

PROSTATIC CALCULI

Prostatic calculi are rare in dogs, and their significance is unknown. They are typically small and are often identified as an incidental finding.[134]

REFERENCES

1. Evans H, Christensen G: The urogenital system. In Evans H (ed): Miller's Anatomy of the Dog. Philadelphia, WB Saunders, 1990, p514.

2. Hamilton D: Anatomy of mammalian male accessory reproductive organs. In Lamming G (ed): Marshall's Physiology of Reproduction. New York, Churchill Livingstone, 1990, p693.
3. Rogers K, et al: Diagnostic evaluation of the canine prostate. Compend Contin Ed Pract Vet 8:799, 1986.
4. Olson P: Disorders of the canine prostate. In: Proceedings of the Annual Meeting of the Society of Theriogenology, Denver, CO, 1984, p46.
5. Dorfman M, Barsanti J: Diseases of the canine prostate gland. Compend Contin Ed 17:791, 1995.
6. Lee C: Role of androgen in prostate growth and regression: Stromal-epithelial interaction. Prostate Suppl 6:52, 1996.
7. Bruschini H, et al: Neurologic control of prostatic secretion in the dog. Invest Urol 15:288, 1978.
8. Rhodes L: The role of dihydrotestosterone in prostate physiology. In: Proceedings of the Annual Meeting of the Society for Theriogenology, Kansas City, MO, 1996, p288.
9. McKerecher G, et al: Dihydrotestosterone and 3-alpha-androstanediol dynamics in the normal, involuted, and hyperplastic canine prostate. Steroids 48:55, 1986.
10. Grino P, et al: Testosterone at high concentrations interacts with the human androgen receptor similarly to dihydrotestosterone. Endocrinology 126:1165, 1990.
11. Chevalier S, et al: Serum and prostate growth-promoting factors for steroid-independent epithelial cells of the adult dog prostate. Prostate 19:207, 1991.
12. Shapiro E, et al: Alpha 2 adrenergic receptors in canine prostate: Biochemical and functional correlations. J Urol 137:656, 1987.
13. Hieble J, et al: Comparison of the alpha-adrenoceptor characteristics in human and canine prostate. Fed Proc 45:2609, 1986.
14. England G, et al: An investigation into the origin of the first fraction of the canine ejaculate. Res Vet Sci 49:66, 1990.
15. Krawiec DR, Heflin D: Study of prostatic disease in dogs: 177 cases (1981–1986). JAVMA 200:1119, 1992.
16. Olson P, et al: Disorders of the canine prostate gland: Pathogenesis, diagnosis, and medical therapy. Comp Contin Ed Pract Vet 9:613, 1987.
17. Barsanti J, Finco D: Prostatic diseases, In Ettinger S, Feldman E (eds): Textbook of Veterinary Internal Medicine, 4th ed. Phiadelphia, WB Saunders, 1995, p1662.
18. O'Shea J: Studies on the canine prostate gland: I. Factors influencing size and weight. J Comp Pathol 72:321, 1962.
19. Ling G, et al: Canine prostatic fluid: Techniques of collection, quantitative bacterial culture, and interpretation of results. JAVMA 183:201, 1983.
20. Barsanti J, et al: Evaluation of diagnostic techniques for canine prostatic diseases. JAVMA 177:160, 1980.
21. Barsanti J: Collection and analysis of prostatic fluid and tissue. In Osborne C, Finco D (eds): Canine and Feline Nephrology and Urology. Media, PA, Williams & Wilkins, 1995, p122.
22. Barsanti JA, Finco DR: Evaluation of techniques for diagnosis of canine prostatic diseases. JAVMA 185:198, 1984.
23. Johnston G, et al: Diagnostic imaging of the male canine reproductive tract. Vet Clin North Am 21:553, 1991.
24. Feeney DA, et al: Canine prostatic disease—comparison of ultrasonographic appearance with morphologic and microbiologic findings: 30 cases (1981–1985). JAVMA 190:1027, 1987.
25. Feeney DA, et al: Dimensions of the prostate and membranous urethra in normal dogs during maximum distension retrograde urethrocystography. Vet Radiol 25:249, 1984.
26. Bell FW et al: Clinical and pathologic features of prostatic adenocarcinoma in sexually intact and castrated dogs: 31 cases (1970–1987). JAVMA 199:1623, 1991.
27. Thrall M: Cytologic diagnosis of canine prostatic disease. J Am Anim Hosp Assoc 21:95, 1985.
28. Smith S: Ultrasound-guided biopsy. Vet Clin North Am 15:1249, 1985.
29. Weaver A: Transperineal punch biopsy of the canine prostate gland. J Small Anim Pract 18:573, 1977.
30. Hager D, et al: Ultrasound-guided biopsy of the canine liver, kidney and prostate. Vet Radiol 26:82, 1985.
31. Berry S, et al: Effects of aging on prostate growth in beagles. Am J Physiol 250:R1039, 1986.
32. Brendler CB, et al: Spontaneous benign prostatic hyperplasia in the beagle: Age-associated changes in serum hormone levels, and the morphology and secretory function of the canine prostate. J Clin Invest 71:1114, 1983.
33. Berry SJ, et al: Development of canine benign prostatic hyperplasia with age. Prostate 9:363, 1986.
34. Cochran RC, et al: Serum levels of follicle stimulating hormone, luteinizing hormone, prolactin, testosterone, 5α-dihydrotestosterone, 5α-androstane-3α, 17β diol, and 17β-estradiol from male beagles with spontaneously induced benign prostatic hyperplasia. Invest Urol 19:142, 1981.
35. Winter M, et al: Induction of benign prostatic hyperplasia in intact dogs by near-physiological levels of 5α-dihydrotestosterone and 17β-estradiol. Prostate 26:325, 1995.
36. Lipowitz AJ, et al: Testicular neoplasms and concomitant clinical changes in the dog. JAVMA 163:1364, 1973.
37. Merk F, et al: Multiple phenotypes of prostatic glandular cells in castrated dogs after individual or combined treatment with androgen. Lab Invest 54:442, 1986.
38. Winter M, Liehr J: Possible mechanism of induction of benign prostatic hyperpla-

sia by estradiol and dihydrotestosterone in dogs. Toxicol Appl Pharmacol 136:211, 1996.

39. Isaacs J, Coffey D: Changes in dihydrotestosterone metabolism associated with the development of canine benign prostatic hyperplasia. Endocrinology 108:445, 1981.

40. DeKlerk DP, et al: Comparison of spontaneous and experimentally induced canine prostatic hyperplasia. J Clin Invest 64:842, 1979.

41. Krawiec DR: Canine prostate disease. JAVMA 204:1561, 1994.

42. Trachtenberg J, et al: Androgen- and estrogen-receptor content in spontaneous and experimentally induced canine prostatic hyperplasia. J Clin Invest 65:1051, 1980.

43. Barsanti J, Finco D: Medical management of canine prostatic hyperplasia. In Bonagura J, Kirk R (eds): Current Veterinary Therapy XII. Philadelphia, WB Saunders, 1995, p1033.

44. Barsanti J: Diseases of the prostate gland. In: Proceedings of the Annual Meeting of the Society of Theriogenology, Montreal, Quebec, 1997, p72.

45. Read RA, Bryden S: Urethral bleeding as a presenting sign of benign prostatic hyperplasia in the dog: A retrospective study (1979–1993). JAVMA 31:261, 1995.

46. Feeney DA, et al: Canine prostatic disease—comparison of radiographic appearance with morphologic and microbiologic findings: 30 cases (1981–1985). JAVMA 190:1018, 1987.

47. Barsanti J, Finco D: Canine prostatic diseases. In Morrow D (ed): Current Therapy in Theriogenology. Philadelphia, WB Saunders, 1986, p553.

48. Freshman J: Effects of drugs and environmental agents on fertility in the stud dog. In: Proceedings of the Annual Meeting of the Society of Theriogenology. San Diego, CA, 1991, p226.

49. Berry S, et al: Effect of age, castration, and testosterone replacement on the development and resoration of canine benign prostatic hyperplasia. Prostate 9:295, 1986.

50. Funke P, et al: Effects of the antioestrogen tamoxifen on steroid-induced morphological and biochemical changes in the castrated dog prostate. Acta Endocrinol 100:462, 1982.

51. Wright P, et al: Medroxyprogesterone acetate and reproductive processes in male dogs. Aust Vet J 55:437, 1979.

52. Bamberg-Thelen B, Linde-Forsberg C: Treatment of canine benign prostatic hyperplasia. J Am Anim Hosp Assoc 29:221, 1993.

53. Takezawa Y, et al: Effects of a new steroidal antiandrogen, TZP-4238 (17 alpha-acetoxy-6-chloro-2-oxa-4, 6-pregnadiene-3, 20-dione), on spontaneously developed canine benign prostatic hyperplasia. Prostate 27:321, 1995.

54. Kawakami E: Effects of oral administration of chlormadinone acetate on canine prostatic hypertrophy. J Vet Med Sci 55:631, 1993.

55. Kawakami E, et al: Comparison of the effects of chlormadinone acetate-pellet implantation and orchidectomy on benign prostatic hypertrophy in the dog. Int J Androl 18:248, 1995.

56. Orima H, et al: Short-term oral treatment of canine benign prostatic hypertrophy with chlormadinone acetate. J Vet Med Sci 57:139, 1995.

57. Shimizu M, et al: Effect of chlormadinone acetate-pellet implantation on the volume of prostate, peripheral blood levels of sex hormones and semen quality in the dog. J Vet Med Sci 57:395, 1995.

58. Laroque P, et al: Quantitative evaluation of glandular and stromal compartments in hyperplastic dog prostates: Effect of 5α-reductase inhibitors. Prostate 27:121, 1995.

59. Cohen S, et al: Comparison of the effects of new specific azasteroid inhibitors of steroid 5-α reductase on canine hyperplastic prostate: Suppression of prostatic dihydrotestosterone correlated with prostate regression. Prostate 26:55, 1995.

60. Juniewicz P, et al: Effect of combination treatment with zanoterone (WIN 49,596), a steroidal androgen receptor antagonist, and finasteride (MK 906), a steroidal 5α-reductase inhibitor, on the prostate and testes of beagle dogs. Endocrinology 133:904, 1993.

61. Laroque P, et al: Effects of chronic oral administration of a selective 5α-reductase inhibitor, finasteride, on the dog prostate. Prostate 24:93, 1994.

62. Cohen SM, et al: Magnetic resonance imaging of the efficacy of specific inhibition of 5alpha-reductase in canine spontaneous benign prostatic hyperplasia. Magn Reson Med 21:55, 1991.

63. Iguer-Ouada M, Verstegen J: Effect of finasteride (Proscar MSD) on seminal composition, prostate function and fertility in male dogs. J Reprod Fertil Suppl 51:139, 1997.

64. Kamolpatana K, Johnston S: Effect of finasteride on serum dihydrotestosterone and testosterone in the dog. In: Proceedings of the Annual Meeting of the Society for Theriogenology, Kansas City, MO, 1996, p141.

65. Juniewicz P, et al: Effects of androgen and antiestrogen treatment on canine prostatic arginine esterase. Prostate 17:101, 1990.

66. Cartee R, et al: Evaluation of drug-induced prostate involution in dogs by transabdominal B-mode ultrasonography. Am J Vet Res 51:1773, 1990.

67. Breslin D, et al: Medical management of benign prostatic hyperplasia: A canine model comparing the in vivo efficacy of alpha-1 adrenergic antagonists on the prostate. J Urol 149:395, 1993.

68. Chang W, et al: Experimentally-induced prostatic hyperplasia in young beagles: A model to evaluate chemotherapeutic effects of gossypol. Res Commun Mol Pathol Pharmacol 92:341, 1996.

69. Leveille RJ, et al: Enhanced radiofrequency ablation of canine prostate utilizing a liquid conductor: The virtual electrode. J Endourol 10:5, 1996.

70. Benjamin D, et al: Histopathologic evaluation of the canine prostate following electrovaporization. J Urol 157:1144, 1997.

71. Harmon W, et al: Transurethral enzymatic ablation of the prostate: A canine model. Urology 48:229, 1996.

72. Selman S, Keck R: The effect of transurethral light on the canine prostate after sensitization with the photosensitizer TIM (II) etiopurpurin dichloride: A pilot study. J Urol 152:2129, 1994.

73. Foster R, et al: High-intensity focused ultrasound in the treatment of prostatic disease. Eur Urol 23(Suppl 1):29, 1993.

74. Gelet A, et al: High-intensity focused ultrasound experimentation on human benign prostatic hypertrophy. Eur Urol 23(Suppl 1):44, 1993.

75. Michel M, et al: Rotoresect: New technique for resection of the prostate: Experimental phase. J Endourol 10:473, 1996.

76. Brendler CB, et al: Spontaneous benign prostatic hyperplasia in the beagle: Age-associated changes in serum hormone levels, and the morphology and secretory function of the canine prostate. J Clin Invest 71:1114, 1983.

77. Ling G, Ruby A: Aerobic bacterial flora of the prepuce, urethra, and vagina of normal adult dogs. Am J Vet Res 39:695, 1979.

78. Dorfman M, Barsanti J: CVT Update: Treatment of canine bacterial prostatitis, In Bonagura J, Kirk R (eds): Current Veterinary Therapy XII. Philadelphia, WB Saunders, 1995, p1029.

79. Cowan L, et al: Effects of castration on chronic bacterial prostatitis in dogs. JAVMA 199:346, 1991.

80. Ling GV, et al: Comparison of two sample collection methods for quantitative bacteriologic culture of canine prostatic fluid. JAVMA 196:1479, 1990.

81. Branan J, et al: Selected physical and chemical characteristics of prostatic fluid collected by ejaculation from healthy dogs and from dogs with bacterial prostatitis. Am J Vet Res 45:825, 1984.

82. Barr F: Percutaneous biopsy of abdominal organs under ultrasound guidance. J Small Anim Pract 36:105, 1995.

83. Rubin S: Managing dogs with bacterial prostatic disease. Vet Med 85:387, 1990.

84. Dorfman M, et al: Enrofloxacin concentrations in dogs with normal prostates and dogs with chronic bacterial prostatitis. Am J Vet Res 56:386, 1995.

85. White RA, Williams JM: Intracapsular prostatic omentalization: A new technique for management of prostatic abscesses in dogs. Vet Surg 24:390, 1995.

86. Glennon J, Flanders J: Decreased incidence of postoperative urinary incontinence with a modified Penrose drain technique for treatment of prostatic abscesses in dogs. Cornell Veterinarian 83:189, 1993.

87. Closa J, et al: What is your diagnosis? Paraprostatic cyst in a dog. J Small Anim Pract 36:114, 1995.

88. Girard C, Despots J: Mineralized paraprostatic cyst in a dog. Can Vet J 36:573, 1995.

89. Lisciandro GR: What is your diagnosis? Large, round mass with intramural mineralization in the mid-to-caudal portion of the abdominal cavity; prostatomegaly. JAVMA 206:171, 1995.

90. Harari J, Dupuis J: Surgical treatments for prostatic diseases in dogs. Semin Vet Med Surg (Small Anim) 10:43, 1995.

91. Cotchin E: Further observations on neoplasms in dogs with particular reference to site of origin and malignancy. Br Vet J 110:274, 1954.

92. Alsaker R: Neoplastic cells in the blood of a dog with prostatic adenocarcinoma. J Am Anim Hosp Assoc 13:486, 1977.

93. Grant C: Carcinoma of the canine prostate. Acta Pathol Microbiol Scand 15:197, 1957.

94. Borthwick R: The signs and results of treatment of prostatic disease in dogs. Vet Rec 89:374, 1971.

95. Taylor P: Prostatic adenocarcinoma in dog and summary of ten cases. Can Vet J 14:162, 1973.

96. O'Shea J: Studies on the canine prostate gland: II. Prostatic neoplasms. J Comp Pathol 73:244, 1963.

97. Weaver A: Fifteen cases of prostatic carcinoma in the dog. Vet Rec 109:71, 1981.

98. Obradovich J, et al: The influence of castration on the development of prostatic carcinoma in the dog: 43 cases (1978–1985). J Vet Intern Med 1:183, 1987.

99. Hargis A, Miller L: Prostatic carcinoma in dogs. Compend Contin Ed 5:647, 1983.

100. Hubbard BS, et al: Prostatic adenocarcinoma in a cat. JAVMA 197:1493, 1990.

101. Hawe RS: What is your diagnosis? Prostatic adenocarcinoma. JAVMA 182:1257, 1983.

102. Hornbuckle W, Kleine L: Medical management of prostatic disease. In Kirk R (ed): Current Veterinary Therapy VII. Philadelphia, WB Saunders, 1980, p1146.

103. Leib M: Squamous cell carcinoma of the prostate gland in a dog. J Am Anim Hosp Assoc 22:509, 1986.

104. Leav I, Ling GV: Adenocarcinoma of the canine prostate. Cancer 22:1329, 1968.

105. Hayden DW, et al: Prostatic hemangiosarcoma in a dog: Clinical and pathologic findings. J Vet Diagn Invest 4:209, 1992.

106. Hayden D, Klausner JS: Prostatic leiomyosarcoma in a dog. J Vet Diagn Invest, in press.

107. Sawczuk I: Primary transitional cell carcinoma of prostatic periurethral ducts. Urology 25:339, 1985.

108. Waters DJ, Bostwick DG: The canine prostate is a spontaneous model of intraepithelial neoplasia and prostate cancer progression. Anticancer Res 17:1467, 1997.

109. Waters DJ, et al: Prostatic intraepithelial neoplasia in dogs with spontaneous prostate cancer. Prostate 30:92, 1997.

110. Hornbuckle WE, et al: Prostatic disease in the dog. Cornell Veterinarian 68:284, 1978.

111. Evans JE Jr, et al: Prostatic adenocarcinoma in a castrated dog. JAVMA 186:78, 1985.

112. Waters DJ, et al: Comparing the age at prostate cancer diagnosis in humans and dogs (letter). J Natl Cancer Inst 88:1686, 1996.

URO

113. Noble D: The development of prostate adenocarcinoma in the Nb rat following prolonged sex hormone administration. Cancer Res 37:1929, 1977.

114. Hoover D, et al: Experimental induction of neoplasia in the accessory sex organs of male Lobund-Wistar rats. Cancer Res 50 1990.

115. Gann P, et al: Prospective study of sex hormone levels and risk of prostate cancer. J Natl Cancer Inst 88:1118, 1997.

116. Meikle AW, et al: Familial factors affecting prostatic cancer risk and plasma sex-steroid levels. Prostate 6:121, 1985.

117. Jackson M, et al: Factors involved in the high incidence of prostatic cancer among American blacks. Prog Clin Biol Res 53:111, 1981.

118. Santen R, et al: Adrenal of male dog secretes androgens and estrogens. Am J Physiol 239:109, 1980.

119. Uno M, et al: Prostatic cancer 30 years after bilateral orchidectomy. Br J Urol 81:506, 1998.

120. Goedegebuure S: Secondary bone tumors in the dog. Vet Pathol 16:520, 1979.

121. Durham SK, Dietze AE: Prostatic adenocarcinoma with and without metastasis to bone in dogs. JAVMA 188:1432, 1986.

122. Lee-Parritz D, Lamb C: Prostatic adenocarcinoma with osseous metastases in a dog. JAVMA 192:1569, 1988.

123. Osborne C: Feline urologic syndrome: A heterogenous phenomenon? J Am Anim Hosp Assoc 20:17, 1984.

124. Barsanti J, Finco D: Canine bacterial prostatitis. Vet Clin North Am 9:679, 1979.

125. Corazza M, et al: Serum total prostatic and non-prostatic acid phosphatase in healthy dogs and in dogs with prostatic diseases. J Small Anim Pract 35:307, 1994.

126. Bell FW, et al: Evaluation of serum and seminal plasma markers in the diagnosis of canine prostatic disorders. J Vet Intern Med 9:149, 1995.

127. McEntee M, et al: Adenocarcinoma of the canine prostate: Immunohistochemical examination for secretory antigens. Prostate 11:163, 1987.

128. Ackerman N: Prostatic reflux during positive contrast retrograde urethrography in the dog. Vet Radiol 24:251, 1983.

129. Feeney DA, et al: Two-dimensional, gray-scale ultrasonography: Applications in canine prostatic disease. Vet Clin North Am Small Anim Pract 15:1159, 1985.

130. Turrel JM: Intraoperative radiotherapy of carcinoma of the prostate gland in ten dogs. JAVMA 190:48, 1987.

131. Hardie E: Complications of prostatic surgery. J Am Anim Hosp Assoc 20:50, 1984.

132. Basinger R: Urodynamic alterations associated with clinical prostatic diseases and prostatic surgery in 23 dogs. J Am Anim Hosp Assoc 25:385, 1989.

133. Mann FA, et al: Use of a retained urethral catheter in three dogs with prostatic neoplasia. Vet Surg 21:342, 1992.

134. Feeney D, Johnston G: Urogenital imaging: A practical update. Semin Vet Med Surg 1:144, 1986.

CHAPTER 173

FAMILIAL RENAL DISEASE IN DOGS AND CATS

Stephen P. DiBartola

Most familial renal diseases result in chronic renal failure at a young age (<5 years), but some are characterized by renal tubular defects (e.g., Fanconi's syndrome in the Basenji) or morphologic abnormalities that result in hematuria (e.g., renal telangiectasia in Pembroke Welsh corgis). A *familial* disease is one that occurs in related animals with a higher frequency than would be expected by chance. *Congenital* diseases are present at birth and may be genetically determined or result from exposure to adverse environmental factors during development. In many familial renal diseases of dogs, the kidneys are thought to be normal at birth but undergo structural and functional deterioration early in life. Some familial renal diseases of dogs probably are examples of renal dysplasia. The term *renal dysplasia* refers to disorganized development of renal parenchyma due to abnormal differentiation that is characterized by the presence of structures in the kidney inappropriate for the stage of development of the animal. Lesions suggestive of renal dysplasia include asynchronous differentiation of nephrons (indicated by persistence of immature or "fetal" glomeruli) and persistent mesenchyme (usually in the medullary interstitium).[1] Persistent metanephric ducts, atypical tubular epithelium, and dysontogenic metaplasia are observed less frequently.

Many familial renal diseases are very variable in severity and rate of progression among individual animals. Most of these diseases are progressive and ultimately fatal, and therapy usually is limited to conservative medical management of chronic renal failure. The mode of inheritance and specific pathogenesis for many of these diseases are unknown. The primary nature of the renal disease and its mode of inheritance, where known or suspected, are listed in Table 173–1.

SIGNALMENT

Familial renal disease has been reported in many breeds of dog (see Table 173–1) and may occur sporadically in mixed breed animals. The clinician should consider the possibility of familial renal disease whenever chronic renal failure occurs in immature or young adult animals. In cats, familial amyloidosis has been characterized in the Abyssinian cat and polycystic kidney disease has been described in the Persian breed.

In most of these diseases there is no clear sex predilection. In Samoyeds, however, hereditary glomerulopathy arises from an X-linked dominant trait. The age at onset of familial renal disease usually is 6 months to 5 years, with many animals presented before 2 years of age. Renal amyloidosis in beagles and English foxhounds and telangiectasia of the Welsh corgi, however, occur in older dogs (≥5 years), whereas polycystic kidney disease in Cairn and West Highland white terriers is detected at a very young age (5 to 6 weeks).

HISTORY AND PHYSICAL FINDINGS

The most common historical findings in dogs and cats with chronic renal failure due to familial renal disease are

TABLE 173–1. FAMILIAL RENAL DISEASES OF DOGS AND CATS

BREED	DISEASE DESCRIPTION	AGE AT PRESENTATION	INHERITANCE	PROGRESSIVE RENAL FAILURE?
Abyssinian cat	Amyloidosis	1–5 yr	Autosomal dominant (incomplete penetrance)*	Yes
Beagle	Amyloidosis	5–11 yr	Unknown	Yes
English foxhound	Amyloidosis	5–8 yr	Unknown	Yes
Oriental shorthair cat	Amyloidosis	<5 yr	Unknown	Variable, severe liver involvement
Shar Pei	Amyloidosis	1–6 hr	Unknown	Yes
Siamese cat	Amyloidosis	<5 yr	Unknown	Variable, severe liver involvement
Basenji	Tubular dysfunction (Fanconi's syndrome)	1–5 yr	Unknown	Variable
Norwegian elkhound	Tubular dysfunction (renal glucosuria)	NR	Unknown	No
Beagle	Unilateral renal agenesis	Incidental finding	Unknown	No
Bull terrier	Basement membrane disorder	<1–10 yr	Autosomal dominant	Yes
Doberman pinscher	Basement membrane disorder	<1–6 yr	Unknown	Yes
English cocker spaniel	Basement membrane disorder	<2 yr	Autosomal recessive	Yes
Samoyed	Basement membrane disorder	<1 yr (males)	X-linked dominant	In males
Bernese Mountain dog	Membranoproliferative glomerulonephritis	2–5 yr	Autosomal recessive*	Yes
Brittany spaniel	Membranoproliferative glomerulonephritis (C3 deficiency)	4–9 yr	Autosomal recessive	Variable
Rottweiler	Glomerular disease	≤1 yr	Unknown	Yes
Norwegian elkhound	Periglomerular fibrosis (primary lesion unknown)	<1–5 yr	Unknown	Yes
Soft-coated Wheaten terrier	Glomerular disease	2–11 yr	Unknown	Yes
Cairn terrier	Polycystic kidneys	6 wk	Autosomal recessive*	NR
West Highland white terrier	Polycystic kidneys	5 wk	Autosomal recessive*	NR
Bull terrier	Polycystic kidneys	<1–2 yr	Autosomal dominant	Yes, valvular heart disease
Persian cat	Polycystic kidneys	3–10 yr	Autosomal dominant	Yes
Alaskan malamute	Renal dysplasia	<1 yr	Unknown	Yes
Chow	Renal dysplasia	<1–5 yr	Unknown	Yes
Golden retriever	Renal dysplasia	<1–3 yr	Unknown	Yes
Lhasa apso and Shih Tzu	Renal dysplasia	<1–5 yr	Unknown	Yes
Miniature schnauzer	Renal dysplasia	<1–3 yr	Unknown	Yes
Soft-coated Wheaten terrier	Renal dysplasia	<1–3 yr	Unknown	Yes
Standard poodle	Renal dysplasia	<1–2 yr	Unknown	Yes
German shepherd	Multiple cystadenocarcinomas	5–11 yr	Autosomal dominant*	Variable
Pembroke Welsh corgi	Telangiectasia	5–13 yr	Unknown	No

*Suspected.
NR = not reported.

URO

1699

anorexia, lethargy, stunted growth or weight loss, polyuria and polydipsia, and vomiting. Other less common client complaints include poor hair coat, diarrhea, foul breath, and nocturia. In the Pembroke Welsh corgi with renal telangiectasia, the most common client complaints are hematuria, dysuria, and apparent abdominal pain. Hematuria also has been reported in German shepherds with multifocal renal cystadenocarcinomas.

Dogs and cats with chronic renal failure due to familial renal disease may be thin and dehydrated. On oral examination, pallor of the mucous membranes, foul odor, and uremic ulceration may be noted. The kidneys usually are small and irregular, with the exception of Cairn and West Highland white terriers and Persian cats with polycystic kidney disease in which the kidneys often are markedly enlarged. Renal pain on palpation may be noted in Welsh corgi dogs with renal telangiectasia. Signs of fibrous osteodystrophy such as "rubber jaw" or pathologic fractures usually are detected in young growing dogs with renal failure. Signs of renal osteodystrophy rarely are apparent in older dogs with renal failure. Blood pressure should be measured and fundic examination performed to evaluate for complications of hypertension (e.g., retinal hemorrhages, retinal detachments).

LABORATORY FINDINGS

The most common laboratory findings in dogs with familial renal disease resulting in chronic renal failure are azotemia, hyperphosphatemia, isosthenuria, and non-regenerative anemia. Serum calcium concentrations in dogs may be normal, decreased, or increased. Hypercalcemia may be more common in young dogs with renal failure than in older ones. Compensated metabolic acidosis also may be observed. The presence of hypercholesterolemia and proteinuria should lead the clinician to suspect primary glomerular disease. Beagles with glomerular amyloidosis and Bernese Mountain dogs with membranoproliferative glomerulonephritis have nephrotic syndrome and proteinuria, but proteinuria is variable and dependent on the extent of glomerular involvement in Abyssinian cats and Shar Pei dogs with familial amyloidosis. Glucosuria is found in Norwegian elkhounds and Basenjis with primary renal tubular disorders.

Juvenile renal disease in the Basenji is an animal model of Fanconi's syndrome in humans and is characterized by glucosuria, proteinuria, isosthenuria, and aminoaciduria. Affected Basenjis also demonstrate decreased fractional reabsorption of phosphate, sodium, potassium, and urate. They may develop hypokalemia and metabolic acidosis with a normal anion gap (hyperchloremic metabolic acidosis). In Welsh corgis with renal telangiectasia, the major laboratory finding is hematuria, but urinary tract infection also may be present. Blood loss anemia is more common than non-regenerative anemia, owing to large amounts of blood that may be lost in the urine. Affected Welsh corgis may develop nephrocalcinosis and calculi, and hydronephrosis may occur if a blood clot or calculus obstructs the ureter.

PATHOLOGIC FINDINGS

Familial renal disease is characterized by the presence of primary dysplastic lesions, compensatory lesions, and degenerative lesions.[1] In many cases, the secondary degenerative lesions overshadow the underlying primary dysplastic lesions, making the correct diagnosis difficult. Primary dys-

plastic lesions that have been observed in some familial renal disease of dogs include immature or "fetal" glomeruli, hyperplasia or adenomatoid proliferation of the medullary collecting ducts, and persistent mesenchyme in the renal medulla. Such changes are most prominent in the Lhasa apso, Shih Tzu, soft-coated Wheaten terrier, standard poodle, chow chow, and miniature schnauzer. Juvenile renal disease in the Samoyed, English cocker spaniel, and bull terrier appears to result from defective glomerular basement membranes and represents animal models of X-linked dominant, autosomal recessive, and autosomal dominant hereditary nephritis in humans, respectively.

Secondary degenerative lesions that are observed commonly in familial renal disease include interstitial fibrosis, interstitial infiltration by mononuclear inflammatory cells, dystrophic mineralization, and cystic glomerular atrophy. The pathologic features of several individual familial renal diseases are presented here.

Abyssinian Cat. Abyssinian cats with familial amyloidosis usually are presented between 1 and 5 years of age. Male and female cats are affected. Amyloid deposits first appear in the kidneys between 9 and 24 months of age; and, in many cats, amyloid deposition leads to chronic renal failure within the first 3 years of life. Amyloid deposition in the kidney may be mild, and some affected cats may live to an advanced age without detection of their amyloid deposits. Proteinuria is a variable clinical finding and reflects the severity of glomerular involvement. Difficulty in determining the mode of inheritance arises from the variability in severity and progression of amyloidosis among affected Abyssinian cats, but the disease appears to be inherited as an autosomal dominant trait with variable penetrance. Amyloid deposits in the kidneys of affected Abyssinian cats contain amyloid protein AA.[2]

The principal pathologic lesions in the kidneys of Abyssinian cats with familial amyloidosis are medullary amyloid deposits, papillary necrosis, chronic tubulointerstitial nephritis characterized by lymphoplasmacytic infiltration and fibrosis, and variable glomerular amyloid deposits. Glomerular amyloidosis is mild and often difficult to detect in many affected cats, but occasionally it can be severe. Medullary amyloid deposition was found in all affected Abyssinians whereas glomerular deposits were found in 75 per cent.[3] Medullary interstitial amyloid deposits interfere with blood flow to the renal papilla, resulting in papillary necrosis and secondary interstitial medullary fibrosis and mononuclear inflammation.[4] Amyloid deposition is not restricted to the kidneys in Abyssinian cats with amyloidosis, and deposits frequently are found in other organs (e.g., adrenal glands, thyroid glands, spleen, stomach, small intestine, heart, liver, pancreas, colon).[3] Amyloid deposits in these other organs, however, do not appear to make an important contribution to the clinical syndrome, which is that of chronic renal failure.

Alaskan Malamute. Chronic renal failure in three sibling Malamute pups (4 to 11 months of age) was associated with histologic evidence of renal dysplasia.[5] The lesions observed included immature ("fetal") glomeruli, cystic glomerular atrophy, glomerular sclerosis, periglomerular fibrosis, adenomatoid hyperplasia of tubules, and persistent mesenchymal tissue.

Basenji. Histologic findings in the kidneys of Basenji dogs with Fanconi's syndrome are not consistent. Non-specific findings include tubular atrophy and interstitial fibrosis. One morphologic marker for this disease may be enlarged, hyperchromatic nuclei in renal tubular cells (renal tubular cell karyomegaly). Affected animals may deteriorate rapidly and die of acute renal failure with papillary necrosis or pyelonephritis.

Beagle. A family of adult beagles developed glomerular amyloidosis and nephrotic syndrome characterized by proteinuria, hypercholesterolemia, and renal failure.[6] Some dogs had mild medullary deposition of amyloid. The amyloid deposits were sensitive to permanganate oxidation, suggesting the presence of amyloid protein AA.

Bernese Mountain Dog. Membranoproliferative glomerulonephritis resembling membranoproliferative glomerulonephritis type I in humans was described in young (2- to 5-year-old) male and female Bernese Mountain dogs.[7, 8] Affected dogs had typical laboratory abnormalities of renal failure as well as marked proteinuria, hypercholesterolemia, and hypoalbuminemia. Pedigree analysis suggested an autosomal recessive mode of inheritance. Ultrastructural lesions included a double-layered glomerular basement membrane and electron-dense deposits primarily in a subendothelial location. Immunoglobulin M and the third component of complement were identified by immunofluorescence in glomeruli of affected dogs. Most of the dogs had high serologic titers against *Borrelia burgdorferi*, but the organism could not be detected immunohistochemically in the tissues of affected dogs. Membranoproliferative glomerulonephritis also has been reported in Brittany spaniels with deficiency of the third component of complement.[9]

Bull Terrier. Familial renal disease leading to chronic renal failure has been reported in bull terriers aged 1 to 8 years.[10, 11] Both male and female dogs are affected, and the disease is inherited as an autosomal dominant trait.[12] It may represent an animal model of the rare dominant form of Alport's syndrome in humans.[13] Proteinuria is an early manifestation and correlated with underlying glomerular lesions in affected bull terriers.[14] Repeated urine protein/creatinine ratios greater than 0.3 are considered supportive evidence of the disease in suspect bull terriers older than 2 years of age but without overt evidence of renal failure.[11, 14]

Light microscopy of affected bull terriers shows thickening and splitting of glomerular basement membranes and less frequent involvement of tubular basement membranes.[10, 14, 15] Familial polycystic kidney disease occurring in association with nodular thickening of the mitral and aortic valves and mitral dysplasia also has been reported in bull terriers.[16] Affected dogs did not have hepatic cysts.

Cairn Terrier. Autosomal recessive polycystic disease in the Cairn terrier is characterized by the presence of multiple cysts throughout the liver and kidneys. Multiple fusiform to cylindrical cysts are present in both the renal cortex and medulla, and these cysts radiate from the capsular surface to the medulla. The renal parenchyma appears normal except for a decrease in the total number of glomeruli. Autosomal recessive polycystic kidney disease also has been reported in young (5-week-old) West Highland white terriers.[17]

Chow. Chronic renal failure in six young related chows (five males and one female) was suggestive of renal dysplasia.[18] Renal failure developed in four dogs by 6 months of age and in two dogs after 1 year of age. Renal dysplasia was suspected based on presence of immature ("fetal") glomeruli and pseudostratified columnar epithelium in renal tubules of some dogs. Secondary renal lesions included cystic glomerular atrophy and radial interstitial fibrosis.

English Cocker Spaniel. Juvenile renal disease in the cocker spaniel is an animal model of autosomal recessive hereditary nephritis in humans.[19, 20] Mutations have been identified in the α3 and α4 type IV collagen genes on chromosome 2 in affected humans, and these loci are candidate genes for the disease in the English cocker spaniel.

The disease affects both male and female English cocker spaniels and manifests itself between 6 and 24 months of age. The earliest detectable abnormality (5 to 8 months of age) is proteinuria, followed by reduced growth rate, impaired urinary concentrating ability, and azotemia (7 to 17 months of age).[19] The primary lesion is thickening and multilaminar splitting of the glomerular basement membrane. This lesion is identical to that observed in Samoyeds with X-linked hereditary nephritis and is similar to lesions observed in bull terriers with hereditary nephritis. The disease ultimately leads to diffuse glomerular sclerosis and periglomerular fibrosis with secondary tubulointerstitial disease and is invariably fatal.

Doberman Pinscher. Diffuse thickening or multifocal irregular thickening with lamellation of the lamina densa have been observed in the glomerular basement membranes of Doberman pinschers with glomerulopathy.[21] Occasionally, deposits of immunoglobulins have been detected in the glomerular capillary wall, but these are thought to result from nonspecific trapping of immune complexes in basement membranes with some underlying structural defect. Unilateral renal aplasia has been observed in some affected female Doberman pinschers. Additional glomerular lesions include lobular accentuation of glomerular capillary loops, increased mesangial matrix, hypercellularity, intraglomerular adhesions, fibroepithelial crescent formation, and periglomerular fibrosis.[21]

English Foxhounds. Renal amyloidosis was reported in related adult English foxhounds.[22] The disease had an acute presentation characterized by renomegaly and papillary necrosis in some affected dogs. Amyloid deposits were sensitive to permanganate oxidation, suggesting the presence of amyloid protein AA.

German Shepherd. German shepherds with bilateral multifocal renal cystadenocarcinomas are presented between 5 and 11 years of age for non-specific signs such as anorexia, weight loss, polydipsia, and gastrointestinal disturbances.[23] Hematuria was observed in approximately 20 per cent and azotemia in approximately 50 per cent of affected dogs. The renal lesions were accompanied by cutaneous and subcutaneous nodules (dermatofibrosis) and multiple uterine leiomyomas in affected female dogs. The disorder is thought to be inherited as an autosomal dominant trait.

Golden Retriever. Chronic renal failure has been reported in young golden retrievers (<3 years of age).[24, 25] Hypercholesterolemia was a common finding despite lack of other evidence of primary glomerular disease in most affected dogs. Hypercalcemia also was common and attributed to increased serum complexed calcium concentration. Cystic glomerular atrophy and periglomerular fibrosis were common histologic lesions whereas immature ("fetal") glomeruli were uncommon. Adenomatoid proliferation of the collecting ducts suggestive of primitive metanephric ducts was observed in several dogs and supports a diagnosis of renal dysplasia. Pyelonephritis occasionally complicated the disease in affected dogs.

Lhasa Apso and Shih Tzu. In the Lhasa apso and Shih Tzu, microscopic findings include a reduced number of glomeruli, glomerular atrophy, and small, immature ("fetal") glomeruli, which are hypercellular and have inconspicuous capillary lumens. Tubular changes include atrophy, dilatation, and epithelial hyperplasia. Interstitial fibrosis is particularly severe in the renal medulla, whereas interstitial inflammation is minimal. To a certain extent, increased interstitial medullary tissue may be persistent mesenchyme and, along with the immature glomeruli, is evidence of a primary renal dysplasia.

Miniature Schnauzer. Chronic renal failure suggestive of renal dysplasia was reported in eight related miniature schnauzers ranging in age from 4 months to 3 years.[26] Immature ("fetal") glomeruli, glomerular sclerosis, and severe interstitial fibrosis were observed.

Norwegian Elkhound. In the Norwegian elkhound, periglomerular fibrosis is an early histologic lesion that may be detected in some dogs before the onset of azotemia. Pathologic findings in dogs with more advanced disease consist of generalized interstitial fibrosis with glomerular sclerosis and atrophy. Tubular changes are mild except in extremely severe cases, in which tubular atrophy, saccular dilatation of the distal tubule and collecting duct, and basement membrane mineralization are noted. Interstitial mononuclear infiltration is recognized only in dogs with advanced disease. Hyperplasia of the collecting ducts also has been observed and may represent a primary dysplastic change, but immature ("fetal") glomeruli have not been observed. Norwegian elkhounds may also develop primary renal glucosuria that is not associated with chronic renal failure.

Persian Cat. In the Persian cat, polycystic kidney disease is inherited as an autosomal dominant trait.[27, 28] Cysts originate from both the proximal and distal tubules, occur both in the renal cortex and medulla, and increase in number and size over time.[29] They can be detected by ultrasound examination of affected kittens as early as 6 to 8 weeks of age, but the absence of cysts at this early age does not preclude their development at a later age. In one study, ultrasound examination had a sensitivity of 75 per cent and specificity of 100 per cent when performed at 16 weeks of age and a sensitivity of 91 per cent and specificity of 100 per cent when performed at 36 weeks of age.[28] Affected Persian cats usually do not develop chronic renal failure until later in adult life (3 to 10 years; average, 7 years), and renomegaly may be an incidental finding on physical examination.

On pathologic examination, there are multiple cysts of varying size in the renal cortex and medulla. Examination of other areas of the kidney may show reduced numbers of glomeruli and interstitial fibrosis. Occasionally, cysts may be found in the liver.[30]

Rottweiler. Chronic renal failure was reported in four related rottweilers (three females and one male) ranging in age from 6 to 12 months.[31] Hypercholesterolemia and high urine protein/creatinine ratios were consistent with a diagnosis of primary glomerular disease. Histologically, cystic glomerular atrophy and irregular thickening of glomerular basement membranes were observed.

Samoyed. Affected male Samoyeds with hereditary nephritis develop proteinuria, glucosuria, and isosthenuria by 2 to 3 months of age and azotemia and overt renal failure by 6 to 9 months of age. Death due to renal failure usually occurs by 12 to 16 months of age.[32] Mesangial thickening, glomerular sclerosis, and periglomerular fibrosis are observed by light microscopy in affected males by 8 to 10 months of age.[33] Affected female dogs develop proteinuria at 2 to 3 months of age but remain clinically normal other than failing to achieve normal adult body weight. This difference in clinical course is a consequence of the X-linked dominant inheritance pattern and results from normal random inactivation of one X chromosome in each cell of the female embryo during development.[34]

Juvenile renal disease in the Samoyed is a hereditary glomerulopathy arising from a mutation in the type IV collagen gene on the X chromosome.[35] At birth, the glomerular basement membranes of affected male Samoyed dogs are morphologically normal but reduplication and bilaminar splitting of the lamina densa are detected by electron microscopy at 1 month of age and progress to multilaminar splitting, thickening, and glomerular sclerosis by 8 to 10 months of age.[36] Affected female dogs have only focal splitting of glomerular basement membranes and do not develop progressive disease.

Proteinuria and progressive renal disease presumably result from wear and tear on glomerular basement membranes weakened by abnormal cross-linking of type IV collagen.[37] Deterioration of basement membranes and onset of renal failure in affected male dogs can be delayed but not prevented by feeding a diet low in protein and phosphorus beginning at 1 month of age.[38]

Shar Pei. Familial amyloidosis resulting in chronic renal failure at a young age (mean, 4 years) occurs in male and female Shar Pei dogs.[39] Proteinuria and laboratory evidence of nephrotic syndrome (e.g., hypoalbuminemia, hypercholesterolemia) variably are present, depending on the severity of glomerular involvement. Some affected Shar Pei dogs had a previous history of episodic joint swelling (usually the tibiotarsal joints) and high fever that resolves within a few days, regardless of treatment.[40, 41] Recurrent fever and joint swelling, culminating in renal failure due to reactive systemic amyloidosis in young Shar Pei dogs may represent an animal model of familial Mediterranean fever in humans. There is some evidence that amyloidosis in the Shar Pei dog is inherited as an autosomal recessive trait.[42]

Affected Shar Pei dogs have moderate to severe renal medullary deposition of amyloid, but only two thirds have glomerular involvement. These findings are similar to those observed in Abyssinian cats with familial amyloidosis. The remaining renal lesions are those of end-stage renal disease. Amino acid sequence analysis has demonstrated that the amyloid deposits in affected Shar Pei dogs contain amyloid A protein.[43] In addition to the kidney, amyloid deposits may be observed in many other organs (e.g., liver, spleen, gastrointestinal tract, thyroid gland). Icterus, hepatomegaly, and rarely hepatic rupture with hemoabdomen may occur in Shar Pei dogs with severe deposition of amyloid in the liver.[44]

Soft-Coated Wheaten Terrier. Pathologic findings in soft-coated Wheaten terriers with juvenile renal disease are suggestive of renal dysplasia.[45, 46] Numerous cystic lesions may be noted grossly in the cortex. Histologically, cortical lesions are segmental, whereas medullary disease is more diffuse. Cortical lesions include interstitial fibrosis, periglomerular fibrosis, cystic glomerular atrophy, decreased numbers of glomeruli, and the presence of immature ("fetal") glomeruli. Adenomatous proliferation of the collecting duct epithelium also is a prominent feature. In another report, protein-losing nephropathy was documented in several soft-coated Wheaten terriers.[47] Laboratory findings were typical of nephrotic syndrome and the underlying renal lesion was membranoproliferative glomerulonephritis. Thus, familial renal disease in the soft-coated Wheaten terrier may take the form of renal dysplasia or membranoproliferative glomerulonephritis. Dogs with renal dysplasia were younger than age 3 years when examined, whereas those with glomerulonephritis were 2 to 11 years of age.

Standard Poodle. In affected standard poodles, cystic glomerular atrophy and large numbers of immature ("fetal") glomeruli are observed, especially in dogs presented at 3 to

4 months of age. The cortical interstitium contains segmental areas of fibrosis, whereas more diffuse lesions occur in the medulla.

Welsh Corgi. Welsh corgis with renal telangiectasia have red to black nodules in the kidneys, especially in the renal medulla adjacent to the corticomedullary junction. Clotted blood often is identified in these lesions and in the renal pelvis. Hydronephrosis (presumably due to ureteral obstruction) occurs in almost half of affected dogs. Similar nodular lesions may be identified in other tissues, including the subcutis, spleen, duodenum, anterior mediastinum, thoracic wall, retroperitoneal space, and central nervous system. Histologically, these lesions are cavernous, blood-filled spaces lined with endothelium, and thrombosis is a frequent finding in the sinuses. These sinuses with their simple endothelial linings may represent vascular malformations rather than benign tumors of vascular origin.

REFERENCES

1. Picut CA, Lewis RM: Microscopic features of canine renal dysplasia. Vet Pathol 24:156–163, 1987.
2. DiBartola SP, Benson MD, Dwulet FE, et al: Isolation and characterization of amyloid protein AA in the Abyssinian cat. Lab Invest 52:485–489, 1985.
3. DiBartola SP, Tarr MJ, Benson MD: Tissue distribution of amyloid deposits in Abyssinian cats with familial amyloidosis. J Comp Pathol 96:387–398, 1986.
4. Boyce JT, DiBartola SP, Chew DJ, et al: Familial renal amyloidosis in Abyssinian cats. Vet Pathol 21:33–38, 1984.
5. Vilafranca M, Ferrer L: Juvenile nephropathy in Alaskan Malamute littermates. Vet Pathol 31:375–377, 1994.
6. Bowles MH, Mosier DA: Renal amyloidosis in a family of beagles. JAVMA 201:569–574, 1992.
7. Reusch C, Hoerauf A, Lechner J, et al: A new familial glomerulonephropathy in Bernese Mountain dogs. Vet Rec 134:411–415, 1994.
8. Minkus G, Breuer W, Wanke R, et al: Familial nephropathy in Bernese Mountain dogs. Vet Pathol 31:421–428, 1994.
9. Cork LC, Morris JM, Olson JL, et al: Membranoproliferative glomerulonephritis in dogs with a genetically determined deficiency of the third component of complement. Clin Immunol Immunopathol 60:455–470, 1991.
10. Robinson WF, Shaw SE, Stanley B, et al: Chronic renal disease in bull terriers. Aust Vet J 66:193–195, 1989.
11. Jones BR, Gething MA, Badcoe LM, et al: Familial progressive nephropathy in young Bull terriers. N Z Vet J 37:79–82, 1989.
12. Hood JC, Robinson WF, Huxtable CR, et al: Hereditary nephritis in the bull terrier: Evidence for inheritance by an autosomal dominant gene. Vet Rec 126:456–459, 1990.
13. Hood JC, Savige J, Hendtlass A, et al: Bull terrier hereditary nephritis: A model for autosomal dominant Alport syndrome. Kidney Int 47:758–765, 1995.
14. Hood JC, Robinson WF, Clark WT, et al: Proteinuria as an indicator of early renal disease in bull terriers with hereditary nephritis. J Small Anim Pract 32:241–248, 1991.
15. Hood JC, Robinson WF, Huxtable CR, et al: Hereditary nephritis in the bull terrier: Evidence for inheritance by an autosomal dominant gene. Vet Rec 126:456–459, 1990.
16. Burrows AK, Malik R, Hunt GB, et al: Familial polycystic kidney disease in bull terriers. J Small Anim Pract 35:364–369, 1994.
17. McAloose D, Casal M, Patterson DF, et al: Polycystic kidney and liver disease in two related West Highland white terrier litters. Vet Pathol 35:77–81, 1998.
18. Brown CA, Crowell WA, Brown SA, et al: Suspected familial renal disease in chow chows. JAVMA 196:1279–1284, 1990.
19. Lees GE, Helman RG, Homco LD, et al: Early diagnosis of familial nephropathy in English cocker spaniels. J Am Anim Hosp Assoc 34:189–195, 1998.
20. Lees GE, Wilson PD, Helman RG, et al: Glomerular ultrastructural findings similar to hereditary nephritis in 4 English cocker spaniels. J Vet Intern Med 11:80–85, 1997.
21. Picut CA, Lewis RM: Juvenile renal disease in the Doberman pinscher: Ultrastructural changes of the glomerular basement membrane. J Comp Pathol 97:587–596, 1987.
22. Mason NJ, Day MJ: Renal amyloidosis in related English foxhounds. J Small Anim Pract 37:255–260, 1996.
23. Lium B, Moe L: Hereditary multifocal renal cystadenocarcinomas and nodular dermatofibrosis in the German shepherd dog: Macroscopic and histopathologic changes. Vet Pathol 22:447–455, 1985.
24. Autran de Morais HS, DiBartola SP, Chew DJ: Juvenile renal disease in golden retrievers: 12 cases (1984–1994). JAVMA 209:792–797, 1996.
25. Kerlin RL, Van Winkle TJ: Renal dysplasia in golden retrievers. Vet Pathol 32:327–229, 1995.
26. Morton LD, Sanecki RK, Gordon DE, et al: Juvenile renal disease in miniature schnauzer dogs. Vet Pathol 27:455–458, 1990.
27. Biller DS, Chew DJ, DiBartola SP: Polycystic kidney disease in a family of Persian cats. JAVMA 196:1288–1290, 1990.
28. Biller DS, DiBartola SP, Eaton KA, et al: Inheritance of polycystic kidney disease in Persian cats. J Hered 87:1–5, 1996.
29. Eaton KA, Biller DS, DiBartola SP, et al: Autosomal dominant polycystic kidney disease in Persian and Persian-cross cats. Vet Pathol 34:117–126, 1997.
30. Stebbins KE: Polycystic disease of the kidney and liver in an adult Persian cat. J Comp Pathol 100:327–330, 1989.
31. Cook SM, Dean DF, Golden DL, et al: Renal failure attributable to atrophic glomerulopathy in four related Rottweilers. JAVMA 202:107–109, 1993.
32. Jansen B, Valli VE, Thorner P, et al: Samoyed hereditary glomerulopathy: Serial clinical and laboratory (urine, serum biochemistry and hematology) studies. Can J Vet Res 51:387, 1987.
33. Jansen B, Thorner PS, Singh A, et al: Animal model of human disease: Hereditary nephritis in Samoyed dogs. Am J Pathol 116:175–178, 1984.
34. Jansen B, Tryphonas L, Wong J, et al: Mode of inheritance of Samoyed hereditary glomerulopathy: An animal model for hereditary nephritis in humans. J Lab Clin Med 107:551–555, 1986.
35. Zheng K, Thorner PS, Marrano P, et al: Canine X chromosome–linked hereditary nephritis: A genetic model for human X-linked hereditary nephritis resulting from a single base mutation in the gene encoding the alpha-5 chain of collagen type IV. Proc Natl Acad Sci U S A 91:3989–3993, 1994.
36. Jansen B, Thorner P, Baumal R, et al: Samoyed hereditary glomerulopathy: Evolution of splitting of glomerular capillary basement membrane. Am J Pathol 125:536–545, 1986.
37. Thorner P, Baumal R, Binnington A, et al: The NC1 domain of collagen type IV in neonatal dog glomerular basement membranes: Significance in Samoyed hereditary nephropathy. Am J Pathol 134:1047–1054, 1989.
38. Valli VE, Baumal R, Thorner P, et al: Dietary modification reduces splitting of glomerular basement membranes and delays death due to renal failure in canine X-linked hereditary nephritis. Lab Invest 65:67–73, 1991.
39. DiBartola SP, Tarr MJ, Webb DM, et al: Familial renal amyloidosis in Chinese Shar Pei dogs. JAVMA 197:483–487, 1990.
40. May C, Hammill J, Bennett D: Chinese Shar Pei fever syndrome: A preliminary report. Vet Rec 131:586–587, 1992.
41. Rivas AL, Tintle L, Kimball ES, et al: A canine febrile disorder associated with elevated interleukin-6. Clin Immunol Immunopathol 64:36–45, 1992.
42. Rivas AL, Tintle L, Meyers-Wallen V, et al: Inheritance of renal amyloidosis in Chinese Shar Pei dogs. J Hered 84:438–442, 1993.
43. Johnson KH, Sletten K, Hayden DW, et al: AA amyloidosis in Chinese Shar-Pei dogs: Immunohistochemical and amino acid sequence analysis: Amyloid. Int J Exp Clin Invest 2:92–99, 1995.
44. Loeven KO: Spontaneous hepatic rupture secondary to amyloidosis in a Chinese Shar Pei. J Am Anim Hosp Assoc 30:577–579, 1994.
45. Eriksen K, Grondalen J: Familial renal disease in soft-coated Wheaten terriers. J Small Anim Pract 25:489–500, 1984.
46. Nash AS, Kelly DF, Gaskell CJ: Progressive renal disease in soft-coated Wheaten terriers: Possible familial nephropathy. J Small Anim Pract 25:479–487, 1984.
47. Littman MP, Giger U: Familial protein-losing enteropathy (PLE) and/or protein-losing nephropathy (PLN) in soft-coated Wheaten terriers. In: Proceedings of the 8th ACVIM Forum, 1990, p 1135.

URO

CHAPTER 174

DISORDERS OF RENAL TUBULES

Joseph W. Bartges

NORMAL PHYSIOLOGY

The nephron, the functional unit of the kidney, consists of a glomerular capillary network, a proximal convoluted tubule, the loop of Henle, a distal convoluted tubule, and a collecting duct. Whereas renal function is often thought of in terms of azotemia, a reflection of glomerular function, tubular function is responsible for the final composition of urine through reabsorption and secretion of compounds (e.g., electrolytes, water). It is also involved in metabolism of hormones (e.g., erythropoietin, renin) and in maintaining systemic acid-base balance.

Tubulopathies can be classified as either isolated or complex and as congenital or acquired. They may involve alteration in carbohydrate, nitrogen, electrolyte, mineral, fluid, and acid-base metabolism. There are several underlying principles of tubulopathies:[1]

1. Tubular disorders involve an abnormality of transport function.
2. Clinical and biochemical abnormalities reflect the site of tubular function.
3. Inherited tubular disorders involve loss of a transport protein or an error of metabolism.
4. Diseases that perturb energy production or structural integrity of tubular cells result in complex disorders.
5. Therapeutic principles are simple and involve replacement of the substance lost in urine or avoidance of the toxic substance.
6. Dose of replacement therapy relates to the altered site. If the altered site is responsible for bulk reabsorption, larger replacement doses will be required than at a site with less reclamation of a lost compound.

ISOLATED TUBULAR DISORDERS

DISORDERS OF CARBOHYDRATE METABOLISM

Glucosuria

Glucosuria Associated With Euglycemia

Glucosuria with normal blood glucose concentrations is termed *renal glucosuria*. Renal glucosuria is uncommon but has been reported in Scottish terriers, Basenjis, mixed breed dogs, as a familial disorder in Norwegian elkhounds, and in dogs with congenital renal disease such as Lhasa apsos and Shih Tzus. Renal glucosuria occurring with normal renal function (primary renal glucosuria) in humans is due to a transport defect either in the brush border membrane or in the transtubular reabsorptive process for glucose. Two forms of this disorder have been described. Type A variant repre-

sents a reduction in both the renal threshold for glucose and maximal rate of glucose reabsorption ($Tm_{glucose}$). Patients with type B glucosuria have a low renal threshold for glucose but a normal $Tm_{glucose}$. Dogs with primary glucosuria have polydipsia and polyuria due to osmotic diuresis induced by glucosuria. Glucosuria may predispose to bacterial or fungal urinary tract infections; therefore, signs of lower urinary tract disease may be present. However, dogs with renal glucosuria may also be asymptomatic. Diagnosis of renal glucosuria is based on documentation of persistent glucosuria without ketonuria and on euglycemia. There is no specific treatment. Hypoglycemia does not occur, and restriction of dietary carbohydrate does not alter urinary glucose excretion. Appropriate antimicrobial therapy is indicated in animals that develop urinary tract infections.

Glucosuria Associated With Hyperglycemia

Any condition resulting in hyperglycemia may result in glucosuria if glomerular filtration of glucose exceeds $Tm_{glucose}$. The $Tm_{glucose}$ is exceeded when blood glucose concentrations exceed 180 to 220 mg/dL in dogs and 260 to 310 mg/dL in cats. Hyperglycemia and glucosuria may occur with diabetes mellitus, pancreatitis, hyperadrenocorticism, central nervous system lesions (variable), pheochromocytoma, and hyperprogesteronemia, or with administration of glucose-containing solutions, glucocorticoids (rarely), adrenocorticotropic hormone, glucagon, progestational compounds, epinephrine, morphine, and phenothiazines.

Pentosuria

Pentosuria occurs in humans because of overflow of pentoses (5-carbon cyclic sugars) from blood into urine.[1] Pentosuria has not been described in dogs or cats either because it does not exist or because glucose oxidase–impregnated test strips are used and so pentosuria is missed.

DISORDERS OF NITROGEN METABOLISM

Aminoaciduria

Amino acids are reabsorbed in the proximal tubule by several major shared transport systems: cyclic and neutral amino acids and glycine, dibasic amino acids, dicarboxylic amino acids, and beta-amino acids. Greater than 95 per cent of filtered amino acids are reabsorbed by the proximal tubule. Aminoaciduria occurs by one of several different defects. First, plasma concentration of an amino acid may be increased as a result of a metabolic defect, which increases the quantity filtered at the glomerulus. If tubular reabsorptive capacity for that amino acid is exceeded, overload amino-aciduria occurs. Second, there could be a defect in the proximal tubule brush border amino acid transport system. Because the amino acid transport systems found in the proximal tubule are in some cases the same as those in the intestine, transport defects may be found simultaneously in both tissues. Third, the proximal tubule cell may take up the amino acid but fail to metabolize it or fail to return it to blood because of a defect in basolateral membrane transport. Lastly, aminoaciduria could arise from a more generalized defect, as in toxic nephropathies and Fanconi's syndrome.

Cystinuria

Cystinuria is an inborn error of metabolism characterized by increased urinary excretion of cystine, which predisposes to cystine urolith formation. Normally, circulating cystine is filtered freely at the glomerulus, and 99 to 100 per cent is actively reabsorbed in the proximal tubule. Decreased tubular reabsorption of cystine and, in some cases, of other amino acids (lysine, glycine, ornithine, arginine) has been observed in dogs with cystine uroliths.[2, 3] Aminoaciduria is associated with low or normal plasma levels of affected amino acids. Some affected dogs have a net secretion of cystine.[4] Decreased tubular reabsorption of cystine and lysine may be due to a membrane transport defect. Jejunal mucosal uptake of cystine is not apparently reduced.[5]

Many breeds of dogs have been reported to develop cystine uroliths, but English bulldogs, Newfoundlands, and dachshunds appear to be predisposed.[6-8] Data contained in published pedigrees from inbred lines of dachshunds, basset hounds, and rottweilers suggest a sex-lined or autosomal recessive pattern of inheritance.[9] Although cystine uroliths have been reported primarily in male dogs, cystine uroliths have been reported in female dogs.[7, 8] Cystine uroliths appear to affect primarily young to middle-aged dogs.[7, 10] Not all cystinuric dogs form uroliths; therefore, cystinuria is a predisposing rather than a primary cause of cystine urolith formation. Uroliths form, in part, because the solubility of cystine decreases in acidic urine, but cystine becomes more soluble in alkaline urine. Cystine uroliths have also been identified in cats.[11, 12] In one cat, renal excretion of cystine, ornithine, lysine, and arginine was increased.[11] Little information is available concerning cystinuria and cystine urolithiasis in cats.

Treatment of cystine uroliths includes use of a low-protein diet, alkalinization therapy, and thiol-containing drugs (see Chapters 175 and 176). Because cystine is an amino acid, consumption of a low-protein diet is associated with less cystine intake and excretion. Cystine is more soluble at a urine pH greater than 7.0; therefore, urinary alkalinization is of benefit in the dissolution and prevention of cystine uroliths. Most low-protein diets are formulated to induce alkaluria. Thiol-containing drugs, such as D-penicillamine and 2-mercaptopropionylglycine (2-MPG), decrease urinary cystine excretion by a thiol disulfide exchange reaction, resulting in compounds that are more soluble than cystine.[8] Thiol-containing drugs may be used for dissolution and prevention of cystine uroliths.

Hypercarnitinuria

Carnitine is a non-essential sulfur-containing amino acid. Although carnitine is reabsorbed in the proximal renal tubule similar to other amino acids, it is less than that for other mammals (approximately 75 per cent reabsorption in dogs compared with more than 90 per cent in other mammals). Dilated cardiomyopathy has been associated with systemic carnitine deficiency.[13] Recently, hypercarnitinuria has been reported to occur in cystinuric dogs in which dilated cardiomyopathy developed.[14] Hypercarnitinuria likely represents a proximal renal tubular transport defect. Treatment of carnitine deficiency includes feeding a diet with adequate or increased carnitine content or supplementation with L-carnitine. The reader is referred to Chapter 116 for further information.

Other Aminoacidurias

Other aminoacidurias have been observed to occur in humans, but they have not been described in dogs or cats.

Uricaciduria

Uric acid is one of several biodegradation products of purine nucleotide metabolism. In most dogs and cats, allantoin is the major metabolic end product; it is the most soluble of the purine metabolic products excreted in urine.[15] However, in some breeds of dogs, such as Dalmatian coach hounds and English bulldogs, uric acid is the major purine metabolite that is excreted in urine.[10] The ability of Dalmatians to oxidize uric acid to allantoin is intermediate between humans and most non-Dalmatian dogs. Humans have a serum uric acid concentration of 3 to 7 mg/dL and excrete 500 to 700 mg of uric acid in their urine per day. Most non-Dalmatian dogs have a serum uric acid concentration of less than 0.5 mg/dL and excrete 10 to 60 mg of uric acid in their urine per day. Dalmatians have a serum uric acid concentration that is two to four times that of non-Dalmatians and excrete more than 400 to 600 mg of uric acid in their urine per day.[16]

Studies of the fate of uric acid in Dalmatians have revealed unique hepatic and renal pathways of metabolism. Of these two metabolic sites, reciprocal allogenic renal and hepatic transplantations between Dalmatians and non-Dalmatians indicate that the hepatic mechanism is quantitatively the most significant. The liver of Dalmatians does not completely oxidize available uric acid, even though it contains a sufficient concentration of uricase. Compared with non-Dalmatians, Dalmatians convert uric acid to allantoin at a reduced rate. It has been hypothesized that their hepatic cellular membranes are partially impermeable to uric acid.[17]

The proximal renal tubules of Dalmatians reabsorb less uric acid than non-Dalmatians; a small amount is secreted by the distal tubules.[18] In non-Dalmatian dogs, 98 to 100 per cent of the uric acid in glomerular filtrate is reabsorbed by the proximal tubules and returned to the liver for further metabolism.

The definitive mechanism of urate urolith formation in Dalmatian dogs remains unknown. Increased uric acid excretion is a risk factor rather than a primary cause. Although all Dalmatians excrete relatively high quantities of uric acid in their urine, apparently only a small percentage form urate uroliths. At one time it was thought that urolith-forming Dalmatians did not excrete greater quantities of uric acid in their urine than non–urolith-forming Dalmatians. However, recent studies indicate that insensitive methods of measurement of urine uric acid concentration were responsible for this conclusion. When steps are taken to ensure that urine uric acid remains in solution, differences in urine uric acid concentrations between non–urolith-forming Dalmatians and urolith-forming Dalmatians may be expected.

URO

Urate uroliths can be dissolved by feeding a diet low in purine and administering a xanthine oxidase inhibitor, allopurinol. Allopurinol impairs the conversion of xanthine to uric acid, resulting in decreased concentrations of uric acid in blood and urine. However, increased concentrations of xanthine in blood and urine may result in xanthine urolith formation. Additional information concerning urate urolithiasis may be found in Chapter 176.

Xanthinuria

Xanthine is a product of purine metabolism and is converted to uric acid by the enzyme xanthine oxidase.[15] Hereditary xanthinuria is a rarely recognized disorder of humans characterized by a deficiency of xanthine oxidase. As a consequence, abnormal quantities of xanthine are excreted in urine as a major end product of purine metabolism. Because xanthine is the least soluble purine naturally excreted in urine, xanthinuria may be associated with urolith formation. In dogs, xanthinuria is usually associated with allopurinol administration. However, we have observed xanthine uroliths in a dog that did not receive allopurinol (Allen H et al, unpublished data),[19] and naturally occurring xanthine uroliths have been reported in three Cavalier King Charles spaniels.[19-21] Naturally occurring xanthine uroliths have also been observed in cats.[12] The mechanism(s) responsible for hyperxanthinuria and xanthine urolith formation in these animals are not known, but hyperxanthinemia was present.

DISORDERS OF MINERAL AND ELECTROLYTE METABOLISM

Calcium

Hypercalciuria may have several causes and increases the risk of calcium (Ca^{2+}) stone formation, particularly calcium oxalate stones. Hypercalciuria may occur due to hypercalcemia, decreased renal tubular reabsorption of Ca^{2+} (renal leak hypercalciuria), increased mobilization of Ca^{2+} from bone (resorptive hypercalciuria), or increased intestinal absorption of Ca^{2+} (absorptive hypercalciuria). Absorptive hypercalciuria may be differentiated from renal leak hypercalciuria by measuring 24-hour urinary Ca^{2+} excretion during a fed and fasted state. Ca^{2+} excretion decreases during food deprivation in dogs with absorptive hypercalciuria but not in dogs with renal leak hypercalciuria. It is thought that miniature schnauzers, and perhaps other breeds, that form calcium oxalate uroliths have absorptive hypercalciuria.[22] Treatment involves dietary modification to minimize urinary Ca^{2+} excretion, including sodium (Na^+) restriction, protein restriction, and alkalinization. Hydrochlorothiazide has also been shown to decrease urinary Ca^{2+} excretion in dogs, but its safety and efficacy in dogs with calcium oxalate uroliths are unknown.[8]

Phosphorus

Phosphate transport disorders resulting in hyperphosphaturia and skeletal disease have been identified in humans.[1] However, in animals, hyperphosphaturia usually occurs as part of a complex tubulopathy.

Magnesium

Renal tubular magnesium (Mg^{2+}) wasting has been observed in some humans with hypomagnesemia. Tetany,

weakness, nausea, and hypocalcemia (due to impaired parathyroid hormone secretion and action) may occur. Treatment with aminoglycoside or cisplatin can cause renal Mg^{2+} and potassium (K^+) wasting, leading to hypomagnesemia and hypokalemia. Treatment of hypomagnesemia consists of oral supplementation with magnesium salts; magnesium oxide is tolerated best.

Sodium and Potassium

Hyperaldosteronism

Increased aldosterone production and secretion stimulates tubular reabsorption of Na^+ and excretion of K^+ and hydrogen (H^+), resulting in hypokalemia and metabolic alkalosis. Hyperaldosteronism may occur as a result of an adrenal tumor or hyperplasia (primary aldosteronism, Conn's syndrome), hyperreninism due to a tumor of the juxtaglomerular apparatus or renovascular hypertension, from Bartter's syndrome (characterized by hyperreninemia, metabolic acidosis, increased secretion of vasodilatory prostaglandins, and normal systemic arterial blood pressure), or from exogenous mineralocorticoid administration. Hyperaldosteronism has been observed in a dog[23] and in cats.[24] Treatment involves removal of the tumor if possible, K^+ supplementation, and administration of K^+-sparing diuretics (spironolactone or triamterene).

Hypoaldosteronism

Hypoaldosteronism due to decreased aldosterone production or decreased responsiveness to aldosterone has been observed in humans. Hyperkalemia and metabolic acidosis occur, and hypertension may be present. This has not been observed to occur in dogs or cats except as part of hypoadrenocorticism.

Renal Tubular Potassium Secretion Defect

Children with this syndrome have decreased renal tubular secretion of K^+, metabolic acidosis, short stature, urinary tract infections, calcium oxalate urolithiasis, hypertension, and weakness. The primary defect appears to be decreased secretion of K^+ with secondary impairment of proximal tubule bicarbonate (HCO_3^-) reabsorption. Chlorothiazide administration, HCO_3^- supplementation, and dietary Na^+ restriction are used to treat this disorder.

DISORDERS OF VITAMIN METABOLISM

Methylmalonic Aciduria Associated With Vitamin B₁₂ Deficiency

Methylmalonic aciduria has been observed in giant schnauzers with intestinal malabsorption of vitamin B_{12} (cobalamin).[25] Vitamin B_{12} deficiency occurs because of absent intrinsic factor vitamin B_{12} receptors in the ileum. The trait appears to be autosomal recessive. Affected puppies exhibit inappetence and failure to thrive between 6 and 12 weeks of age. Megaloblastic anemia occurs. Treatment involves parenteral administration of vitamin B_{12}.

DISORDERS OF WATER METABOLISM

Nephrogenic diabetes insipidus describes any disorder in which there is a structural or functional defect in the ability of the kidneys to respond to antidiuretic hormone (ADH). This hormone induces increased water permeability in the distal tubule and collecting ducts by binding to a peritubular membrane receptor, resulting in activation of specific adenylate cyclases to form cyclic adenosine monophosphate. This compound leads to phosphorylation of other proteins that alter microtubular structures and permit augmented water permeability. Numerous drugs (e.g., furosemide, glucocorticoids, methoxyflurane), toxins (e.g., *Escherichia coli* endotoxin), and conditions (e.g., hypokalemia, hypercalcemia, medullary cystic disease, interstitial nephritis, bacterial pyelonephritis) can result in nephrogenic diabetes insipidus.

Congenital nephrogenic diabetes insipidus is a rare disorder associated with a deficiency of ADH receptors in the distal nephron. Affected animals present at a young age for severe polyuria and polydipsia. Urine is hyposthenuric (urine specific gravity 1.001 to 1.005; urine osmolality is less than 200 mOsm/kg) and does not increase above isosthenuric range during water deprivation. Animals do not respond to exogenous ADH. Treatment consists of massive amounts of water or dietary Na^+ restriction and use of thiazide diuretics (chlorothiazide, 10–20 mg/lb q12h) or hydrochlorothiazide (1–2 mg/lb q12h).[26] Thiazide diuretic administration results in mild dehydration, enhanced proximal renal tubular reabsorption of Na^+, decreased delivery of tubular fluid to the distal nephron, and reduced urine output. Thiazides have been reported to reduce urine output by 20 to 30 per cent in dogs with congenital nephrogenic diabetes insipidus. Inhibitors of prostaglandin synthesis (ibuprofen, indomethacin, aspirin) have been reported to reduce urine volume, increase urine osmolality, and reduce delivery of solute to the distal tubule in humans. Reduction of dietary Na^+ and protein may reduce the amount of solute that must be excreted in urine and may further reduce obligatory water loss and polyuria.

DISORDERS OF ACID-BASE METABOLISM

Renal Tubular Acidosis

Renal tubular acidosis is the name for a rare group of disorders that lead to metabolic acidosis. Two types have been described: decreased HCO_3^- reabsorption (proximal renal tubular acidosis [pRTA], type II), and defective acid excretion (distal renal tubular acidosis [dRTA], type I). Distal RTA associated with development of hyperkalemia resulting from hypoaldosteronism or aldosterone resistance has been termed type IV RTA but represents a type of dRTA.

The kidney maintains normal systemic acid-base balance by conserving HCO_3^- and excreting organic acids. Processes that are crucial in maintaining acid-base balance include proximal reclamation of filtered HCO_3^-, proximal synthesis and medullary recycling of ammonium ion (NH_4^+), and distal secretion of H^+. Distal H^+ secretion occurs in the outer medullary and cortical collecting ducts and the inner medullary collecting duct. For each secreted H^+, a "new" HCO_3^- ion is transferred to the circulation by means of a chloride (Cl^-)/HCO_3^- exchanger across the basolateral membrane. The most important transporter for apical secretion of H^+ is believed to be an electrogenic H^+-ATPase pump. Once secreted into the tubular lumen, passive back-diffusion of H^+ does not occur under physiologic conditions.[27]

Free H^+ ions can be excreted in urine only to a limited degree. They are bound either to filtered buffers to be excreted as titratable acid or to NH_3 to form NH_4^+. Net acid excretion (NAE) by the kidney is given by the equation:

$$NAE = (titratable\ acid\ +\ NH_4^+)\ -$$
$$urinary\ loss\ of\ HCO_3^-.$$

In this equation, the contribution of buffer-bound H^+ excretion is referred to as titratable acid because it is measured by the amount of NaOH required to titrate the urine pH of a 24-hour urine sample to 7.40. The most important buffer is phosphate. In one study, titratable acid in healthy adult beagles varied from 0.05 to 6.0 mmol/kg per 24 hours depending on diet consumed.[28]

The NH_4^+ is generated primarily in the proximal renal tubular cells from metabolism of glutamine. This results in formation of NH_4^+ and alpha-ketoglutarate. Alpha-ketoglutarate can be further metabolized for production of HCO_3^-, which is transported to extracellular fluid. Ammonia is secreted into the tubular lumen, presumably by substituting for H^+ on an internal binding site of the apical membrane Na^+/H^+ exchanger. Greater than 50 per cent of NH_4^+ is subsequently reabsorbed in the thick ascending limb of the loop of Henle by a combination of $Na^+/NH_4^+/2Cl^-$ cotransport and voltage-driven diffusion. This process is referred to as medullary recycling. Active reabsorption of NH_4^+ in the thick ascending limb provides a single effect for counter-current multiplication of NH_4^+ in the renal medulla. Depending on the pH in the renal interstitium, NH_4^+ partly dissociates into NH_3 and H^+. Dissociated H^+ is probably secreted into the lumen of the loop of Henle or collecting duct, converting luminal HCO_3^- remaining after proximal HCO_3^- reabsorption to H_2CO_3. Accumulated medullary NH_3 diffuses to areas with a low NH_3 concentration, including the medullary collecting tubules. Here, NH_3 passively diffuses into the lumen, where it serves as a proton acceptor to form NH_4^+ again. The NH_4^+ is lipid insoluble; therefore it cannot diffuse out of the lumen ("ion trapping") and is secreted in urine. Binding of H^+ by NH_3 in the distal tubular lumen is crucial to maintain a favorable gradient for H^+ secretion and to a lesser extent NH_3 diffusion. Urinary NH_4^+ excretion in healthy adult beagles consuming various diets was 0.45 to 4.0 mmol/kg per 24 hours[28]; and in 8 healthy cats fed four struvite management diets, it was 2.0 to 40 mmol/kg.[29] This ability to alter NH_4^+ excretion allows the kidney to increase acid excretion (NAE).

Not all of NH_4^+ produced by the kidney is excreted in the urine. In steady-state conditions, approximately 50 per cent is shunted to renal veins. The role of disturbances in shunting of NH_4^+ in the development of renal tubular acidosis has not been evaluated.

Urinary loss of HCO_3^- is the final component of the NAE equation. Bicarbonate excretion in healthy adult beagles consuming various diets was 0.07 to 0.25 mmol/kg per 24 hours.[28] Increased loss of HCO_3^- can be a source of decreased NAE even when the mechanisms discussed are fully intact. Normally, 85 to 90 per cent of filtered HCO_3^- is reabsorbed in the proximal renal tubule secondary to glutamine metabolism. Another 2 to 5 per cent is reabsorbed in the loop of Henle. "New" HCO_3^- is added to blood in the process of distal H^+ secretion.

Distal Renal Tubular Acidosis

In dRTA, urine cannot be maximally acidified because of impaired H^+ secretion (and thus HCO_3^- generation) in collecting ducts, and urine pH is typically more than 6.0 despite moderately to markedly decreased plasma HCO_3^- concentration. Urinary tract infection by urease-producing bacteria must be ruled out before the diagnosis of dRTA can be made. Nephrolithiasis, nephrocalcinosis, bone demineralization, and urinary potassium wasting with hypokalemia occur uncommonly. When plasma HCO_3^- concentration is increased to normal by supplementation, urinary fractional excretion of HCO_3^- becomes normal (< 5 per cent).

Four mechanisms are potentially involved in the pathogenesis of dRTA: (1) a defective or partially absent proton pump (secretory defect), (2) an unfavorable electrical gradient for H^+ secretion (voltage defect), (3) back-diffusion of H^+ (permeability defect), and (4) insufficient supply of NH_3 to the distal nephron (NH_3 defect).[27] Type IV dRTA is associated with hyperkalemia and is due to aldosterone deficiency, aldosterone resistance, or use of aldosterone antagonists such as spironolactone. It probably represents a combination of a rate-limited secretory defect, caused by the absence of the direct stimulation by aldosterone of H^+-ATPase and, less importantly, a voltage defect resulting from decreased distal Na^+ reabsorption. Hyperkalemia further adds to these mechanisms by its deleterious effects on NH_4^+ production and transport.

In type IV dRTA, the ability to lower urinary pH is usually maintained. The term *incomplete dRTA* is used for disorders of distal acidification that become symptomatic only under conditions of an increased acid load. The "incompleteness" of acidification may simply be less severe, or increased ammoniagenesis may occur to compensate for decreased distal H^+ secretion.

Diagnosis of dRTA may be made by an ammonium chloride challenge test during which urine pH is monitored using a pH meter before and at hourly intervals for 6 hours after oral administration of 110 mg/kg of ammonium chloride. Normal dogs can reduce their urine pH to 5.0, and cats can reduce their urine pH to 5.5. The amount of HCO_3^- supplementation required to correct metabolic acidosis in humans with dRTA varies but is usually less than that required in pRTA. Alkali supplementation usually ranges from 1 to 5 mEq/kg per day. A combination of K^+ and Na^+ citrate may be preferred over HCO_3^- as the alkali supplement.

Proximal Renal Tubular Acidosis

Proximal RTA results from a disturbance in proximal reclamation of filtered HCO_3^-. Urinary fractional excretion of HCO_3^- is usually more than 15 per cent when plasma HCO_3^- concentration is increased to normal with supplementation. Bicarbonaturia is absent and urine pH is appropriately low when metabolic acidosis is present and plasma HCO_3^- concentration is decreased because distal acidifying ability is functional. When plasma HCO_3^- concentration is decreased, the filtered load of HCO_3^- is reduced and almost all of the filtered HCO_3^- is reabsorbed in the distal tubules, despite the presence of the proximal tubule defect. Thus, pRTA can be viewed as a "self-limiting" disorder in which plasma HCO_3^- stabilizes at a lower than normal concentration after the filtered load falls sufficiently that distal HCO_3^- reabsorption can maintain plasma HCO_3^- at a new but lower steady-state concentration. The metabolic acidosis of pRTA results not only from proximal HCO_3^- loss but also from decreased NH_4^+ excretion, caused by either decreased proximal NH_4^+ synthesis or excessive NH_4^+ shunting to renal veins.[27]

Other abnormalities of proximal tubular function may accompany impaired HCO_3^- reabsorption in pRTA, including defects in glucose, phosphate, Na^+, K^+, uric acid, and amino acid reabsorption. This condition of proximal tubular defects is known as Fanconi's syndrome. Serum K^+ concentration is usually normal at time of diagnosis, but alkali therapy may precipitate hypokalemia and aggravate urinary K^+ wasting, presumably by increasing distal delivery of Na^+ and HCO_3^-.

Diagnosis of pRTA is made by finding a urine pH less than 6.0 and hyperchloremic metabolic acidosis, but a urine pH more than 6.0 and increased urinary fractional excretion of HCO_3^- (> 15 per cent) after plasma HCO_3^- concentration has been increased to normal by alkali administration. Correction of metabolic acidosis by alkali therapy is more difficult in pRTA than in dRTA because of the marked bicarbonaturia that occurs when plasma HCO_3^- concentration is increased to normal. Sodium bicarbonate dosages in excess of 11 mEq/kg per day may be required to correct plasma HCO_3^-, and such therapy may result in hypokalemia. Potassium citrate may be a preferred source of alkali. One 540-mg tablet of potassium citrate will provide 5 mEq of K^+ and 1.7 mEq of citrate, and its metabolism will yield 5 mEq of HCO_3^-.[26]

Renal tubular acidosis is rare in dogs and cats. Both pRTA and dRTA have been observed occasionally. Distal RTA has been reported in cats with pyelonephritis caused by *E. coli*.[30] Clinical signs include polyuria, polydipsia, anorexia, lethargy, enlarged kidneys, and isosthenuria. Distal RTA and hepatic lipidosis were reported in another cat without bacterial urinary tract infection.[31] It may also occur as a consequence of ischemia-induced acute renal failure.[32] Clinical features of pRTA and dRTA are characterized in Table 174–1.

COMPLEX TUBULAR DISORDERS

FANCONI'S SYNDROME

Urinary hyperexcretion of amino acids, phosphate, glucose, HCO_3^-, Ca^{2+}, K^+, and other ions, and proteins of molecular weights under 50,000 daltons, in conjunction with RTA and ADH-resistant polyuria, defines the complex tubulopathy termed *Fanconi's syndrome*.[1] There are inherited and acquired forms of Fanconi's syndrome. The pathogenesis of the syndrome regardless of its cause involves one of two basic mechanisms. The first is that renal tubular membranes become leaky, allowing less efficient reabsorption of solutes. The second hypothesis suggests that the intracellular metabolism of renal tubular cells fails to produce sufficient energy to support transport. Any substance that could be "toxic" and alter renal tubular metabolism, such as heavy metals (e.g., lead, copper, mercury, organomercurials, Lysol, maleic acid) and drugs (e.g., gentamicin, cephalosporins, outdated tetracycline, cisplatin, salicylate) could impair transport processes. Fanconi's syndrome may also occur with malignancies (e.g., multiple myeloma), monoclonal gammopathies, hyperparathyroidism, K^+ depletion, amyloidosis, nephrotic syndrome, vitamin D deficiency, and interstitial nephritis associated with antitubular basement membrane antibodies or as a complication of renal transplantation.

Fanconi's syndrome occurs as a familial disease in Basenjis. Ten to 30 per cent of Basenjis in the United States are affected.[33] Other dogs that have been reported with idiopathic Fanconi's syndrome include border terriers,[34] Norwegian elkhounds,[35] a whippet,[36] a Yorkshire terrier,[37] a Shetland sheepdog,[38] and a mixed breed dog.[39] Fanconi's syndrome also has been reported in a dog with gentamicin-induced acute renal failure,[40] in a dog with primary hypoparathyroidism with concurrent hypovitaminosis D,[41] in a

TABLE 174–1. CLINICAL FEATURES OF PROXIMAL AND DISTAL RENAL TUBULAR ACIDOSIS (RTA)

FEATURE	PROXIMAL RTA	DISTAL RTA
Hypercalciuria	Yes	Yes
Hyperphosphaturia	Yes	Yes
Urinary citrate	Normal	Decreased
Bone disease	Less severe	More severe
Nephrocalcinosis	No	Possible
Nephrolithiasis	Not usually	Yes
Hypokalemia	Mild	Mild to severe
Potassium wasting	Worsened by alkali therapy	Improved by alkali therapy
Alkali required for treatment	>11 mEq/kg/d	<4 mEq/kg/d
Other defects of proximal tubular function*	Yes	No
Reduction in plasma HCO_3^-	Moderate	Variable (can be severe)
Fractional excretion of HCO_3^- with normal plasma HCO_3^- concentration	>15%	<15%
Urine pH during acidemia	<6.0	>6.0
Urine pH after ammonium chloride	<6.0	>6.0

*Decreased reabsorption of sodium, potassium, phosphate, uric acid, glucose, and amino acids.
Modified from DiBartola SP: Renal tubular acidosis. *In* Ettinger SJ, Feldman EC (eds): Textbook of Veterinary Internal Medicine, 4th ed. Philadelphia, WB Saunders, 1995, p 1802.

dog with possible ethylene glycol toxicosis,[42] and in dogs experimentally given 4-pentenoate[43] and maleic acid.[44]

Dogs with Fanconi's syndrome have abnormal fractional reabsorption of many solutes.[45] Reabsorption of glucose, phosphate, and amino acids is abnormal in all affected dogs. Aminoaciduria is generalized in most dogs but occasionally is limited to cystinuria with minor defects in reabsorption of methionine, glycine, and some dibasic amino acids. Many dogs also have variably severe reabsorptive defects for HCO_3^-, Na^+, K^+, and uric acid. Defective reabsorption of Na^+ and phosphate in Basenjis is manifested at approximately 3 years of age, and defective reabsorption of glucose and amino acids is apparent at approximately 4 years of age.[45] The renal tubular disorder in affected Basenjis may be due to a metabolic or membrane defect affecting sodium movement or to increased backleak or to cell-to-lumen flux of amino acids. Isolated brush border vesicles from affected Basenjis showed decreased sodium-dependent glucose uptake but no decrease in cystine uptake.[2] Defective urinary concentrating ability in dogs with Fanconi syndrome represents a form of nephrogenic diabetes insipidus. This defect may precede development of glucosuria. Glomerular filtration rate is normal in some affected dogs and reduced in others.

Clinical findings include polyuria, polydipsia, weight loss, poor hair coat, dehydration, and muscular weakness. The disease usually is identifiable in adult dogs when there is glucosuria and low urine specific gravity with a normal blood glucose concentration. Proteinuria usually is mild. Metabolic acidosis is variable in severity and hyperchloremic in nature, as expected with decreased proximal tubular reabsorption of HCO_3^-. Hypokalemia can occur with long-standing disease and may contribute to muscular weakness in some dogs. Azotemia and hyperphosphatemia are observed in dogs with advanced disease and renal failure. Renal clearance studies to identify reabsorptive defects for electrolytes and amino acids are necessary to differentiate Fanconi's syndrome from primary renal glucosuria. Growth disturbances, metabolic bone disease, and nephrocalcinosis are observed in affected human patients but have not been observed in dogs with Fanconi's syndrome. Hyperchromatic karyomegaly of renal tubular cells is a distinctive renal lesion in affected Basenjis, but its significance is unknown.

Progression of the disease in affected Basenjis is variable. Some dogs develop chronic renal failure within a few months of diagnosis, and others remain stable for several years. Rapid progression and death may result from acute renal failure and papillary necrosis or acute pyelonephritis. Treatment of dogs with Fanconi's syndrome is limited to control of metabolic acidosis, appropriate antibiotic therapy for urinary tract infections, and conservative medical management of chronic renal failure. It may be difficult to control acidosis even with high doses of alkali therapy. This is a consequence of the marked bicarbonaturia that occurs whenever plasma HCO_3^- concentration is increased with replacement to within the normal plasma range. Potassium citrate therapy provides both alkalinization and K^+ supplementation. The veterinarian should strive to maintain a serum HCO_3^- concentration or total carbon dioxide concentration above 12 mEq/L and a serum K^+ concentration of 4 to 6 mEq/L.

REFERENCES

1. Chesney RW, Novello AC: Defects of renal tubular transport. *In* Massry SG, Glassock RJ (eds): Textbook of Nephrology, 3rd ed, vol 1, p 513. Baltimore, Williams & Wilkins, 1995.
2. McNamara PD, Rea CT, Bovee KC, et al: Cystinuria in dogs: Comparison of the cystinuric component of the Fanconi syndrome in Basenji dogs to isolated cystinuria. Metabolism 38:8, 1989.
3. Hoppe A, Denneberg T, Jeppsson JO, et al: Urinary excretion of amino acids in normal and cystinuric dogs. Br Vet J 149:253, 1993.
4. Bovee KC, Segal S: Renal tubule reabsorption of amino acids after lysine loading of cystinuric dogs. Metabolism 33:602, 1984.
5. Holtzapple PG, Bovee KC, Rea CF, et al: Amino acid uptake by kidney and jejunal tissue from dogs with cystine stones. Science 166:1525, 1969.
6. Ling GV, Franti CE, Ruby AL, et al: Urolithiasis in dogs: II. Breed prevalence, and interrelations of breed, sex, age, and mineral composition. Am J Vet Res 59:630, 1998.
7. Case LC, Ling GV, Franti CE, et al: Cystine-containing urinary calculi in dogs: 102 cases (1981–1989). JAVMA 201:129, 1992.
8. Lulich JP, Osborne CA, Bartges JW, et al: Canine lower urinary tract disorders. *In* Ettinger SJ, Feldman EC (eds): Textbook of Veterinary Internal Medicine, 4th ed, vol 2, p 1833. Philadelphia, WB Saunders, 1995.
9. Wallerstrom BI, Wåagberg TI, Lagergren CH: Cystine calculi in the dog: An epidemiological retrospective study. J Small Anim Pract 33:78, 1992.
10. Bartges JW, Osborne CA, Lulich JP, et al: Prevalence of cystine and urate uroliths in English bulldogs and urate uroliths in Dalmatians (1981–1992). JAVMA 204:1914, 1994.
11. DiBartola SP, Chew DJ, Horton ML: Cystinuria in a cat. JAVMA 198:102, 1991.
12. Osborne CA, Lulich JP, Thumchai R, et al: Feline urolithiasis: Etiology and pathophysiology. Vet Clin North Am Small Anim Pract 26:217, 1996.
13. Keene BW, Panciera DL, Atkins CE, et al: Myocardial L-carnitine deficiency in a family of dogs with dilated cardiomyopathy. JAVMA 198:647, 1991.
14. Sanderson SL, Osborne CA, Lulich JP, et al: Carnitine and taurine excretion in 5 dogs with cystinuria. Am J Vet Res 1998, in press.
15. Bartges JW, Osborne CA, Felice LJ: Canine xanthine uroliths: Risk factor manage-

URO

ment. *In* Kirk RW, Bonagura JD (eds): Current Veterinary Therapy, ed XI, p 900. Philadelphia, WB Saunders, 1992.

16. Sorenson JL, Ling GV: Metabolic and genetic aspects of urate urolithiasis in Dalmatians. JAVMA 203:857, 1993.

17. Giesecke D, Tiemeyer W: Defect of uric acid uptake in Dalmatian dog liver. Experientia 40:145, 1984.

18. Roch-Ramel F, Peters G: Urinary excretion of uric acid in nonhuman mammalian species. *In* Kelley WN, Weiner IM (eds): Handbook of Experimental Pharmacology, vol 51, Uric Acid, p 211. Berlin, Springer-Verlag, 1978.

19. Kidder DE, Chivers PR: Xanthine calculi in a dog. Vet Rec 83:228, 1968.

20. van Zuilen CD, Nickel RF, van Dijk TH, et al: Xanthinuria in a family of Cavalier King Charles spaniels. Vet Q 19:172, 1997.

21. Kucera J, Bulkova T, Rychla R, et al: Bilateral xanthine nephrolithiasis in a dog. J Small Anim Pract 38:302, 1997.

22. Lulich JP, Osborne CA, Nagode LA, et al: Evaluation of urine and serum metabolites in miniature schnauzers with calcium oxalate urolithiasis. Am J Vet Res 52:1583, 1991.

23. Breitschwerdt EB, Meuten DJ, Greenfield CL, et al: Idiopathic hyperaldosteronism in a dog. JAVMA 187:841, 1985.

24. Ahn A: Hyperaldosteronism in cats. Semin Vet Med Surg Small Anim 9:153, 1994.

25. Fyfe JC, Giger U, Hall CA, et al: Inherited selective intestinal cobalamin malabsorption and cobalamin deficiency in dogs. Pediatr Res 29:24, 1991.

26. DiBartola SP: Renal tubular disorders. *In* Ettinger SJ, Feldman EC (eds): Textbook of Veterinary Internal Medicine, 4th ed, vol 2, p 1801. Philadelphia, WB Saunders, 1995.

27. Smulders YM, Frissen PHJ, Slaats EH, et al: Renal tubular acidosis: Pathophysiology and diagnosis. Arch Intern Med 156:1629, 1996.

28. Bartges JW, Osborne CA, Felice LJ, et al: Influence of 4 diets on uric acid and ammonia metabolism in healthy beagles. Am J Vet Res 57:324, 1996.

29. Bartges JW, Tarver SL, Schneider C: Comparison of struvite activity product ratios and relative supersaturations in urine collected from healthy cats consuming four struvite management diets. Presented before the Ralston Purina Nutrition Symposium, St. Louis, 1998.

30. Watson AD, Culvenor JA, Middleton DJ, et al: Distal renal tubular acidosis in a cat with pyelonephritis. Vet Rec 119:65, 1986.

31. Brown SA, Spyridakis LK, Crowell WA: Distal renal tubular acidosis and hepatic lipidosis in a cat. JAVMA 189:1350, 1986.

32. Winaver J, Agmon D, Harari R, et al: Impaired renal acidification following acute renal ischemia in the dog. Kidney Int 30:906, 1986.

33. Noonan CH, Kay JM: Prevalence and geographic distribution of Fanconi syndrome in Basenjis in the United States. JAVMA 197:345, 1990.

34. Darrigrand Haag RA, Center SA, Randolph JF, et al: Congenital Fanconi syndrome associated with renal dysplasia in 2 border terriers. J Vet Intern Med 10:412, 1996.

35. Finco DR: Familial renal disease in Norwegian elkhound dogs: Physiologic and biochemical examinations. Am J Vet Res 37:87, 1986.

36. Mackenzie CP, Van Den Broek A: The Fanconi syndrome in a whippet. J Small Anim Pract 23:469, 1982.

37. McEwan NA, Macartney L: Fanconi's syndrome in a Yorkshire terrier. J Small Anim Pract 28:737, 1987.

38. Bovee KC, Joyce T, Blazer Yost B, et al: Characterization of renal defects in dogs with a syndrome similar to the Fanconi syndrome in man. JAVMA 174:1094, 1979.

39. Padrid P: Fanconi syndrome in a mixed breed dog. Mod Vet Pract 69:162, 1988.

40. Brown SA: Fanconi syndrome and acute renal failure associated with gentamicin therapy in a dog. J Am Anim Hosp Assoc 22:635, 1986.

41. Freeman LM, Breitschwerdt EB, Keene BW, et al: Fanconi's syndrome in a dog with primary hypoparathyroidism. J Vet Intern Med 8:349, 1994.

42. Settles EL, Schmidt D: Fanconi syndrome in a Labrador retriever. J Vet Intern Med 8:390, 1994.

43. Boulanger Y, Wong H, Noel J, et al: Heterogeneous metabolism and toxicity of 4-pentenoate along the dog nephron. Ren Physiol Biochem 16:182, 1993.

44. Pouliot JF, Gougoux A, Beliveau R: Brush border membrane proteins in experimental Fanconi's syndrome induced by 4-pentenoate and maleate. Can J Physiol Pharmacol 70:1247, 1992.

45. Bovee KC: Genetic and metabolic diseases of the kidney. *In* Bovee KC (ed): Canine Nephrology, p 339. Philadelphia, Harwal Publishing Company, 1984.

CHAPTER 175

FELINE LOWER URINARY TRACT DISEASES

Carl A. Osborne, John M. Kruger, Jody P. Lulich, David J. Polzin, and Chalermpol Lekcharoensuk

ETIOPATHOLOGIC PARADIGMS

OVERVIEW

During the past three decades, prevailing opinions published in textbooks and journals about the etiology of the symptom complex of recurrent dysuria, pollakiuria, stranguria, hematuria, periuria, and/or urinary outflow obstruction have often been based on poorly defined metabolic, infectious, and dietary ad hoc theories, many of which were apparently extrapolated from studies in other species and some of which were the product of rationalization and creative imagination. Acceptance of the value of a variety of treatments for lower urinary tract diseases (LUTD) was unconsciously reinforced by the fact that many patients had self-limiting disease, whereas in others the signs spontaneously waxed and waned. Our experience has been that the severity of many untreated cases of LUTDs declined within 2 or 3 days, with complete remission in 5 to 10 days.[1–3] In this situation, many forms of treatment appeared to be beneficial provided they were not overtly harmful.

THE BACTERIAL INFECTION ERA

In terms of treatment, one of the most popular theories in the 1960s, 1970s, and 1980s linked many cases of this symptom complex to bacterial infections. The notion that bacteria were involved in feline LUTD was reinforced by false-positive in vitro culture results associated with improper urine collection techniques and failure to quantify bacterial isolates. The idea that bacteria were important etiologic agents was further enhanced by the observation that signs of LUTD often subsided in association with antimicrobial therapy. In retrospect, it is probable that many affected cats without bacterial urinary tract infection (UTI) appeared to respond to antibacterial drugs because they had self-limiting clinical signs of LUTD.

In 1970 Schechter,[4] using proper selection of patients and proper urine collection and culture techniques, found that only about 1 per cent of untreated affected cats had bacterial UTI. This observation indicated that bacterial UTI was an uncommon initiating cause of LUTD, a conclusion subsequently confirmed by several other groups of investigators.[5]

THE VIRAL INFECTION ERA

In a series of studies beginning in the late 1960s, a gamma herpesvirus (subsequently identified as bovine herpesvirus type 4), a calicivirus (feline calicivirus), and a retrovirus (feline syncytium-forming virus) were isolated from urine and tissues of cats with naturally occurring LUTD.[5] After experimental induction of characteristic signs of LUTD in specific pathogen-free (SPF) male kittens with the herpesvirus, it was concluded that these experimental studies demonstrated that the cell-associated herpesvirus was a primary cause of feline urologic syndrome (FUS).[6] A calicivirus was incriminated as having a secondary role as it exacerbated the severity of the disease in cats infected with herpesvirus.

Subsequently, several groups of investigators were unable to isolate the cell-associated herpesvirus or caliciviruses from cats with naturally occurring FUS.[5] However, inability to detect viruses in cats with naturally occurring LUTD must be viewed with caution. Negative findings by various investigators appear to be confounded by improper selection of naturally occurring cases of FUS, the viricidal nature of feline urine, improper handling of samples, and/or insensitive or inappropriate virus detection methods.[5]

The observation of virus-like particles tentatively identified as calicivirus in a substantial number of crystalline-matrix urethral plugs obtained from male cats with naturally occurring urethral obstruction led us to reexamine the roles of viruses in the etiology of naturally occurring LUTD (Fig. 175–1).[7] As a part of a prospective study of the prevalence of calicivirus urinary tract infections in 1998, we isolated a calicivirus from urine obtained from a nonobstructed cat with naturally occurring idiopathic LUTD. Further studies are necessary to determine whether this isolate is causally or coincidentally related to LUTD. However, on the basis of available data, we hypothesize that caliciviruses are causally related to at least some idiopathic cases of LUTD. Refer to: Viral Urinary Tract Infections.

THE STRUVITE UROLITHIASIS ERA

In the early 1970s, the association between dry diets and the "feline urolithiasis syndrome" became a topic of intense discussion. Also in the early 1970s and continuing for the next decade, several groups of investigators experimentally produced magnesium hydrogen phosphate and then magnesium ammonium phosphate uroliths in normal cats by adding various types of magnesium salts to their diets.[8] The cats developed typical signs of LUTD, including urethral obstruction. However, this model did not result in production of the struvite-matrix urethral plugs commonly encountered in cats with naturally occurring urethral obstruction.[9] Nonetheless, as the viral etiology of FUS lost popularity in the late 1970s, the general consensus of many investigators and clinicians was that consumption of dry diets with excessive magnesium was an important primary cause of FUS.

Beginning in 1983, reports from the Minnesota Urolith Center of medical dissolution of naturally occurring sterile

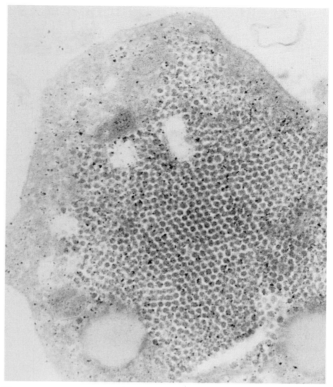

Figure 175–1. Transmission electron micrograph of a section of urethral plug obtained from a 3-year-old domestic longhair cat. Note the virus-like structures contained in an unidentified cell. Original magnification ×80,000.

struvite urocystoliths with modified diets corroborated the importance of dietary risk and protective factors in the etiology of sterile struvite urolithiasis.[10, 11]

In 1985, investigators at the University of California studied normal cats receiving diets containing alkalinizing and acidifying salts of magnesium.[12] Their results shifted the focus of attention from dietary magnesium to alkaline urinary pH as a primary factor involved in the development of struvite crystalluria. Results of these diet-related studies supported the view in that era that many cases of FUS were caused by struvite uroliths and urethral plugs. The pet food industry also responded to these recommendations by placing increased emphasis on development of urine-acidifying diets modified to dissolve and prevent struvite crystalluria. Even now, many adult feline maintenance diets have been modified to minimize struvite crystalluria.[13]

There is abundant evidence that in past years, sterile struvite uroliths and struvite urethral plugs played a prominent causative role in a substantial number of cats with naturally occurring obstructive and nonobstructive LUTD. In addition, dietary factors contributed to both the cause and the treatment or prevention of struvite-related LUTD. As a result of dietary modifications by numerous pet food manufacturers, in the mid-1980s the prevalence of struvite uroliths and struvite urethral plugs began to decline (Fig. 175–2). Although struvite continued to be the primary component in urethral plugs (Fig. 175–3), the frequency with which they formed dramatically declined as evidenced by a parallel decline in the number of perineal urethrostomies performed to minimize recurrent urethral obstruction (Fig. 175–4). Unexpectedly, the decline in struvite-related urolithiasis was associated with a concomitant rise in calcium oxalate uro-

URO

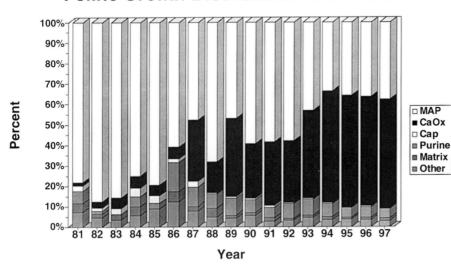

Figure 175–2. Changing trends in mineral composition of feline uroliths submitted to the Minnesota Urolith Center from 1981 to 1997.

lithiasis, but, unexplainably, struvite remained the primary component of urethral plugs (see Figs. 175–2 and 175–3). Refer to: Epidemiology of Uroliths and Urethral Plugs.

THE VESICOURACHAL DIVERTICULA ERA

In the late 1970s and early 1980s, vesicourachal diverticula were cited as playing an etiopathogenic role in some cats with FUS.[14] Surgical removal of the vesicurachal diverticula was popularly recommended. The observation that clinical signs subsided coincidentally with diverticulectomy and lack of studies of the biologic behavior of macroscopic diverticula without surgery reinforced the opinion that diverticulectomy was required to eliminate signs of LUTD associated with this abnormality.

Vesicourachal diverticula were detected by positive contrast radiography in approximately 25 per cent of cats with naturally occurring LUTD.[15] Subsequent clinical studies re-

vealed that most adult-onset macroscopic vesicourachal diverticula were sequelae rather than causes of LUTD.[14, 16] Refer to: Vesicourachal Diverticula.

THE INTERSTITIAL CYSTITIS ERA

In 1994 investigators found some cats with idiopathic forms of LUTD had interstitial cystitis (IC) because they had abnormalities similar to those reported in humans with IC.[17] Human IC is a nonmalignant inflammatory disorder of unknown etiology.[18] In humans, the disease is characterized by dysuria, pain above the pubic region that is relieved by voiding; dysuria; pyuria, hematuria, and/or proteinuria detected by urinalysis; distinctive mucosal lesions called glomerulations detected by cystoscopy; and decreased urine concentrations of glycosaminoglycans. Although IC has affected humans of all ages and both sexes, it is most common in middle-aged white females.

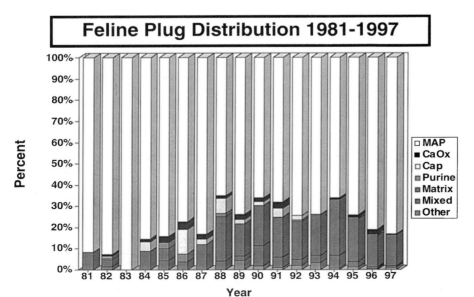

Figure 175–3. Changing trends in mineral composition of feline urethral plugs submitted to the Minnesota Urolith Center from 1981 to 1997.

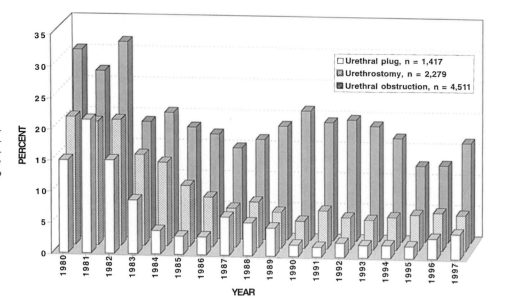

Figure 175–4. Declining frequency of urethral obstructions, urethral plugs, and urethrostomies in 22,908 cats with lower urinary tract disease admitted to 24 veterinary colleges in North America from 1980 to 1997.

In 1997, cats with idiopathic LUTD were reported to have several clinical abnormalities that were similar to those observed in humans with IC, including characteristic cystoscopic findings.[19] Decreased urine concentrations of glycosaminoglycans (GAGs) and increased urinary bladder permeability were also reported.[20] It was recommended that idiopathic LUTD be renamed idiopathic cystitis or feline interstitial cystitis.[17, 21]

The term interstitial cystitis describes clinical manifestations and morphologic changes in the bladder whose cause is idiopathic. Similarities between human IC and idiopathic feline LUTD disorders may represent finite responses of the bladder and urethra to more than one disease process. Further studies designed to compare findings in cats with idiopathic LUTD with those in cats with naturally occurring LUTD of known causes are needed. Also needed are further studies designed to define the specific etiologic relationship between feline idiopathic LUTD and human IC.[22]

In 1994, proponents of the feline IC theory stated that they had encouraging responses to treatment of feline IC with amitriptyline.[17] They also suggested that buspirone and hydrodistention of the bladder may provide relief of signs in some cats. As a result, an increasing number of veterinary practitioners, referral specialists, and academic clinicians are suggesting use of drugs advocated to treat IC in humans in attempts to treat cats with idiopathic LUTD. Like many drugs used in the past, however, these drugs have gained popularity for treatment of nonobstructive LUTD because they are often associated with remission of clinical signs. But the occurrence of two events in consecutive order does not prove a cause-and-effect relationship. In view of the fact that the clinical course of idiopathic feline LUTD is often self-limiting and that use of the drugs may be associated with undesirable side effects, when is the use of these drugs warranted and what is the associated risk-benefit ratio? To prevent repeating errors of the past, we feel that endorsements regarding use of any treatment, including drugs such as amitriptyline, be withheld pending results of prospective randomized double-blind controlled studies designed to evaluate their safety and efficacy in cats with properly confirmed types of naturally occurring LUTD.

FELINE LOWER URINARY TRACT DISEASES ALIAS FELINE UROLOGIC SYNDROME ALIAS FELINE INTERSTITIAL CYSTITIS

In order to minimize the stereotyped approach to treatment of LUTD so prevalent in the past, we continue to urge our colleagues to replace a clinical diagnosis of FUS and FIC with refined diagnostic terms pertaining to sites (e.g., urethra, bladder), causes (e.g., anomalies, urolithiasis, bacteria, fungi, parasites, neoplasms, metabolic disturbances, idiopathic forms), morphologic changes (e.g., inflammation, neoplasia), and pathophysiologic mechanisms (e.g., obstructive uropathy, reflex dyssynergia) whenever possible.[23, 24] Logically, in order to localize and define different causes of feline LUTD, contemporary diagnostic evaluation of each patient is necessary (Table 175–1). If the cause of feline LUTD cannot be identified after appropriate evaluation, we suggest that it be called idiopathic lower urinary tract disease.

INCIDENCE AND PROPORTIONAL MORBIDITY OF LOWER URINARY TRACT DISEASE

INCIDENCE

The incidence of disease is defined as the annual rate of appearance of new cases of disease among the entire population of individuals at risk for the disease. Studies reported in the 1970s and early 1980s estimated the overall incidence of feline LUTDs in the United States and Great Britain to be 0.5 to 1.0 per cent per year.[25, 26] On the basis of this estimate, a quarter-million to a half-million of the 57 million pet cats in the United States[27] are afflicted with some form of LUTD annually.

Although idiopathic disease accounts for the majority of these cases,[15, 19] the actual incidence of idiopathic disease, its rate of recurrence, and the frequency of sequelae are unknown. There have been no contemporary controlled epi-

URO

TABLE 175–1. DIAGNOSTIC PLAN FOR FELINE DYSURIC HEMATURIA

FACTOR	WITH URETHRAL OBSTRUCTION		WITHOUT URETHRAL OBSTRUCTION	
	First or Infrequent Episodes	*Frequent or Persistent Episodes*	*First or Infrequent Episodes*	*Frequent or Persistent Episodes*
Defined history	+ + + + +	+ + + + +	+ + + + +	+ + + + +
Defined physical examination	+ + + + +	+ + + + +	+ + + + +	+ + + + +
Urinalysis (with sediment)*	+ + + + +	+ + + + +	+ + + + +	+ + + + +
Screening, quantitative urine culture*	+ + +	+ + + +	+ + +	+ + + +
Serum chemistry profile (especially SUN, creatinine, K^+, and $T\text{-}CO_2$)	+ + + + +	+ + + + +	+	+ +
Assess lesion(s), site(s), and causes(s)				
Palpation	+ + + + +	+ + + + +	+ + + + +	+ + + + +
Survey radiography	+ + +	+ + + + +	+ + +	+ + + + +
Ultrasonography	+ + +	+ + + + +	+ + +	+ + + + +
Contrast radiography (retrograde urethrocystography or antegrade cytourethrography)	+	+ + + + +	+	+ + + +
Urethrocystoscopy	+ +	+ + + +	+	+ + + +
Analysis of urethral plug or urolith†	+ + + + +	+ + + + +	+ + + + +	+ + + + +
Urine urease activity	+	+ +	+	+ +
Complete blood count	+	+ + +	+	+ + +
Exploratory cystotomy and biopsy‡	Infrequent	±	Infrequent	±
Urine electrolytes, amino acids, purine precursors§	±	±	±	±

*Urine sample preferably collected by cystocentesis; however, cystocentesis commonly causes hematuria.
†If available, submit stones and urethral plugs for quantitative analysis. A portion of plugs may be fixed in formalin for light microscopic analysis.
‡Exploratory cystotomy is indicated only when there is reason to believe that the results will justify the risks to the patient and cost to the client.
§Primarily of value in patients with confirmed uroliths.

demiologic studies designed to evaluate subsets of cats with LUTDs defined on the basis of specific diagnostic criteria.

PROPORTIONAL MORBIDITY RATES AND RATIOS

The incidence of naturally occurring hematuria, dysuria, and/or urethral obstruction in domestic cats should not be confused with the frequency with which such cats are seen in veterinary hospitals (so-called proportional morbidity ratios). As is apparent in the following discussion, proportional morbidity ratios for FUS are not a reliable index of the incidence of FUS.

Proportional Morbidity in the 1970s and 1980s

The proportional morbidity ratio of cats with lower urinary tract disorders was reported to be as high as 10 per cent in the 1970s. However, the most commonly reported frequency in the 1980s was 1 to 6 per cent.[25, 28]

Proportional Morbidity of Lower Urinary Tract Disease at North American Colleges of Veterinary Medicine, 1980 to 1997

Retrospective evaluation of data from 24 colleges of veterinary medicine in North America compiled by workers at the Veterinary Data Base, Purdue University, indicated that from 1980 to 1997, LUTD was diagnosed in 8.0 per cent (22,908 of 286,076) of cats admitted to teaching hospitals (cases were counted only once irrespective of the number of readmissions). The highest rates among the 24 colleges of veterinary medicine were reported from the University of Minnesota (13 per cent), University of Pennsylvania (13 per cent), University of Illinois (9 per cent), University of Tennessee (8 per cent), Cornell University (9 per cent), and the University of Wisconsin (8 per cent). Rates less than the 8 per cent average of all colleges were reported by Tuskegee University (2 per cent), University of Florida (3 per cent), Oklahoma State University (4 per cent), University of Missouri (7 per cent), University of Georgia (6 per cent), and Purdue University (7 per cent).

The wide variance reported by each of these veterinary teaching hospitals emphasizes the need for caution in formulating generalities about proportional morbidity ratios of LUTD on the basis of reports from one center. LUTD is more commonly encountered and/or recognized in veterinary teaching hospitals with special interests in this disease. Although proportional morbidity ratios reported by these centers are unlikely to be representative of veterinary hospitals without a special interest in urology, the frequency with which specific causes of LUTD are recognized by contemporary diagnostic evaluation suggests that specific causes of LUTD are underdiagnosed.

Specific Disease-Related Proportional Morbidity of Lower Urinary Tract Disease

All 24 Colleges of Veterinary Medicine—1980 to 1997

For the 22,908 cats with LUTD, diagnoses included feline urologic syndrome (30 per cent) and undefined urinary tract infection (10 per cent). Unspecified (idiopathic) cystitis was reported in 24 per cent of the patients, urocystolithiasis in 5 per cent, urinary incontinence in 5 per cent, bacterial UTI in 5 per cent, bacterial cystitis in 3 per cent, ruptured urinary bladders in 1 per cent, and neoplasms in 0.3 per cent. Urinary bladder diverticula were observed in less than 0.5 per cent.

Urethral obstruction was encountered in 20 per cent of 22,908 patients, urethrolithiasis (urethral plugs) affected 6 per cent, and urethral strictures affected 2 per cent. Urethral neoplasms, detrusor–urethral reflex dyssynergia, urethral rupture, and prostate neoplasms were all reported in less than 0.1 per cent of the patients.

Five per cent of cats with LUTD died or were euthanized, compared with 8 per cent for other feline diseases. The

TABLE 175–2. FREQUENCY OF DISORDERS IN CATS WITH SIGNS OF LOWER URINARY TRACT DISEASE

DISORDER	1981–1985[19]		1993–1995[24]	
	Male (%)	Female (%)	Male (%)	Female (%)
Nonobstructive LUTD	(n = 47)	(n = 43)	(n = 47)	(n = 62)
Idiopathic	79	58	64	65
Urolith	17	40	9	19
Urolith + UTI	0	2	0	0
UTI	0.04	0	0.02	0
Neoplasia	0	0	4	0
Anatomic defect	NR*	NR†	11§	10§
Behavioral abnormality	NA‡	NA‡	13	6.5
Obstructive LUTD	(n = 51)	(n = 0)		
Idiopathic	29	0	ND	ND
Urethral plug	59	0	ND	ND
Uroliths	10	0	ND	ND
Urolith + UTI	2	0	ND	ND

NA = not applicable; NR = not reported; ND = not determined; LUTD = lower urinary tract disease; UTI = urinary tract infection.

*A urachal diverticulum was identified in nine male cats, and urethral narrowing was identified in four cats with nonobstructive LUTD. These anatomic abnormalities were not considered a primary cause of clinical signs in this study.

†A urachal diverticulum was identified in seven female cats with nonobstructive LUTD. Urachal diverticula were not considered a primary cause of clinical signs in this study.

‡Cats with periuria in the absence of hematuria, pollakiuria, and/or urethral obstructions were excluded from this study.

§Six cats had a urachal diverticulum, five cats had a urethral stricture, and one cat had a malpositioned urethra. Gender of affected cats was not specified. These anatomic abnormalities were considered primary causes of clinical signs in this study.

average period of hospitalization for cats with LUTD was 2 ± 4.5 days.

University of Minnesota—1981 to 1985

Data from the Purdue Veterinary Medical Data Base should be interpreted in the context of retrospective studies. In a prospective clinical study, 141 untreated cats with hematuria, dysuria, urethral obstruction, or combinations of these signs were evaluated by contemporary diagnostic methods. The cats had no concomitant disease of other body systems.

Specific diagnoses were established in 66 of 153 (46 per cent; Table 175–2).[15]

Ohio State University—1993 to 1995

In a prospective clinical study, 109 cats with nonobstructive LUTD were evaluated by contemporary diagnostic methods. Specific diagnoses were established in 29 (27 per cent; see Table 175–2).[19] In addition to a 10-year time span, the Ohio State University (OSU) study differed from the mid-1980 Minnesota study in the following ways: (1) the Minnesota study was designed to include case controls, whereas this was not a feature of the OSU study; (2) cats examined because of urethral obstruction were excluded from the OSU study but were included in the Minnesota study; (3) even though urethral obstruction was an exclusion criterion in the OSU study, some male cats with recurrent LUTD were previously treated by perineal urethrostomy; and (4) cats being treated at the time of the evaluation were apparently not excluded from the OSU study (the exclusion criteria were not reproducibly defined), but cats given any treatment before evaluation were excluded from the Minnesota study (see Table 175–2).[15, 19] Thus, in the OSU Study, treatment may have masked otherwise identifiable causes of LUTD.

Age-Related Proportional Morbidity of Lower Urinary Tract Disease in Cats—1980 to 1997

LUTD is uncommon in immature cats. However, when we encounter LUTD in immature cats, we have a high index of suspicion for bacterial UTI associated with functional or anatomic defects.

FUS, idiopathic cystitis, urocystolithiasis, urethral obstruction, urethral plugs, and urethral strictures were more commonly diagnosed in cats between the ages of 1 and 10 years than in cats younger than 1 or older than 10 years (Fig. 175–5). Further prospective studies are needed to determine whether the frequency of recurrence of urethral obstruction declines after affected cats reach 10 years of age or whether the cats at risk for urethral obstruction are no longer alive.

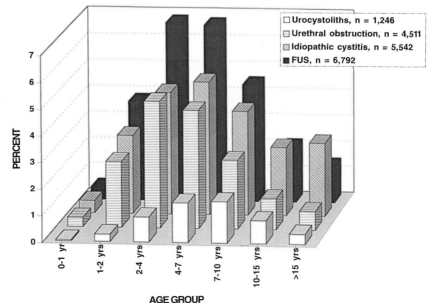

Figure 175–5. Age-specific proportional morbidity rate (per cent) of urocystoliths, urethral obstructions, idiopathic cystitis, and feline urologic syndrome of 286,076 cats admitted to 24 colleges of veterinary medicine in North America from 1980 to 1997.

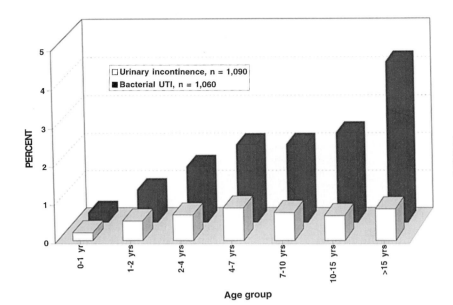

Figure 175–6. Age-specific proportional morbidity rate (per cent) of urinary incontinence and bacterial urinary tract infection of 286,076 cats admitted to 24 colleges of veterinary medicine in North America from 1980 to 1997.

Although bacterial UTI is uncommonly encountered in young adult cats, the prevalence of UTI increases with age (Fig. 175–6). Likewise, the proportional morbidity of urinary incontinence increases with advancing age (see Fig. 175–5).

Gender-Related Proportional Morbidity of Lower Urinary Tract Disease—1980 to 1997

LUTD affected males twice as often as females. Of 22,908 cats diagnosed with LUTD at 24 colleges of veterinary medicine, 7 per cent were nonspayed females, 25 per cent were neutered females, 16 per cent were noncastrated males, and 52 per cent were castrated males.

In females with LUTD the specific causes, from most common to least common, were (1) idiopathic cystitis (30 per cent), (2) urocystolithiasis (8 per cent), (3) urinary incontinence (7 per cent), (4) bacterial cystitis (4 per cent), (5) urethral obstruction (less than 3 per cent), (6) urethroliths (2 per cent), and (7) urethral strictures (<1 per cent).

In males with LUTD the specific causes, from most common to least common, were (1) urethral obstruction (28 per cent), (2) idiopathic cystitis (22 per cent), (3) urethral plugs (8 per cent), (4) urocystoliths (4 per cent), (5) urinary incontinence (3 percent), (6) bacterial cystitis (3 per cent), and (7) urethral strictures (2 per cent).

PRIORITY OF DIAGNOSTIC AND THERAPEUTIC PLANS FOR LOWER URINARY TRACT DISEASES

Micturition encompasses both a storage phase and a voiding phase. During the storage phase of micturition, the urinary bladder, acting as a low-pressure reservoir, is relaxed and fills with urine. Urine is contained in the bladder lumen by resistance generated by muscles in the bladder neck and urethra that function as high-pressure unidirectional valves. During the voiding phase of micturition, muscle in the wall of the bladder contracts, generating high pressure to pump urine through the urethral lumen. Simultaneously, as muscles in the bladder neck and urethra relax, the urethra becomes a low-pressure conduit for urine being voided from the body.

The consequences of a variety of diseases of the lower urinary tract (e.g., urinary bladder and urethra) are dysfunction of the voiding and/or storage phases of micturition. Disorders of the storage phase are characterized by pollakiuria, nocturia, and urinary incontinence. Pollakiuria is often associated with dysuria, stranguria, and hematuria. Disorders of the voiding phase of micturition may result in complete or incomplete retention of urine and overflow (also called paradoxical) urinary incontinence.

We recommend that disorders of the lower urinary tract be localized to disorders of the storage and/or disorders of the voiding phase of micturition. To enhance our ability to detect the underlying cause of various types of micturition disorders in a consistent and cost-effective fashion, we follow a prioritized sequence of diagnostic steps. To summarize, after initial identification of the patient's problems, further diagnostic plans to confirm, localize, and identify the underlying causes of these initial problems encompass the following sequence: (1) initial verification of signs of LUTD, especially those defined by clients; (2) initial localization of LUTD as disorders of the storage phase or the voiding phase of micturition; (3) clinical investigation of the most probable pathophysiologic mechanism(s) associated with the identified problems utilizing the DAMNIT acronym (Tables 175–3 and 175–4); and (4) implementation of diagnostic tests to confirm or exclude the pathophysiologic mechanisms of LUTD thought to be most probable in each patient. By using the DAMNIT acronym, numerous diagnostic *possibilities* can be logically reduced to likely diagnostic *probabilities*.

The following sections describing different types of LUTD are organized according to the DAMNIT scheme of pathophysiologic causes (see Tables 175–3 and 175–4).

DIAGNOSIS AND TREATMENT OF BEHAVIORAL PERIURIA

ETIOPATHOGENESIS (see Table 175–3)

Feline behavioral periuria is defined as functionally normal voluntary elimination of urine at the wrong place (sites

TABLE 175–3. DAMNIT PATHOPHYSIOLOGIC SCHEME OF NONOBSTRUCTIVE CAUSES OF LOWER URINARY TRACT DISEASES

D—Dementia (behavioral)
  • Urination in unusual locations
A—Anomolous and congenital abnormalities
  • Urachal anomalies
  • Phimosis
  • Urethrorectal fistula
M—Metabolic disorders (including nutritional)
  • Uroliths (see Tables 175–5 and 175–7 to 175–14)
N—Neoplasia of urinary bladder
  • Benign
    • Cystadenoma, leiomyoma
    • Fibroma, papilloma
    • Hemangioma
  • Malignant
    • Carcinomas (transitional, squamous, adenocarcinoma)
    • Sarcoma (hemangio-, lympho-, myxo-, rhabdomyosarcoma)
N—Nutritional
  • Diet-sensitive urolithiasis
I—Inflammatory disorders
  • Infectious inflammatory agents
    • Viral
    • Bacterial
    • Fungal
    • Parasitic
    • *Mycoplasma, Ureaplasma*

I—Noninfectious inflammatory disorders
  • Immune mediated?
  • Others
I—Iatrogenic disorders
  • Transurethral catheters used to flush urethra
  • Reverse flushing solutions
  • Damage to mucosa and submucosa
  • Systemic toxicity
  • Cystocentesis-induced hematuria
  • Palpation-induced bladder trauma
  • Urethrocystoscopy complications
  • Postsurgical transurethral catheters
  • Urethrostomy complications
    • Bacterial UTI
  • Antibiotic-induced resistant bacterial UTI
I—Idiopathic
  • Inflammatory (noninfectious)
  • Includes cats suspected of having interstitial cystitis
T—Trauma
  • See iatrogenic disorders
T—Toxins
  • Adverse drug reactions
  • See iatrogenic disorders

UTI = urinary tract infection.

other than the litter box or outdoors) or at the wrong time (nocturia) as defined by the owner. We define the term periuria as urination in inappropriate locations. The causes and management of behavioral disorders associated with functionally normal micturiton are beyond the scope of this discussion but have been described in detail elsewhere.[29, 30] The point emphasized here is that most cats with disorders of the lower urinary tract also void in inappropriate location.[24] LUTDs are not, however, commonly associated with undesirable urine marking (urine spraying).

DIAGNOSIS

Understandably, owners of house cats usually cannot distinguish between periuria associated with behavioral problems, from periuria associated with urge incontinence (unrestrainable detrusor contractions associated with irritative cystourethritis), and periuria associated with urinary incontinence caused by urethral sphincter problems or etopic ureters. Differentiation between primary behavioral periuria and periuria of nonbehavioral or secondary behavioral causes begins with acquisition of relevant history associated with the problem. When possible, the cat should be directly observed during the voiding phase of micturition. Results of the history and physical examination may then be used for cost-effective choice of additional diagnostic procedures (see Table 175–1).

In some cats with LUTD, periuria may not be associated with detectable dysuria, pollakiuria, or gross hematuria. For these cats, additional diagnostics should be considered before concluding that periuria is a primary behavioral disorder.[31]

URO

TABLE 175–4. DAMNIT PATHOPHYSIOLOGIC SCHEME OF OBSTRUCTIVE CAUSES OF LOWER URINARY TRACT DISEASES

D—Developmental and congenital abnormalities
  • Phimosis
  • Persistent uterus masculinus
  • Urethral strictures
  • Phimosis
M—Metabolic disorders (including nutritional)
  • Urethroliths (see Tables 175–5 and 175–7 to 175–14)
  • Crystal-matrix urethral plugs (see Tables 175–6 and 175–15)
N—Neoplastic
  • Transitional cell carcinoma
  • Prostate adenocarcinoma
  • Endometrial adenocarcinoma
N—Nutritional
  • Diet-sensitive urethroliths and matrix-crystal urethral plugs
I Inflammatory disorders
  • Infectious agents
    • Viral
    • Bacterial
    • Fungal
  • Noninfectious
    • Immune mediated

I—Iatrogenic disorders
  • Transurethral catheters used to flush urethra
  • Urethral flushing solutions
    • Damage to mucosa
    • Systemic toxicity
  • Indwelling transurethral catheters, especially open systems (see table 175–18)
  • Ruptured urinary bladder
  • Postsurgical transurethral catheters
  • Urethrostomy complications
    • Bacterial UTI
    • Urethral strictures
  • Antibiotic-induced resistant bacterial UTI
I—Idiopathic
  • Inflammatory (noninfectious)
  • Reflex dyssynergia
  • Primary urethral spasm
T—Trauma
  • See iatrogenic disorders
  • Hypotonic bladder (secondary to overdistention)
T—Toxins
  • Adverse drug reactions

UIT = urinary tract infection.

TREATMENT

Some cats resume urination in appropriate locations when the LUTD has been effectively treated or spontaneously resolves. However, the longer a cat has been voiding in inappropriate locations, the more difficulty is likely to be encountered in training it to resume micturition in acceptable places. In this situation, there is a need to develop strategies to modify abnormal behavior in addition to treatment of the associated disease of the lower urinary tract.[31]

DIAGNOSIS AND TREATMENT OF DEVELOPMENTAL ABNORMALITIES

OVERVIEW

As with other species, congenital abnormalities of the lower urinary tract may be associated with hematuria, dysuria, urinary incontinence, and/or urethral obstruction. However, congenital causes of feline LUTD are uncommonly recognized. Vesicourachal diverticula are an exception to this generality as they have been diagnosed in as many as one of four cats with LUTD. They are worthy of further discussion.

VESICOURACHAL DIVERTICULA

Function and Dysfunction of the Urachus

The urachus is a fetal conduit that allows urine to pass from the developing urinary bladder to the placenta. It becomes nonfunctional at birth. Microscopic remnants of the fetal urachus characterized by microscopic lumens lined by transitional epithelium have been detected at the bladder vertex in healthy adult cats. In a study of 80 feline urinary bladders, more than 40 per cent had microscopic urachal diverticula.[14]

Microscopic remnants persisting in the urinary bladder vertex after birth are usually clinically silent but represent a risk factor for development of macroscopic diverticula of the urinary bladder in adult cats.[14] Abnormal and/or sustained increase of bladder intraluminal pressure associated with feline lower urinary tract disorders may cause enlargement and/or tearing of microscopic diverticula, leading to development of self-limiting macroscopic diverticula of varying size.

Congenital and Acquired Vesicourachal Diverticula

In our experience, radiographically detectable diverticula affecting the vertex of the urinary bladder wall occur in almost one of four adult cats with hematuria, dysuria, and/ or urethral obstruction.[14, 15] They occur twice as often in male (27 per cent) as female (14 per cent) cats without a breed predisposition. The mean age of affected cats at the time of diagnosis in our series was 3.7 years (range 1 to 11 years); clinical signs of LUTD were not observed when the cats were younger than 1 year. The higher frequency of occurrence of vesicourachal diverticula in males is probably related to the higher prevalence of urethral outflow obstruction in males.

There are two etiologically distinct forms of macroscopic vesicourachal diverticula. In cats with the more common form, microscopic remnants of the urachus located at the bladder vertex remain clinically silent until LUTD associated with increased bladder lumen pressure develops. Radiographically detectable acquired vesicourachal diverticula may develop at the bladder vertex as a result of enlargement of these microscopic vesicourachal remnants after onset of increased intraluminal pressure caused by acquired urethral obstruction and/or detrusor hyperactivity induced by inflammation (Fig. 175–7). This hypothesis is supported by the observation that many macroscopic diverticula in cats resolve within 2 to 3 weeks after amelioration of clinical signs of lower tract disease.[16]

Congenital macroscopic vesicourachal diverticula are the second, less common form. Although the exact sequence of events resulting in their formation has not been defined, they appear to be caused by disorders that cause abnormally high or sustained pressure in the bladder lumen. Congenital macroscopic vesicourachal diverticula are typically associated with signs of LUTD in immature cats. In our experience, they do not resolve spontaneously. Persistent congenital macroscopic diverticula predispose to bacterial UTIs. If infections are caused by urease-producing calculogenic microbes (especially staphylococci), infection-induced struvite uroliths often develop.

Diagnosis of Vesicourachal Diverticula

Feline vesicourachal diverticula are best identified by contrast cystography, although extramural diverticula may be identified at the time of celiotomy. Positive antegrade cystourethrography and retrograde positive-contrast urethrocystography are the procedures of choice (see Fig. 175–7). Double-contrast cystography or intravenous urography may also be utilized. Pneumocystography has not been as consistently reliable as positive-contrast cystography in our experience.

Treatment of Vesicourachal Diverticula

Urachal diverticula are an uncommon primary factor in development of feline LUTD. Most macroscopic diverticula

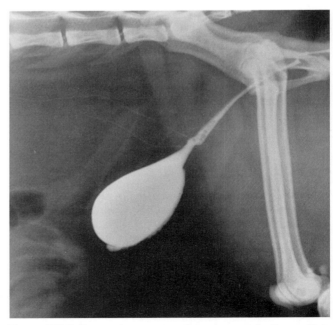

Figure 175–7. Retrograde contrast urethrocystogram of a 5-year-old domestic short-hair cat illustrating a vesicourachal diverticulum and uroliths in the proximal urethra. The urethroliths were flushed back into the bladder lumen. After dissolution of the uroliths with a protocol designed to dissolve sterile struvite, the diverticulum resolved.

of the bladder vertex are sequelae of lower urinary tract dysfunction. Furthermore, most macroscopic diverticula may be self-limiting if the urinary bladder and urethra return to a normal state of function.[3, 32] Acquired diverticula usually heal within 2 to 3 weeks after elimination of the underlying cause of increased intraluminal pressure.[16, 25]

DIAGNOSIS, THERAPY, AND PREVENTION OF METABOLIC ABNORMALITIES: UROLITHS AND URETHRAL PLUGS (see Tables 175–3 and 175–4)

TERMINOLOGY

There are physical and probable etiopathogenic differences between feline uroliths and urethral plugs. Therefore, these terms should not be used as synonyms.

Uroliths are polycrystalline concretions composed primarily of minerals (organic and inorganic crystalloids) and smaller quantities of matrix. Unlike urethral plugs, uroliths are not disorganized precipitates of crystalline material but consist of crystal aggregates with a complex internal structure.

Feline urethral plugs are commonly composed of large quantities of matrix mixed with minerals.[7] However, some urethral plugs are composed primarily of matrix; some consist of sloughed tissue, blood, and/or inflammatory reactants; and a few are composed primarily of aggregates of crystalline minerals. They may form a cast of the urethral lumen, implying rapid formation.

The mineral composition of uroliths and urethral plugs should be used to describe them because most therapeutic regimens have been based on their mineral composition. A variety of different minerals have been identified in uroliths (Table 175–5) and urethral plugs (Table 175–6) of cats.

TABLE 175–5. MINERAL COMPOSITION OF 20,343 FELINE UROLITHS EVALUATED BY QUANTITATIVE METHODS*,†

PREDOMINANT MINERAL TYPE	NUMBER OF UROLITHS	%
Magnesium ammonium phosphate 6H$_2$O	8621	42.4
Magnesium hydrogen phosphate 3H$_2$O	35	0.2
Magnesium phosphate hydrate	13	0.1
Calcium oxalate	9416	46.3
Calcium phosphate	122	0.6
Uric acid and urates	1136	5.6
Xanthine	11	0.1
Cystine	36	0.2
Silica	3	<0.1
Mixed‡	248	1.2
Compound§	487	2.4
Matrix	220	1.1
Urea	6	<0.1
Drug metabolite	2	<0.1
Total	20,343	100%

*Uroliths analyzed by polarizing light microscopy and x-ray diffraction methods.
†Uroliths composed of 70 to 100 per cent of mineral type listed; no nucleus and shell detected.
‡Uroliths did not contain at least 70 per cent of mineral type listed; no nucleus or shell detected.
§Uroliths contained an identifiable nucleus and one or more surrounding layers of a different mineral type.

TABLE 175–6. MINERAL COMPOSITION OF 1901 FELINE URETHRAL PLUGS ANALYZED BY QUANTITATIVE METHODS*,†

PREDOMINANT MINERAL TYPE	NUMBER OF UROLITHS	%
Magnesium ammonium phosphate 6H$_2$O	1493	78.5
Newberyite	12	0.6
Calcium oxalate	23	1.2
Calcium phosphate	24	1.3
Ammonium acid urate	8	0.4
Xanthine	1	<0.1
Sulfadiazine	1	<0.1
Mixed‡	49	2.6
Matrix	290	15.3
Total	1901	100

*Urethral plugs examined by polarizing light microscopy and x-ray diffraction methods.
†Urethral plugs composed of 70 to 99 per cent of mineral type listed; no nucleus and shell detected.
‡Urethral plugs did not contain at least 70 per cent of mineral type listed; no nucleus or shell detected.

EPIDEMIOLOGY OF UROLITHS AND URETHRAL PLUGS

Uroliths

As of mid-1998, the mineral composition of approximately 42 per cent of the naturally occurring uroliths submitted to the University of Minnesota by veterinarians in the United States and Canada was primarily struvite (see Table 175–5). The 42 per cent frequency of naturally occurring struvite uroliths observed in 1998 represents an 8 per cent decrease from 1995, an 18 per cent decrease from 1993, a 37 per cent decrease from 1989, and a 46 per cent decrease from 1984.[25, 33] In contrast, the frequency of feline uroliths composed of calcium oxalate rose from approximately 2 per cent in 1984 to 5.6 per cent in 1989, 27 per cent in 1993, 37 per cent in 1995, and approximately 46 per cent in 1998 (see Fig. 175–2).[25, 33]

Urethral Plugs

As of mid-1998, the mineral composition of approximately 79 per cent of the naturally occurring urethral plugs submitted to the University of Minnesota was primarily struvite (see Table 175–6). The 79 per cent frequency of naturally occurring struvite urethral plugs observed in 1998 represents approximately a 1 per cent increase in the series we reported in 1995, an 11 per cent decrease from 1989, and a 15 per cent decrease from 1984.[25, 33] Although the prevalence of calcium oxalate uroliths has been increasing, the prevalence of calcium oxalate in urethral plugs has always been low (see Figs. 175–2 and 175–3). Struvite has consistently remained the most common mineral in feline urethral plugs.

Clinical Significance

The decline in appearance of naturally occurring struvite uroliths and urethral plugs during the past decade associated with a reciprocal increase in calcium oxalate uroliths may be explained in part by (1) the widespread use of a calculolytic diet designed to dissolve struvite uroliths, (2) modification of maintenance and prevention diets to minimize struvite crystalluria, (3) inappropriate use of diets known to be

URO

effective in dissolving and preventing struvite uroliths and struvite crystalluria in attempt to manage other types of uroliths, and (4) inconsistent follow-up evaluation of the efficacy of dietary management protocols by urinalysis.

The explanation for why the prevalence of feline calcium oxalate uroliths is rising while the prevalence of calcium oxalate in feline urethral plugs is extremely low is not obvious, especially in light of the observation that male gender appears to be a risk factor for calcium oxalate uroliths and struvite urethral plugs. However, the high prevalence of struvite in urethral plugs is of clinical significance in terms of dietary strategies to prevent their formation. The frequency of urethral obstruction of male cats with struvite plugs appears to have been on the decline over the past two decades, in large part, in our opinion, because of widespread utilization of magnesium-restricted, acidifying diets. This has been associated with a dramatic decline in the frequency with which perineal urethrostomies have been performed and an associated decline in the undesirable sequelae of perineal urethrostomies (see Fig. 175–3). Data from 24 colleges of veterinary medicine in North America compiled by workers at the Veterinary Data Base, Purdue University, indicated that 2279 perineal urethrostomies were performed from 1980 to 1997, whereas approximately 12–18 urethrostomy cases per 1000 hospitalized cats per year were reported between 1980 and 1984; only approximately 3–4 cases per 1000 hospitalized cats per year were reported between 1990 and 1997.

RELATIONSHIP OF UROLITHS, URETHRAL PLUGS, AND ACRYSTALLURIC LOWER URINARY TRACT DISEASE: THE FRUIT JELL-O HYPOTHESIS

Most cases of feline LUTD characterized by hematuria, dysuria, pollakiuria, and/or urethral obstruction are related to various forms of noninfectious or infectious inflammation and/or urolithiasis. Various combinations of these two etiologic events may lead to three different but commonly recognized clinical manifestations (Fig. 175–8).[7, 25] Our hypothesis does not encompass all potential causes of feline LUTD (see Tables 175–3 and 175–4).

Acrystalluric Hematuria and Dysuria

Idiopathic inflammation and UTIs with viruses and occasionally bacteria or fungal pathogens lead to production of mucoprotein and inflammatory reactants and the clinical signs of hematuria and dysuria (see Fig. 175–8). Urethral obstruction is an uncommon clinical feature of this form of LUTD because a noncrystalline gel of mucoprotein and inflammatory reactants can usually be voided through the urethral lumen of female and male cats.

Urolithiasis

The initial step in formation of a urine crystal is formation of a crystal nidus (or crystal embryo). This phase of initiation of urolith formation, called nucleation, is dependent on supersaturation of urine with calculogenic crystalloids. The degree of urine supersaturation may be influenced by the magnitude of renal excretion of the crystalloid, urine pH, and/or factors that inhibit crystal formation or crystal aggregation. Noncrystalline proteinaceous matrix substances may also play a role in nucleation in some instances. Unlike urethral plugs, noncrystalline matrix constitutes only a small proportion of uroliths.

Further growth of the crystal nidus is dependent on its ability to remain in the lumen of the excretory pathway of the urinary system, the degree and duration of supersaturation of urine with crystalloids identical to or different from that in the nidus, and physical characteristics of the crystal nidus. If they are compatible with other crystalloids, epitaxial growth with different crystalloids may occur.

The presence of factors that promote crystal formation and growth in urine, in the absence of concomitant but unrelated idiopathic inflammation or infections characterized by production of large quantities of mucoprotein and inflammatory reactants, leads to formation of classical uroliths (see Fig. 175–8 and Table 175–9) In light of the fact that struvite, calcium oxalate, ammonium urate, cystine, and other types of uroliths contain only small quantities of matrix, it is unlikely that formation of large quantities of crystalline material stimulates production of matrix substances by tissues lining the lower urinary tract. Urolithiasis affect-

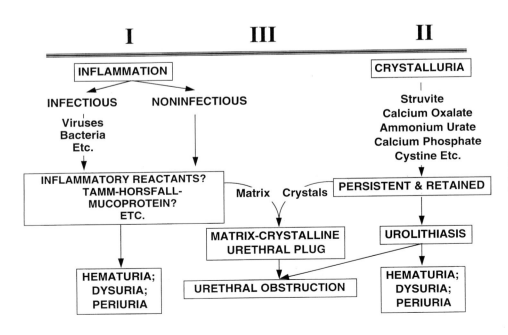

Figure 175–8. Illustration of different manifestations of feline lower urinary tract diseases associated with a single or interacting causes.

TABLE 175–7. BIOLOGIC BEHAVIOR OF FELINE UROLITHS

MINERAL TYPE	RATE OF FORMATION	RATE OF GROWTH	SIZE	NUMBER	FREQUENCY OF RECOGNITION (%)
Sterile struvite	Days to weeks	Rapid	Usually small	Single or multiple	40
Infection-induced struvite	Days to weeks	Rapid	Small to very large	Single or multiple	~2
Calcium oxalate	Months	Slow	Usually small	Often multiple	46
Calcium phosphate	Unknown	Slow	Usually small	Often multiple	0.6
Cystine	Months	Months	Usually small	Single or multiple	0.2
Urates	Unknown	Weeks to months	Usually small; some large	Single or multiple	6
Silica	Unknown (months?)	Unknown	Usually small	Single or multiple	Rare

ing the lower urinary tract is typically characterized by hematuria and dysuria. However, urethral obstruction may occur if small uroliths become lodged in the urethra.

Obstruction with Matrix-Crystalline Urethral Plugs

The concomitant occurrence of urinary tract inflammation (I) and persistent crystalluria (II) may lead to formation of matrix-crystalline plugs (III) that obstruct various portions of the urethra, especially of male cats (see Fig. 175–8). The same type of phenomenon is known to occur during formation of casts in renal tubular lumens. Tamm-Horsfall mucoprotein may form a gel in tubular lumens that traps intact cells (cellular casts), disintegrating cells (granular casts), or lipid droplets (fatty casts). This process of formation of matrix-crystalline urethral plugs could also be compared with the preparation of fruit Jell-O: the matrix (comparable to gelatin) traps various types of crystals (comparable to fruit). In addition to various types of crystals, the matrix may trap red cells, white cells, epithelial cells, bacteria, and cells containing viruses. This hypothesis provides a plausible explanation for the observed association of virus particles or bacteria in matrix-crystalline plugs containing crystals of different mineral compositions (see Table 175–6). Crystalluria per se is an unlikely cause of the production of large quantities of matrix because classic uroliths, which are composed of at least 90 to 95 per cent crystalline material, contain relatively little matrix.

UROLITHS

Biological Behavior of Uroliths

Detection of a urolith is not always justification for surgical management. In cats, small uroliths may remain asymptomatic within the urinary tract (especially the renal pelvis and urinary bladder) for months or years. However, the underlying cause(s) of uroliths and the sequelae of uroliths (partial or total obstruction, UTI) remain potential hazards. In situations in which uroliths are detected fortuitously in asymptomatic patients without significant bacteriuria, minimizing risk factors by medical management and monitoring urolith activity by appropriate procedures are an accepted alternative to surgery. If the uroliths remain inactive, therapy designed to dissolve or remove them is not mandatory. If the uroliths become active, appropriate medical and/or surgical therapy is recommended.

Rate of Formation

The rate of formation of uroliths varies from days to months, being influenced by mineral composition and a variety of risk factors (Table 175–7). Infection-induced struvite uroliths can grow quite rapidly.

When crystals of one mineral type form in urine, they may reduce the amount of lithogenic substances required for crystals of other mineral types to form. The principle involved is called heterogeneous nucleation (or "seeding"), and it operates in the same way as when foreign substances such as suture material or catheters predispose to formation of uroliths. Viewed in this context, a crystal of one mineral type serves as a risk factor for formation of crystals of other types and provides one explanation why macroscopic uroliths may contain more than mineral.

Movement of Uroliths

Small uroliths that form in the urinary bladder may pass into the urethra of male or female cats. Likewise, small renoliths may pass into the ureters. Because of the tendency of uroliths to change in size and position, radiographic evaluation of the urinary system should be repeated if there has been a significant time lapse between diagnosis and surgery scheduled to remove them.

Recurrence

In two retrospective studies of uroliths, recurrence rates of 19 and 37 per cent were reported.[33, 34] Unfortunately, the type of mineral in the recurrent uroliths was not specified. In our experience, sterile and infection-induced struvite uroliths have recurred within weeks to several months after elimination. Cystine urocystoliths also may recur within a few weeks to several months after removal. Calcium oxalate, calcium phosphate (brushite), and ammonium urate uroliths also have an unpredictable tendency to recur, typically within months (rather than weeks) after removal.

Pseudorecurrence

Because many feline uroliths are small, complete surgical removal of all uroliths may be difficult. In a retrospective clinical study at the University of Minnesota, uroliths were detected by radiographs taken within 14 days after cystotomies in 20 per cent of the patients.[35] We call this phenomenon pseudorecurrence. Results of this study emphasize the importance of postsurgical radiography to assess urolith status before evaluating recurrence and/or therapeutic efficacy.

Diagnosis of Uroliths

Physical Examination

Most uroliths in cats cannot be detected by abdominal palpation. For example, in one study of 30 urocystoliths in

URO

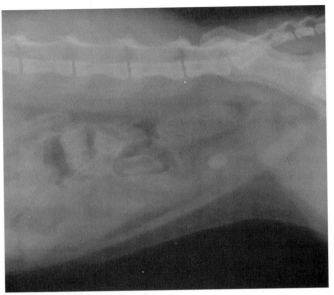

Figure 175–9. Survey radiograph or the lateral aspect of the abdomen of a 3-year-old spayed female domestic short-hair cat. Note the solitary radiodense urolith in the bladder lumen. Urinalysis revealed a pH of 6.5 and struvite crystalluria.

cats, stones were detected by palpation in only three patients.[36] Likewise, it is not possible to detect uroliths located in the renal pelves by palpation through the abdominal wall. Therefore, radiographic and/or ultrasonographic evaluation of the urinary tract is required to detect feline uroliths consistently (Tables 175–8 and 175–9).

Laboratory Findings

Abnormalities detected by urinalysis should lead to a high index of suspicion for urolithiasis and the probable mineral composition of uroliths. In the context of urolithiasis, evaluation of urine pH, crystalluria, specific gravity, and whether or not UTI is caused by urease-producing bacteria is of particular importance.

Cats with portovascular anomalies may have decreased concentrations of serum urea nitrogen, increased concentrations of serum uric acid and bile acids, and hyperammonemia.

In most cats with calcium oxalate and calcium phosphate uroliths, serum concentrations of minerals, including calcium, have been normal. However, mild hypercalcemia (11.1 to 13.5 mg/dL) has been observed with sufficient frequency in cats with calcium oxalate uroliths to warrant routine evaluation of serum total calcium concentration. Cats with calcium oxalate uroliths may have increased serum total carbon dioxide concentrations.

Radiography and Ultrasonography

Objectives. The primary objective of radiographic or ultrasonographic evaluation of patients suspected of having uroliths is to determine their location(s), number, density, and shape (Figs. 175–9 and 175–10; see Tables 175–8 and 175–9 and Fig. 175–7) and to detect predisposing abnormalities.

Size. The radiographic and ultrasonographic appearance of uroliths is influenced by their mineral composition, size, number, and location. Most uroliths larger than 3 mm have varying degrees of radiodensity and therefore can be detected by survey abdominal radiography. Uroliths larger than 1 mm can usually be detected by double-contrast cystography, provided excessive contrast medium is not used. Small uroliths (less than 3 mm) may not visualized by survey radiography. Detection of uroliths smaller than 3 mm by ultrasonography is dependent on the design of transducers and the skill of the ultrasonographer. Hyperechoic material presumed to be crystalline in nature may be detected by ultrasonography. The size and number of uroliths are not a reliable index of the probably efficacy of therapy.

Radiodensity. A diagnosis of radiodense or radiolucent stones should be based on their radiodensity compared with soft tissues and not their radiodensity compared with positive contrast material. Uroliths composed primarily of calcium oxalate, calcium phosphate, magnesium ammonium phosphate, cystine, and silica are typically more radiodense than ammonium urate uroliths (see Table 175–9 and Fig. 175–9).

TABLE 175–8. ADVANTAGES AND DISADVANTAGES OF SURVEY RADIOGRAPHS, DOUBLE-CONTRAST CYSTOGRAPHS, AND ULTRASONOGRAPHY IN ASSESSING UROLITHS

PURPOSE	SURVEY RADIOGRAPHS	DOUBLE-CONTRAST CYSTOGRAPHY	ULTRASONOGRAPHY
Assessment of urethroliths	Yes if radiodense	Indirectly during transurethral catheterization	Poor
Assessment of radiolucent urocystoliths	Unreliable	Yes	Yes
Distinguish blood clot from urocystolith	No	Probably	Yes
Assessment of laminated urocystolith	Best of the three methods	Probably	No
Assessment of other bladder disorders	Unreliable	Yes	Sometimes
Assessment of urocystolith number	Yes (>3 mm)	Yes (>1 mm)	Equipment and observer dependent
Assessment of urocystolith size	Yes (>3 mm)	Yes (>1 mm)	Equipment and observer dependent
Assessment of urocystolith density	Yes (>3 mm)	No	No
Assessment of urocystolith shape	Yes (>3 mm)	Yes (>1 mm)	No (air artifacts)
Immediate postsurgical assessment for uroliths	Yes	Not recommended, risk of iatrogenic UTI	
Risk of air artifact in bladder	No	Yes	No
Risk of iatrogenic bacterial UTI	No	Yes	No
Exposed to ionizing radiation	Yes	Yes	No
Necessity to remove hair	No	No	Often
Our overall choice	Screening	Investigation	Third choice

UTI = urinary tract infection.

TABLE 175-9. "GUESSTIMATING" MINERAL COMPOSITION OF FELINE UROLITHS

MINERAL TYPE	PREDICTORS								
	Urine pH	Crystal Appearance	Urine Culture	Radiographic Density	Radiographic Contour	Serum Abnormalities	Breed Predisposition	Gender Predisposition	Common Ages
Sterile struvite	6.5 to >7.5	Three- to eight-sided colorless prisms	Sterile	+ to + +	Round, sometimes disk shaped	None	None	Female > male	Average 7 years; range 3 months to 22 years
Infection-induced magnesium ammonium phosphate	Neutral to alkaline	Three- to eight-sided colorless prisms	Urease-producing bacteria (*Staphylococcus, Proteus*)	+ to + + (sometimes laminated)	Smooth, round, or faceted; May assume shape of renal pelvis, ureter, bladder, or urethra	None	None	None	Any age
Calcium oxalate	Acid to neutral	Dihydrate salt = colorless envelope or octahedral shape. Monohydrate salt = spindles or dumbbell shape	Negative	+ + + +	Rough or spiculated (dihydrate salt). Small smooth, round (monohydrate salt). Sometimes jackstone	Usually normocalcemic, occasionally hypercalcemic	Burmese, Himalayan, Persian	Males > females	Average 7 years; range 3 months to 22 years
Purines including urates	Acid to neutral	Yellow-brown spherical or thornapple shapes (NH_4^+ urate)	Negative	0 to +	Smooth, (occasionally irregular) round or oval; ± jackstone	Low urea nitrogen in cats with portal-systemic shunts	None	Males = females	Average 6 years; range 5 months to 15 years
Calcium phosphate	Alkaline to neutral (brushite forms in acid urine)	Amorphous or long thin prisms	Negative	+ + + +	Smooth or irregular; round or faceted	Occasional hypercalcemia	None	Females > males	Average 8 years; range 5 months to 19 years
Cystine	Acid to neutral	Flat, colorless hexagonal plates	Negative	+ +	Smooth, (occasionally irregular; round to oval	None	None	Males = females	Average 4 years; range 4 months to 12 years

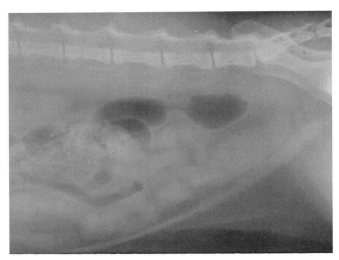

Figure 175–10. Survey radiograph of the lateral aspect of the abdomen of the cat in Figure 175–9 obtained approximately 1 month after initiation of medical therapy to induce sterile struvite urolith dissolution. There are no radiodense uroliths in the urinary tract.

Ammonium urate uroliths are often radiolucent, but some containing other mineral types are somewhat radiodense. Because of significant variation, the radiodensity of uroliths is not itself a reliable index of mineral composition.

Uroliths larger than 3 mm are not commonly radiolucent, except for uroliths composed of 100 per cent ammonium or sodium urate, or uric acid. Many ammonium urate uroliths are marginally radiodense. This may be related to a variable but minor quantity of phosphates and other radiodense minerals in urate uroliths.

Pure matrix uroliths are radiolucent. Blood clots are also radiolucent and may be mistaken for radiolucent uroliths. Radiolucent uroliths may be readily distinguished from blood clots when evaluated by two-dimensional gray-scale ultrasonography. Uroliths are usually in the dependent portion of the bladder lumen, produce sharply marginated shadows containing few echoes, and are associated with acoustic shadowing. Blood clots may be located anywhere in the bladder lumen, typically have an irregular outline and indistinct margins, and are not associated with acoustic shadowing.

Uroliths that appear radiodense on survey radiography may appear to be radiolucent when evaluated by properly performed double-contrast radiography (see Fig. 175–7). This is related to the fact that many uroliths are more radiodense than body tissue but less radiodense than the contrast material.

Determination of Urolith Composition

Knowledge of urolith composition is important because contemporary methods of detection, treatment, and prevention of the underlying causes of urolithiasis are based primarily on knowledge of urolith composition. To promote dissolution of uroliths, we use a protocol that facilitates "guesstimation" of urolith composition (see Table 175–9).

Uroliths may also be retrieved from the urinary bladder without surgical intervention by catching them in an aquarium fishnet placed in the urine stream when the patient is voiding, by collecting them with the aid of a transurethral catheter,[37] or by voiding urohydropropulsion.[38] Stone dissolution or preventive protocols based on quantitative mineral analyses of uroliths typically provide the most consistent therapeutic results.

Although specific mineral types of uroliths often have characteristic shapes, colors, and surface characteristics, the overlap in gross appearance between stones of different mineral types and the fact that some stones contain more than one mineral preclude a specific diagnosis of mineral type on the basis of gross morphologic characteristics of uroliths.

Ammonium Urate Uroliths

Epidemiology

Ammonium urate and uric acid (collectively called purines) constituted approximately 6 per cent of the total (see Table 175–5) of all stones studied. The urinary bladder was the most common site of purine uroliths (88 per cent); the urethra (8 per cent), bladder and urethra (4 per cent), kidneys (less than 1 per cent), and ureters (less than 1 per cent) were less common sites. Males are affected as often as females; the mean age of affected cats was 6.1 ± 3.1 years (range 5 months to 15 years).

Etiopathogenesis

There have been isolated case reports of uric acid and ammonium urate uroliths in cats during the past 20 years.[25] Although portovascular anomalies associated with hyperammonemia and hyperuricemia have been confirmed as the underlying cause in a few cases, the cause(s) of formation of most feline urate uroliths has not been established.[39] We have not been able to determine precisely the cause(s) of feline urate uroliths in our stone series. This problem has been compounded by the difficulty of reproducibly measuring the uric acid concentration in serum and urine by methods commonly used in clinical laboratories. However, formation of ammonium urate uroliths is likely to be associated with several risk factors (Table 175–10).

We have encountered xanthine uroliths in the bladders of 11 cats that were not given allopurinol. One patient was a 15-month-old neutered male domestic long-hair cat. A urolith surgically removed from the urinary bladder was composed of 95 per cent xanthine and 5 per cent uric acid. Another patient was a 9-month-old neutered male domestic short-hair cat with uroliths in the bladder and the urethra. Many crystals resembling uric acid were observed in the urine sediment. Evaluation of a hemogram and serum biochemical profile revealed no abnormalities. Quantitative analysis revealed that the uroliths were composed of 100 per cent xanthine. Evaluation of a urine sample by high-performance liquid chromatography revealed that the uric acid concentration was 3.4 mg/dL and the xanthine concentration 54 mg/dL.

Treatment and Prevention

Medical protocols that consistently promote dissolution of ammonium urate uroliths in cats have not yet been developed. Urocystoliths small enough to pass through the urethra may be removed with the aid of a urinary catheter or by voiding urohydropropulsion.[37, 38] Surgery remains the most reliable method for removing larger, inactive uroliths from the urinary tract.

We induced dissolution of an ammonium urate urocystolith affecting a 3-year-old male castrated domestic short-hair cat with a combination of allopurinol (14 mg/lb/day divided into two equal subdoses) and a diet relatively low

TABLE 175–10. POTENTIAL RISK FACTORS ASSOCIATED WITH AMMONIUM URATE UROLITHIASIS

RISK FACTOR	ETIOPATHOLOGIC DISORDER	PATHOPHYSIOLOGIC MECHANISM
Hyperuricosuria	Hepatic portal vascular anomaly and other forms of hepatic failure	Reduces availability and/or function of hepatic urate oxidase and thereby minimizes conversion of uric acid to allantoin, which is more water soluble
Hyperuricosuria	Excess dietary purine	Promotes hyperuricemia and hyperuricosuria
Hyperuricosuria	Increased nucleic acid breakdown (e.g., lymphoma, leukemia, diffuse tissue destruction)	Results in accelerated metabolism of purines, which are further metabolized to uric acid
Hyperammonuria	Excess dietary protein	Provides additional urea for metabolism to NH_3 and glutamine for conversion to NH_4^+
Hyperammonuria	Metabolic acidosis	Promotes metabolism of glutamine to NH_4^+
Hyperammonuria	Aciduria	Ionizes NH_3 that has diffused into renal tubule lumens; trapped NH_4^+ subsequently excreted
Hyperammonuria	Hypokalemia	Produces intracellular acidosis and subsequent NH_4^+ excretion
Hyperammonuria	Urinary tract infection by microorganisms that produce urease	Promotes conversion of urea in urine to NH_3 and NH_4^+
Aciduria	Acidosis	Decreases solubility of urine uric acid
Decreased urine volume	Intravascular volume depletion	Conservation of water promotes increased urine concentration and urine supersaturation of uric acid. Urine retention provides additional time for crystal nucleation and growth.

in purine precursors. Although allopurinol may be considered to reduce formation of uric acid, additional studies of the efficacy and potential toxicity of allopurinol in cats are required before meaningful generalities are established. Of particular concern is the potential for inducing xanthine uroliths.

Prevention should encompass consumption of diets that are low in purine precursors (e.g., low in liver) and promote formation of less acid urine (pH 7) that is not highly concentrated.

Calcium Oxalate Uroliths

Epidemiology

In our latest series, calcium oxalate uroliths constituted approximately 46 per cent of the total (see Table 175–5). Although calcium oxalate uroliths were located primarily in the urinary bladder (72 per cent), they were also found in various combinations in the kidneys, ureters, and urethra. Four per cent of the calcium oxalate uroliths were voided.

Nephroliths make up approximately 3 per cent of the feline urolith submissions to the Minnesota Urolith Center. Approximately 45 per cent of the nephroliths were composed of calcium oxalate and less than 5 per cent of struvite. Approximately 15 per cent were composed of calcium phosphate.

In our series, male cats (57 per cent) were affected more than females (43 per cent). The mean age of affected cats was 7.3 ± 3.4 years (range 3 months to 23 years) and there was a higher prevalence of calcium oxalate uroliths in Burmese, Himalayan, and Persian breeds.[40, 41]

Etiopathogenesis

Serum Analytes. In most cats with calcium oxalate uroliths, serum concentrations of minerals, including calcium, have been normal. The sequence or sequences of events that promote initiation and growth of calcium oxalate uroliths in normocalcemic cats have not been defined. However, epidemiologic studies have identified several probable risk factors (Table 175–11).

URO

TABLE 175–11. RISK FACTORS ASSOCIATED WITH CALCIUM OXALATE UROLITHIASIS

RISK FACTOR	ETIOPATHOLOGIC DISORDER	PATHOPHYSIOLOGIC MECHANISM
Hypercalciuria	Excess dietary calcium	Results in increased renal clearance of calcium and hypercalciuria
Hypercalciuria	Excess dietary sodium	Enhances renal excretion of calcium
Hypercalciuria	Hypercalcemia	Results in increased renal clearance of calcium and hypercalciuria
Hypercalciuria	Excess vitamin D	Augments intestinal calcium absorption and by suppressing parathyroid hormone promotes calcium excretion
Hypercalciuria	Acidosis	Promotes skeletal mobilization of calcium and inhibits renal tubular reabsorption of calcium
Hypercalciuria	Hypophosphatemia (e.g., hyperparathyroidism)	Stimulates vitamin D production, which augments intestinal calcium absorption
Hyperoxaluria	Excess dietary oxalate	Results in increased renal clearance of oxalate and hyperoxaluria
Hyperoxaluria	Excess vitamin C	Serves as a precursor for oxalate production
Hyperoxaluria	Pyridoxine deficiency	Promotes increased endogenous production of oxalate
Hyperoxaluria	Primary hyperoxaluria	Results in increased endogenous production of oxalate
Hypocitraturia	Idiopathic	Increases urine concentration of calcium ions available to bind with oxalate
Hypocitraturia	Acidemia (e.g., renal tubular acidosis)	Promotes renal tubular utilization of citrate and reduced excretion of citrate
Decreased macromolecular inhibitors?	Inherited disorder?	Minimizes production of glycoproteins capable of inhibiting calcium oxalate crystal growth and aggregation
Decreased urine volume	Intravascular volume depletion	Conservation of water promotes increased urine concentration and urine supersaturation of calcium oxalate. Urine retention provides additional time for crystal nucleation and growth.

Mild hypercalcemia (11.1 to 13.5 mg/dL) has been observed with sufficient frequency to warrant routine evaluation of the serum total calcium concentration in affected patients. Hypercalcemia promotes urinary calcium excretion and may result in precipitation of calcium oxalate crystals. Although primary hyperparathyroidism has been recognized as a cause of hypercalcemia and calcium oxalate uroliths in cats, the underlying cause of hypercalcemia in most cats with calcium oxalate uroliths has not been detected. If hypercalcemia is confirmed in serially obtained serum samples, serum ionized calcium, parathormone, and vitamin D concentrations should be evaluated.

Acidemia and Aciduria. Cats with calcium oxalate urolithiasis typically have acidic urine (urine pH 6.3 to 6.7). Pretreatment blood pH and total carbon dioxide concentration are often reduced (pH 7.3). However, the solubility of calcium oxalate crystals is apparently not directly influenced by urine pH within the physiologic range. The indirect association between aciduria, acidemia, and calcium oxalate urolithiasis may be that acidemia promotes mobilization of carbonate and phosphorus from bones to buffer hydrogen ions. Concomitant mobilization of bone calcium may result in hypercalciuria. Hypercalciuria in turn is a risk factor for calcium oxalate crystals. Results of epidemiologic studies support this association inasmuch as cats with calcium oxalate uroliths were three times more likely then hospitalized cats to have been fed diets that promote urine pH values less than 6.3.[40]

Hyperoxaluria. Primary hyperoxaluria (L-glyceric aciduria) has been encountered in related cats with deficient quantities of hepatic d-glycerate dehydrogenase, an enzyme required for metabolism of oxalic acid precursors.[42] This disorder has been reported to be inherited as an autosomal recessive trait. To date, the clinical manifestations of this metabolic disorder have been primarily related to progressive weakness and acute onset of renal failure in immature (about 4 to 9 months of age) cats. Although the kidneys of affected cats contain birefringent crystals, an association between feline primary hyperoxaluria and calcium oxalate urolithiasis has apparently not yet been reported.

Diet-Related Factors. *Dietary protein* may be a risk factor in calcium oxalate urolithiasis. Consumption of animal protein increases urinary calcium excretion and decreases urinary citric acid excretion (citric acid chelates calcium to form a soluble salt of calcium citrate). One mechanism for protein-mediated hypercalciuria is increased endogenous acid production and thus increased urinary acid excretion. Acidifying metabolites are neutralized by phosphate and carbonate mobilized from bone. Calcium released from bone along with phosphate and carbonate results in hypercalciuria. Increased urine acid excretion is also thought to decrease calcium reabsorption in the distal nephron and increase urine citric acid uptake in the proximal nephron. Dietary protein may also promote hypercalciuria by increasing the glomerular filtration rate.

The interrelationship between dietary calcium, oxalic acid, and phosphorus may also play a role in calcium oxalate urolithiasis. Intestinal hyperabsorption of dietary calcium is recognized as a common cause of hypercalciuria and calcium oxalate urolithiasis in humans. Our observations indicate that excessive gastrointestinal absorption of calcium is an important cause of sustained hypercalciuria in dogs with calcium oxalate urolithiasis.[43] Hence, it may seem logical to restrict dietary calcium to minimize calcium oxalate urolith formation. However, results of studies suggest that dietary calcium restriction increases the risk of calcium oxalate uroliths.

An important relationship exists between gastrointestinal absorption of oxalic acid and calcium. Dietary calcium and oxalic acid form complexes of nonabsorbable calcium oxalate in the intestinal lumen. However, if dietary calcium is reduced without a concomitant reduction in oxalic acid, intestinal absorption of oxalic acid from the intestine followed by increased urinary excretion may occur. Hyperoxaluria is a greater risk factor for calcium oxalate urolith formation than an equivalent increase in urinary calcium concentration because smaller increments of oxalic acid are required for formation of insoluble calcium oxalate. This may explain why humans consuming diets with reduced levels of calcium are at greater risk for calcium oxalate urolith formation than those consuming diets with a higher calcium content.[44] In contrast, consumption of calcium supplements between meals would not alter dietary oxalic acid absorption. In this situation, dietary calcium supplements result in increased absorption and excretion of calcium in urine because it is not bound to intestinal oxalic acid. Thus, oral calcium supplements are a risk factor for calcium oxalate urolith formation.

Dietary phosphorus may also play a role in calcium oxalate urolithiasis. In humans, neutral potassium phosphate lowers urinary calcium excretion. The ability of phosphorus to reduce calcium oxalate urolith recurrence is often attributed to its role in minimizing renal production of calcitriol and enhancing urinary excretion of pyrophosphate, an inhibitor of calcium oxalate salts. Diets deficient in phosphorus may stimulate calcitriol production, which promotes intestinal absorption of both calcium and phosphorus. Therefore, diets designed to minimize calcium oxalate urolith formation should not be designed to restrict phosphorus. Diets deficient in phosphorus may also increase the availability of absorbable calcium in the intestine. Whether dietary phosphorus supplements would minimize calcium oxalate urolith formation in dogs awaits further study.

Dietary oxalic acid may play a role in calcium oxalate urolithiasis. The effect of dietary sources of oxalic acid on naturally occurring feline calcium oxalate uroliths has not been evaluated by controlled studies. Although hyperoxaluria and nephrocalcinosis have been observed in kittens that consumed diets deficient in vitamin B_6, a naturally occurring form of this syndrome has not been observed.[45] Urinary oxalic acid excretion in kittens that consumed diets oversupplemented with vitamin B_6 was similar to that in kittens consuming diets with adequate vitamin B_6.

Dietary potassium may play a role in calcium oxalate urolithiasis. Results of epidemiologic studies of humans, dogs, and cats indicate that diets higher in potassium are less frequently associated with calcium oxalate urolith formation.[46]

Dietary magnesium may play a role in calcium oxalate urolithiasis. It is noteworthy that magnesium has been reported to be a calcium oxalate inhibitor in rats and humans.[8] For this reason, orally administered magnesium is sometimes recommended to prevent recurrence of human calcium oxalate uroliths. The value of supplemental magnesium in cats with calcium oxalate uroliths is unclear.

Urine Concentration and Volume. Diuresis associated with increased fluid intake has been associated with decreased risk of calcium oxalate urolithiasis in people. Likewise, cats consuming canned diets had one third the risk for calcium oxalate urolith formation of cats consuming other dietary formulations. Increased urine volume could minimize formation of uroliths by reducing the concentration of calculogenic substances in urine and by promoting elimination of crystals before they can become large enough to cause clinical disease. Total water consumption is often less in cats fed low-moisture diets, resulting in formation of a lower volume of highly concentrated urine. In addition to the water content of diets, total water consumption and urine concentration and volume may be related to the palatability and caloric density of the diet, fecal water loss in undigested food, and the availability of drinking water.

Inhibitors of Crystal Growth and Aggregation. Nephrocalcin, a glycoprotein identified in human urine that inhibits calcium oxalate crystal growth, has been reported to be defective in urolith-forming humans.[46] Nephrocalcin has also been isolated from eight other vertebrate species, including the dog.[46]

The mechanisms by which nephrocalcin inhibits crystal growth are not completely understood. However, nephrocalcin's hydrophilic and hydrophobic (amphiphilic) nature and film-forming capabilities are probably important factors. It is currently thought that the hydrophilic or charged portion of nephrocalcin becomes anchored to the surface of calcium oxalate crystals, forming a stable two-dimensional film that covers the crystal. In contrast, the hydrophobic portion of nephrocalcin is exposed to urine. Because the hydrophobic portion of nephrocalcin has relatively few charged sites, fewer calculogenic ions in urine can attach to existing calcium oxalate crystals. As a consequence, they have a reduced opportunity to grow or aggregate.

Treatment and Prevention

Overview. Medical protocols that promote dissolution of calcium oxalate uroliths in cats are not yet available. Urocystoliths small enough to pass through the urethra may be removed by voiding urohydropropulsion.[38] Surgery is the only practical alternative for removal of larger active calcium oxalate uroliths. However, some calcium oxalate uroliths, especially those located in the kidneys, may remain clinically silent for months to years. Because of the unavoidable destruction of nephrons during nephrotomy, this procedure is not recommended unless it can be established that the stones are a cause of clinically significant disease. Serially performed urinalyses, renal function tests, serum electrolyte evaluations, and/or radiographic studies are indicated to evaluate the clinical activity of calcium oxalate uroliths.

After urolith removal, medical protocols should be considered to minimize urolith recurrence or to prevent further growth of uroliths remaining in the urinary tract. In general, medical therapy should be formulated in a stepwise fashion, with the initial goal of reducing the urine concentration of calculogenic substances. Medications that have the potential to induce a sustained alteration in body composition of metabolites, in addition to urine concentration of metabolites, should be reserved for patients with active or frequently recurrent calcium oxalate uroliths. Caution must be used so that the side effects of treatment are not more detrimental than the effects of uroliths.

In cats with hypercalcemia, the cause of hypercalcemia (e.g., primary hyperparathyroidism) should be corrected. Whether calcium oxalate uroliths remaining in the patient after appropriate therapy subsequently dissolve is unknown; however, calcium oxalate urolith growth or recurrence is less likely. For patients with normal serum calcium concentrations, the plan should be to identify risk factors for urolith formation (see Table 175–11). Amelioration or control of

the consequences of risk factors should minimize urolith growth and recurrence.

Dietary Considerations. The goals of dietary prevention include (1) reducing calcium concentration in urine, (2) reducing oxalic acid concentration in urine, (3) promoting high concentration and activity of inhibitors of calcium oxalate crystal growth and aggregation in urine, and (4) maintaining a high volume of unconcentrated urine.

What about dietary levels of calcium and oxalic acid? Although reduction of urine calcium and oxalic acid concentrations by reduction of dietary calcium and oxalic acid appears to be a logical therapeutic goal, it is not necessarily a harmless maneuver. Reducing consumption of only one of these constituents (such as calcium) may increase the availability of the other (such as oxalic acid) for intestinal absorption and subsequent urinary excretion. The general consensus of opinion is that restricting dietary calcium is inadvisable unless absorptive hypercalciuria has been documented. Even then, modification of dietary calcium should be accompanied by an appropriate modification of dietary oxalic acid and phosphorus.

What about dietary levels of sodium? Consumption of high levels of sodium may augment renal excretion of calcium. The 24-hour urinary calcium excretion of normal dogs consuming diets with 0.8 percent sodium (dry weight analysis) was comparable to that of dogs with naturally occurring calcium oxalate uroliths.[46] If results are similar in cats, moderate dietary restriction of sodium would be a logical recommendation for active calcium oxalate urolith formers. Oral administration of sodium chloride to induce polyuria and compensatory polydipsia is not recommended.

What about dietary levels of phosphorus? Dietary phosphorus should not be restricted in patients with calcium oxalate urolithiasis because reduction of dietary phosphorus may be associated with activation of vitamin D, which promotes intestinal calcium absorption and subsequent urinary calcium excretion. In addition, pyrophosphate is an inhibitor of calcium oxalate urolith formation. If calcium oxalate urolithiasis is associated with hypophosphatemia and normal serum calcium concentration, oral phosphorus supplementation may be considered. Caution must be used, however, because excessive dietary phosphorus may predispose to formation of calcium phosphate uroliths.

What about dietary levels of magnesium? Increased urine magnesium concentration reduces formation of calcium oxalate crystals in vitro.[47] For this reason, supplemental magnesium has been used to minimize recurrence of calcium oxalate uroliths in humans. However, supplemental dietary magnesium may contribute to formation of magnesium ammonium phosphate uroliths and hypercalciuria. Pending further studies, we do *not* recommend dietary magnesium restriction or supplementation for treatment of calcium oxalate uroliths in cats.

What about dietary levels of protein? Ingestion of foods that contain high quantities of animal protein may contribute to calcium oxalate urolithiasis by increasing urinary calcium and oxalic acid excretion and by decreasing urinary citric acid excretion. Some of these are consequences of obligatory acid excretion associated with protein metabolism.

What about dietary levels of water? The relationship of water content in the diet and formation of uroliths has also been studied in cats by several investigators. Factors involved include dietary moisture, drinking behavior, digestibility of food and its relationship to fecal water loss, and the quantity of sodium chloride in the diet. Because of numerous variables, a cause-and-effect relationship between

URO

dietary moisture, urine volume, and urolithiasis has not been clearly established. Pending further studies, it is logical to recommend consideration of highly digestible, high-moisture diets to minimize recurrence of uroliths.

How should diets be formulated to minimize risk factors for calcium oxalate urolithiasis effectively and safely? For several years, feline diets specifically designed to minimize dietary risk factors for calcium oxalate were unavailable. Therefore, diets designed for management of feline renal failure were recommended to minimize recurrence of calcium oxalate uroliths because they contained reduced quantities of protein and sodium and were formulated to minimize acidosis. However, because they contained reduced quantities of phosphorus and the high-normal range of vitamin D, they were not ideal for management of calcium oxalate urolithiasis.

With contemporary knowledge, diets that minimize calcium oxalate urolithiasis should be formulated to minimize acidosis and should not contain excessive oxalic acid precursors. Likewise, excessive levels of vitamin D (which promote intestinal absorption of calcium) and ascorbic acid (a precursor of oxalate) should be avoided. Diets should contain adequate, but not excessive, quantities of calcium, phosphorus, magnesium, and potassium. The diet should be adequately fortified with vitamin B_6 because vitamin B_6 deficiency promotes endogenous production and subsequent urinary excretion of oxalic acid. Canned diets are preferred to dry formulations to enhance formation of less concentrated urine and to promote increased micturition.

Several diets have been specifically formulated to minimize calcium oxalate urolith recurrence in cats (Prescription Diet Feline c/d-o, Hills Pet Products; Nutritional Urinary Formula Moderate pH/0, Iams Company; Waltham Feline S/0, Waltham; Select Care Feline Modified Formula, Innovative Veterinary Diets). One diet that incorporates many of these features is Prescription Diet c/d-o. To our knowledge, it is the only diet whose manufacturer utilized activity product ratios to verify its ability to promote formation of urine that is undersaturated in calcium oxalate.

Supplemental Citrate. Citric acid inhibits calcium oxalate crystal formation because of its ability to form soluble salts with calcium. This may explain why some humans with abnormally low quantities of urinary citric acid are at risk for development of calcium oxalate uroliths.[47] Oral administration of potassium citrate (approximately 40 mg/lb/day) to human patients has been associated with marked increases in urinary citric acid excretion.[47] Potassium citrate may also be beneficial in the management of calcium oxalate because of its alkalinizing effects. In dogs, chronic metabolic acidosis inhibits renal tubular reabsorption of calcium, whereas metabolic alkalosis enhances tubular reabsorption of calcium.[47] Potassium citrate (Urocit-K) is preferred to sodium bicarbonate as an alkalinizing agent because oral administration of sodium may enhance urinary calcium excretion. We currently recommend a dose of 36 to 50 mg/lb/day (divided into two or three subdoses). The dosage may be titrated by monitoring urine pH with the objective of obtaining values of 7.0 to 7.5.

Supplemental Vitamin B_6. Vitamin B_6 increases the transamination of glyoxylate, an important precursor of oxalic acid, to glycine. Although additional vitamin B_6 was associated with decreased oxalic acid excretion in cats consuming diets deficient in vitamin B_6, the ability of supplemental vitamin B_6 to reduce urinary oxalic acid excretion in cats with calcium oxalate uroliths consuming diets with adequate quantities of vitamin B_6 is unknown. In our hospi-

tal, administration of vitamin B_6 (4.5 mg/lb/day) to a normal cat for 10 days was not associated with decreased urine oxalic acid concentration (1.1 ± 0.1 mmol/L before vitamin B_6 supplementation compared with 1.4 ± 0.2 mmol/L during vitamin B_6 administration).[47]

Thiazide Diuretics. Thiazide diuretics have been recommended to reduce recurrence of calcium-containing uroliths in humans because of their ability to reduce urinary calcium excretion. It has been hypothesized that thiazide diuretics promote mild extracellular volume contraction and thereby promote proximal tubular reabsorption of several solutes, including sodium and calcium.[47]

Although hydrochlorthiazide diuretics may be beneficial in minimizing urinary calcium excretion in humans and dogs (1 to 2 mg/lb by mouth every 12 hours), no data have been provided to indicate their efficacy in cats with calcium oxalate uroliths. Because thiazide diuretic administration can be associated with adverse affects (dehydration, hyopkalemia, hypercalcemia), we cannot yet recommend their routine use pending further evaluation.

Calcium Phosphate Uroliths

Epidemiology

In our current series, calcium phosphate accounted for approximately 1 per cent of the naturally occurring feline uroliths (see Table 175–5) located in the kidneys (32 per cent), ureters (6 per cent), urinary bladder (51 per cent), urethra and bladder (6 per cent), and urethra (2 per cent). Four per cent of calcium phosphate uroliths were voided. Calcium phosphate uroliths occurred more commonly in females (57 per cent) than males (43 per cent). The mean age of affected cats was 8 ± 5 years (range 5 months to 19 years).

Etiopathogenesis

Several risk factors may be associated with calcium phosphate uroliths (Table 175–12). Calcium phosphate uroliths may occur in association with primary hyperparathyroidism in humans and dogs, and this association has also been made in cats.[8]

We have documented nephroliths composed of blood clots mineralized with calcium phosphate. Such mineralized blood clots may be found in renal pelvic diverticula in addition to the renal pelvis and less commonly in the lower urinary tract. Formation of highly concentrated urine in patients with gross hematuria may favor formation of blood clots. In one persistently hematuric patient, such nephroliths remained inactive (did not increase in number or size, cause outflow obstruction, or predispose to bacterial urinary tract infection) over a 3-year period of evaluation.

Treatment and Prevention

Voiding urohydropropulsion may be utilized to remove small calcium phosphate urocystoliths. Surgery remains the most reliable way to remove larger active calcium phosphate uroliths from the urinary tract. However it may be unnecessary for clinically inactive calcium phosphate uroliths.

Patients should be periodically monitored by urinalysis, appropriate radiographic procedures, and, if indicated, laboratory tests on blood and urine. If recurrent urocystoliths are detected when they are small, they may be nonsurgically removed by voiding urohydropropulsion or by aspiration through a urinary catheter.[37, 38] Medical therapy of patients

TABLE 175–12. POTENTIAL RISK FACTORS ASSOCIATED WITH CALCIUM PHOSPHATE UROLITHIASIS

RISK FACTOR	ETIOPATHOLOGIC DISORDER	PATHOPHYSIOLOGIC MECHANISM
Hypercalciuria	Hypercalcemia	Results in increased renal clearance of calcium and hypercalciuria
Hypercalciuria	Excess vitamin D	Augments intestinal calcium absorption and by suppressing parathyroid hormone promotes calcium excretion
Hypercalciuria	Hypophosphatemia (e.g., hyperparathyroidism)	Stimulates vitamin D production, which augments intestinal calcium absorption
Hypercalciuria	Acidosis	Promotes skeletal mobilization of calcium and inhibits renal tubular reabsorption of calcium
Hypercalciuria	Excess dietary calcium	Results in increased renal clearance of calcium and hypercalciuria
Hypercalciuria	Excess dietary sodium	Enhances renal excretion of calcium
Hyperphosphaturia	Excess dietary phosphorus	Results in increased renal clearance of phosphorus and hyperphosphaturia
Alkaline urine	Alkaline urine	Increases urine concentration and saturation of PO_3^{-} by removing hydrogen ions from $H_2PO_4^{-}$ and HPO_4^{2-}
Alkaline urine	Alkaline urine	Reduces solubility of calcium phosphates, except brushite
Decreased urine volume	Intravascular volume depletion	Conservation of water promotes increased urine concentration and increased urine supersaturation of calcium phosphate. Urine retention provides additional time for crystal nucleation and growth.

with recurring calcium phosphate uroliths should then be directed at removing or minimizing risk factors that contribute to supersaturation of urine with calcium phosphate.

If the patient is hypercalcemic, the underlying cause of the hypercalcemia should be identified and eliminated or controlled. Several different medical protocols have been reported to be of value in humans with normocalcemic hypercalciuria. Unfortunately, there has been little clinical experience of use of drugs in dogs and cats with calcium phosphate uroliths. However, medications that can enhance calcium excretion such as glucocorticoids or furosemide and those containing large quantities of sodium should be avoided if possible.

Diets designed to avoid excessive protein, sodium, calcium, and vitamin D may be of benefit. Excessive restriction or supplementation of dietary phosphorus should probably be avoided. Enhancement of urine volume by feeding a canned diet and encouraging water consumption may also be of benefit. Although it is understandably difficult with some patients, fluid intake should be encouraged throughout the day to promote a constantly high urine volume.

With the exception of brushite, calcium phosphates tend to be less soluble in alkaline urine. Acidification would reduce urine concentrations of ionic phosphate (PO_4^{3-}) and hydroxyl ion (OH^-). However, whether such patients would benefit from use of appropriate dosages of acidifiers is unknown. Acidification tends to enhance urine calcium excretion and is a risk factor for calcium oxalate urolith formation. Pending further studies, we are unable to recommend routine use of urine acidifiers for patients with calcium phosphate urolithiasis.

Cystine Uroliths

Epidemiology

In our series of feline cystine uroliths, all but one were composed of 100 per cent cystine (see Table 175–5) All uroliths were obtained from the lower urinary tract (62 per cent came from the bladder, 5 per cent from the bladder and urethra, and 5 per cent from the urethra and 28 per cent were voided). Large radiodense bilateral renoliths subsequently developed in a cat that initially had only urocystoliths. Small nephroliths appeared in another cat. Feline cystine uroliths occurred in males (47 per cent were castrated) and females (41 per cent spayed; 11 per cent intact) with equal frequency. Mean age of cats at the time of diagnosis of cystine urolithi-

asis was 3.6 years (range 4 months to 12.2 years). Most cats were of the domestic short-hair breed (67 per cent) and 17 per cent were Siamese.

Etiopathogenesis

Cystine urolithiasis, a disorder associated with a transport defect for cystine and other basic amino acids, has been extensively studied in humans and dogs. In contrast, there is a paucity of information about cystine urolithiasis in cats. Evaluation of urine amino acid profiles of four affected cats revealed increased levels of arginine, lysine, and ornithine in addition to cystine.

One cat with this pattern of amino aciduria also had other renal tubular defects characterized by normoglycemic glucosuria, hyperkalemia hyponatremia, and hypochloremia. The serum aldosterone concentration in this patient was 10 times higher than the normal reference range. Transient but severe hyperammonemia was recognized in another cystinuric cat on two occasions.

The initial clinical signs of affected cats were characteristic of feline lower tract disease (hematuria, dysuria, pollakiuria, and/or urethral obstruction). Cystine crystalluria was a characteristic finding in urine samples from cats with cystine urocystoliths. Some cats also had struvite and calcium oxalate crystalluria. Hematuria was also a consistent finding. The urine pH of affected cats was variable, ranging from 6.0 to 8.0. Bacterial urinary tract infections were not observed. Cystine uroliths were radiodense (see Table 175–9).

Treatment and Prevention

Medical protocols that consistently promote dissolution of cystine uroliths in cats have not yet been developed. Urocystoliths small enough to pass through the urethra may be removed by voiding urohydropropulsion. Surgery remains the most reliable method for removing larger active uroliths from the lower urinary tract.

We have had the opportunity to monitor the biologic behavior of cystinuria in three cystine urolith–forming cats (two spayed females and one neutered male with a perineal urethrostomy). In these cats, the rate of recurrence of radiographically detectable cystine urocystoliths ranged from 2 weeks to approximately 3 months. We have relied solely on voiding urohydropropulsion to control recurrent urocystoliths in two cats (one male cat with a perineal urethrostomy has had 12 recurrent episodes, and one female cat has had

URO

32 recurrent episodes). In a 2-year-old spayed female domestic short-hair cat, we have reduced the rate of urocystolith recurrence from 2-week intervals to approximately 6-week intervals by daily administration of N-(2-mercaptopropionyl)glycine (2-MPG) at oral dose of 5.4 to 9 mg/lb given every 12 hours. Evaluation of hemograms and serum biochemistry profiles has revealed no adverse effects of 2-MPG therapy in this cat. Detection of the urocystoliths by survey radiography while they are still small has allowed us to remove them by voiding urohydropropulsion. We have used this combination successfully to manage 36 recurrent episodes of cystine urocystoliths in this cat for almost 4 years. In all three cats, analysis of recurrent urocystoliths revealed that they were 100 per cent cystine.

The solubility of cystine is pH dependent. Changes in urine pH that do not result in alkalinity are likely to have minimal effect on cystine solubility. Therefore, recommending consumption of high-moisture alkalinizing diets (such as renal failure diets) is logical. If necessary, a sufficient quantity of potassium citrate or sodium bicarbonate should be given orally in divided doses to sustain a pH of approximately 7.5. Data from studies of other species with cystinuria suggest that dietary sodium may enhance cystinuria.[48] Therefore, potassium citrate may be preferable to sodium bicarbonate as a urine alkalinizer. Further studies are required to evaluate the effect of dietary sodium on urinary excretion of cystine in cats.

Pending further studies, we recommend moist renal failure diets in an attempt to increase urine volume and to minimize formation of acid urine. We have not detected secondary bacterial UTIs in cats with recurrent cystine uroliths.

Struvite Uroliths

Types of Struvite Uroliths

Results of our clinical and experimental studies indicate that three distinct etiologic mechanisms may be responsible for development of clinically significant urinary tract precipitates containing large quantities of struvite.[8] Formation of sterile struvite uroliths (perhaps in association with dietary risk factors) is one type. Formation of "infected" or "urease" struvite uroliths as a sequela of UTI with urease-producing bacteria is a second type. A sterile struvite nidus that predisposes to UTI with urease-producing microbes may result in the formation of an outer layer of infection-induced struvite. Formation of urethral plugs containing a large quantity of matrix in addition to varying quantities of struvite is a third form.

Epidemiology of Struvite Uroliths

At this time, approximately 42 per cent of the naturally occurring uroliths removed from cats contain primarily struvite (see Table 175–5). Although the exact percentage of sterile versus infection-induced struvite uroliths in this series could not be precisely determined, we estimate that at least 90 to 95 per cent were composed of sterile struvite. Sterile struvite uroliths contain less matrix than infection-induced struvite and have other characteristic features. In sterile struvite uroliths, unlike infection-induced ones, bacteria cannot be detected in the matrix by culture, light microscopy, or electron microscopy.

Struvite uroliths occur more commonly in females (55 per cent) than males without breed prevalence. The mean age of affected cats was 7 ± 3.5 years (range 3 months to 22 years). The urinary bladder was the most common site of detection of struvite uroliths; the kidneys, ureters, and urethra were less common sites.

Etiopathogenesis

Experimental Studies of Sterile Struvite Uroliths. Data for cats with induced sterile struvite uroliths indicate that several dietary factors play a role in the etiopathogenesis of naturally occurring sterile struvite uroliths. Of these, factors affecting urine magnesium concentration, urine pH, and urine concentration are of major therapeutic importance.

Naturally Occurring Sterile Struvite Uroliths. A decrease is urine volume and increase in urine specific gravity secondary to decreased water consumption would be a logical risk factor for urolith formation (Table 175–13). Likewise, excessive consumption of food (perhaps associated with ad libitum feeding) would be expected to result in obesity and excretion of excess minerals (some of which could be calculogenic) in urine. Cats maintain magnesium homeostasis by excreting excessive dietary magnesium in their urine.[8] Rather than considering obesity a risk factor for FUS, it is logical that both obesity and urolithiasis may be linked to excessive food consumption.

Naturally Occurring Infection-Induced Struvite Uroliths. Infection of the feline urinary tract with urease-producing microbes (especially staphylococci) may result in the rapid production of magnesium ammonium phosphate uroliths in a fashion identical to that in dogs.[8] Rather than being linked to urinary excretion of excessive quantities of dietary minerals, the etiopathogenesis of infection-induced struvite is linked to microbial urease that hydrolyzes urea. The result is alkalinization of urine associated with large quantities of ammonia and phosphate ion. The difference in etiopathogenesis between infection-induced and sterile struvite uroliths is of great therapeutic significance.

Because cats are innately resistant to bacterial UTI, infection-induced struvite uroliths are far less commonly encountered than sterile struvite uroliths. When encountered, they usually affect cats whose local host defenses have been altered by persistent diseases (e.g., congenital anomalies, neoplasm), perineal urethrostomies, or indwelling urinary catheters. The difference in etiopathogenesis of infection-induced and sterile struvite uroliths is of great therapeutic significance.

Infection-induced struvite often contains a greater quantity of matrix than sterile struvite, presumably as a result of increased production of inflammatory reactants. These uroliths also tend to grow more rapidly and are frequently larger. Urease-producing microbes can be readily cultured form their inner portions and can be detected by light and electron microscopy.

Treatment and Prevention

Sterile Struvite Uroliths. A summary of recommendations for medical dissolution of feline sterile struvite uroliths

TABLE 175–13. SOME POTENTIAL RISK FACTORS FOR FELINE STERILE STRUVITE UROLITHIASIS

DIET	URINE	METABOLIC
Alkalinizing potential	Mineral concentration	Alkalosis?
Reduced moisture content	Urine concentration	Hydration status?
High magnesium	Urine retention	Others?
Reduced protein	Crystallization promoters?	
High phosphorus	Crystallization inhibitors?	
Energy content (low fat)	Others?	
Others?		

TABLE 175–14. SUMMARY OF RECOMMENDATIONS FOR MEDICAL DISSOLUTION OF FELINE STRUVITE UROLITHS

1. Perform appropriate diagnostic studies, including complete urinalyses, quantitative urine culture, and diagnostic radiography. "Guesstimate" urolith composition by evaluation of appropriate clinical data (see Tables 175–5 and 175–9).
2. Initiate dietary management designed to reduce the urine concentration of magnesium and create a pH of approximately 6.3. No other food should be fed to patients consuming calculolytic diets. Monitor urine pH 4 to 8 hours after eating. Urine that is acid at this time is likely to be acid throughout the day.
3. Antimicrobic therapy:
   a. Sterile struvite: Attempt to eradicate or control secondary urinary tract infections with antimicrobial agents. Although control of secondary urinary tract infection is not essential for inducing sterile struvite urolith dissolution, it is warranted to prevent damage to tissues of the urinary tract by bacteria and their metabolites.
   b. Infection-induced struvite: Initiate antimicrobic therapy to eradicate or control urease-positive urinary tract infections. Maintain therapy as long as uroliths can be detected by radiography.
4. Periodically (2- to 4-week intervals) monitor the size of uroliths by survey radiography. Survey radiography is preferable to retrograde contrast radiography to monitor urolith dissolution because use of catheters during retrograde radiographic studies may result in iatrogenic urinary tract infection. Alternatively, ultrasonography or intravenous urography may be considered.
5. Periodic evaluation of urine sediment for crystalluria may be considered. In vivo struvite crystals should not form if therapy has been effective in promoting formation of urine that is undersaturated with magnesium ammonium phosphate.
6. Continue calculolytic diet therapy for at least 1 month after survey radiographic disappearance of uroliths. The rationale is to provide therapy of adequate duration to dissolve small uroliths that cannot be detected by survey radiography.
7. If uroliths increase in size during dietary management or do not begin to decrease in size after approximately 4 to 8 weeks of appropriate medical management, alternative methods should be considered. Difficulty in inducing complete dissolution of uroliths by creating urine that is undersaturated with the suspected calculogenic crystalloid should prompt consideration that (1) the wrong mineral component was identified, (2) the nucleus of the urolith is of different mineral composition than other portions of the urolith, or (3) the owner of the patient is not complying with medical recommendations.

---

is presented in Table 175–14 (see Figs. 175–9 and 175–10). Sterile struvite uroliths can be readily dissolved in cats in an average of 1 month by feeding a canned or dry, high-energy, calculolytic diet (Prescription Diet Feline s/d).[11, 47] The diet is formulated to contain reduced quantities of magnesium and to promote formation of acid urine. It is not restricted in protein. Because of its sodium chloride content and because it is formulated to produce aciduria, neither sodium chloride nor urine acidifiers should be given concomitantly. It should not be given to immature cats because they may develop metabolic acidosis, anorexia, and dehydration. Likewise, this diet should not be given to cats that are acidemic (e.g., postrenal azotemia, primary renal dysfunction); have a positive fluid balance (e.g., cardiac dysfunction, hypertension); or have calcium oxalate, calcium phosphate, urate, cystine, or xanthine uroliths.

Consumption of the struvitolytic diet by cats with struvite uroliths of the lower urinary tract is typically associated with remission of dysuria and pollakiuria within 2 to 3 weeks. Reduction of the magnitude of hematuria and pyuria coincides with remission of clinical signs. Likewise, reduction of urine pH and reduction or elimination of struvite crystalluria occur. At the time abdominal radiography indicates urolith dissolution, urinalysis findings are typically normal.

Uncontrolled clinical studies performed at the University of Minnesota indicate that acidification of urine to a pH of approximately 6.0 to 6.3 and consumption of low-magne-sium diets are effective in preventing recurrence of naturally occurring sterile struvite urocystoliths in male and female cats. No attempt was made to determine whether acidification of urine and/or low-magnesium diets were the major factor(s) responsible for the beneficial results. Excessive consumption of acidifiers may result in metabolic acidosis, which, if prolonged, can result in bone demineralization and increase blood ionized calcium concentration.[47]

If nonacidifying diets are used, urine acidifiers may be mixed with them. Alternatively, acidifiers in tablet form may be given at mealtime. The goal is to reduce postprandial alkalinization of urine. Therefore, the dosage of urine acidifiers should be monitored by evaluation of 4- to 6-hour postprandial urine pH values. Blood bicarbonate or total carbon dioxide values may also be monitored. Acidification adequate to prevent sterile struvite uroliths has been achieved with methionine (approximately 1000 mg/day per cat) or ammonium chloride (approximately 800 mg/day per cat).[47] We prefer methionine because ammonium chloride occasionally causes gastrointestinal signs. Caution should be used to avoid toxic doses of methionine because it has been reported to cause anorexia, ataxia, cyanosis, methemoglobinemia, and Heinz-body anemia in cats.[47]

Systemic overacidification with acidifiers should be prevented. Acidemia is most likely to occur in cats with preexisting renal failure, cats consuming acidifying diets, and immature cats. Long-term overacidification may result in metabolic acidosis, potassium depletion, demineralization of bone, and predispositions to renal dysfunction and calcium oxalate urolithiasis.

Reduction of some risk factors for formation of struvite crystals, including promoting the formation of less alkaline or more acidic urine, is one of several risk factors for calcium oxalate urolithiasis. Therefore, periodic reevaluation of the patient to determine the efficacy of dietary management is recommended. Special emphasis should be placed on evaluation of urine specific gravity, urine pH, and crystalluria. If persistent calcium oxalate crystalluria occurs, appropriate adjustments in management should be made.

Infection-Induced Struvite Uroliths. Probable risk factors for infection-induced struvite urolithiasis include infections with urease-producing microbial pathogens (especially staphylococci), abnormalities in local host defenses of the urinary tract that allow bacterial infections (including perineal urethrostomies), and the quantity of urea (the substrate of urease) excreted in urine. Because of the different etiopathogenic mechanisms involved in formation of sterile and infection-induced struvite uroliths, there are some important differences in dissolution protocols.

In addition to dietary therapy, it is essential to utilize antimicrobics as long as infection-induced struvite uroliths can be detected radiographically. The reason is that viable calculogenic microbes tend to persist in inner portions of the uroliths and may cause a relapse of infection. Control of urease-positive infection in cats with infection-induced struvite uroliths is especially important because current calculolytic diets are not protein restricted. Protein restriction has been avoided because cats normally have a relatively high protein requirement. We emphasize that the protein-restricted struvitolytic diets designed for use in dogs are contraindicated for use in cats. The time required to dissolve staphylococci-induced struvite uroliths in three cats was 79 days (range 64 to 92 days).[11, 47] Eradication or control of infections of the urinary tract caused by urease-producing bacteria is the most important factor in preventing recurrence of most infection-induced struvite uroliths.

URO

Struvite and Calcium Oxalate Urolith Combinations. In situations in which cats have documented occurrences of either calcium oxalate followed by struvite urolithiasis or vice versa, uncontrollable risk factors may be present. The paradox in formulating therapy is that control of some risk factors for struvite urolith formation enhances the risks of calcium oxalate or calcium phosphate urolith formation.

If struvite urolithiasis is associated with a urease-positive UTI, therapy should be devised to eradicate the UTI and prevent its recurrence. We recommend that emphasis be placed on minimizing recurrence of calcium oxalate uroliths, because they cannot be dissolved by medical management. Should struvite uroliths recur, they often can be dissolved by dietary management and, if necessary, antimicrobial agents. This strategy tends to minimize the need for repeated surgical intervention.

For uroliths containing a nidus of calcium oxalate surrounded by layers of struvite, it is probable that the calcium oxalate stones predisposed the patient to infection-induced struvite urolithiasis. Therefore, preventive management should be designed to eradicate the bacterial UTI and to recommend changes in diets to minimize calcium oxalate urolith recurrence.

Monitoring Response to Urolith Treatment and Prevention

Overview

Periodic reevaluation of the patient to determine therapeutic efficacy and safety is recommended. We recommend scheduled reexaminations at 4-week intervals in which serum biochemical profiles and other monitoring procedures may be warranted (Figs. 175–9 and 175–10).

Radiography and Ultrasonography

The number, size, and location of uroliths should be periodically monitored by survey radiography and, if necessary, contrast radiography. Although retrograde double-contrast cystography is more sensitive in identifying small urocystoliths, survey radiography is usually preferable because use of catheters during retrograde radiographic studies may result in iatrogenic UTI. Alternatively, ultrasonography or intravenous urography may be considered.

Urine Examination and Status of Urinary Tract Infection

Monthly evaluation of urine pH, protein, and occult blood with reagent test strips and evaluation of sediment for crystalluria, hematuria, and pyuria are also recommended. Crystals should not form in fresh uncontaminated urine if therapy has been effective in promoting formation of urine that is undersaturated with calculogenic minerals.

Difficulty in eradication of infection while uroliths persist may be related to persistence of viable microbes harbored within the stones that are not exposed to antimicrobial drugs. The concentration of antimicrobial drug may also be a factor. Diet-induced diuresis should also be considered when formulating antimicrobial drug dosages so that a quantity of antimicrobic greater than four times the minimal inhibitory concentration is present in urine.

Duration of Therapy

Because small (less than 3 mm in diameter) struvite uroliths may escape detection by survey radiography or ultraso-nography, we recommend that a calculolytic diet and (if necessary) antimicrobial agents be continued for approximately 1 month after radiographic documentation of urolith dissolution. If urinalysis results are normal, dissolution therapy may be discontinued. This maneuver is likely to prevent rapid recurrence of radiographically detectable uroliths and bacterial UTI after cessation of therapy.

Persistence of Uroliths Despite Therapy

Difficulty in inducing complete dissolution of uroliths by creating urine that is undersaturated with the suspected calculogenic crystalloid should prompt consideration that (1) the wrong mineral component was identified, (2) the nucleus of the uroliths is of different mineral composition than the outer portions, and/or (3) the owner or the patient is not complying with therapeutic recommendations.

Difficulty is also encountered in attempting to induce complete dissolution of a urolith with a nucleus of calcium oxalate or silica and a shell of struvite because the solubility characteristics of these two minerals are dissimilar. However, in our experience, compound uroliths make up only 2.4 per cent of the uroliths formed by cats (see Table 175–9). This phenomenon should be considered if medical therapy seems to be ineffective after initially reducing the size of a urolith. However, if reduction in size of the urolith allows it to pass through the urethra, it may be removed by voiding urohydropropulsion.

URETHRAL PLUGS

Etiopathogenesis

Mineral Composition. Urethral plugs contain varying quantities of minerals in proportion to large quantities of matrix (Figs. 175–11 and 175–12). A variety of different minerals have been identified in urethral plugs of cats, suggesting that multiple factors are involved in their formation (see Table 175–6). The infrequency with which nonstruvite minerals are recognized in urethral plugs suggests that they are not of clinical importance. They are of great conceptual

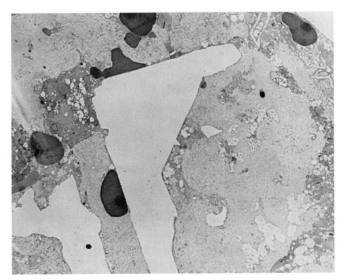

Figure 175–11. Transmission electron micrograph of a section of urethral plug removed from an 11-year-old male Siamese cat. Note the struvite crystals, red blood cells, unidentified cell, and cell fragments trapped in proteinaceous matrix. Original magnification ×3300.

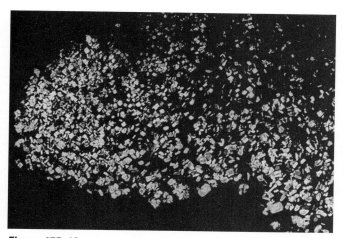

Figure 175–12. Polarizing light micrograph of a urethral plug voided by a 5-year-old neutered domestic medium-hair cat. The plug contains calcium oxalate crystals. Original magnification ×50.

importance, however, because they suggest that any type of crystal may become trapped in plug matrix (Fig. 175–12). This observation is relevant because it suggests that matrix and different crystals play important but distinctly separate roles in the formation of a urethral plug (Fig. 175–12). The mineral composition of urethral plugs should be used to describe them, at least in part, because therapeutic regimens are often influenced by knowledge of their mineral composition.

Matrix Composition. Compared with uroliths, urethral plugs contain large quantities of matrix. Some urethral plugs do not contain crystalline components. Light and transmission electron microscopic evaluation of naturally occurring feline urethral plugs has revealed that noncrystalline components of plugs also include red blood cells, white cells, epithelial cells, spermatozoa, virus-like particles, and bacteria surrounded by amorphous material (See Figs. 175–1 and 175–11).[49] It appears that these structures have been trapped by the amorphous matrix in a manner analogous to fruit in Jell-O (see Fig. 175–8). We emphasize that obstructive urethropathy in male cats may also be caused by one or more intraluminal, mural, or extramural abnormalities located at one or more sites (Table 175–15). Formation of matrix-crystalline plugs appears to be the most common but not the only cause of urethral obstruction (see Fig. 175–11).

Biologic Behavior of Urethral Plugs

There is general agreement that obstruction of urine outflow produces predictable clinical and biochemical abnor-

malities that vary with the duration and degree of obstruction. Systemic abnormalities in fluid, acid-base, and electrolyte balance caused by urethral obstruction probably occur irrespective of the specific cause (e.g., uroliths, plugs, strictures).

Clinical studies indicate that urethral obstruction in male cats may be initiated and maintained at one or more sites by one or a combination of primary, secondary, and iatrogenic causes. Even in instances in which recurrent obstruction is caused by urethral plugs, there have been no studies specifically designed to compare the nature and composition of first-occurrence plugs and recurrent obstructing material.

Diagnosis of Urethral Plugs

Because urethral outflow obstruction may be caused by several different mechanisms in addition to urethral plugs, routine diagnostic evaluation of the patient is warranted (see Table 175–1). In addition to an appropriate history and physical examination, blood and urine samples should be collected prior to administration of diagnostic or therapeutic agents that could alter test results.

A complete urinalysis with special emphasis on evaluation of urine sediment unadulterated with reverse flushing solution is especially valuable. Pretreatment urine samples may be obtained during decompressive cystocentesis.

Survey abdominal radiographs of the lower urinary tract should be obtained before therapy designed to reestablish urethral patency. Results of our clinical studies indicate that although most urethral plugs evaluated in vivo are radiolucent, some are sufficiently radiodense to be detected by survey radiography. The radiodensity of urethral plugs may be influenced by a variety of factors: (1) their size, (2) their location (within or exterior to the bony pelvis), (3) their composition (that is, ratio of mineral to matrix), (4) the quantity of tissue that must be penetrated by x-rays, (5) the mineral type of crystals they contain, and (6) the radiographic technique used to evaluate them.

Quantitative analysis of the mineral components of plugs removed from the urethra should be routine. In addition to mineral analysis, a portion of the plug should be placed in 10 per cent buffered formalin and submitted for light microscopic evaluation. If viral urinary tract infection is suspected, a portion of the plug may be placed in the appropriate fixative and submitted for electron microscopy.

Treatment of Urethral Plugs

Medical Treatment

Irrespective of the cause(s) of urethral obstruction, predictable clinical and biochemical abnormalities subsequently

URO

TABLE 175–15. DIAGNOSTIC RULE-OUTS FOR URETHRAL OBSTRUCTION IN MALE CATS

PRIMARY CAUSES	PERPETUATING CAUSES	IATROGENIC CAUSES

Intraluminal
  Urethral plugs (matrix and/or crystals)
  Urethroliths
  Tissue sloughed from urinary bladder
    and/or urethra
Mural or extramural
  Strictures
  Urethral neoplasms
  Prostate neoplasms
  Reflex dyssynergia
  Anomalies
Combinations
	Intraluminal
	  Increased production of inflammatory reactants,
	    red blood cells, white cells, fibrin, and so forth
	  Sloughed tissue
	
	Mural
	  Inflammatory swelling
	  Muscular spasm
	  Reflex dyssynergia
	  Strictures
	
	Combinations
		Tissue damage
		  Reverse flushing solutions
		  Catheter-induced trauma
		  Catheter-induced foreign body reaction
		  Catheter-induced infection
		Postsurgical dysfunction
		  Strictures
		
		Combinations

develop. They are characterized by systemic deficits and/or excesses in fluid (dehydration), electrolyte (e.g., hyperkalemia, hyperphosphatemia), and acid-base (metabolic acidosis) balance and retention of metabolic wastes (creatinine, urea, other protein catabolites). The magnitude of these systemic abnormalities varies with the degree and duration of obstruction.

Obstructive uropathy that persists longer than about 24 hours usually results in postrenal azotemia. This occurs because increased back pressure induced by obstruction of outflow impairs glomerular filtration, renal blood flow, and tubular function. After obstruction of the urethra of normal cats, death occurs in 3 to 6 days. Damage to the mucosal surface of the urinary bladder may shorten survival time. Despite the potentially catastrophic outcome of urethral obstruction, the biochemical consequences of this disorder are potentially reversible provided appropriate supportive and symptomatic parenteral therapy is given. In severe cases, supportive therapy to correct hyperkalemia, metabolic acidosis, and volume depletion should be initiated immediately after decompression of the excretory pathway by cystocentesis.

The immediate need to remove urethral plugs within hours of their discovery precludes attempts to cause their dissolution over a period of days or weeks. In some instances urethral plugs are repulsed into the bladder lumen. Thus, the question arises, can such plugs be dissolved by medical therapy? Recall that urethral plugs contain a substantially greater quantity of matrix than classical uroliths. It is probable that medical protocols effective in inducing sterile struvite urolith dissolution would also be effective in dissolving the struvite crystalline component of urethral plugs located in the bladder lumen, but such therapy may not result in dissolution of the plug matrix. Calcium oxalate and ammonium urate crystals have been identified in a few naturally occurring feline urethral plugs (see Table 175–10). This accounts for lack of expected response in some patients.

Attempts to dissolve struvite crystals with urine acidifiers or diets designed to promote acid urine should not be initiated in cats with postrenal azotemia. The metabolic sequelae of urethral obstruction, particularly severe metabolic acidosis, must be corrected before diets designed to acidify urine are incorporated in the management plan.

Reestablishment of Urethral Patency

Overview. Obstructive urethropathy may be caused by one or more intraluminal mural, or extramural abnormalities located at one or more sites (see Table 175–15). Reverse flushing solutions may be effective in dissolving urethral plugs but would have no effect on obstructive lesions located in the urethral wall or periurethral tissue. Inability to restore patency by flushing the urethral lumen with a solution should arouse one's suspicion of a mural or periurethral lesion in addition to, or instead of, a firmly lodged urethral plug or urethrolith.

Physical and Anesthesia Restraint. The method of restraint should be designed to facilitate atraumatic aseptic urethral catheterization while minimizing anesthetic risk to the patient. Physical restraint alone or in combination with topical anesthesia may be sufficient for obstructed patients that are particularly docile or severely depressed. Wrapping the cat in a bath towel may help to protect the patient and the assistant.

If local anesthetics are used to anesthetize the urethral mucosa, they should be administered only in a quantity sufficient to accomplish this goal. We do not recommend use of local anesthetic agents as primary reverse flushing solutions because they may induce systemic toxicity if a sufficient quantity is absorbed. Their absorption may be enhanced by damage to the urothelium, and their toxic potential may be enhanced by postrenal uremia.

Because of an increased risk of adverse drug reactions associated with obstructive uropathy, pharmacologic restraint should be avoided when feasible. The risk of adverse drug reactions must be weighed against the possibility of iatrogenic trauma to the urethra in an uncooperative patient. If the disposition of the patient is such that attempts to dislodge the urethral obstruction are likely to be associated with additional damage to the urethra or if there is a high risk of iatrogenic UTI, some form of pharmacologic restraint should be considered. Short-acting barbiturates (thiamylal), propofol, and/or inhalant anesthetics may be considered if general anesthesia is required. Anesthetics must be given cautiously because dosages less than those recommended for patients with normal renal function are required for patients with postrenal azotemia. If ketamine hydrochloride is used, similar caution must be exercised because it is excreted in active form by the kidneys. Low doses of ketamine hydrochloride (0.5 to 1.0 mg/lb given intravenously) and diazepam (0.1 mg/lb given intravenously) have been effective. However, if difficulty is encountered in relieving outflow obstruction, additional quantities of ketamine should be administered with caution.

Correction of Intraluminal Urethral Obstruction. We recommend a step-by-step procedure when attempting to restore the urethral patency of an obstructed male cat.

1. *Gentle massage* of the penis between the thumb and fingers may help to dislodge plugs located in the penile urethra. If necessary, the penis may be manipulated while it is retracted within the prepuce. Plugs located in the preprostatic (abdominal) or membranous (pelvic) urethra may occasionally be dislodged by massaging the urethra per rectum. Although these methods are often ineffective, their simplicity and occasional success make them worth trying before considering cystocentesis or catheterization.

2. Inability of a cat to void urine spontaneously indicates that increasing intraurethral pressure by *digitally compressing the urinary bladder* is unlikely to be effective. However, if this technique is utilized *after* urethral massage, sufficient intraluminal pressure may be generated to dislodge fragments of urethral precipitates (Fig. 175–13). Use caution to prevent iatrogenic damage to the urinary bladder. If UTI is likely, the consequence of inducing vesicoureteral reflux of urine during palpation should be considered because microbes may be forced into the upper urinary tract.

3. In general, *decompressive cystocentesis* should be performed if the aforementioned techniques are ineffective in reestablishing urethral patency (Table 175–16; Fig. 175–14). The *benefits* of performing decompressive cystocentesis before flushing the urethral lumen via a catheter are that (1) a urine sample suitable for analysis and culture is obtained, (2) decompression of an overdistended urinary bladder by removing most (but not all) of the urine provides a mechanism for temporarily halting the continued adverse effects of obstructive urethropathy (irrespective of cause), (3) decompression of an overdistended urinary bladder and proximal urethra may facilitate repulsion of a urethral plug or urolith into the bladder lumen, and (4) the gross character of aspirated urine may provide valuable clues about the nature of the obstructive disorder (intraluminal precipitates of matrix and crystalline material versus extraluminal compression). Urine that contains large quantities of visible pre-

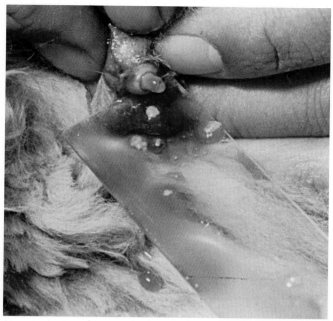

Figure 175–13. A 3-year-old domestic short-hair cat after digital manipulation of the distal urethra and manual compression of the urinary bladder. Fragments of a struvite urethral plug are visible on the microscope slide.

TABLE 175–16. TECHNIQUE OF DECOMPRESSIVE CYSTOCENTESIS

1. Attach a 22-gauge needle to one end of a flexible intravenous extension set, and attach a three-way valve and large-capacity syringe (35 to 60 mL) to the other end. Use of a large-capacity syringe minimizes unnecessary manipulation and therefore reduces the likelihood of trauma to the bladder wall. The intravenous extension set allows one individual to immobilize the urinary bladder and the 22-gauge needle.
2. The 22-gauge needle should be inserted through the ventral or ventrolateral wall of the bladder to minimize trauma to the ureters and adjacent major abdominal vessels (see Fig. 175–14). The needle should be inserted midway between the vertex of the bladder surface and the junction of the bladder with the urethra. This permits removal of urine and decompression of the bladder lumen. If the needle is placed in or adjacent to the vertex of the bladder, it may not remain within the bladder lumen.
3. Excessive digital pressure should not be applied to the bladder wall while the needle is in its lumen lest urine be forced around the needle into the peritoneal cavity. Caution should also be used to prevent laceration of the bladder as a result of movement of the needle. The bladder should be emptied as completely as is consistent with atraumatic technique. Attempting complete evacuation of the bladder lumen is undesirable because the sharp point of the needle may then damage the bladder wall. We recommend that 15 to 20 mL of urine remain in the bladder.
4. If patency of the urethra is not established before the bladder refills with urine or solutions used to flush the urethra, decompressive cystocentesis should be repeated.
5. The need for prophylactic antibacterial therapy after cystocentesis must be determined on the basis of the status of the patient and retrospective evaluation of technique. If subsequent restoration of urethral patency requires intermittent or indwelling catheterization, preventive antimicrobial therapy should be considered after the catheter is removed (see Table 175–18).

cipitates suggests a greater likelihood of reobstruction after subsequent flushing of the urethral lumen.

The potential *risks* of performing decompressive cystocentesis are that (1) it may result in extravasation of urine into the bladder wall and/or peritoneal cavity and (2) it may injure the bladder wall or surrounding structures. Although these complications could be severe in patients with a devitalized bladder wall, in our experience this has been the exception rather than the rule if the majority, but not all, of the urine is removed from the bladder. The key is to remove most but not all of the urine from the bladder lumen and to prevent overdistention of the bladder by serial cystocentesis until adequate urine outflow is restored. Loss of a small quantity of urine into the peritoneal cavity is usually of little consequence, especially if it does not contain pathogens. The

potential of trauma to the bladder and adjacent structures can be minimized by proper technique.

We are not advocating an "always or never" recommendation regarding decompressive cystocentesis. Clinical judgment is required regarding its use in each patient. However, it is preferable to decompress the urinary bladder by cystocentesis (saving an aliquot for appropriate diagnostic tests) before use of reverse flushing procedures in patients likely to have adequate integrity of the bladder wall and in which immediate overdistention of the bladder lumen is not allowed to recur.

4. *Flushing the urethral lumen* with sterilized solutions after urethral catheterization may dislodge urethral plugs and uroliths. However, it is emphasized that urethral obstruction may be caused by a combination of intraluminal precipitates (uroliths or urethral plugs), swelling of the urethral wall, and/or spasm of urethral musculature (Table 175–17).

Reverse flushing solutions should be selected cautiously because accumulation and absorption of large quantities of acid or anesthetic solutions from an inflamed urinary bladder may cause systemic toxicity. In addition, they may damage the coating of glycosaminoglycans that lines the surface of the urothelium. GAGs normally minimize adherence of crystals and microbes to the urethral mucosa.[50] Adherence of crystals to the urothelium is most likely to occur if acidic solutions utilized to dissolve struvite crystals are used. Pending results of further studies, we prefer physiologic saline or lactated Ringer's solution because they are readily available, sterilized, nontoxic, nonirritating, and economical. We do not recommend buffered acetic acid (so-called Walpole's solution). The general guidelines to be followed when reverse flushing feline urethras to reestablish patency are outlined in Table 175–17.

5. Inability to establish adequate urethral patency by use of catheters and reverse flushing should arouse a high index

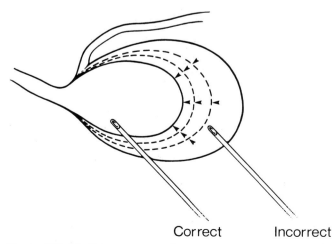

Correct   Incorrect

Figure 175–14. Correct and incorrect sites of insertion of a 22-gauge needle into the urinary bladder for the purpose of removing urine. The correct position permits removal of urine and decompression of the bladder without need for reinsertion of the needle into the bladder lumen (see Table 175–16).

URO

TABLE 175–17. GENERAL GUIDELINES FOR TRANSURETHRAL FLUSHING OF OBSTRUCTED MALE CATS (see Fig. 175–15)

1. Make every effort to protect the patient from iatrogenic complications associated with catheterization of the urethra (especially trauma and urinary tract infection with bacteria).
2. Strive to use meticulous aseptic "feather-touch" technique.
3. Use only sterile catheters.
4. Cleanse the penis and prepuce with warm water before catheterization.
5. Select the shortest Minnesota olive-tipped feline urethral catheter* for initial catheterization of the urethra, and attach it to a flexible intravenous connection set and a syringe.
6. Coat the olive tip with sterile aqueous lubricant.
7. Before insertion of the catheter into the external urethral orifice, the extended penis should be displaced dorsally until the long axis of the urethra is approximately parallel to the vertebral column.
8. Carefully advance the catheter to the site of obstruction. If necessary, replace the short olive-tipped Minnesota needle with a longer one. Record the site of suspected obstruction, because this information may be of value when considering use of muscle relaxants and/or when considering urethral surgery to prevent recurrent obstructions. CAUTION: Never use excessive force when advancing the catheter.
9. Next, flush a large quantity of physiologic saline or lactated Ringer's solution (as much as several hundred mL) into the urethral lumen, and allow it to reflux out the external urethral orifice. When possible, the catheter may be advanced toward the bladder. As a result of this maneuver, the obstructed urethral plugs may be gradually dislodged and flushed around the catheter and out of the urethral lumen. Application of steady but gentle digital pressure to the bladder wall after the urethra has been flushed with physiologic saline or lactated Ringer's solution may result in expulsion of a urethral plug or urolith from the urethral lumen. Excessive pressure should not be used because it may result in trauma to the bladder, reflux of potentially infected urine into the ureters and renal pelvis, and/or rupture of the bladder wall.
10. If the technique outlined in step 9 is unsuccessful, it may be necessary to attempt repulsion of suspected urethral plugs or uroliths back into the bladder lumen by occluding the distal end of the urethra around the olive tip of the catheter before injecting fluid into the urethra. By preventing reflux of solutions out of the external urethral orifice, this maneuver tends to dilate the urethral lumen. If the obstruction persists, an attempt may be made to advance the suspected plug or urolith gently toward the bladder. *Excessive force should not be used.*
11. On occasion it is advantageous to allow the reverse flushing solution to soften the obstructing urethral plugs (this technique is ineffective for most uroliths) before attempting to propel them back into the bladder. Allowing lapse of several hours between attempts to remove firmly lodged plugs by reverse flushing has been effective.

*Minnesota feline olive-tipped urethral catheters are available from EJAY International, P.O. Box 1835, Glendora, California 91740.

of suspicion that the underlying cause is not a urethral plug (see Table 175–15). Appropriate diagnostic procedures should be considered (see Table 175–1). Overdistention of the bladder lumen may be prevented by serial decompressible cystocentesis. We do not recommend surgical intervention to correct obstructive urethropathy in uremic cats unless no reasonable alternative exists.

Care Immediately After Restoration of Urethral Patency

After urine flow has been reestablished by nonsurgical techniques, most of the urine should be removed from the bladder lumen. Removing all the urine from the bladder lumen is unnecessary and inadvisable because trauma associated with such efforts may aggravate the severity of bladder lesions. Manual compression may be used provided it does not require substantial pressure to induce voiding. Manual compression of the bladder is not necessarily the procedure of choice if an overdistended bladder has been recently

decompressed by cystocentesis, as it may result in extravasation of urine into the bladder wall or peritoneal cavity. Alternative methods include use of a catheter and syringe and cystocentesis. Each of these procedures has benefits and risks that must be considered in light of the status of the urinary bladder and urethra of each patient.

If the gross appearance of voided or aspirated urine suggests that reobstruction with intraluminal debris is likely, removal of this material with saline or lactated Ringer's solution flushes of the bladder lumen may be of value in minimizing reobstruction. Particulate material located in the dependent portion of the bladder may be dispersed throughout the bladder lumen by digitally moving the bladder in and up-and-down fashion, which may in turn facilitate aspiration of crystals, inflammatory reactants, and blood clots into the catheter and syringe. Local instillation of antimicrobial agents into the bladder lumen in an attempt to prevent or treat UTI is of unproved value. Unless the bladder wall is hypotonic or atonic, the antimicrobial agent is likely to be voided soon after instillation. If circumstances dictate the need for antimicrobial agents, they should be given orally or parenterally to maximize their effectiveness (Table 175–18).

The urinary bladder should be periodically evaluated after restoration of adequate urethral patency to ensure that urethral obstruction has not recurred and/or that the detrusor muscle is not hypotonic. Micturition induced by gentle digital compression of the bladder may facilitate evaluation of urethral patency.

Although glucocorticoid therapy has been advocated to minimize inflammatory swelling of the urethra, glucocorticoids may aggravate the severity of potentially life-threatening uremia by inducing protein catabolism (via gluconeogenesis) and may predispose the patient to nosocomial bacterial UTI.[51] Likewise, administration of acidifying agents to azotemic cats may aggravate the severity of existing metabolic acidosis.

After relief of urethral obstruction, a transitory obligatory postobstructive diuresis may develop. Even though polyuric cats may consume some water, it is often insufficient to maintain proper fluid balance. Therefore, supplementing water intake by parenteral administration of rehydrating or maintenance fluids may be advisable.

Indwelling Transurethral Catheters

Perspectives. We do not recommend routine use of indwelling urinary catheters in cats after relief of urethral obstruction because they may induce further damage to the urinary tract. Disruption of the GAG coating of the urothe-

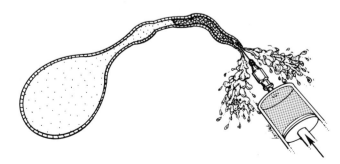

Figure 175–15. Illustration of flushing of a male cat's urethra containing a matrix-crystalline plug. After insertion of a Minnesota olive-tipped catheter, a large quantity of saline is injected into the urethral lumen and allowed to reflux out of the distal urethra (see Table 175–17).

TABLE 175–18. GUIDELINES FOR REDUCING RISK OF CATHETER-INDUCED URINARY TRACT INFECTION

1. Avoid unnecessary catheterization, especially in patients with increased risk for bacterial UTI and its sequelae (e.g., patients with diseases of the lower urinary tract; diseases associated with polyuria; and diabetes mellitus).
2. Urinary catheterization should be performed by trained personnel.
3. If there is need for prolonged catheterization, atraumatic intermittent brief catheterization is often preferable to indwelling catheterization.
   a. If single brief catheterization is required for high-risk patients, consider prophylactic administration of an antibiotic excreted in high concentration in urine, and administer it 8 to 12 hours before and 2 to 3 days after catheterization. Adequate concentration of the drug should be in the urine before catheterization.
   b. Choose antimicrobial agents most likely to be effective against nosocomial pathogens known to be present in the hospital environment.
   c. Collect a urine sample by cystocentesis 2 to 3 days after catheterization to detect nosocomial UTI at a subclinical stage of development.
   d. If UTI is present, select an antimicrobial drug on the basis of susceptibility tests and administer it for an appropriate period.
4. Indwelling transurethral catheters.
   a. Select indwelling urethral catheters constructed of materials least likely to cause irritation and inflammation of the adjacent mucosa.
   b. Thoroughly cleanse the external genitalia, and insert the catheter using aseptic technique.
   c. Avoid overinsertion of catheters to minimize damage to the bladder.
   d. Avoid open catheters; maintain a closed system.
   e. Avoid prolonged use of indwelling catheters.
   f. Prevent retrograde flow of urine from the collection receptacle by positioning it below the level of the patient.
   g. Try to avoid inducing diuresis during indwelling catheterization, especially if an "open" system is used.
   h. Avoid giving prophylactic antimicrobial drugs in an attempt to prevent UTI unless the duration of catheterization is less than 2 to 3 days. Even when indwelling catheters are used for a short period, waiting until the catheter is removed before antimicrobic therapy is often best.
   i. During longer duration of use of indwelling catheters, avoid administration of antibiotics unless evidence of UTI associated with morbidity is detected. Although antibiotics may decrease the frequency and delay the onset of UTI, there is high risk of promoting development of infectious bacteria that are resistant to multiple antimicrobial drugs.
   j. If catheter-induced infection develops and remains asymptomatic, treat the infection after removal of the catheter.
   k. Remove the catheter as soon as possible. At the time of catheter removal, perform a urinalysis, quantitative urine culture, and antimicrobial susceptibility test.
   l. If UTI is confirmed after the catheter is removed, initiate therapy with an appropriate antimicrobial drug and continue giving for at least 10 to 14 days.
   m. If infection with more than one bacterial species occurs and if the pathogens have different drug susceptibilities, treat the bacteria most likely to be virulent first. Then select the drug most likely to eliminate the remaining pathogens.
   n. Remove and, if appropriate, replace indwelling catheters that are grossly contaminated.
   o. Unless the benefits outweigh the risks, treatment with corticosteroids should not be given to patients with indwelling catheters. In most instances, the risk of UTI outweights the potential benefit of reducing catheter-induced inflammation with corticosteroids.

UTI = urinary tract infection.

lium as a result of indwelling urethral catheters may promote adherence of microbes and UTI. Disruption of the GAG coating may also facilitate adherence of crystals to the urothelium, facilitating their growth and/or aggregation.

Catheter-induced nosocomial UTIs are common, especially in cats with preexisting disease of the lower tract, because catheters interfere with host defenses against ascending migration of bacteria through the urethral lumen. Even when closed catheter systems are used, catheters permit bacteria to ascend via the interface between the catheter and the mucosal surface. Bacteria may also adhere to the surface of urinary catheters and initiate growth of biofilms composed of bacteria, bacterial glycocalices, Tamm-Horsfall protein, and struvite crystals.[52] These biofilms may shield the bacteria they contain from antimicrobics, resulting in treatment failures. Nosocomial bacterial UTIs are especially prevalent in cats with LUTD and have the potential to cause significant morbidity including pyelonephritis, renal failure, and septicemia. Therefore, unnecessary use of urinary catheters should be avoided (Table 175–18)!

Indications for Indwelling Transurethral Catheters. The likelihood that a cat will voluntarily resume adequate voiding after restoration of urethral patency may be assessed by evaluation of: 1) the caliber of the urine stream during the voiding phase of micturition, 2) the abundance of material in urine with the potential to occlude the urethral lumen, and 3) the adequacy of detrusor tone immediately after relief of urethral obstruction. Indwelling urinary catheters may be indicated after relief of urethral obstruction to: 1) facilitate measurement of the urine formation rate during intensive care of critically ill cats, 2) promote recovery of detrusor atony by maintaining an empty bladder, and 3) prevent recurrence of urethral obstruction caused by urine

precipitates or mural abnormalities in high-risk patients (see Table 175–12). Indwelling catheters are often unnecessary if: 1) the cat has a good urine stream during the voiding phase of micturiton, 2) there is a functional detrusor muscle, and 3) urine does not contain particulate matter that could reobstruct the urethral lumen.

Rupture of the Urinary Bladder

Overview. A diagnosis of rupture of the urinary bladder is usually best confirmed by positive-contrast cystography or positive-contrast urethrocystography. Surgical repair has generally been considered the definitive treatment for rupture of the urinary bladder. Although this recommendation is logical, there have apparently been no studies to compare surgical versus medical therapy of bladder wall rents by controlled clinical trials.

Clinical Experiences with Nonuremic Patients. While evaluating feline LUTD, we have observed leakage of contrast medium from the maximally distended bladder lumen into the peritoneal cavity on several occasions. Affected cats had hematuria and dysuria but did not have a bacterial UTI. Some had urethral outflow obstruction, but none had postrenal uremia at the time of radiography. In two obstructed male cats, the bladder wall was ruptured during attempts to reestablish urethral patency. In most cases, we could not ascertain the site(s) of discontinuity of the bladder wall by evaluation of positive-contrast radiography. We managed all cases successfully by nonsurgical therapy.[53]

In our opinion, medical management of iatrogenic rupture of the urinary bladder may be considered provided (1) there is no evidence of an underlying atraumatic lesion (e.g., neoplasm) that predisposed the bladder to rupture, (2) the

URO

bladder wall is not hypotonic and unable to contract, (3) there is no reason to believe that the wound edges are devitalized, (4) there is no evidence of significant urosepsis, (5) there are no other complications requiring celiotomy, and (6) the patient can be appropriately monitored for a sufficient time. When the bladder lumen contains only a small volume of urine, contraction of the bladder musculature often quickly seals the site of disruption. Urine and contrast agents that have accumulated in the peritoneal cavity are rapidly absorbed and excreted by the kidneys. If the cat is pollakiuric and has a completely patent urethral lumen, it may be unnecessary to use an indwelling transurethral catheter to prevent filling of the bladder with urine. However, if gentle palpation, ultrasonography, or radiography reveals distention of the bladder lumen with urine, a closed indwelling transurethral catheter system may be used to minimize distention of the bladder wall. A decision to utilize antibiotics to prevent bacterial UTI should be made on a case-by-case basis but in general is a logical safety precaution. Provided clinical and laboratory findings typical of uroperitoneum and postrenal azotemia do not develop, indwelling catheters may be removed after 3 to 6 days. Prior to the removal of the catheter, a low-pressure positive contrast cystogram to evaluate bladder wall integrity should be made.

Clinical Experience with Uremic Patients. Spontaneous rupture of the urinary bladder and clinically significant uroperitoneum secondary to urethral outflow obstruction are uncommon. They usually occur in association with overzealous or incorrect attempts to restore urethral patency. In this setting, patients typically have postrenal uremia associated with varying degrees of fluid, electrolyte, and acid-base imbalances. Compared with nonuremic cats with rupture of the urinary bladder, patients with postrenal uremia before bladder rupture often decline rapidly. If the obstruction of urine outflow has been present for several days, the integrity of the entire overdistended bladder wall may be severely compromised.

Initial management should be designed to correct the polysystemic consequences of postrenal uremia, especially hyperkalemia, acidemia, and dehydration. When fluid, electrolyte, and acid-base disorders have been corrected and the patient's vital signs have been stabilized, patency of the urethra should be reestablished. An indwelling urethral catheter (closed system) may be used to minimize continued loss of urine into the peritoneal cavity. If necessary, a peritoneal dialysis type of catheter may be placed in the abdomen to facilitate removal of fluid from the peritoneal cavity. As soon as the patient's overall condition has been stabilized, the specific nature and timing of additional diagnostic procedures and surgical or medical therapy should be considered. When formulating diagnostic and therapeutic plans, care must be used not to overlook consideration of the initial cause(s) of urethral outflow obstruction, the site and size of the rent in the bladder wall, and the time-related trends of change in the status of associated clinical abnormalities.

Surgical repair of a large rent in the bladder wall is certainly consistent with conventional knowledge and clinical wisdom. However, we have also observed remission of uroperitoneum and postrenal uremia in cats with iatrogenic bladder rupture. Therapy consisted of restoration of urine outflow, intermittent abdominocentesis, and supportive and symptomatic treatment of postrenal uremia.

If rupture of the bladder has occurred as a result of an underlying disease that has altered the integrity of the tissues of the bladder wall, repair without surgical intervention would seem to be unlikely.

Dysfunctional Urinary Bladder

Severe and/or prolonged distention of the urinary bladder caused by obstruction of urine outflow may cause impaired capacity of the detrusor muscle to contract during the voiding phase of micturition. The underlying cause is thought to be related to disruption of specialized portions of bladder smooth muscle cells (so-called tight junctions) that normally transmit neurogenic impulses from smooth muscle pacemaker cells. In this situation, the cat has impaired ability to empty the bladder completely. Voiding can usually be induced by manual compression applied through the abdominal wall.

When urethral patency has been reestablished, therapy designed to maintain relatively low pressure within the bladder lumen often results in restoration of adequate detrusor function. One option is trial therapy with bethanechol, a parasympathomimetic (muscarinic) agent. This drug may enhance detrusor contractility. The suggested oral dosage for cats is 1.25 to 2.5 mg given every 8 hours (Table 175–19).[54] If the desired effect does not occur within a few days, the dose may be increased incrementally up to 5 to 7.5 mg every 8 hours, provided harmful side effects do not occur (e.g., excessive salivation, abdominal cramping, vomiting, and/or diarrhea).

Because bethanechol can also increase urethral resistance by its nicotinic effects on smooth muscle in the proximal urethra, it may be given with phenoxybenzamine. Phenoxybenzamine is an alpha-adrenergic antagonist that facilitates relaxation of smooth muscle in the proximal urethra (oral dose = 0.1 mg/lb every 12 hours (see Table 175–19).[54] Alternatively, an indwelling catheter whose tip is located within the bladder lumen may be utilized. Periodic attempts to induce voiding by manual compression of the urinary bladder may also be considered, provided they do not result in a marked increase in intraluminal pressure.

If an indwelling urinary catheter is utilized to minimize accumulation of urine within the bladder, the previously described precautions designed to prevent catheter-induced injury should be considered. In addition to orally administered antimicrobial agents, irrigation of the bladder lumen with antimicrobial solutions may be considered, provided a sufficient quantity of the agent will remain in the bladder long enough to have a beneficial effect. Sterilized solutions should be injected in volume sufficient to allow contact with all portions of the bladder mucosa.

Persistent Urethral Outflow Resistance

After restoration of urethral patency as confirmed by transurethral catheterization, induced voiding, or contrast radiography, impaired flow of urine through the urethra may persist. This may be related to one or more primary, predisposing or perpetuating causes (see Table 175–15). One cause is inflammatory swelling induced by trauma during attempts to remove plugs or stones from the urethra. This problem can be expected to resolve within a few days provided there is no persistent periurethral extravasation of urine.

Another possibility is spasm of smooth or skeletal muscles surrounding the urethra. The frequency with which this type of abnormality occurs and its responsiveness to smooth and skeletal relaxants have not been extensively characterized. In a pilot study of six cats with urethral obstruction of undetermined cause, urodynamic studies indicated that urethral muscle spasm was not a significant problem after restoration of urethral patency.[55]

TABLE 175–19. DRUGS THAT MAY BE CONSIDERED FOR MANAGEMENT OF FELINE MICTURITION DISORDERS

DESIRED EFFECT	NAME	CLASSIFICATION	SUGGESTED DOSAGE	COMMENTS AND CAVEATS
Decrease detrusor contractility	Propantheline	Cholinergic antagonist	0.1 to 0.2 mg/lb q12–24h	Adverse effects include vomiting, constipation, urine retention; ptyalism
Decrease detrusor contractility; smooth muscle relaxation	Oxybutynin	Antispasmodic Cholinergic antagonist	0.5 to 1.25 mg/cat PO q8–12h	Adverse effects include vomiting, constipation, urine retention; ptyalism
Increase urethral sphincter tone	Testosterone	Reproductive hormone	5 to 10 mg IM prn	Behavioral changes
Increase urethral smooth muscle contractility	Phenylpropanolamine	Alpha-adrenergic agonist	1.5 to 2.2 mg/kg PO q8–12h	Efficacy questionable; contraindicated in cardiac, hypertensive disease
Increase detrusor contractility	Bethanechol	Cholinergic agonist	1.25 to 7.5 mg/cat PO q8h	Adverse effects include ptyalism, vomiting; contraindicated with urinary or gastrointestinal obstruction
Decrease urethral smooth muscle tone	Phenoxybenzamine	Alpha-adrenergic antagonist	2.5 to 7.5 mg/cat PO q12–24h	Adverse effects include hypotension; gastrointestinal irritation
Decrease urethral smooth muscle tone	Prazosin	Alpha-adrenergic antagonist	0.03 mg/kg IV	Hypotension possible
Decrease urethral striated muscle tone	Diazepam	Benzodiazepine Skeletal muscle relaxant	1 to 2.5 mg/cat PO q8H	Adverse effects include sedation, increased appetite, paradoxical excitement possible; rare hepatoxicity
Decrease urethral striated muscle tone	Dantrolene	Direct skeletal muscle relaxant	0.5 to 2.0 mg/kg PO q8h 1.0 mg/kg IV	Adverse effects include sedation, weakness; contraindicated in cardiac, pulmonary, and hepatic disease

Other potential causes of impaired voiding through the urethra include reflex dyssynergia; intraluminal accumulations of sloughed tissue, inflammatory cells, or red blood cells; and reformation of matrix-crystalline urethral plugs.

Urethral strictures may cause persistent outflow resistance in patients with recurrent urethral obstruction. Urethral strictures usually occur as a sequela of catheter trauma induced at the time of treatment of urethral plugs or urethroliths; use of indwelling transurethral catheters, especially those constructed of material that stimulates a foreign body response; and self-trauma. Formation of urethral strictures may be minimized by proper restraint of the patient during urethral catheterization, avoiding use of indwelling urethral catheters when possible, and use of restraint devices to minimize self-trauma. If urethral strictures predispose to clinical signs, corrective surgery should be considered, but not before the lower urinary tract has been evaluated by antegrade cystourethrography or retrograde urethrocystography.

Prevention of Matrix-Crystalline Urethral Plugs

Overview. We emphasize that obstructive urethropathy may occur at different sites and have different causes (see Table 175–15). Therefore the need for and the type of prophylactic therapy should be based on appropriate diagnostic information (see Table 175–3).

Medical Protocols. Because insoluble crystals appear to be an integral component of many matrix-crystalline urethral plugs, use of medical protocols to prevent crystal formation in affected patients is logical. Struvite has been the primary mineral component of most naturally occurring urethral plugs, although other mineral types have been encountered (see Table 175–6). Consult Medical Prevention of Feline Stones.

Surgical Protocols. On occasion, medical procedures designed to correct or prevent recurrent urethral obstruction are ineffective. In these situations, perineal urethrostomies and other surgical procedures designed to bypass the penile urethra are often considered, irrespective of the underlying cause. Contrast antegrade cystourethrography or retrograde urethrocystography should be performed to localize the site(s) of urethral obstruction before considering this technique.

Studies designed to determine the underlying cause(s) of naturally occurring lower urinary tract signs *before* and *after* urethral surgery suggest that urethrostomies may be associated with significant short-term and long-term complications.[56] They include bacterial UTIs, abnormal urethral pressure profiles, and urethral strictures. If staphylococcal UTIs develop as a result of surgical removal of the penile urethra and associated local host defense mechanisms, infection-induced struvite urocystoliths may subsequently develop.

DIAGNOSIS AND TREATMENT OF NEOPLASTIC DISORDERS

ETIOPATHOGENESIS

Although a variety of benign and malignant neoplasms of the lower urinary tract have been observed in cats (see Tables 175–3 and 175–4), transitional cell carcinomas account for approximately 50 percent. They are typically encountered in older cats with dysuria and intermittent or persistent hematuria. They may be associated with secondary bacterial UTIs. Transitional cell carcinomas are often invasive, infiltrating adjacent tissue. Because of the infrequency with which they occur, they are commonly misdiagnosed and mistreated as other forms of LUTD.

Adenocarcinomas of the prostate have been reported as causes of urethral obstruction in a few cats. We encountered a prostate adenocarcinoma in a dysuric 6-year-old male Domestic Longhair cat that caused partial obstruction of the prostate urethra. We have encountered a uterine adenocarcinoma that invaded and partially occluded the urethra of a dysuric adult female cat.

DIAGNOSIS

Occasionally, neoplastic cells may be observed by light microscopy in fresh or properly preserved urine sediment. Samples collected by catheterization are more likely to yield neoplastic cells than samples collected by cystocentesis. Lavage of the bladder lumen and cytospin preparations may increase the yield of neoplastic cells.

URO

Contrast radiography and/or ultrasonography often reveals space-occupying masses protruding into the bladder lumen and/or marked thickening and irregularity of the bladder wall. If the mass is at the trigone, contrast urography may reveal varying degrees of ureteral and bladder neck outflow obstruction. Positive-contrast urethrocystography of patients with urethral neoplasms may reveal varying degrees of luminal outflow obstruction and anatomic distortion of the urethra. Survey radiography of the chest may reveal evidence of neoplastic metastasis.

TREATMENT

Surgical extirpation of the neoplastic tissue together with an appropriate margin of adjacent tissue without severely compromising bladder function remains the treatment most likely to be successful. Unfortunately, resection of malignant lower urinary tract neoplasms has been associated with a high rate of recurrence.

DIAGNOSIS AND TREATMENT OF INFECTIOUS INFLAMMATORY DISORDERS

VIRAL URINARY TRACT INFECTIONS

Etiopathogenesis

Viruses have been implicated as causative agents of some forms of naturally occurring feline LUTD (see Tables 175–3 and 175–4).[5] See "The Virus Infection Era."

Diagnosis

Establishing a cause-and-effect relationship between viruses and various forms of feline LUTD is dependent on identifying and localizing the viruses in urinary tract tissues. Unfortunately, virus-induced disease cannot be distinguished from LUTD of other causes on the basis of clinical signs, clinical laboratory data, and light microscopic evaluation of tissues.[5] In general, diagnostic criteria for viral infections include isolation and identification of viral agents; direct demonstration of virus particles, viral antigens, or viral nucleic acids in tissues or body fluids; and/or detection and quantification of specific viral antibodies. Specific details of the diagnosis of viral UTI have been summarized elsewhere.[5] Since these procedures are not routinely available to most practicing veterinarians, the most practical step is to exclude other known causes of hematuria, dysuria, and urethral obstruction.

Treatment

Interest in antiviral chemotherapeutic and biologic agents has grown considerably. However, antiviral agents available for clinical use are relatively few in number and are limited in their antiviral specificity.[27] Antiviral agents have not been evaluated in cats with LUTD.

Management of feline LUTD suspected to be caused by viral agents has been limited to supportive and symptomatic care given during the course of clinical signs. It is noteworthy that clinical signs of hematuria and dysuria in many nonobstructed cats with the idiopathic form of LUTD spontaneously subsided approximately 7 to 10 days after diagnosis.[1, 2] Regardless of whether viruses have causative roles in idiopathic LUTD, these observations emphasize the unpredictability with which signs of feline LUTD undergo remission.

BACTERIAL URINARY TRACT INFECTION

Etiopathogenesis

Initial episodes of LUTD in young adult cats usually occur in the absence of significant numbers of detectable aerobic bacteria.[5, 57] In prospective diagnostic studies of male and female obstructed and nonobstructed cats, aerobic bacterial UTIs were identified in less than 3 percent of patients (see Table 175–2)[15, 19, 58] The infrequency with which aerobic bacteria have been isolated from urine of young adult and middle-aged cats during the initial phases of LUTD is related to highly effective local host defense mechanisms in this species.[57]

Although bacterial UTI is uncommonly encountered in young adult cats, the prevalence of UTI increases with age (see Fig. 175–5). Among 22,908 cats with LUTD, bacterial cystitis was diagnosed in 3 (males) to 4 (females) percent. The frequency with which bacterial UTI has been recognized in geriatric cats with LUTD should prompt appropriate diagnostic evaluation in this population of clinical patients.

When bacterial UTI has been detected in cats, it usually is a secondary or complicating factor rather than a primary etiologic factor. Local urinary tract defenses against bacterial infection are frequently compromised in cats with various forms of naturally occurring nonbacterial LUTD, especially if the episode is associated with urethral obstruction.

Use of indwelling transurethral catheters is associated with a high prevalence of secondary or complicating bacterial UTI. In studies of normal cats and cats with induced LUTD, catheter-induced bacteriuria was detected in 33 percent of cats after 1 day of catheterization and in 50 to 83 percent after 5 days of indwelling catheterization.[59] Bacterial UTI is also a common sequela in cats after perineal urethrostomies.

Diagnosis

A diagnosis of bacterial UTI in cats with LUTD should be based on urinalysis and quantitative urine culture. Although urinalysis findings of hematuria, pyuria, and proteinuria are consistent with bacterial infection, a diagnosis of bacterial UTI should not be based on these findings alone. In a prospective study of cats with naturally occurring LUTD, hematuria and pyuria were detected in 20 per cent of cats with idiopathic disease, 57 per cent of cats with urethral matrix-crystalline plugs, and 60 per cent of cats with urolithiasis.[15] Conversely, clinical and experimental studies in cats have demonstrated that pyuria may not be observed in urinalyses of cats with confirmed bacterial UTIs.

Quantitative urine cultures provide the most definitive means of confirming and characterizing bacterial UTIs. Detection of 1000 or more colony-forming units (CFU) per mL of urine collected by cystocentesis or catheterization is considered to indicate significant bacteriuria in cats. In urine samples collected by voluntary micturition or manual compression of the urinary bladder, detection of more than 10,000 CFU/mL may be significant. However, results of quantitative cultures of voided urine samples must be interpreted with caution. Studies of normal cats have shown that contamination of voided urine samples may result in colony counts greater than 100,000 per mL.[57]

Considering that bacterial UTIs are uncommon causes of initial episodes of feline LUTD and that most patients with significant bacteriuria have secondary or complicating UTIs, an effort should be made to identify factors that predispose to bacterial UTI. Additional diagnostic procedures that may be considered include survey and contrast radiography, ultrasonography, cystoscopy, exfoliative cytology of urine sediment, serology, and virus isolation. With the exception of neoplasia, which is uncommon in cats, exploratory cystotomies to obtain biopsy specimens do not provide information of therapeutic value. With few exceptions, we do not currently recommend them.

Treatment

Antimicrobial agents remain the cornerstone of therapy for feline bacterial UTIs. However, they should not be given indiscriminately or without clinical follow-up. The infrequency with which bacterial uropathogens are isolated from cats with LUTD emphasizes that routine use of antimicrobial agents in treating LUTD is unnecessary.

Once bacterial UTI has been confirmed, antimicrobials should be selected on the basis of susceptibility tests. Urine should be recultured 3 to 5 days after initiation of therapy to confirm sterilization of urine. Antibiotic therapy should be continued until there is clinical and laboratory evidence of response as determined by clinical signs, urinalysis, and bacterial culture. Prevention of recurrent bacterial UTI may be dependent on correction or control of abnormalities in host defenses.

FUNGAL URINARY TRACT INFECTIONS

Etiopathogenesis

Although uncommonly recognized, fungal UTIs have been reported in cats.[60] Factors predisposing to fungal UTI include local urinary tract or systemic disorders that compromise host urinary tract defenses. In addition, cats with fungal UTI may have been given symptomatic treatment for clinical signs of LUTD. In this context, many forms of therapy currently in vogue for empirical treatment of LUTD represent predisposing factors for fungal UTI. Examples include prolonged antibiotic and/or glucocorticoid administration, aciduria (optimal pH for fungal growth is 5.1 to 6.4), and indwelling transurethral catheters.[60]

Diagnosis

Yeasts observed in urine may be contaminants or pathogens. Identification of yeasts or mycelia in urine sediment of samples collected by cystocentesis eliminates the possibility of contaminants from the lower genitourinary tract samples. Detection of yeasts and fungi in two serial samples collected by voiding should be investigated further. Detection of an inflammatory response (white cells, red blood cells, and proteinuria) provides support for the interpretation that the fungi are pathogens and not contaminants.

Definitive identification of yeasts and fungi is based on their growth on Sabouraud's dextrose agar or cycloheximide-free blood agar. Culture strips designed for detection of Candida spp. may be of value (Microstix-Candida). Uncontested confirmation of fungal UTI requires demonstration of fungal organisms in urinary tract tissues.

Treatment

Because funguria may be transient, risks and benefits of therapy should be assessed for each patient's circumstances.

In patients with asymptomatic fungal UTIs, correcting identifiable predisposing factors and alkalinizing urine to a pH greater than 7.5 with potassium citrate or sodium bicarbonate may be sufficient.[60] We have not been successful in eradicating fungal UTIs with alkalinization of urine alone. Strive to eliminate predisposing factors such as indwelling transurethral catheters, immunosuppresive drugs, and antibiotics.

A more aggressive therapeutic plan may be indicated for patients with symptomatic funguria or asymptomatic patients with debilitating disease. Flucytosine has a narrow range of antifungal activity, limited primarily to yeast-like fungi such as Candidia, Torulopsis, and Cryptococcus. Unfortunately, fungal agents often become resistant to flucytosine, especially when low dosages are used. A dose of 88 mg/lb/day (divided into three or four subdoses) has been empirically suggested for cats.[60] Provided there are no undesirable side effects, this drug may be continued for 2 to 3 weeks beyond resolution of fungal UTI. Because the drug is excreted primarily in urine, appropriate dosage adjustments should be made for patients with azotemic renal failure. Adverse effects include reversible bone marrow depression, hepatic toxicity, and dermatitis.

Amphotericin B is an effective antifungal agent but is often associated with nephrotoxicity. Its use for fungal UTI has been reviewed.[60] Fluconazole may be an alternative to flucytosine and amphotericin B.

Response to treatment should be monitored by serially performed urine fungal cultures. Treatment should be continued until two successive negative urine cultures are obtained at 1- to 2-week intervals.

PARASITIC URINARY TRACT INFECTIONS

Etiopathogenesis

Although parasitic UTIs are quite prevalent in certain regions of the world, parasites are not frequently recognized as causes of feline LUTD in North America. To date, the nematode Capillaria feliscati is the only parasite that has been associated with clinical signs of feline LUTD (see Table 175–7).[5] Lack of clinical signs most likely reflects their low numbers and their superficial attachment to bladder mucosa.

Diagnosis and Treatment

Diagnosis of C. feliscati is based on identification of characteristic ova in urine sediment or visualization of adult worms in the urinary bladder. Ova of C. feliscati are bipolar, measuring 50 to 68 μm in length and 22 to 32 μm in width. Adults are small threadlike worms 13 to 45 mm in length.

Fenbendazole (11 mg/lb every 12 hours for 3 to 10 days) has been suggested.[61]

DIAGNOSIS AND TREATMENT OF URINARY INCONTINENCE

ETIOPATHOGENESIS

Normal Urinary Continence

We define micturition as function of the lower urinary tract that encompasses both a storage phase and a voiding phase. During the storage phase of micturition, the urinary

URO

bladder, acting as a low-pressure reservoir, is relaxed and fills with urine. Even though pressure in the urinary bladder gradually increases, urine remains contained within the bladder lumen because of resistance generated primarily by smooth muscle in the bladder neck and striated muscle in the urethra, which function as high-pressure unidirectional valves.

Low pressure in the bladder lumen is maintained by activity in beta-adrenergic (sympathetic) receptors via the hypogastric nerve and central inhibition of cholinergic (parasympathetic) activity. High pressure in the bladder neck and preprostatic urethra is maintained primarily by activity of alpha-adrenergic (sympathetic) receptors via the hypogastric nerve. High pressure in the postprostatic urethra is sustained primarily by skeletal (urethralis) muscle activated by the pudendal nerve.

During the voiding phase of micturition the bladder becomes a high-pressure pump, expelling urine through the urethral lumen. Simultaneously, the urethra becomes a low-pressure conduit for urine being voided from the bladder because of inhibition of alpha-adrenergic innervation to smooth muscle of the bladder neck and urethra, and inhibition of innervation to the striated urethralis muscle.

Definitions of Different Types of Urinary Incontinence

See Chapter 25.

DIAGNOSIS OF URINARY INCONTINENCE

Most causes of urinary incontinence may be classified as disorders of the storage phase of micturition. The exception is overflow (including paradoxical) urinary incontinence, which is a disorder of the voiding phase of micturition. Urinary incontinence may be: congenital or acquired, neurogenic or non-neurogenic, and constant or intermittent.

DRUGS USED FOR SYMPTOMATIC TREATMENT OF URINARY INCONTINENCE

The safety and efficacy of many drugs commonly used to treat urinary incontinence and other disorders of micturition in cats have not been evaluated by "blinded" controlled clinical trials utilizing patients with naturally occurring disease (Table 175–19). Many dosages have been extrapolated from recommendations derived for other species and personal experience.[54] Therefore, they should be used only with informed consent of clients and with compassionate precautions.

If significant side effects are associated with use of these drugs, they may be minimized by reducing the dose and/or frequency of administration. In this context, client education is important. Undesirable side effects are often associated with less frustration if clients can anticipate them, recognize the difference between nuisance side effects and significant adverse reactions, and be taught how to deal with them if they occur.

CAUSES AND TREATMENT OF ACQUIRED URINARY INCONTINENCE

Idiopathic Incompetence of the Urethral Sphincter. Urethral sphincter incompetence after neutering is less commonly observed in cats than in dogs. A diagnosis of idiopathic urethral incompetence is based on exclusion of other known causes. Estrogens should not be empirically administered to cats with idiopathic urethral sphincter incompetence on the premise that they might help but can do no harm. They may induce estrus, and high doses have the potential to cause bone marrow suppression and blood dyscrasias. Phenylpropanolamine, a nonselective alpha- and beta-adrenergic agonist, may be a safer alternative. The suggested oral dose is 0.7 to 1.0 mg/lb given every 8 hours. Sustained-release capsules of phenylpropanolamine may be considered to reduce dosage frequency provided they are properly compounded by a reputable pharmacy. Adverse events occur and caution is advised for incontinent cats that are hypertensive or have cardiovascular dysfunction.

Testosterone administered intramuscularly was reported to be effective in only one of three male cats.[62]

Trauma. Traumatic lumbar and sacral injuries may cause lower motor neuron dysfunction characterized by urine retention related to detrusor areflexia and secondary overflow incontinence. In severe cases, complete paralysis of the urinary bladder, urethra, rectum, and tail may be present. The prognosis is dependent on the severity of the injury but in severe cases is unfavorable. Several months are often required to assess the degree of reversibility of the neuromuscular dysfunction, during which time the urinary bladder must be emptied by manual compression or intermittent catheterization (Table 175–18).

Detrusor Overdistention. Overflow incontinence associated with impaired contraction of the detrusor muscle can occur as a result of prolonged overdistention of the urinary bladder. The mechanism is thought to be disruption of tight junctions between muscle cells, impairing the coordinated contraction of the detrusor muscle. When observed in cats, it is usually a sequela of urethral obstruction.

Dysautonomia. Feline dysautonomia is an idiopathic polyneuropathy characterized by widespread failure of both the sympathetic and parasympathetic components of the autonomic nervous system.[63] The cause is unknown. Dysfunction of the lower urinary tract is thought to be related to inability to contract the detrusor muscle. Voiding may be easily induced by manual compression of the urinary bladder. Management consists of supportive and symptomatic treatment.[63] Also see Section VI (The Nervous System).

Feline Leukemia–Associated Urinary Incontinence. Acquired incontinence associated with intermittent dribbling of urine during periods of relaxation has been observed in cats that test positive for feline leukemia virus (FeLV). It may be associated with anisocoria.[62, 64] The significance of the association between incontinence and feline leukemia has not been established. The incontinence may be related to urethral incompetence and/or unrestrainable contraction of the detrusor muscle. In one cat with feline leukemia–associated detrusor instability, oral administration of oxybutin chloride (an anticholinergic agent) at a dose of 0.2 mg/lb every 12 hours was associated with resolution of incontinence.[64] For patients that have an unacceptable degree of incontinence that is not responsive to symptomatic use of drugs, chemotherapy has been suggested.[65] We have no experience with use of chemotherapy in this clinical setting.

Iatrogenic Urinary Incontinence. Urethral incompetence is an uncommon neuromuscular complication of perineal urethrostomies. Urinary incontinence associated with acquired ectopic ureters has been reported as a consequence of abdominal surgery.[66]

CAUSES OF CONGENITAL URINARY INCONTINENCE

Ectopic Ureters. Ectopic ureters are less commonly recognized in cats than dogs. Continuous and sometimes intermittent incontinence is usually observed in male or female kittens in which one (50 per cent) or both (50 per cent) ureters terminate in the urethra.[67] In females, ectopic ureters occasionally terminate in the vagina. Hydroureter and pyeloectasia have been observed in approximately half the cases. Ectopic ureters terminating in the urethra may occur without urinary incontinence. Cats with bilateral ureteral ectopia may or may not void urine normally, depending on how much urine flows retrogradely into the bladder lumen. Diagnosis is confirmed by intravenous urography and retrograde contrast urethrography. The prognosis after ureteronephrectomy or transplantation of ectopic ureters terminating in the urinary bladder is usually good, provided concomitant hypoplasia of the urinary bladder or dysfunction of the urethral sphincter mechanism is not also present.

Congenital Incompetence of Urethral Sphincters. Congenital dysfunction of the urethral sphincter mechanism associated with copious incontinence has been observed in female cats.[68] This syndrome is commonly associated with other congenital defects including vaginal aplasia, bladder hypoplasia, ectopic ureters, and renal aplasia. Fair to excellent response to reconstructive surgery has been reported.

Urethrorectal Fistulas. Urethrorectal fistulas, sometimes associated with atresia ani, may cause urinary incontinence in kittens. The disorder is associated with bacterial UTI and feces-stained urethral discharges. The best option for treatment is surgical ligation or removal of the anomalous fistula.

Spinal Anomalies. Congenital paralysis of the bladder and urethra caused by lower motor neuron dysfunction secondary to myelodysplasia and vertebral anomalies may be observed in Manx kittens. Overflow incontinence is associated with urinary retention and may be associated with fecal incontinence, fecal retention, and hindlimb dysfunction. Treatment is palliative and consists of manual expression of the urinary bladder and evacuation of feces from the rectum.

DIAGNOSIS AND TREATMENT OF DYSURIC-HEMATURIC IDIOPATHIC LOWER URINARY TRACT DISEASES

DEFINITION OF IDIOPATHIC LOWER URINARY TRACT DISEASES

In a large percentage of naturally occurring cases of LUTDs, the exact causes of hematuria, pollakiuria, stranguria, periuria (urinating in inappropriate locations), and/or urethral obstruction are still unknown. After appropriate diagnostic evaluation, these cats are classified as having idiopathic LUTDs. Because there is no pathognomonic test or diagnostic procedure, diagnosis of idiopathic LUTD is dependent on exclusion of other known causes. Idiopathic LUTDs are the most commonly recognized cause of hematuria, dysuria, and/or urethral obstruction in male and female cats (see Table 175–2).

ETIOPATHOGENESIS OF IDIOPATHIC LOWER URINARY TRACT DISEASES: CURRENT STATUS

Viruses

In a prospective clinical study designed to detect causes of hematuria, dysuria, and/or urethral obstruction in 141 untreated male and female cats with naturally occurring disease, causative agents (e.g., infectious agents, uroliths, neoplasms) could not be detected in 53 per cent of the cases.[15] Although we were unable to identify viruses in urine of affected patients, no attempt was made to explant tissues for virus isolation. This fact is noteworthy in light of our ability to identify herpesvirus from explanted tissue, but not urine, of cats with induced cell-associated herpesvirus infection.[5] The subsequent course of clinical signs in many of these 77 cats was consistent with a viral etiology. Clinical signs of gross hematuria, dysuria, and pollakiuria resolved spontaneously without treatment.

Virus-like particles morphologically resembling calicivirus were present in a substantial number of crystalline-matrix urethral plugs obtained from male cats with naturally occurring urethral obstruction (see Fig. 175–1).[7] In 1998 we isolated a calicivirus from urine obtained from a nonobstructed cat with naturally occurring idiopathic LUTD. Further studies are necessary to determine whether this isolate is causally or coincidentally related to LUTD. However, on the basis of available data, we hypothesize that caliciviruses are causally related to at least some idiopathic cases of LUTD. Refer to Viral Urinary Tract Infection.

Interstitial Cystitis

With the exception of humans, naturally occurring idiopathic LUTDs have not been well characterized in other species. Interstitial cystitis (IC) is an idiopathic lower urinary tract disorder of humans. It is characterized clinically by pollakiuria, dysuria, lower abdominal pain, normal urinalysis, and distinctive cystoscopic lesions.[18] Proposed causes include bacterial and viral infections, autoimmune disease, mast cell–mediated disease, lymphatic or vascular obstruction, neurogenic disease, endocrinopathies, and defective urinary bladder urothelium.[69] There is no consistently reliable and effective treatment of IC. Although symptomatic treatment may be associated with a decrease in the severity of clinical signs, complete and permanent remission of IC has been rare.

Some cats with idiopathic LUTD have findings similar to those observed in humans with IC. They include increased urinary bladder permeability, decreased urine concentrations of GAGs, characteristic cystoscopic findings, similar gross and light microscopic changes, and lack of consistently effective treatment.[20] These similarities have prompted the hypothesis that feline idiopathic LUTD is an analogue of human IC. Similarities between the two disorders may also be coincidental representing the finite ability of the bladder and urethra to respond to a wide variety of disease processes. See The Insterstitial Cystitis Era.

SIGNALMENT OF CATS WITH IDIOPATHIC LOWER URINARY TRACT DISEASES

Nonobstructive idiopathic LUTD occurs in male and female cats of all ages but more commonly in young to middle-aged cats (mean 3.5 years, range 0.5 to 17.5 years).[15, 19] It is uncommon in cats younger than 1 year and less common in cats older than 10 years (see Fig. 175–4). There are no apparent breed predilections.

CLINICAL MANIFESTATIONS OF IDIOPATHIC LOWER URINARY TRACT DISEASES

Clinical Signs

Periuria, pollakiuria, stranguria, and gross hematuria are the most common clinical signs observed in cats with nonob-

URO

structive idiopathic LUTDs[15, 19] and often precede the obstructive form of the disorder.

Laboratory Findings

Unless complicated by concurrent illness, results of complete blood counts and biochemistry profiles of cats with nonobstructive idiopathic LUTDs are usually normal. Urine obtained from cats with idiopathic LUTDs is usually concentrated and acid. Hematuria and proteinuria in the absence of pyuria or bacteriuria are typical urinalysis findings. Although microscopic hematuria may be a consequence of cystocentesis-induced trauma, the observation of gross hematuria in 81 per cent and microscopic hematuria in 95 per cent of nonobstructed cats with idiopathic LUTDs suggests that hematuria is a prevalent feature of idiopathic LUTDs.

The prevalence, magnitude, and type of crystalluria are variable in cats with idiopathic LUTDs and do not appear to differ from those in unaffected control cats.[15] Struvite crystals have been the most common crystal type identified in urine of cats with idiopathic LUTDs. Undoubtedly, some instances of struvite crystalluria in these patients represent in vitro rather than in vivo formation.

Results of urine culture from cats with idiopathic LUTDs have been negative for aerobic bacteria, *Mycoplasma, Ureaplasma*, and viruses. Most cats with idiopathic LUTDs are seronegative for feline immunodeficiency virus antibodies and FeLV antigen.[15, 70]

Radiography and Ultrasonography

Survey abdominal radiographs of cats with nonobstructive idiopathic LUTD are usually normal. Contrast cystourethrography may be normal or may reveal thickening of the bladder wall, mucosal irregularities, urachal diverticula, and/or urethral narrowing. Ultrasonographic findings of idiopathic LUTDs have not been characterized; however, blood clots and mural irregularities or thickening may be detected.

Cystoscopy

Cystoscopic examination of cats with nonobstructive idiopathic LUTDs may reveal increased mucosal vascularity, superficial urothelial desquamation, and focal areas of submucosal hemorrhage ("glomerulations").[20] Although commonly observed in humans with an idiopathic disorder called interstitial cystitis, glomerulations are nonspecific and may be associated with bacterial, chemical, or radiation cystitis or any other urinary bladder disorder characterized by small bladder capacity.[69] In addition, cystoscopy-induced urothelial trauma may be confused with primary pathologic lesions.

Exploratory Cystotomy and Biopsy

Exploratory cystotomy has been commonly used for diagnostic evaluation of idiopathic LUTDs. With the advent of less invasive means of evaluating the lower urinary tract, the need for cystotomy and surgical biopsy of the urinary bladder for the purpose of establishing a diagnosis has largely been eliminated. Most biopsy samples reveal mucosal erosions and ulcerations and varying degrees of submucosal hemorrhage, edema, and fibrosis. These light microscopic findings are nonspecific and rarely lead to improved therapy. We cannot recommend cystotomy over less invasive diagnostic procedures for establishing a diagnosis of idiopathic LUTD.

BIOLOGIC BEHAVIOR OF IDIOPATHIC LOWER URINARY TRACT DISEASES

Clinical signs of hematuria, dysuria, and pollakiuria in many untreated nonobstructed male and female cats with acute idiopathic LUTDs frequently subside within 5 to 7 days.[1, 2] These signs may recur after variable periods of time and again subside without therapy. Our impression is that recurrent episodes of acute idiopathic LUTDs tend to decrease in frequency and severity over time.[3]

Although recurrent clinical signs in patients with idiopathic LUTDs are often assumed to indicate recurrence of the original disease, recurrent signs may also be the result of a delayed manifestation of the original disease (e.g., spontaneous or iatrogenic urethral stricture) or onset of a different disease associated with clinical manifestations similar to those of the original disorder (such as urolithiasis), or combinations of these.

We have encountered cats with hematuria and dysuria that have persisted for weeks to months and for which a specific cause was not identified. Whether chronic idiopathic LUTDs represent one extreme in the spectrum of clinical manifestations associated with similar etiologic factors or an entirely different mechanism of disease than that associated with acute self-limiting idiopathic disease is unknown.

TREATMENT OF IDIOPATHIC LOWER URINARY TRACT DISEASES

Overview

Because clinical signs associated with this form of the disease are frequently self-limiting and of short duration, any form of therapy might appear to be beneficial as long as it is not harmful. The self-limiting nature of clinical signs in many cats with idiopathic LUTDs underscores the need for controlled prospective double-blind clinical studies to prove the efficacy of various forms of therapy.

Management of cats with nonobstructive idiopathic LUTDs should encompass (1) thorough diagnostic evaluation to exclude other causes of LUTDs, (2) strategies to minimize the frequency of life-threatening sequelae (e.g., urethral obstruction), (3) client education emphasizing the lack of definitive studies and demonstrating the efficacy of proposed therapies, 4) consideration of pharmacologic agents for symptomatic management of persistent clinical signs, and (5) prevention of iatrogenic disease.

The following generalities concerning treatment of nonobstructive forms of feline idiopathic LUTDs have not all been substantiated by experimental and/or clinical investigations. Some of our recommendations are based on our uncontrolled clinical observations and personal opinions. They should be considered within this framework.

Antibacterial Agents

Antibiotics are commonly used for empirical treatment of idiopathic LUTDs. It has been well established that bacterial UTIs are uncommon in young to middle-aged cats with signs of LUTD. Indiscriminate use of antibiotics has probably contributed, to microbial strains with polyresistance to antimicrobics.

Urinary Tract Analgesics

Phenazopyridine, an azo dye that is commonly used as a urinary tract analgesic in humans, has become available as an over-the-counter preparation. Use of phenazopyridine, alone or in combination with sulfa drugs, is contraindicated in cats because they are susceptible to dose-related methemoglobinemia and irreversible oxidative changes in hemoglobin, resulting in formation of Heinz's bodies and anemia.[71]

Skeletal and Smooth Muscle Antispasmodics

Pollakiuria is a common features of feline LUTDs. Inappropriate voiding of urine occurs at low volumes of bladder filling and may be associated with sensations of pain, bladder fullness, and urgency. Presumably, pollakiuria is the result of inflammation-induced stimulation of urinary bladder sacral sensory afferent nerves. Sensations of pain and perception of fullness and urgency induce a premature micturition reflex and subsequent inappropriate or involuntary voiding of small quantities of urine. Because cholinergic parasympathetic efferents are normally responsible for detrusor contraction, anticholinergic agents may logically be considered for symptomatic treatment of pollakiuria and urge incontinence. However, the efficacy of the agents in cats with nonobstructive idiopathic LUTDs has not been established by controlled clinical trials.

The anticholinergic agent propantheline minimizes the force and frequency of uncontrolled detrusor contractions but has a negligible effect on urethral sphincter pressure. Propantheline may reduce the severity of pollakiuria in nonobstructed cats. It has a rapid onset of action. However, care must be taken to prevent urine retention as a result of excessive doses. Other potential adverse effects include tachycardia, vomiting, and constipation. An empirical dose of 0.1 to 0.2 mg/lb orally every 12 to 24 hours has been suggested. Further studies using appropriate doses and maintenance intervals are required to substantiate a beneficial symptomatic effect of propantheline in cats with severe pollakiuria.

Other smooth muscle (oxybutynin, phenoxybenzamine, acepromazine, prazosin) and skeletal muscle (dantrolene, diazepam) antispasmotics have been recommended for the symptomatic management of urethrospasm associated with LUTDs.[71] Although some of these pharmacologic agents produce significant decreases in intraurethral pressure in normal male cats and cats with naturally occurring urethral obstruction,[55, 71] the role of urethral smooth or skeletal muscle spasm in producing clinical signs associated with idiopathic LUTD is unknown. In cats with urethral obstruction of unspecified causes, intraurethral pressures before administration of antispasmodics were not significantly different from those of normal nonobstructed male cats. Similar studies in cats with idiopathic forms of LUTD have not been performed. On the basis of available data, we are unable to recommend smooth or skeletal muscle antispasmodics to treat idiopathic LUTDs.

Anti-Inflammatory Agents

Overview

Lack of specific therapy for cats with idiopathic LUTDs has stimulated interest in anti-inflammatory agents to reduce the severity of clinical signs. However, there have been only a few controlled clinical trials to study the short- and long-term effectiveness of anti-inflammatory agents in the symptomatic treatment of dysuria and hematuria in cats. Hematuria and dysuria in cats with idiopathic LUTDs are often self-limiting.

Glucocorticoids

By virtue of their potent anti-inflammatory properties, glucocorticoids are a logical therapeutic choice to minimize dysuria and hematuria in cats with idiopathic LUTDs. Results of a double-blind placebo-controlled study of untreated male and female cats with idiopathic LUTDs indicate that anti-inflammatory doses of prednisolone (0.44 mg/lb by mouth every 12 hours for 10 days) were of no significant benefit in reducing the magnitude and duration of clinical signs in affected cats.[2] Clinical signs subsided within 1 to 2 days and hematuria and pyuria in 2 to 5 days in both groups. The inconsistency of favorable clinical responses and potential adverse effects associated with glucocorticoids suggest that these agents should be used cautiously, if at all, in cats with idiopathic LUTDs.

Dimethyl Sulfoxide

Dimethyl sulfoxide (DMSO) is an analgesic anti-inflammatory agent with weak antibacterial, antifungal, and antiviral activity.[71] DMSO has been used to treat LUTDs in cats on the basis of its reported efficacy in humans with IC. Dosages and frequency of administration of DMSO have been empirical. Intravesicular instillation of 10 to 20 mL of 10 per cent DMSO was associated with amelioration of clinical signs in three cats with chronic LUTD.[71] However, appropriately controlled clinical trials to evaluate the effectiveness of local instillation of DMSO into the urinary bladder of cats with idiopathic disease have not been reported. In one controlled study of cats with induced chemical cystitis, intravesicular administration of 45 per cent DMSO for 3 days was of no benefit in minimizing bacterial infection or inflammation.[59] Licensed products available to veterinarians contain 90 per cent DMSO and are not pyrogen free; licensed products available to physicians contain 50 per cent DMSO and are pyrogen free. Side effects of intravesicular DMSO administration in normal cats and cats with idiopathic LUTDs have apparently not been evaluated. Pending further studies, we do not recommend its use.

Piroxicam

Piroxicam, a nonsteroidal anti-inflammatory drug, has been empirically suggested to reduce dysuria and pollakiuria in cats with idiopathic LUTDs. The empirical dose is 0.12 mg/lb by mouth every 24 hours. Pending double-blind controlled clinical trials, it is not possible to make recommendations about the safety and efficacy of piroxicam for treating cats with idiopathic LUTDs.

Glycosaminoglycans

Transitional epithelium of the urinary bladder is covered by a thin layer of hydrated extracellular macromolecules called GAGs. Urothelial GAGs play an important role in preventing adherence of microorganisms and crystals to the bladder urothelium and limiting transepithelial movement of urine proteins and other ionic and nonionic solutes.[72] Quantitative or qualitative defects in surface GAGs and subsequent increased urothelial permeability have been hypothesized to be a causative factor in the pathogenesis of feline idiopathic IC.[20]

Oral or intravesicular administration of GAGs is commonly used in humans for management of IC. Pentosan polysulfate sodium (Elmiron) is a semisynthetic low-molecu-

URO

lar-weight heparin analogue that has been shown to reinforce urothelial GAGs and reduce transitional cell injury.[73] Symptomatic remission was observed in approximately one third of human patients with IC treated with oral or intravesicular pentosan polysulfate sodium compared with approximately one fifth of patients treated with a placebo.[74, 75] Prolongation of prothrombin time, epistaxis, gingival bleeding, alopecia, abdominal pain, diarrhea, and nausea have been observed uncommonly in humans treated with pentosan polysulfate sodium. Despite promising results of studies in other species, the safety and efficacy of pentosan polysulfate sodium or other GAG preparations for treatment of feline idiopathic LUTD have not been evaluated by controlled clinical trials. We urge caution in the use of GAGs to treat idiopathic LUTD.

Amitriptyline

Amitriptyline (Elavil) has been advocated for symptomatic therapy of feline idiopathic LUTDs.[76] Amitriptyline is a tricyclic antidepressant and anxiolytic drug with anticholinergic, antihistaminic, anti–alpha-adrenergic, anti-inflammatory, and analgesic properties. Anecdotal reports and limited data suggest that administration of amitriptyline to some cats with chronic idiopathic forms of LUTDs results in amelioration of clinical signs. Consequently, amitriptyline has gained popularity as an agent for symptomatic therapy of feline idiopathic LUTD. As is the case for humans, appropriately controlled clinical studies designed to evaluate the effectiveness of amitriptyline in controlling signs in cats with idiopathic forms of LUTDs have not been reported.

Dose, frequency, and duration of amitriptyline therapy are entirely empirical. A dose of 5 to 10 mg per cat by mouth every 24 hours given at night has been suggested; dosage should be adjusted to produce a slight calming effect on the cat.[76] Sedation, urine retention, neutropenia, thrombocytopenia, weight gain, and an unkempt haircoat have been observed in cats treated with amitriptyline. We urge caution in the use of amitriptyline to treat idiopathic LUTD.

Urohydrodistention

Controlled distention of the urinary bladder during cystoscopy reportedly alleviates clinical signs in some cats with idiopathic LUTDs.[77] However, the efficacy of urohydrodistention has not been evaluated by appropriately controlled clinical trials. Currently, establishing a diagnosis of idiopathic LUTD requires retrograde contrast radiography and/or cystoscopy (both of which distend the urinary bladder). Until other, more specific, markers of idiopathic LUTD are identified, it is difficult to differentiate the beneficial effects of bladder distention for diagnostic purposes from those induced by other forms of therapy.

Stress Reduction

Stress may play a role in precipitating or exacerbating clinical signs associated with idiopathic LUTDs.[20] Stress is an unlikely primary cause of idiopathic LUTDs. Environmental stress may be reduced by minimizing changes in the home, maintaining a constant diet, and providing toys and hiding places.[25]

REFERENCES

1. Kruger JM, Osborne CA: Recurrent nonobstructive idiopathic feline lower urinary tract disease: An illustrative case report. J Am Anim Hosp Assoc 31:312, 1995.
2. Osborne CA, Kruger JM, Lulich JP, et al: Prednisolone therapy of idiopathic feline lower urinary tract disease. A double blind study. Vet Clin North Am 26:563, 1996.
3. Osborne CA, Kruger JM, Lulich JP: Feline lower urinary tract disease: The Minnesota experience. Proceedings 15th Annual ACVIM Forum, San Antonio, 1997, p 338.
4. Schecter RD: The significance of bacteria in feline cystitis and urolithiasis. JAVMA 156:1567, 1970.
5. Kruger JM, Osborne CA: The role of uropathogens in feline lower urinary tract disease. Vet Clin North Am 23:101, 1993.
6. Fabricant CG: Herpesvirus-induced urolithiasis in specific-pathogen-free male cats. Am J Vet Res 38:1837, 1977.
7. Osborne CA, Kruger JM, Lulich JP, et al: Feline matrix-crystalline urethral plugs: A unifying hypothesis of causes. J Small Anim Pract 33:172, 1992.
8. Osborne CA, Lulich JP, Thumchai R, et al; Feline urolithiasis. Etiology and pathophysiology. Vet Clin North Am 26:217, 1996.
9. Finco DR, Barsanti JA, Crowell WA: Characterization of magnesium-induced urinary disease in the cat and comparison with feline urologic syndrome. Am J Vet Res 46:391, 1985.
10. Osborne CA, Abdullahi SU, Polzin DJ, et al: Current status of medical dissolution of canine and feline uroliths. Columbus, OH, 1983 Kal Kan Symposium for the Treatment of Small Animal Diseases, 1983, p 53.
11. Osborne CA, Lulich JP, Kruger JM, et al: Medical dissolution of feline struvite urocystoliths. JAVMA 196:1053, 1990.
12. Buffington CA, Rogers QR, Morris JG, et al: Feline struvite urolithiasis: Magnesium effect depends on urinary pH. Feline Pract 15:29, 1985.
13. Jackson JR, Kealy RD, Lawler DF, et al: Long-term safety of urine acidifying diets for cats. Vet Clin Nutr 2:100, 1995.
14. Osborne CA, Johnston GR, Kruger JM, et al: Etiopathogenesis and biological behavior of feline vesicourachal diverticula. Don't just do something—Stand there. Vet Clin North Am 17:697, 1987.
15. Kruger JM, Osborne CA, Goyal SM, et al: Clinical evaluation of cats with lower urinary tract disease. JAVMA 199:221, 1991.
16. Osborne CA, Kroll RA, Lulich JP, et al: Medical management of vesicourachal diverticula in 15 cats with lower urinary tract disease. J Small Anim Pract 30:608, 1989.
17. Buffington CA, Chew DJ, Dibartola SP: Lower urinary tract disease in cats: Is diet still a cause? JAVMA 205:1524, 1994.
18. Simon LJ, Landis R, Erickson DR, et al: The Interstitial Cystitis Data Base Study: Concepts and preliminary baseline descriptive statistics. Urology 49(Suppl 5A):64, 1997.
19. Buffington CAT, Chew DJ, Kendall MS, et al: Clinical evaluation of cats with nonobstructive urinary tract diseases. JAVMA 210:46, 1997.
20. Buffington CAT, Chew DJ, DiBartola SP: Interstitial cystitis in cats. Vet Clin North Am 26:317, 1996.
21. Buffington CA, Chew DJ: Does interstitial cystitis occur in cats? In Bonagura JD (ed): Current Veterinary Therapy XII. Philadelphia, WB Saunders, 1995, p 1009.
22. Elbadawi A: Interstitial cystitis: A critique of current concepts with a new proposal for pathologic diagnosis and pathogenesis. Urology 49(Suppl 5A):14, 1997.
23. Osborne CA, Johnston GR, Polzin DJ, et al: Redefinition of the feline urologic syndrome. Feline lower urinary tract disease with heterogeneous causes. Vet Clin North Am 14:409, 1984.
24. Osborne CA, Kruger JM, Lulich JP: Feline lower urinary tract disorders. Definition of terms and concepts. Vet Clin North Am 26:169, 1996.
25. Osborne CA, Kruger JM, Lulich JP, et al: Feline lower urinary tract disorders. In Ettinger SJ (ed): Textbook of Veterinary Internal Medicine, 4th ed, Vol 2. Philadelphia, WB Saunders, 1995, p 1805.
26. Lawler DF, Jolin DW, Collins JE: Incidence rates of feline lower urinary tract disease in the United States. Feline Pract 15:13, 1985.
27. AVMA Membership Directory and Resource Guide. American Veterinary Medical Association, Schaumburg, IL, 1997, p 29.
28. Willeberg P: Epidemiology of naturally occurring feline urologic syndrome. Vet Clin North Am 14:455, 1984.
29. Beaver BV: Disorders of behavior. In Sherding RG (ed): The Cat: Diseases and Clinical Management, 2nd ed, Vol 1. Philadelphia, WB Saunders, 1994, p 191.
30. Hart BL: Behavioral and pharmacologic approaches to problem urination in cats. Vet Clin North Am 26:651, 1996.
31. Scrivani PV, Chew DJ, Buffington CAT, et al: Results of double-contrast cystography in cats with idiopathic cystitis: 45 cases (1993–1995). JAVMA 212:1907, 1998.
32. Lewis LD, Chow FHC, Taton GF, et al: Effects of various dietary mineral concentrations on the occurrence of feline urolithiasis. JAVMA 172:559, 1978.
33. Osborne CA, Kruger JM, Lulich JP, et al: Feline lower urinary tract disease: Relationships between crystalluria, urinary tract infections, and host factors. In August JR (ed): Consultations in Feline Internal Medicine. Philadelphia, WB Saunders, 1994, p 351.
34. Hesse A, Sanders G: A survey of urolithiasis in cats. J Small Anim Pract 26:465, 1985.
35. Lulich JP, Osborne CA, Polzin DJ, et al: Incomplete removal of canine and feline urocystoliths by cystotomy. Proceedings 11th ACVIM Forum, Washington, DC, 1993, p 397.
36. Osborne CA, Lulich JP, Kruger JM, et al: Medical dissolution of feline struvite urocystoliths. JAVMA 196:1053, 1990.
37. Lulich JP, Osborne CA: Catheter assisted retrieval of urocystoliths from dogs and cats. JAVMA 201:111, 1992.
38. Lulich JP, Osborne CA, Carlson M, et al: Nonsurgical removal of urocystoliths in dogs and cats by voiding urohydropropulsion. JAVMA 23:660, 1993.

39. Duval D, Barsanti JA, Cornelius LM, et al: Ammonium acid urate urolithiasis in a cat. Feline Pract 23:18, 1995.
40. Kirk CA, Ling GV, Franti CE, et al: Evaluation of factors associated with development of calcium oxalate urolithiasis in cats. JAVMA 207:1429, 1995.
41. Thumchai R, Lulich JP, Osborne CA, et al: Epizootiology evaluation of 3498 feline uroliths: 1982–1992. JAVMA 208:547, 1996.
42. McKerrell RE: Primary hyperoxaluria (L-glyceric aciduria) in the cat. In Grunsell CSG, Raw ME (eds): The Veterinary Annual, 31st ed. London, Blackwell Scientific, 1991, p 180.
43. Lulich JP, Osborne CA, Parker ML, et al: Evaluation of urine and serum analytes in miniature schnauzers with calcium oxalate urolithiasis. Am J Vet Res 52:1538, 1991.
44. Curhan GC, Willet WC, Speizer FE, et al: Comparison of dietary calcium with supplemental calcium and other nutrients as factors affecting the risk for kidney stones in women. Ann Intern Med 126:497, 1997.
45. Bai SC, Sampson DA, Morris JG, et al: Vitamin B_6 requirement of growing kittens. J Nutr 119:1020,1989.
46. Lulich JP, Osborne CA, Thumchai R, et al: Epidemiology of canine calcium oxalate uroliths: Identifying risk factors. Vet Clin North Am, 29:113, 1999.
47. Osborne CA, Lulich JP, Thumchai R, et al: Diagnosis, medical treatment, and prognosis of feline urolithiasis. Vet Clin North Am 26:589, 1996.
48. Osborne CA, Sanderson SL, Lulich JP, et al: Canine cystine urolithiasis: Cause, detection, treatment, and prevention. Vet Clin North Am, 29:193, 1999.
49. Osborne CA, Lulich JP, Kruger JM, et al: Feline urethral plugs: Etiology and pathophysiology. Vet Clin North Am 26:233, 1996.
50. Osborne CA, Kruger JM. Lulich JP, et al: Medical management of feline urethral obstruction. Vet Clin North Am 26:483, 1996.
51. Barsanti JA, Finco DR, Brown SA: The role of dimethyl sulfoxide and glucocorticoids in lower urinary tract diseases. In Bonagura JD (ed): Current Veterinary Therapy, Vol 12. Philadelphia, WB Saunders, 1995, p 1011.
52. Nickel JC, Gristina AG, Coserton JW, et al: Electron microscopic study of an infected Foley catheter. Can J Surg 54:50, 1985.
53. Osborne CA, Sanderson SL, Lulich JP, et al: Medical management of iatrogenic rents in the wall of the feline urinary bladder. Vet Clin North Am 26:551, 1996.
54. Lane IF: Pharmacologic management of feline lower urinary tract disorders. Vet Clin North Am 26:515, 1996.
55. Straeter-Knowlen IM, et al: Urethral pressure response to smooth and skeletal muscle relaxants in anesthetized adult male cats with naturally acquired urethral obstruction. Am J Vet Res 56:919, 1995.
56. Osborne CA, Caywood DD, Johnston GR, et al: Feline perineal urethrostomy: A potential cause of feline lower urinary tract disease. Vet Clin North Am 26:535, 1996.
57. Lees GE: Bacterial urinary tract infections. Vet Clin North Am 26:297, 1996.
58. Senior DF, Brown MB: The role of Mycoplasma species and Ureaplasma species in feline lower urinary tract disease. Vet Clin North Am 26:305, 1996.
59. Barsanti JA, Shotts EB, Crowell WA, et al: Effect of therapy on susceptibility to urinary tract infection in male cats with indwelling urethral catheters. J Vet Intern Med 6:64, 1992.
60. Lulich JP, Osborne CA: Fungal infections of the feline lower urinary tract. Vet Clin North Am 26:309, 1996.
61. Brown SA, Prestwood AK: Parasites of the urinary tract. In Kirk RW (ed): Current Veterinary Therapy, Vol 9. Philadelphia, WB Saunders, 1986, p 1153.
62. Barsanti JA, Downey R: Urinary incontinence in cats. J Am Anim Hosp Assoc 20:979, 1984.
63. Nash AS: Clinical features and management of feline dysautonomia. J Small Anim Pract 28:339, 1987.
64. Lappin MR, Barsanti JA: Urinary incontinence secondary to idiopathic detrusor instability: Cystometrographic diagnosis and pharmacologic management in 2 dogs and a cat. JAVMA 191:1439, 1987.
65. Ling GV: Lower Urinary Tract Diseases of Dogs and Cats. St Louis, CV Mosby, 1995.
66. Allen WE, Webbon PM: Two cases of urinary incontinence in cats associated with acquired vagino-ureteral fistula. J Small Anim Pract 21:367, 1980.
67. Osborne CA, Johnston GR, Kruger JM: Ectopic ureters and ureteroceles. In Osborne CA, Finco DR (eds): Canine and Feline Nephrology and Urology. Philadelphia, Williams & Wilkins, 1995, p 608.
68. Holt PE, Gibbs C: Congenital urinary incontinence in cats: A review of 19 cases. Vet Rec 130:437, 1992.
69. Messing M: Interstitial cystitis and related syndromes. In Walsh PC et al (eds): Campbell's Urology, 6th ed. Philadelphia, WB Saunders, 1992, p 982.
70. Barsanti JA, Brown J, Marks A, et al: Relationship of lower urinary tract signs to seropositivity for feline immunodeficiency virus in cats. J Vet Intern Med 10:34, 1996.
71. Kruger JM, Osborne CA, Lulich JP: Management of nonobstructive idiopathic feline lower urinary tract disease. Vet Clin North Am 26:571, 1996.
72. Parsons CL, Boychuk D, Jones S, et al: Bladder surface glycosaminoglycans: An epithelial permeability barrier. J Urol 143:139, 1990.
73. Parsons CL, Schmidt JD, Pollen J: Successful treatment of interstitial cystitis with sodium pentosanpolysulfate. J Urol 130:51, 1983.
74. Parson CL, Benxon G, Childs SJ, et al: Quantitatively controlled method to study prospectively interstitial cystitis and demonstrate efficacy of pentosanpolysulfate. J Urol 150:845, 1993.
75. Anonymous: Pentosan for interstitial cystitis (letter). Med Lett Drugs Ther 39:56, 1997.
76. Chew DJ, Buffington CAT, Kendall MS, et al: Amitriptyline treatment for severe recurrent idiopathic cystitis in cats. JAVMA 213:1282, 1998.
77. Buffington CAT, Chew DJ: Idiopathic lower urinary tract disease in cats—Is it interstitial cystitis? Proceedings 13th ACVIM Forum, Orlando, FL, 1995, p 517.

URO

CHAPTER 176

CANINE LOWER URINARY TRACT DISORDERS

Jody P. Lulich, Carl A. Osborne, Joseph W. Bartges, and Chalermpol Lekcharoensuk

The lower urinary tract is a specialized organ system devoted to the storage and periodic release of urine. It consists of the urinary bladder and urethra. The portion of the upper urinary tract (ureter) lying within the bladder wall forms the vesicoureteral valve. This unique connection between the ureter and bladder, as well as the large compliance of the urinary bladder, promotes unidirectional flow of urine and protects the upper urinary tract from bacterial invasion and hydronephrosis.

Because the urinary bladder functions as a reservoir for hypertonic urine, it was thought to be impermeable to water; however, a variety of structural as well as functional processes are required to maintain the unique composition of urine. Active transport of urine sodium regulated by aldosterone suggests a functional similarity between the bladder and distal tubules of the kidney. Sodium channels in the urinary bladder wall are regulated by prostaglandins, urokinase, and kallikrein.[1] Although urothelial impermeability has been inferred from the presence of tight junctions between apical cells lining the bladder, inactivation of the glycosaminoglycan layer lining the urinary bladder of rabbits increased urea permeability.[2] These illustrations emphasize that the lower urinary tract performs multiple functions. It serves to preserve fluid and electrolyte balance by maintaining urine composition, protects against pyelonephritis and hydronephrosis, and maintains urinary continence. No other epithelia are known to perform all these functions; therefore, no adequate replacement for the urinary bladder exists.[3, 4] Care must be used to maintain lower urinary tract structure and function by appropriate diagnosis and disease management.

EPIDEMIOLOGY

Between 1980 and 1993, diseases of the lower urinary tract occurred in 3 per cent of dogs (20,001 of 676,668) admitted to the 24 veterinary colleges in North America that register data with the Veterinary Medical Data Base at Purdue University. Of the 20,001 cases of lower urinary tract disease recorded, 57.4 per cent (11,474) occurred in female dogs and 42.4 per cent (8,168) occurred in male dogs. Females had a slight, but significantly higher risk of lower urinary tract disease (95 per cent confidence interval for relative risk = 1.28 to 1.32) than males.

The proportion of dogs evaluated for lower urinary tract disease at veterinary colleges increased with advancing age. Diseases of the urinary bladder and urethra were reported in less than 1 per cent of dogs younger than 1 year of age (Fig. 176–1). By contrast, the proportion with lower urinary tract disease was greater than 6.5 per cent in dogs older than 10 years old.

The three most commonly reported diseases affecting the lower urinary tract were cystitis (40 per cent), urinary incontinence (24 per cent), and urolithiasis (18 per cent). In most cases, the underlying cause of cystitis was not specified; however, bacterial urinary tract infections (UTIs) were diagnosed in half of the cases. The majority of the dogs with urinary incontinence (see Chapter 25) were female (71 per cent, 3,433 of 4,811 dogs), and the majority of female dogs with urinary incontinence were neutered (79 per cent, 2,722 of 3,433 female dogs). In contrast to dogs with urinary incontinence, urolithiasis predominated in males (58 per cent of dogs were male and 42 per cent were female).

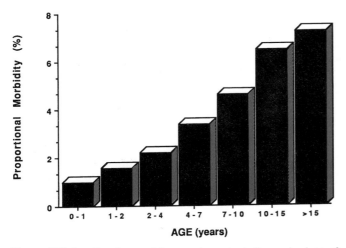

Figure 176–1. Prevalence of lower urinary tract disease in dogs of different ages based on 676,668 dogs admitted to 24 veterinary colleges in North America as entered into the Veterinary Medical Data Base at Purdue University.

PATTERN	LOCATION
Independent of urination	Urethra, genital tract
Beginning of urination	Urethra, genital tract
Throughout urination	Kidney, coagulopathy
End of urination	Urinary bladder

TABLE 176–1. LOCALIZING HEMATURIA

LOCALIZING CLINICAL SIGNS

Clinical signs localizing disease to the lower urinary tract include dysuria, pollakiuria, stranguria, hematuria, and urinary incontinence. Most lower urinary tract diseases lack signs associated with systemic illness. Development of uremia as a result of mucosal tears or obstruction of the lower urinary tract is a notable exception to this generality. Because of close communication with the kidney, systemic signs also result from disease processes that concurrently affect both the lower and upper urinary tracts (see Chapters 23 through 28 and Table 176–1).

DIAGNOSTIC TECHNIQUES FOR LOWER URINARY TRACT DISEASE

EVALUATION OF URINE

Urinalysis. A urinalysis is a simple, inexpensive, specific, and sensitive test for lower urinary tract disorders. A complete urinalysis includes visual inspection of urine, measurement of solute concentration (usually specific gravity), evaluation of chemical constituents (reagent strip), and microscopic examination of urine sediment.[5] Proper interpretation of urinalysis results requires knowledge of the solute concentration of urine and the method of urine collection. For example, a protein determination of 1 + or observation of four leukocytes per high-power field may be normal in a dog with a urine specific gravity of 1.045. In a patient with a urine specific gravity of 1.008, however, the same values should arouse suspicion of disease.

Several methods are used to collect urine. Knowledge of how the sample was collected is helpful to interpret results and localize disease. Cystocentesis is the preferred method because it is a safe, simple, and rapid method of obtaining urine for diagnostic and therapeutic evaluation. Cystocentesis provides samples free of vaginal and preputial contaminants; and when proper technique is used in a relaxed patient, it has virtually no adverse effects. If the urinary bladder is difficult to palpate, ultrasound can be used to guide the cystocentesis needle into the bladder lumen. We routinely use a 1.5-inch 22-gauge needle attached to a dry sterile syringe. Intravenous tubing and a three-way stopcock are attached between the needle and syringe, when large quantities of urine are to be removed.

Voided urine samples (midsteam) can be collected from patients if the urinary bladder cannot be localized or stabilized sufficiently for cystocentesis. Collection of midstream samples minimizes contamination. Collection of samples by voiding is recommended to collect urine from patients with ascites in which sampling of ascitic fluid can be mistaken for urine. Urethral and prostatic diseases may be best evaluated with a voided sample (initial stream) or by comparison of results of analysis of voided and cystocentesis samples. Manual bladder expression or transurethral catheterization of the urinary bladder can be performed. However, urinary catheterization is associated with risk of iatrogenic trauma and nosocomial infection.

Urine Culture. Failure to demonstrate bacteria by urine sediment examination does not rule out bacteriuria. The gold standard for the diagnosis of UTI is quantitative urine culture. Failure to perform urine cultures or failure to properly interpret the results of urine cultures may lead not only to diagnostic error but also to therapeutic failure.

DIAGNOSTIC IMAGING

Radiography is a valuable technique in the diagnosis of lower urinary tract disorders. Although survey radiography is adequate for a diagnosis of radiodense uroliths or for the assessment of bladder position, contrast medium–enhanced procedures are needed for evaluation of mucosal irregularities, diverticula, urine leakage, and radiolucent uroliths. Double-contrast cystography is the preferred technique because it provides the best evaluation of the mucosal surface. The normal empty canine urinary bladder can be moderately distended by injecting 3 mL of fluid or air per pound of body weight; however, palpation of the urinary bladder should be used as the primary method to minimize overdistention during filling. To avoid air embolization, carbon dioxide or nitrous oxide is preferable to air for negative contrast. One report suggested a minimum of three orthrogonal radiographic views to evaluate the bladder: right and left lateral and the ventrodorsal.[5] Superimposition of the vertebral column over the urinary bladder reduces the value of the ventrodorsal view. Therefore, either the right or left oblique view is preferred. Retrograde positive contrast urethrography or voiding cystourethrography will allow visualization of structural defects of the urethra.

Urinary obstruction resulting from radiolucent structures (e.g. urate uroliths, polyps, urethral vales, peduculated neoplasms) is best identified using antigrade positive contrast urography. The bladder is filled with contrast medium by means of transabdominal cystocentesis, transurethral catheterization, and renal excretion after intravenous administration. Once full, the urinary bladder is expressed, forcing urine in a normograde direction to the site of obstruction.

Fluoroscopic evaluation of cystography can assist identification of functional disorders of micturition. Mucosa proliferation and blood clots are best evaluated by ultrasonography. Computed tomography and magnetic resonance imaging are valuable if vascular disorders are suspected.[6]

CYSTOURETHROSCOPY

Cystourethroscopy, although useful and easily performed with appropriate equipment, has not achieved the degree of application that endoscopy has for evaluation of gastrointestinal disease. One explanation for this may be the ease with which lower urinary tract diseases are detected by simpler procedures.

A variety of equipment can be used to visualize the urinary tract. The urethral orifice can be examined with a vaginoscope or otoscope. To evaluate more proximal portions, an arthroscope is easily inserted into the urethral lumen of most dogs. Flexible pediatric bronchoscopes may be used to visualize the urinary bladder.[7] Depending on the size of the urethra in relation to the size of the cystoscope, urethral dilation or pre-pubic percutaneous cystoscopy may be required.[8, 9]

BIOPSY OF THE LOWER URINARY TRACT

Many options are available to obtain tissue for microscopic evaluation. If structures can be palpated abdominally or rectally, they can be aspirated with a needle and syringe. Use of the Franzen needle guide is ideal for transrectal aspiration of urethral or prostatic structures (Fig. 176–2).[10] The advantages of fine-needle aspiration relate to the speed with which samples can be obtained and viewed and a diagnosis established with practically no risk to the patient. When larger tissue samples are required, they can be obtained by catheter biopsy, ultrasound-guided catheter biopsy,[11] cystoscopy, and pinch biopsy or, when the urinary bladder is friable, by celiotomy and core resection. A practical alternative to these procedures is the use of endoscopy biopsy forceps without the endoscope (Fig. 176–3).[12] Routine biopsy forceps can be easily inserted into the urethra of most male and female dogs and female cats (Table 176–2). Diffuse mucosal abnormalities or lesions at the apex of the urinary bladder can be sampled blindly. Localized lesions can be reached with the aid of palpation, cystoscopy, fluoroscopy, or ultrasonography.

OTHER TESTS AND PROCEDURES

Results of hematology tests and serum chemistries seldom indicate abnormalities, except when disease processes extend beyond the lower urinary tract. Bladder wash cytology may be helpful in cases of suspected neoplasia. An alternative to this procedure is detection of basic fibroblastic growth factor,

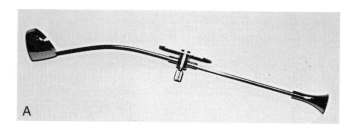

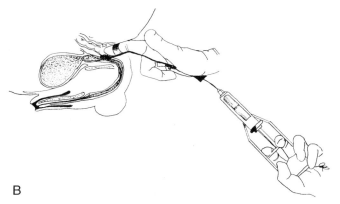

Figure 176–2. Urethral biopsy using Franzen needle guide. *A*, Franzen needle guide (can be obtained from Secureline: 800-847-0670). *B*, Urethral biopsy: (1) Place guide on gloved index finger. If desired, a second glove can be placed over the guide. (2) Introduce index finger and guide into rectum. (3) Locate urethral lesion by palpation. (4) Insert long aspiration needle (with syringe attached) into guide. Continue inserting needle until the tip enters the lesion. (5) Aspirate tissue into needle by pulling back syringe piston. Release piston. For additional samples redirect needle and aspirate. (6) Remove needle, and expel tissue on microscope slide. (7) Stain, mount, and view specimen.

URO

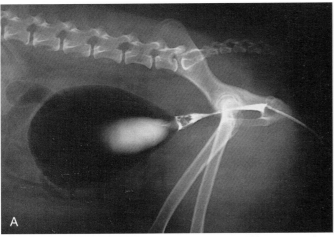
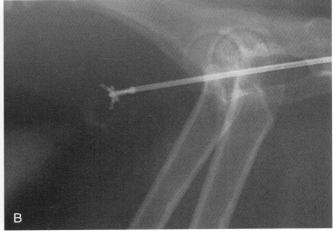

Figure 176–3. Retrograde urethrogram of an 11-year-old American Eskimo dog with a proliferative mass in the neck of the urinary bladder *(A)*. Endoscopy forceps were used to obtain a biopsy of the mass after its position was localized with fluoroscopy *(B)*. Microscopic evaluation confirmed a transitional cell carcinoma.

a marker for transitional cell carcinoma.[13] A commercial kit detecting basic fibroblast growth factor reliably identified dogs with transitional cell carcinoma. Ten per cent of dogs with UTI were also positive for basic fibroblast growth factor. Ultrasound transducers contained within 2-mm diameter catheters can provide endoluminal ultrasonography of the urethra, urinary bladder, ureters, and renal pelvis.[14] Cystometry and urethral profilometry are useful in the diagnosis and prognosis of urinary incontinence.

AVOID CREATING DIAGNOSTIC CHAOS

Once the problem has been defined, diagnostic chaos can be created by relying on information from inappropriately collected samples (Table 176–3). Sometimes conditions of sample collection or client impatience may result in less than ideal sampling. For example, urine samples collected by owners are routinely used to diagnose and monitor urinary disease. However, owners may collect urine in improperly rinsed containers, allow samples to dehydrate, or store samples at improper temperatures. In our hospital, midstream urine collections are commonly adulterated with debris, resulting from the patient stepping into the collection container. For us to expect our clients to achieve cleaner samples is usally too great an expectation. When questionable results occur in samples collected under less than ideal conditions, interpretation of results should encompass the possibility (or probability) that in vitro factors may have influenced the test result. To clarify the ambiguities, the test should be repeated under more suitable conditions.

Once an appropriate sample is collected, verifying the diagnosis requires accurate interpretations of appropriate tests. But not all tests are created equal. In fact, some diagnostic test results should not be relied on at all (Table 176–4).

Before attempting to interpret the significance of results, one should determine whether any medications have been given, the type of diet the patient is receiving, the method of urine collection, the method of urine preservation, and the specific gravity. A common cause of abnormal urinalysis results and potential misdiagnosis is associated with therapy before sample collection.

TABLE 176–2. PERFORMING FORCEPS BIOPSY WITHOUT AN ENDOSCOPE

Obtaining tissue samples using the endoscopy forceps is similar to methods used to obtain gastrointestinal mucosa with an endoscope. Because the endoscope is not inserted into the urethra, other methods, such as palpation or radiography, are needed to localize the lesion and direct the biopsy forceps.

1. Allow the patient to void urine before biopsy. If micturition is difficult owing to partial or complete obstruction, urine can be removed by transurethral catheterization or decompressive cystocentesis.
2. Sedate or anesthetize the patient. For many dogs general anesthesia is not needed. However, mild tranquilization may facilitate urethral catheterization and palpation of the urethra and bladder and will minimize patient discomfort and anxiety.
3. Identify the site for biopsy by palpation, catheterization, and/or radiography.
4. With the grasping unit at the end of the forceps closed, insert the flexible endoscopy forceps (not the endoscope) into the urethra.
5. Advance the forceps until the grasping unit is near the area to be sampled. The tip of the grasping unit can be positioned by abdominal palpation, rectal palpation, radiography, fluoroscopy, or ultrasonography. For most urethral lesions, the biopsy site is easily determined during insertion and advancement of the forceps through the urethral lumen; increased friction and force are often required to advance the forceps at the biopsy site. For diffuse urothelial lesions, the apex of the bladder can be sampled by advancing the forceps to the most cranial portion of the bladder.
6. After the biopsy forceps is properly positioned, open the grasping unit and slightly advance the forceps against the lesion.
7. Close the grasping unit. With the grasping unit closed, the forceps and tissue samples are retracted from the urinary tract.
8. The biopsy sample can be removed from the forceps by lifting the sample from the cup of the grasping unit with a 22- or 25-gauge needle. The sample should then be transferred to formalin for histologic processing.
9. Impression smears for immediate cytologic evaluation can be made before placing the sample in formalin. Tissue samples are first lightly blotted on filter paper or dry gauze pads to remove surface blood. Then impressions are made on glass slides and stained before microscopic evaluation.
10. Several samples should be retrieved to ensure complete representation of the area in question.
11. Administration of antimicrobials is indicated because the integrity of the mucosal surface of the lower urinary tract is damaged by this procedure, further altering normal host defenses.

TABLE 176–3. PRACTICALLY WORTHLESS TESTS

TEST	PURPOSE	RATIONALE	APPROPRIATE ALTERNATIVES
Qualitative urolith analysis	To determine the mineral composition of uroliths	Qualitative tests for mineral analysis are not very accurate (50% false-negative rate and an 18% false-positive rate). These test kits cannot detect silica or drugs in uroliths and cannot distinguish between minerals comprising different layers of the urolith.	Quantitative analysis (optical crystallography, x-ray diffraction, infrared spectroscopy, others)
Survey radiography	To assess Dalmatians and dogs with portovascular shunts for uroliths	Approximately 95% of uroliths in male Dalmatians are composed of purines with the radiographic density of soft tissue and therefore not discernible by survey radiography.	Double contrast cystography or ultrasonography
Abdominal palpation	To exclude uroliths as a cause of lower urinary tract signs	Bladder palpation is an insensitive method of urolith detection (3–20% diagnosed) and is dependent on experience, urolith size, urolith number, and bladder fullness.	Radiography or ultrasonography
Visual test of cloudy urine	For diagnosis of urinary tract infection	Although bacteria, inflammatory cells, and inflammatory proteins result in increased urine turbidity, other substances (i.e., crystals, fat droplets, neoplastic cells, and genital secretions) also cause cloudy urine.	Urine cultures should be performed to verify urinary tract infection
Urine concentrations, fractional excretions, and mineral to creatinine ratios of calcium, phosphorus, magnesium, or urate from random urine samples	For evaluating dogs with uroliths	Concentrations of minerals in urine are affected by type of diet consumed and time of feeding in relation to sample collection. Urine mineral concentrations determined from "spot" urine samples do not correlate with daily mineral excretion.	Twenty-four hour urine samples using previously tested diets or rely on presence of crystalluria to indicate that conditions are favorable for urolith recurrence.

ANATOMIC DISORDERS

URETHRORECTAL FISTULA

Fistulas that connect the lumen of the urogenital tract with the rectum may be congenital or acquired. The paucity with which they have been reported in the veterinary literature probably indicates that they are uncommon. Some dogs are asymptomatic; however, simultaneous passage of urine out of the anus and urogenital tract has been observed. Surgical extirpation of the anomalous fistula was successful in some cases; however, extrapelvic urethral anastomosis was required in one dog. Control of secondary bacterial UTI and urolithiasis is an important consideration in the management of urethrorectal fistulas.[15]

URETHRAL PROLAPSE

Prolapse of the mucosal lining of the distal portion of the urethra through the external urethral orifice occasionally occurs in brachycephalic dogs, especially English bulldogs.

URO

TABLE 176–4. TEST CONDITIONS THAT CAN PRODUCE WORTHLESS RESULTS

TEST CONDITION	CONFOUNDING PRINCIPLES	SOLUTIONS
Urine samples collected by owners	Owners may collect urine in improperly rinsed containers, allow samples to dehydrate, or store samples at improper temperatures. In addition, voided samples may become contaminated with substances from the urethra, genital tract, digestive tract, or bottom of the patient's foot.	Discourage clients from allowing their pet to void urine 3 hours before evaluation. A moderately full bladder will facilitate urine collection by cystocentesis.
Uroliths or urethral plugs submitted in formalin for mineral analysis	Formalin can dissolve and alter the chemical makeup of some minerals, particularly struvite.	When submitting urethral plugs or uroliths for mineral analysis, submit them dry without preservative.
Refrigerated urine samples for assessing "in vivo" crystalluria	As urine cools, solubility decreases and crystals precipitate out of solution.	Evaluate urine sediment shortly after obtaining sample.
Urine specific gravity after therapy	Many therapies (i.e., fluids, glucocorticoids, diet) alter urine specific gravity. Relying on this test after therapeutic intervention may lead to errors in diagnostic interpretation (i.e., verification and localization of azotemia, dehydration, polydipsia).	Urine-specific gravity is the most important part of the urinalysis because all other results are interpreted in relation to this value. Obtain samples before administration of therapeutic agents.

Underlying factors predisposing to urethral prolapse are not known; however, sexual arousal has been incriminated. Physical examination typically reveals a red or purple pea-sized, doughnut-shaped lesion protruding from the end of the penis. It has been suggested that small urethral prolapses may resolve spontaneously in some patients. Most cases have been managed by manual reduction combined with retention sutures or by surgical excision of the prolapsed position of the urethra. When hematuria and trauma are absent, therapy may not be needed, but patients should continue to be monitored.

PERSISTENT URACHUS

The urachus is a fetal conduit that provides communication between the urinary bladder and the allantois (a portion of the placenta). This structure allows varying quantities of fetal urine to pass from the urinary bladder through the urachus to the placenta, where unwanted metabolites are presumable absorbed by the fetal circulation and subsequently excreted in the mother's urine. At the time of birth the urachus is nonfunctional and undergoes substantial atrophy. A persistent urachus occurs if the entire urachal canal remains patent. It is characterized by inappropriate loss of urine through the umbilicus during the storage phase of micturition and expulsion of urine to the exterior through the umbilicus and urethra, during the voiding phase of micturition. Omphalitis and UTI may also occur. Increased intravesicular pressure can apparently convert a closed urachal canal into a patent urachus. The diagnosis of persistent urachus should be confirmed by contrast radiographic procedures. If it is confirmed, the canal should be surgically removed.

VESICOURACHAL DIVERTICULA

Vesicourachal diverticula result from failure of the urachal canal to undergo complete atrophy at its connection to the urinary bladder. They are significant because they predispose to recurrent UTI. By predisposing to UTI, they may indirectly contribute to the formation of magnesium ammonium phosphate uroliths. Failure to remove a diverticulum at the time of urolith removal may result in the recurrence of infection and subsequent recurrence of uroliths. In our experience, vesicourachal diverticula produce no clinical signs unless UTI is present. Occasionally, a vesicourachal diverticulum develops because of increased intravesicular pressure due to obstruction of urine outflow. Vesicourachal diverticula that form as a result of urinary obstruction may heal spontaneously; those that persist should be removed surgically.

URETHRAL STRICTURE

In our experience, most urethral strictures have resulted from improper surgery or improper use of urinary instruments, especially catheters. Use of firm polypropylene catheters and indwelling catheters should be avoided, if possible, because they often cause trauma. Likewise, catheters should not be used to push uroliths back into the urinary bladder. Urethral strictures commonly occur as a sequela to urethrotomy and urethrostomy procedures.

Urethral strictures necessitating repair can be opened along the longitudinal axis over the stricture for a distance of 3 to 4 mm and then closed transversely with absorbable suture. Strictures in the os penis are difficult to repair and may require urethrostomy to restore urine flow.

URETEROCELE

Ureterocele is a congenital abnormality resulting from obstruction of the ureteral orifice and associated cystic dilation of the terminal ureter that may protrude into the urinary bladder and occasionally the urethra. In one reported case, a ureterocele developed as a complication of neoureterocystotomy.[16] Ureteroceles are categorized as orthotopic when the ureter enters the urinary bladder at its normal location or ectopic when the ureter enters the urinary bladder at an aberrant location.

Clinical signs associated with ureteroceles are variable, depending on the type and degree of deformity, but may include dysuria, urinary incontinence, hematuria, chronic UTI, and urinary obstruction. Depending on the location of obstruction, hydroureter, hydronephrosis, and impaired renal function may also be present. Confirming the diagnosis requires contrast radiography and/or ultrasonography.

Clinical abnormalities are minimized or eliminated by reconstruction of the urinary tract. Orthotopic ureteroceles can be incised transurethrally with electrocautery or by celiotomy and cystotomy. Excision of the ureterocele and re-implantation of the ureter is recommended to resolve hydroureter, complete ureteral obstruction, or ectopic ureteroceles.[17, 18]

URINARY TRACT TRAUMA

Etiopathogenesis. Injury to the urinary bladder may be caused by blunt abdominal trauma, penetrating abdominal trauma, overzealous abdominal palpation, overinsertion of rigid urinary catheters, overdistention of the bladder lumen during retrograde contrast urethrocystography, improper placement of peritoneal dialysis catheters containing stylets, improper cystocentesis technique, and careless celiotomy incisions.

Urethral trauma may be caused by penetrating pelvic or os penis fracture fragments, animal bites, bullets, and improper use of urinary instruments. The urethra may be contused, lacerated, partially or totally ruptured, or avulsed from the bladder neck. Male dogs and cats are more commonly affected than are female dogs and cats. In a study of pelvic fractures, rupture of the intrapelvic portion of the urethra occurred in five male dogs (5 per cent).[14] There was no correlation between the severity of pelvic fractures and the occurrence of urinary tract injury. Damage to the urinary tract may be characterized by contusions and lacerations.

Clinical Signs. Contusions and lacerations of the internal lining of the urinary bladder cause varying degrees of hematuria. Dysuria may occur if the lesions stimulate a substantial inflammatory response. Patients with traumatic herniation of the urinary bladder through the abdominal wall will develop the clinical signs related to an impaired ability to void. If the ureters remain patent but the proximal urethra is obstructed, a distended bladder may be palpated in the hernial sac.

Clinical signs associated with rupture of the urinary bladder are variable, depending on the site of the rupture (intraperitoneal and/or extraperitoneal), the size of the rent in the bladder wall, the duration of the rupture, the quantity of sterile or infected urine extravasated into adjacent tissues, and the condition of the patient at the time of rupture. In cases associated with trauma, signs characteristic of shock or disorders caused by trauma to other organs and tissues (especially the bony pelvis) may initially obscure the signs related to the urinary system. Patients with ruptured urinary bladders may or may not be able to void urine, depending on the site and size of rupture and the integrity of neurologic innervation to the bladder and urethra. Some patients will void a small quantity of grossly bloody urine that may contain blood clots, but this finding is not constant. Rectal palpation may reveal evidence of a fractured bony pelvis or obstructive lesions of the urethra (e.g., uroliths, inflammatory or neoplastic thickening).

Transient intraperitoneal extravasation of urine from the bladder as a result of overdistention of the urinary bladder during retrograde contrast urethrocystography or cystocentesis is usually not associated with clinical signs referable to the lower urinary tract. Iatrogenic lesions of this nature are usually self-limiting.

Continuous intraperitoneal extravasation of a significant quantity of urine will induce progressive signs caused by chemical and/or bacterial peritonitis within 8 to 24 hours (anorexia, depression, vomiting, dehydration, abdominal pain characterized by discomfort during palpation and reluctance to walk, and mild to moderate ascites). Rectal temperature may be increased, normal, or decreased. Onset of postrenal azotemia may compound polysystemic signs (depression, anorexia, vomiting, and dehydration). If appropriate therapy is not initiated in patients with intraperitoneal bladder rupture that is associated with severe peritonitis and postrenal azotemia, death typically occurs in 3 to 5 days.

Extraperitoneal extravasation of urine from the urinary bladder may not be associated with localizing signs during early stages. Continuous loss of urine eventually causes signs related to cellulitis including fever, depression, dysuria, and fistulous tracts.

Diagnosis. The most important aspect in the diagnosis of trauma to the urinary tract is to suspect its occurrence in all patients with a history of abdominal or pelvic injury. The location(s) and severity of trauma should be evaluated by retrograde urethrocystography. Using a balloon catheter eliminates the need to insert a catheter beyond the distal urethra and therefore minimizes the chance of further catheter-induced trauma or infection. We recommend the use of a dilute solution (2.5 to 5.0 per cent) of contrast agents commonly used for intravenous urography. Conventional ventrodorsal, lateral, and oblique views should be obtained.

Abdominal paracentesis is helpful to support a diagnosis of intraperitoneal rupture of the urinary bladder. Aspirated fluid typically has a bloody appearance. Comparing the concentration of creatinine in peritoneal fluid reveals a disproportionate elevation when compared with creatinine concentration of serum sampled at the same time. Because of the smaller size of urea and its ability to rapidly equilibrate across membranes, urea nitrogen concentration in peritoneal fluid is usually similar to that of blood and not a sensitive discriminator in the diagnosis of urine leakage.

Therapy. Provided that the cause is removed and all anatomic structures have been realigned, minor lesions usually heal spontaneously (contusions and partial thickness lacerations). Antimicrobial agents may be used to prevent or control infections caused by commensal microbes and conservative medical therapy used to correct metabolic abnormalities associated with urine retention.

Non-surgical procedures may be considered for iatrogenic rupture of the bladder that occurs during retrograde urethro-cystography, for small bladder tears, and for lacerated and partially ruptured urethras. Depending on the size and location of the tear, urinary diversion (urinary catheter, tube cystostomy) may be required for 3 to 10 days. Surgical repair is the treatment of choice for severe trauma, rents in the urinary bladder, or avulsion/transection of the urethra.

UROLITHIASIS

CLINICAL SIGNIFICANCE

Urolith formation is not a specific disease but the sequela to a group of underlying disorders. The urinary system is designed to dispose of wastes in liquid form. However, during urolith formation, sustained alterations in urine composition promote oversaturation of one or more substances eliminated in urine and result in their precipitation and subsequent growth. The fact that urolith formation is erratic and unpredictable emphasizes that several interrelated pathologic and physiologic factors are often involved. Therefore, detection of urolithiasis is only the beginning of the diagnostic process. Essential to urolith eradication and prevention is identification of the diseases and risk factors underlying crystal formation, retention, and growth.

Regardless of the process of urolith formation, they have the potential to disrupt normal urinary tract function, those resulting in clinical signs should be appropriately managed.

PREVALENCE

Between 1980 and 1983 urolithiasis was diagnosed in 0.53 per cent (3,628 dogs). The proportion of dogs admitted to veterinary hospitals in West Germany with urolithiasis was similar (0.5 to 1 per cent).[19] From these data it is difficult to predict the prevalence of urolithiasis for all dogs; however, when the number of dogs registered with the Swedish Kennel Club was compared with the number of dogs that had uroliths removed surgically at several veterinary hospitals in Sweden, the prevalence of urolithiasis was lower (0.23 per cent).[20]

PHYSICAL AND CHEMICAL CHARACTERISTICS

Various terms have been used to describe precipitates that form in urine. Depending on their size and consistency, they have been referred to as crystals, sand, gravel, pebbles, stones, rocks, calculi, and uroliths. The preferred term for microscopic precipitates in urine is *crystals*. Macroscopic precipitates should be referred to as *uroliths*.

Uroliths may be named according to their location (nephroliths, renoliths, ureteroliths, urocystoliths, urethroliths), their shape (smooth, faceted, pyramidal, laminated, mulberry, jack-stone, stag horn, or branched), and, most importantly, their mineral composition. Of over 77,000 canine urolith submissions analyzed at the Minnesota Urolith Center, magnesium ammonium phosphate was the most common (Table 176–5). Uroliths composed of calcium oxalate, urate, cystine, silica, and calcium phosphate occurred less frequently. On occasion, no single mineral predominated; different minerals were mixed together throughout the urolith (mixed uroliths). In other instances, discrete layers of uroliths were composed of different minerals (compound uroliths). Detection, treatment, and prevention of the causes

TABLE 176–5. MINERAL COMPOSITION* OF UROLITHS FROM 77,190 DOGS

PREDOMINANT MINERAL TYPE	NO. OF UROLITHS	%
Magnesium ammonium phosphate	38,299	49.6
Calcium oxalate	24,267	31.4
Urate	6,144	8.0
Cystine	760	1.0
Silica	659	0.9
Calcium phosphate	435	0.6
Compound	5,113	6.6
Mixed	1,464	1.9
Matrix	45	0.1
Drug metabolite	4	0.01
Total	22,142	

*Mineral composition determined by optical crystallography, x-ray spectroscopy, and infrared spectroscopy.

underlying urolith formation depend on knowledge of the composition of all portions of uroliths.

In addition to minerals, uroliths also contain variable quantities of a non-crystalline organic matrix. Substances identified in the organic matrix of uroliths from humans and those produced experimentally in animals included matrix substances A, Tamm-Horsfall mucoprotein (uromucoid), serum albumin, and alpha and gamma globulin.[21] Matrix has been hypothesized by some to represent the skeleton of uroliths. In vitro studies using human urine revealed that Tamm-Horsfall protein is related to formation of calcium oxalate crystals. Although the physical characteristics of uroliths suggest an organized relationship between the matrix skeleton and crystalline building blocks, the role of each component in formation, retention, and growth of uroliths is still poorly understood.

BIOLOGIC BEHAVIOR

Formation. The first step in the development of a urolith is the formation of a crystal nidus (crystal embryo). This phase, called nucleation, depends on supersaturation of urine with lithogenic crystalloids. The degree of supersaturation may be influenced by the magnitude of renal excretion of the crystalloid, urine pH, and crystallization inhibitors in urine. Further growth of the crystal nidus depends on its ability to remain in the urinary tract, the degree and duration of supersaturation of urine with crystalloids identical to or different from that of the nidus, and the physical characteristics of the crystal nidus.

Several theories have been proposed to explain initiation of uroliths and include the precipitation-crystallization theory, the matrix-nucleation theory, and the crystallization-inhibition theory. Each theory emphasizes a single factor; however, they are not mutually exclusive.

Precipitation-Crystallization Theory. This hypothesis incriminates supersaturation of urine with stone-forming crystalloids as the primary event in lithogenesis. In this hypothesis, nucleation (initiation of urolith formation) is considered to be a physicochemical process of precipitation of crystalloids from a supersaturated solution. Urolith formation is thought to be independent of performed matrix or inhibitors of crystallization.

According to this hypothesis, production of urine excessively saturated with one or more urolith-forming crystalloids leads to spontaneous nucleation of the crystalloid. If nucleated crystalloids become trapped in the urinary system during continued supersaturation, uroliths will grow. Mucoprotein matrix is thought to be non-specifically incorporated into uroliths as growth proceeds.

Oversaturation of urine with urolith-forming crystalloids may be associated with the following factors: (1) increased renal excretion of crystalloids as a result of increased glomerular filtration, increased tubular secretion, or decreased tubular reabsorption (e.g., hypercalciuria, hyperuricosuria, hyperoxaluria, cystinuria, xanthinuria); (2) negative body water balance associated with increased tubular reabsorption of water and subsequent urine concentration (e.g., excessive water loss through non-urinary routes, lack of water consumption, habitation in hot, dry climate); and (3) urine pH favoring crystallization (e.g., formation of alkaline urine by urease-producing bacteria, formation of alkaline urine as a result of renal tubular acidosis, formation of alkaline, or less acid or urine as a result of diet or feeding pattern or alkalinizing drugs).

The precipitation-crystallization hypothesis provides a plausible explanation for formation of cystine, urate, and magnesium-ammonium phosphate uroliths. It is also applicable to those patients with oxalate uroliths in which hypercalciuria, hyperoxaluria, hyperuricosuria, or a combination of these can be detected.

Matrix-Nucleation Theory. This hypothesis states that matrix substances are promoters of nucleation, and it implicates pre-formed organic matrix as the primary determinant of lithogenesis. The matrix nucleation theory is based on the assumption that pre-formed organic matrix forms a nucleus that subsequently permits stone growth by precipitation of crystalloids. The theory is somewhat analogous to bone formation in its requirement for organic matrix.

The role of organic matrix in lithogenesis has not been identified with certainty; however, the similarity of the overall composition of matrix from human uroliths of various mineral composition has been used to support this hypothesis.[19] The observation that the specific amino acid composition differed for human uroliths of varied mineral content also supports this hypothesis.[19] Opponents of the matrix nucleation theory cite data indicating that uroliths can acquire a large portion of organic matrix by physical adsorption during urolith growth.

Crystallization-Inhibition Theory. This hypothesis incriminates reduction or absence of organic and inorganic inhibitors of crystallization as the primary determinant of calcium oxalate and calcium phosphate lithogenesis.[22, 23] The theory is based on the fact that several crystalloids, including calcium, are maintained in solution at concentrations significantly higher than is possible in water (i.e., urine is a metastable supersaturated solution).

Summary. Several lines of evidence have been reported to support each hypothesis. None has been completely accepted; however, the balance of evidence suggests the most likely cause of nucleation and formation of a crystal embryo is precipitation from an oversaturated solution. An organic matrix is not required for precipitation, and inhibitors may be more important for growth than for initiation of urolith formation.

Growth. Once a crystal nidus has formed, it may be voided or retained in the urinary tract and subsequently permitted to grow. As with initiation of urolithiasis, the exact events leading to crystal growth have not been identified. Uroliths do not appear to grow haphazardly because they are composed of an orderly arrangement of crystals. It has been suggested that a crystalline nidus may grow by crystal growth, epitaxial growth, or crystal aggregation.

Crystal Growth. Once a nidus has formed, it may develop into a stone of the same composition by a process of crystal growth. The critical factor for crystal growth appears to be sustained urine supersaturation for that crystal species, rather than reduced excretion of crystallization inhibitors. Because pre-formed crystals serve as templates for additional mineral precipitation, crystal growth requires a lower degree of urine supersaturation than crystal formation.

Epitaxial Growth. Growth by epitaxy is growth of one type of crystal on the surface of another type. The physical characteristics of the initiating crystals and the growth crystals must permit proper alignment with respect to each other; thus, growth by epitaxy implies regular alignment of crystals.

Epitaxial growth may plausibly explain why uroliths frequently are of mixed composition. It may represent a heterogeneous form of nucleation. Thus, calcium phosphate may serve as a nidus for epitaxial growth by calcium oxalate. Likewise, a nidus of monosodium urate may support epitaxial growth with calcium oxalate, and brushite (calcium hydrogen phosphate dihydrate) may serve as a nidus for further growth of calcium phosphate or calcium oxalate.

Crystal Aggregation. This hypothesis is based on the supposition that further aggregation of nucleated crystals may be normally inhibited by substances present in urine. In stone formers, crystals may bind to one another, forming large clusters. The aggregates may be detected in urine sediment.

It has been suggested that the crystal aggregation phenomenon distinguishes simple crystalluria, which occurs in most normal animals, from stone formation. In the presence of crystal aggregation inhibitors, crystals that form do not grow but readily pass through the urinary tract. If crystal aggregation inhibitors are deficient or have impaired function, growth by aggregation occurs. This hypothesis is supported by the observation that only individual calcium oxalate crystals are found in normal humans, whereas stone formers often excrete large aggregates of this salt.[24] Substances thought to have crystal aggregation-inhibiting properties for calcium salts include glycosaminoglycans, citrates, pyrophosphates, and diphosphonates.[25, 26]

Growth Versus Time. Although the time required for uroliths to form naturally has not been determined, radiographically detectable struvite uroliths have been induced experimentally in dogs within 2 weeks. We have also induced dissolution of naturally occurring struvite uroliths in dogs and cats in as short a period as 2 weeks.[27, 28] These observations suggest that urolith kinetics for struvite should be conceived in terms of days to weeks rather than months to years.

Sequela to Urolith Formation. Uroliths may spontaneously pass through various parts of the urinary tract, spontaneously dissolve, continue to grow, or become inactive (no growth occurs). Not all persistent uroliths are associated with clinical signs. They can remain inactive. In our experience, most inactive uroliths are not associated with UTI. Nonetheless, if uroliths remain in the urinary tract, dysuria, UTI, partial or total urinary obstruction, and polyp formation are potential sequelae.

UTI is common in dogs with urolithiasis. In most instances, UTI is the cause of struvite urolith formation. However, once uroliths have formed they may contribute to the persistence and spread of infection. In turn, the presence of other urolith types can facilitate initiation of UTI. Factors contributing to the increased risk of UTI include traumatic disruption of the mucosal lining of the urinary bladder, incomplete urine voiding, and sequestration of microorganisms. Infections with urease-producing bacteria can result in the deposition of magnesium ammonium phosphate over other urolith types, confounding diagnostic and management efforts to resolve the initial lithogenic events that are ultimately responsible for disease.

Small uroliths located in the urinary bladder commonly pass into the urethra of male and female dogs during the voiding phase of micturition. Uroliths whose diameter is slightly smaller than that of the dilated proximal urethral lumen commonly are voided to the exterior by female dogs but may lodge behind the os penis of male dogs. Complete obstruction to urine outflow associated with UTI may result in rapid destruction of renal parenchyma and septicemia within days. Persistent obstruction affecting both kidneys, with or without UTI, results in uremia.

Polyp formation has been documented in a few cases of dogs with urocystoliths. The events promoting polyp formation are unknown; however, it is logical to assume that chronic irritation to the urinary bladder mucosa and bacterial infection contribute to mucosal hyperplasia. Although, polyps have been routinely managed surgically, inflammatory polyps have spontaneously regressed after eradication of uroliths and urinary infection (see Fig. 176–5). We have also observed spontaneous dissolution of struvite uroliths in five dogs. It is likely that spontaneous dissolution of infection-induced struvite uroliths is associated with abatement of UTI, rapid formation of large volumes of urine, and decreased urine urea concentration. Spontaneous dissolution of uroliths generally appears to be uncommon.

Recurrence. The likelihood of urolith recurrence after medical or surgical therapy has been unpredictable. The apparent interval between elimination of uroliths and their subsequent detection may be influenced by several factors, including (1) diagnostic methods used to detect urolith recurrence and frequency of examination, (2) failure to remove all uroliths from the urinary tract during surgery, (3) persistence or recurrence of UTI with lithogenic microorganisms, (4) use of non-absorbable suture material that is exposed to the lumen of the urinary tract and therefore serves as a nidus for mineral precipitation, (5) owner or patient noncompliance with therapeutic or prophylactic recommendations, and (6) persistence of factors responsible for urolith initiation at the time of urolith eradication. These variables may account for the wide range of reported recurrence rates for uroliths in dogs (20 to 75 per cent).

In a retrospective clinical survey of 438 dogs surgically treated for urolithiasis, 111 patients had 155 known recurrences. Recurrence was observed in 47 per cent of dogs with cystine uroliths, 33 per cent with urate uroliths, 25 per cent with oxalate uroliths, and 18 per cent with "phosphate" uroliths. Results of a retrospective study on the recurrence rate of calcium oxalate uroliths in dogs indicated that the rate of recurrence increased with the length of time that the dogs were evaluated: 3 per cent recurred after 3 months, 9 per cent after 6 months, 36 per cent after 1 year, 42 per cent after 2 years, and 48 per cent after 3 years.[29]

To date, all clinical studies of recurrence of canine uroliths have been based on post-surgical evaluation. The rate of recurrence after medical dissolution of canine struvite and ammonium acid urate uroliths has not been evaluated in a large population of patients; however, our clinical observations indicate that the rate of recurrence is lower than that associated with surgery. In addition, the time elapsed between recurrent episodes is longer after medical dissolution.

DIAGNOSIS

Urocystoliths should be considered as a probability in dogs with dysuria and hematuria with or without urethral

URO

obstruction. Urinalysis, urine culture, and radiography may be required to different uroliths from UTI, urinary tract neoplasia, polyps, blood clots, and urogenital anomalies.

A variety of methods have been used to evaluate the composition of uroliths, including their gross appearance, crystalluria, radiographic appearance, quantitative analysis, and urolith culture. Of these, quantitative analysis provides the most definitive diagnostic, prognostic, and therapeutic information.

Crystalluria. Crystalluria, by definition, is the appearance of crystals in urine. Proper identification and interpretation of urine crystals is important in formulating medical protocols to dissolve uroliths. Routine laboratory procedures for detection of crystalluria are qualitative not quantitative. Caution must be used in interpreting the significance of crystalluria, because crystal formation can be altered by factors other than the underlying disease process. Variables influencing crystal formation after urine collection include (1) temperature changes, (2) evaporation, (3) pH changes, and (4) technique of specimen preparation (e.g., centrifugation versus non-centrifugation, volume of urine examined). When knowledge of in vivo urine crystal formation and type is especially important, fresh specimens should be examined. Ideally, they should be at body temperature. If this is not possible, they should be evaluated at room temperature rather than after storage by refrigeration.

One must avoid overinterpretation or underinterpretation of the significance crystalluria (Table 176–6). Crystalluria is not synonymous with urolith formation, but it can be considered a useful process to manage a potentially dangerous episode of urinary supersaturation. By forming a large number of small crystals that are rapidly washed out of the urinary tract, crystalluria is a beneficial process. The formation of a clinically significant urolith requires that crystals be retained in the urinary tract and then allowed to grow. Because crystals occur only in urine that is supersaturated with crystallogenic substances, it represents a risk factor for urolithiasis. In most instances, however, crystal formation in an anatomically and functionally normal urinary tract is harmless. Identification of crystals in such patients does not justify therapy. Likewise, treatment of crystalluria in patients with hematuria and dysuria may not be necessary. Other factors (uroliths, UTI, neoplasia) are often the cause of clinical signs of lower urinary tract disease. On the other hand, detection of some types of crystals, or large aggregates of others, may have diagnostic, prognostic, or therapeutic importance. For example, ammonium urate crystalluria may be indicative of portal vascular anomalies or primary hepatic disorders. Calcium oxalate monohydrate and calcium oxalate dihydrate crystalluria may occur in dogs with ethylene glycol toxicity or hypercalcemia; cystine crystalluria is pathognomonic of cystinuria.

Imaging. The primary objective of radiographic or ultrasonographic evaluation of patients is to verify urolith presence, location, number, size, density, and shape. In our experience, the lateral survey radiograph provides sufficient information to exclude the presence of uroliths. Radiograph should include all portions of the urethra, which usually requires taking views more caudal than for routine abdominal evaluation. A lateral double-contrast cystogram can be performed for further verification. Sedation is often unnecessary unless the patient is very dysuric or uncooperative.

The radiographic or ultrasonographic appearance of uroliths is influenced by their size, number, location, and mineral composition. Most uroliths greater than 3 mm have varying degrees of radiodensity and therefore can be detected by survey abdominal radiography or ultrasonography. Uroliths less than 3 mm in size may not be visualized by these techniques. Compared with soft tissue density, uroliths composed of magnesium ammonium phosphate, calcium oxalate, calcium phosphate, silica, and cystine are often radiodense; those composed of urate salts may be radiolucent. It is possible for a urolith to be larger than that depicted by its radiodensity if only a portion of it contains radiodense minerals. This phenomenon is most likely to occur with rapidly growing struvite uroliths.

Serum Chemistry Values. Evaluation of serum chemistry values is helpful in the identification of underlying abnormalities responsible for urolith formation. For example, lower serum concentrations of urea nitrogen commonly occur in dogs with hepatic porto-systemic shunts and urate uroliths. Hypercalcemia has been reported in dogs with primary hyperparathyroidism and calcium oxalate and calcium phosphate uroliths. Absence of changes in serum chemistry values is not a good predictor for eliminating various urolith types.

Urine Chemistry Values. Detection of the underlying mechanisms for specific types of urolithiasis is unavoidably linked to evaluation of the biochemical composition of urine. For best results, 24-hour urine samples should be collected, because determination of fractional excretion of many metabolites in random "spot" urine samples does not accurately reflect 24-hour metabolite excretion. We emphasize that the quantity of metabolites excreted in urine is also influenced by the amount and composition of the diet and by whether urine was collected during fed or fasted conditions.

Analysis of Uroliths. Uroliths can be submitted for analysis in a clean dry container. Submitting uroliths in preservatives or other solutions may alter the physical properties of minerals or dissolve away surface crystals. If multiple uroliths are present, one urolith may be placed into 10 per cent buffered formalin for microscopic examination of matrix.

Because many uroliths contain more than one mineral component, it is important to examine representative por-

TABLE 176–6. WHAT EVERY VETERINARIAN SHOULD KNOW ABOUT CRYSTALLURIA

1. Crystals detected in urine samples collected recently from the patient are a more reliable indication of events occuring in the patient (i.e., in vivo crystalluria). In contrast, crystals detected in stored urine may represent formation after collection (i.e., in vitro crystalluria).
2. Evaluating urine samples collected by owners is not recommended because contamination, increased storage time, changes in pH, and changes in temperature may promote in vitro crystalluria and alter in vivo crystalluria.
3. Analyze fresh urine samples to avoid variables introduced by refrigeration to preserve time.
4. Detection of crystals in fresh urine samples indicates that this urine is able to support additional crystal formation and crystal growth. This is a risk factor for urolith formation.
5. Crystalluria needs to be interpreted in reference to urine concentration (i.e., specific gravity). For example, crystals detected in dilute urine (e.g., 1.006) have a greater significance than the same number of crystals observed in more concentrated urine (e.g., 1.060).
6. Persistent crystalluria is thought to indicate a greater risk for urolith formation than intermittent crystalluria.
7. Numerous crystals are thought to indicate a greater risk for urolith formation than fewer crystals.
8. Aggregates of crystals and crystals of large size are thought to indicate a greater risk for urolith formation than single, small crystals.
9. Crystalluria is not synonymous with urolithiasis. Crystalluria may be detected in dogs without uroliths and absent in dogs with confirmed uroliths.

tions. The mineral composition of crystalline nuclei may be identical to or different from that of the remainder of the uroliths. The nuclei of uroliths should be analyzed separately from their outer layers, because the initiating cause of the urolith is suggested by the mineral composition of the nuclei.

We do not recommend single qualitative chemical analysis of uroliths. The major disadvantage is that it detects only some of the chemical radicals and ions. In addition, the proportion of the different chemical constituents in the urolith cannot be quantified.

In contrast to chemical methods of analysis, physical methods have proven to be far superior for crystalline substances. They also permit differentiation of various subgroups of minerals (i.e., calcium oxalate monohydrate and calcium oxalate dihydrate, or uric acid, ammonium acid urate, and xanthine) and allow semi-quantitative determinations of various mineral components. Physical methods commonly used by laboratories that specialize in quantitative urolith analysis include a combination of polarizing light microscopy, x-ray diffractometry, and infrared spectroscopy. Some laboratories are also equipped to perform elemental analysis with an energy-dispersive x-ray microanalyzer (EDAX) or by neutron activation. On occasion, chemical methods of analysis and paper chromatography may be used to supplement information provided by the physical methods mentioned.

Predicting Mineral Composition Before Urolith Analysis.

Formulating effective medical protocols for urolith dissolution depends on knowledge of the mineral composition of uroliths. This poses a problem without the availability of surgically removed uroliths for analysis. To overcome this problem we recommend a protocol that facilitates determination of the mineral composition of uroliths by recognizing prototypes for mineral types (Table 176–7). Formulation of medical protocols based on the mineral composition of uroliths determined by this protocol is usually associated with a high degree of success in dissolving uroliths, or arresting their growth.[30] Urolith dissolution may be hampered if uroliths are composed of several mineral types of differing solubility characteristics. This is especially true for compound uroliths in which one mineral is completely surrounded by a different mineral. For example, difficulty may be encountered in the dissolution of an ammonium urate urolith (which dissolves more readily in alkaline urine) surrounded by magnesium ammonium phosphate (which dissolves more readily in acidic urine). Dissolution has not been a significant problem in dogs with uroliths composed principally of magnesium ammonium phosphate and small quantities of calcium apatite because the solubility characteristics of these two minerals are similar.

An alternative to predicting mineral composition, small uroliths can be retrieved using a non-surgical method.[31] Once retrieved, uroliths can be quantitatively analyzed. Uroliths located in the urinary bladder or urethra are commonly voided during micturition by female dogs and occasionally by male dogs. Commercially available fish nets designed for household aquariums facilitate collection of uroliths during voiding. Small urocystoliths can also be retrieved for analysis by aspirating them into a urinary catheter (see Fig. 176–4).[32] The only equipment needed to perform this technique is a urinary catheter and a 60-mL syringe. With the patient in lateral recumbency, a wel-lubricated sterile catheter is advanced through the urethra into the bladder lumen. The tip of the catheter is positioned so that it will not interfere with the movement of the bladder wall as fluid is aspirated from the bladder lumen. If the urinary bladder is not distended with urine, it should be moderately distended with physiologic saline solution. Palpation of the urinary bladder per abdomen during distention with saline should be used as the primary method to minimize overdistention. The urine (or saline solution) is then aspirated into the syringe as an assistant vigorously and repeatedly moves the patient's abdomen in an up and down direction. This maneuver causes uroliths located in the dependent portion of the bladder to disperse throughout fluid in the bladder lumen. Small uroliths in the vicinity of the catheter tip may then be sucked into the catheter along with the urine-saline mixture. Best results are obtained when the catheter opening is positioned in the trigone of the urinary bladder. It is also important to aspirate fluid in a steady continuous fashion with the goal of removing all the fluid without having to re-position the catheter. It may be necessary to repeat this sequence of steps several times before a sufficient number of uroliths are retrieved for analysis.

MANAGEMENT

Medical Management. The objective for medical management of uroliths are to promote dissolution or arrest further growth. For therapy to be effective it must induce undersaturation of urine with calculogenic crystalloids. This can be achieved by reducing calculogenic crystalloids, increasing the solubility of crystalloids, and/or increasing the volume of urine. Change in diet is one method available to reduce the quantity of calculogenic crystalloids in urine. Attempts to increase the solubility of crystalloids in urine often include administration of medications designed to change urine pH. As a general rule, salts of basic ions (PO_4^{3-}, CO_3^{2-}) are more soluble in acidic urine because the basic ions uncouple and react with hydrogen ions; the reverse is true for salts of acidic ions. Increasing urine volume decreases the concentration of calculogenic substances. Induction of diuresis is the common method of increasing urine volume; however, the effects of diuresis on urinary excretion of calculogenic minerals and the concentration of crystallization inhibitors has not been investigated in dogs. Nonetheless, increasing urine volume has been beneficial in the medical dissolution of struvite uroliths.

Surgical Removal. Detection of uroliths is not in itself an indication for surgery. Surgical candidates include patients with urolith-induced obstruction to urine outflow that cannot be corrected by non-surgical techniques. This is especially true in patients with urinary tract infection. In this situation, rapid spread of infection and damage to the urinary tract are likely to induce pyelonephritis, renal failure, and septicemia. Therefore, it is important that this combination of disorders be resolved as soon as possible. Surgery should also be considered in dogs with uroliths refractory to medical therapy (calcium oxalate, silica, calcium phosphate) that are too large to be voided through the urethra. In some instances, surgery is needed to manage uroliths because of poor client or poor patient compliance with therapeutic recommendations for medical dissolution. In rare instances, some medical recommendations cannot be continued because of drug or diet intolerance by the patient. For example, we have observed generalized lymphadenopathy, thrombocytopenia, and leukopenia in dogs receiving N-(2-mercaptopropionyl)-glycine to dissolve cystine uroliths. Surgery may represent a convenient alternative. For dogs with certain anatomic defects of the urinary tract (persistent diverticulum or persistent urachus) that may predispose to UTI and uroliths, uroliths

URO

TABLE 176–7. PREDICTING MINERAL COMPOSITION OF UROLITHS

MINERAL TYPE	PREDICTORS								
	Urine pH	*Crystal Appearance*	*Urine Culture*	*Radiographic Density*	*Radiographic Contour*	*Serum Abnormalities*	*Breed Predisposition*	*Gender Predisposition*	*Common Ages*
Magnesium ammonium phosphate	Neutral to alkaline	Four- to 6-sided colorless prisms	Urease-producing bacteria (*Staphylococcus*, *Proteus*, *Enterococcus*, *Mycoplasma*)	+ to ++++	Smooth, round, or faceted; may assume shape of bladder or urethra	None	Miniature schnauzer, bichon frisé, cocker spaniel	Female (>80%)	2–8 yr or younger
Calcium oxalate	Acid to neutral	Dihydrate salt, colorless envelope or octahedral shape; monohydrate salt-spindles or dumbbell shape	Negative	++ to ++++	Rough or spiculated (dihydrate salt); small, smooth, round (monohydrate salt); sometimes jackstone	Occasional hypercalcemia	Miniature schnauzer, Lhasa apso, Yorkshire terrier, miniature poodle, Shih Tzu, bichon frisé	Males (>70%)	5–12 yr
Urate	Acid to neutral	Yellow-brown amorphous shapes or sphericals (ammonium urate)	Negative	– to ++	Smooth, round or oval	Low urea nitrogen and serum albumin in dogs with hepatic portal systemic shunts	Dalmatian, English bulldog, miniature schnauzer, Yorkshire terrier	Males (>85%)	1–4 yr
Calcium phosphate	Alkaline to neutral (brushite forms in acidic urine)	Amorphous, or long thin prisms	Negative	++ to ++++	Smooth, round or faceted	Occasional hypercalcemia	Yorkshire terrier, miniature schnauzer, cocker spaniel	Male (>60%)	7–11 yr
Cystine	Acid to neutral	Flat colorless, hexagonal plates	Negative	+ to ++	Smooth to slightly irregular, round to oval	None	English bulldog, dachshund, basset hound	Male (>90%)	1–8 yr
Silica	Acid to neutral	None observed	Negative	++ to +++	Round center with radial spoke-like projections (jackstone)	None	German shepherd, golden retriever, Labrador retriever, miniature schnauzer	Male (>90%)	4–9 yr

can be removed at the same time these abnormalities are surgically repaired.

Although cystotomy or urethrotomy to remove uroliths is not technically difficult, these surgical procedures have several limitations. Because surgery has little to no effect on urolith formation, persistence of underlying causes often results in a high rate of urolith recurrence. Inability to remove all uroliths or fragments of uroliths also is of great concern. In one retrospective study, all uroliths were not removed by cystotomy from one of every seven dogs and from one of every five cats.[33] These findings indicate that established methods of verifying urolith removal (catheter passage through the urethra, retrograde flushing of the urethra, and visual or tactile inspection of the lumen of the urinary bladder) may be unreliable or inadequately performed. Therefore, post-surgical radiography should be considered in dogs with multiple uroliths to better assess complete urolith removal. In high-risk patients, medical dissolution or other forms of urolith removal may be considered more safe.

Non-surgical Urolith Removal. These non-surgical procedures permit safe and rapid removal of small to moderately sized urocystoliths.[33, 34]

Catheter Urolith Retrieval. Catheter retrieval of uroliths was previously described to remove a few uroliths for quantitative analysis (Fig. 176–4). This technique can also be used to remove all uroliths if their size permits passage through urethral catheters. Catheter retrieval of uroliths is suitable for patients at high risk for anesthesia-related morbidity and mortality because it is easily performed in conscious animals. After urolith retrieval, double contrast cys-

tography should be performed to assess urolith status. To minimize catheter-induced bacterial UTI anti-microbial therapy should be considered immediately before and for an appropriate duration after catheter urolith retrieval.

Voiding Urohydropropulsion. Compared with catheter urolith retrieval, voiding urohydropropulsion has an advantage of removing larger uroliths; however, urolith size is still limited to the size of the dilated urethra.[34] This technique is effective because of our ability to alter the patient's body position before the micturition and to use gravity to assist urolith position (Figs. 176–5 and 176–6).

Voiding urohydropropulsion is commonly performed in anesthetized dogs. No special equipment is needed; however, if the urinary bladder is not distended with urine, it should be moderately distended with physiologic saline solution injected through a transurethral catheter. To minimize overdistention of the urinary bladder during infusion, its size should be subjectively assessed by palpation per abdomen. Next the dog is positioned so that the vertebral column is approximately vertical (see Fig. 176–6). The urinary bladder is then gently agitated in an effort to promote gravitational movement of urocystoliths into the bladder neck. By applying steady pressure to the urinary bladder, urine and uroliths are manually expressed through the urethra into a cup (see Fig. 176–6, insert). If comparison of the number of voided uroliths to those detected previously by radiography indicated that urocystoliths remain within the lower urinary tract, the urinary bladder is again filled with saline solution and manually expressed until uroliths are no longer observed in the expelled saline solution. Before discontinuing the procedure, double-contrast cystography should be performed to determine whether all urocystoliths were removed.

Hematuria is a common complication of this procedure. Unlike surgery, however, visible hematuria often resolves within 4 hours, and dysuria was not induced as a result of voiding urohydropropulsion.

Proper selection of animals for voiding urohydropropulsion will enhance successful removal of urocystoliths. Uroliths larger than the smallest diameter of any portion of the distended urethral lumen are unlikely to be voided. Therefore, voiding urohydropropulsion may not be effective in removal of uroliths lodged in the urethral lumen because the urethra may be incapable of being distended further. Likewise, large uroliths remaining in the urinary bladder after voiding urohydropropulsion may predispose the patient to urethral obstruction. Uroliths composed of magnesium ammonium phosphate, ammonium urate, or cystine that are initially too large to be voided through the urethra can be easily removed once their size is reduced using medical therapy.[28] Urethral dilation has been used to facilitate passage of cystoscopes in female dogs and can be considered to facilitate removal of large uroliths or uroliths through previously strictured sections of urethra.

Lithotripsy. Lithotripsy is the process of breaking uroliths into smaller fragments that can be easily flushed out of the urinary tract or voided by the patient. Two types of lithotripsy have been used to manage uroliths in the lower urinary tract of dogs. The electrohydrolic lithotriptor consists of a spark generator that creates a shock wave at the surface of the urolith that fragments the stone.[35] A pneumatic impactor uses compressed air to drive metal rods into the urolith causing it to fragment.[36] Both lithotriptors require use of a cystoscope for insertion into the bladder lumen and for visualization of uroliths. Extracorporal shock wave lithotriptors appear to be more suitable for fragmenting uroliths residing in the ureter and kidney.[37, 38]

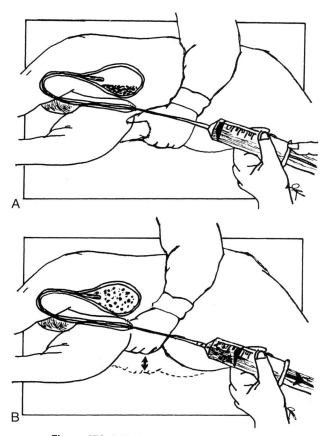

Figure 176–4. Catheter urolith retrieval (see text).

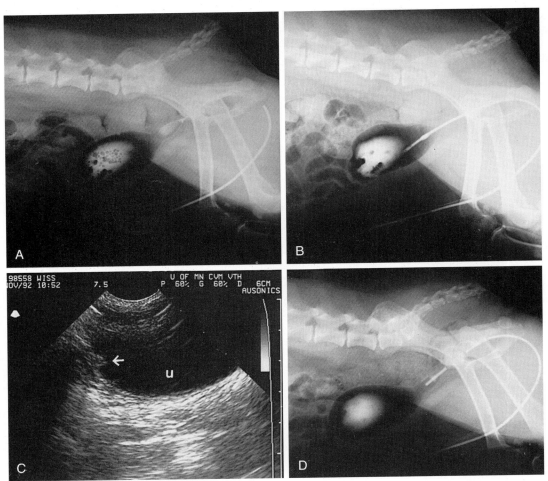

Figure 176–5. Lateral double-contrast cystogram of a 6-year-old male bichon frisé with multiple urocystoliths and mucosal polyps before *(A)* and immediately after *(B)* voiding urohydropropulsion. Ultrasonography *(C)* of the urinary bladder (u) confirmed complete urocystolith removal (mineral composition = 75 per cent calcium oxalate dihydrate, 20 per cent calcium oxalate monohydrate, and 5 per cent calcium phosphate) and mucosal polyp formation *(arrow)*. One month after urolith removal, lateral double-contrast cystogram *(D)* demonstrated spontaneous polyp regression.

STRUVITE UROLITHIASIS

Of 77,190 urolith submissions to our laboratory, magnesium ammonium phosphate was the most common canine urolith analyzed (49.6 per cent). It was also the most common urolith (61 per cent) analyzed in dogs younger than 1 year of age (Table 176–8). No single breed predominated; however, mixed breed (24.8 per cent), miniature schnauzer (11.8 per cent), Shih Tzu (8.6 per cent), and bichon frisé (7.8 per cent) represented more than 50 per cent of the cases. Eighty percent of struvite uroliths occurred in female dogs. Fifty-five percent of the dogs were between 3 and 8 years old (mean = 6 ± 2.9 years).

Etiopathogenesis. Urine must be supersaturated with magnesium ammonium phosphate for struvite uroliths to form. Supersaturation of urine with magnesium ammonium phosphate is associated with UTI caused by urease-producing microbes (especially *Staphylococcus* and *Proteus* spp.) and alkaline urine in most dogs. Clinical studies indicate that in some dogs microbial urease is not involved in formation of struvite uroliths. In this situation, dietary, metabolic, or familial factors may be involved in the genesis of struvite uroliths.

Infection-induced formation of struvite uroliths occurs when urease-producing microbes infect the urinary tract of dogs with sufficient quantity of urea. Such conditions favor formation of struvite, calcium apatite, and carbonate apatite. The following mechanisms are involved:

1. Urease produced by bacteria or *Ureaplasma* hydrolyzes urea to form two molecules of ammonia and a molecule of carbon dioxide. Because urease is not consumed during this reaction, a single urease molecule may catalyze the hydrolysis of multiple urea molecules.

2. The ammonia molecules react spontaneously with water to form ammonium and hydroxyl ions, which alkalinizes urine by reducing its hydrogen ion concentration. Ammonia also damages the glycosaminoglycan lining of the urothelium, increasing the ability of bacteria and crystals to adhere to mucosa. The solubility of struvite (and calcium apatite) decreases in alkaline urine. In addition to alkalinizing urine, the newly generated ammonium ion is available to form magnesium ammonium phosphate crystals.

3. The newly generated molecule of carbon dioxide combines with water to form carbonic acid, which in turn dissociates to form bicarbonate. Anions of carbonate may displace anions of phosphate in calcium apatite crystals to form carbonate apatite crystals.

4. In the progressively alkaline environment induced by

TABLE 176–8. MINERAL COMPOSITION* OF UROLITHS FROM 950 DOGS YOUNGER THAN 1 YEAR OF AGE

PREDOMINANT MINERAL TYPE	NO. OF UROLITHS	%
Magnesium ammonium phosphate	581	61.2
Calcium oxalate	21	2.2
Urate	207	21.8
Cystine	13	1.4
Silica	0	0
Calcium phosphate	27	2.8
Compound	59	6.2
Mixed	40	4.2
Matrix	2	0.2
Drug metabolite	0	0
Total	950	

*Mineral composition determined by optical crystallography, X ray spectroscopy, and infra red spectroscopy.

microbial hydrolysis of urea, dissociation of monobasic hydrogen phosphate (H_2PO_4) results in an increased concentration of dibasic hydrogen phosphate (HPO_4^{2-}) and anionic phosphate (PO_4^{3-}). Given a constant concentration of total phosphate, a change in pH from 6.80 to 7.40 increases the PO_4^{3-} concentration by a factor of approximately six. Anionic phosphate is then available in increased quantities to combine with magnesium and ammonium to form struvite or with calcium to form calcium-apatite.

Recurrent struvite urocystolithiasis has been evaluated in three related English cocker spaniels—a sire and two male offspring from different litters and dams.[39] Episodes of struvite urocystolithiasis were associated with alkaluria but not with bacterial UTI, urease activity in urine, or distal renal tubular acidosis.

Although struvite is less soluble in alkaline than acid urine, the mechanisms of sterile struvite urolith formation in dogs are not clear. Under physiologic conditions associated with alkaluria, urine contains low concentrations of ammonia (and thus ammonium ion). Thus, alkaline urine formed in the absence of ureolysis would not be expected to favor formation of crystals that contain ammonia ion (such as magnesium ammonium phosphate hexahydrate). Clinical studies of naturally occurring urolithiasis in humans support this generalization. Formation of persistently alkaline urine in absence of urease-mediated ureolysis may predispose to formation of uroliths containing hydroxylapatite [$Ca_{10}(PO_4)_6(OH)_2$] but not carbonate apatite.

In vitro studies consisting of addition of magnesium ($MgSO_4$), ammonium (NH_4Cl), or phosphate ($NH_4H_2PO_4$ or NaH_2PO_4) to sterile human urine ranging in pH from 5.0 to 9.6 revealed that struvite crystals could be induced in an acid or an alkaline environment.[40] A high ammonia concentration was not necessary for formation of struvite crystals provided the concentration of $[Mg] \times [NH_4] \times [PO_4]$ was of sufficient magnitude at a given pH. Corresponding studies in vivo have not yet been performed in dogs.

Treatment (Table 176–9). **Control of UTI.** The importance of UTIs caused by urease-producing bacteria in the formation of most struvite uroliths in dogs emphasizes the importance of therapy to eradicate or control these infections. Because of the quantity of urease produced by bacterial pathogens, it may be impossible to acidify urine with urine acidifiers administered in doses that prevent systemic acidosis. Therefore, sterilization of urine appears to be an important objective in creating a state of struvite undersaturation that may prevent further growth of uroliths or that promotes their dissolution.

TABLE 176–9. RECOMMENDATIONS FOR MEDICAL DISSOLUTION OF STRUVITE UROLITHS

Diagnostic plan
1. Perform appropriate diagnostic studies including urinalysis (with sediment examination), quantitative urine culture, diagnostic radiography.
2. Determine mineral composition of voided or retrieved uroliths. If unavailable, predict mineral composition by evaluating clinical data (see Table 176–7).

Therapeutic plan
1. Consider surgical correction, if uroliths obstructing urine flow cannot be dislodged, or if patients with a high risk of urine outflow obstruction cannot be monitored.
2. Eradicate urinary tract infection with appropriate antibiotics. Maintain antimicrobial therapy at the full dose during dissolution of uroliths and for 3 to 4 weeks after dissolution. If urine culture is sterile in patients not previously given antibiotics, antibiotics are not needed.
3. Initiate therapy with a diet designed to dissolve magnesium ammonium phosphate uroliths. No other food, supplements, or treats should be fed. Continue dietary therapy 3 to 4 weeks after radiographically detected dissolution.

Plan to monitor efficacy of therapy
1. Evaluate serial urinalyses. Urine pH should be acidic, urine specific gravity should be low (<1.015), and struvite crystalluria should be absent.
2. Perform urine cultures to determine whether bacteria have been eradicated. They are especially important in patients that are infected before therapy and those that are catheterized during therapy.
3. Perform radiography monthly to assess urolith number, size, and position. If uroliths grow during medical management or do not begin to dissolve in 4 to 8 weeks, alternative methods should be considered (see Fig. 176–6).

For immature dogs
1. Cautiously consider feeding protein-restricted diets to growing dogs.
2. Short-term therapy with calculolytic diets may be considered; however, monitor the patient for evidence of nutritional deficiencies (especially protein malnutrition).
3. Pending further studies, surgery remains the safest means of removing uroliths from immature dogs.

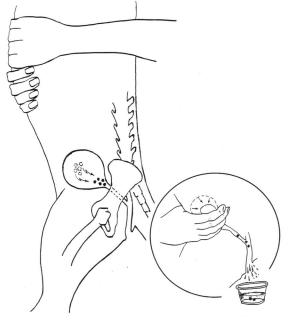

Figure 176–6. Voiding urohydropropulsion (see text). (Adapted from Lulich JP, et al: Nonsurgical removal of uroliths in dogs and cats by voiding urohydropropulsion. JAVMA 203:660, 1963.)

URO

Appropriate antimicrobial agents selected on the basis of susceptibility or minimum inhibitory concentration tests should be used in therapeutic doses. The fact that diuresis reduces the urine concentration of the antimicrobial agent should be considered when formulating antimicrobial dosage. Antimicrobial agents should be administered as long as the uroliths can be identified by survey radiography, because pathogens harbored inside uroliths may be protected from antimicrobial agents. Whereas the urine and surface of uroliths may be sterilized after appropriate antimicrobial therapy, the original infecting organisms may remain viable below the surface of the urolith. Premature discontinuation of antimicrobial therapy may result in relapse of bacteriuria and infection and inhibit further urolith dissolution (Table 176–10).

Urine Acidification. Urine acidification to a pH of approximately 6 has been effective in promoting sterile struvite urolith dissolution; however, addition of urinary acidifiers is often not needed for dogs currently receiving a calculolytic diet (Hill's Prescription Diet s/d), which already promotes formation of acidic urine. Urinary acidifiers should be considered in patients in which calculolytic diet is not tolerated or contraindicated.

Calculolytic Diet. The goal of calculolytic diets is to reduce urine concentration of urea (the substrate of urease), phosphorus, and magnesium. A calculolytic diet (Hill's Prescription Diet Canine s/d) was formulated that contains a reduced quantity of high-quality protein and reduced quantities of phosphorus and magnesium. The diet was supplemented with sodium chloride to stimulate thirst and induce compensatory polyuria. Reduction of hepatic production of urea from dietary protein reduces renal medullary urea concentration and further contributes to diuresis.

The efficacy of the aforementioned diet in dissolving infected struvite uroliths has been confirmed by controlled experimental and clinical studies in dogs.[41] When a combination of a calculolytic diet and antimicrobial agents was given to 11 dogs with naturally occurring urease-positive UTIs and urocystoliths presumed to be composed of struvite, the uroliths dissolved. The mean time required to dissolve urocystoliths was approximately 3 months (range, 2 weeks to 7 months).

When dogs with infection-induced struvite uroliths are fed a calculolytic diet, a marked reduction in the serum concentration of urea nitrogen and slight reductions in the serum concentrations of magnesium, phosphorus, and albumin typically occur.[41] A mild increase in the serum activity of hepatic alkaline phosphatase isoenzyme may also be observed. These alterations in serum chemistry values were not associated with detectable clinical consequence during 6-month experimental studies or during clinical studies. However, they underscore the fact that the diet is designed for

TABLE 176–10. MANAGING REFRACTORY OR INCOMPLETE MAGNESIUM AMMONIUM PHOSPHATE UROLITH DISSOLUTION

CAUSES	IDENTIFICATION	THERAPEUTIC GOAL
Client and patient factors 1. Inadequate dietary compliance	Question owner Persistent struvite crystalluria Serum urea nitrogen >8–12 mg/dL, urine specific gravity >1.010–1.015, during treatment with Prescription Diet Canine s/d	Emphasize need to feed dissolution diet exclusively
2. Inadequate antibiotic administration	Question owner Count remaining antibiotic pills Positive urine culture with same bacterial species and same susceptibility	Emphasize need to administer the full dose of antibiotics Determine whether owner is capable and willing to administer medication Demonstrate a variety of methods to administer medication
Clinician factors 1. Incorrect prediction of mineral type	Analysis of retrieved urolith	Alter therapy based on identification of mineral type
2. Inappropriate antibiotic choice	Positive urine culture with poor susceptibility for chosen antibiotic	Choose antibiotics based on susceptibility testing
3. Inappropriate antibiotic dose for degree of diuresis	Positive quantitative urine culture with same bacterial species and same susceptibility, number of bacteria may be lower	Administer antibiotic at the higher recommended dose, or consider a higher dose than recommended
4. Premature discontinuation of antibiotic	Discontinuing antibiotic before complete urolith dissolution Positive urine culture with same bacterial species and same susceptibility	Prescribe full antibiotic dose for the entire period of urolith dissolution
Disease factors 1. Change in bacterial susceptibility	Positive urine culture with susceptibility results different from previous culture	Choose antibiotic based on susceptibility testing
2. New bacterial infection	Positive urine culture identifying new bacterial species	Choose antibiotic effective against both bacteria Avoid procedures requiring urinary catheterization
3. Compound urolith	Radiographic density of nucleus and outer layer(s) of urolith are different Analysis of retrieved urolith	Alter therapy based on identification of new mineral type Uroliths not causing clinical signs should be monitored for potential adverse consequences (e.g., obstruction, UTI) Clinically active uroliths may require surgical removal; remove small uroliths by voiding urohydropropulsion (see Fig. 176–6)

short-term (weeks or months) dissolution therapy rather than long-term (months to years) prophylactic therapy. Changes in serum urea nitrogen concentration may be used as one index of client and patient compliance with dietary recommendations.

Controlled experimental and clinical studies have confirmed the efficacy of calculolytic diets (Hill's Prescription Diet Canine s/d) in inducing sterile struvite urolith dissolution.[42] Unless secondary UTI develops, antibiotics and urease inhibitors are not required. The time required to induce dissolution of sterile struvite is usually shorter than that required for infection-induced struvite. When the calculolytic diet was given to nine dogs with naturally occurring sterile uroliths presumed to be composed of struvite, uroliths dissolved in a mean time of 6 weeks (range, 1 to 3 months). After management of six episodes of naturally occurring sterile struvite urocystoliths affecting two unrelated male English cocker spaniels with calculolytic diet, the uroliths dissolved in a mean interval of 38.5 ± 12.8 days.[39]

Urease Inhibitors. Experimental and clinical studies of dogs have revealed that administration of microbial urease inhibitors in pharmacologic doses inhibits struvite urolith growth or promotes struvite urolith dissolution. Acetohydroxamic acid (AHA) given orally to dogs, 11.5 mg/lb/day in two divided subdoses, reduces urease activity, struvite crystalluria, and urolith growth.[43] By reducing the pathogenicity of staphylococci it may also reduce the severity of dysuria, bacteriuria, pyuria, hematuria, and proteinuria.

Although larger doses of AHA may dissolve uroliths, they are not recommended, because they may cause reversible hemolytic anemia and abnormalities in bilirubin metabolism.[43] AHA should not be administered to pregnant dogs, because it is teratogenic.[44]

We have not routinely used AHA to promote dissolution of infection-induced struvite uroliths in dogs because calculolytic diet and antimicrobial therapy are efficacious. However, we have used this agent in combination with calculolytic diets and antimicrobial agents for patients that have refractory "urease-producing UTI." If infection-induced struvite uroliths do not dissolve after an appropriate trial of therapy with diet modification and antimicrobial agents, AHA may be added to the therapeutic regimen.

Prevention. *Infection-Induced Struvite Uroliths.* Eradication or control of UTIs caused by urease-producing bacteria is the most important factor in preventing recurrence of most infection-induced struvite uroliths. If recurrent UTI persists, indefinite therapy with prophylactic doses of antimicrobial agents that are eliminated in high concentration in urine is indicated.

In light of the effectiveness of diets inducing dissolution of struvite uroliths, use of dietary modification to prevent recurrence of uroliths is logical and feasible. However, further studies must be performed to evaluate the long-term effects of low-protein calculolytic diets in dogs before reliable recommendations can be established. Because they induce polyuria, varying degrees of hypoalbuminemia, and mild alteration in hepatic enzymes and morphology, we recommend long-term use of severely protein-restricted calculolytic diets only if patients develop recurrent urolithiasis despite augmented fluid intake, urine acidification, and attempts to control infection.

Studies are in progress to evaluate the preventive efficacy of mild to moderate restriction of protein, magnesium, and phosphorus in acidifying diets. Caution must be used when deciding whether to induce prophylactic diuresis in patients with a history of struvite uroliths induced by recurrent UTI.

Although formation of dilute urine tends to minimize supersaturation with calculogenic crystalloids, it tends also to counteract the natural antimicrobial properties of urine. Experimental studies of rats and cats indicate that diuresis tends to minimize pyelonephritis but enhance lower UTI.

Sterile Struvite Uroliths. When compared with patients with infection-induced struvite uroliths in which the UTI has been eradicated or controlled, sterile struvite uroliths have a greater tendency to recur. If the urine pH of patients with sterile struvite urolithiasis remains alkaline, administration of urine acidifiers should be considered. The prophylactic value of concomitant restriction of dietary phosphorus and magnesium has not been determined.

CALCIUM OXALATE

Calcium oxalate uroliths are the second most common urolith analyzed by the Minnesota Urolith Center. At one time, detection of calcium oxalate in uroliths of dogs was considered to be uncommon. For example, in a study of the composition of naturally developing uroliths removed from the urinary tract of 150 miniature schnauzers and submitted to the University of Minnesota before 1981, uroliths composed of calcium oxalate were detected in 6 dogs (4 per cent).[45] The prevalence of dogs with calcium oxalate has increased from 5.3 per cent in 1981 (17 of 320 submissions) to 35.4 per cent in 1997 (5,401 of 15,259 submissions) (see Table 176–1).

Over the past 50 years, the incidence of calcium oxalate uroliths in humans living in the United States has also increased.[46] Global distributions of urolithiasis in humans indicate that calcium oxalate uroliths predominate in the United States and other industrialized, technologically advanced regions of the world. Although originally attributed to the sedentary lifestyle of inhabitants of such countries, increased incidence of calcium oxalate uroliths now is thought to reflect the ability of these more affluent societies to spend disposable income for the consumption of animal protein, which leads to increased urinary excretion of calcium and oxalate. This prompts the question as to whether variables contributing to the increased incidence of calcium oxalate uroliths in humans also influence the incidence of calcium oxalate uroliths in dogs.

Between 1981 and 1997 the Minnesota Urolith Center diagnosed calcium oxalate uroliths in 24,267 dogs. Although calcium oxalate uroliths have been reported in many breeds, 58 per cent of cases were represented by only six breeds; miniature schnauzer (24.1 per cent), Lhasa apso (8.9 per cent), Yorkshire terrier (8.3 per cent), bichon frisé (6.3 per cent), Shih Tzu (5.7 per cent), and miniature poodle (5.2 per cent). An additional 13.1 per cent were reported in mixed breed dogs.

Data from this survey support the hypothesis that some of the factors promoting formation of calcium oxalate uroliths in dogs are inherited.[47, 48] Familial patterns of calcium oxalate urolithiasis and hypercalcemia have been recognized in humans. A genetic basis for recurrent calcium oxalate urolithiasis has been clearly established in humans with primary hyperoxaluria and hereditary distal renal tubular acidosis. Selective breeding of hypercalciuric rats increased the intensity and frequency of hypercalciuria in their offspring and provided evidence for hereditary hypercalciuria.[49] Genetics provide a plausible explanation for the disproportionate increase in calcium oxalate uroliths in commonly affected canine breeds.

URO

Of the 24,263 dogs with calcium oxalate uroliths, 71.2 per cent were male (30.6 per cent were intact and 69.4 per cent were neutered) and 26 per cent were female (12.1 per cent were intact and 87.9 per cent were neutered). Gender was not reported in 2.8 per cent of dogs. In humans, calcium oxalate uroliths also were recognized more frequently in males than females. It has been postulated that women have a lower incidence of calcium oxalate uroliths because of estrogen-dependent increases in urine citrate concentration and estrogen-dependent decreases in urine calcium and oxalate concentrations.

Our data suggest that calcium oxalate uroliths more commonly affect older dogs. Although calcium oxalate uroliths were detected in dogs younger than 1 year of age, the mean age at detection was 8.5 ± 2.9 years. Sixty per cent of dogs with calcium oxalate uroliths were between 6 and 11 years old.

Etiopathogenesis. For uroliths to form, urine must be supersaturated with respect to that crystal system.[50] Following this line of reasoning, calcium oxalate uroliths form as a result of varying combinations of underlying factors that disturb the balance between urine concentrations of potentially lithogenic minerals (calcium and oxalate) and stone inhibitors (e.g., citrate, phosphorus, magnesium, uric acid, Tamm-Horsfall mucoprotein, and nephrocalcin).

Role of Diet

CALCIUM. Intestinal hyperabsorption of calcium is recognized as a common cause of hypercalciuria and calcium oxalate urolithiasis in humans. Our observations indicate that excessive gastrointestinal absorption of calcium is an important cause of sustained hypercalciuria in dogs with calcium oxalate urolithiasis.[51] Based on this observation it may seem logical to restrict dietary calcium to minimize calcium oxalate urolith formation. However, results of recent studies suggest that dietary calcium restriction increases the risk of calcium oxalate uroliths.

An important relationship exists between gastrointestinal absorption of oxalate acid and calcium. Dietary calcium and oxalic acid form complexes of nonabsorbable calcium oxalate in the intestinal lumen. However, if dietary calcium is reduced without a concomitant reduction in oxalic acid, intestinal absorption of oxalic acid from the intestine followed by increased urinary excretion may occur. Hyperoxaluria is a greater risk factor for calcium oxalate urolith formation than an equivalent increase in urinary calcium concentration because smaller increments of oxalic acid are required for formation of insoluble calcium oxalate. This produces a plausible explanation as to why humans consuming diets with reduced levels of calcium are at greater risk for calcium oxalate urolith formation compared with those consuming diets with a higher calcium content.[52] In contrast, consumption of calcium supplements between meals would not alter dietary oxalic acid absorption. In this situation, dietary calcium supplements result in increased absorption and excretion of calcium in urine because it is not bound to intestinal oxalic acid. Thus, oral calcium supplements are a risk factor for calcium oxalate urolith formation.[53]

OXALATE. Hyperoxaluria promotes recurrence of calcium oxalate uroliths because comparatively small increments in oxalate excretion markedly increase the formation of calcium oxalate crystals. Although small quantities of oxalic acid are a common component of many foods, foods such as spinach, rhubarb, peanuts, chocolate, and tea contain large quantities.

Oxalic acid is the metabolic end-product of glyoxylate metabolism. The majority of urine oxalic acid is derived from metabolic pathways; 30 to 40 per cent is derived from the metabolism of ascorbic acid. The remainder is derived from the conversion of glycine and glycolate, compounds primarily derived from dietary protein and sugar (Fig. 176-7). Vitamin B_6 also plays a key role in oxalate metabolism; vitamin B_6 deficiency results in increased formation of oxalic acid and hyperoxaluria.

ANIMAL PROTEIN. Consumption of animal protein is a risk factor for calcium oxalate urolithiasis because it increases urinary calcium excretion and decreases urinary citric acid excretion (citric acid chelates calcium to form a soluble salt of calcium citrate). One mechanism for protein-mediated hypercalciuria is increased endogenous acid production and thus increased urinary acid excretion. Acidifying metabolites are neutralized by phosphate and carbonate mobilized from bone. Calcium released from bone along with phosphate and carbonate results in hypercalciuria. Increased urine acid excretion also is thought to decrease calcium reabsorption in the distal nephron and increase urine citric acid uptake in the proximal nephron. Dietary protein may also promote hypercalciuria by increasing the glomerular filtration rate.

SODIUM. The postulate that reducing dietary sodium would be beneficial in treatment of calcium oxalate urolithiasis was based on the observations that increased sodium consumption by humans was associated with increased urinary sodium and calcium excretion. To determine if dietary sodium altered urine calcium excretion in dogs, we fed six clinically healthy beagles a canned diet with and without sodium chloride supplementation. By using a cross-over study design, each dog was evaluated during both treatments. At the end of each 6-week treatment period, 24-hour urine calcium excretion was determined. Mean urine calcium excretion was lower (0.49 mg/kg/24 hr) when dogs consumed the diet without sodium chloride supplmentation (0.24 per cent sodium on a dry matter basis) compared with urine calcium excretion (1.36 mg/kg/24 hr) during sodium supplementation (1.2 per cent sodium on a dry matter basis). Likewise, urinary calcium and sodium excretion increased in dogs parenterally given isotonic saline, hypertonic mannitol, and hypertonic glucose. These observations are physiologically

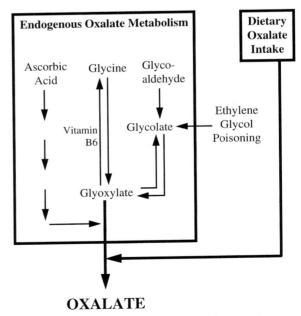

OXALATE

Figure 176-7. Biosynthesis and excretion of oxalate.

sound, because calcium and sodium are absorbed at common sites along the renal tubule. At one time, oral sodium chloride was commonly recommended to minimize urolith recurrence in dogs by promoting thirst and diuresis. However, it is now thought that dietary sodium should be restricted when designing protocols to minimize calcium oxalate urolith recurrence.

PHOSPHORUS. In humans, neutral potassium phosphate (1500 mg/d) lowers urinary calcium excretion. The ability of phosphorus to reduce calcium oxalate urolith recurrence is often attributed to its role in minimizing renal production of calcitriol, and also by enhancing urinary excretion of pyrophosphate, an inhibitor of calcium oxalate salts. Diets deficient in phosphorus may stimulate calcitriol production, which promotes intestinal absorption of both calcium and phosphorus. Therefore, diets designed to minimize calcium oxalate urolith formation should not be designed to restrict phosphorus. Diets deficient in phosphorus may also enhance the availablitiy of absorbable calcium in the intestine. Whether or not dietary phosphorus supplements will minimize calcium oxalate urolith formation in dogs awaits further study.

POTASSIUM. Results of epidemiologic studies in humans, dogs, and cats indicate that diets higher in potassium are less frequently associated with calcium oxalate urolith formation.[48, 53] The beneficial effect of potassium may be due to the high alkali content of many potassium-rich foods, which in turn would be expected to increase urine citric acid, a natural inhibitor of calcium crystals in urine.

WATER. If excessive fluid dilutes crystallization inhibitors, it could paradoxically increase the risk of calcium oxalate formation. However, reducing the urine concentration of lithogenic constituents by increasing urine volume may more than offset the potential detrimental effect of crystallization inhibitors and thus prove to be beneficial. Diuresis associated with increased fluid intake has been associated with decreased risk of calcium oxalate urolithiasis in humans. Likewise, cats consuming canned diets had one third the risk for calcium oxalate urolith formation compared with cats consuming other dietary formulations. It is logical to assume that a similar effect occurs in dogs.

Defective Macromolecular Crystal Growth Inhibitors. In addition to urinary concentration of calculogenic minerals and other ions, crystallization inhibitors have a profound ability to enhance solubility of calcium oxalate. Citrate, glycosaminoglycans, Tamm-Horsfall protein, osteopontin, nephrocalcin, uronic acid–rich protein, and urinary prothrombin fragment are substances identified in human urine that have a high affinity for calcium ions.[54–56a] Preliminary studies of urine obtained from dogs with calcium oxalate uroliths identified defective nephrocalcin.

Normal nephrocalcin is an acidic glycoprotein containing 33 per cent acidic amino acids residues and 5 per cent aromatic and basic amino acid residues. Nephrocalcin has been purified into four isoforms, designated as fractions A through D. Nephrocalcin from humans without uroliths is biochemically different from nephrocalcin in humans with calcium oxalate uroliths. Fractions A and B are strong inhibitors of calcium oxalate crystal growth and abundant in the urine of normal humans. Humans with calcium oxalate urolithiasis excrete reduced quantities of fractions A and B and more of fractions C and D, which are weak inhibitors of calcium oxalate crystal growth.

The exact mechanisms by which nephrocalcin inhibits crystal growth are not completely understood; however, nephrocalcin's amphiphilic nature and film-forming capabili-

ties appear to be important factors. It is hypothesized that the hydrophilic or charged portion of nephrocalcin becomes anchored to the surface of calcium oxalate crystals. Nephrocalcin forms a stable two-dimensional film that is able to cover the crystal. With the hydrophilic portion attached to the crystal surface, the hydrophobic moieties of nephrocalcin are exposed to ions in urine. The hydrophobic regions of nephrocalcin have few charged sites. As a result, few sites of attachment are available for ions in solution (urine). Therefore, calcium oxalate crystal growth by addition of new ions (i.e., minerals) is inhibited.

We characterized nephrocalcin in six clinically healthy beagles without uroliths and seven dogs with calcium oxalate uroliths. Our findings support the hypothesis that dogs with calcium oxalate uroliths have abnormal nephrocalcin. As in humans with calcium oxalate uroliths, the urine of dogs with calcium oxalate uroliths had greater quantities of nephrocalcin fractions C and D and lesser quantities of fractions A and B when compared with the urine of dogs without uroliths. With lesser quantities of fractions A and B, we hypothesize that nephrocalcin from dogs with calcium oxalate uroliths is not an effective inhibitor of crystal growth.

Concurrent Diseases. Diseases promoting urine excretion of calcium and oxalic acid excretion increase the risk of calcium oxalate formation. Calcium oxalate and calcium phosphate uroliths have been reported in several surveys of dogs with primary hyperparathyroidism and hypercalcemia.[58–60] We are unaware of a documented association between calcium oxalate uroliths and paraneoplastic hypercalcemia in dogs with other types of cancer.

In a retrospective case-controlled study of dogs with urolithiasis, dogs with hyperadrenocorticism were 10 times as likely to have uroliths containing calcium.[61] Thirteen of the 16 dogs with calcium-containing uroliths had uroliths composed of calcium oxalate. The mechanism for increased urine calcium excretion is not completely understood. A glucocorticoid-mediated decrease in renal tubular calcium reabsorption has been suggested.[62] Glucocorticoids also increase glomerular filtration rate.

The Reciprocal Relationship Between Calcium Oxalate and Struvite Uroliths. Although the prevalence of canine calcium oxalate uroliths has been increasing, the prevalence of struvite uroliths has declined. In 1981, uroliths were submitted for analysis from 320 dogs; 77.5 per cent of dogs were diagnosed with struvite. By comparison, in 1997 the prevalence of struvite uroliths was 45.4 per cent (6923 of 15,259 submissions), a decline of almost 40 per cent. During this same time period the prevalence of calcium oxalate uroliths has increased by 670 per cent (Fig. 176–8). Several possibilities have been hypothesized to explain the decrease in struvite uroliths occurring with the reciprocal rise in calcium oxalate uroliths. As our understanding of the pathophysiology of struvite uroliths excelled, clinicians have been better able to prevent and dissolve them. As a result, struvite urolith formation and their submission for analysis would have decreased, resulting in a proportional increase in the percentage of calcium oxalate uroliths. Formation of most struvite uroliths in dogs is dependent on prior development of a UTI with urease-producing bacteria. Therefore, improved strategies and antimicrobials for controlling UTI today, as opposed to a decade ago, would contribute to the decreased struvite urolith formation.

Many breeds with a high prevalence of struvite also have a high prevalence for calcium oxalate. However, dogs forming calcium oxalate uroliths were significantly older (8.5 ± 2.9 years) than dogs forming struvite uroliths (6 ± 2.9 years).

URO

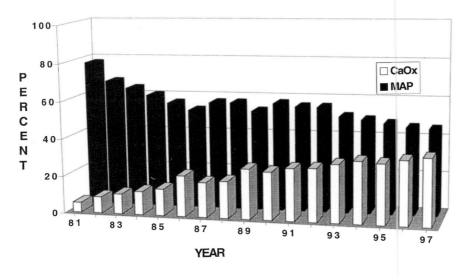

Figure 176–8. Yearly distribution of calcium oxalate and struvite uroliths in dogs (1981–1997).

These observations may help explain why some dogs that formed struvite uroliths previously are at risk for forming calcium oxalate later in life. Perhaps these breeds are at risk for forming all urolith types. This phenomenon could be explained by inadequate or defective production of a universal crystal inhibitor in these breeds of dogs. Likewise, control of some risk factors in dogs that initially form struvite uroliths (e.g., reduced pH, reduced magnesium, and reduced phosphorus) predispose to formation of calcium oxalate uroliths.

Treatment. In contrast to struvite, urate, and cystine uroliths that dissolve when supersaturation of urine with calculogenic substances is abolished, as yet we have been unable to dissolve calcium oxalate uroliths in dogs. Therefore, physically removing calcium oxalate uroliths remains the current method to correct clinically active disease. Surgery is the time-honored method to remove calcium oxalate uroliths from the urinary tract; however, because of the small size and irregular contour of many calcium oxalate uroliths, complete surgical removal of all visible uroliths may be difficult. Alternatively, small urocystoliths can be nonsurgi-

cally removed by aspiration through a transurethral catheter or voiding urohydropropulsion instead of cystotomy.[33, 34] Nephroliths and ureteroliths associated with complete obstruction or progressive deterioration in renal function are indications for their removal. Lithotripsy provides a nonsurgical means of removing calcium oxalate uroliths from kidneys and ureters.[63] In some patients, however, calcium oxalate uroliths are clinically silent, obviating the need for intervention (Fig. 176–9). For those patients in which surgery is not indicated, the clinical status of uroliths should be periodically assessed by urinalyses, renal function tests, radiography, and/or ultrasonography.

Prevention. Therapy designed to decrease urine concentrations of lithogenic minerals and also to increase urine concentrations of stone inhibitors will minimize the recurrence of calcium oxalate uroliths. However, caution must be used so that side effects of treatment are not more detrimental than the effects of uroliths. To avoid overtreatment, we recommend that medical therapy be formulated in a stepwise fashion. To minimize the recurrence of uroliths, we use the following chronologic sequence: (1) evaluate baseline data,

TABLE 176–11. RISK FACTORS TO AVOID TO MINIMIZE CALCIUM OXALATE UROLITH FORMATION

RISK FACTOR	RATIONALE
Calcium supplements independent of meals	Promote excessive urine calcium excretion
Canine treats	In an epidemiologic study, feeding canine treats was associated with calcium oxalate urolithiasis.
Concentrated urine	Decreased urine volume results in increased urine concentration of calculogenic precursors.
Drugs and diets promoting acidosis and acidic urine (e.g., ammonium chloride, methionine, diets to dissolve or prevent struvite uroliths)	Promotes hypercalciuria and decreases citrate excretion
Dry diets	Are associated with formation of more-concentrated urine and higher concentrations of calculogenic minerals
Foods with high protein content	Promote metabolic acidosis, increased urine calcium excretion, and decreased urine citrate excretion
Foods with high oxalate content (see Table 176–5)	Promote increased urine oxalate excretion
Furosemide	Promotes increased urine calcium excretion
Glucocorticoids	Promotes skeletal resorption and increased urine calcium excretion
Human food	In an epidemiologic study, feeding human food was associated with calcium oxalate urolithiasis in dogs.
Restricted availability of urine elimination	Prolonged crystal retention allows crystal growth
Sodium chloride	Promotes increased urine calcium excretion
Vitamin C supplements	Serve as a substrate for conversion to oxalate
Vitamin D supplements	Promote intestinal calcium absorption and subsequent hypercalciuria
Water restriction	Decreased urine volume results in increased urine concentration of calculogenic precursors

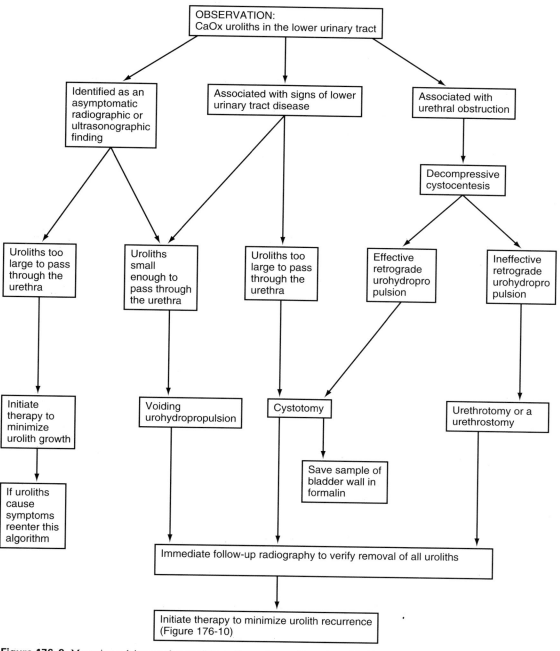

Figure 176–9. Managing calcium oxalate uroliths in the urethra and/or urinary bladder. Consider voiding urohydropropulsion or cystotomy to remove any uroliths remaining in the urinary bladder.

(2) eliminate correctable risk factors, (3) modify the diet, (4) consider pharmacologic intervention, and (5) monitor outcome of therapy (Fig. 176–10).

Evaluate Baseline Data. Serum calcium concentration is needed to identify dogs with hypercalcemia. Hypercalcemia warrants further investigation as to its underlying cause. In dogs with normal serum calcium concentrations, risk factors for urolith formation should be identified and controlled.

Evaluation of serum total carbon dioxide concentrations may be beneficial in as much as acidemia stimulates mobilization of phosphorus and carbonate from bone to buffer acids. Release of calcium at the same time results in hypercalciuria.

Eliminate or Reduce Risk Factors. Some risk factors for

calcium oxalate urolith formation cannot be influenced, such as age, breed, and gender. Other risk factors can be modified, such as medications and nutrient supplements (Tables 176–11 to 176–13). For example, urinary acidifiers are beneficial in preventing struvite urolith formation; however, acid-producing medications are a risk factor for calcium oxalate urolith formation. To minimize calcium oxalate urolith formation in dogs, urinary acidifiers (e.g., ammonium chloride and methionine) should be avoided.

Diuretics have been recommended for dogs with uroliths to reduce the concentrations of minerals in urine by increasing urine volume. However, the effect of diuretic therapy is dependent on the type of diuretic given. Because thiazide diuretics promote renal tubular reabsorption of sodium and

URO

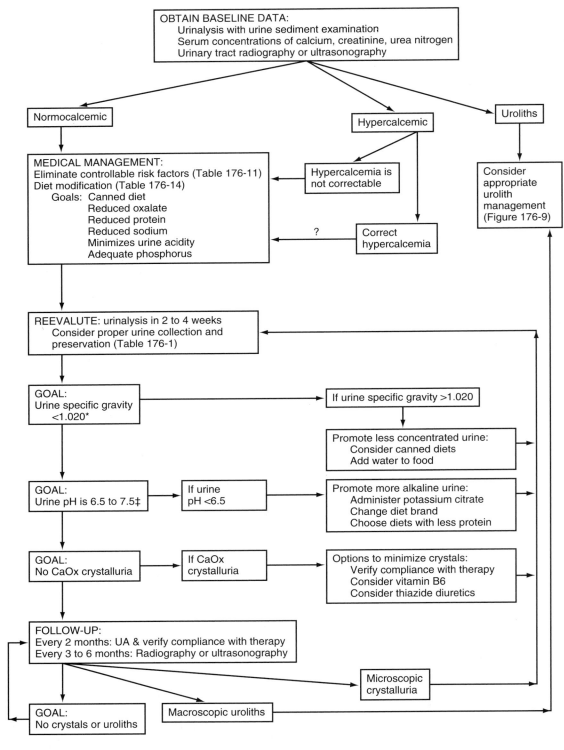

CaOx = calcium oxalate
* In general, the degree to which the urine specific gravity is lowered, will concomitantly lower the concentration
   of calculogenic minerals, which in turn reduces the risk for urolith formation.
‡ In general, formation of alkaline urine is associated with 1) minimizing skeletal calcium release associated with
   bone buffering of metabolic acids and 2) promoting renal tubular reabsorption of calcium and 3) promoting
   renal tubular excretion of citrate.

Figure 176–10. Minimizing calcium oxalate urolith growth and recurrence.

TABLE 176–12. SOME HUMAN FOODS PERMISSIBLE TO FEED TO DOGS WITH CALCIUM OXALATE UROLITHIASIS

Meats
  Eggs
  Poultry

Vegetables
  Avocado
  Cabbage
  Cauliflower
  Mushrooms
  Peas, green
  Radishes
  White potatoes

Fruits
  Avocado
  Banana
  Bing cherries
  Grapefruit
  Green grapes
  Mangos
  Melons: cantaloupe, casaba, honeydew, watermelon
  Plums: green or yellow

Breads, grains, nuts
  Macaroni
  Rice
  Spaghetti

Miscellaneous
  Jellies
  Preserves

Note: These foods have minimal calcium oxalate content.

calcium, they minimize hypercalciuria. However, loop diuretics (e.g., furosemide) promote sodium and calcium excretion and exacerbate hypercalciuria. A safe and effective alternate method of increasing urine volume is feeding canned food instead of dry diets or addition of water to

TABLE 176–13. SOME HUMAN FOODS TO AVOID FEEDING TO DOGS WITH CALCIUM OXALATE UROLITHIASIS

Meats	Fruits
Bologna	Apples
Herring	Apricots
Oysters	Cherries
Salmon	Most berries
Sardines	Peel of lemon, lime, or orange
	Pineapple
Vegetables	Tangerine
Asparagus	
Baked beans	Breads, grains, nuts
Broccoli	Corn bread
Carrots	Fruit cake
Celery	Grits
Corn	Peanuts
Cucumber	Pecans
Eggplant	Soybean
Green beans	Wheat germ
Green peppers	
Lettuce	Miscellaneous
Spinach	Beer
Sweet potatoes	Chocolate
Tofu	Cocoa
Tomatoes	Teas
Milk and dairy products	
Cheese	
Ice cream	
Milk	
Yogurt	

Note: These foods have high calcium oxalate content.

food. Other drugs that are risk factors for calcium oxalate uroliths because they promote calciuresis include sodium chloride, vitamin D, calcium supplements, and glucocorticoids.

Modify Diet. Intestinal hyperabsorption of calcium is recognized as a common cause of hypercalciuria and calcium oxalate urolithiasis in humans. Our observations indicate that excessive gastrointestinal absorption of calcium is an important cause of sustained hypercalciuria in dogs with calcium oxalate urolithiasis.[51] Based on this observation it seems logical to restrict dietary calcium to minimize calcium oxalate urolith formation. However, results of recent studies suggest that dietary calcium restriction increases the risk of calcium oxalate uroliths.

An important relationship exists between gastrointestinal absorption of oxalate and calcium. Dietary calcium in the intestinal lumen complexes with oxalate to form calcium oxalate, which is poorly absorbed. Conversely, if dietary calcium is reduced without a concomitant reduction in oxalate, intestinal absorption of oxalate and its urinary excretion increase.

Although oxalate is a common component of many foods, the majority of urine oxalate is derived from endogenous metabolic pathways (see earlier). Consumption of animal protein is a risk factor for calcium oxalate urolithiasis because it increases urinary calcium excretion and decreases urinary citrate excretion (citrate chelates calcium to form a soluble salt of calcium citrate).

To minimize calcium oxalate urolith recurrence we recommend diets with lower quantities of protein and sodium and adequate phosphorus, magnesium, and potassium. Ideally, diets should not promote acidosis or contain excessive oxalate. Canned diets are preferred over dry formulations because the diuresis associated with increased fluid intake should minimize the concentration of calculogenic substances in urine (Table 176–14).

Pharmacologic Therapy. Detection of persistent calcium oxalate crystalluria or recurrence of uroliths despite diet modification should prompt consideration of adding various drugs to the prevention protocol. Each drug should be incorporated in a stepwise fashion, evaluating urinalyses before selecting additional medications.

In humans, potassium citrate is highly effective in prevention of recurrent calcium oxalate uroliths by forming soluble salts with calcium (e.g., calcium citrate). However, oral administration of up to 150 mg/kg/d of potassium citrate to normal dogs was not associated with a consistent rise in urine citrate concentration. However, a dose-dependent rise in urine pH did occur. Even though, oral administration of potassium citrate may not be associated with a sustained increase in urine citrate concentration in dogs, potassium citrate may be beneficial in management of calcium oxalate because of its alkalinizing effects.

Vitamin B$_6$ has been recommended for management of calcium oxalate uroliths because it reversed hyperoxaluria in kittens fed vitamin B$_6$–deficient diets.[64] We do not generally consider vitamin B$_6$ unless dogs are consuming unfortified diets (human food or owner-made diets) or have maldigestive or malabsorptive disorders.

Thiazide diuretics have been recommended to reduce recurrence of calcium-containing uroliths in humans because of their ability to reduce urine calcium excretion. The exact mechanism(s) by which thiazide diuretics reduce urine calcium excretion is unknown. Because the hypocalciuric response of thiazide diuretics was blocked when volume depletion was prevented by sodium chloride administration in

TABLE 176–14. SOME CANNED DIETS WITH QUALITIES THAT POTENTIALLY MINIMIZE THE RISK FOR CALCIUM OXALATE UROLITH FORMATION IN DOGS

DIET	DIET COMPONENTS (% DRY MATTER)					
	Protein	*Carbohydrate*	*Ca*	*P*	*Na*	*K*
Prescription Diet u/d* (Hill's Pet Products)	11.5	57.4	0.29	0.11	0.25	0.39
Prescription Diet k/d (Hill's Pet Products)	14.8	54.6	0.81	0.11	0.21	0.30
Prescription Diet w/d† (Hill's Pet Products)	16.2	54.3	0.49	0.42	0.26	0.60
NF-Formula (Purina)	16.5	50.36	0.5	0.3	0.24	0.72
Canine Modified Formula (Select Care)	16.8	55.9	0.83	0.35	0.24	0.96
Canine Low Protein (Waltham Veterinary Diets)	17.7	50.5	1.16	0.51	0.59	0.86

*Contains potassium citrate and promotes formation of alkaline urine.
†Considered for dogs with fiber-responsive disorders (e.g., recurrent pancreatitis, hyperadrenocorticism, hyperlipidemia, diabetes mellitus, obesity) and calcium oxalate urolithiasis.

humans, it has been hypothesized that thiazide diuretics promote mild extracellular volume contraction, thereby promoting proximal tubular reabsorption of several solutes, including sodium and calcium. We observed a significant reduction in urine calcium excretion in eight dogs with calcium oxalate urolithiasis after 2 weeks of oral hydrochlorothiazide (1 mg/lb q12 h).

Monitoring Response to Therapy. After selection of a protocol to minimize calcium oxalate recurrence, the safety and efficacy of the protocol must be evaluated. Control of dietary risk factors should reduce urine concentration (e.g., specific gravity), minimize or prevent aciduria (e.g., urine pH), and eliminate crystalluria. We recommend that urinalyses be repeated every 2 to 4 weeks to determine if modifications in therapy achieve these goals (see Fig. 176–10).

The decision to include drug therapy in the prevention protocol requires monitoring not only the effectiveness of the drugs to minimize urolith recurrence but also their potential for adverse effects. Mild hyperkalemia (up to 6.1 mEq/L) has been the only laboratory abnormality that we have observed with higher doses of potassium citrate. Although unassociated with clinical signs, we recommend that the dosage of potassium citrate be reduced or an alternative alkalinizing agent be considered. Although the product insert states that nausea, vomiting, abdominal discomfort, and diarrhea have been reported in humans, we have not observed these adverse effects.

Hypokalemia, hypercalcemia, and dehydration are potential adverse effects of thiazide diuretics. When initiating hydrochlorothiazide therapy, we recommend evaluation of serum electrolyte concentrations within several weeks. If dosages are adjusted, serum electrolytes should be evaluated within 2 weeks.

Because diet modification and drug therapy usually do not eliminate all of the underlying risk factors, complete elimination of all urolith recurrences should not be expected. In our experience, therapy will eliminate urolith recurrence in some dogs and delay urolith recurrence in others. However, the fact that uroliths recur does not always mean that additional surgery will be required. The key to eliminating additional surgery is detection of uroliths when they are small enough to easily pass through the urethral lumen. Small urocystoliths can be quickly and effectively removed by voiding urohydropropulsion in male and female dogs. Therefore, we recommend radiographic imaging of the urinary tract every 3 to 6 months even if patients are asympto-

matic. If patients are re-evaluated only at the time they develop clinical signs associated with uroliths, uroliths are often too large to pass through the urethra (see Fig. 176–10).

Most calcium oxalate uroliths form during a limited span of life. In our experience, urolith formation seems to diminish or fade out with time. Why this occurs is poorly understood. We have observed that as animals age, they are more likely to develop dilute urine. Because dilute urine is likely to be associated with reduced urine concentrations of calcium and oxalate, it may provide one logical explanation for the concomitant reduction in urolith formation.

Therapy should also be interrupted if patients develop more serious diseases in which therapy for uroliths is contraindicated. For example, potassium citrate may promote life-threatening hyperkalemia in dogs that later develop hypoadrenocorticism. Reducing dietary protein is recommended to prevent calcium oxalate urolith recurrence. Protein calories eliminated from commercial diets are often replaced with additional fat calories. Addition of fat to a diet may adversely affect dogs at risk for pancreatitis. Miniature schnauzers, which have a high incidence of calcium oxalate uroliths, also have a high incidence of diseases in which additional dietary fat would be contraindicated (i.e., hereditary hyperlipidemia, hyperadrenocorticism, diabetes mellitus, and pancreatitis). Therefore, formulating preventative therapy in this breed requires special considerations and monitoring to prevent adverse effects of therapy.

Treating Dogs at Risk for Both Calcium Oxalate and Struvite Uroliths. Dogs have formed calcium oxalate uroliths after successful management of struvite uroliths and vice versa. Sometimes, a urolith contains both struvite and calcium oxalate. The paradox in managing patients forming uroliths with both of these minerals is that control of some risk factors for struvite urolith formation (such as pH, magnesium, and phosphorus) predisposes to formation of calcium oxalate uroliths. In this situation, we recommend that emphasis be placed on minimizing recurrence of calcium oxalate uroliths, because calcium oxalate uroliths cannot be dissolved medically (Fig. 176–11).

CANINE AMMMONIUM URATE AND URIC ACID UROLITHIASIS

Etiopathogenesis. Uric acid is one of several biodegradation products of purine nucleotide metabolism. Ammo-

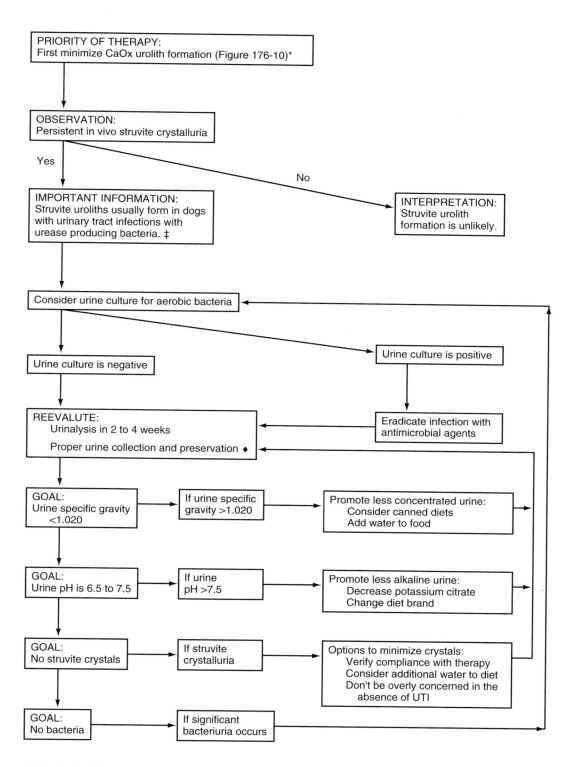

PRIORITY OF THERAPY:
First minimize CaOx urolith formation (Figure 176-10)*

OBSERVATION:
Persistent in vivo struvite crystalluria

Yes

No

INTERPRETATION:
Struvite urolith
formation is unlikely.

IMPORTANT INFORMATION:
Struvite uroliths usually form in dogs
with urinary tract infections with
urease producing bacteria. ‡

Consider urine culture for aerobic bacteria

Urine culture is negative

Urine culture is positive

REEVALUTE:
  Urinalysis in 2 to 4 weeks

  Proper urine collection and preservation ♦

Eradicate infection with
antimicrobial agents

GOAL:
Urine specific gravity
<1.020

If urine specific
gravity >1.020

Promote less concentrated urine:
  Consider canned diets
  Add water to food

GOAL:
Urine pH is 6.5 to 7.5

If urine
pH >7.5

Promote less alkaline urine:
  Decrease potassium citrate
  Change diet brand

GOAL:
No struvite crystals

If struvite
crystalluria

Options to minimize crystals:
  Verify compliance with therapy
  Consider additional water to diet
  Don't be overly concerned in the
     absence of UTI

GOAL:
No bacteria

If significant
bacteriuria occurs

URO

* In those situations where dogs have documented occurrences of both calcium oxalate and struvite uroliths, we
   recommend that emphasis be placed on minimizing recurrence of calcium oxalate uroliths, since this type of
   urolith cannot be dissolved by medical management.
‡ Staphylococcal and proteus are the most common species of bacteria associated with struvite urolith formation
   in dogs.
♦ Evaluating urine samples collected by owners or preserved by refrigeration is not recommended because
   contamination, increased storage time, changes in pH, and changes in temperature promote in vitro crystalluria.

Figure 176–11. Managing dogs at risk for both calcium oxalate and struvite urolith formation.

nium urate (also known as ammonium acid urate and ammonium biurate) is the monobasic ammonium salt of uric acid. It is the most common naturally occurring purine urolith observed in dogs. Other naturally occurring purine uroliths include sodium urate, sodium calcium urate, potassium urate, uric acid dihydrate, and xanthine.

Dalmatians. Dalmatian dogs are predisposed to urate uroliths owing to unique metabolism of purines. The ability of Dalmatians to oxidize uric acid to allantoin is intermediate between humans and non-Dalmatian dogs. Humans have a serum uric acid concentration of 3 to 7 mg/dL and excrete 500 to 700 mg of uric acid in their urine per day.[65] Non-Dalmatian dogs have a serum uric acid concentration of less than 0.5 mg/dL and excrete 10 to 60 mg of uric acid in their urine per day. Dalmatians have a serum uric acid concentration that is two to four times that of non-Dalmatians and excrete 400 to 600 mg of uric acid in their urine per day.[66] Studies of the fate of uric acid in Dalmatians have revealed unique hepatic and renal pathways of metabolism. Of these two metabolic sites, reciprocal allogenic renal and hepatic transplantations between Dalmatians and non-Dalmatians indicate that the hepatic mechanism is quantitatively the most significant.[67] The liver of Dalmatians does not completely oxidize available uric acid, even though it contains a sufficient concentration of uricase. Compared with non-Dalmatians, Dalmatians convert uric acid to allantoin at a reduced rate. It has been hypothesized that hepatic cellular membranes are partially impermeable to uric acid.

The proximal renal tubules of Dalmatians reabsorb less uric acid than those of non-Dalmatians; a small amount is secreted by the distal tubules. In non-Dalmatian dogs, 98 to 100 per cent of the uric acid in glomerular filtrate is reabsorbed by the proximal tubules and returned to the liver for further metabolism. Uric acid in urine of non-Dalmatians is thought to be secreted by the distal tubules.[66]

The definitive cause of urate urolith formation in Dalmatian dogs remains unknown. Increased urate excretion is a risk factor rather than a primary cause. Although all Dalmatians excrete relatively high quantities of urate in their urine, only a small percentage (especially males) form urate stones.[67, 68] At one time, it was thought that stone-forming Dalmatians did not excrete greater quantities of uric acid in their urine than non–stone-forming Dalmatians. However, studies indicate that insensitive methods of measurement of urine uric acid concentration were responsible for this conclusion. When steps are taken to ensure that urine uric acid remains in solution, differences in urine uric acid concentrations between non–urolith-forming Dalmatians and urolith-forming Dalmatians may be expected.

Even though ammonium urate uroliths commonly affect Dalmatian dogs, not all uroliths formed by Dalmatians are composed of ammonium urate. For example, of 387 uroliths formed by Dalmatian dogs, 82 per cent were composed of purines (ammonium urate, sodium urate, uric acid, and xanthine), 7 per cent were of mixed composition, 3 per cent were struvite, 3 per cent were composed of calcium oxalate, 3 per cent were composed of compound uroliths, 1 per cent were composed of cystine, and 1 per cent were composed of matrix.[67]

Non-Dalmatian Dogs. Many breeds of dogs have been affected with urate urolithiasis. Although urate uroliths are commonly encountered in Dalmatian dogs, 30 to 60 per cent of all canine urate uroliths analyzed by quantitated methods are found in other breeds. English bulldogs have a significantly higher incidence of urate urolithiasis compared with other breeds.[67] Clinical evaluation of eight male English bulldogs with confirmed ammonium urate urocystoliths revealed mild elevations in serum uric acid concentration. The size of their livers was normal, as was serum concentration of hepatic enzymes, blood concentration of ammonia, and bromosulphalein retention. Other non-Dalmatian breeds that appear to have a significantly higher incidence of urate urolithiasis based on quantitative analyses are miniature schauzers, Shih Tzus, and Yorkshire terriers.

Urate uroliths of non-Dalmatian dogs have been most frequently recognized in males. They have been detected throughout the lifespan of affected dogs but were most frequently detected in dogs 3 to 6 years of age.[67]

Comparatively little is known about urate lithogenesis in non-Dalmatian dogs that do not have portovascular anomalies. Risk factors for urate lithogenesis in dogs include (1) increased renal excretion and urine concentration of uric acid; (2) increased renal excretion, renal production, or microbial urease production of ammonium ion; (3) low urine pH; and (4) presence of promoters or absence of inhibitors of urate urolith formation.[69]

Regardless of cause, severe hepatic dysfunction may predispose dogs to urate lithogenesis, especially ammonium urate uroliths. Our observations and evidence from other experimental models suggest that prolonged consumption of severely protein-restricted diets may be associated with formation of urate uroliths in dogs.[69] Biochemical and histologic evaluations of these dogs suggest that chronic consumption of diets severely restricted in protein may induce hepatocellular dysfunction and concomitant hyperuricemia. Hepatic cirrhosis has also been reported to be associated with urate uroliths in dogs and other species. However, in our experience, cirrhosis, severely restricted protein diets, and other causes of hepatic dysfunction have been uncommon causes of ammonium urate urolithiasis.

Portovascular Anomalies. A high incidence of ammonium urate uroliths have been observed in dogs with portovascular anomalies. They occur in both males and females and usually are detected before 3 years of age.

Direct communication between the portal and systemic vasculature bypasses blood around the liver, resulting in severe hepatic atrophy and diminished hepatic function. Hepatic dysfunction, in turn, is associated with reduced hepatic conversion of uric acid to allantoin and of ammonia to urea. The predisposition of dogs with portosystemic shunts to urate urolithiasis is probably associated with concomitant hyperuricemia, hyperammonemia, hyperuricuria, and hyperammonuria. Serum uric acid concentrations in 15 dogs with portosystemic shunts that we evaluated were found to be increased. Not all dogs with portosystemic shunts develop concurrent ammonium urate urolithiasis.

Treatment

Dogs Without Portovascular Anomalies. Our current recommendations for medical dissolution of canine ammonium urate uroliths (Table 176–15) include a combination of (1) calculolytic diet, (2) administration of xanthine oxidase inhibitors (allopurinol), (3) alkalinization of urine, and (4) eradication or control of UTIs.

Calculolytic Diets. The goal of dietary modification for patients with uric acid or ammonium urate uroliths is to reduce urine concentration of uric acid, ammonium ion, and hydrogen ion. We use a purine-restricted non-acidifying diet that does not contain supplemental sodium (Prescription Diet Canine u/d, Hill's). When properly used, consumption of this diet by healthy and urate urolith–forming dogs results

TABLE 176–15. SUMMARY OF RECOMMENDATIONS FOR MEDICAL DISSOLUTION OF CANINE AMMONIUM ACID URATE UROLITHS

1. Perform appropriate diagnostic studies, including complete urinalyses, quantitative urine culture, and diagnostic radiography. Determine precise location, size, and number of uroliths. The size and number of uroliths are not a reliable index of probable efficacy of therapy.
2. If available, determine mineral composition or uroliths. If unavailable, predict their composition by evaluation of appropriate clinical data (see Table 176–7).
3. Consider surgical correction if uroliths are obstructing urine outflow and cannot be returned to the urinary bladder.
4. Determine base-line pretreatment serum uric acid concentrations and (if possible) fractional excretion of urine uric acid.
5. Initiate therapy with a low purine calculolytic diet (Prescription Diet Canine u/d). No other food supplements should be fed to the patient.
6. Initiate therapy with allopurinol at a dosage of 15 mg/kg q12h PO (a lesser dose will be required in azotemic patients).
7. If necessary, administer potassium citrate or sodium bicarbonate orally in order to eliminate aciduria. Strive for a urine pH of approximately 7.
8. If necessary, eradicate or control urinary tract infections with appropriate antimicrobial agents. Maintain antimicrobial therapy during, and for an appropriate period after, urate urolith dissolution.
9. Devise a protocol to monitor efficacy of therapy:
   a. Try to avoid diagnostic follow-up studies that require urinary catheterization. If they are required, give appropriate pericatheterization antimicrobial agents to prevent iatrogenic urinary tract infection.
   b. Evaluate serial urinalyses. Urine pH, specific gravity, and microscopic examination of sediment for urate crystals are especially important. Remember, crystals formed in urine stored at room or refrigeration temperatures may represent *in vitro* artifacts.
   c. Serially evaluate the serum uric acid concentrations and (if possible) fractional excretion of urine uric acid.
   d. Evaluate urolith(s) location(s), number, size, density, and shape at approximately monthly intervals. Intravenous urography may be utilized for radiolucent uroliths located in the kidneys, ureters, or urinary bladder. Retrograde contrast urethrocystography may be required for radiolucent uroliths located in the bladder and urethra.
   e. If necessary, perform quantitative urine cultures. They are especially important in patients that are infected before therapy and in patients that are catheterized during therapy.

in substantial reductions in urinary uric acid and ammonia excretion.

Xanthine Oxidase Inhibitors. Allopurinol is a synthetic isomer of hypoxanthine. It rapidly binds to and inhibits the action of xanthine oxidase and thereby decreases production of uric acid by inhibiting the conversion of hypoxanthine to xanthine and of xanthine to uric acid. The result is a reduction in serum and urine uric acid concentration within approximately 2 days and a concomitant but lesser degree of increase in the serum concentrations of hypoxanthine and xanthine. Although allopurinol has a short half-life in humans with normal renal function (approximately 90 minutes), its metabolic derivative oxypurinol is also a xanthine oxidase inhibitor, and it has a half-life of approximately 12 to 16 hours. In mongrel dogs and beagles, the half-life of allopurinol is approximately 2 hours and that of oxypurinol is approximately 4 hours.[70] The biologica half-life in Dalmatians is unknown to us.

The dosage of allopurinol that we have used for dissolution of ammonium urate uroliths in dogs is 7 mg/lb every 12 hours. According to the manufacturer, the drug has been given to normal dogs at this dosage for one year without causing significant abnormalities. We have given this dosage to non-azotemic urate urolith–forming dogs for up to 6 months without detectable consequences. However, when owners supplemented the diet with foods containing purine

precursors, a layer of xanthine formed around ammonium urate uroliths.

Although uncommon, allopurinol has caused adverse side reactions in humans. They include gastrointestinal complaints, rashes, leukopenia, thrombocytopenia, vasculitis, and hepatitis. Other than formation of xanthine uroliths, adverse reactions to allopurinol are apparently uncommon in dogs. We have not detected them and found no reports of their occurrence in dogs in the literature.

Because allopurinol and its metabolites are dependent on the kidneys for elimination from humans, the dosage is commonly reduced in patients with renal dysfunction. Allopurinol has been reported to cause life-threatening erythematous desquamative rash, fever, hepatitis, eosinopenia, and further decline in renal function when given to humans with renal insufficiency. Pending further studies, appropriate precautions should be used when considering use of allopurinol in dogs with primary renal failure.

Alkalinization of Urine. Because ammonium ion and hydrogen ion appear to precipitate urates in dog urine, administration of alkalinizing agents, such as oral sodium bicarbonate or potassium citrate, appear to be of value in preventing acid metabolites from increasing renal tubular production of ammonia. Under physiologic conditions associated with alkaluria, urine contains low concentrations of ammonia and ammonium ion.

The dosage of urine alkalinizers should be individualized for each patient. Preliminary dosages of sodium bicarbonate vary from 10 to 90 grains per day depending on the size of the patient and pre-treatment urine pH values. Alternatively, potassium citrate in wax matrix tablets may be given. Because sodium may combine with uric acid to form sodium urate, potassium citrate may be preferable to sodium bicarbonate as a urinary alkalinizer. Administration of divided doses is suggested to maintain a consistently non-acidic environment in the urinary tract.

The goal of treatment with urine alkalinizers is to maintain a urine pH of approximately 7.0. Higher values (>7.5) should be avoided until it is determined whether or not they provide a significant risk factor for formation of calcium phosphate uroliths. Deposition of a layer of calcium phosphate crystals around existing urate uroliths could impede stone dissolution. Owners may participate in monitoring urine pH with pH paper.

Eradication or Control of UTI. Clinical studies indicate that UTIs in dogs with ammonium urate uroliths usually occur as a consequence of altered local host defenses. These alterations may be caused by urolith-induced trauma to the urothelium, or they may occur as a consequence of catheterization or other invasive diagnostic procedures. Every effort should be made to prevent, eradicate, or control them because they may cause problems of equal or greater severity than the uroliths.

Augmenting Urine Volume. Augmenting urine volume with the goal of decreasing urine uric acid and ammonium concentration, and enhancing urine flow through the excretory pathway, appears to be a logical recommendation. Because the calculolytic diet designed for urate urolith dissolution impairs urine concentrating capacity by decreasing renal medullary urea concentration, additional diuretic agents are not required. Excessive dietary sodium should be avoided, particularly if the urine pH is high, because excessive sodium excretion may cause hypercalciuria. This event may, in turn, cause calcium phosphate crystals to form (see the section on calcium oxalate urolithiasis).

It is of interest that oral sodium chloride given to normal

URO

human volunteers for 10 days did not alter urine uric acid concentration. Long-term administration (up to 3 years) of hydrochlorothiazide to humans with uroliths containing calcium salts resulted in a rise in serum and urine uric acid concentration.

Dogs with Portovascular Anomalies. There apparently have been few studies of the biologic behavior of ammonium urate uroliths in dogs with portovascular anomalies. It is logical to hypothesize that elimination of hyperuricuria and reduction of urine ammonium concentration after surgical correction of anomalous shunts would result in spontaneous dissolution of uroliths composed primarily of ammonium urate. Appropriate clinical studies are needed to prove or disprove this hypothesis. We observed a substantial reduction of urine uric acid concentration in a 3-month-old female miniature schnauzer after surgical correction of an extrahepatic portacaval shunt. Additional clinical studies are needed to evaluate the relative value of calculolytic diets, allopurinol, and/or alkalinization of urine in dissolving ammonium urate uroliths in dogs with portovascular anomalies. The efficacy of allopurinol may be altered in such dogs, because biotranformation of this drug, which has a very short half-life, to oxypurinol, which has a longer half-life, requires adequate hepatic function.

Monitoring Response to Therapy. In our experience, ammonium urate urocystoliths have a propensity to move into the urethra of dogs. This may be related to their small size, their round to ovoid shape, and their smooth surface. If small enough, they readily pass through the urethra. If larger, they often become lodged behind the os penis of males. Owners should be informed of this likelihood and given a written summary of associated clinical findings. In those circumstances in which urethroliths cause clinical signs, they may be easily returned to the bladder lumen by urohydropropulsion.[27] Their physical characteristics that promote their passage into the urethra also facilitate their removal from the urethra.

The size of the uroliths should be periodically monitored by survey and (if necessary) double-contrast radiography. It is more difficult to monitor changes in the size and number of uroliths that are radiolucent. We have successfully used retrograde double-contrast urethrocystography to monitor dissolution of radiolucent urethrocystoliths without causing iatrogenic UTIs.

Urine pH should be monitored at appropriate intervals. Periodic evaluation of urine sediment for crystalluria should also be considered. Ammonium urate crystals should not form in fresh urine if therapy has been effective in promoting formation of urine that is undersaturated with ammonia and uric acid. Reduction of serum urea nitrogen concentration below pre-treatment values (usually < 10 mg/dL in previously non-azotemic patients), reduction of urine specific

TABLE 176–16. MANAGING REFRACTORY OR INCOMPLETE URATE UROLITH DISSOLUTION

CAUSES	IDENTIFICATION	THERAPEUTIC GOAL
Client and patient factors		
1. Inadequate dietary compliance	Question owner Persistent cystine crystalluria Serum urea nitrogen >10–17 mg/dL, urine specific gravity >1.010–1.020, and urine pH <7.0–7.5 during treatment with Prescription Diet Canine u/d (use lower values for canned diet)	Emphasize need to feed dissolution diet exclusively
2. Inadequate allopurinol administration	Question owner Count remaining pills	Emphasize need to administer allopurinol Determine whether owner is capable and willing to administer medication Demonstrate a variety of methods to administer medication
Clinician factors		
1. Incorrect prediction of mineral type	Analysis of retrieved urolith	Alter therapy based on identification of mineral type
2. Excessive allopurinol administration	Xanthine urolith formation	Reduce allopurinol administration in conjunction with appropriate dietary therapy to minimize purine consumption Clinically active uroliths may require surgical removal; remove small uroliths by voiding urohydropropulsion (see Fig. 176–6)
Disease factors		
1. Xanthine urolith formation	Analysis of retrieved urolith Allopurinol administration without concomitant reduction in dietary protein consumption Excessive allopurinol dose	Clinically active uroliths may require surgical removal; remove small uroliths by voiding urohydropropulsion (see Fig. 176–6)
2. Inadequate hepatic function	Hepatic portal systemic shunts should be suspected in breeds other than Dalmatians and English bulldogs Elevated postprandial serum bile acid concentration Microhepatica	Clinically active uroliths may require surgical removal; remove small uroliths by voiding urohydropropulsion (see Fig. 176–6) Repair vascular anomaly
3. Compound urolith	Radiographic density of nucleus and outer layer(s) of urolith are different Analysis of retrieved urolith	Alter therapy based on identification of new mineral type Uroliths not causing clinical signs should be monitored for potential adverse consequences (e.g., obstruction, UTI) Clinically active uroliths may require surgical removal; remove small uroliths by voiding urohydropropulsion (see Fig. 176–6)

gravity (usually < 1.020), and increase in urine pH (usually > 7.0) indicates owner and patient compliance with recommendations to consume the calculolytic diet exclusively (Table 176–16). Reductions in serum and urine uric acid concentrations also indicate compliance with recommendations for dietary and allopurinol therapy.

There is no rigid therapeutic time interval after which response to dissolution therapy is unlikely. The fact that current medical protocols are not designed to induce dissolution of urolith matrix may be a factor that influences dissolution rate. The time required to induce dissolution of nine episodes of urate urolithiasis in our clinical study has ranged from 4 to 40 weeks (mean = 14.2 weeks). If uroliths increase in size during therapy, or do not begin to decrease in size after approximately 8 weeks of appropriate medical therapy, re-evaluation of the diagnosis and/or alternative methods of management should be considered.

Prevention. Prophylactic therapy should be considered for dogs at high risk for recurrent urate uroliths. As a first choice, diets that are restricted in purines and that promote formation of dilute alkaline urine should be considered. If urate crystalluria or hyperuricuria persists, serial evaluation of urine pH to ensure appropriate alkalinization is indicated. If necessary, alkalinizing agents may be added to the protocol. If difficulties persist, allopurinol (3–10 mg/lb/d) may be given. Prolonged administration of high doses (13.5 mg/lb/d) of allopurinol may result in formation of xanthine uroliths.[71, 72] The risk of xanthine urolithiasis is enhanced if dietary purines are not restricted during allopurinol therapy. Therefore, appropriate caution in long-term administration of this drug is indicated. Because it is possible to induce dissolution of recurrent ammonium urate uroliths, it is unnecessary to risk the use of prophylactic protocols that may cause disorders themselves.

CANINE CYSTINE UROLITHIASIS

Etiopathogenesis. Cystine is a non-essential sulfur-containing amino acid composed of two molecules of cysteine. Although the exact mechanism(s) of cystine urolith formation are unknown, oversaturation of urine with cystine is a prerequisite. Canine cystinuria is an inborn error of metabolism characterized by increased urinary excretion of cystine. Normally, circulating cystine is freely filtered at the glomerulus, and 99 to 100 per cent is actively reabsorbed in the proximal tubule. Decreased tubular reabsorption of cystine and in some cases of other amino acids (lysine, gline, ornithine, arginine) has been observed in dogs with cystine uroliths.[73, 74] Aminoaciduria is associated with low or normal plasma levels of affected amino acids. Some affected dogs have a net secretion of cystine.[75] Results of one study of a cystinuric Welsh corgi suggested that decreased tubular reabsorption of cystine and lysine was due to a membrane transport defect.[73] An intestinal transport defect for cystine has also been identified in some cystinuric humans.[76] In one study of cystinuric dogs, two of eight had decreased jejunal mucosal uptake of cystine, lysine, and glycine, but the effect was considered minimal. However, in another study of four cystinuric dogs, a jejunal transport defect was not observed. The observation that some dogs did not have an intestinal transport defect indicates differences between the disease in some dogs and humans with cystinuria. Studies of cystinuric humans suggest that tubular reabsorption of cysteine, the immediate precursor of cystine, is defective. In this situation, two cysteine molecules may combine to form cystine in renal tubular lumen.

Many breeds of dogs have been reported to develop cystine uroliths. Of the uroliths analyzed at our laboratory, cystine occurred most frequently in English bulldogs (21 per cent) and dachshunds (11 per cent). Data contained in published pedigrees from inbred lines of dachshunds, basset hounds, and rottweilers suggest a sex-linked or autosomal recessive pattern of inheritance.[77] Although cystine uroliths have been reported primarily in male dogs, five female dogs with cystine uroliths have been reported, suggesting an autosomal recessive mode of inheritance in some breed.[78–80] We and others have observed that cystine uroliths primarily affect young to middle-aged dogs; 60 per cent of urolith submissions were retrieved from dogs 2 to 7 years old.[67, 77, 81]

Not all cystinuric dogs form uroliths; therefore, cystinuria is a predisposing rather than a primary cause of cystine urolith formation. In a study of five generations of offspring from one Scottish terrier, only one of six cystinuric males formed uroliths.[71] Uroliths form, in part, because the solubility of cystine in urine is pH dependent. Cystine is relatively insoluble in acidic urine but becomes more soluble in alkaline urine.

Treatment. *Current Recommendations.* Current recommendations for dissolution of cystine uroliths consist of reducing the urine concentration of cystine and increasing the solubility of cystine in urine. This may be accomplished by reduction of dietary protein alkalinization of urine, and administration of thiol-containing drugs (Table 176–17).[80]

Dietary Modification. Reduction of dietary protein has the potential of minimizing formation of cystine uroliths. It appears logical that decreased oral intake of methionine, a sulfur-containing amino acid, would result in decreased urinary excretion of cystine. However, experimental studies in humans suggest that the main source of cystine results from

TABLE 176–17. SUMMARY OF RECOMMENDATIONS FOR MEDICAL DISSOLUTION OF CANINE CYSTINE UROLITHS

1. Perform appropriate diagnostic studies including complete urinalysis, quantitative urine culture, and diagnostic radiography. Determine precise location, size, and number of uroliths (size and number of uroliths are not a reliable index of probable efficacy of therapy).
2. If available, determine mineral composition of uroliths. If unavailable, determine their composition by evaluation of appropriate clinical data.
3. Consider surgical correction if uroliths are obstructing urine outflow, or if correctable abnormalities predisposing to current UTI are identified by radiograph or other means.
4. Initiate therapy with calculolytic diet (Prescription Diet Canine canned u/d). No other food or mineral supplements should be fed.
5. Initiate therapy with N-(2-mercaptopropionyl)-glycine (2-MPG), approximately 15 mg/kg q12h PO.
6. If necessary, administer potassium citrate orally (75 mg/kg q12h) to induce alkaluria. Titrate dose to achieve a pH of approximately 7.5.
7. If necessary, eradicate or control UTI with appropriate antimicrobial agents.
8. Devise protocol for follow-up therapy:
   a. Try to avoid follow-up studies that require urinary catheterization, but if they are required, give appropriate peri-catheterization antimicrobial agents to prevent iatrogenic UTI.
   b. Evaluate serial urinalyses. Urine pH, specific gravity, and microscopic examination of sediment for crystals are especially important. Remember, crystals formed in urine stored at room or refrigeration temperature may represent artifacts in vitro.
   c. Perform serial radiography at monthly intervals to evaluate stone location, number, size, density, and shape. Intravenous urography may be utilized for radiolucent uroliths located in the kidneys, ureters, or bladder. Antegrade contrast cystourethrography may be required for radiolucent uroliths in the bladder and urethra.
9. Continue calculolytic diet, 2-MPG, and alkalinizing therapy for approximately 1 month after disappearance of uroliths as detected by radiography.

URO

endogenous metabolism; 96 per cent of ingested methionine is incorporated into body protein. Clinical studies in humans indicate that dietary methionine restriction is associated with limited benefit.

An even more important indirect effect of dietary protein restriction would be a reduction in renal medullary urea concentration and associated reduction in urine concentration of cystine. In addition, reduced oral intake of protein is associated with production of less acidic urine. We have successfully used a protein-restricted, alkalinizing diet (Hill's Prescription Diet Canine canned u/d) in combination with thiol-containing drugs in protocols to dissolve cystine urocystoliths.

Alkalinization of Urine. The solubility of cystine is pH dependent. In dogs, the solubility of cystine at a urine pH of 7.8 has been reported to be approximately double that at a urine pH of 5.0. Changes in urine pH that remain in the acidic range have minimal effect on cystine solubility. Therefore, a sufficient quantity of potassium citrate or sodium bicarbonate should be given orally in divided doses to sustain a urine pH of approximately 7.5. Data derived from studies in cystinuric humans suggest that dietary sodium may enhance cystinuria.[82, 83] Therefore, potassium citrate may be preferable to sodium bicarbonate as a urinary alkalinizer. One protein-restricted diet (Hill's Prescription Diet Canine canned u/d) is formulated to contain potassium citrate as a urinary alkalinizing agent. Further studies are required to evaluate the effect of dietary sodium on urinary excretion of cystine in dogs.

Thiol-Containing Drugs. N-(2-mercaptopropionyl)-glycine (2-MPG) decreases the concentration of cystine by a thiol disulfide exchange reaction resulting in a compound, cysteine-2-MPG disulfide, that is more soluble in urine than cystine.[84] Studies in humans indicate that this drug is highly effective in reducing urinary cystine concentration.[84]

Oral administration of 2-MPG (7 mg/lb q12 h PO) was effective in inducing dissolution of multiple cystine urocystoliths in three of four dogs evaluated (Table 176–18).[85] Dissolution required 2 to 4 months of therapy. One dog developed non-pruritic vesicular skin lesions after 3 months of therapy. One month after reduction of the oral dose of 2-MPG from 7 to 6 mg/lb every 12 hours, the skin lesions healed.

We have induced dissolution of multiple cystine urocystoliths in 18 dogs by a combination of diet (Hill's Prescription Diet Canine canned u/d) and 2-MPG therapy (7–11 mg/lb q12h PO). Urocystoliths dissolved in an average of 85 ± 45 days (range, 29–217 days). Two dogs developed a Coombs-positive regenerative spherocytic anemia that resolved after withdrawal of 2-MPG; one dog was also given prednisone orally.[86]

D-Penicillamine (dimethylcysteine) is a non-metabolizable degradation product of penicillin that may combine with cysteine to form cysteine-D-penicillamine disulfide. The resulting compound has been reported to be 50 times more soluble than free cystine. The cysteine-D-penicillamine complex does not react with cyanide-nitroprusside, as cystine does, providing a mechanism to titrate drug dosage.

Historically, D-penicillamine has been used in the management of cystine uroliths. The most common oral dosage of D-penicillamine for dogs has been 7 mg/lb every 12 hours. Higher doses frequently cause vomiting, and sometimes other undesirable reactions. If nausea and vomiting occur with the aforementioned dose, the drug may be mixed with food or given at mealtime. In some instances, it may be necessary to prevent gastrointestinal disturbances by initiating therapy with low doses and gradually increasing them until the full dosage is reached. In humans, D-penicillamine has been associated with a variety of adverse reactions: fever, lymphadenopathy, arthralgia, skin hypersensitivity re-

TABLE 176–18. MANAGING REFRACTORY OR INCOMPLETE CYSTINE UROLITH DISSOLUTION

CAUSES	IDENTIFICATION	THERAPEUTIC GOAL
Client and patient factors 1. Inadequate dietary compliance	Question owner Persistent cystine crystalluria Serum urea nitrogen >10–17 mg/dL, urine specific gravity >1.010–1.020, and urine pH <7.0–7.5 during treatment with Prescription Diet Canine u/d (use lower values for canned diet)	Emphasize need to feed dissolution diet exclusively
2. Inadequate 2-MPG administration	Question owner Count remaining pills	Emphasize need to administer the full dose of medication Determine whether owner is capable and willing to administer medication Demonstrate a variety of methods to administer medication
Clinician factors 1. Incorrect prediction of mineral type	Analysis of retrieved urolith	Alter therapy based on identification of mineral type
2. Inadequate 2-MPG dose for degree of diuresis	No change in urolith size after 2 months of appropriate therapy	Increase 2-MPG dose to 20 mg/kg q12h
Disease factors 1. Compound urolith	Radiographic density of nucleus and outer layer(s) of urolith are different Analysis of retrieved urolith	Alter therapy based on identification of new mineral type Uroliths not causing clinical signs should be monitored for potential adverse consequences (e.g., obstruction, UTI) Clinically active uroliths may require surgical removal; remove small uroliths by voiding urohydropropulsion (see Fig. 176–6)

2-MPG = N-(2-Mercaptopropionyl)-glycine.

actions, pancytopenia, thrombocytopenia, and immune-complex glomerulonephritis. Because D-penicillamine administration is associated with a higher incidence of side effects that are more severe than those of 2-MPG, we do not recommend its use in the management of cystine uroliths.

Prevention. Because cystinuria is a metabolic defect and because cystine uroliths recur in a high percentage of urolith-forming dogs after surgical removal, prophylactic therapy should be considered. The objectives of prophylactic therapy are to (1) minimize cystine crystalluria, (2) promote alkaluria, (3) promote diuresis, and (4) promote a negative cyanide-nitroprusside test. A protein-restricted, alkalinizing diet (Hill's Prescription Diet Canine canned u/d) or a combination of dietary modification combined with urine alkalinizing therapy may be initiated to reduce urine concentrations of cystine. If necessary, 2-MPG (7 mg/lb q12 h PO) may be added to the regimen.

CALCIUM PHOSPHATE UROLITHS

Calcium phosphate was recognized in less than 1 per cent of submissions to our urolith analysis laboratory. The most common form of calcium phosphate was hydroxyapatite and carbonate apatite (60 per cent). Twenty-five per cent of uroliths submitted were from Yorkshire terriers, mixed breed dogs, miniature schnauzers, and cocker spaniels; no distinguishing trends for gender and age were recognized.

Brushite (CaH_2H_2O) (39.5 per cent) and tricalcium phosphate (0.5 per cent) were less frequently observed. Forty per cent of brushite uroliths were observed in four breeds: Yorkshire terrier, miniature poodle, bichon frisé, and Shih Tzu. Seventy-eight per cent of brushite urolith formers were male, and 73 per cent were between the ages of 5 and 13 years.

Etiopathogenesis. Calcium phosphate is commonly found as a minor component of struvite and calcium oxalate uroliths. Pure calcium phosphate uroliths are infrequently encountered in dogs, and they are usually associated with metabolic disorders such as primary hyperparathyroidism, renal tubular acidosis, and excessive dietary calcium and phosphorus.

Calcium phosphates are less soluble in alkaline urine. Alkaline urine favors dissociation of monobasic phosphate ($H_2PO_4^-$) to dibasic phosphate (HPO_4^{2-}) and phosphate ions (PO_4^{3-}). In humans with urine at a pH greater than 6.9, brushite undergoes rapid transformation into calcium phosphates of a higher calcium-to-phosphate ratio, such as calcium apatite.

The clinical significance of brushite may lie in its association to calcium oxalate urolith formation. As the pH of human urine was increased, the percentage of calcium oxalate dihydrate crystals increased until the pH reached 7; above a pH of 7, calcium phosphate, and not calcium oxalate, crystals were observed.[87] When human calcium oxalate urolith formers were compared with controls, both groups formed urine supersaturated for calcium oxalate; however, only urolith formers produced urine that was supersaturated for brushite.[88] These findings suggest that the heterogenous nucleation of calcium oxalate may occur only after a core of brushite has precipitated.

Treatment and Prevention. The solubility of calcium phosphate in urine depends on (1) calcium ion concentration, (2) inorganic phosphate ion concentration, and (3) hydrogen ion concentration. Because uroliths composed principally of calcium phosphate are most likely to be encountered in dogs

with diseases associated with hypercalcemia or renal tubular acidosis, it is tempting to speculate that correction of the metabolic abnormalities might be associated with formation of urine undersaturated with calcium phosphate. In undersaturated urine, uroliths would be expected to dissolve; however, this has not been the case. Therefore, physical means of urolith removal are often necessary to correct clinically active disease. Nonetheless, correction of underlying abnormalities should minimize urolith recurrence.

In one study of human urolith formers, it was determined that brushite saturation was exclusively determined by the urine concentration of calcium and urine pH.[89] The reader is referred to the section on prevention of calcium oxalate uroliths for further information on methods for reducing urine calcium and to the sections on the treatment and prevention of magnesium ammonium phosphate for further information on methods for reducing urine phosphate and pH. If a specific underlying disorder is not diagnosed, we generally manage calcium phosphate uroliths similar to strategies used for calcium oxalate uroliths, because reducing urine pH promotes excessive urinary calcium excretion.

SILICA

Silica is a compound of the two most abundant elements in the earth's crust, oxygen and silicon. Yet, only 1.3 per cent of uroliths submitted to our laboratory were composed of silica. The majority of submissions were from German shepherds (10.7 per cent), Golden retrievers (8.2 per cent), and Labrador retrievers (8.2 per cent). Ninety-two per cent of dogs with silica uroliths were male, and 55.4 per cent of dogs were between 4 and 9 years old.

Etiopathogenesis. Available clinical information provides a strong link between canine silica uroliths and dietary ingredients. Diets that contain substantial quantities of corn gluten feed or soybean hulls are especially suspect. One explanation for the high prevalence of silica uroliths in German shepherds and other large breed dogs is the frequency with which large breed dogs are fed dry foods that contain relatively large quantities of plant ingredients such as corn gluten feed. Sources of silica (soybean hulls) are sometimes added to reducing diets as a non-nutritive ingredient. An association between the consumption of soil and silica urolith formation in dogs is plausible but has not been demonstrated. Silica uroliths appear to only occur in humans taking antacids (magnesium trisilicate). Diets with a high calcium-to-phosphorus ratio that promote formation of alkaline urine have been considered risk factors for silica uroliths formation in sheep.[90]

Treatment and Prevention. Effective medical protocols to induce dissolution of canine silica uroliths have yet to be developed. Silica formation, induced by feeding tetraethylorthosilicate to rats, was significantly reduced after dietary supplementation with sodium chloride or sodium phosphate.[91] Because initiating and perpetuating causes of silica urolithiasis are not known, non-specific measures to reduce supersaturation of silica have been recommended for their prevention. At this time our recommendations include (1) change of diet (avoid diets containing substantial plant proteins) and (2) increasing urine volume (enhancing water consumption).

COMPOUND UROLITHS

Uroliths consisting of a nucleus of one mineral type and a shell of another type were observed in 6.6 per cent in our

URO

series of uroliths analyzed. Compound uroliths form because factors promoting precipitation of one type of urolith have been superseded by factors promoting precipitation of another mineral. For example, administration of urinary acidifiers to manage struvite uroliths may promote hypercalciuria, resulting in a shell of calcium oxalate or calcium phosphate. Likewise, we have observed a shell of sulfadiazine after administration of sulfonamide antibiotics. Some mineral types may serve as a template for deposition of other minerals. This property may explain why some calcium oxalate uroliths have a nidus of silica. All uroliths predispose to urinary tract infection. If infections by microorganisms that produce urease persist, it is likely that struvite will precipitate over pre-existing uroliths.

Because risk factors that predispose to precipitation of different minerals may vary, management of compound uroliths poses a unique challenge. If possible, dissolution protocols can be initiated to dissolve the outer layer first. Once urolith size shows no further reduction, medical therapy can be initiated to dissolve the inner layers. In some cases, dissolution of the outer layers reduces urolith size sufficiently such that uroliths can be easily removed by voiding urohydropropulsion (see Fig. 176–5). Uroliths refractory to current methods of medical dissolution can be removed surgically.

In the absence of clinical evidence to the contrary, it seems logical to recommend prevention protocols designed principally to minimize recurrence of minerals comprising the nucleus, rather than the shell, of compound uroliths. Follow-up studies include complete urinalysis, urine culture, and radiography.

Unusual and Rare Uroliths

In addition to dissolved minerals, the urinary tract functions to excrete many other substances, especially drug metabolites. Although crystalluria has been reported with a variety of drugs, urolith formation has only been reported with sulfonamide administration. If conditions favor sulfonamide precipitation (acidic urine, concentrated urine), pre-existing uroliths could become surrounded by precipitated drug metabolites, rendering them less amenable to medical dissolution. For this reason, sulfonamide antimicrobials should not be administered to dogs with uroliths. Urinary alkalinization, maintenance of high urinary output, and use of sulfonamide mixtures should be considered when their administration is unavoidable.

Foreign material in the urinary tract has been associated with urolith formation. Foreign material in the lumen of the urinary tract may predispose to urolith formation by favoring urinary tract formation or by serving as a template for heterogeneous nucleation of crystals. Foxtail awns, urinary catheters, bullets, blood clots, necrotic tissue, and suture material have been identified as the nucleus of uroliths. Prevention in some cases may be difficult; however, to avoid suture-induced urolithiasis, we recommend use of nonabsorbable sutures and their placement such that sutures do not penetrate the urinary tract lumen.

CYSTITIS AND URETHRITIS

Cystitis is inflammation of the urinary bladder. Whether diagnosed by clinical description, urinalysis, bacteriologic culture, cystoscopy, or light microscopic tissue evaluation,

signs are usually characterized by varying degrees of dysuria, pollakiuria, and hematuria. Because of the close proximity of the urethra, disease processes affecting the bladder often extend to the urethra.

Many diverse underlying causes can initiate an inflammatory response. Therefore, a diagnosis of cystitis or urethritis is a clinically insufficient description for appropriate patient management, because neither prognosis nor treatment can be applied without a high degree of uncertainty of efficacy or without a high degree of potential error. Some clinically useful classifications of cystitis and urethritis include bacterial, fungal, traumatic, emphysematous, polyploid, granulomatous, drug induced, and idiopathic (Table 176–19).

COMMON MISCONCEPTIONS IN THE DIAGNOSIS AND MANAGEMENT OF CANINE LOWER URINARY TRACT DISEASE

1. Crystalluria is an indication for change of diet. Crystals occur only in urine that is or recently has been supersaturated with crystallogenic substances. Crystalluria represents a risk factor for urolithiasis; however, crystalluria (microlithiasis) is not synonymous with formation of macrouroliths and the clinical signs associated with them, nor is it irrefutable evidence of a urolith-forming tendency. In fact, crystalluria that occurs in individuals with anatomically and functionally normal urinary tracts is usually harmless because the crystals are eliminated before they grow to sufficient size to cause clinical signs. Therefore, the need for dietary change to minimize crystalluria may be premature. On the other hand, detection of some types of crystals (ammonium urate and cystine), detection of large aggregates of crystals, or detection of any form of crystals in patients with confirmed urolithiasis may be of diagnostic, prognostic, and therapeutic importance.

2. Crystalluria causes hematuria and dysuria. Crystals are a common finding from the urinalysis of most normal dogs. It is true that crystalluria may be associated with urolithiasis, and urolithiasis may promote hematuria and dysuria, but crystalluria has not been proven a cause for hematuria and dysuria. Therefore, implicating crystals as the cause of hematuria or dysuria may delay investigation of an appropriate underlying cause (urinary tract infection, urolithiasis, neoplasia) and is likely to be associated with therapeutic failure and unnecessary client costs.

3. Cystotomy guarantees removal of uroliths from the lower urinary tract. Historically, surgery has been considered the only practical method of eliminating uroliths from the lower urinary tract, especially uroliths refractory to medical dissolution. However, success of this technique is variable. In one retrospective study, cystotomy was ineffective in removing all urocystoliths in one of every seven dogs and one of every five cats. These findings indicate that established intraoperative techniques of verifying urolith removal (catheter passage through the urethra, retrograde flushing of the urethra, and visual or tactile inspection of the lumen of the urinary bladder) may be unreliable or inadequately performed. Therefore, post-surgical radiography should be considered in dogs and cats with multiple uroliths. Without this information, it is impossible to distinguish between urolith recurrence and incomplete surgical removal as a cause for recurrent signs.

4. Surgery is needed to manage polyploid cystitis. Polyploid cystitis is an inflammatory condition of the bladder

TABLE 176–19. FORMS OF CYSTITIS AND URETHRITIS

TYPE	DEFINITION	CAUSE	DIAGNOSIS	TREATMENT
Bacterial	Mucosal adherence, replication, and invasion by pathogenic bacteria	Altered structure and/or replication of host defenses	Significant numbers of bacteria determined from bacterial cultures of properly collected urine	Appropriate antimicrobials selected on the basis of susceptibility testing Correct underlying abnormal host defenses
Fungal	Mucosal adherence, replication, and invasion by pathogenic fungi	Altered structure and/or function of host defenses Systemic fungal infections Chronic antimicrobial administration	Demonstration of fungal tissue invasion remains the gold standard by which pathogenic colonization cannot be disputed. Urine sediment examination Urine culture for fungi	Restore normal local host defenses and systemic immunocompetence Some asymptomatic infections will resolve spontaneously Use antimicrobials that achieve high concentrations in urine (flucytosine or fluconazole)
Emphysematous	Intraparenchymal gas within urothelial mucosa	Bacterial fermentation of glucose or other sugars within devitalized bladder wall	Survey radiography: mottling of bladder wall with small gas bubbles	Eradicate UTI Control glucosuria
Granulomatous	Infiltrative disease of mucosa characterized by nodular inflammation	Unknown Chronic bacterial infection plays a significant role in its development	Multifocal nodular aggregates of lymphocytes, plasma cells, and macrophages are commonly identified by microscopic evaluation of tissue samples	Chronic antimicrobial therapy is needed until mucosal irregularities resolve Immunosuppression therapy is contraindicated but can be considered if proliferative lesions fail to regress Intermittent urinary catheterization may be needed to control urethral obstruction
Polyploid	Mucosal polyploid projections of the urothelium	Chronic irritation (e.g., UTI, uroliths) to the urinary bladder, promoting mucosal hyperplasia	Contrast radiography, ultrasonography, cystoscopy, and mucosal biopsy	May spontaneously regress with eradication of the underlying cause If persistent, consider surgical removal
Traumatic	Mucosal irritation, due to blunt, abrading, penetrating, shearing or stretching forces	Urolithiasis, overdistention, bladder herniation, cystotomy, catheterization, etc.	History of trauma, radiography, ultrasonography, cytoscopy	Spontaneous regression with resolution of trauma or obstruction
Parasitic	Mucosal invasion of adult parasites	*Capillaria plica*	Identification of parasite ova (double operculated eggs) via microscopic evaluation of urine sediment Identification of *Dioctaphyma renale* ova or microfiliaria in urine usually indicates infection in other locations (kidney and heart)	Fenbendazole (50 mg/kg q3d), albendazole (50 mg/kg q12h for 14 days), and ivermectin (0.2 mg/kg SC) eliminated eggs in urine In the absence of re-infection (isolation from the intermediate host—earthworms), spontaneous recovery has occurred within 90 days
Drug induced	Bacteriologically sterile infections resulting from drug toxicity	Retrograde flushing solutions or metabolites of cyclophosphamide	History of drug administration	Discontinue drug, promote diuresis, and treat secondary UTI
Idiopathic	Inflammation in which structural abnormalities, infections, cytotoxic drug administration, and trauma to the lower urinary tract has been eliminated	Unknown Inhaled and dietary allergens have been suspected	This diagnosis has been surmised by excluding known causes of bladder infection. Eosinophilic and lymphoplasmacytic infiltration of bladder mucosa are detected in human cases	Antispasmodics (propantheline, oxybutynin, phenoxybenzamine), urinary analgesics (phenazopyridine), sedatives (diazepam, amitriptyline), or mucosal surface glycoprotein replenishers (pentosan polysulfate sodium, cosequin) may minimize dysuria

URO

mucosa characterized by growth of one or more non-neoplastic polyps. Polyps are often associated with chronic urinary tract infection and/or chronic trauma (urolithiasis). In our experience, inflammatory polyps may spontaneously resolve after eradication of infection and/or uroliths. The choice of antimicrobials should be based on results of culture and sensitivity tests. Appropriate antimicrobials should be given for at least 4 to 6 weeks. Prolonged antibiotic therapy may be necessary to prevent recurrence.

5. Corticosteroids are indicated in the management of granulomatous urethritis. Although the cause of granulomatous urethritis is unknown, we believe that chronic bacterial infection plays a significant role in its development. Therefore, therapy should be directed at eradicating and controlling UTIs. Appropriate antimicrobials should be based on results of culture and sensitivity tests and given for at least 4 to 6 weeks, or longer, if needed. Because of the potential adverse effects of immunosuppressive drugs, especially in patients with infection, prednisolone and cyclophosphamide should be reserved for refractory cases.

6. Absence of pyuria and bacteriuria is sufficient evidence to rule out UTI. In most cases, bacteriuria cannot be detected by sediment examination unless concentrations of bacterial rods are greater than 10,000 organisms/mL and concentrations of bacterial cocci are equal to 100,000/mL. Likewise, the degree of inflammation is variable, being influenced by the virulence of invading microorganisms and the host's response. A blunted inflammatory response is common in dogs with hyperadrenocorticism, likely, as a result of excessive endogenous corticosteroid secretion. Therefore, a lack of detection of bacteria in urine sediment is not conclusive evidence to rule out bacteriuria.

7. Persistent alkaluria is an indication for antibiotic administration. Although UTI caused by microorganisms capable of elaborating urease (*Staphylococcus, Proteus, Ureaplasma*, others) result in urine that is alkaline, other physiologic and pathologic processes can also result in alkaluria. After food consumption, alkaline ions are secreted by the kidney to compensate for acid ions secreted in the stomach to aid digestion. The magnitude of the post-prandial alkaline urine tide is proportional to the amount of food consumed. Diets containing alkaline metabolites (vegetables, citrate bicarbonate) also result in formation of alkaline urine. In normally hydrated animals, alkaline urine is associated with disorders promoting metabolic or respiratory alkalosis.

Antibiotics may be indicated, if a high index of suspicion of ureaplasmal UTI is suspected and facilities for ureaplasmal identification are inaccessible. Otherwise, antibiotic administration should be reserved for confirmed bacteriuria.

REFERENCES

1. Jeremy JY, et al: Eicosamoid synthesis by human urinary bladder mucosa: Pathological implications. Br J Urol 59:36, 1987.
2. Parsons CL, et al: Bladder surface glycosaminoglycans: An epithelial permeability barrier. J Urol 143:139–142, 1990.
3. Mcloughlin MA, Walshaw R, Thomas MW, et al: Gastric conduit urinary diversion in normal dogs. Vet Surg 21:25–32, 1992.
4. Fries CL, Binnington AG, Valli VE, et al: Enterocystoplasty with cystectomy and subtotal intracapsular prostatectomy in the male dog. Vet Surg 20:104–112, 1991.
5. Scrivani PV, Leveille R, Collins RL: The effect of patient positioning on mural filling defects during double contrast cystography. Vet Radiol Ultrasound 38:355–359, 1997.
6. Littman MP, Niebauer GW, Hendrick MK: Macrohematuria and life-threatening anemia attributable to subepithelial vascular ectasia of the urinary bladder in a dog. JAVMA 196:1487–1489, 1990.
7. Berearley MJ, Cooper JE: The diagnosis of bladder disease in dogs by cystoscopy. J Small Anim Pract 28:75, 1987.
8. McCarthy TC, McDermaid SL: Prepubic cystoscopy in thge dogs and cat. J Am Anim Hosp Assoc 22:213, 1986.
9. Senior DF: Urethral dilation. In Kirk RW, Bonagura JD (eds): Kirk's Current Veterinary Therapy 11: Small Animal Practice. Philadelphia, WB Saunders, 1992, pp 880–882.
10. Cater HB: Instrumentation and endoscopy. In Walsh PC, Retik AB, Stamey TA, Vaughan Ed Jr (eds): Campell's Urology, 6th ed. Philadelphia, WB Saunders, 1992, pp 339–340.
11. Lamb CR, Trower ND, Gregory SP: Ultrasound-guided catheter biopsy of the lower urinary tract: Technique and results in 12 dogs. J Small Animal Pract 37:413–416, 1996.
12. Lulich JP, Osborne CA: Forceps biopsy of the lower urinary tract. In Kirk RW, et al (eds): Current Veterinary Therapy X. Philadelphia, WB Saunders, June 1999.
13. Allen DK, Waters DJ, Knapp DW, Kuczek T: High urine concentrations of basic fibroblast growth factor in dogs with bladder cancer. J Vet Intern Med 10:231–234, 1996.
14. Goldberg BB, Bagley D, Liu JB, et al: Endoluminal sonography of the urinary tract: Preliminary observations. AJR Am J Roentgen 156:99–103, 1991.
15. Tobias KS, Barbee D: Abnormal micturition and recurrent cystitis associated with multiple congenital anomalies of the urinary tract in a dog. JAVMA 207:191–193, 1995.
16. Martin RA, Harvey HJ, Flanders JA: Bilateral ectopic ureters in a male dog: A case report. J Am Anim Hosp Assoc 21:80–84, 1985.
17. Takiguchi M, Yasuda J, Ochial K, et al: Ultrasonographic appearance of orthotopic ureterocele in a dog. Vet Radiol Ultrasound 38:398–399, 1997.
18. McLoughlin MA, Hauptman JG, Spaulding K: Canine ureteroceles: A case report and literature review. J Am Anim Hosp Assoc 25:699–706, 1989.
19. Hesse A: Canine urolithiasis: Epidemiology and analysis of urinary calculi. J Small Anim Pract 31:599–604, 1990.
20. Wallerstrom, BI, Wagberg TI: Canine urolithiasis in Sweden and Norway: Retrospective survey of prevalence and epidemiology. J Small Anim Pract 33:534–539, 1992.
21. Roberts SR, Resnick MI: Urinary stone matrix. In Wickham JEA, Colin Buck A (eds): Renal Tract Stone: Metabolic Basis and Clinical Practice. New York, Churchill Livingstone, 1990.
22. Asplin J, DeGanello S, Nakagawa YN, Coe FL: Evidence that nephrocalcin and urine inhibit nucleation of calcium oxalate monohydrate crystals. Am J Physiol 261:F824–F830, 1991.
23. Atmani F, Lacour B, Drueke T, Daudon M: Isolation and purification of a new glycoprotein from human urine inhibiting calcium oxalate crystallization. Urol Res 21:61, 1993.
24. Hess B, Nakagawa Y, Coe FL: Inhibition of calcium oxalate crystal aggregation by urine proteins. Am J Phys 257:F99–F106, 1989.
25. Ashby RA, Sleet RI: The role of citrate complexes in preventing urolithiasis. Clin Chim Acta 210:157–165, 1992.
26. Grover PK, Ryall RL, Marshall VR: Calcium oxalate crystallization in urine: Role of urate and glycosaminoglycans. Kidney Int 41:149–154, 1992.
27. Osborne CA, et al: Medical dissolution and prevention of canine and feline uroliths: Diagnosis and therapeutic caveats. Vet Rec 127:369, 1990.
28. Osborne CA, et al: Relationship of nutritional factors to the cause, dissolution, and prevention of canine uroliths. Vet Clin North Am Small Anim Pract 19:583, 1989.
29. Lulich JP, Perrine L, Osborne CA, Unger L: Postsurgical recurrence of calcium oxalate uroliths in dogs. J Vet Intern Med 6:119, 1992.
30. Osborne CA, Lulich JP, Kruger JK, et al: Medical dissolution of feline struvite urocystoliths: Prospective clinical study of 30 cases. JAVMA 196:1053–1063, 1990.
31. Osborne CA, Lulich JP, Unger LK: Nonsurgical retrieval of uroliths for mineral analysis. In Kirk RW, Bonagura JD (eds): Kirk's Current Veterinary Therapy 11. Philadelphia, WB Saunders, 1992, pp 886–888.
32. Lulich JP, Osborne CA: Catheter-assisted retrieval of urocystoliths from dogs and cats. JAVMA 210:111–113, 1992.
33. Lulich JP, Osborne CA, Polzin DP, et al: Incomplete removal of canine and feline urocystoliths by cystotomy. J Vet Intern Med 7:124, 1993.
34. Lulich JP, Osborne CA, Carlson M, et al: Nonsurgical reroval of uroliths in dogs and cats by voiding urohydropropulsion. JAVMA 203:660–663, 1993.
35. Senior DF: Electrohydraulic shock-wave lithotripsy in experimental canine struvite bladder stone disease. Vet Surg 13:143–145, 1984.
36. Grasso M, Loisides P, Beaghler M, Bagley D: Treatment of urinary calculi in a porcine and canine model using the Browne pneumatic impactor. Urology 44:937–941, 1994.
37. Block G, Adams LG, Widmer WR, et al: Use of extracorporeal shock wave lithotripsy for treatment of nephrolithiasis and ureterolithiasis in five dogs. JAVMA 208:531–536, 1996.
38. Bailey G, Burk RL: Dry extracorporeal shock wave lithotripsy for treatment of ureterolithiasis and nephrolithiasis in a dog. JAVMA 207:592–595, 1995.
39. Bartges JW, Osborne CA, Polzin DJ: Recurrent sterile struvite urocystolithiasis in three related cocker spaniels. J Am Anim Hosp Assoc 28:459–469, 1992.
40. Boistelle R, et al: Growth and stability of magnesium ammonium phosphate in acidic sterile urine. Urol Res 12:79, 1984.
41. Abdullahi SU, et al: Evaluation of a calculolytic diet in female dogs with induced struvite urolithiasis. Am J Vet Res 45:1508, 1984.
42. Osborne CA, et al: Struvite urolithiasis in animals and man: Formation, detection, and dissolution. Adv Vet Sci Comp Med 29:1, 1985.
43. Krawiec DR, et al: Effect of acetohydroxamic acid on dissolution of canine uroliths. Am J Vet Res 45:1266, 1984.

44. Baillie NC, et al: Teratogenic effect of acetohydroxamic acid in clinically normal beagles. Am J Vet Res 47:2604, 1986.

45. Klausner JS, Osborne CA, Clinton CW, et al: Mineral composition of urinary tract calculi from miniature schnauzers. JAVMA 178:1082–1083, 1981.

46. Mandel NS, Mandel GS: Urinary tract stone disease in the United States veteran population: II. Geographical analysis of variations in composition. J Urol 142:1516–1521, 1989.

47. Bovee KC, McGuire T: Qualitative and quantitative analysis of uroliths in dogs: Definitive determination of chemical type. JAVMA 185:983–987, 1984.

48. Thumchai R: Epizootiologic evaluation of canine calcium oxalate uroliths 1990–1992: A case-control study. PhD thesis, University of Minnesota, January 1996.

49. Bushinsky DA, Johnston RB, Nalbantian CE, et al: Increases in calcium absorption and retention without elevated serum 1,25(OH)$_2$D$_3$ in genetically hypercalciuric rats. Kidney Int 33:336, 1988.

50. Smith LH: The pathophysiology and medical treatment of urolithiasis. Semin Nephrol 10:31–52, 1990.

51. Lulich JP, Osborne CA, Nagode LA, et al: Evaluation of urine and serum metabolites in miniature schnauzers with calcium oxalate urolithiasis. Am J Vet Res 152:1583–1590, 1991.

52. Curhan GC, Willet WC, Rimm EB, Stampfer MJ: A prospective study of dietary calcium and other nutrients and the risk of symptomatic kidney stones. N Engl J Med 328:833–838, 1993.

53. Curhan GC, Willet WC, Speizer FE, et al: Comparison of dietary calcium with supplemental calcium and other nutrients as factors affecting the risk for kidney stones in women. Ann Intern Med 126:497–504, 1997.

54. Nakagawa Y, Abram V, Parks JH, et al: Urine glycoprotein crystal growth inhibitors, evidence for a molecular abnormality in calcium oxalate nephrolithiasis. J Clin Invest 76:1455–1462, 1985.

55. Nakagawa Y, Ahmed M, Hall SL, et al: Isolation of human calcium oxalate renal stones of nephrocalcin, a glycoprotein inhibitor of calcium oxalate crystal growth: Evidence that nephrocalcin from patients with calcium oxalate nephrolithiasis is deficient in 2-carboxyglutamic acid. J Clin Invest 79:1782–1787, 1987.

56. Hess B: Tamm-Horsfall glycoprotein and calcium nephrolithiasis. Miner Electrolyte Metab 20:393–398, 1994.

56a. Ryall RL: Macromolecules in stones: Promiscuous players, inadequate protectors, or malevolent provocateurs? In Tiselius HG (ed): Renal Stones. Edsbruk, Akademitryck, 1995, pp 9–15.

57. Kajander EO, Ciftcioglu N: Nanobacteria: An alternative mechanism for pathogenic intra- and extracellular calcification and stone formation. Proc Natl Acad Sci USA 95:8274–8279, 1998.

58. DeViries SE, Feldman EC, Nelson RW, Kennedy PC: Primary parathyroid gland hyperplasia in dogs: Six cases (1982–1991). JAVMA 202:1132–1136, 1993.

59. Klausner JS, O'Leary TP, Osborne CA: Calcium urolithiasis in two dogs with parathyroid adenomas. JAVMA 191:1423–1426, 1987.

60. Berger B, Feldman EC: Primary hyperparathryoidism in dogs: 21 cases (1976–1986). JAVMA 191:350–356, 1987.

61. Hess RC, Kass PH, Ward CR: Association between hyperadrenocorticism and development of calcium-containing uroliths in dogs with urolithiasis. JAVMA 212:1889–1891, 1998.

62. Ritz E, Kreusser W, Rambausek M: Effects of glucocorticoids on calcium and phosphate excretion. Adv Exp Med Biol 32:151–156, 1984.

63. Block G, Adams LG, Widmer WR, Lingemen JE: Use of extracorporeal shock wave lithotripsy for treatment of nephrolithiasis and ureterolithiasis in five dogs. JAVMA 208:531–536, 1996.

64. Bai SC, Sampson DA, Morris JG, et al: Vitamin B$_6$ requirements of growing kittens. J Nutr 119:1020, 1989.

65. Williams AW, et al: Uric acid metabolism in humans. Semin Nephrol 10:9, 1990.

66. Foreman JW: Renal handling of urate and other organic acids. In Bovee KC (ed): Canine Nephrology. Media, PA, Harwal, 1984, p 135.

67. Bartges JW, et al: Prevalence of cystine and urate uroliths in English bulldogs and urate uroliths in Dalmatians (1981–1992). JAVMA 204:1914–1918, 1993.

68. Case LC, et al: Urolithiasis in Dalmatians: 275 cases (1981–1990). JAVMA 203:96, 1993.

69. Kruger JM, et al: Etiopathogenesis of uric acid and ammonium urate uroliths in non-Dalmatian dogs. Vet Clin North Am 16:87, 1986.

70. Bartges JW, et al: Influence of allopurinol and two diets on 24-hour urinary excretion of uric acid, xanthine, and ammonia by healthy dogs. J Am Vet Res 56:595–599, 1995.

71. Bartges JW, et al: Canine xanthine uroliths: Risk factor management. In Kirk RW, et al (eds): Current Veterinary Therapy XI. Philadelphia, WB Saunders, 1992, p 900.

72. Ling GV, et al: Xanthine-containing urinary calculi in dogs given allopurinol. JAVMA 198:1935, 1991.

73. McNamara PD, et al: Cystinuria in dogs: Comparison of the cystinuric component of the Fanconi syndrome in basenji dogs to isolated cystinuria. Metabolism 38:8, 1989.

74. Bovee KC: Canine cystine urolithiasis. Vet Clin North Am Small Anim Pract 16:211, 1986.

75. Bovee KC, et al: Renal tubule reabsorption of amino acids after lysine loading of cystinuric dogs. Metabolism 33:602, 1984.

76. Milliner DS: Cystinuria. Endocrinol Metab Clin North Am 19:889, 1990.

77. Wallerstrom BI, et al: Cystine calculi in the dog: An epidemiological retrospective study. J Small Anim Pract 33:78, 1992.

78. Bruhl M: Studie zur Epidemiologie der Urolithiasis bei Hund, Katze und Kaninchen auf der Grundlage infarotspecktroskopischer untersuchungen. Giessen, Justus-Liebig Universitat, 1989.

79. Casal ML, Giger U, Bovee KC, Patterson DF: Inheritance of cystinuria and renal defect in Newfoundlands. JAVMA 207:1585–1589, 1995.

80. Osborne CA, et al: Canine and feline urolithiasis: Relationship of etiopathogenesis to treatment and prevention. In Bojrab MJ (ed): Disease Mechanisms in Small Animal Surgery. Philadelphia, Lea and Febiger, 1992, p 464.

81. Case LC, et al: Cystine-containing calculi in dogs: 102 cases (1981–1989). JAVMA 201:129, 1992.

82. Cystinuria is reduced by low-sodium diets. Nutr Rev 45:79, 1987.

83. Jaeger P, et al: Anticystinuric effects of glutamine and of dietary sodium restriction. N Engl J Med 315:1120, 1986.

84. Singer A et al: Cystinuria: A review of the pathophysiology and management. J Urol 142:669, 1989.

85. Hoppe A, et al: Treatment of clinically normal and cystinuric dogs with 2-mercaptopropionylglycine. Am J Vet Res 49:923, 1986.

86. Osborne CA, et al: Medical dissolution and prevention of cystine urolithiasis. In Kirk RW (ed.): Current Veterinary Therapy 10. Philadelphia, WB Saunders, 1989, p 1189.

87. Martin X, Smith L, Werness PG: Calcium oxalate dihydrate formation in urine. Kidney Int 25:948–952, 1984.

88. Berland Y, Boistelle R, Omer M: Urinary supersaturation with respect to brushite in patients suffering from calcium oxalate lithiasis. Nephrol Dial Transplant 5:179–184, 1990.

89. Ackermann D, Baumann JM: Chemical factors governing the state of saturation towards brushite and whewellite in urine of calcium stone formers. Urol Res 15:63–65, 1987.

90. Stewart SR, Emerick RJ, Pritchard RH: High dietary calcium to phosphorus ratio and alkali-forming potential as factors promoting silica urolithiasis in sheep. J Anim Sci 68:498–503, 1990.

91. Emerick RJ: Chloride and phosphate as impediments to silica urinary calculi in rats fed tetraethylorthosilicate. J Nutr 114:733–738, 1984.

URO

SECTION XV

HEMATOLOGY AND IMMUNOLOGY

CHAPTER 177

REGENERATIVE ANEMIAS CAUSED BY BLOOD LOSS OR HEMOLYSIS

Urs Giger

Anemia is not a diagnosis in itself but is a common clinical sign and laboratory test abnormality in companion animals. Anemia may indicate a specific erythrocyte problem or can be associated with other organ disorders. Anemia and other hematologic abnormalities occur so frequently that a complete blood cell count is generally requested in the diagnostic assessment of any ill patient. Anemia is defined as a decrease in the red blood cell (RBC) mass as expressed by a reduction in number of circulating RBCs, hematocrit, and hemoglobin. Clinical signs result from decreased oxygen-carrying capacity, reduced blood volume, underlying disease, and the adjustments made to increase the efficiency of the erythron. The severity of signs depends on the rapidity of onset, the degree and cause of anemia, and the extent of physical activity (see Chapter 55). An orderly approach to the diagnosis of anemia is usually fruitful. Anemias are classified by pathophysiologic mechanisms, bone marrow response, and RBC indices. In view of the limitations of such subclassification, this chapter reviews regenerative anemias caused by blood loss or hemolysis. Nonregenerative anemias are covered in the next chapter.[1-3]

REGENERATIVE BONE MARROW RESPONSE

The number of erythrocytes present in the circulation is a dynamic equilibrium between the production and delivery of erythrocytes (Fig. 177–1) into the blood circulation and their destruction or loss from circulation. The normal homeostatic mechanisms of the body bring about recovery from anemia by accelerating erythropoiesis. The bone marrow response is regulated by erythropoietin, a lineage-specific hematopoietic growth factor. Erythropoietin synthesis in the renal cortex is induced by anemia, although the actual sensor measures oxygen tension and recognizes only renal hypoxia. This hormone acts on erythroid precursor cells of the bone marrow known as burst-forming units–erythroid (BFU-E) and particularly colony-forming units–erythroid (CFU-E). At maximal stimulation, the bone marrow is capable of producing erythrocytes at 10-fold the normal rate. Erythropoietin also contributes to the maturation from committed erythroid precursors to fully hemoglobinized erythrocytes, which takes approximately 1 week.[1, 3]

RETICULOCYTES

The most useful marker of accelerated erythropoiesis continues to be an increased number of reticulocytes in circula-

tion.[1, 3, 4] Reticulocytes form after extrusion of the pyknotic nucleus of the normoblasts and continue to mature, finally to erythrocytes, in the bone marrow and peripheral blood. Reticulocytes normally reside within the marrow for almost 2 days before they are released into the blood circulation. They continue to synthesize hemoglobin as long as they have functional messenger RNA, which is usually 1 day in circulation. However, during accelerated erythropoiesis, reticulocytes may be released prematurely from the marrow. The so-called stress or shift reticulocytes are macrocytic, less developed, and, therefore, require a longer time to mature to erythrocytes in circulation. Because they contain residual RNA, which can be precipitated into a reticulum network and stained by certain supravital dyes such as new methylene blue or brilliant cresyl blue, reticulocytes can be readily enumerated. The latter stain is particularly suitable as it is relatively free of precipitates. On a stained blood smear, the number of reticulocytes is counted per 500 to 1000 erythrocytes and the reticulocyte result is reported as a percentage of cells examined (number per 100 cells).

Because canine reticulocytes contain strong aggregates, they are relatively easy to count. In contrast, cats produce two types of reticulocytes, namely aggregate and punctate reticulocytes (Fig. 177–2). The aggregate reticulocytes correspond to the reticulocytes seen in dogs and indicate an active regenerative response. After a short maturation time of less

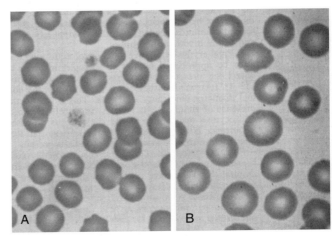

Figure 177–1. Normal uniformity and central pallor of feline *(A)* and canine *(B)* erythrocytes. Wright-Giemsa stain. (From Weiser MG: Erythrocyte responses and disorders. *In* Ettinger SJ, Feldman EC [eds]: Textbook of Veterinary Internal Medicine, 4th ed. Philadelphia, WB Saunders, 1995, p 1866.)

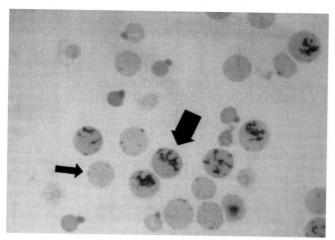

Figure 177–2. Feline reticulocytes and Heinz bodies as visualized with brilliant cresyl blue stain. Round, homogeneous Heinz bodies stain medium blue with this stain. Several aggregate reticulocytes (large arrow) and punctate reticulocytes (small arrow) are present. The reticulum stains dark blue compared to Heinz bodies. (From Weiser MG: Erythrocyte responses and disorders. *In* Ettinger SJ, Feldman EC [eds]: Textbook of Veterinary Internal Medicine, 4th ed. Philadelphia, WB Saunders, 1995, p 1872.)

than a day, these aggregate forms become punctate reticulocytes. On a blood smear stained for reticulocytes, they contain up to 10 individual blue dots, which do not coalesce. As punctate reticulocytes circulate over a period of 1 to 2 weeks and represent a cumulative response, they can reach high percentages. It is therefore best to report either the aggregate reticulocytes only or both separately in cats.

The upper limit of a normal reticulocyte count is often stated as 1 per cent; however, healthy small animals generally have less than 0.4 per cent reticulocytes per 100 erythrocytes. This number is not only increased by enhanced hematopoiesis but also affected by anemia, as it depends on the number of circulating erythrocytes, and the duration of reticulocyte maturation in circulation. Therefore, various adjustments to the reticulocyte count are being used.

If the erythrocyte count is available, the absolute reticulocyte count can be calculated and is less than 40,000/μL in a healthy animal:

$$\frac{\% \text{ reticulocytes} \times \text{RBC}/\mu L}{100} = \text{reticulocytes}/\mu L$$

The absolute reticulocyte count is likely to be adopted as the preferred expression of erythroid regeneration. However, the correction for anemia can also be made on the basis of the patient's hematocrit compared with the average normal packed cell volume (PCV) value (dogs 45 per cent; cats 37 per cent) and is normally less than 0.4 per cent.

$$\% \text{ reticulocytes} \times \frac{\text{patient's PCV}}{\text{normal PCV}} = \frac{\text{corrected}}{\% \text{ reticulocytes}}$$
(dogs 45; cats 37)

Finally, the reticulocyte production index (RPI) also takes into consideration the extended maturation of stress or shift reticulocytes in circulation. The maturation time is taken as 1 day if the PCV is 45 per cent (37 per cent for cats), 1.5 days at 35 per cent (29 per cent), 2 days at 25 per cent (21 per cent), and 2.5 days at 15 per cent (11 per cent) and an RPI less than 1 is considered normal.

corrected reticulocyte % ÷ maturation time = RPI

Several automated hematology analyzers have incorporated staining to detect reticulocytes; however, automated

counts may be falsely increased in the presence of Heinz's bodies and Howell-Jolly bodies as well as punctate reticulocytes.

An increase in absolute reticulocyte count, corrected reticulocyte percentage, or RPI provides the best evidence for a regenerative response. Although not as accurate, other hematologic manifestations may be used to indicate increased erythropoiesis when a reticulocyte count is not available. On a regularly (Wright; Diff-Quik) stained blood smear, polychromatophilic cells represent erythrocytes recently released from the bone marrow. As their blue-grey tint color is due to the presence of RNA, their numbers correlate with the reticulocyte count. When more than one polychromatophilic cell is recognized per microscopic oil immersion field, accelerated erythropoiesis is suggested. Polychromatophilic erythrocytes are often macrocytic, which indicates that these cells are released prematurely from the marrow, thereby contributing greatly to the high mean cell volume (MCV) and red cell distribution width (RDW) as well as anisocytosis of regenerative anemias. It should be noted that macrocytic anemia is not always regenerative but may indicate a maturation problem such as feline leukemia virus (FeLV) infection or folate deficiency in cats.

Nucleated erythrocytes (Fig. 177–3) also known as normoblasts or metarubricytes with variably shrunken nuclei are rarely found in blood of healthy animals (less than 1 per 100 white blood cells). Large numbers may accompany a marked regenerative response in anemic patients. However, nucleated RBCs may also be seen in patients without reticulocytosis because of breakdown of the barrier between marrow and vasculature. In fact, the highest numbers are observed in acute lead poisoning in the absence of anemia. Mild to moderate normoblastosis with nonregenerative anemia may be seen with myeloproliferative disorders, dyshematopoiesis, extramedullary hematopoiesis, hemangiosarcoma, and sepsis. Thus, normoblastosis should not be equated with a regenerative response without confirmation by a reticulocyte count.

If the anemia is characterized as regenerative on the basis of finding a reticulocytosis, bone marrow examination is rarely indicated. In regenerative anemia, the bone marrow cellularity is increased and the ratio of myeloid to erythroid elements in the bone marrow is generally below one. The

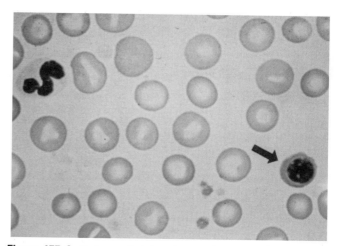

Figure 177–3. Canine nucleated erythrocyte (arrow), anisocytosis, and a few stomatocytes. (From Weiser MG: Erythrocyte responses and disorders. *In* Ettinger SJ, Feldman EC [eds]: Textbook of Veterinary Internal Medicine, 4th ed. Philadelphia, WB Saunders, 1995, p 1866.)

earliest morphologically recognizable erythroid cell is a pronormoblast, and an exponentially increasing number of later erythroid precursors that decrease in size to the pyknotic normoblast indicate normal maturation. Although the erythropoietin response is lineage specific, independent stimulation of thrombopoiesis (iron deficiency) or granulopoiesis (immune-mediated hemolytic anemia) may also be present. Bone marrow examination rarely provides helpful information about an underlying cause or marrow iron deposition in patients with regenerative anemia that would otherwise remain undetected.

BLOOD LOSS ANEMIA

Blood loss anemia occurs whenever a disease process damages vascular integrity sufficiently for RBCs to escape from the intravascular space. The blood loss may be localized to one site, caused by trauma, surgery, tumor, gastrointestinal disorders, or parasites, or generalized in association with a hemorrhagic tendency. Surface bleeding such as petechiae and epistaxis suggests a platelet problem, whereas hematomas and cavity bleedings indicate a coagulopathy. These primary and secondary hemostatic disorders are discussed in other sections. Regardless of the cause, clinical manifestations of blood loss anemia are essentially the same and related to the compensatory mechanisms but depend on the volume of blood loss and onset, that is, whether it is acute or chronic.

ACUTE BLOOD LOSS

Rapid blood loss of major proportions represents a double threat as it decreases the total blood volume and oxygenation of tissue.[4, 5] The total blood volume of dogs and cats is 8 and 6 per cent of the body weight, respectively. Blood donations for transfusion of 4.4 ml/lb body weight, representing 11 to 15 per cent of the blood volume of healthy animals, are generally well tolerated. However, when the hemorrhage exceeds 20 per cent, cardiovascular signs occur. Initial physiologic adjustments are peripheral vasoconstriction and tachycardia. Regional blood flow to skin and spleen is curtailed, a sacrifice designed to protect perfusion of the brain, heart, and viscera. Thus, pallor in acute blood loss anemia is caused not by thinness of blood but by reduced perfusion of the skin and is associated with a prolonged capillary refill time and dry mucous membranes. Besides the redistribution of blood to areas most vulnerable to hypoxemia, the heart rate is increased in an attempt to maintain cardiac output. This high-velocity flow is well tolerated because of vasodilatation in the central and cerebral vascular beds into which most blood is diverted. As the blood loss exceeds 30 to 40 per cent of the original blood volume, the cardiac output falls and hypotension and cardiovascular collapse ensue. The animal becomes immobile and exhibits a rapid, thready pulse and cold skin and extremities. An acute blood loss of 50 per cent within hours results in shock and eventually death before any changes in hematocrit and plasma protein are observed.

If the acute blood loss is more gradual, restoration of the plasma volume can occur, which in turn lowers the hematocrit. Unless fluid is administered, the plasma volume expansion is a relatively slow process. After a sudden, single hemorrhagic event, albumin-containing fluid is mobilized from the extravascular space over a period of 2 to 3 days.

This fluid shift reduces the skin turgor until the fluid deficit is replenished by oral or parenteral fluid intake. Because the associated fall in hematocrit is gradual, the severity of the hemorrhage may be markedly underestimated.

As the anemia is initially normocytic-normochromic and nonregenerative, it could be mistaken for a defective hematopoietic problem. Within a few hours, serum erythropoietin levels are increased and erythropoiesis is stimulated. After 3 days, the anemia becomes macrocytic and regenerative. A maximal reticulocyte response is seen within 4 to 7 days. The corrected reticulocyte count may reach 3 to 10 per cent, which is somewhat less than with hemolytic anemias. In acute anemia, adequate iron stores are generally present but the marrow response may be hampered by limited iron mobilization. In cats, the transient rise in aggregated reticulocytes is followed by a marked sustained increase in punctate reticulocytes over a few weeks. A stress leukogram may also be observed. Although platelets are being consumed at the site of injury, this does not result in a significant thrombocytopenia; to the contrary, acute blood loss is accompanied by a mild reactive thrombocytosis. In case of external blood loss, there is a concomitant loss of plasma proteins including albumin and globulins. Thus, the triad of anemia, hypoproteinemia, and reticulocytosis is considered a hallmark of external blood loss. Other test abnormalities depend on the cause of bleeding. Besides typical clinical signs of hemorrhage, examination of a blood smear for platelets and schistocytes and evaluation of an activated clotting time and buccal mucosal bleeding time may suggest a hemostatic defect that can be confirmed by appropriate laboratory tests.

There are four main objectives in the management of acute blood loss anemia: (1) fluid replacement, (2) prevention of further bleeding, (3) blood transfusion support, and (4) treatment of the underlying disorder. With sudden hemorrhage the immediate effects of volume depletion are more important than the loss of circulating RBCs. Thus, the first requirement is to maintain an adequate blood volume by intravenous infusion of crystalloid fluids (electrolytes), colloid solutions of plasma, hydroxyethylstarch, or whole blood. The choice of fluids depends on the clinical setting, particularly the severity and rate of hemorrhage. With major hemorrhage leading rapidly to shock, losses are primarily from the intravascular space with little change in extra- and intracellular fluid compartments. Crystalloid fluids (isotonic saline or Ringer's lactate) are the first choice. Because crystalloids are rapidly distributed between the intra- and extravascular compartments, they need to be infused in a volume of two to four times the estimated loss. An infusion of crystalloids can rapidly restore circulation, thereby normalizing many hemodynamic parameters.

Within days, intra- and extracellular fluids shift into the intravascular space. For adequate resuscitation of a patient with hemorrhagic hypotension and shock, much larger fluid volumes must be given quickly to replete the fluid compartments and restore circulation. Colloid fluids such as 6 per cent hydroxyethylstarch or dextran 70 solutions produce a volume expansion slightly larger than the volume infused and maintain its effect for as long as a day. As species-specific albumin solutions are not available for small animals, plasma or whole blood transfusions may be used for replacement therapy. Their use should, however, be discouraged unless clotting factors are needed or, because of major blood loss, an oxygen carrier is deemed necessary. A bovine hemoglobin solution has become commercially available that provides oncotic pressure and an oxygen transporter and may therefore prove useful in the emergency management of acute blood loss.[6]

The depletion of the RBC mass after acute blood loss may be difficult to appreciate as the hematocrit falls only as the total blood volume returns to normal by expansion of the plasma volume. Thus, the transfusion trigger is particularly difficult to define in a hemorrhaging patient. Whereas a healthy normovolemic anemic animal at rest may tolerate a hematocrit as low as 10 per cent, signs of hypoxia develop much earlier in a hypovolemic anemic animal. Thus, small animals with precipitous blood loss may be deemed in need of a blood transfusion at hematocrits above 20 per cent. Ten milliliters of whole blood per pound body weight increases the hematocrit by 10 per cent, but fluid shifts and concomitant replacement of fluids may diminish the response. It should be noted that except for isotonic saline, fluids have to be administered through a catheter other than that used for transfusion. If venous access cannot be obtained in severely hypotensive animals, the intraosseous route may be considered as RBCs and fluids rapidly reach the intravascular space. Because canine stored blood or packed RBCs have low 2,3-diphosphoglycerate (DPG) concentrations, which may hamper the oxygen release, some clinicians have advocated the use of fresh blood. However, DPGs are rapidly replenished in canine erythrocytes and, therefore, this may be more of a theoretic concern. As the hemoglobin-oxygen affinity of feline erythrocytes is not DPG dependent, this is not a problem in cats, but closed blood collection systems for storage of feline blood are.

The preceding cardiovascular parameters as well as PCV and total protein are used to monitor the bleeding patient during treatment. When hemorrhage has ceased, the recovery of the red cell mass to normal occurs rapidly within 1 to 2 weeks. Animals with acute blood loss anemia have adequate iron stores and generally do not require supplemental iron to reach an appropriate erythroid bone marrow response.

CHRONIC BLOOD LOSS ANEMIA—IRON DEFICIENCY ANEMIA

Animals have approximately 9 to 22 mg iron per lb body weight and most of the iron is located in erythrocytes as hemoglobin (1 mg iron in 2 mL of blood).[3, 7] In addition, muscle myoglobin and many important enzymes contain heme iron (e.g., cytochromes). Iron is also stored in various tissues, particularly spleen, liver, and bone marrow, as a soluble mobile fraction (ferritin) or insoluble fraction (hemosiderin), depending on the amount available. Transferrin represents the iron transport protein in the plasma and is normally 20 to 60 per cent saturated with iron. As under physiologic conditions iron losses through gut, urine, and skin are negligible, amounting to less than 1 mg/day in small animals, the iron balance is regulated by iron absorption. Iron is absorbed in the ferrous (Fe^{2+}) form as heme iron or nonheme iron by the mucosal cells of the proximal small intestine. The exact control mechanisms have not been elucidated, but absorption increases with diminished storage and increased erythropoietic activity. However, the maximal absorption remains rather limited, only a few milligrams per day.[8]

Chronic external blood loss is the major cause of iron deficiency anemia in small animals and, contrary to common beliefs, results in regenerative anemia. Iron deficiency denotes a deficit in total body iron, which occurs in varying degrees. Iron depletion is present when iron stores are depleted but serum iron and blood hemoglobin concentrations remain normal. In iron-deficient erythropoiesis, serum iron levels are also low but the anemia is only mild. Iron deficiency anemia refers to the most advanced stage, characterized by absent iron stores, low serum iron concentration, low transferrin saturation, and low hemoglobin and hematocrit values.

Chronic external blood loss may result from gastrointestinal hemorrhage, parasitism, and chronic bleeding neoplasia.[9–13] Severe flea infestation can cause substantial blood loss and mortality, particularly in kittens and puppies, as 100 fleas could potentially consume 1 mL of blood daily. Similarly, the quantity of blood loss caused by hookworms and rarely whipworms is proportional to the worm burden and may reach 100 mL/day. Hookworms burrow their heads deeply into the small intestinal wall and suck blood by peristaltic pumping. Chronic or intermittent gastrointestinal blood loss may also result from hemorrhaging gastrointestinal neoplasia including leiomyoma, carcinoma, and lymphoma; bleeding intestinal aneurysm; and ulcerogenic drugs such as glucocorticosteroids, salicylates, and nonsteroidal anti-inflammatory agents. As each regular blood collection (450 mL) removes approximately 200 mg of iron from the body, overzealous blood donations and frequent phlebotomies for diagnostic purposes in small patients may lead to iron deficiency states.

In young animals the iron needed for growth may exceed the supply available from diet and stores, and thus they are particularly at risk for developing an iron deficiency anemia. Because milk is low in iron, nursing animals may become iron deficient. However, with the general use of balanced commercial diets for growing animals, iron deficiency related to inadequate intake alone is rare. Intestinal malabsorption syndromes, such as inflammatory bowel disease in Shar Peis, are associated with iron deficiency states.

Iron deficiency anemia develops over weeks and is almost always insidious, allowing remarkably effective adaptation. The clinical signs are nonspecific and depend more on the rate of the progression than on the extent of the anemia. Even when the hematocrit falls below 5 to 10 per cent, clinical signs of anemia, besides pallor, may not be obvious at rest. The animals may become increasingly fatigued and exercise intolerant and, when stressed, may suddenly decompensate and die. Clinical manifestations include extremely pale mucous membranes, bounding pulses, gallop rhythm, and a systolic flow murmur. The cardiac output is maintained by reduced blood viscosity and vascular resistance (decreased afterload) as well as increased left ventricular filling (increased preload). Thus, chronic anemia causes cardiomegaly through cardiac hypertrophy and dilation and may eventually lead to congestive heart failure.[13] Pica, the craving to eat, chew, or lick unusual substances such as dirt, clay, feces, and metal, is a classical manifestation of iron deficiency. Because iron deficiency is most commonly caused by gastrointestinal blood loss, melena is likely to be present, but occasionally it is intermittent or detected only by the occult fecal blood test. A positive test result for an animal receiving a commercial diet is probably significant. Typical laboratory test abnormalities may provide the first clue to an iron deficiency anemia and possibly an occult intestinal malignancy.

Iron deficiency can produce clinical manifestations independent of anemia because of depletion of iron-containing compounds in nonerythroid tissue resulting in impaired proliferation, growth, and function, including reduced muscle activity, abnormal behavior, and skin and nail changes.

HEM

Severe iron deficiency anemia is characterized by a hypochromic microcytic anemia caused by decreased synthesis of hemoglobin and delayed cell maturation and extra mitosis.[1, 9, 14] On a blood smear the hypochromic cells are readily recognized by the increased central pallor and are reflected by a decreased mean corpuscular hemoglobin concentration (MCHC). In advanced states the red cell corpuscles represent mere rings. Microcytosis is less well appreciated on a blood smear because cell diameter is less affected than cell thickness; these flat, poorly stained cells are called leptocytes and cause a reduced MCV. Anisocytosis is also a recognizable morphologic change and can be quantified by an increased RDW as determined by particle size counters. In addition, iron-deficient erythrocytes appear stiffer and less deformable, presumably because of oxidative damage of membrane proteins. Thus, erythrocyte fragmentation (Fig. 177–4) and increased mechanical fragility and lysis may occur and thereby affect the various erythrocyte indices. However, in the osmotic fragility test, the red cells may be more resistant to destruction in hypotonic salt solutions because of their increased capacity to expand.[1, 8]

Whereas in humans iron deficiency anemia is non- or poorly regenerative,[8] iron deficiency in small animals is usually associated with a pronounced reticulocytosis.[9] The reticulocyte counts may exceed 500,000/µL (10 per cent corrected), presumably because of their delayed maturation. This reticulocytosis greatly contributes to the degree of anisocytosis and high RDW.

The leukocytes are usually normal in number, but slight neutropenia may occur, whereas eosinophilia is seen in parasite-induced anemia. Interestingly, the platelet count is commonly increased to about twice normal and may exceed $1 \times 10^6/\mu L$.[9] Thrombocytosis associated with acute and chronic blood loss is considered reactive, but the exact mechanism remains unexplained. A search for occult blood loss is highly warranted in anemic animals with thrombocytosis. In uncomplicated iron deficiency anemia, the chemistry screening test results are unremarkable except for a low total protein related to concomitant intestinal losses of albumin and globulin.

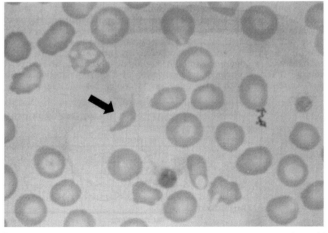

Figure 177–4. Erythrocyte fragmentation and hypochromia in a dog with iron deficiency anemia. Note that a few cells have increased central pallor compared with normal. A small fragment is indicated by the arrow. In addition, several oxidative membrane fusions that appear like vacuoles are present. (From Weiser MG: Erythrocyte responses and disorders. *In* Ettinger SJ, Feldman EC [eds]: Textbook of Veterinary Internal Medicine, 4th ed. Philadelphia, WB Saunders, 1995, p 1870.)

The bone marrow is characterized by mild to moderate erythroid hyperplasia with nuclear distortions. The normoblasts appear small and have scant cytoplasm. After staining the bone marrow aspirate or biopsy section with Prussian blue, one sees dark blue granular material scattered throughout the marrow. In iron deficiency anemia, no stainable iron in the form of deep blue granules is found (hemosiderin appears in the unstained marrow smear as golden refractile granules). However, healthy cats normally store only small amounts of ferritin and hemosiderin in macrophages of their marrow; thus, a lack of positive Prussian blue staining is not diagnostic for iron deficiency, but Prussian blue–positive deposits in marrow exclude iron deficiency.

Serum iron concentrations are usually low, ranging from 5 to 60 µg/dL compared with a normal range of 60 to 230 µg/dL, depending to some extent on the method used.[7] However, serum iron levels are subject to many variables that may cause normal or even high results, including hemolyzed samples, iron supplementation, and recent transfusions. The iron-binding capacity is a measure of the amount of transferrin in circulating blood and may be slightly increased in iron deficiency states; thus, the transferrin saturation is markedly decreased to below 20 per cent (normal 20 to 60 per cent). Serum ferritin concentrations would be expected to be low, but as ferritin is an acute phase protein, values are often increased by coexisting inflammation.

Management of chronic blood loss anemia is directed toward correction of the anemia and iron deficiency states and treatment of the underlying disease. Transfusions with packed RBCs or whole blood are indicated only in cases of severe anemia or in preparation for anesthesia and surgery to correct the gastrointestinal hemorrhage (PCV less than 15 per cent) and signs of tissue hypoxia. As these patients are normovolemic and in a state of high cardiac output, transfusion volumes and rates should be limited to avoid cardiac failure. Volume overload occurs more commonly in cats than in dogs. Correction of the anemia also results in resolution of the cardiomegaly within several weeks. Although ulcerogenic drugs can be withdrawn immediately, control of ecto- and endoparasites as well as any surgical corrections should be undertaken only when the patients have been stabilized.

Once critical care has been provided and the underlying condition has been corrected, iron supplementation is initiated to replenish iron stores. Iron is highly effective in treating iron deficiency. It has, however, no other legitimate therapeutic use as it exerts no beneficial effects in numerous other forms of anemias and may in fact be harmful (exception: animals with chronic renal failure may in fact also experience an iron deficiency state). Iron can be administered orally and parenterally. The oral route is the safest and least expensive. Ferrous sulfate in tablet or liquid form at a dose of 5 mg/lb twice daily along with a meal is effective, although the exact iron requirements have not been established for small animals. Iron fumarate and gluconate may be substituted but other iron preparations are likely not to be effective, may cause gastric irritation, and are not recommended. Treatment has to be continued for weeks to months to correct the iron deficiency state, but iron stores may never be completely replenished.

If oral iron replacement is deemed inappropriate or insufficient or a gastrointestinal disorder prevents iron absorption, parenteral iron may be administered. Iron dextran complex containing 50 mg iron per milliliter can be given intramuscularly or intravenously. (Ferrous chloride is available outside the United States.) After a small dose is injected deep into the muscle to test for hypersensitivity reaction, a maximal dose of 2 mL is administered daily; two thirds of the iron is absorbed from the injection site within days. As 2 mL of blood contains 1 mg iron, blood transfusions also provide an excellent source of iron, but they should be restricted to severely anemic patients.

HEMOLYTIC ANEMIAS

Once the erythrocyte has lost its nucleus and ribosomes, it can no longer synthesize protein. Nevertheless, it survives hundreds of miles of hazardous travel through large and tiny blood vessels with its limited equipment. It is capable of sustaining adequate energy levels through anaerobic glycolysis, maintaining ionic composition, reducing methemoglobin and oxidized glutathione, and resealing its membrane if portions are lost. Despite these capacities, erythrocytes have a finite life span that may be shortened when the environment becomes hostile or when the cell's ability for self-repair becomes impaired. Accelerated erythrocyte destruction is the major mechanism in hemolytic disorders and plays a minor role in many other common anemias.[15]

The normal life span of erythrocytes averages approximately 100 to 120 days in dogs and 70 to 78 days in cats.[2, 3] Although it is rarely done in clinical practice, the erythrocyte life span can be measured directly by two labeling methods. The cohort method depends on the incorporation of an isotopically labeled chemical such as radioactive iron or glycine into newly formed cells. In contrast, the random labeling methods use tracers that bind with all erythrocytes in the circulation and include radiolabeled chromium or cyanate but also nonradioactive biotin.[16] Because chromium elutes from cells readily, the apparent half-life is much shorter, for instance, 20 to 30 days instead of 60 days for normal canine erythrocytes and only 6 to 14 days instead of 37 days for feline cells.[17]

Although the concept of erythrocyte aging and death is well established, the precise mechanisms involved in normal cell senescence are still not clearly defined. There is no single marker to identify aged erythrocytes, but the following factors may contribute to the finite life span of erythrocytes: declining enzyme activities, change in calcium balance, diminished negative membrane charge, repeated oxidative injuries, and binding of complement and naturally occurring autoantibodies against membrane band 3 protein and galactosyl-containing glycolipid.[15, 16]

The erythrocyte life span may be shortened as a result of some intrinsic defect, such as an erythroenzymopathy, or because of some extrinsic mechanism that leads to premature erythrocyte removal, such as antibodies against erythrocytes. These can be distinguished by cross-transfusion studies. When erythrocytes from a healthy animal are transfused to a patient with an extrinsic cause for hemolysis, the donated cells are destroyed as rapidly as the patient's own cells. However, if the patient's corpuscles are removed from the unfavorable environment, they survive normally. In contrast, erythrocytes with an intrinsic defect would be disposed of as rapidly in the patient or a healthy recipient. Such survival studies are generally not required in the evaluation of hemolytic anemias in clinical practice. If needed, the nonradioactive biotin labeling method should be considered.

Erythrocyte destruction may take place either extra- or intravascularly.[1, 3] Extravascular hemolysis is the predominant form and also assumed to be the mode of destruction of senescent erythrocytes in healthy animals. Extravascular destruction refers to erythrophagocytosis by macrophages of the spleen, liver, and bone marrow. Damaged or senescent erythrocytes are prone to enhanced sequestration in these organs. Erythrophagocytosis may be either complete (culling) or partial (pitting). In particular, splenic environment with its low glucose concentration, mild hypoxia, hypercapnea, and relatively low pH can be deleterious to erythrocytes. On the basis of its structure, the canine spleen is more efficient than the feline spleen in removing erythrocytes. Macrophages destroy ingested erythrocytes through proteolytic and lipolytic enzymes.

The heme oxygenase system responsible for hemoglobin degradation is located primarily in phagocytic cells of the spleen, liver, and bone marrow as well as hepatocytes. The globin is broken down to amino acids, which are reused. In heme catabolism, iron becomes liberated and recirculates bound to transferrin in plasma back to the marrow for erythropoiesis, and the protoporphyrin ring opens; carbon monoxide is split off and exhaled and biliverdin forms and is subsequently reduced to bilirubin.

Unconjugated bilirubin is then released into the plasma; it is water insoluble and reversibly binds to albumin (indirect-reacting bilirubin). The albumin-bound bilirubin is readily absorbed by hepatocytes. In the liver bilirubin is conjugated with glucuronic acid to form bilirubin diglucuronide, also known as direct bilirubin. The conjugated bilirubin is excreted via the bile canaliculi into the duodenum, but in the presence of massive heme breakdown, conjugated bilirubin leaks back into the plasma and is also excreted in the urine. Intestinal bacteria in the colon convert the bilirubin to urobilinogens. Most of the urobilinogen is excreted in the feces, but a small amount is reabsorbed. The reabsorbed urobilinogen is readily reexcreted by the liver (enterohepatic recirculation) with a small portion lost in the urine.

The serum bilirubin concentration is an important marker of the rate of hemoglobin metabolism and of hepatobiliary function. Normal serum values, measured by colorimetric methods, do not exceed 0.4 mg/dL and jaundice is not appreciated until the serum bilirubin exceeds 2 mg/dL. One might predict that hemolytic disorders are associated with a greater rise in indirect bilirubin, whereas hepatic failure leads to a larger increase in direct bilirubin. However, as the process to conjugated bilirubin is highly efficient and rapid in small animals, the differential bilirubin determination has not proved helpful in distinguishing hemolytic from hepatic causes of hyperbilirubinemia. Liver function tests are often indicated as hemolysis may be associated with a hepatopathy, for example, immune-mediated hemolytic anemia (IMHA). Furthermore, one might predict that hemolytic disorders are associated with a greater rise in indirect bilirubin, whereas hepatic failure leads to a larger increase in direct bilirubin. Heme can be metabolized by alternative pathways in other tissues (e.g., kidney in dogs). In any case, a rise in heme degradation results in hyperbilirubinuria because of increased urinary excretion of conjugated bilirubin. Bilirubin is readily identified by the diazo reaction on the urine dipstick. Small amounts of bilirubin are normally found in urine from healthy dogs but not cats. Hemoglobinuria may make the bilirubin readings invalid. Bile pigment gallstones, seen in humans with hemolysis, are not observed in small animals.

Less commonly, erythrocytes are lysed within the systemic circulation as a consequence of membrane permeability changes or cellular fragmentation. With intravascular hemolysis, hemoglobin is directly released into the blood, from which it is removed by several mechanisms. Hemoglobin breaks into two alpha-beta dimers and binds to haptoglobin in plasma or further dissociates into heme to form hemopexin and methemalbumin. After these complexes are taken up by macrophages and hepatocytes, hemoglobin and heme are metabolized as described earlier in relation to extravascular hemolysis. Binding prevents excretion of hemoglobin into the urine, but during intravascular lysis, haptoglobin becomes easily depleted. Unbound plasma hemoglobin and heme, some oxidized to methemoglobin in the plasma, may be removed by the liver or excreted through the renal glomeruli. Proximal tubule cells reabsorb and catabolize most of the filtered hemoglobin and heme. Hemoglobinuria ensues when the amount filtered exceeds the limited capacity of the tubular cells to resorb dimers. Although heme pigments may precipitate and form casts in the distal renal tubules, hemosiderinuric tubular necrosis and acute renal failure are rarely observed in small animals with severe and chronic hemoglobinuria.

Thus, intravascular lysis can be readily recognized by the presence of hemoglobinemia, depletion of plasma haptoglobin, and hemoglobinuria. Plasma hemoglobin levels of 10 to 20 mg/dL give plasma an amber coloration, and at 50 to 100 mg/dL the plasma appears reddish. The hemoglobinemia has to be distinguished from artifactual increases in plasma hemoglobin caused by poor blood collection and handling as well as delayed plasma separation. Plasma hemoglobin concentrations can be quantitated spectrophotometrically by an accurate and simple hemoglobinometer (HemoCue).[18] Hemoglobinuria imparts a red-brown color to the urine, reflecting both hemoglobin and methemoglobin. As the urine dipstick identifies only heme (labeled "blood"), hemoglobinuria has to be differentiated from hematuria (whole erythrocytes) by microscopic examination after urine sedimentation. Myoglobinuria associated with massive muscle necrosis can also cause a positive test result but is hardly observed in small animals.

On the basis of the preceding mechanisms of erythrocyte destruction, the clinical features and laboratory test abnormalities of the various hemolytic disorders are similar. Beside the general signs of anemia such as pallor and weakness, characteristic signs of hemolysis are jaundice and pigmenturia. Jaundice is first appreciated on mucous membranes (gingiva and sclera) when the serum bilirubin level exceeds 2 mg/dL, whereas the skin becomes icteric only at higher bilirubin concentrations. Milder and chronic forms of hemolysis may not be associated with jaundice. Pigmenturia caused by hemolysis may be due to hyperbilirubinuria and hemoglobinuria. Hyperbilirubinuria persists in dogs with hemolytic disorders, whereas in cats that appears not to be a constant finding. Hemoglobinuria and hemoglobinemia are hallmark features of intravascular hemolysis and often indicate a more severe disorder. The term hemolytic anemia or hemolytic disorder is limited to conditions in which the rate of erythrocyte destruction is accelerated and the ability of the bone marrow to respond to the stimulus is unimpaired. As indicated in the introduction, hemolytic anemias are generally associated with accelerated erythrocyte production that is unrestricted by iron availability. In fact, the highest reticulocyte counts and most severe erythroid hyperplasias are observed in animals with hemolytic anemias. Thus, hemolytic anemias are regenerative and macrocytic-hypochromic, although in the early stages and in some complicated acquired forms the erythroid response may be poor. In addition, a number of common complex anemias related to insufficient erythrocyte production have a component of accelerated erythrocytic destruction, but it would be misleading to include them here.

The disorders associated with hemolytic anemia have been classified in various ways. The division into acute and chronic forms is of limited usefulness, because acute crises may develop during the course of chronic disorders. Classification based on the site of hemolysis, predominantly within the circulation (intravascular) or within tissue macrophages (extravascular), is of some help, as only a few are associated with overt intravascular hemolysis. However, intravascular lysis may occur only transiently; therefore, the unique manifestations of hemoglobinemia and hemoglobinuria may be missed. Excessive destruction of erythrocytes may occur either because of an intrinsic defect in the cell itself or because of the action of extrinsic factors on normal erythrocytes. Intrinsic defects are generally inherited and the extrinsic ones are acquired. The division into intrinsic and extrinsic or inherited and acquired forms is of pathogenic importance and is most useful as hereditary hemolytic anemias gain greater recognition.

INHERITED ERYTHROCYTE DEFECTS

Several hereditary erythrocyte defects (Table 177–1) have been described in dogs and cats and much new information has emerged over the past decade.[19] The mode of inheritance is autosomal recessive for all described erythrocyte defects, with the exception of feline porphyria, which is inherited as a dominant trait. This is a large heterogeneous group of disorders and most occur rarely. Through inbreeding practices (popular sire, line breeding), certain erythrocyte defects have become common in certain breeds. Unless the affected breeds are closely related, the disease is probably caused by different mutations of the same gene. Erythrocyte-induced defects vary from mild compensated hemolytic to life-threatening anemia. Accurate laboratory tests are now available for many erythrocyte defects to detect affected as well as carrier animals. Some defects represent hematologic curiosities without clinical signs (such as in Akitas and miniature poodles with inconsequential microcytosis and macrocytosis, respectively). Hereditary erythrocyte disorders have been classified into three groups: (1) heme defects and hemoglobinopathies, (2) membrane abnormalities, and (3) erythroenzymopathies. Hereditary production and maturation defects of erythrocytes and other hematopoietic cells are discussed in the next chapter.

HEMOGLOBIN AND RELATED DISORDERS

Dogs and cats apparently have embryonic but no fetal hemoglobin.[2] With the exception of some Japanese dog breeds, only one adult hemoglobin has been found in dogs, but further studies are needed to better characterize canine hemoglobin. Historically, two major adult hemoglobins were described in cats with a large variation of the hemoglobin A/hemoglobin B ratios. Later studies, however, revealed that adult cats have one alpha globin and six different beta globins.[20] With each cat having one to four different beta globins, at least 17 hemoglobin patterns were recognized. In contrast to the common occurrence of thalassemia and sickle cell anemia in humans, no hemoglobinopathies have been documented in dogs and cats.

The physiologically or pathologically generated methemoglobin, which contains heme in the ferric iron (Fe^{3+}) and, therefore, cannot carry oxygen, is reduced to the ferrous form (Fe^{2+}) by the methemoglobin or cytochrome b_5 reduc-

TABLE 177–1. INHERITED ERYTHROCYTE DEFECTS

DEFECTS	BREED	INHERITANCE	PCV (%) (RANGE)	RETICULOCYTE (%) (CORRECTED)	ERYTHROCYTE HALF-LIFE (DAYS)	ERYTHROCYTE MORPHOLOGY	SPECIFIC TESTS	CLINICAL FEATURES
Erythroenzymopathies								
Pyruvate kinase (PK) deficiency	Basenji, beagle, West Highland white and cairn terrier, miniature poodle, dachshund	AR	11–25	10–45	4–9	Polychromasia, echinocytes	DNA test; Abnormal M-PK, PK kinetic and stability and glycolytic intermediates	Hemolytic anemia, myelofibrosis, osteosclerosis
	Abyssinian, Somali, DSH cats	AR	10–33	1–33	U	Polychromasia	DNA test; PK activity <20%	Intermittent hemolytic anemia
Phosphofructokinase (PFK) deficiency	English springer spaniel, cocker spaniel, mixed breed dog	AR	11–18	5–23	4	Polychromasia	DNA test; PFK activity, 8–22%	Inducible hemolytic crises, mild myopathy, pigmenturia
Hemoglobin synthesis defects								
Hemoglobinopathies	None							
Cytochrome-b_5 reductase (Cb_5R) deficiency	Many isolated cases; Dogs, DSH cats	U	High	N	U	Unremarkable	Cb_5R activity, 10–30%; Methemoglobin > 10%	Cyanosis, no anemia, exercise intolerance
Porphyria	Siamese	AD	N	N	U			Anemia, discolored teeth
	DSH cats	AD	N	N	U	Unremarkable	Porphobinogen deaminase deficiency	Discolored teeth, ± anemia
Membrane and other abnormalities								
Elliptocytosis (band 4.1 deficiency)	Mixed breed dog	AR	34	2	16–23	Elliptocytes	Membrane protein electrophoresis	None
Stomatocytosis	Alaskan malamute, miniature schnauzer	AR	N	3–7	6–18	Stomatocytes, polychromasia	Stomatocytes, increased osmotic fragility	Chondrodysplasia in malamutes, none in schnauzers
Increased osmotic fragility	English springer spaniel, mixed breed dog	U	N	2–5	U	Polychromasia, poikilocytosis	Increased osmotic fragility, unknown	Exercise-induced hyperthermia
	Abyssinian, Somali	U	8–35	1–4	U	Macrocytosis	Increased osmotic fragility	Intermittent anemia, splenomegaly
High-potassium erythrocytes	Akita, Japanese mongrels	U	N	N	U	Unremarkable	Increased erythrocyte and serum potassium	None, pseudohyperkalemia
Nonspherocytic hemolytic disorders	Beagle	AR	29–12	8–23	7–15	Polychromasia	Calcium ATPase pump (?)	None, mild anemia
Poikilocytosis	DSH cats	U	7–12	10–30	U	Severe poikilocytosis	Poikilocytosis	Severe anemia
Familial microcytosis	Akita	U	N	N	U	Microcytosis	Erythrocyte indices	None
Familial macrocytosis and dyshematopoiesis	Poodle (miniature and toy)	U	N	N	U	Macrocytes, hypersegmented neutrophils	Macrocytosis, normal osmotic fragility	None, gingivitis

Data collected from references and author's unpublished observations.
N = normal; U = unknown; AR = autosomal recessive; AD = autosomal dominant; DSH = domestic short-hair.

HEM

tase system. Isolated cases of methemoglobinemia associated with methemoglobin reductase deficiency were found among dogs of various breeds and several domestic short-hair cats.[3, 21–23] Affected animals have cyanotic mucous membranes but generally do not exhibit any other clinical signs of hypoxemia unless vigorously exercised. The blood remains dark after air exposure because of the presence of 13 to 52 per cent methemoglobin. In contrast to those with other erythrocyte defects, these animals are not anemic but rather develop a mild erythrocytosis and can have a normal life expectancy. Reducing agents such as methylene blue could be used but are generally not needed.

Defects of heme synthesis known as porphyrias have been reported in anemic Siamese cats and nonanemic domestic short-hair cats with pigmented and pink-fluorescent teeth and bones.

ERYTHROCYTE MEMBRANE–RELATED ABNORMALITIES

The erythrocyte membrane consists of a bilayer affixed to a membrane skeleton, which determines cell shape and reformability. Owing to proteolysis, canine and feline erythrocytes lose their Na^+,K^+-adenosinetriphosphatase (Na^+,K^+-ATPase) during late maturation in the bone marrow.[24] Therefore, erythrocytes have high sodium and low potassium concentrations similar to those of serum electrolytes. Consequently, hyperkalemia generally does not occur after intravascular hemolysis unless stress reticulocytes are lysed. Erythrocytes from Sheiba, Akitas, and some mongrel dogs in Korea and Japan represent an exception as they keep their Na^+,K^+-ATPases and, therefore, have high potassium and low sodium concentrations. Because Akitas' erythrocytes are leaky "in vitro," pseudohyperkalemia may occur if the plasma and serum are not separated from erythrocytes and its clot, respectively.[25]

Elliptocytosis and microcytosis related to cytoskeleton protein band 4.1 deficiency has been described in an inbred, nonanemic mongrel dog.[26] Other erythrocyte membrane defects are far less well defined but are generally characterized by increased osmotic fragility. Stomatocytes are overhydrated, cup-shaped macrocytes that are recognized by a slitlike pallor on a blood film. In the Alaskan malamute, stomatocytosis is associated with a chondrodysplastic dwarfism.[27] Miniature schnauzers with stomatocytosis had no skeletal abnormalities and both breeds had only mild regenerative anemia on the basis of hemoglobin measures with high MCV and low MCHC indices.[28] Furthermore, stomatocytosis and hypertrophic gastritis have been reported in the Drentse partrijshond dog breed (Dutch breed) and a lipid disorder is suspected on the basis of abnormal erythrocyte membrane and plasma phospholipids.[29] A marked osmotic fragility of erythrocytes associated with recurrent anemia, severe splenomegaly, weight loss, lymphocytosis, and hyperglobulinemia but a negative Coombs test has been observed mostly in Abyssinian and Somali cats.[30] Although the cause has not been identified, affected cats with marked splenomegaly may benefit from prednisone treatment and splenectomy. However, the in vitro osmotic fragility of erythrocytes does not improve after treatment.

ERYTHROENZYMOPATHIES

Devoid of a nucleus and mitochondria, erythrocytes generate energy almost exclusively through anaerobic glycolysis, also known as the Embden-Meyerhof pathway. Phosphofructokinase (PFK) and pyruvate kinase (PK) are two key regulatory enzymes of this pathway, but their deficiency results in two distinctly different forms of anemia. The Embden-Meyerhof pathway also plays an important role in an ancillary pathway. The Rapoport-Luebering pathway is responsible for the synthesis of DPG, which influences the oxygen affinity of canine but not feline hemoglobin. (The erythrocyte DPG concentration is very low in cats.[3, 31])

Phosphofructokinase Deficiency

PFK deficiency is characterized by a chronic hemolytic disorder accentuated by hemolytic crises and an exertional myopathy.[32–34] After episodes of excessive panting and barking, extensive exercise, and high temperatures, affected dogs develop dark brown-red urine because of hemoglobinuria and hyperbilirubinuria. These sporadic events are associated with hyperventilation and elevated body temperature, and the ensuing slight alkalemia results in intravascular lysis of PFK-deficient erythrocytes as these cells are more alkaline fragile than normal canine erythrocytes. During these crises, affected dogs may become severely anemic and icteric and exhibit fever, lethargy, and anorexia, which usually resolve within days with supportive care. If situations that trigger hemolytic crises are avoided, PFK-deficient dogs may rarely experience problems and can reach a normal life expectancy. However, they have persistent hyperbilirubinuria and reticulocytosis despite a normal hematocrit because of ongoing hemolysis and a high hemoglobin-oxygen affinity as PFK-deficient erythrocytes contain low DPG levels and, therefore, lead to a relative tissue hypoxia. Furthermore, because affected dogs totally lack PFK activity in muscle, they have a metabolic myopathy characterized by exercise intolerance, occasional muscle cramps, and mildly increased serum creatine kinase activity; thus, they perform poorly as field trial dogs.

This glycolytic enzyme deficiency is common in field trial English springer spaniels in the United States, Great Britain, and Denmark (the true prevalence remains unknown) but has also been reported in bench English springer spaniels as well as a cocker spaniel and a mixed breed dog.[31, 35] It is caused by a missense mutation of the muscle-type PFK gene that results in truncation and instability of the enzyme, thereby leading to a complete muscle-type PFK deficiency.[36] A simple polymerase chain reaction (PCR)–based DNA test accurately diagnoses PFK-deficient and carrier dogs. A small blood sample, buccal swab, or semen is an appropriate source for DNA testing and requires no special handling or shipping. English springer spaniels (and cocker spaniels) with suspicious clinical signs or before field training and breeding should be tested for PFK deficiency.

Pyruvate Kinase Deficiency

The classic erythrocytic PK deficiency initially reported in Basenjis is now seen in several other breeds including beagles, West Highland white and cairn terriers, miniature poodles, toy Eskimo, and dachshund.[31, 37–40] Despite a persistent hemolytic anemia, the clinical signs, except for pallor, are mild. The anemia ranges from about 10 to 26 per cent and is highly regenerative with numerous circulating metarubricytes and reticulocyte counts approaching 95 per cent. An unexplained progressive myelofibrosis and osteosclerosis of the bone marrow develop. It appears likely that the previously described nonspherocytic hemolytic anemia and osteosclerosis in miniature poodles were caused by a PK deficiency.[41] PK-deficient dogs die because of anemia and generalized hemosiderosis with associated hepatic failure before 5 years of age. Splenectomy and prednisone treatment appear unhelpful. Erythrocytes completely lack the adult erythrocyte isozyme form of PK known as R-PK. Instead, they express a fetal M-PK form that is dysfunctional in erythrocytes in vivo. Molecular genetic screening tests are available for the identification of the PK mutation of affected and carrier Basenjis and West Highland white terriers but not yet for others.[42-44] A cumbersome PK enzyme activity test with isozyme characterization is required to define PK deficiency in other breeds. Carriers do not express the M-PK form and have approximately half-normal PK activity; however, differentiation between carriers and homozygous normal dogs on the basis of enzyme activity may not be accurate.

Erythrocytic PK deficiency has also been described in the Abyssinian and Somali breeds as well as a domestic cat.[45] Affected cats have chronic intermittent hemolytic anemia and mild splenomegaly but no osteosclerosis. The anemia is moderately regenerative and no poikilocytosis is seen. Erythrocyte PK activity is severely reduced and there is no M-type PK expression. A deletion caused by a splicing transition in the PK gene has been identified, and a molecular screening test has been made available. Intermittent prednisone therapy and splenectomy appear to ameliorate the clinical signs of intermittent anemia. The oldest living cat reached 13 years of age.

IMMUNE-MEDIATED HEMOLYTIC ANEMIA

IMHA arises when an immune response targets erythrocytes directly or indirectly and hemolytic anemia ensues. Until the antierythrocytic antibodies are identified and the pathogenesis is better understood, the nomenclature and classification of IMHA remain imprecise and sometimes confusing.[46, 47] In primary IMHA no inciting cause can be identified, hence the synonyms idiopathic IMHA and autoimmune hemolytic anemia. In contrast, secondary IMHA is associated with an underlying condition or triggered by an agent. In addition, alloimmune hemolytic anemias such as neonatal isoerythrolysis and hemolytic transfusion reactions are caused by antierythrocytic alloantibodies and are discussed later.

Immune Mechanisms

Regardless of the underlying cause, IMHA results from a breakdown in immune self-tolerance. Because the process of clonal deletion of central tolerance is not capable of completely eliminating all potential self-reacting B cell clones in utero and clonal anergy, another central control mechanism, is not totally efficient in the inactivation of B cells designed to respond to self-antigens, an immune response against erythrocytes may occur. Because some erythrocyte antigens are hidden or cryptic, the appropriate B cell may encounter the antigen only after membrane damage exposes the antigen. An inflammatory or infectious process can also release new antigens into the circulation that cross-react with erythrocyte antigens or attach to the erythrocyte membrane. Furthermore, the appropriate T cell must find the matching B cell and bind via receptor-ligand pairs to activate the respective cell. However, during infection and inflammation, nonspecific activation of lymphocytes can occur, so self-reacting

antibodies may be nonspecifically induced. Finally, impairment of the down-regulation mechanisms such as activated B-cell death by apoptosis through a Fas ligand signal from T cells may allow an active autoimmune response to develop.[46]

Immune destruction of erythrocytes is initiated by the binding of immunoglobulin G (IgG) or IgM antibodies and complement to the surface of erythrocytes. Under most clinical circumstances, immune destruction is an extravascular process that depends on recognition of erythrocytes opsonized with IgG or complement or both by specific receptors on reticuloendothelial cells.

IgG-coated erythrocytes can be destroyed without complement activation because tissue macrophages express receptors that recognize the Fc portion of the IgG molecule. IgG binding by Fc receptors on macrophages can mediate complete phagocytosis, particularly in the red pulp of the spleen. Macrophages with engulfed erythrocytes may be noted by cytologic examination of tissue aspirates. Alternatively, only a portion of the membrane is removed by phagocytes, leaving erythrocytes with a reduced surface area/volume ratio and thereby forming spherocytes. Because the deformability of spherocytes is impaired, these rigid cells are trapped in the spleen and are subsequently destroyed. Erythrocyte-bound IgG1 and IgG3 antibodies have a strong affinity for Fc receptors. Erythrocytes that become heavily coated with IgG can also bind complement. Inasmuch as macrophages also have receptors for complement components C3b and iC3b, the attachment of complement component C3b, iC3b, or both via CR1 and CR3 receptors together with IgG enhances the phagocytic process, particularly of hepatic macrophages (Kupffer's cells). In addition, erythrocytes heavily coated with IgG may activate so much complement that intravascular cytolysis occurs.[47, 48]

In contrast, macrophages do not have receptors for the Fc portion of IgM, and thus the destruction of IgM-coated erythrocytes is mediated by complement. The pentameric structure of IgM is readily able to induce binding and activation of complement on erythrocytes. High IgM antibody titers can generate the cytolytic complex via the classical complement system and, thereby, intravascular hemolysis ensues. However, the IgM antierythrocyte antibodies are more commonly present in sublytic concentrations and full complement activation is prevented by inhibitory regulatory proteins. Nevertheless, some C3b and iC3b are bound to the cell surface, resulting in extravascular destruction of complement-sensitized erythrocytes. Alternatively, erythrocyte-bound complement may be inactivated to C3dg, which no longer impairs erythrocyte survival. Antierythrocyte antibodies inducing hemolysis are generally reactive at body temperature. Only in exceptional cases do cold-acting antibodies (at 4 to 30°C) contribute to in vivo hemolysis and erythrocyte agglutination in cooler, peripheral vasculature.

Underlying Conditions and Predispositions

Historically, in most dogs with IMHA, no underlying condition was ever identified, and thus it was considered to be primary or idiopathic IMHA.[49] However, in later studies of autoimmune hemolytic anemia, probably reflecting more intense investigations, an underlying disease process or trigger could be identified, including drugs and infectious, neoplastic, and immune disorders (Table 177–2). In babesiosis and hemobartonellosis, hemolysis is exaggerated by immune processes. Many chronic infections including abscesses, discospondylitis, pyometra, and pyelonephritis can induce secondary immune disorders including IMHA. A temporal asso-

HEM

TABLE 177–2. EXAMPLES OF UNDERLYING DISORDERS AND TRIGGERS OF IMMUNE-MEDIATED HEMOLYTIC ANEMIA

Infectious
    Viral: FeLV, FIV infection, transient upper respiratory or
      gastrointestinal disease
    Bacterial: various acute and chronic infections (e.g., abscess)
    Parasitic: babesiosis, hemobartonellosis, dirofilariasis, ehrlichiosis
Drugs
    Sulfonamides
    Cephalosporin
    Penicillin
    Vaccines
    Propylthiouracil
    Methimazol
    Procainamide
Neoplasia
    Hemolymphatic: leukemias, lymphoma
    Solid tumors
Immune disorders
    Systemic lupus erythematosus
    Hypothyroidism
    Immunodeficiencies
Genetic predisposition
    American cocker spaniel
    English springer spaniel
    Old English sheepdog
    Irish setter
    Poodle
    Dachshund

FeLV = feline leukemia virus; FIV = feline immunodeficiency virus.

ciation between vaccination and onset of IMHA has also been suggested. In a limited retrospective study, one quarter of all dogs with IMHA of unknown cause were vaccinated within 1 month of onset of clinical signs.[50] As this correlation was associated with modified and killed vaccines against common infectious diseases from different manufacturers, it appears likely that vaccines may trigger or enhance a smoldering immune process rather than be the underlying cause. Although a number of anecdotal reports support a temporal relationship between vaccination and IMHA, no significant association was found in a large-scale study of animal health insurance records from Britain.[51] The higher rate of IMHA during the warmer months from May through August reported in some studies, but not others, may also suggest an infectious cause including tick-borne disorders.[52] The seasonality may vary geographically. The association of IMHA with other immune disorders, including hypothyroidism and immune-mediated thrombocytopenia (ITP), lends support to the hypothesis of a general immune disturbance. IMHA and ITP occurring concurrently are known as Evans' syndrome.[52, 53]

IMHA is the most common reason for hemolytic anemias in dogs. A genetic predisposition is suggested in some dogs by the breed predilection and familial occurrence.[49, 52] American cocker spaniels may represent up to 40 per cent of all dogs. In other canine breeds predisposition is less well documented and may vary geographically. Certain histocompatibility leukocyte antigens have been associated with the occurrence of IMHA in humans. The previously reviewed hereditary erythrocyte defects should also be considered as an important differential diagnosis whenever IMHA is suspected. As with other immune disorders, female dogs appear slightly predisposed, even when spayed. In contrast, IMHA is rarely documented in cats and is generally secondary to FeLV or *Haemobartonella* infections or antithyroidal medication.[54] No breed, gender, or other association has been found in cats.

Clinical Signs of Immune-Mediated Hemolytic Anemia

IMHA may present at any age but is most commonly encountered in young adult to middle-aged dogs. The clinical history is generally brief and vague. An underlying condition may be identified. An episode of vomiting or diarrhea may precede the typical signs of anemia (lethargy, weakness, exercise intolerance, pallor) and hemolysis (pigmenturia, icterus).[45–52] Some animals may be febrile, presumably because of erythrocyte lysis or an underlying disease process. Others develop dyspnea, indicating pulmonary problems either as the underlying disease or as a thromboembolic complication of IMHA.[55] Physical examination may also reveal mild splenomegaly and, less commonly, mild hepatomegaly and lymphadenopathy, which again suggest a secondary cause of IMHA. Furthermore, signs attributable to their underlying disease may predominate, whereas chronic or recurrent signs of IMHA suggest a primary form.

In the rare case of cold-reacting antierythrocytic antibodies, peripheral skin lesions characterized by acrocyanosis and gangrenous necrosis of ear, nose, and tail tip as well as nail beds may be the presenting signs without any evidence of hemolysis.

Routine Laboratory Test Results

The anemia can be mild to life threatening and the hematocrit may drop precipitously after presentation because of active hemolysis. Although a regenerative, macrocytic-hypochromic anemia would be expected, as many as one third of all cases of IMHA are nonregenerative on presentation.[52, 56] The disease course may have been peracute, not yet allowing time to mount a regenerative response. Alternatively, antibodies may be directed against erythroid precursors, thereby removing metarubricytes and reticulocytes, or the IMHA disease process may change the microenvironment of the bone marrow and thereby impair erythropoiesis. Evidence of ineffective erythropoiesis and erythrophagocytosis may be found on cytologic examination of a bone marrow aspirate.[57] Autoagglutination of erythrocytes and spherocytosis are typical findings on blood smears.

Besides erythroid abnormalities, a leukocytosis is often present and can exceed 100,000/μL, mostly because of a mature neutrophilia. Because high white blood cell counts are not generally encountered with anemia, this probably reflects a unique inflammatory and cytokine response specific for IMHA, but concomitant infection and steroid-induced leukocytosis should also be considered. Thus, hyperplasia of erythroid and myeloid cells may be present in the bone marrow. Furthermore, thrombocytopenia related to a concomitant ITP (Evans' syndrome) or disseminated intravascular coagulation (DIC) may occur.[52]

Serum analysis generally reveals a hyperbilirubinemia, and a serum bilirubin concentration above 10 mg/dL has been associated with a grave prognosis.[52] However, serum bilirubin values may be only slightly increased in chronic cases, presumably because of highly efficient and accelerated bilirubin metabolism. Thus, high serum bilirubin values may also indicate a concomitant hepatopathy. In fact, dogs with IMHA often have increased serum liver enzymes even before steroid therapy. The degree of hemoglobinemia—a sign of intravascular hemolysis—can vary drastically and rapidly and is associated with hemoglobinuria. Hyperbilirubinuria is expected as with any other hemolytic anemia; in cats, any degree of bilirubinuria is considered important, whereas larger amounts of bilirubin are generally present in urine of dogs. There may also be evidence of a bacterial cystitis, which may indicate an underlying infectious disease or may occur secondarily because of immunoderegulation or immunosuppressive therapy.

Various imaging studies may be indicated to reveal underlying disease processes, such as neoplasia, and complications of IMHA. Evidence of thromboemboli may be detected on chest radiographs and abdominal ultrasonography as well as at the site of catheters.

Diagnostic Laboratory Test Results

A diagnosis of IMHA requires demonstration of accelerated immune destruction of erythrocytes. Thus, beside documenting a hemolytic anemia, a search for antibodies or complement or both directed against erythrocytes is required; that is, one or more of the following three hallmarks has to be present to reach a definitive diagnosis of IMHA:

1. Marked spherocytosis
2. True autoagglutination
3. Positive direct Coombs test

Spherocytosis. Spherocytes (Fig. 177–5) are spherical erythrocytes that appear microcytic with no central pallor. They result from either partial phagocytosis or lysis and are rigid and extremely fragile in the erythrocyte osmotic fragility test. Because spherocytes have lost some membrane, they do not have any reserves to expand in hypotonic solution. Large numbers of spherocytes are present in approximately two thirds of dogs with IMHA, but small numbers may be seen with hypophosphatemia, zinc intoxication, and microangiopathic hemolysis. Hereditary spherocytosis related to various membrane defects in humans has not been reported in small animals. In cats, spherocytes are difficult, if not impossible, to identify owing to the small size and lack of central pallor of normal feline erythrocytes.

Autoagglutination. Antierythrocytic IgM and, in large quantities, IgG antibodies may cause direct autoagglutination

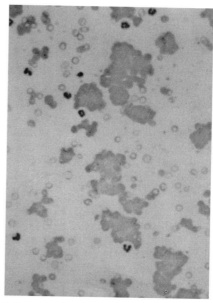

Figure 177–6. Low-magnification view of immune-mediated agglutination of canine erythrocytes on a Wright-Giemsa–stained blood film. (From Weiser MG: Erythrocyte responses and disorders. *In* Ettinger SJ, Feldman EC [eds]: Textbook of Veterinary Internal Medicine, 4th ed. Philadelphia, WB Saunders, 1995, p 1869.)

(Fig. 177–6). Agglutination may be visible to the naked eye when blood (at low hematocrit) is in an ethylenediaminetetraacetic acid (EDTA) tube or placed on a glass slide (macroscopic agglutination) or may become apparent as small clumps of erythrocytes on a stained blood smear or in a saline wet mount (microscopic agglutination). Autoagglutination has to be distinguished from rouleau formation (Fig. 177–7), in which erythrocytes stack up on top of each other. For unexplained reasons, canine erythrocytes have a

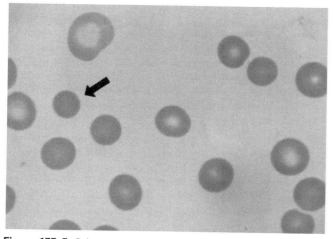

Figure 177–5. Spherocytes in canine blood. A spectrum of sphere injury may be visualized in this field. The largest cells with the greatest central pallor are interpreted as normal or near normal. Complete sphere formation is evident in cells with the smallest diameter and absence of central pallor (arrow). Cells with decreased central pallor and diameter have intermediate sphere injury. Wright-Giemsa stain. (From Weiser MG: Erythrocyte responses and disorders. *In* Ettinger SJ, Feldman EC [eds]: Textbook of Veterinary Internal Medicine, 4th ed. Philadelphia, WB Saunders, 1995, p 1868.)

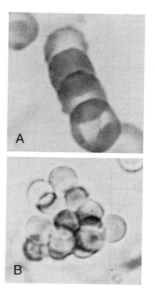

Figure 177–7. *A,* Microscopic wet preparation of canine blood demonstrating rouleau formation. Rouleau must be distinguished from autoagglutination. *B,* Microscopic wet preparation of canine blood exhibiting autoagglutination. Note the clumping of erythrocytes typical of agglutination. (Courtesy of Dr. Dennis J. Meyer. From Thompson JP: Immunologic disorders. *In* Ettinger SJ, Feldman EC [eds]: Textbook of Veterinary Internal Medicine, 4th ed. Philadelphia, WB Saunders, 1995, p 2008.)

HEM

tendency to agglutinate unspecifically in the presence of plasma at lower temperatures. Mixing one drop of blood with one drop of saline may not break up this unspecific form of agglutination. It is, therefore, important to determine whether the agglutination persists after "saline washing," which has been termed true autoagglutination. This is accomplished by adding three times physiologic saline solution to blood after repeated centrifugation and removal of supernatant including the plasma. It should be noted that autoagglutination can interfere with the direct Coombs test and blood typing test.

Direct Coombs Test. The direct Coombs test, also known as the direct antiglobulin test, is used to detect antibodies and/or complement on the erythrocyte surface when the antierythrocyte antibody strength or concentration is too low (subagglutinating titer) to cause spontaneous autoagglutination.[58-60] The so-called incomplete antibodies on erythrocytes together with species-specific antiglobulins against IgG, IgM, and C3b (Coombs reagents) allow antibody bridging and thereby agglutination and/or lysis of coated erythrocytes. Separate IgG, IgM, and C3b as well as polyvalent Coombs reagents are available for dogs and cats. They are added at varied concentrations after washing the patient's erythrocytes free of plasma. The mixture is generally incubated at 37°C, then centrifuged, and supernatant and pellet are analyzed for hemolysis and agglutination, respectively. Performance of the direct Coombs test at lower temperatures (4 and 20°C) is rarely indicated, because cold agglutinins and hemolysins are rarely strong enough and rarely active at near-normal body temperatures (30°C) to cause disease. Cold agglutinins and hemolysins of clinical importance are generally IgM antibodies at high titer with a thermal amplitude that reaches 30°C. Because the same erythrocyte washing procedure is used in the direct Coombs test as in the true autoagglutination test and the end point of the Coombs reaction is agglutination and lysis of erythrocytes, true autoagglutination precludes the performance of a direct Coombs test.

Positive direct Coombs test results are reported as +1 to +4 or in the form of dilutions of the Coombs reagent that cause agglutination and/or lysis; the strength of the Coombs reaction does not necessarily predict the severity of hemolysis. In order to reach a definitive diagnosis of IMHA, the direct Coombs test should be positive, but this does not discriminate between primary and secondary IMHA. Dogs with negative Coombs test results should be reevaluated for other causes of hemolytic anemia. However, a small proportion of dogs may have IMHA despite a negative Coombs test result. False-negative Coombs test results may occur because of insufficient quantities of bound antibodies and for many technical reasons (inappropriate reagents or dilutions). Various techniques have been used to enhance the sensitivity of the direct Coombs test, but none of them have gained wide acceptance in human and veterinary medicine. Furthermore, the test result may be negative in the absence of an inciting agent (e.g., drug). Negative results are also obtained for animals in which the disease is in remission; however, a few days of immunosuppressive therapy are not likely to reverse the test results. In fact, treated animals may still have positive Coombs test results long after the hemolytic anemia resolves. False-positive Coombs test results occur only rarely, for example, after an incompatible transfusion or because of technical problems. Furthermore, some animals may have a positive Coombs test result without evidence of hemolysis.

Little is known about the usefulness of the indirect Coombs or antiglobin test in which the presence of antierythrocyte antibodies in the patient's serum is evaluated with random erythrocytes. Clearly, the indirect Coombs test would remain negative if the antibody is directed against a cryptic or new (drug, parasite) antigen on the erythrocyte surface. Alternatively, a false-positive test result may occur in a dog that has previously been transfused and developed alloantibodies.

Therapy of Immune-Mediated Hemolytic Anemia

Because the severity of IMHA ranges from indolent to life-threatening disease, therapy has to be tailored for each patient and depends in part on whether the IMHA is primary or secondary. Removal of the triggering agent or treatment of the underlying condition can bring the IMHA under control. Thus, in cases of secondary IMHA related to infection, antiprotozoals, antirickettsials, or antibiotics should be instituted. Because of the potential for underlying occult infection and the predisposition to infection because of immunoderegulation associated with IMHA and immunosuppressive therapy, antibiotic therapy is generally indicated. Also, surgical correction of abscesses and other sites of infections may be considered. Nonessential drugs, particularly those implicated in causing an immune reaction, should immediately be withdrawn. Despite these interventions, transfusion and immunosuppressive therapy are probably still required in the initial control of secondary IMHA.

In case of signs of hypoxia with severe anemia and a dropping hematocrit, packed RBC transfusions are beneficial. The increased oxygen-carrying capacity provided by transfused cells may be sufficient to maintain the animal for the few days required for other treatment modalities to become effective. The notion that transfusions are especially hazardous in animals with IMHA has been overemphasized and is not supported by retrospective studies. As the antierythrocytic antibody in IMHA is not an alloantibody, the destruction of transfused cells is no higher than that of autologous erythrocytes. However, even after RBC washing, autoagglutination may hamper accurate blood typing and cross-matching tests; thus, only dog erythrocyte antigen (DEA) 1.1–negative blood should be transfused in dogs (see Chapter 79). If compatible blood is not available, the bovine hemoglobin solution approved by the Food and Drug Administration can be administered and provides increased oxygen-carrying capacity and plasma expansion. In contrast, oxygen inhalation therapy is of little benefit unless the animal is suffering from pulmonary disease such as pulmonary thromboemboli. Thanks to adequate transfusion support, animals with IMHA rarely die because of anemia, but they die because of overwhelming hemolysis and secondary complications such as thromboemboli and infections.

The main goal in the treatment of IMHA is to control the immune response by reducing phagocytosis, complement activation, and antierythrocytic antibody production.[61] Glucocorticosteroids are the initial treatment of choice for IMHA. They interfere with both the expression and function of macrophage Fc receptors and thereby immediately impair the clearance of antibody-coated erythrocytes by the macrophage system. In addition, glucocorticosteroids may reduce the degree of antibody binding and complement activation on erythrocytes and, after weeks, diminish the production of autoantibodies. Oral prednisone or prednisolone at a dose of 0.5 to 1 mg/lb twice daily is the mainstay treatment. Alternatively, oral or parenteral dexamethasone at an equipotent dose of 0.3 mg/lb daily can be used but is probably not more beneficial. A response reflected by a stabilized or even rising hematocrit, appropriate reticulocytosis, and less autoagglutination and spherocytes can be expected within days. As glucocorticosteroid therapy is associated with well-known side effects, the initial dose is then tapered by reducing the amount by one third every 7 to 10 days. Within weeks, a low-dose alternate-day therapy may be reached with minimal steroid side effects. In secondary IMHA with appropriate control of the underlying disease, the tapering can be accomplished more rapidly. Because of the potential for gastrointestinal ulceration by steroids, treatment with misoprostol (2 to 4 μg/lb every 6 hours by mouth), a synthetic analogue of prostaglandin E_1 that inhibits gastric acid secretion, cimetidine (2 to 5 mg/lb every 6 to 12 hours by mouth), and sucralfate may be considered. Despite apparent recovery as judged by reaching a normal hematocrit, animals, particularly those with primary IMHA, may continue to have a positive Coombs test for weeks to months and could obviously have relapses. Such relapses may be controlled by the same treatment as initially used, but a more gradual tapering regimen may be used in which the animal receives prednisone therapy every other day for months.

Other immunosuppressive therapy is warranted when prednisone fails, controls the disease only at persistently high doses, or causes unacceptable side effects. It is generally used together with prednisone but may eventually be used independently. Cytotoxic drugs were historically added first. Cyclophosphamide, an alkylating and potent myelosuppressive agent, has been advocated in cases of fulminant IMHA. However, a randomized limited prospective trial comparing prednisone with a combination of prednisone and cyclophosphamide did not find any beneficial effects of cyclophosphamide in the acute management of IMHA.[62] Retrospective studies with cyclophosphamide and/or azathioprine, an antimetabolite, were similarly disappointing.[63, 64] These cytotoxic drugs inhibit lymphocytes and thereby suppress the antierythrocyte antibody production within weeks. They are, therefore, probably not effective in the acute management of IMHA but may have a place in the long-term control of refractory and relapsing cases. A reasonable regimen for dogs might include either cyclophosphamide at 1 mg/lb every other day or azathioprine at 1 mg/lb once a day or every other day.[64] In addition to the strong myelosuppressive effects of these cytotoxic drugs, leading to reticulocytopenia, neutropenia, and thrombocytopenia, cyclophosphamide can induce a sterile hemorrhagic cystitis and secondary neoplasia. Thus, the risk-versus-benefit ratio should be carefully considered when using these drugs.

Several other immunosuppressive agents have been used on a limited basis in conjunction with prednisone, and anecdotal success has been reported in dogs and humans. As all of these agents interfere with antibody action and macrophage function, they can elicit more immediate effects. Cyclosporine, an expensive but potent immunosuppressive agent most commonly used in preventing graft rejection and graft-versus-host disease in transplant patients, may be beneficial in controlling the immune response in dogs with IMHA. A dose regimen of 5 mg/lb once a day may be used initially, but blood concentrations should be monitored periodically to achieve an effective but safe level. Leflunomide is in a class of agents similar to that of cyclosporine and has been used in a few cases with anecdotal success. Danazol, an androgen derivative, at a dose of 5 mg/lb once a day, may inhibit binding of antibodies and phagocytosis. However, a retrospective study in dogs with IMHA was

disappointing; furthermore, danazol is expensive and may be hepatotoxic.[65] Intravenous human immunoglobulin (IVIG) may be helpful in the short-term treatment of dogs with IMHA, although its mode of action remains unresolved.[66–68] IVIG can block Fc receptors on macrophages, thereby reducing Fc-mediated phagocytosis of IgG-coated erythrocytes; interfere with complement action; and suppress antibody production. Human IVIG binds to canine lymphocytes and monocytes and inhibits erythrocyte phagocytosis.[68] A single IVIG dose of 0.25 to 1 g/lb has been beneficial in some refractory cases as indicated by a rising PCV and reticulocytosis within days, but the response has often been only temporary. Anecdotally, plasmapheresis has also been used as an adjuvant therapy.[69]

Splenectomy may be considered in IMHA patients who do not respond to prednisone and other immunosuppressive therapy, requiring long-term high-dose therapy to remain in remission or suffering, intractable drug side effects. The spleen is a major site of autoantibody production as well as sequestration and destruction of erythrocytes coated with IgG but probably does not affect the clearance of IgM-coated cells. In addition, histologic examination of the spleen may provide evidence of an underlying disease. The response to splenectomy remains to be determined in animals. There is a slight risk of developing overwhelming infections immediately after splenectomy and systemic bacterial infections subsequently. Splenectomy should, therefore, not be performed along with immunosuppressive therapy other than prednisone.

Thrombemboli and DIC are unique serious complications that greatly contribute to the morbidity and mortality of patients with IMHA. Although the pathogenesis remains unknown, venipuncture, catheters, and glucocorticosteroid therapy represent predisposing conditions. Thus far, no study has documented any successful prevention and/or management protocol for these life-threatening hemostatic problems in IMHA. Predisposing factors should, whenever possible, be limited, and adequate perfusion and oxygenation of tissue should be provided with fluids and transfusions. Generally, anticoagulant therapy is instituted only after there is some evidence or suspicion of thromboemboli. Heparin at a dose of 5 to 50 IU/lb subcutaneously every 6 hours or by continuous infusion is the most commonly used drug, and fresh frozen plasma (5 mL/lb every 12 hours) may be administered to replenish dangerously low plasma antithrombin III concentrations (see Chapter 180). Other complications are probably related to drug therapy.

Despite appropriate implementation of these therapeutic strategies, the mortality rate remains high; in fact, there is an impression that the fulminate form of IMHA is more frequently encountered today. Depending on the type of practice (primary to tertiary), mortality rates from 20 to 75 per cent have been reported. Negative prognostic indicators are a rapid drop in PCV, high serum bilirubin levels, nonregenerative anemia, intravascular hemolysis, autoagglutination, and thromboembolic complications.

ALLOIMMUNE HEMOLYTIC ANEMIAS—NEONATAL ISOERYTHROLYSIS AND HEMOLYTIC TRANSFUSION REACTIONS

Erythrocyte alloantibodies, also known as isoantibodies, are specific antibodies directed against erythrocyte antigens (blood types) from the same species but not from the individual producing the antibody.[2] Depending on the species and

HEM

blood group system, these alloantibodies occur naturally (cats) or are produced only after sensitization with a mismatched blood transfusion (dog) and are responsible for neonatal isoerythrolysis (NI) and acute or delayed hemolytic transfusion reactions. Additional information can be found in the chapter on transfusion medicine (see Chapter 79).

In cats, only the AB blood group system has been recognized; it consists of three blood types: type A, type B, and type AB.[2] The inheritance pattern of these blood types is unique and of considerable importance to breeders. The A allele is dominant over the B allele. Thus, only homozygous B/B cats express the type B antigen on their erythrocytes. Type A cats are either homozygous (A/A) or heterozygous (A/B).[70] The rare AB blood type, seen in certain families, is inherited separately as a third allele that is recessive to A and codominant with B.[71] Simple in-practice blood typing cards are available. As a reaction in both test wells could be caused by autoagglutination, type AB test results should be confirmed in a reference laboratory.[72] The prevalence of feline blood types varies geographically and among breeds.[70] All type B cats develop very strong naturally occurring anti-A antibodies with high hemolysin and agglutinin titers (greater than 1:32) after a few weeks of age, whereas type A cats generally develop only weak anti-B antibodies. Type AB cats have no alloantibodies. Thus, acute life-threatening hemolytic transfusion reactions occur during the first mismatched transfusion (as little as 1 mL of blood) and NI is seen in type A and AB kittens born to primiparous type B queens.

Feline NI is caused by maternal anti-A alloantibodies that gain access to the circulation and destroy type A and type AB erythrocytes.[2, 73–75] Thus, type A and type AB kittens from matings between a type B queen and a type A or AB tom are at risk. The proportion of kittens at risk for NI varies from 0 to 25 per cent, depending on the frequency of type B cats, and therefore represents a major and now preventable cause of the neonatal kitten complex in purebred cats.[70] The low-titer anti-B alloantibodies of type A queens have not been associated with NI. Cats, as well as dogs, have an endotheliochorial placenta that is impermeable to immunoglobulins from the mother's serum. However, feline colostrum as well as milk contains high maternal concentrations of immunoglobulins which pass the gastrointestinal tract and are absorbed intact only during the first 16 hours of life.

Thus, type A or type AB kittens produced by type B queens are born healthy. Upon ingestion of colostrum or milk containing anti-A antibodies, the kittens at risk develop clinical signs. They may die suddenly without obvious clinical signs during the first few hours of life. They develop severe pigmenturia, which is readily visible when stimulating the neonates to urinate with a moist cotton ball. These kittens fail to thrive, are reluctant to nurse, become anemic and icteric, and rarely survive the first week of life. Some kittens at risk may have a subclinical course or slough their tail tip at 1 to 2 weeks of age, presumably because of an agglutinin-induced occlusion. The severity of clinical signs depends on the amount of colostral antibodies ingested before the kitten's ability to digest proteins and closure of the gut to intact proteins and varies from kitten to kitten, between queens and litters, and even within a litter. NI can be confirmed by typing the queen and kitten or the tom if the kitten died with suspicious signs.

Because of the acute disease course, treatment of NI is rarely successful. Foster nursing by a type A queen or with milk replacer, transfusion, and supportive care may be attempted. During the first day, when anti-A alloantibodies could still be absorbed, washed type B blood may be preferred, but thereafter type A blood is appropriate and may be best administered by the intraosseous route. However, NI can be readily prevented by (1) blood typing queen and tom and mating type B queens only to type B toms or (2) foster nursing type A and AB kittens born to type B queens for the first 24 hours. This can be accomplished by placing the kittens at risk with a type A queen (exchange only if the type A queen's kittens are older than 1 day) or feeding a commercial milk replacer. Either all kittens of a litter at risk are removed from the type B queen or umbilical cord blood or blood from the jugular vein of the kittens is typed with the typing card or cross-matched with anti-A plasma from the queen, thereby providing an opportunity to leave the type B kittens with the queen. Although maternal passive immunity does not appear to be essential in most cattery situations, 1 to 3 mL of serum from a type A cat may be administered intraperitoneally or subcutaneously to kittens receiving a milk replacer.

More than a dozen blood group systems have been described in dogs and are referred to as DEA followed by a number.[2, 72, 76] For all blood groups other than the DEA 1 system, erythrocytes from a dog can be positive or negative (e.g., DEA 4 positive or negative). The DEA 1 system, however, has at least two subtypes: DEA 1.1 (also known as A_1) and DEA 2 (A_2). Thus, the dog's erythrocytes can be DEA 1.1 positive or negative and DEA 1.1 negative erythrocytes can be DEA 1.2 positive or negative. The most antigenic and, therefore, most important blood type is DEA 1.1, for which blood typing cards are available. An autoagglutination test card has been added, as autoagglutinating samples appear like DEA 1.1 positive.[72] True autoagglutination precludes typing. Typing for DEA 1.2, 3, 4, 5, and 7 is provided only by Midwestern Blood Services. In contrast to cats, dogs do not have clinically important naturally occurring alloantibodies but can develop them after mismatched transfusions, particularly anti–DEA 1.1 antibodies in DEA 1.1–negative dogs. Thus, NI is not a clinical problem in dogs unless the bitch has previously received blood products, and acute hemolytic transfusion reactions are encountered only when a dog receives a blood transfusion four or more days after the first transfusion.[76, 77] They can be prevented by cross-matching all dogs that have been previously transfused even when using the same donor. Furthermore, delayed hemolytic transfusion reactions characterized by a more rapid then anticipated drop of the hematocrit may be observed 1 to 2 weeks after a (first) transfusion because of the development of new antibodies. As most reactions are directed against the DEA 1.1 antigen, DEA 1.1–negative as well as untyped dogs should never receive any blood products from DEA 1.1–positive donors. Furthermore, some hemolytic reactions may be caused by use of expired, inappropriately stored, and contaminated blood. In case of acute hemolytic transfusion reactions, the transfusion has to be stopped immediately and shock and supportive therapy provided. Glucocorticosteroid administration has not been proven to be effective in the prevention and treatment of hemolytic transfusion reactions.

INFECTION-ASSOCIATED HEMOLYSIS

Hemolytic anemia may develop upon exposure to several parasitic, bacterial, and viral agents because of the direct action of the infecting agent or its products on erythrocytes.

Few rickettsial and protozoal organisms are capable of infecting erythrocytes directly and causing severe hemolytic anemia (Table 177–3). Other infectious agents may induce a hemolytic component indirectly along with other major clinical signs. Thus, any infection may trigger the production of humoral antibodies against host erythrocytes, and, together with an activated complement and phagocytic system, the rate of erythrocyte destruction may be markedly accelerated. Cats in particular have an inflammation-associated shortened survival of erythrocytes caused by an abscess, surgery, or trauma.[78] Furthermore, during bacterial (e.g., *Leptospira, Clostridium, Streptococcus, Staphlycoccus*) septicemia, specific hemolysins can be produced and result in hemolytic anemia. For instance, alpha toxin released during clostridial sepsis is a lecithinase that can attack erythrocyte membrane lipids, leading to erythrocyte fragmentation. Additional information on these infectious diseases can be found in Section IV.

Hemobartonellosis

Hemobartonellosis in cats, also known as feline infectious anemia, is caused by *Haemobartonella felis*, an epicellular rickettsial parasite of erythrocytes.[79] *H. felis* is classified in the family Anaplasmataceae, is distinctly different from *Bartonella*, but is genetically similar to *Mycoplasma*. The natural transmission of *H. felis* still remains unclear, although bloodsucking ectoparasites are considered to be major vectors. Iatrogenic infection can occur via blood transfusion from carrier cats. In addition, *H. felis* may be transmitted by oral ingestion of infected blood or from queens to their newborns. Finally, because cat bite abscesses often precede hemobartonellosis by a few weeks, particularly in male cats that roam outdoors, this may represent another form of transmission.

H. felis is considered an opportunistic organism that causes illness only under predisposing conditions. Approximately half of the cats with hemobartonellosis are FeLV positive and infection with both agents exaggerates the severity of the anemia, whereas concurrent infection with feline immunodeficiency virus (FIV) does not appear to worsen the anemia. Although viral infections, abscesses, systemic illnesses, and trauma (including surgery) are apparent predisposing factors, such conditions may not be identifiable in each case.[80, 81]

The pathogenesis of hemobartonellosis can be divided into parasitic incubation, acute parasitemia, and recovery or carrier stage.[82] One week to months after infection, cats, when stressed, develop an acute parasitemic phase that results in mild to severe anemia. This stage is characterized by cyclic parasitemia and often lasts for weeks to months unless death caused by massive parasitemia and anemia ensues earlier. Parasitized erythrocytes lose their deformability as well as elicit an immune response and are, therefore, rapidly sequestered and phagocytized in spleen and other tissues. However, sequestered erythrocytes may shed the parasites and reenter the blood circulation. Although cats may recover by mounting an immune response against the parasites, they cannot completely clear the infection and thus they remain carriers indefinitely by harboring some *H. felis* organisms in macrophages.

Feline hemobartonellosis is associated with a gradual to precipitous drop in hematocrit that results in clinical signs of anemia. Cats are lethargic, weak, and inappetent, and cyclic fevers occur during the transient periods of parasitemia. Pale but only rarely icteric mucous membranes are noted. Splenomegaly and weight loss may develop gradually.

At present, a diagnosis of feline hemobartonellosis can be made only by recognizing *H. felis* organisms on erythrocytes in a blood smear. Blood needs to be collected before treatment and sometimes repeatedly. Blood smears should be prepared shortly after collection as organisms may detach. Any Romanowsky-type blood stain (e.g., Wright-Giemsa, Diff-Quik) may be used. *H. felis* organisms appear as blue-staining ring, rod, or coccoid forms on the surface of erythrocytes. They need to be differentiated from Howell-Jolly bodies, other parasites, basophilic stippling, and staining artifacts. New methylene blue and reticulocyte stains are inappropriate as *H. felis* may be confused with punctate reticulocytes and Heinz bodies, and fluorescent stains provide no advantages. Parasitized erythrocytes become spherical. Erythrophagocytosis by monocytes and tissue macrophages (e.g., bone marrow or splenic aspirates) as well as autoagglutination of parasitized erythrocytes may be observed, and the direct Coombs test at 37°C is often positive, supporting the major role of immune destruction. Because of the cyclic nature of the parasitemia, absence of organisms does not rule out an infection. No serologic tests are presently available, but a PCR-based test to detect *H. felis* DNA may aid in the diagnosis in the near future.[83] An apparent therapeutic response to doxycycline is insufficient for a definitive diagnosis of hemobartonellosis. Furthermore, *H. felis* may be incidentally discovered in carrier cats with other diseases.

Infected cats are treated with tetracycline products for 3 weeks.[79] Doxycycline at a dose of 2.5 mg/lb twice a day is the preferred product as it needs to be administered only twice daily and appears to cause fewer side effects such as

HEM

TABLE 177–3. HEMOLYSIS ASSOCIATED WITH INFECTION

DISEASE AND ORGANISM	HOST	VECTOR	SPECIAL DEMOGRAPHICS	THERAPY
Hemobartonellosis				
Haemobartonella felis	Cat	Blood, fleas(?)	Worldwide	Doxycycline
Haemobartonella canis	Dog	Blood, ticks	Worldwide	Doxycycline
Babesiosis				
Babesia canis vogeli	Dog	Ticks	United States	Imidocarb
Babesia canis?			Europe, Asia	
Babesia canis rossi			South Africa	
Babesia canis gibsoni	Dog	Ticks	United States, Africa, Asia	Imidocarb
Babesia felis	Cat	?	Africa	Imidocarb
Babesia felis	Cat	?	India	Imidocarb
Cytauxzoonosis				
Cytauxzoon felis	Cat (bobcats reservoir)	Ticks?		Generally fatal, imidocarb, diminazene

fever, anorexia, and hepatopathy. The parasitemia resolves immediately and a clinical response is seen within days. None of the tetracyclines clear the infection completely; thus, treated cats remain carriers, although relapses appear uncommon and have not been documented experimentally. Severely anemic cats may also benefit from blood transfusion from a blood type–compatible donor. Furthermore, because of the immune-mediated mechanism involved, treatment with prednisone at 0.5 to 1.0 mg/lb twice a day is indicated, particularly to inhibit the erythrophagocytosis.

In contrast to cats, dogs rarely have hemobartonellosis. It is caused by *Haemobartonella canis*, which can be transmitted by the brown dog tick (which also serves as a reservoir) and infected blood.[84] Unless dogs are splenectomized or have other serious illness and splenic dysfunction, infected dogs do not develop clinical signs of anemia. On stained blood smears *H. canis* differs from *H. felis* in that *H. canis* often forms chains across the surface of erythrocytes. Infected dogs with anemia are treated as described for cats and probably also remain latently infected.

Cytauxzoonosis

Fatal cytauxzoonosis has been sporadically reported in cats in south central and southeastern states of the United States and in Africa.[85, 86] It is caused by *Cytauxzoon felis*, a piroplasm of the family Theileriidae. In *C. felis*'s life cycle schizonts develop to merozoites in mononuclear phagocytes, whereas the erythrocytic piroplasms are the terminal chronically infected stage. Wildcats, particularly the bobcat (*Lynx rufus*), appear to be the natural reservoir for *C. felis* in North America and ticks probably serve as vectors; thus, cats with access to tick-infected wooded areas during the summer months are mostly at risk.

After an incubation period of days to weeks, the course of illness is rapidly progressive and leads to death in less than a week. Affected cats develop fever, anemia, icterus, pigmenturia, and dyspnea. The rapid multiplication of the protozoa in tissue and destruction of parasitized erythrocytes result in organ dysfunction, particularly of lungs, and hemolytic anemia, respectively, leading to hypoperfusion, hypoxia, and DIC. Only extremely rarely does a cat recover from the acute illness. A diagnosis is reached by documenting the protozoa in erythrocytes on a Wright-Giemsa–stained blood smear. They appear classically as signet ring–shaped blue forms, although other oval, tetrad, and dot forms may also be observed. Up to 5 per cent of the erythrocytes may be parasitized, each with one piroplasm. Serologic and direct fluorescent antibody tissue tests have been developed but are not commercially available. Supportive fluid therapy and administration of the carbanilide compound diminazene or imidocarb may be attempted, but cytauxzoonosis remains generally fatal.

Babesiosis

Whereas *Haemobartonella* and *Cytauxzoon* are important infectious agents in cats, babesiosis is a major cause of acute hemolytic anemia in dogs.[87] *Babesia canis* and *B. gibsoni* are the only two hematozoan species that infect dogs, but strains of *B. canis* have been proposed on the basis of geographic range and pathogenesis. In the United States, canine babesiosis occurs most commonly in the southern states, but endemic areas have also been found farther north.[88] Puppies younger than 8 months of age and greyhounds appear to be more susceptible to *Babesia* infection,

and, depending on the degree of tick control, few to all of the greyhounds in a kennel may be seropositive. Feline babesiosis has not been reported in the United States.

Ixodid ticks serve as major vectors, although transplacental transmission and transfer via blood transfusion have also been documented. Ticks must feed a minimum of 2 days to pass sporozoites via saliva into the blood circulation of the host. *Babesia* are engulfed by erythrocytes, in which they multiply into merozoites that infect other erythrocytes. A host immune response is elicited that may clear the infection. In fact, most infected dogs in the United States do not become ill but remain carriers.

After a 10- to 12-day incubation period, infected dogs may, however, develop severe hemolytic anemia, hypotensive shock, and a multiple organ dysfunction syndrome.[88–91] Although direct parasite damage contributes to the anemia, a secondary immune-mediated hemolytic anemia appears more important. Autoagglutination and a positive direct Coombs test result are commonly encountered.[92] Furthermore, infected dogs often have thrombocytopenia and leukocytosis. Besides the typical signs of anemia, fever, vomiting, lymphadenopathy, and splenomegaly may be noted. Although the hemolysis is mostly extravascular, signs of intravascular hemolysis may also be observed. The erythrocytic osmotic fragility is increased in vitro. Finally, a variety of other atypical signs, DIC, and death may occur because of multiple organ failure.

Babesiosis is diagnosed by blood smear examination or immunodiagnostics.[87] Single or pairs of large piriform organisms in erythrocytes are characteristic of *B. canis*, whereas singular intracellular organisms are probably *B. gibsoni*. As only few erythrocytes are generally parasitized, examination of erythrocytes in or below the buffy coat or of blood collected from an ear prick may improve the chances of finding the organism. The indirect fluorescent antibody test and enzyme-linked immunosorbent assay are most helpful in the diagnosis of babesiosis, although dogs seen early in the disease course are serologically negative and a few dogs may remain negative. Because of some serologic cross-reactivity, *B. canis* and *B. gibsoni* may be differentiated only by examination of parasites. Finally, dogs infected with *B. gibsoni* may have false-positive reactions for *Toxoplasma*, *Neospora*, and *B. canis*.

Imidocarb dipropionate as a single intramuscular injection of 3.5 mg/lb clears *B. canis* and probably *B. gibsoni* infection.[87] In addition, it has prophylactic activity for 6 weeks, eliminates the infectivity of ticks for up to 4 weeks, and is effective against *Ehrlichia canis*, a common dual infection. The few side effects are thought to be related to the anticholinergic effects of the drug and include hypersalivation, gastrointestinal signs, and dyspnea. In addition, supportive care to correct dehydration, anemia, and acidosis is important.[93] Treatment with immunosuppressive doses of prednisone is also indicated for 2 to 3 weeks in order to control the immune-mediated hemolytic component. Tick control is important in preventing spread in a kennel. A vaccine against *B. canis* is available in Europe.[94] All prospective blood donors should be tested for *Babesia* by serology and blood smear examination. Splenectomy of blood donors to increase the likelihood of finding parasites is not generally recommended.

CHEMICAL-INDUCED HEMOLYTIC ANEMIA

Many compounds including chemical agents, drugs, and food components and additives can induce oxidative damage to erythrocytes leading to a hemolytic anemia.[95] Many of these agents are derivatives of aromatic organic compounds (Table 177–4). In some cases, the chemical itself acts as an oxidative agent, but more often the compound or its metabolite interacts with oxygen to form free radicals and peroxides (see Chapter 80). Extracellularly produced oxidants injure the membrane, whereas oxidants generated intracellularly attack hemoglobin as well as membrane structures. Thus, a single agent may inflict erythrocyte injury and thereby hemolysis and reduced oxygen delivery to tissue by one or all three of the following:

1. Oxidation of heme iron resulting in methemoglobin production

2. Oxidative denaturation of hemoglobin leading to Heinz body formation

3. Membrane damage causing impaired deformability and ion transport

METHEMOGLOBINEMIA

Methemoglobin is the form of hemoglobin in which the heme iron has been oxidized from the ferrous (Fe^{2+}) to the ferric (Fe^{3+}) state and is, therefore, unable to bind and transport oxygen.[3] Normally, approximately 3 per cent of hemoglobin is oxidized daily by spontaneous oxidation of oxyhemoglobin and oxidant generation in regular metabolic pathways. This is a reversible process as methemoglobin is being continuously reduced by the reduced nicotinamide adenine dinucleotide (NADH) cytochrome-b_5 reductase enzyme in erythrocytes, thereby keeping the blood methemoglobin concentration below 1 per cent. Methemoglobin can accumulate because of a hereditary deficiency of the cytochrome b_5 reductase enzyme, as described earlier in this chapter, or because of exposure to oxidative agents. Dogs and cats with a genetic predisposition are at extreme risk of developing a life-threatening methemoglobinemia. Although many compounds are capable of inducing methemoglobin formation, benzocaine-containing skin products and laryngeal or nasopharyngeal sprays, phenazopyridine (a urinary

TABLE 177–4. OXIDATIVE DAMAGE–INDUCED HEMOLYTIC ANEMIA, HEINZ BODY ANEMIA, AND METHEMOGLOBINEMIA

Food components
  Onions
  Garlic
  Broccoli
  Propylene glycol (semimoist food)
Drugs
  Acetaminophen
  Benzocaine (skin ointment, Cetacaine spray)
  Phenazopyridine (urinary tract analgesic)
  Methylene blue (old urinary antiseptic)
  Phenacetin
  Vitamin K_3
  DL-Methionine
Chemicals
  Naphthalene
Heavy metals
  Zinc
  Copper
Feline disorders associated with Heinz body formation
  Diabetes mellitus ± ketoacidosis
  Hepatic lipidosis
  Hyperthyroidism
  Lymphoma and other neoplasms

tract analgesic), and acetaminophen produce severe methemoglobinemia in cats within minutes to hours of exposure.

For several reasons, cats appear more susceptible to oxidative agents. Feline hemoglobin contains 8 to 10 reactive sulfhydryl groups that are easy targets for oxidation, whereas other species' hemoglobins have maximally 4 sulfhydryl groups. Furthermore, the drug-metabolizing steps are restricted in cats. They cannot conjugate drugs with glucuronides and their sulfate conjugation and glutathione pathways are rapidly saturated and depleted. Thus, instead of excreting acetaminophen as a glucuronide conjugate, cats produce reactive metabolites through mixed function oxidase activities that damage erythrocytes, leading to methemoglobinemia and Heinz body anemia.[96] In fact, as little as a baby acetaminophen tablet (65 mg) may be lethal to a debilitated cat, whereas 10-fold higher doses are required to induce toxicity characterized by hepatic failure in other species.

Although methemoglobin is quantified in EDTA-anticoagulated blood spectrophotometrically in commercial laboratories, simple spot tests can indicate the presence of clinically important methemoglobinemia. If a tube of blood or drop of blood on a filter paper remains brown after exposure to air (oxygen), whereas the control sample turns red, the patient's blood methemoglobin concentration exceeds 10 percent of the total hemoglobin. At this level the mucous membranes appear cyanotic, but serious clinical signs are not appreciated until the methemoglobin level reaches 50 per cent. Exercise intolerance, lethargy, dyspnea, ataxia, and coma develop and death ensues when the methemoglobin concentration exceeds 70 per cent. Besides the clinical signs related to hypoxia, cats intoxicated with acetaminophen develop facial edema and hypersalivation.

Heinz Body Anemia

Heinz bodies represent irreversibly denatured and precipitated hemoglobin in erythrocytes. Eccentrocytes may be noted instead and are characterized by shifting of hemoglobin to one side of the cell, leaving a clear moon-shaped zone outlined by membrane. The conformational changes of the globin chains caused by oxidation of the hemoglobin sulfhydryl groups and oxidative membrane damage result in binding and clustering of precipitated hemoglobin on the membrane. Heinz bodies containing erythrocytes are rigid, have decreased deformability, and therefore may lyse or be removed from the circulation by macrophages. When passing through the spleen, Heinz body–containing erythrocytes are retained in the meshwork and phagocytized as a whole (culled) or only the Heinz bodies are removed (pitting). However, because of large openings in the venous sinus walls, the feline spleen has poor pitting function. Heinz body hemolytic anemia has been associated with a variety of conditions, many of which also cause methemoglobinemia and membrane injury. Ingestion of dietary onions—raw, cooked, or dehydrated (onion powder) and usually as part of table scraps fed by owners—can result in up to 90 percent Heinz body formation within a day followed by hemolysis leading to severe anemia by 5 days.[97, 98] Several thiosulfates in onion extracts have been implicated in producing Heinz bodies but only minimal amounts of methemoglobin. Onion toxicity occurs more commonly in dogs than cats and the susceptibility appears to vary among individuals. Administration of various drugs, including methylene blue, DL-methionine, phenacetin, and vitamin K_3 (above 2.5 mg/lb/day) can lead to Heinz body hemolytic anemia. The previously mentioned agents acetaminophen, benzocaine-containing products, and phenazopyridine that induce severe methemoglobinemia can also cause Heinz body formation. Furthermore, increased numbers of Heinz bodies have been associated with various organ disorders in cats, including hyperthyroidism, lymphoma and other cancers, and diabetes mellitus, particularly in the presence of ketoacidosis.[99]

Membrane Injury

Many oxidative agents directly cause membrane lipid peroxidation, cross-linking and clustering of cytoskeleton proteins, and impaired ion transport function. These membrane injuries result in severe intra- and extravascular hemolysis, sometimes without much Heinz body and methemoglobin formation. For instance, naphthalene, the active ingredient in old-fashioned mothballs or crystals as well as toilet bowl deodorizers, is an important poison in small animals, causing intravascular hemolysis, vomiting, seizures, and hepatopathy.[100] Hemolytic anemia has also been associated with acute zinc toxicity in dogs that swallowed zinc-containing objects such as zinc nuts and bolts from animal carriers, U.S. pennies minted since 1983 (98 percent zinc by weight), and zinc oxide ointments.[101, 102] As these objects are retained in the stomach, the gastric acid liberates zinc and zinc is absorbed. The mechanism by which zinc causes life-threatening intravascular hemolysis remains uncertain, but few Heinz bodies and spherocytes have been found. Besides identifying the metal object by radiographs, the diagnosis can be confirmed by documenting increased serum zinc concentrations (above 5 parts per million; samples must be submitted in plastic tubes for analysis). Similarly, acute copper toxicosis may result in severe intravascular hemolysis and some methemoglobinemia. It has been associated with fulminant hepatic failure caused by copper storage in Bedlington terriers (see Chapter 144). In contrast, lead toxicity is generally not associated with hemolysis, but large numbers of nucleated RBCs and gastrointestinal and neurologic signs are observed.

Treatment of oxidative hemolytic anemias includes immediate removal of the oxidative agent, use of antioxidants, transfusion, and supportive care. Vomiting is induced only if the substance has just been ingested and activated charcoal may be administered. Metallic objects such as pennies and nuts are best removed by gastroscopy or gastrotomy. In case of severe anemia and/or methemoglobinemia, transfusion with packed RBCs is indicated, whereas oxygen therapy hardly improves tissue oxygenation. The anemia nadir is often not reached for several days, but thanks to the generally observed strong regenerative response, recovery from anemia is swift. Severe methemoglobinemia can be corrected with one slow intravenous injection of methylene blue (0.44 mg/lb). Methylene blue acts as an electron donor for an alternative, otherwise nonfunctional methemoglobin reductase. In cats with acetaminophen intoxication, either oral or intravenous N-acetylcysteine (Mucomyst) at an initial dose of 64 mg/lb followed by seven treatments of 32 mg/lb every 8 hours should be administered. As the drug of choice, N-acetylcysteine increases the sulfate availability for conjugation of acetaminophen and provides cysteine for glutathione regeneration and metabolism of toxic metabolites of acetaminophen. Treatments with other agents such as sodium sulfate to add sulfide, cimetidine to inhibit cytochrome P-450, and ascorbic acid as antioxidants have been proposed but have not been shown to provide additional benefits. Because of the effect of oxidative substances on other organ systems including gastrointestinal tract, liver, and central nervous system, animals may continue to show clinical signs after correction of the anemia and methemoglobinemia and require additional supportive care. Furthermore, care should be taken to avoid any reexposure to these and other toxins.

Hypophosphatemia-Induced Hemolysis

Severe hypophosphatemia causing hemolysis in dogs and cats has been associated with diabetes mellitus, hepatic lipidosis, and primary hyperparathyroidism as well as with enteral and parenteral hyperalimentation (starvation-refeeding syndrome) and oral administration of phosphate-binding antacids.[103–105] During insulin, fluid, and bicarbonate treatment of (ketoacidotic) diabetic animals, the phosphate value in plasma declines precipitously. Hypophosphatemia occurs because of intracellular phosphate shifts, enhanced renal losses, and reduced intestinal absorption of phosphate. In addition to myopathy and cardiac and neurologic dysfunction, acute hemolytic anemia, characterized by a rapid drop in PCV and mild intravascular lysis and Heinz body formation, is observed in animals with hypophosphatemia. On the basis of experimental data, serum phosphorus concentrations would need to be less than 1 mg/dL (normal 2.9 to 7 mg/dL) to cause hemolysis, but in clinical practice hemolysis occurs with phosphate values less than 2.5 mg/dL. Serum phosphate measurements may underestimate the phosphate depletion in these disease states and can erroneously be higher because of hemoglobinemia and hyperbilirubinemia. The pathogenesis of the hypophosphatemia-induced anemia is probably related to depletion of erythrocytic ATP, DPG (in dogs), and reduced glutathione, which leads to decreased deformability and increased osmotic fragility as well as susceptibility to oxidative injury. As discussed in relation to canine erythrocyte PFK deficiency, DPG-depleted erythrocytes are extremely alkaline fragile and have a high hemoglobin oxygen affinity, thereby contributing to intravascular hemolysis and tissue hypoxia in dogs but not in cats. Furthermore, thrombocytopenia and platelet and leukocyte dysfunction have been documented experimentally in dogs.

Hypophosphatemic animals need to receive oral or parenteral phosphate supplementation. Aggressive intravenous phosphate therapy is often needed in severely hypophosphatemic and anorexic or vomiting animals. An initial sodium or potassium phosphate dosage of 0.005 to 0.015-0.03 mmol/lb/h appears safe and effective, but serum phosphorus and calcium concentrations should be measured every 6 hours and the dose should be adjusted and route switched to oral when appropriate. Potential complications of intravenous phosphate supplementation include hypocalcemia, acute renal failure, and dystrophic soft tissue calcification and should be immediately corrected by stopping the phosphate infusion and initiating infusion of a calcium gluconate. Oral supplementation with a normal balanced diet, skim milk, or commercial phosphate products is preferred in cases of mild hypophosphatemia, and prophylactic phosphorus supplementation should always be considered when treating severe diabetes mellitus or hepatic lipidosis.

MICROANGIOPATHIC HEMOLYTIC ANEMIA

A large variety of conditions may cause physical damage to erythrocytes that leads to cell fragmentation and intra- as well as extravascular hemolysis.[106] In case of water intoxication associated with near drowning in fresh water, erythrocytes undergo hypotonic lysis similar to the swelling and lysis of erythrocytes in the in vitro osmotic fragility test.

Heat stroke and severe burns can inflict thermal injury to erythrocytes. Heart valve disease as well as cardiovascular implants and intravenous catheters can induce mechanical damage to erythrocytes as much as dirofilariasis, particularly in the form of the caval syndrome (see Chapter 119). In addition, other endothelial damage caused by vasculitis, hemangiosarcoma and other tumors, various splenic diseases or torsion, and liver disease can injure erythrocytes. A hemolytic-uremic syndrome characterized by acute renal failure, platelet activation leading to thrombocytopenia and thrombosis, and microangiopathic hemolytic anemia has been described in dogs. Similarly, DIC is associated with a fragmentation hemolysis (see Chapter 180). A diagnosis of microangiopathic hemolysis that is often subclinical and rarely causes overt intravascular hemolytic anemia is made by identifying the triggering condition and characterizing schistocytes (schizocytes). These are erythrocyte fragments that appear on blood smears as small, misshapen, often triangular or helmet-shaped structures. Schistocytes are important even in small numbers and cannot be fabricated by poor blood smear preparation. On the other hand, schistocytes are observed with a variety of other anemias including chronic iron deficiency states and zinc intoxication. Concomitantly, thrombocytopenia and coagulopathy are often present. Besides supportive care, therapy is directed at the underlying disease and control of DIC. Blood component therapy should be considered. The prognosis is guarded to poor if the underlying disease cannot be corrected.

REFERENCES

1. Jain NC: Schalm's Veterinary Hematology. Philadelphia, Lea & Febiger, 1986.
2. Again NS, Board PG: Red Blood Cells of Domestic Animals. Amsterdam, Elsevier, 1983.
3. Harvey JW: The erythrocyte: Physiology, metabolism and biochemical disorders. In Kaneko JJ et al (eds): Clinical Biochemistry of Domestic Animals, 5th ed. New York, Academic Press, 1997, p 157.
4. Weiser MG: Erythrocyte responses and disorders. In Ettinger S, Feldman E (eds): Textbook of Veterinary Internal Medicine. Philadelphia, WB Saunders, 1995, p 1864.
5. Hillman RS: Erythrocyte disorders: Anemias due to acute blood loss. In Williams WJ, Beutler E, Erslev AJ, Lichtman MA (eds): Hematology, 4th ed. New York, McGraw-Hill, 1990, p 700.
6. Rentko V, et al: A clinical trial of a hemoglobin based oxygen carrying (HBOC) fluid in the treatment of anemia. ACVIM Proceedings, 1996, p 759.
7. Smith JE: Iron metabolism and its disorders. Physiology, metabolism and biochemical disorders. In Kaneko JJ et al (eds): Clinical Biochemistry of Domestic Animals, 5th ed. New York, Academic Press, 1997, p 223.
8. Fairbanks VF, Beutler E: Iron deficiency. In Williams WJ, Beutler E, Erslev AJ, Lichtman MA (eds): Hematology, 4th ed. New York, McGraw-Hill, 1990, p 482.
9. Harvey JW, et al: Chronic iron deficiency anemia in dogs. J Am Anim Hosp Assoc 18:946, 1982.
10. Weiser G, O'Grady MR: Erythrocyte volume distribution analysis and hematologic changes in dogs with iron deficiency anemia. Vet Pathol 20:230, 1983.
11. French TW, et al: A bleeding disorder (von Willebrand's disease) in a Himalayan cat. JAVMA 190:437, 1987.
12. Fulton R, et al: Electronic and morphologic characterization of erythrocytes of an adult cat with iron deficiency anemia. Vet Pathol 25:521, 1988.
13. Yaphé W, et al: Severe cardiomegaly secondary to anemia in a kitten. JAVMA 202:961, 1993.
14. Fulton R, et al: Electronic and morphologic characterization of erythrocytes of an adult cat with iron deficiency anemia. Vet Pathol 25:251, 1988.
15. Deiss A: Destruction of erythrocytes. In Lee GR, et al (eds): Wintrobe's Clinical Hematology, 10th ed. Baltimore, Williams & Wilkins, 1999, p 267.
16. Christian JA, et al: Senescence of canine biotinylated erythrocytes: Increased autologous immunoglobulin binding occurs on erythrocytes aged in vivo for 104 to 110 days. Blood 82:3469, 1993.
17. Giger U, Bucheler J: Transfusion of type-A and type-B blood to cats. JAVMA 198:411, 1991.
18. Callan MB, et al: Evaluation of an automated system for measurement of hemoglobin in animals. Am J Vet Res 53:1760, 1992.
19. Giger U: Hereditary erythrocyte disorders. In Bonagura J (ed): Kirk's Current Veterinary Therapy XIII. Philadelphia, WB Saunders, in press.
20. Kohn B, et al: Polymorphism of feline β-globins studied by high performance liquid chromatography. Am J Vet Res 59:830, 1998.
21. Harvey JW, et al: Methemoglobin reductase deficiency in dogs. Comp Haematol Int 1:55, 1991.
22. Harvey JW, et al: Methemoglobin reductase deficiency in a cat. JAVMA 205:1290, 1994.
23. Giger U, et al: Familial methemoglobin reductase deficiency in domestic shorthair cats. Proceedings, First International. Feline Genetic Disease Conference, Philadelphia, 1998.
24. Inaba M, Maede Y: Na,K-ATPase in dog red cells. J Biol Chem 261:16099, 1986.
25. Degen M: Pseudohyperkalemia in Akitas. JAVMA 290:541, 1987.
26. Smith JE, et al: Hereditary elliptocytosis with protein band 4.1 deficiency in the dog. Blood 61:373, 1983.
27. Fletch SM, et al: The Alaskan malamute chrondrodysplasia (dwarfism-anemia) syndrome: A review. J Am Anim Hosp Assoc 11:353, 1975.
28. Brown DE, et al: Erythrocyte indices and volume distribution in a dog with stomatocytosis. Vet Pathol 31:247, 1994.
29. Slappendel RJ, et al: Normal cations and abnormal membrane lipids in the red blood cells of dogs with familial stomatocytosis–hypertrophic gastritis. Blood 84:904, 1994.
30. Kohn B, et al: Hemolytic anemia caused by increased osmotic fragility of erythrocyte cells. ACVIM Proceedings, 1996, p 760.
31. Giger U: Inherited erythrocyte phosphofructokinase and pyruvate kinase deficiency. In Schalm's Veterinary Hematology. Baltimore, Williams & Wilkins.
32. Giger U, et al: Inherited phosphofructokinase deficiency in dogs with hyperventilation-induced hemolysis: Increased in vitro and in vivo alkaline fragility of erythrocytes. Blood 65:345, 1985.
33. Giger U, Harvey JW: Hemolysis caused by phosphofructokinase deficiency in English springer spaniels: Seven cases (1983–1986). JAVMA 191:453, 1987.
34. Harvey JW, et al: Effect of 2,3-diphosphoglycerate concentration on alkaline fragility of phosphofructokinase deficient canine erythrocytes. Comp Biochem Physiol B Biochem Mol Biol 89:105, 1998.
35. Giger U, et al: Inherited phosphofructokinase deficiency in the American cocker spaniel. JAVMA 201:1569, 1992.
36. Smith BF, et al: Molecular basis of canine muscle type phosphofructokinase deficiency. J Biol Chem 271:20070, 1996.
37. Searcy GP, et al: Animal model: Pyruvate kinase deficiency in dogs. Am J Pathol 94:689, 1979.
38. Giger U, Noble NA: Determination of erythrocyte pyruvate kinase deficiency in basenjis with chronic hemolytic anemia. JAVMA 198:1755, 1991.
39. Chapman BL, Giger U: Inherited pyruvate kinase deificiency in the West Highland white terrier. J Small Anim Pract 31:610, 1990.
40. Schaer M, et al: Pyruvate kinase deficiency causing hemolytic anemia with secondary hematochromatosis in a Cairn terrier. J Am Anim Hosp Assoc 28:233, 1992.
41. Randolph JF, et al: Familial nonspherocytic hemolytic anemia in poodles. Am J Vet Res 47:687, 1986.
42. Whitney KM, et al: Molecular basis of canine pyruvate kinase deficiency. Exp Hematol 22:866, 1994.
43. Whitney KM, Lothrop CD: Genetic test for pyruvate kinase deficiency in basenjis. JAVMA 207:918, 1995.
44. Skelly B, et al: A six base pair insertion causes erythrocyte pyruvate kinase (PK) deficiency in the West Highland white terrier. Am J Vet Res, in press.
45. Giger U, et al: Molecular basis of erythrocyte pyruvate kinase deficiency in cats. Blood 90:2701, 1997.
46. Thomas AT: Autoimmune hemolytic anemias. In Lee GR, et al (eds): Wintrobe's Clinical Hematology, 10th ed. Baltimore, Williams & Wilkins, 1999, p 1233.
47. Parker CJ, Foerster J: Mechanism of immune destruction of erythrocytes. In Lee GR, et al (eds): Wintrobe's Clinical Hematology, 10th. ed. Baltimore, Williams & Wilkins, 1999, p 1191.
48. Corato A, et al: Proliferative responses of peripheral blood mononuclear cells from normal dogs and dogs with autoimmune haemolytic anaemia to red blood cell antigens. Vet Immunol Immunopathol 59:191, 1997.
49. Jones DRE, Gruffydd-Jones TJ: The haematological consequences of immune-mediated anemia in the dog. Comp Haematol Int 1:83, 1991.
50. Duval D, Giger U: Vaccine-associated immune-mediated hemolytic anemia in the dog. J Vet Intern Med 10:290, 1996.
51. Elliott J: Annual booster vaccinations. Is there an association with immune-mediated problems? J Small Anim Pract 38:179, 1997.
52. Klag AR, et al: Idiopathic immune-mediated hemolytic anemia in dogs: 42 cases (1986–1990). JAVMA 202:783, 1993.
53. Jackson ML, Kruth SA: Immune-mediated hemolytic anemia and thrombocytopenia in the dog: A retrospective study of 55 cases diagnosed from 1969 through 1983 at the Western College of Veterinary Medicine. Can Vet J 26:245, 1985.
54. Peterson ME, et al: Propylthiouracil-associated hemolytic anemia, thrombocytopenia, and antinuclear antibodies in cats with hyperthyroidism. JAVMA 187:46, 1984.
55. Klein MK, et al: Pulmonary thromboembolism associated with immune-mediated hemolytic anemia in dogs: Ten cases (1982–1987). JAVMA 195:246, 1989.
56. Jonas LD, et al: Nonregenerative form of immune-mediated hemolytic anemia in dogs: 42 cases (1986–1990). JAVMA 23:201, 1987.
57. Walton RM, et al: Bone marrow cytological findings in 4 dogs and a cat with hemophagocytic syndrome. J Vet Intern Med 10:7, 1996.
58. Barker RN, et al: Red cell–bound immunoglobulins and complement measured by an enzme-linked antiglobin test in dogs with autoimmune haemolysis or other anaemias. Res Vet Sci 54:170, 1993.
59. Barker RN, et al: Autoimmune haemolysis in the dog: Relationship between

anaemia and the levels of red blood cell bound immunoglobulins and complement measured by an enzyme-linked antiglobin test. Vet Immunol Immunopathol 34:1, 1993.

60. Barker RN, Jones DRE: Effects of papain on the agglutination of canine red cells with serum antibodies. Res Vet Sci 55:156, 1993.

61. Miller E: Immunosuppressive therapy in the treatment of immune-mediated disease. J Vet Intern Med 6:206, 1992.

62. Mason NJ, et al: Evaluation of combined cyclophosphamide and prednisone versus prednisone alone in the treatment of canine immune mediated hemolytic anemia. ACVIM Proceedings, 1997, p 130.

63. Burgess KE, et al: Immune mediated hemolytic anemia in dogs: A retrospective study of 60 cases treated with cyclophosphamide. ACVIM Proceedings, 1995, p 143.

64. Allyn ME, Troy GC: Immune mediated hemolytic anemia—A restrospective study: Focus on treatment and mortality (1988–1996). ACVIM Proceedings, 1997, p 131.

65. Miller E: Danazol therapy for the treatment of immune mediated hemolytic anemia in dogs. ACVIM Proceedings, 1997, p 130.

66. Scott-Moncrieff JCR: Treatment of nonregenerative anemia with human gamma-globulin in dogs. JAVMA 206:1895, 1995.

67. Scott-Moncrieff JCR, et al: Intravenous administration of human immune globulin in dogs with immune-mediated hemolytic anemia. JAVMA 210:1623, 1997.

68. Reagan WJ, et al: Effects of human intravenous immunoglobulin on canine monocytes and lymphocytes. Am J Vet Res 59:1568, 1998.

69. Matus RE, et al: Plasmapheresis as adjuvant therapy for autoimmune hemolytic anemia in two dogs. JAVMA 186:691, 1985.

70. Giger U, et al: Frequency and inheritance of A and B blood types in feline breeds of the United States. J Hered 82:15, 1991.

71. Griot-Wenk M, et al: Biochemical characterization of the feline AB blood group system. Anim Genet 24:401, 1993.

72. Giger U: Blood typing and crossmatching to assure compatible transfusions. In Bonagura J (ed): Kirk's Current Veterinary Therapy XIII. Philadelphia, WB Saunders, in press.

73. Hubler M, et al: Feline neonatal isoerythrolysis in two litters. J Small Anim Pract 28:833, 1987.

74. Giger U: Feline neonatal isoerythrolysis: A major cause of the fading kitten syndrome. ACVIM Proceedings, 1991, p 347.

75. Casal ML, et al: Transfer of colostral antibodies from the queen to the neonatal kitten. Am J Vet Res 57:1653, 1996.

76. Giger U, et al: An acute hemolytic transfusion reaction caused by dog erythrocyte antigen 1.1 incompatibility in a previously sensitized dog. JAVMA 206:1358, 1995.

77. Callan MB, et al: Hemolytic transfusion reactions in a dog with an alloantibody to a common antigen. J Vet Intern Med 9:277, 1995.

78. Weiss DJ, Krehbiel JD: Studies of the pathogenesis of anemia of inflammation: Erythrocyte survival. Am J Vet Res 44:1830, 1983.

79. Harvey JW: Hemobartonellosis. In Greene CE (ed): Infectious Diseases of the Dog and Cat. Philadelphia, WB Saunders, 1998, p 166.

80. Grindem CB, et al: Risk factors for Haemobartonella felis infection in cats. JAVMA 196:96, 1990.

81. Bobade PA, et al: Feline haemobartonellosis: Clinical haematological and pathological studies in natural infections and the relationship with feline leukaemia virus. Vet Res 122:32, 1988.

82. Harvey JW, Gaskin JM: Experimental feline haemobartonellosis. J Am Anim Hosp Assoc 13:28, 1977.

83. Messick JB, et al: Development and evaluation of a PCR based assay for detection of Haemobartonella felis infection in cats and differentiation using restriction fragment length polymorphism. J Clin Microbiol 36:462, 1998.

84. Lester SJ, et al: Haemobartonella canis infection following splenectomy and transfusion. Can Vet J 36:444, 1995.

85. Hoover JP, et al: Cytauxzoonosis in cats: Eight cases (1985–1992). JAVMA 205:455, 1994.

86. Kier AB, Greene CE: Cytauxzoonosis. In Greene CE (ed): Infectious Diseases of the Dog and Cat. Philadelphia, WB Saunders, 1998, p 470.

87. Taboada J: Babesiosis. In Greene CE (ed): Infectious Diseases of the Dog and Cat. Philadelphia, WB Saunders, 1998, p 473.

88. Taboada J, et al: Seroprevalence of babesiosis in greyhounds in Florida. JAVMA 200:47, 1992.

89. Abdullah AS, et al: Clinical and haematological findings in 70 naturally occurring cases of canine babesiosis. J Small Anim Pract 31:145, 1990.

90. Kontos VJ, Koutinas AF: Clinical observations in 15 spontaneous cases of canine babesiosis. Canine Pract 22:30, 1997.

91. Jacobson LS, Clark IA: The pathophysiology of canine babesiosis: New approaches to an old puzzle. J S Afr Vet Assoc 65:134, 1994.

92. Adachi K, et al: Immunologic characteristics of anti–erythrocyte membrane antibody produced in dogs during Babesia gibsoni infection. J Vet Med Sci 57:121, 1995.

93. Jacobson LS, Swan GE: Supportive treatment of canine babesiosis. J S Afr Vet Assoc 66:95, 1995.

94. Schetters TH, et al: Vaccination of dogs against Babesia canis infection. Vet Parasitol 73:35, 1997.

95. Christopher MM, et al: Erythrocyte pathology and mechanism of Heinz body–mediated hemolysis in cats. Vet Pathol 27:299, 1990.

96. Savides MC, et al: The toxicity and biotransformation of single doses of acetaminophen in dogs and cats. Toxicol Appl Pharmacol 74:26, 1984.

97. Harvey JW, Rackear D: Experimental onion-induced hemolytic anemia in dogs. Vet Pathol 22:387, 1985.

98. Robertson JE: Heinz body formation in cats fed baby food with onion powder. ACVIM Proceedings, 1997, p 131.

99. Christopher MM: Relationship of endogenous Heinz bodies to disease and anemia in cats: 120 cases. JAVMA 194:1089, 1989.

100. Todisco V, et al: Hemolysis from exposure to naphthalene mothballs. N Engl J Med 325:1660, 1991.

101. Latimer KS, et al: Zinc-induced hemolytic anemia caused by ingestion of pennies by a pup. JAVMA 195:77, 1989.

102. Luttgen PJ, et al: Heinz body hemolytic anemia associated with high plasma zinc concentration in a dog. JAVMA 197:1347, 1990.

103. Willard MD, et al: Severe hypophosphatemia associated with diabetes mellitus in six dogs and one cat. JAVMA 190:1007, 1987.

104. Adams LG, et al: Hypophosphatemia and hemolytic anemia associated with diabetes mellitus and hepatic lipidosis in cats. J Vet Intern Med 7:266, 1993.

105. Justin RB, Hohenhaus AE: Hypophosphatemia associated with enteral alimentation in cats. J Vet Intern Med 9:228, 1995.

106. Martinez J: Microangiopathic hemolytic anemia. In Williams WJ, Beutler E, Erslev AJ, Lichtman MA (eds): Hematology, 4th ed. New York, McGraw-Hill 1990, p 657.

CHAPTER 178

NON-REGENERATIVE ANEMIA

Susan M. Cotter

Evaluation of a patient with anemia of unknown cause starts with a thorough history, including vaccination status, diet, travel, life-style, duration of signs, drug or toxin exposure, prior or current illnesses, and similar illnesses in housemates or relatives (Fig. 178–1). The physical examina-tion is then conducted, including evaluation for icterus, petechiae, and stool color; determination of heart rate and rhythm; evaluation of size of lymph nodes, liver, and spleen; and palpation of the abdomen for masses. In males, the testicles are palpated for tumors.

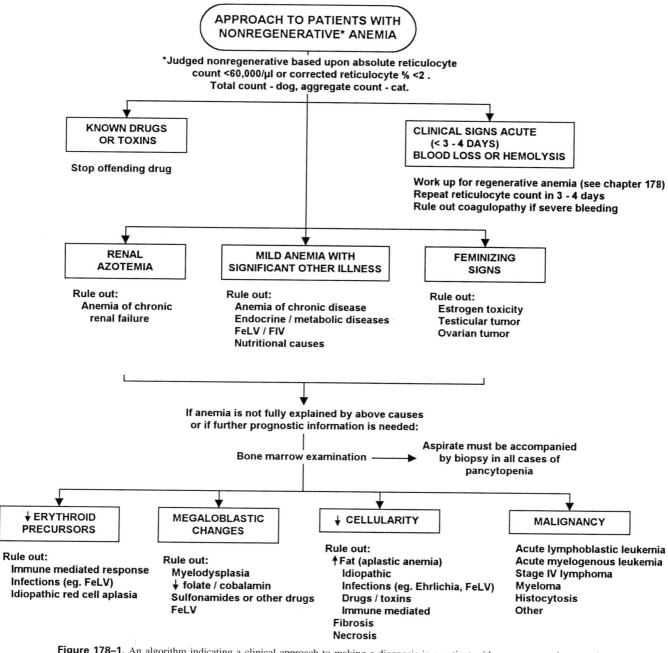

Figure 178–1. An algorithm indicating a clinical approach to making a diagnosis in a patient with non-regenerative anemia. Absolute reticulocyte count/μL = (number of reticulocytes/100 RBCs) $\times$ RBC count/μL. Corrected reticulocyte percent = (patient's Hct/normal Hct) $\times$ (number of reticulocytes/100 RBCs). Conventional normal Hct in the dog is 45% and cat is 37%.

HEM

If the cause of the anemia is still not evident, an important determination will then be whether the anemia is regenerative or non-regenerative. The reticulocyte count provides objective evidence as to whether the marrow is responding appropriately. Assuming that anemia has been present for longer than 3 to 4 days, the absence of reticulocytosis is indicative of non-regenerative anemia. Because the onset of non-regenerative anemia is usually gradual, the anemia is often severe by the time the patient becomes symptomatic. Compensatory mechanisms to improve oxygenation of tissues such as increased 2,3-diphosphoglycerate in dogs and increased heart and respiratory rates in both dogs and cats are in place. For example, if an animal had lost over 50 per cent of its red cell volume acutely, one would expect obvious clinical signs related to hemorrhage or hemolysis, whereas if this same loss occurred from decreased production of red cells, clinical signs would be minimal or absent. Another clue that an anemia might be non-regenerative is concurrent leukopenia or thrombocytopenia, or both (pancytopenia), indicative of damage to the marrow.

Nucleated red cells may be present in the blood of anemic patients regardless of whether or not an anemia is regenerative (Fig. 178–2). One must avoid the temptation to consider circulating nucleated red cells as "immature" cells indicative of an active marrow response. On the contrary it is more likely an abnormal, non-beneficial response.

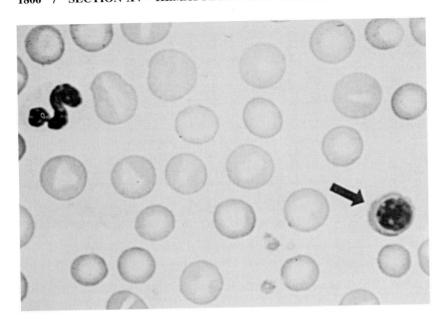

Figure 178–2. Nucleated erythrocyte (arrow), Wright-Giemsa stain. (From Weiser MG: Erythrocyte responses and disorders. *In* Ettinger SJ, Feldman EC [eds]: Textbook of Veterinary Internal Medicine, 4th ed. Philadelphia, WB Saunders, 1995, p 1867, with permission.)

Non-regenerative anemia can be caused by exogenous factors affecting the marrow or by primary marrow failure (Table 178–1). To produce normal red cells, the marrow must have an adequate number of pluripotent stem cells, appropriate hematopoietic growth factors to which stem cells and committed progenitors are capable of responding, a favorable microenvironment, and adequate nutrition. If anything is missing or if suppressive or toxic factors are present, such as drugs, autoantibodies affecting progenitors, or unknown substances such as those secreted by leukemic cells, adequate numbers of normally functioning red cells cannot be produced.

TABLE 178–1. CAUSES OF NON-REGENERATIVE ANEMIA

Acute blood loss or hemolysis (first 3–4 days)
Anemia of chronic disease/inflammation
Chronic renal failure
Deficiencies (rare)
   Folate, cobalamin, iron (usually regenerative)
   Malnutrition
Metabolic diseases
   Hypothyroidism, other endocrine deficiencies
   Hyperestrogenism (iatrogenic or neoplasia)
   Liver disease
Immune mediated
Infections
   Retroviruses
   Ehrlichiosis
   Parvoviruses
Drugs/toxins (see Table 178–3)
Radiation
Pure red cell aplasia
   Most immune mediated
   Idiopathic
Aplastic anemia
   Infections/drugs/toxins
   Immune mediated
   Idiopathic
Necrosis or sclerosis of the marrow
Myelofibrosis
Myelodysplasia
Acute lymphoblastic or acute myelogenous leukemia
Myeloma
Malignant histiocytosis
Other malignancy

Overall, most anemias of small animal patients are non-regenerative. Dogs or cats with any debilitating or chronic illness commonly have a mild anemia, known as anemia of chronic disease or inflammation. In cats, non-regenerative anemia also occurs secondary to infection with retroviruses.

Non-regenerative anemias often have a worse prognosis than do regenerative anemias; however, non-regenerative anemia secondary to renal failure, metabolic, or deficiency diseases or to a treatable chronic illness may be fully reversible because the marrow in each case is normal. When the marrow has been damaged by drugs, toxins, infectious agents, or radiation, the anemia may be irreversible.

Hematologic findings in most non-regenerative anemias include absolute reticulocyte counts less than 60,000/μL or corrected reticulocyte counts less than 2 per cent. In cats, the counts refer to aggregate reticulocytes, which, like those of dogs, persist in the circulation for about 24 hours. About 5 per cent of red cells in normal cats are punctate reticulocytes. These increase more slowly and often to higher levels after loss of red cells. They persist for an additional 1 to 2 weeks before subsiding.[1] Because of this delay in both appearance and maturation they are not an accurate indicator of current marrow activity. Sometimes in mild regenerative anemias aggregate reticulocytes are not released into the circulation, and only punctate reticulocytes increase. Despite this, most laboratories report only aggregate reticulocyte counts in cats. Non-regenerative anemia is usually normocytic normochromic, except it may be macrocytic in some cats with anemia secondary to feline leukemia virus (FeLV) or myelodysplasia and, rarely, in dogs with certain toxins or deficiencies. Microcytosis is seen with iron-deficiency anemia, which is usually regenerative. Macrocytosis is normal in some poodles, and microcytosis is normal in Akitas and Shebas; when these dogs become anemic, indices must be interpreted with caution.

ANEMIA OF CHRONIC DISEASE (ANEMIA OF INFLAMMATORY DISEASE)

The most common cause of anemia in dogs and cats is anemia of chronic disease, which accompanies infection, neoplasia, and other debilitating diseases. The anemia is mild to moderate in severity and develops slowly over 2 to 3 weeks, with the hematocrit seldom dropping below 25 per cent in dogs. Because feline red cells have a shorter life span than those of dogs, the hematocrit may drop more quickly in cats and to a greater degree, perhaps as low as 15 per cent. The anemia is usually normocytic normochromic, but in rare cases it may be microcytic and hypochromic, leading to confusion with iron deficiency. Generally, the abnormalities associated with the underlying disease overshadow the anemia, which is often asymptomatic.

Several factors are involved in the pathogenesis of anemia of chronic disease. Cytokines are a family of peptides that include interleukins, interferons, tumor necrosis factor, and certain hematopoietic growth factors. They are secreted by fibroblasts, endothelial cells, lymphocytes, macrophages, and some hematopoietic cells in response to infections and other tissue injury. Some cytokines as well as bacterial by-products such as endotoxin can inhibit erythropoiesis.

Chronic diseases are associated with impairment of transfer of storage iron from macrophages back to hematopoietic tissue. Normally, iron is released into the plasma, bound to transferrin, and transported back to the marrow to be incorporated into newly developing red cell precursors. Because 95 per cent of the iron used for red cell production comes from reutilization of senescent red cell iron, a delay in release of iron from macrophages limits the availability of iron. The sequestered iron is taken up by apoferritin in macrophages to form ferritin, the storage form of iron (Fig. 178–3).[2] Excessive iron remains in the marrow, and serum ferritin is normal to high, especially in dogs. Serum ferritin concentrations correlate reasonably well with total body stores of iron, and species-specific assays have been validated for use in dogs but are not readily available for clinical practice. Serum iron is decreased in anemia of chronic disease, but the iron-binding capacity (transferrin) does not increase. The iron saturation of transferrin is low to normal. As aptly stated by Babior and Stossel, the red cells then find themselves in Coleridge's ancient mariner's predicament, except that what they need and cannot get is iron, not water.[2]

Whether this decrease in serum iron is in any way beneficial to the patient is not clear. It has been suggested that part of the pathogenicity of bacteria is to compete with the host for iron; by making iron unavailable to the bacteria, the host can overcome the infection. If this does play a role in elimination of pathogenic bacteria, it is probably a minor one.

Secretion of erythropoietin is decreased as well as the response to erythropoietin of committed red cell progenitors, the earlier burst-forming units (BFU-E), and the later colony-forming units (CFU-E). Red cells that are produced have shortened survival, possibly because of increased uptake of red cells by activated macrophages in the spleen. An immune mechanism may also be involved in decreased red cell survival. Cats with experimentally induced anemia of chronic disease had evidence of IgG on red cells and increased phagocytosis by macrophages.[3]

Several studies of anemia of chronic disease have been conducted in animals.[3, 4] Inflammation was induced by subcutaneous injection of an irritant resulting in abscess formation. In dogs, anemia developed after 2 to 3 weeks, whereas in cats the hematocrit decreased from 9 to 15 per cent over approximately 1 week.[4] Much of this loss was caused by destruction of red cells, as determined by chromium release assays. In these cats, serum iron concentrations decreased over the same time period and erythropoietin concentrations did not increase. Although shortened red cell life span was

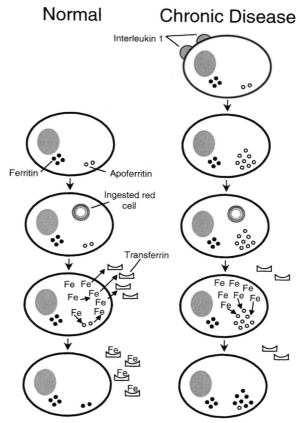

Figure 178–3. Proposed basis for the anemia of chronic disease. In inflammatory states, a cytokine is released that stimulates the synthesis of apoferritin by mononuclear phagocytes. As a result, some of the iron released into the phagocyte during the breakdown of ingested red cells is not secreted into the plasma, its usual fate, but instead is taken up by the extra apoferritin to form ferritin, the storage form of iron. Iron stores are thereby increased at the expense of the iron supply available for red cell production. (From Babior BM, Stossel TP: Hematology, A Pathophysiological Approach, 2nd ed. New York, Churchill Livingstone, 1990, p 55, with permission.)

thought to be the major cause of the initial drop in hematocrit, it obviously was not the only cause because an appropriate erythropoietin and reticulocyte response failed to develop, thus inhibiting an expected marrow response to the red cell destruction.

A similar response was demonstrated inadvertently in a study of the reticulocyte response to blood loss in normal cats (Figs. 178–4 and 178–5).[1] In this study, blood (13.6 mL/lb) was removed from 6 cats and the hematocrit and reticulocyte counts were monitored over the next month. As expected, reticulocytosis and recovery of hematocrit occurred in five cats, but one developed signs of a mild upper respiratory tract viral infection 5 days after blood loss. The aggregate reticulocyte count dropped abruptly to zero and did not increase until signs of the infection subsided. The punctate reticulocytes remained stable for the duration of the 6-day illness and then increased. This shows not only the effect of inflammation but also that anemia of chronic disease may be multifactorial, depending on both the underlying disease and other superimposed factors. These might include malnutrition, chronic blood loss through repeated blood sampling or gastrointestinal losses, renal failure, consumption coagulopathy, drugs used in treatment, or even marrow infiltration with malignant cells.

HEM

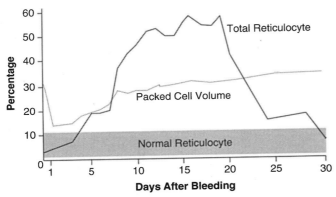

Figure 178–4. Mean percent total (aggregate plus punctate) reticulocyte response and packed cell volume in five normal cats after removal of 30 mL blood/kg body weight. The initial reticulocyte response is followed by a period of stable values reflecting the maturation of reticulocytes from aggregate to punctate to mature red cells. Most reticulocytes were punctate, with less than 1 per cent aggregate present at any time. (Adapted from Cramer DV, Lewis RM: Reticulocyte response in the cat. JAVMA 160:61, 1972, with permission.)

If the anemia is severe, a secondary cause must be sought because typically the hematocrit in anemia of chronic disease ranges from the low end of the reference range to 10 to 15 per cent below it and is rarely severe enough to cause clinical signs. Specific treatment of anemia of chronic disease is neither necessary nor beneficial. Iron supplementation should not be used. If the underlying disease is reversible, the hematocrit will return to normal.

ANEMIA SECONDARY TO CHRONIC RENAL DISEASE

Erythropoietin is produced normally by peritubular endothelial cells in the renal cortex at a rate inversely proportional to the oxygen content of the blood. It most effectively stimulates the later committed erythroid progenitors, CFU-E, and at higher concentrations also stimulates the earlier BFU-E. When renal failure becomes chronic, production of erythropoietin decreases and anemia ensues. Erythropoietin concentration may be low or normal in an anemic animal when one would expect that an appropriate response should

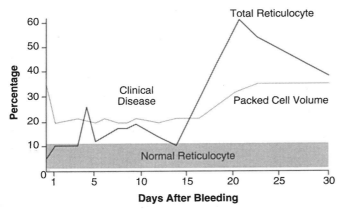

Figure 178–5. The same information as in Figure 178–4 in a single cat that developed a viral upper respiratory tract infection from days 5 through 11 after removal of 30 mL blood/kg body weight showing a temporary halt to red blood cell production. (From Cramer DV, Lewis RM: Reticulocyte response in the cat. JAVMA 160:61, 1972, with permission.)

be an increased concentration. The presence or absence of anemia can be a clue in determining whether renal failure is acute or chronic. In some cases, especially in cats, the clinical signs of anemia rather than those of renal failure are the reason that the patient is brought to the veterinarian. In a survey of feline red cell transfusions given at Tufts University, renal failure was one of the most common reasons for transfusion.

Chronically azotemic patients may become anemic for additional reasons, including decreased life span of red cells, blood loss from gastric ulcers, and abnormal platelet function. If the blood urea nitrogen level is elevated disproportionately to that of creatinine, this could be an indication of gastrointestinal blood loss. Proposed causes of decreased red cell survival include decreased utilization of the hexose monophosphate shunt, resulting in oxidative damage to red cells, and toxic effects of urea, phenols, and other retained substances. The oxidative damage to feline red cells may be evident by the presence of Heinz bodies. In cats with chronic renal failure, those with circulating Heinz bodies were more anemic than those without Heinz bodies.[5] A protective effect of the retention of phosphorus in renal failure is the increase in 2,3-diphosphoglycerate in dogs, which improves oxygen delivery to tissues despite a reduced red cell mass.

Treatment with recombinant erythropoietin has been of significant benefit to human patients with chronic renal failure. Although progression of renal failure continues, the quality of life improves as the need for red cell transfusions is removed. Recombinant human erythropoietin (r-HuEPO) has also been used with some success in comparable canine and feline patients. The structures of erythropoietins of these species are similar but not identical to that of humans. When dogs and cats are treated with r-HuEPO at a starting dose of 70 units/lb three times per week, reticulocytosis is usually evident by the end of the first week and the hematocrit is corrected within 3 to 4 weeks. Because of increased demands on the marrow for erythropoiesis, iron supplementation is indicated at least until the hematocrit is stabilized. Decreased concentrations of serum iron have been documented in approximately 30 per cent of these patients.[6] Ferrous sulfate, 100 to 300 mg/d for dogs and 50 to 100 mg/d for cats, can be given orally. Because iron can irritate the stomach, patients must be monitored carefully. Because of species differences in erythropoietin and because r-HuEPO is suspended in human albumin, allergic reactions or anti-erythropoietin antibodies may develop in up to 50 per cent of dogs and cats any time from 4 weeks to several months into treatment and require the treatment be stopped.[7] Because antibodies react also against endogenous erythropoietin, long-term transfusion therapy may be required. In some patients the antibodies decline over time, but repeated therapy is less likely to be successful.

Administration of H_2 blockers such as cimetidine or ranitidine helps to minimize the risk of additional blood loss through ulceration of the gastrointestinal tract. Anabolic steroids such as oxymetholone or hematinics have minimal if any benefit in reversing anemia secondary to renal failure.

ANEMIA SECONDARY TO NUTRITIONAL DEFICIENCIES

Lack of production of red cells can be the result of general malnutrition or decreased concentrations of iron or vitamins critical to normal red cell production.

IRON

Although iron-deficiency anemia is often classified as a non-regenerative microcytic hypochromic anemia, most cases are regenerative, caused by slow chronic or intermittent blood loss, often from the gastrointestinal tract.[8] Because of continued oral iron intake, the marrow responds with reticulocytosis. In *rare* instances in dogs or cats in which iron deficiency is truly nutritional, marrow response is blunted. Because significant iron is present in a normal meat-containing diet of dogs and cats, only a highly abnormal diet would cause a nutritional iron deficiency.

FOLATE AND COBALAMIN

Folate is required for synthesis of three of the four base pairs in DNA. The vitamin is initially inert and is activated by means of dehydrofolate reductase to tetrahydrofolate and is then incorporated into nucleic acid. The marrow is significantly affected by inhibition of DNA synthesis. In most tissues, cell division occurs only as needed for repair, whereas synthesis of hematopoietic cells occurs constantly. All cell lines of the marrow are affected, but morphologic changes are most evident in erythroid precursors. The granulocytic precursors are also affected, resulting in giant band or hypersegmented neutrophils. Despite the decrease in DNA synthesis in folate deficiency, RNA and protein synthesis remains normal. Asynchrony of maturation (megaloblastosis) occurs in that the nucleus of erythroid precursors matures more slowly than does the cytoplasm. Skipped mitoses result in enlarged mature red cells and an increased mean corpuscular volume.

Because of the abnormality in production, some precursors do not survive the development process and die while still in the marrow. The end result is ineffective hematopoiesis seen in the blood as variable combinations of anemia, neutropenia, and thrombocytopenia.

A deficiency of cobalamin (vitamin B_{12}) can cause a clinical and hematologic picture identical to that of folate deficiency. Cobalamin functions in folate metabolism and in degradation of fatty acids, so that deficiency causes megaloblastosis and neurologic abnormalities. In humans, a deficiency of cobalamin is usually caused by a lack of gastric production of intrinsic factor and is called pernicious anemia. Intrinsic factor, in the presence of increased pH in the duodenum, attaches to cobalamin and subsequently to specific receptors on mucosal cells in the ileum, allowing for absorption. In dogs and cats, intrinsic factor is produced in the pancreas, rather than in the stomach.[9] Removal of seven eighths of the stomach, the duodenum, and 30 cm of the jejunum from normal dogs did not result in macrocytic anemia.[10]

Folate is present in most foods and synthesized by intestinal bacteria, so nutritional deficiency is rare.[11] Cobalamin is also present in the normal dog or cat diet. Folate and cobalamin deficiencies have been produced by feeding artificial diets to dogs and cats. Anemia from folate deficiency occurred after 2 to 4 months in dogs, but much longer was required for clinical signs of cobalamin deficiency to occur because of prolonged hepatic storage. The anemia in both deficiencies was not overtly macrocytic as described in humans. Instead, it was normocytic normochromic with some macrocytes seen on blood smears and magaloblastosis in the marrow.[12]

Abnormalities in folate or cobalamin have been documented in certain maldigestion, malabsorption, or bacterial overgrowth syndromes in dogs and cats.[13] Malabsorption or exocrine pancreatic insufficiency (EPI) results in folate or cobalamin deficiency only in severe chronic cases. The lack of intrinsic factor in EPI may contribute to the finding of low cobalamin concentrations, because concentrations remain low even after enzyme replacement therapy.[14] Folate may be increased in EPI because of enhanced absorption secondary to decreased intestinal pH.[15] In dogs with intestinal bacterial overgrowth, cobalamin may be decreased because of bacterial utilization and folate increased because of production by bacteria. Anemia is not present in these situations unless the condition is severe and prolonged. Diagnosis is by finding decreased serum folate or cobalamin concentrations. Successful treatment of the underlying disease would allow folate or cobalamin concentrations to normalize. Supplementation can be used in severe deficiencies.

An autosomal recessive inherited malabsorption of cobalamin has been described in giant schnauzers.[16] This rare defect is caused by an absence of the receptor for the intrinsic factor–cobalamin complex in the ileal brush border. A chronic non-regenerative anemia (PCV, 21 to 33 per cent) and neutropenia (1760 to 4400/μL) are present. A similar condition occurs in border collies and is suspected in Shar Pei dogs.[12] Treatment is parenteral cobalamin given intermittently for life (0.5–1 mg IM daily for 7 days, then every 3 to 6 months as needed).

Certain chemotherapeutic drugs inhibit folate. Methotrexate inhibits dihydrofolate reductase and at high doses can cause megaloblastic anemia. It is sometimes used with citrovorum factor, a reduced folate that bypasses the block. Hydroxyurea, which inhibits DNA synthesis, causes a mild-to-moderate macrocytic anemia in dogs and humans. This anemia, which has megaloblastic changes in the marrow, resembles the anemia of folate or cobalamin deficiency but is not associated with a decrease in either. Other chemotherapeutic drugs that may induce folate deficiency are 5-fluorouracil and cytarabine.

Megaloblastic anemia has occasionally been seen in dogs treated with anticonvulsive agents primidone, phenytoin, or phenobarbital.[17] A combination of phenytoin and primidone caused macrocytic anemia, neutropenia with hypersegmented neutrophils, and thrombocytopenia in a dog, but in a later series of dogs treated with these same drugs, these abnormalities were not observed. The true prevalence is not known but is probably uncommon. Fenbendazole and quinidine have also been implicated as causes of macrocytic anemia in isolated cases.

Macrocytic, non-regenerative anemia occurs in cats with FeLV infection and in dogs or cats with myelodysplasia. Here, skipped mitoses and ineffective hematopoiesis are the probable mechanisms. Treatment of these patients with folate or cobalamin is of no benefit because serum concentrations are normal. Macrocytosis is seen as an inherited condition in some families of poodles. These dogs have mean corpuscular volumes ranging from 85 to 95 fL (normal, 60–77 fL) but are not anemic and have no clinical signs of illness even though some megaloblastosis is present in the marrow. No treatment is indicated.

OTHER DEFICIENCIES

Experimentally induced copper, niacin, vitamin B_6, or riboflavin deficiency resulted in non-regenerative anemia in the dog, but these are unlikely causes of naturally occurring anemia.[12]

HEM

ANEMIA SECONDARY TO METABOLIC DISORDERS

A mild normocytic normochromic anemia (hematocrit, 28 to 35 per cent) is present in 30 to 50 per cent of hypothyroid dogs.[18] Increased target cells may be seen occasionally on blood smears because of changes caused by increased red cell membrane cholesterol. The anemia, which is usually not symptomatic, may be secondary to decreased oxygen consumption because of slowed metabolism. Thyroid supplementation results in resolution of the anemia.

Mild anemia may also be associated with hypopituitarism, hypoadrenalcorticism, decreased growth hormone, and pregnancy. In pregnant animals, the red cell mass is probably normal but the plasma volume is slightly increased. Anemia in animals with hepatic disease may be caused in part by a decrease in adenosine triphosphate, resulting in a shortened red cell life span, but anemia of chronic disease may play a role as well.

NON-REGENERATIVE ANEMIA—IMMUNE MEDIATED

Most immune-mediated destruction of red cells occurs within the periphery—either intravascular or extravascular hemolysis, with reticulocytosis, a positive Coombs' test, and spherocytosis. Some cases are so acute that sufficient time (3 to 4 days) has not elapsed to allow for reticulocytosis. These acute hemolytic anemias initially appear to be non-regenerative but usually have other signs of hemolysis such as hemoglobinemia or icterus.

In other cases, reticulocytes and even earlier red cell precursors are destroyed in the marrow. These patients, usually dogs, may have a gradual onset of normocytic normochromic non-regenerative anemia. The bone marrow may show erythroid hypoplasia or evidence of erythrophagocytosis (intramedullary destruction of cells). Increased numbers of lymphocytes and plasma cells may be present, implying an immune response.

Serum from human and canine patients with red cell aplasia has suppressed in vitro growth of erythroid precursors.[19] Eight dogs with non-regenerative anemia and decreased red cell precursors in the marrow were studied. A serum IgG inhibitor directed against CFU-E was found in three of five that were Coombs negative and one of three that were Coombs positive. These antibodies were not likely to be alloantibodies (directed against foreign blood group antigens) because none of the dogs had received prior transfusions. Autologous marrow taken from one dog after recovery was inhibited from growing in vitro when incubated with autologous serum taken at the time of illness.

Diagnosis of the non-regenerative form of immune-mediated hemolytic anemia may be relatively easy if the dog is Coombs positive or has spherocytosis, but in other cases it may be made only by excluding other causes of non-regenerative anemia. A bone marrow aspirate can be done to rule out other causes of ineffective erythropoiesis. If no other cause is found, treatment of presumed immune-mediated etiology is warranted. Prednisone is generally used first and other drugs such as azathioprine, cyclophosphamide, or cyclosporine are added if needed. In one review, 42 per cent of dogs responded to prednisone alone whereas 75 per cent responded to prednisone and cyclophosphamide.[20] Intravenous human immunoglobulin was successful when given to five dogs with non-regenerative anemia as an infusion (0.5–0.7 g/lb) over 6 to 12 hours.[21] All had a rapid response, and the two dogs that had relapses were successfully re-treated. A mild thrombocytopenia (32,000–89,000/μL) occurred in some dogs, and thromboembolism has been a concern. Just as the onset of the nonregenerative form of immune-mediated hemolytic anemia may have a slow, insidious onset, the response to treatment may also be slow. Red cell precursors must be restored before the hematocrit can rise, and this may take 1 to 2 weeks or longer if antibody persists.

INFECTIONS

RETROVIRUSES

Feline leukemia virus commonly causes a severe, usually nonregenerative anemia, which may be macrocytic or normocytic and normochromic (Table 178–2). Whenever macrocytic anemia occurs without reticulocytosis in a cat, FeLV infection should be suspected. Macrocytosis is often associated with abnormalities in the marrow (myelodysplasia). Macrocytic non-regenerative anemia occurs to a lesser extent, if at all, with feline immunodeficiency virus (FIV) infection. In long-term experimental FeLV and FIV infections only cats with FeLV developed macrocytic anemia.[22] Those infected with FIV were observed over several years, and most remained asymptomatic or developed only mild anemia. FIV is more likely to suppress granulocytic progenitors than erythroid progenitors in marrow cultures.[23]

Retroviruses cause anemia by several mechanisms. The virus may directly suppress the marrow. Coexisting infections in immunosuppressed cats lead to anemia of chronic disease. Anemia may also be secondary to coexisting marrow abnormalities such as fibrosis, dysplasia, or malignancy. Essentially, FeLV can affect any or all hematopoietic cell lines and cause suppression (cytopenias), abnormal maturation, or malignant transformation. It has been reported that approximately 70 per cent of anemic cats (hematocrit < 20 per cent) are FeLV positive.[24] This was equivalent to the frequency at that time of viremia in cats with lymphoma and leukemia. Some cats with latent FeLV infection may develop hematopoietic malignancy; perhaps they could also develop anemia. Subsequent to those studies, the prevalence of FeLV has decreased in cats in the United States because testing, and to a lesser extent vaccination, has eliminated infection in most catteries, shelters, and multicat households.[25] The incidence of anemia has probably decreased as well, although current epidemiologic studies have not been done.

The pathogenesis of FeLV-associated anemia is complex. The three subgroups (A, B, and C) had different effects in experimental infection of kittens.[26] Subgroup A caused a transient macrocytic anemia with a regenerative marrow

TABLE 178–2. MECHANISMS OF FELINE LEUKEMIA VIRUS–INDUCED ANEMIA

Non-regenerative anemia
  Red cell aplasia
  Anemia of chronic disease
  Aplastic anemia
  Myelodysplasia
  Myelofibrosis
  Acute leukemia (lymphoblastic or myelogenous)
Regenerative anemia (rare)
  Immune mediated
  Recovery from prior anemia

response; subgroup B did not cause any disease. Subgroup C, which, like B, arises from A by recombination with endogenous feline gene sequences, induced fatal red cell aplasia. Subgroup C has also been associated with naturally occurring anemia in both viremic and nonviremic cats.[27] When virus was inoculated into neonatal kittens, approximately 90 per cent became viremic and anemic about 5 weeks later.[28] When the same viral inoculation was given to kittens 4 to 8 weeks old, only 1 of 22 (4.5 per cent) became anemic within 12 weeks of inoculation. When the marrow of neonatally infected kittens was grown in culture, both BFU-E and CFU-E were found to be depleted.[28, 29] Despite the drastic reduction of erythrogenesis, myeloid development remained normal. The mechanism of impairment was thought to be direct inhibition of erythroid progenitors by viral gene products or interaction with lymphoreticular cells, especially T cells, which normally produce necessary hematopoietic growth factors. Because FeLV infects erythroid progenitors, it is also possible that a host immunopathologic response against infected cells could cause their destruction, but evidence for this is lacking. Anemia induced experimentally by FeLV-C is not associated with a clonal expansion of T cells.[30] In addition, T cells from cats with FeLV-induced anemia did not inhibit in vitro erythroid colony growth of normal or autologous marrow.

When presented with an FeLV-positive cat with non-regenerative anemia, one must first search for other co-existing systemic problems. Fever was present in approximately 25 per cent of anemic FeLV-positive cats, even though the virus itself does not cause fever.[24] Successful treatment of co-existing problems such as respiratory infections or hemobartonellosis could result in spontaneous improvement in the anemia. About half of a group of FeLV-positive anemic cats had circulating nucleated red cells even though no correlation was found between the number of nucleated red cells and the magnitude of the reticulocyte count.[24] These cats, like many FeLV-negative cats, commonly exhibit pica by eating litter or licking rusty objects. This is not an indication of iron deficiency; in fact, FeLV-positive anemic cats usually have normal or elevated serum iron concentrations. Iron supplementation not only fails to improve the anemia, it may cause anorexia, gastric upset, and even iron overload, especially if transfusions are given as well.

Many FeLV-positive anemic cats die or are euthanized because of refractory anemia, a few develop leukemia or myelodysplasia, and a few recover. Of 100 FeLV-positive anemic cats, only 29 were treated for longer than 2 weeks.[24] Eight of those recovered, and all remained viremic. Reasons for euthanasia included concerns about prognosis, cost of treatment, or danger to other household cats. Those treated received antibiotics for coexisting infections, and some received corticosteroids. Whether response to corticosteroids implied an immune-mediated cause is unknown.

So far the only evidence for response to biological response modifiers such as *Propionibacterium acnes* or interferons is anecdotal, and many of the cats that responded also received other medications. In one study, oral interferon alfa showed no benefit compared with a saline placebo in clinically ill viremic cats. A similar group improved when treated with intraperitoneal Staph protein A, but the benefit was lost when Staph protein A was followed by interferon.[31] Although it seems unlikely that interferon would inhibit the efficacy of Staph protein A, further studies are needed.

RICKETTSIAL INFECTIONS

Anemia is commonly present in dogs with ehrlichiosis and is usually non-regenerative unless associated with hem-

orrhage from thrombocytopenia, or if hemolysis from concurrent babesiosis is present. The marrow may be hypercellular with an increased myeloid:erythroid ratio in the acute phase, but the chronic phase is characterized by pancytopenia and hypoplasia of the marrow except for plasmacytosis, which is regularly present. Most canine ehrlichiosis in the United States is caused by *Ehrlichia canis*, which infects primarily monocytes. Recently, a granulocytic ehrlichiosis has been described in dogs in the eastern part of the United States possibly associated with *E. equi* or *E. ewingii*.[32] In New York and New England the prevalence of both human and canine granulocytic ehrlichiosis may be increasing. Platelets seem to be primarily affected, but a normocytic normochromic anemia and sometimes polyarthritis may occur as well.

Babesiosis in dogs usually causes a hemolytic anemia, but occasionally the anemia may be non-regenerative.

Hemobartonellosis in cats may sometimes be associated with non-regenerative anemia. In these cases, the organism may be an opportunist, affecting immunosuppressed or debilitated cats. These cats should be tested for retroviruses or other abnormalities. Even if only occasional *Haemobartonella* organisms are seen in a non-regenerative anemia, the organisms may be contributing to the anemia and should be treated.

HYPERESTROGENISM

Elevated estrogen concentration interferes with stem cell differentiation and results in pancytopenia and marrow aplasia (aplastic anemia). Estrogen concentrations may be increased because of endogenous or iatrogenic causes. The toxic effects of estrogen in dogs are well known and have been studied best in cases of overdose of estrogens, especially estradiol cyclopentylpropionate, which has been used in the past to prevent pregnancy or treat prostatic hyperplasia.[33] When sequential hemograms have been performed, neutrophilia occurs in the first 2 to 3 weeks, followed by neutropenia, thrombocytopenia, and anemia. Those dogs that recovered did so after 30 to 70 days; however, most affected dogs died.

Hyperestrogenism has been seen in male dogs with testicular tumors and rarely in female dogs with granulosa cell tumors of the ovary. In a report of 209 testicular tumors, 60 were Sertoli cell tumors, 62 were seminomas, and 87 were interstitial cell tumors.[34] Ten cases of pancytopenia occurred, 8 with Sertoli cell tumors and 1 each with seminoma and interstitial cell tumor. Eight of these 10 dogs showed signs of feminization, and seven of the involved testes were abdominal. The dog with the seminoma had an XY karyotype but a uterus masculinus and was the only one of the 10 pancytopenic dogs to recover.

An estrogen-induced, often fatal pancytopenia occurs related to the estrous cycle of female ferrets. They may remain in nearly a constant state of estrous from March to August if not induced to ovulate. For this reason ovariohysterectomy should be performed on all young female pet ferrets that are not to be bred.

DRUGS AND TOXINS

Toxins such as benzene, phenol, organophosphate, and chlorinated hydrocarbon insecticides can suppress all cell lines of the marrow, although the number of reported cases

HEM

in pets is low. Drugs have been implicated more commonly (Table 178–3).

Anticancer drugs including alkylating agents, anthracyclines, and antimetabolites are myelosuppressive. Neutropenia is most likely to occur because the neutrophil life span in the circulation is only a few hours and constant replacement is needed. In more severe cases, platelets may decrease as well, but because of the long life span of circulating red cells (90–120 days), cessation of production for a short time does not cause a significant drop in hematocrit.

Nitrosoureas (e.g., carmustine, lomustine) have been considered to be especially cytotoxic to the more slowly dividing stem cells, whereas most other chemotherapeutic drugs affect only the more actively dividing cells such as myelocytes. With most myelosuppressive drugs the neutrophil nadir occurs 5 to 7 days after a drug is given and recovers 2 or 3 days later. Loss of myelocytes can quickly be reversed by increased production of earlier granulocytic precursors. When early progenitors or stem cells are killed, recovery takes longer and cumulative permanent marrow damage is more likely. Clinical use of lomustine in dogs has not caused the delayed nadir and prolonged recovery commonly observed in humans, although repeated doses have resulted in a progressive thrombocytopenia, which sometimes has been permanent.[35] Anemia has not been a significant problem. One dog treated for 6 months with melphalan suddenly developed pancytopenia, which persisted for 9 months before resolution, despite withdrawal of all myelosuppressive therapy. A study in cats receiving busulfan showed incomplete stem cell recovery up to 6 years after the drug was stopped.[36] The number of pluripotent stem cells is fixed at birth with no mechanism for new ones to be produced.

Phenylbutazone has been a significant cause of irreversible aplasia of the marrow in dogs, even at recommended doses used for relatively short periods of time, or after weeks to months. Delayed metabolism or clearance of phenylbutazone has been observed in some human patients suffering aplastic anemia after treatment, but this has not been investigated in affected dogs. A single case of marrow suppression caused by another non-steroidal anti-inflammatory drug meclofenamic acid was reported in a dog.[37] It is best to avoid using these drugs in dogs because other effective and safer alternatives exist. If phenylbutazone is used, owners should be advised of the potential risks. Periodic monitoring of the hemogram is not likely to be helpful because significant

TABLE 178–3. DRUGS CAUSING NON-REGENERATIVE ANEMIA OR PANCYTOPENIA

Cancer chemotherapy*
  Alkylating agents—cyclophosphamide, melphalan, busulfan, chlorambucil
  Antibiotics—doxorubicin, mitoxantrone, dactinomycin
  Antimetabolites—methotrexate, cytarabine
  Others—carboplatin, nitrosoureas, hydroxyurea
Estrogen
  Estradiol cyclopentylpropionate (ECP)
Non-steroidal anti-inflammatory drugs
  Phenylbutazone, meclofenamic acid
Antibacterials
  Sulfonamides, trimethoprim, cefazedone, cefadroxil, chloramphenicol
Anticonvulsants
  Phenobarbital, primidone, phenytoin
Other drugs
  Albendazole, fenbendazole, propylthiouracil, methimazole, quinidine, griseofulvin, thiacetarsamide

*Most cause neutropenia ± thrombocytopenia rather than anemia.

damage to the marrow may have already occurred by the time changes are evident on the hemogram.

Chloramphenicol causes a dose-dependent marrow suppression, more severe in cats than dogs. The irreversible idiosyncratic marrow aplasia seen in humans has not been reported in dogs or cats. Because aplastic anemia has occurred in humans after minimal exposure, one must consider the risks to pet owners handling oral preparations and gloves should be worn when the drug is given. Safer antibiotics are available for most canine and feline infections, so chloramphenicol is rarely the antibiotic of choice.

Sulfonamides, especially those containing trimethoprim, act as folate antagonists, causing normocytic normochromic anemia without megaloblastosis and, in rare cases, aplastic anemia.[38]

Other drugs that have been associated with marrow suppression are listed in Table 178–3. Albendazole and fenbendazole caused reversible cytopenias in dogs and cats treated for parasites.[37, 39] A dose-dependent marrow suppression had previously been demonstrated in beagles during drug development.

Anticonvulsants such as phenobarbital, primidone, and phenytoin have caused neutropenia, thrombocytopenia, or pancytopenia.[17, 40] Methimazole has caused reversible leukopenia and thrombocytopenia in up to 20 per cent of cats treated for hyperthyroidism.[41] Despite this, it has fewer adverse hematologic effects than the previously used propylthiouracil.

Griseofulvin has caused aplastic anemia in cats, especially those infected with retroviruses. Because immunosuppression predisposes to ringworm infection, these cats are also the most likely to receive the drug. Alternative treatments should be used if possible.

The mechanisms of marrow damage from drugs may be direct toxicity to progenitors, immune-mediated destruction, or interference with enzymes or other hematopoietic factors. Any animal presenting with red cell aplasia or pancytopenia should be evaluated for exposure to toxins or drugs, and whenever possible these should be eliminated. Depending on the offending agent, recovery may be rapid or the effect may be irreversible.

PURE RED CELL APLASIA

Pure red cell aplasia is defined as a non-regenerative, normocytic normochromic anemia with a selective reduction of erythroid precursors in the marrow. Many cases are idiopathic, but after renal failure and drugs and toxins are ruled out, the most common cause in dogs is probably immune mediated. In cats, FeLV is probably the most common cause. In humans, thymomas and occasionally other malignancies may cause pure red cell aplasia, but this syndrome has not been reported in dogs or cats.[42]

APLASTIC ANEMIA

Pancytopenia is defined as a decrease in red cells, granulocytes, and platelets in the blood. Aplastic anemia is defined as pancytopenia with decreased production of all three cell lines in the marrow and replacement with fat. With aplastic anemia, typically less than 25 per cent of the marrow is composed of hematopoietic cells, primarily lymphocytes and plasma cells.

A bone marrow core biopsy is required for the diagnosis

of aplastic anemia. If an aspirate only is performed, the sample may appear hypocellular, but it may not be obvious whether this was sampling error or true aplasia. Aspirates are most useful for morphologic evaluation of individual cells, but biopsies are needed to determine the degree of cellularity and presence or absence of infiltration with fat or fibrous connective tissue (myelofibrosis).

Many disease processes can interfere temporarily or permanently with the viability of the pleuripotent stem cell, resulting in aplastic anemia. Affected animals are at risk for bacterial sepsis from granulocytopenia or bleeding from thrombocytopenia. In most cases, neutropenia occurs first, then thrombocytopenia, and finally anemia. The hematocrit may fall more quickly if significant bleeding occurs. Some lymphocytes may persist in the blood and marrow, but often lymphopenia is present as well, with only long-lived memory cells surviving.

Most cases of aplastic anemia are idiopathic. In humans, a correctable cause is identified in less than 10 per cent of cases but some physical, chemical, and biologic causes are recognized.[43] Ionizing radiation at doses over 7 Gy will cause permanent aplasia of the marrow. This is unlikely to occur in dogs or cats because whole-body irradiation is rarely used clinically except in preparation for bone marrow transplantation. Some cases in humans, dogs, and perhaps cats appear to be immune mediated. Antibodies or T-cell suppression could be directed against stem cells or factors promoting their growth. Some human cases have responded to corticosteroids alone or with immunosuppressive drugs such as cyclosporine or anti-thymocyte globulin. Relapses have sometimes occurred when treatment was stopped. A few human patients given very aggressive immunosuppression in preparation for bone marrow transplantation have had recovery of their own marrow.[43]

A syndrome of reversible aplastic anemia has been observed at Tufts University in seven dogs younger than 2 years of age. In these dogs, the marrow recovered in as short a time as 2 to 3 weeks or as long as 4 to 5 months after diagnosis. Drugs, toxins, and vaccines were ruled out as potential causes. Most of these dogs received non-myelosuppressive immunosuppressive drugs such as prednisone alone or, in two dogs, prednisone and cyclosporine. An immune-mediated or possibly a viral cause was suspected but not proven.

In cats, FeLV commonly causes red cell aplasia or aplastic anemia. In humans, viruses such as hepatitis, herpes (Epstein-Barr virus), or parvovirus (B19) have been implicated as causes of red cell aplasia or aplastic anemia. Those persons affected often have some underlying abnormality causing increased proliferation and shortened life span of red cells. For example, humans with sickle cell anemia have ongoing rapid turnover of red cells. Superimposed infection with parvovirus stops red cell production and the hematocrit drops rapidly as circulating cells are destroyed and not replaced.

Feline parvovirus (panleukopenia) causes in vitro inhibition of both granulocytic and erythroid progenitor cells.[44] Parvoviruses grow best in rapidly dividing cells such as marrow and intestinal epithelium. Recovery occurs as antibodies develop except in immunosuppressed patients in whom prolonged aplasia may occur. Although neither canine nor feline parvoviruses have been proven to cause aplastic anemia, it is tempting to speculate that a parvovirus could have an effect in dogs or cats similar to that seen in humans.

Aplastic anemia caused by drugs or toxins is treated by withdrawal of the offending agent, and supportive care is begun. Aggressive appropriate antibiotic therapy is used whenever fever or other signs of infection occur. In this situation, immunosuppressive drugs are probably of no benefit and may increase the risk of sepsis.

In idiopathic aplastic anemia, immunosuppression should be tried because of the possibility of an immune-mediated cause. Corticosteroids are often used initially because myelosuppressive drugs such as azathioprine or cyclophosphamide increase the risk of bacterial sepsis. An alternative choice, although of unproven benefit in veterinary medicine, would be cyclosporine, which can be given orally at doses of 4.5 mg/lb per day in dogs and every 12 hours in cats. Absorption is improved if cyclosporine is administered with a fatty meal or if a microemulsion formulation (Neoral) is used. Because of variable absorption, trough concentrations should be measured periodically with a recommended whole-blood concentration of 200 to 300 ng/mL. Adverse effects described in dogs include anorexia, vomiting, diarrhea, weight loss, gingival hyperplasia, papillomatosis, hirsutism, and trembling when trough concentrations approach 400 ng/mL.[45]

Androgens or other anabolic steroids are rarely of benefit. Hematopoietic growth factors such as erythropoietin and granulocyte colony-stimulating factor are generally of only transient benefit in humans and do not alter the course of the disease. The same is probably true in dogs and cats, although granulocyte colony-stimulating factor can be used short term if life-threatening sepsis occurs.

The prognosis for aplastic anemia is better for children in whom the cause may be viral than it is in adults in whom it is often irreversible, or intermittent and progressive. The syndrome of either self-limiting or steroid-responsive aplastic anemia in young dogs implies that the same may be true in dogs. Bone marrow transplantation offers the best chance of permanent recovery in humans with aplastic anemia. Some human patients undergo a transition of aplastic anemia to leukemia, suggesting a genetic fragility or susceptibility.

BONE MARROW STROMAL DISORDERS

MARROW NECROSIS

Marrow necrosis may occur possibly secondary to thrombosis or circulatory failure in cases of sepsis, endotoxemia, drug toxicity, malignancy, or viral infection. Pancytopenia would be seen only in severe diffuse cases. Diffuse marrow necrosis is a rare phenomenon, and it could be reversible if the underlying cause were removed.[46]

OSTEOSCLEROSIS

Osteosclerosis, which can be observed radiographically as increased bone density, has been reported rarely as an end-stage, irreversible change in chronic marrow abnormalities such as pyruvate kinase deficiency in the dog or FeLV infection in the cat.

MYELOFIBROSIS

Myelofibrosis is probably another manifestation of end-stage marrow failure (Fig. 178–6). In humans, cytogenetic evidence exists that a specific syndrome of myelofibrosis with myeloid metaplasia of the spleen and liver is associated with a clonal (malignant) expansion of granulocyte precur-

HEM

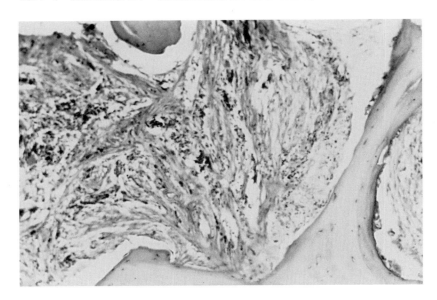

Figure 178–6. Histologic section of a bone marrow biopsy specimen on a cat with myelofibrosis. Most of the marrow space inside of the cortical bone is replaced by fibrous connective tissue at the expense of hematopoietic precursors. (Hematoxylin and eosin, × 400.)

sors and a reactive (non-malignant) proliferation of fibroblasts.[2] Excessive platelet-derived growth factor has been implicated in the stimulation of fibroblast production. Affected humans have moderate to severe splenomegaly and a leukoerythroblastic response in the blood characterized by immature granulocytes, nucleated red cells, morphologically abnormal red cells, and platelets. Eventually, pancytopenia develops as fibrosis fills the marrow. Some of the abnormal cells in the blood may come from the spleen or may be released from the marrow because of disrupted architecture.

Normally, the yolk sac is the initial site of hematopoiesis in the embryo. Later, the liver and then the spleen take over during fetal development, and by the time of birth the marrow has become the primary site of hematopoiesis. The spleen, and occasionally the liver, may revert to its previous role in situations such as myelofibrosis or dysplasia. This phenomenon is referred to as myeloid metaplasia or extramedullary hematopoiesis (EMH). The cat especially may have significant splenomegaly because of EMH. Unfortunately, the spleen is not an efficient producer of hematopoietic cells and EMH is seldom of any benefit in producing adequate numbers of hematopoietic cells. In fact, it may even be detrimental in that the very large spleen may remove more blood cells than it produces through the mechanism of hypersplenism.

A few patients are cured by bone marrow transplantation, suggesting that the primary problem involves the stem cell rather than the fibrous response, which may regress in patients having successful bone marrow transplantation. How myelofibrosis in dogs and cats fits into this picture is not known. Probably most cases are secondary to chronic primary problems, such as FeLV infection.

MYELODYSPLASIA

Myelodysplasia has a spectrum ranging from chronic non-regenerative anemia sometimes with other cytopenias to a "pre-leukemic" state with gradually increasing numbers of blasts in the marrow.[47] In some patients, acute leukemia eventually occurs. Despite peripheral cytopenias, the marrow is usually hypercellular. The reason for the disparity is that hematopoiesis is ineffective and many abnormal cells die while still in the marrow. Iron stores are increased in the

marrow as a result of loss of erythroid precursors. Cats normally have no stainable iron in the marrow, so any visible iron may imply increased turnover of erythroid precursors, perhaps combined with anemia of chronic disease. The red cells are frequently macrocytic but without reticulocytosis (Fig. 178–7). Megaloblastic changes are present in the marrow. These include slowed maturation of nuclei with relatively more mature cytoplasm, especially of erythroid cells.

In human patients, specific chromosomal abnormalities imply that myelodysplasia is a clonal disorder. Myelodysplasia occurs frequently in cats, often in association with FeLV infection, and rarely in dogs. Progression to leukemia is noted infrequently in animals, probably because so many are euthanized soon after diagnosis.

Treatment of myelodysplasia is primarily supportive with transfusions as needed. Even though it is considered to be a clonal or premalignant disorder, chemotherapy has not proven beneficial in humans; instead, it has increased morbidity and mortality. If the cytopenias are mild, affected cats can often survive comfortably for weeks to months, and a few recover spontaneously.

Erythropoietin concentrations are elevated in anemic human myelodysplasia patients; the same is true in the few cats tested. Despite this, treatment with erythropoietin has raised the hematocrit and decreased the transfusion requirements both in human and a few feline patients.[48] One such cat was treated for 4 weeks at 68 U/lb three times weekly before any sign of response was observed.

HEMATOPOIETIC MALIGNANCY

Leukemias are divided into acute and chronic because of significant differences in clinical presentation, treatment, and prognosis. The hematocrit is usually normal at the time of diagnosis of chronic lymphocytic or myelogenous leukemia, whereas pancytopenia is usually present in acute leukemias, often but not always with circulating blasts. The marrow however, is usually filled with blasts (myelophthisis) at the time of diagnosis of all forms of acute leukemia. These blasts are characterized by uncontrolled growth, failure of normal maturation and function, inappropriate infiltration of normal tissues (especially the spleen), and inhibitory effects on normal hematopoiesis. Previously it was thought that

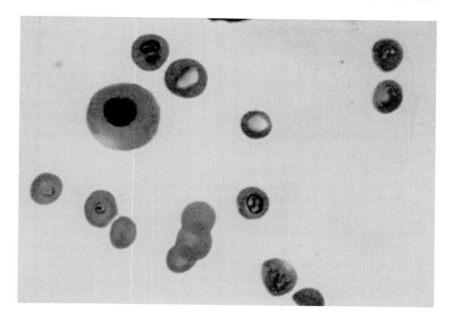

Figure 178–7. Disturbed erythroid maturation in myelodysplasia. The nucleated erythrocyte is unusually large and fully hemoglobinized yet has a retained pyknotic nucleus. (From Weiser MG: Erythrocyte responses and disorders. *In* Ettinger SJ, Feldman EC [eds]: Textbook of Veterinary Internal Medicine, 4th ed. Philadelphia, WB Saunders, 1995, p 1890, with permission.)

neoplastic cells in the marrow simply crowded out normal cells, but some soluble factor produced by the blasts is now known to inhibit in vitro growth of hematopoietic progenitors. In fact, cytopenias and hypoplasia of hematopoietic precursors in the marrow may be observed before significant proliferation of the malignant clone.[49] Regardless of the cell of origin of acute leukemia, human, canine, and feline patients usually are lethargic from non-regenerative anemia, fever or other signs of bacterial infection because of neutropenia, and petechiae or mucosal bleeding because of thrombocytopenia. One exception is that the erythroid (M6) subgroup of acute myelogenous leukemia may, especially in cats, be associated with large numbers of circulating nucleated red cells despite the presence of non-regenerative anemia. The diagnosis of acute leukemia may be obvious if numerous circulating blasts are present; however, they are absent in many patients, and examination of the marrow is necessary to differentiate leukemia from other causes of pancytopenia. The subclassification, treatment, and prognosis are discussed in Chapter 98.

Other malignant diseases that may infiltrate the marrow and cause non-regenerative anemia or pancytopenia are malignant histiocytosis and myeloma. Anemia is also a frequent complication of extensive malignancy of any type. This may be caused by some factor produced by malignant cells, perhaps in combination with some blood loss or anemia of chronic disease.

GENERAL TREATMENT CONSIDERATIONS

TRANSFUSION

For most patients with severe non-regenerative anemia, transfusion of red cells gives immediate relief from clinical signs. Red cells should be given when signs of tachycardia, tachypnea, and weakness are present, rather than at some pre-specified hematocrit. Even in a compensated chronic anemia the hematocrit should not be allowed to drop below 12 to 15 per cent. Some patients, especially those with coexisting heart or lung disease, may require transfusion at a higher hematocrit. Transfusion should not be withheld because of concern that raising the hematocrit will further

suppress erythropoiesis. Transfusion rarely raises the hematocrit to a normal level, so erythropoietin should still be produced. Because these patients may require multiple transfusions, appropriate typing and cross-matching becomes increasingly important over time.

In aplastic anemia, platelet support may be considered, especially for small dogs in which an adequate number of platelets can be obtained from a large donor. The decision to give platelets should be made based on the severity of bleeding rather than giving platelets prophylactically to thrombocytopenic patients. The efficacy of a platelet transfusion is measured by checking a platelet count within 1 hour after transfusion. For a 60-lb patient, platelets from 500 mL of blood would be expected to raise the platelet count by $10,000/\mu L$, assuming no ongoing losses from bleeding or consumption.[50]

Platelet transfusions may need to be repeated every 2 to 3 days if bleeding persists. For cats and large dogs, in which adequate platelet transfusions are difficult to supply, fresh whole blood will provide some platelets as well as red cells. Keeping the hematocrit greater than 20 per cent will also shorten the bleeding time in thrombocytopenic patients.[51] Thus, red cells not only raise the hematocrit but also minimize bleeding if platelets are not available. Dogs become refractory to platelets after repeated transfusions because they develop antibodies to histocompatibility antigens on platelet membranes.

Granulocyte support is impractical because large numbers need to be given one to two times daily. Granulocytes have been collected from human donors by pheresis, but this procedure is rarely used now because other measures such as reverse isolation, hematopoietic growth factor support, and antibiotics are used instead. Short term benefit may be obtained from granulocyte colony-stimulating factor in dogs and cats, but this eventually fails because of antibody formation. Recovery is dependent on regeneration of the marrow.

BONE MARROW TRANSPLANTATION

Because the recovery rate from idiopathic aplastic anemia is low, bone marrow transplantation (BMT) is considered the best chance for cure of those human patients who do not

HEM

respond to immunosuppressive drugs. The techniques for BMT are well known in dogs because the procedures were developed in dogs before the first humans were treated. In a practical sense, however, BMT is available for dogs or cats only in a few specialized settings.[52] The technique of the transplant is simple in that marrow withdrawn from the donor is given intravenously to the recipient. Stem cells find their way to the marrow and repopulate. Difficulties in veterinary medicine include finding a compatible donor because siblings may be difficult to find and only one in four will be compatible. Testing for histocompatibility is not readily available. In addition, the supportive care and transfusion support required during the 3 to 4 weeks before engraftment occurs can be extensive. Even with a compatible donor, graft-versus-host disease (GVHD) can cause significant morbidity and even death. Graft-versus-host disease is the result of transplanted immune cells mounting an immune response against the recipient of the marrow. Signs of GVHD include diarrhea, hepatic failure, and skin lesions.

Cats appear to have fewer side effects and respond to BMT better than dogs.[52] If BMT is an option for a dog or cat with aplastic anemia, a decision has to be made early, because each transfusion given to the potential recipient before BMT increases the chance of development of antibodies that will interfere with successful engraftment of the marrow.

REFERENCES

1. Cramer DV, Lewis RM: Reticulocyte response in the cat. JAVMA 160:61, 1972.
2. Babior BM, Stossel TP: Hematology, A Pathophysiological Approach, 2nd ed. New York, Churchill Livingstone, 1990, p 39.
3. Weiss DJ, McClay CB: Studies on the pathogenesis of the erythrocyte destruction associated with the anemia of inflammatory disease. Vet Clin Pathol 17:90, 1998.
4. Weiss DJ, Krehbiel JD: Studies of the pathogenesis of anemia of inflammation: Erythrocyte survival. Am J Vet Res 44:1830, 1983.
5. Christopher M: Relation of endogenous Heinz bodies to disease and anemia in cats: 120 cases (1978–1987). JAVMA 194:1089, 1989.
6. Cowgill LD, et al: Use of recombinant human erythropoietin for management of anemia in dogs and cats with renal failure. JAVMA 212:521, 1998.
7. Randolph T, et al: Comparison of the biologic activity and safety of recombinant canine erythropoietin to recombinant human erythropoietin in normal beagle dogs (abstract). In Proceedings of the 16th ACVIM Forum, San Diego, 1998.
8. Smith JE: Iron metabolism in dogs and cats. Compend Contin Ed 14:39, 1992.
9. Batt RM, Horadagoda NU: Gastric and pancreatic intrinsic factor mediated absorption of cobalamin in the dog. Am J Physiol 257:9341, 1989.
10. Jain NC: Schalm's Veterinary Hematology. Philadelphia, Lea & Febiger, 1986, p 655.
11. Myers S, et al: Macrocytic anemia caused by naturally-occurring folate deficiency in the cat. Vet Pathol 32:547, 1995.
12. Jain NC: Depression or hypoproliferative anemia. In: Essentials of Veterinary Hematology. Philadelphia, Lea & Febiger, 1993, p 210.
13. Williams DA: Cobalamin and folate in feline malabsorption (abstract). In: Proceedings of the 16th ACVIM Forum, San Diego, 1998.
14. Simpson K, et al: Effect of exocrine pancreatic insufficiency on cobalamin absorption in dogs. Am J Vet Res 50:1233, 1989.
15. Sherding RG, et al: Diseases and surgery of the exocrine pancreas. In Birchard SJ, Sherding RG (eds): Saunders Manual of Small Animal Practice. Philadelphia, WB Saunders, 1994, p 768.
16. Fyfe JC, et al: Inherited selective intestinal cobalamin malabsorption and cobalamin deficiency in dogs. Pediatr Res 29:24, 1991.
17. Bunch SE, et al: Hematologic values and plasma and tissue folate concentrations in dogs given phenytoin on a long-term basis. Am J Vet Res 51:1865, 1990.
18. Nelson RW: Disorders of the thyroid gland. In Nelson RW, Couto CG (eds): Essentials of Small Animal Internal Medicine, 2nd ed. St. Louis, Mosby–Year Book, 1998, p 703.
19. Weiss DJ: Antibody-mediated suppression of erythropoiesis in dogs with red blood cell aplasia. Am J Vet Res 47:2646, 1986.
20. Gilmour M, et al: Investigating primary acquired pure red cell aplasia in dogs. Vet Med, December: 1199, 1991.
21. Scott-Moncrieff JC, Reagan WJ: Human intravenous immunoglobulin therapy. Semin Vet Med Surg (Small Anim) 12:178, 1997.
22. Hofmann-Lehmann R: Parameters of disease progression in long-term experimental feline retrovirus (feline immunodeficiency virus and feline leukemia virus) infections: Hematology, clinical chemistry, and lymphocyte subsets. Clin Diagn Lab Immunol 4:33, 1997.
23. Linenberger ML, et al: Marrow accessory cell infection and alterations in hematopoiesis accompany severe neutropenia during experimental acute infection with feline immunodeficiency virus. Blood 85:94, 1995.
24. Cotter SM: Anemia associated with feline leukemia virus infection. JAVMA 175:1191, 1979.
25. Cotter SM: Feline leukemia virus. In Greene C (ed): Infectious Diseases of the Dog and Cat, 3rd ed. Philadelphia, WB Saunders, 1998, p 71.
26. Hoover EA, et al: Erythroid hypoplasia in cats inoculated with feline leukemia virus. J Natl Cancer Inst 53:1271, 1974.
27. Jarrett O, et al: Interaction between feline leukemia virus subgroups in the pathogenesis of erythroid hypoplasia. Int J Cancer 34:283, 1984.
28. Boyce JT, et al: Feline leukemia virus–induced erythroid aplasia: In vitro hemopoietic culture studies. Exp Hematol 9:990, 1981.
29. Onions D, et al: Selective effect of feline leukemia virus on early erythroid precursors. Nature 296:156, 1982.
30. Abkowitz JJ, et al: Lymphocytes and antibody in retrovirus-induced feline pure red cell aplasia. J Natl Cancer Inst 78:135, 1987.
31. McCaw DL: Immunomodulation therapy for FeLV: A comparison of two agents (abstract). In: Proceedings of the 16th ACVIM Forum, San Diego, 1998.
32. Goldman EE, et al: Granulocytic ehrlichiosis in dogs from North Carolina and Virginia. J Vet Intern Med 12:61, 1998.
33. Gaunt SD, Pierce KR: Effects of estradiol on hematopoietic and marrow adherent cells of dogs. Am J Vet Res 47:906, 1986.
34. Morgan RV: Blood dyscrasias associated with testicular tumors in the dog. J Am Anim Hosp Assoc 18:970, 1982.
35. Moore A, Tufts University School of Veterinary Medicine, personal communication, 1998.
36. Abkowitz JL, et al: Behavior of feline hematopoietic stem cells years after busulfan exposure. Blood 82:2096, 1993.
37. Weiss DJ, Klausner JS: Drug-associated aplastic anemia in dogs: Eight cases (1984–1988). JAVMA 196:472, 1990.
38. Trapanier LA: Sulfonamide hypersensitivity in the dog (abstract). In: Proceedings of the 16th ACVIM Forum, San Diego, 1998.
39. Meyer EK: Adverse events associated with albendazole and other products used for treatment of giardiasis in dogs. JAVMA 213:44, 1998.
40. Jacobs G, et al: Neutropenia and thrombocytopenia in 3 dogs treated with anticonvulsants. JAVMA 212:681, 1998.
41. Peterson ME, et al: Methimazole treatment, 262 cats with hyperthyroidism. J Vet Intern Med 2:150, 1988.
42. Erslev AJ, Soltan A: Pure red-cell aplasia: A review. Blood Rev 10:20, 1996.
43. Young NS, Maciejewski J: The pathophysiology of acquired aplastic anemia. N Engl J Med 336:1365, 1997.
44. Kurtzman GJ, et al: Feline parvovirus propagates in cat bone marrow cultures and inhibits hematopoietic colony formation in vitro. Blood 74:71, 1989.
45. Vaden SL: Cyclosporine and tacrolimus. Semin Vet Med Surg 12:161, 1997.
46. Weiss DJ, et al: Bone marrow necrosis in the dog. JAVMA 187:54, 1985.
47. Duncan JR, et al: Veterinary Laboratory Medicine, 3rd ed. Ames, Iowa State University Press, 1977, p 72.
48. Stasi R, et al: Response to recombinant human erythropoietin in patients with myelodysplastic syndromes. Clin Cancer Res 3:733, 1997.
49. Zucker S: Anemia in cancer. Cancer Invest 3:249, 1985.
50. Cotter SM: Clinical transfusion medicine. In Cotter S (ed): Comparative Transfusion Medicine. San Diego, Academic Press, 1991, p 187.
51. Escolar G, et al: Experimental basis for the use of red cell transfusion in the management of anemic-thrombocytopenic patients. Transfusion 28:406, 1988.
52. Gasper PW, et al: Bone marrow transplantation: Update and current considerations. In Bonagura J (ed): Kirk's Current Veterinary Therapy XI. Philadelphia, WB Saunders, 1992, p 493.

CHAPTER 179

PLATELETS AND VON WILLEBRAND'S DISEASE

Rafael Ruiz de Gopegui and Bernard F. Feldman

Platelets are anuclear 3- to 5-μm cytoplasmic disks essential to the initiation of the healing process. Endothelial cells and adequate numbers of functional platelets are the integral components of primary hemostasis. Following endothelial cell perturbation, there is vascular constriction, platelet adhesion, and platelet aggregation—the primary hemostatic sequence, and the beginnings of the healing process. Platelets are also essential to endothelial function. When platelets are insufficient in terms of number or function, endothelial cell viability is compromised.

PHYSIOLOGY

Platelet Structure. Platelet integrins are heterodimeric membrane molecules with the ability to integrate extracellular and cytoplasmic compartments, allowing interaction between extracellular molecules and intracellular actin. The integrins are composed of alpha and beta subunits. Combinations of these subunits form specific receptors (located in the alpha chain) that bind various ligands and mediate cell-cell and cell-matrix interactions. The five major platelet

integrins are $\alpha_2\beta_1$ (glycoprotein [GP] Ia/IIa, collagen Type I and III receptor), $\alpha_5\beta_1$ (GP Ic/IIIa, fibronectin receptor), $\alpha_6\beta_1$ (laminin receptor), $\alpha_{IIb}\beta_3$ (GP IIb/IIIa, fibrinogen, von Willebrand's factor [vWf], and fibronectin receptor), and $\alpha_v\beta_3$ (GP VnRα/IIIa vitronectin receptor).[1–3]

Platelet Activation. Platelet activation, the biochemical changes resulting in platelet initiation of hemostasis, may be stimulated by platelet agonists: collagen, adenosine diphosphate (ADP), epinephrine, platelet activating factor acether (PAF-acether), thrombin, and arachidonic acid. Thrombin binds irreversibly to platelet GP V.[4] Collagen and thrombin initiate the phosphoinositide pathway and eicosanoid pathway by activation of phospholipase A and phospholipase C (Figs. 179–1 and 179–2). Phospholipase A activation generates arachidonic acid (from platelet membrane phospholipids) and leads to thromboxane A (TXA$_2$) release—the most potent platelet aggregant. Phospholipase C activation is a G protein–mediated process that generates inositol-1,4,5-triphosphate and diacylglycerol. G protein is a messenger or transporting protein found in the platelet membrane responsive to thrombin. Diacylglycerol activates protein kinase C and contributes to arachidonic acid generation. Inositol-

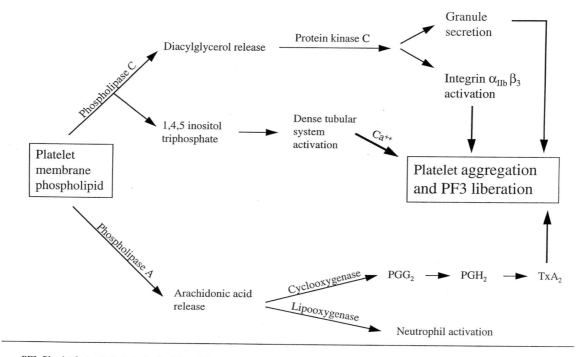

PF3: Platelet factor 3; Ca++: ionized calcium; PG: prostaglandin; Tx: thromboxane

Figure 179–1. Platelet activation by thrombin and collagen.

HEM

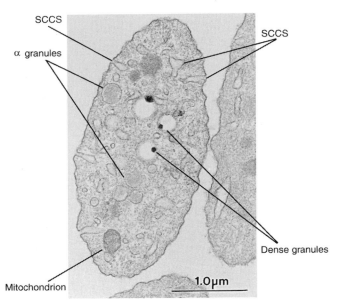

Figure 179–2. Transmission electron micrograph of a canine platelet (magnification: 27,600 ×). Organelles seen include alpha granules (α), dense granules (d), surface connected canaliculi system (SCCS), and mitochondria (m). (Courtesy of Prem J. Handagama, B.V.Sc., Ph.D., University of California, San Francisco.)

1,4,5-triphosphate mobilizes calcium ions from the platelet-dense tubular system. Ionized calcium binds calmodulin and activates calmodulin-dependent protein kinase II and subsequently myosin light chain kinase.[5] Calmodulin regulates platelet membrane calcium movement. Inositol-1,4,5-triphosphate also activates phospholipase A. As a result, the discoid platelet changes to a spherical shape as platelet pseudopods—filopodia—form. In addition, platelet membrane fluidity increases with reorientation of the phosphatidylserine residues to the outer surface. This phenomenon is calmodulin-, protein kinase C–, and intracellular calcium–dependent.[6] Platelet morphology and biochemistry are thus altered, with the resultant expression of the ligand function of integrin $\alpha_{IIb}\beta_3$ and fusion of granules with the open canalicular system, followed by two release reactions: release of dense granule contents, and lysosome and alpha granule degranulation (see Fig. 179–2). Platelet adhesion to the subendothelium is mediated by adhesion proteins, including vWf (the major adhesion protein), which binds to platelet surface GP Ib-IX (GPIb) and to integrin $\alpha_{IIb}\beta_3$ to mediate normal platelet aggregation under high shear rate conditions such as occurs in larger vasculature. Platelet aggregation requires fibrinogen binding, which is also mediated by integrin $\alpha_{IIb}\beta_3$. The common amino acid sequence within this ligand necessary for binding to the receptor is Arg-Gly-Asp (also known as the RGD sequence). Finally, activated platelets expose platelet Factor 3 (PF3), a membrane phospholipid that binds coagulation Factors V, VIII, and X, accelerating thrombin formation. This results in activation of other platelets, acceleration of platelet aggregation, and degranulation, causing amplification of coagulation processes and thrombin generation. Fibrin(ogen) degradation products (FDPs), specifically fragments D and E, have high affinity for platelet membranes, inducing platelet dysfunction through platelet granule release and platelet aggregation inhibition.[7]

Inflammation activates hemostasis through neutrophil activation (inducing platelet aggregation, inactivation of hepa-

TABLE 179–1. PLATELET DEVELOPMENTAL SEQUENCE

Pluripotent stem cell
Burst forming unit megakaryocyte
Colony forming unit megakaryocyte
Megakaryoblast
Promegakaryocyte
Mature megakaryocyte
Productive megakaryocyte
Platelet shedding—direct or pseudopodia

rin-dependent serine proteases and the protein C pathway),[8] monocyte expression of tissue factor (TF; a major procoagulant), complement activation (inducing platelet procoagulant activity), and cytokine release, which induces endothelial TF expression and endothelial changes that are more receptive to coagulation.[9]

Thrombopoiesis. The thrombopoietic sequence can be found in Table 179–1. Megakaryoblasts undergo nuclear division by endomitosis to develop the polyploid (up to 64N) megakaryocyte. Then platelets are shed in bone marrow sinusoids by pseudopod-like formations from megakaryocytes or through surface blebbing. Megakaryocytes may also be found in extramedullary locations, including peripheral blood (2 to 7/μL), spleen, liver, heart, kidneys, and lungs.[10] Thrombopoiesis is induced by thrombopoietin (formerly called c-Mpl ligand), which stimulates all stages of megakaryocytopoiesis and maturation. As megakaryocytes increase in number and size, so do platelet numbers. Platelet production is also stimulated to a lesser extent by interleukin-6 (IL-6), interleukin-11 (IL-11), and erythropoietin.[11, 12] Thrombopoietin synthesis occurs in liver and bone marrow and numerous other disparate sites and seems to be down-regulated by platelet mass.[13]

CLINICAL APPROACH TO PLATELET DISORDERS

Clinical Signs. Hemostatic disorders may induce spontaneous or prolonged hemorrhage. Clinical signs associated with platelet pathology include petechiation, purpura, and/or ecchymosis (Table 179–2). Clinical history must be exhaustive to determine whether the disorder is acquired or congenital and to determine the possible etiology (e.g., drug administration, vaccination status, arthropod parasitism). The presence of a primary process such as liver disease, renal

TABLE 179–2. CLINICAL SIGNS ASSOCIATED WITH HEMOSTATIC DISORDERS

PRIMARY HEMOSTATIC DEFECTS: ENDOTHELIAL CELLS, PLATELETS	COAGULOPATHIES: FACTOR ABNORMALITIES	NONSPECIFIC CLINICAL SIGNS
Ecchymosis	Hemarthrosis	Epistaxis
Petechia	Hematoma	Hematemesis
Purpura	Hemoptysis	Hematochezia
		Hematuria
		Melena
		Prolonged hemorrhage
		Spontaneous hemorrhage

Hemostatic disorders may induce spontaneous or prolonged hemorrhage. Other clinical signs may be associated with depression, anorexia, hyperthermia, and pallor.

TABLE 179–3. TESTS RELATED TO PLATELET FUNCTION

TEST	FUNCTION
Glass bead adhesion	Platelet adherence
Clot retraction	Tests functional integrin $\alpha_{IIb}\beta_3$
Fibrin and fibrinogen degradation products	Inhibit platelet aggregation
Plasma vWf:antigen (vWf:Ag) quantification	Platelet adherence
Serotonin secretion	Platelet granule secretion
Aggregation	Platelet response to agonists
Determination of membrane integrins	Platelet inherited membrane defects
Electron microscopy	Platelet morphologic dysplasia

failure, infection, or neoplasia must be ruled out or confirmed.

Laboratory Testing. Laboratory tests may be used to obtain a definitive diagnosis and to monitor selected therapy. Primary hemostasis involves evaluation of endothelial cell function, platelet function, and platelet mass. Primary hemostasis may be partially assessed by determining platelet numbers and platelet size (mean platelet volume, or MPV; in immune-mediated thrombocytopenia, MPV will initially be decreased and become increased as the process becomes regenerative).[14] If appropriate platelet numbers are present, a bleeding time (BT) test may further determine the adequacy of the vascular response and of platelet function. Prolonged BT in this clinical setting suggests thrombocytopathia or vascular dysfunction—endothelial cell dysfunction. We recommend the buccal mucosal bleeding time (BMBT) test using a standard bleeding time device. If platelet numbers are abnormal, especially when there is thrombocytopenia, further characterization may be achieved by means of (1) bone marrow megakaryocyte examination to determine platelet production status; (2) bone marrow megakaryocyte direct immunofluorescence for the diagnosis of immune-mediated thrombocytopenia; (3) platelet-bound immunoglobulin G (IgG) and serum platelet-bindable antibodies (which requires flow cytometry using either EDTA-anticoagulated blood or serum); and (4) the PF3 test to reveal ongoing platelet destruction (not specific). Specific tests to diagnose an underlying or primary disease are listed in Table 179–3. Morphologic abnormalities of platelets and platelet granules require examination by electron microscopy. Fibrinogen, essential for platelet function and especially for platelet aggregation, must be quantitated before further platelet function tests are performed. Fibrinogen may be quantified by heat precipitation or more accurately by the von Clauss method, which evaluates functional fibrinogen[15] (Figs. 179–3 and 179–4).

THROMBOCYTOPENIA

Infectious Thrombocytopenias (Table 179–4). Rocky Mountain spotted fever (RMSF) is caused by *Rickettsia rickettsii* and is transmitted by *Dermacentor andersoni* and *Dermacentor variabilis* (and other Ixodidae). This organism affects host endothelial cells, resulting in necrotizing vasculitis and hemostatic dysfunction. The altered endothelium induces platelet and fibrinolytic activation, causing thrombocytopenia with clinically evident petechiae and, potentially, consumption coagulopathy (disseminated intravascular coagulation, or DIC).

Canine ehrlichiosis is an acute, subacute, or chronic tick-transmitted disease (*Rhipicephalus sanguineus*) caused by *Ehrlichia canis* that affects platelet number (thrombocytopenia can be a peracute or chronic effect) and function. Other cell lines are often concurrently affected. Presentation and severity of the disease are influenced by ehrlichial strain, immune status, age, and potentially breed. Terminal pancytopenia may be observed more frequently in German shepherds.[16] Initial clinical signs are nonspecific and may include fever, depression, oculonasal discharge, anorexia, and generalized reactive lymphadenopathy. Hemorrhage, including epistaxis (frequently unilateral), and mucosal petechiae or purpura may be present during the acute phase but become more evident in the more severe chronic phase. Pulmonary, ocular, nervous system, digestive tract, and articular disease may also be associated with canine ehrlichiosis. Hematologic signs vary with the evolution of the disease. Lymphocytosis, monocytosis, nonregenerative anemia, and marrow megakaryocytic hyperplasia (this can be a relative megakaryocytic hyperplasia) with peripheral thrombocytopenia are observed in the acute and mild chronic phases. The severe chronic phase is characterized by pancytopenia due to bone marrow hypoplasia. In the acute phase, seemingly appropriate megakaryocyte numbers may be observed in bone marrow preparations. Diagnosis is based on direct observation of *E. canis* morulae and ehrlichia species–specific indirect immunofluorescence (IFA), Western immunoblot serology, dot-blot enzyme-linked immunosorbent assay (ELISA) serology, polymerase chain reaction (PCR), or cell culture reisolation. Treatment includes specific use of tetracyclines (doxycycline 4.5 mg/lb per day orally) for a minimum of three weeks or imidocarb dipropionate (2.3 mg/lb intramuscularly as a single dose, with a second administration two weeks later if indicated); the latter is used especially when there is concurrent babesiosis. Other supportive therapies include intravenous polyionic fluids and transfusion of blood products.[17] The mechanism of thrombocytopenia depends on the stage of the disease: platelets are consumed or sequestered during the acute phase of the disease, and platelet production is decreased in the chronic phase. In the acute phase, prolonged BT (even when platelet numbers are only modestly reduced) and altered platelet aggregation may be observed, indicating platelet dysfunction potentially induced by antiplatelet anti-

TABLE 179–4. KNOWN CAUSES OF INFECTIOUS THROMBOCYTOPENIA

GENERAL CAUSE	SPECIFIC CAUSE	SPECIES AFFECTED
Virus	Adenovirus	Dog
	Coronavirus	Cat
	Herpesvirus	Dog
	Paramyxovirus	Dog
	Parvovirus	Dog, cat
	Retrovirus	Cat
Bacteria	*Rickettsia rickettsii*	Dog
	Ehrlichia spp.	Dog, cat
	Haemobartonella spp.	Cat, dog
	Leptospira spp.	Dog
	Salmonella spp.	Dog, cat
	Other	Dog, cat
Protozoa	*Leishmania* spp.	Dog
	Toxoplasma gondii	Cat
	Cytauxzoon felis	Cat
	Babesia spp.	Dog
Fungus	*Candida albicans*	Dog
	Histoplasma capsulatum	Dog
Metazoa	*Dirofilaria inmitis*	Dog, cat

HEM

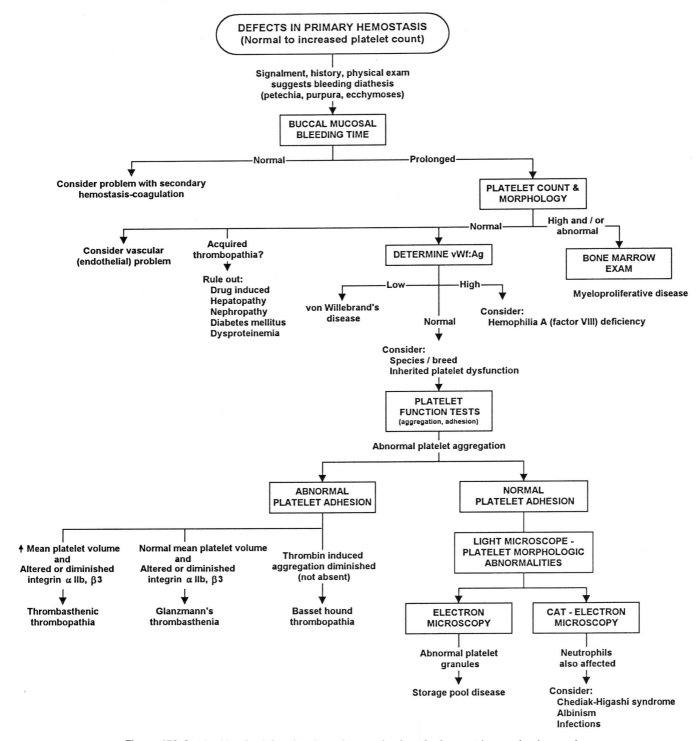

Figure 179–3. Algorithm for defects in primary hemostasis when platelet count is normal to increased.

body interaction with platelet membrane glycoproteins (integrins). Polyclonal hyperglobulinemia is a frequent feature after the acute phase of the disease; however, serum hyperviscosity has also been described in chronic canine ehrlichiosis due to monoclonal gammopathy.[18, 19] It should be noted that in a clinical setting, noninfectious thrombocytopenia usually does not have significant anemia as an associated process. Thrombocytopathy, in addition to thrombocyto-

penia, may be suspected when anemia is found with modest thrombocytopenia.

Ehrlichia platys is the etiologic agent causing canine infectious cyclic thrombocytopenia. The disease is characterized by one- to two-week parasitemic episodes, during which morulae may be observed in canine platelets (Fig. 179–5), alternating with thrombocytopenic episodes caused by peripheral destruction of the parasitized platelets.[20] Platelet

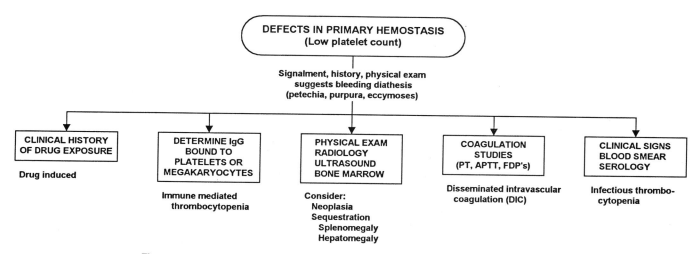

Figure 179–4. Algorithm for defects in primary hemostasis when platelet count is decreased.

counts may be severely decreased, and hemorrhage is often clinically evident. Dual infections with *E. canis* and *E. platys* are common, and immunologic compromise of the dog owing to concurrent infections such as babesiosis or leishmaniasis (and potentially the virulence of the *E. platys* strain) may affect the severity and presentation of the infection. It must be noted that *E. platys* infection may be subclinical. *Ehrlichia equi* and *Ehrlichia ewingii* are the causative agents of canine granulocytic ehrlichiosis. The infection may induce thrombocytopenia and polyarthritis, among other clinical signs, in dogs. Morulae may be observed in neutrophils. Combined infection with other *Ehrlichia* spp. may occur.[21, 22] *E. risticii* is a causative agent of equine ehrlichiosis but may also infect dogs and cats. Ehrlichial infection in cats is characterized by anemia, leukopenia, thrombocytopenia, and dysproteinemia and may also be induced by *E. canis.*[23] *Ehrlichia chaffeensis,* the agent of human ehrlichiosis, is closely related to *E. canis,* but marked thrombocytopenia was not observed in experimentally infected dogs.[24]

Haemobartonella canis, the causative agent of canine haemobartonellosis, is transmitted primarily by *Rhipicephalus sanguineus.* Thrombocytopenia, in addition to anemia, may be found in this disease.[25]

Feline cytauxzoonosis is a tick-transmitted disease, caused by *Cytauxzoon felis,* that may induce severe thrombocytopenia. Effective therapy has not been described as yet, and the prognosis is quite poor.[26]

Viral diseases potentially causing thrombocytopenia include canine adenovirus type 1, herpesvirus, paramyxovirus, canine parvovirus, feline leukemia virus (FeLV), feline immunodeficiency virus (FIV), feline infectious peritonitis (FIP) virus, feline panleukopenia virus, and perhaps modified live distemper virus vaccination.[27] Viremia may also induce thrombopathia in small animals. Peripheral immune-mediated platelet destruction is an important mechanism to explain thrombocytopenia observed in canine distemper. Canine paramyxovirus infects platelets, causing platelet degeneration and phagocytosis by hepatic Kupffer's cells.[28] Bone marrow thrombopoiesis (as well as erythropoiesis and myelopoiesis) may be decreased.[29] Modified paramyxovirus vaccine–induced thrombocytopenia has been related to viral neuraminidase. Levamisole administration has been suggested to prevent platelet neuraminidase-induced aggregation.[30]

Bacterial infections such as salmonellosis and lep-tospirosis and miscellaneous causes of endotoxemia and sepsis may induce thrombocytopenia, often as a result of DIC. Thrombocytopenias may also be induced by fungal diseases such as histoplasmosis and disseminated candidiasis.[31, 32] Leishmaniasis and dirofilariasis induce vasculitis and subsequent thrombocytopenia and thrombopathia. Toxoplasmosis may induce thrombocytopenia in the cat. A reverse transcriptase–producing infectious agent has been suggested as a causative agent of canine thrombocytopenia.[33]

Immune-Mediated Thrombocytopenia (IMT). Immune-mediated thrombocytopenia (idiopathic) is the most frequent cause of severe thrombocytopenia in the dog. Platelet life span is markedly decreased. Antiplatelet antibodies attach to the platelet surfaces and induce destruction by the mononuclear phagocyte system (MPS). The etiology of primary IMT remains unclear, but the presence of antiplatelet antibodies has been related to neoplasia, infection, drugs, and autoimmune diseases.[34] Thrombopoiesis is increased in most cases of IMT. However, antibody-mediated megakaryocyte damage, megakaryocytic hypoplasia, or aplasia may occur, significantly worsening the prognosis.[35] Although unusual in terms of clinical presentation, IMT has also been described in the cat. Notably, megakarocytic hypoplasia occurs in feline IMT.[36, 37]

The hemorrhagic tendency observed in IMT is related to both decreased platelet numbers and platelet dysfunction.

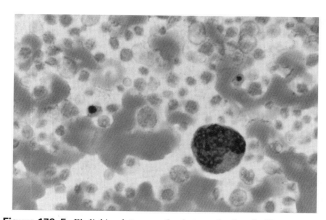

Figure 179–5. *Ehrlichia platys* morulae in two platelets (buffy coat smear, magnification: 5000 ×; Diff-Quik stain).

HEM

The addition of serum from an animal with IMT has been observed to impair platelet aggregation in platelets from normal dogs in in vitro testing.[38]

The diagnosis of IMT is often based on exclusion—based on finding unexplained severe thrombocytopenia—and by microthrombocytosis as determined by MPV, at least in the acute stage. The confirmation of antiplatelet antibodies may be attempted indirectly by estimating the PF3 serum concentration or directly by ELISA, radioimmunoassay (RIA), IFA, and flow cytometry techniques. Specificity and sensitivity of all these tests in canine medicine are not yet optimal.[39] Platelet-bound IgG determination requires flow cytometry of EDTA-anticoagulated blood. When platelet counts are below 5000/μL, this determination may be unreliable. Determination of platelet-bindable antibodies may be attempted by serum flow cytometry.[40] Evidence of IgG binding to the platelet membrane (potentially to integrin $\alpha_{IIb}\beta_3$) indicates IMT, regardless of etiology. True primary "autoimmune" thrombocytopenia is difficult to prove in a clinical setting. Bone marrow examination may reveal megakaryocyte damage. This may be confirmed by direct IFA. Immune-suppressive therapy with glucocorticoids (prednisone 0.45 mg/lb per day) combined with azathioprine (0.45 mg/lb per day) is indicated. Both these drugs are administered and reduced in tandem. Transfusion therapy is not indicated unless used before splenectomy or any other surgical therapy in severely thrombocytopenic dogs. Splenectomy in IMT is not particularly successful.[41] Platelet transfusions are often ineffectual, as transfused platelets are quickly destroyed. In addition, more than several units of platelets may be required for the same animal, and the risk of developing platelet alloantibodies can be enhanced by platelet administration. The administration of an anabolic steroid as well as glucocorticoids and fresh whole blood has been described in dogs with IMT and nonregenerative anemia,[42] but we consider steroid use ineffectual. Other therapeutic options include other chemotherapeutic agents, plasmapheresis, or human gamma globulin administration.[43]

Drug-Induced Thrombocytopenia.[44–50] Impaired platelet production, consumption, or destruction may be induced by drugs (Table 179–5). The diagnosis of drug-induced thrombocytopenia may be based on clinical history of drug administration, unexplained thrombocytopenia, and return of platelet count toward the reference interval after the drug in question is discontinued (unless irreversible myelosuppression has occurred). Thrombocytopenia should recur after reexposure to the same drug. The immediate discontinuation of the suspected drug is the first goal of treatment. Glucocorticoid therapy or blood product administration may be considered if either an immune-mediated mechanism is observed or hemorrhage is ongoing and significant.

Severe side effects of estrogen therapy include aplastic pancytopenia—severe thrombocytopenia, anemia, and leukopenia. Clinical signs include debilitation, mucosal petechiae, ecchymosis, pale mucous membranes, and hemorrhagic diarrhea. The prognosis is poor if thrombocytopenia lasts for more than two weeks. Although anemia and thrombocytopenia can often be treated, death due to leukopenia—neutropenia—is common. Treatment with nonestrogenic anabolic steroids, lithium, and blood products is recommended.[51] Cytokine therapy, specifically use of granulocyte colony stimulating factor (5 μg/kg [2.25 μg/lb] per day subcutaneously), may be considered.[52]

Thrombocytopenia Due to Platelet Sequestration. The spleen normally contains approximately 30 per cent of circulating platelets. Platelet sequestration is frequently

TABLE 179–5. DRUGS INDUCING THROMBOCYTOPENIA

Antibiotics	Antineoplastic Agents
Cephalothin	Azathioprine
Chloramphenicol	Bleomycin
Erythromycin	Chlorambucil
Methicillin	Cyclophosphamide
Novobiocin	Cytosine arabinoside
Oxytetracycline	Doxorubicin
Penicillin	5-Fluorouracil
Rifamycin	L-Asparaginase
Ristocetin	6-Mercaptopurine
Streptomycin	Propylthiouracil
	Vinblastine
Antimicrobials	Vincristine
Dapsone	
Dinitrophenol	**Cardiovascular Drugs**
Isoniazid	Digitoxin
Organic arsenicals	Digoxin
Quinacrine	Hydralazine
Quinine	L-Dopa
Sulfonamides	Methyldopa
Trimethoprim-sulfamethoxazole	Nitroglycerin
	Quinidine
Anticonvulsants	
Methylhydantoin	**Diuretics**
Paramethadione	Thiazide derivatives
Phenacetamide	
Phenobarbital	**Hormones**
Trimethadione	Estrogens
Anti-Inflammatory Drugs	**Miscellaneous**
Acetaminophen	Chlorpheniramine
Acetylsalicylic acid	Colchicine
Gold sodium thiomalate	Desipramine
Indomethacin	Diazepam
Phenylbutazone	Dilantin
Prednisolone	Ethanol
Steroids	Hypoglycemic agents
	Levamisole
	Lidocaine
	Para-aminosalicylic acid
	Protamine sulphate
	Unfractioned heparin

associated with splenomegaly, but hepatomegaly may also induce thrombocytopenia. *Babesia gibsoni* infection in the dog may be an example of thrombocytopenia associated with splenomegaly. However, other mechanisms are also involved, including platelet consumption and immune-mediated platelet destruction.[53]

Thrombocytopenia Due to Platelet Consumption. In contrast to IMT, platelet activation leads to platelet consumption as platelets adhere to various surfaces and platelet aggregation is triggered. Platelet activation is frequently induced by inflammatory mechanisms or when hemostatic inhibition is defective. It must be noted that thrombopathia and coagulopathy may coexist. Examples include protein-losing processes, vasculitis, neoplasia, and DIC.

Thrombocytopenia Due to Neoplasia. Sarcomas, carcinomas, and lymphoproliferative and myeloproliferative disorders, among other neoplastic diseases, have frequently been associated with thrombocytopenia.[54] Pathogenic mechanisms may include[55] (1) sequestration of platelets in splenic, hepatic, and large vascular tumors; (2) decreased platelet production in bone marrow myelophthisis or myelodysplasia, in estrogen-secreting tumors (Sertoli's cell neoplasia, granulosa cell tumor, FeLV), and as the result of chemotherapy; (3) platelet consumption in DIC, platelet-tumor interaction, and microangiopathy; (4) platelet loss in tumor-associated hemorrhage; and (5) immune-mediated platelet and/or megakaryocyte destruction suggested to be associated with some canine neoplasias such as liposarcoma, benign mixed mammary neoplasia, mast cell neoplasia, hemangiosarcoma, nasal adenocarcinoma, and fibrosarcoma, where positive direct immunofluorescence testing of megakaryocytes was reported.[56]

DISORDERS OF THROMBOPOIESIS

Bone Marrow (Megakaryocyte) Hypoplasia. Specific immune-mediated megakaryocyte destruction without alteration of other hematopoietic cell series is an infrequent finding. Other causes of bone marrow hypoplasia include idiosyncratic drug reaction, radiation, viral infection, toxemia, and the chronic severe phase of canine ehrlichiosis.

Megakaryocyte Dysplasia. Dysmegakaryocytopoiesis is indicated by decreased numbers of megakaryocytes; megakaryocytes with nonlobed, large nuclei or multiple small nuclei; and dwarf megakaryocytes (also termed micromegakaryocytes) in the blood and bone marrow, sometimes associated with marrow dysplastic (preleukemic) states.[10] FeLV infection may induce thrombocytopenia and macrothrombocytosis as a result of dysthrombopoiesis.[57]

Myeloproliferative Disorders. Essential thrombocythemia is a clonal disorder originating from a pluripotent stem cell. This disorder has been described in the cat[58] and in the dog[59, 60] and is characterized by marked thrombocytosis and bone marrow megakaryocytic hyperplasia. Despite this, megakaryoblasts make up less than 30 per cent of bone marrow total cellularity. No circulating megakaryoblasts and micromegakaryocytes are observed. Anemia and splenomegaly due to extramedullary hematopoiesis are also clinically absent.[61] Spurious elevations of serum potassium have been described in dogs with essential thrombocythemia.[62] Gastrointestinal hemorrhage due to impaired platelet function and hyposplenism may be observed. Splenectomy is contraindicated. The hematologic criteria used in humans include persistent platelet count over 600,000/μL, bone marrow megakaryocytic hyperplasia, appropriate red cell mass and adequate bone marrow iron storage (with increase of hemoglobin <1 g/dL after 1 month of administered iron), absence of bone marrow collagen, absence of splenomegaly and leukoerythroblastic reaction, absence of causes of secondary (reactive) thrombocytosis, and absence of the Philadelphia chromosome.

Megakaryocytic leukemias described in the veterinary literature entail a confusing array of terms and descriptions. Although the terminology is confusing, therapy is probably similar. The term megakaryocytic myelosis includes megakaryocytic leukemia and megakaryoblastic leukemia. The difference between essential thrombocythemia and megakaryocytic myelosis is the presence of megakaryoblasts in the circulation or a megakaryoblast predominance in bone marrow greater than 30 per cent of the total marrow nucleated cell population.[63] Acute myeloid leukemia (formerly megakaryoblastic leukemia, acute megakaryoblastic leukemia, or one type of acute myelogenous leukemia) is megakaryoblastic infiltration of the bone marrow exceeding 30 per cent of the total marrow nucleated cellularity. Neoplastic cells tend to be acetylcholinesterase-, alpha-naphthyl acetate esterase–, naphthol AS acetate esterase–, GP IIIa–, and vWf-positive and alkaline phosphatase–, acid phosphatase–, myeloperoxidase–, alpha-naphthyl butyrate esterase–, naphthol AS-D chloroacetate esterase–, and Sudan-negative. Other features of the disease include neoplastic infiltration of lymph nodes, liver, and spleen; circulation of micromegakaryocytes and undifferentiated megakaryoblasts in peripheral blood; and thrombocytopenia, thrombocytosis, or pancytopenia. Abnormally shaped platelets and hypogranular or agranular platelets may be observed in blood smears. Thrombopathia and subsequent hemorrhagic tendency may be anticipated.[64, 65] Megakaryocytic leukemia is characterized by infiltration of bone marrow with megakaryocytes in different stages of maturation, but megakaryoblasts are less than 30 per cent of bone marrow cellularity and there is marked thrombocytosis (greater than 10^6 platelets/μL) with bizarre platelets and megakaryocytes. Also, nonregenerative anemia and megakaryocyte infiltration of other anatomic locations such as spleen, liver, and lymph nodes may occur. Megakaryocyte alpha granules and demarcation membrane systems may be observed by electron microscopy, suggesting morphologically appropriate cells acting in an inappropriate manner.[66] There is no distinctive or particularly effective therapy described for these disorders. Hydroxyurea (23 mg/lb orally twice daily and given to effect) has been used (see Chapter 98).

THROMBOCYTOSIS

Primary Thrombocytosis. Myeloproliferative disorders such as megakaryocytic leukemia and essential thrombocythemia induce thrombocytosis, whereas megakaryoblastic leukemia may induce unpredictable platelet quantitative changes.

Secondary Thrombocytosis. Secondary or reactive thrombocytosis is an increase of platelet count beyond the reference interval. "In reactive thrombocytosis, the megakaryocyte count is increased in the bone marrow, and the platelet count is directly proportional to the megakaryocytic mass and indirectly proportional to the mean megakaryocytic volume. . . . In thrombocythemia the platelet count is unrelated to megakaryocyte volume, and megakaryocyte size is not decreased."[67] Secondary thrombocytosis may be physiologic, as when platelet mobilization from the spleen and lungs is induced by exercise and adrenaline. Mast cell neoplasia, adenocarcinoma, lymphocytic leukemia, erythremic myelosis, osteosarcoma, gingival carcinoma, and squamous cell carcinoma induce increases in platelet numbers. Reactive and transient thrombocytosis may occur after myelosuppressive therapy, overcompensated DIC, and acute tumor hemorrhage. *Vinca* alkaloid administration induces marked thrombocytosis in the dog (up to 2×10^6/μL). Thrombotic risk may also increase with this therapy. Transitory thrombocytosis may be observed 36 hours to 10 days after acute hemorrhage and/or surgical trauma, with platelet counts returning to the reference interval in two weeks. Thrombocytosis can also occur after splenectomy. Iron deficiency or chronic blood-loss anemia causes reactive thrombocytosis as a result of the increased secretion of erythropoietin. Reactive thrombocytosis has been observed in canine bleeding gastrointestinal tumors (leiomyoma, adenocarcinoma, fibrosarcoma), urinary tract tumors, and hookworm infection. Primary erythrocytosis in people may be accompanied by thrombocytosis but is infrequently observed in the dog and cat.[65] Inflammation, infection, hyperadrenocorticism, and glucocorticoid administration may also induce varied degrees of thrombocytosis.

PLATELET FUNCTIONAL DISORDERS

Inherited Thrombopathias (Table 179–6). Chédiak-Higashi syndrome (CHS) is an autosomal recessive disease

HEM

TABLE 179–6. INHERITED THROMBOPATHIAS

NAME	SPECIES	BREED	SIGNS	DIAGNOSIS	THERAPY	MECHANISM
Chédiak-Higashi syndrome	Cat	—	Albinism, infections	↑ BT, ↓ PA, ↓ DG, neutrophil dysfunction	Platelet transfusion	Deficient dense granules
Storage pool disease	Dog	American cocker spaniel	Severe hemorrhage	↑ BT, ↓ PA, ↓ PS	Platelet transfusion	Deficient platelet granules
von Willebrand's disease	Dog, cat	54 canine breeds and mixed breeds: Doberman pinscher and Scottish terrier overrepresented	Nonspecific; three types described in veterinary medicine with different degrees of severity	↑ BT, ↓ vWf	Cryoprecipitate transfusion	Defective vWf
Basset hound hereditary thrombopathia	Dog	Basset hound	Nonspecific	↑ BT, ↓ ↓ PA*	Topical thrombin application	Altered regulation of cAMP-phosphodiesterase
Canine thrombasthenic thrombopathia	Dog	Otterhound	Nonspecific	↑ BT, ↓ PA, ↓ PAD, ↓ CR, ↑ ↑ MPV	Platelet transfusion	Abnormal platelet size and abnormal integrin $\alpha_{IIb}\beta_3$
Glanzmann's thrombasthenia	Dog	Great Pyrenees, Spitz	Nonspecific	↑ BT, ↓ ↓ PA, ↓ PAD, ↓ CR	Platelet transfusion	Abnormal integrin $\alpha_{IIb}\beta_3$
Cyclic hematopoiesis	Dog	Grey collie	Infections, cytopenias	↑ BT, ↓ ↓ PA	Platelet transfusion	Dense granule defect and phospholipase C defect

*Thrombin-induced platelet aggregation reduced but not absent. It also happens in Spitz thrombopathia.

↑ = increased; ↓ = decreased; ↓ ↓ = severely decreased; ↑ ↑ = severely increased; vWf = von Willebrand's factor; BT = bleeding time; PA = platelet aggregation; PS = platelet granule secretion; PAD = platelet adhesion; CR = clot retraction; DG = platelet dense granules; MPV = mean platelet volume; cAMP = cyclic adenosine monophosphate.

reported in cats as well as cattle, rats, minks, foxes, and other animals. Collagen-, ADP-, and epinephrine-induced platelet aggregation is markedly impaired. Some animals are deficient in platelet dense granule contents. The defect may include partial ocular albinism and enhanced susceptibility to bacterial infection owing to neutrophil dysfunction. Cats with CHS have platelet storage pool deficiency and prolonged bleeding times owing to the platelet abnormality. Platelet transfusion can effectively correct this abnormality. The half-inactivation time of donor platelets in CHS cats was 3.5 days. Current treatments for storage pool deficiency are deamino-8-D-arginine vasopressin (DDAVP), cryoprecipitate, bone marrow transplantation, and platelet transfusion.[68]

Platelet storage pool disease has been described in American cocker spaniel dogs. Platelet aggregation and secretion were impaired. The hemorrhagic tendency was severe and required platelet transfusions.[69] A thrombopathia resembling storage pool deficiency has been described in two domestic shorthair cats with defective platelet aggregation and a higher than normal platelet ATP-ADP ratio.[70, 70a]

Von Willebrand's disease (vWd), initially known as pseudohemophilia, was first described in 1926. Von Willebrand's factor (vWf) was first identified in 1971 by Zimmermann et al.[71] and designated Factor VIII–related antigen (FVIIIR:Ag), based on the immunologic method used for identification. vWf is a multimeric adhesive glucoprotein composed of 270-kilodalton polypeptide subunits linked by disulfide bonds. The factor is synthesized and assembled by megakaryocytes and endothelial cells. Endothelial cells may release the factor into the vascular tree or into the subendothelial matrix, where it is bound to collagen.[72] In contrast, platelet and megakaryocyte vWf is packaged in platelet alpha granules. Release of stored vWf from endothelial Weibel Palade bodies is induced by histamine, vasopressin, thrombin, fibrin, and estrogens. Thereafter, stored vWf from platelet alpha granules may be released by platelet aggregating agent stimuli such as collagen, ADP, PAF, adrenaline, and thrombin. vWf is necessary as a carrier of the Factor VIII molecule,

supporting its function by prolonging its circulatory half-inactivation time.

There are three types of vWd in dogs (Table 179–7). Type I may be inherited as an autosomal dominant trait with incomplete (or variable) penetrance.[73] Inheritance of vWf deficiency in Doberman pinschers may be consistent with a single gene defect in which each normal allele produces half the total amount of vWf produced when both alleles are normal, and each defective allele produces less than 15 canine units of vWf/dL. Thus, dogs with low plasma vWf concentrations may be homozygous for the defective allele, whereas dogs with midrange plasma vWf concentrations may be heterozygous for the defect.[74] It has been suggested that the mutation responsible for type I vWd of Dobermans is a "splice site mutation," with alternative splicing occurring 90 to 95 per cent of the time. As a consequence, clinically affected dogs can only be homozygous for the defect (vWf between 10 and 20 per cent of normal), and carrier dogs have 30 to 100 per cent of normal concentrations of vWf. Based on these percentages, it should be noted that it is difficult to separate carrier from "normal" individuals. Thus, if homozygous "normals" range from 50 to 150 per cent, there is overlap. The overlap between "normals" and carriers has not yet been defined.[74a] Type II vWd, observed in German wirehaired Pointers, has an autosomal recessive mode of inheritance.[75] Type III vWd also has an autosomal recessive mode of inheritance and is observed in Shetland sheepdogs, Scottish terriers, and other canine breeds.[76] Heterozygous dogs with type III vWd have reduced vWf activities, below 50 per cent, whereas homozygous type III dogs have undetectable vWf activities.[77] Hemophilia (A or B) and vWd may be detected concurrently in dogs.[78] Factor XII deficiency, nonspherocytic hemolytic anemia, and vWd have been described in a family of miniature poodle dogs.[79]

Accurately assessing the true frequency of canine vWd is difficult because many hemorrhagic episodes may go unnoticed and some dog owners might not report the occurrence of hemorrhagic episodes. Feline vWd may be considered

TABLE 179–7. CANINE VON WILLEBRAND'S DISEASE

TYPE	INHERITANCE	CLINICAL SIGNS	LMWM vWf	HMWM vWf	FREQUENCY
I	Autosomal	Variable	Decreased	Decreased	High
II	Autosomal recessive	Severe	Decreased	Undetectable	Very low
III	Autosomal recessive	Severe	Undetectable	Undetectable	Moderate

LMWM vWf = von Willebrand's factor low molecular weight multimers; HMWM vWf = von Willebrand's factor high molecular weight multimers.
Modified from Ruiz de Gopegui R, Feldman BR: von Willebrand's disease. © Springer-Verlag London Ltd. Reproduced with permission from Comp Haematol Int 7:187, 1997.

anecdotal, as described in a male Himalayan cat with a history of hemorrhagic episodes. The cat had undetectable vWf antigen, reduced Factor VIII activity, and moderately prolonged activated partial thromboplastin time (APTT).[80]

There are no confirmed reports of acquired vWd in the dog, but immune-mediated or neoplastic conditions have been observed to induce secondary vWd in people. There is no conclusive evidence of abnormal primary hemostasis as a consequence of canine hypothyroidism.[81] In addition, a genetic predisposition for hypothyroidism has been recognized in some canine breeds with a relatively high incidence of vWd; included are the Airedale terrier, golden retriever, dachshund, Doberman, poodle, Shetland sheepdog, and miniature schnauzer.[82] The relationship between vWd and hypothyroidism must be considered tentative at this time.

The severity and location of hemorrhage are variable in vWd. Mucosal hemorrhages may include prolonged estrual or puerperal hemorrhage (vulvar hemorrhage), urethral hemorrhage, hematuria, melena, hematochezia, gingival hemorrhage, and epistaxis. Nonmucosal hemorrhages observed in vWd includes prolonged bleeding after trauma (surgical trauma or wounds), excessive bleeding with nail cutting, subcutaneous hematoma, hemothorax, hemarthrosis, subarachnoid space hemorrhage,[83] and neonatal umbilical bleeding. Chronic bloody ear infections, abortions, and stillbirths have also been described in canine vWd.[84] In a large study, the most common site of mucosal bleeding in Scottish terriers and Shetland sheepdogs was the oral or nasal cavity; in Dobermans, it was the urogenital tract.[85] Clinical signs in type I vWd are mild to moderately severe and may require transfusion therapy. Clinical signs in type II vWd are often severe, including prolonged gingival bleeding, prolonged hemorrhage after surgery, and epistaxis.[86] In type III vWd, clinical signs tend to be most severe. Hemorrhage is mostly spontaneous and involving the oral mucosa.[87]

Clinically significant vWd is best determined by the BMBT. Quantitation of vWf—done for breeding purposes—is based on antigenic vWf determination by either Laurell "rocket" electroimmunoassay (EIA)[88, 89] or, more accurately, ELISA. The required sample is *nonhemolyzed* citrated platelet poor plasma. Venous blood samples (nine parts of blood to one part 3.8 per cent trisodium citrate) are centrifuged at 1000 g for 10 minutes in plastic containers at room temperature. The plasma is then removed with a plastic pipette and stored in plastic vials with plastic stoppers below −20°C.[90] The assays are often referred to as determinations of vWf:Ag, because they are based on immunologic tests. Multimeric analysis by either crossed immunoelectrophoresis or sodium dodecyl sulphate (SDS)–agarose gel electrophoresis may further characterize the type of vWd.[91, 92] Multimeric analysis allows a qualitative assessment of vWf. The different size vWf multimers are separated into detectable protein bands by SDS-agarose electrophoresis and visualized by autoradiography or enzyme-conjugated secondary

antibodies.[93, 94] Concentration of vWf is expressed as a percentage or in canine units (CU) per deciliter; both measures are considered equivalent. Dogs with vWf below 36 CU/dL are considered at risk of hemorrhage. Normal dogs exceed 70 CU/dL, equivocal dogs are between 50 and 70 CU/dL, carrier dogs (with few or no clinical signs) are between 36 and 50 CU/dL, and severely affected dogs are below 16 CU/dL.[83] Dogs that have approximately 100 CU/dL correspond to 6 μg/mL of vWf in plasma, within the reference interval observed in people.[92] Diagnosis of vWd may be attempted by assessment of vWf biologic activity in terms of impaired primary hemostasis (the BMBT is preferred); reduced platelet adhesion (glass bead platelet retention); abnormal platelet agglutination (ristocetin and botrocetin platelet agglutination); and reduced Factor VIII activity (FVIII determination), increased FVIII-vWf ratio, and prolonged APTT. Although these abnormalities are sometimes observed in human vWd, the FVIII abnormalities are inconsistent in dogs. The determination of BMBT should be part of the basic hemostatic profile and is often the first laboratory finding increasing suspicion of vWd. Bleeding time may be the best way to assess the clinical expression of vWd. Bleeding times approaching the upper limit of established reference intervals should be viewed with suspicion, as potentially severe hemorrhage can occur in these animals.

Transfusion therapy is indicated in severe forms of canine vWd if low plasma vWf concentration is detected or hemorrhage is occurring. To raise plasma concentrations deficient in vWf over 35 CU/dL, cryoprecipitate is the treatment of choice. The advantage of cryoprecipitate is the low volume needed to infuse a large quantity of vWf (dosage is 1 unit/22 lb body weight as needed). If cryoprecipitate is not available, fresh frozen plasma (3 to 5 mL/lb body weight every 8 to 12 hours) or fresh whole blood (5 to 12 mL/lb per day) is indicated, especially if marked hemorrhage has occurred.[95] DDAVP (0.45 μg/lb intravenously or subcutaneously) increases vWf activity and botrocetin cofactor activity in normal dogs 10 minutes after administration, with an anticipated duration of at least two hours.[96] The nasal spray preparation of DDAVP apparently was effective both in treating bleeding episodes and when used prophylactically for minor surgical procedures in several human patients.[97] In surgical patients with clinical vWd, phenothiazine tranquilizers should be avoided. Subcutaneous administration of DDAVP 30 minutes before surgery (0.45 μg/lb subcutaneously is the recommended dosage; 0.4 to 1.5 μg/lb in 1 to 2 mL of saline may be considered) may prevent profuse bleeding in some dogs.[98] The response to DDAVP in dogs requiring sodium pentobarbital anesthesia is equally effective when DDAVP is given either before or after the anesthetic.[99]

Basset hound hereditary thrombopathia has been confused by some basset hound owners and veterinary professionals with vWd. Basset hound hereditary thrombopathia has an autosomal inheritance trait. Affected dogs may have dif-

HEM

fering clinical presentations, depending on the severity. Epistaxis, gingival bleeding, and petechiae are common clinical signs. Bleeding times are variably prolonged. Platelet aggregation is severely impaired with the exception of thrombin-induced aggregation, which is diminished but not absent. An enzymatic regulatory defect of cAMP-phosphodiesterase is suggested; elevated concentrations of cAMP are observed in thrombopathic platelets. Quantitatively normal platelet integrin $\alpha_{IIb}\beta_3$ is present, resulting in appropriate fibrinogen binding and clot retraction. Appropriate fibrinogen binding and clot retraction differentiate this defect from human Glanzmann's thrombasthenia. Topical use of thrombin has been proposed to control posttraumatic cutaneous hemorrhage in dogs afflicted with this disease.[100, 101] Similar defects have been described in cats and in the American foxhound.[102]

Canine thrombasthenic thrombopathia is an autosomal inherited disorder described in otterhounds. This defect resembles Bernard-Soulier syndrome in people, because affected dogs have a significant subpopulation (30 to 80 per cent) of giant platelets. However, it also resembles Glanzmann's thrombasthenia, because GP Ib is increased and integrin $\alpha_{IIb}\beta_3$ is reduced compared with normal dogs. Platelet adhesion, aggregation (induced by all agonists), and clot retraction are deficient in affected dogs.

Glanzmann's thrombasthenia (GT) is a congenital defect of integrin $\alpha_{IIb}\beta_3$, with subsequent impairment of platelet aggregation and clot retraction that can be quantitative (types I and II) or qualitative (type III). One case has been described in an Alaskan malamute.[103] Type I GT is an intrinsic platelet defect in which integrin $\alpha_{IIb}\beta_3$ is quantitatively reduced. It was recently described in a female Great Pyrenees dog.[3] Petechiae in the oral cavity and on the skin of the abdomen and severe gingival bleeding and epistaxis were present. Collagen-, ADP-, thrombin-, and PAF-induced platelet aggregation and clot retraction were markedly impaired. Spitz thrombopathia (Glanzmann's type III) is an intrinsic platelet defect in which integrin $\alpha_{IIb}\beta_3$ is qualitatively altered, resulting in inability of the complex to express ligand binding function. Two female dogs with type III GT had chronic epistaxis and gastrointestinal and gingival bleeding. Platelet aggregation induced by ADP, collagen, and PAF was absent, and thrombin-induced platelet aggregation was altered.[104]

Cyclic hematopoiesis of the grey collie, most often associated with neutropenia and thrombocytopenia, also presents a platelet dense granule defect. Phospholipase C is deficient in platelets of affected dogs.[105]

Acquired Thrombopathia. Platelet function defects can be drug induced or secondary to disease. Most acquired thrombocytopathies are not single-system disorders. Often they are related to thrombocytopenia or to secondary coagulation disorders.

Antithrombotic drug therapy includes antiaggregants and anticoagulants with platelet inhibitory effects (Table 179–8). It should be noted that acetaminophen does not have antithrombotic effects. Experimental administration of phospholipid solutions with PF3 activity has been attempted in aspirin-induced thrombopathia in the dog. Phospholipid infusion has been considered an alternative therapy for platelet disorders (thrombocytopenia and thrombopathia), but the efficacy and safety of this therapy have not yet been established.[106] Glucocorticoids may inhibit primary hemostasis, but the inhibitory effects of aspirin have been experimentally ameliorated using glucocorticoids (in terms of shortened bleeding time) in the dog, an interesting contradiction.[107] The administration of plasma expanders such as high-molecular-weight

TABLE 179–8. DRUGS ASSOCIATED WITH PLATELET DYSFUNCTION

Inhibitors of Arachidonic Acid Metabolism (Nonsteroidal Anti-Inflammatory Drugs)	*Antithrombotic Drugs With Miscellaneous Mechanisms*
Acetylsalicylic acid	Ticlopidine
Ibuprofen	Ridogrel
Indomethacin	Clopidogrel
Phenylbutazone	Dazoxiben
	Unfractioned heparin
Stimulators of Adenyl Cyclase and Guanylyl Cyclase	*Other Drugs*
Prostaglandin E_1	Chondroitin sulfate
Prostacyclin (PGI_2)	Ampicillin
Prostaglandin D_2	Penicillin G
Nitrous oxide	Carbenicillin
Nitroglycerin	Gentamicin
Nitroprusside	Antihistamines
	Estrogens
Calcium Antagonists	Glycerol guaiacolate
Verapamil	Halothane
Nifedipine	Lidocaine
Diltiazem	Phenothiazines
	Procaine
Phosphodiesterase Inhibitors	Propranolol
Dipiridamol	Sulfonamides
Methylxanthines	

This table is not all-inclusive. The number of new antithrombotic drugs inhibiting platelet function keeps growing.

dextran in dogs impairs hemostasis by inducing dilution of vWf and Factor VIII.[108] Chondroprotective agents may also be included among antithrombotic agents. Degenerative joint disease therapy includes chondroitin sulfate (a sulfated proteoglycan that acts as an ATIII cofactor), an inhibitor of platelet aggregation.[109–111]

In liver disease, platelet surface GP Ib can be reduced and FDPs such as fibrin-induced D-dimer and fibrinogen E fragments increased, interfering with platelet aggregation. Liver failure may induce hyperammonemia. Ammonia is incorporated in the hepatic urea cycle, yielding L-arginine. The concentration of L-arginine may also lead to elevated nitrous oxide production and impaired platelet function.[112]

Increased thrombotic risk and impaired primary hemostasis have been reported in human and canine nephrotic syndrome. Platelet aggregation may be impaired owing to an imbalance between PGI_2 and TXA_2 synthesis; platelet adhesion and aggregation are also diminished owing to low-molecular-weight degradation products expressing an RGD sequence. These may accumulate in uremia and bind to $\alpha_{IIb}\beta_3$, resulting in reduced platelet aggregation. Recently, diminished concentrations of platelet nucleotides ATP and ADP have been observed in chronic renal failure in human patients. This was consistent (and coincident) with increased thrombin and plasmin activation. Low concentrations of thrombin may partially activate platelets and induce endothelial secretion of PGI_2 and nitrous oxide. Plasmin may also degrade vWf—and platelet receptors of vWf—and alter arachidonic acid mobilization from platelet phospholipids.[113]

Paraproteins produced in lymphoproliferative disorders can, in theory, coat circulating platelets and impair their adhesiveness and aggregating capability.[114] Essential thrombocythemia and myeloproliferative-induced thrombocytosis can induce both bleeding tendencies and thrombotic tendencies. Hemangioma or hemangiosarcoma may induce thrombocytopenia and thrombocytopathia in dogs. Transfusion of fresh whole blood may be considered before debulking surgery. Acquired vWd due to neoplasia in people has been described.[115]

In immune-mediated thrombopathia, antiplatelet antibodies may damage platelet membranes and cause release of platelet granule contents, affecting platelet function, specifically platelet aggregation. Integrin $\alpha_{IIb}\beta_3$ is highly immunogenic and thus is potentially the most frequent target antigen in IMT.

DIC, producing both thrombocytopenia and thrombocytopathia, is associated with numerous clinical conditions. Depending on the activation rate of the hemostatic system, DIC may occur as an acute and life-threatening event or as a chronic form without severe thrombosis and hemorrhage. DIC may be initiated by a single cause or by multiple causes occurring sequentially or simultaneously. Pathologic processes that may cause DIC include intravascular hemolysis, bacteria, viruses, protozoal infections, metazoal infections, obstetric complications, gastric dilatation–volvulus, diabetes mellitus, neoplasia, traumatic shock, heat stroke, severe hepatopathy, snake and arthropod venoms, and pancreatitis.[116] DIC may be considered an uncontrolled burst of thrombin generation and activity. This massive activation overwhelms hemostatic inhibitors, depletes procoagulants and platelet numbers, induces thrombosis, and, as a final result, severely damages tissues. Thrombus formation and subsequent ischemia and necrosis may activate an enhanced fibrinolytic response, which would impair platelet function and deplete coagulation factors.

REFERENCES

1. Fitzgerald LA, Philips DR: Structure and function of platelet membrane glycoproteins. In Kunicki TJ, George JN (eds): Platelet Immunobiology. Philadelphia, Lippincott, 1989, pp 9–30.
2. Elangbam CS, et al: Cell adhesion molecules—update. Vet Pathol 34:61, 1997.
3. Boudreaux MK: Platelets and coagulation: An update. Vet Clin North Am Small Anim Pract 26:1065, 1996.
4. Venturini CM, Kaplan JE: Thrombin induces platelet adhesion to endothelial cells. Semin Thromb Hemost 18:275, 1992.
5. Ido M, et al: Ca^{2+}-dependent activation of the 33-kDa protein kinase transmits thrombin receptor signals in human platelets. Thromb Haemost 76:439, 1996.
6. Dandona P, et al: Calcium, calmodulin and protein kinase C dependence of platelet shape change. Thromb Res 81:163, 1996.
7. Wintrobe MW, et al: Clinical Hematology. Philadelphia, Lea & Febiger, 1981, pp 104–162.
8. Nguyen P, et al: Mechanisms of the platelet aggregation induced by activated neutrophils and inhibitory effect of specific PAF receptor agonists. Thromb Res 78:33, 1995.
9. Esmond CT: Possible involvement of cytokines in diffuse intravascular coagulation and thrombosis. Baillieres Clin Haematol 7:453, 1994.
10. Jain NC: The platelets. In Essentials of Veterinary Hematology. Philadelphia, Lea & Febiger, 1993, pp 105–133.
11. Wolf RF, et al: Erythropoietin potentiates thrombus development in a canine arterio-venous shunt model. Thromb Haemost 77:1020, 1997.
12. Levin J: Thrombopoietin—clinically realized? N Engl J Med 336:434, 1997.
13. McCarty JM, et al: Murine thrombopoietin mRNA levels are modulated by platelet count. Blood 86:3668, 1995.
14. Northern J, Tvedten HW: Diagnosis of microthrombocytosis and immune-mediated thrombocytopenia in dogs with thrombocytopenia: 68 cases (1987–1989). JAVMA 200:368, 1992.
15. Ruiz de Gopegui R: Determinación de parámetros hematológicos y hemostáticos en el conejo para modelos experimentales. Proceedings of the 2nd Symposio de la SECAL, Bellaterra (Barcelona), Spain, 1992.
16. Nyindo M, et al: Cell-mediated and humoral immune responses of German shepherd dogs and beagles to experimental infection with Ehrlichia canis. Am J Vet Res 41:250, 1980.
17. Iqbal Z, Rikhhsa Y: Reisolation of Ehrlichia canis from blood and tissues of dogs after doxycycline treatment. J Clin Microbiol 32:1644, 1994.
18. Hibler SC, et al: Rickettsial infections in dogs. Part II. Ehrlichiosis and infectious cyclic thrombocytopenia. Compend Contin Ed Vet Pract 8:106, 1986.
19. Harrus S: Platelet dysfunction associated with experimental acute canine ehrlichiosis. Vet Rec 139:290, 1996.
20. Harvey JW, et al: Cyclic thrombocytopenia induced by a Rickettsia-like agent in dogs. J Infect Dis 137:182, 1978.
21. Woody BJ, Hoskins JD: Ehrlichial diseases of dogs. Vet Clin North Am Small Anim Pract 21:75, 1991.
22. Goldman E, et al: Granulocytic ehrlichiosis in dogs. Vet Clin Pathol 26:54, 1997.
23. Peavy GM, et al: Suspected ehrlichial infection in five cats from a household. JAVMA 210:231, 1997.
24. Dawson JE, Ewing SA: Susceptibility of dogs to infection with Ehrlichia chaffeensis causative agent of human ehrlichiosis. Am J Vet Res 53:1322, 1992.
25. Hoskins JD: Canine haemobartonellosis, canine hepatozoonosis, and feline cytauxzoonosis. Vet Clin North Am Small Anim Pract 21:129, 1991.
26. Hoover JP, et al: Cytauxzoonosis in cats: Eight cases (1985–1992). JAVMA 205:455, 1994.
27. McAnulty JF, et al: Thrombocytopenia associated with vaccination of a dog with modified-live paramyxovirus vaccine. JAVMA 186:1217, 1985.
28. Axthelm MK, et al: Canine distemper virus–induced thrombocytopenia. Am J Vet Res 48:1269, 1987.
29. Kraft W, et al: Thrombozytopenie bei Feliner Infektioser Panleukopenie. Kleintierpraxis 25:129, 1980.
30. Pineau S, et al: Levamisole reduces the thrombocytopaenia associated with myxovirus infection. Can Vet J 21:82, 1980.
31. Breitschwerdt EB: Infectious thrombocytopenia in dogs. Compend Contin Ed Vet Pract 10:1177, 1988.
32. Clinkenbeard KD, et al: Thrombocytopenia associated with disseminated histoplasmosis in dogs. Compend Contin Ed Vet Pract 11:301, 1989.
33. Breitschwerdt EB, et al: Preliminary characterization of a novel infectious cause of thrombocytopenia in dogs. J Vet Intern Med 6:124, 1992.
34. Mackin A: Canine immune-mediated thrombocytopenia. Part I. Compend Contin Ed Vet Pract 17:353, 1995.
35. Gaschen FP, et al: Amegakaryocytic thrombocytopenia and immune-mediated haemolytic anemia in a cat. Comp Haematol Int 2:175, 1992.
36. Joshi BC, et al: Autoimmune thrombocytopenia in a cat. J Am Anim Hosp Assoc 15:585, 1979.
37. Cain GR, et al: Immune-mediated hemolytic anemia and thrombocytopenia in a cat after bone marrow transplantation. Vet Pathol 25:162, 1988.
38. Kristensen AT, et al: Platelet dysfunction associated with immune-mediated thrombocytopenia in dogs. J Vet Intern Med 8:323, 1994.
39. Kristensen AT, et al: Comparison of microscopic and flow cytometric detection of platelet antibody in dogs suspected of having immune-mediated thrombocytopenia. Am J Vet Res 55:1111, 1994.
40. Lewis D: Update on autoimmune diseases in dogs and cats. Proceedings of the Continuing Education Northwest Veterinary Symposium, Seattle, 1996.
41. Kristensen AM, Feldman BF: Blood banking and transfusion medicine. In Ettinger SJ, Feldman EC (eds): Textbook of Veterinary Internal Medicine, 4th ed. Philadelphia, WB Saunders, 1995, pp 347–360.
42. Holloway SA, et al: Prednisolone and danazol for treatment of immune-mediated anemia, thrombocytopenia, and ineffective erythroid regeneration in a dog. JAVMA 197:1045, 1990.
43. Mackin A: Canine immune-mediated thrombocytopenia. Part II. Compend Contin Ed Vet Pract 17:515, 1995.
44. Cockburn C, et al: A retrospective study of sixty-two cases of thrombocytopenia in the dog. Southwest Vet 37:133, 1986.
45. Handagama P, et al: Immune-mediated thrombocytopenia in the dog. Can Pract 12:25, 1985.
46. Bloom JC, et al: Gold-induced immune thrombocytopenia in the dog. Vet Pathol 22:492, 1985.
47. Davis VM: Hapten-induced, immune-mediated thrombocytopenia in a dog. JAVMA 184:976, 1984.
48. Peterson ME, et al: Propylthiouracil-associated hemolytic anaemia, thrombocytopenia, and antinuclear antibodies in cats with hyperthyroidism. JAVMA 184:806, 1984.
49. Atwell RB, et al: Suspected drug-induced thrombocytopenia associated with levamisole therapy in a dog. Aust Vet J 57:91, 1981.
50. Handagama P, Feldman BF: Thrombocytopenia and drugs. Vet Clin North Am Small Anim Pract 18:51, 1988.
51. Castellan E, et al: Toxicite iatrogene des estrogenes chez le chien. Rev Med Vet 144:285, 1993.
52. Ogilvie GK: Hematopoietic growth factors: Frontiers for cure. Vet Clin North Am Small Anim Pract 25:1441, 1995.
53. Nagata H: Mechanism of thrombocytopaenia in dogs infected with Babesia gibsoni. Jpn J Vet Res 41:36, 1993.
54. Grindem CB, et al: Epidemiolgic survey of thrombocytopenia in dogs: A report on 987 cases. Vet Clin Pathol 20:38, 1991.
55. Helfand SC: Platelets and neoplasia. Vet Clin North Am 18:131, 1988.
56. Helfand SC, et al: Immune-mediated thrombocytopenia associated with solid tumors in dogs. J Am Anim Hosp Assoc 21:787, 1985.
57. Boyce JT, et al: Feline leukemia virus–induced thrombocytopenia and macrothrombocytosis in cats. Vet Pathol 23:16, 1986.
58. Hammer AS, et al: Essential thrombocythemia in a cat. J Vet Intern Med 4:87, 1990.
59. Hopper PE, et al: Probable essential thrombocythemia in a dog. J Vet Intern Med 3:79, 1989.
60. Evans RJ, et al: Essential thrombocythemia in the dog and cat: A report of four cases. J Small Anim Pract 23:457, 1982.
61. Tablin F, et al: Ultrastructural analysis of platelets and megakaryocytes from a dog with probable essential thrombocythemia. Vet Pathol 26:289, 1989.
62. Mandell CP, et al: Spurious elevation of serum potassium in two cases of thrombocythemia. Vet Clin Pathol 17:32, 1988.
63. Degen MA, et al: Thrombocytosis associated with a myeloproliferative disorder in a dog. JAVMA 194:1457, 1989.
64. Cain GR, et al: Platelet dysplasia associated with megakaryoblastic leukemia in a dog. JAVMA 188:529, 1986.
65. Cobaltzky F, et al: Acute megakaryoblastic leukemia in one cat and two dogs. Vet Pathol 30:186, 1993.

HEM

66. Holscher MA, et al: Megakaryocytic leukemia in a cat. Feline Pract 13:8, 1983.
67. Jain NC: Qualitative and quantitative disorders of platelets. In Schalm's Veterinary Hematology. Philadelphia, Lea & Febiger, 1986, pp 466–480.
68. Cowles BE, et al: Prolonged bleeding time of Chediak-Higashi cats corrected by platelet transfusion. Thromb Haemost 67:708, 1992.
69. Callan MB, et al: Platelet storage pool disease in American cocker spaniels. Proceedings of 11th ACVIM Forum, Washington, DC, 1993, p 940.
70. Callan MB, Giger U: Bleeding caused by platelet disorders in cats. Proceedings of 15th ACVIM Forum, Lake Buena Vista, FL, 1997.
70a. Callan MB: Unpublished observations, 15th ACVIM Forum, Lake Buena Vista, FL, 1997.
71. Zimmermann TS, et al: Immunologic differentiation between classic hemophilia (Factor VIII deficiency) and von Willebrand's disease. With observations on combined deficiencies of antihemophilic factor and proaccelerin (Factor V) and on an acquired circulating anticoagulant against antihemophilic factor. J Clin Invest 40:244, 1971.
72. Ruggeri ZM, Ware J: The structure and function of von Willebrand's factor. Thromb Haemost 67:594, 1992.
73. Littlewood JD: Inherited bleeding disorders of dogs and cats. J Small Anim Pract 30:140, 1989.
74. Moser J, et al: Inheritance of von Willebrand's factor deficiency in Doberman pinschers. JAVMA 209:1103, 1996.
74a. Internet Web site, 1997: http://www.vetgen.com.
75. Brooks M, et al: Plasma von Willebrand's factor antigen concentration as a predictor of von Willebrand's disease status in German wirehaired Pointers. JAVMA 209:930, 1996.
76. Raymond SL, et al: Clinical and laboratory features of a severe form of von Willebrand's disease in Shetland sheepdogs. JAVMA 197:1342, 1990.
77. Stokol T, Parry BW: Stability of canine Factor VIII and von Willebrand's factor antigen concentration in the frozen state. Res Vet Sci 59:156, 1995.
78. Feldman DG, et al: Hemophilia B (Factor IX deficiency) in a family of German shepherd dogs. JAVMA 206:1901, 1995.
79. Randolph JF, et al: Factor XII deficiency and von Willebrand's disease in a family of miniature poodles. Cornell Vet 76:3, 1986.
80. French TW, et al: A bleeding disorder (von Willebrand's disease) in a Himalayan cat. JAVMA 190:437, 1987.
81. Panciera DL: Does abnormal hemostasis occur in canine hypothyroidism? Canine Pract 22:31, 1997.
82. Forrester SD, Monroe WE: Diseases of the thyroid gland. In Leib ME, Monroe WE (eds): Practical Small Animal Internal Medicine. Philadelphia, WB Saunders, 1997, pp 1027–1043.
83. Stokol T, et al: von Willebrand's disease in Doberman dogs in Australia. Aust Vet J 72:257, 1995.
84. Dodds WJ: Inherited bleeding disorders. Can Pract 6:49, 1978.
85. Brooks M, et al: Epidemiologic features of von Willebrand's disease in Doberman pinschers, Scottish terriers, and Shetland sheepdogs: 260 cases (1984–1988). JAVMA 200:1123, 1992.
86. Brooks M, et al: Severe, recessive von Willebrand's disease in German wirehaired Pointers. JAVMA 209:926, 1996.
87. Stokol T, et al: von Willebrand's disease in Scottish terriers in Australia. Aust Vet J 72:404, 1995.
88. Schlink GT, Johnson GS: A sensitive autoradiographic procedure for Factor VIII–related antigen in canine plasma. Vet Clin Pathol 12:21, 1983.
89. Benson RE, et al: Efficiency and precision of electroimmunoassay for canine Factor VIII–related antigen. Am J Vet Res 44:399, 1983.
90. Stokol T, Parry B: Stability of von Willebrand's factor and Factor VIII in canine cryoprecipitate under various conditions of storage. Res Vet Sci 59:152, 1995.
91. Bass AI, et al: Crossed immunoelectrophoretic pre-peak of canine Factor VIII–related antigen. Thromb Res 20:343, 1980.
92. Johnson GS, et al: Canine von Willebrand's disease. A heterogeneous group of bleeding disorders. Vet Clin North Am Small Anim Pract 18:195, 1988.
93. Miller MA, et al: A modified SDS agarose gel method for determining FVIII von Willebrand's factor multimers using commercially available reagents. Thromb Res 39:777, 1985.
94. Brosstad F, et al: Visualization of von Willebrand's factor multimers by enzyme-conjugated secondary antibodies. Thromb Haemost 55:276, 1986.
95. Ruiz de Gopegui R, Feldman BF: Use of blood and blood components in canine and feline patients with hemostatic disorders. Vet Clin North Am Small Anim Pract 25:1387, 1995.
96. Kraus KH, et al: Multimeric analysis of von Willebrand's factor before and after desmopressin acetate (DDAVP) administration intravenously and subcutaneously in male beagle dogs. Am J Vet Res 48:1376, 1987.
97. Rose EH, Aledort LM: Nasal spray desmopressin (DDAVP) for mild hemophilia A and von Willebrand's disease. Ann Intern Med 114:563, 1991.
98. Locke K: Severe haemorrhage in Doberman dogs with von Willebrand's disease and its control during surgery. Aust Vet J 71:263, 1994.
99. Johnstone IB, Crane S: Failure of sodium pentobarbital anesthesia to alter 1-desamino-8-D-arginine vasopressin–induced elevations of plasma Factor VIII/von Willebrand's factor in normal dogs. Can J Vet Res 52:416, 1988.
100. Patterson WR, et al: Absent platelet aggregation with normal fibrinogen binding in basset hound hereditary thrombopathy. Thromb Haemost 62:1011, 1989.
101. Estry DW, et al: Basset hound hereditary thrombopathy: An inherited disorder with defective platelet aggregation despite normal fibrinogen binding and receptor mobility. Comp Haematol Int 5:227, 1995.
102. Dodds WJ: Inherited hemostasis disorders. Proceedings of the Continuing Education Northwest Veterinary Symposium, Seattle, 1996.
103. Dodds WJ: Familial canine thrombocytopathy. Thromb Diath Haemorrh Suppl 26:241, 1967.
104. Boudreaux MK, et al: Identification of an intrinsic platelet function defect in Spitz dogs. J Vet Intern Med 8:93, 1994.
105. Lothrop CD, et al: Characterization of platelet function in cyclic hematopoietic dogs. Exp Hematol 19:916, 1991.
106. Nolte P, et al: A study on the efficacy of a phospholipid solution in dogs with aspirin-induced thrombocytopathy. JAVMA 41:385, 1994.
107. von Ammelounx U, et al: Untersuchung zur Wirksamkeit von Kortison bei gesunden Hunden mit physiologischen Thrombozytenzählen, aspirininduzierten Blutungszeitverlängerungen und bei Hunden mit thrombozytopenischen Krankheitsbilden. Berl Munch Tierärztl Wochenschr 100:124, 1987.
108. Concannon KT, et al: Hemostatic defects associated with two infusion rates of dextran 70 in dogs. Am J Vet Res 53:1369, 1992.
109. McNamara PS, et al: Hematologic, hemostatic, and biochemical effects in dogs receiving an oral chondroprotective agent for thirty days. Am J Vet Res 57:1390, 1996.
110. Catafalmo JL, Dodds WJ: Hereditary and acquired thrombopathias. Vet Clin North Am Small Anim Pract 18:185, 1988.
111. Rao GH, Rao AT: Pharmacology of platelet activation-inhibitory drugs. Indian J Physiol Pharmacol 38:69, 1994.
112. Shinya H, et al: Hyperammonemia inhibits platelet aggregation in rats. Thromb Res 81:195, 1996.
113. Mezzano D, et al: Hemostatic disorder of uremia: The platelet defect, main determinant of the prolonged bleeding time, is correlated with indices of activation of coagulation and fibrinolysis. Thromb Haemost 76:312, 1996.
114. Ruiz de Gopegui R, et al: Paraprotein-induced defective haemostasis in a dog with IgA (kappa-light chain) forming myeloma. Vet Clin Pathol 23:70, 1994.
115. Mohri H, et al: Acquired type 2A von Willebrand's disease in chronic myelocytic leukemia. Hematopathol Mol Hematol 10:123, 1996.
116. Ruiz de Gopegui R, et al: Disseminated intravascular coagulation: Present and future perspective. Comp Haematol Int 5:213, 1995.

CHAPTER 180

COAGULOPATHIES AND THROMBOSIS

Marjory Brooks

Hemostasis is the body's defense mechanism for controlling blood loss from damaged blood vessels. The hemostatic process involves complex interactions between endothelial cells, platelets, leukocytes, and plasma proteins at the site of vascular damage. These interactions result in formation of a platelet aggregate, generation of a fibrin clot, and initiation of inflammatory and fibrinolytic pathways that culminate in tissue and vessel repair. Effective hemostasis must be rapid and localized; too much hemostasis causes thrombosis and too little causes persistent bleeding. Maintenance of an appropriate balance depends on integration of inhibitors and activators of hemostasis.

PHYSIOLOGY OF HEMOSTASIS

PRIMARY HEMOSTASIS

The initial phase of hemostasis consists of a series of interactions between platelets and the site of endothelial cell disruption, culminating in assembly of a platelet aggregate (Fig. 180–1, top).[1] Exposure of subendothelium triggers conformation changes in von Willebrand's factor, an adhesive plasma protein that acts to link platelets to the site of vessel injury. After platelets adhere to subendothelium, they undergo shape change, form intraplatelet bridges, and release agonist compounds from storage organelles. Ultimately, platelet aggregates cover the zone of vascular damage to form a hemostatic plug. Activated platelets provide membrane surfaces and binding sites for assembly of the procoagulant enzyme complexes that promote formation of a fibrin clot in the secondary phase of hemostasis.

SECONDARY HEMOSTASIS

Blood Clotting Cascade

The coagulation cascade consists of a series of enzymatic reactions culminating in cleavage of plasma fibrinogen to form cross-linked fibrin at the site of vessel injury (see Fig. 180–1, middle).[2] All procoagulant factors and cofactors participating in the coagulation cascade are synthesized in the liver and circulate in plasma in inactive forms. Factors II (prothrombin), VII, IX, and X are serine protease proenzymes that undergo a vitamin K–dependent posttranslational modification (gamma carboxylation) before they are secreted from hepatocytes. The presence of gamma-carboxyglutamic acid residues on these factors is critical for their interaction with cell membranes via calcium ion binding.[2] These factors assemble on a membrane surface with their respective substrates and regulatory protein (tissue factor) or procoagulant cofactors (factors VIII and V) as they assume enzymatically

active configurations known as "prothrombinase" or "tenase" complexes (Fig. 180–2).

The principal initiating event of coagulation is mediated by tissue factor, a transmembrane glycoprotein absent from quiescent endothelium.[1, 2] Tissue trauma exposes cells to the vascular compartment that express high levels of tissue factor. In addition, endothelial cells and monocytes are induced to express tissue factor by mediators of inflammation including endotoxin, interleukin, tumor necrosis factor, and complement.

Tissue factor initiates coagulation when it binds to factor VII and forms an active complex (TF-FVIIa) (Fig. 180–3). This complex interacts with factors IX and X to generate the active factors IXa and Xa. If appropriate membrane surfaces and receptors are present, tenase and prothrombinase complexes assemble and ultimately convert prothrombin to its active form thrombin (IIa). Thrombin binds to plasma fibrinogen and cleaves fibrinopeptides A and B, with resultant formation of soluble fibrin monomers. Fibrin monomers polymerize, and in the final step of clot formation, factor XIIIa covalently links polymers to produce insoluble, cross-linked fibrin (see Fig. 180–3).

Thrombin promotes many of the procoagulant reactions of the clotting cascade (see Fig. 180–3). Although TF-FVIIa initiates coagulation in vivo, sustained generation of fibrin apparently requires acceleration of the coagulation cascade by thrombin-mediated formation of an active intrinsic tenase complex.[1]

Inhibitors of Coagulation

Fibrin clot generation must be restricted to the site of vessel damage. Physiologic inhibitors act to localize and dampen the procoagulant reactions of the clotting cascade (Table 180–1). Antithrombin is the major plasma inhibitor of the serine protease factors.[3] Its main inhibitory effects are on thrombin and factors Xa and IXa. Antithrombin blocks the reactive site of these factors through formation of a 1:1 enzyme-inhibitor complex, detected in plasma as thrombin-antithrombin complexes. Serine protease inhibitors of lesser significance include heparin cofactor II, alpha$_2$-macroglobulin, and alpha$_1$-proteinase inhibitor.

Tissue factor pathway inhibitor (TFPI) regulates the tissue factor–mediated pathway of coagulation.[4] Sustained generation of factor Xa is prevented by binding of TFPI to the factor Xa catalytic site and the TF-FVIIa complex. TFPI is a glycoprotein that circulates in plasma bound to lipoproteins, and it is also released from activated platelets.

The protein C–protein S pathway is the third major physiologic inhibitor of coagulation.[1] Its anticoagulant mechanism is initiated when thrombin binds to the endothelial cell surface receptor thrombomodulin. This binding promotes

Pathway: Primary Hemostasis

Endpoint: Platelet Aggregate

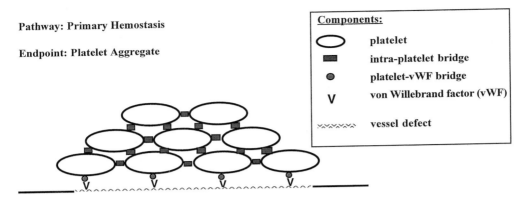

Pathway: Secondary Hemostasis (Coagulation)

Endpoint: Fibrin Clot

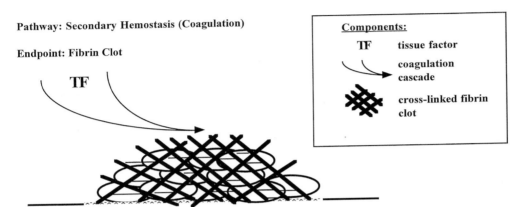

Figure 180–1. Hemostatic pathways.

Pathway: Fibrinolysis

Endpoint: Fibrin degradation

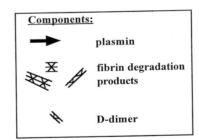

thrombin cleavage of protein C to its active form (APC) and association of APC with its cofactor, protein S. The APC–protein S complex catalyzes inactivation of factors Va and VIIIa. Proteins C and S are vitamin K–dependent plasma glycoproteins.

Pharmacologic and pathologic inhibitors of coagulation also exist (see Table 180–1).[5, 6] Heparin's anticoagulant activity results from its ability to accelerate the rate of complex formation between antithrombin and activated serine proteases. Coumarin and indanedione derivatives block vitamin K recycling, which results in synthesis of descarboxy serine protease zymogens that are unable to form tenase and prothrombinase complexes. Newer classes of anticoagulant agents include hirudin, a specific inhibitor of thrombin, and low-molecular-weight heparins that specifically enhance antithrombin's anti-Xa activity. Pathologic inhibitors of coagulation include fibrin degradation products that interfere with fibrin cross-linkage and antibodies directed against specific coagulation factors or phospholipid and protein components of cell membranes.

FIBRINOLYSIS

The reactions initiating platelet aggregation and fibrin clot formation simultaneously trigger local activation of fibrinolysis. In this process, vascular patency is restored by degradation of fibrin by the proteolytic enzyme plasmin to release cross-linked fibrin degradation products (see Fig. 180–1, bottom).[1]

Plasmin circulates in plasma as a proenzyme, plasminogen. The serine protease enzymes tissue-type plasminogen activator (t-PA) and urokinase-type plasminogen activator (u-PA) are the major physiologic activators of plasminogen (Fig. 180–4).[7] Tissue-type plasminogen activator is produced

Active Extrinsic Tenase Complex

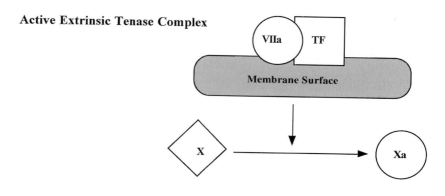

Active Tenase Complex

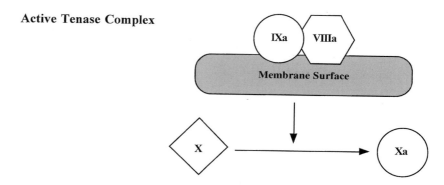

Figure 180–2. Active factor complexes.

Active Prothrombinase Complex

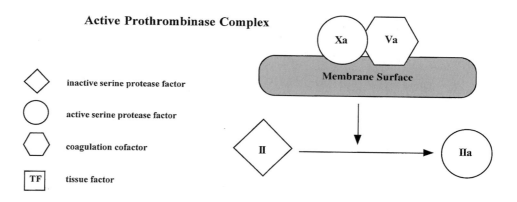

and released from endothelial cells. Bioactivity of t-PA is largely localized to the intravascular compartment by its high affinity for fibrin. Fibrin-bound t-PA has high catalytic efficiency in cleaving plasminogen, resulting in formation of plasmin on the surface of fibrin and efficient in situ degradation of fibrin.

Urokinase-type plasminogen activator is produced in the kidney. In contrast to t-PA, u-PA functions predominately in the extravascular space and its action is not enhanced by fibrin binding. In vivo, u-PA is activated by prekallikrein (PK) and high-molecular-weight kininogen (HK), plasma zymogens that also mediate release of the proinflammatory vasoactive peptide bradykinin. Factors XI, XII, and PK cleave plasminogen directly with low efficiency and in vitro promote coagulation through activation of the tenase complex.[8]

Plasmin's cleavage of fibrin releases a series of cross-linked fragments known as fibrin degradation products or fibrin split products (see Fig. 180–4). The smallest cross-linked fragment is a dimer (D-dimer). Physiologic fibrinolysis occurs only at sites of fibrin-bound plasmin. In disease states, systemic activation of plasminogen causes cleavage of fibrinogen and fibrin.[9] Fibrinogen cleavage forms a series of degradation products but no cross-linked complexes and no D-dimer.

Fibrinolysis is modulated by two different plasma protease inhibitors, one reactive with plasmin and one reactive with t-PA (see Fig. 180–4). The main antiplasmin, alpha$_2$-antiplasmin, is a rapid inhibitor of free plasmin but has limited activity toward fibrin-bound plasmin. Antiplasmin also interferes with plasminogen binding to fibrin. The major physiologic inhibitor of t-PA is plasminogen activator inhibitor 1 (PAI-1). This inhibitor is present in plasma and platelets and rapidly reacts with t-PA and u-PA.[7]

HEM

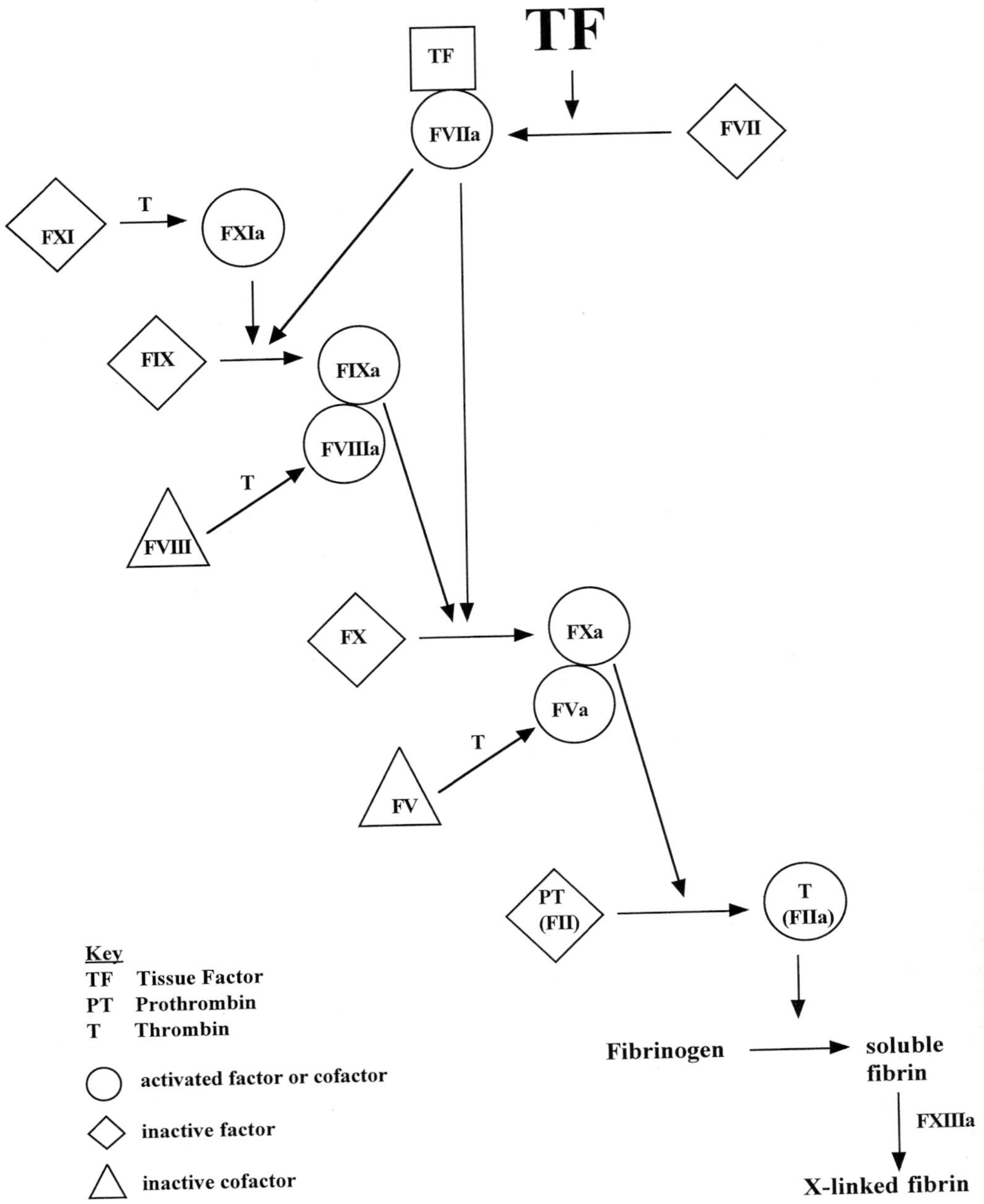

Figure 180–3. Blood coagulation pathway.

REGULATION OF HEMOSTASIS

Vascular endothelium plays a key role in regulating hemostasis.[1, 2] Injury or pathologic states disrupt hemostatic balance by inducing expression of endothelial receptors that promote activation of platelets and coagulant proteins. At the same time, the antithrombotic and anticoagulant properties of intact endothelium are lost.

Clotting factor activity requires phospholipid and membrane surfaces. Platelet aggregates and TF provide these surfaces at sites of vessel injury. Prothrombinase activity generates thrombin, which acts via positive feedback to sustain coagulation and via proteins C and S to inhibit coagulation. Systemic generation of fibrin is limited by dilution of active factors as blood flows away from sites of vessel injury and by rapid antithrombin neutralization.

Fibrinolysis occurs preferentially at sites of fibrin genera-

tion because plasminogen and t-PA are incorporated in developing clots. Fibrin-bound t-PA activates plasminogen, and the action of plasmin is restricted to the surface of fibrin by its plasma inhibitor, antiplasmin. Endothelial cells secrete PAI-1, preventing activation of plasmin at sites of intact endothelium.

The stimulus of tissue injury that triggers hemostasis simultaneously initiates inflammation, complement activation, and wound healing.[1, 2, 8] Many cytokines and chemical messengers are common to these processes, and damaged endothelial cells and activated platelets express receptors for the cellular mediators of inflammation, neutrophils and monocytes.

Hemorrhage or thrombosis results from imbalance of regulators and effectors of hemostasis. Some elements of these complex systems remain undefined, and species differences complicate veterinary application of tests and treatment de-

TABLE 180–1. COAGULATION INHIBITORS

INHIBITOR	CLASS	ACTION
Physiologic inhibitors		
Antithrombin	Serine protease inhibitor (serpin), synthesized in liver	Plasma protein, inactivates factors IIa, IXa, Xa
Tissue factor pathway inhibitor	Kunitz-type inhibitor, synthesized in endothelium	Plasma lipoprotein bound, inhibits TF–factor VIIa and factor Xa
Protein C	Serine protease (protein C), synthesized in liver	Vitamin K–dependent plasma proteins, inhibit factors Va and VIIIa
Protein S		
Pharmacologic inhibitors		
Heparin	Glycosaminoglycan, up to 30 kDa	Enhances antithrombin activity
Low-molecular-weight heparin	Glycosaminoglycans, 4–6 kDa	Enhance anti-Xa action of antithrombin
Warfarin, superwarfarins	Coumadin-indanedione inhibitors of vitamin K epoxide reductase	Vitamin K antagonists, prevent activation of factors II, VII, IX, X
Hirudin	Polypeptide, native and recombinant forms	Specific binding to thrombin's active site
Pathologic inhibitors		
FDP	Fibrin degradation products	Interfere with fibrin polymerization
Factor inhibitors	Antibodies	Specific binding to individual clotting factors
Lupus anticoagulants	Antibodies	Binding to phospholipid, cause in vitro prolongation of clotting time

veloped for human beings. Nevertheless, new understanding of hemostatic mechanisms hold promise for improving management of hemostatic defects.

DIAGNOSIS OF HEMOSTATIC DISORDERS

BLEEDING DISORDERS

Bleeding is a common clinical problem. The broad differential for each patient is blood loss from damaged or diseased blood vessels versus a defect impairing the normal hemostatic process (Fig. 180–5).[9, 10] Vascular integrity is tested primarily by inspection, either visually or using diagnostic aids (e.g., endoscopy, radiography, ultrasonography, computed tomographic scanning). Disorders that cause blood loss from normal blood vessels include traumatic or surgical injury and erosion or infiltration from neoplastic, inflammatory, or granulomatous lesions. Causes of hemorrhage from abnormal vessels (vasculopathies) are usually identified by means of serology and biopsy to define specific inflammatory, toxic, endocrine, or degenerative disease.

Hemostatic disorders are classified as failure of platelet plug assembly (primary hemostatic defects), failure of fibrin clot formation (secondary hemostatic defects), or fibrinolytic defects (see Fig. 180–5). The combination of clinical signs,

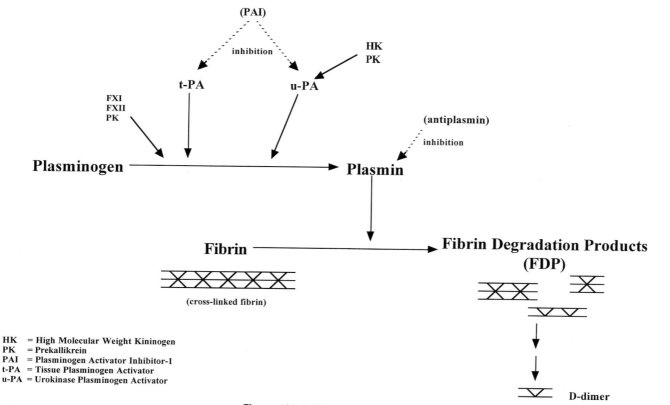

HK = High Molecular Weight Kininogen
PK = Prekallikrein
PAI = Plasminogen Activator Inhibitor-1
t-PA = Tissue Plasminogen Activator
u-PA = Urokinase Plasminogen Activator

Figure 180–4. Fibrinolytic pathway.

HEM

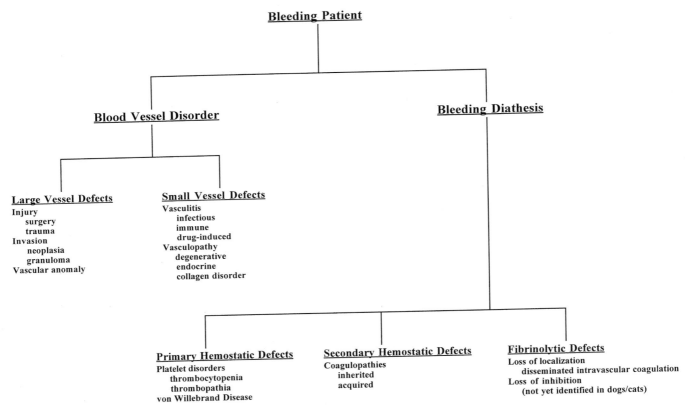

Figure 180–5. Differential diagnosis of the bleeding dog or cat.

history, and screening tests differentiates primary from secondary hemostatic disorders in most cases. Primary hemostatic disorders typically cause petechiae, ecchymoses, and bleeding from mucosal surfaces. Signs suggestive of coagulopathy include hematoma formation, hemarthrosis, and bleeding into pleural and peritoneal spaces. Prolonged bleeding from sites of surgery and trauma is common to all hemostatic defects.

Quick Assessment Tests

Results of platelet count, in vivo bleeding time, and activated clotting time (ACT) tests provide preliminary evidence of a bleeding diathesis. Platelet count and buccal mucosal bleeding time are measures of primary hemostasis. A low platelet count confirms thrombocytopenia, and a long bleeding time in the presence of a normal platelet count indicates platelet dysfunction or von Willebrand's disease (see Chapter 179).

The ACT is a screening test for secondary hemostasis. It is a functional test, measuring the in vitro time for fibrin clot formation.[11] The ACT is sensitive to deficiency or dysfunction of all clotting factors, with the exception of factor VII. Deficiency of PK or HK also causes prolongation of ACT. The test may be technically difficult to perform in cats and small dogs. Sampling from the jugular vein is not recommended, because animals that have severe coagulopathies may develop hematoma and subsequent upper respiratory obstruction. If the ACT is prolonged (or the test is not performed), coagulation defects should be defined through evaluation of coagulation screening tests.[11, 12]

THROMBOTIC DISORDERS

Thrombosis and thromboemboli develop in association with diseases that cause blood stasis, vascular endothelial injury, or hemostatic imbalance.[5, 13] Thrombi may form at any site in the cardiovascular system including heart, arteries, veins, and microcirculation. Clinical signs are caused by organ dysfunction referable to obstruction of blood flow by thrombi or distant embolization of thrombotic material.[5, 13–15] Aortic thromboembolism is typically associated with signs of renal failure or hindlimb paresis and paralysis. Peripheral vein thrombosis often causes signs of dyspnea when thromboemboli travel to the right side of the heart and subsequently lodge in the pulmonary arterial bed. In some animals, arterial and venous thrombosis and pulmonary thromboemboli occur simultaneously.[14]

Diagnostic and therapeutic practices differ for venous and arterial thrombotic disorders.[9, 13, 15] A combination of noninvasive and invasive studies is used to visualize the extent of local thrombosis or distant thromboembolization in people (Table 180–2). The most readily applicable of these procedures to veterinary medicine include angiography, blood gas analysis, echocardiography, thoracic radiography, and ultrasonography. All of these tests have limitations in availability, cost-effectiveness, and predictive utility. Imaging studies require anesthesia, and contrast agents used for angiography may evoke adverse reactions. For these reasons, in vitro tests are also used to try to predict or confirm the presence of thrombosis.[13, 16]

LABORATORY TESTS OF COAGULATION AND THROMBOSIS

Sample Collection

Sample quality is critical for accurate hemostasis testing.[10, 11, 17] Activation of the coagulation cascade or fibrinolytic system affects all subsequent in vitro measures of the individual components of these pathways. Repeated probing of

TABLE 180–2. DIAGNOSTIC TESTS TO LOCALIZE THROMBOSIS AND THROMBOEMBOLI

TEST	APPLICATION
Angiography (I)*	Visualization of filling defects caused by arterial thrombosis or PTE
Arterial blood gas analysis (I)	Identification of hypoxemia and hypocarbia associated with PTE
Echocardiography (N)	Diagnosis of primary cardiac disease and visualization of intracardiac thrombus
IPG (impedance plethysmography) (N)	Detection of obstruction in proximal leg veins by changes in electrical resistance
Thoracic radiography (N)	Identification of nonspecific changes associated with PTE (hyperlucency, small vessels, pleural effusion, alveolar infiltrates)
Ultrasonography (N) (Doppler ultrasound)	Visualization of cardiac, arterial, and venous thrombosis and emboli
Venography (I)	Visualization of vessel obstruction caused by occlusive thrombi
Ventilation perfusion scanning (N)	Indirect evidence of PTE by identifying regions of lung with normal airflow and segmental perfusion defects

*I = invasive test; N = noninvasive test; PTE = pulmonary thromboembolism.

the venipuncture site, drawing blood through a hematoma, and use of excessive vacuum are likely to expose tissue factor, cause turbulent blood flow, stimulate platelet release, and ultimately activate and consume hemostatic proteins. Hemolysis and clot formation are obvious signs of activation, and samples that are hemolyzed or clotted during collection are not accurate indicators of in vivo hemostasis.

Sample activation is prevented by using clean venipuncture technique to collect freely flowing blood directly into a vacuum tube or syringe containing premeasured citrate anticoagulant (Fig. 180–6). Citrate concentrations of 3.2 and 3.8 per cent appear to be acceptable alternatives,[17] but it is ideal to follow the testing laboratory's recommendations. Plasma collected in ethylenediaminetetraacetic acid (EDTA) or heparin anticoagulant is not suitable for clotting time tests. Serum (or plasma placed in clot activator tubes) is depleted of fibrinogen and many other hemostatic proteins and is therefore invalid for hemostasis testing.

In order to retain maximal activity of labile factors, citrated whole blood should be centrifuged as soon as possible after collection and the supernatant plasma transferred to a siliconized glass or plastic tube.[11, 12] Each testing laboratory's recommended procedures for transport should be followed.

Assay systems optimized for testing hemostasis in human beings may not be appropriate for testing animals because of differences among species in enzyme reaction kinetics and variable cross-reactivity of antibody reagents.[18, 19] Overnight courier services provide rapid transport, and it is preferable to send samples to veterinary testing laboratories that use species-specific validated assays, controls, and reference ranges.

Coagulation Screening Tests

Coagulation screening tests are functional assays, measuring the in vitro time for fibrin clot formation in a sample of the patient's plasma. These tests utilize reagents that specifically activate groups of factors or systems within the coagulation cascade (Fig. 180–7).[12]

The activated partial thromboplastin time (aPTT) is a test of the intrinsic and common system factors. The test reagent contains particulate activators and phospholipids that support in vitro activation of the "contact group" factors consisting of factor XII, PK, and HK.

The prothrombin time (PT) tests the extrinsic and common system factors. The test reaction is initiated using a tissue thromboplastin reagent that activates factor VII.

The thrombin clotting time (TT or TCT) measures the rate of fibrin clot formation after addition of thrombin reagent to the patient's plasma. The test is sensitive to deficiency or dysfunction of fibrinogen. Fibrinogen concentration is measured using functional assays involving thrombin time, quantitative methods for detecting fibrinogen antigen, or a semiquantitative method using heat precipitation.[12]

Prolongation of clotting time in one or more screening tests indicates a coagulation disorder. The pattern of abnormalities depends on which individual factor or pathway is involved. Additional clotting time tests (see Fig. 180–7) and/or individual clotting factor assays can be performed to establish a definitive diagnosis.[9–12]

Coagulation Factor Analyses

Specific procoagulant activity of individual clotting factors can be measured in modified aPTT or PT assays on the basis of a fibrin clot endpoint.[12] A different test method utilizes chromogenic substrates, with spectrophotometric detection of color change as the end point. Regardless of methodology, coagulant activity is calculated on the basis of the activity of a standard plasma. Reaction kinetics vary among species, and factor activities in animals should be calculated from same-species standards in order to obtain accurate results throughout physiologic and pathologic ranges.[11, 19]

Coagulation Inhibitor Assays

Antithrombin, TFPI, and proteins C and S are the major inhibitors of coagulation (see Table 180–1). Antithrombin activity in animal plasma can be measured in a chromogenic substrate assay.[3] Assays for TFPI and proteins C and S are not routinely available. The anticoagulant effects of heparin and coumadin are measured using aPTT and PT assays, respectively. Chromogenic substrate assays that measure anti-Xa and anti-IIa activity have been developed for monitoring heparin and low-molecular-weight heparins in human beings.[20]

Pathologic coagulation inhibitors include antibodies that bind to clotting factors or to procoagulant phospholipid and glycoprotein membrane antigens.[6] These antibodies are detected in mixing studies, in which inhibitor plasmas prolong the clotting time when combined with normal species plasma. Antiphospholipid (APL) antibodies are detected in lupus anticoagulant assays, test systems that have a low phospholipid concentration.[6] Paradoxically, APL antibodies are associated with thrombotic disorders.[9, 13]

Fibrinolytic Pathway Tests

Commercial chromogenic substrate assay kits can be used to measure the activity of plasminogen and its major inhibitor, antiplasmin, in animal plasmas.[18] At present, there are no tests for routine measurement of canine and feline PAI and t-PA. Fibrin and fibrinogen degradation products and D-dimer can be detected using commercial latex agglutination kits.[19, 21] These kits contain antibodies directed against human degradation fragments. Cross-reactivity of each kit's antibodies should be confirmed before use in animals.

HEM

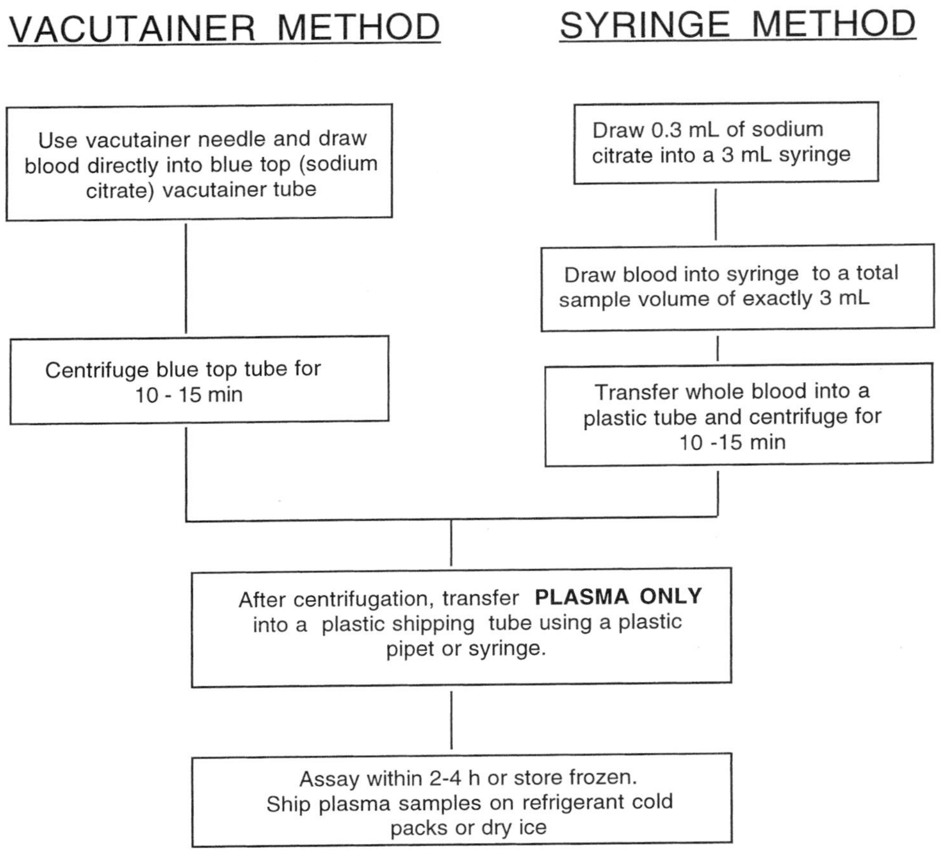

VACUTAINER METHOD   SYRINGE METHOD

```
┌─────────────────────────────┐        ┌─────────────────────────────┐
│ Use vacutainer needle and   │        │ Draw 0.3 mL of sodium       │
│ draw blood directly into    │        │ citrate into a 3 mL syringe │
│ blue top (sodium citrate)   │        └─────────────────────────────┘
│ vacutainer tube             │                      │
└─────────────────────────────┘        ┌─────────────────────────────┐
              │                         │ Draw blood into syringe to  │
              │                         │ a total sample volume of    │
              │                         │ exactly 3 mL                │
              │                         └─────────────────────────────┘
┌─────────────────────────────┐                      │
│ Centrifuge blue top tube    │        ┌─────────────────────────────┐
│ for 10 - 15 min             │        │ Transfer whole blood into   │
└─────────────────────────────┘        │ a plastic tube and          │
                                        │ centrifuge for 10 -15 min   │
                                        └─────────────────────────────┘
```

┌───┐
│ After centrifugation, transfer **PLASMA   │
│ ONLY** into a plastic shipping tube using a │
│ plastic pipet or syringe.   │
└───┘

┌───┐
│ Assay within 2-4 h or store frozen.   │
│ Ship plasma samples on refrigerant cold   │
│ packs or dry ice   │
└───┘

Figure 180–6. Blood sample collection flow chart.

All coagulation screening tests, factor activity and factor inhibitor assays, tests of fibrinolysis and vWF:Ag determination require PLASMA not serum for valid assay.

1. Citrate anticoagulant is suitable for all assays.
2 . The ratio of citrate to whole blood is critical. Use in an exact ratio of 1 part citrate to 9 parts blood
(examples)
0.2 ml citrate + 1.8 ml blood = 2.0 ml total sample volume
0.3 ml citrate + 2.7 ml blood = 3.0 ml total sample volume
0.4 ml citrate + 3.6 ml blood = 4.0 ml total sample volume

Markers of Thrombosis

Thrombosis results from activation of platelets and thrombin and is accompanied by fibrinolysis. Many of the immunoassays used to detect granular constituents released from activated platelets or cleavage products of prothrombin and fibrinogen do not demonstrate cross-reactivity with the corresponding animal proteins.[22] Plasma markers that may be useful for predicting or confirming thrombosis in animals include thrombin-antithrombin complexes, D-dimer, and soluble fibrin monomer.[19, 22]

COAGULATION DISORDERS

ACQUIRED FACTOR DEFICIENCIES

Acquired coagulation disorders are most often caused by liver failure (production defect), vitamin K deficiency (activation defect), or disseminated intravascular coagulation (DIC) (consumption and localization defect).[10, 11] Signs of coagulopathy may also accompany drug therapy, neoplasia, amyloidosis, and immune-mediated disease. Acquired coag-

ulopathies cause simultaneous deficiency of many factors rather than specific deficiency of a single factor. Coagulation screening tests are often sufficient for diagnosis; in more complicated cases, screening test results indicate which specialized tests should be performed (Fig. 180–8).

The liver is the primary site of synthesis and clearance of coagulation factors. Diseases that cause a reduction in functional hepatic mass may cause factor deficiency or dysfunction. These diseases include hepatic necrosis, cirrhosis, portosystemic shunt, and cholestasis.[9, 11, 23] The coagulopathy accompanying liver disease rarely causes spontaneous hemorrhage; more frequently, bleeding complications occur after liver biopsy or surgery. Coagulation screening tests are useful for identifying subclinical coagulopathies before invasive procedures. Liver disease is associated with abnormal hemostasis via other mechanisms including vitamin K deficiency, DIC, platelet dysfunction, and abnormal clearance of plasminogen activators and fibrin degradation products.

Vitamin K deficiencies result from inadequate intestinal absorption or impaired intrahepatic recycling.[9-11] Conditions associated with decreased vitamin K absorption include biliary obstruction, cholestasis, infiltrative bowel disease, chronic oral antibiotic administration, and pancreatic insuf-

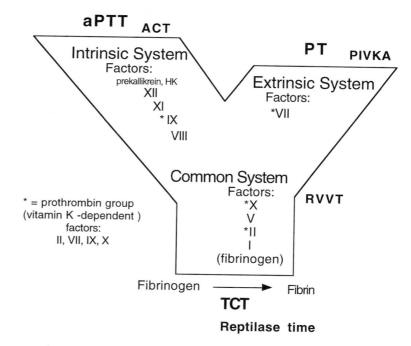

Figure 180–7. Coagulation screening tests.

Tests:	Detects deficiency/dysfunction of:
aPTT	Prekallikrein, HK, factors XII, XI, IX, VIII, X, V, II, I
ACT	Prekallikrein, HK, factors XII, XI, IX, VIII, X, V, II, I
PT	Factors VII, X, V, II, I
PIVKA	Factors VII, X, V, II, I
RVVT	Factors X, V, II, I
TCT	Factor I (fibrinogen)
fibrinogen	Factor I (fibrinogen)
Reptilase time	Factor I (fibrinogen)

Abbreviations:
ACT = activated clotting time
aPTT = activated partial thromboplastin time
HK = high molecular weight kininogen
PIVKA = proteins induced by vitamin K absence or antagonism
PT = prothrombin time
RVVT = Russell viper venom time
TCT = thrombin clotting time

ficiency. Anticoagulant rodenticide ingestion is the most common cause of clinically severe coagulopathy caused by vitamin K deficiency. These rodenticides irreversibly block activity of the recycling enzyme, vitamin K epoxide reductase. Clinical signs of abnormal hemorrhage occur 1 to 2 days after ingestion of a toxic dose, and the anticoagulant effect of second-generation poisons lasts for up to 6 weeks. Because of the short half-life of factor VII, its activity is reduced before signs of hemorrhage are clinically obvious. Moderate to marked deficiencies of all vitamin K–dependent factors coincide with onset of bleeding.

A dilutional coagulopathy may occur if massive, acute blood loss is treated with stored blood products and crystalloid or colloid infusion. High-molecular-weight colloids (hetastarch, dextran) and the newer hemoglobin-based oxygen carrier (Oxyglobin) prolong in vitro clotting time and should be used cautiously for treating patients with acquired or inherited coagulopathies. Other drugs that may cause coagulopathy include beta-lactam and sulfaquinoxaline antibiotics and overdoses of heparins or coumadin.

Signs of hemorrhage associated with amyloidosis, neoplasia, and immune-mediated disease are caused by multiple defects including vasculopathy, DIC, and clotting factor inhibition.

INHERITED FACTOR DEFICIENCIES

Inherited coagulation disorders are caused by mutations in genes coding for specific coagulation factors.[9, 11] New, spontaneous mutations can arise in any purebred or mixed-breed animal and are most often propagated when asymptomatic carriers are bred. Specific coagulant activity assays establish a definitive diagnosis of an inherited factor deficiency (see Fig. 180–8) and provide the basis for designing treatment and disease screening strategies.

Molecular genetic analyses have uncovered many different mutations responsible for factor deficiencies in human families and ethnic groups. Preliminary studies in animals indicate similar molecular genetic heterogeneity.[24] Factor deficiencies can be classified on the basis of inheritance pattern, results of coagulation tests, and breed occurrence (Table 180–3).

HEM

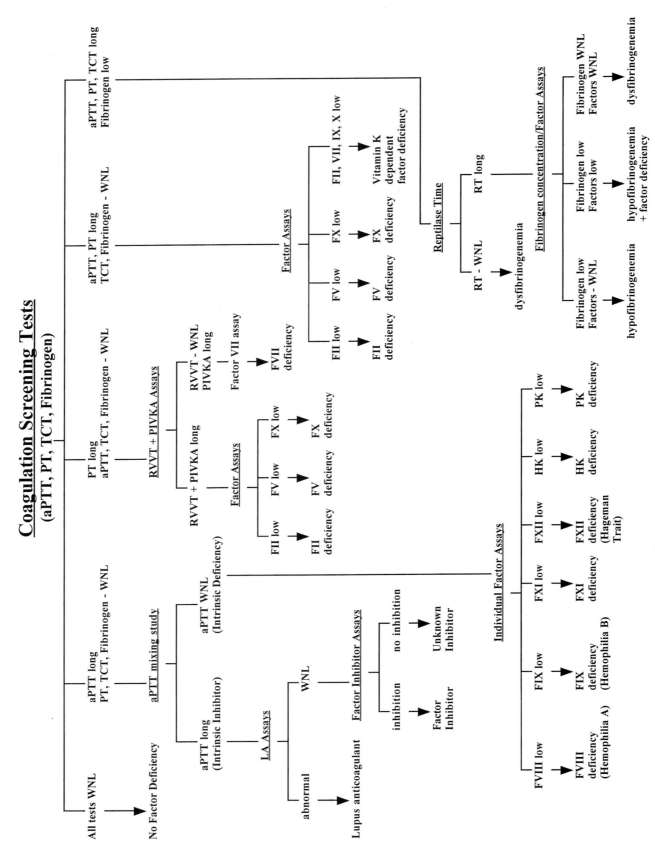

Coagulation Screening Tests
(aPTT, PT, TCT, Fibrinogen)

Figure 180–8. Diagnosis of coagulation factor deficiencies.

TABLE 180–3. INHERITED FACTOR DEFICIENCIES

FACTOR (DEFECT)	INHERITANCE PATTERN	COAGULATION SCREEN RESULTS*	AFFECTED BREEDS
Fibrinogen (dysfibrinogenemia)	Autosomal	Long aPTT, PT, TCT, low fibrinogen	Canine: borzoi, Bernese Mountain Dog, Bichon Frise, collie
II (hypoprothrombinemia)	Autosomal	Long aPTT, PT TCT, fibrinogen WNL	Feline: DSH, DLH† Canine: Boxer, English cocker spaniel
VII (factor VII deficiency)	Autosomal	Long PT aPTT, TCT, fibrinogen WNL	Canine: beagle, malamute Feline: DSH
VIII (hemophilia A)	X-linked recessive	long aPTT PT, TCT, fibrinogen WNL	Canine: German shepherd, many breeds and mixed breeds Feline: DSH, DLH, Havana Brown Siamese, Persian
IX (hemophilia B)	X-linked recessive	Long aPTT PT, TCT, fibrinogen WNL	Canine: many breeds and mixed breeds Feline: DSH, DLH, Himalayan, British Shorthair
X (factor X deficiency)	Autosomal	Long aPTT, PT, RVVT TCT, fibrinogen WNL	Canine: American cocker spaniel, Jack Russell terrier Feline: DSH
XI (factor XI deficiency)	Autosomal	Long aPTT PT, TCT, fibrinogen WNL	Canine: English springer spaniel, Kerry blue terrier
XII (Hageman trait)	Autosomal recessive	Long aPTT PT, TCT, fibrinogen WNL	Canine: Shar Pei, miniature poodle Feline: DSH, DLH

*aPTT = activated partial thromboplastin time; PT = prothrombin time; TCT = thrombin clotting time; WNL = within normal limits.
†DLH = domestic long haired; DSH = domestic short haired.

X-Linked Factor Deficiencies

Hemophilia is the most common inherited coagulation factor deficiency.[9, 11, 24] There are two forms: hemophilia A, caused by factor VIII deficiency, and hemophilia B, caused by factor IX deficiency. The genes for coagulation factors VIII and IX are carried on the X chromosome but are not genetically linked. Expression of both forms of hemophilia is recessive; a single functional gene is sufficient to prevent clinical signs of a bleeding diathesis. Hemophilic males inherit an abnormal gene from their dams and express a bleeding tendency. Female carriers have one normal and one abnormal gene and are clinically normal. Clinical severity of hemophilia correlates with in vitro factor activity. Severe hemophilia is most often propagated by carrier females. Males affected with mild hemophilia may survive to reproductive age, and the possibility of transmission from sire to daughter must be accounted for in familial test programs.

Autosomal Factor Deficiencies

Specific deficiencies of factors XII, XI, X, VII, and II and fibrinogen have been described in dogs and cats (see Table 180–3).[11, 24] The genes coding for these factors are autosomal; therefore males and females express and transmit these traits with equal frequency. Although deficiency of any of these factors causes prolongation of in vitro clotting time, the clinical severity associated with deficiencies varies between factors. Factor XII deficiency is a common defect in cats, yet it does not cause an in vivo bleeding diathesis.[11]

TREATMENT OF COAGULATION DISORDERS

Specific diagnosis and treatment of the primary disease are the basis for management of acquired coagulopathies. Transfusion is the mainstay for controlling or preventing hemorrhage in animals that have inherited coagulopathies and may be indicated for initial stabilization of acquired defects. Transfusion of blood components is the most efficient and safest use of blood products (Table 180–4).[25] Human clotting factor concentrates should not be used because they induce an antibody response when transfused in animals and are much more expensive than animal plasma products.

Management practices that help to reduce transfusion requirements include peripheral rather than jugular vein catheterization, oral rather than parenteral drug administration, cage confinement, and avoidance of invasive procedures. Vitamin K deficiency is treated using vitamin K_1 (not vitamin K_3).[11] A parenteral dose of vitamin K_1 (2.2 mg/kg subcutaneously) followed by 1.1 mg/kg every 12 hours is usually sufficient for initial therapy, with correction of coagulopathy within 1 to 2 days. After stabilization, dogs and cats poisoned by ingestion of second-generation rodenticides can be treated using a tapering dosage schedule of oral vitamin K_1 (1.1 mg/kg every 12 hours for 2 weeks; 1.1 mg/kg every 24 hours for 2 weeks; 0.5 mg/kg every 24 hours for 2 weeks).

THROMBOTIC DISORDERS

Thrombosis accompanies many common acquired disease conditions (Table 180–5), although the pathophysiology is not well defined.[14, 26] In general, thrombus formation is favored by conditions of blood stasis, vascular injury, and hemostatic imbalance or hypercoagulability.[13] In human medicine, heritable hypercoagulable states have been attributed to deficiencies of the anticoagulants antithrombin and proteins C and S, plasminogen deficiency, and mutations in the genes for factors V and II.[27] These defects have not been identified in animals.

Cardiac dysfunction, especially feline cardiomyopathy, is often associated with intracardiac and arterial thrombosis.[28] Atherosclerosis is uncommon in animals but has been described in hypothyroid dogs with arterial thrombosis.[14] Femoral artery thrombosis, believed to be caused by vascular disease, occurs in Cavalier King Charles spaniels and probably has a genetic basis.[29]

All of the other primary disease conditions listed in Table 180–5 have been associated with combined venous and arterial thrombosis or pulmonary thromboembolism (PTE).[14, 26, 30] Severe endothelial cell damage and hypertension accompany PTE caused by heartworm disease and its treatment. Neoplasia and systemic inflammatory disorders may cause

HEM

TABLE 180–4. BLOOD COMPONENT THERAPY*

PRODUCT	VOLUME	FREQUENCY	INDICATIONS
Packed red cells	6–10 mL/kg	q12–24h	Anemia
Fresh plasma	6–12 mL/kg	q8–12h	Inherited and acquired clotting factor deficiencies, von Willebrand's disease, disseminated intravascular coagulation, hypoproteinemia, hypoglobulinemia
Fresh-frozen plasma			
Frozen plasma	6–12 mL/kg	q8–12h	Hypoproteinemia, hypoglobulinemia
Cryoprecipitate	1 unit† per 10 kg	q4–12h	Hemophilia A (factor VIII deficiency), dysfibrinogenemia, hypofibrinogenemia von Willebrand's disease
Cryosupernatant‡	6–12 mL/kg	q8–12h	Hemophilia B (factor IX deficiency)
			Inherited factor II, VII, X, XI deficiency
			Anticoagulant rodenticide toxicity
			Hypoproteinemia, hypoglobulinemia

*Transfuse plasma products at initial rate of 1 to 2 mL/min for all patients and a maximum rate of 3 to 6 mL/min for adult dogs with normal cardiac function.
†One unit = cryoprecipitate prepared from 200 mL of fresh-frozen plasma.
‡Supernatant plasma remaining after cryoprecipitate preparation.

thrombosis via endothelial damage or release of mediators that trigger DIC. Thrombosis accompanies diseases that cause protein loss and has been attributed to concomitant loss of antithrombin.[31] These diseases include glomerulonephritis, amyloidosis, chronic interstitial nephritis, and inflammatory enteropathies. Thrombosis is also seen in conditions of cortisol excess such as Cushing's disease and steroid therapy for neurologic or immune-mediated disease.

Detailed examinations of coagulation inhibitors, fibrinogen, fibrinolysis, and markers of thrombosis are needed to characterize thrombosis in these diseases and other complex disease syndromes such as immune hemolysis and diabetes.

TREATMENT OF THROMBOTIC DISORDERS

Treatment of thrombosis includes specific therapy to correct the primary disease process and supportive care to alleviate signs of hypoxemia and loss of tissue perfusion. Case reports have described the successful use of more aggressive therapy, including fibrinolytic agents and anticoagulant drugs.[32, 33] Rigorous controlled trials are needed to determine the best therapy for different thrombotic syndromes.

The fibrinolytic agents streptokinase and t-PA are most likely to benefit patients with signs of massive pulmonary embolism, cardiogenic shock, or ischemic neuromyopathy.[5, 34] Potential complications of these agents include bleed-

TABLE 180–5. DISEASE CONDITIONS ASSOCIATED WITH THROMBOSIS

Cardiac disease
  Hypertrophic cardiomyopathy
  Dilated cardiomyopathy
  Congestive heart failure
Corticosteroid therapy
Endocrine disease
  Hyperadrenocorticism
  Hypothyroidism
  Diabetes mellitus
Heartworm disease
Immune-mediated disease
  Immune-mediated hemolytic anemia
  Systemic lupus erythematosus
  Lymphocytic enteritis
Neoplasia
Pancreatitis
Renal disease
  Glomerulonephritis
  Amyloidosis
  Chronic interstitial nephritis

ing, embolization of thrombi, and hyperkalemia.[28, 34] Venous thromboembolism in people has been treated with streptokinase (250,000-U bolus dose intravenously, followed by constant-rate infusion [CRI] of 100,000 U per hour for up to 72 hours) or t-PA (CRI of 100 mg over 2 hours).[34] A recommended streptokinase dosage for dogs is 90,000 U intravenously over 1/2 hour, followed by CRI of 45,000 U per hour for 7 to 12 hours.[32] Recombinant t-PA (alteplase) has been used as a series of two to ten bolus intravenous injections (1.1 mg/kg every 1 hour) to treat aortic thrombosis in dogs.[33] Animals undergoing fibrinolytic therapy should be closely monitored for signs of metabolic imbalance or hemorrhage, including serial determination of fibrinogen and fibrin degradation products.

Anticoagulation with heparin followed by oral coumarin (warfarin) therapy is standard treatment of venous thrombosis in people.[5, 34] The recommended therapeutic target range of heparin prolongs aPTT to 1.5 to 2 times the control value. Warfarin doses are adjusted according to clotting time in the PT assay, expressed as an international normalized ratio (INR) to account for laboratory variation in assay reagents and techniques.[35] The target therapeutic INR is 2 to 3. The information needed to calculate INR, the validity of this data transformation, and the optimal therapeutic ranges for heparin and warfarin have not been determined for animals. Heparin has been used for prophylaxis and treatment of venous thrombosis in dogs at 200 to 500 U/kg subcutaneously every 8 hours, with a target dosage to prolong aPTT to 1.5 to 2 times the pretreatment value. Warfarin has been used in dogs at 0.22 mg/kg every 12 hours and in cats at 0.5 mg per cat every 24 hours, with a target dosage to prolong PT to 1.25 to 1.5 times the pretreatment value.[32, 36]

New anticoagulant and antithrombotic agents minimize the complications of hemorrhage and delayed wound healing associated with current regimens and simplify drug administration and monitoring.[5, 34] Specific drugs include low-molecular-weight heparins, hirudins, and antiplatelet drugs that bind to surface glycoproteins and prevent aggregation.[5, 20]

DISSEMINATED INTRAVASCULAR COAGULATION

DIC is a complex disease syndrome caused by systemic, rather than localized, coagulation and fibrinolysis.[37] Many common diseases are capable of triggering DIC through widespread endothelial cell damage or release of tissue thromboplastins that concurrently activate thrombin and plasmin (Fig. 180–9). The DIC process is dynamic; organ

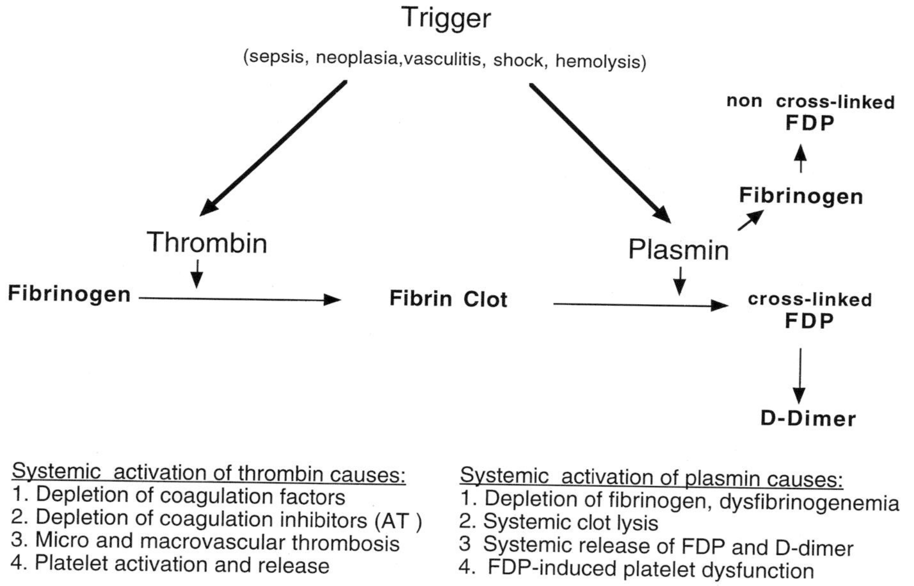

Trigger

(sepsis, neoplasia, vasculitis, shock, hemolysis)

Figure 180–9. Disseminated intravascular coagulation.

non cross-linked
FDP

Thrombin

Plasmin

Fibrinogen

Fibrinogen ————————→ Fibrin Clot ————————→ cross-linked
FDP

↓

D-Dimer

Systemic activation of thrombin causes:
1. Depletion of coagulation factors
2. Depletion of coagulation inhibitors (AT)
3. Micro and macrovascular thrombosis
4. Platelet activation and release

Systemic activation of plasmin causes:
1. Depletion of fibrinogen, dysfibrinogenemia
2. Systemic clot lysis
3 Systemic release of FDP and D-dimer
4. FDP-induced platelet dysfunction

failure caused by thrombosis and severe bleeding occur sequentially or simultaneously. The clinical signs of DIC are therefore highly variable and depend on the underlying disease and the shifting balance between thrombosis and hemorrhage.

The hemorrhagic phase of acute or fulminant DIC often causes signs of petechiae, ecchymoses, and bleeding from multiple sites, including venipuncture and catheter sites. Bleeding may be less obvious or absent in thrombotic or chronic compensated DIC. The diagnosis of DIC is based on a combination of clinical signs and laboratory findings (see Fig. 180–9).[9, 37, 38]

Successful treatment of DIC requires identification and specific treatment of the primary disease and supportive care to correct circulatory and metabolic derangements. Transfusion is indicated to replace red blood cells or hemostatic proteins in patients with severe signs of hemorrhage (see Table 180–4). Heparin is used for its anticoagulant effect if signs of thrombosis predominate, and in some cases administration of plasma products and heparin is needed to restore hemostatic balance.

REFERENCES

1. Rock G, Wells P: New concepts in coagulation. Crit Rev Clin Lab Sci 34:475, 1997.
2. Furie B, Furie BC: Molecular and cellular biology of blood coagulation. N Engl J Med 326:800, 1992.
3. Williamson LH: Antithrombin III: A natural anticoagulant. Compend Contin Educ 13:100, 1991.
4. Broze GJ: Tissue factor pathway inhibitor. Thromb Haemost 74:90, 1995.
5. Ewensteim BM: Antithrombotic agents and thromboembolic disease. N Engl J Med 337:1383, 1997.
6. Sallah S: Inhibitors to clotting factors. Ann Hematol 75:1, 1997.
7. Bu G, et al: Cellular receptors for the plasminogen activators. Blood 83:3427, 1994.
8. Schmaier AH: Contact activation: A revision. Thromb Haemost 78:101, 1997.
9. Blomberg DJ: The pathologist as a clinical consultant for hemostasis in the community hospital. Clin Lab Med 13:951, 1993.
10. Brooks M: Coagulation disorders. In Birchard SJ, Sherding RG (eds): Saunders Manual of Small Animal Practice. Orlando, FL, WB Saunders, 1994, p 164.
11. Dodds WJ: Hemostasis. In Kaneko JJ (ed): Clinical Biochemistry of Domestic Animals. San Diego, Academic Press, 1989, p 274.
12. Palkuti HS: Hemostasis: Part II. Investigation of the coagulation factors by use of qualitative and quantitative assay techniques. Focus 48:109, 1982.
13. Comp PC: Overview of the hypercoagulable states. Semin Thromb Hemost 16:158, 1990.
14. Van Winkle TJ, et al: Clinical and pathological features of aortic thromboembolism in 36 dogs. Vet Emerg Crit Care 3:13, 1993.
15. Goldhaber SZ: Pulmonary embolism. N Engl J Med 339:93, 1998.
16. Mannucci PM, Giangrande PLF: Detection of the prethrombotic state due to procoagulant imbalance. Eur J Haematol 48:65, 1992.
17. Johnstone IB: The importance of accurate citrate to blood ratios in the collection of canine blood for hemostatic testing. Can Vet J 34:627, 1993.
18. Lanevschi A, et al: Evaluation of chromogenic substrate assays for fibrinolytic analytes in dogs. Am J Vet Res 57:1124, 1996.
19. Karges HE, et al: Activity of coagulation and fibrinolysis parameters in animals. Arzneimittelforschung 44:793, 1994.
20. Weitz JI: Low-molecular-weight heparins. N Engl J Med 337:688, 1997.
21. Bick RL, Baker WF: Diagnostic efficacy of the D-dimer assay in disseminated intravascular coagulation (DIC). Thromb Res 65:785, 1992.
22. Ravanat C, et al: Cross-reactivity of human molecular markers for detection of prethrombotic states in various animal species. Blood Coagul Fibrinolysis 6:446, 1995.
23. Lisciandro SC, et al: Coagulation abnormalities in 22 cats with naturally occurring liver disease. J Vet Intern Med 12:71, 1998.
24. Brooks M: Hereditary bleeding disorders (abstract). Proceedings of the 16th Annual ACVIM Forum, American College of Veterinary Internal Medicine, San Diego, 1998, p 424.
25. Kristensen AT, Feldman BF: General principles of small animal blood component administration. Vet Clin North Am Small Anim Pract 25:1277, 1995.
26. Keyes ML, et al: Pulmonary thromboembolism in dogs. Vet Emerg Crit Care 3:23, 1993.
27. Bertina RM, Rosendaal FR: Venous thrombosis—Interaction of genes and environment. N Engl J Med 338:1840, 1998.
28. Pion PD: Feline aortic thromboemboli and the potential utility of thrombolytic therapy with tissue plasminogen activator. Vet Clin North Am Small Anim Pract 18:79, 1988.
29. Buchanan JW: Femoral artery occlusion in Cavalier King Charles spaniels. JAVMA 211:872, 1997.
30. Palmer KG, et al: Clinical manifestations and associated disease syndromes in dogs with cranial vena cava thrombosis: 17 cases (1989–1996). JAVMA 212:220, 1998.
31. Green RA, Kabel AL: Hypercoagulable state in three dogs with nephrotic syndrome: Role of acquired antithrombin III deficiency. JAVMA 181:914, 1982.
32. Ramsey CC, et al: Use of streptokinase in four dogs with thrombosis. JAVMA 209:780, 1996.
33. Clare AC, Kraje BJ: Use of recombinant tissue-plasminogen activator for aortic thrombolysis in a hypoproteinemic dog. JAVMA 212:539, 1998.
34. Ginsberg JS: Management of venous thromboembolism. N Engl J Med 335:1816, 1996.
35. Cunningham MT, et al: The reliability of manufacturer-determined, instrument-specific international sensitivity index values for calculating the international normalized ratio. Am J Clin Pathol 102:128, 1994.
36. Smith SA: Warfarin treatment in small animal patients (abstract). Proceedings of the 16th Annual ACVIM Forum, American College of Veterinary Internal Medicine, San Diego, 1998, p 440.
37. Bick RL: Disseminated intravascular coagulation and related syndromes: A clinical review. Semin Thromb Hemost 14:299, 1988.
38. Feldman BF: Disseminated intravascular coagulation: Antithrombin, plasminogen, and coagulation abnormalities in 41 dogs. JAVMA 179:151, 1981.

HEM

CHAPTER 181

LEUKOCYTE CHANGES IN DISEASE

Gary J. Kociba

GRANULOCYTE PRODUCTION AND KINETICS

Neutrophils, eosinophils, and basophils are produced in the bone marrow by a process of cellular proliferation and maturation. The neutrophil is the predominant granulocyte cell in the marrow. The proliferation, differentiation, and maturation steps from a myeloblast to a segmented granulocyte take about 6 days in dogs.[1] For interpretive purposes, the neutrophils in the marrow compartment often are divided into two compartments.[2] The proliferating pool consists of myeloblasts, progranulocytes, and myelocytes. The maturation and storage pool contains the non-dividing granulocytes, including metamyelocytes, bands, and segmented cells. The pool of granulocytes in the marrow of a normal dog represents about a 5-day supply of neutrophils under steady-state conditions.[3] The most differentiated cells in the marrow are the most deformable and have acquired or altered the appropriate receptors for release from the hematopoietic space. Therefore, segmented neutrophils are preferentially released over band neutrophils or neutrophilic metamyelocytes. This is an advantage because the segmented neutrophil has more effective phagocytic and bactericidal functions than less mature cells. The proliferation and maturation of granulocytic precursors is under the control of glycoprotein growth factors, including granulocyte colony-stimulating factor (G-CSF), granulocyte-macrophage colony-stimulating factor (GM-CSF), and a number of short-range signals generated by stromal elements collectively referred to as the hematopoietic microenvironment.[4] The bone marrow has a high production rate that is finely modulated under steady-state conditions. The production rate can be markedly expanded in response to inflammatory stimuli.

NEUTROPHIL POOLS AND RESPONSES

The leukocytes in the blood are divided into two dynamic pools with those in the axial blood flow designated as the circulating pool and those intermittently loosely associated with the walls of blood vessels called the marginated pool. In normal dogs the marginated neutrophil pool is about equal in size to the circulating pool, whereas in cats the marginated neutrophil pool of cats is two to three times larger than the circulating pool. When blood samples are collected for hemograms, the only granulocyte compartment that is directly sampled is the circulating pool. Based on data from the circulating pool and knowledge of leukocyte responses and the disease processes, predictions are made about the expected changes in other granulocyte compartments. It is important to recognize that neutrophils spend only a short time in the bloodstream, with a half-life of about 7 hours

under normal conditions.[1] The half-life is considerably shorter in inflammatory disease, with the bloodstream serving as a conduit from the marrow to the inflammatory lesion. Neutrophils do not re-enter the bloodstream from the tissues. A schematic presentation of changes in these granulocyte compartments in physiologic leukocytosis and in inflammatory disease is presented in Figure 181–1.

LEFT SHIFT

A left shift refers to an increase in immature neutrophils, especially bands, in the blood. It is a sign of an inflammatory response with release of immature cells in addition to segmented neutrophils from the maturation and storage compartment of the marrow. If the inflammatory lesion is large or severe, neutrophilic metamyelocytes, neutrophilic myelocytes, and even small numbers of progranulocytes and myeloblasts might be part of the left shift.

The criteria for classification of cells as segmented neutrophils versus band neutrophils are slightly variable. With human blood films, neutrophils are classified as segmented when the nuclear lobes are connected by thin membranous filaments. If chromatin is still evident in the constrictions between nuclear lobes, the cells are classified as bands. If these criteria are applied to feline or canine blood, disproportionate numbers of bands are noted in normal animals. Laboratories that process human blood along with veterinary samples frequently report greater numbers of band neutrophils, a factor that must be considered in interpreting left shifts. Veterinary laboratories use slightly different criteria for classification of segmented neutrophils and bands of dogs and cats. Neutrophils with constrictions of the nuclear membrane to 50 per cent or less of the width of the rest of the nucleus are classified as segmented neutrophils (Fig. 181–2).[2] Obviously, these criteria are subject to variation in interpretation among different technologists. Regardless of the criteria used, it should be recognized that the variation in classification of band neutrophils is quite large. When monitoring animals with inflammatory disease, changes in the concentration of band neutrophils in serial samples might not always correlate with changes in the patient. The changes in severity of a left shift could be related to variations in classification of bands by different technologists performing the differential leukocyte counts.

Regenerative Left Shift

A regenerative left shift refers to a neutrophilic leukocytosis with an increase in immature neutrophils but with segmented neutrophils still the predominant cell type. This response should elicit a search for an inflammatory lesion if

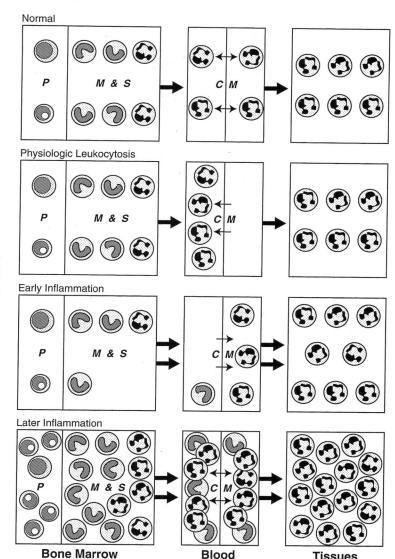

Figure 181–1. Changes in neutrophils in various compartments in physiologic leukocytosis and inflammation. P = proliferating pool; M & S = maturation and storage pool; C = circulating pool; M = marginated pool. (From Kociba GJ: Leukocytosis and leukopenia. *In* Proceedings of the 20th Waltham Symposium on Oncology and Hematology. Vernon, CA, Waltham, USA, 1996, p 106.)

Normal

Physiologic Leukocytosis

Early Inflammation

Later Inflammation

Bone Marrow   **Blood**   **Tissues**

the cause is unknown (Table 181–1). In general, the degree of left shift should correlate with severity of the lesion. Left shifts usually are best monitored as the absolute concentration of bands in the blood. The following general guidelines can be applied to interpretation of neutrophilic responses in animals with left shifts:

CONCENTRATION OF IMMATURE NEUTROPHILS	INTERPRETATION
<300/μL	Normal
>600/μL	Inflammation
>5000/μL	Marked inflammation
>Segmented neutrophils	Degenerative left shift; guarded prognosis

In animals monitored with serial hemograms, drainage or removal of an inflammatory focus may cause a dramatic increase in neutrophilia. For example, in a dog with pyometra the neutrophilia increases after ovariohysterectomy because the prolonged inflammation has induced granulocytic hyperplasia in the marrow and neutrophils are being released at a high rate but the emigration site has been removed.[2]

Severe neutrophilia with a regenerative left shift is not always related to infectious causes. For example, neutrophilia can be associated with either immune-mediated or infectious arthritis. Neutrophilia with counts up to 80,000/μL may accompany immune-mediated hemolytic anemia. Nevertheless, extreme neutrophilia should prompt a search for inflammatory lesions and attempts should be made to exclude infectious causes.

Degenerative Left Shift

A degenerative left shift refers to a condition with a decreasing leukocyte count with a greater concentration of immature neutrophils than segmented neutrophils in the blood (Fig. 181–3). Usually the leukocyte count is normal to subnormal in degenerative left shifts, reflecting a depletion of reserves of granulocytes in the marrow. A degenerative left shift is associated with a poor prognosis. Severe systemic disease or overwhelming infections with septicemia should be considered as potential causes. One exception is noted in dogs or cats in the early stages of recovery from a disease

HEM

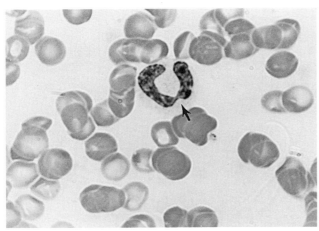

Figure 181–2. Neutrophil of a dog. This cell is classified as a segmented neutrophil because the width of the nucleus at the constriction *(arrow)* is less than 50 per cent of the width of the rest of the nucleus.

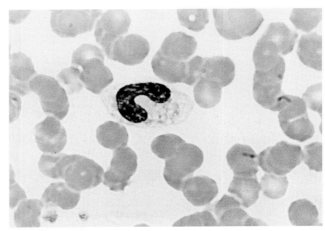

Figure 181–3. Band neutrophil of a dog with a degenerative left shift. Mild cytoplasmic vacuolation and basophilia are also present.

with destruction of hematopoietic precursors in the marrow. An example is feline parvovirus infection with virus-mediated destruction of marrow precursors. If the animal recovers, the immature bands and metamyelocytes may predominate because they are the only cells available for release as granulocytes are generated in the marrow.

In septicemia or other severe systemic diseases, damage to endothelial cells of vascular sinuses in the marrow may remove the barrier that restrains hematopoietic precursors within the marrow compartment. When increased nucleated erythrocytes are released along with neutrophils in a left shift the term *leukoerythroblastic response* is sometimes applied. Leukoerythroblastic responses have been associated with severe systemic diseases, including sepsis, neoplasia, and some forms of physical injury, but are not specific.

PHYSIOLOGIC NEUTROPHILIA

Physiologic leukocytosis is recognized as a mature neutrophilia and lymphocytosis without other causes. Epinephrine release associated with exercise, fear, or excitement causes a transient shift of neutrophils from the marginated pool to the circulating pool. This can increase the concentration of neutrophils to up to double the resting levels, with the changes generally lasting less than an hour, although the changes may last 3 hours after exercise.[9] The total leukocyte

TABLE 181–1. CAUSES OF NEUTROPHILIA

Excitement, exercise
Corticosteroids—endogenous or exogenous
Bacteria—especially staphylococci and streptococci
Rickettsia
Selected viruses—feline calicivirus, feline rhinotracheitis
Fungi—systemic or localized
Parasites—hepatozoonosis of dogs, toxoplasmosis, tick bites
Physical injury—burns, trauma, surgery, frostbite
Metabolite injury—uremia
Hemolysis
Immune-mediated arthritis
Neoplasms—squamous cell carcinoma, other carcinomas, rectal
    polyp, some sarcomas[5–8]
Venoms
Canine granulocytopathy syndrome (CD11/CD18 defect of Irish
    setters)

number in the vascular compartment is unchanged so a mature neutrophilia with no left shift is expected. Similar shifts from the marginated pool of lymphocytes and other marginated cells occur with the net result of an increased leukocyte concentration but no major change in the relative proportions of the various leukocytes. The changes are more dramatic in cats because of the larger size of the marginated pool of neutrophils and lymphocytes in this species.

STRESS LEUKOGRAM

Most dogs and cats develop a consistent change of leukocytes under the influence of increased glucocorticoids of either exogenous or endogenous sources. The expected changes include a neutrophilia without a left shift, lymphopenia, and low or absent eosinophils.[10] In dogs, but usually not as consistently in cats, monocytosis also occurs under steroid influence. The total leukocyte count is variable, but average responses result in a leukocytosis with leukocyte concentrations in the range of 15,000 to 25,000/μL. The neutrophilia is related to an initial release of neutrophils from the marrow, decreased tissue migration, and shift from marginal to circulating pools. The neutrophilia does not impart greater resistance to infections because the cells have inhibited functions. Lymphopenia is related to steroid-induced apoptosis and redistribution of lymphocytes. The eosinopenia is related to egress from the blood and decreased stimuli for release of eosinophils from the marrow.

Glucocorticoid-induced lymphopenia and decreased eosinophils are often found in association with inflammatory responses, resulting in the combination of neutrophilia with a left shift and monocytosis with lymphopenia and eosinopenia.

INFLAMMATION

In inflammatory diseases, neutrophils selectively emigrate to the inflammatory site. The shear stress related to blood flow is initially overcome by selectins, a group of adhesive molecules expressed on the membranes of leukocytes and endothelial cells. Cytokines including tumor necrosis factor-alpha and interleukin-1 produced by cells at the site upregulate the expression of E-selectin by endothelial cells. The intermittent binding of L-selectin on the surface of neutrophils to E-selectin and P-selectin on endothelial cells causes the neutrophils to selectively roll along the endothelium.[11] Neutrophil rolling is a prerequisite for high-affinity adherence of neutrophils to the endothelium, a process involving members of the beta$_2$ integrin family of molecules on leukocytes binding to intercellular adhesion molecules (ICAM-1, ICAM-2) on vascular endothelium. ICAM-1 and ICAM-2 expression and/or affinity is upmodulated by high concentrations of inflammatory stimuli in the region.[12] The beta$_2$ integrins of leukocytes are heterodimers of a constant beta subunit (CD18) and distinct alpha subunits, CD11a (of LFA-1), CD11b (of Mac-1), and CD11c (of p150,95).[13] The CD11b, CD18 heterodimer plays a primary role in binding activated neutrophils to endothelial cells. After binding and flattening, the neutrophils extend pseudopods between endothelial cells and emigrate to the inflammatory site. Chemotaxis, the directional movement of cells toward a concentration gradient, plays a role in emigration. Chemotactic factors include complement components (C5a), lipoxygenase pathway products (leukotrienes), chemokines,[14] and cytokines. A transient (hours) neutropenia may develop as neutrophils leave the vascular compartment. This is followed by an increased release of neutrophils from the bone marrow. As the release rate increases, band neutrophils also are released, creating a left shift. In general, the degree of left shift is proportional to the inflammatory stimulus. The total neutrophil count reflects a combination of factors, including bone marrow reserves, the egress rate from the vascular compartment, the severity of the stimulus, and the size and distribution of the inflammatory lesions.

In instances in which bacteria or other agents that induce neutrophilia are not cleared from the tissues continuous elaboration of inflammatory mediators results in hyperplasia of granulocytic precursors in the marrow and severe neutrophilia (Fig. 181–4). If the leukocyte count is extremely high (>100,000/μL for dogs or 75,000/μL for cats), this reaction is called a leukemoid response because of the similarity to the extreme leukocytosis associated with chronic granulocytic leukemia. Leukemoid responses are distinguished from granulocytic leukemia by finding the inflammatory lesion. In instances in which inflammatory lesions cannot be found, autologous neutrophils can be labeled with technetium-99m and reinfused, followed by external imaging of radioactivity at suspected sites to localize the lesion.[15] Cytoplasmic vacuolation and basophilia and Döhle bodies in neutrophils also support the diagnosis of leukemoid reaction over leukemia.

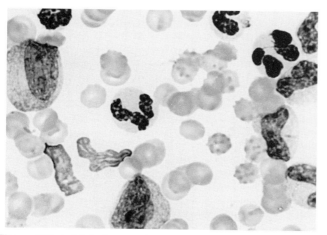

Figure 181–4. Marked neutrophilic leukocytosis with regenerative left shift including neutrophilic myelocytes in a dog with pyometra.

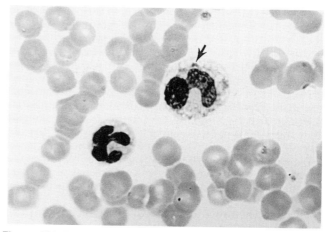

Figure 181–5. Morphologic abnormalities in neutrophils of a dog with inflammatory disease. Note the cytoplasmic vacuolation and basophilia, increased size of the band neutrophil, and Döhle bodies *(arrow)*.

MORPHOLOGIC ABNORMALITIES

Under conditions of enhanced neutrophil turnover rate, a number of morphologic abnormalities may occur in neutrophils. These changes are often called "toxic changes," but most they reflect shortened production times with incomplete maturation in the marrow compartment rather than degeneration. They include Döhle bodies, cytoplasmic vacuolation and basophilia, toxic granulation, and giant neutrophils (Fig. 181–5). Most of these changes reflect intense marrow stimulation and shortened maturation times in the marrow. Döhle bodies are pale blue-grey bodies in the cytoplasm that represent aggregates of endoplasmic reticulum. They are less significant in cats because they are seen in some normal cats and cats with minor inflammation. Cytoplasmic vacuolation may be an acquired defect associated with rapid synthesis, but similar changes can occur in vitro from prolonged exposure to ethylenediamine tetraacetic acid.[16] Cytoplasmic vacuolation occurs in the neutrophils of some cats on high dosages of chloramphenicol (60–120 mg/kg/d, intramuscularly).[17] Cytoplasmic basophilia is associated with conditions with enhanced neutrophil turnover. The intense stimulation of granulopoiesis results in the release of cells, with increased residual cytoplasmic ribonucleic acid imparting the basophilia. Toxic granulation is relatively rare in small animals and represents retention of the blue-purple staining of primary granules formed in the progranulocyte stage. Under normal conditions, the primary granules are diluted by divisions after primary granule synthesis ceases at the progranulocyte stage and by loss of the intense staining of the primary granules as the cells mature. Giant forms of neutrophils are sometimes seen in the recovery stage of diseases representing cells that skipped a mitotic division under intense stimulation of marrow precursors. Overall, these morphologic abnormalities should be interpreted as evidence of enhanced neutrophil turnover that usually correlates with severe inflammatory disease. Combinations of these changes may correlate with more severe disease.

HYPERSEGMENTATION

Lobation of the nuclei of neutrophils is progressive with increased lobes noted in conditions with prolongation of the

HEM

interval in the bloodstream. The average neutrophil in canine or feline blood has three nuclear lobes with fewer than 5 per cent with five lobes. With decreased egress under the influence of corticosteroid hormones, an increased number of neutrophils with four or five lobes are detected. Hypersegmentation is associated with human vitamin B_{12} or folate acid deficiency. Dramatic changes do not appear to accompany these deficiencies of dogs and cats, although occasional hypersegmented neutrophils have been described in giant schnauzers with a defect in vitamin B_{12} absorption.[18] Poodles with erythrocyte macrocytosis have a mild increase in hypersegmented neutrophils, but the change is not as dramatic as the increase in mean corpuscular volume and erythrocytes with multiple Howell-Jolly bodies or atypical nuclear fragments.[19]

Senescent neutrophils with apoptotic nuclei with condensed pyknotic nuclear lobes are rarely noted in normal blood. Apoptotic neutrophils are increased in heat stroke, and a few may be noted under the influence of corticosteroids or other conditions with decreased rates of emigration from the vascular component.

LEUKOCYTE INCLUSIONS

Occasionally, cytoplasmic inclusions are detected in leukocytes that might provoke clues to a specific diagnosis of a disease.

Yeasts

Histoplasma capsulatum yeasts are sometimes detected in monocytes or neutrophils of animals with disseminated histoplasmosis.[20] They are uniform, round-to-oval 2- to 4-μm, lightly stained organisms with a darker central area (Fig. 181–6). Often, multiple yeasts are clustered in the same cell. Budding forms can be visualized in occasional organisms. Buffy coat smears with concentrated leukocytes can be used to increase the probability of finding these inclusions.

Parasites

Hepatozoon canis gametocytes rarely are detected in the cytoplasm of neutrophils or monocytes. In endemic areas, hepatozoonosis may be suspected because of a marked neu-

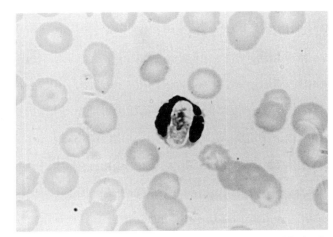

Figure 181–7. Gametocyte of *Hepatozoon canis* in a neutrophil of a dog.

trophilia (20,000–200,000/μL) with a left shift. A mean leukocyte concentration of 85,700/μL was noted in one retrospective study.[21] The gametocytes usually are not found in many cells (<0.1 per cent) but are large, oval, clear blue–staining organisms that are about 5 × 11 μm (Fig. 181–7). Occasionally, up to 5 per cent of the cells can contain gametocytes. A higher percentage of infected neutrophils appears to be more common in the endemic regions of the Mediterranean basin.

Rickettsial Agents

Morulae of rickettsial agents may occur in neutrophils or monocytes (Fig. 181–8). The inclusions are usually 2- to 6-μm blue to blue-grey cytoplasmic morulae with 4 to 20 punctate elementary bodies.

Ehrlichia canis is found in a few monocytes in the acute phase of infection, but only 4 per cent of 221 dogs in one study had detectable organisms in blood cells, making this an unreliable method for diagnosis.[22] Inclusions of *Ehrlichia equi*, *Ehrlichia ewingii*, or human granulocytotropic Ehrlichia sp. may be found in 1 to 5 per cent of neutrophils or rare eosinophils in canine granulocytic ehrlichiosis.[23] Ehrlichial inclusions have been detected in monocytes of a few cats.[24]

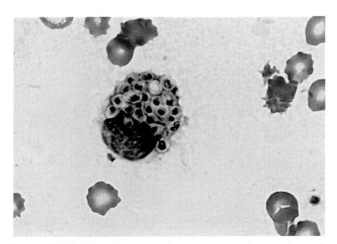

Figure 181–6. *Histoplasma capsulatum* yeasts in the cytoplasm of a macrophage in the bone marrow of a dog.

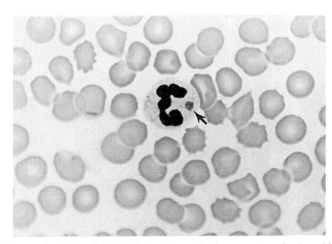

Figure 181–8. Ehrlichial inclusion *(arrow)* in the cytoplasm of a dog with granulocytic ehrlichiosis.

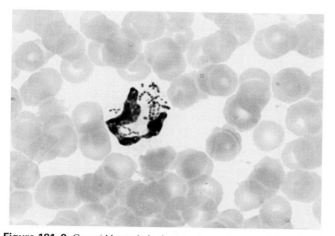

Figure 181–9. Coccoid bacteria in the cytoplasm of a dog with septicemia.

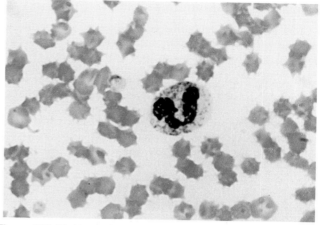

Figure 181–11. Neutrophil with distinctive cytoplasmic azurophilic granules in a neutrophil of a cat with mucopolysaccharidosis VII.

Bacteria

Bacteria may be found in the cytoplasm of neutrophils (Fig. 181–9) in the terminal stages of septicemia but are not commonly detected.

Viruses

Canine distemper cytoplasmic inclusions are rarely noted in neutrophils, lymphocytes, monocytes, and sometimes erythrocytes of viremic dogs with acute distemper.[25] The round to irregular-shaped inclusions vary in staining from pale blue to pink to magenta depending on the stain used (Fig. 181–10).

Non-infectious Inclusions

Lysosomal Storage Diseases

Neutrophils, lymphocytes, eosinophils, and monocytes of cats or dogs with mucopolysaccharidosis (MPS) VI or MPS VII contain numerous pink-purple granules that stain metachromatically with toluidine blue (Fig. 181–11).[26] Granules may be noted in MPS I, but they are usually less distinct than in MPS VI and MPS VII. Metachromatic granules are suggestive of mucopolysaccharidoses but can be observed in

neutrophils and lymphocytes of animals with other storage defects such as subtle staining of granules in GM_2 gangliosidosis. The "distinctive" azurophilic granules are not always prominent and may not be apparent especially in some Diff-Quik–stained slides. Vacuolated leukocytes are noted in some storage defects, but they often are not prominent. Lymphocytes and monocytes of cats with mannosidosis contain numerous clear vacuoles.[26] Vacuolated lymphocytes are noted in GM_1 gangliosidosis of dogs and cats (Fig. 181–12).[27] Specific diagnoses are based on assays for the specific deficient enzymes.

Atypical Granulation of Neutrophils of Birman Cats

An autosomal recessive defect in neutrophil granules has been described in Birman cats.[28] It is common, with 46 per cent of 78 cats of the original report affected. The neutrophils have prominent fine eosinophilic granules that resemble the staining of azurophilic granules. No clinical abnormalities or defects in neutrophilic function have been detected. It is suspected that some alteration in contents of lysosomal granules leads to the increased affinity for acidic dyes.

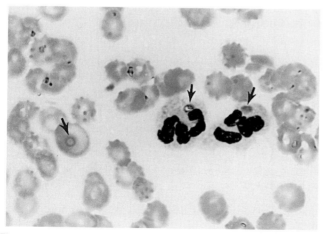

Figure 181–10. Inclusions of canine distemper *(arrows)* in the cytoplasm of neutrophils and one erythrocyte of a dog.

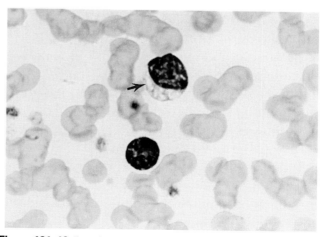

Figure 181–12. Lymphocyte with cytoplasmic vacuolation *(arrow)* associated with GM_1 gangliosidosis.

Chédiak-Higashi Syndrome

Chédiak-Higashi syndrome is an inherited defect characterized by defective microtubule assembly and abnormal fusion of cytoplasmic granules in a number of cells, including leukocytes.[29] It occurs in Persian cats with smoke-blue coat color and yellow-green irises. The pale diluted coat and iris color are related to abnormal granulation of melanocytes. The neutrophils contain atypical, slightly large, red to magenta cytoplasmic granules (Fig. 181–13). Eosinophils also have abnormal granulation. The cats have a mild bleeding tendency related to a deficiency of adenosine diphosphate, adenosine triphosphate, and serotonin in platelets. Neutrophil counts are slightly low, although the counts are usually still in the normal reference range.[30] Although mink and other species with a similar disease have a predisposition to bacterial disease, most affected cats are resistant.

Döhle Bodies

Döhle bodies represent aggregates of endoplasmic reticulum that develop under conditions of rapid leukocyte turnover. They may occur in clinically normal cats but are more significant in dogs, where they indicate rapid leukocyte turnover.

Sideroleukocytes

Sideroleukocytes are neutrophils or monocytes that contain hemosiderin inclusions or stainable iron in the cytoplasm. Sideroleukocytes occasionally are noted in the blood of dogs with hemolytic anemia related to intravascular hemolysis.[31] The hemosiderin granules are irregular-shaped golden-brown inclusions that stain positively for iron with Prussian blue or Perls' stain. In Romanowsky-stained films, blood pigment will sometimes stain blue-black before processing of the phagocytized iron to hemosiderin.

NEUTROPENIA

Neutropenias can be related to increased margination and egress from the blood in inflammatory disease, decreased production due to injury to marrow precursors, or increased destruction due to immune-mediated processes (Table 181–2). Neutrophils are decreased in the early stages of a variety

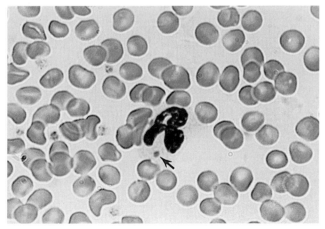

Figure 181–13. Large cytoplasmic granules *(arrow)* in the neutrophil of a cat with Chédiak-Higashi syndrome.

TABLE 181–2. CAUSES OF NEUTROPENIA

Viruses—canine and feline parvovirus, infectious canine hepatitis, feline leukemia virus, feline immunodeficiency virus
Ehrlichiosis
Gram-negative septicemia
Drugs—estrogen or stilbestrol in dogs,[47] anticancer drugs, chloramphenicol[17] or griseofulvin[48] in cats, meclofenamic acid,[49] phenylbutazone,[49] quinidine,[49] or thiacetarsamide in dogs (idiosyncratic), cephalosporins,[50] trimethoprim-sulfadiazine,[51] methimazole,[52] phenobarbital[53]
Irradiation
Hyperestrogenism (Sertoli cell tumor of dogs)[54]
Cyclic hematopoiesis[55]
Myelophthisis (leukemia, myelofibrosis, or granulomatous myelitis)

of inflammation, but this neutropenia is usually not recognized because it is transient and occurs before animals are presented for evaluation. In diseases with depletion of marrow reserves, a degenerative left shift is associated with the neutropenia and is a grave prognostic sign. Neutropenia in parvovirus infection is caused by destruction of hematopoietic precursors in the marrow. If the dog or cat recovers from parvovirus infection, neutrophilia in the blood and granulocytic hyperplasia in the marrow develops within a week. In the recovery phase, a large left shift with release of atypical cells may be seen as the marrow is maximally stimulated to produce granulocytes. Neutrophilic precursors have a high replicative rate, making them susceptible to some viruses and many cytotoxic anticancer agents. Granulocytopenia is the dose-limiting toxicity of many chemotherapeutic drugs. Some investigators recommend that when neutrophil counts dip below 3000/μL in the blood of animals on chemotherapy, consideration must be given to delaying or lowering the dose until neutrophil numbers increase.[32] Neutrophil counts less than 1000/μL should promote close monitoring for signs of sepsis and the use of prophylactic bactericidal antibiotics.[32] Neutropenia has been associated with either feline leukemia virus and/or feline immunodeficiency virus infections in field studies of cats[33] and transient neutropenia has been documented in cats with experimental infections with feline immunodeficiency virus[34] but persistent neutropenia is rarely noted in experimental infections with either virus.[35]

Recombinant canine granulocyte colony-stimulating factor (rcG-CSF) at a dosage of 2.5 μg/kg twice daily has been effective in stimulating granulopoiesis in normal and neutropenic dogs.[36, 37] When given to cats at a dosage of 5 μg/kg per day, rcG-CSF induced a sustained neutrophilia for a 42-day period of treatment without significant clinical signs of toxicosis.[38] In another study, rcG-CSF induced neutrophilia and enhanced neutrophil function in normal cats and cats with Chédiak-Higashi syndrome.[39] Administration of recombinant canine granulocyte-macrophage–stimulating factor to normal dogs induced neutrophilia and a dose-dependent thrombocytopenia related to destruction of platelets in the liver and spleen.[40]

Unfortunately, rcG-CSF is not commercially available, leading to the use of recombinant human G-CSF (rhG-CSF). At doses of 10 to 100 μg/kg per day, rhG-CSF is effective in inducing neutrophilia in dogs for at least 14 days.[41] The development of neutralizing antibodies to the recombinant or endogenous colony-stimulating factors is of concern when non–species-specific G-CSF is used.[42, 43] In some instances, dogs treated with rhG-CSF develop antibodies to rhG-CSF that induce neutropenia and cross-react with rcG-CSF and neutralize both human and canine G-CSF in vitro. The neutropenia may persist for up to 4 months after discontinuation of rhG-CSF administration. The risk of the development of neutralizing antibodies to rhG-CSF in dogs and cats under immunosuppression is not defined but may be less than in normal animals, leading to the short-term use of rhG-CSF in neutropenic dogs and cats.[44]

Cyclic neutropenia can be induced in dogs with cyclophosphamide.[45] The cyclophosphamide-induced injury to granulocytic precursors can cause oscillation of neutrophil counts on an 11- to 13-day cycle. This cycle length is reminiscent of the 10- to 12-day cycle in cyclic hematopoiesis of grey collies, but the oscillations are not dramatic. Cyclic neutropenia also has been noted in a few cats infected with feline leukemia virus.[46] The cycles in cats were less consistent, ranging from 8 to 16 days. Prednisolone therapy appeared to stop the cycling in two cats.

If neutropenia is of unknown causes and persists for more than 1 week, bone marrow biopsy is recommended to evaluate for aplastic anemia, leukemic infiltrates, or myeloproliferative diseases. Idiopathic neutropenias may be asymptomatic in some animals and appear to be more common in cats than dogs. If recurrent infections accompany the neutropenia, a careful search for causes is warranted. If none is found, the remote possibility of immune-mediated neutropenia should be considered. Immune-mediated neutropenia is not a well-documented entity in dogs or cats. The diagnosis should be supported by demonstration of anti-neutrophil antibodies either in serum or on neutrophils and a shift to less mature precursors in the marrow compartment. If a therapeutic trial with immunosuppressive doses of glucocorticoids is considered for an animal with neutropenia, it should be noted that steroid inhibition of leukocyte function may predispose to infectious diseases.

ESTROGEN-INDUCED MYELOTOXICITY

A single dose of estradiol cyclopentylproprionate can induce myelotoxicity in dogs.[56] The changes follow a unique pattern, with thrombocytosis peaking at 5 to 7 days, followed by a precipitous decline in platelets to thrombocytopenic levels with a nadir at 2 to 3 weeks (Fig. 181–14). If the dog recovers, a rebound thrombocytosis occurs at about week 4. Neutrophilia develops and peaks at levels that may exceed 50,000/μL at 2 to 3 weeks, followed by a decline to neutropenic levels. Pancytopenia, anemia, and generalized hypo-

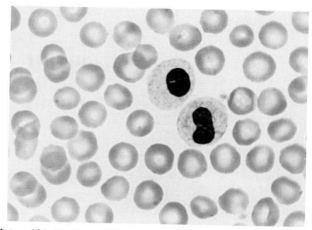

Figure 181–15. Neutrophils with round to indented nuclei but condensed nuclear chromatin in a dog with Pelger-Huët anomaly.

plasia of the marrow are usually apparent by 3 to 4 weeks after exposure. With supportive care and treatment, some affected dogs will recover over the course of 1 to 3 months. Marked variation in susceptibility to estrogen toxicity appears to occur in dogs with marrow hypoplasia induced at doses varying from 0.16 to 0.70 mg/kg. Granulocyte/macrophage progenitors are decreased in the neutropenic phase of the disease. The mechanism of suppression is unknown. In mice, estrogen-mediated effects on the production of regulatory factors produced by thymic epithelial cells or lymphocytes may play a role.[57] Hyperestrogenism related to Sertoli cell tumor or an ovarian tumor in dogs occasionally induces a similar aplastic anemia of insidious onset.[54, 58]

INHERITED DEFECTS INVOLVING NEUTROPHILS

Pelger-Huët Anomaly

This is an inherited disorder of dogs and cats characterized by hyposegmentation of granulocytes.[59, 60] Nuclei of neutrophils are round to bilobed but have condensed chromatin similar to that of normal segmented neutrophils (Fig. 181–15). Usually the abnormality is discovered as a serendipitous finding on a hemogram when the cells are classified as immature neutrophils ranging from neutrophilic myelocytes to bands with few segmented neutrophils. The neutrophils appear to have normal function with no predisposition to infectious diseases noted in the affected heterozygotes. The defect has been detected in domestic short-haired cats and a wide variety of dog breeds but may be more common in hounds. The disease is transmitted as an autosomal dominant. In cats, the affected animals are heterozygotes, with the homozygous form usually lethal. In a similar disease in rabbits and a single cat, the homozygous form also was associated with skeletal defects. Acquired forms of neutrophil hyposegmentation do occur and are called pseudo–Pelger-Huët anomaly. Pseudo–Pelger-Huët anomaly has been associated with diseases with enhanced proliferation of neutrophils. Usually some segmented neutrophils are noted and the changes disappear with treatment of the inflammatory disease.

Cyclic Hematopoiesis

Cyclic hematopoiesis is an autosomal recessive disease of stem cells of grey collie dogs.[61] The associated diluted coat

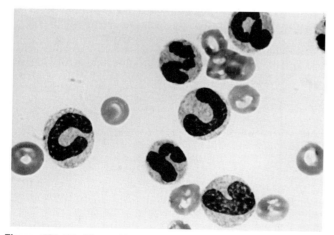

Figure 181–14. Neutrophilia with a left shift and thrombocytopenia in blood of a dog with estrogen toxicity.

color (different from blue merle) is pathognomonic for the disease. Some collie pups have transient diluted coat color but can be differentiated from grey collies by normal color intensity on the nose. Affected pups usually are smaller and weaker than unaffected littermates. The disease is characterized by severe neutropenia, usually with associated fever and illness lasting for 3 to 5 days and recurring at 10- to 12-day intervals. Monocytosis (up to 20,000/µL) is prominent during the later stages of the neutropenic intervals. Neutrophilia with a regenerative left shift occurs after the neutropenia. Cyclic fluctuations of reticulocytes and platelets also occur, but the decreases in these elements do not coincide with the neutropenia. The dogs are predisposed to bacterial diseases during the neutropenic phases and to amyloidosis secondary to the chronic bacterial infections.[62] Only 2 per cent of affected dogs survive to 1 year of age. Antibiotics and supportive therapy may extend the life of affected animals, but most succumb to the secondary diseases within a few years. The molecular basis of the defect has not been defined but appears to involve a defect in the G-CSF signal transduction pathway distal to the G-CSF receptor binding step.[63] The cycle can be interrupted by experimental treatments with endotoxin, lithium carbonate, or recombinant human G-CSF.[64] Bone marrow transplantation with stem cells from normal littermates corrects the defect.[65]

Canine Granulocytopathy Syndrome (Leukocyte Adhesion Protein Deficiency)

An autosomal recessive defect with defective bactericidal activity was described in a colony of Irish setters with life-threatening bacterial infections.[66] Diseases included omphalophlebitis, suppurative dermatitis, gingivitis, lymphadenopathy, pododermatitis, and osteomyelitis. The dogs had persistent leukocytosis (25,000–540,000/µL) with neutrophilia with regenerative left shifts. Hypersegmented nuclei were noted in neutrophils, which could imply a defect in emigration from the blood. The disease was attributed to defective bactericidal activity.[67] In subsequent studies, Irish setters with clinical features and hematologic findings that were very similar were described.[68, 69] These dogs had defective adhesion related to deficiencies of beta$_2$ integrins as detected with antibodies to CD11b and to CD18, the common beta subunit of the beta$_2$ integrins. Defects included diminished adherence to nylon wool, impaired ingestion of particles opsonized with zymosan or IgG, and decreased chemiluminescence in response to C3b-opsonized particles. The leukocytosis likely reflects the defect in binding to endothelial cells and migration into tissues. Fever, lymphadenopathy, and hypergammaglobulinemia are common findings associated with the recurrent bacterial infections. Antibiotic therapy is effective in combating the infections, but most animals die at a few months of age.

Inherited Malabsorption of Vitamin B₁₂

Selective malabsorption of vitamin B$_{12}$ has been observed in giant schnauzers.[18] The animals failed to thrive, with signs apparent by 6 to 12 weeks of age. Mild neutropenia and hypersegmented neutrophils were observed, suggesting a possible defect in neutrophil production, but macrocytic anemia was not observed as expected in vitamin B$_{12}$ deficiency of humans.

Canine X-Linked Severe Combined Immunodeficiency

This disease has been recognized as an enhanced susceptibility to bacterial, fungal, and protozoal agents in the basset hound and at least one Cardigan Welsh corgi.[70] The abnormalities often emerge as levels of maternal antibodies decline. The affected males fail to thrive and may develop fatal diarrhea caused by *Cryptosporidium*, an opportunist. Maturation of the T-cell population is defective, but T-cell numbers may be normal. IgM levels are normal, but IgA and IgG levels are low to absent. Lymphocyte numbers are usually in the low end of reference ranges. The molecular defects involve mutations in the gene for the interleukin-2 receptor gamma chain.

Weimaraner Neutrophil Defect

A metabolic defect in oxidative killing of bacteria has been recognized in Weimaraner dogs.[71] The affected dogs have repeated episodes of fever, bacterial infections, and inflammatory lesions. Most of the affected dogs develop bacterial infections with foci of granulomatous inflammation. The animals have decreased IgG and IgM concentrations in serum and defective chemiluminescent responses. The exact nature of the defect is unknown.

Doberman Pinscher Neutrophil Defect

A defect in bacterial killing by neutrophils has been reported in related Doberman pinschers with histories of recurrent respiratory tract infections.[72] The exact nature of the defect is unknown. The neutrophils have reduced capacity for reduction of nitroblue tetrazolium. Most bacterial infections respond to bactericidal antibiotics.

OTHER DEFECTS OF NEUTROPHIL FUNCTION

Recurrent bacterial infections in young animals with normal or increased neutrophil numbers should raise suspicion of a neutrophil function defect. Abnormalities in adherence, chemikinesis, phagocytosis, or bactericidal functions may predispose to bacterial infections. A number of tests of neutrophil function have been applied to leukocytes of dogs and cats.[73] Most of the tests have a large coefficient of variation, and some leukocytes functions are enhanced by priming in the presence of mediators of inflammation, making interpretation difficult.[74] Ideally, these tests would be performed in a comprehensive battery to evaluate various aspects of neutrophil function. It is recommended that animals be referred to specialized laboratories for evaluation for suspected leukocyte function defects. Acquired defects of neutrophil function have been associated with poorly regulated diabetes mellitus,[75] hepatozoonosis,[76] protothecosis,[77] pyoderma,[78] and feline leukemia virus infection.[79] Most of the acquired defects are mild and do not require specific treatment.

LYMPHOCYTES

Cells with morphologic characteristics of lymphocytes have a wide variety of functions in the immune system. One distinct difference in lymphocyte kinetics is the fact that lymphocytes, especially T lymphocytes, are recirculated. Changes in lymphocyte concentration in the blood may reflect variations in production, recirculation, or destruction.

Lymphocytosis may be associated with immune responses, especially those with prolonged immune stimulation (Table 181–3). The increases usually are modest, although marked

TABLE 181–3. CAUSES OF LYMPHOCYTOSIS

Physiologic (epinephrine, fear, excitement, exercise)
Prolonged immune stimulation
    Protozoa
    Fungi
    Ehrlichia
    Postvaccinal response (acute response)
Hypoadrenocorticism
Leukemia (chronic lymphocytic leukemia, acute lymphocytic leukemia, lymphoma)

TABLE 181–4. CAUSES OF LYMPHOPENIA

Corticosteroid hormones (endogenous or exogenous)
Viruses
    Canine distemper
    Feline leukemia virus
    Infectious canine hepatitis
    Feline immunodeficiency virus
    Parvovirus (canine or feline)
Chylothorax
Lymphangiectasia

increases occasionally occur in young animals. Blood parasites and other protozoan diseases may be associated with lymphocytosis. The increased lymphocytes appear to be secondary to the immune stimulation from the persistent organisms. Lymphocytosis occurs in some dogs and cats with hypoadrenocorticism but not consistently enough to be reliable. Lymphocytosis was noted in 20 per cent of cats and 11 to 20 per cent of dogs with hypoadrenocorticism.[80] The lack of lymphopenia and eosinopenia in a stressed dog or cat may support a concern about hypoadrenocorticism.

Variable increases in small to medium-sized lymphocytes occur with chronic lymphocytic leukemia. Lymphocyte concentrations in excess of 20,000/μL with greater than 90 per cent small lymphocytes are compatible with chronic lymphocytic leukemia. Lymphocyte counts between 8,000 and 20,000/μL are difficult to interpret because tests for clonality of the population or specific markers are not widely available; retesting in a few weeks is warranted because reactive lymphocytosis related to immune stimulation is usually transient. Lymphocytosis with blasts present in the blood should prompt consideration of the possibility of acute lymphoblastic leukemia or bone marrow involvement with lymphoma. Many dogs with lymphoma have a small number of immature lymphocytes present on blood films. Involvement of the marrow may be detectable in core biopsy specimens in more than 50 per cent of dogs at the time of diagnosis of lymphoma.[81]

Reactive lymphocytes with deeply basophilic non-granular cytoplasm and larger nuclei with fine chromatin are commonly associated with diseases with immune stimulation. They are sometimes called immunoblasts. Atypical large lymphocytes with fine chromatin and faint nucleoli are noted in the blood of cats with haemobartonellosis or in dogs or cats in the recovery stage from severe inflammatory diseases. Occasionally, a dramatic lymphocytosis with numerous reactive lymphocytes are noted as a sequel to vaccination in young animals.

Lymphocytosis of large granular lymphocytes often is neoplastic, but reactive large granular lymphocytosis occurs in some inflammatory diseases and has been associated with *Ehrlichia canis* infection in dogs.[82]

Lymphopenia most frequently reflects apoptosis and redistribution of lymphocytes in response to increased concentrations of endogenous or exogenous glucocorticoids (Table 181–4). This is a common, non-specific change related to the stress response in a variety of diseases. Viruses such as distemper, parvo, or infectious canine hepatitis that infect lymphocytes may induce lymphopenia by direct injury of lymphopoietic cells. The mechanism of feline leukemia virus or feline immunodeficiency virus–induced lymphopenias are not as well defined but appear to involve apoptosis. Feline leukemia virus infection causes a decrease in both CD4[+] and CD8[+] lymphocytes.[35] Feline immunodeficiency virus infection induces a significant decrease in the ratio of CD4[+]/

CD8[+] lymphocytes. This change mostly reflects a loss of CD4[+] lymphocytes.[83] In chylothorax or lymphangiectasia, the lymphopenia likely involves a combination of factors but sequestration or drainage of cells and fluid can contribute by interfering with the recirculation of lymphocytes.

EOSINOPHILS

Eosinophilia usually develops in response to specific stimuli. The causes are diverse (Table 181–5) and include parasitic diseases, allergies, other hypersensitivity reactions, and a variety of tissue injuries.[84] Eosinophils contribute to host defense by participating in killing some parasites, ameliorating inflammatory responses by inactivating chemical mediators, and participating in anti-tumor responses. The eosinophilia associated with parasitic infections is T-cell dependent and is mediated by soluble factors including interleukin-3, especially interleukin-5, and GM-CSF.[85] Parasitic diseases with extensive tissue contact are most likely to be associated with eosinophilia. Eosinophils produce some products that can damage host tissue, so their role varies from a beneficial response to a foreign agent or abnormal cell to a mediator of tissue injury depending on the specific conditions. In asthma, eosinophils appear to be major effector cells for damage to airway epithelium. In the tissues, eosinophils tend to be localized beneath the epithelial lining of the gastrointestinal tract, respiratory tract, skin, and uterus, where they are positioned to respond to foreign agents. The degree of eosinophilia appears to relate more to the individual responsiveness of an animal, previous sensitization, and the nature of the specific agent rather than to parasitic load or the extent of tissue injury. Eosinophilic responses in

TABLE 181–5. CAUSES OF EOSINOPHILIA

Parasites
    Heartworms
    Intestinal parasites—nematodes, trematodes, protozoa
    Lung parasites
    Ectoparasites
Allergies—especially flea bite hypersensitivity
Asthma
Upper respiratory tract diseases
Chronic rhinitis, sinusitis
Neoplasms—mast cell tumor, lymphoma, carcinomas
Feline leukemia virus (rare isolates that might involve recombinations of feline leukemia virus with endogenous sequences)[93]
Gastrointestinal disease (especially cats)
Pulmonary infiltrates with eosinophilia
Eosinophilic granuloma complex
Hypereosinophilic syndrome
Estrus
Dermatitis
Hypoadrenocorticism

HEM

German shepherds are often more dramatic than in other breeds. Airway washings should be performed when efforts to identify causes of eosinophilia have been unproductive to help exclude asthma or response to lung parasites. Mild eosinophilic components of inflammatory reactions associated with upper respiratory tract infections are common, especially in cats, and should not be assigned undue specificity for asthma or response to parasites. In eosinophilia, the number and size of eosinophilic granules varies and a few vacuoles may be noted in the cytoplasm of the eosinophils. The heterogeneity and vacuolation appears to be related to the presence of a less dense population of eosinophils that correlates with a primed or an activated phenotype.

Eosinophils of the greyhound often have prominent cytoplasmic vacuolation.[86] Eosinophilia is occasionally associated with neoplasia, including mast cell tumor, fibrosarcoma, mammary carcinoma, and lymphoma.[87–91] The mechanism of the tumor-associated eosinophilia has not been defined in most instances in dogs and cats, although interleukin-5 and interleukin-2 production by the tumor cells is suspected. Hypereosinophilic syndrome can be associated with marked eosinophilia with varying degrees of eosinophilic left shifts in cats.[92] The syndrome frequently includes intestinal thickening, with tissue infiltrates of eosinophils present in the gut, lymph nodes, spleen, liver, and a variety of other tissues. The disease is not always clearly separable from eosinophilic leukemia.[93]

Eosinopenia is difficult to define because most reference ranges for dogs and cats extend to zero. Most commonly, eosinopenia is used in the description of hemograms with no eosinophils as part of a stress leukogram. Corticosteroid hormones inhibit the release of histamine from mast cells, thereby decreasing the stimuli for release of eosinophils from the marrow. Eosinophils are decreased non-specifically in many acute infections, reflecting corticosteroid effects.

BASOPHILS

Basophils are present in very low numbers or are absent in the blood of normal dogs and cats. Basophils contain proteoglycans and histamine and appear to play a role in immune-mediated reactions, especially anaphylaxis and the induction of immediate hypersensitivity reactions or hypersensitivity responses to parasites or allergens. Basophils play an important role in hypersensitivity to arthropod bites.[94] Basophilia is most often associated with eosinophilia (Table 181–6). In endemic regions, dirofilariasis should always be considered in dogs with concurrent eosinophilia and basophilia. Basophilia is sometimes associated with mast cell tumors, although the connection between the two is not defined. Most textbooks mention alterations in lipid metabolism as a cause of basophilia, but this association is weak at best. In theory, heparin from granules of basophils is involved in the activation of lipoprotein lipase for transfer of triglycerides across cell membranes. Basopenia is not a defined entity because the range extends to zero in normal dogs and cats.

TABLE 181–6. CAUSES OF BASOPHILIA

Parasitism
Hypersensitivity reactions
Hypothyroidism
Mast cell tumor
Granulocytic leukemia

TABLE 181–7. CAUSES OF MONOCYTOSIS

Acute or chronic (including granulomatous) inflammation
  Intracellular—bacteria, especially mycobacteria or *Brucella*
  Protozoans
  Feline infectious peritonitis
  Foreign-body reactions
  Immune-mediated arthritis
  Fungal diseases
Corticosteroid hormones (dogs)
Recovery from neutropenia
  Cyclic hematopoiesis
  Parvovirus infection
Hemolytic disease
Canine granulocytopathy

MONOCYTES

The monocyte is a bone marrow–derived cell that is involved in the phagocytosis and killing of bacteria, viruses, fungi, and protozoa. In the tissues, monocytes differentiate under the influence of local environmental factors into free or fixed macrophages of the mononuclear phagocyte system. They are important scavengers of damaged cells and particulate debris. Macrophages derived from monocytes play important roles in immune responses, regulation of inflammation, and regulation of hematopoiesis. Monocytosis is associated with chronic inflammatory diseases, but it should be recognized that monocytosis can occur within hours as an early change in the same diseases that cause neutrophilia (Table 181–7). Monocytes are pleomorphic cells ranging in size from cells the size of neutrophils to large cells up to 20 μm in diameter. Monocyte precursors in the marrow compartment are often difficult to identify by light microscopy but include monoblasts and promonocytes. Monocytes have a shorter marrow transit time than neutrophils, allowing monocyte responses to emerge much earlier than neutrophilia after diseases with depletion of marrow reserves or injury to marrow precursors.

PROGNOSTIC INDICATORS IN LEUKOCYTE RESPONSES

A degenerative left shift characterized by a decreasing leukocyte count and greater numbers of immature neutrophils than segmented neutrophils indicates depletion of marrow reserves and is a grave prognostic sign. Although less reliable, neutrophil counts greater than 100,000/μL in dogs or cats raise concern because they suggest severe inflammatory disease, with prolonged stimulation of granulopoiesis resulting in granulocytic hyperplasia in the bone marrow. The high rate of neutrophil turnover raises concern about potential depletion of marrow reserves.

In inflammatory diseases, a decreasing left shift indicates decreased stimuli for release of neutrophils from the marrow and is a positive sign. Increasing lymphocyte and eosinophil counts in convalescence are good prognostic signs indicating decreasing glucocorticoid release from the adrenal glands.

MAST CELLS

The detection of mast cells on blood films should always elicit a search for mast cell tumors with potential for metastasis to the bone marrow. Mast cells are rarely detected on buffy coat smears from normal dogs. Mast cells are occasionally noted in the blood of dogs with inflammatory diseases. Acute enteritis, especially parvoviral enteritis, is a common cause of mastocytemia, although mast cells have been associated with other severe systemic inflammatory diseases.[95] Buffy coat smears of dogs with inflammatory skin diseases may contain a few to many mast cells. In a series of buffy coat smears from 100 dogs with skin inflammation, 13 samples contained one or more mast cells on four slides examined.[96] Systemic mastocytosis is a unique mast cell neoplasia often associated with mast cell leukemia of cats.[97] Splenomegaly and vomiting are the most consistent findings, but anemia and mastocytemia are also common. The mast cells usually appear well differentiated. Most affected cats are negative for feline leukemia virus. Splenectomy improves the animals comfort and may prolong survival of the cats without mastocytemia. Prognosis is poor for cats with mastocytemia.

ACUTE MYELOID LEUKEMIA

Acute myeloid leukemia includes neoplastic diseases of precursors of granulocytes, monocytes, erythrocytes, or megakaryocytes. These diseases are clinically indistinguishable. Pale mucous membranes and hemorrhages related to thrombocytopenia, hepatomegaly, and splenomegaly are relatively common findings. Leukocytosis, thrombocytopenia, and anemia are the most frequent hematologic findings. Blasts are detected in the blood in 98 per cent of the cases but exceed 30 per cent of the leukocytes in only a little more than a third of the cases. Definitive diagnosis and classification require bone marrow biopsy, with documentation of more than 30 per cent blasts in the marrow.[98] Cytochemical staining is often required for confirmation of the myeloid lineage of blasts, particularly when the distinction between lymphoid and myeloid cells is uncertain.[99–101] Acute myeloid leukemia usually has a short clinical course, often with unrewarding responses to chemotherapy. In cats, a high percentage of acute myeloid leukemias are associated with feline leukemia virus infection.

Acute myeloid leukemia is subdivided into the following categories:

M0—a cell type with restricted myeloid differentiation containing peroxidase-positive granules as demonstrated with electron microscopy and/or immunophenotyping.

Myeloblastic leukemia with maturation (M1)—greater than 90 per cent of the nucleated cells in the marrow are myeloblasts with minimal differentiation to neutrophils and eosinophils.

Myeloblastic leukemia with maturation (M2)—myeloblasts constitute more than 30 per cent but less than 90 per cent of all nucleated cells (Fig. 181–16). Granulocytic differentiation is apparent usually with disproportionate numbers of progranulocytes; monocytes may be increased but are less than 20 per cent of the non-erythroid nucleated cells in the marrow.

Promyelocytic leukemia (M3)—this category is reserved for leukemias with numerous progranulocytes with distinctive prominent cytoplasmic granules. This human disease has a bleeding tendency related to enhanced fibrinolysis. This disease has not yet been described in dogs or cats.

Myelomonocytic leukemia (M4)—myeloblasts and monoblasts constitute more than 30 per cent of all nucleated cells with more than 20 per cent differentiated granulo-

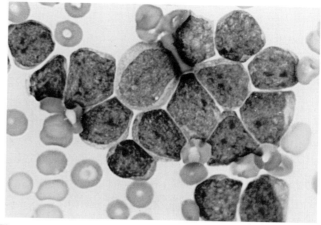

Figure 181–16. Myeloblasts and granulocytic precursors of a dog with acute myeloid leukemia with granulocytic differentiation (M2).

cytes and more than 20 per cent monocytes (Fig. 181–17).

Monocytic leukemia (M5)—cells have monocytic differentiation. This category is subdivided into M5a, with monoblasts and promonocytes accounting for more than 80 per cent of non-erythroid cells (Fig. 181–18), and M5b, with more than 30 per cent but less than 80 per cent monoblasts and promonocytes. Granulocytes must be less than 20 per cent to differentiate category M5 from M4.

Erythroleukemia (M6)—This category includes many of the leukemias that formerly were classified as erythremic myelosis or erythroleukemia. In M6, the erythroid component constitutes more than 50 per cent of all nucleated cells but monoblasts and myeloblasts combined are less than 30 per cent of all nucleated cells. When erythroid cells are excluded from the count, monoblasts combined with myeloblasts are more than 30 per cent. A designation of M6Er is applied when there is more than 30 per cent of combined monoblasts, myeloblasts, and rubriblasts, but rubriblasts are predominant. Granulocytic and monocytic differentiation also may be present in M6 or M6Er leukemia.

Megakaryoblastic leukemia (M7)—bone marrow contains

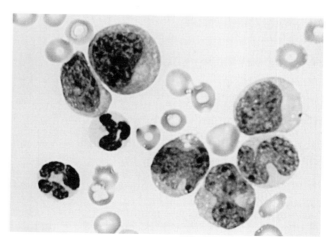

Figure 181–17. Granulocytic and monocytic cells of a dog with acute myeloid leukemia with granulocytic and monocytic differentiation (myelomonocytic; M4).

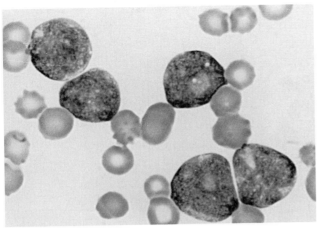

Figure 181–18. Monoblasts of a dog with acute myeloid leukemia with monoblastic differentiation (M5a).

more than 30 per cent megakaryoblasts with variable differentiation of the large blasts to megakaryocytes. Stains for von Willebrand factor and/or glycoprotein IIIa are helpful for confirmation of the megakaryocytic cell type.[102, 103]

MYELODYSPLASIA

When the blast number is disproportionately increased but less than 30 per cent of all nucleated cells in the marrow, chronic myeloid leukemia or myelodysplasia may be suspected.[104] Usually the marrow is hypercellular, but occasionally a hypocellular marrow with asynchronous developmental morphologic abnormalities involving erythroid, granulocytic, or megakaryocytic cells is noted. The disease may be classified as erythrodysplasia or myelodysplasia according to the predominant cell type that is affected. Mild myelofibrosis may be associated with the myelodysplasia. Leukopenia is common in the blood and may reflect increased apoptosis of precursors within the marrow compartment. Dysplasia usually implies an abnormal proliferation of cells without conclusive evidence of neoplasia, but many human myelodysplasias are clonal disorders. A high percentage of myelodysplasias represent preleukemias. In cats, about 70 per cent of the myelodysplasias of cats were positive for feline leukemia virus.

CHRONIC MYELOID LEUKEMIA

The criteria for diagnosis of chronic myeloid leukemia are not well established and overlap with criteria for myelodysplasia. In contrast to human chronic myeloid leukemia with the distinctive translocation known as the Philadelphia chromosome, no markers for this disease in dogs or cats have been described. These leukemias are characterized by a marked neutrophilic leukocytosis and/or monocytosis without evidence of inflammatory disease and without prominent dysplastic changes in the marrow precursors. If marked monocytosis accompanies the neutrophilia, chronic myelomonocytic leukemia must be considered. Some chronic myeloid leukemias have such prominent differentiation toward the eosinophilic or basophilic series to be designated as eosinophilic or basophilic chronic myeloid leukemia. Cyto-

chemical staining for omega-exonuclease may be helpful in confirming the identity of immature basophils.[105]

ACUTE UNDIFFERENTIATED LEUKEMIA

This designation is used for leukemias with a predominance of blasts but no distinctive morphologic or cytochemical feature that allows further classification at this time. Undifferentiated leukemias of cats with unusual pseudopodia and uncertain lineage, previously classified as reticuloendotheliosis, are included in this category.

ACUTE LYMPHOBLASTIC LEUKEMIA

This is a rapidly progressive neoplastic disease of lymphoblasts (Fig. 181–19). In a series of 30 cases, the median age of affected dogs was 5.5 years with a range of 1 to 12 years.[106] The male-to-female ratio was 3:2. Lymphocytosis with a predominance of lymphoblasts in the blood is diagnostic. Cytochemical markers for lymphoblasts are lacking, but reagents are available for immunophenotypic characterization of lymphoid precursors.[107] Genetic analysis may be used to identify cell lineage and clonality by demonstrating rearrangements of the immunoglobulin or T-cell receptor genes.[108] If the leukocyte count is normal or leukopenia is present, bone marrow biopsy is required to document replacement by lymphoblasts. Anemia, thrombocytopenia with petechiae, and splenomegaly are common. Lymphadenopathy may be noted, but marked enlargement supports a diagnosis of lymphoma with involvement of bone marrow. In dogs, the immunophenotype of a limited number of acute lymphoblastic leukemias has been T cell or null cell.[109] The prognosis is poor. Treatment requires aggressive chemotherapy, and remissions often are short lived. Median survival in dogs with complete or partial remissions was 120 days.

LEUKEMIA OF GRANULAR LYMPHOCYTES

These are leukemias of subsets of lymphocytes with abundant cytoplasm and azurophilic cytoplasmic granules (Fig. 181–20).[110] One subset is of T-cell origin and expresses CD3 on its cell membranes whereas the other is of natural killer

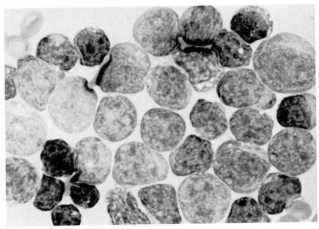

Figure 181–19. Lymphoblasts and a few differentiated lymphocytes of a dog with acute lymphoblastic leukemia.

cell origin. The cells have distinctive eosinophilic to amphophilic granules in the cytoplasm.[111] The granules vary markedly in size and number and occasionally may be difficult to distinguish from mast cell granules in instances when the granules stain more basophilic. The granules should stain for beta-glucuronidase and acid phosphatase and have been demonstrated to contain perforin in some species. The leukemia may be associated with lymphoma in dogs or cats. In cats, lymphoma of large granular lymphocytes frequently involves the intestine or mesenteric lymph nodes.[112] In dogs, leukemia of large granular lymphocytes usually behaves like an aggressive lymphoid leukemia. The survival time is short for lymphoblastic leukemia involving granular lymphocytes despite treatments. A few cases of chronic lymphocytic leukemia involving granular lymphocytes have been detected in dogs. The affected cells are small to medium-sized lymphocytes with condensed chromatin and small numbers of reddish-purple cytoplasmic granules. The biologic behavior of the chronic lymphocytic leukemia of granular lymphocytes is not well defined but appears to be similar to other forms of chronic lymphocytic leukemia with a protracted course even without treatment.

CHRONIC LYMPHOCYTIC LEUKEMIA

Chronic lymphocytic leukemia frequently is first recognized as an incidental finding of lymphocytosis on a hemogram. In a series of 22 cases in dogs, the median age was 10 to 12 years.[113] Most of the cells in the blood are small to medium-sized lymphocytes with normal morphology (Fig. 181–21). No more than 5 per cent immature lymphocytes are expected. Anemia, neutropenia, or thrombocytopenia is not expected in the early stages of the disease and, when present, is milder than expected with acute lymphoblastic leukemia. When lymphocytosis is detected, a hemogram should be obtained in 3 to 4 weeks to confirm persistence of the lymphocytosis and to allow time for regression of reactive lymphocytosis. Dogs without anemia, thrombocytopenia, or organomegaly and leukocyte counts less than 60,000/μL may not require treatment. The cells have a slow turnover rate, which leads to a more indolent course, even untreated. The mean survival time after diagnosis and chemotherapy of dogs with chronic lymphocytic leukemia was 452 days. In occasional dogs, a blast crisis with transformation to prolymphocytic or lymphoblastic leukemia or lym-

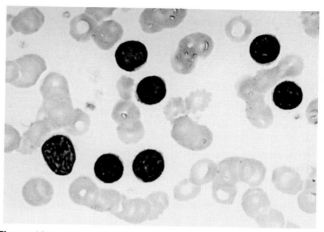

Figure 181–21. Lymphocytes with normal condensed nuclear chromatin of a dog with chronic lymphocytic leukemia.

phoma (Richter's transformation) occurs in the later stages of the disease. Splenomegaly may be present, but lymphadenopathy is usually mild or absent until late in the disease. Bone marrow replacement by the lymphocytes eventually occurs and may induce cytopenias that require treatment. About 50 per cent of patients have monoclonal gammopathies. Immune-mediated hemolytic anemia may be a secondary disease. A few dogs with chronic lymphocytic leukemia with granular lymphocyte phenotype have been detected, but no distinctive biologic behavior has been associated with this phenotype. Of the few cases of canine chronic lymphocytic leukemia in which the neoplastic lymphocytes have been typed, most have been of T-cell origin.[109] This contrasts to human chronic lymphocytic leukemia and canine lymphoma, which typically are of B-cell origin, and conflicts with the association with monoclonal gammopathies.

MALIGNANT HISTIOCYTOSIS

Malignant histiocytosis is a rapidly progressive and inevitably fatal disease of dogs and rarely of cats.[114–116] Lethargy, weight loss, respiratory disease, neurologic disease, hepatosplenomegaly, lymphadenopathy, and anemia are the most common clinical signs. The disease is more frequent in Bernese Mountain dogs, golden retrievers, and rottweilers. Males are more commonly affected than females. This disease is believed to be a proliferative disorder of histiocytic cells. The neoplastic cells are large pleomorphic round cells with abundant slightly granular eosinophilic cytoplasm and large round-to-pleomorphic nuclei with increased mitoses and moderate anaplasia. Multinucleated giant cells are common. Erythrophagocytosis may be prominent in the cells in the spleen, lymph nodes, and bone marrow. Immunohistochemical demonstration of lysozyme and alpha$_1$-antitrypsin is helpful in supporting a macrophage origin. Unpublished observations by Moore at the University of California at Davis suggest that the cells have the immunophenotype of activated Langerhans' cell histiocytes.[117] The relationship of malignant histiocytosis to benign systemic histiocytosis of Bernese Mountain dogs and the histiocytic sarcoma of flat-coated retrievers is not well defined, but these diseases may form a spectrum of histiocytic proliferative disorders.

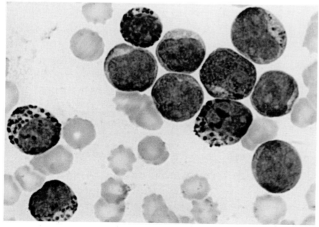

Figure 181–20. Lymphoblasts with distinctive cytoplasmic granules of a dog with leukemia of granular lymphocytes.

REFERENCES

1. Jain NC: Essentials of Veterinary Hematology. Philadelphia, Lea & Febiger, 1993, pp 222–307.

HEM

2. Latimer KS: Leukocytes in health and disease. *In* Ettinger SJ, Feldman EC (eds): Textbook of Veterinary Internal Medicine: Diseases of the Dog and Cat, 4th ed. Philadelphia, WB Saunders, 1995, pp 1892–1929.

3. Boggs DR: The kinetics of neutrophilic leukocytes in health and disease. Semin Hematol 4:359, 1967.

4. Raskin RE: Myelopoiesis and myeloproliferative disorders. Vet Clin North Am Small Anim Pract 26:1023, 1996.

5. Chinn DR, Myers RK, Mathews JA: Neutrophilic leukocytosis associated with metastatic fibrosarcoma in a dog. JAVMA 186:806, 1985.

6. Lappin MR, Latimer KS: Hematuria and extreme neutrophilic leukocytosis in a dog with renal tubular carcinoma. JAVMA 192:1289, 1988.

7. Madewell BR, Wilson DW, Hornoff WJ: Leukemoid blood response and bone infarcts in a dog with renal tubular adenocarcinoma. JAVMA 197:1623, 1990.

8. Thompson JP, Christopher MM, Ellison GW: Paraneoplastic leukocytosis associated with a rectal adenomatous polyp in a dog. JAVMA 201:737, 1992.

9. Ilkiw JE, Davis PE, Church DB: Hematologic, biochemical, blood gas, and acid-base values in greyhounds before and after exercise. Am J Vet Res 50:583, 1989.

10. Moore GE, Mahaffey EA, Hoenig M: Hematologic and serum biochemical effects of long-term administration of anti-inflammatory doses of prednisone in dogs. Am J Vet Res 53:1033, 1992.

11. Zimmerman GA, Prescott SM, McIntyre TM: Endothelial cell interactions with granulocytes: Tethering and signaling molecules. Immunol Today 13:93, 1992.

12. Lawrence MB, Springer TA: Leukocytes roll on a selectin at physiologic flow rates: Distinction from and prerequisite for adhesion through integrins. Cell 65:859, 1991.

13. Larson RS, Springer TA: Structure and function of leukocyte integrins. Immun Rev 114:181, 1990.

14. Rollins BJ: Chemokines. Blood 90:909, 1997.

15. Moon ML, Hinkle GN, Krakowka GS, et al: Scintigraphic imaging of technetium 99m–labeled neutrophils of the dog. Am J Vet Res 49:950, 1988.

16. Gosset KA, Carakostas MC: Effect of EDTA on morphology of neutrophils of healthy dogs and dogs with inflammation. Vet Clin Pathol 13:22, 1984.

17. Watson ADJ, Middleton DJ: Chloramphenicol toxicosis in cats. Am J Vet Res 39:1199, 1978.

18. Fyfe JC, Jezyk PF, Giger U: Inherited selective malabsorption of vitamin B_{12} in giant schnauzers. J Am Hosp Assoc 25:533, 1989.

19. Schalm OW: Erythrocyte macrocytosis in miniature and toy poodles. Canine Pract 3:55, 1976.

20. Van Steenhouse JL, DeNova RC: Atypical *Histoplasma capsulatum* infection in a dog. JAVMA 188:527, 1986.

21. McIntire DK, Vincent-Johnson N, Dillon AR, et al: Hepatozoonosis in dogs: 22 cases (1989–1994). JAVMA 210:916, 1997.

22. Goldman EE, Breitschwerdt EB, Grindem CB, et al: Granulocytic ehrlichiosis in dogs. J Vet Intern Med 12:61, 1998.

23. Ewing SA, Dawson JE, Panciera RJ, et al: Dogs infected with human granulocytotropic *Ehrlichia* spp. J Med Entomol 34:710, 1997.

24. Peavy GM, Holland CJ, Dutta SK, et al: Suspected ehrlichial infection in five cats from a household. JAVMA 210:231, 1997.

25. McLaughlin BG, Adams PS, Cornwell WD: Canine distemper viral inclusions in blood cells of four vaccinated dogs. Can Vet J 26:368, 1985.

26. Alroy J, Freden GO, Goyal V, et al: Morphology of leukocytes from cats affected with α-mannosidosis and mucopolysaccharidosis VI (MPS VI). Vet Pathol 26:294, 1989.

27. Barker WG, Blakemore WF, Dell A, et al: GM_1 gangliosidosis (type 1) in a cat. Biochem J 235:151, 1986.

28. Hirsch VM, Cunningham TA: Hereditary anomaly of neutrophil granulation in Birman cats. Am J Vet Res 45:2170, 1984.

29. Kramer JW, Davis WC, Prieur DJ: The Chédiak-Higashi syndrome of cats. Lab Invest 36:554, 1977.

30. Prieur DJ, Collier LL: Neutropenia in cats with the Chédiak-Higashi syndrome. Can J Vet Res 51:407, 1987.

31. Gaunt SD, Baker DC: Hemosiderin in leukocytes of dogs with immune-mediated hemolytic anemia. Vet Clin Pathol 15:8, 1986.

32. Kisseberth WC, MacEwen EG: Complications of cancer and its treatment. *In* Withrow SJ, MacEwen EG (eds): Small Animal Clinical Oncology, 2nd ed. Philadelphia, WB Saunders, 1996, pp 129–132.

33. Shelton GH, Linenberger ML, Grant CK: Hematologic manifestation of feline immunodeficiency virus infection. Blood 76:1104, 1990.

34. Yamamoto JK, Sparger E, Ho EW, et al: Pathogenesis of experimentally-induced feline immunodeficiency virus infection in cats. Am J Vet Res 49:1246, 1988.

35. Hoffman-Lehmann R, Holznagel E, Ossent P, Lutz H: Parameters of disease progression in long-term experimental feline retrovirus (feline immunodeficiency virus and feline leukemia virus) infections: Hematology, clinical chemistry, and lymphocyte subsets. Clin Diagn Lab Immunol 4:33, 1997.

36. Mishu L, Callahan G, Alleban Z, et al: Effects of recombinant canine granulocyte colony stimulating factor on white blood cell production in clinically healthy and neutropenic dogs. JAVMA 200:1957, 1992.

37. Ogilvie GK, Obradovich JE, Cooper MF, et al: Use of recombinant canine granulocyte colony stimulating factor to decrease myelosuppresion associated with the administration of mitoxantrone in the dog. J Vet Intern Med 6:44, 1992.

38. Obradovich JE, Ogilvie GK, Stradler-Morris S, et al: Effect of recombinant canine granulocyte colony stimulating factor on peripheral blood neutrophil counts in normal cats. J Vet Intern Med 7:65, 1993.

39. Colgan SP, Gasper PW, Thrall MA, et al: Neutrophil function in normal and Chédiak-Higashi syndrome cats following administration of recombinant canine granulocyte colony-stimulating factor. Exp Hematol 20:1229, 1992.

40. Nash RA, Burstein SA, Storb R, et al: Thrombocytopenia in dogs induced by granulocyte-macrophage colony-stimulating factor: Increased destruction of circulating platelets. Blood 86:1765, 1995.

41. Schuening FG, Storb R, Goehle S, et al: Effect of recombinant human granulocyte colony stimulating factor on hematopoiesis of normal dogs and on hematopoietic recovery after otherwise lethal total body irradiation. Blood 74:1308, 1989.

42. Keller P, Smalling R: Granulocyte colony stimulating factor: Animal studies for risk assessment. Int Rev Exp Pathol 34:173, 1993.

43. Reagan WJ, Murphy D, Battaglino M, et al: Antibodies to canine granulocyte colony-stimulating factor induced persistent neutropenia. Vet Pathol 32:374, 1995.

44. Henry CJ: Clinical use of rhG-CSF. Proceedings of the 15th ACVIM Forum, Lake Buena Vista, FL, 1997, pp 565–566.

45. Morley A, Stohlman F: Cyclophosphamide-induced cyclical neutropenia. N Engl J Med 282:643, 1970.

46. Swenson CL, Kociba GJ, Okeefe DA: Cyclic hematopoiesis associated with feline leukemia virus infection in two cats. JAVMA 191:93, 1987.

47. Gaunt SD, Pierce KR: Effects of estradiol on hematopoietic and marrow adherent cells of dogs. Am J Vet Res 47:906, 1986.

48. Shelton GH, et al: Severe neutropenia associated with griseofulvin therapy in cats with feline immunodeficiency virus infection. J Vet Intern Med 4:317, 1990.

49. Weiss DJ, Klausner JS: Drug-associated aplastic anemia in dogs: Eight cases (1984–1988). JAVMA 196:472, 1990.

50. Bloom JC, Lewis HB, Sellers TS, et al: The hematologic effects of cefonicid and cefazedone in the dog: A potential model of cephalosporin hematotoxicity in man. Toxicol Appl Pharmacol 90:135, 1987.

51. Weiss DJ, Adams LG: Aplastic anemia associated with trimethoprim-sulfadiazine and fenbendazole administration in a dog. JAVMA 191:1119, 1987.

52. Peterson ME, Kintzer PP, Hurvitz AI: Methimazole treatment of 262 cats with hyperthyroidism. J Vet Intern Med 2:150, 1988.

53. Jacobs G, Calvert C, Kaufman A: Neutropenia and thrombocytopenia in three dogs treated with anticonvulsants. JAVMA 212:681, 1998.

54. Sherding RG, Wilson GP, Kociba GJ: Bone marrow hypoplasia in eight dogs with Sertoli cell tumor. JAVMA 178:497, 1981.

55. Lund JE, Padgett GA, Ott RL: Cyclic neutropenia in grey collie dogs. Blood 29:452, 1967.

56. Crafts RC: The effects of estrogens on the bone marrow of adult female dogs. Blood 3:276, 1948.

57. Luster MI, Boorman GA, Korach KS, et al: Mechanisms of estrogen-induced myelotoxicity: Evidence of thymic regulation. Int J Immunopharmacol 6:287, 1984.

58. McCandlish IAP, Munro CD, Breeze RG, et al: Hormone producing ovarian tumors in the dog. Vet Rec 105:9, 1979.

59. Latimer KS, Rakich PM, Thompson DF: Pelger-Huët anomaly in cats. Vet Pathol 22:370, 1985.

60. Latimer KS, Kircher IM, Lindl PA, et al: Leukocyte function in Pelger-Huët anomaly of dogs. J Leukocyte Biol 45:301, 1989.

61. Campbell KL: Canine cyclic hematopoiesis. Comp Contin Ed 7:57, 1985.

62. DiGiacomo RF, Hammond WP, Kunz LL, Cox PA: Clinical and pathologic features of cyclic hematopoiesis in grey collie dogs. Am J Pathol 111:225, 1983.

63. Avalos BR, Broudy VC, Ceselski SK, et al: Abnormal response to granulocyte colony stimulating factor (G-CSF) in canine cyclic hematopoiesis is not caused by altered G-CSF receptor expression. Blood 84:789, 1994.

64. Lothrop CD, Warren DJ, Souza LM, et al: Correction of canine cyclic hematopoiesis with recombinant human granulocyte colony-stimulating factor. Blood 72:1324, 1988.

65. Jones JB, Yang TJ, Dale JB, Lange RD: Canine cyclic hematopoiesis: Marrow transplantation between littermates. Br J Haematol 30:215, 1975.

66. Renshaw HW, Chatburn C, Bruan GM, et al: Canine granulocytopathy syndrome: Neutrophil dysfunction in a dog with recurrent infections. JAVMA 166:443, 1975.

67. Renshaw HW, Davis WC, Renshaw SJ: Canine granulocytopathy syndrome: Defective bactericidal capacity of neutrophils from a dog with recurrent infections. Clin Immunol Immunopathol 8:385, 1977.

68. Giger U, Boxer LA, Simpson DJ, et al: Deficiency of leukocyte surface glycoproteins Mol, LFA-1, and Leu M5 in a dog with recurrent bacterial infections: An animal model. Blood 69:1622, 1987.

69. Trowald-Wigh G, Hakanssun L, Johannisson A, et al: Leukocyte adhesion protein deficiency in Irish setter dogs. Vet Immunol Immunopathol 32:261, 1992.

70. Somberg RL, Pullen RP, Casal ML, et al: A simple nucleotide insertion in the canine interleukin-2 receptor gamma chain results in X-linked combined immunodeficiency disease. Vet Immunol Immunopathol 47:203, 1995.

71. Couto CG, Krakowka S, Johnson G, et al: In vitro immunologic features of Weimaraner dogs with neutrophil abnormalities and recurrent infections. Vet Immunol Immunopathol 23:103, 1989.

72. Breitschwerdt EB, Brown TT, DeBuysscher EU, et al: Rhinitis, pneumonia, and defective neutrophil function in the Doberman pinscher. Am J Vet Res 48:1054, 1987.

73. Stickle JE: The neutrophil: Function, disorders, and testing. Vet Clin North Am Small Anim Pract 26:1013, 1996.

74. Thomson MK, Jenson AL, Skak-Nielson et al: Enhanced granulocyte function in a case of chronic granulocytic leukemia in a dog. Vet Immunol Immunopathol 28:143, 1991.

75. Latimer KS, Mahaffey EA: Neutrophil adherence and movement in poorly and well-controlled diabetic dogs. Am J Vet Res 45:1498, 1984.
76. Ibrahim ND, Rahamathulla PM, Njoku CO: Neutrophil myeloperoxidase deficiency associated with canine hepatozoonosis. Int J Parasitol 19:915, 1989.
77. Rakich PM, Latimer KS: Altered immune function in a dog with disseminated prototothecosis. JAVMA 185:681, 1984.
78. Latimer KS, Prasse KW, Mahaffey EA, et al: Neutrophil movement in selected canine skin diseases. Am J Vet Res 44:601, 1983.
79. Kiehl AR, Fettman MJ, Quackenbush SL, et al: Effects of feline leukemia virus infection on neutrophil chemotaxis in vitro. Am J Vet Res 48:76, 1987.
80. Kintzer PP, Peterson ME: Primary and secondary canine hypoadrenocorticism. Vet Clin North Am Small Anim Pract 27:349, 1997.
81. Raskin RE, Krehbiel JD: Prevalence of leukemia blood and bone marrow in dogs with multicentric lymphoma. JAVMA 194:1427, 1989.
82. Weiser MG, Thrall MA, Fulton R, et al: Granular lymphocytosis and hyperproteinemia in dogs with chronic ehrlichiosis. J Am Anim Hosp Assoc 27:84, 1991.
83. Tompkins MB, Nelson PD, English RV, et al: Early events in the immunopathogenesis of feline retroviral infections. JAVMA 199:1311, 1991.
84. Center SA, Randolph JF, Erb HN, et al: Eosinophilia in the cat: A retrospective study of 312 cases (1975–1986). J Am Anim Hosp Assoc 26:349, 1990.
85. Sanderson CJ: Interleukin-5, eosinophils, and disease. Blood 79:3101, 1992.
86. Jain NC: The eosinophils. In Schalm's Veterinary Hematology, 4th ed. Lea & Febiger, Philadelphia, 1986, p 731.
87. O'Keefe DA, Couto CG, Burke-Schwartz C, et al: Systemic mastocytosis in 16 dogs. J Vet Intern Med 1:75, 1987.
88. Bortnowski HB, Rosenthal RC: Gastrointestinal mast cell tumors and eosinophilia in two cats. J Am Anim Hosp Assoc 28:271, 1992.
89. Couto CG: Tumor-associated eosinophilia in a dog. JAVMA 184:837, 1984.
90. Losco PE: Local and peripheral eosinophilia in a dog with anaplastic mammary carcinoma. Vet Pathol 23:536, 1986.
91. Sellon RK, Rottman JB, Jordan HL, et al: Hypereosinophilia associated with transitional cell carcinoma in a cat. JAVMA 201:591, 1992.
92. Hendrick M: A spectrum of hypereosinophilic syndromes exemplified by six cats with eosinophilic enteritis. Vet Pathol 18:188, 1981.
93. Lewis MG, Kociba GJ, Rojko JL, et al: Retroviral-associated eosinophilic leukemia in the cat. Am J Vet Res 46:1066, 1985.
94. Halliwell REW, Schemmer KR: The role of basophils in the immunopathogenesis of hypersensitivity to fleas (Ctenocephalides felis) in dogs. Vet Immunol Immunopathol 15:203, 1987.
95. Stockham SL, Basel DL, Schmidt DA: Mastocytemia in dogs with acute inflammatory diseases. Vet Clin Pathol 15:1621, 1986.
96. Cayette SM, Mcmanus PM, Miller WH, et al: Identification of mast cells in buffy coat preparations from dogs with inflammatory skin diseases. JAVMA 206:325, 1995.
97. Liska WD, MacEwen EG, Zaki FA, et al: Feline systemic mastocytosis: A
review and results of splenectomy in seven cats. J Am Anim Hosp Assoc 15:589, 1979.
98. Jain NC, Blue JT, Grinden CB, et al: A report of the leukemia study group: Proposed criteria for classification of acute myeloid leukemia in dogs and cats. Vet Clin Pathol 20:63, 1991.
99. Jain NC: Clinical-pathological findings and cytochemical characterization of myelomonocytic leukemia in 5 dogs. J Comp Pathol 91:17, 1981.
100. Grindem CG, Stevens JB, Perman V: Cytochemical reactions in cells from leukemic dogs. Vet Pathol 23:103, 1986.
101. Facklam NR, Kociba GJ: Cytochemical characterization of feline leukemic cells. Vet Pathol 23:155, 1986.
102. Colbatzky F, Hermans W: Acute megakaryoblastic leukemia in one cat and two dogs. Vet Pathol 30:816, 1993.
103. Pucheu-Haston CM, Camus A, Taboada J, et al: Megakaryoblastic leukemia in a dog. JAVMA 207:194, 1995.
104. Blue JT, French TW, Krane JS: Non-lymphoid hematopoietic neoplasia in cats: A retrospective study of 60 cases. Cornell Vet 78:21, 1988.
105. Mears EA, Raskin RE, Legendre AM: Basophilic leukemia in a dog. J Vet Intern Med 11:92, 1997.
106. Matus RE, Leifer CE, Macewen EG: Acute lymphoblastic leukemia in the dog: A review of 30 cases. JAVMA 183:859, 1983.
107. Moore PF, Rossetto PV, Danilenko DM, et al: Monoclonal antibodies specific for canine CD4 and CD8 define functional T-lymphocyte subsets and high density expression of CD4 by canine neutrophils. Tissue Antigens 40:75, 1992.
108. Momoi Y, Nagase M, Okamoto M, et al: Rearrangements of immunoglobulin and T-cell receptor genes in canine lymphoma/leukemia cells. J Vet Med Sci 55:775, 1993.
109. Grindem CB: Blood cell markers. Vet Clin North Am Small Anim Pract 26:1043, 1996.
110. Loughran TP: Clonal diseases of large granular lymphocytes. Blood 82:1, 1993.
111. Wellman ML, Couto CG, Starkey RJ: Lymphocytosis of large granular lymphocytes in three dogs. Vet Pathol 26:158, 1989.
112. Wellman ML, Hammer AS, DiBartola SP, et al: Lymphoma involving large granular lymphocytes in cats: 11 cases (1982–1991). JAVMA 201:1265, 1992.
113. Leifer CE, Matus RE: Chronic lymphocytic leukemia in the dog: 22 cases (1974–1984). JAVMA 189:214, 1986.
114. Wellman ML, Davenport DJ, Morton D, et al: Malignant histiocytosis in four dogs. JAVMA 187:919, 1985.
115. Rosin A, Moore P, Dubielzig R: Malignant histiocytosis in Bernese Mountain Dogs. JAVMA 188:1041, 1986.
116. Court EA, Earnest-Koons KA, Barr SC, et al: Malignant histiocytosis in a cat. JAVMA 203:1300, 1993.
117. Moore PF, Schrenzel MD, Olivry T, et al: Canine cutaneous histiocytoma is an epidermotropic Langerhans cell histiocytosis that expresses CD1 and specific β_2-integrin molecules. Am J Pathol 148:1699, 1996.

CHAPTER 182

NON-NEOPLASTIC DISORDERS OF THE SPLEEN

C. Guillermo Couto and Rance M. Gamblin

HEM

The spleen constitutes the single largest component of the mononuclear phagocytic system and is directly interposed between the portal and the systemic circulation. Its unique anatomic and functional features make it prone to undergo both neoplastic and non-neoplastic pathologic changes in a wide variety of disease processes. Neoplastic disorders of the spleen are discussed elsewhere in this text (see Chapters 98 and 100).

PHYSIOLOGY

Hematopoiesis occurs in the spleen, as does filtration and phagocytosis. The spleen serves as a blood reservoir and is important in iron metabolism and in immunology. All these splenic functions are equally important in maintaining homeostasis. Greater detail of splenic anatomy and physiology is found in a previous edition of this text.[1]

SPLENIC MASSES

DEFINITION AND NOMENCLATURE

The term *splenic mass* (or *localized splenomegaly*) refers to a localized palpable enlargement of the spleen. Most splenic masses are round and irregular and can be found in the left cranial or mid-ventral areas.

Splenic masses are more common than diffuse splenic enlargement in dogs, whereas the opposite occurs in cats.[2–7] Splenic masses can be classified as neoplastic and non-neoplastic. Neoplastic splenic masses are discussed in Chapters 98 and 100. Non-neoplastic splenic masses include primarily hematomas and abscesses, with the former being more common.[5, 6, 8]

Splenic hematomas represented the most common splenic mass in 42 dogs splenectomized at the Veterinary Teaching Hospital–Ohio State University, accounting for 33 per cent of all splenic lesions. In other studies, hematomas were diagnosed in approximately 10 per cent of dogs treated by splenectomy, based on samples submitted to diagnostic laboratories for histopathologic evaluation.[5, 6] Splenic hematomas are extremely rare in cats.[7] Most dogs with splenic hematomas are relatively healthy, do not have acute splenic ruptures or develop hemoabdomen, and lack clinically relevant hematologic or hemostatic abnormalities.[8, 9] In most dogs with hematomas, no underlying causes predisposing to intrasplenic bleeding can be found, although hematomas occasionally occur in dogs with splenic lymphoma.

SPLENOMEGALY

DEFINITION

The term *splenomegaly* refers to diffuse enlargement of the spleen.

PATHOGENESIS

Splenic enlargement can result from inflammatory changes (i.e., splenitis), lymphoreticular hyperplasia, congestion, or infiltration with abnormal cells or substances (e.g., amyloidosis) (Table 182–1).

Inflammatory Splenomegaly

Inflammatory changes within the spleen usually result in diffuse enlargement of this organ. Most disorders associated with splenitis are infectious. In addition to lymphoreticular hyperplasia (see later), splenic changes in splenitis include hematogenous infiltration with inflammatory cells (e.g., neutrophils, eosinophils). It is important to classify the splenitis according to the predominant cell type, because different etiologic agents are associated with the different forms.

Suppurative (neutrophilic) splenitis is usually acute or subacute, although chronic suppurative changes of the spleen can also occur. When discrete cavitated lesions filled with pus occur in the spleen, the term *splenic abscess* is preferred. Diseases associated with suppurative splenitis include penetrating wounds to the abdomen, migrating foreign bodies (e.g., plant awns), hematogenous dissemination of bacterial infections (e.g., subacute bacterial endocarditis, septicemia with pyogenic organisms, tuberculosis), bacterial infections secondary to splenic torsion (see later), protozoal infections

(e.g., toxoplasmosis), and certain viral diseases (e.g., acute infectious canine hepatitis), among others[2] (see Table 182–1).

Eosinophilic infiltrates in the spleen have been observed in association with the hypereosinophilic syndrome in cats

TABLE 182–1. CLASSIFICATION OF SPLENOMEGALY IN DOGS AND CATS

TYPE	SPECIES
Inflammatory Splenomegaly	
SUPPURATIVE SPLENITIS	
Penetrating abdominal wounds	C, D
Migrating foreign bodies	C, D
Bacterial endocarditis	C, D
Septicemia	C, D
Splenic torsion	D
Toxoplasmosis	C, D
Mycobacteriosis	D, C
Infectious canine hepatitis (acute)	D
NECROTIZING SPLENITIS	
Splenic torsion	D
Splenic neoplasia	D
Infectious canine hepatitis (acute)	D
Salmonellosis	D, C
EOSINOPHILIC SPLENITIS	
Eosinophilic gastroenteritis	D, C?
Hypereosinophilic syndrome	C
LYMPHOPLASMACYTIC SPLENITIS	
Infectious canine hepatitis (chronic)	D
Ehrlichiosis (chronic)	D
Pyometra	D, C
Brucellosis	D
Hemobartonellosis	D, C
GRANULOMATOUS SPLENITIS	
Histoplasmosis	D, C
Mycobacteriosis	D, C
Leishmaniasis	D
PYOGRANULOMATOUS SPLENITIS	
Blastomycosis	D, C?
Sporotrichosis	D
Feline infectious peritonitis	C
Hyperplastic Splenomegaly	
Bacterial endocarditis	D
Brucellosis	D
Discospondylitis	D
Systemic lupus erythematosus	D
Hemolytic disorders (see text)	D, C
Congestive Splenomegaly	
Pharmacologic (tranquilizers, anticonvulsants)	D, C
Portal hypertension	D, C
Splenic torsion	D
Infiltrative Splenomegaly	
NEOPLASTIC	
Acute and chronic leukemias	D, C
Systemic mastocytosis	D, C
Malignant histiocytosis	D
Lymphoma	D, C
Multiple myeloma	D, C
Metastatic neoplasia	D, C
NON-NEOPLASTIC	
Extramedullary hematopoiesis	D, C?
Hypereosinophilic syndrome	C
Amyloidosis	D

C = cat; D = dog.

and with eosinophilic gastroenteritis in dogs.[2, 9] However, because these proliferative changes may not be inflammatory, they are discussed under Infiltrative Splenomegaly.

Lymphoplasmacytic splenitis, commonly referred to as lymphoreticular hyperplasia or hyperplastic splenomegaly, occurs in association with subacute or chronic infectious disorders such as infectious canine hepatitis, canine ehrlichiosis, pyometra, brucellosis, and hemobartonellosis, among others (see Table 182–1).[2]

Granulomatous splenitis occurs in some systemic mycoses (e.g., histoplasmosis) and mycobacterial infections. Pyogranulomatous splenitis also occurs in association with systemic mycoses such as blastomycosis and sporotrichosis and in some viral infections such as feline infectious peritonitis (see Table 182–1).[2]

Necrotizing splenitis caused by gas-forming anaerobes has been reported in the dog in association with splenic torsion and with splenic lymphoma[2] and observed in dogs with isolated splenic torsion and gastric dilatation-volvulus complex involving the spleen and in dogs with splenic hemangiosarcoma.[10] Coagulation necrosis of the spleen with associated inflammation can also be seen in dogs with infectious canine hepatitis and in dogs and cats with salmonellosis.[10, 11, 12]

Hyperplastic Splenomegaly

The spleen commonly reacts to blood-borne antigens and to red blood cell destruction with hyperplasia of mononuclear phagocytic and lymphoid cells. This hyperplasia has been referred to as "work hypertrophy" because it usually results in varying degrees of splenic enlargement.[2, 9]

Hyperplastic splenomegaly appears to be common in dogs with subacute bacterial endocarditis and chronic bacteremic disorders such as discospondylitis and brucellosis.[13, 14] It has been recognized for some time that red blood cell phagocytosis by the splenic mononuclear phagocytic cells in humans leads to hyperplasia of this cell population, resulting in splenomegaly.[2] The same seems to occur in dogs and cats with certain hemolytic disorders, including immune-mediated hemolytic anemia, drug-induced hemolysis, pyruvate kinase deficiency anemia, phosphofructokinase deficiency anemia, familial nonspherocytic hemolysis in poodles, Heinz body hemolysis, and hemobartonellosis.

Congestive Splenomegaly

The spleen in the dog and the cat has great capacity to store blood, and under normal circumstances it stores between 10 and 20 per cent of the total blood volume. Because of the smooth muscle relaxation of the splenic capsule, tranquilizers and barbiturates increase blood pooling; pooling of blood in an enlarged spleen can account for up to 30 per cent of the total blood volume.[2] Portal hypertension can also lead to congestive splenomegaly; however, splenic congestion secondary to portal hypertension does not appear to be as common in dogs and cats as it is in humans.[15] Causes of portal hypertension that may lead to splenomegaly in small animals are listed in Table 182–1, and ultrasound usually demonstrates markedly distended splenic, portal, and/or hepatic veins.

Splenic torsion, either isolated or associated with the syndrome, commonly results in marked splenomegaly due to congestion[16–18] (see Chapter 136). Splenic torsion can occur independent of the GDV syndrome. Most affected dogs are of large, deep-chested breeds, primarily Great Danes and German shepherds.[16–18] Clinical signs can be either acute or chronic. Acute splenic torsion usually causes abdominal pain and distention, vomiting, depression, and anorexia. Dogs with chronic splenic torsion display a wide variety of clinical signs, including anorexia, weight loss, intermittent vomiting, abdominal distention, polyuria and polydipsia, pigmenturia (due to hemoglobinuria), and abdominal pain. Physical examination usually reveals marked splenomegaly.

Radiographic findings in dogs with splenic torsion include loss of abdominal detail, displacement of other abdominal viscera, identification of the spleen in an abnormal location or shape, splenomegaly, or splenic gas.[18] When the spleen location and shape can be identified as abnormal, the spleen appears folded into a C shape in the central abdomen on lateral radiographic views.[18] Ultrasonographic evaluation of these patients may reveal the presence of greatly distended splenic veins and a diffuse hypoechoic splenic pattern.[17]

Hematologic abnormalities include anemia, presence of target cells, leukocytosis with regenerative left shift, leukoerythroblastosis, and, occasionally, a positive direct Coombs' test.[9, 10] Disseminated intravascular coagulation appears to be a common complication in dogs with torsion of the spleen.[9, 10] A high percentage of dogs with splenic torsion have hemoglobinuria, possibly as a consequence of intravascular or intrasplenic hemolysis.[2, 9, 10] The treatment of choice for dogs with splenic torsion is splenectomy.

Infiltrative Splenomegaly

Infiltration of the spleen with neoplastic cells constitutes one of the most common causes of splenomegaly in small animals[6, 7, 9] (see Chapters 98 and 100). Non-neoplastic causes of infiltrative splenomegaly are less common. Although splenic extramedullary hematopoiesis (EMH) is common in dogs, it rarely results in detectable splenomegaly.[19] In a series of 28 dogs and 5 cats with splenomegaly or splenic masses in which fine-needle aspiration cytology was used for diagnosis, EMH was found in 8 dogs (28 per cent) but in none of the cats.[19] Splenic EMH has also been observed in dogs with pyometra, immune-mediated hemolysis, immune-mediated thrombocytopenia, infectious diseases, and a variety of malignant neoplasms.[9, 10]

Another disorder that commonly results in prominent splenomegaly is the hypereosinophilic syndrome (HES) of cats, a disease characterized by peripheral blood eosinophilia, bone marrow hyperplasia of the eosinophil precursors, and multiple organ infiltration by mature eosinophils.[20, 21] Clinical signs and physical examination findings in cats with HES include diarrhea, vomiting, anorexia and weight loss, lethargy, cutaneous lesions, hepatomegaly, splenomegaly, emaciation, thickened bowel loops, presence of intra-abdominal masses, and occasional cutaneous lesions. Clinicopathologic abnormalities include marked eosinophilia (range: 2100 to 41,000 cells/μL) and hyperplasia of eosinophil precursors in the bone marrow. Histopathologic changes consist mainly of infiltration of various tissues with mature eosinophils. Therapy with immunosuppressive doses of corticosteroids in 6 of 7 cats reported in the literature resulted in variable response and survival times ranging from 1 week to 22 months.[2]

REFERENCES

1. Couto CG, Hammer AS: Diseases of the lymph nodes and spleen. In Ettinger SJ, Feldman EC (eds): Textbook of Veterinary Internal Medicine, 4th ed. Philadelphia, WB Saunders, 1995, p 1930.
2. Couto CG: Diseases of the lymph nodes and the spleen. In Ettinger SJ (ed):

HEM

Textbook of Veterinary Internal Medicine, 3rd ed. Philadelphia, WB Saunders, 1989.

3. Hammer AS, Couto CG: Diagnosing and treating canine hemangiosarcoma. Vet Med 87:188, 1992.

4. Hammer AS, Couto CG (eds): Disorders of the lymph nodes and the spleen. *In* Sherding RG (ed): The Cat—Diseases and Clinical Management, 2nd ed. New York, Churchill Livingstone, 1994, p 671.

5. Johnson KA, Powers BE, Withrow SJ, et al: Splenomegaly in dogs: Predictors of neoplasia and survival after splenectomy. J Vet Intern Med 3:160, 1989.

6. Spangler WL, Culbertson MR: Prevalence, type, and importance of splenic diseases in dogs: 1,480 cases (1985–1989). JAVMA 200:829, 1992.

7. Spangler WL, Culbertson MR: Prevalence and type of splenic diseases in cats: 455 cases (1985–1991). JAVMA 201:773, 1992.

8. Wrigley RH, Konde LJ, Park RD, Lebel JL: Clinical features and diagnosis of splenic hematomas in dogs: 10 cases (1980–1987). J Am Anim Hosp Assoc 25:371, 1989.

9. Couto CG: A diagnostic approach to splenomegaly in cats and dogs. Vet Med 85:220, 1990.

10. Couto CG, Hammer AS: Unpublished observation, 1993.

11. Greene CE: Infectious canine hepatitis. *In* Greene CE (ed): Clinical Microbiology and Infectious Diseases of the Dog and Cat. Philadelphia, WB Saunders, 1984, p 406.

12. Greene CE: Enteric bacterial infections. *In* Greene CE (ed): Clinical Microbiology and Infectious Diseases of the Dog and Cat. Philadelphia, WB Saunders, 1984, p 617.

13. Calvert CA, Greene CE: Cardiovascular infections. *In* Greene CE (ed): Clinical Microbiology and Infectious Diseases of the Dog and Cat. Philadelphia, WB Saunders, 1984, p 220.

14. Greene CE, George LW: Canine brucellosis. *In* Greene CE (ed): Clinical Microbiology and Infectious Diseases of the Dog and Cat. Philadelphia, WB Saunders, 1984, p 646.

15. Johnson SE: Portal hypertension: I. Pathophysiology and clinical consequences. Compend Contin Ed 9:741, 1987.

16. O'Neill JA: Managing an unusual case of splenic torsion. Vet Med 80:35, 1985.

17. Konde LJ, Wrigley RH, Lebel JL, et al: Sonographic and radiographic changes associated with splenic torsion in the dog. Vet Radiol 30:41, 1989.

18. Stickle RL: Radiographic signs of isolated splenic torsion in dogs: Eight cases (1980–1987). JAVMA 194:103, 1989.

19. O'Keefe DA, Couto CG: Fine-needle aspiration of the spleen as an aid in the diagnosis of splenomegaly. J Vet Intern Med 1:102, 1987.

20. Center SA: Eosinophilia in the cat: A retrospective study of 312 cases (1975–1986). J Am Anim Hosp Assoc 26:349, 1990.

21. Scott DW, Randolph JF, Walsh KM: Hypereosinophilic syndrome in a cat. Feline Pract 15:22, 1985.

SECTION XVI

JOINT AND SKELETAL DISORDERS

CHAPTER 183

JOINT DISEASES OF DOGS AND CATS

Niels C. Pedersen, Joe P. Morgan, and Philip B. Vasseur

Disorders involving the joints of dogs and cats are etiologically diverse and divisible into two major categories: (1) noninflammatory and (2) inflammatory (Table 183–1). With the exception of some congenital metabolic disorders, noninflammatory joint disease is confined to the articulations. Inflammatory joint disorders are usually systemic in nature. The major discriminator between these two classes of joint disease is the outpouring of neutrophils into the synovial fluid in the latter.

NON-INFLAMMATORY JOINT DISEASE

Non-inflammatory joint disorders include degenerative joint disease (primary or secondary), traumatic joint disease, luxations and subluxations, meniscal disorders, sesamoid bone disorders, neuropathic arthropathies, developmental arthropathies, arthropathies secondary to inborn errors of metabolism, dietary arthropathies, and neoplasms involving the joints.

DEGENERATIVE JOINT DISEASE (OSTEOARTHRITIS, OSTEOARTHOSIS)

Degenerative joint disease (DJD) is the most common non-inflammatory arthropathy of humans and animals; it is a disorder of movable joints and is characterized grossly by fragmentation and loss of articular cartilage and radiographi-

TABLE 183–1. CLASSIFICATION OF JOINT DISORDERS OF THE DOG AND CAT

I. Noninflammatory joint disease
  A. Degenerative joint disease
    1. Idiopathic (primary)
    2. Secondary
  B. Traumatic joint disease
    1. Damage to the articular cartilage
    2. Damage to soft tissue supporting the joint
      a. Sprains
      b. Tendon contractures
  C. Luxations and subluxations
    1. Appendicular joint instabilities
      a. Shoulder joint
      b. Elbow joint
      c. Carpal joint
      d. Tarsal joint
      e. Hip joint
      f. Stifle joint
        1. Total luxation
        2. Rupture of cranial cruciate ligament
    2. Temporomandibular instabilities
      a. Temporomandibular dislocations
      b. Temporomandibular luxations
    3. Instabilities of the spinal articulations
  D. Meniscal disorders
    1. Meniscal tears
    2. Meniscal calcification
  E. Neuropathic arthropathies
  F. Developmental arthropathies
    1. Conformational abnormalities
    2. Chondrodystrophy
    3. Physeal disorders
    4. Limb shortening
    5. Osteochondrosis
    6. Elbow dysplasia (incongruity)
      a. Medial coronoid process disease
      b. Ununited anconeal process
      c. Osteochondritis of medial humeral condyle
    7. Ununited anconeal process in chondrodystrophic breeds
    8. Hypoplasia of the coronoid process
    9. Hip dysplasia
    10. Patellar luxations
    11. Aseptic necrosis

  G. Arthropathies resulting from inborn errors of metabolism
    1. Hemophilia A
    2. Scottish fold arthropathy
  H. Neoplastic arthropathies
    1. Primary
      a. Synovioma
      b. Osteogenic sarcoma
II. Inflammatory joint disease
  A. Infectious arthritis
    1. Bacterial
    2. Spirochetal arthritis
    3. Bacterial L-forms
    4. Mycoplasmal arthritis
    5. Rickettsial and ehrlichial arthritis
    6. Viral arthritis
    7. Fungal arthritis
    8. Protozoal arthritis
  B. Noninfectious arthritis
    1. Immunologic
      a. Deforming or erosive arthritis
        1. Rheumatoid arthritis of dogs
        2. Polyarthritis of greyhounds
        3. Feline chronic progressive polyarthritis (rheumatoid form)
      b. Periosteal proliferative arthritis
        1. Feline chronic progressive polyarthritis (Reiter's form)
      c. Nondeforming or nonerosive arthritis
        1. Idiopathic nondeforming arthritis
        2. Nondeforming arthritis associated with chronic infectious diseases
        3. Nondeforming arthritis associated with other immune diseases
          a. SLE
          b. Meningitis
          c. Familial Mediterranean fever
          d. Juvenile cellulitis
      4. Nondeforming arthritis associated with neoplasia
      5. Enteropathic arthritis
      6. Plasmacytic-lymphocytic synovitis
      7. Drug-induced arthritides

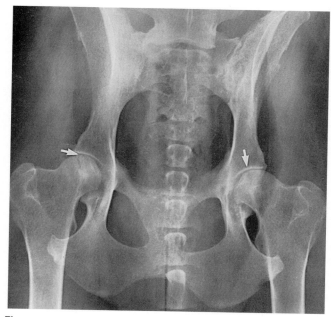

Figure 183–1. Primary joint disease. Ventrodorsal radiograph of the pelvis of a 13-year-old German shepherd dog that had recently developed pain in the hindlegs. Note the normal shape of the femoral heads and acetabular cups. However, increased sclerosis (arrow) in the subchondral bone and marked narrowing of the joint space (arrow) are seen. These are radiographic changes that can be detected as the articular cartilage wears thin with age. Because of the lack of a particular developmental or traumatic insult to the joint, this is called primary joint disease.

cally by narrowing of the joint space, sclerosis of subchondral bone, bone modeling, osteophytes at joint margins, and enthesophyte formation at the attachment of soft tissues.[1] DJD is particularly frequent in dogs[1, 2] but also occurs in many older cats. The disorder exists in two forms, primary (idiopathic) and secondary. The lesions of DJD are due ultimately to the limited ability of cartilage to regenerate and maintain itself despite the cumulative effects of aging, wear and trauma, genetic predisposition, and other unknown factors. Regardless of underlying conditions, the prevalence of DJD increases with age, usually occurring in dogs and cats aged 10 years or older. There is a strong tendency for involvement of large weight-bearing joints.

Idiopathic Degenerative Joint Disease

By definition, idiopathic (or primary) DJD occurs without known predisposing causes (Fig. 183–1). The line between idiopathic and secondary DJD is a fine one, however, and as more knowledge is gained about DJD in general, more of what is now called idiopathic DJD will be classified as secondary. For instance, "primary DJD" has been observed in grossly normal-appearing non-coxofemoral joints in dogs with hip dysplasia,[3] leading to one theory that hip dysplasia is a systemic rather than focal disease.[4] To determine whether dogs with dysplastic hips also had abnormalities in other joints, the composition of cartilage from the shoulder joints of young Labrador retrievers classified as having a low, moderate, or high risk of developing canine hip dysplasia was compared.[5] The fibronectin content of cartilage from the craniolateral region of the humeral head was found to increase as the risk for hip dysplasia increased, indicating that normal-appearing joints of dogs with hip dysplasia are not entirely normal.

DJD occurring without clinical, anatomic, or radiographic evidence of predisposing conditions is surprisingly frequent in dogs and some cats. Twenty per cent of randomly selected dogs were found to have degenerative disease of the stifle joint at autopsy and no predisposing causes could be found in over 60 per cent of these animals.[6] Two additional studies also concluded that primary DJD was a common entity, often involving the shoulder joint of old dogs, both large and small in stature.[7] Primary DJD has been observed in the elbow joint of dogs under similar circumstances but at a lower frequency.[2] One of the most detailed longitudinal studies of primary DJD involved the shoulder joints of 149 colony-reared beagles, a breed without overt predisposing causes.[8] Radiographs and clinical examinations revealed no abnormalities during the first few years of life, but subchondral sclerosis, remodeling of the shoulder joint contour, formation of periarticular enthesophytes, and ossification of soft tissue attachments became progressively evident with age.

Secondary Degenerative Joint Disease

Secondary DJD is the most common cause of clinical lameness in dogs and cats. Secondary degenerative changes result from abnormal force on normal joints or from normal force on abnormal joints (Table 183–2).[9] The net effect of these pathologic forces is to hasten cartilage loss. Secondary

TABLE 183–2. CONDITIONS THAT PREDISPOSE TO DEGENERATIVE JOINT DISEASE

I. Abnormal concentration or direction of force on normal articulation
  A. Malalignment (intra-articular cause)
    1. Epiphyseal malformation
      a. Post-traumatic
      b. Congenital
    2. Elbow joint incongruity
    3. Hip dysplasia
    4. Ligamentous
      a. Ruptured cruciate ligament
      b. Ruptured teres ligament
  B. Malalignment (extra-articular cause)
    1. Inequality of leg length (acquired, congenital)
    2. Achondroplasia
    3. Congenital valgus or varus deformities
    4. Fractures with healing in a malaligned position
    5. Premature epiphyseal closures (e.g., radius curvus)
    6. Acquired carpal and tarsal subluxations and luxations
  C. Loss of protective sensory reflexes
    1. Neuroarthropathy
    2. Repeated intra-articular injections of steroids or use of analgesic drugs
  D. Miscellaneous
    1. Obesity
    2. Excessive activity (working dogs, e.g., cattle or sheep dogs, hunting dogs, racing dogs, sled dogs)
II. Normal concentration of force on abnormal articulation
  A. Normal concentration of force on abnormal cartilage
    1. Osteochondrosis
    2. Transchondral fractures
    3. Meniscal tears, discoid menisci, meniscal calcification
    4. Loose bodies in joint
    5. Preexisting arthritis (septic, immunologic, chronic hemarthrosis)
    6. Metabolic abnormalities (chondrocalcinosis, mucopolysaccharidosis, hypervitaminosis A)
  B. Normal concentration of force on normal cartilage supported by weakened subchondral bone
    1. Osteonecrosis (aseptic necrosis, osteomyelitis)
    2. Osteoporosis
    3. Osteomalacia
    4. Osteitis fibrosa (primary or secondary hyperparathyroidism, pseudohyperparathyroidism)
  C. Normal concentration of force on normal cartilage supported by stiffened subchondral bone

DJD resembles idiopathic disease in its final form, but the pace of cartilage destruction is faster and the lesions are often more severe. The clinical and radiographic abnormalities of the predisposing condition are also superimposed on those of uncomplicated degeneration. In fact, virtually all of the non-inflammatory and inflammatory joint disorders listed in Table 183–1 can have some component of DJD. Hence, DJD is discussed here in general, but readers are referred to individual sections for additional manifestations of known and unknown predisposing causes.

Clinical Signs of Degenerative Joint Disease

The clinical signs of DJD in dogs and cats are similar, regardless of whether it is idiopathic or secondary. Some abnormality in gait or function may precede signs referable to actual joint degeneration by months or years. The earliest common sign is a reluctance of the animal to perform certain tasks or maneuvers without obvious signs of stiffness or lameness. In the next stage, lameness and stiffness occur after periods of sustained activity or after brief overexertion, and the clinical signs often disappear after several days. As the degeneration becomes more severe, stiffness may be most pronounced after periods of rest, and the animals appear to "warm out" of their lameness or stiffness. Cold and damp weather often increase the severity of clinical signs. Stiffness and lameness are fairly constant features in the final stages of the disease, although the severity of signs may still be influenced by environmental factors. Affected animals may show signs of increased irritability and reclusiveness and may snap or bite when approached or touched.

Marked gross deformities of the joints are uncommon in idiopathic DJD, but animals with congenital or acquired predisposing conditions often develop severe changes. Gross deformities consist of an increase in the dimensions of the joint caused by the marginal new bone formation and modeling, enthesophyte production, thickening of the joint capsule, and destruction of the articular surfaces. Subluxation or luxation may occur in larger joints, especially the hip and stifle. Loss of range of motion leading to periarticular ankylosis of the joint is noted in severely affected joints. Palpable swelling of the joints caused by effusions can occur in larger dogs with severe disease but is uncommon in smaller dogs and cats. Redness and heat in the area of the joint are not present. Restrictions of the range of motion and crepitus are frequently seen in advanced cases.

Radiographic Signs of Degenerative Joint Disease

Primary degenerative joints are morphologically normal with superimposed characteristic changes; these changes are usually bilaterally symmetric. Unlike the primary degenerative joint, joints with secondary degenerative joint disease also manifest underlying structural, functional, and anatomic abnormalities characteristic of the predisposing condition. For instance, degenerative changes in a hip joint secondary to hip dysplasia (instability) or femoral head necrosis (collapse of the underlying bone matrix) are radiologically distinct from each other and from those in a hip joint that is undergoing primary degeneration.

The manner of presentation of the radiographic changes is dependent on the joint involved. The hip joint is a ball-and-socket joint that is easily positioned for radiographic examination, and changes involving the femoral head, acetabulum, and joint space are easily seen. Because of changes in weight bearing, the femoral neck undergoes modeling related to change in stress lines early in the disease process. In contrast, the radiocarpal joint has motion primarily in one plane and manifests only limited radiographic changes, the width of the joint space is difficult to evaluate, and changes in the subchondral bone may be difficult to ascertain. Likewise, other joints have specific patterns of presentation of change associated with DJD. Eburnation, or increased density of subchondral bone, is a prominent finding of DJD and indicates that articular cartilage is wearing thin. The subchondral bone assumes stress that had previously been absorbed by the cartilage. This change can be visualized regardless of positioning for the radiographic study and may be uniform in distribution or limited to one part of the subchondral bone, indicating sites of stress localization.

Narrowing of the joint space is a second radiographic finding. Unless the degree of change is severe, however, narrowing may be noted in dogs only in weight-bearing or simulated weight-bearing studies. The joint space may narrow equally throughout the joint or narrow more prominently on one side of the joint than the other. The degree of cartilage loss and narrowing can become so severe that there is actual contact between the two opposing surfaces of subchondral bone.

A characteristic feature of DJD is new bone formation, a response to joint instability. This may be in the form of periarticular lipping resulting from new bone formation at soft tissue attachments (enthesophytes) (Fig. 183–2). Enthesophyte formation may follow ligamentous injury and precede any major changes in joint cartilage or subchondral bone. There is not always a close relationship between the degree of new bone formation and articular cartilage damage.

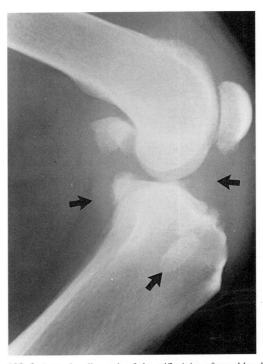

Figure 183–2. Lateral radiograph of the stifle joint of an older dog with secondary joint disease. Radiographic signs seen most clearly are thickening of the joint capsule (arrow) and joint effusion in the area of the fat pad just caudal to the patellar ligament (arrow). Periarticular new bone is noted on the distal patella and tibial plateau. Soft tissue calcification is noted lateral to the proximal tibia (arrow). Subchondral sclerosis is present but difficult to evaluate in this single projection.

Another feature of DJD, particularly noted in the stifle joint of dogs, is secondary subluxation or joint instability. The degree of instability or subluxation is most obvious in weight-bearing studies. Different degrees of subluxation can be present. Most obvious is craniad displacement of the tibia resulting from injury to the cranial cruciate ligament. Another sign of instability is a lateral or medial shifting of bone with formation of reactive periarticular lipping, the new bone being an attempt to provide stabilization of the joint. In addition to a simple lateral or medial displacement, a degree of rotation is often noted. These findings, when observed in joints such as the stifle, may be related to concomitant injury to the ligaments or menisci.

Attrition or wearing away of the subchondral bone can be seen on the weight-bearing surface in cases of severe arthrosis. Attrition of bone is a radiographic finding indicative of severe DJD and can become so extensive that it is referred to as modeling. This results from severe alterations in the lines of stress through the bones and is often associated with an increase in the width of both subchondral and cortical bone on one side. The shadow of the cortical bone on the opposite side is thinner than usual, indicating a decrease in the lines of stress imposed through that part of the bone. Modeling is usually more pronounced on the dependent articular surface.

Calcification is a common finding associated with chronic DJD. It may be intra-articular, within the synovial membrane, or in the joint capsule. Most calcified nodules represent foci of cartilaginous metaplasia in the synovium that undergo endochrondal ossification to form synovial osteochondromas. Others may begin as fragments of cartilage or bone. Calcified tissues without other radiographic findings of DJD usually occur early in the course of joint disease.

Subchondral cysts are frequently present in DJD in dogs and cats but are difficult to detect because of new bone formation peripherally. The cysts have sharp borders, and the surrounding subchondral bone is sclerotic. Frequently, the cysts appear to open into the joint space, but in other cases a thin layer of subchondral bone lies between the cyst and the joint space.

In cases of advanced DJD, especially involving the hip joint of dogs, radiographic changes are so extensive that the original cause of the joint disease, such as hip dysplasia, aseptic necrosis, or acetabular fracture, may be difficult to determine. Magnetic resonance imaging (MRI) arthrography is being utilized to identify early features of joint diseases in humans and animals; it is especially useful for more subtle lesions involving cartilage and subchondral bone and disorders such as osteochondrosis.[10–13]

Clinicopathologic Features of Degenerative Joint Disease

The quantity of synovial fluid in degenerating joints ranges from normal to copious. Copious effusions are seen in larger joints, particularly the elbow and stifle. Such accumulations of synovial fluid can be more or less persistent, or they can become apparent after a period of overexertion or vigorous exercise. In cases in which the synovial fluid is increased in quantity, it is often thin or watery owing to dilution with edema fluid. The mucin quality remains normal, however, because there is no depolymerization of the hyaluronic acid.

Debris from the degenerative cartilage matrix and microhemorrhage in soft tissue initiates a sterile synovitis that leads to increased numbers of macrophages in the fluid,

although total cell counts rarely exceed 5000 cells/μL. Polymorphonuclear neutrophils are not generally seen in numbers exceeding 5 per cent. Synovial fluid from degenerative joints is sometimes yellow tinged because of hemosiderin pigments originating from microhemorrhage in the deeper layers of the synovium.

Attempts have been made in both human and veterinary medicine to develop blood-, urine-, or synovial fluid–based tests that would measure breakdown products of cartilage. Five categories of substances are being investigated as potential biologic markers of arthritis: (1) constituents of the extracellular matrix, (2) degradative proteolytic enzymes, (3) cytokines, (4) nitric oxide, and (5) autoantibodies to cartilage breakdown products.[14–17] Radioimmunoassays for osteocalcin; enzyme-linked immunosorbent assays (ELISAs) for keratan sulfate, chondroitin sulfate, and hyaluronan; and tests for antibodies against collagen I and II have all been studied in normal dogs and dogs with various arthropathies. The consensus is that none of these tests has the desired specificity or sensitivity to be clinically useful.

Treatment of Degenerative Joint Disease

The treatment of DJD involves the following steps: (1) adequate periods of daily rest, (2) avoidance of overexertion of affected joints, (3) reduction in weight if the animal is obese, (4) properly administered exercise, (5) relief of pain by analgesic and anti-inflammatory drugs, and (6) orthopedic operative procedures to relieve pain, regain motion, or correct stressful deformities or instabilities.

Adequate rest of animals with DJD is important for several reasons; excessive use of damaged joints can aggravate clinical signs and, more important, can accelerate the joint destruction. Dogs with severe joint disease cannot be expected to function in the same manner as they did before they developed the problem. Although dogs with advanced DJD should receive adequate rest and avoid strenuous exercise, they should not be allowed to become invalids. Properly administered and controlled exercise is important in maintaining muscle tone and keeping joints limber.[18] Controlled exercise can consist of defined periods of walking with the owner interspersed with short periods of rest or other controlled periods of play, swimming, or similar activities. As the disease becomes more advanced and less activity is tolerated, the amount of exercise should be reduced. Unfortunately, the amount of rest or exercise that an animal can tolerate is difficult to assess. Many dogs are so eager to please their masters that they overexert themselves. In addition, some dogs forgo any considerations of pain because of sheer enjoyment of the activity, such as hunting, jogging, playing, or hiking with the owner or working with livestock. As a rule, any activity that causes the animal to become acutely lame for a period afterward is excessive and should be curtailed or diminished.

Analgesic and anti-inflammatory drugs are often necessary to control pain in severely affected dogs and in a smaller proportion of severely affected cats. Before instigating chronic drug therapy, owners should be made aware of the fact that complete remission of signs is unlikely and that treatment becomes less effective as the degenerative process worsens. It is interesting to note that most people do not expect miraculous improvements in their own DJD with drug treatment but expect their pets with the same condition to return to normal.

A large number of analgesic nonsteroidal anti-inflammatory drugs (NSAIDS) have been developed for the treatment

MSJ

of DJD in humans, but relatively few have application to dogs and cats. Buffered types of aspirin, at a dose of 12 to 25 mg/lb (25 to 50 mg/kg) body weight divided into two or three daily doses for dogs and 12 mg/lb (25mg/kg) once every other day for cats, can afford significant relief to some animals with minimal gastric toxicity.[19] Aspirin is much more effective at higher dosages, but unfortunately gastric toxicity is almost inevitable. Unfortunately, many NSAIDS used in humans for the treatment of DJD are toxic for dogs and cats.[20] Naproxen and ibuprofen have been associated with severe gastric ulceration in dogs.[21, 22] Indomethacin is also considered more gastrotoxic to dogs than humans. A caution has been reported regarding the use of the anti-inflammatory agent diclofenac in dogs.[23] Acetaminophen is extremely toxic to cats.

Phenylbutazone has been widely used in the past by veterinarians to treat dogs with DJD. For chronic use in dogs, the dosage is 40 mg/kg divided three times a day for the first 48 hours and then decreased to the lowest effective amount.[19] The total daily dosage should not exceed 800 mg, regardless of the size of the animal. Bone marrow suppression can be a side effect of prolonged high-level usage of the drug. Phenylbutazone is reportedly effective in cats with severe DJD; Food and Drug Administration (FDA) approval, however, is for dogs and not cats.

Carprofen (Rimadyl) is the newest NSAID to be used in dogs.[24] Carprofen is a propionic acid–derived NSAID that has anti-inflammatory, analgesic, and antipyretic activity. In animals, carprofen is as potent as indomethacin and more potent than aspirin or phenylbutazone, but carprofen appears to be safer than most other NSAIDs. In one study, 70 dogs were included in a randomized, controlled, multicenter trial to test the efficacy of carprofen (2.2 mg/kg body weight by mouth every 12 hours) for relief of clinical signs associated with DJD.[25] Thirty-six dogs received carprofen, and 34 received a placebo. Response was gauged by comparing results of force plate examination, by a graded lameness examination performed before and immediately after 2 weeks of treatment, and by a subjective assessment of the dog's post-treatment condition by owners and participating veterinarians. Dogs treated with carprofen were 3.3 times more likely to have a positive response than dogs treated with the placebo. The improvement was 3.5 times when judged by veterinary evaluation and 4.2 times by owner evaluation. Subsequent experience with the treatment of large numbers of dogs over longer periods of time demonstrated a low incidence of severe liver toxicity.[26] Therefore, dogs receiving long-term carprofen treatment should have periodic liver screens.

Prednisolone or prednisone should be considered only for advanced disease and when significant relief cannot be achieved with other drugs. It is given at an initial dosage of 2 mg/kg once daily for several days to either dogs or cats, followed by a chronic maintenance dose that should not exceed 1 mg/kg every other day. In addition to usual side effects, there is evidence that corticosteroids may actually hasten the degenerative process, so what is gained in the short term may be lost, and more, in the long term. Intra-articular injections of steroids should be avoided.

One of the most controversial treatments for DJD involves so-called chondroprotectants, which first became popular in veterinary medicine for horses.[27] These products, usually containing polysulfated glycosaminoglycan, glucosamine sulfate, and/or chondroitin sulfate, are representative of a trend in human and veterinary medicine toward "alternative" therapies with nutritional supplements (nutriceutics)

instead of pharmaceutics.[28] In theory, chondroprotectants work by enhancing the regenerative functions of chondrocytes and in so doing either impede cartilage destruction or even initiate cartilage healing. Although they are widely prescribed by veterinarians, we are skeptical. Anecdotal reports of their benefits are numerous but do not take into account the placebo effect. Motivated owners readily anthropomorphize their desires for improvement to their pets. A double-blind, controlled clinical study was performed to compare the response of 84 adult dogs affected with hip dysplasia to a placebo and three different dosages of polysulfated glycosaminoglycan, 2.2, 4.4, and 8.8 mg/kg, intramuscularly, every 3 to 5 days for a total of eight injections.[28a] Response to treatment was analyzed on the basis of changes in lameness, range of motion, and pain on manipulation of the hip joints. The differences in clinical improvement between the four treatment groups were not statistically significant. In a randomized double-blind crossover study of 21 dogs with hip dysplasia and secondary DJD, oral glucosamine or glycosaminoglycan given according to the manufacturer's instructions provided no significant relief over placebo as judged by lameness grade, range of coxofemoral joint motion, or owner's functional assessment.[29] With careful dosing and surveillance of untoward gastrointestinal effects, NSAIDs, and not chondroprotectants, are still the drugs of first choice in the treatment of DJD.[30]

Surgery should be used selectively in animals with severe DJD. Fusion of joints such as the elbow, carpus, or hock is occasionally warranted to help relieve pain and restore some use to the limb. Femoral head ostectomy or the insertion of a prosthetic joint can be effective in selected animals with painful and badly diseased hip joints. Some types of joint instability resulting from ligament damage or rupture can be corrected surgically. Obviously, this must be done before secondary degenerative changes become too extensive. In situations in which pieces of cartilage or osteophytic bone have become free within the joint cavity, surgical removal is necessary. Reactive new bone should not be excised, except where it breaks into the joint cavity or impinges on tendons or nerves.

TRAUMATIC JOINT DISEASE

Joint trauma in dogs and cats is usually accidental. Joint trauma can result from the surrounding bones, damage to the cartilage, or damage to soft tissue structures supporting the joints. Of these injuries, bone fractures are the easiest to diagnose; damage to the cartilage and soft tissue is more difficult to localize.[31, 32]

Damage to Articular Cartilage

Damage to the articular cartilage can occur as a result of acute or chronic trauma.[33, 34] Cartilage damage usually accompanies bone fractures or luxations, but because cartilage damage cannot be assessed on radiographs, it may go undetected or be minimized in importance. In a small proportion of traumas, cartilage damage may occur in the absence of bone changes. Such cases may be mistaken for sprains. Even with good bone reconstruction, damaged cartilage heals poorly and post-traumatic DJD months or years later is a frequent sequela. Chronic cartilage damage leading to post-traumatic DJD is less frequent. Dogs that constantly jump down from heights can develop severe bilateral post-traumatic DJD of the front paws. The term canine spavin has been used to describe an exercise-related hock lesion of racing greyhounds.[35, 36]

Damage to Soft Tissues Supporting the Joint

Sprains. Injuries to soft tissues supporting the joints have been termed "sprains." Sprains result from microtrauma to vascular (hemorrhage, edema), ligamentous (separations, tears), bursal, and synovial structures. They are relatively common in dogs, and it is a diagnostic challenge to differentiate them from more serious entities.

Tendon Contractures. Tendon contractures are a sequela of direct damage to associated muscles or their blood supply. The damage results in atrophy and fibrous replacement of the involved muscles and contracture of the associated tendon or tendons. Tendon contractures can result in lameness, gross stiffening of the involved limbs, or immobilization of joints in severe cases. Most tendon contractures are probably traumatic in origin. Sectioning of the contracted tendon is often unsuccessful in correcting the abnormality in the case of the semitendinosus tendon contractures and helpful in the case of infraspinatus tendon contractures. Contracture of the tendons closing the lower jaw may be a sequela of the temporal and mandibular myopathies (eosinophilic, plasmacytic-lymphocytic, and idiopathic) of canines. Affected dogs have a progressive closing of the jaw to the point where they cannot open their mouths to eat. The prognosis for recovery of adequate lower jaw function is good with the use of long-term corticosteroid therapy.

Tenosynovitis. A unilateral, and occasionally bilateral, chronic bicipital tenosynovitis has been described in 29 dogs. Affected dogs have intermittent or progressive weight-bearing lameness, which worsens after exercise. Characteristic signs include pain upon palpation of the biceps tendon within the intertubercular groove and sclerosis or enthesophytosis of the intertubercular groove on radiographs. Synovial fluid changes are consistent with DJD. Medical treatment, consisting of injection of methylprednisolone acetate into the biceps tendon and its synovial sheath, was successful in about one third of the cases. Poor responders were treated surgically with tenodesis of the biceps tendon.[37]

LUXATIONS AND SUBLUXATIONS

Appendicular Joint Instabilities

Luxations and subluxations can involve virtually any joint of the appendicular and axial skeleton. They can be caused by acute trauma[38] or by developmental and acquired problems that affect the stability of the joint. The diagnosis of complete luxation is clinically and radiographically quite easy, whereas subluxations are more difficult to diagnose and require knowledge of normal radiographic anatomy (Fig. 183–3). Subluxations can best be diagnosed by taking radiographs in weight-bearing, simulated weight-bearing, or flexed and extended positions. Joints that require such positioning include the carpus, tarsus, and stifles. Distraction is used in the hips of animals with dysplasia. It is important to note the presence of small fragments originating from the articular surface or periarticular margin; small avulsion or chip fragments frequently accompany luxations or subluxations of certain joints such as the hip or elbow of the dog.

One form of subluxation is associated with the three main developmental diseases of the elbow joint: ununited anconeal process, medial coronoid process disease, and osteochondritis dissecans of the medial aspect of the humeral condyle. These are probably caused by abnormal development of the ulnar trochlear notch (see later under Elbow Dysplasia).

Gradual degeneration and weakening of the supporting ligaments of the carpus have been observed in older, obese dogs. Breeds apparently predisposed to this condition are the Doberman, collie, Shetland sheepdog, Samoyed, and Labrador retriever. Degeneration of supporting ligaments leads to subluxation and eventual luxation of the carpal joints. Involvement of the tarsal joints in a similar process is occasionally observed in the same breeds. This condition, especially if it involves both carpal and tarsal joints, is often mistaken for canine rheumatoid arthritis. Radiographs do not show erosive changes; synovial fluid, except for a mild increase in mononuclear cells, is normal. The treatment for the earlier stages of the disease consists of strict weight loss and judicious exercise; complete luxations are best treated by surgical fusion.

The usual underlying cause of hip luxation is dysplasia. Other causative factors are traumatic and include avulsion fracture of the ligament of the head of the femur and a fractured dorsal rim of the acetabulum. Luxation of the normal hip joint involves rupture of the ligament of the femoral head and the joint capsule. The luxating forces, usually abduction with external rotation or strong adduction, force the head craniodorsally. The altered appearance of the pelvic region and the apparent discrepancy in leg length may make diagnosis obvious.

Rupture of the cranial cruciate ligament is common in middle-aged and older dogs, especially in overweight, seden-

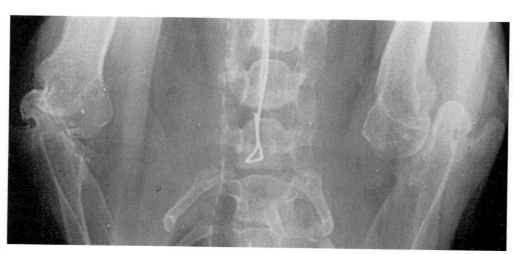

Figure 183–3. Congenital luxation. Both humeral heads were displaced medially at birth. With skeletal maturation, extensive modeling of both the humeral heads and the glenoid cavities occurs. The result is a severe deforming osteoarthrosis.

tary, household pets; spayed females are at the highest risk. It is less common in cats. Although the rupture is usually acute, progressive degeneration of the ligament usually precedes the rupture.[39] There is a tendency for the opposite limb ligament to rupture within a year or so of the first. Gradual stretching of the ligaments of the stifle, associated with cranial drawer movement, is a common feature of plasmacytic-lymphocytic gonitis of the dog (see later). Joint instability caused by rupture of the cranial cruciate ligament eventually leads to DJD and damage to the medial meniscus. (Fig. 183–4). The rate at which degenerative changes occur is proportional to the weight and the activity of the animal. In dogs weighing less than 15 kg and cats, a rest period of 12 to 16 weeks is sufficient to resolve many cases.

Although approximately one half of dogs and most cats with ruptured cranial cruciate ligaments regain adequate use of the leg without surgery, spontaneous recovery should not always be relied upon. Larger dogs are less likely to recover spontaneously and more apt to develop secondary DJD; surgery is therefore a more desirable option.

Temporomandibular Instabilities

Traumatic temporomandibular luxations occur in both dogs and cats and are often associated with fractures. Temporomandibular luxations of dogs, unassociated with trauma, can be of two types. In one type, there is rostral movement of the mandible with malocclusion of the jaw and interference with mouth opening. The second and more common type is associated with open mouth locking that occurs after hyperextension of the jaw and lasts for several seconds or persists until manually reduced. Reduction can be achieved by hyperextending the jaw while placing inward pressure on the displaced mandibular condyle. The condition has been described mainly in young basset hounds but has also been seen in Irish setters, Weimaraners, Dalmatians, and Boxers.[40] Prevention of jaw locking in these dogs is accomplished by excising part of the zygomatic arch on the side of the lockup. Radiographic examination usually differentiates between the various types of temporomandibular joint instabilities and articular fractures.

Instabilities of the Spinal Articulations
(see Chapter 106)

MENISCAL DISORDERS

A torn medial meniscus accompanies 50 per cent of cranial cruciate ligament ruptures. Failure to remove all or part of the damaged meniscus can cause lameness to persist after cruciate ligament surgery. Meniscal tears are often manifested by a click during walking or on passive flexion and extension of the stifle joint.[41]

NEUROPATHIC ARTHROPATHY

Neuropathic arthropathy is secondary to conditions that diminish normal pain, stretch, and proprioceptive reflexes. These changes result in a relaxation of supporting structures, chronic hyperextension and hyperflexion, and loss of neuromuscular and tendon reflexes that prevent the limb from being placed too forcefully on the ground. Clinical and experimental observations support the view that neurogenic arthropathy in dogs and cats is not easily induced by neurogenic deficits alone. If there is preexisting joint disease, it is accelerated by diminished pain and by neuromuscular, neurotendinous, and proprioceptive deficits.

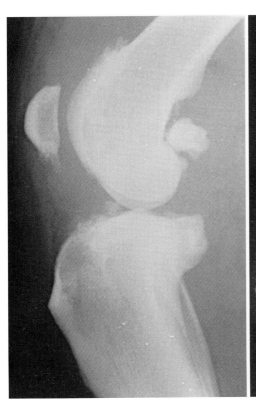
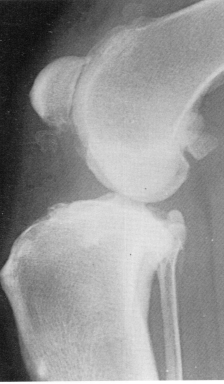

Figure 183–4. Osteoathrosis, chronic (cranial cruciate ligament disease). Modeling changes are prominent on the tibial plateau as a result of cranial displacement of the tibia. Periarticular osteophytes and enthesophytes result from the joint instability.

DEVELOPMENTAL ARTHROPATHIES

Conformational Abnormalities

Abnormalities in the angulation of bones of the limbs can put great stress on adjacent joints and result in ligamentous degeneration and DJD, especially in larger, athletic animals. Conformational abnormalities can be acquired or congenital. Straight stifle conformation and valgus and varus deformities of the elbow, stifles, tarsus, and carpus all occur in dogs and to a much lesser extent in cats. Excessive plantigrade positions of the distal forelimbs or hindlimbs are also occasionally seen in both species. Three types of conformational abnormalities have been described that affect only the femoral head and neck: (1) coxa valga, (2) coxa vara, and (3) increased anteversion. Coxa valga can lead to subluxation of the hip, and increased anteversion is associated with gait abnormalities, joint laxity, and pain. Increased anteversion is most often seen in giant breeds such as Saint Bernards, Newfoundlands, and Irish wolfhounds. These hip disorders can be corrected surgically.[42]

Chondrodystrophy

Chondrodystrophy is inherent and considered normal in bulldogs, pugs, Pekingese, basset hounds, dachshunds, and similar breeds. Chondrodystrophy in some breeds, such as the Alaskan malamute and German shepherd dog, is considered highly undesirable. Chondrodystrophic animals demonstrate angular deformities of the limb joints, and the cartilage surfaces vary greatly in structure. These changes predispose the joints to degenerative changes.

Metaphyseal (Growth Plate) Disorders

Conformational abnormalities of the limbs can result from damage to the physes of immature animals. Such damage usually results in cessation of the longitudinal bone growth normally contributed by the injured growth plate. The damage may result in delayed growth of the entire growth plate, delayed growth of a portion of the growth plate, or complete cessation of growth. Given these scenarios, a range of errors of growth may occur. Although closure of a growth plate might be ascertained through comparison with the opposite limb, delayed growth would be evident only by measurement of the affected bone; the growth plate would remain open as seen on the radiographs. The ultimate outcome is dependent on (1) the particular growth plate involved and its contribution to the total growth of the bone; (2) the age and breed of the animal, which determine how much the growth is affected; (3) the method of surgical reduction (if damaged by fracture); (4) the type of injury that caused the damage; and (5) the involvement of infection as a complicating factor.[43]

Limb Shortening

Fractures with overriding of fragments, if not properly treated, can result in shortening of the limb upon healing. To compensate for the limb shortening, the angulations of the pelvic or thoracic girdle and distal and proximal joints are altered, which in turn predisposes these joints to degenerative changes. If fractures are repaired so that rotation of the distal segment occurs upon healing, degenerative changes can occur in distal and proximal joints because of abnormal stresses imposed by the resulting malformation.

Osteochondrosis

Osteochondrosis, or dyschondroplasia, is a systemic disease with common multifocal disturbances of endochondral ossification; it occurs in many species of domestic animals and is characterized by retention of avascular cartilage in physical and metaphyseal growth areas. Osteochondrosis is an important cause of both transient and permanent lameness in dogs. It is not a problem in cats. Joint pain, gait abnormalities, and lameness usually indicate that the cartilage overlying the area of osteochondrosis has separated. When the cartilage flap separates, the condition is referred to as *osteochondritis dissecans*. This allows joint fluid to come in contact with subchondral bone, which is quite painful.

Osteochondrosis affects a number of joints but in particular the caudal aspect of the humeral head,[11] the lateral and medial femoral condyles of the stifle[44] (Fig. 183–5), the medial portion of the humeral condyle, and the medial ridge of the talus.[45–47] It has also been reported to affect the lateral trochlear ridge of the talus, usually in rottweilers. The condition is bilateral in one third or more cases, although the lesion in one limb may predominate clinically. Osteochondrosis lesions may be found in more than one anatomic location in the same animal, often in association with hip or elbow dysplasia. Osteochondrosis becomes microscopically apparent at 4 to 6 months of age but is clinically inapparent. After separation of the cartilage flap, clinical signs of lameness or subtle gait abnormalities develop. Clinical signs persist and permanent lameness may manifest over a longer period of time as a result of secondary DJD.

The clinical findings of osteochondritis dissecans include lameness, an altered gait (if bilateral), a decrease in the range of motion of the affected joint, and pain on hyperextension and hyperflexion. Crepitation may be evident during manipulation of the joint. There may or may not be muscle atrophy, depending on the duration of the lameness. If the humeral head is affected, the infraspinatus and supraspinatus muscles are often atrophied. Joint effusion and joint capsule thickening along the affected side are early signs of elbow, stifle, and hock joint involvement. They are not palpable in the shoulder joint because of the heavy muscle cover. A special complication of osteochondritis dissecans occurs when a piece of fragmented cartilage enters the synovial tendon sheath of the biceps muscle (shoulder), the long digital extensor or popliteus muscles (stifle), or the flexor hallucis longus muscle (tibial-tarsal joint). This may lead to a severe and painful tenosynovitis.

Osteochondrosis has been studied for over 60 years, and although our knowledge of the disease has greatly increased, the ultimate cause remains elusive. Dogs are genetically predisposed to osteochondrosis, but environmental factors such as rapid body growth, heavy weight, and high energy level of the diet may influence how the disease is manifested. Genetically predisposed dogs may be phenotypically abnormal or normal. The phenotypic expressions of osteochondrosis, elbow dysplasia, and hip dysplasia are all affected by nutrition. Puppies that are subjected to overnutrition by excess consumption and oversupplementation develop osteochondrosis at a higher incidence and with greater severity.[48] On the basis of studies of pigs and horses and observations of dogs and cattle, local ischemia secondary to defects in cartilage canal blood supply is thought to be the key factor in the initiation of lesions of osteochondrosis.[49, 50] Local ischemia leads to zones of epiphyseal cartilage that are particularly prone to stress-induced necrosis. Therefore, the weight of the dog, the joint in question, the congruity or

MSJ

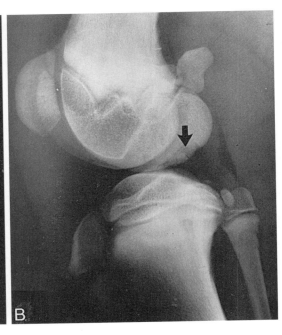

Figure 183–5. Caudocranial and lateral projections of the stifle joint of an immature dog with a large lucent lesion in the lateral condyle of the femur that is characteristic of osteochondrosis in this region.

incongruity of opposing articular surfaces, and the types of activities all affect the final outcome. After death of these deeply situated chondrocytes, the surrounding cartilage matrix fails to mineralize, and blood vessels from the subchondral bone do not invade areas that are unmineralized. Consequently, the osteogenic mesenchyme that accompanies these vessels does not penetrate the cartilage and normal ossification fails to occur. Trauma, whether major or minor, to the overlying articular cartilage leads to separation and cleft formation, clinical signs of pain and lameness, and other chronic sequelae.

All changes in the osteochondrotic lesion after the development of the area of chondromalacia are secondary events. At one extreme in this morphologic spectrum are animals in which the lesion resolves spontaneously. The subchondral capillary bed is able to invade the area of chondromalacia and reestablish normal enchondral ossification. The result is a delay in the modeling of the developing articular surface, seen radiographically as a flattening of the subchondral bone.

Lesions, even when radiographically apparent, may subsequently resolve. More commonly, the early lesion progresses to osteochondritis dessicans. Grossly, the early lesion in the humeral head is outlined by a discoloration of the cartilage in the affected area. Percussion of the area is normal at first and indicates that there has been no separation of the cartilage from the subchondral bone. In advanced lesions, a loosened area of cartilage tears partially away from the defective osteochondral junction and forms a flap. Loose cartilage flaps may remain in position, may gradually fragment and become completely absorbed, or may separate and be nourished by the joint fluid and become loose cartilage bodies (joint "mice"). Some cartilage fragments attach themselves to the synovium, where they can become vascularized and ossified, forming osteochondromas. The lesion is demonstrated radiographically by an irregular-appearing subchondral surface, a focal defect in the subchondral bone (see Figure 183–5), and varying degrees of increased bone density surrounding the defect. The subchondral defect usually appears as a large crater-like lesion. Free mineralized fragments are sometimes identified on survey radiographs. Cartilage flaps can be detected on arthrograms. Secondary

DJD with the development of abnormally shaped epiphyses is seen in the chronic stages of the clinical disorder.

Treatment ranges from simple rest to surgical curettage of the subchondral lesion and removal of any free bodies. When the onset of clinical signs is late (7.5 to 9 months) and the radiographic lesions are small, conservative treatment is warranted. However, rest as therapy is contraindicated, because the lesion heals better with pressure from the opposing surface. The defect fills in with granulation tissue and changes into a form of fibrocartilage with use. The joint contour can be reestablished grossly in this manner, although it is without normal morphology. The ingrowth of granulation tissue is inhibited by the cartilage flap, which is often the case for animals with early onset of clinical signs (4 to 6 months of age) and animals with large radiographic lesions. To hasten the filling of the defect with granulation tissue and to minimize secondary degenerative changes in these more severe cases, surgical removal of the flap and curettage of the defect are often advisable.[51] The value of arthroscopic surgery for this lesion in dogs has been claimed.[52]

Elbow Dysplasia

The term elbow dysplasia was previously applied to a poorly understood disorder of the elbow joint manifested by acute pain and dysfunction and/or chronic progressive DJD. The disorder is particularly common in rottweilers, Labrador retrievers, and Bernese Mountain Dogs, in which its incidence is under genetic control.[53] Rapid growth and genetic predisposition are important. The lesions constituting elbow dysplasia are joint instability in association with (1) ununited anconeal process, (2) medial coronoid process disease, and (3) osteochondrosis of the medial humeral condyle. One theory is that elbow dysplasia is yet another secondary manifestation of osteochondrosis. Work on developmental anomalies of the elbow joint suggested trochlear notch incongruities as critical in the pathogenesis of this condition.[54] In this theory, all three developmental lesions of the elbow result from faulty development of the trochlear notch of the ulna that creates an incongruity between the articular surfaces of the proximal ulna and the distal humerus. The existence of joint incongruity can best be demonstrated on lateral radiographic views with the elbow in slight extension (Fig. 183–6).

Medial Coronoid Process Disease. The diseased medial coronoid process may be cartilaginous and attached, cartilaginous with a fissure, cartilaginous and separated, or it may be ossified and attached, ossified with a fissure, or ossified and separated. The process, whether cartilaginous or ossified, may be malformed. The fragmented coronoid process is the most frequent developmental disease of the canine elbow.[55] A genetic predisposition is present in large and intermediate-sized breeds such as the German shepherd dog, rottweiler, Labrador retriever, Saint Bernard, and Bernese Mountain Dog.

The clinical findings of medial coronoid process disease are lameness, an abnormal gait (if bilateral), and a subtle to moderate resistance to passive flexion and extension of the elbow. This is infrequently accompanied by crepitation. In chronic cases, thickening of the joint capsule, joint effusion, and muscle atrophy are also seen. The lameness or abnormal gait is often characterized by excessive supination of the front paws on extension of the limb. The animal may also hold the elbows bowed out or tucked inward. In severe cases, the owner may notice that the animal wants to sit or lie down a great deal, plays less than other dogs its age, or can barely walk around the block.

The early diagnosis of medial coronoid process disease is usually based on age, breed, clinical findings, and characteristic radiographic features. Radiographic findings include (1) joint incongruity, (2) secondary new bone formation, and (3) progressive secondary DJD. The exact status of the medial coronoid process is usually not determined radiographically.

The treatment of medial coronoid process disease in the past has often involved surgical removal of the malformed fragment. However, the only controlled study of surgical treatment of a fragmented coronoid process showed much better initial results in the medically versus surgically treated population and no difference in results of the two treatments after 9 months.[56] Weight control, coupled with medical treat-ment and the animal's natural inclination to limit stress on the joint, is probably the therapy of choice.

Ununited Anconeal Process in Non-Chondrodystrophic Breeds. An ununited anconeal process in non-chondrodystrophic breeds tends to occur between the ages of 4 and 6 months, at which time the bones are incompletely ossified. It tends to occur in breeds and individuals that have a separate center of ossification for the anconeal process. German shepherd dogs and some individuals of other breeds may have such separate ossification centers. Bone fusion of the anconeal process with the proximal ulna usually takes place by 4 months of age; however, union does not always occur, especially in the German shepherd dog. Instead, a cleavage line develops in the anconeal physis, separating the anconeal process from the ulna.

The presenting disease signs of ununited anconeal processes include a variable degree of lameness of one or both front limbs or an altered gait. There is often lateral positioning of the elbow and paw by the affected animal. Crepitation and pain may be evident upon flexion and extension of the elbow joint and on deep palpation of the olecranon fossa. Joint capsule thickening, joint effusion, and muscle atrophy of the limb occur in dogs with chronic secondary DJD. Radiographic examination reveals the presence of a radiolucent line between the anconeal process and the ulna (see Fig. 183–6).

Removal of the loose process lessens chronic irritation within the joint and may reduce the degree of lameness. Surgery does not alter the joint instability and the basic underlying incongruity of the joint. Reattachment of the loose anconeal process with a lag screw is also of doubtful value and may even be contraindicated because it does not consider the original malformed trochlea. Ulnar osteotomy into the trochlear notch changes the incongruity of the joint and permits bone fusion of the ununited fragment.

Osteochondritis Dissecans of the Medial Condyle of the Humerus. This is the final lesion associated with the syndrome of elbow incongruity in the dog. It is probably due to increased pressure exerted by the medial coronoid process on the opposing trochlear cartilage. This pressure

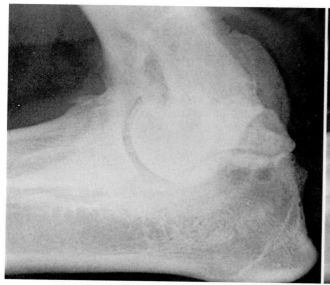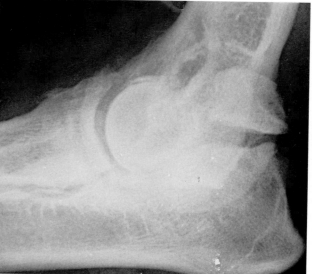

Figure 183–6. Elbow dysplasia. Ununited anconeal process and failure of development of the medial coronoid process characterize the elbow dysplasia on an extended lateral view of the elbow joint. Note the movement of the ununited fragment between the flexed and extended views.

can interfere with normal endochondral ossification and exposes the more deeply situated chondrocytes to undue stress. Lateral radiographs show a flattening of the outline of the humeral condyle. The actual defect is best localized on a craniocaudal view. The lesion on the medial trochlea of the distal humerus is readily seen on gross inspection of the joint but is often confused with a "kissing" lesion. It is located in a thin area and is a part of the DJD. Treatment of osteochondritis dissecans consists of flap removal and curettage of the lesion. The prognosis depends on the size of the lesion, the degree of faulty development of the ulnar trochlear notch, and the other parts of the disease triad that are present. In general, a progressive osteoarthrosis is expected.

Ununited Anconeal Process in Chondrodystrophic Breeds

A loose anconeal process can also develop in some of the larger chondrodystrophic breeds, primarily the basset hound and the English bulldog. However, this is not an ununited process but a true fracture of the process caused by the distal (downward) subluxation of the anconeal process as a result of lagging longitudinal growth of the distal ulnar physis in these breeds. Healing of this fracture can occur at 4 to 5 months of age after cutting of the radioulnar ligament and freeing of the ulna from the distal pull of the radius. This procedure may not be successful in older dogs and removal of the process is recommended.

Hip Dysplasia

Hip dysplasia is a developmental disease identified in most breeds of dogs. It tends to occur more frequently, however, in larger, well-fed, faster growing breeds. The development of hip dysplasia is strongly influenced by complex genetic factors[4] and affects dogs of both sexes with equal frequency. The specific etiology is not known. It has also been described in purebred cats.

Dysplastic dogs are born with normal hip joints that subsequently undergo progressive structural alterations. The following structural anomalies are identified either pathologically or radiographically: joint laxity; shallow acetabular cavities; subluxation; swelling, fraying, and rupture of the round ligament of the femoral head; erosion of the articular cartilage with eburnation of subchondral bone; modeling of the acetabular rim; flattening of the femoral head; and periarticular osteophyte production and enthesophyte formation (Fig. 183–7).[57]

Environmental and nutritional factors, however, are involved in the expression of the abnormal phenotype.[57, 58] There is a debate about whether the fundamental cause is intrinsic or extrinsic to the hip joint. Proponents of an intrinsic cause believe that the primary change occurs in the development of the coxofemoral joint itself. Proponents of an extrinsic cause believe that hip abnormalities are secondary to physical anomalies or inadequacies in the muscles that support the coxofemoral joint during development.[59] Whatever the cause, the end result is a joint that is unstable and predisposed to degeneration.

Hip dysplasia is diagnosed early by measurements of joint laxity and later by the appearance of more gross radiographic changes (see Fig. 183–7). Joint laxity has been quantitated by use of a distraction index (DI), a measure of passive hip joint laxity.[60] Studies of German shepherds indicate that DI should not be measured before 4 months of age, and for breeding dogs DI should be remeasured after maturity to confirm the results obtained at earlier ages.[61] Joint laxity, as measured by the DI, may be the most accurate early indicator of hip dysplasia in certain breeds.[62] Rottweilers and German shepherd dogs between 12 and 40 months old were evaluated for DJD using standard hip-extended-view radiographs; the influences of age, sex, weight, and DI on the risk of developing DJD were also compared. In contrast, in rottweilers, the DI was the only statistically significant predictor of the risk of developing DJD of the coxofemoral joint.

There are considerable variations in the severity of the clinical signs, time of onset of structural changes, age at which clinical signs appear, rate of disease progression, and degree of pain and impaired mobility. Because joint laxity is the earliest sign of hip dysplasia, gait abnormalities without overt lameness or stiffness may precede DJD by many months. DJD may occur within the first year of life, but many animals show no clinical or radiographic signs until later. There is poor correlation between clinical and radiographic signs. The changes noted radiographically are asymmetric in their presentation in over one fourth of the dogs examined. The reliability of preliminary evaluations in determining the ultimate hip status increased significantly as age at the time of preliminary evaluation increased, regardless of whether dogs received a preliminary evaluation of normal or dysplastic.

The treatment of hip dysplasia is mainly palliative and varies with the stage of the disease. Young dogs with unstable hips and no visible signs of DJD are prone to bouts of acute lameness after exercise or strenuous activity. Rest and analgesics for several days are often sufficient to treat the condition. In subsequent stages characterized by considerable pain and minimal degenerative changes, rest, restriction of activities that put stress on the hips, and analgesic drugs may prove adequate. In dogs with more advanced disease, restricted activity and analgesics may not be sufficient to provide relief of pain. At this point, most dogs show prominent radiographic signs of DJD. Sectioning of the pectineus muscle or tendon in the puppy may afford relief from pain. The procedure does not prevent the progression of degenerative changes but rather releases painful pressure on the capsule of the hip joints. The procedure is not without controversy, and although some individual investigators advocate its use wholeheartedly, others are more reserved.[42, 63]

A variety of additional surgeries or variations on surgeries have been suggested. Femoral head ostectomies can be effective in some dogs with advanced disease.[64] Dogs with intractable hip pain but without significant disease in other joints or neurologic problems are the best candidates. The most attractive treatment for advanced hip dysplasia is total hip replacement. Although this procedure is becoming practical from a technical aspect, the cost of the surgery has limited its use. Complications include infection, luxation, and implant loosening.[65]

Reduction in the phenotypic expression of hip dysplasia has been well documented. In one study, 8-week-old Labrador retriever littermates were paired according to gender.[66] All dogs received the same diet for the 5-year study period, but one dog of each pair was fed ad libitum and the other was fed 75 per cent of the amount eaten the previous day by its partner. Radiographic evaluations of coxofemoral joints for frequency and severity of DJD were made when dogs were 4 and 6 months and 1, 2, 3, and 5 years old. Radiographic evaluation for secondary DJD indicated greater frequency and increased severity in the ad libitum–fed group of dogs.

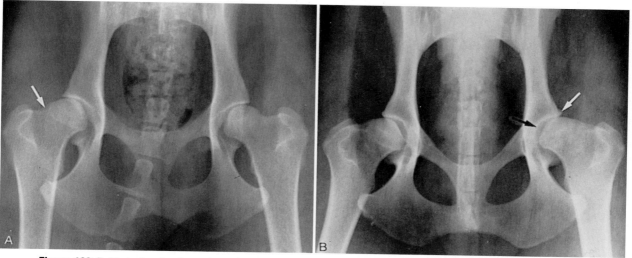

Figure 183–7. Ventrodorsal radiographs of the pelves of two dogs with minimal remodeling of the femoral neck (arrow) *(A)*, lipping of the acetabular rim (arrow) *(B)*, filling of the depths of the acetabulum with bone (black arrow), and subluxation that are characteristic of hip dysplasia.

The ultimate control of hip dysplasia in dog populations has been by genetic selection of dogs for radiographically normal hips. The Orthopedic Foundation for Animals has evaluated hip radiographs of many breeds since 1974. The percentage of dogs born between 1989 and 1992 that were classified as having excellent hip joint phenotype (15,289 of 143,668; 10.64 per cent) was significantly higher than that of dogs born between 1972 and 1980 (9960 of 127,310; 7.82 per cent). Improvement was significantly higher for male than female dogs. Such studies may be biased, however, because there is a strong disincentive to submit radiographs from dogs that are dysplastic. However, an increase in excellent scores in the total population of dogs submitted for evaluation of less than 3 per cent although significant, was not inspiring.[67] This small improvement may have reflected poor breeder application of test results. Although breeding of dogs with the best hips decreases the incidence of dysplasia, it is obvious that phenotypic selection for a polygenic trait does not eliminate the problem, even if rigorously applied. It is hoped that more accurate DNA-based genetic tests will be able to pinpoint more accurately animals that will not pass on the trait.

Patellar Luxation

Patellar luxation is an orthopedic problem of varied etiology. Patellar luxation related to valgus or varus deformities can be congenital or can be acquired by virtue of femoral fractures that have healed with improper alignment. The most common cause, however, is medial congenital patellar luxation occurring in toy breeds of dogs.

The treatment of patellar luxation depends mainly on the severity of the condition. Many toy breeds with patellas that dislocate only occasionally can be treated conservatively with surgical procedures designed to reinforce the lateral ligamentous attachments to the patella. In more severe cases this surgery should be accompanied by surgically deepening the trochlear groove. Repositioning of the tibial crest is also done in more severe cases.

Aseptic Necrosis of the Femoral Head

Aseptic necrosis of the femoral head (Legg-Calvé-Perthes disease) frequently occurs without an apparent predisposing cause in adolescent dogs (mean age 7 months) of toy and small breeds, such as toy poodles and Yorkshire terriers. For undetermined reasons, a major portion of the blood supply to the capital epiphysis of the femur is compromised and the ischemic portion undergoes necrosis. Affected dogs demonstrate muscle atrophy, shortening of the affected leg, pain on passive movement of the hip joint, and in some cases crepitation of the hip joint. Radiographic findings include irregular density and flattening of the femoral head in combination with DJD (Fig. 183–8). Femoral head and neck excision is indicated when conservative treatment fails to lead to clinical improvement within 4 weeks.

ARTHROPATHIES RESULTING FROM INBORN ERRORS OF METABOLISM

Hemophilia A

Lameness is one of the most common clinical signs in humans and dogs with congenital coagulation defects but is less common in cats. The arthropathy of hemophilia A is caused by chronic hemorrhage into joints induced by clinical or subclinical trauma. Larger weight-bearing joints such as the elbows and stifles are more likely to be involved, and larger and more active dogs have more problems than smaller, less active dogs. The effusion of blood into the joint cavity resulting from synovial or subsynovial hemorrhage provokes an acute inflammatory reaction. The synovial membrane thickens and undergoes villous hypertrophy, and hyperplasia of the intimal layer and infiltration of lymphocytes, macrophages, and plasma cells occur. The reaction subsides after several days to weeks, but each subsequent hemorrhagic episode leads to further synovial fibrosis and hemosiderosis. The most significant sites of injury are the articular cartilage and the subchondral bone. Injury to the articular cartilage is caused by granulation tissue covering the articular cartilage that arises from the synovium and from the subchondral bone. Synovial fluid may be frankly bloody during bouts of hemorrhage or xanthochromic with excess numbers of macrophages at other times. Nonspecific joint capsule distention is the earliest radiographic lesion in dogs with factor VIII deficiency–associated arthropathy.

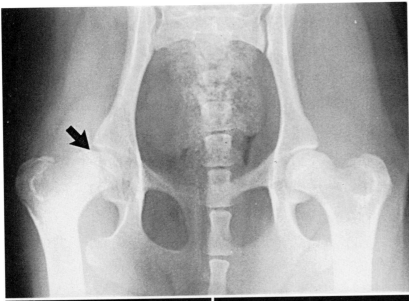

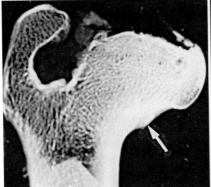 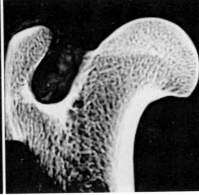

Figure 183–8. Ventrodorsal radiograph of the pelvis shows the fragmentation within the femoral head typical of aseptic necrosis of the femoral head or Legg-Calvé-Perthes disease (black arrow). Radiographs of thin bone sections show the fragmentation and collapse of the affected femoral head and the compensatory thickening of the femoral neck (white arrow). The figure on the lower right shows the normal opposite hip.

Arthropathy Associated With Scottish Fold Cats

The Scottish fold breed of cats is characterized by its abnormally shaped and folded ears. This folding is due to an abnormality in the ear cartilage caused by a simple autosomal dominant gene (*Fd*).[68] Cats that are heterozygous (*Fdfd*) for the folding gene manifest mainly ear abnormalities. In contrast, cats that are homozygous for the defect (*FdFd*) develop generalized cartilage abnormalities manifested by a shortening and thickening of bones of the spine (including the tail) and limbs and a progressive arthropathy of most true joints. A short, squat, appearance of the body, tail, and limbs is the earliest indication that the cat is homozygous for the defect. As the joints become involved, progressive lameness and stiffness are evident. An occasional Scottish fold that is heterozygous for the folding gene, and therefore with normal body conformation, may develop milder forms of arthropathy.

The radiographic changes are bilaterally symmetric and evident in the true joints of the spine and lower limbs. The bones of the spine, tail, and limbs are shorter and thicker than normal. The joints of the feet, especially of the hindlimbs, are most severely affected. There is massive formation of new bone that often bridges the joints; the new bone has a smooth margin but a typical trabecular pattern. Underlying joint structure is difficult to determine because of the overlying bone proliferation.

Treatment is mainly medical, with the judicious use of appropriate NSAIDS. Surgery to remove excessive bone growths may help improve the mobility of selected joints.

NEOPLASTIC ARTHROPATHIES

Primary Neoplastic Arthropathies

Synovial Cell Sarcoma. Synovial cell sarcoma, or synovioma, is by far the most common primary joint tumor in animals. These tumors occur most frequently in middle-aged dogs (6 to 8 years old) and occur less commonly in cats.[69] Synovial cell sarcomas in dogs and cats typically involve a major limb joint, usually the stifle or the elbow joint. Initially, the animals have lameness, at which time radiographic changes may be absent. With time, however, bone surrounding the joint becomes quite lytic (Fig. 183–9). Synovial cell sarcomas tend to grow rapidly and spread slowly by metastasis to local lymph nodes. They tend to spread aggressively at the site of origin, and the accepted treatment is limb amputation.

Osteogenic Sarcoma. The osteogenic sarcoma, or osteosarcoma, is a frequent cause of lameness in large and giant breeds of dogs and rarely invades through subchondral bone into the adjacent joint. When found in long bones, it is important in the differential diagnosis of lameness in giant breeds of dogs.

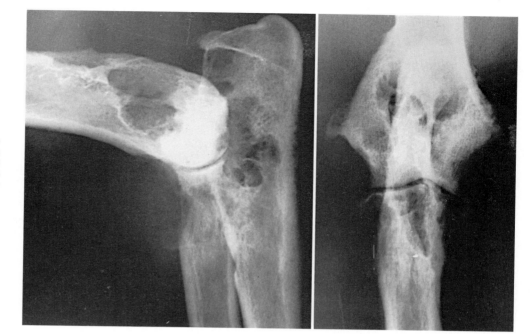

Figure 183–9. Neoplastic joint disease. Multiple destructive lesions in more than one bone are diagnostic of synovial cell sarcoma. Note the absence of bone response to the tumors.

INFLAMMATORY JOINT DISEASE

This major form of joint disease is characterized by inflammatory changes in the synovial membrane and synovial fluid and by systemic signs of illness such as fever, leukocytosis, increased erythrocyte sedimentation rate, elevated levels of phase reactants, hyperfibrinogenemia, lymphadenopathy, malaise, and anorexia. The etiology of inflammatory joint disease of animals is diverse and includes both infectious and noninfectious causes.

INFECTIOUS ARTHRITIS

Joints, both appendicular and vertebral (particularly degenerated disks), are common destinations for blood-borne microbial pathogens. The synovium has a rich blood supply, which perfuses the synovial membrane via myriads of long looping capillaries. Many branching vessels also supply the subchondral bone. The high blood flow to the synovium and subchondral bone is essential for the dissipation of heat and the diffusion of large amounts of nutrients and waste products to and from chondrocytes in the avascular cartilage. The synovium has additional functions, including phagocytosis. As one of the most important phagocytic tissues, the synovium becomes a common site for the trapping and localization of blood-borne microbes and immune complexes.

Blood-borne pathogens are also more likely to localize in joints that have been damaged by some other disease process. Degenerative joints, because they are so common, are particular targets. Therefore, larger dogs, older dogs, and proximal rather than distal joints are more likely to be affected. The pattern of infectious joint disease is more likely to be monarticular (one joint) or pauciarticular (two to five joints) than polyarticular (six or more joints), and shoulders, elbows, hips, stifles, and degenerating intravertebral disks are more apt to be involved than smaller joints. Infectious arthritis, in particular bacterial, is also more likely to occur in male dogs. Males suffer from prostatic infections, which are a common source of bacteria. Joints with septic arthritis are often painful on palpation. Redness and swelling of the overlying skin and soft tissue may be present.

Infectious discospondylitis, both bacterial and fungal, is often found at the lumbosacral junction characterized by disk degeneration in large-breed dogs with chronic genitourinary infectious disease. The disease in the disk space is characterized by disk space collapse and endplate destruction.

Infectious arthritis is uncommon in cats compared with dogs. Urinary tract and skin infections are relatively rare in cats, and acquired heart valve disease is almost nonexistent. Joint disease, in particular DJD, also occurs much less frequently and is milder in cats than dogs. Cats also appear to have a great deal more systemic resistance than dogs to a large number of microbial pathogens, ranging from bacteria to fungi and protozoa.

Bacterial Arthritis

Local Infection. Bacteria may gain entrance to the joint through penetrating wounds, from contiguous sites of infection in bone or soft tissue, or from the bloodstream. Surgical contamination and nonsterile injections into the synovial cavity are other sources of sepsis.

Hematogenous Infection. Bacteria may also gain entrance to the joints from infectious foci within the blood vascular system itself (e.g., heart valves or the umbilical vein) or be carried by the blood from infected organs. Bacterial septicemias in puppies are often associated with *Streptococcus canis* pharyngitis with abscessation of the retropharyngeal lymph nodes occurring during the first 2 weeks of life. Queens or bitches with postparturient uterine or mammary gland infections can infect their young orally shortly after birth. If this leads to a systemic infection, joint abscessation may occur. One of the most common sources of blood-borne bacterial infections is the genitourinary tract, followed by the skin, oral cavity, and respiratory tract. Prostatitis, cystitis, pyelonephritis, pyodermas, and oral infections can all be accompanied by septicemia. Infections involving the genitourinary tract and pelvic lymph nodes of dogs have a unique propensity for localizing in the degenerating intervertebral disks. The infection usually enters the disk in a retrograde fashion through the vertebral veins, which also drain the pelvic organs. Like true appendicular joints, intervertebral disks that are diseased in some other manner are more likely targets for infection than normal disks.

Organisms commonly involved in joint infections in dogs include staphylococci, streptococci, *Erysipelothrix*, *Corynebacterium*, coliforms, *Pasteurella*, *Salmonella*, and occasionally *Brucella*.[70] In cats, the usual offending organisms are *Pasteurella multocida* and hemolytic strains of *Escherichia coli*. The type of organism involved in the joint infection has some clinical significance. Staphylococci and some coliforms cause rapid destruction of the articular cartilage, whereas organisms such as *Erysipelothrix* and streptococci may be present in the joint without causing significant cartilage damage. As a rule, organisms that cause severe cartilage damage also cause toxic or degenerative changes in neutrophils present in the synovial fluid.

Synovial fluid from septic joints is frequently bloody, which differentiates it from that of most noninfectious joint disorders. The fluid contains large numbers of neutrophils, but the absolute count, although high, is similar to the neutrophil count in the synovial fluid from nonseptic, inflamed joints. The presence of toxic, ruptured, and degranulated neutrophils should make one suspicious of a bacterial infection. Infection should not be ruled out when neutrophils in the synovial fluid appear normal, however. If other clinical signs are suggestive, a joint tap should be performed.

Early radiographic findings include thickened synovial membrane, distended joint capsule with displacement of adjacent fascial planes, and a slight widening of the joint space caused by joint effusion. Radiolucent intra-articular shadows representing intra-articular fat pads may disappear because of the accumulation of exudate within the joints. The early signs of infection may also be masked or confused by preexisting signs of DJD. Therefore, infection should not be ruled out when radiographic changes are not detected.

A radiographic finding more commonly noted in the later stages is a fine, faintly identifiable, periosteal proliferation on the bones adjacent to the joint space (Fig. 183–10). This type of reactive periostitis is not to be confused with the prominent, better defined, periarticular bone spurs that develop in DJD or after trauma. Aspiration of the joint at this time is still necessary to reach a positive diagnosis. After the period of early soft tissue swelling and inflammation, and depending on the organism involved, the process expands with destruction of the articular cartilage (see Fig. 183–10) and resulting loss of width of the joint space. Narrowing of the joint space is often unappreciated because of the unwillingness of the animal to bear weight on the leg. If the disease is not controlled, it may quickly lead to an osteomyelitis in the adjacent bones and a widening of the joint space as it fills with debris and exudate. It is difficult to give time intervals from the time of onset for the various stages of bacterial arthritis. This is because of differences in the pathogenicity of the organisms, the manner of inoculation, host immunity, and the type of superimposed treatment that may delay (inappropriate or inadequate antibiotic therapy) or hasten (immunosuppressive drugs) the development of the pathologic process.

Complications of infectious arthritis include osteomyelitis, fibrous or bony ankylosis, and secondary joint disease. An osteomyelitis is present as soon as the articular cartilage is breached and the infectious process enters the subchondral bone. This compounds the severity of the disease and makes the prognosis more guarded. If the articular cartilage has been damaged, fibrotic or bony ankylosis can occur. This is a logical consequence, because the destruction of the cartilage exposes the subchondral bone and simulates a condition like that of a fracture. An abscess frequently forms within the exudate and debris, preventing bone fusion from occurring across the joint space. In these cases, reactive bone bridges the joint, leaving a radiolucent cavity around the abscess.

The treatment of bacterial arthritis is dependent on the isolation and identification of the organism and on the determination of antibiotic sensitivities. Direct culture of synovial fluid is indicated whenever possible; culture from synovial biopsies is no more accurate.[70] In order to maximize the chances of isolating the offending organism, blood and urine cultures should probably be conducted at the same time as joint fluid cultures. Most microbes reach the joints via the blood, and the urinary tract is the source of infection in almost one half of these dogs. Any bacteria that are isolated from blood and/or urine should be considered representative of what is present in the joint. Whenever possible, bactericidal antibiotics should be used. Most antibiotics penetrate the vascular bed of an inflamed joint, so systemic treatment is usually effective. Local infusions of antibiotics can be used when a single joint is involved. In this situation, antibiotics are most effective if they are infused almost continuously and associated with drainage. Generally, antibiotics are given for periods of 2 weeks or more after the signs of infection have disappeared. In the case of bacterial endocarditis, antibiotic treatment may have to be continued longer (see Chapter 113).

Spirochetal Arthritis

Lyme disease is thoroughly reviewed in Chapter 86. Lyme disease is caused by the spirochete *Borrelia burgdorferi*. The disease has been reported in many parts of the world in humans and veterinary species such as dogs, horses, and cattle.[71] *Borrelia* replicates locally in the skin at the site of inoculation for periods of 2 to 5 months. After this time, the infection can become systemic, with the organism localizing in the synovial membrane, heart, and central nervous system. Clinical signs in the dog, when they occur, are most apt to be joint related. An acute, sometimes severe, transient mono- or pauciarthritis occurs from 50 to 90 days after infection (mean 66 days), almost exclusively in the limb closest to the tick bite. This acute arthritis occurs mainly in the dogs that seroconvert most rapidly; animals that seroconvert later (after 90 days) usually remain asymptomatic or demonstrate only mild clinical signs. The volume and cellularity of synovial fluid in infected joints are increased, with the predominant cells being nondegenerate neutrophils.[72] Organisms are most easily identified by polymerase chain reaction (PCR) in skin from the same quadrant as the arthritis and from the synovium of the affected joint(s).[73, 74]

There is no doubt that Lyme borreliosis is vastly overdiagnosed in both human and veterinary medicine. Only one fifth or less of humans diagnosed with Lyme disease by their physicians actually meet the criteria for active disease,[75] and the situation appears similar for dogs.

The main differential diagnoses of Lyme arthritis in dogs are other tick-borne arthritides (i.e., rickettsial or ehrlichial diseases) and immune-mediated arthritis. The high incidence of immune-mediated arthritis makes this differential important. Immune-mediated arthritis is usually polyarticular

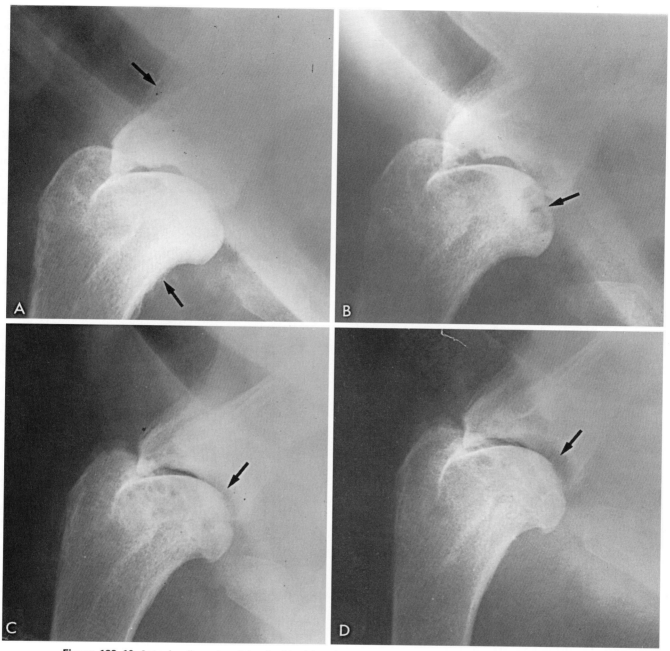

Figure 183–10. Lateral radiographs of the shoulder joint of an 8-year-old male German shepherd dog with progressive infectious arthritis and osteomyelitis, characterized by periosteal new bone response (arrow) and destructive lesions in the humeral head (arrow) and glenoid cavity. Radiographs were obtained *(A)* on the day of the first examination and *(B)* 2 months, *(C)* 1 year, and *(D)* 16 months after the first examination.

and occurs most commonly in pedigreed dogs; it also occurs with equal frequency in *Borrelia* or *Rickettsia* endemic and nonendemic areas. Titers can be helpful when dealing with dogs outside endemic areas but have to be interpreted with caution in regions where tick-borne infections are highly endemic. Rickettsial or ehrlichial arthritis is usually associated with thrombocytopenia. When there is doubt about whether an arthritis is due to tick-borne agents or immune mediated, it is prudent to treat the animal first with tetracycline or doxycycline for at least 5 days before instituting immunosuppressive drug therapy. If the arthritis is due to spirochetes or rickettsia, a favorable response is expected after 48 to 96 hours.[76]

Bacterial L-Forms

L-forms are cell wall–deficient bacteria. They are differentiated from *Mycoplasma* by their ability to revert to their parent cell wall state with time in culture. L-form infections are most common in cats and are usually manifested by fistulating subcutaneous wounds, which frequently spread to local and distant joints by local extension and hematogenously. Destruction and complete luxation of affected joints have been observed. Infections often occur on the lower limbs, indicating bite wounds as a possible source. Infections of spay incisions and iatrogenic infection with contaminated ointments have also been reported. Although the infection is

MSJ

often confined to a single cat, cat-to-cat transmission has been observed among cats in one household.[77] The diagnosis is usually one of exclusion; the exudate is mucinous, slightly cloudy, and odorless; there is no visible evidence of an infectious agent on routine cultures or special stains of exudate or tissues; and there is no response to antibiotics other than tetracycline.

Mycoplasmal Arthritis

A mycoplasmal arthritis can result from the systemic spread of organisms from localized sites of inapparent infection in the respiratory passages, oropharynx, conjunctival membranes, or urogenital tract. Although common in food animals, systemic spread of *Mycoplasma* leading to arthritis is uncommon in both the dog and cat and usually associated with immunocompromise.

Rickettsial and Ehrlichial Arthritis

Organisms in the family Rickettsiaceae, genera *Rickettsia* and *Ehrlichia,* have been increasingly associated with disease in dogs in all parts of the world where the appropriate tick hosts are found (please see Chapter 86 for a complete review of these conditions).

R. rickettsii infection of dogs is often subclinical. However, in severe cases a systemic vasculitis may occur. Polyarthritis is a prominent feature of this vasculitis.

Canine ehrlichiosis occurs in acute and chronic stages, both of which may be asymptomatic, mild, or severe. Acute disease, when apparent, is often associated with fever, depression, lymphadenopathy, and various hematologic abnormalities that always include thrombocytopenia. A nonerosive polyarthritis is often seen in the acute stages of infection as a prominent or secondary feature. Arthritis may also be seen in chronically ill animals but is much less likely to be one of the major complaints. Exact clinical signs also depend on the species of *Ehrlichia*. *E. platys* infection in the United States is reported to be subclinical unless concomitant with other tick-borne diseases; however, more virulent forms of the organism have been identified in the southeastern United States and in other countries.[78, 79] Granulocytic ehrlichiosis (*E. ewingi, E. equi*) is more likely to be manifested initially by polyarthritis than monocytic (*E. canis, E. chaffiensis*) or platelet-associated (*E. platys*) ehrlichiosis.

The suspicion of rickettsial and ehrlichial arthritis is generally based on a history of tick exposure; the triad of fever, lymphadenopathy, and thrombocytopenia; and positive antibody titers to one or more ehrlichial species. Granulocytic species of *Ehrlichia* are usually visible on blood smears, as are the various isolates of *E. platys*. The monocytic species of *Ehrlichia* and *R. rickettsii* are more difficult to visualize in blood or tissue aspirates. The serologic responses to *R. rickettsii, E. platys,* and *E. equi* tend to be unique to each, but the antibodies to *E. canis* and *E. chaffeensis* are strongly cross-reactive. *E. ewingii* is serologically related to *E. canis* and *E. chaffeensis* but distinct from *E. equi* and *E. platys*. The PCR is being increasingly used for both diagnosis and speciation.

The major differential diagnosis for rickettsial or ehrlichial arthritis is immune-mediated joint disease. The same steps should be taken in diagnosing rickettsial or ehrlichial infections as described for Lyme borreliosis; however, thrombocytopenia is an added diagnostic feature of the former. If there is doubt about whether the joint disease is infectious or immunologic, it is prudent to treat first with tetracycline or

doxyclycline for several days while awaiting serologic tests and before embarking on immunosuppressive drug therapy. Combined antibiotic and steroid therapy may also be justified as primary therapy; glucocorticoids given at the same time as antibiotics delayed recovery from experimental Rocky Mountain spotted fever in dogs but did not seem to worsen disease signs.[82]

The treatment of choice for rickettsial or ehrlichial infections is tetracycline and related antibiotics such as doxycycline.[83] Acute-stage infections show definite improvement within 48 hours, and therapy should be continued for an additional 10 to 14 days. Chronic *E. canis* infections, especially when bone marrow damage is substantial, respond poorly and much more slowly to tetracycline therapy. Imidocarb dipropionate may be a preferable treatment for such chronic infections.[84]

Viral Arthritis

A fleeting and sometimes persistent arthropathy is a symptom of many acute viral diseases of humans. It usually occurs in the convalescent period after mumps virus, coxsackievirus, or adenovirus infections.[85] Because animals show signs of pain only when joint inflammation is relatively severe, the degree to which arthropathy complicates acute viral diseases in animals is unknown.

A transient (48 to 72 hours) limping syndrome has been observed after natural and experimental feline calicivirus (FCV) infection. Affected kittens are usually febrile, hyperesthetic, and, in about 40 per cent of cases, manifest ulcers on the tongue or palate. This limping syndrome has been observed commonly after immunization with vaccines containing live FCV. Synovial fluid from affected joints often contains increased numbers of macrophages, many of which contain phagocytized neutrophils.[86, 87]

A mild to moderately severe synovitis has also been observed in cats with the effusive form of FIP. Although the synovial inflammation appears to be relatively severe in some cats with FIP, only a small proportion of affected cats show signs of lameness.

A transient rheumatologic syndrome has been observed after live virus vaccination in people and dogs. An acute systemic vasculitis, starting with gastrointestinal signs and evolving into hypertrophic osteodystrophy and lameness, has been associated with routine vaccinations in Weimaraners. The persistence of distemper virus in joints has been implicated in rheumatoid arthritis of dogs.[88]

Fungal Arthritis

Fungal arthritis is infrequent in dogs and cats. It can occur as an extension of a fungal osteomyelitis or as a primary granulomatous synovitis, with the former occurring more commonly. *Coccidioides immitis, Blastomyces dermatitidis, Histoplasma capsulatum,* and *Cryptococcus neoformans* are the most frequently encountered organisms.

Protozoal Arthritis

Visceral leishmaniasis, caused by organisms in the *Leishmania donovani* complex, is a chronic systemic macrophage proliferative-infiltrative disease of humans and some species of animals. The organism is transmitted by various species of blood-sucking sandflies of the genus *Phlebotomus*; the dog is a principal reservoir for the organism in Mediterranean countries and in parts of Asia. Most infected dogs are asymptomatic or exhibit relatively mild skin disease, and the infection cycle is maintained when sandflies feed from dogs. More severely affected dogs show variable signs of fever, malaise, weight loss, lymphadenopathy, hepatosplenomegaly, anemia, renal disease, enteritis, dermatopathy, and polyarthritis.[89] The arthritis, when observed, is often polyarticular and is associated with mild to moderately severe radiographic signs of periosteal proliferation and destruction. The synovial membrane is infiltrated by large numbers of macrophages filled with leishmanial bodies. Affected dogs should be treated for several months with a combination of organic antimonials and allopurinol, with or without levamisole immunostimulation.

NONINFECTIOUS ARTHRITIS

The noninfectious arthritides of animals can be classified into two general groups depending on the nature and etiology of the disorder (see Table 183–1): (1) arthritis of apparent immunologic cause and (2) crystal-induced arthritis. Crystal-induced arthritis, such as gout or pseudogout, is extremely uncommon in dogs and cats, but immune-mediated joint disease, especially in the dog, occurs at high frequency.

Arthritis of Apparent Immunologic Cause

Deforming or Erosive Arthritis

Canine Rheumatoid Arthritis. Canine rheumatoid arthritis is a well-documented clinical entity.[90] It is an uncommon condition, occurring in approximately 2 per 25,000 dogs examined at the authors' hospital. This disorder occurs mainly in small or toy breeds of dogs 8 months to 8 years of age. Canine rheumatoid arthritis is manifested initially as a shifting lameness with soft tissue swelling around involved joints. Within several weeks or months, the disease localizes in particular joints and characteristic radiographic signs develop. Joint involvement is more severe in the carpal and tarsal joints, although in individual dogs the elbow, stifle, shoulder, and hip joints may show similar radiographic signs. Involvement of the apophyseal joints and costovertebral articulations rarely progresses to the point of causing radiographic changes. In exceptional cases, however, only involvement of the vertebral articulations occurs. The disease is often accompanied by fever, malaise, anorexia, and lymphadenopathy in the earlier stages. Renal amyloidosis can be a complication of long-standing disease that is inadequately controlled.[91]

The earliest radiographic changes consist of soft tissue swelling and loss of trabecular bone density in the area of the joint. Lucent cystlike areas are frequently seen in the subchondral bone. The prominent lesion is a progressive destruction of subchondral bone in the more central areas as well as marginally at the attachment of the synovium.[90] Both narrowing and widening of the joint spaces are identified radiographically as a result of cartilage erosion and destruction of subchondral bone (Fig. 183–11). Subluxation, luxation, and deformation occur most frequently in the carpal, tarsal, and phalangeal joints and occasionally in the elbow and stifle joints. Fibrous ankylosis can occur in advanced cases, particularly in the intercarpal and intertarsal joint space. Soft tissue calcification and atrophy accompany disuse osteoporosis and other radiographic findings. In chronic disease, the ends of bone become atrophied.

Hemograms are normal or reflect the generalized inflammatory process with leukocytosis, neutrophilia, and hyperfibrinogenemia.[90] Serum electrophoresis often shows hypoalbuminemia and variable elevation in alpha$_2$ and gamma globulins. Rheumatoid factors, that is, autoantibodies against sterically altered (e.g., immune-complexed) antibodies, are the hallmark of human rheumatoid arthritis; they are present at high titer in about three fourths of affected people. Rheumatoid factors probably serve a function in cross-linking immune complexes and aiding in their clearance by phagocytes. They are detectable, therefore, in many diseases in which chronic immune complexing occurs. Although rheumatoid factor tests are of definite value in the diagnosis of human rheumatoid arthritis, we have not found them to be either sensitive or specific enough for routine diagnostic use, let alone use as a sole diagnostic tool. Studies have confirmed that rheumatoid factors are present only at low titer and in only about one fourth of dogs with rheumatoid arthritis; they are also present with a similar titer and incidence in unclassified polyarthritis, heartworm disease, pyometra, leishmaniasis, and systemic lupus erythematosus (SLE).[92, 93] Antinuclear antibodies (ANAs) are sometimes detected in dogs with rheumatoid arthritis but not nearly as often as in SLE.

Synovial fluid changes are indicative of an inflammatory synovitis, with an elevated total cell count, a high proportion of neutrophils in the synovial fluid cell population, and a variable decrease in the quality of the mucin clot. Ragocytes (neutrophils that have ingested immune complexes), as described in human rheumatoid arthritis, are not usually seen. A characteristic finding in canine rheumatoid arthritis is the presence in synovial fluid of mononuclear cells containing immunoglobulin G (IgG), with only occasional cells containing C3 protein.[90] These mononuclear cells may produce the immunoglobulin or ingest it from the synovial fluid.

The characteristic pathologic lesions consist of a villous hyperplasia of the synovial membrane with lymphoid and plasma cell infiltrates. Infiltration cells destroy articular cartilage starting at the margins of the joint. A pannus of granulation tissue also invades the surface of the cartilage. In the central regions of the joint, cartilage destruction is caused by a pannus arising from granulation tissue in the underlying marrow cavity. Ankylosis in advanced lesions is common in the intercarpal and intertarsal joints. The dense lymphoid and plasma cell infiltrate in the synovium and the destruction of articular cartilage differentiate rheumatoid arthritis from the synovitis seen in the nonerosive types of arthritis. The large numbers of lymphocytes and plasma cells in the synovium suggest the presence of a local antigenic stimulus and a type IV or delayed-type hypersensitivity reaction; the nature of the antigen that evokes this reaction is unknown.

Canine rheumatoid arthritis responds only temporarily to systemic corticosteroids. Aspirin has no appreciable therapeutic benefit, probably because the disease is much more severe and rapidly progressive in dogs than in humans. If the condition is recognized before severe joint damage occurs, it can usually be arrested with combination immunosuppressive drug therapy. This type of therapy is covered in detail in the discussion of drug therapy of immune-mediated arthritides. In dogs with advanced deformities, immunosuppressive drug therapy may have to be combined with arthrodesis of selected joints. Arthrodesis is not warranted if the disease process cannot first be successfully halted with drug therapy.

Polyarthritis of Greyhounds. A semierosive polyarthritis in greyhounds occurs in different parts of the world.[94] Disease appears in animals from 3 to 30 months of age and

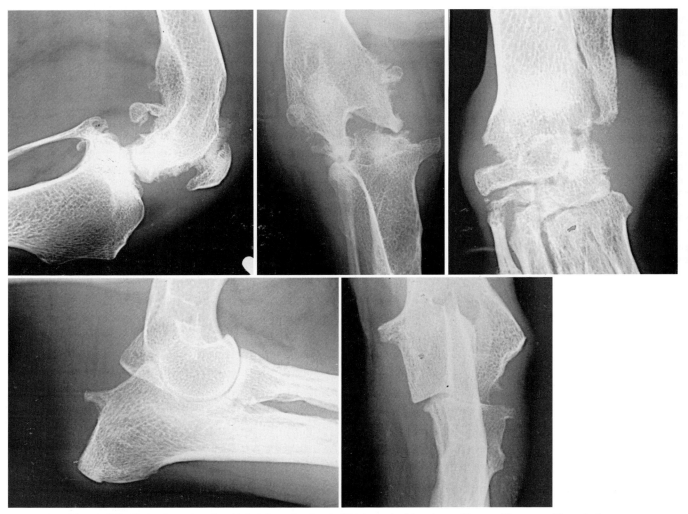

Figure 183–11. Radiographs of multiple joints of a female Welsh corgi with a 1-year history of lameness. The soft tissue swelling, periarticular subchondral erosions, formation of cystlike subchondral lucencies, and subluxation and deformity of the joints are typical of noninfectious erosive (rheumatoid) arthritis of the dog.

most frequently attacks the proximal interphalangeal, carpal, tarsal, elbow, and stifle joints. The shoulder, hip, and atlanto-occipital joints are less frequently involved. A tenosynovitis may be an accompanying feature. The synovial membrane is edematous and hyperemic in the early course of the disease and may be covered with a fine layer of fibrin. The synovial fluid is cloudy and yellowish and often contains fibrin tags. In later stages, a lymphocyte and plasma cell infiltrate is seen in the synovial lining. Peripheral lymph nodes are enlarged and hyperactive. Pannus formation and marginal subchondral erosions are seen to a limited extent. Destruction of articular cartilage occurs in some joints but is often not associated with pannus formation. Gross deformities and radiographic changes are not as apparent as those seen in canine rheumatoid arthritis but appear more pronounced than those described for nonerosive joint disease. This polyarthritis should be treated in the same manner as idiopathic nonerosive polyarthritis of dogs, which it most closely resembles.

Feline Chronic Progressive Polyarthritis (Erosive Form). This form of disease is a less common variant of feline chronic progressive polyarthritis, which is discussed in the next section. This rare disease is insidious in onset, and affected cats remain amazingly mobile until the joint

destruction is quite advanced. The first abnormalities noted are often deformities of the carpal, metacarpophalangeal, metatarsophalangeal, and interphalangeal joints. Radiographic signs of erosion of the margins and central parts of the subchondral bone in these joints precede joint instability and deformities. Proliferation of bone adjacent to affected joints can be identified, but proliferative bone findings are minor in degree, whereas destructive signs are excessive. Synovial fluid from involved joints is abnormal and demonstrates a slight to moderate elevation of white cells. Neutrophils, lymphocytes, and synovial macrophages are present in varying proportions.

Periosteal Proliferative Arthritis

Feline Chronic Progressive Polyarthritis (Periosteal-Proliferative Form). Feline chronic progressive polyarthritis occurs exclusively in male cats; the common age at onset is 1.5 to 4.5 years.[95] The disease occurs acutely with high fever, severe joint pain, stiffness that usually starts in the tarsal and carpal joints, and pronounced lymphadenopathy that is regional to the inflamed joints. Radiographic signs, which progress from osteoporosis to periosteal new bone formation and ankylosis, ensue over the next weeks to months. After the first few weeks, the fever tends to subside, and the disease takes a more chronic progressive course. This is manifested ultimately by severe generalized stiffness, muscle atrophy, weight loss, and gross bone enlargements in joint areas. Mild subluxation of the carpal and tarsal joints is sometimes seen in chronic cases.

Chronic progressive polyarthritis of cats is not caused by identifiable bacteria or *Mycoplasma,* but it is etiologically linked to feline syncytium-forming virus (FeSFV), a common retrovirus infection.[95] All cats with this disease are serologically and virologically positive for this infection. Initial reports of this disease also described a relationship with feline leukemia virus (FeLV), which was present in one third of the animals. With the virtual elimination of FeLV from indoor pet cats, most cases of feline chronic progressive polyarthritis are FeLV negative, suggesting that FeLV is not essential in the pathogenesis. The arthritis cannot be reproduced with FeSFV isolated from diseased cats, however. It has been postulated, therefore, that the arthritis is an uncommon disease manifestation of FeSFV that occurs in certain male cats and that may be potentiated by FeLV. The feline disease resembles human Reiter's arthritis in these respects; Reiter's disease occurs predominantly in men with the human leukocyte antigen HLA-B27.

Synovial fluid contains a greatly increased number of neutrophils. The fluid is usually yellow tinged and cloudy. The hemogram is variable, with leukocytosis predominating. Serologic tests for FeSFV are invariably positive, but the high background incidence of this infection among normal cats limits its specificity. Affected cats should also be tested for FeLV, because cats with both viruses have a much worse prognosis.

Immunosuppressive drugs, usually corticosteroids and cyclophosphamide, are used to treat the disease. Corticosteroids alone lessen the severity of the disease and slow the course but do not halt its progression. Combination immunosuppressive drug therapy, usually prednisolone and cyclophosphamide, has been successful in achieving a remission in about half of the cats treated, but recurrences and drug refractoriness are common when therapy is diminished or discontinued. Therefore, drug therapy should not be lessened or discontinued in cats that are in remission. If there is an underlying FeLV-associated bone marrow suppression, cytotoxic drugs cannot be used to full effectiveness and the prognosis is poor.

Nondeforming or Nonerosive Arthritis

A nonerosive, noninfectious arthritis occurs in the dog and cat, and although it is etiologically diverse, it is probably mediated by similar immunopathologic mechanisms.[96] The presenting clinical signs of this type of arthritis are similar whether it is idiopathic or associated with secondary infectious disease, SLE, neoplasia, inflammatory bowel disease, or drug hypersensitivity. The joint disease tends to be cyclic in nature; has a predisposition for smaller distal joints, the carpus and tarsus in particular; and can occur in the monarticular (rare), pauciarticular (uncommon), or polyarticular (common) form. Radiographic changes, even after many months of joint disease, tend to be minimal or nonexistent and are limited to soft tissue swelling. Biopsies of the synovial membranes show a nonvillous hyperplasia, sparse mononuclear cell infiltrates, moderate neutrophil infiltrate, and fibrin exudation. Marginal erosions and pannus formation are not prominent features in these diseases.

Regardless of the associated disease processes that lead to arthritis, the joint disease is believed to be due to deposition of immune complexes in the synovial membrane with resultant type III immune (i.e., vasculitis) reaction. In idiopathic nondeforming arthritis, the origin and nature of the antigen in the complexes are unknown; the antigens in SLE are of nuclear origin; the antigen in enteropathic arthritis probably originates from the inflamed bowel; and antigens in arthritis secondary to chronic infectious disease or neoplasia originate from the offending microorganisms or from the tumor cells.

Idiopathic Nondeforming Arthritis. Idiopathic nondeforming arthritis is by far the most common disorder of dogs with immune-mediated arthritis. It is termed idiopathic because there is no evidence of an underlying disease. This disorder occurs most predominantly in purebred dogs. Although there is a feeling that medium and larger sporting-type breeds are more affected, the condition has also been observed in many small breeds. A possible association between immune-mediated thyroiditis and hypothyroidism may exist; the numerous breeds that suffer from hypothyroidism are among the breeds most commonly affected with idiopathic nondeforming arthritis. An idiopathic nondeforming polyarthritis has also been recognized in cats but much less frequently than in dogs.

The disease is usually manifested in animals 1 to 6 years of age but is not unusual in puppies, adolescents, and older dogs. The initial history is one of cyclic fever, during which malaise, anorexia, lameness, or generalized stiffness is noted. The fever is most pronounced in dogs with polyarticular disease. In severely affected dogs, periods of remission are usually incomplete, in which case the disease can be debilitating. Generalized muscle atrophy and disproportionate atrophy of the temporal and masseter muscles are frequently seen. This atrophy is due in part to disuse, but in many cases the disease process also involves the muscles or nerves.

During the most severe stages of the disease, swelling and heat in distal joints are sometimes detected. Generalized lymphadenopathy may be noted in varying degrees. During periods of disease activity, a leukocytosis with neutrophilia and hyperfibrinogenemia is often observed. Polyarticular involvement is the most common presentation, with the dogs showing generalized stiffness and reluctance to move their spine, tail, or limbs. Toy breeds, which often have severe generalized arthritis, can become virtually immobile, making it difficult to tell whether the joints are the source of the problem or the immobility is due solely to depression. Radiographic abnormalities are usually not present, except for an increase in the amount of periarticular soft tissue related to inflammation or fibrosis. It is important always to take a sample of synovial fluid from dogs with DJD changes but without obvious predisposing disorders or with an atypical pattern of joint involvement.

Diagnosis is made by consideration of the clinical history of an antibiotic-unresponsive cyclic fever, malaise, and anorexia, upon which is superimposed stiffness or lameness. The cyclic nature of the disease complicates diagnosis, because affected dogs may appear to respond favorably to antibiotic therapy when the improvement is due to coincidental cyclic variation of the inflammatory process. Synovial fluid analysis is imperative even if there are no signs of joint pain, swelling, and reddening. Synovial fluid from affected individuals contains from 5000 to 100,000 or more white cells per microliter. The predominant cells in the fluid are the neutrophils; these cells appear nontoxic and with normal granulation. The fluid is sterile for bacteria, viruses, *Mycoplasma,* and *Chlamydia*. Serologic abnormalities such as the LE-cell phenomenon, ANA, and rheumatoid factor are absent. Blood cultures are negative for bacteria, and there are no signs of primary infectious processes in other areas of the body.

Treatment involves the use of glucocorticoids alone or in combination with more potent immunosuppressive drugs (see later). Complete remission of signs can usually be achieved. From 30 to 50 per cent of the dogs have recurrences of illness after the drug therapy is discontinued.

Nondeforming Arthritis Associated With Chronic Infectious Diseases. A nondeforming arthritis has been associated with subacute bacterial endocarditis; pyometra; discospondylitis; chronic *Acitinomyces* infections in the chest, abdomen, or paravertebral musculature; chronic salmonellosis; heartworm disease; urinary tract infections; and severe periodontitis. These infections are often difficult to pinpoint, and the arthritis may be the primary or sole presenting complaint. Radiographic features are limited to soft tissue swelling. It is important, therefore, to make a thorough search for secondary infections every time a nonerosive type of arthritis is found. This is especially important because immunosuppressive drugs are inevitably used to treat cases in which infection is unrecognized. Joint involvement in this type of disorder is usually monarticular or pauciarticular and has a predisposition for the carpal and tarsal joints. Because the organisms involved in the primary disease process cannot be identified in the synovial membrane, it is likely that the joint disease is also of immune complex origin.

Nondeforming Arthritis Associated With Other Immune Disorders

Systemic Lupus Erythematosus. SLE is recognized in virtually all animal species, but its incidence is highest in purebred species such as purebred dog and cats. There is some confusion about what constitutes SLE in animals. If human criteria were strictly adhered to, most dogs with "SLE" would not qualify. Cats, however, manifest SLE much like that in humans.[97] Dogs tend to have one or two systemic signs, often polyarthritis, but skin, hematologic, central nervous system, and renal manifestations are less important.[96] Hematologic abnormalities in the dog, such as thrombocytopenia or hemolytic anemia, have occurred in only 10 to 20 per cent of the total cases of SLE that the authors have diagnosed and tended to occur as the primary disease manifestation rather than part of a broader disease syndrome. SLE in cats is more systemic in nature, with dermatitis, conjunctivitis, oral ulcers, psychoses, fever, lymphadenopathy, cytopenias, polyarthritis, and a progressive glomerulonephritis being commonly observed. Although polyarthritis is a frequent feature of SLE in both dogs and cats, it is more apt to be the predominant clinical manifestation in dogs. Signs of polyarthritis in cats are often masked, and joint inflammation is often detected only upon routine synovial fluid screening for vague signs or fever of unknown origin.

One of the characteristic diagnostic features of SLE in all species is the presence of ANA in the blood. However, the titers of ANA are much lower than in humans and there is a high background of ANAs at low titer in normal individuals (especially in the cat). ANAs often appear during the acute courses of infectious diseases such as FeLV, feline immunodeficiency virus (FIV), and FIP infections of cats. Because ANA titers are generally lower in dogs and cats and may occur in normal animals and individuals with other illnesses, ANA tests should be interpreted in terms of the whole clinical picture. A positive ANA, regardless of titer, is not by itself diagnostic of SLE, but a low titer in the presence of other characteristic features of the illness may still be significant.

The basic screening test for all ANAs is the indirect immunofluorescence assay using various types of cells as substrates. This test is referred to as the fluorescence ANA or FANA test. The exact nuclear antigen to which the antibody is directed can alter the pattern of fluorescence, that is, homogeneous, speckled, rim, or nucleolar. Using more specific tests, canine ANAs were found to be restricted to the IgG class and reactive against a narrow range of nuclear antigens, that is, histones H1, H2A, H3 and H4.[98]

As with virtually all immune-mediated arthritides, care must be taken to exclude underlying causes of disease (e.g., infections, drugs, neoplasia). A nonerosive polyarthritis has been observed in subacute bacterial endocarditis (SBE) in humans and dogs, and indeed the entire syndrome of SBE can mimic SLE. Chronic bacterial endocarditis can lead to continuous low-grade damage to parenchymal organs, high levels of circulating immune complexes, and a heightened responsiveness of the host's immune system. In humans and animals this may result in the production of ANAs and rheumatoid factors. Rheumatoid factors are made in response to persistent immune complex production. This phenomenon is important, because if such animals are mistakenly diagnosed as having SLE or rheumatoid arthritis, they are treated with immunosuppresive drugs, with potentially serious consequences.

Polyarthritis and Meningitis. Meningitis, secondary to an idiopathic arteritis (polyarteritis), is becoming increasingly common in many breeds of dogs. The primary manifestation is almost always meningitis, with intense neck pain, reluctance to move, and fever. The diagnosis is usually based on the typical clinical signs, age, breed, and inflammatory cerebrospinal fluid, and little attention is given to joint fluid abnormalities. However, joint inflammation involving one or more distal limb joints is not infrequent in these dogs.

The classic form of the immune-mediated meningitis occurs in young beagles, Boxers, pointers, and rottweilers. The disease is usually manifested at 6 to 9 months of age by cyclic attacks of fever, depression, and extreme neck pain lasting for 3 to 7 days, interspersed with periods of normalcy lasting a few days to several weeks. After several cycles of the disease, the attacks become milder and less frequent. Self-cure usually occurs in several weeks or months. Inflammation of one or more distal joints may accompany each attack, although signs of joint disease are usually overshadowed by the neck pain.

A more severe form of this disease is seen in young adult Bernese Mountain Dogs, Akitas, and Weimaraners. Signs of meningitis usually occur in early adulthood and are also cyclic in nature. Although steroid responsive, the meningitis is more apt to become chronic and require long-term treatment. Self-cures after several cycles, as in the classic form of the disease, are less frequent. A pauci- or polyarticular arthritis can be an accompanying feature of the illness. The particularly severe form of the disease is seen in Akita puppies.[99] Both meningitis and polyarthritis are clinically apparent; response to immunosuppressive drug therapy is only partial, and most affected animals are euthanized before 1 year of age.

Familial Mediterranean Fever. Familial Mediterranean fever is a human disorder characterized by recurrent fever of unknown origin, renal amyloidosis, and evidence of peritonitis, pleuritis, and/or synovitis. An analogous syndrome has been described in Chinese Shar Pei dogs.[100] Affected dogs showed elevated levels of interleukin-6 in serum and hypergammaglobulinemia when compared with normal controls. Affected dogs that were 2 years old or older frequently suffered from renal failure associated with amyloidosis and swollen joints.

Juvenile Cellulitis and Arthritis. Four of 15 dogs diagnosed with juvenile cellulitis (juvenile pyoderma, puppy strangles) had signs of joint pain in addition to the characteristic facial inflammation and submandibular lymphadenopathy.[101] Synovial fluids from three of the four dogs with joint pain revealed suppurative arthritis and were negative for bacterial growth on culture. Concurrent treatment with antibiotics and prednisone was highly effective in curing both facial and joint lesions.

Nondeforming Arthritis Associated With Neoplasia.

A sterile polyarthritis has been observed in some dogs and cats with overt or latent neoplastic processes. The signs of polyarthritis may precede the signs of cancer or may be a minor to major component of the overall disease syndrome.

Enteropathic Arthritis.

Enteropathic arthritis is frequently associated with diseases such as ulcerative colitis and regional enteritis in humans. The cause of arthritis is unknown, but it is thought that either the bowel disease and joint disease share a common etiology or antigenic products released into the blood from the inflamed bowel have some effect on the synovium. Hepatopathic arthropathy, which has been seen in several dogs with chronic active hepatitis and cirrhosis, is also a type of enteropathic arthritis. In this disease, antigenic material from the bowel probably gains access to the general bloodstream, because it is not being removed from the portal blood by the reticuloendothelial tissue of the liver.

Plasmacytic-Lymphocytic Gonitis.

A synovitis is observed in less than 10 per cent of dogs undergoing surgery for cranial cruciate ligament (CCL) rupture. This subclass of dogs tends to be younger than the usual dogs with CCL ruptures and they are often purebred animals of medium-sized breeds such as the rottweilers. The synovitis leads to pronounced joint laxity and instability, often manifested by cruciate ligament damage and instability. The synovium is grossly thickened, edematous, and reddish-yellowish tinged. The synovial fluid is cloudy, less viscous, yellow tinged, and contains from 5000 to 20,000 white cells per microliter with 10 to 40 per cent of these being neutrophils. Unlike those in other inflammatory joint diseases, the predominant cell is often a small lymphocyte. The fluid is sterile for known microorganisms. Radiographic changes, when present, are minimal and include soft tissue swelling and periosteal proliferative changes. Erosive changes are absent or slight. These features may be related to the preexisting instability caused by ligament weakness. Synovial biopsies show an intense lymphocytic-plasmacytic infiltrate and synovial hypertrophy that is sometimes villous. Subchondral erosions are minimal or absent.

The etiology of this disorder is unknown, and it is still uncertain whether the peculiar synovitis leads to the cruciate ligament laxity or rupture or is merely a secondary immune reaction by the host to the degenerating ligament. In favor of the latter etiology, CCL reconstruction is sometimes curative in these dogs. Significantly increased levels of serum anti–native collagen type II antibody, as assessed by ELISA, have also been measured in dogs with diverse joint diseases such as rheumatoid arthritis, infective arthritis, primary DJD, and CCL rupture.[102] In favor of the cruciate disease being secondary to some immune disorder: (1) proper immunosuppressive drug therapy early in the course of the disease often renders affected animals sound, (2) the subset of dogs with

this form of CCL rupture is different from the older, sedentary, overweight spayed female dogs that develop classic ligament degeneration, (3) breeds of dogs that suffer from this disorder tend to be the breeds that are afflicted by other immunologic diseases, and (4) inflammation can sometimes be detected in joints other than the affected stifles.

Regardless of the ultimate cause, it would be prudent to treat atypical cases of CCL rupture with inflammatory synovial fluids medically as early in the disease course as possible and to augment or replace medical treatment with surgery in more advanced cases or in animals that fail to respond medically. Medical treatment would be the same as for other immunologic arthritides.

Drug-Induced Arthritis.

Drug-induced vasculitides, usually manifested by acute skin and joint involvement, are becoming increasingly common in dogs, especially as the proportion of purebred animals increases.[103] The most common drug hypersensitivity is to trimethoprim-sulfa, although we have observed identical disease after the use of penicillins, erythromycin, lincomycin, and cephalosporins. Drug reactions involve the deposition of drug-antibody complexes around blood vessels in different areas of the body. The drug may act directly as an antigen or may combine with host proteins as haptens to form neoantigens.

Polyarthritis is only one feature of the disease syndrome; fever, lymphadenopathy, and various types of macular-papular or bullous-type hemorrhagic rashes frequently accompany the disease. Joint fluid contains large numbers of nondegenerative neutrophils. The first sign of the allergic reaction tends to occur 10 to 21 days after drug treatment is initiated for some other condition. This is the time period during which sensitization occurs. Alternatively, drug reactions may occur within hours of administering a drug that had been used safely in the past. Affected dogs become acutely febrile, stiff, and sore and develop a generalized rash. The rash can take several forms, but individual lesions on the skin are clearly of a vascular origin with hemorrhagic blistering, focal necrosis with hemorrhage, severe focal petechiation, and so forth. Additional features may include lymphadenopathy, polymyositis, anemia, glomerulonephritis, focal retinitis, leukopenia, and thrombocytopenia. The diagnosis is readily apparent if the clinician connects drug treatment with the onset of an acute vasculitis syndrome involving primarily skin and joints. This linkage may be missed, especially if it is assumed that the condition is merely an extension of the condition for which the treatment was prescribed. There is rapid resolution of signs upon discontinuation of drug treatment, although whirlpool baths and glucocorticoids may be required to speed the healing of the skin lesions.

Treatment of Immune-Mediated Arthritides

The first imperative is to determine whether the arthritis is associated with some significant underlying disease process. When inciting diseases are present, treatment should be concentrated on the underlying cause first and the immune arthritis second. The objective of therapy should be complete remission, which correlates with the disappearance of synovial fluid abnormalities and not just a return to some perception of "outward normalcy." Allowing the joint disease to simmer slowly during inadequate treatment can lead to secondary DJD over a period of months or years. Moreover, accepting less than complete remission does the animal an unkindness, because even more clinical improvement can be expected with total remission.

Treatment of Idiopathic Polyarthritis, Systemic

Lupus Erythematosus, Plasmacytic-Lymphocytic Synovitis. A clinically acceptable reduction of joint inflammation can be achieved with glucocorticoids alone in about one third of cases. A higher percentage can be treated with glucocorticoids alone if the dosage is kept high and the therapy continued over long periods of time. The side effects of such long-term high-dose therapy are so great, however, that combination drug therapy is preferable.

Dogs started with glucocorticoids alone should receive prednisone or prednisolone at 1.5 mg/lb (3.0 mg/kg) daily (one fifth of this daily dosage for dexamethasone) if they are over 30 to 40 pounds (15 to 20 kg) in weight and 2 mg/lb (4 mg/kg) if they are smaller. The total daily dosage may be divided morning and night for the first 2 weeks to help limit acute side effects. The animals should be carefully reexamined 2 weeks later. This examination should include both a history of therapeutic response and synovial fluid analysis. Care must be taken to tap only the joints that were previously inflamed; only a single joint needs to be sampled at the reexamination. If the synovial fluid is greatly improved (cell count less than 4000/mm^3 and most of the cells mononuclear), the glucocorticoid therapy is likely to be effective by itself. It then becomes a matter of slowly decreasing the glucocorticoid dosage at 2-week intervals. The goal is to have the animal in full remission with no more than 0.5 mg/lb (1 mg/kg) prednisone or prednisolone every other day. The interval between the instigation of therapy and attainment of this dosage level varies from animal to animal but is usually 4 to 10 weeks. Glucocorticoid dosages should not be decreased unless there is a progressive improvement in synovial fluid total cell and neutrophil counts from one 2-week examination period to the next. If clinical signs reappear before maintenance levels of glucocorticoids are reached, the animals should be treated with combination drug therapy. If clinical signs and synovial fluid values return to normal with maintenance therapy, the animal should be treated for at least 2 to 3 more months before being weaned from all glucocorticoids.

If there is not a substantial improvement in both clinical signs and joint fluid abnormalities by the second week of high-dose glucocorticoid therapy, combination drug therapy is probably indicated. Animals that require high-dose glucocorticoids to maintain remission are also candidates for combination drug therapy. Dogs that cannot tolerate initial high-dose glucocorticoid therapy will also benefit from combination therapy. Cytotoxic drugs work synergistically with glucocorticoids and can reduce by one half or more the initial dosages of glucocorticoids. Combination drug therapy always refers to the use of a glucocorticoid along with one or more other immunosuppressive drugs. Non-steroid immunosuppressives usually do not work well by themselves, but when used with the previously described regimen of glucocorticoid therapy, bring about complete remission in 2 to 16 weeks. Non-steroidal immunosuppressive drugs are discontinued 1 to 3 months after complete remission is achieved. Remission is defined by both the disappearance of clinical signs and normal synovial fluids. Remission can usually be maintained after this time with 0.5 mg/lb (1.0 mg/kg) body weight prednisolone or prednisone every other day. At this point the therapeutic regimen is the same as that described originally for glucocorticoids alone. If clinical signs and/or synovial fluid abnormalities reappear with glucocorticoids alone, combination immunosuppressive drug therapy should be reinstated and maintained indefinitely.

Of the various nonsteroidal immunosuppressive drugs, cyclophosphamide and the thiopurines (azathioprine, 6-mercaptopurine) are currently the drugs of choice. As more experience is gained with newer immunosuppressants, such as leflunomide, this may change. Cyclophosphamide, a nitrogen mustard, works by its cross-linking effect on DNA. It is a potent inhibitor of both T and B cell–related immune responses and is active against resting as well as dividing cells. Azathioprine is cleaved by the liver to two molecules of 6-mercaptopurine, the active ingredient. 6-Mercaptopurine is a purine antagonist and has its major effect against RNA synthesis and rapidly dividing cells. It is a potent inhibitor of cellular and to a lesser extent humoral immunity. Cyclophosphamide is often preferable to the thiopurines in initiating a remission, but because of the high incidence of sterile hemorrhagic cystitis associated with the chronic (more than 4 months) use of this drug in dogs, the thiopurines are preferred for long-term maintenance in dogs when combination drug therapy is necessary. Thiopurines can be used for remission induction therapy but take longer than cyclophosphamide to have the same effect. These are only general rules, however. Individual animals may respond much better to thiopurines and glucocorticoids than to cyclophosphamide and glucocorticoids.

The dosage of cyclophosphamide that is most satisfactory is 1.2 mg/lb (2.5 mg/kg) body weight for dogs less than 22 pounds (10 kg) and cats, 1 mg/lb (2 mg/kg) for animals from 20 to 50 pounds (10 to 25 kg), and 0.8 mg/lb (1.75 mg/kg) for larger animals. This dosage is given orally once daily on 4 consecutive days of each week or every other day. Cyclophosphamide should always be administered with glucocorticoids because of their strong synergy. Glucocorticoids are given as outlined previously or, if necessary, at one half the dosages listed for glucocorticoids alone. It is important that cyclophosphamide not be used much longer than 4 months in dogs because of potential problems with sterile hemorrhagic cystitis. This is not a complication with cats. The cystitis is initially manifested by frequent and painful urination and microscopic hematuria. The hematuria becomes grossly apparent if therapy is continued. If the drug is discontinued when signs first appear, the dysuria resolves spontaneously in 4 to 8 weeks. If a cytotoxic drug such as cyclophosphamide is required to maintain remission, a thiopurine should be substituted for cyclophosphamide after the fourth month. If the animal was previously found to be poorly responsive to thiopurines, another mustard compound such as chlorambucil can be substituted for the cyclophosphamide. In our experience, chlorambucil is not as effective for induction therapy but may be adequate for maintenance of remission. The combination of prednisolone and chlorambucil is particularly good for SLE in cats.

Azathioprine and 6-mercaptopurine are both given to dogs at a dosage of 1.0 mg/lb (2.0 mg/kg) body weight orally daily for the first 2 to 3 weeks, then at this dosage every other day (usually on alternating days with the glucocorticoids). In dogs heavier than 50 pounds (25 kg), the dosage of azathioprine should be reduced to 0.8 mg/lb (1.75 mg/kg) per day. Azathioprine or 6-mercaptopurine should always be administered with glucocorticoids, as for cyclophosphamide. The drug is much more toxic in cats than in dogs and should probably be used at one fourth or less of the small-dog dosage and with close monitoring of the complete blood count. Bone marrow and immune suppression associated with long-term combination drug therapy is not a problem with proper dosages. Malignant skin tumors (melanomas and fibrosarcomas) are a complication of chronic (many years) therapy in dogs, and oral squamous cell carcinomas are a potential complication of long-term combination therapy in cats.

Complete blood counts are determined for all animals receiving cyclophosphamide or azathioprine, beginning 2 weeks after the initiation of treatment. If the white blood cell count falls to 6000/mm^3 and the platelet count below 125,000/mm^3, the cytotoxic drug dosage should be reduced by one fourth. If the white blood cell count falls below 4000/mm^3 and the platelet count below 100,000/mm^3, cytotoxic drugs should be discontinued for 1 week and then reinstated at one half of the previous dosage. The thiopurines are more likely to be associated with bone marrow suppression than cyclophosphamide. Thiopurine-induced bone marrow suppression usually occurs from 4 to 6 weeks after beginning treatment, whereas cyclophosphamide often takes many months.

Leflunomide is a new immunosuppressive drug that works through the inhibition of pyrimidine biosynthesis and protein tyrosine kinase activity.[104] It has proved highly effective for the treatment of rheumatologic diseases and allograft or xenograft rejection in humans and animals.[105, 106] Leflunomide has also been highly effective in the treatment of conventional drug refractory immune cytopenias and inflammatory central nervous system disorders in dogs.[107] The initial dose is 4 mg/kg once daily by month for dogs; there is considerable variability in uptake, so after several days the dosage is adjusted to achieve plasma trough levels of about 20 μg/mL. Leflunomide is intestinally necrotizing to dogs when used at higher dosages. The drug appears to be safe for cats. The immunosuppressive effect of leflunomide is synergistic with that of prednisolone, cyclosporine, cyclophosphamide, and azathioprine. Leflunomide differs from cyclophosphamide and azathioprine in that it can often sustain remission of immunologic disorders in the absence of corticosteroids.

It is important to use synovial fluid analysis to determine when complete remission has been achieved. Dogs and cats may return to near clinical normalcy with treatment but still demonstrate mild synovial inflammation. If low-grade inflammation is allowed to persist, DJD gradually occurs and complicates the overall clinical picture. It is prudent, therefore, to select several joints that initially showed inflammatory changes and reexamine fluid from these joints periodically during drug therapy.

If, during drug therapy, there is a drastic change in the clinical appearance of the lameness, immediate reevaluation of the status of the joint disease is imperative. The authors have seen dogs that developed septic arthritis or severe DJD months after being treated for immune-mediated arthritis. It is a grave mistake to reinstitute or intensify drug therapy on the presumption that it is the same disorder.

Treatment of Rheumatoid Arthritis. In order to avoid permanent joint damage, canine rheumatoid arthritis should be treated early and aggressively. Combination drug therapy is therefore essential, usually with prednisolone and azathioprine. Azathioprine is preferred to cyclophosphamide because therapy is often lifelong. Gold salt therapy has been used for the treatment of canine rheumatoid arthritis. It is not effective in inducing remission and usually requires the concurrent use of a glucocorticoid. Leflunomide has shown great promise in rheumatoid arthritis in people and immune-mediated cytopenias and encephalitides in dogs.[106]

Treatment of Enteropathic Arthritis. The overlying enteric disease should be the primary target of treatment. The arthritis can be controlled with minimal treatment, such as aspirin, provided the bowel disease can be controlled.

Immunosuppressive drugs are indicated only when the bowel disease can be controlled by their use. In some cases, immunosuppresive drugs can actually worsen the overlying colitis and can also make the joint disease worse.

REFERENCES

1. Olsson SE: Degenerative joint disease (osteoarthrosis): A review with special reference to the dog. J Small Anim Pract 12:333, 1971.
2. Alexander JW: Osteoarthrosis (degenerative joint disease) in the dog. Canine Pract 6(1):31, 1979.
3. Olewski JM, et al: Degenerative joint disease: Multiple joint involvement in young and mature dogs. Am J Vet Res 44:1300, 1983.
4. Lust G: An overview of the pathogenesis of canine hip dysplasia. JAVMA 210:1443, 1997.
5. Farquhar T, et al: Variations in composition of cartilage from the shoulder joints of young adult dogs at risk for developing canine hip dysplasia. JAVMA 210:1483, 1997.
6. Tirgari M, Vaughan MC: Arthritis of the canine stifle joint. Vet Rec 96:394, 1975.
7. Ljunggren GL, Olsson SE: Osteoarthrosis of the shoulder and elbow joints in dogs: A pathologic and radiographic study of a necropsy material. J Am Vet Radiol Soc 16:33, 1975.
8. Morgan JP, et al: Primary degenerative joint disease of the shoulder in a colony of beagles. JAVMA 190:531, 1987.
9. Mitchell NS, Cruess RL: Classification of degenerative arthritis. Can Med Assoc J 117:763, 1977.
10. Van Bree H, et al: Magnetic resonance arthrography of the scapulohumeral joint in dogs, using gadopentetate dimeglumine. Am J Vet Res 56:286, 1995.
11. Van Bree H: Evaluation of subchondral lesion size in osteochondrosis of the scapulohumeral joint in dogs. JAVMA 204:1472, 1994.
12. Bohndorf K: Osteochondritis (osteochondrosis) dissecans: A review and new MRI classification. Eur Radiol (1):103, 1998.
13. Kippenes H, Johnston G: Diagnostic imaging of osteochondrosis. Vet Clin North Am Small Anim Pract 28:137, 1998.
14. Fife RS, et al: The presence of cartilage matrix glycoprotein in serum as determined by immunolocation analysis is not a sensitive indicator of "early" osteoarthritis of the knee. J Lab Clin Med 117:332, 1991.
15. Scher DM, et al: Biologic markers of arthritis. Am J Orthop 25:263, 1996.
16. Arican M, et al: Hyaluronan in canine arthropathies. J Comp Pathol 111:185, 1994.
17. Arican M, et al: Osteocalcin in canine joint diseases. Br Vet J 152:411, 1996.
18. Millis DL, Levine D: The role of exercise and physical modalities in the treatment of osteoarthritis. Vet Clin North Am Small Anim Pract 27:913, 1997.
19. Booth NH: Non-narcotic analgesics. In Jones LM, et al (eds): Veterinary Pharmacology and Therapeutics, 4th ed. Ames, Iowa State University Press, 1977, p 351.
20. Romatowski J: Comparative therapeutics of canine and human rheumatoid arthritis. JAVMA 185:558, 1984.
21. Daehler MH: Transmural pyloric perforation associated with naproxen administration in a dog. JAVMA 189:694, 1986.
22. Spyridakis LK, et al: Ibuprofen toxicosis in a dog. JAVMA 188:918, 1986.
23. Rupp C, Suter PF: Kurmitteilung an Tierarzte betreffend moglicher Nebenwirkungen von Diclofenac (voltaren) bei hunden. Schweiz Arch Tierheilkd 127:660, 1985.
24. Fox SM, Johnston SA: Use of carprofen for the treatment of pain and inflammation in dogs. JAVMA 210:1493, 1997.
25. Vasseur PB, et al: Randomized, controlled trial of the efficacy of carprofen, a nonsteroidal anti-inflammatory drug, in the treatment of osteoarthritis in dogs. JAVMA 206:807, 1995.
26. MacPhail CM, et al: Hepatocellular toxicosis associated with administration of carprofen in 21 dogs. JAVMA 212:1895, 1998.
27. Caron JP, et al: Results of a survey of equine practitioners on the use and perceived efficacy of polysulfated glycosaminoglycan. JAVMA 209:1564, 1996.
28. Kelly GS: The role of glucosamine sulfate and chondroitin sulfates in the treatment of degenerative joint disease. Altern Med Rev 3:27, 1998.
28a. de Haan JJ, et al: Evaluation of polysulfated glucosaminoglycan for the treatment of hip dysplasia in dogs. Vet Surg 23:177, 1994.
29. Huber DJ, et al: A clinical evaluation of oral glucosamine and glucosaminoglycans as a treatment for canine hip dysplasia. Vet Orthop Soc Abstracts, 1996.
30. Klee S, Ungemach FR: [Pharmacotherapy of degenerative joint diseases in dogs.] Tierarztl Prax 26:1, 1998.
31. Hickman J: Greyhound injuries. J Small Anim Pract 16:455, 1976.
32. Prole JHB: Greyhound injuries. Correspondence. J Small Anim Pract 17:197, 1976.
33. Rendoano VT, Abdinoor D: Management of intra- and extra-articular extremity gunshot wounds. J Am Anim Hosp Assoc 13:577, 1977.
34. Renegar WR, Stoll SG: Gunshot wounds involving the canine carpus: Surgical management. J Am Anim Hosp Assoc 16:233, 1980.
35. Salazar I, et al: Spavin: A proposed term for a non–fracture associated canine hock lesion. Vet Rec 115:541, 1984.
36. Prole JHB: Canine spavin (correspondence). Vet Rec 115:607, 1984.
37. Stobie D, et al: Chronic bicipital tenosynovitis in dogs: 29 cases (1985–1992). JAVMA 207:201, 1995.

MSJ

38. McLaughlin RM Jr: Traumatic joint luxations in small animals. Vet Clin North Am Small Anim Pract 25:1175, 1995.
39. Whitehair JG, et al: Epidemiology of cranial cruciate ligament rupture in dogs. JAVMA 203:1016, 1993.
40. Robins G, Grandage J: Temporomandibular joint dysplasia and open-mouth jaw locking in the dog. JAVMA 171:1072, 1977.
41. Flo GL, DeYoung D: Meniscal injuries and medial meniscectomy in the canine stifle. J Am Anim Hosp Assoc 14:683, 1978.
42. Nunamaker DM, Newton CD: Canine hip disorders. In Bojrab MJ (ed): Current Techniques in Small Animal Surgery. Philadelphia, Lea & Febiger, 1975, p 437.
43. Llewellyn HR: Growth plate injuries—Diagnosis, prognosis and treatment. J Am Anim Hosp Assoc 12:77, 1976.
44. Harari J: Osteochondrosis of the femur. Vet Clin North Am Small Anim Pract 1:87, 1998.
45. Mason TA, et al: Osteochondrosis of the elbow joint in young dogs. J Small Anim Pract 21:641, 1980.
46. Johnson KA, et al: Osteochondrosis in the hock joints in dogs. JAAHA 16:103, 1980.
47. Fitch RB, Beale BS: Osteochondrosis of the canine tibiotarsal joint. Vet Clin North Am Small Anim Pract 28:95, 1998.
48. Richardson DC, Zentek J: Nutrition and osteochondrosis. Vet Clin North Am Small Anim Pract 28:115, 1998.
49. Carlson CS, et al: Osteochondrosis of the articular–epiphyseal cartilage complex in young horses: Evidence for a defect in cartilage canal blood supply. Vet Pathol 32:641, 1995.
50. Weiss S, Loeffler K: [Histological study of cartilage channels in the epiphyseal cartilage of young dogs and their relationship to that of osteochondrosis dissecans in the most frequently affected locations.] Dtsch Tierarztli Wochenschr 103(5):164, 1996.
51. Berzon JL: Osteochondritis dissecans in the dog: Diagnosis and therapy. JAVMA 175:796, 1979.
52. van Bree HJ, Van Ryssen B: Diagnostic and surgical arthroscopy in osteochondrosis lesions. Vet Clin North Am Small Anim Pract 28:161, 1998.
53. Swenson L, et al: Prevalence and inheritance of and selection for elbow arthrosis in Bernese Mountain Dogs and rottweilers in Sweden and benefit:cost analysis of a screening and control program. JAVMA 210:215, 1997.
54. Thomson MJ, Robins GM: Osteochondrosis of the elbow: A review of the pathogenesis and a new approach to treatment. Austr Vet J 72:375, 1995.
55. Boulay JP: Fragmented medial coronoid process of the ulna in the dog. Vet Clin North Am Small Anim Pract 28:51, 1998.
56. Bouck GR, et al: A comparison of surgical and medical treatment of fragmented coronoid process and osteochondritis dessicans of the canine elbow. Vet Comp Orthop Traumatol 8:172, 1995.
57. Morgan JP, Stephens M: Radiographic Diagnosis and Control of Canine Hip Dysplasia. Ames, Iowa State University Press, 1986.
58. Fries CL, Remedios AM: The pathogenesis and diagnosis of canine hip dysplasia: A review. Can Vet J 36:494, 1995.
59. Cardinet GH 3rd, et al: Association between pelvic muscle mass and canine hip dysplasia. JAVMA 210:1466, 1997.
60. Smith GK, et al: Evaluation of risk factors for degenerative joint disease associated with hip dysplasia in dogs. JAVMA 206:642, 1995.
61. Smith GK, et al: Reliability of the hip distraction index in two-month-old German shepherd dogs. JAVMA 212:1560, 1998.
62. Popovitch CA, et al: Comparison of susceptibility for hip dysplasia between rottweilers and German shepherd dogs. JAVMA 206:648, 1995.
63. Wallace LJ, et al: Pectineus tendon or muscle surgery for treatment of clinical hip dysplasia in the dog. In Bojrab MJ (ed): Current Techniques in Small Animal Surgery. Philadelphia, Lea & Febiger, 1975, p 443.
64. Bonneau NH, Breton L: Excision arthroplasty of the femoral head. Canine Pract 8:13, 1981.
65. Olmstead ML: Canine cemented total hip replacements: State of the art. J Small Anim Pract 36:395, 1995.
66. Kealy RD, et al: Five-year longitudinal study on limited food consumption and development of osteoarthritis in coxofemoral joints of dogs. JAVMA 210:222, 1997.
67. Kaneene JB, et al: Retrospective cohort study of changes in hip joint phenotype of dogs in the United States. JAVMA 211:1542, 1997.
68. Robinson R, Pedersen NC: Normal genetics, genetic disorders, developmental anomalies, and breeding programs. In Pedersen NC: Feline Husbandry. American Veterinary Publications, Goleta, CA, pp 75–76, 1991.
69. Madewell BR, Pool R: Neoplasms of joints and related structures. Vet Clin North Am 8:511, 1978.
70. Montgomery RD, et al: Comparison of aerobic culturette, synovial membrane biopsy, and blood culture medium in detection of canine bacterial arthritis. Vet Surg 18:300, 1989.
71. Popovic N, et al: [The importance of Lyme borreliosis in veterinary medicine.] Glas Srp Akad Nauka [Med] 43:277, 1993.
72. Kornblatt AN, et al: Arthritis caused by Borrelia burgdorferi in dogs. JAVMA 186:960, 1985.
73. Straubinger RK, et al: Borrelia burgdorferi migrates into joint capsules and causes an up-regulation of interleukin-8 in synovial membranes of dogs experimentally infected with ticks. Infect Immun 65:1273, 1997.
74. Salinas-Melendez JA, et al: Detection of Borrelia burgdorferi DNA in human skin biopsies and dog synovial fluid by the polymerase chain reaction. Rev Latinoam Microbiol 37:7, 1995.
75. Reid MC, et al: The consequences of overdiagnosis and overtreatment of Lyme disease: An observational study. Ann Intern Med 128:354, 1998.
76. Horowitz HW, Wormser GP: Doxycycline revisited: An old medicine for emerging diseases (letter). Arch Intern Med 158:192, 1998.
77. Carro T, et al: Subcutaneous abscesses and arthritis caused by a probable bacterial L-form in cats. JAVMA 194:1583, 1989.
78. Harrus S, et al: Clinical manifestations of infectious canine cyclic thrombocytopenia. Vet Rec 141:247, 1997.
79. Mathew JS, et al: Characterization of a new isolate of Ehrlichia platys (Order Rickettsiales) using electron microscopy and polymerase chain reaction. Vet Parasitol 68:1, 1997.
80. Goldman EE, et al: Granulocytic ehrlichiosis in dogs from North Carolina and Virginia. J Vet Intern Med 12:61, 1998.
81. Cowell RL, et al: Ehrlichiosis and polyarthritis in three dogs. JAVMA 192:1093, 1998.
82. Breitschwerdt EB, et al: Prednisolone at anti-inflammatory or immunosuppressive dosages in conjunction with doxycycline does not potentiate the severity of Rickettsia rickettsii infection in dogs. Antimicrob Agents Chemother 41:141, 1997.
83. Breitschwerdt EB, et al: Doxycycline hyclate treatment of experimental canine ehrlichiosis followed by challenge inoculation with two Ehrlichia canis strains. Antimicrob Agents Chemother 42:362, 1998.
84. Matthewman LA, et al: Further evidence for the efficacy of imidocarb dipropionate in the treatment of Ehrlichia canis infection. J S Afr Vet Assoc 65:104, 1994.
85. Bayer AS: Arthritis associated with common viral infections. Mumps, coxsackievirus, and adenovirus. Postgrad Med 68:55, 1980.
86. Pedersen NC, et al: A transient febrile limping syndrome of kittens caused by two different strains of feline calicivirus. Feline Pract 13:26, 1983.
87. Church RE: Lameness in kittens after vaccination. Vet Rec 125:609, 1989.
88. May C, et al: Immune responses to canine distemper virus in joint diseases of dogs. Br J Rheumatol 33:27, 1994.
89. Chapman WL Jr, Hanson WL: Leishmaniasis. In Greene CE (ed): Clinical Microbiology and Infectious Disease of the Dog and Cat. Philadelphia, WB Saunders, 1984, p 764.
90. Pedersen NC, et al: Noninfectious canine arthritis: Rheumatoid arthritis. JAVMA 169:295, 1976.
91. Colbatzky F, et al: AA-like amyloid deposits confined to arthritic joints in two dogs with rheumatoid arthritis. J Comp Pathol 105:331, 1991.
92. Chabanne L, et al: IgM and IgA rheumatoid factors in canine polyarthritis. Vet Immunol Immunopathol 39:365, 1993.
93. Nielsen OL: Detection of IgM rheumatoid factor in canine serum using a standardized enzyme-linked immunosorbent assay. Vet Immunol Immunopathol 34:139, 1992.
94. Woodard JC, et al: Erosive polyarthritis in two greyhounds. JAVMA 198:873, 1991.
95. Pedersen NC, et al: Feline chronic progressive polyarthritis. Am J Vet Res 41:522, 1980.
96. Pedersen NC, et al: Noninfectious canine arthritis: The inflammatory, nonerosive arthritides. JAVMA 169:304, 1976.
97. Pedersen NC, Barlough JE: Systemic lupus erythematosus in the cat. Feline Pract 19:5, 1991.
98. Monestier M, et al: Autoantibodies to histone, DNA and nucleosome antigens in canine systemic lupus erythematosus. Clin Exp Immunol 99:37, 1995.
99. Dougherty SA, et al: Juvenile-onset polyarthritis syndrome in Akitas. JAVMA 198:849, 1991.
100. Rivas AL, et al: A canine febrile disorder associated with elevated interleukin-6. Clin Immunol Immunopathol 64:36, 1992.
101. White SD, et al: Juvenile cellulitis in dogs: 15 cases (1979–1988). JAVMA 195:1609, 1989.
102. Bari AS, et al: Anti-type II collagen antibody in naturally occurring canine joint diseases. Br J Rheumatol 28:480, 1989.
103. Giger U, et al: Sulfadiazine-induced allergy in six Doberman pinschers. JAVMA 186:479, 1985.
104. Zielinski T, et al: Leflunomide, a reversible inhibitor of pyrimidine biosynthesis? Inflamm Res 44(Suppl 2):S207, 1995.
105. Waer M: The use of leflunomide in transplantation immunology. Transpl Immunol 4:181, 1996.
106. Mladenovic V, et al: Safety and effectiveness of leflunomide in the treatment of patients with active rheumatoid arthritis. Results of a randomized, placebo-controlled, phase II study. Arthritis Rheum 38:1595, 1995.
107. Gregory CR, et al: Leflunomide effectively treats naturally-occurring immune mediated and inflammatory diseases of dogs that are unresponsive to conventional therapies. International Canine Immunogenetics and Immunologic Disease Conference Abstract University of California, Davis, July 31–August 2, 1998.

CHAPTER 184

SKELETAL DISEASES

Kenneth A. Johnson and A.D.J. Watson

Animals with bone disease may have signs of lameness, deformity, or dysfunction that could be confused with, or complicated by, joint, muscle, or neurologic disorders. Therefore, a systematic approach is necessary in evaluating animals with these signs. The expertise of a radiologist and a bone pathologist is often invaluable in establishing a diagnosis. Traumatic injuries should also be considered in the differential diagnosis but are not discussed here, as excellent descriptions exist elsewhere.[1] Some bone diseases that also affect joints are described in Chapter 183.

The precise etiology of many bone diseases that affect dogs and cats is unknown. Furthermore, some conditions have multiple etiologies, such as the congenital, heritable, and metabolic disorders. This makes logical classification difficult. An etiologic system is used here for want of a better alternative.

BONE PATHOPHYSIOLOGY

STRUCTURAL ORGANIZATION OF BONE

Bone is a living tissue with several important functions, including storage of calcium, phosphorus, and other minerals. Bones act as a series of levers that facilitate the action of muscles and joints in movement, and they provide support and protection for other body systems. In addition, bone marrow is the source of hematopoiesis and osteogenic precursor cells.[2] Bones are structurally composed of compact (cortical) and cancellous (trabecular) bone (Fig. 184–1).[3] The microstructural units of cortical bone are osteons that in cross section have concentric layers of collagen fibers and a central canal. Trabeculae of cancellous bone have a three-dimensional lattice arrangement and large intertrabecular spaces containing hemopoietic or fatty marrow tissue. Long bones have several distinct regions: diaphysis, metaphysis, and epiphysis (see Fig. 184–1). In growing animals, each epiphysis contains one or more ossification centers, is covered by hyaline cartilage on the articular surface, and is separated from the metaphysis by the physis or growth plate.[4]

Bone cells are derived from two separate cell systems: the stromal fibroblastic (osteoblasts and osteocytes) and hemopoietic (osteoclasts) systems.[2, 5] During bone formation, osteoblasts synthesize collagenous matrix called osteoid, which is mineralized to become bone. Osteoblasts entrapped in newly forming bone become osteocytes. At sites of normal skeletal growth and remodeling, osteoblasts are derived from determined osteoblast precursor cells that reside in bone marrow stroma, endosteum, and periosteum. In injury or disease, inducible osteogenic precursor cells derived from other mesenchymal tissues, such as muscle and fibrous tissue, can be stimulated to differentiate to osteoblasts and form extraperiosteal ectopic bone. Osteoblasts can form several different types of bone.[3] Lamellar bone, which has collagen fibers in a parallel array, is found in osteons and mature trabecular bone. Formation of lamellar bone requires a preexisting matrix, such as calcified cartilage matrix (so-called endochondral ossification) or old bone that has been partially removed by osteoclastic resorption. Woven bone is characterized by the random orientation of its collagen fibers. It can be deposited de novo, without preexisting bone or cartilage, and is formed when new bone is laid down rapidly in growth, fracture repair, and bone disease.[6] Normally it is remodeled to lamellar bone, but it may persist in rapidly growing osteogenic tumors.

Osteoclasts are large, multinucleate cells formed by fusion of circulating mononuclear cells. They are found on the surface of bone trabeculae and within remodeling osteons and are responsible for bone removal during growth, modeling, and remodeling of the skeleton. Osteoclasts erode mineralized bone first by solubilizing mineral, then digesting the protein.[5] This leaves concave pits in the bone surface, called Howship's lacunae. Formation and resorption of bone are regulated systemically by parathyroid hormone, calcitonin, and vitamin D (see Chapter 149). The principal action of parathyroid hormone is to activate osteoclastic bone resorption and increase blood calcium concentration. Osteoblasts have parathyroid hormone receptors, but osteoclasts do not. The increase in osteoclast number and activity induced by parathyroid hormone is mediated by osteoblasts via a complex coupling mechanism involving several cytokines, including interleukins and tumor necrosis factor.[5, 7]

BONE GROWTH AND DEVELOPMENT

Growth of the axial and appendicular skeleton is primarily by endochondral ossification at the physes. Most physeal

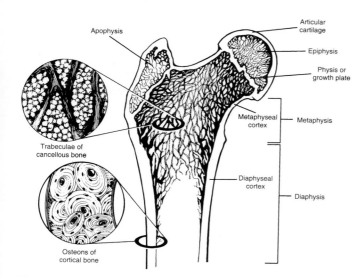

Figure 184–1. Regions and microstructure of an immature proximal femur.

Apophysis

Trabeculae of cancellous bone

Osteons of cortical bone

Articular cartilage

Epiphysis

Physis or growth plate

Metaphyseal cortex — Metaphysis

Diaphyseal cortex

Diaphysis

MSJ

growth is longitudinal, but the zone of Ranvier and subperiosteal appositional growth contribute circumferential expansion as well. Physes have various zones that reflect chondrocytic structure and metabolic activity, but the transition between zones is gradual (Fig. 184–2). Once formed, each chondrocyte remains in a fixed anatomic location throughout its life and there accomplishes all its functions.[8, 9] The two most prominent stages involve proliferation and hypertrophy (including mineralization of matrix) before tissue resorption during vascularization. Most of the longitudinal growth of a physis is due to the 10-fold increase in chondrocyte volume that is maximal in the hypertrophic zone. The final height of a hypertrophic chondrocyte is 40 μm and so, for example, the daily generation of eight new chondrocytes produces approximately 320 μm of physeal growth per day.[8] Defects in any part of the sequence, such as incomplete chondrocyte maturation, cause dwarfism or disordered bone growth (see Fig. 184–2).

MODELING OF BONE

Modeling is the process in which the contours of expanding bones are molded and sculpted during growth. Within the metaphysis, the primary spongiosa is modeled to secondary spongiosa, which in turn is resorbed to form the marrow cavity of the shaft. Simultaneously, bone diameter decreases rapidly in the metaphyseal "cutback zone" as redundant bone is removed by subperiosteal osteoclastic resorption. In modeling, bone formation rates are frequently unequal to resorption rates, but unlike remodeling, bone formation is not dependent on resorption to precede it.[10] Modeling can correct the shape of malunited fractures, deformities, and bone subjected to altered loading, as predicted by Wolff's law. However, because the modeling process is closely coupled to growth, it is usually less effective after maturity.[10]

NORMAL AND PATHOLOGIC BONE REMODELING

Remodeling is the process in which bone renews itself throughout life.[10] It always follows the sequence activation → resorption → formation, and the packets of cells at a remodeling site are collectively called bone multicellular units (Figs. 184–3 and 184–4).[10, 11] Remodeling occurs in three bone envelopes: the periosteal surface, the endosteal-trabecular (cancellous bone) surface, and the osteonal (intracortical) surface (see Figs. 184–3 and 184–4). In normal remodeling, bone formation equals resorption, whereas in bone disease a pathologic imbalance of resorption and formation results in osteopenia of cortical and cancellous bone (see Figs. 184–3 and 184–4). Bones subjected to disease, trauma, or disuse exhibit a response termed the regional acceleratory phenomenon, in which the number of activated bone multicellular units increases suddenly.[10] This results in increased cortical porosity and trabecular thinning that reaches a peak at approximately 2 to 3 months; it may take up to a year to be reversed, during which time resorption sites are refilled with new bone (Fig. 184–5).[12]

DIAGNOSIS OF BONE DISEASE

HISTORY AND SIGNS

Initially, it is important to establish the age, breed, and sex of a dog or cat as these factors may be associated with increased risk of a particular disease. Common complaints from owners are lameness, deformity, difficulty in rising, and reluctance to exercise. One must ascertain the duration and intensity (shifting, constant, intermittent, worsening) of the problem, any known trauma, and any previous illness, medication, or surgery, as well as response to therapy. The owner should be asked whether the problem is exacerbated

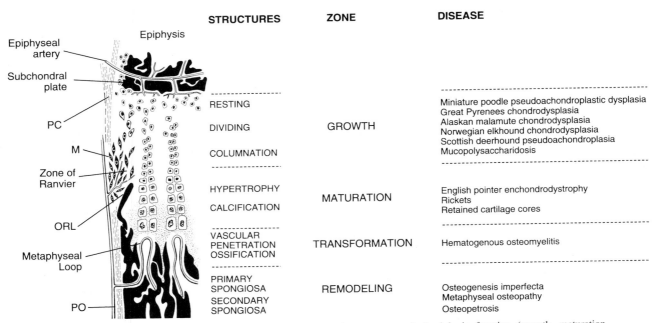

Figure 184–2. The physis divided on the basis of histologic structure and physiologic function (growth, maturation, transformation, and remodeling). Regions affected by some diseases of growth and remodeling are indicated. In the zone of Ranvier, undifferentiated mesenchymal cells (M) give rise to chondroblasts. The periosteum (PO) and perichondrium (PC) are continuous in this region. The metaphyseal cortex also extends into this region, becoming the osseous ring of Lacroix (ORL), which acts as a peripheral restraint to the cell columns but does not impede latitudinal growth of the adjacent zone of Ranvier. (Adapted from Ogden JA: Skeletal Injury in the Child, 2nd ed. Philadelphia, WB Saunders, 1990, p 37.)

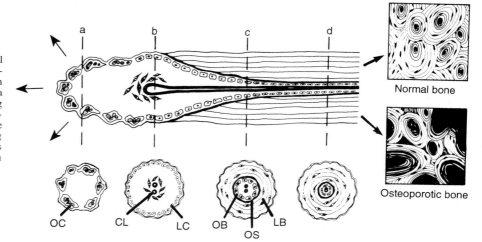

Figure 184–3. Remodeling osteon in cortical bone shown in longitudinal section. Components of this bone multicellular unit are shown in four transverse sections on the lower level: a = cutter cone with osteoclasts (OC) resorbing bone; b = capillary loop (CL) with undifferentiated lining cells (LC) in the quiescent zone between resorption and formation; c = closing cone with centripetally advancing osteoblasts (OB), separated by an osteoid seam (OS) from radially deposited new lamellar bone (LB); d = completed osteon (haversian system).

by exercise or rest and whether swelling, drainage, or apparent pain has been noticed. Recognition of similar problems in related animals may indicate heritable disease. The type and quantity of foods, vitamins, and minerals fed should be determined.

PHYSICAL EXAMINATION

In conjunction with the normal physical examination, special attention is paid to lameness and gait abnormalities and the musculoskeletal system (see Chapter 22).[13, 14] Visual appraisal might detect abnormalities in limb length and symmetry. The bony prominences and distal limb bones should be palpated to detect pain, swelling, dyssymmetry, or crepitus. By comparison with the contralateral limb, muscle atrophy or altered range of joint motion may be identified. Each abnormality alone is rather nonspecific but aids in region localization. Before proceeding with sedation and radiography, further testing should be considered to exclude neurologic disease as a contributing factor (see Chapters 106, 108, and 109).

RADIOLOGY

Radiology is the most useful method for routine noninvasive evaluation of skeletal lesions. To appreciate subtle lesions, radiographs must be excellent. Two or more views are always needed, with the limb properly positioned. Comparison with radiographs of the contralateral limb or a radiographic atlas is useful in distinguishing real bone lesions from anatomic and breed variations.[15]

Bone has a limited number of ways of responding to injury or disease. Lesions should be characterized according to changes in bone density, size, shape, or contour; type of margination; nature of any periosteal reaction; region of bone involved; and soft tissue changes.[16–18] The finding of a particular response, such as periosteal new bone, is not necessarily diagnostic of a specific disease (Table 184–1). Abnormalities could result from traumatic, neoplastic, infectious, idiopathic, or other processes. When considered in conjunction with signalment, history, and physical abnormalities, radiographic findings may lead to a diagnosis or a list of diagnostic alternatives. At this point, it is valuable to consult descriptions of various bone diseases, to evaluate the

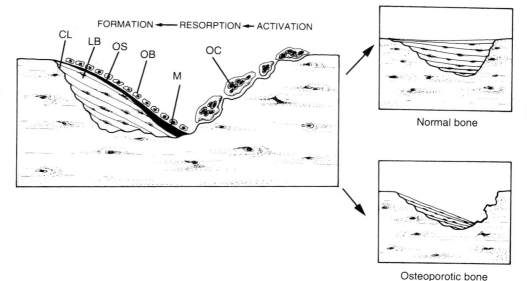

Figure 184–4. Trabecular bone remodeling with the components of bone multicellular unit: osteoclasts (OC), nonmineralized matrix (M), osteoblasts (OB), osteoid seam (OS), new lamellar bone (LB), and cement line (CL) separating it from original bone. Normally, formation equals resorption, but in diseases that cause osteoporosis, bone formation is inadequate or defective.

MSJ

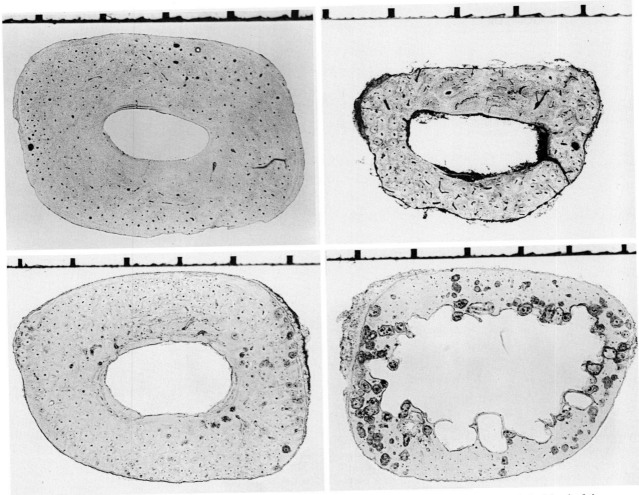

Figure 184–5. Undecalcified cross sections of right and left canine metacarpal bones sectioned at a standard level of the bone. The right forelimb was immobilized for 4 months in a non–weight-bearing situation.[12] Top row: In young adult dogs, the bone loss was primarily from the periosteal envelope. Bottom row: In old adult dogs the net loss of bone occurred primarily from the endosteal envelope. Earlier samples from the same group of animals showed increased activation of all bone envelopes with profound intracortical porosity, reflecting the regional acceleratory phenomenon caused by disuse. By 4 months the regional acceleratory phenomenon had died out, and the intracortical pores filled with new osteons, returning the intracortical envelope to near normal. (Figures courtesy of H. K. Uhthoff.)

possibilities, and to decide what further tests are indicated. Tests that are directed at confirming the most likely diagnosis, yet are least invasive and involve low morbidity, are done first.

NUCLEAR IMAGING

Scintigraphy is highly sensitive in detecting skeletal lesions but is generally not specific for etiology.[19, 20] After a radiopharmaceutical, usually technetium 99m–labeled methylene diphosphonate (^{99m}TcMDP), is injected intravenously, it is incorporated into sites of new bone formation and remodeling and in regions of increased blood flow. The distribution of radionuclide in bone is detected with a gamma camera and is an indication of skeletal metabolic activity, complementing the structural information from radiographs. In cases of lameness in which physical examination and radiographs are unremarkable, scintigraphy may pinpoint a region of increased uptake in bone or a joint. Further procedures such as computed tomography, biopsy, culture, or

surgical exploration would then be needed to determine the cause of the "hot spot."

Tumor metastases in bone have a characteristic multifocal distribution, detectable by scintigraphy before they are seen on radiographs.[20] Although scintigraphy also detects primary bone tumors, it is seldom needed for their diagnosis. Scintigraphy with ^{99m}TcMDP may help detect osteomyelitis before radiographic signs appear, but it is not specific for the disease.

COMPUTED TOMOGRAPHY

High-resolution computed tomography provides excellent cross-sectional images of lesions not found with radiographs. Its greatest application in the musculoskeletal system has been in evaluating the complex anatomy of skull, spine, and pelvis; in delineating boundaries of tumors involving soft tissues or bone; and in detecting early bone destruction.[21] For bone tumors this information allows more precise presurgical planning for en bloc resection of cranial and pelvic

TABLE 184–1. RADIOLOGIC SIGNS OF SOME COMMON BONE DISEASES

Bone loss
  Generalized and diffuse
    Primary hyperparathyroidism
    Renal secondary hyperparathyroidism
    Nuritional secondary hyperparathyroidism
    Disuse osteoporosis
  Thin cortices
    Primary hyperparathyroidism
    Renal secondary hyperparathyroidism
    Nuritional secondary hyperparathyroidism
    Disuse osteoporosis
    Neoplasia
    Osteomyelitis
    Bone cyst
  Focal
    Osteomyelitis
    Neoplasia
    Bone cyst
    Multifocal: myeloma, lymphosarcoma, metastases
  Cystic
    Congenital bone cysts
    Aneurysmal bone cysts
    Subchondral bone cysts
    Central giant cell granuloma
Bone production
  Cortical
    Osteopetrosis
    Trauma
    Remodeling of deformity
    Fracture healing
  Medullary
    Enostosis
    Myelosclerosis
    Osteomyelitis
    Sequestration
    Neoplasia
    Infarcts
    Fracture healing
  Periosteal
    Hypervitaminosis A
    Mucopolysaccharidosis
    Multiple cartilaginous exostosis
    Enostosis
    Metaphyseal osteopathy
    Craniomandibular osteopathy
    Secondary hypertrophic osteopathy
    Osteomyelitis
    Neoplasia
    Trauma

*Adapted from Allan GS: Radiographic signs of diseases affecting bone. Proceedings No 87, Orthopaedic Surgery in Dogs and Cats, The University of Sydney Postgraduate Committee in Veterinary Science, 1986, p 247.

lesions and for limb salvage in appendicular lesions (Fig. 184–6).[22–24]

MAGNETIC RESONANCE IMAGING

Advantages of magnetic resonance imaging are that high-resolution, serial, multiplanar images of skeletal soft tissues, such as ligament, tendon, menisci, and articular cartilage, can be obtained without the use of ionizing radiation. However, because this imaging modality relies on detection of changes in the orientation of mobile tissue protons within a strong magnetic field, the signal intensity of mineralized bone matrix is low. Contours of bone are mainly defined by adjacent soft tissues (periosteum, endosteum, fat, articular cartilage, and bone marrow). Subtle lesions of metaphyseal cancellous bone can be appreciated, as can displacement, compression, and invasion of soft tissue by expansile osse-

ous lesions. However, cortical bone lesions are better visualized using computed tomography.

CHEMISTRY

Estimation of blood calcium and inorganic phosphate concentrations and of alkaline phosphatase activity is occasionally useful in diagnosing bone disease. These variables are maintained within reference ranges in many skeletal diseases. Validated assays for canine parathyroid hormone and parathyroid hormone–related protein may be useful in hypercalcemic disorders (see Chapter 149).

HEMATOLOGY

Alterations in the hemogram may be consistent with acute osteomyelitis, but the hemogram is usually unremarkable in chronic osteomyelitis and other bone diseases.

BIOPSY AND HISTOPATHOLOGY

Histologic examination of a representative bone biopsy specimen is the most reliable way to establish a diagnosis, especially when the radiographic signs are not highly characteristic of a particular disease. Biopsy may be necessary to distinguish malignant from benign neoplasia, osteomyelitis, developmental lesions, and degenerative conditions. It also specifically identifies tumor type and grade, establishes the prognosis, and may dictate appropriate treatment. For various reasons, mistakes are frequent at this stage of the investigation. The most common pitfall is inappropriate sampling and submission of a biopsy specimen that is reactive bone formed secondarily to the actual disease. Because processing of bone for histology can take a week or more, such an outcome can be frustrating and misleading.

Closed needle biopsies of medium to large, solid, solitary lesions of appendicular long bones can be obtained using a 4-inch, 8- or 11-gauge Jamshidi bone biopsy needle (Sherwood Medical Company) (Fig. 184–7).[25] Although relatively small tissue cores are obtained, histopathologic evaluation of biopsies is 92 per cent accurate in differentiating neoplas-

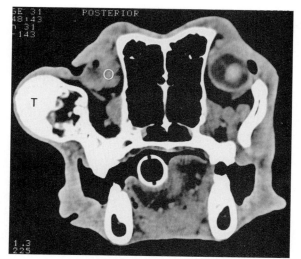

Figure 184–6. Computed tomographic image of an osteoma (T) of the zygomatic arch that caused ocular (O) displacement.

MSJ

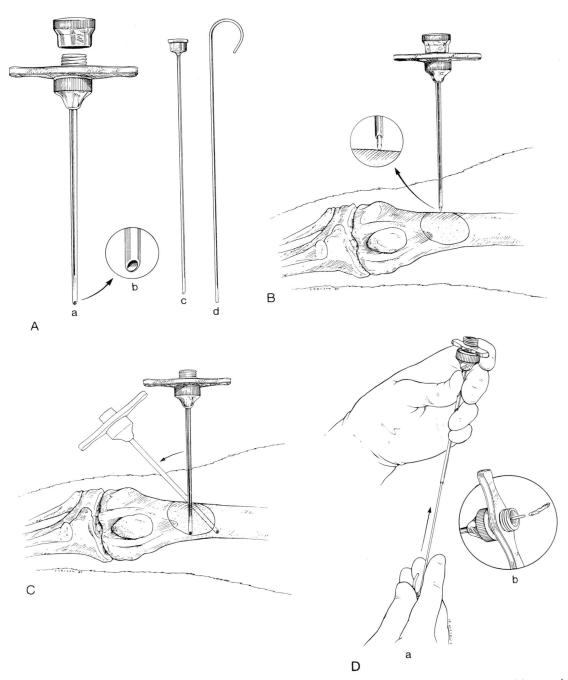

Figure 184-7. Jamshidi bone biopsy technique. *A,* Jamshidi-type bone biopsy needle: cannula and screw-on cap (a), tapered point (b), pointed stylet (c) to advance cannula through soft tissue, and probe (d) to expel specimen from cannula. *B,* With the stylet locked in place, the cannula is advanced through soft tissue until bone is reached. Inset is a close-up of the needle about to penetrate cortex. *C,* The stylet is removed, and the bone cortex is penetrated with the cannula. The cannula is withdrawn, and the procedure is repeated with redirection of the needle. *D,* The probe is inserted into the tip of the cannula (a), and the specimen is expelled through the cannula base (b). (From Powers BE, et al: Jamshidi needle biopsy for diagnosis of bone lesions in small animals. JAVMA 193:205, 1988.)

tic from non-neoplastic disease and 82 per cent accurate in identifying tumor type or specific disease such as osteomyelitis.[25] This method involves less postsurgical morbidity (pain, hematoma, infection, tumor seeding, pathologic fracture) than incisional biopsy. Carefully evaluate the radiograph to ensure that the biopsy specimen is obtained from the center of the lesion and dense reactive bone is avoided. The skin puncture site and biopsy tract must be situated so that they can be subsequently excised if the lesion is surgically resected. Two or three cores of tissue should be obtained by redirecting the needle through the same skin opening. Needle orientation can be guided with image intensification or radiography. Jamshidi needle biopsy is not suitable for lesions of small bones or lesions with recent pathologic fractures, as there may be significant hematoma in the latter. For cystic and fluid-filled lesions or those associated with extensive osteolysis and tumor necrosis, an open incisional wedge biopsy through a limited surgical approach might be necessary. Bone that appears abnormal can also be collected with a bone curette, taking care to avoid mutilating the specimen.

For investigation of diseases affecting growth and endochondral ossification, physeal biopsy specimens can be obtained percutaneously from the greater tubercle of the humerus with a Jamshidi needle.[26] For suspected metabolic bone diseases, larger specimens of cancellous bone should be collected with an 8-mm Michele trephine from the iliac crest or by excision of a segment of rib or distal ulnar diaphysis.[27]

The surgical borders of lesions excised en bloc are labeled with India ink for examination by the pathologist to ensure tumor-free margins.[28] Specimens can also be radiographed using nonscreen film or industrial film in a Faxitron cabinet system. Biopsy specimens are fixed in neutral buffered formalin for 6 to 24 hours; they must not be frozen.[6] Large bone specimens should be cut into 5-mm slabs to ensure proper fixation.[6] If osteomyelitis is suspected, a portion of the biopsy material should be separated for bacteriologic culture before the remainder is fixed in formalin. Bone specimens that cannot be cut with a scalpel are decalcified in 10 per cent formic acid before they are embedded in paraffin. Rapid decalcification in strong acids or excessive decalcification destroys cellular detail and renders the biopsy nondiagnostic. Nondecalcified bone biopsy specimens embedded in methyl methacrylate and sectioned with a sledge microtome are needed for diagnosis of some metabolic bone diseases.[29] Histologic evaluation of bone is rather specialized and requires the expertise of a pathologist with special interest and training. Most pathologists want to review the clinical data and radiographs before making a diagnosis.

CYTOLOGY

Cytologic examination of fluids and exudates obtained by sterile aspiration is valuable in early detection of acute osteomyelitis, before obvious radiographic changes occur in bone.

MICROBIOLOGY

Isolation and identification of bacteria are helpful in confirming a diagnosis of osteomyelitis, and in vitro susceptibility testing aids in antimicrobial drug selection. Cultures of pus from externally draining tracts are less than 50 per cent accurate in identifying the pathogens causing osteomyelitis, because the tracts become colonized by skin organisms and gram-negative bacteria. The best source of information on the bacteria involved is cultures of fluid collected by sterile aspiration or pus, necrotic tissue, and sequestra collected during surgical débridement.

Aerobic and anaerobic cultures should be obtained routinely, because anaerobic bacteria are involved in up to 60 per cent of bone infections in small animals.[30] Samples for aerobic culture, which should be plated out on agar within 10 to 15 minutes, are collected into a sterile container. Specimens for anaerobic culture require special handling because exposure to air for a few minutes kills sensitive anaerobes and prevents subsequent isolation. Fluid for anaerobic culture can be collected into a syringe if air is expelled and the needle capped with a rubber stopper.

When the anticipated delay in plating out samples exceeds 15 minutes, tissue samples and swabs should be placed into a reduced Cary-Blair, solidified anaerobic holding medium (BBL Port-A-Cul tubes) to exclude oxygen. Both aerobes and anaerobes may be isolated from specimens kept in anaerobic media because most aerobic bacteria are facultative anaerobes.

CONGENITAL BONE DISORDERS

Embryonic and postnatal skeletal development is complex and exquisitely susceptible to errors. Skeletal growth disorders that are apparent at birth or manifest later in young animals are of two main types: generalized dysplasias and localized malformations of individual bones. Some are caused by inherited defects and sporadic mutations, and some are due to teratogens and unidentifiable embryopathies. In humans, more than 100 such disorders, mostly inherited, have been listed in the Paris Nomenclature for Constitutional Disorders of Bone.[31] This classification is based on specific clinical, genetic, radiologic, histologic, and biochemical features. Animal diseases are not sufficiently characterized to allow complete adoption of the Paris system,[32] although some general groupings are possible (Table 184–2). Generalized dysplasias are described later with developmental and genetic disorders or with joint diseases (see Chapter 183); dysostoses are considered here.

Dysostoses include malformations of individual bones either singly or in combination. They can involve the craniofacial region, the axial bones (see Chapter 106), and extremities. Embryonic limb bud development commences with a

TABLE 184–2. SOME CONGENITAL SKELETAL DISORDERS OF SMALL ANIMALS*

Osteochondrodysplasias (abnormalities of cartilage and/or bone growth and development)
 Defects of growth of tubular bone or spine
  Multiple epiphyseal dysplasia: beagle
  Pseudoachondrodysplasia: miniature poodle, Scottish deerhound
  Chondrodysplasia: Alaskan malamute, cocker spaniel, English pointer, Great Pyrenees, Norwegian elkhound
  Ocular-skeletal dysplasia: Labrador retriever, Samoyed
  Pelger-Huët anomaly: cats
  Scottish fold osteochondrodysplasia: cats
 Disorganized development of cartilage and fibrous components
  Multiple cartilaginous exostoses (osteochondromatosis)
  Enchondroma
  Fibrous dysplasia
 Abnormalities of density, cortical diaphyseal structure, or metaphyseal molding
  Osteogenesis imperfecta
  Osteopetrosis
Primary metabolic abnormalities
 Vitamin D–dependent rickets
 Mucopolysaccharidosis
 Fucosidosis
 GM gangliosidosis
 Gaucher's disease
Dysostoses with malformation of individual bones, singly or in combination
 Hemimelia
 Phocomelia
 Amelia
 Syndactyly
 Polydactyly
 Ectrodactyly
 Segmental hemiatrophy

Adapted from Sharrard WJW: Pediatric Orthopaedics and Fractures, 3rd ed. London, Blackwell Scientific Publications, 1993.

projection of mesoderm covered by ectoderm that has an inductive apical ectodermal ridge. Subsequently, the individual bones form from cartilage anlagen and then secondary centers of ossification.[4] Three mesodermal rays (ulnar, radial, and central) contribute to pectoral limb formation; disturbances of one or more rays result in perturbations of the corresponding components of bone and associated soft tissue. Except for a few heritable disorders, most dysostoses in dogs and cats occur sporadically.

HEMIMELIA, PHOCOMELIA, AMELIA

In these conditions there is congenital absence of portions of the normal structures in an extremity. Hemimelia is either longitudinal (paraxial), with absence of the ulnar, radial, or central regions in the forelimb, or transverse, with the distal portion of the limb completely absent.

Radial agenesis is the most common paraxial hemimelia in cats and dogs. It is usually unilateral and sporadic. Bilateral radial agenesis might be an inherited autosomal recessive trait in Chihuahua dogs.[32] In radial agenesis, the radius is partially or completely absent and the ulna is shorter, thickened, and curved (Fig. 184–8). The radial carpal bone and first digit are often absent as well. Lack of a radial head support allows humeroulnar subluxation, and the range of elbow motion is reduced. The metacarpus deviates into varus, severely impairing limb function. One hypothesis is that radial agenesis and other hemimelias are a consequence of neural crest injury because limb bud embryopathies often have a segmental pattern that corresponds to the distribution of the segmental sensory nerves.[33] Treatment of radial agenesis by reconstructive surgery has rarely been successful, and amputation may be necessary. Another, less common paraxial hemimelia is tibial agenesis.[32]

Complete absence of a distal portion of a limb (congenital amputation) can be caused by transverse hemimelia, strangulation by constrictive bands, or in utero accidents.[34] In young animals presented with missing limbs, the cause may be impossible to determine as postnatal trauma can also cause amputations.

In phocomelia, an intercalary segment of limb is missing. In severe cases the paw with rudimentary digits is attached to the trunk like a seal flipper. In a golden retriever with unilateral radial and ulnar phocomelia, the limb was too short to function for locomotion, but the dog used it for balance.[35] Proximal femoral focal deficiency is a phocomelia with a missing segment of femur. In humans, this is usually a unilateral defect that is not inherited.[36] A young Dalmatian with proximal femoral focal deficiency had unilateral hindlimb shortening and muscle atrophy that became accentuated with further growth.[37] Radiographically, bone in the intertrochanteric, neck, and head regions of the femur was absent, and there was marked femoral shortening.

Amelia is complete absence of one or more limbs. Two kittens with bilateral hindlimb amelia have been reported.[32] Most animals affected by amelia probably die or are euthanized at birth.

SYNDACTYLY

Two or more digits are fused in a bony or soft tissue union in syndactyly.[6, 32] This is not clinically important in pets, and surgery is generally unwarranted unless the deformity causes lameness.[38] Congenital synostosis of adjacent metatarsal bones is a variation on digital fusion (Fig. 184–9).

POLYDACTYLY

Polydactyly is the presence of extra digits, usually on the medial side of the paw in dogs and cats. There is an inherited syndrome of skeletal defects including polydactyly and syndactyly in Australian shepherd dogs.[6] An X-linked gene was suspected. In cats, polydactyly is an inherited autosomal dominant trait.[32] Multiple hindlimb dewclaws in Great Pyrenees have similar inheritance. In Saint Bernard dogs, dewclaws may be associated with anomalous tarsal bones. Some have a large curved bone that seems to be an extension of the central tarsal bone on the medial side of the proximal row of tarsal bones (Fig. 184–10). These tarsal anomalies

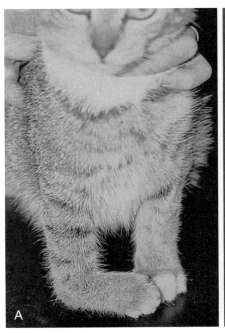
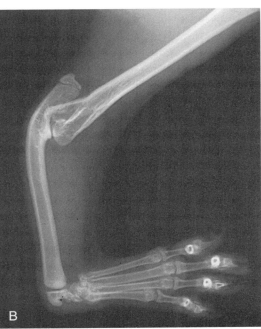

Figure 184–8. Kitten with radial agenesis. *A,* Radial agenesis and a 90-degree varus angulation of the metacarpus. *B,* The radius and radial carpal bone are absent. The proximal ulna is misshapen, the distal ulna thicker than normal, and the carpus malarticulated. (From Winterbotham EJ, et al: Radial agenesis in a cat. J Small Anim Pract 26:393, 1985.)

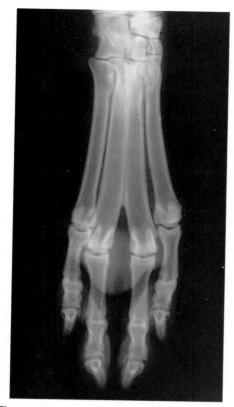

Figure 184–9. Congenital metatarsal bone synostosis.

occur bilaterally, are not associated with clinical signs, and are probably inherited.

ECTRODACTYLY

Often called split-hand or lobster-claw deformity, ectrodactyly is caused by incomplete fusion of the three rays or absence of the central ray.[36] Classically, the third metacarpal bone and digit are absent, producing a deep cleft that divides the paw into radial and ulnar parts, but many variations occur. The third metacarpal bone may be present and hypoplastic, and neighboring digits and metacarpal bones may be absent or hypoplastic.[39–41] The cleft between metacarpal bones may terminate just below the carpus or extend proximally through the carpus, separating radius and ulna entirely (Fig. 184–11).[39–41] Asynchronous radial and ulnar growth can contribute to the structural disorder at the carpus. Fifty per cent of affected dogs have concomitant congenital elbow luxation. In dogs it is usually an isolated deformity without breed predilection, but it may be inherited in cats.[6, 32] Function can be improved by reconstructive surgery or arthrodesis.[39]

SEGMENTAL HEMIATROPHY

Hemiatrophy is a misnomer because the condition is actually limb hypoplasia rather than atrophy of a normal structure. The affected forelimb is noticeably shorter and slimmer, especially in the antebrachium and paw.[42] An affected golden retriever also had darker pigmentation of skin and hair of

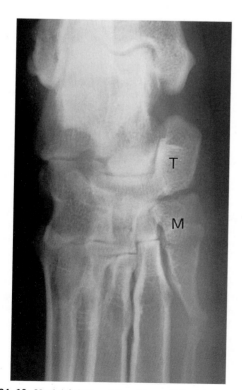

Figure 184–10. Vestigial first metatarsal bone (M) and dewclaw and an anomalous tarsal bone (T) extending medially from the central tarsal bone in a Saint Bernard.

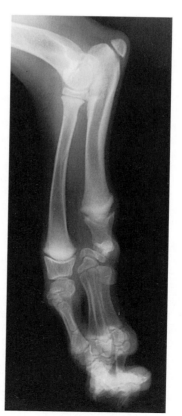

Figure 184–11. Forelimb of 12-week-old mixed-breed dog with ectrodactyly.

MSJ

the abnormal limb and horny keratinization of pads and nails but no pain or discomfort.[35] Radiographically, the carpal bones were smaller, and the numbered carpal bones were misshapen. The metacarpal bones were 3 cm shorter than contralateral bones and half normal diameter. This is a sporadic deformity and probably not inherited. It must be distinguished from atrophy that follows long-term limb immobilization.[12] A similar type of distal hypoplasia of metacarpus and digits is seen in immature dogs, subsequent to accidental trauma or surgery involving the antebrachium.[35] Ilizarov limb lengthening may be indicated if shortening impairs function.

DEVELOPMENTAL AND GENETIC BONE DISORDERS

OSTEOPETROSIS

Defective osteoclastic resorption of bone is the principal feature of osteopetrosis. In growing bones, failure of normal bone modeling results in accumulation of primary spongiosa, so that the diaphysis remains filled with bone and a marrow cavity does not form. Affected bones have a "marbled" densely homogeneous radiographic appearance, but they are actually quite fragile. There are many forms of osteopetrosis. Osteoclasts may be absent, present in reduced numbers, or defective in their ability to resorb bone.[6] The disorder is rare and not well characterized in dogs or cats.[6, 43] Idiopathic acquired osteopetrosis of adult cats was characterized by thickening of diaphyseal cortices and vertebral bodies.[43] Feline leukemia virus also produces medullary sclerosis and nonregenerative anemia in growing cats, probably through infection of hemopoietic precursor cells from which osteoclasts arise.[6]

OSTEOGENESIS IMPERFECTA

Osteogenesis imperfecta is a syndrome caused by a group of heritable diseases that are characterized by excessive bone fragility, osteopenia, and increased susceptibility to fracture. Fractured bones form callus and heal, but unless fractures are stabilized adequately, malunion and deformities occur.[44, 45] Radiographically, there can be signs of generalized osteopenia, thinning of diaphyseal cortices, and multiple fractures in various stages of union. The fundamental defect in humans is abnormal type I collagen production, mostly caused by mutations of collagen genes *COL1A1* and *COL1A2* that normally code for procollagen synthesis.[44] Structural defects in the pro-alpha1 or pro-alpha2 collagen chains of one or more incorrect amino acids may preclude normal triple helix assembly.[46] In bone, the resulting type I collagen fibrils are thin and fail to mineralize normally, which causes bone to be brittle. Osteogenesis imperfecta occurs rarely in dogs and cats, and the mode of heritability and exact biochemical defects are unknown.[32, 45, 47] Young animals may be brought to veterinarians for multiple fractures, with minimal or no trauma. Some may also have dentinogenesis imperfecta (seen as pink teeth), stunted growth, and apparent weakness.[47] Diagnosis of osteogenesis imperfecta is made by analysis of type I collagen from cultured skin fibroblasts.[47] However, the more common causes of osteopenia, including renal and nutritional secondary hyperparathyroidism, need to be eliminated first.

MUCOPOLYSACCHARIDOSIS

The mucopolysaccharidoses are a group of genetic lysosomal storage diseases caused by different specific defects in lysosomal enzymes that are normally involved in metabolism of glycosaminoglycan.[48] Compounds usually degraded by these enzymes accumulate intracellularly, interfering with cellular function and producing a characteristic set of clinical signs. Several mucopolysaccharidosis (MPS) subtypes have been characterized in cats (MPS I, VI, and VII) and dogs (MPS I, II, IIIA, and VII), but severity of skeletal abnormalities is variable among these subtypes.

Feline MPS VI is due to decreased activity of the enzyme arylsulfatase B, leading to intracellular accumulation and urinary excretion of excess dermatan sulfate.[48, 49] It is an autosomal recessive, inherited disease affecting cats of Siamese ancestry. Clinical features become evident from age 8 weeks and include small head and ears, flattened face, corneal clouding, pectus excavatum, growth retardation, skeletal deformity, and neurologic abnormalities. Affected cats have a crouching gait and manipulation of joints and cervical spine is painful. There is no primary central nervous system involvement, and hindlimb paresis or paralysis results from spinal cord compression secondary to focal bone proliferation into the spinal canal and intervertebral foramina. Radiographic features include epiphyseal dysplasia, thinning of long-bone cortices, generalized osteopenia, bilateral coxofemoral subluxation, secondary osteoarthritis, and vertebral fusion.[50] Osteopenia is progressive and is due to functional impairment of osteoblasts and decreased bone formation.[51] Diagnostic confirmation is provided by demonstration of excess dermatan sulfate in urine using a toluidine blue spot test, presence of metachromatic granules in blood neutrophils with Wright-Giemsa stain, and measurement of arylsulfatase B activity in leukocytes.[48, 49] Identification of a mutation causing feline MPS VI has allowed development of a polymerase chain reaction–based screening method to detect carrier cats.[52] Recombinant enzyme replacement may be effective therapy, but treatment must commence early in life, before significant lesions have developed.[53]

Feline MPS I has been described in white domestic shorthaired cats. It is an autosomal recessive disease caused by decreased activity of alpha-L-iduronidase.[48, 54] Clinical features are similar to those of MPS VI, but facial dysmorphia may not be as striking as in Siamese. Also, metachromatic granules are absent from toluidine blue–stained leukocytes. Radiographic features are similar to those of MPS VI, except that epiphyseal dysplasia and dwarfism are absent. Neurologic abnormalities related to spinal cord compression by bone proliferation occurs relatively later, after age 2 years. Excretion of dermatan sulfate and heparin sulfate in urine is detectable by the Berry spot test.[54] MPS I has also been reported in dogs. Affected animals are dwarfed and have swollen painful joints, glossoptosis, corneal clouding, and progressive motor and visual deficits.[48] Radiographic features include epiphyseal dysgenesis, periarticular bone proliferation, and enlargement of femoral diaphyses.[48, 55] Long-term therapy with recombinant alpha-L-iduronidase may result in some improvement in clinical signs in affected dogs.[56]

MPS II was described in a 5-year-old male Labrador retriever that had coarse facial features, macrodactyly, generalized osteopenia, progressive neurologic deterioration, and a positive urine test for glycosaminoglycan.[57] Iduronate-2-sulfatase activity in cultured dermal fibroblasts was deficient. MPS IIIA caused by decreased sulfamidase activity has been reported in two adult wire-haired Dachshund littermates in which the principal signs were of progressive neurologic disease.[58]

Canine MPS VII caused by beta-glucuronidase deficiency was first reported in mongrel dogs.[59] Affected dogs appear normal at birth, but by age 2 to 3 months they develop hindlimb paresis and have a disproportionately large head, flattened face, swollen lax joints, bowed limbs, dorsoventrally flattened rib cage, and corneal clouding.[48, 59, 60] Radiographic features include bilateral coxofemoral luxation, abnormally shaped carpal and tarsal bones, generalized epiphyseal dysplasia, cervical vertebral dysplasia, and platyspondylisis. Peripheral leukocytes contain granular inclusions, and urinary excretion of chondroitin sulfate is increased.[48, 60] A molecular diagnostic test can be used to distinguish phenotypically normal MPS VII carrier dogs from homozygous normal dogs.[61] Feline MPS VII was also reported in a 12-week-old male kitten that had abdominal distention and difficulty walking.[62] The kitten had facial dysmorphism, plump paws, and corneal clouding. Peripheral leukocytes contained metachromatic granules and no beta-glucuronidase activity, and urinary excretion of glycosaminoglycan was increased.

DWARFISM

Various disorders causing small stature in dogs and cats listed in Table 184–3 are reviewed in other chapters. Considered here are endocrinopathies (hyposomatotropism and hypothyroidism) and skeletal dysplasias that are more commonly associated with dwarfism in small animals.

Pituitary Dwarfism

Hypopituitarism and consequent dwarfism is an inherited autosomal recessive condition in German shepherd dogs and Carnelian bear dogs; it has also been described in other dog breeds (Weimaraner, spitz, toy pinscher) and cats.[63] A cystic, vestigial adenohypophysis is present in many affected German shepherds but a few have either a hypoplastic or normal-appearing pituitary gland. The syndrome is dominated by effects of hyposomatotropism, but deficiency of other adenohypophyseal hormones can lead to degrees of accompanying secondary hypothyroidism, hypoadrenocorticism, and hypogonadism. Affected animals are usually recognizable by the age of 2 or 3 months. They grow slowly but retain near-normal body proportions. The soft puppy haircoat is retained initially, but symmetric alopecia and hyperpigmentation develop with age. Accompanying abnormalities

TABLE 184–3. SOME CAUSES OF SMALL STATURE IN DOGS AND CATS

ENDOCRINE	NONENDOCRINE
Hyposomatotropism	Malnutrition
Hypothyroidism	Malassimilation
Hypoadrenocorticism	Portal systemic shunt
Hyperadrenocorticism	Cardiovascular defects
Diabetes mellitus	Glycogen storage disease
	Skeletal dysplasia
	Mucopolysaccharidosis
	Hydrocephalus
	Renal disease

Modified from Feldman EC, Nelson RW: Canine and Feline Endocrinology and Reproduction, 2nd ed. Philadelphia, WB Saunders, 1996.

described include abnormal behavior (aggression, fear biting), delayed dental eruption, short mandible, cardiac disorders, cryptorchidism, megaesophagus, and testicular atrophy or estral abnormalities.

Radiographically, limb bones are shortened, with delayed closure of growth plates in some cases but not in others. Epiphyses may show disordered and incomplete calcification, suggesting hypothyroidism. Hormonal testing can be undertaken to confirm the diagnosis if necessary. Most pituitary dwarf animals can be expected to remain small for life. However, two unusual cases with typical clinical features at 10 weeks of age grew steadily and appeared normal when 1 year old.[64] Both had normal hormonal test results, indicating that growth hormone secretion ideally should be evaluated in suspected cases to clarify the prognosis. Replacement therapy with growth hormone (if available and economical), and thyroxine or glucocorticoid if indicated, could be considered, but the long-term prognosis is poor.[63] A promising alternative approach involves chronic progestin administration to induce growth hormone production from mammary ductular cells of affected dogs of either sex.[65]

Congenital Hypothyroidism

Skeletal development is abnormal in congenital hypothyroidism, which is rare in dogs and cats. Cases are usually encountered sporadically in various breeds, but some familial occurrences are known: secondary hypothyroidism with autosomal recessive inheritance in giant schnauzers,[66] primary dyshormonogenesis with autosomal recessive inheritance in Abyssinian cats,[67] thyroid unresponsiveness to thyroid-stimulating hormone (TSH) with autosomal recessive inheritance in Japanese cats,[68] and thyroid unresponsiveness to TSH in related Scottish deerhounds.[69, 70]

Abnormalities may be detectable by the age of 1 or 2 months. Affected animals are disproportionate dwarfs, with short limbs and spine, a blocklike trunk, and a broad and short skull. The radiographic features are epiphyseal dysgenesis and delayed skeletal maturation (Fig. 184–12). Nonskeletal findings include delayed dental eruption, macroglossia, lethargy, mental dullness, persistent puppy haircoat progressing to thinning and alopecia, mild nonregenerative anemia, and hypercholesterolemia. Thyroid gland enlargement can accompany congenital dyshormonogenesis[71] but is absent if a hypothalamic-pituitary defect is causing thyroid understimulation[72] or thyroids are unresponsive to TSH.

A low blood plasma thyroxine concentration is expected, but results of thyroid stimulation tests differ, depending on whether the defect is of thyroidal, pituitary, or hypothalamic origin (see Chapter 151). The plasma growth hormone response to provocative stimuli may be suppressed.[66, 72] Treatment with thyroxine can reverse many of the abnormalities but should commence early and continue for life.

Skeletal Dysplasias (Osteochondrodysplasias)

Osteochondrodysplasias are disorders characterized by abnormalities of growth or development of bone, cartilage, or both (see Table 184–2). Disorders of this type have been reported in several breeds of dogs. Table 184–4 summarizes the better-characterized entities. Most have a known or suspected genetic basis and autosomal recessive inheritance is common. They frequently cause disproportionate dwarfism, with discrepant development of axial and appendicular skeleton producing reduced limb length relative to the trunk (Fig. 184–13).

MSJ

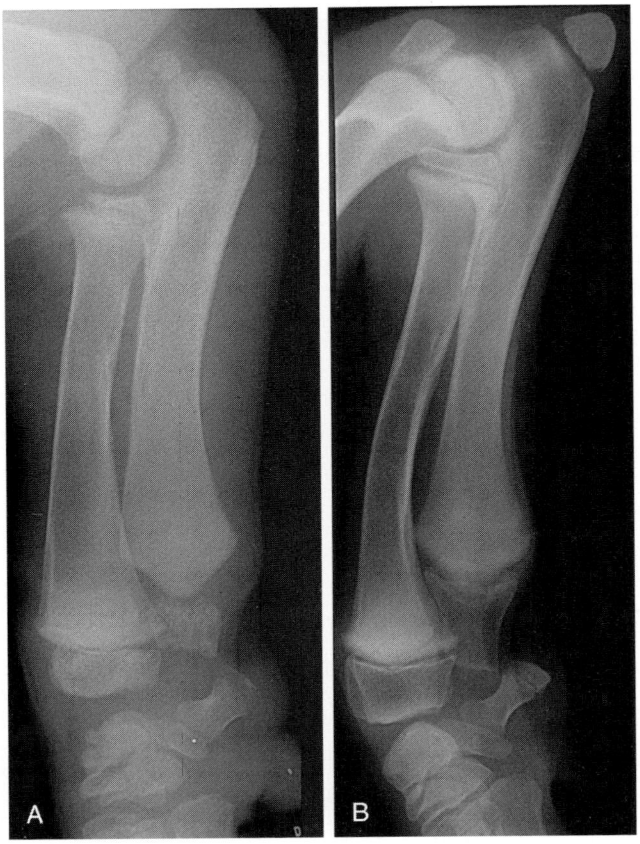

Figure 184–12. *A,* Forelimb of 15-week-old Great Dane with features of congenital hypothyroidism. Note the disordered and irregular ossification of epiphyses (epiphyseal dysgenesis) in humerus, radius, and ulna; the absence of an olecranon apophysis; and delayed skeletal maturation. *B,* Normal Great Dane of similar age for comparison. (Courtesy of R. B. Lavelle.)

Another type of genetic dwarfism occurs in achondroplastic dog breeds, such as bulldog, Boston terrier, Pekingese, pug, and Shih Tzu. These animals have been bred selectively for achondroplasia and thus have shortened maxilla, depressed nasal bridge, flared metaphyses, and short bowed limbs as part of accepted breed standards.[32] Hypochondroplastic breeds, such as basset hound, beagle, dachshund, Dandie Dinmont terrier, Scottish terrier, Skye terrier, and Welsh corgi, also have similarly shaped legs as a breed characteristic, although their skulls are normal.[32]

These forms of dwarfism differ from the nonpathologic, mutant, proportionate reduction in stature that occurs in miniature and toy breeds and that may have led to establishment of some new breeds; for example, the whippet is a miniature of the greyhound.

RETAINED CARTILAGE CORES

In young large- and giant-breed dogs, cartilage cores sometimes form in the metaphysis of the distal ulna. Physeal hypertrophic chondrocytes fail to mature and mineralize adjacent matrix and accumulate in long columns in the primary spongiosa.[89] The etiology of the disorder is not understood. In Great Dane pups, formation of cartilage cores in the distal ulnar and tibial metaphyses was associated with feeding diets containing three times the recommended content of calcium.[90]

Radiographically, there is a central, radiolucent core of cartilage 5 to 10 mm wide and 2 to 6 cm long extending from distal ulnar physis into metaphyseal bone (Fig. 184–14). Lesions are usually bilateral. They may be an asymptomatic, incidental radiographic finding or may be associated with varying degrees of growth retardation after age 5 months. Retarded ulnar growth causes relative shortening of the ulna, valgus and rotation of the paw, cranial bowing of the radius, and carpal and elbow subluxation (see Fig. 184–14).

CRANIOMANDIBULAR OSTEOPATHY

Craniomandibular osteopathy occurs mainly in young West Highland white, Scottish, cairn, Boston, and other terriers and occasionally in nonterrier breeds.[91] Autosomal recessive inheritance is known in West Highland white terriers,[92] and a hereditary predisposition may exist in Scottish terriers. However, the sporadic occurrence in unrelated breeds suggests that other etiologic factors are also involved. Canine distemper virus infection of bone is a possibility.[91]

The condition is usually recognized at age of 3 to 8 months, when affected pups develop mandibular swelling, drooling of saliva, prehension difficulties, pain on opening the mouth, or combinations of these signs. The clinical course may fluctuate, with periods of remission and exacerbation. Abnormal physical findings comprise firm, often painful, swelling of mandible, temporomandibular region, or both areas. Periods of pyrexia occur in some cases. Restricted jaw movements and atrophy of masticatory muscles may be obvious in severely affected dogs. Mandibular swelling without pain or eating difficulties occurs in some dogs, especially of larger breeds.

Radiographic changes are generally bilateral but often asymmetric, with irregular bone proliferation involving the mandible and tympanic bulla–petrous temporal bone areas in about 50 per cent of cases. However, changes can be confined to the mandible (33 per cent of cases) (Fig. 184–15) or the tympanic bulla–petrous temporal region (13 per cent). The calvarium and tentorium ossium are often thickened (Fig. 184–16) and other skull bones are sometimes affected. Concurrent long-bone lesions resembling later stages of metaphyseal osteopathy have been observed in a few terriers with craniomandibular osteopathy.

The diagnosis is straightforward in cases with typical clinical and radiographic features. Routine laboratory tests are unlikely to be helpful. Bone biopsy may be useful in atypical cases, such as in dogs of rarely affected breeds with lesions confined to the mandible, especially if unilateral. The histopathology involves resorption of existing lamellae, proliferation of coarse trabecular bone beyond normal periosteal boundaries, replacement of marrow spaces by vascular fibrous stroma, and infiltration at the periphery of new bone by inflammatory cells. A mosaic pattern of irregular cement lines is present in the new primitive bone.[93]

Craniomandibular osteopathy is self-limiting. Abnormal bone proliferation eventually slows and becomes static at about 1 year of age. Lesions then tend to regress, although radiographic abnormalities or impaired prehension sometimes persists. Anti-inflammatory drug treatment can reduce pain and discomfort, but the effect on lesions is unknown. The prognosis is guarded when extensive changes affect the tympanic-petrous temporal areas and adjacent mandible. Ankylosis and adhesions may then develop, permanently restricting jaw movements and eating. Rostral hemimandibulectomy can be a useful salvage procedure in these cases.[35]

TABLE 84–4. OSTEOCHONDRODYSPLASIAS: CLINICAL AND RADIOLOGIC SIGNS, AND INHERITANCE PATTERN

Alaskan malamute chondrodysplasia[6, 73]
Short limbs, bowed forelegs, carpal joints enlarged, paws deviated laterally. Ulna growth plate thickened, irregular, and flared. Associated hemolytic anemia. Autosomal recessive trait, complete penetrance, variable expression.

Beagle multiple epiphyseal dysplasia[6, 73]
Short limbs, enlarged joints, kyphosis. Stippled mineralization of epiphyses, especially femur and humerus, disappears by 5 months. Vertebrae short. Dysplastic hips. Osteoarthropathy in adults. Autosomal recessive trait.

Bull terrier osteochondrodysplasia[74]
Abnormal hindleg gait, femoral neck fractures. Nonossified foci in femoral necks and metaphyses of long bones. Some long bones distorted. Dwarfing not noted. Littermates affected but inheritance not known.

English pointer enchondrodystrophy[6, 75, 76]
Short limbs, bowed forelegs, abnormal locomotion. Wide irregular growth plates. Possibly inferior prognathism. Probable autosomal recessive trait.

Great Pyrenees chondrodysplasia[6, 73, 77]
Very short limbs, forelegs bowed with valgus deformity. Body length reduced slightly. Flared, flattened metaphyses. Poorly developed epiphyses and cuboidal bones. Vertebrae poorly ossified and irregular. Autosomal recessive trait.

Irish setter hypochondroplasia[78]
Mildly short limbs and spine, variable radius or ulna bowing and carpal valgus. Growth plates, epiphyses, and metaphyses radiographically normal. Autosomal recessive trait.

Labrador retriever ocular-skeletal dysplasia[6, 79]
Short limbs, prominent elbows and carpi, paws deviated laterally, hindlegs hyperextended. Tubular bones short and wide, cortices thin, metaphyses flattened and flared, increased metaphyseal opacity. Epiphyses and cuboidal bones large and misshapen. Hip dysplasia, abnormal elbows. Cataracts, retinal dysplasia, and detachment. Autosomal trait, recessive effect on skeleton, incompletely dominant on eye.

Miniature poodle multiple enchondromatosis[80, 81]
Short bowed limbs, femoral neck fractures. Lucent areas extending from growth plates into metaphyses and some diaphyses. Diaphyses distended and distorted. Ribs and vertebrae also affected. Sternum lacked bone. Autosomal, nondominant trait.

Miniature poodle multiple epiphyseal dysplasia[73]
Similar to disorder in beagle. Inheritance unknown, but two of three affected were littermates.

Miniature poodle pseudoachondroplasia[6, 73]
Poor growth, abnormal gait. Short, bent legs, enlarged joints. Possible inferior prognathism. Vertebrae short, limb bones short and thick with bulbous ends. Stippled densities in epiphyses. Ossification complete by 2 years of age, but limbs remained short and deformed. Probable autosomal recessive trait.

Norwegian elkhound chondrodysplasia[6, 73]
Shortened body, disproportionately short limbs, especially forelegs, which may be bowed. Metaphyses flared and flattened, with denser band. Ventral vertebral bodies irregular, delayed union of vertebral endplates. May have glucosuria. Autosomal recessive trait.

Samoyed ocular-skeletal dysplasia[6, 82, 83]
Short forelegs, varus deformity of elbows, valgus of carpi, premature closure of ulnar growth plates, bowed radii. Domed forehead. Cataracts, retinal detachment, hyaloid artery remnants, eosinophilia. Autosomal recessive trait.

Scottish deerhound pseudoachondroplasia (osteochondrodysplasia)[84, 85]
Retarded growth, short bowed limbs, exercise intolerance, small head, short trunk, lax joints, kyphosis. Vertebrae and long bones short, epiphyseal ossification irregular and delayed. Later osteopenia, severe deformity.

Scottish fold osteochondrodysplasia (osteodystrophy)[86–88]
Folded ears, tail inflexible with thick base. Short and malformed metacarpal, metatarsal, and phalangeal bones. Painful plantar exostoses on tarsal-metatarsal bones. Secondary ankylosing arthroplasty of carpal and tarsal joints. Caudal vertebrae short and thick with widened endplates. Physeal cartilage thickened in some areas with isolated islands of chondrocytes, suggesting inadequate or delayed cartilage maturation. Autosomal dominant trait.

MULTIPLE CARTILAGINOUS EXOSTOSES

In rare instances these benign lesions (osteochondromatosis, multiple hereditary osteochondromas) occur in dogs and cats as single or multiple exostoses. The disorder may be inherited as an autosomal dominant trait in humans, horses, and dogs.[94, 95] Protuberances consist of cancellous bone covered by a cap of hyaline cartilage and arise in the metaphyseal region of bones formed by endochondral ossification. With continued physeal growth and elongation of long bones, exostoses may be finally located in the diaphysis. Lesions develop and grow most rapidly in immature animals, becoming senescent at maturity. Malignant transformation of exostoses to chondrosarcoma occurs rarely in aged animals.[96]

The etiology is unknown. One hypothesis is that congenital or acquired defects in the perichondrial ring allow an island of physeal cartilage to be pinched off and trapped in metaphyseal bone. This physeal cartilage continues to grow radially, giving rise to exostoses. However, this does not explain the similar lesions found occasionally in nonskeletal sites, such as tracheal cartilages.

Superficially located exostoses may be palpable. Signs may include paresis caused by progressive spinal cord compression in young animals (see Chapter 106) or pain related to impingement of exostoses on adjacent tissues.[97] Radio-graphically, lesions are rounded to cauliflower-like in outline, with a smooth thin shell of cortical bone (Fig. 184–17). They protrude above the bone contour and may extend into the medullary cavity. Internally, exostoses have well-defined bone trabeculae that are continuous with the medullary cavity, and diaphyseal cortex in the region is interrupted by the lesion. Adjacent bones such as ulna and metacarpals may be deformed by expanding exostoses (see Fig. 184–17). Biopsies of solitary exostoses are performed to allow differentiation from neoplastic lesions. Surgical excision of exostoses that are causing spinal cord compression or lameness is recommended (see Chapter 106).[97] All exostoses should be monitored for malignant transformation.

IDIOPATHIC BONE DISORDERS

ENOSTOSIS

Enostosis (panosteitis, eosinophilic panosteitis) is a relatively common disease causing lameness in medium, large, and giant-breed dogs, especially the German shepherd dog.[98] Two thirds of affected dogs are male. The age of onset is 6 to 18 months; older dogs are affected rarely. Lameness is acute in onset, not associated with trauma, and intermittent

MSJ

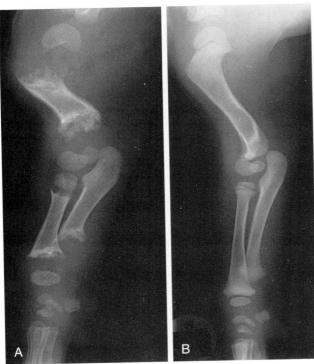

Figure 184–13. *A*, Radiograph of a 5-week-old Alaskan malamute with chondrodysplasia. Physeal cartilage is widened and adjacent metaphyseal bone roughened and irregular. *B*, Radiograph of a normal littermate of the same age for comparison.

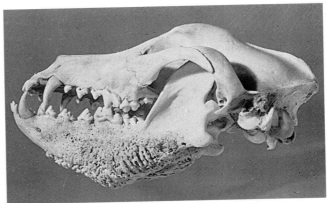

Figure 184–15. Macerated skull of a Doberman pinscher with craniomandibular osteopathy. Note extensive bone changes involving mandible. Tympanic bullae, petrous temporal bones, and temporomandibular joint regions were unaffected in this case. (From Watson ADJ, et al: Craniomandibular osteopathy in Doberman pinschers. J Small Anim Pract 16:11, 1975.)

in one or more limbs. Each episode of lameness lasts 2 to 3 weeks, but with recurrent bouts, enostosis may persist for 2 to 9 months. Other signs in early stages include anorexia, lethargy, pyrexia, and weight loss. On physical examination, pain is detected on deep palpation of affected bones. Bones commonly affected are the ulna, humerus, radius, femur, and tibia. Ilium, metatarsal, and other bones are rarely affected. The disease begins in the medullary bone marrow, in the region of a nutrient foramen. The etiology is unknown:

genetic predisposition, hemophilia, bacterial infection, vascular abnormality, metabolic disease, allergy, hyperestrogenism, and endoparasitism have been proposed, but the evidence for most of these is scant.[98] Viral infection is considered to be a likely cause on the basis of clinical features of the disease, transmission experiments, and in situ hybridization demonstration of virus in bone cells of dogs infected with canine distemper virus.[98, 99]

Three radiographic stages are recognizable.[98] The first stage, with medullary radiolucency related to bone marrow degeneration, is seen infrequently. Most often detected is the second stage (Fig. 184–18). A granular, hazy increased radiopacity that begins in the region of the nutrient foramen may extend to fill the entire medullary cavity. Formation of new endosteal bone and a thin layer of smooth periosteal bone are secondary changes. In the final stage, most bones return to normal appearance, but some have residual thickening of medullary trabeculae and cortical deformity. Histopathologically, lesions are characterized initially by replacement of normal marrow by fibrous tissue, followed by

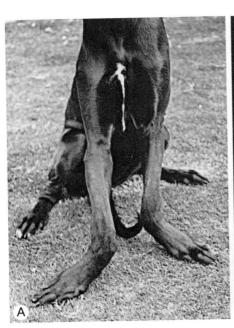

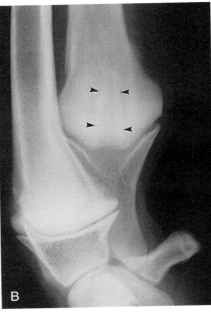

Figure 184–14. *A*, Seven-month-old Great Dane with bilateral forelimb deformities caused by retained cartilage cores in the distal ulnar physes. *B*, Radiograph demonstrating retained cartilage core (arrows) extending from distal ulnar physis into the metaphysis. (From Johnson KA: Retardation of endochondral ossification at the distal ulnar growth plate in dogs. Aust Vet J 57:474, 1987.)

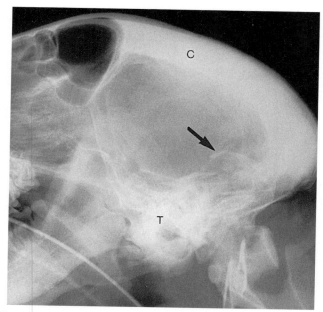

Figure 184–16. Skull of Scottish terrier with craniomandibular osteopathy. The tympanic bulla–petrous bone area (T) shows dense sclerotic bone changes. Note thickened calvarium (C) and tentorium osseum (arrow).

excessive remodeling of cortical and medullary bone in the affected areas, with endosteal new bone formation generally more prominent.[98] Basenjis and West Highland white terrier dogs with inherited pyruvate kinase deficiency can develop intramedullary osteosclerosis, but, unlike enostosis, new trabecular bone formation is uniform throughout the medullary cavity.[100]

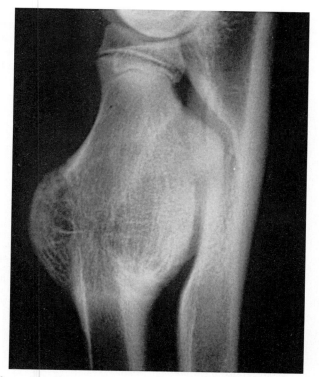

Figure 184–17. Radiograph demonstrating a solitary multiple cartilaginous exostosis-type lesion in the forelimb of a young dog. Note the expansile lesion of the proximal radius, causing malalignment of the radius and attenuation of adjacent ulna. (Courtesy of R. B. Lavelle.)

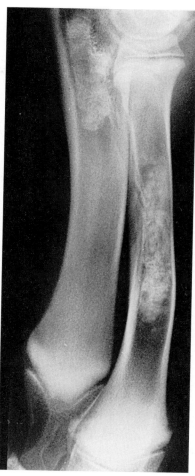

Figure 184–18. Radiograph of a forelimb of a young Great Dane with enostosis, showing patchy intramedullary densities in proximal ulna and midradius. (From Watson ADJ: Diseases of muscle and bone. *In* Whittick WG [ed]: Canine Orthopaedics, 2nd ed. Philadelphia, Lea & Febiger, 1990, p 674. Courtesy of D. M. Turner.)

Enostosis may occur concurrently with developmental diseases such as ununited anconeal process and osteochondritis dissecans, and it may be difficult to determine which disease is causing the lameness. Leukocytosis and eosinophilia occur inconsistently in affected dogs; serum chemistry is unremarkable. Enostosis is self-limiting, usually by age 18 months, but analgesic or nonsteroidal anti-inflammatory drugs may help alleviate pain and lameness.

METAPHYSEAL OSTEOPATHY

Metaphyseal osteopathy (hypertrophic osteodystrophy) is a disease of young rapidly growing dogs of the larger breeds, with onset usually at about 3 to 4 months of age (range 2 to 8 months).[91, 101] Affected pups develop metaphyseal swelling and pain, accompanied by depression, inappetence, and variable pyrexia. Some cases recover within a few days, but others have one or more relapses during the following weeks before finally recovering. In a few instances, repeated relapses and consequent pain, cachexia, and debility necessitate euthanasia. Unexplained deaths have been observed rarely.

Radiographic changes occur especially in metaphyses of limb bones and are usually bilateral. Scapulae and ribs may

MSJ

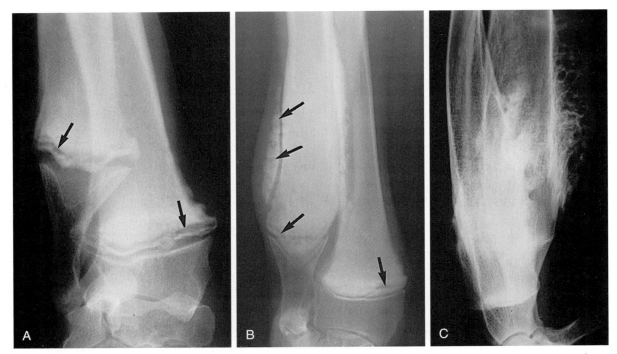

Figure 184–19. Radiographs of metaphyseal osteopathy. *A,* Early stage with irregular radiolucent zone (arrows) separated from the physis by a narrow radiopaque band. *B,* Later stage with radiolucent metaphyseal zones (bottom two arrows) adjacent to the physes still evident. Periosteal new bone and soft tissue mineralization (top two arrows) adjacent to the metaphyseal cortex. *C,* Inactive stage with residual diaphyseal deformity and spiculated periosteal exostoses.

also be affected. In the early stage, an irregular radiolucent zone is present in the metaphysis, separated from the normal-appearing growth plate by an opaque band (Fig. 184–19*A*). Surrounding soft tissue may be swollen. Later radiographs may show metaphyseal enlargement with irregular periosteal new bone formation, although not all affected dogs develop these changes (Fig. 184–19*B*). When the disease is no longer active, bone changes undergo repair and remodeling, but some diaphyseal distortion and exostoses may remain (Figs. 184–19*C* and 184–20).

Hematologic and biochemical tests contribute little to the diagnosis, although neutrophilia, monocytosis, and lymphocytopenia can occur during active disease, reflecting stress and inflammation. The principal histologic changes involve the primary spongiosa of metaphyses, with acute suppurative osteomyelitis, necrosis, trabecular microfractures, and defective bone formation. Trabecular resorption produces the radiolucent metaphyseal zone. The opaque band near the growth plate results from trabecular collapse and secondary bone formation. Periosteal thickening, with subperiosteal fibrosis and inflammation, periosteal new bone formation, and/or extraperiosteal dystrophic calcification, may be seen.[101]

The cause of metaphyseal osteopathy is unknown. Suggestions implicating hypovitaminosis C, overnutrition, or copper deficiency have not been substantiated. Attempts to identify a causative infectious agent or to transmit the disease have not been successful. However, canine distemper virus RNA has been detected within bone cells of dogs with metaphyseal osteopathy, suggesting a role of this virus in the etiopathogenesis.[102] Other circumstantial evidence supports this[101–103]: (1) metaphyseal osteopathy may be accompanied or preceded by respiratory or gastrointestinal signs; (2) dental enamel hypoplasia, a sequel to distemper infection, was found in two dogs with metaphyseal osteopathy; (3) three of seven dogs inoculated with blood from dogs with metaphy-

seal osteopathy developed distemper; and (4) typical bone changes have developed in some pups 10 to 14 days after inoculation with live distemper virus vaccine. However, the osteosclerotic metaphyseal lesions found in a series of dogs clinically affected with distemper differed macroscopically, radiographically, and histologically from metaphyseal osteopathy.[104] At present, the relationship between distemper virus, metaphyseal osteopathy, and other hyperostotic bone diseases (craniomandibular osteopathy and enostosis) remains uncertain. Metaphyseal osteopathy has been reported

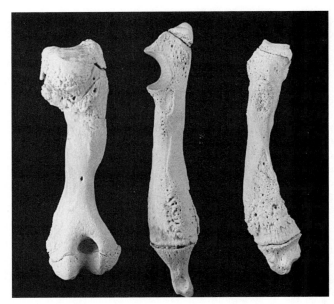

Figure 184–20. Humerus, ulna, and radius of a young giant-breed dog that suffered metaphyseal osteopathy. Note the severe deformities and periosteal new bone.

in littermates of several breeds, but there is little evidence of an inherited predisposition and most cases are sporadic, affecting isolated pups in a litter.

There is no specific treatment for metaphyseal osteopathy. Dietary imbalances or excesses should be avoided and an anti-inflammatory analgesic given as needed to reduce pain. Good nursing care may be required to avoid dehydration, undernutrition, and pressure sores.

CALVARIAL HYPEROSTOSIS

An unusual hyperostosis affecting frontal and parietal bones was reported in two unrelated bull mastiffs.[101] From age 6 months there was progressive outward thickening of the calvarium (the cranial cavity was unaffected) with pyrexia, lymphadenopathy, and eosinophilia. The swelling stabilized at maturity, then regressed. The lesion was a subperiosteal hyperostosis with initial deposition of new woven bone followed by secondary osteonal remodeling. Similarities were noted with cases of craniomandibular osteopathy, inherited pyruvate kinase deficiency, and human infantile cortical hyperostosis.[100, 105, 106]

POLYOSTOTIC PERIOSTITIS

An idiopathic polyostotic periostitis resembling human infantile cortical hyperostosis was described in a young adult West Highland white terrier.[106] Features were pyrexia, joint and bone enlargement and pain, restricted joint movements with crepitus, and periosteal new bone formation on long bones, pelvis, and scapulae.

SECONDARY HYPERTROPHIC OSTEOPATHY

In secondary hypertrophic osteopathy (pulmonary hypertrophic osteoarthropathy), firm nonedematous swelling develops in all four limbs, usually in response to intrathoracic disease, most often neoplasia. Of 180 canine cases, 98 per cent had intrathoracic disease, and 92 per cent of these had either metastatic lung neoplasia or primary tumors of lung or thoracic esophagus.[107] A few dogs had pneumonitis, endocarditis, or dirofilariasis. Of four cases lacking intrathoracic disease, three had urinary rhabdomyosarcoma and one had hepatic carcinoma. Because of the association with neoplasia, secondary hypertrophic osteopathy occurs mostly in older animals. There is no breed or gender predilection in dogs. The disorder is rare in cats.

Signs related to limb changes often precede signs of thoracic disease but can begin simultaneously with or after thoracic signs. Affected animals are stiff and reluctant to move. There is swelling of all limbs, which are warm, firm, and may be painful. Thoracic disease may be manifested by cough, dyspnea, abnormal lung sounds, or cardiac displacement. Abnormal laboratory findings, if any, are related to the underlying intrathoracic disease.

Radiographic changes are characteristic: soft tissue swelling of distal extremities initially, then periosteal new bone formation as irregular nodules perpendicular to the cortex or smoother parallel deposits (Fig. 184–21). Bone changes begin distally and may spread proximally to involve humerus and scapula, femur and pelvis. Ribs and vertebrae are sometimes affected. On histologic examination, the bones are surrounded by highly vascular, dense connective tissue containing numerous thick-walled arteries. The osteogenic layer

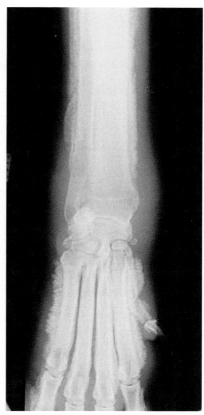

Figure 184–21. Radiograph of distal forelimb of a dog with secondary hypertrophic osteopathy. Periosteal new bone growth with a nodular appearance affecting the metacarpals and digits and smoother deposits on the radius and ulna are seen. Adjacent soft tissues are thickened.

of the periosteum is hyperplastic and overlies maturing and remodeling trabecular bone.

The pathogenesis of secondary hypertrophic osteopathy involves increased blood flow to the distal extremities, then overgrowth of connective tissue and subsequent osteoneogenesis. This seems to involve a neural reflex originating in the thorax and affecting connective tissue and periosteum of the limbs. The efferent pathway apparently involves nerve fibers that leave the lung near the bronchi and join the vagus in the mediastinum. The nature of the efferent connection, whether neural or hormonal, is unknown. Regression of secondary hypertrophic osteopathy may follow removal of the source of afferent impulses by excision of the lung lesion or interruption of the afferent fibers by peribronchial dissection or vagotomy. There may be an alternative afferent pathway from parietal pleura along intercostal nerves, because regression has sometimes followed thoracotomy and section of intercostal nerves or extensive resection of a neoplasm of the thoracic wall. The rare association with intra-abdominal lesions is more obscure.

Treatment should be directed against the underlying thoracic disease, using appropriate medical or surgical methods. Successful resection of lung lesions by lobectomy or pneumonectomy can quickly remove pain, soft tissue swelling, and lameness. The bone abnormalities usually regress gradually over several months. When complete removal of lung lesions is not possible, the skeletal signs may be ameliorated by removal of larger lesions even if multiple small lesions remain. Relief may also follow intrathoracic vagotomy on the same side as the lesion or on the more affected side if metastases are bilateral.

MEDULLARY BONE INFARCTION

Medullary bone infarcts do not cause clinical signs in dogs. They affect older dogs and are usually found in conjunction with osteosarcoma and, occasionally, skeletal fibrosarcoma or renal adenocarcinoma.[108, 109] Bone infarcts are characterized radiographically by numerous, irregularly demarcated areas of increased radiopacity in the medullary cavities of one or more bones (Fig. 184–22). The densities obliterate medullary cavities to varying degrees. Any bone may be affected, but infarcts are mainly found distal to elbow and stifle.[108]

The pathogenesis of the disorder is unknown, and it does not seem to be due to metastatic tumor cell dissemination. However, intramural collagen deposition causes occlusion of nutrient arteries, hypoxia and widespread necrosis of medullary soft tissues and bone, and new bone proliferation on endosteum and medullary trabeculae.[108] Common causes in humans are dysbaric conditions, fat embolization, hyperadrenocorticism, hyperviscosity, hemoglobinopathy, and anemia. Medullary bone infarcts should be differentiated from enostosis, bacterial and fungal osteomyelitis, and metastatic neoplasia.

BONE CYST

Benign cystic bone lesions, either monostotic or polyostotic, are uncommon in dogs and cats. Young dogs of larger

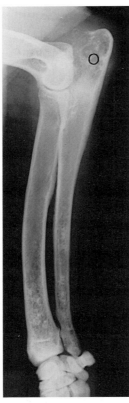

Figure 184–22. Radiograph demonstrating medullary bone infarction in an aged dog with osteosarcoma (O) of the olecranon. The multiple areas of medullary sclerosis in the radius and ulna are infarcts.

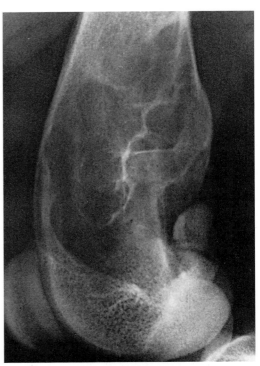

Figure 184–23. Bone cyst in distal femur of a young Doberman pinscher. The lesion has an expansile, lytic appearance, with thinning of overlying cortex. Bony ridges or partitions are evident internally.

breeds are affected most often, with Doberman pinschers and German shepherds overrepresented.[95, 110] Males are affected twice as often as females. The etiology is unknown but may involve intramedullary metaphyseal hemorrhage, local disturbance of bone growth, or other factors.[107] Heritable factors might also be implicated, as lesions occurred in three Doberman pinscher littermates and in three Old English sheepdog littermates and both parents.[95]

Bone cysts may be subclinical until they are large or fracture with trauma. Pain, lameness, and local swelling may then ensue. The lesions occur in metaphyses and adjacent diaphyses of long bones, sparing growth plates and epiphyses. The distal radius and/or ulna is affected most often. The cysts are lined by a thin membrane and contain fluid that may be blood tinged. Radiographically, the lesions are lytic and expansile, with thinned cortex and little or no periosteal reaction. There may be one (so-called unicameral cysts) or several chambers, partially divided by bony ridges or partitions (Fig. 184–23).

Alternative diagnoses are atypical bone neoplasia, aneurysmal bone cyst, and fibrous dysplasia of bone. Fine-needle aspiration biopsy and cytologic examination may be useful: only a benign bone cyst is likely to be fluid filled, although the other lesions may contain areas of cystic degeneration or hemorrhage. If uncertainty persists, surgical biopsy and histopathologic study are indicated. To stimulate healing of bone cysts, surgery has been advocated, using drainage, curettage, bone grafting, and external support to prevent fractures. Some untreated cysts heal without surgery, although pathologic fracture of cystic bone is a risk.[111]

ANEURYSMAL BONE CYST

Aneurysmal bone cyst is a non-neoplastic lesion that results in considerable local bone destruction. Although common in humans, it is rare in dogs and cats. Lesions arise in ribs, pelvis, scapula, spine, and metaphyses of long bones in young adults and geriatric animals.[112, 113] The cause is unknown, but tumors, developmental abnormalities, and trauma-induced hemorrhage causing venous obstruction or arteriovenous shunts in bone marrow have been suggested as initiating factors.[6] Localized partial disruption of medullary blood flow results in endosteal bone resorption and outward displacement of the periosteum. The periosteum forms successive layers of woven bone that are resorbed as the lesion expands, producing the appearance of a ballooning aortic aneurysm.[6] Blood-tinged fluid and fibrovascular tissue fill the lesion, which has a honeycomb appearance with huge vascular channels. Radiographically, it appears as a large expansile cyst, with minimal internal trabecular septation, surrounded by thin rim of mineralized soft tissue or bone. A triangle of laminated periosteal new bone (Codman's triangle) forms at the junction between cyst and adjacent normal diaphyseal bone. Some have an underlying tumor (osteosarcoma, giant cell tumor) that complicates diagnosis. Signs may be suddenly exacerbated by neoplastic erosion of vessels and intralesional hemorrhage or by fracture.[113] Uncomplicated lesions have a good prognosis when treated by en bloc resection, amputation, or curettage.[114] Nonresectable lesions in humans are irradiated to stop bleeding and lesional growth, but postirradiation sarcoma can ensue.

SUBCHONDRAL BONE CYST

Subchondral bone cysts are benign lesions in subchondral bone between growth plate and articular cartilage.[115] They are usually lined with synovium and occasionally communicate with the articular synovial membrane. Radiographs show a single or multilocular radiolucent defect with well-circumscribed borders. They are common in horses and pigs and usually a manifestation of osteochondrosis.[6] This association was also noted in a dog.[115]

FIBROUS DYSPLASIA

Fibrous dysplasia is a rare fibro-osseous lesion of bone believed to be of developmental origin.[6] It affects mainly young or newborn animals and may be monostotic or polyostotic. The lesions are expansile and may cause problems of disfigurement, compression, or obstruction of adjacent structures or bone weakness and fracture (Fig. 184–24). Monostotic lesions have been reported in the jaw or infraorbital bone of dogs and in mandible, maxilla or distal ulna of cats.[116, 117] Fibrous dysplasia, aneurysmal bone cysts, and benign bone cysts are distinct entities but have been confused in the veterinary literature.[118]

The lesions have marked homogeneous radiopacity and are composed of firm, grey fibrous tissue that is gritty when cut. Histologically, they consist of fibrous connective tissue stroma containing spicules of woven bone replacing normal osseous tissue. Cavities of various size containing clear or bloody fluid may be scattered throughout.[6] Two cats had lesions that were resected, and both were free of recurrence 4 years later.[116]

CENTRAL GIANT CELL GRANULOMA

This rare, non-neoplastic lesion affects the tooth-bearing regions of maxilla and mandible of young dogs.[119] Trauma-

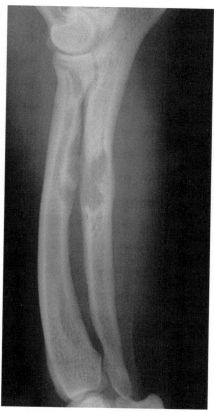

Figure 184–24. Radiograph demonstrating fibrous dysplasia in the ulnar diaphysis, with secondary lysis and new bone formation in adjacent radial cortex. (Courtesy of P. A. Manley.)

associated intraosseous hemorrhage seems to be an initiating factor. Radiographically, the lesion is a rounded to ovoid, expansile, uniloculated radiolucency, well demarcated from surrounding tissue by a thin rim of smooth nonreactive bone. Adjacent teeth may lose their lamina dura and be displaced, but tooth root resorption is rare. The center of the lesion consists of tan-colored soft tissue composed mainly of loose fibrovascular stroma containing pleomorphic mesenchymal cells and numerous large, irregular multinucleated giant cells. These cells arise from mesenchymal tissue and are neither osteoclasts nor involved in bone resorption. The lesions resemble giant cell tumors histologically. The latter are potentially malignant tumors that cause extensive destruction at the ends of long bones. As central giant cell granuloma is rare, diagnosis should be confirmed by biopsy. Treatment is by curettage or en bloc resection.[116, 119]

METABOLIC, NUTRITIONAL, AND ENDOCRINE BONE DISORDERS

The term metabolic bone disease is used here to encompass various conditions that cause a generalized reduction in bone mass, or *osteopenia*. Osteopenia can be categorized into excessive bone resorption, or *osteolysis*, as occurs in hyperparathyroid states, and defective bone formation. The latter is further subdivided into insufficient formation of osteoid, or *osteoporosis*, and defective mineralization of osteoid, or *rickets-osteomalacia*.

Major causes of metabolic bone disease involve nutritional and/or hormonal processes. The more important causes dis-

MSJ

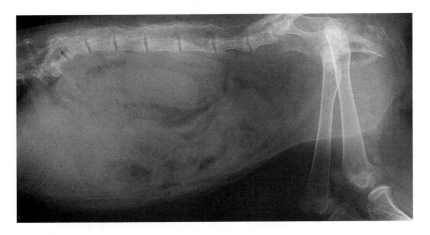

Figure 184–25. Radiograph of the abdomen of a kitten with nutritional secondary hyperparathyroidism. Note poor contrast in radiopacity between bones and soft tissues such as liver and kidneys. The cortices of long bones are thin, vertebrae are lucent, and the vertebral column is deformed in the thoracolumbar area.

cussed here are nutritional secondary hyperparathyroidism, rickets, renal osteodystrophy, and hypervitaminosis A. Other metabolic bone diseases that rarely produce clinical signs related to bone are mentioned briefly.

NUTRITIONAL SECONDARY HYPERPARATHYROIDISM

Nutritional secondary hyperparathyroidism is a metabolic disorder in which bone production is normal but osteopenia results from excessive bone resorption. It is caused by diets providing excess phosphate and/or insufficient calcium.[95] Affected animals have usually been fed mainly meat and/or organ tissue. This provides adequate phosphate but insufficient calcium, and Ca/P ratios are about 1:16 to 1:35,[120] in contrast to the recommended 1.2:1 for dogs and 1:1 for cats. Added cow's milk provides insufficient calcium to correct the imbalance. The imbalance induces hypocalcemia, which increases secretion of parathyroid hormone. Increased parathyroid activity tends to normalize blood calcium and inorganic phosphate concentrations by promoting mineral resorption from bone, enhancing intestinal calcium absorption, and facilitating renal phosphate excretion and calcium retention (see Chapter 149). However, continued ingestion of the defective diet sustains the hyperparathyroid state and causes progressive skeletal demineralization and consequent clinical signs.

Nutritional secondary hyperparathyroidism causes clinical disease in pups and kittens of all breeds but also occurs occasionally in adults. Signs in young animals are lameness, reluctance to stand or walk, and skeletal pain. Costochondral junctions and metaphyses may appear swollen, and pyrexia is sometimes present. Bone fractures can follow relatively mild trauma. Limb deformity may be evident. Paresis or paralysis may result from vertebral compression, and constipation may follow pelvic collapse. Effects are less dramatic in adults, but generalized osteopenia and skeletal pain are sometimes seen, and resorption of alveolar bone may cause loosening and loss of teeth.

Radiographically, decreased bone density and thin cortices are seen, with or without fracturing (Fig. 184–25). Growth plates are normal, but metaphyses may be mushroom shaped. An area of relative radiopacity occurs in the metaphyses adjacent to growth plates, representing the area of primary mineralization, and may be best appreciated in the distal radius and ulna (Fig. 184–26).

Blood biochemical tests are of little value in confirming nutritional secondary hyperparathyroidism. The calcium concentration is usually within the reference range because of compensatory changes. Concentrations of inorganic phosphate and alkaline phosphatase may appear high but should be interpreted carefully because growing animals often have higher values than adults.

Affected animals should be confined for the first few weeks of treatment to reduce the risk of fractures and deformity. A good-quality, nutritionally complete commercial ration should be fed. For all but mildly affected cases, sufficient calcium carbonate should be added to produce a calcium/phosphorus ratio of 2:1. This is maintained for 2 to 3 months, after which the supplement is withdrawn. Oversupplementation with calcium should be avoided. For se-

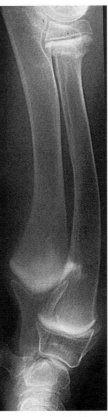

Figure 184–26. Radiograph of the foreleg of a pup with nutritional secondary hyperparathyroidism. Bone is abnormally radiolucent and cortices are thin. Growth plates are normal but relatively radiopaque zones are present in the adjacent metaphyses, representing areas of primary mineralization of osteoid.

verely affected cases parenteral administration of calcium (for example, 10 to 30 mL of 10 per cent calcium gluconate solution by slow intravenous infusion daily for 3 days) may help reduce pain and lameness initially, but it does little to correct the calcium deficiency. A nonsteroidal anti-inflammatory drug might be useful for short-term analgesia. The prognosis is generally good unless skeletal deformity and disability are marked.

RICKETS

Clinical cases of rickets are rare in dogs and cats. Rickets and its adult equivalent, osteomalacia, occur when insufficient calcium and/or phosphorus is available for mineralization of newly formed osteoid. The more likely causes of rickets in dogs and cats are hypovitaminosis D (dietary deficiency),[121] inborn error in vitamin D metabolism,[122] or low availability of minerals from the diet (inadequate concentration, impaired absorption). Dogs and cats do not synthesize cholecalciferol (previtamin D_3) in skin exposed to ultraviolet light and are mainly dependent on dietary intake.[123-125]

Affected animals may be lame and reluctant or unable to walk. Fractures or bending of long bones can occur. Enlargement of costochondral junctions and metaphyses may be evident. Other possible abnormalities are delayed dental eruption, weakness, listlessness, and neurologic signs (excitability, tremor, convulsion, coma) related to hypocalcemia. Potential blood test abnormalities include low calcium, low inorganic phosphate, increased alkaline phosphatase, increased parathyroid hormone, and low 25-hydroxycholecalciferol (the storage form of vitamin D).[121, 122, 126]

Characteristic radiographic findings are axial and radial thickening of growth plates and cupping of adjacent metaphyses (Fig. 184–27). The distal ulnar growth plates are consistently the most severely affected, and this finding reflects a failure of mineralization of cartilage that is being produced at the normal rate. Additional findings are osteopenia, thin cortices, and bowed diaphyses.

When dietary deficiency is suspected, therapy requires a regular diet with adequate and not excessive amounts of calcium, phosphorus, and vitamin D.[121, 126] The regimen described for nutritional secondary hyperparathyroidism would be appropriate. Treatment with dihydrotachysterol was effective in a dog in which an inborn error in vitamin D metabolism was suspected.[122]

RENAL OSTEODYSTROPHY

Renal osteodystrophy is an osteopenic disorder that results from chronic renal failure. This complex abnormality involves both hyperparathyroidism (excessive bone resorption) and rickets-osteomalacia (impaired osteoid mineralization). Hyperparathyroidism results from impaired renal excretion of phosphate and consequent hyperphosphatemia. This lowers the blood calcium concentration, increases parathyroid gland activity, and induces bone resorption. Although this tends to normalize blood calcium concentrations, the hyperparathyroid state is maintained by persisting hyperphosphatemia. Concurrently, synthesis of 1,25-dihydroxyvitamin D declines because of reduced functional renal mass (see Chapter 169). This and other metabolic derangements lead to severe depression of enteric calcium absorption, impaired mineralization of osteoid, and thus rickets-osteomalacia.

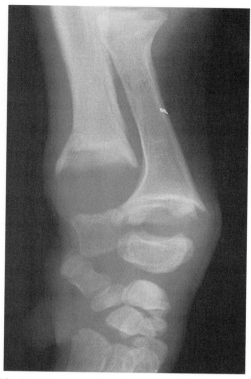

Figure 184–27. Radiograph of the foreleg of a 12-week-old Saint Bernard with rickets. Enlarged physes and cupping of adjacent metaphyseal bone are features of rickets. (From Johnson KA, et al: Vitamin D–dependent rickets in a Saint Bernard dog. J Small Anim Pract 29:657, 1988.)

The syndrome is dominated by signs of renal failure and uremia. Bone disease is more likely to be recognized clinically in growing dogs or, rarely, cats with early-onset renal failure. Changes may be most evident in the head. The mandible and maxilla may be pliable and swollen owing to bone resorption and fibrosis, and teeth may be malaligned, loose, or lost. Skeletal pain, fractures, and bowing of long bones can also occur. Osteopenia of the mandible and maxilla leads to enhanced radiographic contrast between teeth and bone, and teeth may appear almost unsupported by bony tissue. Treatment is reviewed in Chapter 169.

HYPERVITAMINOSIS A

Prolonged intake of excessive vitamin A supplements or ingestion of mainly liver diets can cause osteopathy. The major findings in older cats are extensive, even confluent, exostoses and enthesophytes involving cervical and cranial thoracic vertebrae (Fig. 184–28). Enthesophytes may also form around limb joints, especially shoulder or elbow, which may reflect increased sensitivity of tendon, ligament, and joint capsule attachments to the effects of tension (see Fig. 184–28).[107, 127]

The lesions are painful in the early stages and may ankylose, causing neck stiffness and abnormal posture. Associated clinical signs are lethargy, depression, irritability, poor grooming, lameness, and gingivitis.[107] Experimental vitamin A toxicosis in young animals depressed chondrocyte and osteoblast activities, which produced thin bone cortices, retarded long-bone growth, and loose or lost teeth in kittens.[127, 128] Puppies had joint pain, thin cortices, and retarded bone growth.[129]

MSJ

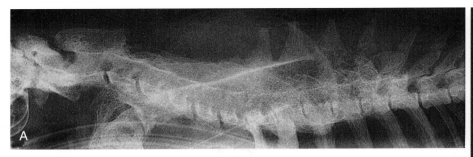

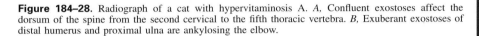

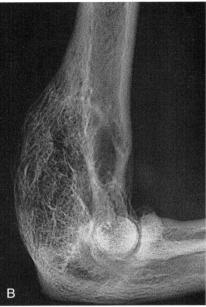

Figure 184–28. Radiograph of a cat with hypervitaminosis A. *A,* Confluent exostoses affect the dorsum of the spine from the second cervical to the fifth thoracic vertebra. *B,* Exuberant exostoses of distal humerus and proximal ulna are ankylosing the elbow.

Treatment necessitates avoiding the source of vitamin A. Mature cats improve clinically, but rigidity resulting from ankylosis is likely to remain despite bone remodeling. Bone growth may be retarded permanently in young animals.[127]

OTHER ENDOCRINE AND NUTRITIONAL BONE DISORDERS

Primary Hyperparathyroidism

With uncontrolled hyperplastic or neoplastic proliferation of parathyroid tissue, excessive secretion of parathyroid hormone may cause increased bone remodeling and skeletal demineralization. This could lead to lameness, pain, fractures, vertebral collapse, loose or lost teeth, and pliable, possibly swollen jaw bones (Fig. 184–29). However, the predominant findings are usually related to hypercalcemia[130] and include polydipsia, polyuria, listlessness, incontinence, weakness, inappetence, and urocystolithiasis (see Chapter 149).

Humoral Hypercalcemia of Malignancy

With certain neoplasms, especially lymphosarcoma or adenocarcinoma of the anal sacs in dogs, widespread skeletal demineralization ensues through the humoral action of parathyroid hormone–related protein.[130, 131] Although skeletal dysfunction can occur as with primary hyperparathyroidism, findings are usually dominated by changes related to the underlying tumor and the effects of hypercalcemia (see Chapters 97 and 149).

Hyperadrenocorticism

Chronic glucocorticosteroid excess related to iatrogenic excess or naturally occurring hyperadrenocorticism causes osteopenia. Retarded growth and delayed growth plate closure may occur in young dogs,[132] and spontaneous fractures and increased prevalence of intervertebral disk disease have been suggested.[133] Osteopenia in naturally occurring canine hyperadrenocorticism is attributable primarily to decreased

bone formation; bone resorption is apparently normal, although parathyroid hyperplasia is present in some cases (see Chapter 154).[133]

Hypogonadism

Hypogonadism, whether a developmental defect or produced surgically, can delay growth plate closure.[6] In dogs, closure was delayed by neutering in both sexes, and the extended growth period resulted in longer radius and ulna in all males, and in bitches neutered at 7 weeks.[134] Gonadectomy in cats delayed distal radial physeal closure but did not affect bone length.[135]

Hepatic Osteodystrophy

Severe hepatic disease can produce rickets-osteomalacia related to malassimilation of fat and vitamin D (and secondarily of calcium) and impaired production of 25-hydroxyvitamin D.[136] Osteoporosis may also occur because of diminished hepatic protein synthesis.[136] Although well recognized in human patients, hepatic osteodystrophy has yet to be characterized in dogs and cats.

Anticonvulsant Osteodystrophy

Prolonged high-dose anticonvulsant therapy with primidone, phenytoin, or phenobarbital can cause osteodystrophy in human epileptics.[136] These drugs induce hepatic enzymes that enhance catabolism and excretion of vitamin D, resulting in calcium malabsorption, hypocalcemia, secondary hyperparathyroidism, and osteomalacia. Phenytoin also directly inhibits intestinal calcium transport and bone resorptive responses to parathyroid hormone and vitamin D metabolites.[136] The significance of these changes in dogs or cats is unknown.

Hypovitaminosis A

Vitamin A is important for growth, maturation, and remodeling of bone. Hypovitaminosis A decreases osteoclastic

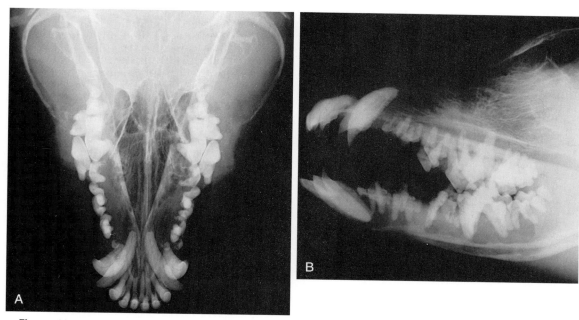

Figure 184–29. Radiograph of an aged keeshond with parathyroid adenoma and hyperparathyroidism, with profound osteopenia of the skull and mandible. *A,* In the ventrodorsal view, there is osteolysis of the zygomatic arch, maxilla, facial bones, and mandible. *B,* In the lateral view, there is loss of the lamina dura and mandibular cortex, except for the thin ventral cortex.

activity and impedes bone remodeling, causing long bones to be deformed. Affected animals are usually lame. The condition is probably rare.[107, 137]

Hypervitaminosis D

Skeletal demineralization follows massive intake of vitamin D or its active metabolites or analogs. Although osteopenia, bone deformation, and retarded growth are possible, the major clinical effects are related to hypercalcemia and soft tissue mineralization.[129] Correcting intakes of vitamin D, calcium, and phosphate should resolve the bone problems, but soft tissue damage may persist.

Zinc-Responsive Chondrodysplasia

This form of dwarfism occurs in Alaskan malamutes and possibly other northern breeds.[137] Affected dogs have short, bowed legs; flared, irregular, thickened growth plates; and coarse, disorganized metaphyseal trabeculae. Hemolytic anemia with macrocytosis, hypochromia, and stomatocytosis is also present. Lifelong supplementation with zinc sulfate or gluconate was suggested.[137]

Copper Deficiency

Lameness and bone fragility can occur in dogs receiving copper-deficient diets.[6] Radiographic features are thickened growth plates and flared metaphyses, with osteopenia and epiphyseal slipping in severe cases. Histologically, there is thickening of the zone of hypertrophic chondrocytes plus disorganization and collapse of the primary spongiosa.[138] The condition is rare.

Lead Poisoning

Although skeletal signs are absent in plumbism, lead lines are seen radiographically in bones of some affected imma-ture dogs. The lines are radiopaque bands in metaphyses adjacent to growth plates of long bones (Fig. 184–30). They result from accumulation of thick mineralized trabeculae at these sites because of impaired osteoclastic activity. The presence of lead itself adds little to the radiopacity.

Overnutrition in Growing Dogs

Provision of balanced diets in excess of recommended daily intake, or feeding diets that contain greater than the recommended content of protein, energy, minerals, or vitamins, has been referred to as overnutrition or overfeeding. Experimental studies of young growing Great Danes found that feeding of an excessively supplemented diet was associated with development of wobbler syndrome, enostosis, osteochondrosis, and metaphyseal osteopathy.[139] Subsequently, it was found that diets with excessive protein content have no adverse effects on skeletal development.[140] However, Great Dane puppies fed a diet containing triple the recommended calcium requirement had increased absorption and retention of calcium. In addition, these dogs had disturbed endochondral ossification, osteochondrosis, retained cartilage cores, radius curvus syndrome, and stunted growth.[90, 141, 142] Young Great Danes fed ad libitum with a balanced commercial diet initially had greater increases in body weight and height than littermates fed a restricted (two thirds of the caloric intake) diet.[126] However, the restricted puppies later had a period of catch-up growth, and by age 7 months their long bones were of identical length.[126] Restricted feeding (25 per cent reduction in total intake) of a balanced diet limited the incidence and severity of osteoarthritis secondary to hip dysplasia in Labrador retriever dogs.[143] Accordingly, overfeeding and oversupplemented diets should be avoided in growing pups. Ad libitum feeding is not recommended because it does not result in larger adult dogs, and it increases the risk of orthopedic problems such as hip dysplasia.[126, 143]

MSJ

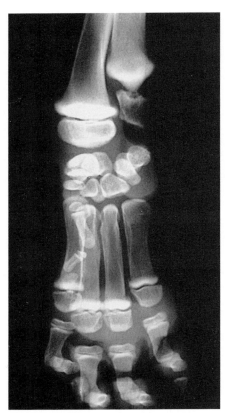

Figure 184–30. Radiograph of the distal forelimb of a puppy with lead poisoning. Radiopaque bands are present in metaphyses adjacent to growth plates.

NEOPLASTIC BONE DISEASE[144]

Neoplasia of the skeletal system can be categorized into primary bone tumors, metastatic bone tumors, tumors of soft tissues extending into adjacent bone, and benign bone tumors.[144] In one study, bone neoplasia had a prevalence of 6.5 cases per 1000 canine patients.[145]

PRIMARY BONE NEOPLASIA

Osteosarcoma

Osteosarcoma constitutes 85 to 90 per cent of all primary bone tumors in large (>20 kg) dogs, and approximately 9000 dogs develop osteosarcoma annually in the United States.[144, 146] The etiology of osteosarcoma is not known, although the association of the tumor with metaphyseal bone suggests that derangement of bone growth or differentiation may result in neoplastic transformation.[144] Aberrant stimulation of stem cells by locally acting hormones and cytokines may lead to neoplasia.[144] Mutation and inactivation of the *p53* tumor suppressor gene is associated with development of canine osteosarcoma, suggesting that some dogs may be genetically predisposed.[147] Primary bone sarcomas have also been rarely reported after internal fixation of fractures and total hip arthroplasty.[148, 149] Osteosarcomas account for about 90 per cent of fracture-associated sarcomas but less than 1 per cent of all osteosarcomas. Time of occurrence after the initial surgery is approximately 5 to 7 years.

Seventy-five per cent of large dogs with osteosarcoma have the primary tumor in the appendicular skeleton.[146] The most common sites are, in descending order, distal radius, proximal humerus, distal femur, and proximal tibia. Other less common sites are metacarpal and metatarsal bones, ulna, and distal tibia. Large or giant-breed dogs are particularly predisposed to appendicular osteosarcoma, and there is a slight predilection for males over females. The average age of occurrence is 7 years, although a bimodal distribution has been suggested with an additional peak at 2 years.[144] Young dogs with high-grade osteosarcoma seem to develop metastases more quickly than older dogs.[146] At the time of diagnosis, 90 per cent of dogs with osteosarcoma already have microscopic tumor spread that is undetectable by the initial diagnostic evaluation.[146] Skeletal neoplasms in small dogs (<15 kg) present some differences: less than 50 per cent are osteosarcoma, a higher proportion involve the axial skeleton, and metastatic bone neoplasia is more prevalent (25 per cent versus less than 5 per cent).[150]

Osteosarcoma of the spine, skull, and pelvis develops less commonly than appendicular osteosarcoma. Osteosarcoma accounts for approximately 10 per cent of all oral tumors and is the most common tumor of ribs and other flat bones.[144, 151, 152]

Diagnosis of Osteosarcoma

Any large dog presented with acute lameness should be thoroughly evaluated to rule out osteosarcoma. The radiographic appearance of osteosarcoma varies, but typical patterns are mixed osteolysis and proliferation and periosteal reaction (Fig. 184–31).[153] A presumptive diagnosis of primary bone tumor can be made given circumstances of a large-breed dog with a bone lesion with a typical radiographic appearance in a preferred site. As a routine, thoracic radiographs, with right and left lateral views and a ventrodorsal view, should be examined for pulmonary metastasis. Other sites such as caudal abdominal lymph nodes, liver,

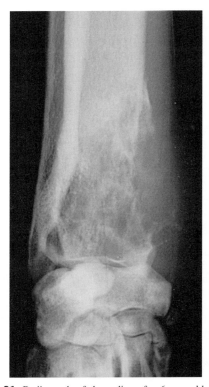

Figure 184–31. Radiograph of the radius of a 6-year-old rottweiler that has osteosarcoma.

and spleen can be evaluated by ultrasonography. Evaluation of blood biochemistry and cell counts may be advisable because adjunctive treatment with antineoplastic drugs may affect renal function and bone marrow.

Multicentric or polyostotic osteosarcoma occurs in up to 5 to 10 per cent of affected dogs and must be considered.[154] Evaluation of dogs using bone imaging techniques revealed that the degree of radionuclide uptake in the primary tumor correlated with the onset of metastasis after amputation.[155] Such information, if confirmed, may be useful as a prognostic factor.

Although most bone neoplasms in dogs are osteosarcoma, definitive diagnosis requires biopsy as described earlier in this chapter. Preoperative biopsy is not essential if limb amputation is the only option for lesions that have fractured or extensively invaded surrounding soft tissues. A sample of the lesion should nevertheless be submitted after amputation to confirm the diagnosis. Otherwise, all bone lesions that have radiographic features of neoplasia should have biopsies performed because many alternative diagnoses exist. Fungal osteomyelitis may resemble osteosarcoma and should be considered in endemic areas.[153] Other lesions suggestive of systemic fungal infections (e.g., draining wounds, pulmonary opacity) should be thoroughly evaluated (see Chapter 93).

Therapy and Prognosis for Osteosarcoma

Improvements have been made in the management of dogs with osteosarcoma in the past two decades, providing options that may prolong survival and maintain a functional, pain-free limb.[156] However, the overriding consideration in treating dogs with osteosarcoma is that 90 per cent die with metastatic disease despite long-term control of the primary tumor. After it has been confirmed that there are no detectable metastases, the next step is excision of the primary tumor by amputation or a limb-sparing technique. Before considering amputation, thorough orthopedic and neurologic examinations are performed to ensure that no concurrent problem exists that would make tripedal ambulation problematic. Also owners are counseled about postamputation care. Dogs that undergo limb amputation without further treatment do well for an average of 5 months; 11 per cent survive 1 year, and 2 per cent survive 2 years, with pulmonary metastasis the most likely eventuality.[146] Dogs that develop osteosarcoma of the spine, pelvis, or ribs are also at high risk of developing metastases, although most affected dogs are euthanased for problems related to the primary tumor.[151, 157–159] The prognosis appears more favorable with mandibular osteosarcoma, with 1-year survival rate of 71 per cent after partial mandibulectomy.[152]

Numerous reports suggest improved survival after amputation if cisplatin is administered.[160] Survival rates vary with the report, but most indicate median survival of 9 to 14 months and 1- and 2-year survival rates of 35 to 60 per cent and 20 to 25 per cent, respectively. This represents a doubling of median survival times after amputation without chemotherapy.

Carboplatin, a related second-generation platinum compound that is less nephrotoxic and does not require prehydration or diuresis, and doxorubicin may both be as effective as cisplatin in controlling osteosarcoma metastasis.[161, 162] Protocols for use of antineoplastic drugs in osteosarcoma appear in Chapter 101. One promising strategy for controlling metastatic disease is to use cisplatin chemotherapy followed by immunotherapy with a macrophage stimulator delivered selectively to macrophage by liposomes.[163] Results to date are encouraging, but further studies are necessary.

Limb-sparing techniques may provide a pain-free, functional limb for dogs with tumors of the distal radius or the ulna.[156] Other sites are problematic because of biomechanical limitations and postoperative infection of allografts. The limb-sparing technique is best performed by an experienced surgeon at a referral center. Metastases still limit success of this procedure and adjuvant drug treatment is recommended before, during, or after surgery. Implantation of sustained-release, cisplatin-impregnated polymer into the graft site may help reduce local tumor recurrence.[156]

Palliative radiation of the primary lesion provides pain relief for dogs with osteosarcoma that cannot undergo amputation or limb-sparing.[164] Relatively high radiation doses are delivered in three fractions (each of 8 to 10 Gy) over a 3-week period. This strategy minimizes inconvenience and discomfort caused by acute radiation reactions. Pain relief is maintained for 4 to 6 months. Intramedullary cisplatin chemotherapy provided effective localized control in two of four dogs with advanced-stage osteosarcoma unable to withstand amputation or limb-sparing surgery.[165] Other treatments, such as anti-inflammatory agents, do not offer consistent benefits for extended periods without complications.

Other Primary Bone Tumors

Other primary bone tumors that occur in dogs and cats include chondrosarcoma, fibrosarcoma, hemangiosarcoma, multilobular osteochondrosarcoma, lymphoproliferative neoplasia, and liposarcoma. Difficulty can arise in classifying bone sarcomas when the section contains no osteoid, the bone matrix material that characterizes the tumor as osteosarcoma.[6] Lack of osteoid in the section raises the question of whether the section truly represents the entire tumor and whether it should thus be classified as an undifferentiated or other type of sarcoma. Such a diagnosis may warrant review of the biopsy and radiographs with the pathologist or a second opinion, as the diagnosis may be confounded by other prominent cell types and the existence of several subcategories of osteosarcoma.

Chondrosarcomas of appendicular bone are rare.[166] The majority of canine chondrosarcomas affect the axial or flat bones, representing the second most common type of primary bone tumor.[151] The metastatic rate is not accurately known. Treatment options include resection of the affected site with adequate margins and reconstruction. Median survival of 15 dogs with primary rib chondrosarcomas after en bloc resection was nearly 3 years.[151]

Fibrosarcomas originating in bone are rare, and little information about their biologic behavior is available. Limited data indicate that appendicular bone fibrosarcomas are of medullary origin and arise in diaphyseal or metaphyseal regions.[167] Radiographic appearance is similar to that of osteosarcoma, and definitive diagnosis requires sufficient biopsy material to eliminate osteosarcoma as a possibility. One review of primary skeletal fibrosarcomas resulted in reclassification of many of these tumors as osteosarcoma.[167] Complete excision is the treatment of choice, and amputation or limb-sparing options may be considered. The role of adjuvant antineoplastic drugs in management of skeletal fibrosarcomas is unclear; however, metastases occur to a wide variety of tissue sites. Fibrosarcomas of the axial skeleton have been reported, but the site of origin can be difficult to determine as fibrosarcomas of soft tissue origin often invade bone.

Hemangiosarcoma arising from a primary bone site occurs rarely in dogs and cats.[168] The diagnosis must be confirmed by biopsy, and confusion about the diagnosis is generally a problem only if the site of bone involvement is one usually associated with osteosarcoma.[144] A thorough evaluation should be conducted to detect metastases. Abdominal ultrasonography and thoracic radiography should be included, and bone scintigraphy may be indicated. The main treatment considerations include management of the primary site with wide surgical excision and adjuvant antineoplastic drugs for probable metastases. This may involve use of doxorubicin, vincristine, and cyclophosphamide in a repetitive, 3-week treatment course (see Chapter 101), but treatment response data are limited.

Multilobular osteochondrosarcoma (multilobular osteoma, multilobular tumor of bone, chondroma rodens, calcifying aponeurotic fibroma) is an infrequent tumor of bone that has a predilection for the skull.[169, 170] It produces a hard bony mass with a characteristic radiographic pattern described as nodular, stippled, and coarsely granular.[169] This tumor occurs in middle-aged and older dogs and usually involves the mandible, maxilla, or cranium. In a study of 34 affected dogs treated by wide surgical excision, 47 per cent had local recurrence and 56 per cent developed metastasis at median intervals of 797 and 542 days, respectively.[169]

Lymphoproliferative disorders can involve bone.[171–173] Multiple punctate, radiolucent lesions are the most commonly reported description of lymphoid infiltration. Myeloma can involve the entire skeleton, producing osteopenia and numerous "punched-out" lesions. Systemic chemotherapy is indicated to control lymphoproliferative diseases, but radiation may be helpful for isolated lesions.

FELINE BONE NEOPLASIA

Primary bone cancer is much less prevalent in cats than in dogs. Osteosarcoma accounts for 90 per cent of bone cancers in cats.[171] No clear pattern of anatomic sites exists, but metaphyses are most frequently involved and lesions are primarily lytic. There is limited information regarding the biologic behavior of feline osteosarcoma, but metastasis is uncommon and survival for several years is possible after amputation.[171] There is no recommended chemotherapy for cats with nonresectable osteosarcoma. Radiation therapy may be useful for reduction of bone pain and tumor control, either after surgery or before surgery for tumors of the axial skeleton.

METASTATIC BONE NEOPLASIA

The most frequently reported metastases to bone are from carcinomas of mammary gland, thyroid, and prostate and epithelial neoplasms.[174] Secondary bone tumors are recognized less often than in humans.

BENIGN BONE TUMORS AND BONE LESIONS RESEMBLING TUMORS

Benign tumors of bone are rare in dogs and cats. Osteoma, ossifying fibroma, chondroma, and several others have been reported.[22, 175] Wide surgical resection is curative if the location permits. Irradiation of inoperable tumors may produce regression or stabilization, but responses may be protracted because of slow cell turnover in these tumors.[144]

Non-neoplastic conditions of bone, such as bone cysts, that may be confused with primary bone cancer are important differentials. Bone cysts are discussed earlier in this chapter.

BONE INFECTION

Bone infection (osteomyelitis) may be bacterial, fungal, or possibly viral (see Metaphyseal Osteopathy) in origin. Beta-lactamase–producing *Staphylococcus* causes approximately 50 per cent of cases of bacterial osteomyelitis, often as monomicrobial infections.[30] Polymicrobial infections may have mixtures of *Streptococcus* and gram-negative bacteria (*Escherichia coli*, *Pseudomonas*, *Proteus*, and *Klebsiella*) and sometimes anaerobic bacteria. More common anaerobic isolates are *Actinomyces*, *Peptostreptococcus*, *Bacteroides*, and *Fusobacterium*.[176] Anaerobes are especially common in bite wound infections. *Nocardia*, *Brucella canis*, and tuberculosis cause osteomyelitis in rare instances.[144] Mycotic genera that cause osteomyelitis include *Coccidioides*, *Blastomyces*, *Histoplasma*, *Cryptococcus*, and *Aspergillus*. Fungal osteomyelitis is often a component of disseminated mycotic infections that occur in certain specific regions of the world. Diagnosis and treatment of deep mycoses are discussed in Chapter 93.

PATHOPHYSIOLOGY

Bacterial contamination of bone can occur with open fractures, surgery, bite wounds, foreign body penetration, gunshot injury, extension from soft tissue, and hematogenous spread. However, the simple presence of bacteria in bone is insufficient to cause osteomyelitis. Bone is relatively resistant to infection unless there is concurrent soft tissue injury, bone necrosis, sequestration, fracture instability, implanted foreign material, altered host defenses, or some combination of these.[177, 178] In chronic infections, sequestra of cortical bone become colonized by bacteria, surrounded by exudate, remain avascular, and may persist for long periods. New bone formed by periosteum (involucrum) incompletely encapsulates the focus of infection and sequestrum. Exudate draining from the bone follows sinus tracts that discharge through skin openings generally in a more dependent location. Osteomyelitis is exacerbated by fracture and instability. Cortical bone at the fracture site is resorbed because of infection and interfragmentary motion, and this causes further widening of the fracture gap and additional instability.

Extraneous material (wood, soil, asphalt, and surgical implants) may incite a foreign body response, interfere with local host defense mechanisms, and provide a nidus for infection.[177, 179] Bacteria have unique mechanisms for bonding to surfaces of implanted foreign material. Initially, the surfaces of implants become coated with matrix and serum proteins, ions, cellular debris, and carbohydrates (Fig. 184–32).[180] One of these proteins, fibronectin, is especially important in bacterial binding to biomaterial. Staphylococci and other gram-positive bacteria possess numerous cell membrane receptors for binding to fibronectin on implant surfaces.[180] Gram-negative bacteria are less effective at binding and have pili and fimbriae that specifically bind cellular proteins, matrix proteins, and glycolipids.[180] Bacteria also bind to exposed collagen matrix proteins (sialoprotein) and hydroxyapatite crystals of damaged bone.[180, 181]

Once adherent, bacteria have two important mechanisms

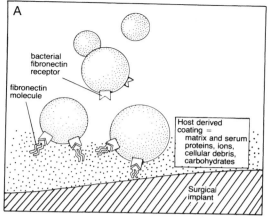

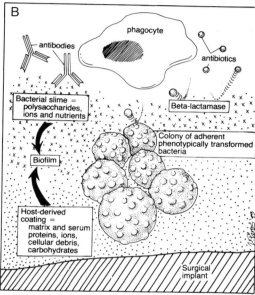

Figure 184–32. Mechanisms of bacterial persistence in chronic osteomyelitis. *A,* Foreign material such as surgical implants become coated with host-derived material containing fibronectin that binds with membrane receptors of contaminating bacteria. *B,* Adherent staphylococci and some other bacteria produce a slime that, together with the host-derived material, is called biofilm. Biofilm increases bacterial adhesion, protects bacteria from phagocytes and antibodies, and may also contain beta-lactamase. In addition, some adherent bacteria are phenotypically transformed to more virulent strains. (From Johnson KA: Osteomyelitis in dogs and cats. JAVMA 205:1882, 1994.)

that ensure their persistence: slime production and phenotypic transformation.[180, 182] Adherent staphylococci and some other bacteria produce a slime composed of extracellular polysaccharide, ions, and nutrients. Slime, together with host-derived material (matrix and serum proteins, ions, cellular debris, and carbohydrate), envelops bacterial colonies and is called biofilm or glycocalyx (see Fig. 184–32). Biofilm is a virulence factor, because it increases bacterial adhesion, shields bacteria from phagocytes and antibodies, and modifies drug susceptibility.[180] Most antimicrobial drugs diffuse through biofilm, but biofilm may contain high concentrations of beta-lactamase, which protects some bacteria. In addition to providing physical protection, biofilm causes adherent bacteria to transform phenotypically to more virulent strains that are more resistant to antimicrobial drugs than when they are tested in vitro.[180]

The metaphyses of long bones are commonly affected in young animals with acute hematogenous osteomyelitis. These regions may be especially vulnerable because capillary endothelium therein is discontinuous, allowing extravasation of erythrocytes and possibly bacteria.[183] When local defenses are compromised, osteomyelitis may ensue. This probably accounts for the development of lesions suggesting metaphyseal osteomyelitis in Irish setter pups with leukocyte adhesion protein deficiency and Border collies with neutropenia caused by impaired release of neutrophils from bone marrow (Fig. 184–33).[184, 185]

DIAGNOSIS

Acute osteomyelitis may produce signs of systemic illness including pyrexia, inappetence, dullness, and weight loss, together with neutrophilia and left shift. Heat, pain, and swelling in muscle and periosteum surrounding the infected bone may be evident. In chronic osteomyelitis, abscessation with single or multiple sinus tracts is a prominent sign. Lymphadenopathy, muscle atrophy, fibrosis, and contracture accompany chronic disease, but hematologic alterations are uncommon.

Radiographs are usually necessary for diagnosis. In acute osteomyelitis, soft tissue swelling is present but there are no osseous changes, except perhaps in young animals with acute metaphyseal osteomyelitis. In chronic osteomyelitis, periosteal new bone forms early and tends to be extensive, spiculated, and radially orientated. Bone resorption produces cortical thinning, medullary lysis, and rounding of fractured bone ends (Fig. 184–34). In young animals, the diaphyseal cortex may be entirely resorbed and replaced by a shell of involucrum. The finding of sequestra is virtually diagnostic for osteomyelitis. Sequestra may be small and obscured by surrounding bone but should always be suspected in cases of persistent bone infection. Contrast radiography may help delineate sinuses and foreign bodies. A water-soluble con-

MSJ

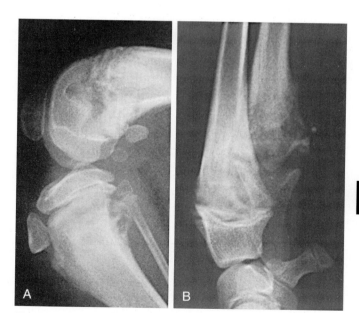

Figure 184–33. Polyostotic metaphyseal osteomyelitis in a Border collie pup that had persistent neutropenia. *A,* Disruption of metaphyseal architecture of distal femur and proximal tibia, with irregular areas of radiolucency and sclerosis, and some periosteal new bone adjacent. *B,* Similar changes are evident in distal ulna and radius.

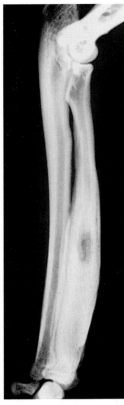

Figure 184–34. Radius of a cat with chronic osteomyelitis caused by anaerobic bacteria. At the focus of infection there is cortical and medullary bone lysis. The diaphysis is thickened by periosteal new bone, formed in response to the infection.

trast medium (10 to 20 mL of meglumine diatrizoate [Urografin], 76 per cent) is injected slowly through a Foley catheter into each sinus. Incomplete delineation of sinuses is a problem. Radionuclide imaging may also be useful. Isolation of bacteria from suspected bone infections should be attempted to confirm the diagnosis and determine the in vitro drug susceptibility. The diagnosis can usually be made from the history, physical examination, radiology, microbiology, or some combination of these.

TREATMENT

Contrary to long-held beliefs, most antimicrobial drugs penetrate bone well. However, osteomyelitis can be difficult to treat because of factors discussed under Pathophysiology. Beta-lactam agents (penicillins, cephalosporins), tetracyclines, and aminoglycosides readily traverse the capillary membrane in normal and infected bone and are widely distributed in interstitial fluid.[186] Peak tissue concentrations of these drugs are reached 25 to 45 minutes after intravenous administration in normal and infected bone, and concentrations in bone closely reflect those in blood.[186] Therefore factors other than drug penetration (such as toxicity, administration routes, in vitro susceptibility, and cost) should dictate drug selection (see Chapters 73 and 74). Acute bacterial osteomyelitis may be cured by 4 to 6 weeks of antimicrobial drug therapy, provided there is limited bone necrosis and no fracture. However, in chronic osteomyelitis, drug treatment is futile without surgical intervention to remove sequestra and débride necrotic tissue.[178] Débridement wounds are left open to heal by secondary intention, protected with sterile dressings, and irrigated daily with sterile physiologic saline. Fractures must be stabilized and bone defects grafted with autologous cancellous bone. Treatment of chronic osteomyelitis is invariably prolonged and expensive and may be frustrated by episodes of recurrence. Treatment of recurrent osteomyelitis may necessitate a further search for sequestra, repeated débridement and drainage, reassessment of fracture stability, and reevaluation of microbiology and antimicrobial drug therapy.

REFERENCES

1. Piermattei DL, Flo GL: Handbook of Small Animal Orthopedics and Fracture Treatment, 3rd ed. Philadelphia, WB Saunders, 1997.
2. Beresford JN: Osteogenic stem cells and the stromal system of bone and marrow. Clin Orthop 240:270, 1989.
3. Martin RB, Burr DB: Structure, Function, and Adaptation of Compact Bone. New York, Raven Press, 1989.
4. Ogden JA: Skeletal Injury in the Child. Philadelphia, WB Saunders, 1990.
5. Mundy GR, Roodman GD: Osteoclast ontogeny and function. In Peck WA (ed): Bone and Mineral Research 5. New York, Elsevier Science Publishers, 1987, p 209.
6. Palmer N: Bones and joints. In Jubb KVF, Kennedy PC, Palmer N (eds): Pathology of Domestic Animals, 4th ed. San Diego, Academic Press, 1993, p 1.
7. Gowen M: Cytokines and Bone Metabolism. Boca Raton, FL, CRC Press, 1992.
8. Hunziker EB, et al: Quantitation of chondrocyte performance in growth-plate cartilage during longitudinal bone growth. J Bone Joint Surg Am 69:162, 1987.
9. Ogden JA, Rosenberg LC: Defining the growth plate. In Uhthoff HK, Wiley JJ (eds): Behavior of the Growth Plate. New York, Raven Press, 1988, p 1.
10. Frost HM: Intermediary Organization of the Skeleton. Boca Raton, FL, CRC Press, 1986.
11. Eriksen EF: Normal and pathological remodeling of human trabecular bone: Three dimensional reconstruction of the remodeling sequence in normals and in metabolic bone disease. Endocr Rev 7:379, 1986.
12. Jaworski ZFG, Uhthoff HK: Disuse osteoporosis: Current status and problems. In Uhthoff HK (ed): Current Concepts in Bone Fragility. Berlin, Springer-Verlag, 1986, p 181.
13. Schrader SC, et al: Diagnosis: Historical, physical and ancillary examinations. In Olmstead ML (ed): Small Animal Orthopedics. St Louis, CV Mosby, 1995, p 3.
14. Sumner-Smith G: Gait analysis and orthopedic examination. In Slatter D (ed): Textbook of Small Animal Surgery, 2nd ed. Philadelphia, WB Saunders, 1993, p 1577.
15. Schebitz H, Wilkens H: Atlas of Radiographic Anatomy of the Dog and Cat, 4th ed. Philadelphia, WB Saunders, 1986.
16. Biery DN: Orthopaedic radiology. In Newton CD and Nunamaker DM (eds): Textbook of Small Animal Orthopaedics. Philadelphia, JB Lippincott, 1985, p 133.
17. Stowater J: Aggressive versus nonaggressive bone lesions. In Thrall DE (ed): Textbook of Veterinary Diagnostic Radiology. Philadelphia, WB Saunders, 1986, p 12.
18. Allan GS: Radiographic signs of diseases affecting bone. Proceedings No. 87, Orthopaedic Surgery—Dogs and Cats. The University of Sydney, Postgraduate Committee in Veterinary Science, 1986, p 247.
19. Murray IPC: Skeletal scintigraphy in the investigation of disorders of bone. In Murray RO, et al (eds): The Radiology of Skeletal Disorders, 3rd ed. Edinburgh, Churchill Livingstone, 1990, p 1859.
20. Lamb CR: Bone scintigraphy in small animals. JAVMA 191:1616, 1987.
21. Adams JE: Computed tomography—Application to musculoskeletal disease. In Murray RO, Jacobson HG, Stoker DJ (eds): The Radiology of Skeletal Disorders, 3rd ed. Edinburgh, Churchill Livingstone, 1990, p 1943.
22. Johnson KA, et al: Zygomatic osteoma with atypical heterogeneity in a dog. J Comp Pathol 114:199, 1996.
23. Straw RC, et al: Partial and total hemipelvectomy in the management of sarcomas in nine dogs and two cats. Vet Surg 21:183, 1992.
24. Straw RC, Withrow SJ: Limb-sparing surgery for dogs with bone neoplasia. In Slatter DJ (ed): Textbook of Small Animal Surgery, 2nd ed. Philadelphia, WB Saunders, 1993, p 2020.
25. Powers BE, et al: Jamshidi needle biopsy for diagnosis of bone lesions in small animals. JAVMA 193:205, 1988.
26. Breur GJ, et al: Percutaneous biopsy of the proximal humeral growth plate in dogs. Am J Vet Res 49:1529, 1988.
27. Ching SV, Norrdin RW: Histomorphometric comparison of measurements of trabecular bone remodeling in iliac crest biopsy sites and lumbar vertebrae in cats. Am J Vet Res 51:447, 1990.
28. Rochat MC, et al: Identification of surgical biopsy borders by use of India ink. JAVMA 201:873, 1992.
29. Baron R, et al: Processing of undecalcified bone specimens for bone histomorphometry. In Recker RR (ed): Bone Histomorphometry: Techniques and Interpretation. Boca Raton, FL, CRC Press, 1983, p 13.

30. Muir P, Johnson KA: Anaerobic bacteria isolated from osteomyelitis in dogs and cats. Vet Surg 21:463, 1992.
31. Sharrard WJW: Pediatric Orthopaedics and Fractures, 3rd ed. London, Blackwell Scientific Publication, 1993.
32. Jezyk PF: Constitutional disorders of the skeleton in dogs and cats. In Newton CD, Nunamaker DM (eds): Textbook of Small Animal Orthopaedics. Philadelphia, JB Lippincott, 1985, p 637.
33. Winterbotham EJ, et al: Radial agenesis in a cat. J Small Anim Pract 26:393, 1985.
34. Schultz VA, Watson AG: Lumbosacral transitional vertebra and thoracic limb malformations in a Chihuahua puppy. J Am Anim Hosp Assoc 31:101, 1995.
35. Johnson KA: Unpublished data.
36. Goldberg MT: The Dysmorphic Child. An Orthopedic Perspective. New York, Raven Press, 1987.
37. Battison JR: Proximal femoral focal deficiency in a Dalmatian pup. Vet Rec 102:86, 1978.
38. Richardson EF, et al: Surgical management of syndactyly in a dog. JAVMA 205:1149, 1994.
39. Keller WG, Chambers JN: Antebrachial metacarpal arthrodesis for fusion of deranged carpal joints in two dogs. JAVMA 195:1382, 1989.
40. Montgomery M, Tomlinson J: Two cases of ectrodactyly and congenital elbow luxation in the dog. J Am Anim Hosp Assoc 21:781, 1985.
41. Montgomery RD, et al: Ectrodactyly. JAVMA 194:120, 1989.
42. Hardie EM, et al: Segmental hemiatrophy in a dog. JAVMA 186:1315, 1985.
43. Kramers P, et al: Osteopetrosis in cats. J Small Anim Pract 29:153, 1988.
44. Gertner JM, Root L: Osteogenesis imperfecta. Orthop Clin North Am 21:151, 1990.
45. Cohn LA, Meuten DJ: Bone fragility in a kitten: An osteogenesis imperfecta–like syndrome. JAVMA 197:98, 1990.
46. Prockop DJ: Mutations that alter the primary structure of type I collagen. J Biol Chem 265:15349, 1990.
47. Campbell BG, et al: Clinical signs and diagnosis of osteogenesis imperfecta in three dogs. JAVMA 211:183, 1997.
48. Bennett D, May C: Joint diseases of dogs and cats. In Ettinger SJ, Feldman EC (eds): Textbook of Veterinary Internal Medicine, 4th ed. Philadelphia, WB Saunders, 1995, p 2032.
49. Haskins ME, et al: Spinal cord compression and hindlimb paresis in cats with mucopolysaccharidosis VI. JAVMA 182:983, 1983.
50. Konde LJ, et al: Radiographically visualized skeletal changes associated with mucopolysaccharidosis VI in cats. Vet Radiol 28:223, 1987.
51. Byers S, et al: Age related changes in trabecular bone in normal and mucopolysaccharidosis type VI vertebrae (abstract). Proceedings of 44th Annual Meeting, Orthopaedic Research Society, 1998, 634.
52. Yogalingam G, et al: Feline mucopolysaccharidosis type VI. Characterization of recombinant N-acetylgalactosamine 4-sulfatase and identification of a mutation causing the disease. J Biol Chem 271:27259, 1996.
53. Byers S, et al: Effect of enzyme replacement therapy on bone formation in a feline model of mucopolysaccharidosis type VI. Bone 21:425, 1997.
54. Haskins ME, et al: The pathology of the feline model of mucopolysaccharidosis I. Am J Pathol 112:27, 1983.
55. Shull RM, Walker MA: Radiographic findings in a canine model of mucopolysaccharidosis I. Changes associated with bone marrow transplantation. Invest Radiol 23:124, 1988.
56. Kakkis ED, et al: Long-term and high-dose trials of enzyme replacement therapy in the canine model of mucopolysaccharidosis I. Biochem Mol Med 58:156, 1996.
57. Wilkerson MJ, et al: Clinical and morphologic features of mucopolysaccharidosis type II in a dog: Naturally occurring model of Hunter syndrome. Vet Pathol 35:230, 1998.
58. Fischer A, et al: Sulfamidase deficiency in a family of Dachshunds: A canine model of mucopolysaccharidosis IIIA (Sanfilippo A). Pediatr Res 44:74, 1998.
59. Haskins ME, et al: Beta-glucuronidase deficiency in a dog: A model of human mucopolysaccharidosis VII. Pediatr Res 18:980, 1984.
60. Patterson DF, et al: Is this a genetic disease? J Small Anim Pract 30:127, 1989.
61. Ray J, et al: Molecular diagnostic tests for ascertainment of genotype at the mucopolysaccharidosis type VII locus in dogs. Am J Vet Res 59:1092, 1998.
62. Gitzelmann R, et al: Feline mucopolysaccharidosis VII due to beta-glucuronidase deficiency. Vet Pathol 31:435, 1994.
63. Feldman EC, Nelson RW: Canine and Feline Endocrinology and Reproduction, 2nd ed. Philadelphia, WB Saunders, 1996, p 38.
64. Randolph JF, et al: Delayed growth in two German shepherd dog littermates with normal concentrations of growth hormone, thyroxine and cortisol. JAVMA 196:77, 1990.
65. Kooistra HS, et al: Progestin-induced growth hormone (GH) production in the treatment of congenital GH deficiency in two dogs (abstract). Proceedings 7th Annual Congress European Society of Veterinary Internal Medicine, 1997, p 125.
66. Greco DS, et al: Congenital hypothyroid dwarfism in a family of giant schnauzers. J Vet Intern Med 5:57, 1991.
67. Jones BR, et al: Preliminary studies on congenital hypothyroidism in a family of Abyssinian cats. Vet Rec 131:145, 1992.
68. Tanase H, et al: Inherited primary hypothyroidism with thyrotrophin resistance in Japanese cats. J Endocrinol 129:245, 1991.
69. Zerbe CA, et al: Congenital hypothyroidism in Scottish deerhounds (abstract). Proceedings, 6th Annual Vet Med Forum. ACVIM, 1988, 721.
70. Robinson WF, et al: Congenital hypothyroidism in Scottish deerhound puppies. Aust J Vet 63:386, 1988.
71. Sjollema BE, et al: Congenital hypothyroidism in two cats due to defective organification: Data suggesting loosely anchored thyroperoxidase. Acta Endocrinol (Copenh) 125:435, 1991.
72. Mooney CT, Anderson TJ: Congenital hypothyroidism in a boxer dog. J Small Anim Pract 34:31, 1993.
73. Sande RD, Bingel SA: Animal models of dwarfism. Vet Clin North Am Small Anim Pract 13:71, 1982.
74. Watson ADJ, et al: Osteochondrodysplasia in bull terrier littermates. J Small Anim Pract 32:312, 1991.
75. Whitbread TJ, et al: An inherited enchondrodystrophy in the English pointer dog. A new disease. J Small Anim Pract 24:399, 1983.
76. Lavelle RB: Inherited enchondrodystrophic dwarfism in English pointers. Aust Vet J 61:268, 1984.
77. Bingel SA, Sande RD: Chondrodysplasia in five Great Pyrenees. JAVMA 205:845, 1994.
78. Hanssen I, et al: Hypochondroplastic dwarfism in the Irish setter. J Small Anim Pract 39:10, 1998.
79. Carrig CB, et al: Inheritance of associated ocular and skeletal dysplasia in Labrador retrievers. JAVMA 193:1269, 1988.
80. Matis U, et al: Multiple enchondromatosis in the dog. Vet Comp Orthop Traum 4:144, 1989.
81. Krauser K: Multiple enchondromatosis in the dog. Vet Comp Orthop Traum 4:152, 1989.
82. Meyers VN, et al: Short-limbed dwarfism and ocular defects in the Samoyed dog. JAVMA 183:975, 1983.
83. Aroch I, et al: Haematological, ocular and skeletal abnormalities in a Samoyed family. J Small Anim Pract 37:333, 1996.
84. Breur GJ, et al: Clinical, radiographic, pathologic, and genetic features of osteochondrodysplasia in Scottish deerhounds. JAVMA 195:606, 1989.
85. Breur GJ, et al: Cellular basis of decreased rate of longitudinal growth of bone in pseudoachondroplastic dogs. J Bone Joint Surg Am 74:516, 1992.
86. Jackson OF: Congenital bone lesions in cats with fold-ears. Bull Feline Advis Bur 14:2, 1975.
87. Mathews KG, et al: Resolution of lameness associated with Scottish fold osteodystrophy following bilateral ostectomies and pantarsal arthrodeses: A case report. J Am Anim Hosp Assoc 31:280, 1995.
88. Malik R, et al: Osteochondrodysplasia in Scottish Fold cats. Aust Vet J 77:85, 1999.
89. Johnson KA: Retardation of endochondral ossification at the distal ulnar growth plate in dogs. Aust Vet J 57:474, 1981.
90. Goedegebuure SA, Hazewinkel HAW: Morphological findings in young dogs chronically fed a diet containing excess calcium. Vet Pathol 23:594, 1986.
91. Watson ADJ, et al: Craniomandibular osteopathy in the dog. Compend Contin Educ Pract Vet 17:911, 1995.
92. Padgett GA, Mostovsky UV: Animal model: The mode of inheritance of craniomandibular osteopathy in West Highland white terriers. Am J Med Genet 25:9, 1986.
93. Riser WH: Canine craniomandibular osteopathy. In Bojrab MJ (ed): Disease Mechanisms in Small Animal Surgery, 2nd ed. Philadelphia, Lea & Febiger, 1993, p 892.
94. Peterson HA: Multiple hereditary osteochondromata. Clin Orthop 239:222, 1989.
95. Watson ADJ: Diseases of muscle and bone. In Whittick WG (ed): Canine Orthopedics, 2nd ed. Philadelphia, Lea & Febiger, 1990, p 657.
96. Doige CE: Multiple cartilaginous exostoses in dogs. Vet Pathol 24:276, 1987.
97. Caporn TM, Read RA: Osteochondromatosis of the cervical spine causing compressive myelopathy in a dog. J Small Anim Pract 37:133, 1996.
98. Muir P, et al: Panosteitis. Compend Contin Educ Prac Vet 18:29, 1996.
99. Mee AP, et al: Detection of canine distemper virus in bone cells in the metaphysis of distemper-infected dogs. Bone Miner Res 7:829, 1992.
100. Chapman BL, Giger U: Inherited erythrocyte pyruvate kinase deficiency in the West Highland white terrier. J Small Anim Pract 31:610, 1990.
101 Muir P, et al: Hypertrophic osteodystrophy and calvarial hyperostosis. Compend Contin Educ Prac Vet 18:143, 1996.
102. Mee AP, et al: Canine virus transcripts detected in the bone cells of dogs with metaphyseal osteopathy. Bone 14:59, 1993.
103. Malik R, et al: Concurrent juvenile cellulitis and metaphyseal osteopathy—An atypical canine distemper virus syndrome? Aust Vet Pract 25:62, 1995.
104. Baumgartner W, et al: Metaphyseal osteosclerosis in young dogs with naturally occurring distemper. Eur J Vet Pathol 2:23, 1996.
105. Staheli LT, et al: Infantile cortical hyperostosis (Caffey's disease). JAMA 203:96, 1968.
106. Baker JR, Lewis DG: Bone disease in a dog similar to infantile cortical hyperostosis (Caffey's disease). Vet Rec 97:74, 1975.
107. Newton CD, Biery DN: Skeletal diseases. In Ettinger SJ (ed): Textbook of Veterinary Internal Medicine, 3rd ed. Philadelphia, WB Saunders, 1989, p 2378.
108. Dubielzig RR: Medullary bone infarction in dogs. In Newton CD, Nunamaker DM (eds): Textbook of Small Animal Orthopaedics. Philadelphia, JB Lippincott, 1985, p 615.
109. Madewell BR, et al: Leukemoid blood response and bone infarcts in a dog with renal tubular adenocarcinoma. JAVMA 197:1623, 1990.
110. Hunt GB, et al: What is your diagnosis? JAVMA 199:1071, 1991.
111. Dueland RT, Van Enkevort B: Lateral tibial head buttress plate: Use in a pathological femoral fracture secondary to a bone cyst in a dog. Vet Comp Orthop Traum 8:200, 1995.
112. Biller DS, et al: Aneurysmal bone cyst in a rib of a cat. JAVMA 190:1193, 1987.

113. Pernell RT, et al: Aneurysmal bone cyst in a six-month-old dog. JAVMA 201:1897, 1992.
114. Duval JM, et al: Surgical treatment of an aneurysmal bone cyst in a dog. Vet Comp Orthop Traum 8:213, 1995.
115. Basher AWP, et al: Subchondral bone cysts in a dog with osteochondrosis. J Am Anim Hosp Assoc 24:321, 1988.
116. Halliwell WH: Tumorlike lesion of bone. In Bojrab MJ (ed): Disease Mechanisms in Small Animal Surgery, 2nd ed. Philadelphia, Lea & Febiger, 1993, p 932.
117. Wilson RB: Monostotic fibrous dysplasia in a dog. Vet Pathol 26:449, 1989.
118. Di Meo A, et al: Polyostotic fibrous dysplasia in a dog. Vet Comp Orthop Traum 11:112, 1998.
119. Johnson KA, et al: Maxillary central giant cell granuloma in a dog. J Small Anim Pract 35:427, 1994.
120. Lewis LD, et al: Small Animal Clinical Nutrition, 3rd ed. Topeka, Mark Morris Associates, 1987, p A4.
121. Malik R, et al: Rickets in a litter of racing greyhounds. J Small Anim Pract 38:109, 1997.
122. Johnson KA, et al: Vitamin D–dependent rickets in a Saint Bernard dog. J Small Anim Pract 29:657, 1988.
123. How KL, et al: Dietary vitamin D dependence of cat and dog due to inadequate cutaneous synthesis of vitamin D. Gen Comp Endocrinol 96:12, 1994.
124. How KL, et al: Photosynthesis of vitamin D_3 in cats. Vet Rec 134:384, 1994.
125. Hazewinkel HAW: Nutrition in relation to skeletal growth deformities. J Small Anim Pract 30:625, 1989.
126. Hazewinkel HAW: Nutrition in Orthopedics. In Bojrab MJ (ed): Disease Mechanisms in Small Animal Surgery, 2nd ed. Philadelphia, Lea & Febiger, 1993, p 1119.
127. Herron MA: Hypervitaminosis A. In Bojrab MJ (ed): Disease Mechanisms in Small Animal Surgery, 2nd ed. Philadelphia, Lea & Febiger, 1993, p 876.
128. Nutrient Requirements of Cats, revised ed. Washington, National Academy Press, 1986, p 22.
129. Nutrient Requirements of Dogs, revised ed. Washington, National Academy Press, 1985, p 23.
130. Feldman EC, Nelson RW: Canine and Feline Endocrinology and Reproduction, 2nd ed. Philadelphia, WB Saunders, 1996, p 455.
131. Rosol TJ, et al: Parathyroid hormone (PTH)–related protein, PTH, and 1,25-dihydroxyvitamin D in dogs with cancer-associated hypercalcemia. Endocrinology 131:1157, 1992.
132. Feldman EC, Nelson RW: Canine and Feline Endocrinology and Reproduction, 2nd ed. Philadelphia, WB Saunders, 1996, p 187.
133. Norrdin RW, et al: Trabecular bone morphometry in beagles with hyperadrenocorticism and adrenal adenoma. Vet Pathol 25:256, 1988.
134. Salmeri KR, et al: Gonadectomy in immature dogs: Effects on skeletal, physical, and behavioural development. JAVMA 198:1193, 1991.
135. Stubbs WP, et al: Effects of prepubertal gonadectomy on physical and behavioral development in cats. JAVMA 209:1864, 1996.
136. Buckley JC: Pathophysiologic considerations of osteopenia. Compend Contin Educ Pract Vet 6:552, 1984.
137. Kronfeld DS: Nutrition in orthopaedics. In Newton CD and Nunamaker DM (eds): Textbook of Small Animal Orthopaedics. Philadelphia, JB Lippincott, 1985, p 655.
138. Read R, et al: The matrix components of the epiphyseal growth plate and articular cartilages from dogs treated with ammonium tetrathiomolybdate, a copper antagonist. Aust J Exp Biol Med Sci 64:545, 1986.
139. Hedhammar A, et al: Overnutrition and skeletal disease. An experimental study in growing Great Dane dogs. Cornell Vet 64(Suppl 5):1, 1974.
140. Nap RC, et al: Growth and skeletal development in Great Dane pups fed different levels of protein intake. J Nutr 121:S107, 1991.
141. Hazewinkel HAW, et al: Influences of chronic calcium excess on the skeletal development of growing Great Danes. J Am Anim Hosp Assoc 21:377, 1985.
142. Hazewinkel HAW, et al: Calcium metabolism in Great Dane dogs fed diets with various calcium and phosphorus levels. J Nutr 121:S99, 1991.
143. Kealy RD, et al: Five-year longitudinal study of limited food consumption and development of osteoarthritis in coxofemoral joints of dogs. JAVMA 210:222, 1997.
144. Johnson KA, et al: Skeletal diseases. In Ettinger SJ, Feldman EC (eds): Textbook of Veterinary Internal Medicine, 4th ed. Philadelphia, WB Saunders, 1995, p 2077.
145. Johnson JA, et al: Incidence of canine appendicular musculoskeletal disorders in 16 veterinary teaching hospitals from 1980 through 1991. Vet Comp Orthop Traum 7:56, 1994.
146. Spodnick GL, et al: Prognosis for dogs with appendicular osteosarcoma treated by amputation alone: 162 cases (1978–1988). JAVMA 200:995, 1992.
147. Johnson AS, et al: Mutation of the p53 tumor suppressor gene in spontaneously occurring osteosarcomas of the dog. Carcinogenesis 19:213, 1998.
148. Murphy ST, et al: Osteosarcoma following total hip arthroplasty in a dog. J Small Anim Pract 38:263, 1997.
149. Stevenson S: Fracture-associated sarcoma. Vet Clin North Am Small Anim Pract 21:859, 1991.
150. Cooley DM, Waters DJ: Skeletal neoplasms in small dogs: A retrospective study and literature review. J Am Anim Hosp Assoc 33:11, 1997.
151. Pirkey-Ehrhart N, et al: Primary rib tumors in 54 dogs. J Am Anim Hosp Assoc 31:65, 1995.
152. Straw RC, et al: Canine mandibular osteosarcoma: 51 cases (1980–1992). J Am Anim Hosp Assoc 32:257, 1996.
153. Roberts RE: Radiographic examination of the musculoskeletal system. Vet Clin North Am Small Anim Pract 13:19, 1983.
154. Berg J: Bone scintigraphy in the initial evaluation of dogs with primary bone tumors. JAVMA 196:917, 1990.
155. Forrest LJ, et al: Relationship between quantitative tumor scintigraphy and time to metastasis in dogs with osteosarcoma. J Nucl Med 33:1542, 1992.
156. Straw RC, Withrow SJ: Limbsparing surgery versus amputation for dogs with bone tumors. Vet Clin North Am Small Anim Pract 26:135, 1996.
157. Hammer AS, et al: Prognostic factors in dogs with osteosarcomas of the flat or irregular bones. J Am Anim Hosp Assoc 31:321, 1995.
158. Heyman SJ, et al: Canine axial skeletal osteosarcoma. A retrospective study of 116 cases (1986–1989). Vet Surg 21:304, 1992.
159. Veterinary Cooperative Oncology Group: Retrospective study of 26 primary tumors of the osseous thoracic wall in dogs. J Am Anim Hosp Assoc 29:68, 1993.
160. Berg J: Canine osteosarcoma: Amputation and chemotherapy. Vet Clin North Am Small Anim Pract 26:111, 1996.
161. Berg J, et al: Results of surgery and doxorubicin chemotherapy in dogs with osteosarcoma. JAVMA 206:1555, 1995.
162. Bergman PJ, et al: Amputation and carboplatin for treatment of dogs with osteosarcoma: 48 cases (1991–1993). J Vet Intern Med 10:76, 1996.
163. MacEwen EG, Kurzmann ID: Canine osteosarcoma. Amputation and chemoimmunotherapy. Vet Clin North Am Small Anim Pract 26:123, 1996.
164. Siegel S, Cronin KL: Palliative radiotherapy. Vet Clin North Am Small Anim Pract 27:149, 1997.
165. Hahn KA, et al: Intramedullary cisplatin chemotherapy: Experience in four dogs with osteosarcoma. J Small Anim Pract 37:187, 1996.
166. Boudrieau RJ, et al: Chondrosarcoma of the radius with distant metastasis in a dog. JAVMA 205:580, 1994.
167. Wesselhoeft Ablin L, et al: Fibrosarcoma of the canine appendicular skeleton. J Am Anim Hosp Assoc 27:303, 1991.
168. Jennings PB, et al: Bone haemangiosarcoma in a young Belgium malinois. J Small Anim Pract 31:349, 1990.
169. Dernell WS, et al: Multilobular osteochondrosarcoma in 39 dogs: 1979–1993. J Am Anim Hosp Assoc 34:11, 1998.
170. Hay CW, et al: Multilobular tumour of bone in an unusual location in the axilla of a dog. J Small Anim Pract 35:633, 1994.
171. Ogilvie GK, Moore AS: Managing the Veterinary Cancer Patient. Trenton, Veterinary Learning Systems, 1995.
172. Shell L, et al: Generalized skeletal involvement of a hematopoietic tumor in a dog. JAVMA 194:1077, 1989.
173. Roger KS, et al: Lymphosarcoma with disseminated skeletal involvement in a pup. JAVMA 195:1242, 1989.
174. Durham SK, Dietze AE: Prostatic adenocarcinoma with and without metastasis to bone in dogs. JAVMA 188:1432, 1986.
175. McGlennon NJ: The musculoskeletal system. In White RAS (ed): Manual of Small Animal Oncology. Cheltenham, British Small Animal Veterinary Association, 1991, p 265.
176. Johnson KA, et al: Osteomyelitis in dogs and cats caused by anaerobic bacteria. Aust Vet J 61:57, 1984.
177. Fossum TW, Hulse DA: Osteomyelitis. Semin Vet Med Surg (Small Anim) 7:85, 1992.
178. Johnson KA: Osteomyelitis in dogs and cats. JAVMA 205:1882, 1994.
179. Nelson DR, et al: The promotional effect of bone wax on experimental Staphylloccus aureus osteomyelitis. J Thorac Cardiovasc Surg 99:977, 1990.
180. Gristina AG, et al: Molecular mechanisms of musculoskeletal sepsis. In Esterhai JL, et al (eds): Musculoskeletal Infection. Park Ridge, IL, American Academy of Orthopaedic Surgeons, 1992, p 13.
181. Ryden C, et al: Selective binding of bone matrix sialoprotein to Staphylococcus aureus in osteomyelitis. Lancet 2:515, 1987.
182. Proctor RA: The staphylococcal fibronectin receptor: Evidence for its importance in invasive infections. Rev Infect Dis 9(Suppl 4):S335, 1987.
183. Johnson KA: Treatment of osteomyelitis, discopondylitis and septic arthritis. In Bonagura JD (ed): Kirk's Current Veterinary Therapy XII. Philadelphia, WB Saunders, 1995, p 1200.
184. Trowald-Wigh G, et al: Leucocyte adhesion protein deficiency in Irish setter dogs. Vet Immunol Immunopathol 32:261, 1992.
185. Allan FJ, et al: Neutropenia with a probably hereditary basis in Border collies. N Z Vet J 44:67, 1996.
186. Fitzgerald RH, et al: Pathophysiology of osteomyelitis and pharmacokinetics of antimicrobial agents in normal and osteomyelitic bone. In Esterhai JL, et al (eds): Musculoskeletal Infection. Park Ridge, IL, American Academy of Orthopaedic Surgeons, 1992, p 387.

APPENDICES

APPENDIX 1

CLIENT INFORMATION SERIES

Neuro
Disk disease **1919**
Seizures **1920**

Cancer
Chemotherapy **1921**
Hemangiosarcoma **1922**
Lymphoma **1923**
Mast cell tumor **1924**
Osteosarcoma **1925**
Squamous cell carcinoma in cats (solar induced) **1926**
Vaccine induced sarcoma in cats **1927**
Mammary tumors **1928**

Endocrine
Cushing's disease **1929**
Diabetes mellitus **1930**
Hyperthyroidism in cats **1931**
Hypothyroidism **1932**

Reproduction
Birth control alternatives **1933**
Breeding management of the bitch **1934**
Whelping in the bitch **1935**
Dystocia **1936**
Pyometra **1937**

GI
Colitis **1938**
Chronic active hepatitis in dogs **1939**
Dentistry **1940**
Flatulence **1941**
Gastrointestinal food allergies **1942**
GDV **1943**
Hepatic lipidosis in cats **1944**
Managing PEG tubes and feeding tubes **1945**
Megaesophagus **1946**
Non-neoplastic infiltrative bowel disease **1947**
Pancreatitis **1948**

Heart
Cardiomyopathy **1949**
Collapsing trachea **1950**
Congenital heart disease **1951**
Congestive heart failure due to mitral/tricuspid valvular fibrosis **1952**
Heartworm disease **1953**
Feline asthma **1954**
Pneumonia **1955**

Infections
FeLV, FIV **1956**
FeLV vaccinations in cats **1957**
Parvovirus in dogs **1958**
Distemper **1959**

Immune-mediated
Immune-mediated hemolytic anemia and/or thrombocytopenia **1960**
Immune-mediated joint disease **1961**
Von Willebrand disease **1962**

Kidney
Chronic renal failure **1963**
Chronic and/or recurring urinary tract infections **1964**
Ethylene glycol toxicity (radiator fluid) **1965**
Urinary stones **1966**
Urinary tract disease **1967**

Rx
Steroid therapy **1968**
Antibiotics **1969**

Skin
Demodecosis **1970**
Fleas **1971**
Food hypersensitivity **1972**
Inhalant skin allergies (atopy) **1973**
Otitis externa **1974**

Disk Disease ■ Richard A. LeCouteur

The spinal column is made up of a number of small bones called vertebrae that are lined up like building blocks. A hole in the center of each vertebra forms a tunnel in which the spinal cord lies. The spinal cord is extremely important as it carries the messages from the brain to the rest of the body. The spinal cord is extremely delicate, and being surrounded by the bony vertebrae helps to protect it. Between each pair of vertebrae, just underneath the spinal cord, is a little cushion, called an intervertebral disk. Disks cushion the vertebrae from one another and provide flexibility to the spine during movement.

As a part of the normal aging process, these disks deteriorate, resulting in so-called disk disease. Normally, each disk consists of an outer fibrous ring and an inner gelatinous center (a good analogy would be a jelly doughnut). With age this "doughnut" changes in its consistency: the outer fibrous ring becomes fragmented and the inner "jelly" center hardens to a consistency of hard cheese. The fragmented outer fibrous ring may no longer be able to hold this hard center in place, and movement of the vertebrae on either side may suddenly squeeze the disk out of its normal position. Unfortunately, this material usually moves upward and comes to rest against the spinal cord, bruising it in the process. This "slipping" of the disk often occurs explosively, causing significant damage to the spinal cord and pain to the animal. In this abnormal position the disk presses against the spinal cord, causing further damage.

This type of disk disease may occur in dogs and cats of any age or breed but occurs most commonly in the "short-legged" breeds (e.g., dachshund, French bulldog, Welsh corgi, Pekingese) and some other small breeds such as the poodle and cocker spaniel. It may also occur in larger breeds of dog, including Doberman pinschers.

The parts of the spine most commonly affected by "slipped" disks are the neck and the middle to lower back. When a disk "slips" out of place and pushes against the spinal cord, it usually causes the animal significant back pain and frequently the damage to the spinal cord interferes with the normal functions of the front and/or rear legs (depending on the location of the disk rupture). In addition to being in pain, the affected dog or cat may be lame, uncoordinated, and/or paralyzed.

These symptoms (pain, incoordination, and possibly paralysis) indicate that the dog or cat has a problem affecting the spinal cord but not the exact location or cause of the problem. Disk disease, a tumor of the spine, or an infection of the spine may all produce similar symptoms. Tests are needed to determine the exact location and cause of the problem and to decide on the appropriate therapy. In order to accomplish this, the patient must be anesthetized for x-rays and collection of fluid from around the spinal cord. "Myelography" is an x-ray study in which a special dye is injected into the fluid surrounding the spinal cord. This then allows any disk material pushing against the cord to be identified on the x-rays. Analysis of the fluid around the spinal cord helps to rule out other causes of the problems such as infection.

In most cases disk disease is a problem requiring surgery to remove the disk material compressing the spinal cord. Occasionally, animals with disk disease are not treated by means of surgery. In these animals, strict cage confinement and immobilization are used. Usually this approach is used for a first bout of back pain in animals that do not have problems walking. Although strict cage confinement does not correct the spinal cord compression, it may temporarily reduce some of the pain and swelling around the spinal cord and permit the ruptured disk to "heal." As time goes on, it is not uncommon for animals treated without surgery to suffer repeated bouts of pain, lameness, and paralysis as additional disk material slips and compresses the spinal cord. With each bout of disk disease the spinal cord suffers additional *permanent* damage. Surgical removal of disk material from the spinal canal is the only treatment that provides rapid and maximal recovery of spinal cord function.

Cortisone administration to animals with disk disease is of therapeutic value only during the first 8 hours after the initial spinal cord injury. Current scientific evidence does not support the use of cortisone beyond this time. Furthermore, the adverse effects of cortisone (e.g., stomach ulcers) must always be kept in mind.

The surgery used most frequently to remove disk material from around the spinal cord is called a laminectomy. For animals undergoing a laminectomy, the speed of recovery and the extent to which normal function of the legs is regained depend on many factors, including the degree of the damage to the spinal cord and the length of time that the spinal cord has been compressed by the disk material. Animals exhibiting severe neurologic signs (e.g., depressed feeling in their toes), a rapid onset of symptoms (hours), and a long period of time before surgery generally have a prolonged recovery period and may have varying degrees of permanent damage.

APP

Seizures ■ Michael Podell

The diagnosis and treatment of seizure disorders in small animals are similar in many respects to the diagnosis and treatment of other ailments: a historical problem arises, a proper diagnosis is made to confirm the condition, and therapy is started to treat the underlying disease and/or signs of the disease. In seizure disorders, however, unlike other diseases, a long period of normal activity may occur between the seizure events. Even during these normal periods, serious conditions may still be present as the cause of the seizures. Knowing which animals are at the highest risk for such problems is helpful in planning the proper tests and treatment.

First, your veterinarian wants to be sure that an epileptic seizure has occurred and, if so, the seizure type(s) manifested. An *epileptic seizure* is the clinical sign of excessive, abnormal activity in the brain and the clinical features can be separated into three components. The *aura* is the initial manifestation of a seizure. During this time period, which can last from minutes to hours, animals can exhibit recurrent pacing or licking, excessive or unusual salivation or vomiting, and/or even unusual psychic events such as excessive barking or increased or decreased attention seeking. Some owners even report that they know their dog is going to have a seizure days in advance by changes in the animal's behavior. The *ictal* period is the actual seizure event, manifested by involuntary muscle tone or movement and/or abnormal sensations or behavior, usually lasting from seconds to minutes. After the ictal event is the *postictal* period. During this time, an animal can exhibit unusual behavior, disorientation, inappropriate bowel or bladder activity, excessive or depressed thirst and appetite, and actual neurologic problems, such as weakness and blindness.

Seizure types can be classified into two major categories: *partial* and *generalized*. Partial seizures are the result of a focal abnormal electrical event in the brain. This seizure type is associated with a higher prevalence of focal disease, such as a tumor. Animals with *simple partial* seizures have a sudden change in activity without any change in awareness, such as twitching of facial muscles. Animals with *complex partial* seizures often show bizarre behavioral activity, such as "fly-chasing" behavior patterns. Generalized seizures are either *convulsive* ("grand mal") or *nonconvulsive* ("petit mal") seizures. Generalized convulsive seizures are by far the most common seizure type seen in animals and are characterized by impaired consciousness coupled with symmetric stiffening, paddling, or even loss of movement of the limb muscles. The major form of nonconvulsive seizure is the "absence" variety, manifested as a "spacing-out" episode. The severity of the seizure does not necessarily match the cause, as dogs with brain tumors may have mild partial seizures and dogs with primary epilepsy may have severe generalized seizures.

The second level of assessment is the diagnosis of the cause of the seizures. Just as a cough signals a problem in the airway, a seizure tells us there is a problem in the brain, but not the cause. The goals of a diagnostic evaluation are to determine the underlying cause, evaluate the chance for recurrence, and establish whether medication is necessary for treatment. *Primary epileptic seizure (PES)* is diagnosed if no underlying cause of the seizure can be identified (idiopathic). This term is often reserved for inherited epilepsy in

people, but the genetic component of epilepsy is difficult to determine in many animals. Breed-related inherited epilepsy in the dog has been documented in beagle, Belgian Tervuren, keeshond, dachshund, and Siberian husky dogs. Other breeds with a high prevalence of an inherited component of their seizures are German shepherd, border collie, Irish setter, and golden retriever dogs. A diagnosis of PES is most common in large breed dogs 1 to 5 years of age and/or when the interval between the first and the second seizure event is long (>4 weeks). *Secondary epileptic seizure (SES)* is the direct result of an abnormal brain structure. The conditions involved include developmental brain problems, inflammation, tumors, or strokes. An animal is categorized as having *epilepsy* if recurrent PES or SES is diagnosed, indicating the presence of a chronic brain disorder. *Reactive epileptic seizure (RES)* is a reaction of the normal brain to transient systemic insults or physiologic stresses. A patient with recurring RES is not defined as having epilepsy, as there is not a primary chronic brain disorder underlying the seizure activity. An underlying identifiable cause (SES or RES) of the seizures is suspected in dogs that have an initial seizure when they are younger than 1 or older than 5 years of age, the initial interval between the first and second seizure events is less than 4 weeks, or a partial seizure is the first observed seizure. Cats, in general, do not suffer as frequently from seizures as dogs. When cats have seizures, there is a high likelihood that an underlying problem in the brain (SES) is present, such as inflammation, stroke, or tumor.

Maintaining a seizure-free status without unacceptable adverse effects is the ultimate goal of antiepileptic drug (AED) therapy. This optimal balance is achieved in less than half of epileptic people and, probably, just as many dogs. Before starting AED treatment, owners and veterinarians should have a realistic idea of what to expect over the course of therapy. First and foremost is that seizure control does not equal elimination. Decreasing the number and severity of seizures and postictal complications, while increasing the time period between seizures, is a realistic goal. Once treatment is started, you should realize that there is a daily treatment regimen, reevaluations are required, and there is a potential for emergency situations to arise, along with the inherent risks of the drug.

The decision to start AED therapy is based on the underlying cause, seizure type and frequency, and postictal effects. An acceptable AED is one that can be given two to three times per day, has documentable benefit, is well tolerated, and has few side effects. The two AEDs most widely used in the dog and cat are phenobarbital and potassium bromide. Bromide has the benefit of a reduced chance of liver toxicity but may not be as effective as phenobarbital for stopping all types of seizures or work as quickly. Periodic measurements of the amount of drug present in the bloodstream are necessary to determine that an acceptable level of medication is present. At the same time, blood tests to evaluate liver function may be necessary. These periodic evaluations are important in trying to maximize the benefit of drug therapy while monitoring for early detection of possible complications. Treating each animal as an individual, applying the philosophy that seizure prevention is better than intervention, and consulting your veterinarian to help formulate or revise treatment plans increase chances of success.

Chemotherapy ■ Susan A. Kraegel

WHAT IS CHEMOTHERAPY?

The use of a drug or chemical to treat any illness is chemotherapy, but this term commonly refers to the use of drugs in the treatment of cancer. The goal of chemotherapy in companion animals is either to increase the life span or to improve the quality of life for the animal with cancer.

HOW DOES CHEMOTHERAPY WORK?

Cancer can be defined as a rapid, uncontrolled growth of cells. Anticancer drugs work by blocking cell growth and division. Different drugs interfere with different steps in these processes. In many cases, a combination of drugs is the most effective way to kill the cancer cells.

HOW IS CHEMOTHERAPY GIVEN?

Most anticancer drugs are given by mouth or by injection. The route chosen depends on the type of drug and the type of cancer.

HOW LONG WILL MY PET RECEIVE CHEMOTHERAPY?

The length of time and frequency of drug administration depend on the kind of cancer being treated and how well the therapy is tolerated by the patient. Treatment may be given daily, weekly, or monthly.

AM I AT RISK OF EXPOSURE TO THESE DRUGS?

Yes. Most anticancer drugs are very potent and must be handled with care. Some are "carcinogens" and can cause cancer with prolonged exposure. With orally administered drugs, it is important that the pills or capsules are kept out of reach of children in childproof containers. When handling these drugs, the owner should wear latex or polyvinyl gloves to avoid unnecessary exposure. With oral and injectable drugs, the urine and feces of the animal may be contaminated with active drug compounds for several days after adminis-tration. Always avoid contact with the urine and feces of animals receiving chemotherapy. Wear latex or polyvinyl gloves to clean up accidents or the litter box. Rinse exposed surfaces well.

WILL MY PET EXPERIENCE SIDE EFFECTS?

Maybe. Veterinarians try to choose drug doses and combi-nations that cause the fewest side effects. Ideally, the animal receiving chemotherapy does not even realize that he or she is ill. The drugs used in chemotherapy, however, are ex-tremely potent and side effects can occur. The potential for side effects must be balanced against the benefits of the chemotherapy and the side effects of the cancer if left untreated. Choosing chemotherapy for your pet is an individ-ual decision.

WHAT KINDS OF SIDE EFFECTS OCCUR?

Side effects arise because the normal cells in the body are also exposed to the anticancer drug. The most sensitive normal cells are found in the blood, gastrointestinal tract, skin, and reproductive system. Consequently, potential side effects include infection, bleeding, decreased appetite, vom-iting, diarrhea, thin haircoat or skin color changes, and sterility. Rare side effects associated with specific drugs include bladder discomfort, kidney damage, and heart fail-ure. The most serious side effect is overwhelming infection leading to death.

WHAT ARE THE MOST COMMON SIDE EFFECTS?

The most common side effect reported by owners is that the pet seems to be "off" for a day or two. This might mean that the pet has slightly less energy or seems less excited than normal about eating. Less commonly, the pet may skip a meal or two, have one episode of vomiting or diarrhea, or seem lethargic. Unfortunately, there is no way to predict which pet will develop the most serious reactions. The animal receiving chemotherapy needs to be watched closely and taken to his or her veterinarian at the first sign of illness.

APP

Hemangiosarcoma in the Dog ■ Mona P. Rosenberg

Hemangiosarcoma is an aggressive cancer that arises from blood vessels. The cancer can be found anywhere in the body (because blood vessels occur throughout the body). Hemangiosarcoma is most commonly found in the spleen, liver, and heart. Prognosis is determined by the location of the disease. Although any breed of dog can develop hemangiosarcoma, certain breeds of dogs appear to be at higher risk, such as the German shepherd, English setter, and golden retriever. We do not know what triggers the growth of this type of cancer.

Symptoms of hemangiosarcoma are usually determined by the location of the disease. Many dogs with the cancer in an internal organ show signs of intermittent or persistent weakness or even collapse. This is due to a variety of factors. Because the cancer is producing abnormal blood vessels, these vessels tend to be very weak and prone to leaking. Further growth leads to rupture of one of these cancerous vessels, resulting in loss of blood. As the spleen is the internal organ most commonly affected by this cancer and is an organ that filters the blood, if one of the abnormal blood vessels ruptures, this allows the "spilling" of blood from the spleen into the abdominal cavity. Rapid loss of blood causes weakness or collapse. If only a small amount of blood is lost, the episode of weakness can be transient, as that blood can be reabsorbed into the body. If a large amount of blood is lost, the weakness is so profound that the dog may collapse. This can be an emergency situation. Distention of the belly may also be observed because of the large volume of free blood in the abdominal cavity. If the cancer is on the heart, this bleeding occurs into the sac that surrounds the heart, resulting in a compromise of the heart's ability to pump blood effectively. This also can cause weakness and potential collapse.

A further problem exists when the cancerous blood vessel ruptures. The release of blood into a body cavity carries with it cancer cells, effectively resulting in bathing of the cavity with cancer cells. This, along with the ease with which cancer cells break off from the abnormal blood vessels and thus gain access to the rest of the body through the bloodstream, results in rapid dissemination of cancer throughout the body. This spread of cancer to distant sites is termed "metastasis." It is this widespread metastasis that makes hemangiosarcoma so "aggressive" and bad. Often the cancer has metastasized before any clinical signs are evident.

When hemangiosarcoma is diagnosed (or suspected), a number of diagnostic tests will be performed to *stage* your dog's cancer. Staging allows your veterinarian and the veterinary oncologist to educate you further about your dog's disease, allowing you to make informed decisions regarding treatment. A chest x-ray will be performed to evaluate the size of the heart and the lungs and look for metastasis. A complete blood count, chemistry profile, and urinalysis will be obtained to assess your dog's overall health status. We may perform a coagulation blood panel to evaluate the ability of your dog's body to clot blood. We may also perform an ultrasound examination of the abdomen and/or the heart in search of metastasis. Other tests may be recommended, depending on individual circumstances.

Treatment for hemangiosarcoma involves two different modalities. The first is often surgery to remove the primary tumor. Sometimes, if multiple sites of metastases are found during the diagnostic testing, surgery will be of no benefit. Whenever we are dealing with cancers that have a high potential to metastasize, we use chemotherapy.

Fortunately, chemotherapy in dogs and cats is very different from "chemo" in people. Because our focus is on quality of life for our pets, this is an important factor; we never want the treatment to be worse than the disease. There are various reasons why chemo is better tolerated in pets, but the most important factor is psychologic. Your dog does not know he has cancer. He also does not know the drugs make people sick, so he does not *anticipate* that he will get sick. Human cancer patients suffer from a phenomenon called anticipatory vomiting, but dogs do not have this problem. This is not to say that some dogs may not have any side effects caused by the chemo, but in the few dogs that do show side effects, the signs are typically mild and transitory. Most breeds of dogs do not lose their hair (they have fur, which grows differently from hair). Your veterinarian or cancer specialist will discuss possible side effects with you at greater length.

Unfortunately, hemangiosarcoma is not curable. Dogs with internal organ involvement who are treated with surgery live an average of only 2 months. Dogs who do not have identifiable metastasis at the time of surgery and who are treated with chemotherapy live a median of 6 to 10 months. (Median survival means that 50 per cent of dogs live less than this time and 50 per cent live longer.) Some dogs with demonstrable metastasis may also respond to chemotherapy, providing a prolonged quality of life compared with dogs that are not treated at all. Dogs with this type of cancer located in the subcutaneous tissues (just under the skin) live a median of about 6 months with surgery alone. No studies have been performed on use of chemotherapy for this anatomic location. Hemangiosarcoma can also occur on the skin of dogs. This appears to be a form of cancer induced by exposure to the sun and carries a much better prognosis than the internal form of the disease. Surgical removal of the skin form, provided it did not arise as a metastasis from the more aggressive form, provides a disease-free interval of about 1.5 years. New lesions can continue to form, however, because of previous or continued sun damage and exposure.

New types of treatments are being investigated continuously in the hope of improving the response rate of dogs with this disease. Again, quality of life is always the main goal, and this can often be achieved by working closely with your veterinary team.

Lymphoma ■ Susan A. Kraegel

Lymphoma is a cancer of a specific white blood cell called the lymphocyte. Lymphocytes are found throughout the body in blood and tissues and act to protect the body from infection. Lymphocytes are the major cells found in lymph nodes or "glands." In lymphoma, the cancer cells invade and destroy normal tissues. The most common site for lymphoma is the lymph nodes, but lymphoma cells, like lymphocytes, can grow anywhere in the body. In most dogs and cats with lymphoma, the cancer cells are present in multiple lymph nodes and tissues.

Chemotherapy is the treatment of choice for almost every dog and cat with lymphoma. Chemotherapy is the administration of drugs by injection or by mouth to kill cancer cells. The chemotherapeutic drug circulates throughout the body. This is important for lymphoma because the cancer cells are in many places at once. Surgery and radiation therapy are less useful in lymphoma because these treatment methods attack cancer cells at only one site.

The goal of chemotherapy for animals with lymphoma is to induce a complete "remission" by killing most of the cancer cells. "Remission" means that all symptoms of the cancer have temporarily disappeared. Animals with lymphoma that are in complete remission look like normal animals by all tests. They do not have any signs of cancer, and all masses or lumps have disappeared. They eat, drink, and run just as they did before they developed cancer. Some of the cancer cells do survive in an animal in complete remission, but the numbers are too small to detect. Eventually, these few cells will grow and the cancer will become evident again. When this happens the animal is said to be "out of remission." Sometimes a second remission can be achieved with additional chemotherapy. Eventually, the cancer cells will become resistant or insensitive to all drugs and cause the dog or cat to die.

Veterinarians use many different drugs and drug combinations called "protocols" to treat lymphoma in dogs and cats. No one knows the "best" treatment, and many protocols give similar results. In general, the longest survival times are reported for protocols that use a combination of drugs and include more expensive drugs.

Although chemotherapy does not cure dogs and cats with lymphoma, in most it does extend the quantity and quality of life. About 80 to 90 per cent of dogs with lymphoma attain a complete remission with an average survival of 1 year, and 25 per cent of dogs live 2 years. For cats, the remission rate is lower, with about 50 per cent attaining a complete remission, but cats who achieve only partial remission also feel better according to owners. The average survival for cats is 7 to 10 months.

Veterinarians use chemotherapy to give dogs and cats with lymphoma a good quality of life with minimal side effects. Most dogs and cats with lymphoma feel good even though they are receiving chemotherapy. The potential for side effects does exist, however, and varies with the protocol used. The most common side effects include decreased energy, decreased appetite, vomiting, and diarrhea. Occasionally, more severe side effects occur, and in rare cases an animal receiving chemotherapy will die as a result of treatment. Unfortunately, the only way to know whether an animal is going to have a drug reaction is to give the drug. Some animals never get sick during chemotherapy, but others are very sensitive to the drugs. If your pet has a serious reaction, the drugs or doses your pet receives may be individually adjusted to maintain a good quality of life.

As an owner, you can help your pet with lymphoma by watching the pet closely after each treatment. Chemotherapy will suppress your pet's immune system and make him or her more susceptible to infections. These infections generally arise from bacteria that normally live in the intestinal tract and on the skin, not from the environment. Signs of an infection may include loss of appetite, vomiting, diarrhea, decreased activity, or depression. Phone your veterinarian immediately if your pet appears ill while receiving chemotherapy. These signs are usually only brief reactions to the drugs, but prompt treatment can often prevent more serious side effects from developing.

APP

Mast Cell Tumors in Dogs ■ Mona P. Rosenberg

Mast cell tumors are common on or just under the skin of dogs. Any breed of dog can develop a mast cell tumor (MCT), but certain breeds are predisposed, including Boxers, bulldogs, pugs, Boston terriers, golden retrievers, and cocker spaniels. Mast cells are normal cells within the body that are responsible for responding to allergic reactions. For example, if you are stung by a bee and the area becomes red, hot, and itchy, it does so because mast cells infiltrate into the area, releasing a variety of substances including histamine, causing these symptoms. Other than hereditary factors, we do not know why dogs develop these tumors.

Your veterinarian may have diagnosed this tumor on the basis of a procedure called fine-needle aspiration. This is a minimally invasive technique that involves sticking a needle into the tumor, sucking a few cells out, and smearing the cells on a slide for a pathologist to evaluate under a microscope. This procedure is not painful to your dog and allows us to make a diagnosis in most cases. It does not, however, allow us to predict the biologic behavior of ("prognose") MCTs; surgical removal of the tumor followed by the use of a grading system is required. Location of the MCT is also of prognostic significance. Knowing that we are dealing with an MCT before surgery can be helpful, because MCTs are notorious for sending out long, finger-like projections of cells into the surrounding tissue. This means we must surgically remove a wider margin of "normal" tissue surrounding any visible tumor in an attempt to remove all the microscopic "fingers."

Grade I or well-differentiated MCTs are the least aggressive of the three classes. If we are able to surgically excise the entire tumor (the pathologist will comment that the margins of tissue removed are "clean" or free of cancer cells), the incidence of recurrence is typically small, with 93 per cent of dogs being disease free at 1 year. "Metastasis" or spread of this form of MCT to distant, internal locations is unusual.

Grade II or intermediately differentiated MCTs are more aggressive than their grade I counterparts. An as yet unidentified percentage of dogs with this form of MCT develop metastasis of their cancer to internal organs, typically to the bone marrow, spleen, or local lymph node. Provided there has been no spread of the cancer, 50 per cent of dogs with completely excised grade II or intermediately differentiated MCTs develop recurrence within 10 months of diagnosis; if no recurrence is detected in this period of time, there is a very good chance that the dog will survive for 5 years free of tumor.

Grade III or poorly differentiated MCTs carry a very poor prognosis, with 97 per cent of dogs succumbing to their cancer by 1 year. This is due to the high rate of metastasis or spread of the cancer to internal organs.

Mast cell tumors in the groin behave similarly to grade III MCTs, regardless of their histologic grade. It is not currently understood, but a high potential for metastasis has been consistently observed. Some oncologists believe that

MCTs in the armpits and mucocutaneous junctions (e.g., lip margins, vulva, anus) can be quite malignant as well.

Once a dog is diagnosed with a MCT, several diagnostic tests are recommended. First, a complete blood count, biochemical profile, and urinalysis are performed to ensure that your dog exhibits no negative effects of the cancer in his or her system. Sometimes, a blood test called a buffy coat test is performed. This test looks for mast cells circulating through the bloodstream. This test is useful if it is positive, but it is often negative even if the cancer has spread; thus, it is not very sensitive. The next step is to grade the cancer if this has not yet been done. Again, this can be done only by surgically removing all or part of the tumor. Once the tumor grade is known, a decision regarding further testing and treatment can be made. If the local lymph node is enlarged, it will be aspirated to look for cancer cells. If the MCT has been graded as intermediate or poorly differentiated (grade II or III), aspiration of the bone marrow and the spleen is advised. This is the most sensitive technique for determining whether the cancer has metastasized. Unfortunately, dogs with mast cell cancer in the bone marrow or the spleen have a very poor prognosis; many dogs live only 90 days from the time of diagnosis because of the effects of the cancer cells on the body. Sometimes, even in dogs with advanced disease, treatment can improve both the quality and quantity of life. Your veterinarian may refer you to a cancer specialist for the testing or further discussion of your options for treatment.

Treatment for dogs with MCTs is dependent on the grade of tumor and results of testing. Dogs with grade I tumors that have been completely excised (removed) are not typically treated with any additional therapy. The "gold standard" of treatment for dogs with grade II MCTs, because of their moderate incidence of local recurrence even with complete surgical excision, is radiation therapy. We also recommend using radiation therapy to treat grade I and II tumors that cannot be completely excised, provided there is no evidence of metastasis. Eighty-eight per cent of dogs with incompletely excised grade II tumors survive for 5 years without disease when treated with radiation therapy.

For dogs with grade III MCTs, dogs with MCTs in the groin, or dogs that have been diagnosed with systemic spread of their mast cell cancer, drug therapy is often recommended. These drugs include diphenhydramine (Benadryl) and cimetidine (Tagamet) to counteract the effects of histamine on the body and prednisone and other chemotherapy drugs to attempt to kill the cancer cells. These drugs are usually well tolerated by dogs. Signs of terminal stages of the cancer include lethargy and gastrointestinal signs such as vomiting, diarrhea, and poor appetite.

Our goal for all cancer patients is that their quality of life be excellent; we never want the treatment to be worse than the disease. This goal is often achieved by working as a close team with your veterinarian and often a board-certified cancer specialist.

Osteosarcoma ■ Susan A. Kraegel

Osteosarcoma is the most common type of bone cancer in dogs. This cancer most often affects large, middle-aged dogs weighing more than 40 pounds. Osteosarcoma can occur in any bone (e.g., rib, skull, toe) but the most common sites are the ends of leg bones, especially at the wrist, shoulder, knee, and hip. The causes of osteosarcoma are unknown, but genetics and microscopic injury to the ends of the bone during growth play a role.

Osteosarcoma begins in the bone but spreads to the lungs and other organs early in the course of disease, even before the initial cancer in the bone is detected. This spread of cancer is called metastasis. In 5 per cent of dogs with osteosarcoma, these metastases are visible on a chest x-ray when the dog is first brought in for the bone cancer. In over 90 per cent of the dogs with osteosarcoma, these metastases are present but are too small to be seen on the initial x-ray. They are termed "micrometastases."

The first sign of osteosarcoma is generally lameness caused by pain from the cancer. The lameness may come and go and vary in severity from dog to dog. In some dogs the leg may fracture at the cancer site. As the cancer grows, a swelling at the site will also develop, which you may be able to feel or see.

X-rays are the first step in identifying bone cancer. X-rays can only suggest the diagnosis on the basis of the appearance of the bone. X-rays of the chest are also recommended to search for metastases.

Biopsy of the abnormal bone is the only way to diagnose bone cancer absolutely. Side effects of biopsy can include pain, bleeding, and, rarely, fracture of the diseased bone. In 10 to 20 per cent of cases, biopsy may fail to diagnose the cancer, so negative results should be evaluated carefully.

Osteosarcoma is a very aggressive form of cancer in dogs. Oncologists (cancer treatment specialists) have not found a cure. Treatment of both the cancer in the bone and the metastases, however, can give many dogs months to years of good-quality life. Amputation and chemotherapy are the ideal treatment for dogs with osteosarcoma. The amputation removes the primary cancer and also relieves the bone pain. Most dogs are walking the day after amputation and running soon after. Three-legged dogs have been known to herd cattle and compete in field trials and generally enjoy the same activities as four-legged dogs. The chemotherapy slows down but does not eliminate the metastases. The chemotherapy currently recommended by most oncologists is usually given once every 3 weeks for four treatments. Most dogs tolerate chemotherapy well and experience only a day or two of mild lethargy or decreased appetite after each treatment. Potentially serious side effects after chemotherapy are uncommon but can include poor to no appetite, vomiting, diarrhea, blood infection, kidney damage, or heart damage. With amputation and chemotherapy, 50 per cent of dogs are alive at 12 months and 15 to 20 per cent are alive at 2 years. Almost all dogs eventually die from osteosarcoma.

Amputation without chemotherapy provides only pain relief. The metastases continue to grow until they cause death. Only fifty per cent of dogs are alive 4 months after amputation alone and 5 to 10 per cent are alive at 1 year.

In rare cases, amputation may not be advised by your veterinarian. Dogs with preexisting disease in other legs or severe obesity may not do well after amputation. One option for these dogs is limb-sparing surgery instead of amputation. This is generally possible only when the cancer is in the front limb in the bone called the radius. With this procedure, the cancerous bone is removed, replaced with bone from a dead dog, and the wrist joint is fused so that it cannot bend. Recovery takes 1 to 2 months and infections are common. Survival times are the same as for amputation. For dogs unable to benefit from surgery at all, radiation therapy may be offered as a treatment to relieve pain. Radiation is given over a 3-week period and reduces but does not eliminate pain in about 30 per cent of dogs. The improvement lasts for about 4 to 5 months in these dogs. This therapy increases the likelihood that a dog will break the limb at the cancer site.

Dogs who do not receive any therapy for osteosarcoma are in pain and have a poor quality of life. This pain continues to progress and, according to people with bone cancer, is severe and uncontrollable. Common painkillers do not work. Euthanasia is generally the only humane choice.

APP

Solar-Induced Squamous Cell Carcinoma in Cats ■ Mark M. Smith

Squamous cell carcinoma is a cancerous disease that most commonly involves skin. Fair-skinned people tend to be predisposed to this type of cancer after chronic, excessive exposure to sunlight. Likewise, white or light-colored cats are also susceptible to squamous cell carcinoma. Solar-induced squamous cell carcinoma usually occurs in areas with little hair coverage that are chronically exposed to sunlight. The most common area affected in cats is the ear tip.

This disease occurs in older cats and may first become apparent in summer, when sunlight exposure is greatest. The first symptom of this disease that you will notice is reddening of the ear tip. Other early signs of this disease include mild hair loss and flaking of skin on the ear tip. Usually the first impression is that your cat has psoriasis, in which the skin seems scaly and inflamed. If caught early, these clinical signs may be indicative of the precancerous form of the disease known as actinic dermatitis. A small skin biopsy is required to differentiate precancerous actinic dermatitis from squamous cell carcinoma. It is best to perform the biopsy procedure early because the clinical lesions of squamous cell carcinoma are subtle and similar to this form of dermatitis. One or both ears may be affected. If only one ear is diseased, the other should be monitored closely because it may also acquire the disease in the future.

Early, effective treatment of precancerous lesions may prevent the onset of squamous cell carcinoma. Treatment for actinic dermatitis includes sun restriction, especially during times of peak solar intensity; water-resistant sunscreens with sun protection factor (SPF) 15 or greater applied to the ear tips twice daily; topical steroid application; and possibly oral steroid or anti-inflammatory therapy. The drug etretinate may also be used to alleviate symptoms. The effect of etretinate is to decrease inflammation and skin flaking while normalizing skin cell metabolism. Medical therapy is not effective for lesions that advance to squamous cell carcinoma, underlining the importance of early diagnosis for suspicious lesions.

Surgical removal of squamous cell carcinoma of the ear tip (partial pinnectomy) is most effective when performed as soon after diagnosis as possible. Early intervention decreases the amount of the ear that must be removed, because the lesion is smaller. Early surgical removal also decreases the incidence of spread of the cancer to the lymph nodes near the ear. There are different surgical methods that are effective in removing the cancer. With cryosurgery, like frostbite, the ear tip is frozen. The frozen tissue dies and is removed. Although this method may be effective, it is sometimes difficult to control the precise area of tissue freezing. Freezing an inadequate area may lead to recurrence of the cancer, and excessive freezing may result in an unsightly appearance and be associated with excessive scar and deformation of the remaining ear. Laser surgery is available in veterinary medicine, but the equipment is expensive and may be available only at special referral facilities. Laser surgery provides precise removal of the cancer with minimal, if any, side effects. Finally, traditional surgical methods may be used to remove the cancer. The procedure is similar to ear cropping in dogs, in which part of the ear is removed with scissors and the skin edges are sutured together. In cats with squamous cell carcinoma of the ear tip, the veterinarian caring for the pet will remove the cancerous ear tip *and* about one-quarter inch of normal-appearing ear. A small amount of normal-appearing ear is removed to ensure that the entire cancer has been removed. You should insist that a pathologist evaluate the excised tissue to make sure that the cancer has been completely removed. If the biopsy shows that the cancer has not been completely removed, further surgery should be performed. Incomplete removal of the cancer at the initial surgery is not the fault of your veterinarian. Microscopic evaluation of the tissue after special processing is required to determine whether cancer cells are present in the tissue. The naked eye is not able to make this determination. Cats tolerate the surgery well, and healing should progress without complication. The healed surgery area will have more hair than the ear tip, which will aid in preventing recurrence of the cancer. Preventive care should be continued after successful surgery.

In summary, prevention of precancerous actinic dermatitis is recommended by limiting the outdoor activity of white or light-colored cats to periods of nonpeak solar intensity. Appropriate sunscreens should be applied to the ear of predisposed cats who are outdoors during periods of peak solar intensity. If your cat is diagnosed with actinic dermatitis, it should be treated aggressively in the hope of preventing cancer. Progression of actinic dermatitis to squamous cell carcinoma requires surgery to remove the cancer. Because of availability and financial considerations, most cats with this form of cancer receive treatment consisting of traditional surgery. The appearance of your cat's ear after surgery will depend on the extent of the disease. The ear may simply appear rounded at the tip or require complete removal. If the entire ear is removed, your cat will still be loved and cute with a striking resemblance to "E.T." of movie fame. Either result is far better than uncontrolled spread of cancer to deeper tissues of the head.

Vaccine-Induced Sarcoma in Cats ■ Susan A. Kraegel

A vaccine-induced sarcoma is a connective tissue cancer that occurs where a vaccine has previously been given. Vaccine-induced sarcoma is a rare consequence of vaccination in cats. It does not occur in dogs. This disease was first recognized in the late 1980s and early 1990s. During this time, many new feline vaccines were developed and vaccination of cats became more common than it had been previously. The goal of these changes was to improve the health of cats. At the same time, however, veterinary pathologists noticed more sarcomas at the sites where vaccines are generally given in cats: between the shoulders, on the back legs, and over the back.

Studies were done to determine the cause of this phenomenon. The studies showed that the majority of cats do not get cancer from vaccination. Only 1 in 1000 to 1 in 10,000 cats develop a tumor at a vaccination site. The tumors were found to occur more commonly with vaccines for rabies and feline leukemia virus but the brand of vaccine did not make a difference. The risk was over twice as high when two or more vaccines were given in the same location. Finally, there was no way to predict which cats would develop cancer at a vaccination site.

The exact cause of cancer arising from vaccination remains a mystery. A vaccine normally works by causing irritation or inflammation at the vaccination site. One theory is that in rare cats, normal cells at the vaccination site divide abnormally and mutate. A cell that accumulates many mutations will divide uncontrollably and become a sarcoma.

Vaccine-associated sarcomas in cats are aggressive tumors. They may develop as early as 2 months or as late as 3 to 4 years after vaccination. They grow deep into muscles and fat, with long "fingers" of cancer cells extending well beyond any visible mass. These fingers of cancer are invisible to the naked eye and can be seen only under the microscope. The sarcoma will grow back after surgery unless every single cancer cell is removed, including the microscopic fingers around the mass.

Vaccine-induced sarcomas can be cured with surgery if they are found and treated while they are still small. The surgery must be aggressive to remove every cancer cell. When the tumor occurs on the leg, for instance, the leg must be amputated. Three-legged cats have a normal lifespan and an active, happy life if the cancer has been detected early.

Sometimes the vaccine-induced sarcoma is not found until it is big or it occurs in a location where aggressive surgery is difficult. Then, radiation therapy combined with surgery may help the cat to live several years. Radiation therapy may be given before or after the surgery. Radiation therapy takes 3 to 4 weeks and may make the cat tired. Temporary skin irritation and hair loss around the tumor site are common. When radiation is given over the chest area, lung irritation is possible.

Chemotherapy can shrink vaccine-induced sarcomas but cannot cure this type of cancer. Side effects depend on which drugs are used. Many cats experience increased lethargy and decreased appetite for a day or two after chemotherapy. In rare cases, the loss of appetite may last a week or more and be accompanied by vomiting or diarrhea.

Veterinarians and owners must work as a team to fight vaccine-induced sarcomas. To prevent sarcomas, veterinarians give each vaccine at a separate site when multiple vaccines are needed. To help ensure that successful treatment will be possible, veterinarians give the vaccines known to cause sarcomas in the back legs. In this way, should a cat be extremely unlucky and develop a tumor, it can be completely removed by amputation. The most important thing an owner can do to is to find the tumors when they are very small. This means that any time your cat gets a hard lump in a vaccination site more than 1 month after the vaccine is given, you should have your veterinarian examine your cat. These simple measures prevent cats from dying of a vaccine-induced sarcoma while making sure that important infectious diseases can still be prevented by vaccination.

APP

Canine Mammary Tumors ■ Deborah W. Knapp

Tumors of the mammary gland are the most common tumors of female dogs. Mammary tumors have been reported to occur in approximately 2 of 1000 female dogs. Approximately half of canine mammary tumors are malignant or cancerous, meaning that they have the potential to spread to other parts of the body. The remaining mammary tumors are benign.

Most mammary tumors become apparent as lumps in the mammary gland area, typically in older dogs. Other conditions can result in enlarged or lumpy mammary glands, and a biopsy with microscopic evaluation of the tissue removed by a trained pathologist is needed to make a diagnosis of benign or malignant mammary tumors. Malignant mammary tumors, also referred to as "mammary cancer," can be subclassified as various types of carcinomas, adenocarcinomas, malignant mixed tumors, or less commonly sarcomas.

When a malignant mammary tumor is diagnosed in a dog, it is appropriate to perform a series of tests to "stage" the cancer, which means simply to determine whether the tumor has metastasized (spread) and the extent of the spread. These tests include radiographs ("x-rays") of the thorax and abdomen and ultrasonography of the abdomen. The most common sites of mammary cancer metastasis are the lymph nodes and lung. These tests allow detection of tumor nodules in the lungs, lymph nodes, and other organs. It must be noted, however, that nodules smaller than a few millimeters (less than approximately 1/4 inch) will not be detected by these tests. Therefore, microscopic tumor cells and very small cancer nodules cannot be detected or ruled out by these tests. Currently, noninvasive tests are not available to rule out microscopic spread of the cancer.

Surgical removal of the tumor(s) is the treatment of choice for benign mammary tumors and for malignant mammary tumors that have not spread beyond the mammary tissue and adjacent lymph nodes. Most benign mammary tumors are curable by surgery. Approximately half of malignant mammary tumors are cured by surgery. This is possible because some malignant (cancerous) mammary tumors in the dog do not spread very quickly and can be removed before they spread. "Radical" mastectomy has not been shown to be any more effective than more limited surgery. Tumors that are larger than 3 cm and tumors that are of higher grade (as classified by the pathologist) are more likely to recur (70 per cent recurrence at 1 year) than smaller tumors and tumors of a lower histopathologic grade (30 per cent recurrence at 1 year).

After surgical removal of a malignant mammary tumor, your dog should be examined by your veterinarian periodically to determine whether the tumor has recurred either in the mammary area or at another location in the body. An example of a typical reexamination schedule would be rechecks at 1, 3, 6, 9, 12, 18, and 24 months after surgery. These rechecks could include a complete physical examination, radiographs, and ultrasonography.

An effective chemotherapy protocol for canine mammary cancer has not been defined. A small percentage of dogs have had partial remission with drugs such as doxorubicin (Adriamycin) or cisplatin. Because surgery alone is successful in many cases and chemotherapy has not been successful in many cases, chemotherapy is usually reserved for tumors that cannot be removed surgically. Radiation therapy has not been studied to any extent in dogs with mammary tumors.

It is important to note that mammary cancer can be prevented in the dog by early ovariohysterectomy (spaying). The risk of developing mammary tumors in dogs has been reported to be 0.05 per cent for dogs spayed before the first estrus, 8 per cent for dogs spayed after the first estrus and before the second estrus, and 26 per cent for dogs spayed after the second estrus. Therefore, dogs that are not going to be used for breeding purposes should undergo early ovariohysterectomy.

o,p'-DDD Treatment of Pituitary Cushing's Syndrome ■ Edward C. Feldman

Hyperadrenocorticism (Cushing's syndrome) refers to a clinical condition that results from having excess cortisone in the system. A minority of dogs with this disease have a tumor in one of the two glands that produce cortisone (the adrenal glands). Your dog, like more than 80 per cent of dogs with the naturally acquired form of this disease, has a small tumor at the base of the brain in an area called the pituitary gland. The pituitary gland controls adrenal function. A tumor in the pituitary can cause excess demand for cortisone production, which, in turn, causes excess cortisone throughout the body and results in symptoms recognized by owners ("pituitary-dependent" Cushing's syndrome). The most common symptoms of Cushing's syndrome in dogs include excess urination and water consumption, a voracious appetite, hair loss, muscle weakness, a "potbellied" appearance, panting, thin skin, and lethargy. Virtually all dogs with Cushing's syndrome have at least one or two of these signs, but it would be uncommon for a dog to have all these symptoms. By evaluating a variety of test results, your veterinarian has diagnosed your dog as having pituitary-dependent Cushing's. Now, treatment with *o,p'*-DDD has been recommended.

During World War II, scientists did research on the insecticide DDT in an attempt to create an extremely toxic form. One of the forms of DDT created was *o,p'*-DDD (Lysodren; mitotane), a chemical that can destroy the cortisone-producing cells of adrenal glands in dogs. The drug has been used successfully in thousands of dogs with Cushing's, but you must remember that it is a "poison" and that it must be used appropriately. The protocol we use in treating dogs with this drug is straightforward. A day or two before starting treatment, begin feeding your dog one third of its normal food allotment twice daily (each 24 hours it should receive a total of two thirds of the normal amount). This should make your dog even more hungry, but this is just for a brief time (we do not recommend use of this drug in dogs with a poor appetite). After 1 or 2 days of reduced feeding, begin giving the *o,p'*-DDD at a dose of 25 mg/kg of body weight twice daily (a dog weighing 22 pounds would receive one-half tablet twice daily; the tablets contain 500 mg). The drug should be given immediately *after* the dog eats. So, feed the dog, note how long it takes to finish the meal, and then give the medication (the drug is absorbed best from a stomach containing food).

The key to treating these dogs is watching them eat and knowing when to stop giving the *o,p'*-DDD. As long as their appetite is ravenous, give the medication. As soon as you see *any reduction in appetite*, STOP giving the drug. Reduction in appetite may be noted as the dog taking longer to finish the meal; eating half of the food, wandering away for a drink, and then finishing; or simply looking up at the owner once or twice before finishing. In other words, we do not want the dog to stop eating entirely, we wish to see a "reduction" in appetite as a signal to stop the medication. Other signals include reduced water intake, vomiting, diarrhea, and listlessness, but appetite reduction usually precedes these more worrisome symptoms. Most dogs respond to this drug in 5 to 9 days, a few respond in as little as 1 to 3 days, and some may take longer than 14 days.

No dog should receive *o,p'*-DDD for more than 8 days without being tested for the effect of the drug. The test is done by your veterinarian and takes 1 to 2 hours. We typically start the treatment on a Sunday and plan the recheck test 8 days later (Monday), and more than 85 per cent of owners have stopped medication on the Thursday, Friday, Saturday, or Sunday before the test is performed on Monday. When the *o,p'*-DDD has been demonstrated to have had an effect, the dog can be returned to a normal amount of food. The dog will continue to receive *o,p'*-DDD for the rest of its life. The initial maintenance dose is usually approximately 50 mg/kg per week (a 22-pound dog would receive one-half tablet twice weekly). That dose is likely to be increased or decreased on the basis of testing performed 1 month after maintenance treatment has been started and testing performed every 2 to 4 months thereafter. The average dog (11.5 years old when the syndrome is diagnosed) treated in this manner lives about 30 months (some live a few weeks and some 6 to 10 years). The dogs with the longest survival have owners who are committed to helping their pet, diligent veterinarians, and luck. Close observation and frequent veterinary rechecks can only help in the long-term management of these dogs.

APP

Diabetes Mellitus in Dogs and Cats ■ Edward C. Feldman

All consumed food is eventually converted to sugar, the energy source for every organ in the body and for every cell in every organ. If too much food is consumed, the extra calories can be stored by the body for later conversion to sugar. Sugar is carried in the blood to all areas of the body, and any cell that is in need of sugar simply uses the sugar present in the blood. How do cells move sugar into their interior from the bloodstream? A substance called *insulin*, produced by an organ located in the abdomen (the pancreas), is the key that allows cells to obtain sugar from the bloodstream. Insulin is necessary for life.

People, dogs, and cats who do not have insulin have a disease called *diabetes mellitus*. Diabetes mellitus is an extremely common disease in people, dogs, and cats. There are two common forms of diabetes. The form in which an individual has absolutely no insulin has several names: insulin-dependent diabetes mellitus (IDDM), type I diabetes, and juvenile-type diabetes. The other form occurs when an individual has insulin but either does not have enough or has a condition that interferes with insulin function. It has several names: non–insulin-dependent diabetes mellitus (NIDDM), type II diabetes, adult-onset diabetes. Approximately 10 per cent of people with diabetes mellitus have type I disease and 90 per cent have type II. Approximately 60 per cent of diabetic cats have type I and 40 per cent type II. Virtually 100 per cent of dogs with diabetes mellitus have type I disease.

What happens when an individual has diabetes mellitus? Without sugar constantly being removed from the blood by cells everywhere in the body, the diabetic person, dog, or cat has more and more sugar accumulate in the blood. Eventually, so much sugar accumulates that it begins to "spill over" into the urine through the kidneys along with water. Therefore, diabetics urinate large volumes. In dogs and cats, sometimes the first thing that an owner observes is that the pet is no longer "housebroken" or the pet cat begins urinating outside the litter box. Because the volume of fluid lost into the urine of diabetics is excessive, they make up for these losses by drinking more and more water. Because cells throughout the body have lost their access to sugar, they begin to "starve." Individual cells do not see the lack of insulin, they see only a lack of energy (sugar). Therefore, messages are sent out for energy (sugar) and the diabetic begins to eat more and more. Cells still have no access to the sugar, so additional messages for energy are sent out and the body begins to break down fat and muscle for energy (the components of fat and muscle can be converted to sugar by the liver). Although it makes sense to create more energy, the body still cannot use the sugar resulting from this process. The symptoms common to all diabetics now become obvious: they *drink excessively, urinate excessively, eat excessively,* and *lose weight.*

When a dog or cat is brought to a veterinarian for any or all of the symptoms known to be associated with diabetes, the diagnosis is quite easily made. Testing is necessary, however, because there are other diseases that cause all or some of the same symptoms. However, once the diagnosis is made, the real problems begin. Treating diabetes mellitus is not easy. It takes skill by the veterinarian, commitment by the owner, and some luck. The cornerstones of treating type II diabetic people include weight loss, exercise, and changes in diet to increase fiber content and to decrease simple sugars. If these factors do not help enough, pills can be given. Use of all these treatments rarely helps type I diabetic people. Type I diabetic people, like 100 per cent of diabetic dogs and 80 to 90 per cent of diabetic cats, require insulin by injection to live. All diabetic dogs and cats do best with good commercial pet food given in two equal-sized meals (cats that tend to "graze" all day should be allowed to continue feeding that way). High-fiber foods may be of benefit but are not critical.

Unfortunately, although insulin has been available to treat diabetics for more than 70 years, it must still be given by injection. Your veterinarian will teach you how to give injections to your pet. It is understood that this can be quite intimidating for owners and that your pet will feel the needles. However, once you have done this for a few weeks, you will become quite competent and your pet will accept the tiny pinpricks. Don't give up! Your pet can live an extremely healthy life despite requiring insulin. There are several different kinds of insulin. Regular (R; crystalline) insulin is the most potent and the shortest acting; Ultralente (U) is the least potent and the longest acting; protamine zinc insulin (PZI) is similar to Ultralente; neutral protamine Hagedorn (NPH; N) insulin is less potent and longer acting than regular but more potent and shorter acting than Ultralente; and Lente (L) is 30 per cent regular and 70 per cent Ultralente and has effects similar to those of NPH. One insulin may not work satisfactorily in your pet but another may work well. It takes time to determine which insulin and which insulin dose are best for an individual cat or dog. Whereas most cats and dogs respond best to insulin given twice daily (do not try to give the insulin exactly every 12 hours; it is not necessary), some do well with only one injection per day.

Remember the most important goal in treating a diabetic dog or cat: we want the pet to be happy and stable. No diabetic pet becomes absolutely normal. Finally, regardless of treatment, virtually 100 per cent of diabetic dogs (not cats) develop cataracts and become blind within the first 6 to 24 months; this is inevitable and not a reflection of the job you have done in treating your pet.

Hyperthyroidism in Cats ■ Edward C. Feldman

The thyroid is a two-lobed gland located in the neck of people, dogs, cats, and other animals, one lobe located on each side of the trachea (windpipe). The thyroid produces thyroid hormone, a substance that is transported via the blood to every cell in the body. The primary function of thyroid hormone is to control the rate at which cells function: too much thyroid hormone makes cells work very fast and too little causes cell function to slow down. Low thyroid function *(hypothyroidism)* is relatively common in dogs and quite rare in cats. Excess thyroid function *(hyperthyroidism)* is rare in dogs but is one of the most common diseases diagnosed in cats 8 years of age and older.

Each cat may respond to hyperthyroidism a little differently, causing abnormalities to vary from cat to cat. Among the most common owner observations are weight loss; increases in appetite; patchy hair loss or failure to groom (some cats have been observed to pull their hair out); and increases in water intake, urine output, and activity (cats may be persistently restless or nervous). Vomiting and diarrhea (some cats have bulky stools and others produce unusually large amounts of stool) are a little less common. Relatively uncommon but well-documented problems are panting, difficulty breathing, loss of appetite, listlessness, changes in behavior, and seeking cool places.

It is not known exactly why cats develop hyperthyroidism. About 15 per cent of hyperthyroid cats have a single thyroid tumor (not a cancerous tumor), and about 80 per cent have excess activity in both lobes (a benign condition called hyperplasia). Only 3 to 5 per cent of hyperthyroid cats have a malignant (cancerous) thyroid tumor. The diagnosis of hyperthyroidism, regardless of cause, is relatively easy. Most hyperthyroid cats have too much thyroid hormone (thyroxine or "T_4") in their blood, and this can be confirmed with a blood test. A small percentage of hyperthyroid cats do not have a "diagnostic" blood T_4 level, and in this situation your veterinarian may wish to repeat the test a few days or a few weeks later, use a different T_4 test (called the "free" T_4 test), or have a *thyroid scan* performed. All these tests are excellent and each tends to complement the others. The T_4 and the free T_4 tests can be performed almost anywhere, but the scan requires special facilities and is not available everywhere. Nevertheless, if your veterinarian believes your cat has this condition, the diagnosis of hyperthyroidism is usually relatively easy and relatively inexpensive to confirm.

Three common treatments are available for managing hyperthyroidism in cats. Each treatment has advantages and disadvantages. Your veterinarian will explain the choices to you and allow you to decide what is best for you and your cat. Hyperthyroid cats that are not treated tend to become more and more ill, whereas treatment will usually either return your cat to a reasonable state of good health or cure your cat. One treatment option is the use of an oral (pill) medication called methimazole that works by preventing the thyroid gland from creating T_4. The drug is readily available and not extremely expensive. The major negative aspect of this drug is that some cats are not the best pill takers. The drug usually works best when given at least twice daily at total daily doses of 7.5 to 10 mg; it may cause side effects (vomiting, loss of appetite), especially if the first doses are too high (we start at 2.5 mg twice daily), but some of the less common side effects are more worrisome (liver damage; decreases in red cells, white cells, and platelets [cells that help blood to clot]; and some cats severely lacerate their own faces by scratching uncontrollably when given the drug). Although these side effects are alarming, they are not common, and we still use the drug for virtually every hyperthyroid cat we treat (see the end of this sheet).

Another therapy is surgery to remove the abnormal thyroid gland(s). Surgery is not difficult, does not require fancy equipment, is not terribly expensive, resolves the hyperthyroidism quickly, and can cure your cat permanently. The negative aspects of surgery are that it does require anesthesia and many hyperthyroid cats are older cats with other problems that could complicate the anesthesia; during the surgery, glands called the parathyroid glands (necessary for life) could be accidentally removed; and, like any treatment, it is not always successful.

The third treatment option is the use of radioactive iodine. Iodine is the primary ingredient of thyroid hormone. Iodine that is radioactive can destroy abnormal thyroid cells. This is an extremely effective treatment that resolves the hyperthyroidism quickly, requires no anesthesia and no pills, and almost never results in hypothyroidism. The negative aspects of this form of treatment are that sophisticated facilities are needed (this treatment is not available everywhere) and that is usually requires 7 to 14 days of hospitalization for the cat to eliminate all the radioactivity in urine and feces (otherwise people might become exposed to this radioactivity).

It is important to understand that all three treatments are excellent and all three have their negative aspects. It is also important to understand that the blood supply to the kidneys will decrease after successful treatment for hyperthyroidism. We use the pills before surgery or radioactive iodine because the effect of pills is reversible. If the kidneys are damaged by decreasing thyroid hormone levels, a permanent form of treatment (surgery, radioactive iodine) is avoided. If the thyroid hormone levels decrease and the kidneys are not harmed, permanent treatment is an option.

Canine Hypothyroidism ■ J. Catharine R. Scott-Moncrieff

Hypothyroidism is the clinical condition caused by thyroid hormone deficiency. The thyroid hormones, thyroxine (T_4) and triiodothyronine (T_3), are produced by the thyroid glands, which are located in the neck on either side of the trachea. Thyroid hormones influence the metabolism of most of the organs in the body. Deficiency of thyroid hormone results in a decreased metabolic rate, which may cause a wide variety of clinical signs. "Decrease in metabolic rate" means that the speed at which cells function or "work" slows down. For example, the heart rate slows, mental function slows, and body temperature decreases. Decreased secretion of thyroid hormones by the thyroid gland may be due to inflammation (thyroiditis) or progressive failure (atrophy) of the thyroid glands. In rare cases, thyroid tumors may cause hypothyroidism.

Hypothyroidism is the most common endocrine disease of the dog. Breeds that are predisposed to developing hypothyroidism include the golden retriever and the Doberman pinscher, but any breed of dog may be affected.

The most common clinical signs of hypothyroidism are weight gain, cold intolerance, lethargy, and a variety of skin problems. The most common skin abnormalities include hair loss, changes in hair color and quality, and predisposition to skin infections. Other less common clinical signs include abnormalities of the reproductive and nervous systems.

A diagnosis of hypothyroidism is made by measurement of thyroid hormone concentrations (T_3, T_4, and free T_4) in the blood. If thyroid hormone concentrations are low, other tests may be performed to determine whether the decrease is due to a thyroid gland problem or to the effects of other diseases or medications. These additional tests may include measurement of thyroid-stimulating hormone (TSH) and measurement of a variety of antithyroid antibodies. In some cases, it is necessary to use trial therapy with thyroid hormone supplementation to confirm the diagnosis of hypothyroidism.

Fortunately, hypothyroidism is a disease that is easily treated. Treatment involves daily or twice-daily oral medication with synthetic thyroxine. Treatment is usually started with two treatments per day, one in the morning and one in the evening. When the clinical signs have resolved, the treatment can be reduced to one dose per day in many dogs. In most cases, treatment is required for the life of the dog.

It may take several weeks for the clinical signs of hypothyroidism to resolve. An increase in activity level is usually observed after 1 to 2 weeks of treatment. It usually takes longer for skin problems to resolve, but improvement should be observed within 6 to 8 weeks. In some cases the skin may actually appear worse for the first 1 to 2 weeks of treatment as the old haircoat is shed. If a dog was experiencing reproductive or neurologic problems, it may take several months of treatment for complete resolution of the problems.

Clinical signs of excessive supplementation with thyroid hormone include nervousness, weight loss, and increased drinking or increased urination. These signs are rare, but if they occur it is important to call your veterinarian for adjustment of the dose.

In order to establish that the dose of thyroid hormone supplementation is appropriate, it is recommended that blood samples be collected for measurement of thyroid hormone concentrations 1 to 2 months after the start of treatment. The results of these tests are used to adjust the dose of thyroid hormone supplementation. Then it is usually necessary to measure thyroid hormone concentrations only once a year or if clinical signs of hypothyroidism recur.

Birth Control Alternatives ■ Autumn P. Davidson

Neutering, ovariohysterectomy (spaying) of females or castration of males, remains the most effective, least expensive, safest, and permanent method of birth control for pets. The procedures are well tolerated by dogs and cats and are routinely performed in most veterinary hospitals, and both dogs and cats can have the surgery as young as 6 to 8 weeks of age.

The only valid reason to avoid neutering as a birth control method is that the pet has value as a breeding animal. A valuable breeding animal has desirable physical and behavioral traits for its (pure) breed. This animal should have undergone appropriate testing and found not to have evidence of any known genetic defects. In addition, the owner of that pet must be willing and able to take responsibility for managing breeding, whelping or queening, weaning, socializing, and placing the offspring produced. Breeding dogs and cats is not a financially rewarding undertaking—much the opposite! Financial setbacks are common, raising puppies and kittens can be quite time consuming, and finding desirable homes for the offspring is a major responsibility. The pet overpopulation problem is a gigantic and serious reality in the United States that underscores the need for responsible breeding. Breeding animals should be neutered for health reasons when their reproductive careers are complete. Neutered animals have the same capacity to perform as hunting, herding, and guard animals. Breast cancer is at least as common in dogs and cats as in people, and spaying a female before her first "heat" virtually eliminates risk of breast cancer in dogs and cats. Spaying between the first and second cycles dramatically decreases the risk of breast cancer. Obviously, spaying also eliminates risk of diseases of the ovaries or uterus, which are relatively common. Prostate and testicular diseases are also common, and neutering of males decreases the risk of these problems as well. Neutered animals should be fed approximately 25 per cent fewer calories to prevent obesity; otherwise, their physique remains normal. Urinary incontinence occasionally occurs in spayed female dogs. This condition is treatable.

Alternatives to neutering for temporary birth control in pets are few. Most products available in the United States are not licensed for use in pets or are not recommended for pets intended for breeding. None have current application to the male. Birth control in females is accomplished by preventing estrous cycles or interrupting pregnancy establishment. Estrous cycles can be prevented in bitches or queens by appropriate administration of commercially available vet-erinary progestin or testosterone compounds. Progestin compounds work to prevent estrous cycles by keeping the female in a "pregnant-like" condition. Unfortunately, the administration of progesterone to an intact (unspayed) bitch or queen can cause uterine wall disease, leading to the later development of a severe and potentially life-threatening uterine infection called "pyometra" or infertility. Progesterone medications can also cause or contribute to the development of serious diseases (diabetes, growth hormone disorders) and anatomic problems (mammary masses, gallbladder disorders). Therefore, we do not recommend the use of progestogens to prevent estrous cycles. Testosterone-like compounds prevent estrous cycles in bitches by keeping the female in an anestrus-like (no ovarian activity) condition. Behavioral side effects (aggression), tearing of the eyes, malodorous skin, liver problems, and subfertility during subsequent estrous cycles are common consequences of the use of testosterone compounds. Clearly, these are not ideal compounds for use in valuable breeding animals.

Methods for preventing estrous cycles by administering synthetic hormones with fewer side effects or immunizing the animal against egg membranes or endogenous hormones have not been perfected to the point where they are commercially available. Methods for preventing pregnancy by interfering with egg travel in the fallopian tubes or embryo implantation in the uterus with estrogen compounds are not recommended because of their potential for causing life-threatening bone marrow suppression (the bone marrow is the sole source of red and white blood cells and cells that help clotting, called platelets). Estrogens may also promote later development of pyometra, clearly undesirable in an animal intended for breeding. Application of newer human birth control agents, such as carbergoline and mifepristone, in pets is limited by availability in the United States, but these agents have the best promise for providing effective birth control with minimal side effects.

The best current nonpermanent method for preventing pregnancy in the bitch or queen is simply to prevent breeding (copulation) by confining the individual indoors, away from intact (un-neutered) males. Bitches should be let into an enclosed yard only with direct supervision or on leash for the entire time when copulation could occur. This could be as long as 3 weeks. A veterinarian can determine when the bitch's cycle is complete by performing vaginal cytology. Queens must be kept isolated from toms during their entire period of receptivity, as they ovulate after copulation.

APP

Breeding Management of the Bitch ■ Autumn P. Davidson

The canine estrous cycle consists of four phases: anestrus (the period when the dog appears the same as any spayed female), proestrus (the period when the female attracts males, the vulva is enlarged, and there is vaginal bleeding but she refuses to breed), estrus (the period of breeding), and diestrus (the period of pregnancy). The interestrous interval (period between apparent heat cycles) normally varies from 4.5 to 10 months in duration, with 7 months being the average. Remember, all normal dogs have the period of "pregnancy" (the ovaries work as if pregnancy exists) after estrus, even when not pregnant.

A bloody vaginal discharge (of uterine origin) signals that the female is no longer in anestrus and that she is in proestrus. This bloody vaginal discharge may cease before the start of estrus, may change to a clear or straw-colored discharge before the start of estrus, or may persist throughout estrus. Your veterinarian can evaluate vaginal cytology smears (cells easily obtained from your dog's vagina with a cotton-tipped swab), which will help distinguish a vaginal discharge related to normal ovarian activity from one caused by a problem such as trauma. During diestrus, the normal bitch again becomes refractory to breeding and less attractive to males, the vaginal discharge becomes mucoid before stopping, and enlargement of the vulva slowly resolves.

Primiparous (maiden) bitches should have a veterinary examination before breeding to ascertain general health and, specifically, to rule out any problems that would arise during breeding or whelping, such as vaginal strictures. In general, if the bitch is healthy, we recommend that the owner observe one normal proestrus and estrus before having the dog bred. This confirms that she is healthy and also provides her with time to mature before undergoing the rigors of pregnancy and nursing a litter. Screening tests for genetic diseases common to your breed and *Brucella canis* testing should be done. Vaginal cultures are not necessary for healthy bitches.

If a normal cycle has been observed, the recommendations for breeding should be straightforward. One option is to bring the female to the male when her vaginal cytology shows more than 50 per cent "superficial" cells. Alternatively, within 2 to 4 days of first noticing a bloody vaginal discharge, the bitch should be taken to the home of a dominant male (do not use a stud dog) to observe her behavior. The question asked is simple: Is she willing to allow mounting and breeding? A leash and handler should control the male and another person should control the female. Ideally, the female is brought to the male when she is unwilling to breed (too soon). If this is true, she can then be returned to the male every 24 to 72 hours for observation. Whenever she appears willing to allow breeding, she should be taken to the stud and bred every other day *as long as she will allow breeding*. Alternatively, she can be bred every third day. Breeding less frequently is discouraged for a young healthy female that has never had a litter.

If only one or two breedings are allowed, if frozen or chilled semen is to be used, if there is a history of failure to conceive despite use of a proven sire, if there is a history of not being willing to breed, if artificial insemination is to be used, or if there are any other serious concerns, ovulation timing techniques should be utilized. These involve combining information gained from a series of smears from the vagina (vaginal cytology) and a series of blood tests assessing female hormones. The most commonly tested hormone is progesterone. Another hormone, luteinizing hormone (LH), can also be used but requires daily testing. Vaginal cytology is initiated during the first few days after vaginal bleeding is first seen and is performed every other day. Your veterinarian, a technician, or you can obtain the vaginal smears, and then the technician or veterinarian evaluates them. They help to determine whether the ovaries are working correctly and may help to tell when breeding should begin. Vaginal cytology determines when blood testing should begin. Progesterone assays are extremely helpful in determining when breeding should occur. When more than 50 per cent of the epithelial cells are cornified (superficial cells), progesterone levels should be checked every 48 hours (daily LH testing could begin at this time as well). The bitch is most fertile and should be bred 2, 4, and 6 days after progesterone begins to rise or after the "surge" in LH is demonstrated. Natural breedings with "ties" always provide the best chance of the bitch becoming pregnant. A "tie" means that the male and female are actually stuck together, and this can last from 5 minutes to as long as an hour. Duration of a tie is not critical, but the development of a tie for any length of time is quite important. Artificial insemination using a fertile dog and proper timing can also be highly successful. Normal gestation is 64 to 66 days from the day after progesterone begins to increase or after the LH rise or 56 to 58 days from the first day of diestrus.

Whelping in the Bitch ■ Margaret V. Root Kustritz and Autumn P. Davidson

Whelping usually occurs with relatively few problems. Dogs can usually deliver their puppies with little help from owners. This sheet is intended to provide information to help you decide when an abnormality is present. Most dogs whelp about 63 days after breeding (normal range, 58 to 71 days). To determine exactly when the dog is due, determine her first day of diestrus (day 1) with vaginal cytology and she will whelp on day 56, 57, or 58; alternatively, start taking your dog's rectal temperature two to four times daily, starting about 55 days after breeding. To take your dog's rectal temperature, you can use a human oral thermometer. Lubricate it with a little petroleum jelly, make sure the thermometer bulb is totally within the anus, and leave it in for at least 1 minute. When the dog's temperature falls to below 100°F (usually below 99°F), she should begin to whelp within 24 hours and will probably begin in 4 to 6 hours. You should have a place set aside for her that is warm and private. She may pick a place for herself and start nesting behavior there as she nears whelping. It is useful to have on hand clean towels, iodine, thread or dental floss, a postal or small food scale, vanilla ice cream, and your veterinarian's phone number.

Labor starts with a long stage in which the uterine contractions begin, the birth canal relaxes, and the cervix opens. The abdominal contractions may not be visible, but your dog may appear nervous or restless, pant, or vomit. This stage lasts 6 to 12 hours. The second stage is the actual birth of the puppies. You will usually see fetal tissues protruding before you actually see a pup born. Remember, breech deliveries are normal. The puppies are born covered by a membrane that the dog ruptures with her teeth. She also bites through the umbilical cord of each pup. Abdominal contractions are evident at this stage, but it is usually best to leave the bitch alone. Dogs can voluntarily stop giving birth if they are disturbed, so you should make sure she is in a quiet place. When you first see the hard abdominal contractions signaling the second stage of labor, you should give your dog 2 hours to have the first pup. Once you see fetal tissues protruding, she should have a pup within 30 minutes. When she starts delivering, allow 2 hours between pups. Most dogs have a pup every 30 to 60 minutes; some may have several and then rest a while before finishing. If you are unsure about whether whelping is progressing normally, please call your veterinarian. The third and final stage of labor is that of expelling the placenta or afterbirth. The dog usually expels the placenta for each pup after it is born and sometimes expels two placentas after delivering two pups. You should clean these away; there is no good physiologic reason for allowing the bitch to eat them. Trying to count these is notoriously unreliable, but you can try.

You may need to help the pups if the mother does not. Do not try to pull a puppy if it appears to be stuck, as it is easy to harm the pups. If the mother does not clean the pups, you should dry them with a towel, wipe clear all fluid from the nose and mouth, and rub the puppies vigorously. If the bitch does not sever the umbilical cord, you will have to do it. Wait for 5 to 10 minutes and then tie the umbilical cord in two places with thread or dental floss. The closest tie should be 1 to 2 inches from the pup's body. Cut between the two ties, dipping the end of the cord in iodine. Leave the pups with the bitch; even though she may not let them nurse, they need her warmth and physical contact. Many bitches will eat a special treat such as vanilla ice cream while whelping. Vanilla ice cream is good for bitches during whelping as it provides energy and calcium.

After whelping is completed, make sure all the pups nurse within 12 to 18 hours. The first milk they receive is important in providing them with immunity to many common diseases. It is also important to make sure the puppies are warm enough; they should be kept in an environment at about 85°F for the first several weeks of life. Be careful in your use of heating pads or heat lamps; it is easy to burn the pups. The mother may have a green to red-brown vulvar discharge for up to 3 weeks after whelping. This is normal and is of no concern as long as it is not foul smelling and she seems fine otherwise. Inspect the mother's mammary glands daily to check for the presence of milk, any abnormal swellings, and pain. Please call you veterinarian if you have any concerns. The puppies should be weighed at birth and daily thereafter. They may lose a small amount of weight the first day but should gain steadily after that, doubling their birth weight by 10 to 14 days of age. Following is a checklist of reasons to call your veterinarian for help (also see the handout on dystocia):

- The dog has started labor and is not progressing within the time limits just listed.
- The rectal temperature dropped more than 24 hours ago and the dog has not started labor.
- The dog appears ill, depressed, feverish, fatigued.
- You have trouble getting the puppies to breathe early on or to suckle later.
- You are not sure if the dog has finished whelping.
- You have any particular concerns or questions.

A novel approach to canine obstetric monitoring involves the use of external monitoring devices to detect and record uterine activity and fetal heart rates.* These devices can be used in the home setting or the veterinary clinic to transmit recorded information by modem to obstetric personnel capable of interpretation and subsequent consultation with the attending veterinarian and owner. Sensors detect changes in intrauterine and intra-amniotic pressures, as well as Doppler monitoring of fetal heart rates. The presence of normal prelabor uterine activity can be detected, often before behavioral clues exist, allowing recognition of stage 1 labor. Because the bitch's drop in body temperature can be missed, this detection of early labor can be valuable. The use of uterine and fetal monitors allows the veterinarian to manage labor medically with knowledge of the presence of fetal distress and allows the administration of oxytocin and calcium to be directed and tailored to each bitch. Absolute indications for cesarian section could be detected with monitoring before fetal death or maternal compromise occurs. Overall, the anxiety level of breeders is diminished and the level of participation of the veterinarian improved. The cost to the client of monitoring is less than the price of one puppy.

APP

---

*Veterinary Perinatal Services, (888) 281-4867.

Dystocia in the Bitch ■ Autumn P. Davidson

Dystocia can be defined as inability to expel neonates through the birth canal from the uterus. Dystocia is not uncommon in the bitch and can have several causes. The diagnosis of dystocia should be made and treatment instituted in an expedient fashion. An incorrect diagnosis of dystocia may result in an unnecessary caesarian section, but failure to recognize or prioritize dystocia usually results in loss of puppies and perhaps even the dam.

Dystocia can occur as a consequence of problems with the dam's uterus or birth canal or with the fetus. The diagnosis of dystocia should be based on the presence of any of the following criteria:

1. *Failure of the dam to initiate labor at term.* Bitches can be considered over term at more than 70 to 72 days from the first breeding, more than 58 to 60 days of diestrus, or more than 66 days from the luteinizing hormone (LH) surge or initial rise in progesterone during estrus.

2. *Failure of the dam to enter stage 1 labor* beyond 24 to 36 hours after a detectable drop in rectal temperature to less than 99 to 100°F *or to proceed from stage 1 to stage 2 labor* within 24 hours.

3. *Failure of the dam to complete delivery of all fetuses in a timely fashion.* Delivery should occur within 30 minutes to 1 hour of active labor (visible abdominal efforts) or 4 to 6 hours of intermittent labor.

4. *Fetal distress* (unborn puppies with slow heart rates, stillborns).

5. *Maternal distress* (excessive pain or systemic illness), green or copious vaginal bleeding.

6. *Irreversible history of dystocia* (pelvic canal abnormalities, mismatch between fetal and maternal size) or radiographic evidence of fetal malposition.

Your veterinarian's diagnosis of dystocia is based on taking an accurate history, including reproductive history, ovulation timing, and breeding dates, and performing a careful physical examination including a digital pelvic examination for the presence of vaginal abnormalities and the presence of a fetus in the birth canal. A handheld Doppler device, abdominal ultrasonography, and x-rays can be helpful in assessing fetal viability, litter size, and fetal position. A blood test to measure calcium and glucose levels may be helpful in identifying metabolic disorders contributing to dystocia.

Uterine abnormalities contributing to the development of dystocia include uterine inertia, abnormalities associated with fetal fluids, and herniation or torsion of a uterine horn. Uterine inertia, failure of the uterine muscle to contract in an effective manner, can be primary or secondary. Primary uterine inertia is multifactorial, with genetic, mechanical, hormonal, and physical components. Bitches exhibiting primary inertia fail to proceed into an effective labor pattern, and cesarian section is indicated. Bitches exhibiting secondary inertia fail to complete expulsion of all fetuses because of exhaustion of the uterine muscle. Medical management can be attempted, with adequate fetal monitoring, but cesarian section may be necessary. Intravenous glucose-containing solutions and oxytocin ("pit") and calcium injections can be administered in appropriate doses. Generally, minute doses of oxytocin are adequate (0.25 to 4.0 units per dog). Spastic, uncoordinated contractions of the uterus occur if oxytocin is administered too rapidly or at too high a dose. Uterine contractions interfere with fetal oxygen supply by compressing placentas. Oxytocin should be administered only with veterinary guidance. Abnormalities of fetal or placental fluids include hydrops, an excessive accumulation of allantoic fluid associated with each fetus, causing the fetal unit to be markedly oversized. Rarely, underproduction of fetal fluids occurs, resulting in dystocia caused by lack of lubricating fluids.

Disorders of the birth canal contributing to dystocia include pelvic abnormalities such as narrowing resulting from a healed fracture or congenital disorders and vaginovulvar abnormalities such as strictures. Successful natural breedings can occur despite the presence of septate (vertical) bands in the vaginal vault. Unfortunately, subsequent vaginal delivery of fetuses is usually impaired. Strictures should be detected by the veterinarian at the time of the soundness examination, before breeding. Anular (circular) strictures are often detected at the time of breeding, as they often interfere with the ability to attain a natural tie. These should be repaired before breeding. Bitches with unusually small vulvar openings may require a partial episiotomy to deliver puppies vaginally.

Fetal causes of dystocia include fetal oversize; fetal anomalies; and abnormal fetal position, presentation, or posture. Fetal oversize can occur with prolonged gestation in abnormally small litters (especially if there is a single pup) and is the most common fetal cause of dystocia. Fetal anomalies such as anasarca and hydrocephalus (abnormalities of body fluid distribution) can cause a mismatch between the size of the birth canal and that of the fetus. Because both anterior (head-first) and posterior (breech) presentations are normal in the bitch, only a transverse (sideways) presentation is associated with dystocia and is rare. Puppies are normally positioned with the fetal backbone adjacent to the top surface of the uterus. Malpositioning can cause mild dystocia. Abnormalities of posture, normal being fully extended, are the second most frequent fetal cause of dystocia. Malpositioning of the head, forelimbs, or hindlimbs of the canine fetus is not readily corrected with the use of forceps, traction, or digital manipulation because of the limitations of the size of the birth canal of the bitch.

Pyometra ■ Autumn P. Davidson

Pyometra is a progesterone-mediated uterine disorder in bitches and queens. Progesterone is the female hormone that works to maintain pregnancy. All normal female dogs are naturally exposed to tremendous concentrations of progesterone during the 45 to 75 days that follow the period of breeding (the period called diestrus). Progesterone places the nonpregnant uterus at risk for bacterial infection. These bacteria are normally found in the vagina but have infected the uterus by migrating through the cervix. A bacterium called *Escherichia coli* is the most common cause of pyometra in both bitches and queens. The incidence of pyometra is thought to be greater in the bitch than the queen because dogs are exposed to natural progesterone more frequently than cats. An increased incidence of pyometra is associated with estrogen administration in the bitch. Therefore, estrogen should not be used as a treatment for "mismate" in dogs. Administration of progesterone to queens can also precipitate pyometra. Progesterone compounds should not be used as anti-inflammatory or behavior-modifying drugs in intact queens.

Pyometra can occur with or without vaginal discharge, depending on the ability of uterine contents to flow through an open (patent) or closed cervix. Closed cervix pyometra is more serious because some of these dogs become ill before an owner realizes there is a problem. In contrast, dogs with "open cervix" pyometra can be recognized as having a problem earlier because they usually have an obvious, malodorous, pus-colored vaginal discharge before they become seriously ill. Dogs with closed cervix pyometra may suffer from uterine rupture, which can be as critical and life threatening as when people have a ruptured appendix. In addition to the vaginal discharge, the classic clinical signs of pyometra include partial to complete loss of appetite, fever, lethargy, weight loss, an unkempt appearance, vomiting and diarrhea, and excessive thirst and urination. Blood and urine tests are consistent with infection and may indicate involvement of other organs that can be harmed by this severe disease. Abdominal x-rays and ultrasonography can be useful in confirming the diagnosis. Although it is rare, pyometra can occur in one uterine horn with pregnancy in the other.

The best, least expensive, most reliable, quickest, and easiest treatment for pyometra, after stabilization of your dog or cat with intravenous fluids and antibiotics, is the spay (ovariohysterectomy). This would not be the first and best treatment only if your pet is younger than 6 years of age and a valuable breeding bitch or queen. Medical treatment of open cervix pyometra, using prostaglandin $F_{2\alpha}$ ($PGF_{2\alpha}$) and appropriate antibiotics, has been successful in both the bitch and queen. Antibiotics alone are almost never success-ful in completely resolving pyometra. $PGF_{2\alpha}$ causes emptying of uterine contents and a lowering of blood progesterone levels. The presence of live fetuses should be ruled out by use of ultrasonography before treatment because the drug causes abortion and because the treatment is not usually successful if there are any remnants of previous pregnancies in the uterus. Those dogs and cats should be spayed, as should any dog or cat that is extremely ill. The $PGF_{2\alpha}$ treatment should never be used for an extremely ill dog or cat.

Bitches and queens may need to be hospitalized for the $PGF_{2\alpha}$ treatment to enable administration of adjunct supportive care, such as intravenous fluids and antibiotics, and to permit monitoring of adverse effects and outcome of treatment. The treatment protocol includes 5 to 7 days of injections. Most can be treated on an outpatient basis because dogs and cats treated with $PGF_{2\alpha}$ should never be critically ill. Predictable physical reactions that occur after the administration of this drug include restlessness, panting, salivation, vomiting, diarrhea, urination, and dilatation of the pupils (bitch and queen) and grooming, lordosis, and kneading (queens). These reactions usually resolve within 5 to 60 minutes. After each subsequent injection, the reactions diminish in severity and duration. Reactions are rarely considered severe enough to warrant discontinuation of the drug.

A successful short-term response, defined as resolution of the signs of pyometra, may not be evident at the completion of $PGF_{2\alpha}$ treatment. At the time of release from the hospital, bitches and queens should have an improved appetite and normal rectal temperature. However, the abnormal vaginal discharge may be completely gone or may persist for another 5 to 10 days. Reexaminations should be scheduled for 7 and 14 days after completion of treatment. At 2 weeks after treatment, there should be little or no vaginal discharge and the pet should be otherwise healthy. Abdominal x-rays or ultrasonography can be used to evaluate reduction in uterine size compared with that on previous examinations. Persistence of problems suggests that retreatment be considered. A second series of injections for recurrent pyometra can be successful and may be considered if the condition of the bitch or queen permits. A successful long-term response is defined as a return to normal estrous cycles and, if bred, conception and carrying a litter to term. Breeding at the next estrus is recommended to avoid potential complications after progesterone's effects on a nonpregnant uterus. Prostaglandins do not resolve underlying uterine wall disease. The overall successful conception rate after $PGF_{2\alpha}$ treatment has been reported to be 40 to 82 per cent in bitches and 85 per cent in queens.

APP

Colitis ■ Albert E. Jergens

Colitis refers to inflammation of the colon (e.g., large intestine) with any of a variety of causes. Colitis is a relatively common problem in pets and may be caused by reactions to food, gastrointestinal parasites, bacterial or fungal infections, benign infiltrative diseases (such as inflammatory bowel disease), and even neoplasia (cancer). The most common symptoms of colitis include straining to defecate, bright red blood on the stool, fecal mucus, and increased frequency of defecation. Most animals are alert, active, and have normal appetites in spite of having colitis. Occasionally, they have diseases affecting both the small intestine and colon, which may cause vomiting, alterations in appetite, and/or weight loss.

Diagnosis of colitis is based on the patient's history and findings of the physical examination by your veterinarian and selected diagnostic tests. Puppies and kittens are particularly prone to acute colitis caused by dietary indiscretion (eating garbage), parasites, and bacterial infections, which may be spread from animal to animal. Most of these disorders cause abrupt symptoms prompting veterinary attention. Parasites are easily diagnosed by your veterinarian, who can do so by examining fecal material under a microscope. Rectal swabs for cytologic examination or bacterial fecal cultures may also be recommended. Other diseases, such as fungal infections (e.g., histoplasmosis), inflammatory bowel disease, and neoplasia, occur mostly in adult animals and are characterized by symptoms that have been present for several weeks to months. These animals usually require hospitalization and a more in-depth diagnostic evaluation to confirm a diagnosis. Careful rectal examination is performed in all animals and may provide important clues to the cause of inflammation.

Therapeutic trials in animals suspected of having parasitic or dietary causes of colitis are reasonable. Some parasites (such as whipworm infestation in dogs) are difficult to detect. Your veterinarian may treat your pet with medication to kill this or other suspected parasites. If bacterial infection caused by *Clostridium perfringens* is suspected, treatment with an antibiotic is often useful. Pets that have dietary causes of colitis usually respond favorably to being fed "bland" or hypoallergenic diets. These nutritionally complete diets are highly digestible and reduce the workload of the gut. Fiber supplementation is also beneficial in promoting healing and repair of colonic tissue. A variety of prescription foods or recipes for homemade diets that are appropriate for your pet are available from your veterinarian.

Animals that fail to respond to symptomatic therapy and those having chronic symptoms require additional diagnostic testing. These tests may include blood work, urinalysis, radiographic imaging procedures, and tissue biopsy. Endoscopic examination of the colon (e.g., colonoscopy, which is an examination of the inside of the colon with a scope and light) with mucosal biopsy provides the most definitive diagnosis in most cases. Your pet may require hospitalization before the procedure for bowel cleansing. The colonoscopy is performed while your pet is anesthetized or sedated. The results of endoscopic biopsy will guide treatment recommendations by your veterinarian and provide useful information about the likelihood of cure or recurrence. Regardless of the cause, dietary modification with a hypoallergenic diet and fiber supplementation are beneficial for most dogs and cats with chronic colitis.

Chronic Hepatitis in the Dog ■ Richard E. Goldstein

Chronic hepatitis is a syndrome in dogs that can result from many different disease processes. It means that the liver has undergone or is undergoing "inflammation" and/or "necrosis." Inflammation is an invasion into the liver from the bloodstream of different types of white cells that are active in the immune system; necrosis refers to the death of large numbers of liver cells. The invasion of white cells of the immune system and cell death can be a result of previous damage to the liver by infectious agents, such as viruses or bacteria, or of toxic damage. Such damage can be caused by poisons ingested by the dog or the accumulation of substances made by the body. A primary attack of the immune system against the liver cells can also cause inflammation and cell death, a condition known as "autoimmune" disease. Cancer can result in similar liver damage, but if cancer is identified in the liver, the term chronic hepatitis is not used. The term "chronic" means that the damaging process has been going on for some time, at least a number of weeks. In contrast, an "acute" hepatitis has most likely gone on for just a few days. Unfortunately, the chance for complete recovery is less in chronic hepatitis than in acute disease.

Chronic hepatitis can occur in any breed of dog, male or female, and at any age, although most dogs are middle aged to older. Certain breeds are predisposed to this condition. Therefore, although the exact mechanism of disease in unknown, genetics most likely plays a role in the development of this problem in those breeds. Bedlington terriers, and in some instances West Highland white terriers and Skye terriers, may develop chronic hepatitis as a result of accumulation of copper in the cells of their liver. Affected Bedlington terriers are not able to eliminate copper from the liver because of a well-defined genetic defect. The high concentrations of copper damage the liver cells, resulting in what can be severe chronic hepatitis. Doberman pinschers and cocker spaniels (American and English) are also commonly diagnosed with chronic hepatitis. Cocker spaniels are frequently affected at a young age and are usually diagnosed when they are 1 to 4 years old. Unfortunately, cocker spaniels also tend to be severely affected, and many dogs die within 1 month of diagnosis despite therapy. Although this grave prognosis is true for the majority of cases, some dogs with luck and aggressive treatment live much longer.

The symptoms associated with this condition vary greatly as a result of the multiple functions of the liver. The common signs may include a mild to marked decrease in appetite, lethargy, vomiting, and diarrhea. The dog may also drink more and urinate more, have a swollen belly filled with fluid, and have a yellow (jaundiced) tinge to his or her skin, ears, and gums. Occasionally, dogs exhibit strange behavioral or neurologic signs such as severe lethargy, depression, aggression, blindness, standing in corners or pressing their heads into walls or corners, and sometimes even loss of consciousness, seizures, and coma.

Liver disease is suspected from the dog's symptoms and the physical examination performed by the veterinarian. Confirmation of liver dysfunction is achieved with a variety of blood tests. Imaging techniques such as x-rays or abdominal ultrasonography are also commonly used to assess the size and appearance of the liver. Dogs with chronic hepatitis tend to have a small liver. A liver biopsy is the only definitive way to diagnose chronic hepatitis. A biopsy can be performed surgically or through the skin with a special needle under ultrasound guidance. The information obtained by performing the biopsy is necessary for the veterinarian in determining the type and severity of liver disease that the dog has, as well as allowing an accurate assessment of the dog's condition and the determination of appropriate treatment. The potential benefits and risks and precautionary measures that should be taken before the biopsy procedure vary from case to case and should be discussed with your veterinarian.

The treatment of chronic hepatitis is complex and is determined on the basis of the severity and type of disease process in the liver as well as the clinical signs exhibited by the dog. Hospitalization, fluid therapy, and supportive care may be necessary in severe cases. Medications commonly used in this disorder include antibiotics, immunosuppressive or anti-inflammatory agents, medications to prevent ulceration of the stomach and intestines, diuretics to increase urination and promote fluid loss, and low-protein diets. Additional medications are also used in specific instances, such as in dogs whose disease is associated with copper accumulation or in dogs showing neurologic signs. Unfortunately, despite appropriate treatment, this condition is usually not curable. Many dogs, though, can be kept relatively free of clinical signs and have a good quality of life for months and even years with therapy. Your veterinarian will need to recheck your dog's clinical state and blood work frequently and make changes in the therapeutic regimen as needed.

APP

Dental Disease in Dogs and Cats ■ M. J. Lommer and F. J. M. Verstraete

Periodontal disease (problems in the area around the teeth) is one of the most common health problems in companion animals. It is estimated that 80 per cent of dogs and 70 per cent of cats older than 3 years of age suffer from some level of periodontal disease. Just as in the human mouth, the process begins with plaque, which is made of salivary proteins and bacteria. The bacteria irritate the gum, causing an inflammatory reaction, which is known as gingivitis. If the plaque is removed by toothbrushing, the gingivitis resolves and the gums return to normal. If the plaque is not removed, it hardens into "tartar" or "calculus." The calculus provides a rough surface for even more plaque to accumulate. Bad breath may be noted. Inflammation continues in the gums and can also affect any bone in the area, resulting in destruction of the bone around the tooth roots. Eventually, the teeth become loose and may fall out.

In addition to tooth loss, periodontal disease has other, more serious, consequences. The millions of bacteria present in an unhealthy mouth can spread to other parts of the body, such as the heart, lungs, kidneys, and liver, causing disease in these vital organs. In small breed dogs with tiny jawbones, the bone destruction caused by periodontal disease can weaken the jawbone enough to cause a fracture.

The good news is that periodontal disease is completely preventable! Removing the plaque reverses the inflammatory process in the gingiva and restores the gums to health. As we know from our own experience, plaque removal is best achieved by brushing the teeth. Dog and cat teeth are not as close together as ours are, so flossing is not necessary. However, in order to be effective, brushing must be done *every day.* A soft-bristled toothbrush with a small head is the best tool for removing plaque from your dog's or cat's teeth. Special pet toothpaste is available in flavors such as "malt," "poultry," and "seafood" to help your pet enjoy the experience. Human toothpaste should not be used, because pets do not like the mint flavor and because the foaming agents in human toothpaste can cause stomach upset if pets swallow the toothpaste. Because dogs and cats rarely get caries (cavities), fluoride is not necessary. Feeding special diets such as Hill's T/D and encouraging chewing activity with toys such as the Dental Kong also help reduce plaque accumulation.

Daily toothbrushing, special diets, and chewing activity help prevent plaque from hardening into calculus. Once calculus is present, however, a professional cleaning is required. Although the bone destruction caused by periodontal disease cannot be reversed, the inflammatory process can be stopped or slowed with proper treatment. Routine periodontal treatment involves sonic or ultrasonic scaling above *and* below the gumline. Because your veterinarian cannot simply tell your pet to "hold still," these procedures require that your pet be placed under anesthesia. Anesthesia always has inherent risks. However, your veterinarian is experienced and the risk related to anesthesia is minimal. To further minimize this risk to your pet, your veterinarian may recommend blood and other tests prior to sedation. These are done before anesthesia to reveal any problems that may not be obvious from a physical examination. Dental x-rays are important to determine the amount of bone destruction present. Teeth with significant bone loss may benefit from periodontal surgery. Extraction is usually recommended for teeth with little bone support remaining.

In addition to periodontal disease, cats can develop "resorptive" lesions, which can lead to pain and difficulty eating. These lesions are sometimes called "cavities," but they do not result from bacteria and sugars as people's cavities do. Cells such as the ones responsible for removing deciduous (baby) tooth roots become activated and start to attack permanent teeth. The result is destruction of large amounts of the tooth and exposure of the nerve, or pulp, inside the tooth. Pain may be evident in behavior such as pawing at the face, dropping food, drooling, or reluctance to eat. The areas of destruction can be seen on careful examination of the teeth and with the use of dental x-rays. Resorptive lesions cannot be filled like human cavities, as the cells continue to work under the filling to destroy the remaining tooth. The current recommendation for affected teeth is extraction. At this time, because we do not know why the cells become activated, there is no known way to prevent resorptive lesions. Regular examinations by your veterinarian will help to detect these lesions early, before they cause significant pain to your cat.

By brushing your pet's teeth every day and scheduling regular examinations with your veterinarian, you can provide your companion with a lifetime of fresh breath, clean teeth, healthy gums, and strong jawbones. In addition, you will be helping to keep your pet pain free and in overall good health.

Flatulence ■ W. Grant Guilford

Flatulence refers to the anal passage of intestinal gas. It is also known by many other names, including "farting," "passing wind," and "passing gas." Flatulence more commonly affects dogs than cats and is most often observed in inactive dogs that spend long periods indoors.

It is normal for dogs to pass gas in small quantities at infrequent intervals. However, persistent passage of excessive quantities of gas is abnormal. Excessive flatulence usually results from intolerance of one or more components of the pet's diet. This intolerance is most often due to the feeding of a diet of inferior quality containing ingredients of poor digestibility. These ingredients pass through the intestinal tract without being absorbed and end up in the large intestine (colon and rectum), where bacteria ferment them to produce gas. Some of these gases do not smell, whereas others, particularly those derived from the fermentation of proteins and fats, smell badly. Flatulence can also occur when a dog eats excessive quantities of food, overwhelming the ability of its gastrointestinal tract to digest the food. Furthermore, some dogs are born without the ability to digest certain ingredients in their diets. For example, many dogs (and cats) have difficulty digesting lactose in milk. Other dogs have trouble digesting some legumes such as soy. Fortunately, flatulence resulting from legumes can be successfully reduced by a variety of manufacturing techniques. Another cause of flatulence is greedy eating resulting in the ingestion of large quantities of air. Once ingested, air has to be removed from the gastrointestinal tract either by burping or by flatulence.

Although flatulence is usually normal, on occasion it can herald more serious gastrointestinal disease, particularly of the small bowel or pancreas. You should seek veterinary advice if the measures listed below fail to control flatulence, if gaseousness appears to be causing your pet abdominal discomfort, or if the flatulence is associated with concurrent vomiting or diarrhea. All of these signs suggest more serious gastrointestinal disease.

The management of flatulence begins with a change to a high-quality (highly digestible) diet without excessive fat content. Suitable commercial products are available from most of the major manufacturers. Alternatively, owners can prepare a homemade diet composed of highly digestible protein and carbohydrate sources such as cottage cheese and rice appropriately balanced with vitamins and minerals. Homemade diets are less desirable than commercial diets because their long-term use is often associated with nutritional deficiencies or excesses. Ensuring regular exercise is also helpful because it promotes regular defecation. Reducing the dog's gulping of air by avoiding situations that provoke nervousness and by discouraging greedy eating, for instance, by ensuring that the dog does not have to compete for food, may also be helpful. In the rare event that dietary manipulation is not successful in controlling flatulence, call your veterinarian, because a diagnostic investigation of your pet's digestive system may be required. Alternatively, your veterinarian may suggest a trial with medications that reduce gas production by assisting digestion, absorbing gas, or assisting the passage of gas.

APP

Gastrointestinal Food Allergies ■ Michael D. Willard

An allergy is an immune-mediated reaction that harms the body instead of protecting it. Examples of such reactions include fatal human reactions to a single bee sting or eating a single strawberry. These are called "hypersensitivity" reactions. Certain types of reactions by the body (depending on the type of hypersensitivity reaction, of which there are four) cause an exaggerated response that produces excessive irritation (inflammation) or decreases the size (constriction) of vessels or airways. The substances that mediate these reactions (antibodies and lymphocytes) are programmed to respond to specific substances called antigens. Antigens that cause hypersensitivity reactions are usually proteins or carbohydrates, and they may be found in almost anything, including food. Depending on where the hypersensitivity reaction takes place and how many antibodies or lymphocytes are involved, the consequences may vary from sudden, life-threatening episodes to delayed ones that cause inflammation in just one part of the body. In dogs and cats, most hypersensitivity reactions that result from eating foods cause either skin disease (characterized by scratching) or various gastrointestinal (GI) signs such as diarrhea and/or vomiting. Sometimes both the skin and the GI tract are affected in animals that have a food allergy, but many animals with food hypersensitivity have either skin or GI signs but not both.

The GI signs of food allergy sometimes occur immediately after eating (i.e., immediate-type hypersensitivity reactions). However, food allergy in pets is more commonly a "delayed" hypersensitivity reaction, meaning that the consequences arise hours or days after eating the food and then persist for hours or days after each exposure. Because most pets eat the offending antigens every day, GI signs tend to be more or less constant. There is seldom a clear-cut association between eating and the onset of signs, making it hard to determine that eating a particular food is causing the disease. To help diagnose this problem, we can look for microscopic changes on small pieces of intestine obtained by doing surgery or by passing a long instrument from the outside into the stomach. However, changes that suggest allergy (i.e., eosinophilic inflammation) are usually a form of inflammation. Inflammation caused by food allergies usually resembles that caused by other diseases. The best way to diagnose a food allergy is to feed the pet a hypoallergenic diet (i.e., a therapeutic dietary trial) and see if the problems disappear.

When performing a therapeutic trial for a food allergy, the diet must be carefully chosen. Because there is no one diet that is hypoallergenic for all pets, one must design or find a diet that is appropriate for each animal. The pet may be allergic to almost any component of its current diet; therefore, we want foodstuffs that the pet has not eaten before. We usually choose a diet that (1) contains as few ingredients as possible, (2) contains foodstuffs that we know the pet has not eaten in the past (and hence is unlikely to be allergic to), and (3) contains foodstuffs that we know hardly ever cause allergic reactions (e.g., potato, rice). Because some patients that are allergic to multiple antigens require a strict hypoallergenic diet, homemade diets are sometimes needed. Although inconvenient and restrictive, they are often the most successful in treating the allergy. Most homemade diets are not balanced but are adequate for use in mature animals for the 2 to 4 months when the animal is having the trial. We have to make many assumptions when we choose these diets, and it is possible that the pet is allergic to something unexpected. When such a dietary trial is begun, it is imperative that absolutely *nothing* else be fed. Even flavored pills or toys can contain enough antigens to cause signs of food allergy to persist. The dietary trial must be performed long enough to allow the clinical signs of delayed-type hypersensitivity to disappear. Some patients evidence improvement within a day of dietary change, whereas others require 4 to 8 weeks before improvement is seen. If a patient has a dietary allergy, it may have a genetic predisposition to allergy and may eventually become allergic to the ingredients of the hypoallergenic diet that it responded to well at first. Other tests have been tried in order to determine what dietary components a pet is sensitive to. As of this writing, these tests have not always correlated well with the results of dietary trials.

Gastric Dilatation-Volvulus ■ W. Grant Guilford

Gastric dilatation-volvulus is otherwise known as "bloat," "stomach torsion," or "twisted stomach." The cause of the condition is unknown. It can have tragic consequences and result in death in as short a time as 2 to 3 hours. The stomach bloats as a result of rapid accumulation of gas. Eventually, the distended stomach rotates around its supporting ligaments, trapping the gas and choking off its own blood supply. The distended stomach presses on the chest, making it difficult for the dog to breathe, and compresses large veins in the abdomen, preventing blood from returning to the heart. The difficulty in breathing and the poor blood flow eventually result in collapse and death unless treatment is prompt.

Treatment of gastric dilatation-volvulus is successful in up to 70 per cent of cases if the owners recognize the signs of the disease promptly. The most important sign is distention of the abdomen. If the abdomen becomes drum tight, the diagnosis is almost certain. Other signs include loss of appetite, frequent retching, abdominal pain, distress, and eventually collapse. Treatment begins with rapid intravenous fluid therapy (to replenish lost fluid and improve blood flow) and decompression of the bloated stomach. Decompression of the gas-filled stomach is usually performed by placing a needle directly into the stomach through the abdominal wall or by passing a tube into the stomach via the mouth. Drugs may be required, including antibiotics, drugs to help prevent shock, and drugs to reduce damage to the stomach lining. When the dog is in as fit a state for surgery as possible, it is anesthetized and operated on to return the stomach to the normal position. In addition, the surgeon will attempt to suture the stomach to the abdominal wall in the correct position in the hope of preventing a further bout of bloat. This is called a "gastropexy." Without this procedure the likelihood of recurrence of the bloat is as high as 80 per cent. If the surgery reveals extensive areas of dead stomach, the likelihood of the dog surviving the postoperative period is very low. Sadly, in this situation, a veterinarian may advise euthanasia of the dog on the operating table in order to avoid further suffering.

The postoperative period is full of risk for dogs with bloat. Abnormal beats of the heart are common postoperatively, as are life-threatening problems such as severe ulcers or holes (perforations) in the stomach and bowel, pancreas or liver damage, infections, and excessive blood clotting. For this reason, dogs usually remain at the veterinary clinic under close observation for several days after the surgery.

Prevention of gastric dilatation-volvulus is difficult because the underlying cause or causes of the disease are unknown. However, some risk factors that predispose a dog to develop bloat have been recognized. Avoidance of these risk factors (where possible) minimizes the likelihood of the disease occurring. Knowledge of these factors is important if you own a large, deep-chested dog because dogs with this type of conformation are predisposed to the disease (e.g., Great Danes, Saint Bernards, Weimaraners, Irish setters, Dobermans, German shepherds). Risk factors that have been identified in some (but not all) studies include eating only one meal per day (this leads to a larger stomach size than eating two or more meals), eating faster, and a nervous temperament. It is also prudent to avoid exercising dogs when their stomach is full. Many predisposed dogs have the disease precipitated by a stressful event, so owners should be particularly vigilant for the disease at such times.

APP

Hepatic Lipidosis in Cats ■ Richard E. Goldstein

Hepatic lipidosis, or fatty liver, is a common syndrome characterized by excess fat accumulation in the liver of cats. It can occur in cats of any age or breed and may affect more females than males. Hepatic lipidosis classically occurs after a period of anorexia (loss of appetite) of at least 2 weeks duration. When an additional disease state is found to be the cause of the anorexia, the hepatic lipidosis is defined as "secondary." The term "primary" or "idiopathic" hepatic lipidosis is used when an additional disease state cannot be identified. This is the case in approximately 50 per cent of cats diagnosed with the disorder. Obesity before the period of anorexia increases the chances of a cat developing clinical hepatic lipidosis. The decrease in appetite causing secondary hepatic lipidosis can occur for a variety of reasons. The more common of the predisposing disease states are diabetes mellitus, pancreatitis (inflammation of the pancreas), cancer, and other liver diseases. Behavioral or stress-related causes of anorexia are also common; they include the owners being away on vacation, family members leaving or new people or pets being introduced into the household, boarding, and dietary changes. Unfortunately, once this disease develops, cats feel ill and may not begin to eat again even if the initial cause of their loss of appetite has been eliminated. Without aggressive medical intervention, this vicious circle can lead to death in over 90 per cent of the cats.

Cats are unique in their tendency to develop this disorder. Excessive amounts of fat are broken down from the cat's peripheral fat storage tissue during fasting. This fat is then transported to the liver. The liver should then process this fat and export it to the rest of the body in a new form. In cats that develop hepatic lipidosis this process is impaired and the rate of fat export from the liver is much slower than the rate of fat intake, resulting in liver fat accumulation. Damage to the liver is caused by swelling of liver cells filled with fatty deposits as well as additional processes.

Symptoms commonly seen with this syndrome are anorexia, weight loss, lethargy, vomiting, jaundice (yellow tinge to the skin, inside of the ears, and gums), and occasionally behavioral or neurologic signs such as excessive drooling, blindness, semicoma or coma, and seizures. The suspicion that a cat is suffering from liver disease is confirmed by physical examination and appropriate abnormalities in blood work. Imaging techniques such as x-rays or ultrasound examination of the abdomen are helpful in demonstrating the size and appearance of the liver, as well as ruling out other disease states. The definitive diagnosis of hepatic lipidosis requires visualization of fat globules in liver cells obtained via liver biopsy or needle aspiration.

The treatment of hepatic lipidosis varies depending on its severity and the existence of other diseases. Prevention is extremely important. Any anorexic cat, especially if obese, should be seen by a veterinarian. Thus, the development of hepatic lipidosis can be caught in its early stages or prevented entirely with appropriate therapy. Hospitalization, fluid therapy, and supportive care may be required initially when the disease develops. Additional therapy such as antibiotics, vitamin K, and the treatment of other diseases may also be necessary.

The cornerstone of therapy, the only way to reverse the process of fat accumulation in the liver, is aggressive feeding to supply your cat with his or her full caloric requirements. Offering different diets and appetite-stimulating medications may induce a cat to eat in the initial phases of anorexia but will most likely not be of benefit once clinical signs of hepatic lipidosis develop. Force feeding is usually not a good idea. Even with the most cooperative cat, it is virtually impossible to feed adequate amounts in this fashion. Cats also seem to develop food aversions rapidly, and the association between food and the unpleasant experience of forcing may delay the cat's return to eating. Therefore, in the clinical phase of the disease the only reliable treatment option is tube feeding.

The use of long-term tube feeding has changed the outcome in this disease from over 90 per cent mortality to less than 30 per cent. There are three types of feeding tubes commonly used for this disease. A tube placed through the nose into the stomach or esophagus can be used temporarily. Long-term feeding is achieved with a tube surgically placed in the esophagus or, more commonly, a tube surgically or endoscopically placed through the body wall directly into the stomach. A commercially available maintenance diet is used for most cats. Your veterinarian will supply you with a feeding plan aimed at meeting your cat's nutritional requirements. Additional medications to control vomiting are sometimes necessary. Frequent rechecks with your veterinarian will be required to assess the tube location, possible infection, your cat's clinical state, and blood work. Liver parameters usually improve within 2 to 8 weeks after initiating feeding. Oral food should not be offered until that time. Once your cat begins to eat, tube feedings can be gradually reduced over a few weeks and eventually discontinued. Most cats' tubes can be removed 3 to 4 months after placement. In cats with idiopathic hepatic lipidosis recurrence is rare, and the cats that recover go on to live normal lives.

Managing PEG Tubes and Feeding Tubes ■ Theresa M. Ortega and Marcella F. Harb-Hauser

Feeding tubes allow continued feeding of an animal when it has a mouth, jaw, throat, esophageal, stomach, liver, kidney, or pancreatic disorder that causes loss of appetite or prevents normal eating, swallowing, or digestion. There are several different types of feeding tubes, all of which have an external feeding port connected to a tube that ends in the gastrointestinal tract. *Nasoesophageal, nasogastric,* and *nasojejunal* tubes enter one of the nostrils, pass through the nose and throat, and end in the esophagus, stomach, or small intestine (jejunum), respectively. *Pharyngostomy* tubes enter the throat (pharynx) and *esophagostomy* tubes enter the esophagus; both end in the esophagus. *Gastrostomy* tubes enter the left abdominal wall directly into the stomach. "PEG" tubes (percutaneous endoscopic gastrostomy tubes) are gastrostomy tubes that have been placed using endoscopy. "Button" tubes are short gastrostomy tubes that have only an external feeding port at the entrance into the body wall and no external feeding tube. *Jejunostomy* tubes enter the abdominal wall and end in the small intestine (jejunum). Feeding tubes are secured to the body with sutures, bandages, tube stents, or elastic stockinette or fishnet material. An Elizabethan collar (or "E-collar") is usually placed around your pet's neck to prevent it from removing the tube.

HOW TO FEED (FOLLOW THIS ORDER)

Prepare and warm the food and medications as directed by your veterinarian. Attach an empty syringe to the external feeding port. Release or open any external tube clamps (some gastrostomy tubes have a clamp that should be closed between changing syringes and between meals). Aspirate the tube with an empty syringe to check for residual food or fluid left over from the previous feeding. Return any of the aspirated food or fluid back into the tube. If more than half of the volume of the previous feeding is aspirated, skip this feeding.

With nasal tubes, administer about 3 mL of water and watch for signs of coughing or breathing problems; if either of these occurs, *do not* give any medication or any food. If liquid medications are to be given at the time of meal feeding, attach the medication syringe to the feeding port and administer all the medications before feeding. Attach a food syringe to the feeding port and administer the food slowly over 5 to 10 minutes so that your pet can adapt to an enlarging stomach. If your pet begins to drool or seems uncomfortable, feed more slowly. (If these signs worsen or your pet vomits during the feeding, stop feeding.) Flush the tube with 5 to 10 mL of water (at room or body temperature). This will help prevent tube clogging. *Every time you finish administering medication or food through the tube, you must flush the tube with water.* Close any tube clamps (if present). Detach the empty water syringe and close the external feeding port.

TUBE CARE

NASOESOPHAGEAL OR NASOGASTRIC TUBES

When feeding, check the tube position and security on the face and nose. Also check for irritation of the face and nose (redness, swelling, hair loss, nasal discharge, or sneezing). Gently remove any debris from the nostril and tube using a warm, moist cotton ball, gauze, or cloth.

PHARYNGOSTOMY, GASTROSTOMY, AND JEJUNOSTOMY TUBES

Check the tube position daily by locating the external mark placed on the tube by your veterinarian. Also check the insertion site for redness, swelling, discharge, or pain. It is normal for a thin rim of pink or red tissue to grow outward to the skin of the insertion site. Clean the insertion site with an antiseptic solution recommended by your veterinarian, and clean debris on the tube with a warm, moist cotton ball, gauze, or cloth. After cleaning, place antiseptic ointment and gauze over the insertion site. All of these activities should be performed *daily*.

CLOGGED FEEDING TUBES

Check for kinks in the external tube and make sure the tube clamp is open (if present). Massage the external tube to loosen any material in the tube. Flush and aspirate the tube with water. If it flushes but food cannot be administered, check the tip of the feeding syringe; the syringe tip (versus the tube) may be obstructed. If water flushing does not relieve the obstruction, leave water in the tube, and attempt to flush again in 20 minutes. Finally, place cola or other carbonated drink in the tube, leave in place for 20 minutes, and attempt to flush again.

WHEN TO CALL THE HOSPITAL

1. The tube position has changed or the tube is no longer secure or falls out any time. *Call immediately.*
2. The insertion site or sutured skin is excessively irritated, swollen, painful, or infected.
3. The tube cracks or rips, or its attachments (feeding port, external stent) become detached.
4. Your pet coughs or develops breathing problems. *Call immediately.*
5. Your pet vomits, develops a fever, or becomes more lethargic.
6. The tube clogs (even if you can clear it). Your veterinarian may wish to change the feeding formulation.

FEEDING INSTRUCTIONS

In a mixer, blend _____ (mL or cups) of _____ (type of food) with _____ (mL or cups) of water until the consistency is smooth. Food can be blended and stored in the refrigerator for up to 3 days. Feed _____ (mL) of the food mixture slowly over 5 to 10 minutes, _____ times daily. After each feeding, flush the tube with _____ mL of water.

APP

Megaesophagus ■ Michael D. Willard

The esophagus is a long, muscular tube that connects the back of the mouth (pharynx) to the stomach. The opening of the esophagus into the pharynx is close to where the windpipe (trachea) enters the pharynx. The purpose of the esophagus is to transport swallowed food and water to the stomach. To do this, the esophagus normally uses a squeezing movement behind the food (peristalsis) to propel the material into the stomach within a few seconds after it is swallowed. After swallowing, the normal esophagus is empty and resembles a collapsed hose.

Megaesophagus refers to a syndrome in which the esophagus is weak and flaccid and subsequently becomes much larger than normal (hence the term *mega*esophagus). This occurs because the weak, flaccid esophagus has no tone and does not propel ingested air, food, and water into the stomach; rather, these items stay in the esophagus and stretch it out of shape (dilatation). This syndrome is much more common in dogs than in cats and can occur in dogs of any age. There are many causes of this weakness, but the consequences tend to be similar regardless of cause. Affected pets usually regurgitate fluid and/or food. Regurgitation is much like vomiting, except that vomiting involves ejecting material from the stomach and intestines whereas regurgitation involves emptying material from the esophagus or the back of the mouth. Regurgitation related to megaesophagus may occur soon after eating or hours later. Dogs may or may not lose weight, depending on how much food ultimately reaches the stomach.

The most devastating side effect of this syndrome is having food, water, and saliva leak into the windpipe (trachea) and the lungs (this leakage is called aspiration), subsequently causing pneumonia (i.e., infection of the lungs). Because the esophagus and the trachea enter the pharynx so close to each other, it is easy for this to happen. In some instances, the dog has signs of aspiration (i.e., cough, labored breathing, and/or fever) despite the owner never seeing evidence of regurgitation. This is because the dog may regurgitate the material into its mouth and then reswallow it or inhale it without ever having that material ejected from the mouth. If only small amounts of material are aspirated into the windpipe, cough will be the most obvious problem. This cough may be moist or dry. If larger amounts are inhaled and material reaches the lungs, pneumonia may occur, causing fever and labored breathing. Dogs can die from severe aspiration pneumonia. Sometimes nasal discharge occurs when regurgitated material is pushed from the pharynx into the back of the nose. If large amounts of material are aspirated and reach the lungs, the dog can develop sudden, severe pneumonia and they can even die from asphyxiation. Such a sudden death may occur any time, even if the dog has not been regurgitating for several weeks or months.

Megaesophagus is diagnosed by taking radiographs (x-rays) of the chest, often after feeding a contrast agent (material visible on an x-ray) such as barium. It is important to obtain these radiographs because there are other problems that cause clinical signs resembling those of megaesophagus but require very different therapy (in some cases surgery).

Because of the potentially devastating side effects of megaesophagus, it is wise to look for an underlying cause. Underlying causes are found only 15 to 25 per cent of the time; however, finding such a cause may allow the veterinarian to treat the cause of the megaesophagus (which tends to be more successful) instead of the signs (which often fails to prevent aspiration). If an underlying cause cannot be found (termed "idiopathic" megaesophagus), then symptomatic therapy is provided. This consists of trying to help food traverse the diseased esophagus and reach the stomach. If food does not remain in the esophagus, it cannot be regurgitated and aspirated. Although there is substantial dog-to-dog variation, one generally makes the dog stand on its hindlegs when it eats, so that it is as nearly vertical to the ground (and like a person) as possible. The dog should remain in this position for 5 to 10 minutes after eating. In doing this, we hope that gravity will help pull the food down into the stomach. Gruels are often fed in the hope that they will "slide" down the esophagus more easily than dry foods; however, some patients tolerate dry food or canned foods better than gruels. Feeding several small meals a day is usually preferred to feeding one or two large meals. Sometimes, drugs such as cisapride help diminish regurgitation.

Rarely, a tube can be placed through the skin and wall of the abdomen directly into the stomach (i.e., gastrostomy tube) so that the dog may be fed and watered without anything having go through the esophagus. This feeding technique does not eliminate all aspiration (the dog is still swallowing saliva), but it can help diminish aspiration. Gastrostomy tubes may allow dogs with idiopathic megaesophagus to live a nearly normal life, except for their manner of being fed and watered.

Non-Neoplastic Infiltrative Bowel Diseases ■ Albert E. Jergens

Non-neoplastic (noncancerous) infiltrative bowel diseases are a group of disorders that cause infiltration of the gastrointestinal tract with inflammatory cells. Broadly speaking, there are two major causes: inflammatory bowel disease and fungal or algal infections. The significance of these disorders is that they cause chronic debilitating disease, and they are reliably diagnosed only by gastrointestinal tract biopsy. The cause(s) and therapy of these disorders are widely divergent.

Inflammatory bowel disease is the most common cause of intractable vomiting and diarrhea in dogs and cats. Although the exact cause of inflammatory bowel disease is unknown, inflammatory cells probably infiltrate the gut in response to dietary or bacterial challenges. The inflammatory bowel disease disorders may strike anywhere in the gastrointestinal tract, but the small intestine and large intestine are primarily affected. Middle-aged pets are most often diagnosed with this disease. The most common symptoms include vomiting, diarrhea, loss of appetite, and weight loss, but symptoms may vary depending on the severity of inflammation and the extent of gut involvement. A diagnosis of inflammatory bowel disease is one of exclusion (everything else is ruled out, leaving only this diagnosis) and requires ruling out many other diseases that may cause intestinal inflammation.

Baseline diagnostic tests that may be recommended by your veterinarian include multiple fecal examinations, routine blood work (to test the kidneys, liver, etc.), urinalysis, radiographic imaging procedures, thyroid testing (in cats), and tests for feline viral diseases (e.g., feline leukemia virus, feline immunodeficiency virus). Surgical or endoscopic biopsy of the intestine is required to confirm the presence of inflammatory cells and to exclude other diseases that mimic inflammatory bowel disease. Therapy for inflammatory bowel disease includes the use of anti-inflammatory drugs to combat gut inflammation and use of a hypoallergenic diet to reduce the workload on the gut. Your pet is likely to require several weeks to months of drug and/or dietary therapy and to require a hypoallergenic diet indefinitely. Most animals with inflammatory bowel disease respond favorably to therapy; however, relapses should be expected.

Fungal or algal infections are caused by various organisms that are introduced into the gastrointestinal tract, inciting an inflammatory response to their presence. Histoplasmosis is the most frequently diagnosed fungal infection affecting the gastrointestinal tract of animals (primarily dogs). Infection with the fungus generally causes intractable diarrhea. Other symptoms may include loss of appetite, weight loss, fever, labored breathing, and enlargement of the lymph nodes. Diagnosis requires detecting the organisms (contained within inflammatory cells) in rectal scrapings or in surgical or endoscopic biopsy specimens of the intestines. Current blood tests for histoplasmosis are unreliable. Therapy usually consists of antifungal drugs given over several months. The prognosis varies with the extent of disease activity. Animals with severe symptoms or widespread disease generally fail to respond to therapy.

Pythiosis and protothecosis are rare fungal and algal infections that cause infiltrative gastrointestinal disease in animals. Both diseases are most common in dogs, and both preferentially affect the large intestine, causing diarrhea, weight loss, and generalized debilitation. Diagnosis is made only by demonstrating the organisms in affected gastrointestinal tract tissues. Surgical removal of all infected tissue, if possible, is the preferred treatment for pythiosis. There is presently no effective therapy for protothecosis.

APP

Pancreatitis ■ David A Williams

The pancreas is the organ in the abdomen that is responsible for producing the enzymes that digest food before its absorption and for producing the hormone insulin, which regulates blood glucose concentrations and prevents diabetes mellitus. Pancreatitis is inflammation of the pancreas and develops when the enzymes produced and stored within the pancreas become active and start to digest the pancreas itself. Many factors can trigger this abnormal self-digestion of the pancreas. In human beings pancreatitis is most commonly caused by gallstones and excessive alcohol consumption, factors that are not important in dogs and cats. Other causes of pancreatitis include various drugs and toxins, conditions such as shock and trauma that affect the supply of oxygen to the pancreas, genetic factors, dietary factors, excessive fat in the bloodstream, and tumors or parasites in the pancreatic duct system. In many cats and dogs with pancreatitis no evidence of any of these predisposing factors can be found, and the cause is unknown.

The clinical signs of pancreatitis are highly variable, probably reflecting the great variation in digestive enzyme activation that may be present in any individual dog or cat. Diagnosis of pancreatitis is usually suspected from the history and clinical signs (usually depression, poor or no appetite, and vomiting) and a suggestive pattern of abnormalities on routine blood testing. Confirmation of the diagnosis (and elimination of other diseases that cause similar clinical signs) may be difficult and usually requires special blood testing, radiographic and ultrasonographic examination of the abdomen, and sometimes direct examination and biopsy of the pancreas at surgery.

Once a diagnosis has been made, it is important to remember that pancreatitis is a highly unpredictable disease of widely varying severity, and it is difficult or impossible to give a prognosis. If the underlying cause is known and can be corrected (for example, exposure to a toxin, side effect of a drug, ingestion of a meal high in fat), supportive care and fluid therapy for a couple of days are usually followed by complete recovery. Overweight pets are more likely to have severe pancreatitis and to have a protracted recovery or even fatal complications.

Most dogs and cats with uncomplicated pancreatitis probably recover naturally after a single episode and do well as long as high-fat foods are avoided. Many dogs recover fully after an isolated episode of severe pancreatitis. Unfortunately, in some pets life-threatening signs accompanying severe acute fulminating pancreatitis lead to death in spite of aggressive supportive measures. In other cases, relatively mild or moderate chronic or recurrent pancreatitis persists despite all therapy, and the pet either dies in an acute severe exacerbation of the disease or undergoes euthanasia because of failure to recover and the expense of long-term supportive care.

Special care usually includes intravenous fluid therapy and provision of good nutritional support by tube feeding if vomiting is not too severe. If vomiting is severe, food may be withheld for a few days in an attempt to "rest" the pancreas. Because such starvation may not be tolerated well, long-term (particularly in cats) intravenous feeding or feeding through a tube placed in the intestine may be recommended.

Despite much research, there are no "magic" drugs to treat pancreatitis. We try to remove the cause if it is known. A goal is to keep your pet comfortable, well nourished, and well hydrated. It is important to be aggressive with supportive medical care and to do everything possible to prevent the pancreas from starting to digest itself. In many patients this approach is successful, but it is not possible to predict which animals will do well.

When dogs and cats recover from pancreatitis, no special treatment is required other than to avoid known risk factors, particularly fatty foods and obesity. In a few patients (especially miniature schnauzers) pancreatitis smolders, sometimes without obvious clinical signs, and the pancreas may gradually be destroyed. If the pancreatic cells producing digestive enzymes are destroyed, your pet may eventually require special enzymes to be added to meals in order to digest food and prevent weight loss and diarrhea. If the pancreatic cells producing insulin are destroyed, diabetes mellitus may develop and insulin therapy may be required. Fortunately, these complications of pancreatitis are uncommon.

Canine and Feline Cardiomyopathy ■ Stephen J. Ettinger

Cardiomyopathy is the name applied to an abnormality of heart muscle function. The heart's pumping ability is diminished, resulting in such signs as inability to exercise; fatigue; fainting; fluid collection in the lungs, abdomen, and limbs; or emboli (clots that arise in the heart and travel to the kidney, brain, or legs). Although some patients with cardiomyopathy do not develop clinical signs, others experience rapid progression of their disease or sudden death. The causes of cardiomyopathy include genetic predisposition, infections, toxic causes (drugs and chemical compounds), specific dietary insufficiencies, and unknown causes. Whereas some cases are entirely reversible, others are not and are treated with various levels of success.

Three major forms of cardiomyopathies occur in the canine and feline species. In *dilated cardiomyopathy*, the heart muscle is weak and flaccid (floppy). This condition is associated with a reduction in heart muscle function during contraction (systole) and a decrease in forward flow of blood. Subsequent upper heart chamber (left atrial) enlargement is associated with backup of blood and then fluid into the lungs (pulmonary edema).

Hypertrophic cardiomyopathy is a thickening of the lower heart muscle chambers (ventricles). The results are inappropriate heart function, obstruction of blood flow from the heart into the circulation, and enlargement of the upper heart chambers (atria). This abnormality is called diastolic dysfunction, a condition in which the heart fails to relax fully, fill, and then empty. The resulting backup of pressures into the lung is responsible for the clinical signs of respiratory distress, coughing, and systemic emboli (blood clots).

Unclassified or restrictive cardiomyopathies are unidentified disease conditions in which heart problems are associated with severely enlarged upper chambers and diminished pumping ability. The clinical signs resemble those of hypertrophic cardiomyopathy. Although not thickened, the ventricular muscle is dysfunctional and the heart is unable to fill and then pump adequately.

Cardiomyopathies are seen in both dogs and cats. The form in dogs is usually dilated, whereas hypertrophic and unclassified forms are identified most often in cats. The diagnosis of cardiomyopathy is based on a history of weakness, coughing, panting, fainting, or fluid collection around the lungs and in the abdominal cavity. Weight loss occurs, and seizures associated with fainting may occur. Emboli (clots) can result in blood vessel blockage, sudden lameness, and cold painful limbs. Clinical signs usually develop suddenly, often without apparent prior illness. In addition to these signs, the diagnosis depends on abnormalities found at the physical examination. Irregularities occur in the heart's rhythm and rate, and abnormal heart sounds (murmurs) are heard with the stethoscope. Radiographs (x-rays) of the chest show heart enlargement. Evaluation of the blood may identify complicating organ problems. The electrocardiogram can diagnose an irregular heart rhythm and substantiate heart enlargement. Ultrasound examination of the heart confirms the suspicion of cardiomyopathy. Dilatation of the heart cavity, poor contractility of the heart muscle, and left atrial enlargement occur with dilated cardiomyopathy. Thickening of the heart muscle, obstruction of the flow of blood into the circulation, and left atrial enlargement identify hypertrophic cardiomyopathy. Normal muscle thickness with disturbed function and enlarged left atria indicates restrictive cardiomyopathy.

Treatment varies with the type of cardiomyopathy. Dilated cardiomyopathies, indicative of a loss of contractile heart strength, require medications to improve strength (digitalis), to remove excess fluid accumulation (diuretics), and to counteract abnormal hormone levels that contribute to heart failure (angiotensin-converting enzyme inhibitors). A low-salt diet is important to reduce sodium levels and subsequent water retention. Nutrients such as taurine and carnitine may be required to counteract specific deficiencies. Manual removal of excess fluid accumulation is sometimes necessary.

Treatment of hypertrophic and unclassified cardiomyopathies requires drugs to allow the ventricular muscle to relax. This improves heart filling and blood flow to the body. Beta-adrenergic blocking agents or calcium channel blocking agents are often used for this purpose. Removal of excess fluids from the body (diuretics) and sometimes manual removal of fluid from the chest space are necessary to improve comfort. Low-salt diets to counteract salt and water retention are indicated but may be difficult to achieve with a finicky and ill cat. Aspirin is used to reduce the likelihood of blood clot formation within the heart. Antiarrhythmic agents to control irregularities of the heart's rate and rhythm are called upon at times, as are nutritional supplements (taurine and/or carnitine) in known deficiencies.

The prognosis for survival with cardiomyopathies varies from poor to good. Once cardiomyopathy has been recognized, much of the damage to the heart muscle has already occurred. The result is congestive heart failure, the signs and symptoms of which may be treated for a variable period of time (often 3 to 12 months, which is equivalent to 3 to 5 years in a human). Although the pet may enjoy a period of good health and comfort, the long-term prognosis continues to indicate that heart failure will recur. As a result, the pet will become less responsive to medical intervention. Surgery is not yet an option for any form of cardiomyopathy.

APP

Collapsing Trachea ■ Stephen J. Ettinger

Collapsing trachea occurs most often in middle-aged to older dogs. The diagnosis is suggested by a honking cough precipitated by activity, excitement, or water drinking. Nonproductive coughing may occur without a stimulus. Signs vary and include mild to severe panting, respiratory distress, and bluish discoloration of the mucous membranes (cyanosis). Abdominal breathing efforts result in tense abdominal muscles.

Dogs are frequently overweight but may be thin. A heart murmur associated with valvular heart disease is often encountered because both problems occur in aging dogs.

Collapsing trachea results when the windpipe (tracheal) cartilages soften. The trachea (windpipe) should resemble a relatively firm garden hose. Viewed on end, the windpipe is a U-shaped structure with a tight membrane covering the top. Where cartilage softens, it collapses and widens at the top. The membrane then drapes (collapses) loosely, blocking the inside of the "hose." This results in an inability to bring air into or out of the trachea and lungs during breathing.

Complications of this disease include lung problems, heart disease and/or failure, enlarged liver, and chronic kidney insufficiency. Dental infections, other infections, and obesity aggravate the disease.

The diagnosis of collapsing trachea, initially historical, is substantiated when a veterinarian can cause your pet to cough by digital manipulation of the neck. Radiographs (x-rays) identify changes in the trachea during both inspiration and expiration.

The diagnostic evaluation includes laboratory sampling of the blood to identify causal or complicating medical problems, motion studies of the trachea and lung during respiration, endoscopic examination of the windpipe and throat, and evaluation of abdominal organ enlargement.

There are four components of treating collapsing trachea. During the acute phase, respiratory distress and severe bouts of coughing are ameliorated with drugs that relax the trachea and lung and sedate the pet. Fluid congestion is relieved with diuretic drugs, and short-term anti-inflammatory agents minimize swelling and tissue irritation. Antibiotics are utilized if there is an infection. Cough suppressants temporarily relieve discomfort. Cough suppressants (narcotic derivatives) may be used in a lifelong schedule for some pets with collapsing trachea.

Later, drugs that relieve bronchial constriction and spasm are utilized along with products to reduce anxiety and overstimulation. Anticough medications are used orally as necessary. Corticosteroid anti-inflammatory drugs may be helpful during episodes of acute exacerbation of the coughing.

Problems requiring simultaneous medical care that compromise the tracheal syndrome include recurrent pulmonary or pharyngeal infections, dental disease, and swelling of lymph tissue in the pharynx and tracheal region. Weight control is important.

Evaluation of thyroid function may be indicated. Liver enlargement, secondary to fatty infiltration or other disease, adversely affects the outcome of this disease. Many smaller dogs are simultaneously affected with heart disease. Your veterinarian understands how these conditions interact. Diagnosing and treating both may significantly improve the long-term prognosis.

Surgical correction of a collapsing trachea may be considered in young dogs when the trachea is collapsed in the neck region. Older dogs, those with complicating medical problems, and those with most of the trachea affected are not candidates for surgery.

The prognosis remains good for many pets with early-developing collapsing trachea, but the condition can be a serious, life-threatening problem when severe respiratory distress occurs. Bouts of severe coughing and respiratory distress negatively affect a good prognosis. The client should be made aware of the frustrating nature of therapy for these pets. Unless properly informed that coughing is likely to continue to occur to some degree, on and off, the client may become frustrated and seek additional care.

Congenital Heart Disease ■ Stephen J. Ettinger

Your pet was born with a congenital heart defect. Congenital defects are abnormalities that occur in the developing fetus and are usually recognized soon after birth. If the defect is too severe, the embryo dies before birth. Other situations, not as severe, allow embryo development to birth, and the pet can live until the defect interferes with normal functioning (here, the cardiovascular system). Most congenital defects are first recognized at or near the time of weaning when the pet is taken to the veterinarian for a first examination. Sometimes these problems may not be identified until later in life. Congenital defects are most often the result of abnormalities in the genetic makeup of the pet. The abnormal genes may or may not be present in other members of the litter but are carried by the mother and/or father, sometimes without compromising their health. Other causes of congenital defects include exposure to radiation, toxins, or physical events that occurred during the animal's embryonic stage.

There are numerous ways to classify congenital heart defects, but for simplicity we will consider them in four major categories: (1) obstruction of blood flow within the heart; (2) abnormal communication between the two sides of the heart, increasing the blood flow from the left (systemic) to the right (lung) side of the heart; (3) abnormal communications sending blood in the opposite direction of flow, from the right (lung) to the left (systemic) side of the heart; and (4) vessel (vascular) abnormalities that obstruct a body part and interfere with normal function.

Obstruction of blood flow within the heart includes conditions such as pulmonic, mitral, or aortic valvular stenosis. Valvular obstruction is caused by a narrowing of an area of blood flow, decreasing circulation from the heart to some part of the body. These conditions vary from mild to severe. They may be minimal and require no care. However, in other cases, medication only, opening the obstruction with a special catheter, or surgical correction may be needed. Surgery, although commonly performed in humans, is both difficult and infrequent in veterinary medicine.

Blood may flow abnormally from the left to the right side of the heart because of a hole between the two sides of the heart that did not close during embryonic formation. One such condition, patent ductus arteriosus (PDA), is a remnant of normal embryonic heart function. If PDA is diagnosed early, it may be corrected surgically and the pet may be able to lead a normal life. Other conditions such as ventricular or atrial septal defects involve a hole between two chambers of the heart. Closure of septal defects requires open heart cardiopulmonary bypass surgery, which is infrequently performed in veterinary medicine.

Blood flow from the right to the left side of the heart without passing through the lungs is very abnormal and quite uncommon. Thus, a serious communication problem exists that results in unoxygenated blood being transported to the body. Such a situation usually does not allow the pet to live beyond early adulthood. Because of the complicated nature of these problems, open heart surgery is rarely an available option. Surgical procedures may be available at teaching and specialty clinics to treat such problems.

Persistent aortic arch, peripheral arteriovenous shunts, and cor triatriatum are heart problems that are the result of abnormal vessels interfering with normal blood flow. These conditions can usually be corrected surgically if identified early, before complicating problems develop to preclude normal life.

Because many congenital heart defects are thought to be due to genetic problems that can be passed from one generation to the next, veterinarians recommend that animals with such conditions be neutered at an early age to prevent breeding and the dissemination of defective genes to a new generation. Some congenital heart defects may be surgically corrected; others are effectively dealt with for variable periods using medication. Regrettably, most congenital heart defects have a poor long-term prognosis. It is sad for the owner and for the pet to suffer needlessly. In selected circumstances, euthanasia may be recommended if the pet is unable to maintain a good quality of life.

A number of more complicated congenital heart defects are not covered in this handout. If such a situation exists in your pet, your veterinarian will be able to discuss it with you and will probably refer you to a specialist with additional training and diagnostic equipment.

A congenital heart defect is suspected after a thorough physical examination has been performed. The electrocardiogram helps to identify the presence of abnormal heart chamber size as well as irregularities of the heart's rate and/or rhythm. Radiographs (x-rays) are needed to visualize abnormalities in the size and appearance of the heart, vessel, and lung structures. The ultrasound (echocardiogram) examination is a direct, noninvasive means of looking inside the heart's walls to measure the size of the heart's four chambers and to identify abnormalities (qualitatively and quantitatively) in blood flow. Occasionally, more invasive procedures such as cardiac catheterization (passing small tubes into the heart and blood vessels and injecting dye) or surgical evaluation may be recommended.

APP

Canine Valvular Insufficiency and Congestive Heart Failure ■ Stephen J. Ettinger

Valvular insufficiency occurs when damaged and thickened valves develop within the heart of small and midsize dogs. Value problems are unusual in larger breed dogs and in cats but they may develop. In the small breeds of dogs, valvular insufficiency begins in midlife and progresses slowly. The disease is associated with thickening and shortening of the valve components that separate the upper (atria) from the lower (ventricles) parts of the heart. Remember, normally blood flows in only one direction. If the valves fail to close completely when the heart contracts, blood moves forward but some leaks backward. Clinical signs vary depending on whether the right and/or left side of the heart is affected and whether heart enlargement presses on the windpipe. Fluid accumulates when the heart fails to pump enough blood to the body and instead the blood is transmitted backward from the heart to the lung or body.

Owners of pets with valve problems see inappropriate panting, heavy breathing, diminished exercise ability, fatigue, cough, and occasionally fainting. The cough usually starts at night and progresses to daytime as well, particularly when associated with exercise. Retching and nonproductive gagging follow the cough. When the right side of heart is affected, fluid may accumulate around the lungs, making it difficult to breathe, and in the abdomen, making it swell.

Abnormal heart sounds heard with a stethoscope suggest the need for an electrocardiogram (ECG) to identify heart enlargement or irregularities of the heart's rhythm. Radiographs (x-rays) can demonstrate heart enlargement and/or inappropriate fluid accumulation. Blood testing can identify hormonal, kidney, or other internal medical problem. An ultrasound examination (echocardiography) accurately pictures enlarged heart chambers, abnormalities of valve structure, and the heart's pumping ability. These tests assess heart function and severity of the disease and identify the need for therapy.

A number of treatments are used for pets with valvular heart disease, including exercise restriction. Walking is good exercise. Digitalis is a medication used to strengthen the heart and to treat some irregularities of its rhythm. It maintains a slower and more effective heart muscle contraction. Signs of digitalis excess include loss of appetite, lethargy, vomiting, and diarrhea. ECG monitoring permits the veterinarian to supervise the pet's progress. Diuretic agents are commonly given to remove excess water accumulation from the body and can cause increased water drinking and urination. Diuretics can induce weakness, dehydration, and blood salt abnormalities. Alterations in electrolyte (salt) levels are identified through periodic testing of the pet's blood. Angiotensin-converting enzyme inhibitors (ACEIs) are drugs that improve the body's ability to reduce salt and water retention, to reduce high blood pressure, and to limit the effect of hormones that adversely affect heart muscle. Given in excess, ACEI drugs cause malaise, blood salt disturbances, loss of appetite, and possibly kidney damage. Antiarrhythmic agents may be given to stabilize the cardiac rate and rhythm. Drugs to decrease blood pressure and nutritional supplements may be required for specific conditions.

In order to control the symptoms of heart failure, low-salt (sodium) diets may be suggested. Excess sodium is normally removed by the kidney, but this does not occur as effectively in heart failure. Commercial low-salt diets, varying from moderate to extreme restriction, are effective in preventing salt and water retention. These diets are recommended only after heart failure has been diagnosed. A modest reduction in salt intake may be indicated before the onset of heart failure. If the pet refuses to eat a commercial diet, low-salt foods can be prepared by the owner under veterinary direction. It is important to emphasize that mixing low-salt diets with regular (high-salt) diets or feeding snacks high in sodium is not recommended.

Longevity and quality of life in dogs with this disease vary with the severity of the valve damage and the amount of blood leakage into the upper chambers of the heart. Concurrent medical conditions, age, and the physical status of the pet play a large role in determining the animal's prognosis. Clinical signs are progressive, and although they may be decreased, they never entirely resolve. Medical therapy can enhance the quality of life of the pet as well as increase life expectancy. Dogs with left-sided valvular heart disease treated with medication and a low-salt diet have an average life expectancy of about 9 months from the time heart failure begins. Abdominal fluid accumulation and body emaciation are signs of right-sided heart failure. Regularly removing the extra fluid may increase life expectancy. Surgical replacement of the valves is not an option in dogs at this time.

Canine Heartworm Disease ■ Clarke Atkins

Heartworm disease (HWD) refers to the condition caused by the parasite *Dirofilaria immitis*, carried by mosquitoes and affecting dogs, cats, and ferrets. In the United States, it is a major problem in the Southeast, East, and the Mississippi River valley.

PARASITE AND LIFE CYCLE

The adult worm is large, up to 12 inches long, and lives predominantly in the pulmonary arteries (PAs, the large vessels that carry blood to the lungs from the heart). When an infection consists of both male and female mature worms, reproduction occurs with resultant microscopic circulating baby forms called microfilariae (L1). These are an important part of the life cycle because they allow infection of other animals to occur and, when found upon microscopic examination of the blood, allow the diagnosis of HWD. For transmission of heartworms (HWs) to occur, a mosquito sucks blood containing L1 from infected dogs. The L1 develops in the mosquito, becoming infective in about 2 weeks. The mosquito then transmits the infective larvae to another dog. Further development occurs with migration to the heart and PAs 3 to 4 months later. Adult HWs are thought to live for 5 to 7 years.

CLINICAL SIGNS

From 1 to over 200 HWs may reside in the heart and PAs. The PAs become thickened and inflamed, increasing the work of the heart as it pushes blood past the worms into the lungs. In addition, the lungs themselves become inflamed. Mild infestations may produce no signs. The earliest clinical signs are typically exercise intolerance, cough, and weight loss. More severe signs may include severe cough, labored breathing, and heart failure (usually manifested as abdominal swelling). Once HWD has reached this stage, the dog may die.

DIAGNOSIS

The diagnosis can be made by finding L1 in blood. An enzyme-linked immunosorbent assay (ELISA, a test that identifies proteins [antigens] produced by adult female HWs) readily detects infections with two or more adult females. A diagnosis may also be suspected on the basis of radiographs (x-rays).

TREATMENT

ADULTICIDAL THERAPY

After tests to ensure that a dog is healthy enough, arsenical drugs are used to kill adult HWs. A newer, more expensive agent (melarsomine) is safer than arsenamide (Caparsolate), allowing gradual destruction of HWs so that the lungs can gradually "clean up" the infection. Both drugs can cause irritation at the site of injection and could damage the liver and kidneys. By far the greatest concern is dead HWs, producing a severe reaction in the lungs 1 to 3 weeks after administration. This can be prevented or minimized with melarsomine given in three doses (one initially and two

separated by 24 hours in 1 month) and by severely restricting exercise for at least 1 month after adulticidal therapy. *Exercise restriction is imperative after adulticidal therapy!*

Therapy with steroids may be needed to reduce lung inflammation and resultant cough but is typically discontinued before adulticidal therapy. Aspirin may be used to reduce the vascular damage caused by HWs but is controversial.

MICROFILARICIDAL (L1) THERAPY

After killing the adult worms, the L1 forms should be killed, thereby lessening the risk to other pets. A dosage of ivermectin, milbemycin, or moxidectin can be given approximately 6 weeks after the adults have been killed. Although often effective, this treatment may produce severe reactions. An alternative is to use ivermectin at lower doses, thereby gradually eliminating L1 over about 6 months. This may be done before or after the adulticide and adverse reactions are rare. Ideally, the pet is closely observed the day of the first dose with either method.

PREVENTION

Heartworm infection is clearly better prevented than treated. Prevention is instituted at 6 to 8 weeks of age or as soon thereafter as climatic conditions dictate. Prevention of HWD can be accomplished by daily administration of diethylcarbamazine (DEC) or monthly administration of ivermectin, milbemycin, or moxidectin. Although each of these drugs is effective when given as directed, even brief lapses in DEC therapy may result in infection. The monthly drugs, however, provide protection despite lapses of up to a month. Both DEC and monthly drugs are extraordinarily safe if administered before infection but may produce severe, even fatal, reactions if administered to dogs with L1. Such reactions are more severe with DEC. Heartworm testing should be performed in *all* dogs older than 6 months of age (if there has been seasonal potential for exposure) before institution of preventative.

SEASONAL AND GEOGRAPHIC CONSIDERATIONS

There are areas in the United States in which no HW preventative is necessary. In the deep South and California, preventative is typically administered all year. In the North, the season is shorter; DEC is used from the first mosquito sighting until 2 months after the first hard frost, and the monthly drugs should be administered from the onset of mosquito season until 1 month after the first hard frost. Your veterinarian knows the appropriate preventative schedule for your region.

YEARLY TESTING

Yearly testing is required for dogs receiving DEC because of the potential for adverse reactions in dogs that become infected and are restarted with preventative. The need for yearly testing with monthly treatment is less certain. Many veterinarians still advocate yearly testing because pets may not receive or may not swallow the necessary preventatives. If it is certain that the medication is administered and swallowed for the entire HW season, then testing every 2 years is an option.

APP

Feline Bronchitis ("Feline Asthma") ■ Carol Norris

Feline bronchitis, commonly called feline asthma, is a disease in cats affecting the smaller airways that branch off the windpipe (trachea). These branches, called bronchi, allow the transport of air into and out of the lungs. When the bronchi become obstructed because of constriction or contraction of the muscles in the walls of these airways, the inflammation or irritation of the airways, or excessive secretions that plug the insides of the airways, the end result is an impaired ability to bring oxygen into the lungs for delivery to the rest of the body. Although the term "asthma" is commonly used to describe this syndrome in cats, this term is somewhat misleading. Asthma, in people, specifically refers to the reversible constriction of muscles in the walls of the bronchi. Some cats have true asthma, whereas others have bronchitis. Bronchitis is associated with inflammation and swelling of the walls of the bronchi that cause a narrowed passageway and airway obstruction by plugs of mucus or other secretions, which also narrows these tubes. Bronchitis can be acute (short duration) and associated with reversible changes in the structure of the airways or chronic (long duration, usually more than 2 to 3 months) and associated with permanent, irreversible changes in the airways. Bronchitis and asthma can occur at the same time and can be caused by bacterial infections, parasites, allergies, or inhaled irritants; in many cases, the underlying cause cannot be found.

The most common signs of bronchitis in cats include constant, cyclic, or seasonal coughing; difficulty breathing; and/or wheezing. Episodes of coughing can mimic vomiting; some owners think their cats are vomiting up hairballs when they are truly having a coughing fit followed by retching. Breathing may be rapid or require excessive effort; some severely affected cats may breathe with their mouths open. If you cat ever displays any of these symptoms, it should be promptly taken to your veterinarian for further evaluation, as these signs are a warning of potentially serious disease. These signs are not specific for bronchitis and can also be seen with many other diseases including heart failure, pneumonia, and lung cancer.

In the diagnosis of feline bronchitis by your veterinarian, the first test is usually to take a radiograph (x-ray) of the chest. Second, your veterinarian may recommend obtaining a sample of cells from the trachea and bronchi to examine under a microscope and to culture for any infectious organisms. It is also common to check the blood and feces for parasites (heartworm and lung worm, respectively).

There are several principles to follow in the treatment of feline bronchitis. First, any underlying disease (for example, bacterial or parasitic infection) must be appropriately diagnosed and treated. Second, changes must be made in the cat's environment, since cats with bronchitis often have sensitive, hyperactive airways, and inhalation of irritating particles from the environment can cause worsening of their disease. Consequently, it is strongly recommended that their exposure to smoke (cigarette or fireplace), dusts (cat litter, carpet fresheners, flea powder), and sprays (insecticides, hair spray, perfumes, and cleaning products) be eliminated or minimized. Third, weight reduction in obese cats should be attempted under the supervision of a veterinarian. Finally, medication should be given to treat the airway obstruction directly. Two classes of drugs are commonly prescribed: bronchodilators (examples include theophylline, aminophylline, and terbutaline) and steroids (examples include prednisone, dexamethasone, and methlyprednisone). Bronchodilators help to dilate or open the airways by relaxing the muscular walls. Common side effects of bronchodilators in cats can include gastrointestinal upset, restlessness, and lethargy. Steroids decreases the inflammation and swelling of the airway walls. Side effects in cats are uncommon but may include behavioral changes.

It is important that your cat have regular rechecks with your veterinarian, as the doses of the medications commonly need to be adjusted. Prognosis is variable for this disease. If the underlying cause can be identified and successfully treated or eliminated, the prognosis is excellent. If permanent damage to the airways has occurred, the disease cannot be cured. With proper medical management, clinical signs can be controlled and the damage to the bronchi can be stopped or slowed. Some cats suffering severe asthma attacks can die despite intensive medical efforts.

Pneumonia ■ Alfred M. Legendre

Pneumonia is an inflammation of the lungs. It is rare in cats and less common in dogs than in people. There are many types of pneumonia, with bacterial and fungal infections being the most common. The dog's lungs are not very susceptible to primary bacterial pneumonia, but prior lung damage predisposes them to secondary invasion by bacteria. The canine distemper virus causes severe damage to the cells lining the respiratory tract of dogs, making the lungs more susceptible to bacterial infection and pneumonia.

A common type of pneumonia is aspiration pneumonia, which occurs when dogs vomit and inhale that material into their lungs. Aspiration may occur when animals vomit after surgery because anesthetic drugs depress the swallowing reflexes. Aspiration pneumonia may be caused by a condition called megaesophagus. In megaesophagus, there is abnormal movement of the esophagus (the tube that connects the mouth with the stomach), allowing food to accumulate instead of moving into the stomach. This pool of food and saliva is constantly regurgitated into the mouth and some of the material goes down the trachea into the lungs. Some diseases of the nerves that control swallowing can also allow entry of food into the lungs. The inhaled food contains bacteria and sometimes stomach acid that cause inflammation.

Dogs with pneumonia are usually brought to the veterinarian because of coughing, loss of appetite, depression, and difficulty breathing. They often have a fever. Lung sounds heard with a stethoscope are increased because of the abnormal pus and fluid in the airways. The effort required to breathe gives an indication of the severity of the lung infection.

Identification of the cause of the pneumonia is necessary for optimal treatment. Chest radiographs (x-rays) are required for accurate diagnosis of pneumonia. Fungal pneumonias have a typical pattern of inflammation that helps differentiate them from bacterial pneumonia. In megaesophagus, there is an enlarged esophagus and the lung inflammation occurs in the lower part of the lungs. Diagnosis of bacterial pneumonia secondary to distemper is difficult. Additional tests for distemper should be done in dogs whose vaccinations are not current. Bacterial pneumonia can also be secondary to tumors and foreign bodies, such as pieces of grass.

A complete blood count is helpful in assessing the severity of the lung inflammation and identifying secondary diseases. Obtaining pus and fluid from the airways is important in identifying the organism causing the problem. The type of bacteria and its antibiotic sensitivity determine the antibiotic needed. People can cough up a sputum sample for testing, but dogs are not as cooperative. A procedure known as a percutaneous (going through the skin) tracheal washing is an effective and relatively safe way to obtain material from the trachea and bronchi. A local anesthetic in the skin allows painless passage of a small tube through the skin of the neck into the trachea or windpipe. Fluid is injected through the tube to dilute the thick material in the airways, which can be sucked into a syringe. During the 2 to 3 days required for the bacterial test to be completed, an antibiotic likely to be effective may be started. This antibiotic may need to be changed when the culture results are obtained.

Antibiotics or antifungal drugs are the mainstay of bacterial and fungal pneumonia treatment, respectively. Dogs with severe respiratory difficulties may require oxygen treatment to improve their breathing. Nebulization of a fine water mist can help keep the airway moist, loosen thick mucus, and help the lungs remove debris through coughing.

The outcome of pneumonia in dogs depends on the cause of the pneumonia and the severity of the infection. There must be enough lung capacity to maintain an adequate oxygen supply to the body for at least 2 to 3 days until the antibiotics can begin to work. Primary pneumonias without underlying disease are usually treated successfully. The prognosis for aspiration pneumonia depends on the ability to correct the cause of the vomiting and on the severity of the pneumonia. Pneumonias secondary to distemper or similar viral diseases have a guarded prognosis. At least half of dogs with distemper develop seizures because of the effects of the virus on the brain.

APP

Feline Immunodeficiency Virus ■ Alfred M. Legendre

Feline immunodeficiency virus (FIV) was first identified in an immunosuppressed cat in 1986. FIV is a lentivirus (slow virus), so named because of the slow development of disease. FIV is of the same family of viruses as human immunodeficiency virus (HIV), which causes acquired immunodeficiency syndrome (AIDS) in people. It is important to remember that FIV is infectious only to cats.

Immunodeficiency related to FIV infection occurs most often in free-roaming, male cats older than 6 years. Transmission of FIV is usually through cat bites incurred when fighting. Defense of territory explains the higher incidence of disease in male cats. FIV is occasionally transmitted to kittens by their mothers.

Random testing of cats seen by veterinarians shows a healthy cat prevalence of 1 to 2 per cent in the United States and up to 12 per cent in Japan, where most cats are kept outside and are not neutered. Twelve to 40 per cent of sick cats are infected with FIV. Once cats develop FIV infection, they are infected for life. Studies of frozen serum samples from 20 years ago show that the prevalence of FIV infection has not changed.

Cats with FIV, like people with HIV, have an acute phase of illness that begins 4 to 6 weeks after a bite from an infected cat. Most cats develop fever, depression, and enlarged lymph nodes that last from weeks to months. These symptoms are usually mild enough that owners rarely notice. Kittens infected as newborns may die in the acute phase. After recovery from the acute phase, these cats may appear completely normal for 3 years or more. During this asymptomatic period, the FIV virus is gradually destroying the immune system, limiting the ability to fight infection.

When the immune dysfunction is relatively mild, cats have bacterial and viral infections commonly seen in cats, such as mouth infections, abscesses, chronic nasal and eye discharges, skin infections, ear infections, and diarrhea. FIV-infected cats have ringworm at three times the expected rate. These infections respond to the usual treatment, but not as well as expected, and often recur after treatment is completed.

FIV can also affect the bone marrow, causing anemia. Parasitic diseases such as toxoplasmosis that normally cause only mild signs become life threatening. The FIV has an affinity for brain tissue and can produce personality changes. Shy cats may become aggressive and outgoing cats may hide. Malignancy of lymph node cells (lymphosarcoma) may develop. Cats infected with FIV are also more likely to develop kidney failure.

When immune depression is severe, cats may develop opportunistic infections (infections that do not usually occur in that species) such as demodectic mange seen in dogs. During the later stages, standard treatments are not effective because they require the help of the immune system to resolve infections. Nevertheless, immunosuppressed cats may live a year or longer if treated.

When FIV is suspected, a blood test can be done. A negative test usually excludes a diagnosis of FIV, but an early infection (first 2 months) could be missed. A positive test with appropriate signs is quite reliable, but an occasional false-positive test can occur. A Western blot test (a more specific and definitive test) of blood confirms the diagnosis.

A positive test for FIV is not a reason for euthanasia. A study of newly diagnosed FIV-infected cats showed that 7 of 11 cats were still alive 2 years later. We rarely know when cats become infected. A cat with early infection may have 3 or 4 more years of disease-free life. FIV-positive cats should be kept indoors for the safety of other cats and to limit their exposure to disease.

The response to treatment of FIV-infected cats depends on the degree of immune suppression. There are no good antiviral drugs for the cat. Azidothymidine (AZT), a drug used in people to inhibit virus reproduction, works against the FIV virus but has significant toxicity in the cat. There are other promising drugs but they are not yet available. Most of the illness in FIV-infected cats results from secondary bacterial infections that can be controlled with antibiotics. Antibiotics can prolong the cat's life in spite of a poorly functioning immune system.

Prevention with vaccination would be helpful but, as in people, an effective vaccine has not yet been developed.

Feline Leukemia Virus Vaccinations in Cats ■ Alfred M. Legendre

Feline leukemia virus (FeLV) is a communicable agent in cats that is usually transmitted through virus-infected saliva via cat fight wounds, mutual grooming, or sharing food and water dishes. The most hazardous situation for FeLV transmission is a multicat household in which a large number of cats are crowded into a limited space. The virus causes a fatal infection through development of malignancy or depression of immunity (inability to fight infection) with the development of secondary diseases. The virus lives only a few days in the environment and is easily killed by common detergents and disinfectants. Thus, most of the risk of transmission is due to direct contact between cats.

Most cats with FeLV infection die within 2 or 3 years of the time of infection. The most common problem is depression of the immune system, which makes the cat susceptible to a variety of secondary infections. Cats may have persistent and recurring abscesses, chronic mouth infections, chronic respiratory diseases, diarrhea, and poor appetite. The virus can also suppress the cells of the bone marrow that produce red and white blood cells. Red blood cell suppression produces severe anemia. Suppression of the white blood cells needed for prevention of bacterial invasion allows the development of uncontrollable infections.

Development of malignancies is also a major concern in FeLV-infected cats. FeLV was originally identified in 1964 in Scotland in catteries where there was an epidemic of malignancies. It was later found that months to years after infection, many cats develop malignancies of the cells of the lymph nodes and the bone marrow. When these malignant cells are found in the blood, the malignancy is called a leukemia. These malignancies can also be found in many organs including the bone marrow, chest, kidneys, liver, and intestinal tract (called lymphoma). There is no treatment to eliminate FeLV; only supportive care and treatment of the secondary bacterial infections with antibiotics are possible. Some of the malignancies induced by FeLV can be controlled with chemotherapeutic drugs for a few months to a year or longer.

Fortunately, there are vaccines that are quite effective in preventing FeLV infection. Young cats are more susceptible to infection than adult cats and should be vaccinated before they come in contact with possible FeLV carrier cats. The current recommendation is an initial vaccine after 9 weeks of age and a second booster dose 3 weeks to a month later. Yearly booster vaccines are recommended for cats at risk.

Only killed virus vaccines are available for vaccinating cats against FeLV because of concerns that a modified live virus in a vaccine could undergo a mutation into a potentially dangerous virus. Killed virus vaccines of any type can cause the development of a tumor called a fibrosarcoma. This is an aggressive malignancy of fibrous tissue that develops in response to inflammation at the site of vaccination. The rate of development of malignancies at vaccine injection sites is estimated to be 1 in 5000 doses of vaccine given. In cats that are exposed to FeLV, outside cats, and cats that come in contact with cats that go outside, the infection rate for FeLV is 2 per 100. In these cats, the benefits of vaccination far outweigh the possible problems of vaccine-induced tumors. In cats very unlikely to be exposed, the risk/benefit ratio of vaccination is less evident. Cats that are kept strictly indoors are not at risk for infection if other cats in the same household are not infected with FeLV and all cats in the household are kept indoors.

There are a number of in-office blood tests that your veterinarian can perform to identify FeLV-infected cats. Cats in multiple-cat households should be checked to be sure they are not carriers of FeLV. All new cats introduced into the household must be quarantined for 3 months and checked twice for FeLV infection before being admitted into the household. Checking cats in the household and preventing the entry of infected cats are effective in developing an FeLV-free environment where vaccination is not necessary.

FeLV infection is a lethal infection of cats that can be readily prevented. All cats at risk should be vaccinated regularly.

APP

Parvovirus in Dogs ■ Alfred M. Legendre

Parvovirus infection, commonly called "parvo," is a disease of dogs that affects the intestinal tract and causes vomiting, diarrhea, fever, and decreased ability to fight infection. It is especially severe in puppies. Doberman pinschers and rottweilers are more susceptible and have more severe signs of parvo than other breeds, but puppies of any breed or mixed breed puppies can die from this disease.

Parvo is a relatively new disease entity in dogs that was first identified in the late 1970s. The virus did not exist before that time. It is believed that this is a disease caused by a virus of the cat or other species that adapted itself to dogs. When the virus first emerged, dogs of all ages became infected. Now that the disease is in its second decade, usually only young dogs are infected. This is because the virus is so contagious and so commonly found in the environment that most older dogs have become immune through vaccination or infection early in life.

Oral intake of virus-infected materials transmits the infection to susceptible dogs. Parvovirus multiplies in the intestinal tract of infected dogs, and a billion virus particles per teaspoon of stool can be passed during an infection. The virus is sturdy and persists in the environment for at least 6 months. It is impossible to eliminate the virus from contaminated soil without killing all vegetation. For inside facilities, thorough washing and rinsing followed by careful application of a chlorine bleach solution containing 1 ounce of bleach per quart of water is needed. Avoid skin and eye contact with the bleach solution.

Infection of puppies usually results from exposure to contaminated soil, and signs of disease are seen from 4 to 14 days after exposure. The initial signs are depression, loss of appetite, and fever. Vomiting and blood-streaked diarrhea develop within 1 or 2 days. These signs progress quickly to dehydration and death in severely affected dogs. Puppies 6 to 8 weeks of age have a higher death rate than older dogs. The age of onset of infection depends on exposure to the virus as well as the pups' level of antibodies against parvovirus. Bitches that are immune by vaccination or previous exposure to the virus pass some of their antibodies to their puppies in milk. Depending on the amount of antibodies passed to the puppies, the antibodies protect them for a few weeks to as long as 3 months. The puppies' bodies gradually degrade or break down the antibodies and the puppies must then produce their own immunity to be protected.

The initial damage to the body in parvo occurs because the virus destroys the cells in which it reproduces. Unfortunately, there is no antivirus treatment at this time. Treatment of dogs infected with parvo depends on the severity of the infection. Dogs with mild infections can recover with nursing care, but those with severe infection become severely dehydrated. These dogs require intravenous fluid to maintain their hydration because they are unable to take in fluids and are losing large amounts of fluid in the vomiting and diarrhea. In addition to the fluid loss, the virus destroys the lining cells of the intestinal tract, which allows bacteria from the intestine to enter the body. When this bacterial invasion occurs (septicemia), antibiotics must be given to kill the bacteria in the bloodstream. In addition to allowing bacterial entry into the bloodstream, the parvovirus damages the bone marrow, where white blood cells are produced. Neutrophils, a specific type of white blood cell necessary for destroying invading bacteria, are severely reduced in numbers. Immune dysfunction causes some dogs with parvo to die in spite of extensive treatment with fluid and antibiotics.

The best approach to parvo is prevention of disease with vaccination. Puppies should be started on vaccines at 6 weeks of age and exposure to infected environments should be minimized until the vaccination series is complete. Puppies should be vaccinated every 2 to 3 weeks until 16 weeks of age. The long course of vaccination is necessary because of the maternal antibodies passed from the mother to the pups. Although these antibodies protect against infection, they also interfere with an effective response to vaccination. Low levels of maternal antibodies interfere with vaccination but may not protect puppies from infection. Advances in parvovirus vaccines have resulted in improved vaccines that provide effective protection despite some maternal antibodies. It is advised that the exposure of puppies be minimized until vaccines given at 16 weeks of age have been administered.

Canine Distemper ■ Alfred M. Legendre

Canine distemper is a disease that primarily affects the lungs, intestinal tract, and nervous system of dogs. Among the virus-induced diseases in dogs, the mortality rate of distemper is second only to that of rabies. The virus is highly contagious and is passed directly from dog to dog by close contact. The virus is easily killed by detergents and heat. The virus dies within minutes in a warm environment but can persist for weeks at near-freezing temperatures.

Young, unvaccinated dogs 3 to 6 months of age are most often infected with distemper. Nasal discharges containing virus are aerosolized by sneezing, thereby spreading the virus. The virus establishes itself in the nasal passages of a susceptible dog, multiplies, and spreads through the body. Dogs develop a fever a week after infection but this fever may not be noticed. Two weeks after infection, the virus produces severe damage to the cells of the nasal passages, eyes, lungs, and intestinal tract. These damaged tissues commonly become secondarily infected with bacteria. This combined infection with virus and bacteria produces loss of appetite, fever, snotty nose, thick discharge from the eyes, pneumonia, and diarrhea. The virus infects the pads of the feet, producing a hard, scaly thickening referred to as "hard pad" disease. The virus also damages the immune system, thereby interfering with the body's ability to fight off the infection.

If the bacterial component of the infection can be controlled with antibiotics, the dogs will appear normal for 2 to 3 weeks until signs of brain and spinal cord disease occur. Half of the dogs with distemper develop neurologic disease. The canine distemper virus is attracted to and grows well in nervous tissue. The damage done to the brain and spinal cord results in epileptic seizures and localized seizures of the head often called "chewing gum fits." Damage to the spinal cord can produce weakness and paralysis. Nerve damage may also produce involuntary twitching of the legs. Most dogs with neurologic disease die or are euthanized.

Making a definite diagnosis of distemper can be difficult if the dog does not develop the typical snotty nose–pneumonia syndrome. After the initial 14 days of the infection, the virus is difficult to identify in swabs of infected tissues. Increasing antibody titers against distemper in dogs that have not been vaccinated strengthen the suspicion of distemper. It is especially difficult to diagnose distemper in dogs with nervous system signs that have not had the other typical signs of distemper.

Currently, no drugs are available to treat the distemper virus, so treatment with antibiotics is aimed at controlling the secondary bacterial infection. The antibiotic treatment relieves many of the signs of disease but does not prevent the virus from entering and damaging the brain and spinal cord. Nursing care; good-quality, palatable food; and a stress-free environment are helpful in improving appetite and general well-being. Because the treatment options are limited, prevention by vaccination is the prime strategy.

Vaccines against distemper should be started when puppies are weaned. If the mother has been vaccinated or recovered from an exposure to distemper, she will pass protection (antibodies) against distemper to her puppies in her milk. These maternal antibodies protect the pups for a few weeks after birth. The amount of antibodies passed from the mother to her pups depends mainly on the level of the mother's antibodies. The antibodies not only protect the pups from distemper but also interfere with the pups' response to vaccination. As long as the pups have maternal antibodies, they cannot be successfully vaccinated.

By 6 weeks of age, half of the litters of pups no longer have enough antibodies to interfere with vaccination. As the pups grow, the antibodies obtained from the dam are gradually broken down, and by 13 weeks of age more than 95 per cent of the pups are susceptible to distemper and can be protected by vaccination. It is not economically feasible to measure antibodies in the pups, so a vaccine schedule has been developed to protect pups optimally against distemper. Vaccines should be started soon after weaning, at 6 to 7 weeks of age, and given every 2 to 3 weeks until the puppies are 14 weeks of age. The pups should be kept away from other dogs until the vaccination schedule is complete. This scheme of vaccination has proved effective in preventing this lethal disease.

APP

Immune-Mediated Hemolytic Anemia and Immune-Mediated Thrombocytopenia ■ Carol Norris

Immune-mediated hemolytic anemia (IMHA) and immune-mediated thrombocytopenia (ITP) are diseases in which the body's own immune system attacks its red blood cells (IMHA) or platelets (ITP). Symptoms that develop are caused by a massive, often sudden, depletion of red blood cells or platelets. One of the major functions of red blood cells is to carry oxygen from the lungs to all other tissues in the body. When there are inadequate numbers of red blood cells (anemia), the body becomes starved for oxygen. As the pet owner, you may notice depression, listlessness, panting, loss of appetite, weakness, or reluctance to exercise in your pet.

The major function of platelets is to help form blood clots to stop bleeding. Destruction of large numbers of platelets can result in pinpoint bleeding in the skin or gums or may appear as nosebleeds. Less commonly, blood can be seen in the stool (which takes on a black appearance if it is digested or a bright red appearance if it is not) or urine. Severe anemia can result from excessive bleeding. Occasionally, IMHA and ITP occur together.

IMHA and ITP are more commonly seen in dogs than cats. It is believed that cocker spaniels, toy and miniature poodles, and Old English sheepdogs are breeds predisposed to develop IMHA. The latter two breeds and standard poodles are also at increased risk for developing ITP. Most affected dogs are middle-aged females. No breed or sex predilection is appreciated in cats. You should remember, however, that these conditions can develop in any dog or cat of any age, either sex, neutered or not. There is no scientific evidence that these diseases are caused by anything you feed your pet or by where your pet lives.

Both IMHA and ITP can be classified as ''primary'' or ''secondary.'' In primary disease, no underlying cause of the immune destruction can be found after an exhaustive clinical and laboratory evaluation. In comparison, secondary IMHA or ITP occurs when the immune system inadvertently destroys its own red blood cells or platelets secondary to an immune attack directed against an underlying condition such as cancer, infection, a drug, or toxin exposure. If an underlying condition is present, it is critical to attempt to correct that problem while simultaneously treating the immune disease.

Treatment of IMHA and ITP relies on suppressing the immune system's attack against the red blood cells and platelets, respectively. The medication most commonly prescribed to shut off the immune system is a steroid hormone called *prednisone*. Side effects of this drug in dogs include an increase in water intake and urination, an increase in appetite, and panting; cats tend not to have significant side effects. Therapy must be continued until there is laboratory evidence that anemia has resolved and there is no ongoing destruction of red blood cells or platelets. This requires frequent recheck examinations to monitor the success of therapy. If the immune system has been adequately suppressed, the dosage of prednisone can be slowly tapered (often over a period of several months) and ultimately discontinued. Generally, most veterinarians like to check a dog or cat immediately before each decrease in prednisone dose. These frequent rechecks are extremely important. If inadequate suppression of the immune system occurs, additional drugs such as *cyclophosphamide*, *azathioprine*, or *cyclosporine* may be tried. These drugs can have more severe side effects than prednisone, so it is important to talk to your veterinarian about the potential risks of each medication and what problems you need to look for.

In some dogs and cats, the destruction of red blood cells or platelets is so severe that a life-threatening anemia can occur. Blood transfusions may be necessary to stabilize these pets until the bone marrow can keep up with the demand for red blood cells and platelets and until the drugs suppressing the immune attack have had time to work.

Prognosis for both diseases is highly variable and depends on the underlying cause if one is present, complications related to the disease or drug therapy, and the response to treatment. Relapses can occur months to years after the initial episode. Overall, if there is no severe underlying illness or significant complications and if your pet responds to therapy, prognosis for both diseases is generally good.

Immune-Mediated Arthritis ■ David Feldman

Your pet has been diagnosed with immune-mediated arthritis. Symptoms typically include reluctance to walk or move and/or painful, swollen joints. There are two broad types of this condition, one caused by infection in the body (less common) and one caused by "autoimmunity" (more common). Both cause fever and both appear similar to the pet owner and to the veterinarian. It is important to differentiate between the two types of disease because the treatment for one is in direct opposition to that for the other. When immune-mediated arthritis is caused by infection in the body, the infection is usually not in the joints themselves. Rather, the infection is often deep seated in the body, for example, in the uterus or prostate, on a heart valve, in a kidney, on the spine, or elsewhere. The infection may also be body wide, such as those that result from the bite of a tick, such as Lyme disease, or those caused by internal fungal infections. Minor or superficial infections in the body do not usually cause this disease. The presence of inflamed joints resulting from an infection elsewhere in the body is similar to the human condition of "achy joints" in the presence of influenza (a human lung infection). In this instance, the infectious virus itself attacks the lungs, yet the body's immune system that fights off the infection attacks the joints as "innocent bystanders," making them sore and inflamed. Typical tests to find the source of internal infection would include a thorough physical examination, routine screening of blood and urine samples, and a bacterial culture of the urine. More advanced testing may be indicated depending on the specific case and your geographic area and may include radiographs (x-rays) or ultrasound examination of the body, serologic (blood) tests for the presence of an infectious disease, and/or a bacterial culture of the blood or spinal fluid. In all cases, an analysis of the fluid that bathes the joints (synovial fluid) is necessary to make the diagnosis of immune-mediated arthritis (either type). A small needle placed into the joint after the pet has been given a light sedative is all that is needed to collect a sample. Analysis of this fluid can aid the veterinarian in determining whether an infectious or autoimmune condition exists. Usually, however, the diagnosis is made by reviewing all test results and relating them to the patient's history and physical examination findings. When the infection in the body (if present) resolves, either through antibiotic treatment by the veterinarian or spontaneously, the inflammation in the joints (arthritis) almost always resolves permanently as well.

If a thorough examination and testing have not identified a source of infection in the body, the condition is termed "autoimmune" arthritis. An autoimmune disease is one in which the body's immune system (the circulating white blood cells and molecules that fight infection) has malfunctioned. Instead of performing its intended job, the immune system has been misdirected and has begun attacking parts of the body itself. In autoimmune arthritis the attack occurs at the lining of the joints. The reason for this misdirected attack is not clear but could be related in some way to the animal's genetic makeup. Certain breeds of dogs are prone to this condition, and there is an age group and gender association. A typical dog with this disease is a 2- to 6-year-old, large, female "sporting" breed dog. However, almost any age, breed, or sex of dog or cat may develop this disease. A particularly debilitating form of this disease, rheumatoid arthritis, typically affects aging, smaller to toy breeds of dogs. Autoimmune arthritis may occur by itself or may be part of an attack on several areas of the body, such as systemic lupus. Lupus is a generalized autoimmune disease in which the immune system attacks not only the joints but also the skin, kidneys, nervous system, blood cells, or other organs. The cause of lupus is not known but is presumed to be at least partially genetic.

Treatment for this form of the disease involves "turning off" or suppressing the immune system, thereby alleviating the inflammation in the joints. The drug most commonly used for this purpose is prednisone (cortisone). Prednisone itself is usually enough to treat the disease effectively. Common side effects of prednisone include increased water drinking, increased urination, increased appetite, weight gain, and panting. These effects are bothersome but not serious and should dissipate when the dose of the medication is decreased. Sometimes more potent immunosuppressive drugs need to be added to the protocol. In this case, care must be taken to avoid too much weakening of the immune system. This requires careful monitoring and regular blood checks by the veterinarian. In approximately 50 per cent of animals treated, the medication is eventually withdrawn over a period of many weeks to months and the prognosis is excellent. The remainder of affected animals have relapses with symptoms during gradual withdrawal of medication. Most of these relapsing cases are managed effectively with some tolerable dosage of medicine that needs to be continued for the long term or indefinitely. The goal of therapy in chronic or relapsing cases is to administer the minimum effective dose to control symptoms. This minimizes some potentially troubling side effects of the medication.

APP

Von Willebrand's Disease ■ Rafael Ruiz de Gopegui and Bernard F. Feldman

Von Willebrand's disease (vWd), a bleeding disorder, is the most common hereditary disease of dogs and people. Erik von Willebrand first described the disease more than 70 years ago. He called it pseudohemophilia because both women and men were affected. True hemophilia affects males. This genetic disease can be carried by the sire or dam and results from a deficiency of a protein called von Willebrand's factor (vWf), produced primarily by cells lining the walls of blood vessels. The function of vWf is to avoid and prevent bleeding by allowing small cells in the blood, called platelets, to "stick" to the walls of injured blood vessels and form a physical barrier to bleeding. The resulting mass of platelets is termed the platelet "plug." Von Willebrand's factor allows platelets to "stick" to the injured portion of a vessel wall and to stick to other platelets. Deficiency of vWf may result in bleeding. This deficiency may cause your dog to bleed without obvious trauma or to bleed for a long time after trauma. You may have observed red urine, blood in feces, bleeding from the dog's nose or gums, prolonged vaginal bleeding associated with the female heat period, or red spots in the skin or in mucous membranes.

Von Willebrand's disease occurs in many canine breeds (more than 50) and in mixed breed dogs but is more frequently observed in some breeds such as the Doberman pinscher, Scottish terrier, or Shetland sheepdog. Most breeds (the Doberman pinscher is an example) suffer a type of vWd (type I) that is the most common but least severe form of the disease. The severity of vWd is related to the quantity of active vWf. Many dogs look healthy and do not exhibit any bleeding tendencies—or bleeding may be so mild that it is not noticed—but are carriers of the defect and transmit the disease to their puppies. Therefore, both the dam and sire should be tested before breeding. In contrast, Scottish terriers, some shelties, and German pointers (in Europe these dogs are known as German Bracke and Drathaar) may have more severe forms of vWd, types II and III vWd. In these dogs, veterinarians are not able to identify carriers of the defect and can only detect severely affected dogs.

To diagnose vWd, your veterinarian may perform some blood clotting tests to demonstrate that there is a disorder resulting in bleeding. The best screening test, a test that suggests vWd, is the buccal mucosal bleeding time (BMBT). This test requires a tiny, painless cut in the inside of the lip. If the BMBT is prolonged and platelet numbers are normal, platelet dysfunction is suggested. For specific diagnosis of vWd, the vWf plasma concentration must be determined. This test requires that a specially handled blood sample be shipped to a laboratory specializing in testing for vWd. This test cannot be performed in ill dogs, dogs who are severely stressed, dogs recently exercised, female dogs in heat, or very young puppies.

Von Willebrand's disease cannot be cured, but vWf deficiency can be treated by blood or blood product transfusion to resolve ongoing hemorrhage (bleeding). Affected dogs do not require continuous transfusions. If they have suffered trauma resulting in hemorrhage or if surgery is required for any reason, transfusion therapy may be required. There is also a drug, a form of vasopressin, that acts on vessel wall cells, potentially increasing liberation of vWf for a short time. It may be used in type I vWd–affected dogs before surgery and may prevent or control bleeding. Apparently, this drug works better in people than in dogs and may be of little or no help in some dogs. Therapy with this drug is worth trying as it has few significant side effects.

Finally, if you already know your dog has vWd or the parents, grandparents, or littermates of your dog have a bleeding disorder, do not forget to give this information to your veterinarian. It is also important to know your dog's vWd status and to avoid drugs (aspirin is one example) that prevent platelets from functioning normally. These drugs in combination with vWd may result in severe hemorrhage. Your veterinarian may take special precautions before and during surgical procedures in dogs with vWd.

Chronic Renal Failure ■ David J. Polzin

Renal failure (kidney failure) occurs when kidney function has deteriorated to such a degree that the kidneys can no longer perform their normal functions of excreting wastes, maintaining water and electrolyte balance, and producing hormones. Renal failure occurs in acute or chronic forms. Acute renal failure is of recent onset and is potentially reversible. In contrast, chronic renal failure has been present for months to years at the time of diagnosis and is irreversible. Dogs and cats with chronic renal failure cannot be cured, but their clinical signs can often be managed successfully.

Kidneys are composed of many small functional units called nephrons (approximately 190,000 in cats and approximately 400,000 in dogs). Dogs, cats, and humans are normally born with such an abundance of nephrons that signs of kidney failure do not become apparent until more than two thirds of the nephrons have been damaged. Because of this redundant kidney tissue, it is possible to donate a kidney for transplantation and survive. On the other hand, surplus nephrons make it difficult to detect chronic kidney diseases until they are well advanced. As a consequence, chronic kidney failure is often an insidious condition that remains unrecognized until it is severe. Because kidney disease is often quite advanced at the time of initial diagnosis, the initiating cause of chronic renal failure can rarely be established. Although chronic renal failure occurs most often in older dogs and cats, renal failure is not simply a result of aging.

The earliest signs of renal failure are typically thirst (polydipsia) and increased urine volume (polyuria). These signs result from inability of the diseased kidneys to form concentrated urine. Other common early signs include weight loss, poor haircoat, and an increasingly selective appetite. Further decline in kidney function results in progressive inability to excrete waste products, leading to retention of toxic wastes in blood and tissues in the body. This is called uremia (literally, urine in the blood). Prominent clinical signs of uremia include loss of appetite, vomiting, ulcers in the mouth, "uremic" (foul ammonia smelling) breath, weakness, and lethargy. Other important effects of renal failure include anemia (caused by inability of failing kidneys to produce erythropoietin, the hormone responsible for making red blood cells) and high blood pressure. Anemia worsens the weakness, lethargy, and loss of appetite of dogs and cats with chronic renal failure, and high blood pressure may cause sudden blindness, strokelike signs (such as mental dullness, sudden behavioral changes, coma, or seizures), or injury to the kidneys and heart.

Diagnosis of chronic renal failure is confirmed by laboratory evaluation of your pet's blood and urine. A urine test can help determine whether the kidneys can form concentrated urine and provide evidence of other urinary tract problems such as urinary tract infections. Blood tests used to evaluate kidney function include blood urea nitrogen (BUN) and serum creatinine concentrations. Because the kidneys excrete urea and creatinine, increases in urine and creatinine concentrations in blood indicate decreased kidney function. These tests are usually done together because they provide different information. The serum creatinine concentration is the more specific test for kidney function, and treatment and other factors may influence the BUN. In addition to evaluating kidney function, other tests may be used to evaluate your pet for anemia, electrolyte and acid-base abnormalities, nutrition, and hypertension. Ultrasound examination and x-rays may also be used to evaluate kidney disease.

Fortunately, most dogs and cats can be treated, providing a good quality of life for months or years. Treatment for chronic renal failure is tailored to the unique clinical requirements of each pet but may include a special diet (e.g., limiting protein, phosphorus, and salt intake); hydration therapy; and medications designed to control clinical signs (such as poor appetite, nausea, and vomiting), acid-base and electrolyte disturbances, anemia, and hypertension. Consumption of excess protein may make some pets ill because the waste products of protein metabolism are excreted by the kidneys and are retained in renal failure. Dehydration (abnormal depletion of body fluids) is a special threat to pets with renal failure, and they may deteriorate if episodes of vomiting, diarrhea, or inadequate water intake are not dealt with promptly. Water should never be withheld from dogs and cats with renal failure.

In humans, renal failure is most often managed by dialysis (hemodialysis or peritoneal dialysis) or renal transplantation. Chronic hemodialysis and peritoneal dialysis have thus far not proved to be satisfactory options for dogs and cats with chronic renal failure because they are expensive and fail to provide an acceptable quality of life. Renal transplantation is an expensive but potentially useful option for selected cats but has not met with similar success in dogs. Renal transplantation is best reserved for cats that can no longer be managed by standard medical therapy.

APP

Chronic and/or Recurrent Urinary Tract Infections ■ Gerald V. Ling

Urinary tract infection (UTI, cystitis) refers to a condition in the urinary bladder (sometimes also involving the kidneys) caused by infection, usually with bacteria. In people, the condition is most often seen in women and girls, but in dogs it is common in both males and females. UTI is uncommon in cats. In people the signs of UTI often include fever, feeling sick, back pain, lower abdominal (bladder) cramping, an uncontrollable urge to urinate frequently, and passage of small amounts of urine. Blood is sometimes present in the urine. Dogs most often have *no signs* that can be seen by either the owner or the veterinarian. When signs are present in dogs, they include an obvious need to urinate more frequently than normal (frequent attempts to urinate on walks, asking to be let outside more often). Cats may use the litter box more often than is normal and may spend more time in the litter box. Both dogs and cats may be seen to pass bloody urine. Some owners may notice that their pet has increased thirst or a change in the odor of its urine when UTI is present.

Your veterinarian can make a diagnosis of UTI by taking a small sample of urine from your pet. The sampling procedure may involve introducing a catheter into the bladder through the pet's urethra, but is most easily done by inserting a small needle on a syringe into the bladder through the abdomen from the outside. This can easily be accomplished by your veterinarian with essentially no pain or risk to your pet. The urine sample must be obtained in a sterile manner that does not result in contamination of the sample by bacteria from outside the urinary tract. For this reason, owner-obtained samples of urine (catch samples) are not appropriate for determination of the presence or absence of UTI.

Your veterinarian will analyze the urine (urinalysis) and examine a small amount of the urine under a microscope. If bacteria and/or white blood cells (WBCs, "pus cells") are seen during this examination, your veterinarian will suggest that the urine be cultured. In some instances your veterinarian will send the urine sample to a laboratory for examination and/or culture. If bacteria are grown on culture, it means that an infection is present and an antibiotic "sensitivity test" may be performed on the bacteria. This determines the antibiotics to which the infection is most sensitive. In this way, your veterinarian can select the right antibiotic to kill the infection. It may take 2 or 3 working days before complete information is available to your veterinarian.

The antibiotic that your veterinarian selects will usually be in pill, capsule, or liquid form for oral use (for you to give to your pet). Depending on the antibiotic, you will need to give medicine to your pet from once to three times each day for at least 2 weeks (sometimes longer than 2 weeks but rarely shorter). Your veterinarian, or a technician who works at your veterinary hospital, can show you how to give the antibiotic to your pet and can answer any questions you have regarding the technique involved, side effects of the antibiotic, and so on.

Your veterinarian should reculture your pet's urine *during the second week of antibiotic treatment.* This culture is to be certain that the antibiotic is working to kill the bacteria causing the UTI. The results should be negative (no bacterial growth). A second reculture *10 to 14 days after completion of treatment* is also recommended. Results of this culture tell your veterinarian whether, as sometimes happens, the UTI has come back after treatment. If the result of this culture is also negative, your pet is not likely to have another UTI, at least in the near future. If infection is present, however, at either recheck, a new antibiotic susceptibility test must be performed and, in all likelihood, a new antibiotic selected on the basis of results of the test.

If the pet has three or more episodes of UTI in the course of 1 year, the infections are said to be recurrent. In this special and uncommon case, after an infection has been eliminated (culture-negative urine), a daily dose of an antibiotic is often given on a long-term basis (6 months is recommended) to prevent future episodes of UTI. This low-dose, preventive treatment is usually effective in preventing future UTI. Frequent urine cultures are necessary, however, to verify this fact for the individual pet.

It is not known why pets have UTI. It is known that certain diseases, certain types of medicines, and certain breeds of dogs are associated with UTI more often than normal. It is also known that it is important to recognize and treat UTI because, if left untreated, UTI can cause serious kidney ailment and bladder stones, as well as potentially serious infections in other parts of the body.

Ethylene Glycol (Radiator Fluid) Toxicity ■ Denise A. Elliott

Ethylene glycol is the principal ingredient of radiator fluid that is responsible for antifreeze poisoning in dogs and cats. Antifreeze poisoning is most common in the fall and spring, when radiator fluid is inadvertently abandoned in streets and garages after automobile radiator fluid is changed. Antifreeze is colorless, odorless, and has a sweet taste that dogs and small children find appealing and will readily drink. Cats are less likely to drink unknown fluids. It is suspected that cat poisoning occurs after cats have walked through antifreeze and ingest it when they clean their feet. As little as a teaspoon of antifreeze is sufficient to cause death in cats and a tablespoon is all that is required to poison dogs.

Poisoning classically proceeds through three stages. Absorption after ingestion is rapid and initial signs occur within 30 minutes to 12 hours. Ethylene glycol is an alcohol; hence during the initial phase the animals appear "drunk" and consequently exhibit many of the classical signs associated with alcohol intoxication: staggering, stumbling, and incoordination. Vomiting, nausea, extreme thirst, and frequent urination are also observed. Some animals simply sleep through this period and owners are not aware that poisoning has occurred. At the end of the first phase, the clinical signs resolve and the animal appears to have recovered. The second phase of intoxication occurs 12 to 24 hours after poisoning. The heart rate and breathing rate are rapid, but this is rarely noticed by owners. Unfortunately, most dogs and cats poisoned with antifreeze are not recognized until the third stage, when kidney damage becomes apparent and kidney (renal) failure occurs. Ethylene glycol is converted by the liver to more toxic substances (metabolites) that are responsible for the majority of injury to tissues including the kidney, liver, lungs, and heart. Signs of kidney failure include severe depression, vomiting, and diarrhea. The kidneys stop producing urine and toxins normally excreted by the kidney build up in the body, resulting in a life-threatening situation.

Early diagnosis of poisoning is often difficult because of an inadequate history and the nonspecific clinical signs, which can mimic those of many other conditions. A high index of suspicion is vital for rapid diagnosis, and it is important not to rule out ethylene glycol poisoning because the owner has not seen the pet exposed to radiator fluid. Laboratory findings are often the key to making the diagnosis. Tests that support a diagnosis of ethylene glycol poisoning are available to your veterinarian.

Treatment involves preventing absorption from the stomach, increasing removal from the body, and preventing the alteration of ethylene glycol to its more toxic components. If poisoning is witnessed, vomiting should be induced immediately and the stomach cleaned out with activated charcoal. Your veterinarian will need to give intravenous fluid solutions. Additional treatment depends on the stage of the disease. If the animal is not in kidney failure, drugs to stop the metabolism of ethylene glycol or methods for directly removing the ethylene glycol and its metabolites from the body are indicated. Ethanol (alcohol) and 4-methylprazole (fomepizole; Antizol-Vet) stop the metabolism of ethylene glycol; however, these drugs must be administered within several hours of poisoning and are ineffective when kidney damage had occurred. An effective dose of 4-methylprazole to stop the conversion of ethylene glycol has not been identified for cats, so its use is not recommended in cats. Peritoneal dialysis and hemodialysis are two techniques with which the poisons may be removed from the body.

If the animal is in kidney failure, techniques to support kidney function are required. Medications to encourage the kidney to produce urine are administered but are often futile, and advanced techniques such as peritoneal dialysis or hemodialysis that replace the function of the failing kidneys may be necessary. Both of these procedures require referral to a speciality center. Support must be provided until the kidneys can heal, which may take several weeks to months, and in some animals the damage is too severe and recovery is not possible. In these patients, kidney transplantation may be indicated to replace the crippled kidneys.

The most common problem caused by antifreeze poisoning is sudden kidney failure, and it is associated with a high death rate. The prognosis for animals to recover from acute kidney failure is poor; however, the prognosis has improved with the advent of hemodialysis, which provides support until the kidneys can regenerate. Antifreeze poisoning is a deadly disease. Prevention requires public awareness and responsible disposal of radiator fluid. The advent of less toxic antifreeze compounds such as propylene glycol will reduce the frequency of antifreeze poisoning in companion animals.

APP

Urinary Stones: Cause, Treatment, Prevention ■ Carl A. Osborne

Does your dog or cat have urinary stones? Perhaps you know them by the name kidney stones or bladder stones. They form in the urinary tract of all kinds of animals and in humans. Urinary stones are rock-hard structures. Stones in the urinary tract cause problems because this system is designed to eliminate body wastes in liquid form, whereas the intestinal tract is designed to eliminate wastes in solid form. In animals and in humans, urinary stones are often called "calculi," from the Latin word for stone. It is the same Latin word used in the mathematical term calculus, as stones were at one time used for counting. The word "lith" as in "urolith" is from the Greek word for stone. The prefix "uro-" is a Greek term referring to the urinary tract. Thus, a urolith is a urinary tract stone that may be located in the kidneys (nephrolith; nephro is Greek for kidney), ureters (ureterolith), urinary bladder (urocystolith), or urethra (urethrolith).

Have you ever wondered why stones form in the urinary tract? The process is a complicated one, but basically stones form because certain waste products present in urine increase in concentration to a point at which they precipitate as microscopic crystals. If these crystals remain in the urinary tract and grow, they become large enough to see with the unaided eye. With time, the stones may fill the space in the urinary tract normally occupied by urine.

All urinary stones contain two major components—minerals (which typically constitute about 95 per cent of a stone) and nonmineral matrix (typically about 5 per cent of a stone). The matrix can be thought of as a kind of mortar that may help to cement minerals together. Because stones are composed primarily of minerals, their number, location, and size can usually be detected by x-ray studies or ultrasound studies.

Do all urinary stones have the same mineral composition? The answer is no. The most common types of minerals in urinary stones formed by dogs and cats are magnesium ammonium phosphate (also called struvite), calcium oxalate, calcium phosphate, ammonium urate, cystine, and silica. Sometimes stones contain more than one type of mineral. On occasion, the center of a urolith may be composed of one type of mineral (for example, calcium oxalate), whereas outer layers are composed of a different mineral (especially struvite).

Determining the types of minerals in stones is important because different mineral types occur as a result of fundamentally different causes. Therefore, urinary stones should not be considered a single disease but rather a potential consequence of several underlying risk factors. Treatment and/or prevention of stone formation depends on identifying their mineral composition. In addition, evaluation of your pet's diet, blood analysis, and urine composition analysis are important steps in formulating recommendations for stone treatment and prevention.

How can urinary stones be effectively treated? Options include various types of surgery and various types of nonsurgical therapy designed to dissolve stones in the urinary tract. Which treatment is best? The risks and benefits of medical versus surgical therapy must be considered for each pet. Complete obstruction of the flow of urine through the urinary tract should be regarded as an emergency.

Although surgical removal is an effective method that may immediately eliminate uroliths, surgery alone is associated with several limitations, including (1) persistence of the underlying causes of stones and therefore a high rate of recurrence of uroliths after surgery, (2) risks inherent in general anesthesia and the type of surgery performed, and (3) inability to remove all uroliths during surgery. For these and other reasons (that is, the urolith is asymptomatic), medical dissolution of some types of uroliths may be considered.

The objectives of medical dissolution of uroliths are to stop further stone growth and/or to promote stone dissolution by correcting or controlling underlying abnormalities. For medical dissolution therapy to be effective, it must reduce the urine concentration of minerals that have precipitated to form the stone. This usually involves a change in diet and in addition often includes administration of specific drug.

The size and number of uroliths as such do not dictate the likelihood of response to dissolution therapy. There has been success in dissolving uroliths that are small and large, single and multiple. However, the rate of dissolution is related to the size and surface area of the urolith exposed to urine. Just as one large ice cube dissolves more slowly than an equal volume of crushed ice, one large urolith dissolves more slowly than an equal volume of many smaller uroliths.

Uroliths tend to recur. Prevention of recurrent uroliths that reduces the need for medical therapy and/or surgery is therefore cost effective. In general, prevention strategies are designed to eliminate or control the underlying causes of various types of uroliths. When causes cannot be identified, preventive therapy is usually designed to minimize risk factors associated with formation of all stones. Recommendations commonly include dietary modifications and sometimes administration of drugs.

Does Your Cat Have Lower Urinary Tract Disease? ■ Carl A. Osborne

Has your cat ever suffered from a disorder of the lower urinary tract? Cats occasionally develop such problems, and the signs include frequent urination, straining to urinate, bloody urine, and at times inability to urinate.

In order to recognize and properly treat lower urinary tract diseases (LUTDs), it is helpful to have a conceptual understanding of the structure and function of the urinary tract. The normal urinary tract of a cat consists of two identical kidneys. Urine formed by the kidneys passes into pliable tiny muscular tubes called ureters. The ureter from each kidney is connected to the urinary bladder. The bladder is like a balloon. Rhythmic one-directional contractions of the ureter walls transport urine formed by the kidneys into the bladder for temporary storage. Urine contained in the urinary bladder can be voided out of the cat's body through a tube larger than the ureters. This cylindrical muscular tube is called the urethra. Urine is normally retained in the bladder primarily by resistance in the urethra caused by muscular tone. When the bladder becomes filled with urine, however, the muscular wall of the bladder contracts while the muscles in the urethral wall relax. The result is complete ejection of urine stored in the bladder.

What are the clinical signs of diseases of the bladder and urethra (or LUTDs)? They include difficult urination, bloody urine, crystals in urine, and urethral obstruction that causes complete inability to move urine from the bladder through the urethra to the outside. These signs may have different causes. Thus, there is a need for evaluation of each cat as an individual to determine the proper form of treatment and prevention. Possible causes of LUTDs include urinary stones, bacterial and viral infections, birth defects, trauma, tumors, and neuromuscular diseases. In more than 50 per cent of cats, it may not be possible to determine the underlying cause(s).

To determine the underlying cause of LUTDs, the veterinarian examines your cat, takes a medical history, and also performs urinalyses (tests on the urine) on urine samples that have not been altered by previous treatment. X-ray and ultrasound studies may be needed to locate the exact site(s) of the problem and to identify the causes of persistent or frequently recurring signs. Identifying the site and cause of urethral obstruction is especially important if some form of urethral surgery is being considered.

Although a variety of disorders can cause obstruction of the urethra (especially in male cats), no matter what the cause, complete obstruction results in dysfunction of both kidneys that, if not quickly corrected, ultimately causes death. Untreated cats usually die within 3 to 5 days after the onset of obstruction. Why is complete obstruction of the urethra life threatening? Death results from retention of wastes, especially potassium and metabolic acids, in the bloodstream. However, the retention can be reversed by eliminating the obstruction and by correcting the abnormalities in blood.

How should LUTDs be managed? Specific treatment of LUTDs should be directed at the underlying causes, only some of which are currently known. Of course, detecting known causes calls for appropriate evaluation and diagnosis. In the case of a cat with urethral obstruction, the treatment depends on the cause, site, degree, and duration of the obstruction.

To treat a bacterial infection, a veterinarian should prescribe appropriate antibiotics and eliminate or control problems in the normal body defense system. For cases of urinary stones, either medical dissolution protocols or surgical procedures may be considered.

Treatment of difficult urination and bloody urine not associated with identifiable causes remains a puzzle. Fortunately, the signs of many cats with this form of LUTD usually subside on their own. Unfortunately, the signs are unpredictably recurrent. Because specific therapy is unavailable, veterinarians often recommend therapy to treat the symptoms. When evaluating the success of various treatments, we must be careful. Many disorders in humans and animals are self-limiting, meaning that our bodies' defense systems eliminate the diseases. Examples of self-limiting human diseases include the common cold and many gastrointestinal problems involving vomiting and diarrhea. In these cases, a treatment may seem beneficial as long as it is not harmful. A similar situation occurs in some cats with LUTDs. However, your veterinarian may recommend changes in diet, litter boxes, water availability, environment, or medications. Close communication between you and your veterinarian regarding the benefit or lack of benefit of any treatment trial will be valuable after you closely observe your cat. Remember, there is no "cure." Also remember that inability of a cat to urinate is a medical emergency that requires immediate veterinary attention.

APP

"Steroid" Therapy ■ Edward C. Feldman

In Latin, "kidney" is "renal" and "next to" is "ad." There is a small organ next to each kidney called the adrenal. The adrenals have various functions, including the production of "steroids," which enter the bloodstream and are distributed to cells everywhere in the body. Steroids do a number of jobs that are vital. In other words, without steroids, a person, dog, or cat would die. In addition to being produced naturally, steroids are manufactured and sold as medicine for a variety of conditions. The most popular steroids used by veterinarians are those called glucocorticoids. The drugs in this category include prednisone, prednisolone, methylprednisolone, triamcinolone, dexamethasone, and others. When given by injection, pill, or as a topical cream, steroids have specific effects, dictating the diseases for which they are commonly used.

Steroids can have potent anti-inflammatory effects and are often used for dogs and cats with severe allergic conditions such as flea allergy dermatitis, in which the allergic condition causes so much irritation that animals begin to bite at their skin and can hurt themselves. As you know, there are additional allergic conditions for which steroids are beneficial, including asthma-like diseases, food allergies, bee stings, and many others. Steroids are useful for chronic arthritis, especially in older dogs with problems such as hip dysplasia. "Disk disease" of the spine can result in severe pain or paralysis. A "bulging" or "slipped" disk causes trauma to the spinal cord or nerves that, in turn, causes inflammation, swelling, and damage to those structures. Steroids can reduce the harmful inflammation and swelling while giving the body a chance to heal.

Steroids can also suppress the immune system. The immune system fights infection. However, there are conditions in which the immune system is overzealous. In these conditions, the immune system may begin to fight and destroy normal cells. These are often called "autoimmune" diseases and can include anemia, destruction of cells that allow blood to clot (thrombocytopenia), joint diseases, and kidney diseases. In these conditions, steroids are given to stop the immune system and, by accomplishing this, stop the destruction of normal cells needed for a healthy existence. Steroids can also be effective in fighting some, but not all, cancers.

Steroids are not "strong" medicines. They are drugs with which veterinarians have become quite familiar. For these reasons, steroids are extremely popular, being used for relatively minor problems and sometimes for serious life-threatening diseases. For most conditions, veterinarians begin dogs or cats on relatively high doses in order to achieve certain desired effects. Once these effects have been accomplished (usually in days to weeks), the most common treatment protocols involve slowly decreasing the amount of steroid given each day. The reasons for decreasing or "tapering" the dose are at least twofold. First, by decreasing the dose while completing frequent rechecks, your veterinarian can determine whether the condition being treated has remained under control. Sometimes the steroid dose can be decreased slowly and then stopped. However, there are other conditions or situations in which one dose controls the condition but a lower dose fails to keep the problem in check. If this occurs, your veterinarian can simply raise the dose again to see whether the disease again responds. With some dogs and cats, this trial-and-error approach to increasing and decreasing dosages of steroids goes on for months. This is common and, although frustrating, is often to be expected. The second advantage of tapering steroid doses is that it allows the body to adapt to their withdrawal. Some dogs and cats can become "addicted" to steroids, and if the drug is stopped too quickly, the dog or cat can become ill. So, slow tapering over time is the correct method for discontinuing this form of treatment, even if your veterinarian no longer considers the steroids necessary.

In addition to the many beneficial attributes of steroids, there are some potential problems associated with their use. In dogs especially, steroids cause some annoying side effects. Some of these are extremely common and will definitely be worrisome to you but do not cause permanent harm to the dog. These side effects include dramatic increases in thirst, hunger, and urine volume. Some previously housebroken dogs produce so much urine that they cannot wait to be taken outside and urinate in the home. Other side effects include panting, muscle weakness, and lethargy. With long-term use of steroids, dogs can begin to lose hair from their trunk but usually not from their head or legs. Both dogs and cats can develop a "potbellied" appearance. All these side effects are completely reversible and diminish when the steroid dose is decreased or stopped. There are also more worrisome side effects. Because of the suppression of the immune system, steroid-treated dogs and cats are prone to infection. These infections can become severe and life threatening. This complication is not common but it can arise. An even less common problem is ulcers of the stomach and/or intestine, especially if your pet is given steroids in the treatment of any form of paralysis.

Finally, steroids do not always work. They may fail over time or they may never work in the first place. If they fail to do the job for which they were given, your veterinarian is likely to recommend different and often more potent medication. These new medications are often given with steroids so that the drugs can work together for more effect than either can have alone.

Antibiotics ■ Etienne Côté

"Antibiotics" are medications that either kill or prevent the multiplication of bacteria. These drugs are used in the treatment of bacterial infections involving almost any part of the body. Penicillins and sulfonamides are some of the first antibiotics ever used and were distributed after World War II. Since then, hundreds of other antibiotics have been developed.

The beneficial effects of antibiotics range from the mildly helpful to the lifesaving. It is possible for bacterial infections that are not controlled by the body's own defenses to spread within the affected tissue by local invasion or even to spread to the rest of the body through the bloodstream. Judicious use of antibiotics can prevent or eliminate bacterial infections that could otherwise become life threatening. Prescribing these drugs is based on the concern that without antibiotics, the animal may sustain an increasingly severe bacterial infection. Whether the risk of progressive infection is great enough to warrant the cost, owner effort, and potential side effects of antibiotic treatment is an important assessment that your veterinarian must make before deciding whether or not to prescribe these medications.

Antibiotics are unable to fight viral or other nonbacterial types of infections such as yeast (fungal infections). They are prescribed to treat "primary" bacterial infections (those caused purely by bacteria) or "secondary" infections (those caused by bacteria that settle in parts of the body that have first been damaged and made vulnerable by other conditions).

A major stumbling block in using antibiotics is antibiotic resistance. Many bacteria have developed antibiotic resistance, meaning that the bacteria are unaffected by the antibiotic and continue to multiply in tissues, continuing the "infection." This means the infection spreads even though an antibiotic is being given. Because of antibiotic resistance, *it is crucial that the full course of an antibiotic be given as prescribed, even when the visible signs of illness are improving or are gone.* If antibiotics are stopped prematurely, bacteria that are partially resistant to the antibiotic survive and multiply, creating increasingly resistant (and harder to eliminate) strains of bacteria.

Choosing the right antibiotic is an important decision made by your veterinarian. The reason that so many different antibiotics exist is that each has a different "profile" for reaching specific tissues in the body and eliminating certain types of bacteria. Antibiotics work through ingenious mechanisms by which bacterial cells are damaged or killed while normal cells in your dog or cat are spared. These mechanisms include inhibition of bacterial cell wall production (penicillins), inhibition of bacterial protein synthesis (tetracyclines, chloramphenicol), and inhibition of bacterial DNA synthesis (fluoroquinolones). Ideally, an antibiotic is chosen on the basis of the results of a laboratory test known as a *bacterial culture and sensitivity* test. This test determines which bacteria are present in an infection and which antibiotics are most effective against those specific bacteria.

An antibiotic can also be chosen "empirically" (i.e., on the basis of the veterinarian's experience) and then changed if there is no improvement in the condition of your pet. In such situations, veterinarians choose an antibiotic that they have found to work well against certain types of infection. If the infection continues even after the full course of antibiotics is given, further testing is warranted to determine whether a different antibiotic would be better or whether a completely different problem may actually be present, masquerading as a bacterial infection.

Whereas individual bacteria are so small as to be invisible to the naked eye, large accumulations of bacteria and infected tissue can form fluid-filled pockets of pus called *abscesses.* When an infection forms an abscess, antibiotics alone rarely fix the problem because they cannot eliminate such high numbers of bacteria. If an abscess exists, it must often be lanced or surgically drained. Then antibiotics can be expected to help resolve the infection.

Like any medication, antibiotics have the potential to cause adverse effects. Even though antibiotics are commonly used, adverse reactions remain a rare occurrence. One of the more common adverse reactions is mild digestive upset such as vomiting or diarrhea, which usually stops after the antibiotic is discontinued. The first step in dealing with any perceived adverse effect of antibiotics is to discuss the problem with your veterinarian. An alternative type of antibiotic or other medication may then be chosen instead, or medical testing may be needed for further definition of the animal's illness.

APP

Canine Demodicosis ■ Terese C. DeManuelle

Demodicosis is a disease caused by *Demodex canis*, a mite that normally lives in the hair follicles of dogs. These mites pass from the bitch to the nursing pups at about 3 days of age. The mite spends its entire life on the dog and it is not considered contagious to other dogs, cats, or humans. Because of genetic factors and/or disorders of the immune system, the number of mites on the skin may increase dramatically and lead to the development of lesions. The clinical signs associated with demodicosis are highly variable and may include hair loss, redness of the skin, and recurring bacterial skin infections.

There are two forms of demodicosis: juvenile onset and adult onset. They are additionally classified as either "localized" or "generalized." The disease is generalized if two or more feet are affected; if five or more small circular areas of hair loss, scale, and redness are seen; or if an entire body region is affected. Dogs with generalized demodicosis should not be bred because the defect in the immune system that allows them to develop the disease is believed to be inherited.

Dogs with juvenile-onset demodicosis are younger than 18 months of age at the onset of clinical signs. The localized form of the disease is considered benign and should not be treated because about 80 per cent of these dogs naturally control their own mite population within 2 to 3 months. Some develop generalized juvenile-onset demodicosis with hair loss, crusting, and irritation affecting the entire body. In addition to genetic and immunologic factors, nutritional status, parasitic infections, heat cycles, and other diseases are considered potentiating causes.

Adult-onset generalized demodicosis (dogs older than 18 months of age) is a serious disease because it may be an indication of internal disease that is altering or suppressing the immune system. Many of these dogs have received corticosteroids for a prolonged period of time. Clinical signs are similar to those in the juvenile-onset generalized form of demodicosis. Diagnostic tests may be performed to investigate an underlying cause, such as hyperadrenocorticism (excess cortisone production or administration), hypothyroidism, systemic disease or organ dysfunction, and cancer. Chemotherapy or other immunosuppressive drug therapy may also lead to the development of adult-onset generalized demodicosis.

Demodicosis is usually diagnosed by obtaining deep skin scrapings and visualizing the mites under a microscope. The presence of more than one adult mite or of immature forms indicates disease. In some breeds, such as the Chinese Shar Pei, and in dogs with chronic disease, especially of the feet, a skin biopsy may be necessary to diagnose demodicosis.

Generalized demodicosis is a serious disease and must be treated aggressively with drugs to control the mites and the secondary bacterial skin infections. Treatment of generalized demodicosis consists of identification and correction of possible underlying diseases that have allowed the mites to proliferate as well as specific therapy for the mites and treatment of accompanying secondary bacterial infections. Most treatments for demodicosis require months of intensive therapy. It is not unusual for your veterinarian to prescribe an extended course of oral antibiotics to treat the deep bacterial skin infections that frequently accompany demodicosis. Other treatments are available for demodicosis, but amitraz (Mitaban) is the only treatment for demodicosis that is approved by the U.S. Food and Drug Administration. In any treatment plan for demodicosis, corticosteroids (topical or systemic) are contraindicated.

Your veterinarian may recommend that Mitaban dips initially be performed in the veterinary hospital by qualified personnel to ensure that the treatment is performed correctly as well as to observe for side effects. Medium-haired and long-haired dogs should be clipped every 3 to 4 weeks to facilitate adequate penetration of the Mitaban dip. Dogs should be bathed with a benzoyl peroxide shampoo before each dip. The dip is mixed with water according to the instructions given by your veterinarian in a well-ventilated room or outdoors. Rubber gloves should be worn and, using a sponge, the mixture applied thoroughly to saturate the skin. The dip should be applied with the dog standing in a washtub as the dip runoff is reapplied with a sponge for a full 15 minutes. It is important to treat the facial area, ears, and feet as these regions are commonly affected by demodicosis. Dogs that have demodicosis affecting the feet should stand in the dip preparation for a minimum of 15 minutes. *The dip should not be rinsed off.* Allow the dog to air dry. Your dog should not be allowed to become wet (including the feet) between Mitaban treatments, as this washes off the medication. This procedure should be repeated as directed by your veterinarian. A new mixture must be prepared for each treatment because the drug is unstable when exposed to light and air; for the same reason, any remaining dip should be discarded. The side effects of Mitaban include lethargy, skin irritation, itchiness, loss of appetite, and occasional vomiting or diarrhea. Side effects are more commonly seen in small dogs, especially the toy breeds. If side effects are observed, your veterinarian should be notified.

Other drugs can help in the treatment of demodicosis. These systemic drugs are ivermectin (Ivomec/Stromectol 1 per cent) and milbemycin (Interceptor). If your dog has not received heartworm preventive on a regular basis, your veterinarian needs to perform a blood test for heartworm disease before administration of either of these drugs. The side effects of ivermectin and milbemycin include decreased appetite, lethargy, weakness, dilated pupils, tremors, vomiting, coma, and death. Usually the more serious side effects occur with ivermectin, but they may also occur with milbemycin. The side effects are rare and usually resolve with discontinuation of the drug. Collies, Shetland sheepdogs, Old English sheepdogs, Australian shepherds, border collies, or their crosses should not be treated with ivermectin.

Your dog needs to be evaluated by your veterinarian every 4 to 8 weeks. Skin scrapings are obtained at each visit and treatment usually continues until two or three consecutive skin scrapings have been negative. Treatment is discontinued at this time, and your dog is reevaluated every 3 months for 1 year. Your dog is not considered "cured" until 1 year has passed without visualization of mites on skin scrapings. A small percentage of dogs have chronic demodicosis and may require lifelong therapy.

Fleas and Flea Allergy Dermatitis ■ Terese C. DeManuelle

Flea allergy is the most common cause of itching and scratching in dogs and cats. When a flea bites your pet, it injects a small amount of saliva into the skin. Dogs and cats can develop an allergy to a protein in the flea saliva and react with severe itching and scratching. This itching sensation may last for up to 2 weeks after the last flea bite. In the adult dog, the most commonly observed signs of flea allergy are biting and scratching around the rump, tail base, and groin areas ("hot spots"). Puppies and cats may manifest flea allergy in a variety of ways. In cats, you may see areas of hair loss and scratching or notice excessive grooming, but more often you may feel small scabs and bumps around the neck and down the back (miliary dermatitis). In puppies, itching and rash may affect the whole body.

It may seem confusing to be told that your dog or cat has flea allergy dermatitis if you almost never see fleas. When your pet is itchy, he or she has a remarkable capacity to chase and subsequently eat these fleas before you can see them! However, you may find evidence that fleas have been biting your pet by using a fine comb and brushing out the "flea dirt" that they leave behind. This dirt looks like small black dots and consists mostly of dried blood in the excrement of the flea. If you put some flea dirt on moist paper, it dissolves and leaves streaks of blood.

The only good long-term safe therapy for flea allergy dermatitis is to keep your pet from being bitten by fleas. This may seem like an impossible task, but it is not.

RECOMMENDATIONS FOR FLEA CONTROL

Flea control must involve all areas of infestation. This means killing the fleas on your pets *and* in your house and yard. Treating only once kills the adults and some preadults but results in recurrence of infestation when the resistant eggs hatch or pupae leave their cocoons. Adequate flea control involves a three-pronged attack. All aspects of this attack must be maintained or the flea will break through your lines of defense. These recommendations will assist you in control, but you should remember that they are simply guidelines to follow. The flea control program you use must be tailored to your individual situation.

FLEA CONTROL ON YOUR PET

DOGS

An adulticide product for flea-allergic pets or households with flea-allergic pets is recommended. Several new "spot-on" formulations are available that are safe and offer great convenience of application. These products have been shown to be effective when used as instructed by your veterinarian and are not absorbed into your pet's bloodstream. Imidacloprid (Advantage) and fipronil (Frontline) are two such products. Permethrin-pyriproxifen (BioSpot) is also available for dogs only. These products are applied by parting the hair between the shoulder blades and down the back and applying small amounts of liquid to the skin. Application frequency varies with the product and bathing needs. They are not applied more frequently than every week and are most often applied every 3 to 4 weeks. It is recommended that you not bathe your dog the day of or 1 day after application of the spot-on treatment. In addition, Frontline is formulated as a spray. Frontline products and permethrin are also effective for the dog tick. The use of a pyrethrin-based daily spray or foam product may be recommended for your pet. These products are used when animals are bathed often with therapeutic shampoos or are frequent swimmers.

CATS

If you own cats, they must be involved in the flea control program even if they are not exhibiting any problems, or they can carry the fleas to your house, yard, and dogs. Cats are more sensitive to the chemicals in flea preparations, and some products used on dogs cannot be used on cats. For cats, Advantage and Frontline in the cat formulation are safe and easy to use. They are applied in a similar fashion as to dogs. Their application also varies from weekly to 4-week intervals.

JUVENILE FLEA STAGES

Several life cycle stages occur before a flea becomes a biting adult. Decreasing the numbers of immature (juvenile) fleas can be an excellent way to help prevent adult fleas and thus flea bites. Several products interrupt the life cycle of the flea and are used in combination with on-animal treatments to decrease the flea burden of your pet quickly and effectively. Pyriproxifen is a juvenile flea growth hormone imitator that is stable in sunlight and is available in environmental treatments (Nylar, Knockout). Pyriproxifen is also available in a collar for cats (Knockout) that is effective for 13 months, as well as a water-based spot-on

formulation (Breakthru! IGR Stripe-on) for cats and in combination with permethrin as a spot-on formulation or spray for dogs. An Ovitrol collar is a breakaway collar available for cats and dogs that contains only methoprene and is effective for up to 12 months.

All of these synthetic hormones are quite safe. They prevent the adult female flea from laying live eggs and prevent immature fleas from developing into adults. Lufenuron (Program) is an oral medication available for both dogs and cats that is given monthly with food. As the adult female flea feeds on the dog or cat, she lays eggs that cannot hatch. Lufenuron is also available in a combination pill with a monthly heartworm preventive (Sentinel). An injectable product containing lufenuron is available for cats that is administered once every 6 months. It may take up to 6 months for the flea problem in your environment to be eliminated unless this approach is combined with on-animal control. Many other forms of flea control have been scientifically shown to be ineffective. Flea shampoos kill the adult fleas but have virtually no residual effect and do not prevent reinfestation once they are rinsed off. Flea collars alone are ineffective because they are not able to sustain high enough concentrations of insecticide over the animal's entire body. Electronic flea collars; brewer's yeast; garlic; vitamin B tablets; and extracts of eucalyptus, tea tree oil, or pennyroyal are not flea repellent and provide no protection for your pet. Flea combs, although helpful, are similar in effect to the use of flea shampoos alone and do not prevent reinfestation.

SIGNS OF TOXICITY

All flea control products are potentially toxic and may produce unexpected side effects. Toxicity may result from accidental overdose or unexpected sensitivity. If you suspect that your animal is reacting adversely to a flea control product, stop using the product and consult your veterinarian immediately. If the reaction occurs immediately after application, the product should be rinsed off thoroughly and the animal brought to the veterinarian for evaluation. Insecticides can be toxic to people, and all products should be handled carefully, avoiding direct contact as much as possible. Keep all products out of the reach of children.

FLEA CONTROL IN YOUR HOUSE

House treatments need to be concentrated on "source points," which are areas where your pets spend most of their time. If you choose to utilize professional exterminators, they should use a combination of an adulticide to kill the adult fleas and an insect growth regulator for the juvenile stages, such as methoprene (Precor—indoor only) or pyriproxifen (Nylar), which may be used inside and outside. If you choose to perform your own environmental control, a premise spray that contains an adulticide and an insect growth regulator is recommended for house treatment. Flea bombs and foggers are inadequate to control fleas as they do not go around corners or under furniture, where fleas hide. Treatment should be repeated as instructed on the product label. Other ways to lessen the flea burden in the home include thorough vacuuming of all source points in the house followed by disposal of the vacuum bag and washing all animal bedding weekly in hot water with drying at high heat for 20 minutes.

FLEA CONTROL IN YOUR YARD

In some cases, when you live in an area conducive to year-round flea reproduction out of doors and when the use of on-animal and preadult products has proved inadequate, yard treatment may be necessary. It is important to focus on areas where your pets spend most of their time and where immature fleas may develop. Typically, fleas survive and reproduce in shaded, moist areas that contain plant, sand, or organic debris (e.g., under decks and bushes). Either a professional exterminator or you must treat for fleas in your yard. You can treat the yard yourself by purchasing malathion or diazinon from your local hardware store. These chemicals can be purchased in a container that you connect to your garden hose for easy spraying of the focal areas where fleas may accumulate. These yard treatments should be performed as instructed on the product label. Pyriproxifen (Nylar), an insect growth regulator, may also be used in the yard in some states. Another product available for outdoor use is a parasitic nematode (Bioflea) that can be applied to areas of damp soil. These worms seek and destroy flea larvae. Label directions must be followed closely for this product to be effective.

SPECIAL CONSIDERATIONS

Pregnant women, small children, or debilitated individuals should not be involved in the application of chemicals on animals or in the house.

APP

Food Hypersensitivity ■ Terese C. DeManuelle

Food hypersensitivity is an uncommon skin disorder in dogs and cats that is caused by an allergic reaction to food. The component of the food that the animal reacts to is usually a protein source (beef, chicken, egg, cow's milk) but it may be a minor component (preservative, additive, dye). Because this is an acquired disease, the animal has often been fed the food for months to years before the onset of the disease.

The most common sign of food allergy is an intense, nonseasonal itch. In dogs, the itch tends to be generalized, but the ears, face, and feet may be more severely affected. Some dogs may exhibit signs of recurrent ear disease as the only manifestation of food allergy. Food allergy in cats usually affects the face and neck, and the itch may be so severe that the animal scratches itself until it bleeds. Up to 15 per cent of animals with food hypersensitivity have accompanying gastrointestinal signs (vomiting and/or diarrhea). In both dogs and cats, the disease may be poorly responsive to glucocorticoids (steroids). The majority of dogs with food hypersensitivity manifest clinical signs before 3 years of age, but the disease may occur at any age.

The diagnosis of food allergy involves a food elimination trial. There is currently no other accurate test to determine whether your pet has food allergy. It is believed that animals may react to allergens in their food for up to 6 weeks or more; therefore a restrictive diet must be given for up to 10 weeks. Because food allergy is an acquired disease (a food component becomes allergenic after being fed), only foods that the animal has never eaten before may be used. One protein source and one carbohydrate source are chosen and all other foods are discontinued. Cats may eat a single protein source for the elimination trial. Your veterinarian will base the trial diet on what your pet has eaten in the past. Therefore, it is important to be complete when relating your animal's diet history.

During a food elimination trial, only that diet is fed. Treats, rawhide chews, dog biscuits, pig ears, chew hooves, vitamin pills, food supplements, or unapproved medications (including some heartworm preventives) should not be given. Your veterinarian may change the heartworm preventive that your pet is receiving to a nonflavored pill for the duration of the trial period. You may not use cheese, hot dogs, and so forth to disguise medication during the diet trial. Treats must consist of the same ingredients used in the diet trial. Outdoor cats must be kept away from other food sources to have a successful food trial. It may be necessary to confine them indoors for the duration of the food trial. Please exercise caution if you have other pets and make certain that the pet receiving the trial diet never has an opportunity to eat any of the other animals' food (or even lick their bowl). One morsel of another type of food has the potential to invalidate the entire elimination diet trial and could necessitate commencement of a different diet for 10 weeks. The other animals in the household could also be fed the elimination diet. Inform everyone in the household that your pet is receiving a special diet. It is important to be diligent when your pet is on walks to ensure that ingestion of foodstuffs does not occur. Simply changing the brand of dog food (even to diets that are described as "hypoallergenic") is not equivalent to an elimination diet. Most dog foods share similar protein, grain meal, preservatives, and/or dye sources and contain many potentially allergenic ingredients in order to be fully balanced.

Your veterinarian will recommend a protein (e.g., fish, pork, tofu, lamb, pinto beans, rabbit, venison, duck) and a carbohydrate (e.g., potato, rice, oatmeal) in a ratio of one cooked pound of protein to six cups of cooked carbohydrate. Flavorings other than salt, pepper, and garlic may not be used (no oils, butters, or cooking spray). Many clients find it easier to prepare the diet in bulk (e.g., 1 week at a time) and freeze the diet in measured daily rations. Approximately one cup is fed per 10 pounds of body weight daily. Switch gradually to the new diet over a period of 3 to 5 days by giving more of the new diet and less of the old diet each day.

Some animals may have loose stools while receiving the trial diet. Your pet may develop vomiting, diarrhea, or constipation or may refuse to eat the new diet. Cats may begin to develop a serious liver disease if they do not eat for 2 days or more. Do not allow your cat to go without eating for more than 2 days, and consult your veterinarian if any of the other problems occur before giving up or changing the diet. Cats may be especially difficult to coax to eat the trial diet. If your veterinarian approves, certain baby foods may be used for cats for the elimination diet.

It is advisable to keep a daily diary during the trial so that progress may be monitored. Many clients use a calendar to record the level of itchy behavior (scale of 1 to 10) in conjunction with the body areas the pet is targeting. In the event that your pet refuses to eat the elimination diet, your veterinarian may recommend a commercial prescription limited-antigen diet. It is important that during the elimination diet no corticosteroids (pills, drops, or creams) are administered to your pet, as these drugs may cloud the assessment of the response to the trial diet.

The elimination diet is not a balanced diet and it is not recommended that pets continue to eat the diet for longer than 10 weeks without veterinary supervision. It is not necessary for your pet to exhibit 100 per cent improvement while receiving the diet; 50 per cent improvement may be sufficient to demonstrate response to the diet trial. It is important to remember that up to 30 per cent of food-hypersensitive dogs may exhibit multiple allergies (flea allergy, environmental allergies); therefore, the response to the diet may be partial. The confirmation of food hypersensitivity is definitively determined by dietary rechallenge. It is important to avoid changes in bathing, ear treatments, oral medications. The original diet should be slowly reintroduced over 3 to 5 days and the pet monitored for increases in itching, which should return within 14 days. If the itching returns, stop feeding the original diet and revert back to feeding the elimination trial diet until your pet returns to normal. If your pet is diagnosed with a food hypersensitivity, your veterinarian will work closely with you to try to select a commercial diet that contains ingredients to which your pet is not allergic. In rare instances, pets may react to all commercial diets and must receive a home-cooked diet. Your veterinarian may consult veterinary nutritional specialists (usually located at veterinary colleges) who can provide a recipe that completely balances the home-cooked diet.

Canine Atopic Dermatitis ■ Sandra Merchant

Atopic dermatitis (allergic dermatitis, inhalant dermatitis, atopy) is an inherited predisposition to develop allergic symptoms after repeated exposure to some otherwise harmless substance, an "allergen" such as dust, dust mites, grasses, or pollen. Most dogs begin to show their allergic signs between 1 and 3 years of age. A few dogs may show clinical symptoms at 6 months of age. It is also unusual to see clinical symptoms start after 7 years of age. Because of the hereditary nature of the disease, several breeds, including golden retrievers, most terriers, Irish and English setters, Lhasa apsos, dalmatians, bulldogs, beagles, miniature schnauzers and Chinese Shar Peis, are more commonly "atopic."

Atopic animals usually rub, lick, chew, bite, or scratch at their feet, muzzle, ears, armpits, or groin, causing hair loss and reddening and thickening of the skin. In some cases, several offending substances can "add" together to cause an animal to itch where each individual substance alone would not be enough to cause an itching sensation. These substances include not only airborne allergens (e.g., pollens) but also allergens in food and allergens from parasites (e.g., fleas) and itching caused by bacterial or yeast infections of the skin. Sometimes, eliminating some but not all of the problems may cause a dog's or cat's itchiness to go away. Therefore, it is important to treat any other problems that could be making your pet itch while dealing with allergy.

Diagnosis of atopic dermatitis is based on clinical signs (areas of itching) and an *initial* seasonality to the skin problem. However, many dogs soon begin to scratch and rub year round. Specific therapy is based on the results of a skin test or blood test to detect reaction to the specific allergic substance.

Treatment can include avoidance of the substance, therapy to control the itching (symptomatic therapy), or specific therapy (desensitization vaccine) in an attempt to desensitize your pet to the specific substances to which he or she is found to be allergic.

Complete avoidance of the allergic substance may not be practical, but decreased exposure may be feasible. If your pet is allergic to pollen, decreasing the outdoor exposure especially at dusk and dawn is helpful. Your pet should never be walked through fields with high grass or weeds and should not be outside when the lawn is cut. If your pet has an allergy to fungi or molds, it should not be keep in rooms with high moisture levels (bathroom or laundry room) or allowed to be in areas of increased dust (crawl spaces under the house). Control of house dust or mites in the home can be a major undertaking, consisting of removing carpeting, covering mattresses, regular washing of the bedding, high-efficiency vacuuming, avoiding stuffed toys, and frequent damp mopping of the areas most frequented by your pet.

Antihistamines and fatty acids, when given in combination, can decrease the itching sensation in about 10 to 20 per cent of atopic pets. Your pet can take antihistamines and fatty acids for life with no long-term problems. The only side effect usually seen with antihistamines is drowsiness. Several different types of antihistamines may need to be tried to find the one that works the best. These two combined therapies (antihistamines together with fatty acids) should be given a few months before a decision is made concerning their effectiveness.

Products applied topically to the skin (shampoos, cream rinses, leave-on conditioners, gels, lotions, sprays) with anti-itch properties may also be of benefit. These products usually need to be applied daily (sprays, gels, lotions) or a few times weekly (shampoos, cream rinses, leave-on conditioners). It is most important that your pet be bathed in cool water because warm or hot water increases the itching sensation.

Steroids (e.g., prednisone, cortisone) can also be used to alleviate the itch. However, these drugs have potential side effects and are reserved for pets for which other therapy is not possible or is ineffective or to control a severe itch for a short period of time.

Desensitization vaccines can be formulated for your pet on the basis of results of a skin test or blood test. These vaccines are usually given for the lifetime of your pet. After an initial series of injections, periodic boosters are needed (every few weeks). Sixty to 80 per cent of animals improve with these vaccines. However, desensitization takes time. Improvement may not be seen for 3 to 6 months or longer. If results are not seen in 9 to 12 months, a reevaluation of the vaccine usage is necessary.

Allergies are a lifelong problem and tend not to just go away. The best chance for success is realized when you can spend the time and effort in utilizing symptomatic therapy only on your pet or while your pet is undergoing the process of desensitization. Only by trial and error can the optimal therapy be formulated. *Time and patience are the keys!*

APP

Otitis Externa ■ Sandra Merchant

Otitis externa is an inflammation or infection of the outer (external) ear canal. Many factors can cause or contribute to the development of otitis externa in dogs and cats. Parasites (e.g., ear mites, ticks), foreign bodies (e.g., grass awns, dried medication, dried wax, displaced hairs), allergic disease (canine atopic dermatitis, food allergy), and diseases causing abnormal skin renewal time (keratinization disorders) have all been implicated as factors that can cause otitis externa.

Factors that predispose an animal to develop otitis externa include ear structure (e.g., long floppy ears, heavily haired ears, long narrow ear canals), errors in treating or cleaning ears (aggressive use of Q-Tips deep in the ear canal), and diseases that obstruct the ear canal (growths, swelling of the ear canal tissue). Factors that usually cannot cause otitis externa by themselves but can be a significant problem in need of treatment are bacterial and yeast ear infections. Sometimes, in long-standing cases of otitis externa, problems can be seen in the ear past the ear drum (middle ear—otitis media), and these problems also need to be treated.

It is most important to recognize that many factors may come together in development of your pet's ear problem. Recognition and subsequent treatment of all factors are the keys to successful clinical management of the otitis externa.

A variety of tests may need to be performed, including examination of the discharge from your pet's ear under a microscope, bacterial culture of the discharge from your pet's ear, blood testing or skin testing for allergy, a dietary change to determine whether a food allergy is the cause of your pet's ear disease, and x-rays of the skull to aid in diagnosing middle ear problems.

One or more in-hospital ear cleaning procedures may need to be performed on your pet. This may be as simple as ear cleaning requiring just a few minutes with no or minimal sedation to more involved ear cleaning requiring more time and general anesthesia.

The goal of complete resolution of your pet's ear disease depends heavily on your ability to clean and medicate your pet's ears, follow through with therapy based on the results of the various tests, and faithfully return your pet for serial reevaluations at your veterinarian's clinic.

Recurrent otitis externa that is not managed properly can cause chronic irreversible changes in the ear canal, most notably a narrowing of the ear canal diameter. This narrowing does not allow medication or ear cleaning solution into the affected area and also does not allow the normal ear wax secretions to exit from the ear canal. Even though your pet's ear may seem to be improved (less discharge, less smell, less discomfort), the ear disease may not be completely resolved and premature discontinuation of therapy can be detrimental to the chances of final resolution of the ear problem.

Sometimes, the underlying problem cannot be found or corrected. In these cases, a maintenance cleaning and medicating protocol may need to be formulated for your pet. If this protocol is followed, many cases of ear disease can be controlled with minimal time and effort on your part and minimal discomfort for your pet.

Appropriate cleaning is a vital part of the overall program for appropriately addressing ear disease. The ear canal should be thoroughly cleaned of all debris before any medication is instilled in the canal. Your pet may object to having its ears cleaned initially, but better acceptance is usually seen with time. If your pet's ear canal is red and uncomfortable at the beginning of treatment, gentle but thorough cleaning helps. After filling the ear canal with the ear cleaning solution, massage of the canal helps loosen the debris and discharge. The debris can then be massaged up from the base of skull (where the ear meets the head) to a cotton ball that is seated firmly in the opening of the canal. This procedure should be repeated until debris is no longer recovered on the cotton ball. Medication is then placed in the canal and massaged down to the base of the ear. Q-Tips should never be used to clean the ear, except on the outer ear folds. The key to successful cleaning is being consistent and thorough.

Reevaluations at the clinic are also a vital part of successful clinical management. Your pet's ears may appear normal to you but may need continued medication and cleaning for complete resolution of the inflammation or infection. In addition, especially in chronic cases of otitis externa, a maintenance cleaning or medicating protocol may need to be formulated on the basis of the information obtained from the reevaluation visits.

APPENDIX 2

CONGENITAL DEFECTS OF THE CAT

Johnny D. Hoskins

GUIDE TO CONGENITAL DEFECTS OF CATS

CONDITION	BREEDS AFFECTED	REMARKS
Body Wall		
Conjoined twins		An anomaly in which two embryos or parts of embryos are attached to one another; both may be fully formed and attached at the head, thorax, or abdomen (often called Siamese twins); in other situations only one part is duplicated; kittens with two faces (diprosopus), two heads (dicephalus), or two tails
Hernia		
Diaphragmatic, peritoneopericardial and pleuroperitoneal		Peritoneopericardial hernias are more common than pleuroperitoneal hernias; presenting signs depend on amount of displaced tissue contained in the hernia
Hiatal		Defect of the phrenoesophageal liagment that allows displacement of the gastroesophageal junction forward into the thoracic cavity
Inguinal		Defect in formation of the aponeuroses of the inguinal ring and linea alba
Umbilical		Failure of normal closure of the umbilical ring; increasing abdominal pressure with advancing age forces the omentum or occasionally the intestines into the defect
Pectus excavatum		Intrusion of the sternum into the thorax; the ventral ends of the ribs turn medially to join dorsally the displaced sternebrae
Bones and Joints		
Achondroplasia		Muscle weakness and atrophy, especially of hindlimbs; limbs extremely shortened at birth; kittens usually die between 1 and 4 months of age; associated defects include storage disease of the liver and ascites
Amelia		Leglessness
Brachydactyly		Reduced size and function of outer toes
Brachury (short tail)		Condition that occurs in normally long-tailed breeds
Craniofacial abnormalities	Burmese	Commonly referred to by breeders as "head deformity"; abnormalities are often severe and incompatible with life; kittens that survive are genetic carriers of the head deformity abnormalities
Cranioschisis		Soft spots in the cranium (skull fissures); defects are apparently calvarium developmental abnormalities or persistent fontanelles
Dimelia		Duplication of an entire limb
Ectrodactyly		Agenesis of all or part of the digits of a forepaw
Ectromelia		Condition in which the scapula is the only bone of the forelimb present
Forelimb and hind limbs, arrested development	Scottish fold	Kangaroo cats; forelimbs are short, hindlimbs are long; females affected
Hip dysplasia	Siamese and other breeds	Deformity of coxofemoral joint attributed to disparity between development of the primary muscle mass and the skeleton
Osteoporosis		Condition caused by abnormal bone resorption but radiographically uniformly dense bones; kittens usually present as swimmers
Patellar luxation	Devon rex	Condition resulting from alteration of structures that maintain the normal position of patella; usually medial, being unilateral or bilateral; onset usually evident at an early age
Peromelus ascelus		Agenesis of hindlimbs
Polydactyly		Reappearance of first digit on the hindlimbs
Radial hemimelia		Complete lack of development of the radius evident as a unilateral or bilateral problem at an early age; lack of radial support for the carpus medially results in medial deviation of the paw
Sacrocaudal dysgenesis	Manx and other breeds	Malformation of sacrocaudal vertebrae
Syndactyly		Fusion of digits; single digit present
Tail, kinked		Kink is between coccygeal vertebrae at the connection of the anulus fibrosus of the bodies of the vertebrae; defect usually toward the end of the tail; corrective surgery ineffective

GUIDE TO CONGENITAL DEFECTS OF CATS *Continued*

CONDITION	BREEDS AFFECTED	REMARKS
Vertebral anomalies		Hemivertebrae are shortened or misshapen vertebrae that occur when the right and left halves of the vertebral body develop asymmetrically or fail to fuse (most common site is T7-9 area); block or fused vertebrae occur when there is incomplete segmentation of two or more adjacent vertebrae; butterfly vertebrae result because of persistence or sagittal cleavage of the notochord, leading to a sagittal cleft in the vertebral body; spinal cord compression often occurs with these vertebral anomalies
	Cardiovascular System	
Aortic stenosis		Subvalvular most common form; a ridge of fibrocartilaginous tissue is located below the aortic valve; valvular and supravalvular less common
Atrial anomalies		Seldom recognized as individual anomalies and are usually with other cardiac defects; another atrial defect is cor triatriatum, which results from persistence of the embryonic eustachian valves within the right atrium
Endocardial fibroelastosis	Burmese, Siamese	Characterized by proliferation of elastic and collagenous fibers within the endocardium; left atrium and ventricle usually exclusively involved; kittens develop lesions during the first days of life and grow slowly, may die; aortic stenosis may be present
Mitral valve malformation		Dilatation of the mitral anulus, anomalies of valve leaflets, and altered chordae tendineae and papillary muscles
Patent ductus arteriosus	Siamese, Persian, and other breeds	Condition occurring when the normal fetal vessel (ductus arteriosus) that shunts blood past the nonfunctional fetal lungs into the aorta fails to close within the first 2 to 3 days of life; associated with multiple heart defects, including septal and valvular defects
Persistent atrial standstill	Siamese, Burmese, domestic shorthair	Bradycardia of persistent atrial standstill does not respond to atropine; symptomatic cats must be treated by permanent pacemaker implantation
Persistent right aortic arch		Aorta originates from right fourth aortic arch rather than left; communication with ligamentum arteriosus results in esophageal blockage
Pulmonic stenosis		Narrowing or obstruction between the right ventricle and pulmonary trunk; although stenosis may occur in supravalvular, valvular, or subvalvular area, pulmonary stenosis attributable to valvular dysplasia is most common
Tetralogy of Fallot		Tetralogy of Fallot includes ventricular septal defect, right ventricular outflow obstruction, hypertrophy of the right ventricle, and dextropositioned aorta that accept blood from both ventricles
Tricuspid valve dysplasia		A spectrum of abnormalities, including anomalies of valve cusps, chordae tendineae, papillary muscles, and valvular tissue; enlargement of right atrium and ventricle occurs secondary to valvular incompetence
Ventricular preexcitation syndrome		An isolated abnormality that occurs in association with anatomic congenital defects
Ventricular septal defect		Usually a single defect located high in the septum just below the tricuspid and aortic valves
	Digestive System	
Anorectal defects		Imperforate anus, segmental aplasia, rectovaginal fistula, rectovestibular fistula, anovaginal cleft, and rectal urethral fistula; of these defects, imperforate anus is the most common
Brachygnathia		Upper jaw is longer than the lower jaw
Cleft palate–cleft lip complex	Siamese	Cleft lip usually occurs as a unilateral defect in the lip or in the floor of the nostril; cleft palate may be identified as offset palatal rugae on the roof of the oral cavity, incomplete fusion of the soft palate, or oronasal fistula through a cleft palate
Cricopharyngeal achalasia		Failure of cricopharyngeus muscle and part of the thyropharyngeus muscle to relax and thus permit a food bolus to move from the pharynx into the cranial esophagus
Dentition, abnormal		Disorders affecting dentition include anodontia (absence of one or more teeth), retained deciduous teeth, supranumerary teeth, dens in dente, and shape abnormalities
Lymphangiectasia, intestinal		Malformation of the lymphatic system that contributes to clinical signs reflective of protein-losing enteropathy
Intestinal anomalies		Congenital defects of intestinal tract include atresia or duplication of an intestinal sgement; usually incompatible with life unless surgically corrected
Meckel's diverticulum		Sacculation or appendage of the ileum derived from an unobliterated yolk stalk
Megacolon		Dilatation, elongation, and hypertrophy of the colon with absence of myenteric plexus; chronic constipation, abdominal distention, and anorexia presenting complaints

GUIDE TO CONGENITAL DEFECTS OF CATS *Continued*

CONDITION	BREEDS AFFECTED	REMARKS
Megaesophagus, idiopathic	Siamese and other breeds	Characterized by primary motor system disturbances of the esophagus that result in abnormal or unsuccessful transport of ingesta between the pharynx and stomach; may be associated with feline dysautonomia (Key-Gaskell syndrome—a progressively fatal autonomic polyneuropathy of young cats)
Microcheilia		Reduced oral fissure
Prognathism	Burmese, Persian (accepted breed standard)	Upper jaw is shorter than lower jaw
Pyloric stenosis	Siamese	Characterized by a narrow pyloric canal but not associated with muscular hypertrophy of the pylorus as in the dog

Ear

Deafness	Most often in white cats with blue eyes, occasionally white cats with other color eyes	Lack of or loss of the sense of hearing; congenital deafness is most common type; may be partial or complete and affect only one ear or both ears; unilateral deafness is most common form; of the electrodiagnostic techniques used for determining extent of deafness, recording of brain stem auditory evoked potentials and impedance audiometry are most frequently used; hearing loss occurs secondary to degeneration, hypoplasia, or aplasia of the spiral organ of the inner ear
Folded ears	Scottish fold	Often associated with skeletal abnormalities of the tail and lower extremities, particularly shortening of the coccygeal vertebrae; claws frequently overgrow
Four ears		Bilateral small extra pinnas on the sides of the head; often associated with microphthalmia and micrognathia

Endocrine and Metabolic Systems

Diabetes insipidus		Hypothalamic-neurohypophyseal in origin; signs in kittens are usually restricted to polyuria and polydipsia
Diabetes mellitus		May become evident as early as first 6 months of life; pancreatic lesions include atrophy of beta cells and associated noninflammatory atrophy of a few acinar cells; affected individuals usually exhibit failure to grow in addition to the polyphagia and soft or diarrheic stools
Hyperchylomicronemia	Domestic shorthair, Himalayan, Persian, Siamese	Results from enzyme deficiency, lipoprotein lipase; signs result from the fasting hyperlipemia, lipemia retinalis, and peripheral neuropathy
Hypoparathyroidism		Results from absence of parathyroid tissue; signs are related to the presence of severe hypocalcemia, signs classically include muscle tremors, twitches, and tetany
Hypothyroidism		Results from thyroid dysgenesis, circulating thyroid hormone transport abnormalities, dyshormonogenesis, congenital thyroid-stimulating hormone deficiency, and severe iodine deficiency; congenital defects probably cause early kitten death and thus go unrecognized
Neonatal hypoglycemia		Occurs during the nursing period because of inadequate glycogen or protein substrate stores or immature liver enzyme systems; also occurs from failure to adapt to fasting during the post weaning period; signs are related to severity
Porphyria	Domestic shorthair, Siamese	Overproduction of porphyrins with accumulation in bones and teeth and excretion in feces and urine; color is brown, turning red under a fluorescent light

Eye

Aberrant canthal dermis		Encroachment of dermis at the nasal canthus on bulbar and palpebral conjunctiva
Agenesis of the eyelid	Domestic shorthair, Persian	Absence of varying segments of the eyelid margin, usually temporal one third of the upper eyelid
Anophthalmos		Complete absence of the globe
Aphakia		Congenital absence of the lens; usually occurs with other ocular defects
Blepharophimosis		Abnormal narrowing of the space between the eyelids
Cataracts	Domestic shorthair, Persian, Birman, Himalayan	In animals younger than 6 months of age are classified as either congenital or juvenile; congenital cataracts are present at birth, although they may not be noticed until 6 to 8 weeks of age, and may be inherited or secondary to in utero influences, so it is essential to question the owner regarding presence of cataracts in the sire, dam, previous litters, or their pedigrees; juvenile cataracts develop from newborn period until 6 years of age; heredity is major factor, although other causes may contribute to juvenile cataract formation; course of juvenile cataracts usually progressive, but rate at which progression occurs varies; complete opacification of the lens may occur in less than 1 year after diagnosis; if functional vision is present, congenital or juvenile cataracts in kittens may undergo spontaneous resorption within the first year
Corneal dystrophy	Manx, domestic shorthair	Typically manifested early in life, usually bilateral, and shows a preference for the central cornea

APP

GUIDE TO CONGENITAL DEFECTS OF CATS *Continued*

CONDITION	BREEDS AFFECTED	REMARKS
Dermoid	Birman, Burmese, domestic shorthair	First noticed as skinlike appendage soon after the eyelids open; usually involves cornea and lateral limbal area and affects one eye or both
Districhiasis		Extra row of eyelashes that protrude from orifices of meibomian glands within the intermarginal space of the eyelid; upper, lower, or both eyelids may be involved
Divergent strabismus		First noted when eyelids open; normal ocular alignment develops during the second postnatal month
Ectopic cilia	Siamese	Abnormal location for cilia
Enophthalmos		Recession of the globe within the orbit; most often associated with microphthalmos
Entropion	Persian	Inward deviation of the eyelid; lower eyelid is more commonly affected because of poorly formed tarsal plate
Glaucoma	Siamese, domestic shorthair	Pressure increase occurring within the first year of life is rare
Heterochromia	Persian, Angora	Variation in iris color; occurs commonly in subalbinotic animals; variations in tapetal development and degree of pigmentation in the retinal pigment epithelium and choroid may occur simultaneously
Iris cyst		Identified by their spherical shape and tendency to be attached at the pupillary margin
Microcornea		Affected eyes have more bulbar conjunctiva exposed medially and laterally but no apparent visual problems
Microphakia	Domestic shorthair, Siamese	Margin of the abnormally small lens along with elongated ciliary processes in microphakia may be seen after pupillary dilatation
Microphthalmos		Failure of the globe to develop to normal size; characterized by varying degrees of enophthalmos with or without other ocular defects; commonly associated with other ocular defects including colobomas, persistent pupillary membranes, cataract, equatorial staphylomas, choroidal hypoplasia, retinal dysplasia and detachment, and optic nerve hypoplasia; vision often impaired
Nystagmus, spontaneous	Siamese	Results from an anomalous visual pathway development
Optic nerve colobomas		Pits or excavations in the optic disk; may occur as a single lesion or accompany multiple ocular defects
Optic nerve hypoplasia, aplasia	Domestic shorthair	Poor vision is common in bilaterally affected animals, although owners usually fail to recognize the vision deficit while the animal is with its siblings; unilateral lesions often incidental findings, as the kitten compensates with the unaffected eye; affected eyes exhibit sluggish to absent direct pupillary light reflexes; resting pupil size may be larger than normal; affected optic disk often less than half its normal size, its center is depressed, and periphery is pigmented
Persistent pupillary membranes		Arise from anterior iris surface and represent remnants of embryonic vascular system
Pupillary anomalies		Ventronasal, notchlike defect (coloboma) in pupillary border results in keyhole-shaped pupil; eccentric pupil (corectopia) may accompany multiple ocular defects
Retinal degeneration, atrophy	Siamese, Persian, Abyssinian	Initial retinal lesions appear as focal areas of tapetal hyperreflectivity; later, lesions coalesce into diffuse retinal degeneration
Retinal dysplasia		Characterized by folds in outer retinal layers and by retinal rosettes, in which variably differentiated retinal cells are arranged around central lumen; more severe forms of retinal dysplasia may demonstrate retinal detachment attributable to subretinal fluid accumulation; may occur alone or in association with other congenital ocular defects
Strabismus, convergent	Siamese	Results from a limited ability to process spatially coordinated binocular information, an ability on which normal ocular alignment depends
Tapetal hypoplasia		Lack of visible tapetum and uniform reddish brown fundus reflex evident
Trichiasis		Condition in which otherwise normal eyelashes are deviated from their normal position, allowing contact between the deviated eyelash and the cornea

Hematopoietic, Immune, and Lymphatic Systems

CONDITION	BREEDS AFFECTED	REMARKS
Anasarca		Affected individuals with anasarca have generalized subcutaneous edema and fluid accumulation
Anomaly of neutrophil granulation	Birman	Neutrophils have fine eosinophilic granules that resemble primary granules; neutrophil function in affected cats is normal
Chédiak-Higashi syndrome	Persian and other breeds	Characterized by partial oculocutaneous albinism (lightly colored irides and fundic hypopigmentation), enlarged granules in leukocytes and melanocytes, early development of cataracts, and a bleeding tendency
Coagulation protein disorders Factor XII		Not associated with a bleeding diathesis; affected individuals may be predisposed to infection and/or thrombosis

GUIDE TO CONGENITAL DEFECTS OF CATS *Continued*

CONDITION	BREEDS AFFECTED	REMARKS
Factor IX (hemophilia B)	British shorthair, Siamese, domestic shorthair	Sex-linked hemorrhagic disorder; excessive bleeding from umbilical cord is common sign; hemarthrosis, gingival bleeding during tooth eruption, and spontaneous hematoma formation are other typical manifestations
Factor VIII:C (hemophilia A)		One of the most common inherited coagulopathies; defect in cats is mild compared with that in other species; bleeding tendencies are same as for factor IX deficiency
Factor VIII (von Willebrand's disease)	Himalyan and other breeds	Attributable to defective or deficient factor VIII–related antigen (von Willebrand's factor); bleeding tendencies are same as for factor IX deficiency
Lymphedema		Primary lymphedema attributable to developmental abnormalities within lymphatic system; lymphatic channels may be aplastic, hypoplastic, or hyperplastic; lymph nodes may be normal, hypocellular, or absent; characterized by soft, pitting, nonpainful edema of one or more extremities, usually involving hindlimbs; rarely, abdominal or pleural effusions may develop
Mucopolysaccharidosis	Domestic shorthair, Siamese	Results from deficiencies of α-L-iduronidase (mucopolysaccharidosis I) and arylsulfatase B (mucopolysaccharidosis VI); granules in neutrophils are commonly seen in mucopolysaccharidosis VI and stain with toluidine blue; granules in neutrophils seen in mucopolysaccharidosis I do not stain with Wright's stain or toluidine blue but may be present ultrastructurally; excessive glycosaminoglycans can be detected in the urine of cats with both types of mucopolysaccharidosis by the toluidine (Berry) spot test
Pelger-Huët anomaly		Decreased lobulation of granulocytic cells; abnormal nuclear shape may contribute to reduced cell mobility and abnormal chemotaxis; not all affected animals have chemotactic defects, and none has increased risk of infection
Thrombopathia		Intrinsic platelet disorder; affected animals exhibit signs typical of quantitative and qualitative platelet defects, including epistaxis, gingival bleeding, and petechiation; characterized by abnormal fibrinogen receptor exposure and impaired dense granule release
Thymic aplasia	Birman	Affected individuals with thymic atrophy can be detected within 1 to 3 months of age; signs include stunted growth, chronic wasting, and suppurative pneumonia
Thymic branchial cyst		Arises from remnants of branchial pouch epithelium, the embryonic precursor of thymic tissue; occurs in thymus or subcutis of the neck

Liver

CONDITION	BREEDS AFFECTED	REMARKS
Biliary atresia		Failure of the biliary tract to develop creates incomplete functional connection between liver and duodenum
Gallbladder anomalies		Congenital malformations include trilobed or biloped gallbladders; development of two separated gallbladders with cystic ducts united in a common duct; ductular bladders developing as supernumerary vesicles derived from either hepatic, cystic, or common bile ducts; and trabecular bladders derived from vesicular outgrowths of liver trabeculae
Hepatic cysts		May be parenchymal or ductal in origin; most are of ductular origin, arising from one or more primitive bile ducts lacking connection with biliary tract and subsequently developing into retention cysts
Intrahepatic arterioportal fistulas		Result from failure of the common embryologic anlage to differentiate; contribute to portal hypertension and shunting through multiple portosystemic collaterals and ascites
Portosystemic venous shunts Intrahepatic		Most often remnant of fetal ductus venosus that remains patent; other large intrahepatic venous communications may be present; ductus venosus is embryonic venous channel originating from umbilical vein that traverses liver and drains into left hepatic vein and then into caudal vena cava
Extrahepatic	Domestic shorthair and longhair, Himalayan, Persian, Siamese	Left gastric vein is frequently the shunting vessel in the cat; shunt may also occur between portal vein and postcava or between portal vein and azygous vein; complete absence of portal vein entry into liver is unusual

Nervous System

CONDITION	BREEDS AFFECTED	REMARKS
Cranial dysraphism		Defects occurring because of faulty closure of the neural tube; conditions that may be seen in association with cranial dysraphism include anencephaly (brain is absent at birth or more commonly only the basal nuclei and cerebellum are well developed), exencephaly (brain is exposed as result of congenital cleft in skull), cranium bifida (open cleft in skull), encephalocele and meningocele (brain or meninges, respectively, protrude through congenital cleft in skull), and cyclopia (developmental anomaly characterized by single orbital fossa, with either complete or partial agenesis of the globe)

APP

GUIDE TO CONGENITAL DEFECTS OF CATS *Continued*

CONDITION	BREEDS AFFECTED	REMARKS
Cerebellar hypoplasia		Uniform forms of cerebellar hypoplasia in which clinical signs of cerebellar dysfunction are present at birth and do not progress; most commonly associated with feline panleukopenia virus infection
Hydrocephalus	Simaese and other breeds	Excessive accumulation of cerebrospinal fluid within the skull; the terms *internal* and *external* denote excess fluid within or outside the ventricular system, respectively; congenital forms may occur because of structural defects that either obstruct cerebrospinal fluid outflow at the mesencephalic aqueduct or impede cerebrospinal fluid absorption
Lysosomal storage diseases		
Ceroid lipofuscinosis	Siamese	Results from unknown enzyme deficiency
GM$_1$ gangliosidosis	Siamese, Korat, domestic shorthair	Results from enzyme deficiency, β-galactosidase
GM$_2$ gangliosidosis	Domestic shorthair, Korat	Results from enzyme deficiency, β-hexosaminidase; neuronal degeneration results from an excessive accumulation of GM$_2$ ganglioside in the cerebral cortex; seen at 2 to 4 months of age; manifested as incoordination, tremors, and quadriplegia
Globoid cell leukodystropy	Domestic shorthair	Results from enzyme deficiency, β-galactocerebrosidase; demyelinating leukoencephalopathy characterized by progressive deterioration; onset at 2 weeks of age; signs include a piercing cry, ataxia, and visual impairment; opisthotonos and hindlimb paralysis precede death at 6 weeks of age
Glycogenosis	Domestic shorthair, Norwegian forest	Results from enzyme deficiency, α-glucosidase
Mannosidosis	Domestic shorthair, Persian	Results from enzyme deficiency, α-mannosidase
Metachromatic leukodystrophy	Domestic shorthair	Results from enzyme deficiency, arylsulfate
Mucopolysaccharidosis I	Domestic shorthair, Siamese, Korat	Results from enzyme deficiency, α-L-iduronidase
Mucopolysaccharidosis VI	Siamese	Results from enzyme deficiency, arylsulfate B
Sphingomyelinosis	Domestic shorthair, Siamese, Balinese	Results from enzyme deficiency, sphingomyelinase
Narcolepsy-cataplexy		Excessive daytime sleep (narcolepsy); periods of acute muscular hypotonia often seen in association with narcolepsy (cataplexy)
Neuroaxonal dystrophy	Tricolor breeds	Marked axonal distention (axonal spheroids) in central nervous system; signs are typical of cerebellar disease which usually begin at 5 to 6 weeks of age and progress in affected kittens
Neuropathy	Birman	Diffuse loss of myelinated fibers in peripheral nerves, spinal cord, and cerebellum resulting in paraparesis between 8 and 10 weeks of age
Spina bifida	Manx, Maltese and crossbred Siamese, rare in other breeds	Closure defect of vertebral arches, sometimes associated with dysplasia or protrusion of the meninges and/or spinal cord; signs are taillessness, a hypermetric gait, and fecal and urinary incontinence
Spongiform encephalopathies	Egyptian Mau	Manifested by multifocal neurologic dysfunction and marked vacuolation of central nervous system white matter
Vestibular disorders	Siamese, Burmese	Affected animals have signs of vestibular dysfunction, including head tilt, circling, and rolling at birth or within a few weeks; defect may be unilateral or bilateral; signs do not progress or resolve although some compensation may occur

Neuromuscular System and Muscles

Fibrodysplasia ossificans progressiva		Characterized by progressive stiffness of gait, with enlargement of proximal limb musculature; radiography reveals multiple mineralized densities within the affected musculature
Hereditary myopathy	Dexon rex	Characterized by progressive ventroflexion of the head and neck, dorsal protrusion of the scapulas, megaesophagus, generalized appendicular weakness, and fatigability; may be first noted at 3 weeks of age and older
Myasthenia gravis	Siamese, domestic shorthair	Leads to failure of neuromuscular transmission because of congenital deficiency of acetylcholine receptors in postsynaptic membrane; may be first noted at 6 to 9 weeks of age and older
Nemaline myopathy		Affected cats first show stilted gait, reluctance to walk, and simultaneous advancement of pelvic limbs (hypermetric gait) at 6 to 18 months of age
X-linked muscular dystrophy	Siamese, European and domestic shorthair	Affected cats first show stilted gait and simultaneous advancement of pelvic limbs (bunny hop) at 6 to 9 weeks of age

Reproductive System

Amastia		Absence of mammae
Aplasia of the duct system		Failure of any part of testicular duct system to develop results in impaired transportation of spermatozoa to urethra, accumulation of sperm proximal to obstruction, and potential development of sperm granuloma and testicular degeneration
Chimeras		
True hermaphrodite		True hermaphrodites have both ovarian and testicular tissue present in same individual; true hermaphrodite chimeras have either XX/XY or XX/XXY chromosome constitutions, enlarged clitoris, little testicular tissue, and external female appearance

GUIDE TO CONGENITAL DEFECTS OF CATS *Continued*

CONDITION	BREEDS AFFECTED	REMARKS
XX/XY chimeras with testes		External genital opening with cranially displaced vulvalike structure, hypoplastic penis contained in vulva-like structure, no external scrotum or testes (testes are located near caudal pole of kidneys), and bicornuate uterus
Chromosomal number abnormalities XXY syndrome	Tricolor cats	Recognized readily in tortoiseshell cats; normal male external phenotype with abnormal chromosome constitution has small testes with seminiferous tubular dysgenesis and no evidence of spermatogenesis
XO syndrome		Occurs in females that have normal phenotype and not cycled by 24 months of age
Triple-X syndrome		Occurs in females that have normal phenotype, underdeveloped genitalia, and not cycled by 24 months of age
Cryptorchidism		Normally, feline testes descend to scrotum by 10 days after birth; if both testes are not within the scrotum by 8 weeks of age, diagnosis of cryptorchidism is warranted; both males and females may carry gene for cryptorchidism and pass to offspring; heterozygous males, heterozygous females, and homozygous females are phenotypically normal carriers; only homozygous males are cryptorchid
Hypospadias		Abnormality in location of urinary orifice, being ventral and proximal to normal site in glans penis; urinary orifice may be located in glans penis (mild hypospadias), the penile shaft (moderate hypospadias), or penoscrotal junction, scrotum, or perineum (severe hypospadias); may be accompanied by cryptorchidism, scrotal abnormalities, persistent müllerian structures, and intersexuality
Os penis deformity		May result in deviation of penis and, depending on severity, inability to retract penis fully into preputial sheath; persistent exposure of portion of glans penis results in desiccation, trauma, or necrosis
Ovarian agenesis		Absence of one or both ovaries
Ovarian hypoplasia		Abnormal development of the ovarian germinal epithelium; results in sterility; may be unilateral or bilateral and usually first noticed soon after puberty
Prepuce anomaly		Abnormal shortening of prepuce results in persistent exposure of glans penis; may result in desiccation, trauma, or necrosis
Pseudohermaphroditism Female		Female hermaphrodite has XX chromosome constitution and ovaries but internal or external genitalia are masculinized
Male		Male hermaphrodite has XY chromosome constitution and testes but internal or external genitalia are to some degree those of female
Testicular hypoplasia		Abnormal development of the seminiferous tubular germinal epithelium; results in oligospermia or azoospermia and sterility; may be unilateral or bilateral and usually first noticed soon after puberty
Umbilical cord aplasia		Lack of development of a umbilical cord
Vaginal atresia		Absence or closure of the vagina
Vulvar atresia		Absence of the vulva
Respiratory System		
Bronchial cartilage hypoplasia		Seen during first several months of life, usually as severe respiratory distress
Bronchoesophageal fistula		Connection between esophagus and airways that may allow saliva and ingested material to enter into lungs
Laryngeal hypoplasia		Incompletely developed larynx; signs, when present, vary with degree of laryngeal narrowing
Nares, agenesis	Burmese	Predisposes to laryngeal collapse by causing formation of a partial vacuum with inspiration; dyspnea, mouth breathing, and snoring sounds are common
Tracheal collapse		Occurs because malformations of tracheal rings cause dorsoventral flattening of trachea
Unilateral agenesis of lung		Absence of lung on one side of thorax or a lung lobe
Skin		
Alopecia universalis	Sphinx, Canadian hairless	Generalized lack of hair coverage; adnexal abnormalities concurrently not present
Aplasia cutis (epitheliogenesis imperfecta)		Discontinuity of squamous epithelium; present at birth as glistening red, well-demarcated defect in skin; defect is covered with one to three layers of flat to cuboidal epithelium and a stroma devoid of all adnexa
Cutaneous asthenia (Ehlers-Danlos syndrome, dominant collagen dysplasia, dermal fragility syndrome, dermatosparaxis)	Himalayan and other breeds	Connective tissue disease characterized by loose, hyperextensive, and abnormally fragile skin easily torn by minor trauma

APP

GUIDE TO CONGENITAL DEFECTS OF CATS *Continued*

CONDITION	BREEDS AFFECTED	REMARKS
Hypotrichosis	Sphinx, Cornish and Devon rexes, Mexican hairless, Siamese, Birman	Incomplete ectodermal defect in that affected individuals have remnants of hair follicles and other epidermal appendages in skin; small amount of hair present at birth is lost by 2 weeks of age; hair regrows again at 6 weeks with complete loss by 6 months of age; only guard hairs and down hairs develop
Nevi		Circumscribed developmental defect in skin; when nevus forms a hyperplastic mass, it is referred to as hamartoma; various other types include sebaceous, hyperpigmented epidermal, and mucocutaneous angiomatous nevi
Rex mutant	Rex	Kittens have wavy, wooly hair; adults develop short, curly plush hair; guard hairs and vibrissae are absent or normal
Seborrhea oleosa	Persian	Recognized in kittens days or weeks after birth; greasy and scaly haircoat with rancid odor
Tricolor coats		Tricolored cats possess white, black, and orange hairs blended together (tortoiseshell) or in large patches (calico)

Urinary System

CONDITION	BREEDS AFFECTED	REMARKS
Ectopic ureter		May occur unilaterally or bilaterally and may be associated with other urinary tract anomalies; affected individuals, mostly females, have history of incontinence since birth or weaning
Malposition of urinary bladder (pelvic bladder)		Caudal malposition of urinary bladder; may be cause of urinary incontinence and is associated with other urinary tract abnormalities
Renal defects		
Agenesis or absence of kidneys		Can be unilateral or bilateral and is usually accompanied by associated ureteral aplasia; right kidney is more commonly affected than the left; is fatal if bilateral and a recognized cause of fading kitten syndrome
Amyloidosis	Abyssinian	Renal function in affected individuals varies depending on degree and duration of renal involvement; advanced signs of renal failure eventually occur and are typically associated with severe proteinuria and hypoproteinemia
Fusion (horseshoe) kidney		Fusion of embryonic kidneys; usually incidental finding and not associated with reduced renal function
Polycystic kidneys	Persian	Characterized by variable number of fluid-filled cysts in renal parenchyma, ranging from extremely small to massive; affected individuals may be asymptomatic or show evidence of rapidly progressing renal failure
Primary hyperoxaluria	Domestic shorthair	Signs result from acute renal failure caused by renal tubular deposition of oxalate crystals in combination with profound generalized lower motor neuron weakness
Renal duplication		Usually an incidental finding and not associated with clinical signs of altered renal function
Renal ectopia		Arrest in normal embryonic ascent of kidney; kidney appears as caudal abdominal mass within pelvis or in sublumbar area; usually incidental finding and not associated with reduced renal function
Urachal anomalies		Vary from complete persistence of urachus with communication between urinary bladder and umbilicus to blind cysts to cranioventral urachal diverticulum
Ureterocele		Dilatation of submucosal segment of intravesical ureter resulting in bulging of dilated segment into urinary bladder
Urethral anomalies		Include hypospadias (urethral opening on underside of penis or on perineum), imperforate urethra, ectopic urethra, urethral aplasia (associated with penile aplasia), duplicate urethra, and urethrorectal fistula
Urinary bladder anomalies		Include exstrophy of urinary bladder (absence of ventral abdominal body wall and ventral bladder wall), duplication of urinary bladder, and agenesis of urinary bladder

APPENDIX 3

CONGENITAL DEFECTS OF THE DOG

Johnny D. Hoskins

GUIDE TO CONGENITAL DEFECTS OF DOGS

CONDITION	BREEDS AFFECTED	REMARKS
	Body Wall	
Conjoined twins		An anomaly in which two embryos or parts of embryos are attached to one another; both may be fully formed and attached at the head, thorax, or abdomen (often called Siamese twins); in other situations only one part is duplicated; puppies with two faces (diprosopus), two heads (dicephalus), or two tails
Hernia		
Diaphragmatic, peritoneopericardial and pleuroperitoneal	Weimaraner, German shepherd	Peritoneopericardial hernias are more common than pleuroperitoneal hernias; presenting signs depend on amount of displaced tissue contained in the hernia
Hiatal	Brachycephalic breeds and Chinese Shar Pei	Defect of the phrenoesophageal ligament that allows displacement of the gastroesophageal junction forward into the thoracic cavity
Inguinal	Basset hound, cairn terrier, basenji, Pekingese, West Highland white terrier	Defect in formation of the aponeuroses of the inguinal ring and linea alba
Umbilical	Airedale terrier, basenji, Pekingese, pointer, Weimaraner	Failure of normal closure of the umbilical ring; increasing abdominal pressure with advancing age forces the omentum or occasionally the intestines into the defect
Pectus excavatum	Many breeds	Intrusion of the sternum into the thorax; the ventral ends of the ribs turn medially to join dorsally the displaced sternebrae
	Bones and Joints	
Achondroplasia		
Appendicular	Basset hound, dachshund, miniature poodle, Scottish terrier	Cartilage of epiphyseal plate grows in irregular directions and is scant
Axial	Poodle, Scottish terrier	Chondrodystrophia fetalis
Anury	Cocker spaniel, English bulldog	Absence of one to all caudal vertebrae
Bone cysts	Doberman pinscher	Single or multilocular fluid-filled spaces found in the metaphyseal, epiphyseal, or diaphyseal regions of long bones
Brachydactyly	Many breeds	Reduced size and function of outer toes
Brachury (short tail)	Beagle, cocker spaniel, English bulldog, toy griffon	Condition that occurs in normally longer tailed breeds
Carpal subluxation	Labrador retriever, Irish setter	Condition that occurs bilaterally and is limited to the carporadial joints; appears when puppies begin to walk at about 3 weeks of age
Cartilaginous exostosis	German shepherd, Alaskan malamute, Yorkshire terrier	Radiographically visualized as localized osteochondromatous outgrowths protruding from long bones, scapula, ilium, cervical and thoracic vertebrae, metatarsus, and phalanges
Cervical calcinosis circumscripta	Great Dane	Calcinosis masses typically attach to tendons inserting on lateral processes of C4 and C5 just below muscle; histopathologic examination reveals dense collagen, granulomatous reaction, and islands of trabecular bone and marrow
Cervical vertebral instability (wobbler syndrome)	Basset hound, Doberman pinscher, English sheepdog, fox terrier, Great Dane, Irish setter, Rhodesian ridgeback, Saint Bernard	Condition that exists when the ventral spinal canal is narrower dorsoventrally than the dorsal canal between C3 and C7; deformed vertebral bodies result in spinal neurosis; in basset hounds, a malformed C2–3 may be involved
Chondrodysplasia (dwarfism)	Alaskan malamute, Shetland sheepdog, Labrador retriever	Stunted forelegs, lateral deviation of paws, and sloping top line attributable to impaired endochondral bone growth
Craniomandibular osteopathy	West Highland white terrier, Scottish terrier, cairn terrier, Labrador retriever, Great Dane, Doberman pinscher, English bulldog, Boxer	Proliferations of bones of skull and mandible that reduces jaw motion
Cranioschisis	Cocker spaniel	Soft spots in the cranium (skull fissures); defects are apparently calvarium developmental abnormalities or persistent fontanelles
Dimelia	Many breeds	Duplication of an entire limb
Ectromelia	Pointer	Condition in which the scapula is the only bone of the forelimb present

APP

GUIDE TO CONGENITAL DEFECTS OF DOGS *Continued*

CONDITION	BREEDS AFFECTED	REMARKS
Elbow dysplasia (see ununited anconeal process)		
Elbow luxation	Yorkshire terrier, Boston terrier, miniature poodle, English bulldog, Pomeranian, Chinese pug	Results from an embryonic failure in formation of intra-articular ligaments
Epiphyseal dysplasia	Beagle, poodle	Characterized by stippling defects of the epiphyseal sites; abnormal movement of the hindlimbs and a swaying gait result
Foramen magnum dysplasia	Chihuahua, cocker spaniel, Skye terrier	Characterized by malformation of the occipital bone with enlargement of the foramen magnum and exposure of the cerebellum and brain stem; hydrocephalus may be present
Hip dysplasia	Primarily large and giant breeds; also cocker spaniel and Shetland sheepdog	Deformity of coxofemoral joint attributed to disparity between development of the primary muscle mass and the skeleton; onset of hip dysplasia most frequent at 5 months of age
Legg-Calvé-Perthes disease (aseptic femoral head necrosis)	Small breeds, including Manchester terrier, Pekingese, poodle, Chinese pug, schnauzer, wirehaired fox terrier	Characterized by increase in trabecular bone of the femoral head followed by aseptic necrosis secondary to ischemia; revascularization of the bone is followed by demineralization
Lumbosacral malarticulation (stenosis)	German shepherd	Condition in which compression is created on the cauda equina; attributable to subluxation, stenosis, or spondylosis of the lumbosacral articulation
Mucopolysaccharidosis	Miniature pinscher, Plott hound, mixed breed	Condition that results in epiphyseal dysplasia, decreased long bone growth, dysostosis, degenerative joint disease, hepatomegaly, large tongue, and corneal clouding
Odontoid process dysplasia (nonunion with C2)	Chihuahua, Pekingese, Pomeranian, poodle, Yorkshire terrier	Condition that results in atlantoaxial subluxation; signs vary from neck pain to quadriplegia
Osteoporosis	Dachshund	Condition caused by abnormal bone resorption but radiographically uniformly dense bones; puppies usually present as swimmers
Panosteitis (enostosis)	German shepherd, basset hound, and other breeds	Excessive formation of bone in various states of maturity of the ulna, humerus, radius, femur, and tibia, and excessive osteoblastic activity with formation of new bone by fibrous metaplasia; radiographically evident as opacity in the area of the nutrient foramen, intermittent leg lameness at 6 to 12 months of age
Patellar luxation	Toy and miniature breeds	Condition resulting from alteration of structures that maintain the normal position of patella; usually medial, being unilateral or bilateral; onset usually evident at 4 to 6 months of age
Polydactyly	Many breeds	Reappearance of first digit on the hindlimbs
Radial agenesis	Many breeds	Complete lack of development of the radius evident as a unilateral or bilateral problem at an early age; lack of radial support for the carpus medially results in medial deviation of the paw
Radial dysplasia (premature closure of radius)	Many breeds	When the distal radial physis prematurely closes, one side of the radius usually continues to grow while the other side closes; resultant deformity is angulation of the carpus and metacarpal bones toward the closed side; closure of the proximal radial physis results in progressive separation of the radial head from the distal humerus
Short spine	Greyhound, Shiba Ina	Abnormal development produces short vertebral column, kyphosis, and scoliosis; high shoulders and back sloping sharply to the tail are seen
Shoulder luxation	Chihuahua, griffon, Cavalier King Charles spaniel, miniature pinscher, miniature poodle, Pomeranian, wirehaired fox terrier	First occurs at 3 to 4 months of age; in severely affected individuals, may lead to medial shoulder luxation at an early age; radiographs confirm shoulder luxation if a flexed and rotated view of the shoulder region is taken
Spina bifida	Beagle, English and French bulldog, Boston terrier, Chinese pug	Condition resulting from defective fusion of vertebral arches
Syndactyly	Many breeds	Fusion of digits; single digit present
Ulnar dysplasia (premature closure of ulna)	Many breeds	When the distal ulnar physis closes prematurely, majority of ulnar lengthening stops while the radius grows unabated; the resultant deformity is progressive bowing and twisting of the radius, as the ulna acts as a bowstring
Ununited anconeal process (elbow dysplasia)	German shepherd, Labrador retriever, basset hound, French bulldog, Great Dane, bull mastiff, Great Pyrenees, Irish wolfhound, Weimaraner, Newfoundland	Failure of normal fusion of anconeal process to diaphysis of ulna; may be unilateral or bilateral; stunted and usually loose process contributes to elbow joint laxity and synovitis that produce progressive arthritic changes; frequently inapparent until secondary arthritis has occurred
Vertebral anomalies	Boston terrier, English and French bulldogs, Pomeranian, Chinese pug, German shorthaired pointer, Yorkshire terrier	Hemivertebrae are shortened or misshapen vertebrae that occur when the right and left halves of the vertebral body develop asymmetrically or fail to fuse (most common site is T7–9 area); block or fused vertebrae occur when there is incomplete segmentation of two or more adjacent vertebrae; butterfly vertebrae result because of persistence or sagittal cleavage of the notochord, leading to a sagittal cleft in the vertebral body; spinal cord compression often occurs with these vertebral anomalies

GUIDE TO CONGENITAL DEFECTS OF DOGS *Continued*

CONDITION	BREEDS AFFECTED	REMARKS
Cardiovascular System		
Aortic stenosis	Newfoundland, Boxer, German shepherd, German shorthaired pointer, golden retriever, rottweiler	Subvalvular most common form; a ridge of fibrocartilaginous tissue is located below the aortic valve; valvular and supravalvular less common
Atrial anomalies	Boxer and other breeds	Seldom recognized as individual anomalies and are usually with other cardiac defects; another atrial defect is cor triatriatum, which results from persistence of the embryonic eustachian valves within the right atrium
Endocardial fibroelastosis	Many breeds	Characterized by proliferation of elastic and collagenous fibers within the endocardium; left atrium and ventricle usually exclusively involved
Mitral valve malformation	Great Dane, German shepherd, English bulldog, Chihuahua, bull terrier, golden retriever, Newfoundland	Dilatation of the mitral anulus, anomalies of valve leaflets, and altered chordae tendineae and papillary muscles
Patent ductus arteriosus	Poodle, Pomeranian, collie, German shepherd, Shetland sheepdog, English springer spaniel, keeshond, Maltese, bichon frisé, Yorkshire terrier	Condition occurring when the normal fetal vessel (ductus arteriosus) that shunts blood past the nonfunctional fetal lungs into the aorta fails to close within the first 2 to 3 days of life
Persistent atrial standstill	English springer spaniel	Bradycardia of persistent atrial standstill does not respond to atropine; symptomatic dogs must be treated by permanent pacemaker implantation
Persistent right aortic arch	German shepherd, Irish setter, Great Dane	Aorta originates from right fourth aortic arch rather than left; communication with ligamentum arteriosus results in esophageal blockage
Pulmonic stenosis	Beagle, English bulldog, Chihuahua, fox terrier, Samoyed, miniature schnauzer, keeshond, mastiff, Boxer, Newfoundland	Narrowing or obstruction between the right ventricle and pulmonary trunk; although stenosis may occur in supravalvular, valvular, or subvalvular area, pulmonary stenosis attributable to valvular dysplasia is most common
Stenosis of atrioventricular bundle (bundle of His)	Chinese pug	Individuals with stenosis of atrioventricular bundle have syncopal attacks that begin during the first several months of life
Tetralogy of Fallot	Keeshond, English bulldog	Tetralogy of Fallot includes ventricular septal defect, right ventricular outflow obstruction, hypertrophy of the right ventricle, and dextropositioned aorta that accepts blood from both ventricles
Tricuspid valve dysplasia	Great Dane, Weimaraner	A spectrum of abnormalities, including anomalies of valve cusps, chordae tendineae, papillary muscles, and valvular tissue; enlargement of right atrium and ventricle occurs secondary to valvular incompetence
Ventricular preexcitation syndrome	Many breeds	An isolated abnormality that occurs in association with anatomic congenital defects
Ventricular septal defect	English bulldog, English springer spaniel, keeshond	Usually a single defect located high in the septum just below the tricuspid and aortic valves
Digestive System		
Anorectal defects	Many breeds	Atresia ani, segmental aplasia, rectovaginal fistula, rectovestibular fistula, anovaginal cleft, and rectal urethral fistula; of these defects, imperforate anus is the most common
Brachygnathism	Many breeds, Brussels griffon, dachshund, Chinese Shar Pei	Upper jaw is longer than the lower jaw
Cleft palate–cleft lip complex	Brachycephalic breeds, beagle, cocker spaniel, dachshund, Shetland sheepdog, schnauzer, Labrador retriever, German shepherd	Cleft lip usually occurs as a unilateral defect in the lip or in the floor of the nostril; cleft palate may be identified as offset palatal rugae on the roof of the oral cavity, incomplete fusion of the soft palate, or oronasal fistula through a cleft palate
Cricopharyngeal achalasia	Toy breeds	Failure of cricopharyngeus muscle and part of the thyropharyngeus muscle to relax and thus permit a food bolus to move from the pharynx into the cranial esophagus
Dentition, abnormal	Many breeds	Disorders affecting dentition include anodontia (absence of one or more teeth), retained deciduous teeth, supranumerary teeth, dens in dente, and shape abnormalities
Elongated soft palate	Brachycephalic breeds, affenpinscher, chow chow	Disorder contributes to exercise and heat intolerance and abnormal oropharyngeal function
Enteropathy	Chinese Shar Pei	Defect in small intestinal mucosal function associated with bouts of intermittent diarrhea and poor weight gain or weight loss
Esophageal diverticula	Many breeds	Segments of the esophagus typically involved with diverticula are areas just cranial to the thoracic inlet and diaphragm; periodic diverticularization of the esophagus at the thoracic inlet is considered to be a normal finding for most young English bulldogs
Lymphangiectasia, intestinal	Many breeds, Norwegian Lundehunde	Malformation of the lymphatic system that contributes to clinical signs reflective of protein-losing enteropathy
Intestinal anomalies	Many breeds	Congenital defects of intestinal tract include atresia or duplication of an intestinal sgement; usually incompatible with life unless surgically corrected
Meckel's diverticulum	Many breeds	Sacculation or appendage of the ileum derived from an unobliterated yolk stalk

APP

GUIDE TO CONGENITAL DEFECTS OF DOGS *Continued*

CONDITION	BREEDS AFFECTED	REMARKS
Megaesophagus, idiopathic	Great Dane, German shepherd, Irish setter, dachshund, miniature schnauzer, wirehaired fox terrier, Labrador retriever, Chinese Shar Pei	Characterized by primary motor system disturbances of the esophagus that result in abnormal or unsuccessful transport of ingesta between the pharynx and stomach
Microcheilia	Schnauzer	Reduced oral fissure
Parotid salivary gland, enlargement of	Dachshund	Affected individuals present with enlarged parotid salivary glands and hypersalivation (profuse drooling)
Prognathism	Brachycephalic breeds	Upper jaw is shorter than lower jaw
Pyloric stenosis (antral pyloric hypertrophy)	Boxer, Boston terrier	Probably caused by excessive secretion of the gastrointestinal hormone, gastrin, which is produced by the G cells in the stomach wall and has a potent trophic effect on pyloric circular smooth muscle as well as the mucosa
Selective cobalamin malabsorption	Giant schnauzer, border collie	Defect in transport of intrinsic-cobalamin complex receptor to the ileal brush border membrane resulting in malabsorption of cobalamin
Wheat-sensitive enteropathy	Irish setter	Defect in small intestinal mucosal function associated with dietary sensitivity to gluten in wheat
	Ear	
Deafness	Akita, American Staffordshire terrier, Australian heeler and shepherd, border collie, Australian cattle dog, beagle, Boston terrier, Boxer, border collie, bull terrier, catahoula leopard dog, American cocker spaniel, collie, Dalmatian, dappled dachshund, Doberman pinscher, Dogo Argentino, English setter and bulldog, foxhound, fox terrier, German shepherd, Great Dane, Great Pyrenees, Ibizan hound, Jack Russell terrier, kuvasz, Maltese, miniature pinscher, toy and miniature poodles, Old English sheepdog, papillon, pointer, Rhodesian ridgeback, rottweiler, Saint Bernard, schnauzer, Scottish and Sealyham terriers, Norwegian dunkerhound, Shetland sheepdog, Shropshire terrier, Siberian husky, Walker American foxhound, West Highland white terrier	Lack of or loss of the sense of hearing; congenital deafness is most common type; may be partial or complete and affect only one ear or both ears; unilateral deafness is most common form in dogs; of the electrodiagnostic techniques used for determining extent of deafness, recording of brain stem auditory evoked potentials and impedance audiometry are most frequently used; hearing loss occurs secondary to degeneration, hypoplasia, or aplasia of the spiral organ of the inner ear
External ear canal, malformations of	Brachycephalic breeds	Incomplete development of canals or may be shorter, more tortuous than normal, or atretic
Pinna, malformations of	German shepherd, wirehaired terrier, collie, Irish setter	Deviations in size and shape typical for breed, such as gross variations in the size of the pinna (macrotia, microtia) or its complete absence (anotia)
	Endocrine and Metabolic Systems	
Adrenal hyperplasia	Great Dane	Deficiency in one of the enzymes (17-hydroxylase) necessary for cortisol synthesis; signs include poor growth and those of glucocorticoid deficiency
Diabetes insipidus	Miniature poodle, German shepherd, Boston terrier, Norwegian elkhound, schnauzer, German shorthaired pointer	Can be hypothalamic-neurohypophyseal or nephrogenic in origin; hypothalamic-neurohypophyseal diabetes insipidus is the most common; signs in puppies are usually restricted to polyuria and polydipsia
Diabetes mellitus	Keeshond, golden retriever, whippet, West Highland white terrier, Alaskan malamute, standard poodle, Old English sheepdog, Doberman pinscher, miniature schnauzer and pinscher, schipperke, German shepherd, Labrador retriever, Finnish spitz, Manchester terrier, English springer spaniel, chow chow, mixed breeds	May become evident as early as 2 to 6 months of age; pancreatic lesions include atrophy of beta cells and associated noninflammatory atrophy of a few acinar cells; affected individuals usually exhibit decreased rate of growth in addition to the polyphagia, polyuria, and soft or diarrheic stools
Dysbetalipoproteinemia	Miniature schnauzer	Defective synthesis of apolipoprotein; signs include abdominal distress and seizures
Glycogen storage disease	German shepherd	Results from enzyme deficiency, amylo-1,6-glucosidase; signs reflect severity of hypoglycemia
Hyperchylomicronemia	Miniature schnauzer	Results from enzyme deficiency, lipoprotein lipase; signs include abdominal distress and seizures with onset
Hypoadrenocorticism	Many breeds	Signs caused by deficiency of glucocorticoids or deficiency of mineralocorticoids and glucocorticoids; congenital hypoplasia of the adrenal glands probably causes early puppy death and thus goes unrecognized

GUIDE TO CONGENITAL DEFECTS OF DOGS *Continued*

CONDITION	BREEDS AFFECTED	REMARKS
Hypothyroidism	Giant schnauzer, Scottish deerhound	Results from thyroid dysgenesis, circulating thyroid hormone transport abnormalities, dyshormonogenesis, congenital thyroid-stimulating hormone deficiency, and severe iodine deficiency; congenital defects probably cause early puppy death and thus go unrecognized
Neonatal hypoglycemia	Toy breeds	Occurs during the nursing period because of inadequate glycogen or protein substrate stores or immature liver enzyme systems; also occurs from failure to adapt to fasting during the postweaning period; signs are related to severity
Pituitary dwarfism	German shepherd, toy pinscher, Weimaraner, spitz, Karelian bear dog, giant schnauzer	Caused by deficiencies of growth hormone and sometimes other adrenohypophyseal hormones; signs include proportional limb-to-trunk dwarfism, prognathism, altered mentality, delayed eruption of permanent teeth, retained puppy coat leading to eventual alopecia, and suppressed immune responses
Primary parathyroid hyperplasia	German shepherd	Affected individuals develop signs at 2 weeks of age, including stunted growth, muscular weakness, polyuria, and polydipsia
Urea cycle defect (citrullinemia)	Golden retriever, beagle	Results from urea cycle enzyme deficiency, argininosuccinate synthetase; signs include vomiting, seizures, and altered mentation

Eye

CONDITION	BREEDS AFFECTED	REMARKS
Aberrant canthal dermis	Many breeds	Encroachment of dermis at the nasal canthus on bulbar and palpebral conjunctiva
Agenesis of the eyelid	Many breeds	Absence of varying segments of the eyelid margin, usually temporal one third of the upper eyelid
Aniridia	Many breeds	Near or complete absence of iris
Anophthalmos	Many breeds	Complete absence of the globe
Anterior uveal cysts	Boston terrier, golden retriever	Arise from the pigmented epithelium of the posterior surface of iris and occasionally from the ciliary body
Aphakia	Saint Bernard	Congenital absence of the lens; usually occurs with other ocular defects
Blepharophimosis	Many breeds	Abnormal narrowing of the space between the eyelids
Cataracts	Afghan hound, Akita, Alaskan malamute, American cocker spaniel, beagle, basenji, Boston terrier, Cavalier King Charles spaniel, Australian shepherd, Chesapeake Bay retriever, chow chow, collie, Doberman pinscher, English cocker spaniel, German shepherd, golden retriever, Labrador retriever, Bedlington and Sealyham terriers, Old English sheepdog, miniature schnauzer, rottweiler, Samoyed, Siberian husky, Staffordshire terrier, poodle, Welsh springer spaniel, West Highland white terrier	In animals younger than 6 months of age are classified as either congenital or juvenile; congenital cataracts are present at birth, although they may not be noticed until 6 to 8 weeks of age, and may be inherited or secondary to in utero influences, so it is essential to question the owner regarding presence of cataracts in the sire, dam, previous litters, or their pedigrees; juvenile cataracts develop from newborn period until 6 years of age; heredity is major factor, although other causes may contribute to juvenile cataract formation; course of juvenile cataracts usually progressive, but rate at which progression occurs varies; complete opacification of the lens may occur in less than 1 year after diagnosis; if functional vision is present, congenital or juvenile cataracts in puppies usually undergo spontaneous resorption within the first year
Collie eye anomaly	Smooth- and rough-coated collies, border collie, Shetland sheepdog, Australian shepherd	Characterized by an array of posterior segment abnormalities; included in order of increasing severity are choroidal hypoplasia, optic nerve and scleral colobomas, and retinal detachment
Corneal dystrophy	Afghan hound, Airedale terrier, bichon frisé, Cavalier King Charles spaniel, Shetland sheepdog, rough-coated collie, beagle, Siberian husky, Samoyed, American cocker spaniel, Boston terrier, Chihuahua	A non-inflammatory corneal opacity present in one or more of the corneal layers; usually bilateral
Dacryops	Basset hound	Embryonic malformation of the lacrimal excretory ducts or associated lacrimal glands
Dermoid	Saint Bernard, German shepherd, dachshund, Dalmatian	First noticed as skinlike appendage soon after the eyelids open; usually involves temporal cornea and conjunctiva and affects one eye or both
Districhiasis	Airedale terrier, English bulldog, toy and miniature poodles, cocker spaniel, Pekingese, Boxer, Alsatian, Shetland sheepdog, Bedlington and Yorkshire terriers, Shih Tzu, Chinese pug, Saint Bernard	Extra row of eyelashes that protrude from orifices of meibomian glands within the intermarginal space of the eyelid; upper, lower, or both eyelids may be involved
Divergent strabismus	Brachycephalic breeds	First noted when eyelids open; normal ocular alignment develops during the second postnatal month
Dyscoria	Many breeds	Abnormally shaped pupil
Ectropion	Cocker spaniel, Saint Bernard, bloodhound, basset hound	Everted, allowing exposure of underlying bulbar conjunctiva; affected animals tend to display mucopurulent exudation and hyperemia of exposed conjunctiva and diminished Schirmer tear test values

GUIDE TO CONGENITAL DEFECTS OF DOGS *Continued*

CONDITION	BREEDS AFFECTED	REMARKS
Enophthalmos	Saint Bernard, Great Dane, Doberman pinscher, golden retriever, Irish setter	Recession of the globe within the orbit; most often associated with microphthalmos
Entropion	Many breeds	Inward deviation of the eyelid; lower eyelid is more commonly affected because of poorly formed tarsal plate
Glaucoma	Beagle, basset hound, American and English cocker spaniel, poodle, Samoyed, Bouvier des Flandres, Siberian husky, Alaskan malamute, wirehaired terrier, Norwegian elkhound, cairn terrier, West Highland white terrier, chow chow, miniature poodle, Chinese Shar Pei, Samoyed	Pressure increase occurring within the first year of life is rare, despite the existence of congenital iridocorneal abnormalities
Hemeralopia (day blindness)	Alaskan malamute	Affected individuals are visually impaired in daylight but function well at night and on overcast days; ocular fundus appears normal
Heterochromia iridis	Merled collie, Shetland sheepdog, Australian shepherd, harlequin Great Dane, Siberian husky, Alaskan malamute, Dalmatian, American foxhound, Norwegian dunker hound	Variation in iris color; occurs commonly in subalbinotic animals; variations in tapetal development and degree of pigmentation in the retinal pigment epithelium and choroid may occur simultaneously
Imperforate lacrimal punctum	Bedlington terrier, cocker spaniel, Sealyham terrier	Opening of the nasolacrimal drainage system fails to develop, resulting in epiphora
Iridocorneal abnormalities	Many breeds	Congenital mesodermal remnants occur in the iridocorneal angle in basset hounds
Iris cyst	Many breeds	Identified by their spherical shape and tendency to be attached at the pupillary margin
Lens coloboma	Many breeds	Notch defect in lens
Lenticonus	Many breeds	Conical protrusion of lens
Microcornea	Basenji, collie, Saint Bernard, miniature schnauzer, Australian shepherd, poodle	Affected eyes have more bulbar conjunctiva exposed medially and laterally but no apparent visual problems
Microphakia	Saint Bernard, beagle	Margin of the abnormally small lens along with elongated ciliary processes in microphakia may be seen after pupillary dilatation
Microphthalmos with colobomas	Australian shepherd, merled Shetland sheepdog, harlequin Great Dane	Large equatorial staphylomas, up to 20 diopters deep, are evident
Microphthalmos	Australian shepherd, Great Dane, beagle, collie, Borzoi, Portuguese water dog, Shetland sheepdog, dachshund, miniature schnauzer, Old English sheepdog, akita, Cavalier King Charles spaniel, Bedlington and Sealyham terriers, Labrador retriever, Doberman pinscher	Failure of the globe to develop to normal size; characterized by varying degrees of enophthalmos with or without other ocular defects; commonly associated with other ocular defects including colobomas, persistent pupillary membranes, cataract, equatorial staphylomas, choroidal hypoplasia, retinal dysplasia and detachment, and otic nerve hypoplasia; vision often impaired
Optic nerve colobomas	Collie, Shetland sheepdog, Australian shepherd, basenji	Pits or excavations in the optic disk occur as part of the collie or sheltie eye anomaly or as single lesions
Optic nerve hypoplasia, micropapilla	Beagle, dachshund, collie, Irish wolfhound, German shepherd, Great Pyrenees, Saint Bernard, miniature and toy poodles, Belgian sheepdog, Tervuren, English cocker spaniel	Poor vision is common in bilaterally affected animals, although owners usually fail to recognize the vision deficit while the animal is with its siblings; unilateral lesions often incidental findings, as the puppy compensates with the unaffected eye; affected eyes exhibit sluggish to absent direct pupillary light reflexes; resting pupil size may be larger than normal; affected optic disk often less than half its normal size, its center is depressed, and periphery is pigmented
Persistent hyperplastic primary vitreous	Doberman pinscher, Staffordshire terrier, standard schnauzer	Characterized by presence of fibrovascular membrane on posterior lens surface; results from persistence of hyaloid vasculature coupled with proliferation of mesoderm within the arborizing vascular tunic surrounding the lens
Persistent pupillary membranes	Basenji, chow chow, collie, Pembroke Welsh corgi, mastiff, and other breeds	Arise from anterior iris surface and represent remnants of embryonic vascular system
Polycoria	Many breeds	Presence of more than one pupil
Progressive retinal atrophy	Collie, Irish setter, Norwegian elkhound, miniature schnauzer, Cardigan Welsh corgi, English and American cocker spaniels, Labrador retriever, Tibetan terrier	Disorder affecting retinal photoreceptor layer; animals first demonstrate visual deficits in dim lighting; progressive loss of day vision then occurs, followed by total blindness and dilated pupils; retinal appearance varies with stage of disorder
Progressive retinal degeneration	Borzoi, papillon	First occurs at 6 months of age; initial retinal lesions appear as focal areas of hyperreflectivity in extreme peripheral tapetum; later, lesions coalesce into diffuse retinal degeneration
Pupillary anomalies	Many breeds	Ventronasal, notchlike defect (coloboma) in pupillary border results in keyhole-shaped pupil; eccentric pupil (corectopia) may accompany multiple ocular defects in Australian shepherd

GUIDE TO CONGENITAL DEFECTS OF DOGS *Continued*

CONDITION	BREEDS AFFECTED	REMARKS
Retinal dysplasia	English springer spaniel and toy spaniel, Labrador and golden retrievers, Bedlington terrier, bearded collie, border collie, American cocker spaniel, beagle, Akita, Cavalier King Charles spaniel, Chesapeake Bay retriever, clumber spaniel, collie, bullmastiff, German shepherd, puli, Australian shepherd, mastiff, English cocker spaniel, Sealyham and Tibetan terriers, Samoyed, Newfoundland, Norwegian elkhound, Doberman pinscher, Old English sheepdog, rottweiler, Yorkshire and Airedale terriers, standard schanuzer, Sussex spaniel, Cardigan and Pembroke Welsh corgi, Petit Basset Griffon Veneen, soft-coated wheaten terrier, afghan hound	Characterized by folds in outer retinal layers and by retinal rosettes, in which variably differentiated retinal cells are arranged around central lumen; more severe forms of retinal dysplasia may demonstrate retinal detachment attributable to subretinal fluid accumulation; may occur alone or in association with other congenital ocular defects
Retinal folds	Collies and other breeds	Usually appear in nontapetal portion of the fundus; believed to be caused by transient growth differential between inner and outer layers of optic cup and usually disappear when dogs are about 6 months of age
Retinopathy	Belgian sheepdog	Visual deficit seen as early as 8 weeks of age; vision disturbed in bright and dim light
Stationary night blindness	Tibetan terrier, briard	Night blindness first evident by 6 weeks of age; fundus of the briard appears normal, and low-level illumination demonstrates increased tapetal granularity in the Tibetan terrier; Tibetan terrier may subsequently develop progressive retinal atrophy
Tapetal hypoplasia	Beagle	Lack of visible tapetum and uniform reddish brown fundus reflex evident
Trichiasis	Many breeds	Condition in which otherwise normal eyelashes are deviated from their normal position, allowing contact between the deviated eyelash and the cornea

Hematopoietic and Lymphatic Systems

CONDITION	BREEDS AFFECTED	REMARKS
Anasarca	English bulldog	Affected individuals with anasarca have generalized subcutaneous edema and fluid accumulation
Coagulation protein disorders		
Factor XII	Standard and miniature poodles, German shorthaired pointer	Not associated with a bleeding diathesis; affected individuals may be predisposed to infection and/or thrombosis
Factor XI	English springer spaniel, Great Pyrenees, Weimaraner, Kerry blue terrier	Severe factor XI deficiency characteristically a minor bleeding diathesis that becomes major after trauma or surgery
Factor X	American cocker spaniel, Jack Russell terrier	Individuals homozygous for gene usually stillborn or die within first weeks of life from massive pulmonary and/or abdominal hemorrhage; heterozygotes have mild to severe bleeding tendency
Factor IX (hemophilia B)	Many breeds	Sex-linked hemorrhagic disorder; excessive bleeding from umbilical cord or tail or feet at the time of tail-docking and dew-claw removal is common sign; hemarthrosis, gingival bleeding during tooth eruption, and spontaneous hematoma formation are other typical manifestations
Factor VIII (hemophilia A)	Many breeds	One of the most common inherited hemorrhagic disorders; bleeding tendencies are same as for factor IX deficiency
Factor VIII (von Willebrand's disease)	Many breeds	Attributable to defective or deficient factor VIII–related antigen (von Willebrand's factor), is most common inherited bleeding disorder; bleeding tendencies are same as for factor IX deficiency
Factor VII	Beagle, miniature schnauzer, Alaskan malamute, Boxer, bulldog	Usually not accompanied by detectable bleeding, although affected individuals may experience bruising or prolonged bleeding after surgery
Factor II	English cocker spaniel, Boxer	Disorders of prothrombin including detectable bleeding tendencies, usually epistaxis and gingival bleeding
Factor I	Saint Bernard, Vizsla, Russian wolfhound	Affected individuals with dysfibrinogenemia or hypofibrinogenemia experience mild bleeding manifested by lameness and epistaxis; challenge with surgery or trauma results in life-threatening bleeding
Erythrocyte defects		
Pyruvate kinase deficiency	Basenji, beagle, West Highland white terrier, cairn terrier	Premature red blood cell destruction and moderate to severe anemia with evidence of red blood cell regeneration
Stomatocytosis	Alaskan malamute, miniature schnauzer, Drentse patrijshond	Stomatocytes and polychromasia in association with autosomal recessive–transmitted chondrodysplasia in Alaskan malamutes
Familial nonspherocytic anemia	Miniature poodle	Markedly regenerative red blood cell response, hepatosplenomegaly, and bone marrow myelofibrosis and osteosclerosis
Nonspherocytic hemolytic disorders	Beagle, poodle	Mild anemia and polychromasia

APP

GUIDE TO CONGENITAL DEFECTS OF DOGS *Continued*

CONDITION	BREEDS AFFECTED	REMARKS
Phosphofructokinase deficiency	English springer spaniel, American cocker spaniel	Results in primary hemolytic disorder with appropriate bone marrow response (reticulocytosis)
Glucose-6-phosphate dehydrogenase deficiency	Weimaraner	Generally no anemia or polychromasia
Cytochrome b_5 reductase deficiency	Many breeds	May have no anemia, cyanosis, and exercise intolerance
Elliptocytosis	Mixed breed	Attributable to decrease in red blood cell membrane protein, a protein band 4.1 deficiency; affected red blood cells are mechanically unstable, resulting in mild to moderate regenerative hemolytic anemia
Increased osmotic fragility	English springer spaniel	May have no anemia, polychromasia, poikilocytosis, and exercise-induced hyperthermia
High-potassium erythrocytes	Akita, Japanese mongrel	No anemia but increased erythrocyte and serum potassium (pseudohyperkalemia)
Familial microcytosis	Akita	No anemia but prominent microcytosis
Cyclic hematopoiesis	Silver grey collie	Intermittent cytopenias usually present
Selective cobalamin malabsorption	Giant schnauzer	Usually have moderate anemia, nonregenerative megaloblasts, hypersegmented neutrophils, cachexia, and dementia
Familial macrocytosis and dyshematopoiesis	Miniature and toy poodles	No anemia, macrocytosis, hypersegmented neutrophils, and normal osmotic fragility
Lymphedema	English bulldog, Old English sheepdog, German shepherd, Borzoi, Labrador retriever, Great Dane, poodle, Belgian and Tervuren shepherds	Primary lymphedema attributable to developmental abnormalities in lymphatic system; lymphatic channels may be aplastic, hypoplastic, or hyperplastic; lymph nodes may be normal, hypocellular, or absent; characterized by soft, pitting, nonpainful edema of one or more extremities, usually involving hindlimbs; rarely, abdominal or pleural effusions may develop
Methemoglobinemia	Borzoi, English setter	Results from enzyme deficiency, NADH-methemoglobin reductase; affected animals have evidence of cyanosis, brownish mucous membranes and dark brownish blood that does not turn red on exposure to oxygen, and exercise intolerance
Thrombasthenic thrombopathia	Otterhound, Great Pyrenees	Intrinsic platelet disorder; defect distinguished by presence of bizarre, giant platelets and reductions in membrane glycoproteins II and III; platelets fail to support normal clot retraction, have reduced retention on glass bead surfaces, and fail to aggregate normally in response to adenosine diphosphate, collagen, and thrombin
Thrombopathia	Basset hound, spitz	Intrinsic platelet disorder; affected animals exhibit signs typical of quantitative and qualitative platelet defects, including epistaxis, gingival bleeding, and petechiation; characterized by abnormal fibrinogen receptor exposure and impaired dense granule release
Thymic branchial cyst	Many breeds	Arise from remnants of branchial pouch epithelium, the embryonic precursor of thymic tissue; occur in thymus or subcutis of the neck

Immune System

CONDITION	BREEDS AFFECTED	REMARKS
Combined immunodeficiency	Basset hound, Cardigan Welsh corgi	Affected individuals develop severe bacterial skin infections, stomatitis, and otitis within first few weeks of life and have lymphopenia, depressed T-lymphocyte function with low serum immunoglobulin A (IgA) and IgG and variable IgM concentrations
Complement deficiency	Brittany spaniel	Absence of complement 3 and impaired function of phagocytes
Cyclic hematopoiesis	Collie, cocker spaniel, Pomeranian	Basis for cyclic hematopoiesis is bone marrow stem cell defect resulting in cyclic fluctuation in neutrophils, reticulocytes, and thrombocytes from the bone marrow; additional defects in lysosomal function result in decreased bactericidal capacity of neutrophils; respiratory, umbilical, and septicemic infections are common
Granulocytopathy	Irish setter, Doberman pinscher, Weimaraner	Defect in neutrophilic bactericidal capacity; affected individuals are stunted, have recurrent bacterial infections, and require continual antibiotic therapy
Pelger-Huët anomaly	Many breeds	Decreased lobulation of granulocytic cells; abnormal nuclear shape may contribute to reduced cell mobility and abnormal chemotaxis; not all affected animals have chemotactic defects, and none has increased risk of infection
Pneumocystosis	Dachshund	Most cases occur in animals younger than 6 months of age with suspected congenital immunodeficiency
Selective IgA deficiency	German shepherd, beagle, Chinese Shar Pei, Airedale terrier	Affected animals have low or undetectable serum or secretory IgA concentrations or both and experience chronic recurrent upper and lower respiratory infections, otitis externa, and dermatitis; despite selective low IgA levels in many related animals, some animals are not symptomatic
Thymic anomaly	Weimaraner, Mexican hairless dog	Affected individuals with thymic atrophy can be detected within 1 to 3 months of age; signs include stunted growth, chronic wasting, and suppurative pneumonia; additional defects noted include decreased growth hormone concentration and T-cell function

GUIDE TO CONGENITAL DEFECTS OF DOGS *Continued*

CONDITION	BREEDS AFFECTED	REMARKS
Liver and Pancreas		
Biliary atresia		Failure of the biliary tract to develop creates incomplete functional connection between liver and duodenum
Copper-associated hepatopathy	Bedlington and West Highland white terriers, Doberman pinscher	Age-related accumulation of copper in hepatic lysosomes associated with chronic active hepatitis; in the Bedlington terrier, only dogs homozygous for the trait accumulate copper in the liver; in other breeds, copper accumulation probably related to degree of active liver disease
Gallbladder anomalies	Many breeds	Congenital malformations include trilobed or biloped gallbladders; development of two separated gallbladders with cystic ducts united in a common duct; ductular bladders developing as supernumerary vesicles derived from either hepatic, cystic, or common bile ducts; and trabecular bladders derived from vesicular outgrowths of liver trabeculae
Hepatic cysts	Cairn terrier and other breeds	May be parenchymal or ductal in origin; most are of ductular origin, arising from one or more primitive bile ducts lacking connection with biliary tract and subsequently developing into retention cysts
Hepatoportal microvascular dysplasia	Cairn terrier	Multiple microscopic intrahepatic shunts that may be asymptomatic or cause signs comparable to those of congenital portosystemic venous shunts
Intrahepatic arterioportal fistulas	Many breeds	Result from failure of the common embryologic anlage to differentiate; contribute to portal hypertension and shunting through multiple portosystemic collaterals and ascites
Pancreatic hypoplasia	German shepherd, Doberman pinscher, Irish setter, beagle, Labrador retriever, Saint Bernard	Associated with generalized reduction in pancreatic exocrine (acinar) cells, but the islets of Langerhans remain intact
Portosystemic venous shunts Intrahepatic	Doberman pinscher, golden and Labrador retrievers, Irish setter, Samoyed, Irish wolfhound, Australian cattle dog	Most often remnant of fetal ductus venosus that remains patent; other large intrahepatic venous communications may be present; ductus venosus is embryonic venous channel originating from umbilical vein that traverses liver and drains into left hepatic vein and then into caudal vena cava
Extrahepatic	Miniature schnauzer, Maltese, poodle, Yorkshire terrier, dachshund	Shunt between portal vein and postcaval or between portal vein and azygous vein; complete absence of portal vein entry into liver is unusual
Urea cycle enzyme deficiency	Golden retriever, beagle	Significant reductions in urea cycle enzyme argininosuccinate synthetase lead to inability to handle endogenous ammonia and signs of hepatic encephalopathy
Nervous System		
Afghan myelopathy	Afghan hound	Demyelination with accompanying myelomalacia occurs predominantly in dorsal funiculi of caudal cervical spinal cord, all funiculi of thoracic segments, and ventral funiculi of the lumbar area
Ataxia of fox terriers	Smooth-haired and Jack Russell fox terriers	Progressive demyelination of spinal cord segments, especially spinal cord segments of the pelvic limbs
Cranial dysraphism	Many breeds	Defects occurring because of faulty closure of the neural tube; conditions that may be seen in association with cranial dysraphism include anencephaly (brain is absent at birth or more commonly only the basal nuclei and cerebellum are well developed), exencephaly (brain is exposed as result of congenital cleft in skull), cranium bifida (open cleft in skull), encephalocele and meningocele (brain or meninges, respectively, protrude through congenital cleft in skull), and cyclopia (developmental anomaly characterized by single orbital fossa, with either complete or partial agenesis of the globe)
Cerebellar abiotrophies	Kerry blue terrier, Gordon setter, and other breeds	Loss of vital, nutritional substances; cerebellum is normal in gross appearance, but marked depopulation involving principally Purkinje cells is present; other areas of brain may be affected
Cerebellar hypoplasia	Chow chow, Irish setter, wirehaired fox terrier	Uniform forms of cerebellar hypoplasia in which clinical signs of cerebellar dysfunction are present at birth and do not progress
Cerebellar vermis hypoplasia	Boston terrier and bull terrier	Caudal cerebellar vermis is preferentially hypoplastic, although other portions of cerebellum are often hypoplastic to lesser degree and some have concomitant hydrocephalus
Degenerative changes in cerebellum	Airedale terrier, Finnish harrier, Bernese mountain dog, bull mastiff, rough-coated collie, Irish setter, miniature poodle, beagle, Labrador retriever	Other breed-specific syndromes in which there are degenerative changes in the cerebellum alone or together with other areas of the central nervous system occur; clinical signs in some cases are progressive, whereas in others they are apparently static
Demyelination of miniature poodles	Miniature poodle	Progressive demyelination involving principally the spinal cord leads to paraparesis at 2 to 4 months of age and subsequently tetraplegia
Epilepsy	Beagle, Belgian and Tervuren shepherds, keeshond, collie, dachshund, poodle, German shepherd, setters, retrievers, spaniels	Recurrence of seizures; genetic predisposition in several dog breeds, but potential heritable basis for epilepsy include beagle, Belgian and Tervuren shepherds, German shepherd, and keeshond

APP

GUIDE TO CONGENITAL DEFECTS OF DOGS *Continued*

CONDITION	BREEDS AFFECTED	REMARKS
Hydrocephalus	Maltese, Yorkshire terrier, English bulldog, Chihuahua, Lhasa apso, Chinese pug, toy poodle, Pomeranian, cairn and Boston terriers, Pekingese	Excessive accumulation of cerebrospinal fluid within the skull; the terms *internal* and *external* denote excess fluid within or outside the ventricular system, respectively; congenital forms may occur because of structural defects that either obstruct cerebrospinal fluid outflow at the mesencepalic aqueduct or impede cerebrospinal fluid absorption
Hypertrophic neuropathy	Tibetan mastiff	Affected individuals have prominent concomitant demyelination and remyelination that occur at 8 weeks of age and progress to tetraparesis
Hypomyelination, dysmyelination	Chow chow, Welsh springer spaniel, Samoyed, Weimaraner, Bernese mountain dog, lurcher, golden retriever, Dalmatian	Reduced (hypomyelination) and abnormal (dysmyelination) of the central nervous system occurs, suggesting that the responsible lesion may involve either failed or delayed differentiation of oligodendrocytes
Lissencephaly	Lhasa apso, Irish setter, wirehaired fox terrier	Marked reduction or absence of cerebral gyri; may occur as single entity or concurrently with cerebellar hypoplasia, cyclopia, and hydrocephalus
Lysosomal storage diseases Ceroid lipofuscinosis	English setter, cocker spaniel, Chihuahua, dachshund, Saluki, border collie	Results from unknown, perhaps *p*-phenylenediamine, enzyme deficiency
Fucosidosis	English springer spaniel	Results from enzyme deficiency, α-L-fucosidase
GM$_1$ gangliosidosis	Beagle, English springer spaniel, Portuguese water dog	Results from enzyme deficiency, β-galactosidase
GM$_2$ gangliosidosis	German shorthaired pointer, Japanese spaniel	Results from enzyme deficiency, β-hexosaminidase
Globoid cell leukodystropy	Cairn and West Highland white terriers, poodle, bluetick hound, beagle, basset hound, Pomeranian	Results from enzyme deficiency, β-galoctocerebrosidase
Glucocerebrosidosis	Dalmatian	Results from enzyme deficiency, β-glucosidase
Glycogenosis	Silky terrier	Results from enzyme deficiency, α-glucosidase
Sphingomyelinosis	German shepherd, poodle	Results from enzyme deficiency, sphingomyelinase
Motor neuronopathies	Brittany spaniel, collie, Swedish Lapland, rottweiler, pointer, Great Dane	Degeneration of previously differentiated ventral horn cells of the spinal cord (spinal abiotrophies)
Myelodysplasia	Weimaraner, Samoyed, Dalmatian, rottweiler	Refers collectively to anomalies involving spinal cord, vertebral column, and skin subsequent to faulty closure of neural tube; meninges (meningocele), spinal cord or roots (myelocele), or both (meningomyelocele) may protrude through defective fusion of the vertebral arch (spina bifida); neural lesions may be noted; spinal clefts (myeloschisis) may communicate with dilated central canal (hydromyelia) or cystic spaces within spinal parenchyma (syringomyelia)
Narcolepsy-cataplexy	Doberman pinscher, Labrador retriever, miniature poodle, dachshund, beagle, Saint Bernard, Airedale terrier, Afghan hound, Irish setter, Welsh corgi, Alaskan malamute, rottweiler, English springer spaniel, giant schnauzer	Excessive daytime sleep (narcolepsy); periods of acute muscular hypotonia often seen in association with narcolepsy (cataplexy)
Neuroaxonal dystrophy	Shetland sheepdog, rottweiler, Chihuahua, Ibizan hound	Marked axonal distention (axonal spheroids) in central nervous system; signs manifested reflect predominant location of axonal spheroids within central nervous system
Neuronal abiotrophy	Swedish Lapland dog	Thoracic or pelvic limb weakness at 5 to 7 weeks of age that progresses to tetraparesis within 1 to 2 weeks
Neuronal degeneration	Cocker spaniel	Occurs in young cocker spaniels; causes ataxia, tremors, abnormal behavior, and seizures by several months of age
Neuronopathy	Cairn terrier	Pelvic limb weakness begins between 12 and 24 weeks of age and progresses to tetraparesis over 2 months, and head tremor present
Neuropathies	German shepherd, Alaskan malamute, rottweiler, golden retriever, Tibetan mastiff	Loss of nerve fibers leads to paraparesis and progresses to tetraparesis and esophageal or laryngeal paralysis
Peripheral vestibular disorders	German shepherd, English cocker spaniel, Doberman pinscher, Shetland sheepdog, Akita, beagle	Absence of signs of central vestibular disease in affected animals suggests that developmental lesions affecting peripheral labyrinth are involved; affected animals have signs of peripheral vestibular dysfunction, including head tilt, circling, and rolling at birth or within a few weeks
Progressive axonopathy	Boxer	Affected individuals have axons that are markedly enlarged in both peripheral and central nervous system; pelvic limb ataxia typically begins at 2 months of age; other neurologic dysfunctions are noted as disease progresses
Pug encephalitis	Chinese pug, similar condition in Yorkshire terrier and Maltese	Affected individuals have signs principally of forebrain dysfunction, including seizures, attitude change, and circling; marked, predominantly mononuclear pleocytosis is noted in affected animals
Sensory neuronopathies and neuropathies	Dachshund, German shorthaired and English pointers, border collie, Siberian husky	Loss of sensory nerve fibers, neuronal cell bodies, or both, results in pelvic limb ataxia and/or hyporeflexia, urinary incontinence, gastrointestinal dysfunction, loss of conscious proprioception, depressed pain sensation, and self-mutilation of extremities

GUIDE TO CONGENITAL DEFECTS OF DOGS *Continued*

CONDITION	BREEDS AFFECTED	REMARKS
Spinal muscular atrophy	German shepherd, pointer, rottweiler, Brittany spaniel	Loss of functional motor neurons in spinal cord or brain stem leads to paraparesis that progresses to tetraparesis
Spongiform encephalopathies	Labrador retriever, Samoyed, silky terrier, Dalmatian	Manifested by multifocal neurologic dysfunction and marked vacuolation of central nervous system white matter

Neuromuscular System and Muscles

Dermatomyositis	Collie, Shetland sheepdog	Idiopathic inflammation of skin and muscles; family history of syndrome exists; almost all individuals with skin lesions have some degree of muscle involvement; signs range from mild symmetric temporalis muscle atrophy to generalized muscle atrophy and weakness; megaesophagus and trismus can develop in severely affected individuals
Familial myoclonus	Labrador retriever	Episodes of marked muscular hypertonicity that begins at 3 weeks of age; extensor rigidity and opisthotonos become more pronounced upon stimulation
Labrador retriever myopathy	Labrador retriever	Progressive degenerative myopathy first noted at 3 to 4 months of age as stiffness of gait and simultaneous advancement of pelvic limbs (bunny hop); signs do not progress significantly in some dogs beyond 6 to 8 months of age
Myasthenia gravis	Jack Russell and smooth-coated fox terriers, English springer spaniel, Samoyed	Leads to failure of neuromuscular transmission because of congenital deficiency of acetylcholine receptors in postsynaptic membrane; may be first noted at 6 to 9 weeks of age and older
Myotonia	Chow chow, Great Dane, Staffordshire terrier, Rhodesian ridgeback, cocker spaniel, Labrador retriever, Samoyed, West Highland white terrier	Persistent muscle contraction subsequent to either voluntary contraction or stimulation; prominent stiffness of gait noted when affected animals first become ambulatory and lessens with further exercise, being worse in pelvic limbs
Scotty cramp	Scottish terrier, Dalmatian	Characterized by paroxysms of muscular hypertonicity; episodes usually begin at 6 to 8 weeks of age and are generally precipitated by fear or excitement
X-linked muscular dystrophy	Irish terrier, golden retriever, Samoyed, rottweiler, Belgian shepherd	Occurs homologous with Duchenne's muscular dystrophy in humans; only affected males and homozygous females first show stilted gait and simultaneous advancement of pelvic limbs (bunny hop) at 8 to 10 weeks of age

Reproductive System

Aplasia of the duct system	Many breeds	Failure of any part of testicular duct system to develop results in impaired transportation of spermatozoa to urethra, accumulation of sperm proximal to obstruction, and potential development of sperm granuloma and testicular degeneration
Chimeras True hermaphrodite	Many breeds	True hermaphrodites have both ovarian and testicular tissue present in same individual; true hermaphrodite chimeras have either XX/XY or XX/XXY chromosome constitutions, enlarged clitoris, little testicular tissue, and external female appearance
XX/XY chimeras with testes	Old English sheepdog	External genital opening with cranially displaced vulva-like structure, hypoplastic penis contained in vulva-like structure, no external scrotum or testes (testes are located near caudal pole of kidneys), and bicornuate uterus
Chromosomal number abnormalities XXY syndrome		Not recognized as readily as in tortoiseshell cats, normal because the haircoat color paradox does not signal its presence; normal male external phenotype with a 79,XXY chromosome constitution has small testes with seminiferous tubular dysgenesis and no evidence of spermatogenesis
XO syndrome	Doberman pinscher	Occurs in females that have normal phenotype and not cycled by 24 months of age
Triple-X syndrome	Airedale terrier	Occurs in females that have normal phenotype, underdeveloped genitalia, and not cycled by 24 months of age
Chromosomal sex abnormalities	Many breeds	Dogs have 78 chromosomes, including the X and Y chromosomes; affected phenotypic males and females with abnormal sex chromosome constitutions, except chimeras and mosaics, have underdeveloped genitalia; with few exceptions, individuals are sterile
Cryptorchidism	Toy and miniature poodles, Pomeranian, Yorkshire and cairn terriers, dachshund, Chihuahua, Maltese, Boxer, Pekingese, English bulldog, miniature schnauzer, Shetland sheepdog, Siberian husky	Normally, canine testes descend to scrotum by 10 days after birth; if both testes are not within the scrotum by 8 weeks of age, diagnosis of cryptorchidism is warranted; both males and females may carry gene for cryptorchidism and pass to offspring; heterozygous males, heterozygous females, and homozygous females are phenotypically normal carriers; only homozygous males are cryptorchid
Hypospadias	Boston terrier and other breeds	Abnormality in location of urinary orifice, being ventral and proximal to normal site in glans penis; urinary orifice may be located in glans penis (mild hypospadias), the penile shaft (moderate hypospadias), or penoscrotal junction, scrotum, or perineum (severe hypospadias); may be accompanied by cryptorchidism, scrotal abnormalities, persistent müllerian structures, and intersexuality

APP

GUIDE TO CONGENITAL DEFECTS OF DOGS *Continued*

CONDITION	BREEDS AFFECTED	REMARKS
Os penis deformity	Many breeds	May result in deviation of penis and, depending on severity, inability to retract penis fully into preputial sheath; persistent exposure of portion of glans penis results in desiccation, trauma, or necrosis
Persistent penile frenulum	Many breeds	Persistence of band of connective tissue extending from ventral tip of glans penis to either prepuce or ventral surface of penis
Prepuce anomaly	Many breeds	Abnormal shortening of prepuce results in persistent exposure of glans penis; may result in desiccation, trauma, or necrosis
Pseudohermaphroditism Female	Many breeds	Female hermaphrodite has XX chromosome constitution and ovaries but internal or external genitalia are masculinized
Male	Miniature schnauzer, poodle, Pekingese	Male hermaphrodite has XY chromosome constitution and testes but internal or external genitalia are to some degree those of female
Testicular hypoplasia	Many breeds	Abnormal development of the seminiferous tubular germinal epithelium; results in oligospermia or azoospermia and sterility; may be unilateral or bilateral and usually first noticed soon after puberty
Vaginal prolapse	Large breeds	Protrusion of edematous vaginal tissue into vaginal lumen, often through vulva of intact female during time of estrogen stimulation
XX sex reversal	Cocker spaniel, beagle, Chinese pug, Kerry blue terrier, Weimaraner, German shorthaired pointer	Animals in which chromosomal and gonadal sex do not agree are called *sex reversed*; dogs with XX sex reversal have 78,XX chromosome constitution and varying amounts of testicular tissue in gonad; individuals are XX true hermaphrodites or XX males and have mild to severe gonadal masculinization

Respiratory System

CONDITION	BREEDS AFFECTED	REMARKS
Bronchial cartilage hypoplasia	Pekingese	Seen during first several months of life, usually as severe respiratory distress
Bronchoesophageal fistula	Many breeds	Connection between esophagus and airways that may allow saliva and ingested material to enter into lungs
Laryngeal hypoplasia	Skye terrier and brachycephalic breeds	Incompletely developed larynx; signs, when present, vary with degree of laryngeal narrowing
Laryngeal paralysis	Bouvier des Flandres, Siberian husky, Dalmatian	Failure of larynx to abduct during inspiration produces muted bark and soft, moist cough; later, roaring sound of inspiratory dyspnea becomes dominant sign
Pulmonary emphysema	Many breeds	Abnormally large airspaces occur distal to terminal bronchi; affected individuals may show signs of respiratory distress as early as 6 weeks of age
Primary ciliary dyskinesia	English pointer, English springer spaniel, border collie, English setter, Dalmatian, Doberman pinscher, Chihuahua, golden retriever, Old English sheepdog, chow chow, bichon frisé, rottweiler, Chinese Shar Pei, Norwegian elkhound	Abnormally functioning cilia of respiratory epithelium, resulting in reduced mucociliary clearance of respiratory secretions, inhaled particles, and infectious agents
Stenotic nares	Brachycephalic breeds and Chinese Shar Pei	Predisposes to laryngeal collapse by causing formation of a partial vacuum with inspiration; dyspnea, mouth breathing, and snoring sounds are common
Tracheal collapse	Brachycephalic and miniature breeds, especially Chihuahua, poodle, Pomeranian	Occurs because malformations of tracheal rings cause dorsoventral flatting of trachea
Tracheal hypoplasia	Brachycephalic breeds and Chinese Shar Pei	Inadequate growth of tracheal rings; commonly associated with secondary respiratory tract infections

Skin

CONDITION	BREEDS AFFECTED	REMARKS
Acanthosis nigricans	Dachshund	Cutaneous reaction pattern of acanthosis nigricans characterized by bilateral axillary hyperpigmentation, lichenification, and alopecia
Acral mutilation syndrome	German shorthaired and English pointers	Sensory neuropathy that results in progressive mutilation of distal extremities; begins as biting and licking at paw(s) with hindlimbs being most severely involved
Acrodermatitis	American bull terrier	At birth, affected individuals have skin pigmentation lighter than normal, are physically weak, cannot chew or swallow well, and have retarded growth; by 6 weeks of age, skin lesions appear on footpads, ears, and muzzle and around all body orifices
Alopecia universalis	American hairless terrier, beagle	Generalized lack of hair coverage; adnexal abnormalities concurrently not present
Aplasia cutis (epitheliogenesis imperfecta)	Many breeds	Discontinuity of squamous epithelium; present at birth as glistening red, well-demarcated defect in skin; defect is covered with one to three layers of flat to cuboidal epithelium and a stroma devoid of all adnexa
Black hair follicular dysplasia	Black and white mixed breeds, bearded collie, basset hound, papillon, schipperke, dachshund	Defective haircoat found only in black haircoat regions; includes hypotrichosis; fractured, stubby hairs lacking normal sheen; and periodic scaliness of skin

GUIDE TO CONGENITAL DEFECTS OF DOGS *Continued*

CONDITION	BREEDS AFFECTED	REMARKS
Collagen disorder of the footpads	German shepherd	All footpads are soften than normal, often tender; discrete ulcers may develop on one or more pads, especially the carpal and tarsal pads; lesions contain multifocal areas of collagenolysis and neutrophilic inflammation
Color mutant alopecia	Doberman pinscher, Irish setter, chow chow, dachshund, standard poodle, Great Dane, greyhound, whippet, basset hound, Boston terrier, Chihuahua	Ectodermal defect of color mutants characterized by partial alopecia, dry lusterless haircoat, scaliness, and papules; defects in melanization and cortical structure of affected hairs also occur
Cutaneous asthenia (Ehlers-Danlos syndrome, dominant collagen dysplasia, dermal fragility syndrome, dermatosparaxis)	Beagle, dachshund, Boxer, Saint Bernard, German Shepherd, English springer spaniel, greyhound	Connective tissue disease characterized by loose, hyperextensive, and abnormally fragile skin easily torn by minor trauma
Cutaneous mucinosis	Chinese Shar Pei	Produces peculiar puffed face appearance favored in some breed lines and contributes to thickness of multiple skin folds
Cutaneous vasculopathy	German shepherd	Vasculitis and collagenolysis of nose, ear margins, and paw pads
Dermatomyositis	Collie, Shetland sheepdog, Pembroke Welsh corgi, Australian cattle dog, chow chow, German shepherd	Idiopathic inflammation of skin and muscles; family history of syndrome exists; early skin lesions favor locations over bony prominences that are especially exposed to trauma; almost all individuals with skin lesions have some degree of muscle involvement
Dermoid sinus	Rhodesian ridgeback, Shih Tzu, Boxer	Neural tube defect resulting from incomplete separation of skin and neural tube during embryonic development; sinus is tubular indentation of skin extending from dorsal midline as blind sac ending in subcutaneous tissue or extending through spinal canal to dura mater
Digital hyperkeratosis	Irish terrier, Dogues de Bordeaux	Hyperkeratosis of the footpads of all four paws develops at an early age; affected pads tend to fissure, become secondarily infected, and are painful
Ectodermal defect	Miniature poodle, whippet, cocker spanial, Belgian shepherd, Lhasa apso, Yorkshire terrier, miniature poodle	Affected individuals are born with two thirds of normally haired parts of body exhibiting hairlessness; hairless skin is extremely thin and contains no cutaneous appendages
Epidermal dysplasia	West Highland white terrier	Familial defect in keratinization that first presents as erythema and pruritus of extremities and ventrum, progressing to severe hyperpigmentation and seborrhea
Epidermolysis bullosa	Collie, Shetland sheepdog	Probably a mild form of canine familial dermatomyositis in which muscle lesions are inapparent
Hypotrichosis	Beagle, Yorkshire terrier, Labrador retriever, Lhasa apso, Irish water spaniel, toy poodle, French bulldog	Incomplete ectodermal defect in that affected individuals have remnants of hair follicles and other epidermal appendages in skin; in some cases, may be confined to certain hair color pattern; hypotrichosis may also develop after birth as a delayed-onset trait
Ichthyosis	West Highland white terrier, American pit bull terrier, Boston terrier, Doberman pinscher	Extreme hyperkeratosis on all or part of skin and exaggerated thickening of digital, carpal, and tarsal pads; present at birth and becomes progressively more severe with age
Lethal acrodermatitis	English bull terrier	Characterized by growth retardation, acrodermatitis, pyoderma, paronychia, diarrhea, pneumonia, and abnormal behavior that results in death usually before 15 months of age
Lichenoid-psoriasiform dermatosis	Springer spaniel	Asymptomatic, generally symmetric, erythematous, lichenoid papules and plaques initially noted on pinnae and in external ear canal and inguinal region; with time, lesions become more hyperkeratotic and spread to face, ventral trunk, and perineal area
Nevi	German shepherd, miniature poodle and schnauzer, Shetland sheepdog	Circumscribed developmental defect in skin; when nevus forms a hyperplastic mass, it is referred to as hamartoma; various other types include sebaceous, hyperpigmented epidermal, and mucocutaneous angiomatous nevi
Partial alopecia	Chinese crested dog, Mexican hairless dog, Chihuahua, Abyssinian sand dog, Turkish naked dog, Peruvian hairless dog, Xoloitzcuintli	These breeds are bred specifically for varying degrees of alopecia and as such become accepted standard
Seborrhea, congenital	English springer spaniel	Affected individuals born with dry skin and discolored hair; patches of hyperkeratosis and scale then develop, and adherent scale and debris accumulate on hair shafts
Tyrosinase deficiency	Chow chow	Changes in color of tongue, buccal mucosa, and portions of hair shaft are result of deficiency of tyrosinase, the enzyme necessary in chemical reactions that produce melanin
Tyrosinemia	German shepherd	Early-age onset of eye and skin lesions with mental retardation; serum tyrosine levels are elevated because of deficiency of cytosolic hepatic tyrosine aminotransferase; inflammatory response to tyrosine crystals deposited in tissue results in eye and possibly skin lesions
Vitiligo	Doberman pinscher, rottweiler, Belgian shepherd, Tervuren and German shepherds, Old English sheepdog, dachshund	Loss of skin pigment, especially around nose, lips, buccal mucosa, and facial skin; footpads and nails as well as haircoat may be affected

APP

GUIDE TO CONGENITAL DEFECTS OF DOGS *Continued*

CONDITION	BREEDS AFFECTED	REMARKS
Urinary System		
Ectopic ureter	Siberian husky	May occur unilaterally or bilaterally and may be associated with other urinary tract anomalies; affected individuals, mostly females, have history of incontinence since birth or weaning
Malposition of urinary bladder (pelvic bladder)	Doberman pinscher	Caudal malposition of urinary bladder; may be cause of urinary incontinence and is associated with other urinary tract abnormalities
Renal defects		
Agenesis or absence of kidneys	Many breeds	Can be unilateral or bilateral and is usually accompanied by associated ureteral aplasia; is fatal and a cause of fading puppy syndrome
Amlyoidosis	Chinese Shar Pei, beagle	Renal function in affected individuals varies depending on degree and duration of renal involvement; advanced signs of renal failure eventually occur and are typically associated with severe proteinuria and hypoproteinemia
Cystinuria	Dachshund, basset hound, English bulldog, Chihuahua, Yorkshire and Irish terriers, Newfoundland	Caused by specific defect in renal tubules; results in defective resorption of certain amino acids including cystine
Familial renal disease	Basenji, cocker spaniel, Doberman pinscher, Lhasa apso, Shih Tsu, rottweiler, chow chow, Norwegian elkhound, Samoyed, bull and soft-coated wheaten terrier, standard poodle, Chinese Shar Pei, Newfound-land, Bernese mountain dog	Renal function in affected individuals varies depending on degree and duration of renal involvement; polyuria and polydipsia, anorexia, lethargy, weight loss or inability to gain weight, and eventually nonregenerative anemia, azotemia, skeletal changes, gastrointestinal signs occur in most of affected individuals
Fanconi's syndrome	Basenji	Caused by resorptive defect in proximal nephron leading to glycosuria, aminoaciduria, proteinuria, phosphaturia, renal tubular acidosis, and resorptive abnormalities of sodium, potassium, and urate
Fusion (horseshoe) kidney	Many breeds	Fusion of embryonic kidneys; usually incidental finding and not associated with clinical signs
Polycystic kidneys	Cairn terrier	Characterized by variable number of fluid-filled cysts in renal parenchyma, ranging from extremely small to massive; affected individuals may be asymptomatic or show evidence of rapidly progressing renal failure
Primary hyperoxaluria	Tibetan spaniel	Signs result from acute renal failure caused by renal tubular deposition of oxalate crystals
Renal duplication	English bulldog	Usually an incidental finding and not associated with clinical signs of altered renal function
Renal ectopia	Many breeds	Arrest in normal embryonic ascent of kidney; kidney appears as caudal abdominal mass within pelvis or in sublumbar area; usually incidental finding and not associated with clinical signs
Renal glucosuria	Norwegian elkhound	Isolated tubular defect for resorption of glucose; may predispose affected individuals to urinary tract infection
Urachal anomalies	Many breeds	Vary from complete persistence of urachus with communication between urinary bladder and umbilicus to blind cysts to cranioventral urachal diverticulum
Ureterocele	Many breeds	Dilatation of submucosal segment of intravesical ureter resulting in bulging of dilated segment into urinary bladder
Urethral anomalies	Many breeds	Include hypospadias (urethral opening on underside of penis or on perineum), imperforate urethra, ectopic urethra, urethral aplasia (associated with penile aplasia), duplicate urethra, and urethrorectal fistula
Urinary bladder anomalies	English bulldog, Doberman pinscher	Include exstrophy of urinary bladder (absence of ventral abdominal body wall and ventral bladder wall), duplication of urinary bladder, and agenesis of urinary bladder

INDEX

Note: Page numbers in *italics* refer to illustrations; page numbers
followed by t indicate tables.

AB blood group system, 353, *353,* 1798
Abdomen, distention of, 137–139, *138*
  liver disease and, 1273t, 1276
  fluid in. See *Ascites.*
Abducens nerve, anatomy of, 664t
  examination of, 562–566, *564,* 567t
Abelcet, for blastomycosis, 462
  for fungal infection, 456, 475t
Abortion, induced, 1544–1548, *1547*
  spontaneous, 1527–1528, 1592
Abrus precatorius, toxicity of, 364–365
Abscesses, of anal sacs, 1266–1267
  of brain, 556, 583, 591
  of dental pulp, 1135, 1136
  of liver, 1337
    ultrasonography of, 1292
  of lung, 1065, 1065t
  of prostate, 1692–1693
  of skin, 36–37, 39, 391t, 398–399
  of spleen, 1858
  periodontal, 1129
  subcutaneous, 63, 65
Abyssinian, renal amyloidosis in, 1699t, 1700,
  1982t
Acanthamoeba infection, polysystemic, 416
Acanthomatous epulis, 1114, *1115,* 1117
Acanthosis nigricans, 1994t
Acarbose, for diabetes, 1448
Acariasis. See *Mite infestation.*
Accelerated idioventricular rhythms, 816
Accessory nerve, anatomy of, 664t
  examination of, 563, 567t
Acemannan, for feline immunodeficiency virus
    infection, 437, 437t
  for feline leukemia virus infection, 430
Acepromazine, as tranquilizer, in heart failure,
    733–734
  in lung infection, 1065t
  in pulmonary edema, 1065t, 1082
  cardiac effects of, echocardiography of, 842–
    843, 845t
  for tick paralysis, 673
  for vascular neuropathy, 679
Acetaminophen, 318
  for pain, 24t, 25
  toxicity of, to liver, 1327, 1331–1332
Acetic acid, in ear cleansing, for otitis externa,
    989t, 994, 996
Acetylcholine, in gastric acid secretion, 1156,
    1156
  receptors of, in myasthenia gravis, 675–676
N-Acetylcysteine, for acetaminophen toxicity, to
    liver, 1332
  for hemolytic anemia, 1802
Achalasia, cricopharyngeal, 1145, 1976t, 1985t
  esophageal, vs. idiopathic megaesophagus,
    1149

Achondroplasia, 1975t, 1983t
  and dwarfism, 1898
  maxillofacial development in, 1123–1124
  narrow pelvic canal in, and dystocia, 1534
Acid citrate dextrose, in blood storage, 350, 350t
Acidophil cell hepatitis, 1306–1307, 1330–1331
Acidosis, fluid therapy in, 330t
  hyperkalemia in, 342
  in renal disease, prevention of, diet in, 270
  metabolic, in renal failure, acute, 1624, 1629
    chronic, 1640, 1652
  renal tubular, 1707–1708, 1709t
    and hyperchloremia, 234
  respiratory, blood gas analysis in, 1039
Aciduria, 1605
  renal tubular disorders and, 1704–1706, 1709
Acinar atrophy, pancreatic, and exocrine
    insufficiency, 1355, *1355,* 1359
Acoustic reflex testing, in deafness, 1001
Acquired immunodeficiency syndrome (AIDS),
    cat scratch disease with, 382, 386
Acral mutilation, 669, 1994t
Acrodermatitis, 48, 1994t, 1995t
Acromegaly (hypersomatotropism), 1370–1373,
    1370–1373
  and cardiomyopathy, 914
  and obesity, 71
  polyphagia with, 105
Acrylamide, toxicity of, to peripheral nerves,
    673t
ACTH. See *Adrenocorticotropic hormone.*
Actigall, for cholangiohepatitis, 1310
  for liver disease, 1304
Actinic dermatitis, and carcinoma, client
    information on, 1926
  of pinna, 988–991, 989t
Actinic keratosis, and nasal carcinoma, 1019,
    1020
Actinomycosis, 391t, 395
  and enteritis, 1219
  and meningitis, spinal, 616
Actisite, for periodontitis, 1132
Acupuncture, 366–373
  diagnosis in, 366–367, *367*
  for intervertebral disk disease, *370,* 373, 634
  for pain, 25
  in cancer management, 374–375, 375t
  in small animal practice, *370–372,* 370–373
  meridians in, 367–369, *368*
  working mechanism of, 369–370
Acutrim, for urinary dysfunction, 320, 1739t
Acyclovir, for feline herpesvirus infection, 447
Addison's disease, 1488–1498. See also
    Hypoadrenocorticism.
Adenine arabinoside, for feline infectious
    peritonitis, 441
Adenitis, sebaceous, 48

Adenocarcinoma. See *Carcinoma.*
Adenocard, for arrhythmia, 826t, 828t, 831–832
Adenoma, of rectum, 1260–1262
  parathyroid. See *Hyperparathyroidism.*
  perianal, 1267–1268
  pituitary, 584t
    and hyperadrenocorticism, 1462
  rectal, 1254, *1254*
Adenomatous polyposis coli gene, in
    carcinogenesis, 478–479
Adenosine, for arrhythmia, 826t, 828t, 831–832
Adenosine triphosphatase, in heart failure, 704t
Adenovirus infection, and hepatitis, 419, 419t,
    1306, 1330
  and tracheobronchitis, 419t, 419–420
Adhesins, in periodontal disease, 1128
Adrenal glands, anatomy of, 1488
  disorders of, neurologic signs of, 551
  hyperfunction of, 1460–1487. See also *Hypera-
    drenocorticism.*
  hypofunction of, 1488–1498. See also *Hypoad-
    renocorticism.*
  hypoplasia of, 1986t
  steroid production in, 307–308, *308*
Adrenergic receptors, drugs blocking. See *Beta
    blockers.*
  steroid effects on, 311
Adrenocorticotropic hormone, ectopic production
    of, paraneoplastic, 503
  in hyperadrenocorticism, 1486
    in stimulation test, *1469,* 1469–1471, 1470t,
    1485
  in hypoadrenocorticism, 1489, 1496, 1498
    in stimulation test, 1495, 1498
  in steroid production, 307, *308*
Adriamycin. See *Doxorubicin.*
Advantage, in flea control, client information on,
    1971
Aelurostrongylus abstrusus infestation, of lung,
    1065t, 1070
Afghan hound, myelopathy in, 1991t
Afterload, in cardiac output, 693
  in heart failure, assessment of, 708
Agalactia, 1538
Agar-disk diffusion test, 303
Agglutination tests, in hemolytic anemia,
    immune-mediated, *1795,* 1795–1796
Aggression, glucocorticoids and, 316
  in cats, 160t, 160–162, *161,* 1597, 1597t
  in dogs, 156–158, *157,* 158t
  sleep-associated, 152
Aging, and adverse drug reactions, 322–323
  and deafness, 1001
  and drug disposition, 296
  and tremors, 141
Agleristone, in abortion induction, 1545
AIDS, cat scratch disease with, 382, 386

Airway. See also specific structures, e.g.,
    Trachea.
  maintenance of, in cardiopulmonary resuscita-
      tion, 190
Alanine aminotransferase, in
    hyperadrenocorticism, 1464–1465
  in hyperthyroidism, 1403t, 1403–1404
  in hypoadrenocorticism, 1493–1494
  in liver disease, 1279, 1279t, *1282*
  inflammatory, 1299, 1300
Albendazole, for *Filaroides hirthi* infestation, of
    lung, 1070
  for giardiasis, of small intestine, 1222
  for parasitosis, of urinary tract, 1779t
  for protozoal infection, 410t
Albumin, blood level of, decreased. See
    Hypoalbuminemia.
  in cerebrospinal fluid, 574t, 575
  in fluid therapy, 327, 329, 331, 331t, 339t
  in liver disease, 1278t, 1284
  in pancreatitis, 1354
  in systemic inflammatory response syndrome,
      327
  in urine, *101*
Albuterol, for bronchopulmonary disease, 1056,
    1059t
Alcohol, ethyl, for ethylene glycol toxicity, 361,
    1626t
  injection of, for hyperthyroidism, 1415
  for hyperparathyroidism, 1391
  methyl, toxicity of, 361
Aldactazide (spironolactone/hydrochlorothiazide),
    for edema, pulmonary, with hypertrophic
    cardiomyopathy, 908
  with hepatic failure, 1302t
Aldosterone, deficiency of, 1490, *1490,*
    1495–1496. See also *Hypoadrenocorticism.*
  excess of, and hypokalemia, 225, *226*
  renal tubular dysfunction in, 1706
  in heart failure, 700–701, 702t, 703
Algal infection, intestinal, 1219
  client information on, 1947
Aliasing, in echocardiography, 841, *842*
Alimentary tract. See *Gastrointestinal tract* and
    specific structures, e.g., *Esophagus.*
Alkaline phosphatase, in hepatitis, chronic, 1300
  in hyperadrenocorticism, 1465, 1471
  in hyperthyroidism, 1403t, 1404
  in liver disease, 1279t, *1282,* 1282–1283
Alkalosis, fluid therapy in, 330t
  metabolic, in acute renal failure, 1624, 1629
Alkaluria, 1605
  with urinary tract infection, 1780
Alkylating agents, in cancer therapy, 488
Allergy, and cough, 163t, 165
  and dermatitis, 1973
  and otitis externa, 989t, 992, 996
  client information on, 1942, 1971–1973
  flea infestation and, 1971
  to drugs, 324–325
  to food, 251–252, *252,* 1230–1232, 1231t,
      1942, 1972
    and otitis externa, 992
    and pruritus, 32–34, 33t, 34t
    clinical features of, 253–254, *254*
    diagnosis of, 255–256, *256*
    in inflammatory bowel disease, 1251
    management of, 256–257
  with pruritus, 32, 33, 33t, 34t, 36
  with zinc deficiency, 48–49
Alloimmune hemolytic anemia, 1797–1798
Allopurinol, for leishmaniasis, 410t, 415
  for urate urolithiasis, 1724–1725, 1773, 1775
Alopecia, 29–31, *30*
  and hyperpigmentation, 58

Alopecia *(Continued)*
  and hypopigmentation, 57
  chemotherapy and, 487
  congenital, 1981t, 1994t, 1995t
  in hypothyroidism, 1421
  of pinna, nonpruritic, 987t, 988
Alpha₁-protease inhibitor, fecal assay for, 1207
Alpha-bungarotoxin, in diagnosis of myasthenia
    gravis, 675–676
Alpha-fetoprotein, in liver disease, 1285
Alpha-fucosidosis, 3t, 1992t
  and peripheral neuropathy, 670
Alpha-glucosidase deficiency, 1290, 1992t
Alpha-L-iduronidase deficiency, in
    mucopolysaccharidosis, 1979t, 1980t
  skeletal abnormalities with, 1896
  spinal cord dysfunction with, 638
Alpha-mannosidase deficiency, 1980t
Alpha-tocopherol. See *Vitamin E.*
Alprazolam, for behavioral disorders, 156, 158t
Alsatian, giant axonal neuropathy in, 667
Alteplase, for thromboembolism, 1840
Aluminum compounds, for renal failure, 319,
    1650–1651
Alveolar bone, loss of, in periodontal disease,
    1128–1130, *1130, 1131*
Alveoli, in atelectasis, 1088
Amalgam, in dental restoration, 1140–1141
Amanita species, toxicity of, 364, 1329, 1332
Amastia, 1980t
Amebiasis, of large intestine, 1245–1246
  of small intestine, 408–410, 409t, 410t
  polysystemic, 416
Amelia, 1894, 1975t
Ameloblastoma, 1114
Ameroid constrictor, for portosystemic shunt,
    1314, 1315
Amikacin (Amiglyde), concentration of, and
    bacterial susceptibility, 303t
  dosage of, in renal failure, 1649t
  for bacteremia, with liver disorders, 1335
  for lung infection, 1065t
Amiloride, for pulmonary edema, with mitral
    insufficiency, 793
Amine precursor uptake and decarboxylation
    tumors, and gastric ulcers, 1166
Amines, vasoactive, in food, adverse reactions
    to, 253
Amino acids, blood level of, in liver disease,
    1278t, 1284–1285
  branched-chain, for hepatic encephalopathy,
      1334
  in diet, 237, 239t
    in gastrointestinal disorders, 259
    in hepatic disease, 260
  in parenteral nutrition, 281, 282, 282t
  in urine, 1704–1705
    in Fanconi's syndrome, 1709
Aminophylline, for cough, 165t
  for respiratory disorders, with heart failure,
      734
  for tracheal disease, 1043t
5-Aminosalicylic acid, for inflammatory bowel
    disease, 1250
Amiodarone, for arrhythmia, 824t–826t, 828t,
    830
  in cardiopulmonary resuscitation, 192t, 193
Amitraz, for demodicosis, 62
  client information on, 1970
  for mange, notoedric, 61
  pinnal, 988, 989t
  for scabies, 61
  toxicity of, 357
Amitriptyline, for behavioral disorders, in cats,
    160, 160t

Amitriptyline *(Continued)*
  in dogs, 156, 158t
  for pain, 24t, 25
  for urinary tract disorders, idiopathic, 1746
Amlodipine, for arrhythmia, 824t, 830, 831
  for hypertension, 182
    in renal failure, 1653–1654
Ammonia, blood level of, in liver disease, 1278t,
    1286, 1286–1287
  in renal tubular acidosis, 1707, 1708
Ammonia biurate crystalluria, in liver disease,
    1291
Ammonium urate, in urolithiasis, in cats, 1723t,
    1724–1725, 1725t
  in dogs, 1758t, 1770–1775, 1773t, 1774t
Amoxicillin, concentration of, and bacterial
    susceptibility, 303, 303t
  dosage of, in renal failure, 1649t
  for bacterial infection, 391t
  for *Helicobacter* infection, with gastritis, 1164
  for intestinal bacterial overgrowth, with histo-
      plasmosis, 464
  for lung infection, 1065t
Amphimerus pseudofelineus infestation, of
    pancreas, 1363t, 1364
Amphotericin B, dosage of, in renal failure,
    1649t
  for blastomycosis, 456, 462
  for central nervous system infection, 593t
  for coccidioidomycosis, 467–468
  for cryptococcosis, 471
  for fungal infection, 454–456, 475t
  for leishmaniasis, 410t, 415
  toxicity of, to kidney, 455–456, 1616
Ampicillin, concentration of, and bacterial
    susceptibility, 303t
  dosage of, in renal failure, 1649t
  for bacteremia, with liver disorders, 1335
  for bacterial infection, 391t
  for central nervous system infection, 593t
  for hepatic encephalopathy, 1333, 1334t
  for lung infection, 1065t
Amprolium, for protozoal infection, 410, 410t
Amputation, congenital, 1894
  for osteosarcoma, 1911
Amrinone, for cardiomyopathy, 884
  for heart failure, 732–733
  for hypotension, 184t, 185
Amyloidosis, of kidneys, and proteinuria,
    100–101, *101*
  clinical findings in, 1669t, 1669–1670
  congenital, 1982t, 1996t
  diagnosis of, 1670–1672, *1670–1672*
  familial, 1698, 1699t, 1700–1702
  pathogenesis of, 1667–1669, 1668t
  treatment of, 1674
  of liver, 1323, 1337
  of pancreas, in islet cell destruction, 1439,
      1440
Anabolic steroids, for anemia, in renal failure,
    1655
Anafranil, for behavioral disorders, in cats, 160t
  in dogs, 156, 158t
Anal sacs, anatomy of, 1257
  impaction of, 1266–1267
  tumors of, 1267
Anal sphincter, disorders of, and incontinence,
    133, 134, *134,* 134t
Analgesia, acupuncture and, 369–370
Analgesics, for urinary tract disorders,
    idiopathic, 1744–1745
  over-the-counter, 318
  with adrenal surgery, for hyperadrenocorti-
      cism, 1475–1476
Anaphylaxis, food allergy and, 253

Anaphylaxis (Continued)
  hydroxyethyl starch and, 334
  hyperimmune serum and, in treatment of tick
    paralysis, 673
  hypotension in, 184t
Anasarca, congenital, 1978t, 1989t
Ancobon. See Flucytosine.
Anconeal process, ununited, 1871, 1871, 1872,
  1984t
Ancylostomiasis, of large intestine, 1246
  of small intestine, 1220–1221, 1221t
  of spinal cord, 647
  zoonotic, 387
Anemia, 198–203
  and weakness, 10–11
  aplastic, 201, 202t, 203, 1812–1813
    and epistaxis, 214
    estrogen therapy and, 1822
  blood loss and, 1786–1789, 1788
  bone marrow in, regenerative response in,
    1784, 1784–1786, 1785
    stromal disorders in, 1813–1814, 1814
    transplantation of, 1815–1816
  chemical toxicity and, 1811–1812
  chronic disease and, 1806–1808, 1807, 1808
  cyanosis with, 207
  diagnosis of, 198t, 199–200, 200t, 1804–1806,
    1805, 1806, 1806t
    differential, 200–203, 201, 202t
  drug toxicity and, 504, 1812, 1812t
  familial nonspherocytic, 1989t
  feline leukemia virus and, 427, 429
  hemolytic, 198–200, 200t, 201, 202t, 1789–
    1803
    chemical toxicity and, 1800–1802, 1801t
    erythrocyte defects and, inherited, 1790–
      1793, 1791t
    hypophosphatemia and, 1802
    immune-mediated, 199, 200t, 1793–1798,
      1794t, 1795
      client information on, 1960
    infection-associated, 1798–1800, 1799t
    microangiopathic, 1802–1803
  hyperestrogenism and, 1811
  in renal failure, 1640–1641, 1808
    management of, 1654–1656
  leukemia and, 1814–1815
  liver disease and, 1291
  metabolic disorders and, 1810
  myelodysplasia and, 1814, 1815
  non-regenerative, 1804–1816
  nutritional deficiencies and, 1808–1809
  paraneoplastic, 503–504, 504
  pure red cell aplasia in, 1812
  retroviral infection and, 1810t, 1810–1811
  rickettsial infection and, 1811
  transfusion for, 1655, 1815
Anencephaly, 1979t
Anesthesia, before catheterization, for urethral
  obstruction, 1734
  cardiac arrest during, acupuncture for, 372,
    372
  for biopsy, of liver, 1296, 1296t
  for gonadectomy, prepubertal, 1541
  intolerance to, liver disease and, 1273t, 1275–
    1276
  local, for pain, 23, 24t
  respiratory arrest during, acupuncture for, 372,
    372
Anestrus, 1510, 1510, 1514–1516, 1516, 1587
  prolonged, in cat, 1591, 1595
    in cystic endometrial hyperplasia, 1524,
      1524–1525
    in dog, 1562, 1562
  shortened, 1525

Aneurysm, arterial, 968, 969
Aneurysmal bone cysts, 539, 1904–1905
Angiitis, arterial, 972–974
Angiocardiography, of cardiomyopathy, dilated,
  910, 910
  hypertrophic, canine, 889–890, 890
    feline, 899–901, 902, 904, 904
  of patent ductus arteriosus, 748, 750
  of pulmonic insufficiency, congenital, 773,
    774
  of pulmonic stenosis, congenital, 762, 764,
    765
  of subaortic stenosis, 770, 771
  of tetralogy of Fallot, 782, 782
  of thromboembolism, 916, 917
  of ventricular septal defect, 758, 759
Angioedema, 37, 39
  food allergy and, 253–254
Angiogenesis, in tumor metastasis, 481–482, 482
Angiography, in congenital heart disease,
  741–742
  of arteriovenous fistula, 970–971
  of brain, 576
  of vena cava, 974, 975, 976
Angiomatosis, bacillary, in cat scratch disease,
  382
Angiostrongylus cantonensis infestation, of
  spinal cord, 647
Angiostrongylus vasorum infestation, of lung,
  1065t, 1070
Angiotensin, in heart failure, 700, 702t, 703
Angiotensin-converting enzyme inhibitors, for
  cardiomyopathy, dilated, 883, 884
    hypertrophic, 905–907
  for glomerulonephritis, 1673
  for heart failure, 713–714, 718–723, 720t
  for hypertension, 182
    in dirofilariasis, 949t
    in renal failure, 1653–1654
  for mitral insufficiency, 793
  toxicity of, to kidney, 1617
Aniridia, 1987t
Anisocoria, feline immunodeficiency virus
  infection and, 436, 436
  in neurologic examination, 658–661, 659t,
    660t
Anisocytosis, 1785, 1785
  in anemia, 200t
Ankylosing spondylitis, 651
Anodontia, 1122
Anophthalmos, 1977t, 1987t
Anorexia, 102–104, 104
  and cachexia, 73
  and hypokalemia, 223–225
  hydralazine and, in heart failure, 724
  in renal failure, 1635, 1636t
    management of, 1648, 1648
  liver disease and, 1273t, 1276
  paraneoplastic, 499–501
  with ptyalism, 108
Anosmia, and anorexia, 103
Anoxia, and neurologic dysfunction, 586
Antacids, for gastric ulcers, 1168
Anthelminthics, for small intestinal parasitosis,
  1220, 1221, 1221t
Antiarrhythmic drugs, 822–832. See also
  Arrhythmia.
Antibiotics, 301–307. See also specific drugs,
  e.g., Clindamycin.
  adverse reactions to, hepatic disease and, 323t
    renal disease and, 323t, 324
  aminoglycoside, concentration of, and clinical
    outcome, 304
  ionization of, 295
  and colitis, 1245

Antibiotics (Continued)
  and diarrhea, 1245
  client information on, 1969
  dosage of, in renal failure, 1649, 1649t
  effectiveness of, local factors in, 302
  elimination of, 297, 298
  for bacteremia, with liver disorders, 1335
  for bacterial infection, 391t
    of small enteritis, 1217, 1218
    with arthritis, 1876
  for bacterial intestinal overgrowth, 1224, 1225
    with pancreatic exocrine insufficiency,
      1363t, 1363–1364
  for bronchial asthma, 1058, 1059t
  for bronchiectasis, 1057, 1059t
  for bronchitis, 1056, 1059t
  for central nervous system infection, 592, 593t
  for cholangiohepatitis, 1310
  for cough, 165t, 166
  for diarrhea, 1215
  for discospondylitis, 625
  for endocarditis, 798–799
  for hepatic encephalopathy, 1333, 1334t
  for inflammatory bowel disease, 1227
  for intracellular infection, 302
  for osteomyelitis, 1914
  for otitis externa, 990t, 995, 996
  for otitis media, 990t, 999
  for parvovirus infection, of small intestine,
    1216
  for periodontal disease, 1132–1133
  for prostatitis, 1693
  for pyoderma, 46, 46t, 47
  for pyometra, 1554
  for stomatitis, 1119
  for urinary tract disorders, idiopathic, 1744
  for urinary tract infection, 1682–1686, 1684,
    1685t
    client information on, 1964
    in susceptibility testing, 1681–1682
  in artificial insemination, 1574
  in cancer therapy, 488
  in surgery, prophylactic use of, 306–307
  minimum inhibitory concentration of, and clin-
    ical outcome, 304, 304–305
  selection of, 302–304, 303t
  tissue penetration of, 301–302
  tissue-directed therapy with, 302
  toxicity of, to kidney, 1616
Antibodies, in cerebrospinal fluid, 574t, 575
Anticholinergic drugs, for gastritis, 1162
Anticoagulants. See also Heparin and Warfarin.
  for glomerulonephritis, 1672t, 1674
  for thromboembolism, 917
    in hemolytic anemia, immune-mediated,
      1797
  for thrombosis, 1840
  in blood storage, 350, 350t
  in rodenticides, toxicity of, 359–360
Anticonvulsants, 577. See also Seizures.
  and hyperadrenocorticism, vs. Cushing's syn-
    drome, 1470
  and osteodystrophy, 1908
  effect of, on liver enzyme concentrations,
    1279, 1283
  toxicity of, and anemia, 1812
    to liver, 1307
Antidepressants, for behavioral disorders, in cats,
  160, 160t
  in dogs, 156, 158t
  for pain, 24t, 25
Antidigitalis antibody fragments, for glycoside
  toxicity, 365
Antidiuretic hormone (vasopressin), endogenous,
  in heart failure, 701

Antidiuretic hormone (vasopressin) *(Continued)*
  for hemorrhagic disorders, in renal failure, 1639
  for von Willebrand's disease, 1825
  in diabetes insipidus, 1374–1379, *1375, 1378*
  in polyuria, deficiency of, 85t, 85–89, *86*, 87t, 88t
    with water deprivation testing, 88t, 1604
  inappropriate secretion of, paraneoplastic, 503
Antiemetics, over-the-counter, 319
Antifreeze. See *Ethylene glycol.*
Antifungal drugs, 454–457, *457*, 475t. See also specific agents, e.g., *Fluconazole.*
Antigen presentation, in small intestine, *1194*, 1194–1195, *1195*
Antihistamines, for atopic dermatitis, client information on, 1973
  over-the-counter, 319
Anti-inflammatory drugs, for brain disorders, 577
  for inflammatory bowel disease, 1227
  nonsteroidal, and stomach ulcers, 1165–1166
    for degenerative joint disease, 1865–1866
    for fever, 9
    for pain, 24, 24t, 25
  steroidal, 307–317. See also *Corticosteroids.*
Antimetabolites, in cancer therapy, 489
Antineoplastons, in cancer therapy, 377
Antinuclear antibodies, in joint inflammation, in synovial fluid, 80
  with systemic lupus erythematosus, 1882
  methimazole and, in treatment of hyperthyroidism, 1411
Antiplatelet drugs, for thromboembolism, 917–918
Antirobe. See *Clindamycin.*
Antispasmodics, for urinary tract disorders, idiopathic, 1745
Antithrombin, 1830, 1833t
Antithyroglobulin antibodies, in hypothyroidism, 1425
Antizol-Vet, for ethylene glycol toxicity, 361
Antrum, of stomach, anatomy of, 1155, *1155*
  hypertrophy of, and outlet obstruction, *1169*, 1169–1170
  in motility, 1158
Anuria, in acute renal failure, 1623
Anury, 1983t
Anus, anatomy of, 1257–1258
  atresia of, 1264
  congenital defects of, 1976t, 1985t
  disorders of, and fecal incontinence, 1268, 1268t, 1269
  diagnosis of, 1258t, 1258–1259
  function of, 1258
  furunculosis of, 1264–1266
  rectal prolapse through, 1262–1263
  stricture of, 1263–1264
  tumors of, 1267–1268
Anxiolytics, for heart failure, 733–734
Aorta, aneurysm of, 968, *969*
  coarctation of, 786
  echocardiography of, 852–853, 856t, 858
  in tetralogy of Fallot, *754*, 780–782, *782*
  thrombosis of, chondrosarcoma and, *967*
  transposition of, with pulmonary artery, 783–784
Aortic arch, malformation of, and esophageal compression, 1145
  right, persistent, 784–785, *785*, 1976t, 1985t
Aortic atresia, 783, *783*
Aortic insufficiency, 796
  client information on, 1952
  murmur with, 172, 174
Aortic regurgitation, congenital, 773–774

Aortic regurgitation *(Continued)*
  echocardiography of, 857t, 871
Aortic stenosis, and syncope, 15
  auscultation of, 739t
  congenital, 1976t, 1985t
  echocardiography of, 866–869, *868*
    in blood pressure measurement, 847, 847t
  murmur with, 172, 174
  subvalvular, 768–772, *769–772*
    auscultation of, 739t
    cardiac catheterization in, 742, *743*
    clinical findings in, 769–771, *770–772*
    echocardiography of, continuous-wave, *844*
    in hypertrophic cardiomyopathy, 887–888, *888*
    management of, 771–772
    murmur with, 172, 174
    natural history of, 771
    pathology of, 768–769, *769*
Aortic valve, blood flow through, echocardiography of, *842*, 843–845, 845t
  in hypertrophic cardiomyopathy, 898, *899*
Aorticopulmonary septal defect, 785–786
Apathetic hyperthyroidism, 1403
Apexification, in endodontic treatment, 1139
Aphakia, 1977t, 1987t
Apicoectomy, in endodontic treatment, 1140
Aplasia cutis, 1981t, 1994t
Aplastic anemia, *201*, 202t, 203, 1812–1813
  and epistaxis, 214
  estrogen therapy and, 1822
Apnea, during sleep, 154
Apoptosis, in carcinogenesis, 479–480
Appetite, changes in, with diarrhea, 122, 122t
  excessive, 104–107, 105t, *106*
    in pancreatic exocrine insufficiency, 1358–1359
    with cachexia, 73
  loss of. See *Anorexia.*
APUDomas, and gastric ulcers, 1166
Aqueous humor, disorders of, and vision loss, 17, 17t
Arachidonic acid, in diet, 240
  in platelet activation, 1817, *1817*
Arachnids. See also specific infestations, e.g., *Demodicosis.*
  in skin infestation, 59t, 60–62, *62*
Arachnoid cysts, and spinal cord dysfunction, 645–647, *646*
Argasid ticks, in skin infestation, 59t, 61
Arginase, in liver disease, 1279–1280
Arginine, for hepatic encephalopathy, 1335
  in diet, 239t
Arginine vasopressin. See *Antidiuretic hormone.*
Arnica, in cancer management, 378t
Arrhythmia, adenosine for, 826t, 828t, 831–832
  amiodarone for, 824t–826t, 828t, 830
  beta blockers for, 824t–826t, 827–830, 828t, 829t
  bretylium for, 184t, 824t, 826t, 830
  calcium channel blockers for, 824t–826t, 828t, 829t, 830–831
  digitalis glycosides for, 826t, 828t, 829t, 831
  disopyramide for, 825, 825t, 826t, 828t
  drugs for, 822–832
    classification of, Sicilian gambit, 823–824, 825t, 826t
    Vaughn-Williams, 823, 824t
  edrophonium for, 832
  electrocardiography of, 800–822. See also *Electrocardiography.*
  flecainide for, 824t, 826t, 827
  ibutilide for, 830
  in cardiomyopathy, dilated, 879, 880, *880*, 880t

Arrhythmia *(Continued)*
  drugs for, 885
  hypertrophic, 898, 905
  right ventricular, *912*, 912–913
  in digitalis toxicity, 729–730
  in heart failure, 706
  in hypotension, 184t, 185
  in mitral insufficiency, 790, 794–795
  isoproterenol for, 828t
  lidocaine for, 824t–826t, 826, 828t
  mexiletine for, 824t–826t, 826, 827, 828t
  pacemakers for, 832t, 832–833
  phenylephrine for, 832
  procainamide for, 824t–826t, 825–826, 829t
  propafenone for, 824t, 826t, 827, 829t
  quinidine for, 824t–826t, 824–825, 829t
  radiofrequency ablation for, 832
  respiratory sinus, 809–810, *810*
  sotalol for, 824t–826t, 829t, 830
  tocainide for, 824t–826t, 826–827, 829t
  with gastric dilatation and volvulus, 1173–1174
Arsenamide. See *Thiacetarsamide.*
Arsenic, toxicity of, 363
Arteries. See also specific vessels, e.g., *Pulmonary artery.*
  aneurysms of, 968, *969*
  inflammation of, 972–974
  occlusion of, 964t, 964–968, *965*, 965t, *967*
  pseudoaneurysm of, 968–969
  pulses in, 174–177, *175, 176*
  spasticity of, 974
Arteriography, of arteriovenous fistula, hepatic, 1318
  of brain, 576
Arterioportal fistulas, 1979t, 1991t
Arteriosclerosis, 971–972, *972*
Arteriovenous fistula, 969–971, *970, 971*
  hepatic, 1317–1318, 1979t, 1991t
    and portosystemic shunt, 1316
    ultrasonography of, 1292
Arteritis, with meningitis, and arthritis, 1882
  spinal, steroid-responsive, 621–622
Arthritis, acupuncture for, 372
  classification of, 77–79, 78t
  degenerative, 1862–1866, *1863*, 1863t, *1864*
  diagnosis of, 79, *79*, 79–80
  immune-mediated, 77–80, 78t, *79*, 1879–1883, *1880*
    client information on, 1961
    treatment of, 1883–1885
  infectious, 1875–1879, *1877*
  obesity with, 71
Arthrocentesis, in arthritis, 79, *79*, 1879
  in degenerative joint disease, 1865
Arthropod bites, and granuloma, 37
Artificial insemination, 1574–1577, *1576*
  client information on, 1934
  semen collection for, 1571–1572
Arylsulfatase deficiency, in metachromatic leukodystrophy, 1980t
  in mucopolysaccharidosis, 1979t, 1980t
  skeletal abnormalities with, 1896
  spinal cord dysfunction with, 638
Ascites, 137–139, *138*
  biliary tract disorders and, 1342, 1344
  in dirofilariasis, 941, 943, *945*
  in peritonitis, feline infectious, 440t, 440–441
  liver disease and, 1276, 1277
  with heart failure, abdominocentesis for, 733
  with hepatic failure, management of, 1302t
  with hepatic venous outflow obstruction, 1318–1319
  with lymphangiectasia, of small intestine, 1229, *1229*

Ascites (Continued)
with mitral insufficiency, 790
with pericardial constrictive disease, 934
with protein-losing enteropathy, 1202
with weakness, 11
Ascorbic acid (vitamin C), for acetaminophen toxicity, to liver, 1332
for methemoglobinemia, in naphthalene toxicity, 357
in diet, 240
in orthopedic developmental disorders, 248
Aseptic necrosis, of femoral head, 1873, 1874, 1984t
L-Asparaginase, in cancer therapy, 489
for lymphoma, 511t
Aspartate aminotransferase, in hypoadrenocorticism, 1493–1494
in liver disease, 1279, 1279t, 1282
Aspergillosis, 473, 473–475, 475t
and rhinitis, 1018–1019
computed tomography of, 1009–1012, 1013, 1014
of lung, 1068
Aspiration, and pneumonia, 1084–1086, 1085
client information on, 1955
with dysphagia, 114, 115
fine-needle, in cytology, 52
Aspirin, 318
angiotensin-converting enzyme inhibitors with, 719
for degenerative joint disease, 1866
for glomerulonephritis, 1672t, 1674
for pain, 24t, 25
for thromboembolism, arterial, 968
in cats, 917–918
pulmonary, in dirofilariasis, 949t
in cancer management, 378t
Asthenia, 10
cutaneous, 1981t, 1995t
Asthenozoospermia, 1579–1580
Asthma, bronchial, 1057–1058, 1058t, 1059t
client information on, 1954
Astigmata mites, 59t, 61. See also Mite infestation.
Astrocytes, feline immunodeficiency virus in, 434
Astrocytoma, 584, 584t, 585t
Astrovirus infection, 451
Asystole, ventricular, in cardiopulmonary arrest, 192
Ataxia, 142–143
hereditary, 629, 1991t
in brain disorders, 560
in spinal cord disorders, 611
in lesion localization, 613–615
Atelectasis, 1088
Atenolol, for arrhythmia, 824t, 827, 828t, 830
for cardiomyopathy, dilated, 911
hypertrophic, 905–907
for hypertension, 182
for hyperthyroidism, 1412
for subaortic stenosis, 772
for tachyarrhythmia, with mitral insufficiency, 794–795
Atherosclerosis, 971–972, 972
Atlantoaxial joint, subluxation of, 615, 615–616, 616, 1984t
Atopic dermatitis, and pruritus, 32, 33, 33t, 34t, 36
client information on, 1973
with zinc deficiency, 48–49
Atopy, and otitis externa, 992
Atrial extrasystoles, 810–811, 811
Atrial fibrillation, electrocardiography of, 812–813, 813

Atrial fibrillation (Continued)
with dilated cardiomyopathy, 879, 880, 880, 880t
Atrial flutter, electrocardiography of, 812, 812
Atrial gallop, 170
Atrial natriuretic peptide, in heart failure, 701
Atrial septal defect, 750–759
auscultation of, 739t
client information on, 1951
clinical findings in, 755, 755–756, 756, 854t
management of, 758–759
natural history of, 758
pathogenesis of, 751, 753
pathophysiology of, 751–752
Atrial standstill, electrocardiography of, 820, 821
persistent, 914, 1976t, 1985t
Atrial tachycardia, electrocardiography of, 811–812, 812
Atridox, for periodontitis, 1132
Atrioventricular bundle, conduction blocks of, 817, 817–819
stenosis of, 1985t
Atrioventricular myopathy, 890–891
Atrioventricular node, junctional, in rhythm disturbances, 813, 813
Atrioventricular valves. See Mitral valve and Tricuspid valve.
Atrium, anomalies of, 1976t, 1985t
left, echocardiography of, 850t, 851, 854–857, 856t, 859
enlargement of, and bronchial compression, 1059, 1060, 1060
with mitral insufficiency, 788–790, 789, 791
rupture of, mitral insufficiency and, 795
right, echocardiography of, 856t, 858–859, 859, 862
hemangiosarcoma of, and pericardial effusion, 928, 932, 932–933
Atropine, for arrhythmia, 828t
for bradyarrhythmia, with hypotension, 184t
for insecticide toxicity, 359
for organophosphate toxicity, with megaesophagus, 1150t
in anesthesia, for prepubertal gonadectomy, 1541
in cardiopulmonary resuscitation, 192t
with electrocardiography, in sinus bradycardia, 809
in vagal inhibition, 806, 807
Attitudinal reactions, in neurologic examination, 561, 561–562, 562
Audiometry, impedance, in deafness, 1001
Auditory evoked responses, brain stem, 575
in deafness, 1001–1002
Aujeszky's disease (pseudorabies), 423, 595
in cats, 451–452
ptyalism in, 108
Autoimmunity, and arthritis, client information on, 1961
and hypopigmentation, 55, 57
and skin erosions, 40t, 43
in hypoadrenocorticism, 1489
Autosomal genetic defects, 2, 3, 3t. See also Genetic defects.
Axid (nizatidine), for gastric motility disorders, 1176
for gastric ulcers, 1168
for gastrinoma, 1506, 1506t
Axillary nerve, injury to, signs of, 663t
Axis, articulation of, with atlas, subluxation of, 615, 615–616, 616, 1984t
Axons, in neuroaxonal dystrophy, congenital, 642, 1980t, 1992t
in peripheral nerves, 662, 662, 665–666

Axons (Continued)
loss of, in developmental disorders, 667–668, 1992t
Ayurvedic treatment, for cancer, 376, 377t
Azathioprine, for anemia, paraneoplastic, 504
for arthritis, immune-mediated, 1884–1885
for glomerulonephritis, 1672, 1672t
for hepatitis, chronic, 1301
for inflammatory bowel disease, 1227, 1250–1251
for thrombocytopenia, immune-mediated, 1822
paraneoplastic, 505
Azidothymidine (AZT), for feline immunodeficiency virus infection, 437, 437t
PIND-ORF derivative of, for feline leukemia virus infection, 431
Azoospermia, 1578–1579
Azotemia, amphotericin B and, 455–456
definition of, 1600
diuretics and, in heart failure, 715, 717
etiology of, 1615, 1616t
in renal failure, 1641
dietary management of, 271t, 272, 272t
AZT, for feline immunodeficiency virus infection, 437, 437t
PIND-ORF derivative of, for feline leukemia virus infection, 431
Azulfidine. See Sulfasalazine.

B lymphocytes, in colonic mucosal immunity, 1239
in inflammation, steroid effects on, 310–311
in small intestinal immune response, 1195
Babesiosis, and anemia, hemolytic, 1799t, 1800
non-regenerative, 1811
polysystemic, 414
screening for, in blood donors, 348
zoonotic, 383t
Babinski reflex, testing of, 570
Bacillary angiomatosis, in cat scratch disease, 382
Bacillus piliformis infection, and enteritis, 1218–1219
Baclofen, for urine retention, 95t
Bacteremia. See Sepsis.
Bacteria, as leukocyte inclusions, 1847, 1847
in large intestine, normal, 1239
in small intestine, normal, 1193
overgrowth of, 1223t, 1223–1225, 1224t
and pancreatic exocrine insufficiency, 1356–1357, 1363t, 1363–1364
tests for, 1211–1212
with histoplasmosis, 464
in urine, 1609, 1609–1611, 1611t
in vagina, normal, 1518–1519, 1559, 1560t, 1567
Bacterial infection, 390–407, 391t. See also specific diseases, e.g., Salmonellosis.
and arthritis, 1875–1878, 1877
and cholangiohepatitis, 1309
and cystitis, 1778, 1779t
and discospondylitis, with spinal cord dysfunction, 624, 625
and endocarditis, 796–799, 797
echocardiography of, 857t
murmur with, 172
and fetal loss, 1527
and granuloma, 37
and meningitis, 597, 603–604, 605, 606
cerebrospinal fluid examination in, 574, 574t
spinal, 616–618, 618t
and metritis, 1536

IND

Bacterial infection (*Continued*)
  and myositis, 686–687
  and otitis externa, 990t, 993, 996
  and otitis media, 990t, 997–999
  and pyometra, in cystic endometrial hyperplasia, 1549, 1554
  and rhinitis, 1018
    with epistaxis, 215
  and sepsis, with liver disorders, 1335–1336
  and thrombocytopenia, 1821
  and urethritis, 1778, 1779t
  antibiotics for, 301–307, 303t, *304*, 391t. See also *Antibiotics* and specific drugs, e.g., *Tetracycline.*
  in epidermal dysplasia, in West Highland white terrier, 48
  of biliary tract, 1342–1344
  of bone, 306, 1912–1914, *1913, 1914*
  of joints, 306
  of large intestine, 1241, 1243–1245
  of liver, and abscess, 1337
  of lung, 1063–1066, 1065t
  of prostate, 1689t, 1692–1693, *1693*
  of root canal, 1135
  of skin, and abscesses, 391t, 398–399
    and erosions, 40t, 40–42
    and ulcers, 40t, 40–42
    antibiotics for, 305
  of small intestine, 1217–1219, *1218*
    fecal examination for, 1207
  of trachea, 1041–1042
  of urethra, 1593–1594
  of urinary tract, 1678–1686. See also *Urinary tract, infection of.*
  subcutaneous, 63, 65
  with herpesvirus infection, 446–447
Bacterial plaque, periodontal, 1127–1130, 1129t, *1129–1131,* 1130t
  removal of, 1130–1133
Bacteroides infection, antibiotics for, 303, 305
Balanoposthitis, with preputial discharge, 84, 84t
Balantidiasis, of large intestine, 1246
  of small intestine, 408–411, 409t, 410t
Balloon valvuloplasty, for pulmonic stenosis, 766, 767, *767*
  for subaortic stenosis, 772
Band keratopathy, in hyperparathyroidism, 1380
Barberry bark, in cancer management, 378t
Barium, in contrast radiography, of esophagus, 1143
    with fistula, 1147
    with stricture, 1148, *1149*
  of gastric ulcers, 1167
  of small intestine, 1208, *1209*
Baroreflex control, in heart failure, 700
Bartonellosis, 391t, 399
  screening for, in blood donors, 349
  zoonotic, 382–386, 399
Baruria, 1604
Basal cell tumors, of skin, 51, 525
Basement membrane, renal, disorder of, in bull terrier, 1699t, 1701
  tumor invasion through, *482,* 482–483
Basenji, enteropathy in, 1228
  gastritis in, 1165
  renal tubular dysfunction in, 1699t, 1700–1701
Basophilia, 1852, 1852t
  cytoplasmic, 1845, *1845*
  in dirofilariasis, 947
  in leukemia, 515t, 515–516
Basophils, production of, 1842
Basrani's classification, of tooth fractures, 1137, 1137t
Basset hound, thrombopathia in, 1824t, 1825–1826, 1990t

Bats, rabies in, 388
Baylisascariasis, zoonotic, 386–387
Baypamun, for feline leukemia virus infection, 431
Baytril. See *Enrofloxacin.*
Beagle, renal amyloidosis in, 1699t, 1701, 1996t
Bedlington terrier, hepatic copper accumulation in, 5, 1304–1305, *1305,* 1991t
Bee stings, hepatic reaction to, 1329
Behavior, changes in, after prepubertal gonadectomy, 1540–1541
  in hyperthyroidism, 1401
  liver disease and, 1273t, 1276
  rabies and, 423, 450
  disorders of, in cats, 158–162, *159,* 160t, *161*
    and urination, in inappropriate location, 1716–1718, 1717t
    in mating activity, 1594–1595, 1597, 1597t
  in dogs, 156–158, *157,* 158t
  postparturient, 1538–1539
Benazepril, for cardiomyopathy, dilated, 883
    hypertrophic, 905–907
  for heart failure, 720t, 723
  for hypertension, 182
Bence Jones proteins, in multiple myeloma, 516–519
Benylin DM (dextromethorphan), for cough, 165t, 319
  in heart failure, 734
  in tracheal disease, 1043t
Benzocaine, for skin disorders, 319
Benzodiazepine receptor antagonists, for hepatic encephalopathy, 1334
Benzodiazepines, for behavioral disorders, 156, 158t
Bernese Mountain dog, glomerulonephritis in, 1699t, 1701
  histiocytosis in, 520–521, *521*
  of lung, 1078
Besnoitia infection, enteric, 408, 409t
Beta blockers, for arrhythmia, 824t–826t, 827–830, 828t, 829t
  for cardiomyopathy, dilated, canine, 884–885
    feline, 911
    hypertrophic, canine, 890
    feline, 905, 907
  for hyperthyroidism, 1412
  for myocardial infarction, 905, 907
  for subaortic stenosis, 772
Beta-catenin, in carcinogenesis, 478–479
Beta-cell neoplasia, pancreatic, 1429–1438. See also *Insulinoma.*
Betadine (povidone-iodine), for anal sacculitis, 1266
  for otitis externa, 989t, 995
Beta-galactocerebrosidase deficiency, in globoid cell leukodystrophy, 1992t
Beta-galactosidase deficiency, in gangliosidosis, 589, 590t, 1980t, 1992t
Beta-glucosidase deficiency, in glucocerebrosidosis, 1992t
Beta-glucuronidase deficiency, in mucopolysaccharidosis, skeletal abnormalities with, 1897
Beta-hexosaminidase deficiency, in gangliosidosis, 1992t
Beta-lactam antibiotics, concentration of, and clinical outcome, 304
Betamethasone, dosage of, 313t
  potency of, 312t, 312–313
Bethanechol, for bladder dysfunction, 95t, 96, 1738, 1739t
  in dysautonomia, 680
Bicarbonate, for diabetes mellitus, with ketoacidosis, 1444t, 1445

Bicarbonate (*Continued*)
  for ethylene glycol toxicity, 361
  for hyperkalemia, 342
    in renal failure, 1628, 1628t
  for metabolic acidosis, in renal failure, 1629, 1652
  in cardiopulmonary resuscitation, 192t
  in gastric physiology, 1157
  in renal tubular acidosis, 1707, 1708
Biceps reflex, testing of, 568, *568*
Biceps tendon, inflammation of, 1867
Biguanides, for diabetes mellitus, 1449–1451
Bile, in reflux gastritis, 1165
Bile acids, in liver disease, 1278t, *1288,* 1288–1290
Bile salts, unconjugated, in small intestinal disorders, 1211
Biliary tract, anatomy of, 1340, *1341*
  atresia of, 1979t, 1991t
  cholestasis in, and hyperlipidemia, 290
    with sepsis, 1336–1337
  cysts of, 1322
  disorders of, and jaundice, 211–212
    diagnosis of, *1341,* 1341–1342
  inflammation of, with hepatitis, 1308–1311, *1309,* 1342, 1343
  obstruction of, 1342
    ultrasonography of, 1292
  physiology of, 1340–1341
  rupture of, *1342,* 1343–1344
  tumors of, *1320,* 1320–1322, 1343
Bilirubin, elevated blood level of, diagnosis of, *211,* 211–212
  pathophysiology of, 210–211
  in hemolytic anemia, 1789, 1790
    immune-mediated, 1794–1795
  in liver disease, 1276, 1278t, *1287,* 1287–1288
  in urinalysis, 1606
Bilirubinuria, 96, 99
  in liver disease, 1291
Biofield therapy, in cancer management, 376
Biopsy, in discospondylitis, 625
  in hypothyroidism, 1426
  of bone, 1891–1893, *1892*
  of bone tumors, 536
  of brain, 576–577
  of cutaneous masses, 37–39, *38*
  of gastric ulcer, 1167
  of intestines, in diarrhea, *124,* 125, 126
  of kidney, 1612–1613, *1613*
    in acute renal failure, *1621,* 1621–1622
    in amyloidosis, *1671,* 1671–1672, *1672*
    in glomerulonephritis, 1665, *1665,* 1671
  of liver, 1294–1298, *1295,* 1296t
    client information on, 1939
    in acute disorders, 1331
    in copper-associated hepatopathy, 1304, *1305*
    in hepatitis, 1300–1301, 1310
    in hyperadrenocorticism, 1471
    in microvascular dysplasia, 1315–1316
  of lung tumors, primary, 1074–1075
  of lymphoma, *509,* 509–510
  of muscle fibers, 685t, 686
  of nasal cavity, in epistaxis, 216
    in nasal discharge, 197
    rostral access for, 1013–1016
  of prostate, 1689–1691, *1690, 1691*
  of rectal tumors, 1261–1262
  of respiratory system, 1038
  of sarcoma, of bone, 1911
    of soft tissue, *530,* 530–531
  of skin, 51–55, *52,* 53t, *54*
    in food allergy, 1231, 1231t

Biopsy *(Continued)*
    in hyperpigmentation, 58
    in hypopigmentation, *56,* 57
    in neoplasia, 523–524
    of small intestine, 1212t, 1212–1213, *1213,*
      1213t
      in food allergy, 1231, 1231t
      in inflammatory bowel disease, 1225, 1226,
        1226
      in lymphangiectasia, 1229, *1230*
    of stomach, 1159
    of urinary tract, 1749, *1749, 1750,* 1750t
    in idiopathic disorders, 1744
BioSpot, in flea control, client information on,
    1971
Biotin, in diet, 239t
Birman cat, neuropathy in, 668, 1980t
    neutrophil granulation in, 1847, 1978t
Birth. See *Parturition.*
Bisacodyl, for constipation, 132t
Bismuth subsalicylate, for diarrhea, 318–319,
    1215
    for *Helicobacter* infection, with gastritis, 1164
Black's classification, of dental caries, 1137,
    1137t
Bladder, anomalies of, 1982t, 1996t
    cancer of, 541–542
    detrusor dysfunction in, urethral obstruction
      and, 1738, 1739t
    disorders of, and incontinence, 89–92, *91,*
      1742
      and urine retention, 93t, 93–96, *94,* 95t
      with lumbosacral vertebral stenosis, 638
    distention of, in hyperkalemia, 228, *229*
    diverticula of, 1712, *1718,* 1718–1719, 1752
    endoscopy of, 1744, 1749
    incision of, for lithiasis, 1778
    inflammation of, 1778–1780, 1779t
      idiopathic, 1743
      incidence of, 1748
      interstitial, 1712–1713
    malposition of, 1982t
    needle drainage of, decompressive, before ure-
      thral plug removal, 1734–1735, *1735,*
      1735t
    paralysis of, with spinal disorders, 373
    rupture of, urethral obstruction and, 1737–
      1738
    trauma to, 1752–1753, 1778, 1779t
Blastoma, of spinal cord, 640
Blastomycosis, 458–462, *459–461*
    amphotericin B for, 456, 462
    and spinal meningitis, 616
    geographic distribution of, 453, *454*
    of lung, 459, *459–461,* 1067, *1067, 1068*
Blebs, pleural, with pneumothorax, 1109, *1109,*
    1110
Bleeding. See *Hemorrhage.*
Blepharitis, and conjunctivitis, 66
    systemic disease and, 984
Blepharophimosis, 1977t, 1987t
Blessed thistle, in cancer management, 378t
Blindness, acute onset of, 17t, 17–20, 18t, *19*
    congenital, day, 1988t
      night, 1989t
    hypertension and, 180, *181,* 182
      with hyperadrenocorticism, 1466
    renal failure and, 1639
Block vertebrae, and spinal cord compression,
    621
Blood, disorders of, congenital, 1978t–1979t,
    1989t–1990t
    feline immunodeficiency virus infection
      and, 435
      liver disease and, 1291

Blood *(Continued)*
    in anemia, 198–203, 1784–1816. See also *Ane-*
      mia.
    platelets in. See *Platelets.*
    pooling of, in splenomegaly, 1858t, 1859
Blood gases, analysis of, 1038–1039, *1039*
Blood groups, in transfusion, 353, *353,* 1798
Blood pressure, arterial, determinants of, 175
    decreased. See *Hypotension.*
    increased. See *Hypertension.*
    measurement of, 179, 183–185
      echocardiographic, 847t, 847–848
      intracardiac, in congenital heart disease,
        742, 742–743, *743*
    overload in, and heart failure, 694, *695, 696*
Blood transfusion, adverse reactions to,
    354–355, 1797–1798
    blood groups in, 353, *353,* 1798
    collection for, 348t, 348–349, 349t
    components in, 351–353, *352*
    crossmatching before, 353–354, 354t
    for anemia, erythrocytes in, 1796
      in renal failure, 1655
      non-regenerative, 1815
    for coagulation disorders, 1839, 1840t
    for purpura, 222
    for von Willebrand's disease, 1825
    storage for, 349–351, *350,* 350t
    technique of, 354
Blood urea nitrogen. See *Urea nitrogen.*
Blood vessels. See also *Arteries, Veins,* and
    specific vessels, e.g., *Jugular vein.*
    constriction of, in heart failure, 701, 702t, *703*
    disorders of, and nervous system injury, 556
      cutaneous, congenital, 1995t
    in tumor metastasis, 481–483, *482*
    inflammation of, arterial, 972–974
      immune-mediated, of lungs, 1065t, *1072,*
        1072–1073, *1073*
      in brain, infection and, 591
      pinnal, 989t, 991
    malformations of, and spinal cord disorders,
      652–653
    peripheral, disorders of, 964, 964t
    tumors of, benign, and spinal cord disorders,
      652–653
Blood volume, overload in, and heart failure,
    694–696, *697*
Blood-brain barrier, disruption of, cerebrospinal
    fluid evaluation in, 572
    drug penetration across, 577
    in prevention of infection, 591
Blue morning glory, toxicity of, 365
Bogbean, in cancer management, 378t
Bombesins, 1502
Bone(s), calcium loss from, cancer and, 501
    cysts of, 539, 1904, *1904*
      aneurysmal, 539, 1904–1905
      congenital, 1983t
      subchondral, 1905
    development of, 1887–1888, *1888*
    disorders of, congenital, 1893t, 1893–1896,
      1894, 1895
      in cats, 1975t, 1976t
      in dogs, 1983t, 1984t
      developmental, 1896–1899, 1897t, *1898,*
        1899t, *1900, 1901*
        nutrition in, 245–250, *246,* 249t, *250*
      diagnosis of, 1888–1893, *1891,* 1891t, *1892*
      metabolic, 1905–1909, *1906–1910*
    endochondral ossification defect of, and
      growth failure, 74
    fibrous dysplasia of, 1905, *1905*
    hyperostosis of, diffuse idiopathic, and spinal
      cord dysfunction, *623,* 623–624

Bone(s) *(Continued)*
    hypertrophy of, paraneoplastic, 503, *503*
      secondary, *1903,* 1903–1904
    in aspergillosis, 474
    in blastomycosis, 459–460, *461*
    in calvarial hyperostosis, 1903
    in coccidioidomycosis, 465, 466, *467*
    in enostosis, 1899–1901, *1901,* 1984t
    in hyperparathyroidism, with hyperphospha-
      temia, in chronic renal failure, *1642,*
      1642–1643
    in metaphyseal osteopathy, 1901–1903, *1902*
    in multiple myeloma, 517–519, *518*
    infarction of, medullary, 1904, *1904*
    infection of, 1912–1914, *1913, 1914*
      antibiotics for, 306
      vertebral, and spinal cord dysfunction, 624–
        626, *625, 626*
    loss of, in periodontal disease, 1128–1130,
      1130, 1131
    modeling of, 1888
    polyostotic periostitis of, 1903
    remodeling of, 1888, *1889, 1890*
    structure of, 1887, *1887*
    tumors of, 535–540, *1910,* 1910–1912
      radiotherapy for, 491, 497t
Bone marrow, disorders of, and anemia,
    200–203, *201,* 202t, 1813–1814, *1814*
      feline leukemia virus and, 427, 429
    erythropoiesis in, *1784,* 1784–1786, *1786*
    evaluation of, in hypercalcemia, 1388
      in polycythemia, 206
      in purpura, 220, *221*
    hypoplasia of, 1823
    in leukemia, 1853–1855, *1853–1855*
    leukocyte production in, 1842
    toxicity to, chemotherapy and, 485t, 485–487,
      486
      estrogen and, with neutrophilia, 1849, *1849*
    transplantation of, for anemia, 1815–1816
      for genetic disorders, 5
Borborygmus, 135–136, 1201
Bordetella bronchiseptica infection, and
    tracheobronchitis, 1043
Boric acid, toxicity of, 357
Borna disease virus infection, 450–451
Borreliosis, 391t, 396–397
    and arthritis, 1876–1877
    and glomerulonephritis, 1670
    and meningitis, spinal, 616
    erythema chronicum migrans in, 28
    zoonotic, 384
Botanical medicine, in cancer management, 377,
    378t
Botulism, 391t, 398
    and peripheral neuropathy, 672
Bouvier des Flandres, laryngeal paralysis in,
    669, 1994t
Bovine spongiform encephalopathy, 451, 599
Bowel. See *Colon* and *Small intestine.*
Bowen's disease, crusting in, 51
Boxer, axonopathy in, progressive, 668, 1992t
Brachial plexus, avulsion injury of, 678
    injury to, signs of, 663t
    neuritis in, 674–675
    tumors in, 640
Brachury, 1983t
Brachydactyly, 1975t, 1983t
Brachygnathia, 1976t, 1985t
Brachytherapy, for cancer, 491, *491, 492*
Bradyarrhythmia, in hypotension, 184t
Bradycardia, in Branham's test, for arteriovenous
    fistula, 970
    in renal failure, 1623
    sinus, electrocardiography of, 809, *810*

IND

Brain. See also *Nervous system, central.*
  abscess of, 556, 583, 591
  blood flow to, decreased, and syncope, 13t, 13–16, *14*
  disorders of, 552–599
    and seizures. See *Seizures.*
    and vision loss, 17, 18t
    biopsy in, 576–577
    cerebrospinal fluid examination in, 572–575, 574t
    classification of, 555–556
    degenerative, 589–590, 590t
    developmental, 586–588
    disseminated, rapid-onset, 586
    electrodiagnostic tests in, 575
    feline immunodeficiency virus and, 434–436, *436*, 599
    history in, 552t, 552–555, 553t, *553–555*
    idiopathic, with vestibular disease, 582
    imaging in, 575–576
    in coma, 144t–146t, 144–147, *145*
    in hypernatremia, 230, 232
    in listeriosis, 594
    in rabies, 594–595
    in spongiform encephalopathy, 599
    inflammatory, 590–598, 593t
    neurologic examination in, 556–559, 557t, *558, 559*
      general observations in, 559t, 559–560, *560*
      interpretation in, 571–572, *572*
      of cranial nerves, 562–566, *563–565*, 567t
      of gait, 559t, 560–561
      of postural reactions, 559t, *561*, 561–562, *562*
      of spinal segmental reflexes, 566–571, *567–572*, 571t
      of stance, 559t, 560
    paraneoplastic, 506, 506t
    parasitic, 582
    trauma and, 578–580, *579, 580*, 581t
    treatment of, principles of, 577
    tremor syndromes in, 598–599
    vascular, 580–582
    with liver disease. See *Encephalopathy, hepatic.*
  herniation of, 144, 144t
  lesions of, and anisocoria, 660t
  lymphoma of, treatment of, 512
  tumors of, 577, 583–586, 584t, 585t
    radiotherapy for, 494, 497t
Brain natriuretic peptide, in heart failure, 701
Brain stem, auditory evoked responses of, 575
  in deafness, 1001–1002
  disorders of, reticular activating system in, 559
    signs of, 557, 557t
    trauma to, prognosis of, 580, 581t
Branched-chain amino acids, for hepatic encephalopathy, 1334
Branchial cyst, of thymus, 1979t, 1990t
Branham's bradycardia sign, arteriovenous fistula and, 970
Breath tests, for small intestinal disorders, 1211, 1224
Breathing. See *Respiration.*
Breeding. See *Reproductive system.*
Brethine (terbutaline), for bronchopulmonary disease, 1059t
  for tracheal disease, 1043t
Bretylium, for arrhythmia, 824t, 826t, 830
  ventricular, with hypotension, 184t
  in cardiopulmonary resuscitation, 192t, 193
Brevibloc (esmolol), for arrhythmia, 824t, 827, 828t, 830

Brevibloc (esmolol) *(Continued)*
  supraventricular, with hypotension, 184t
Briard dogs, hypercholesterolemia in, 291
Bricanyl (terbutaline), for bronchopulmonary disease, 1059t
  for tracheal disease, 1043t
Brittany spaniel, spinal muscular atrophy in, 667, 1993t
Brodifacoum, toxicity of, 359–360
Bromethalin, toxicity of, 360
Bromocriptine, for pseudopregnancy, 1526
  in abortion induction, 1546, 1547, *1547*
  in inhibition of lactation, 1596
  in prolactin suppression, in estrous cycle management, *1515, 1516, 1516*
  with sterilization, 1543
Bronchi, cartilage of, hypoplasia of, 1981t, 1994t
  compression of, 1059–1060, *1060*
  disorders of, and asthma, 1057–1058, 1058t, 1059t
    in ciliary dyskinesia, 1058–1059, 1059t
  foreign bodies in, 1060
  left main stem, compression of, with mitral insufficiency, 792–793
  mineralization of, 1060–1061
Bronchiectasis, 1057, *1057*, 1059t
Bronchitis, 1055–1057, 1059t
  client information on, 1954
  endoscopy in, 1037, *1037*, 1038t
  infectious, with tracheitis, 1043t, 1043–1044
Bronchoalveolar lavage, 1038
  in tracheal disorders, 1042
Bronchodilators, for heart failure, 734
  for pneumonia, bacterial, 1064
  for tracheal collapse, 1043t, 1048–1050
Bronchoesophageal fistula, 1060, 1994t
Bronchopneumonia, bronchoscopy of, 1038t
Bronchoscopy, 1037, *1037*, 1038t
  in tracheal disorders, 1041, 1051–1053
Brucellosis, 391t, 394–395
  and fetal loss, 1527
  and reproductive disorders, 1518
  zoonotic, 383t
Bruises, diagnosis of, 220, *221*
  pathophysiology of, 218–220, 219t
  treatment of, 220–222
Brush border, of small intestine, anatomy of, *1184*, 1186
  diseases of, 1197, 1197t, *1198*
Brushite, in urolithiasis, 1758t, 1777
Buccal mucosa, inflammation of, periodontal disease and, 1129
Bucindolol, for arrhythmia, 827
Buckbean, in cancer management, 378t
Bulbourethral glands, anatomy of, 1586
Bull mastiff, cerebellar degeneration in, with hydrocephalus, 589
Bull terrier, acrodermatitis in, 48, 1994t, 1995t
  renal basement membrane disorder in, 1699t, 1701
Bullae, of pinna, 987t, 991
Bullous disease, of lungs, 1083–1084
Bumetanide, for heart failure, 714
Bundle branch block, 817–818, *820, 821*
  with atrial fibrillation, 812
Bundle of His, conduction blocks of, 817, *817–819*
  stenosis of, congenital, 1985t
α-Bungarotoxin, in diagnosis of myasthenia gravis, 675–676
Buparvaquone, for protozoal infection, 410t
Bupivacaine, for pain, 23, 24t
Buprenorphine, cardiac effects of, echocardiography of, 842–843, 845t
Burkitt's lymphoma, 481

Burmese cats, hypokalemia in, with periodic paralysis, 225
Burst-forming units, erythroid, 1784
Buspirone (BuSpar), for behavioral disorders, in cats, 160, 160t
  in dogs, 156, 158t
Butorphanol, for bronchopulmonary disease, 1056, 1059t
  for cough, 165t
    with heart failure, 734
  for pain, 24t, 25
    in vascular neuropathy, 679
  for pancreatitis, 1353, 1363t
  for tracheal disease, 1043t
  in anesthesia, for liver biopsy, 1296t
  in sedation, for blood donation, 349
Butterfly vertebrae, and spinal cord compression, 621

Cabergoline, for pseudopregnancy, 1526
  in abortion induction, 1546, 1547, *1547*
  in estrous cycle management, 1516, 1595
  in inhibition of lactation, 1596
  with sterilization, 1543
Cachectin, in heart disease, 265
  in hyperthermia, 7, 7t
Cachexia, 72–74, *73*
  in heart disease, 265–266, 706
    with weakness, 11
  paraneoplastic, 499–501
Cadherins, in carcinogenesis, 478–479
Cairn terrier, neuronopathy in, progressive, 666, 1992t
  polycystic kidneys in, 1699t, 1701, 1996t
Calciferol. See *Vitamin D.*
Calcification, in degenerative joint disease, *1864*, 1865
Calcinosis, cutaneous, 36, 37
  ulcers in, 40t, 42
Calcinosis circumscripta, and spinal cord compression, 619, *619*
  cervical, congenital, 1983t
Calcitonin, excess of, in orthopedic developmental disorders, 246
  for rodenticide toxicity, 360
Calcitriol. See *Vitamin D.*
Calcium, blood level of, decreased. See *Hypocalcemia.*
  elevated. See *Hypercalcemia.*
  challenge test with, in gastrinoma, 1505
  for hyperphosphatemia, in renal failure, 1651
  for uterine inertia, in dystocia, 1532
  in diet, 239t
    in orthopedic developmental disorders, 246, 249t, 1909
    in urolithiasis, calcium oxalate, 1726, 1764
      calcium phosphate, 1728, 1729, 1729t
    in hyperparathyroidism, with bone loss, 1906–1907
    with hyperphosphatemia, in renal failure, *1642*, 1642–1643
  in urine, in renal tubular dysfunction, 1706
Calcium channel blockers, for arrhythmia, 824t–826t, 828t, 829t, 830–831
  for cardiomyopathy, dilated, 884, 885
    hypertrophic, canine, 890
      feline, 905, 906
Calcium chloride, in cardiopulmonary resuscitation, 192t
Calcium gluconate, for hyperkalemia, 342
  in renal failure, 1628, 1628t
Calcium oxalate, in urinary calculi. See *Urinary tract, lithiasis of.*

Calcium phosphate, in urinary calculi, in cats, 1723t, 1728–1729, 1729t
   in dogs, 1758t, 1777
Calculus (calculi), in urinary tract. See *Urinary tract, lithiasis of.*
   of prostate, 1696
   periodontal, 1127, 1131–1132
Calicivirus infection, 448–449
   and arthritis, 1878
   and rhinitis, 1018
   of respiratory tract, 1063
   of urinary tract, 1711
Calico cat, testicular hypoplasia in, 3, 1981t
Caloric test, in coma, 145–146
Calories, in diet. See *Energy.*
Calvarium, hyperostosis of, 1903
Campylobacteriosis, 391t, 391–392
   and colitis, 1244
   and enteritis, 1217
   zoonotic, 383t
Cancer, 477–546. See also *Tumors* and specific types, e.g., *Lymphoma.*
   and adrenocorticotropic hormone production, ectopic, 503
   and anemia, 503–504, *504*
   and antidiuretic hormone secretion, inappropriate, 503
   and cachexia, 499–501
   and erythrocytosis, 502–503
   and fever, 505–506
   and hypercalcemia, *501*, 501–502, 1385, *1385*, *1386*, 1388
   and hypergammaglobulinemia, 505
   and hyperparathyroidism, surgery for, 1389, *1389*
   and hypertrophic osteopathy, 503, *503*
   and hypocalcemia, 502
   and hypoglycemia, 502
   and leukocytosis, 504–505
   and thrombocytopenia, 505, 505t
   and weakness, 12
   client information on, 1921–1928
   endocrine, 501
   feline leukemia virus and, client information on, 1957
   management of, acupuncture in, 374–375, 375t
      alternative therapy in, 374–379, 375t, 377t–379t
      ayurvedic, 376, 377t
      biofield therapy in, 376
      chemotherapy in, 484–489, 485t, *486*, 487t. See also *Chemotherapy.*
      and anemia, non-regenerative, 1812, 1812t
      chiropractic care in, 375
      homeopathic medicine in, 376
      massage in, 375–376
      naturopathic medicine in, 376–377
   metastasis of, biology of, 481–483, *482*
   neurologic complications of, 506, 506t, 549t, 551
   peripheral, 677–678
   of bladder, 541–542
   of esophagus, 1147
   of prostate, 542–543
   of testicles, 543–544
   onset of, biology of, 478–481, 479t
   paraneoplastic syndromes with, 498–506
      pulmonary neoplasia and, 1073–1074
   radiation therapy for, 489–496. See also *Radiation therapy.*
Candidiasis, 475
Cannabis sativa, toxicity of, 365
Canthus, aberrant dermis on, 1977t, 1987t

Caparsolate. See *Thiacetarsamide.*
Capillaria aerophila infestation, and rhinitis, 1018
   of lung, 1065t, 1070
Capillaria feliscati infestation, of urinary tract, 1741
Capillaries, fluid dynamics in, 325–327, *326, 327*
   in cyanosis, 206–208, 207t
Capnocytophaga canimorsus infection, zoonotic, 383t
Captopril, for heart failure, 718–720, 720t
   for hypertension, in renal failure, 1654
Carafate. See *Sucralfate.*
Carbam. See *Diethylcarbamazine.*
Carbamate insecticides, toxicity of, 359
Carbamide peroxide, for otitis externa, 989t, 994
Carbenicillin, for central nervous system infection, 593t
Carbimazole, for hyperthyroidism, 1408t, 1411–1412
   before surgery, 1412–1413
Carbohydrates, absorption of, from small intestine, 1187–1188, *1189*
   digestion of, in small intestine, 1187, 1187t, *1188*
   in diet, in diabetes mellitus, 261
      in enteral nutrition, 280t, 281t
      in hepatic disease, 260
      in parenteral nutrition, 281, 282t
      intolerance to, 253
   metabolism of, disorders of, and glucosuria, 1704
      and pentosuria, 1704
   in liver disease, 1290
Carbon dioxide, in smoke inhalation, 1087
Carbon monoxide, in smoke inhalation, 1087
Carboplatin, for bladder cancer, 542
   for osteosarcoma, 536
      after amputation, 1911
   for squamous cell carcinoma, nasal, 1020, *1021*
   in cancer therapy, 485t, 486, 489
      with radiotherapy, 495, 496
Carboxyhemoglobin, in inhalation injury, 1087
Carcinogenesis, 478–481, 479t. See also *Cancer.*
Carcinoid tumors, intestinal, 1508
Carcinoma. See also *Cancer.*
   nasal, 1019–1021, *1021*
   of anal sacs, 1267
   of biliary tract, 1320–1322
   of colon, *1253,* 1253–1254
   of ear, otitis externa and, 996–997
   of esophagus, 1147
   of kidney, in German shepherd, 1699t, 1701
   of mouth, *1115,* 1115–1118, *1116,* 1117t
   of ovaries, and prolonged estrus, 1523, *1523*
   of pancreas, 1364
   of prostate, 1694–1696, *1695, 1696*
   of rectum, *1253,* 1253–1254, 1260–1262
   of salivary glands, 1119
   of skin, crusting in, 51
      squamous cell, 42, 524–525
   of small intestine, 1234–1235
   of stomach, 1176, 1177
   of thyroid, radioactive iodine for, 1414–1415
   of tonsils, 1029
   parathyroid, and hyperparathyroidism, 1392
   perianal, 1268
   radiotherapy for, 497t
   solar-induced, client information on, 1926
Cardia, of stomach, anatomy of, 1155, *1155*
Cardiac arrest, during sleep, 154
   in anesthesia, acupuncture for, 372, *372*
   with pulmonary arrest, 189, 192

Cardiac arrest *(Continued)*
   resuscitation from, 190t, 190–193, *191,* 192t
Cardiac tamponade, mitral insufficiency and, 795
   pericardial disorders and, 924–925, *926*
   treatment of, 931–933, *933*
Cardiac vector, in electrocardiography, 801–802, *802*
Cardiomyopathy, acromegaly and, 914
   and thromboembolism, 914–918, *915–917*
   atrial standstill with, 914
   carnitine deficiency and, 264–265, 877–878
   classification of, 896, 898t
   client information on, 1949
   dilated, canine, 874–886
      diagnosis of, 879–883, 880t, *880–882*
      pathogenesis of, 876–878
      pathology of, *875,* 875–876, *876*
      pathophysiology of, 878–879
      prevalence of, 874–875, *875*
      prognosis of, 886
      treatment of, 883–885
      feline, 908–912, *909, 910*
   doxorubicin and, 914
   echocardiography of, 857t
   feline, 896–918
   hypertension and, 914
   hyperthyroidism and, 913–914, 1403
   hypertrophic, and pericardial effusion, *935,* 935–936
      canine, 886–890, *887–890*
      feline, 896–903
         clinical findings in, 899–902, *901,* 901t, *902*
         differential diagnosis of, 902
         etiology of, 896
         pathology of, 898, *900*
         pathophysiology of, 896–898, *899*
         prevalence of, 896, *897*
         prognosis of, 902–903
         treatment of, 905–908
   hypothyroidism with, 1422, 1426–1427
   in heart failure, 711
   left ventricular moderator bands in, 913, *913*
   myocarditis and, 877, 914
   neoplastic infiltration and, 914
   restrictive, canine, 890
      feline, 903–905, *904,* 908
   right ventricular, arrhythmogenic, *912,* 912–913
   taurine deficiency and, 263–264, 908–912, *909, 910*
   unclassified, feline, 913
Cardiomyoplasty, for dilated cardiomyopathy, 885
Cardiomyotomy, for megaesophagus, 1151
Cardiopulmonary arrest, 189, 192
   resuscitation from, 190t, 190–193, *191,* 192t
Cardizem. See *Diltiazem.*
Caries, dental, Black's classification of, 1137, 1137t
Carmustine, toxicity of, and anemia, 1812
Carnitine, deficiency of, and cardiomyopathy, 264–265, 877–878
   for hepatic encephalopathy, 1335
Carotid artery, occlusion of, 967, *967*
Carotid sinus, compression of, in electrocardiography, 806, *807*
Carprofen, for degenerative joint disease, 1866
   for fever, 9
   for pain, 24t, 25
   toxicity of, to liver, 1308, 1327–1328
Carpus, luxation of, 1867
   subluxation of, congenital, 1983t
Carrisyn, for feline immunodeficiency virus infection, 437, 437t

Carrisyn (Continued)
for feline leukemia virus infection, 430
Cartilage, articular, trauma to, 1866–1867
bronchial, hypoplasia of, 1981t, 1994t
in osteochondrosis, 1869–1870, 1870
with nutritional imbalances, 245–250, 246, 249t, 250
retained cores of, 1898, 1900
Cartilage products, in cancer management, 377
Cartilaginous exostoses, congenital, 1983t
multiple, 539, 540, 1899, 1901
and spinal cord disorders, 642–643
Carvediol, for arrhythmia, 827
for cardiomyopathy, dilated, 885
Castor bean plant, toxicity of, 365
Castor oil, for constipation, 132
Castration. See Sterilization.
Casts, in urine, 1608, 1609, 1609
Cat scratch disease, 382–386, 399
Cataplexy, congenital, 1980t, 1992t
Cataracts, and vision loss, 17, 17t
congenital, 1977t, 1987t
diabetes and, 985, 1458
systemic disease and, 985
β-Catenin, in carcinogenesis, 478–479
Catheterization, for urolith removal, 1759, 1759
in oxygen supplementation, 1062, 1062
of bladder, for urethral obstruction, 95, 96, 1734–1737, 1736, 1737t
in urinary tract infection, in diagnosis, 1680
of heart, in atrial septal defect, 756
in cardiomyopathy, dilated, 880–881
in congenital disease, 742, 742–743, 743
cyanotic, 780
in patent ductus arteriosus, 748, 749, 749
in pulmonic stenosis, congenital, 742, 743, 762
in subaortic stenosis, congenital, 742, 743, 770–771
in ventricular septal defect, 758
Catpox, 450
Cauda equina, in sacrocaudal dysgenesis, 645, 1975t
lesions of, localization of, 614–615
Cauda equina syndrome, with lumbosacral stenosis, 636t, 636–638, 638, 639
Cavities, dental, Black's classification of, 1137, 1137t
Cecocolic intussusception, 1252, 1252
Cefadroxil, for staphylococcal pyoderma, 46t
Cefalexin, for central nervous system infection, 593t
Cefazolin, concentration of, and bacterial susceptibility, 303t
prophylactic use of, with surgery, 306–307
Cefotaxime, concentration of, and bacterial susceptibility, 303t
for central nervous system infection, 593t
Cefoxitin, concentration of, and bacterial susceptibility, 303t
Celiac artery, anatomy of, 1155
Cells, fluid dynamics in, 325–327
infection within, antibiotics for, 302
Cellulitis, juvenile, 36, 37
and arthritis, 1883
of pinna, 991
Cemento-enamel junction, anatomy of, 1127, 1127
Central venous pressure, measurement of, 184
Cephalexin, dosage of, in renal failure, 1649t
for lung infection, 1065t
for otitis media, 990t, 999
for staphylococcal pyoderma, 46t
Cephalosporins, concentration of, and clinical outcome, 304

Cephalosporins (Continued)
for meningitis, spinal, 618
prophylactic use of, with surgery, 306–307
Cephalothin, concentration of, and bacterial susceptibility, 303t
dosage of, in renal failure, 1649t
for lung infection, 1065t
Cephapirin, for central nervous system infection, 593t
Cephulac, for constipation, 132
Cerebellum. See also Brain.
abiotrophy of, 589
congenital disorders of, 1991t
degeneration of, with hydrocephalus, in bull mastiff, 589
disorders of, and ataxia, 142
signs of, 557, 557t, 559, 559t
hypoplasia of, 587–588, 1980t
Cerebrospinal fluid, examination of, in brain disorders, 572–575, 574t
in brain neoplasia, 584–585, 585t
in cerebrovascular disorders, 581
in degenerative myelopathy, 623
in distemper, 574t, 626
in globoid cell leukodystrophy, with spinal cord demyelination, 628
in meningitis, bacterial, 603–604
spinal, infectious, 617, 618
with arteritis, corticosteroid-responsive, 621–622
in meningoencephalomyelitis, granulomatous, 628
in peritonitis, feline infectious, 627
in spinal cord disorders, 610
in spinal cord hemorrhage, 629
in spinal neoplasia, 641
in hydrocephalus, 587
in intra-arachnoid cyst, 645–646
Cerebrovascular occlusion, and stroke, 966
Cerebrum. See Brain.
Ceroid lipofuscinosis, 589, 590t, 1980t, 1992t
Cerumen, in otitis externa, 989t, 994
Cervix uteri, cancer of, papillomavirus and, 481
Cesarean section, indications for, 1536
Charcoal, activated, for digoxin toxicity, 730
for insecticide toxicity, 359
for rodenticide toxicity, 360
Chédiak-Higashi syndrome, 1823–1824, 1824t, 1978t
neutrophil inclusions in, 1848, 1848
Chemet, for lead toxicity, 362
Chemical injury, and anemia, 1800–1802, 1801t, 1811–1812
and carcinogenesis, 481
Chemodectoma, 1096
and pericardial effusion, 928, 930, 933
Chemonucleolysis, for intervertebral disk extrusion, 634–635
Chemoreceptor trigger zone, in vomiting, 118–119
Chemotherapy, 484–485, 485t
client information on, 1921–1923
drug selection in, 488–489
for bladder cancer, 541–542
for brain tumors, 586
for hemangiosarcoma, 1922
for leukemia, lymphoblastic, 514–515
for lymphoma, 510–512, 511t, 1923
for oral tumors, 1117
for pancreatic islet cell tumors, 1437
for sarcoma, of soft tissue, 532, 534
for skin tumors, mast cell, 527
for spinal cord tumors, 642
for squamous cell carcinoma, of skin, 525
for thyroid tumors, with hyperthyroidism, 1417

Chemotherapy (Continued)
strategies in, 487–488
toxicity of, 485t, 485–487, 486, 487t
and anemia, 504, 1812, 1812t
with surgery and radiation, 495–496
Chest. See Thorax.
Cheyletiellosis, 59t, 62, 62
and pruritus, 32, 33t, 34, 34t
and scaling dermatosis, 49
Cheyne-Stokes respiration, in metabolic encephalopathy, 548
Chigger infestation, and pruritus, 33t
Chimeras, sexual developmental disorders in, 1582–1583, 1583, 1980t–1981t, 1993t
Chinaberry, toxicity of, to liver, 1329
Chiropractic care, in cancer management, 375
Chitin synthetase inhibitors, for fungal infection, 457
Chlamydia psittaci infection, and abortion, 1592
and conjunctivitis, 66
zoonotic, 384t
Chlorambucil, in cancer therapy, for lymphocytic leukemia, 514–515
for lymphoma, 511t
for multiple myeloma, 518
Chloramphenicol, dosage of, in renal failure, 1649t
for bacterial infection, 391t
for bronchopulmonary disease, 1056, 1057, 1059t
for central nervous system infection, 593t
for lung infection, 1065t
toxicity of, and anemia, 1812
Chlorhexidine, for anal sacculitis, 1266
for oral disorders, with renal failure, 1629, 1630t
for otitis externa, 989t, 994
Chloride, absorption of, from intestine, 1192, 1193, 1193
blood level of, decreased, 234
elevated, 234
in hypoadrenocorticism, 1491–1492, 1492t
clearance of, in renal function assessment, 1604t, 1605
in diet, 239t
in heart disease, 265t
Chlormadinone acetate, for prostatic hypertrophy, 1692
Chlorothiazide, for diabetes insipidus, 1707
Chlorpheniramine, with hydrocodone, for cough, 165t
Chlorphenoxy compounds, in herbicides, toxicity of, 363
Chlorpromazine, for hemobartonellosis, 407
for vomiting, in gastritis, 1161
in renal failure, 1629, 1630t
Cholangiohepatitis, 1308–1311, 1309, 1342, 1343
Cholangitis, 1342, 1343
drug toxicity and, 1272–1274
Cholecalciferol. See Vitamin D.
Cholecystitis, 1341–1344, 1342, 1343
Cholecystography, in liver disease, 1291
Cholecystokinin, 1500–1501, 1503
Choledyl SA, for cough, 165t
Cholelithiasis, 1341–1344, 1343
Cholestasis, and hyperlipidemia, 290
and jaundice, 211–212
with sepsis, 1336–1337
Cholesterol, blood level of, elevated, 286–291. See also Hyperlipidemia.
in hyperadrenocorticism, 1465
metabolism of, 284–286, 285t, 285–287
in liver disease, 1290
Cholestyramine, for digoxin toxicity, 730

Choline, in diet, 239t, 240
Chondrodysplasia, 1983t
    zinc-responsive, 1909
Chondrodystrophy, 1869
    and growth failure, 74
    pulmonary mineralization in, 1088
Chondroprotectants, for degenerative joint
    disease, 1866
Chondrosarcoma, 538, 1911
    and aortic thrombosis, 967
Chordae tendineae, rupture of, with pulmonary
    edema, in mitral insufficiency, 794
Choriomeningitis, lymphocytic, zoonotic, 384t
Chorionic gonadotropin, human. See
    Gonadotropin, human chorionic.
Chorioretinitis, distemper and, 418
    systemic disease and, 985, 986t
Choroid plexus tumor, 584t, 585t
Chow, renal dysplasia in, 1699t, 1701
Chromosomal disorders, 2–3, 3t. See also
    Genetic defects.
    in sexual development, 1581–1585, 1582–
    1584, 1981t, 1993t
Chronic relapsing neuropathy, 674
Chylomicrons, elevated blood level of, 286–291.
    See also Hyperlipidemia.
    metabolism of, 284, 285, 285t, 286
Chylothorax, 187, 188–189, 1102, 1103, 1103,
    1104, 1105t, 1107, 1107–1108
Chymopapain, for intervertebral disk extrusion,
    634–635
Cilastatin, with imipenem, for lung infection,
    1065t
Cilia, ectopic, congenital, 1978t
Ciliary dyskinesia, 1058–1059, 1059t, 1994t
Cimetidine, for esophagitis, 1148, 1149, 1150t
    for gastric acid secretion, in pancreatic exo-
        crine insufficiency, 1362, 1363t
    for gastric ulcers, 1167–1168
        in renal failure, 1629, 1630t
        with coagulopathy, in acute liver disorders,
            1335
        with steroid therapy, for hemolytic anemia,
            1797
    for gastrinoma, 1506, 1506t
    for gastroesophageal reflux, 1152
    with maintenance steroid therapy, 315
Ciprofloxacin, concentration of, and bacterial
    susceptibility, 303t
Circling, brain injury and, 560, 560
    listeriosis and, 594
Circumanal gland adenoma, 1267–1268
Cirrhosis, copper-associated, 1304–1306, 1305
    diagnosis of, 1299–1301, 1300
Cisapride, for gastric motility disorders, 1175
    for gastritis, in renal failure, 1629, 1630t
    for gastroesophageal reflux, 1152
    for megaesophagus, 1150–1151
    for urine retention, 95t, 96
Cisplatin, and gastritis, 1162
    for bladder cancer, 541–542
    for osteosarcoma, 536, 537
        after amputation, 1911
    in cancer therapy, 485t, 486, 487, 487t, 489
        with radiotherapy, 495, 496
    toxicity of, to kidney, 1616–1617
Citrate, for calcium oxalate urolithiasis, 1728,
    1769
    for metabolic acidosis, in renal failure, 1652
Citrate phosphate dextrose adenine, in blood
    storage, 350, 350t
Citrullinemia, 1987t
Clavulanic acid, with amoxicillin, concentration
        of, and bacterial susceptibility, 303t
    for lung infection, 1065t

Clavulanic acid (Continued)
    with ticarcillin, for Pseudomonas aeruginosa
        infection, in otitis externa, 996
Cleft lip, 1976t, 1985t
Cleft palate, 1976t, 1985t
Clindamycin, concentration of, and bacterial
    susceptibility, 303t
    dosage of, in renal failure, 1649t
    for bacterial infection, with feline immunode-
        ficiency virus infection, 437, 437t
    for bronchopulmonary disease, 1057, 1059t
    for neosporosis, with myositis, 687
    for protozoal infection, 410, 410t
Clitoris, anatomy of, 1586
Clofazimine, for bacterial infection, 391t
Clomipramine (Clomicalm), for behavioral
        disorders, in cats, 160t
    in dogs, 156, 158t
Clonazepam, for sleep disorders, 155
Cloprostenol, in abortion induction, 1546, 1547,
    1547
Clorazepate, for behavioral disorders, 156, 158t
Clostridium botulinum infection, 391t, 398
    and peripheral neuropathy, 672
Clostridium difficile infection, and colitis, 1245
Clostridium infection, and enteritis, 1218
    antibiotics for, 303
Clostridium perfringens infection, and colitis,
    1241, 1243–1244
    diagnosis of, 1241
    and enterotoxicosis, with diarrhea, 125, 126
    and hemorrhagic gastroenteritis, 1162
Clostridium piliforme infection, and Tyzzer's
    disease, 392
Clostridium tetani infection, 391t, 398, 604
Clotrimazole, for aspergillosis, 474, 475t,
    1018–1019
Cloxacillin, for central nervous system infection,
    593t
Coagulation, disorders of, 1836–1839, 1837,
    1838, 1839t, 1840t
    and arterial thrombosis, 964–965
    and epistaxis, 214t, 214–215, 216
    and hemoptysis, 217, 217t
    and hemorrhage, with spinal cord disorders,
        628, 629
    and purpura, 218–220, 219t, 221
    and thromboembolism, 915, 917–918
    congenital, 3t, 5, 1978t–1979t, 1989t
    dextran and, 333
    glomerular disease and, 1675, 1676
    hydroxyethyl starch and, 334
    in hemophilia, 3t, 1839, 1839t, 1979t, 1989t
        and arthropathy, 1873
    in von Willebrand's disease, 3t, 5, 1824t,
        1824–1825, 1825t, 1979t, 1989t
        client information on, 1962
        testing for, in blood donors, 348
    liver disease and, 1278t, 1285–1286, 1335
    oxypolygelatin and, 332
    with hypothyroidism, 1422
    with vitamin K deficiency, in pancreatic exo-
        crine insufficiency, 1358, 1363t
    disseminated intravascular, 965–966, 1840–
        1841, 1841
    and epistaxis, 214
    in hemolytic anemia, immune-mediated,
        1797
    paraneoplastic, 505, 505t
    platelet dysfunction in, 1827
    physiology of, 1829–1833, 1830–1833, 1833t
Coarctation, of aorta, 786
Cobalamin. See Vitamin B12.
Coccidian infection. See Protozoal infection.
Coccidioidomycosis, 465–468, 466–468

Coccidioidomycosis (Continued)
    and meningitis, spinal, 616, 618
    geographic distribution of, 453, 454
    lufenuron for, 457, 475t
    of lung, 465, 466, 466, 1067–1068
Cocker spaniel, hepatitis in, 1306
    renal basement membrane disorder in, 1699t,
        1701
Codeine, for pain, 24t, 25
    for tracheal disease, 1043t
    in cancer management, 378t
Coenzyme Q-10, for dilated cardiomyopathy,
    885
Colace, for constipation, 132t
Colchicine, for amyloidosis, of kidneys, 1668,
    1674
    of liver, 1323, 1337
    for fibrosis, of liver, 1304
Colchicum, in cancer management, 378t
Cold, exposure to, and frostbite, of pinna, 991
Coley's toxin, in cancer management, 377
Colitis, acute, 1247
    bacterial infection and, 1243–1245
    chronic, treatment of, 1251
    client information on, 1938
    eosinophilic, 1248
    idiopathic, 1247–1251, 1248, 1248t, 1249,
        1249t
    in renal failure, 1637
    liver disorders with, 1336
    lymphocytic-plasmacytic, 1247–1248, 1248,
        1248t, 1249t
    ulcerative, and arthritis, 1883, 1885
    histiocytic, 1249, 1249
Collagen, in footpad disorder, congenital, 1995t
Collagen dysplasia, dominant, 1981t, 1995t
Collie, eye anomaly in, 17, 1987t
Colloids, in fluid therapy, 329t, 329–331,
    331t–333t. See also Fluid therapy.
Coloboma, 1978t, 1988t
Colon, 1238–1254. See also Gastrointestinal
    tract.
    anatomy of, 1238, 1238–1239
    bacterial infection of, 1241, 1243–1245
    bleeding in, and melena, 127t, 127–129
    cancer of, genetic mutation and, 479
    disorders of, and diarrhea, 122, 122t, 126
        and fecal incontinence, 1268, 1268t, 1269
        and tenesmus, 132–133, 133t
        and vomiting, 118t, 119–121, 120
        congenital, 1976t
        diagnosis of, 1240t, 1240–1243, 1241–1243,
            1242t, 1243t
        with pancreatitis, 1254
        with spinal cord disorders, 1254
    electrolyte absorption from, 1192, 1193
    enlarged, and abdominal distention, 137
        perineal herniorrhaphy with, 1260
    fluid transport in, 1240
    fungal infection of, 1246–1247
    in constipation, 129–132, 130t, 131, 132t,
        1252–1253
    in irritable bowel syndrome, 1200, 1200t,
        1252
        food reactions in, 254
    intussusception of, 1251–1252, 1252
    microflora of, 1239
    motility of, 1239–1240, 1240t
    mucosal immunity in, 1239, 1239t
    parasitosis of, 1241, 1245, 1245–1246, 1246
        migration of, to lung, 1071
    scintigraphy of, in liver disease, 1291–1292
    tumors of, 1253, 1253–1254
Colonoscopy, 1238, 1242–1243, 1243t
    in diarrhea, 125, 126

IND

Colony-forming units, erythroid, 1784
Color mutant alopecia, 1995t
Color-flow Doppler echocardiography, 835t, *848*, 848–849. See also *Doppler echocardiography.*
  of heart disease, congenital, 741
  of pulmonic stenosis, congenital, 765, *766*
Coma, 144–147, *145*, 145t, 146t
  hypernatremia and, 230, 232
  myxedema and, 1422, 1426
Combined immunodeficiency, 3t, 1990t
  neutrophils in, 1850
Compazine (prochlorperazine), for vomiting, in gastritis, 1629, 1630t
  in renal failure, 1629, 1630t
Complement, congenital deficiency of, 1990t
Composite materials, in dental restoration, 1141
Compound 1080/1081, toxicity of, 360
Computed tomography, in atlantoaxial subluxation, 615, *616*
  in hyperadrenocorticism, 1473
  in spinal neoplasia, 641, *641*
  of bone disorders, 1890–1891, *1891*
  of brain, 576
  of mediastinum, 1093–1094, *1094*
  of nasal cavity, 1009–1012, *1011–1015*
  of nasal tumors, 1022, 1023, *1023*
  of pericardial effusion, 931
Conduction disorders, cardiac, 816–820, *817–821*
  with excitation disorders, 820–822, *822, 823*
  in deafness, 1001
Coneflower, in cancer management, 378t
Conformation, abnormalities of, 1869
Congenital defects, in cats, 1975t–1982t
  in dogs, 1983t–1996t
Conjoined twins, 1975t, 1983t
Conjunctiva, changes in, systemic disease and, 984–985
Conjunctivitis, 66–69, *67*
  radiation injury and, in nasal tumor therapy, 1022
Conocybe filaris, toxicity of, 364
Conofite, for *Malassezia* infection, in otitis externa, 990t, 996
Consciousness, altered states of, 144t–146t, 144–147, *145*
  hypernatremia and, 230, 232
  myxedema and, 1422, 1426
Constipation, 129–132, 130t, *131*, 132t
  drugs for, 131, 132t, 319–320
  hypothyroidism and, 1252–1253
  megacolon and, 129–132, 1253
  perineal hernia and, 1259
Contraception, *1542*, 1542–1544
  client information on, 1933
  prepubertal gonadectomy in, 1539–1541
Contrast echocardiography, 835t, 838–839, *841*. See also *Echocardiography.*
Contrast radiography. See also *Radiography.*
  of arterial occlusion, 967, *967*
  of esophagus, 1143, *1144*
    fistula in, 1147
    stricture in, 1149, *1149*
  of gastric ulcers, 1167
  of osteomyelitis, 1913–1914
  of portosystemic shunts, congenital, 1313, *1313*
    multiple acquired, 1317, *1317*
  of skull, in brain disorders, 576
  of small intestine, 1208, *1209*
Contusion, pulmonary, 1084
Convalleria majalis, toxicity of, 365
Convulsions. See *Seizures.*

Coombs' test, in hemolytic anemia, 199, 1796
Coonhound paralysis, 673–674
Copper, deficiency of, and bone fragility, 1909
  hepatic accumulation of, 1299, 1299t, 1304–1306, *1305*, 1991t
    treatment of, 261, 1301–1304, 1303t
  in diet, 239t
    in orthopedic developmental disorders, 247
  toxicity of, 362
    and hemolytic anemia, 1802
    in Bedlington terrier, 5, 1304–1305, *1305*
Cor pulmonale, in dirofilariasis, 937–938, 942
Cor triatriatum, 778–779
Cordarone (amiodarone), for arrhythmia, 824t–826t, 828t, 830
  in cardiopulmonary resuscitation, 192t, 193
Corgi, renal telangiectasia in, 1698, 1699t, 1703
Cori's disease, 1322, 1323
  and myopathy, 689
Cornea, disorders of, and vision loss, 17, 17t
  congenital, 1977t, 1987t, 1988t
  in glaucoma, 69
  inflammation of, *67*, 69
    herpesvirus infection and, 446
    systemic disease and, 984–985
    with conjunctivitis, 66
      radiation injury and, in nasal tumor therapy, 122
Corneal reflex, in cranial nerve examination, 566, 567t
Cornifying epithelioma, cutaneous, 525
Coronary arteries, anomalies of, with pulmonic stenosis, 760, *762*
  disease of, with hypercholesterolemia, in hypothyroidism, 290
  sclerosis of, 971, 972, *972*
Coronavirus infection, 419t, 422
  and enteritis, 1217
  and peritonitis, 438–443, 440t, *442*
Coronoid process, medial, developmental defect of, 1871, *1871*
Corticosteroids. See also specific drugs, e.g., *Dexamethasone.*
  adrenal production of, 307, *308*, 1461, 1488–1490, *1490*
    deficiency of, 1489–1490, 1496–1498. See also *Hypoadrenocorticism.*
    excessive, 1460–1487. See also *Hyperadrenocorticism.*
  and leukocyte changes, 1844
  and pancreatitis, 1350
  and polyuria, 1374, *1375*
  and stomach ulcers, 1166
  and thyroid hormone deficiency, 1424
  anti-inflammatory effects of, 310–311
  catabolic effects of, 311
  client information on, 1968
  contraindications to, 316
  dosage of, in renal failure, 1649t
  effect of, on liver enzyme concentrations, *1282*, 1282–1284
  for allergic skin disease, 36
  for arthritis, 1884
  for aspiration pneumonia, 1086
  for brain tumors, 585
  for bronchial asthma, 1058, 1059t
  for central nervous system inflammation, 592–593, 593t
  for cerebral edema, 147
    after trauma, 579
    with seizures, 150t
  for cholangiohepatitis, 1310
  for cough, 165t, 166
  for degenerative joint disease, 1866
  for demyelinating neuropathy, acquired, 674

Corticosteroids *(Continued)*
  for dirofilariasis, 943, 949t, 951, 960, 961
  for distemper, with myelitis, 626
  for eosinophilic disease, of lungs, 1065t, 1072
  for eosinophilic granuloma complex, 1118
  for esophageal stricture, 1149
  for gastritis, eosinophilic, 1163
    with lymphocytic-plasmacytic infiltrates, 1163
  for glomerulonephritis, 1673
  for granulomatous meningoencephalomyelitis, 628
  for hemolytic anemia, immune-mediated, 1796–1797
    infection-associated, 1800
  for hepatitis, 1301
  for hyperadrenocorticism, in screening test, 1470–1472, *1471*, 1485–1486
  for hypothyroidism, with neurologic signs, 551
  for inflammatory bowel disease, 1227, 1250, 1251
  for intervertebral disk protrusion, 634
  for intracranial pressure elevation, 577
  for lung disorders, 1065t
  for lymphangiectasia, small intestinal, 1230
  for megaesophagus, 1150, 1150t
  for meningitis, spinal, 618
    with arthritis, 621–622
    with feline infectious peritonitis, 627
  for myositis, immune-mediated, 687
  for otitis externa, 989t, 995
  for pancreatic exocrine insufficiency, 1363t, 1364
  for pancreatic islet cell tumors, 1434, 1434t, 1435, 1435t, 1437
  for pancreatitis, 1354
  for pansteatitis, 29
  for polyarthritis, periosteal proliferative, 1881
  for pulmonary thromboembolism, 1079–1080
  for shock, 315, 316
    with gastric dilatation and volvulus, 1172
  for spinal cord trauma, 315–316, 648–649
  for spondylomyelopathy, cervical, 620–621
  for thrombocytopenia, 1822
  for tremor, 598–599
  for urethritis, 1780
  for urinary tract disorders, idiopathic, 1745
  for vasculitis, of lungs, 1065t, 1072, *1072, 1073*
  in abortion induction, 1547–1548
  indications for, 312t, 312–313
  maintenance therapy with, 314–315
  production of, 307–308, *308*
  receptors of, 308–310, *310*
  renal effects of, 311
  route of administration of, 313t, 313–314, 314t
  side effects of, 316
  structure of, 308, *309*
  withdrawal of, 316–317
Corticotropin-releasing hormone, in steroid production, 307, *308*
Cortinarius species, toxicity of, 364
Cortisol. See *Hydrocortisone.*
Cortisone, for intervertebral disk disease, 1919
  potency of, 312t
Cortrosyn. See *Adrenocorticotropic hormone.*
Corynebacterium equi infection, 391t, 396
Coughing, and syncope, 16
  causes of, 162–163, 163t
  diagnosis of, 163–165, *164*
  drugs for, over-the-counter, 319
  tracheal disorders and, 419t, 419–420, 1043t, 1043–1044

Coughing (Continued)
    treatment of, 165t, 165–166
    with heart failure, 706, 734
Coumadin. See Warfarin.
Coupage, for pneumonia, 1064
Cowpox, in cats, 450
Coxiella burnetii infection, 385t, 407
Crackles, respiratory, 1035, 1035t
Cramps, in Scottish terrier, 588
Cranial nerve(s), anatomy of, 664t
    examination of, 562–566, 563–565, 567t
    fifth, inflammation of, 680
        motor dysfunction in, 582
    second. See Optic nerve.
    seventh, inflammation of, 680–681
        paralysis of, 582–583, 1000
    third, palsy of, and anisocoria, 660t
Craniofacial defects, 1975t
Craniomandibular osteopathy, 1898, 1900, 1901,
    1983
Cranioschisis, 1975t, 1983t
Cranium, congenital defects of, 1975t, 1983t
    osteopathy of, with mandibular osteopathy,
        1898, 1900, 1901, 1983t
    radiography of, in brain disorders, 575–576
        in hydrocephalus, 587
Creatine kinase, in skeletal muscle disorders,
    686, 688
Creatinine, blood level of, in
        hyperparathyroidism, 1381t, 1385
    in renal failure, and prognosis, 1645
        increased, in hypoadrenocorticism, 1492,
            1492
    clearance of, in renal failure, and drug dosage
        changes, 1649, 1649t
    in glomerular function testing, clearance of,
        1602t, 1602–1603
    serum level of, 1602, 1602, 1602t
    in urine, ratio of, to cortisol, in hyperadreno-
        corticism, 1469, 1469
        to protein, 100, 101
Crenosoma infestation, of lung, 1065t,
    1070–1071
Cribriform plate, anatomy of, 1003, 1003
Cricopharyngeal achalasia, 1145, 1976t, 1985t
Crossbite, anterior, 1125–1126
Crossed extensor reflex, testing of, 570–571,
    571, 571t
Crossmatching, for blood transfusion, 353–354,
    354t
Crowns, in dental restoration, 1141
Cruciate ligament, cranial, rupture of,
    1867–1868
Crusting, 47, 49–51, 50
Cryoprecipitate, transfusion of, 351
    for von Willebrand's disease, 1825
Cryptococcosis, 468–471, 469, 470
    and encephalitis, 597
    and gastric outlet obstruction, 1170
    nasal, 1019
    of lung, 1068
    with feline immunodeficiency virus infection,
        437, 437t
    zoonotic, 383t
Cryptorchidism, in cat, 1593, 1597t, 1597–1598,
    1981t
    in dog, 1584–1585, 1993t
Cryptosporidiosis, and diarrhea, 125
    of small intestine, 408–411, 409t, 410t, 1222
    zoonotic, 383t
Crypts of Lieberkühn, 1238–1239
Crypt-villus units, of small intestine, 1183, 1184,
    1193
Crystalloids, in fluid therapy, 328–329, 329t,
    330t. See also Fluid therapy.

Crystalluria, 99, 1609–1610, 1610, 1611
    ammonia biurate in, in liver disease, 1291
    and urolithiasis, 1756, 1756t
    management of, 1778
Crystodigin, for heart failure, 730–731
Ctenocephalides fleas, in skin infestation, 59,
    59t, 60
Cushing's syndrome, 1460–1487. See also
    Hyperadrenocorticism.
Cutaneovisceral reflex, in acupuncture, 366
Cuvier's duct, atrophy of, and pericardial
    defects, 925–927
Cyanosis, evaluation of, 207–208, 208, 209,
    209t, 210t
    in congenital heart disease, 779–784, 781–784
        evaluation of, 780
        in aortic atresia, 783, 783
        in double outlet right ventricle, 783
        in pulmonary atresia, 782–783, 783
        in tetralogy of Fallot, 780–782, 781, 782
        in transposition of great arteries, 783–784
        in tricuspid atresia, 783, 784
        pathophysiology of, 779–780
    pathophysiology of, 206–207, 207t
    treatment of, 209–210
Cycad palm, toxicity of, to liver, 1329
Cyclic hematopoiesis, 1824t, 1826, 1990t
    neutrophils in, 1849–1850
Cyclophosphamide, and neutropenia, 1849
    dosage of, in renal failure, 1649t
    for arthritis, 1884, 1885
    for glomerulonephritis, 1672, 1672t
    for hemolytic anemia, 1797
    for lung tumors, 1065t
    for lymphoma, 510, 511, 511t
    for multiple myeloma, 518, 519
    in cancer therapy, 485t, 486–488
Cyclopia, 1979t
Cyclosporine, for anemia, aplastic, 1813
    hemolytic, 1797
    for bronchopulmonary disease, 1059t
    for glomerulonephritis, 1672, 1672t
    for inflammatory bowel disease, 1251
Cylindruria, 1609
Cyproheptadine, for bronchopulmonary disease,
    1059t
Cyst(s), and spinal cord compression, 643
    intra-arachnoid, 645–647, 646
    synovial, 652
    mediastinal, 1093, 1093, 1095
    of biliary tract, 1322
    of bone, 539, 1904, 1904
        aneurysmal, 539, 1904–1905
        congenital, 1983t
        subchondral, 1905
    of gallbladder, 1344
    of iris, congenital, 1978t, 1988t
    of kidney, in polycystic disease, 1698, 1699t,
        1700–1702
    of liver, 1322, 1322
        congenital, 1979t, 1991t
        ultrasonography of, 1292
    of prostate, 1689t, 1693–1694
    of thymus, branchial, 1979t, 1990t
    ovarian, and anestrus, 1525
        and infertility, 1562, 1562, 1564–1565
        follicular, 1564–1565
            and prolonged estrus, 1521, 1523, 1523–
                1524, 1524
    pericardial, congenital, pathophysiology of,
        927–928
    subcutaneous, 36, 37
    uveal, anterior, 1987t
Cystadenocarcinoma, renal, 1699t, 1701
Cysteine, in diet, 239t

Cystic disease, of lungs, 1083–1084
Cystic endometrial hyperplasia. See
    Endometrium, cystic hyperplasia of.
Cystic mucinous hypertrophy, of gallbladder,
    1344
Cystine, in urinary calculi, in cats, 1723t,
    1729–1730
    in dogs, 1758t, 1775t, 1775–1777, 1776t
Cystinuria, 3t, 1705, 1996t
Cystitis, 1778–1780, 1779t
    idiopathic, 1743
    incidence of, 1748
    interstitial, 1712–1713
Cystocentesis, decompressive, before urethral
    plug removal, 1734–1735, 1735, 1735t
Cystoisospora infection, enteric, 408–410, 409t,
    410t
Cystoscopy, in idiopathic disorders, 1744
Cystotomy, for lithiasis, 1778
Cystourethroscopy, 1749
Cytauxzoonosis, and hemolytic anemia, 1799t,
    1800
    and thrombocytopenia, 1821
    polysystemic, 414–415
Cytochrome b_5, in hemolytic anemia,
    1790–1792, 1791t
Cytochrome b_5 reductase deficiency, 1990t
Cytokines, in anemia, of chronic disease, 1807,
    1807
    in hyperthermia, 7, 7t, 8
    in inflammation, steroid effects on, 311
    in periodontal disease, 1128
Cytoplasmic basophilia, 1845, 1845
Cytoplasmic vacuolation, 1845, 1845
Cytotec (misoprostol), for gastrinoma, 1506,
    1506t
    for stomach ulcers, in renal failure, 1629,
        1630t
    with steroid therapy, for hemolytic anemia,
        1797
Cytoxan. See Cyclophosphamide.

Dachshund, sensory neuropathy in, 669, 1992t
Dacryops, 1987t
Dalmatian, laryngeal paralysis in, 668, 1994t
    urate urolithiasis in, 1772
Danazol, for hemolytic anemia, 1797
Dancing Doberman disease, 679–680
Dandelion, in cancer management, 378t
Dantrolene, for bladder dysfunction, 1739t
    for urine retention, 95t
Dapsone, for bacterial infection, 391t
Datura species, toxicity of, 365
Daylily, toxicity of, 364
DEA blood group system, in transfusion, 353,
    1798
Deafness, 1000t, 1000–1002
    congenital, 1977t, 1986t
    furosemide and, in heart failure, 715
Débridement, for osteomyelitis, 1914
DEET, toxicity of, 357
Defibrillation, cardiac, 193
Deglutition, disorders of, 114, 114t, 115,
    1026–1029
    physiology of, 1025, 1026
Dehydration, diuretics and, in heart failure,
    716–717
    fluid therapy for, 337, 339t
    in hypernatremia, 228–232, 230t, 231
    in neonate, 244
    in renal failure, and hypovolemia, 1622, 1623t
        management of, 1652
    parvovirus infection and, 445

Delivery. See *Parturition.*
Deltalin. See *Vitamin D.*
Demerol, for pancreatitis, 1353, 1363t
Demodicosis, 59t, 61–62
  after glucocorticoid therapy, 316
  and hyperpigmentation, 57, 58
  and otitis externa, 989t, 990t, 993
  and pruritus, 32, 33t, 34, 34t
  client information on, 1970
  skin lesions in, 28
Demyelination, congenital, 588, 1991t, 1992t
  of peripheral nerves, 674
  of spinal cord, in globoid cell leukodystrophy, 627–628
  in leukoencephalomyelopathy, 636
Denervating disease, distal, 679
Dens, of axis, in atlantoaxial subluxation, *615,* 615–616, *616,* 1984t
Dentin, fracture of, 1137t, 1137–1140, *1138*
Dentistry. See *Teeth.*
Deoxyribonucleic acid (DNA), damage to, in carcinogenesis, 479–481
  radiation effects on, in cancer therapy, 489–490
  testing of, in genetic defects, 5
Depo-Provera. See *Medroxyprogesterone.*
L-Deprenyl, for hyperadrenocorticism, 1482
Dermacentor ticks, as vectors, of Rocky Mountain spotted fever, 616
  bites of, and paralysis, 672–673
Dermal fragility syndrome, 1981t, 1995t
Dermanyssus gallinae mite infestation, 59t, 61
Dermatitis, acral lick, 36, 37
  actinic, and carcinoma, client information on, 1926
  of pinna, 988–991, 989t
  and crusting, 49–50, *50*
  and pruritus, 32–36, 33t, 34t, *35*
  atopic, client information on, 1973
    with zinc deficiency, 48–49
  glucagonoma and, *1507,* 1507–1508
  granulomatous, periadnexal multinodular, 520
  itraconazole and, 457, *457*
  necrolytic, superficial, liver disease and, 28, 1272, 1337
Dermatomyositis, 26
  and megaesophagus, 1150t
  congenital, 1995t
  erosions in, 43
  hypopigmentation in, 55, 57
  ulcers in, 43
Dermatophytosis, 49
  zoonotic, 383t
Dermatosis, lichenoid-psoriasiform, congenital, 1995t
Dermatosparaxis, 1981t, 1995t
Dermoid, ocular, congenital, 1978t, 1987t
Dermoid cyst, of spinal cord, 643
Dermoid sinus, 1995t
Desmopressin. See *Antidiuretic hormone.*
Desoxycorticosterone, for hypoadrenocorticism, 1496–1498
  after adrenalectomy, 1487
Detrusor muscle. See also *Bladder.*
  dysfunction of, and incontinence, 1742
  and urine retention, 93, 93t, 94, *94*
  urethral obstruction and, 1738, 1739t
Devil's ivy, toxicity of, 364
Dexamethasone, and stomach ulcers, 1166
  dosage of, 313t, 314, 314t
  effect of, on liver enzyme concentrations, 1282, *1282*
  for arthritis, 1884
  for central nervous system inflammation, 592–593, 593t

Dexamethasone *(Continued)*
  for cerebral edema, 147
    with seizures, 150t
  for hemolytic anemia, 1796–1797
  for hepatitis, 1301
  for hyperadrenocorticism, in screening test, 1470–1472, *1471,* 1485–1486
    with surgery, 1475
  for intracranial pressure elevation, 577
  for otitis externa, 995
  for pancreatic islet cell tumors, 1435, 1435t
  for shock, 316
    with gastric dilatation and volvulus, 1172
  for spinal cord trauma, 315–316
  in abortion induction, 1547–1548
  in cardiopulmonary resuscitation, 192, 192t
  potency of, 312t, 312–313
  structure of, *309*
Dexatrim (phenylpropanolamine), for urinary tract dysfunction, 320, 1739t
Dextran, in fluid therapy, 329t, 329–333, 331t, 332t
  for shock, with gastric dilatation and volvulus, 1172
Dextromethorphan, for cough, 165t, 319
  in heart failure, 734
  in tracheal disease, 1043t
Dextrose, for hyperkalemia, 342
  for pancreatic islet cell tumors, 1434–1436, 1435t
  in parenteral nutrition, 281, 282t
Diaβeta, for diabetes mellitus, 1449
Diabetes insipidus, 1374–1379
  and hypernatremia, 228–230
  central, 85t, 85–87, *86,* 87t
  congenital, 1977t, 1986t
  diagnosis of, *1377,* 1377–1378
  nephrogenic, 85t, *86,* 87t, 1706–1707
  pathogenesis of, 1374–1377, *1375, 1376*
  signs of, 1377
  treatment of, 1378–1379
Diabetes mellitus, 1438–1459
  after excision of insulinoma, 1436
  and cataracts, 985, 1458
  and growth hormone excess, 1371, *1372, 1373, 1373*
  and hypernatremia, 228
  classification of, 1438–1441
  client information on, 1930
  complications of, 1457–1459
  congenital, 1977t, 1986t
  diagnosis of, *1442,* 1442–1444, 1443t
  etiology of, *1439,* 1439t, 1439–1440, *1440*
  exercise in, 1448–1449
  hyperadrenocorticism with, 1483
  hyperlipidemia in, 289–290
  hypokalemia in, 225
  hypothyroidism with, 1422
  liver enzymes in, 1284
  obesity with, 71, 72
  pathophysiology of, 1441–1442
  peripheral neuropathy in, 671
  prognosis of, 1459
  treatment of, diet in, 261, 1447–1448, 1448t
    insulin in, 1451–1457
      adjustment of, 1453–1455
      complications of, 1455–1457, 1456t, *1457*
      monitoring of, 1452–1453, 1453t
      with surgery, 1455
    oral hypoglycemic drugs in, *1449,* 1449–1451, *1450*
    with ketoacidosis, 1444t, 1444–1447
Diacylglycerol, in platelet activation, 1817, *1817*
Dialysis, for renal failure, acute, 1631t, 1631–1632

Dialysis *(Continued)*
  chronic, 1646, 1658–1659
  peritoneal, in pancreatitis, 1354
Diaphragm, displacement of, 1100
  hernia through, 1098–1099, *1099*
    congenital, 1975t, 1983t
    perineal, 1259–1260
    peritoneopericardial, 784
      congenital, 925–927, *927, 935, 936,* 1975t
  paralysis of, 1100
Diarrhea, acarbose and, in diabetes, 1448
  astrovirus and, 451
  causes of, 1182, 1183t
  classification of, 121–123, 122t
  diagnosis of, 123–126, *124*
  fiber-responsive, 1252
  in adverse food reactions, 253, 254
  in colitis, 1247
    bacterial, 1243–1245
  in histoplasmosis, 463, 464
  in pancreatic exocrine insufficiency, 122–123, 125, 1359
  in pancreatitis, 1254
  in renal failure, 1637
  liver disease and, 1273t, 1275
  management of, 126
    over-the-counter drugs in, 318–319
  parvovirus and, 420–421, 445
  reovirus and, 451
  rotavirus and, 451
  small intestinal disorders and. See *Small intestine.*
Diazepam, for behavioral disorders, 160, 160t
  for bladder dysfunction, 1739t
  for Scotty cramp, 588
  for seizures, 150t, 151t
    with coma, 147
  for tremor, 599
  for urine retention, 95t
  in anesthesia, before catheterization, for urethral obstruction, 1734
  in sedation, for blood donation, 349
    for liver biopsy, 1296t
  toxicity of, to liver, 1328
Diazoxide, for pancreatic islet cell tumors, 1434t, 1437
Dichlorphenamide, for glaucoma, with blastomycosis, 462
Dicloxacillin, dosage of, in renal failure, 1649t
Dideoxycytidine, for feline leukemia virus infection, 431–432
Dieffenbachia species, toxicity of, 364
Diestrus, *1510,* 1510–1514, *1514, 1515,* 1520–1522
Diet, adverse reactions to, clinical features of, 253–254, *254*
  diagnosis of, 255–257, *256*
  types of, 251–253, *252*
  and intestinal gas, 136
  and obesity, 70, *71,* 72
  as aid to management, of cancer, 377–378, 379t, 500–501
    of cardiomyopathy, 911–912
    of crystalluria, 1778
    of diabetes mellitus, 261, 1447–1448, 1448t
    of diarrhea, 1215, 1252
    of eosinophilic gastritis, 1163
    of gastric motility disorders, 1175
    of gastrointestinal disorders, 258–260
    of glomerulonephritis, 1672t, 1673–1674
    of heart disease, 262–268, 264t–268t
    of hepatic copper accumulation, 1303t, 1304
    of hepatic disorders, 260–261

Diet (Continued)
of hepatic encephalopathy, 1332–1335, 1333t
of hepatic failure, 1302t
of hip dysplasia, 1872
of inflammatory bowel disease, 1227, 1249t, 1249–1250
of megaesophagus, 1150
of mitral insufficiency, 794
of pancreatic islet cell tumors, 1434, 1434t, 1436–1437
of perineal hernia, 1260
of periodontal disease, 1134
of portosystemic shunt, congenital, 1313–1314
of renal disease, 269–271, 271t, 272t, 273–274
of renal failure, 271t, 271–273, 273t, 274t
  acute, 1630–1631
  chronic, 1646–1648, 1647t, 1648
    with hyperphosphatemia, 1650
    with hypokalemia, 1651
of short-bowel syndrome, 1236
of small intestinal lymphangiectasia, 1230
of urinary calculi, 271t, 272t, 274
  calcium phosphate, 1729
  cystine, 1775–1777, 1776t
  struvite, 1731, 1731t, 1762–1763
  urate, 1772–1773, 1773t, 1774t
deficiencies of, and anemia, 1808–1809
  management of, 236, 237
disorders of, and diarrhea, 1214
  and gastritis, 1160, 1161
  and growth failure, 74–77, 75t, 76
  and hyperparathyroidism, 1396
    bone loss in, 1906, 1906–1907
  and hypokalemia, 223–225
  and nervous system injury, 555–556
  and weakness, 12
excessive intake of, and bone growth disorders, 1909
fat in, and hyperlipidemia, 290–291
for kittens, 241–244, 243t
for puppies, 241–242, 244
in anorexia, 102–104, 104
in cachexia, 72–74, 73
in calcium oxalate urolithiasis, 1726–1728, 1764, 1764–1765, 1766t, 1769, 1769t
in constipation, 129, 130t
in diarrhea, 123
in fecal incontinence, 135
in food allergy. See Allergy, to food.
in food intolerance, 1233
in gluten-sensitive enteropathy, 254, 1232–1233, 1986t
in hepatic lipidosis, 1329, 1330
in orthopedic developmental disorders, 245–250, 246, 249t, 250
in pancreatic exocrine insufficiency, 1357–1358, 1361, 1362
in pancreatitis, 1349, 1353, 1354
in polyphagia, 104–107, 105t, 106
in ptyalism, 108
in vomiting, 118t, 119
intake in, 236
palatability of, 236
recommendations for, 236–240, 239t
sensitivity to, and inflammatory bowel disease, 1251
support of, client information on, 1944, 1945
  enteral, 275–281, 276, 278, 279, 279t–281t
  parenteral, 281–282, 282t
  patient selection for, 275
toxins in, and hemolytic anemia, 1800–1801, 1801t

Diethylcarbamazine, for Crenosoma infestation, of lung, 1065t, 1071
  preventive use of, against dirofilariasis, 950t, 954–955
    against intestinal parasitosis, 1221t
  toxicity of, to liver, 1307–1308
Diethylstilbestrol, and vaginal bleeding, vs. prolonged estrus, 1523
  for prostatic hypertrophy, 1691–1692
Diethyltoluamide, toxicity of, 357
Diff-Quik staining, 52
Diffuse idiopathic skeletal hyperostosis, and spinal cord dysfunction, 623, 623–624
Diflucan. See Fluconazole.
Digestion, pancreatic enzymes in, 1345–1346, 1346t
  physiology of, in small intestine, 1187, 1187t, 1188, 1189
    in stomach, 1156, 1156–1159
Digibind, for digoxin toxicity, 730
Digitalis, for arrhythmia, 826t, 828t, 829t, 831
  for heart failure, 713, 714, 726–731
  toxicity of, 365, 729–730
    and syncope, 16
Digitoxin, for heart failure, 730–731
Digits, anomalies of, 1894–1895, 1895, 1983t, 1984t
  hyperkeratosis of, congenital, 1995t
  tumors of, 525
Digoxin, dosage of, in renal failure, 1649t
  for arrhythmia, 826t, 828t, 831
  for cardiomyopathy, dilated, 884, 911
    hypertrophic, 906
  for heart failure, 713, 714, 726–730
    congestive, in dirofilariasis, 949t
  for hypotension, 184t
  for mitral insufficiency, 793
Dihydrotachysterol, for hypoparathyroidism, 1397–1398, 1398t
1,2-Dihydroxymethane. See Ethylene glycol.
1,25-Dihydroxyvitamin D. See Vitamin D.
Dilacor XR. See Diltiazem.
Dilantin (phenytoin), and osteodystrophy, 1908
  for arrhythmia, 829t
  for digitalis toxicity, 730, 829t
Diltiazem, for arrhythmia, 824t–826t, 828t, 830, 831
  supraventricular, with hypotension, 184t
  for cardiomyopathy, hypertrophic, in cats, 906, 907
    in dogs, 890
  for pulmonary hypertension, in dirofilariasis, 949t
  for tachyarrhythmia, with mitral insufficiency, 794–795
  in cardiopulmonary resuscitation, 192t, 192–193
Dimelia, 1975t, 1983t
Dimenhydrinate, with D-penicillamine, for lead toxicity, 362
Dimethyl sulfoxide, for amyloidosis, of kidneys, 1674
  of liver, 1323
  for urinary tract disorders, idiopathic, 1745
  with fluocinolone, for otitis externa, 989t, 995, 996
Dimethylcysteine (D-penicillamine), for cystine urinary calculi, 1776–1777
  for lead toxicity, 362
Dinoprostum, in abortion induction, 1546
Dioctyl sodium sulfosuccinate, for otitis externa, 989t, 994
Dipetalonema reconditum, microfilariae of, vs. Dirofilaria immitis, 939t
Diphenhydramine, for anaphylaxis, 184t

Diphenoxylate, for diarrhea, 1215
Diphenylhydantoin (phenytoin), and osteodystrophy, 1908
  for arrhythmia, 829t
  for digitalis toxicity, 730, 829t
Diptera infestation, 59t, 60
Dipylidiasis, of small intestine, 1221, 1221t
  zoonotic, 383t
Dipyridamole, for glomerulonephritis, 1673
Dipyrone, for fever, 9
Diquat, toxicity of, 363
Dirofilariasis, 937–961
  and dyspnea, 169
  and hemoptysis, 217, 218
  and pulmonary thromboembolism, 1078, 1080
  and weakness, 13
  client information on, 1953
  clinical significance of, 941–943, 942, 943t, 944t, 945–947
  diagnosis of, in cats, 956–958, 956–960
    in dogs, 943–947, 944t, 945–947
  heartworm life cycle in, 937, 937–938, 938, 938t
  history in, 947, 956
  of spinal cord, 647
  pathology of, 939t, 939–941, 940, 941, 947
  physical examination in, 947, 956
  prevention of, 954–955, 961
  reaction to, 939, 939, 939t
  resistance to, 938t, 938–939, 939, 941–942
  risk factors for, 955
  signs of, 955t, 955–956
  treatment of, in cats, 949t, 950t, 960–961
    in dogs, 948t–951t, 948–952, 951
      complications of, 952, 952–954, 953
      evaluation of, 954
  zoonotic, 383t
Disaccharides, intolerance to, 253
Discoid lupus, 55, 57
Discospondylitis, and spinal cord dysfunction, 624–626, 625, 626
Disks, intervertebral, disorders of, acupuncture for, 371, 373
  and spinal cord compression, 630, 630–633, 631, 633
    treatment of, 633–635
  client information on, 1919
  radiography of, in lumbosacral vertebral stenosis, 637, 639
Disopyramide, for arrhythmia, 825, 825t, 826t, 828t
Disseminated intravascular coagulation. See Coagulation, disseminated intravascular.
Distemper, 418–419, 419t
  and encephalitis, 595–596
  and megaesophagus, 1150t
  and myelitis, 626–627
  and neurologic disorders, 604
  and respiratory disease, 1063
  cerebrospinal fluid examination in, 574t
  client information on, 1959
  in leukocyte inclusions, 1847, 1847
Distichiasis, 1978t, 1987t
Diterpene acids, in cancer management, 378t
Dithiazanine iodide, for dirofilariasis, 951
Diuretics, for ascites, with protein-losing enteropathy, 1202
  for cardiomyopathy, dilated, canine, 883
    feline, 911
  for diabetes insipidus, nephrogenic, 1707
  for edema, in brain trauma, 579–580
    pulmonary, 1065t, 1082–1083
      with cardiomyopathy, hypertrophic, 906–908
      with mitral insufficiency, 793

Diuretics *(Continued)*
　　with hepatic failure, 1302t
　　for heart failure, 713–717
　　　vs. low-sodium diet, 263
　　　with mitral insufficiency, 794
　　for intracranial pressure elevation, 577
　　for renal failure, 1627
　　for urolithiasis, calcium oxalate, 1728
　　　preventive use of, 1769–1770
Diverticula, esophageal, 1145–1146
　　congenital, 1985t
　　Meckel's, 1976t, 1985t
　　vesicourachal, 1712, *1718,* 1718–1719, 1752
DMSO. See *Dimethyl sulfoxide.*
DNA, damage to, in carcinogenesis, 479–481
　　radiation effects on, in cancer therapy, 489–490
　　testing of, in genetic defects, 5
Doberman pinscher, dancing disease in, 679–680
　　hepatic copper accumulation in, 1305–1306
　　neutrophil defect in, 1850, 1971t
　　renal basement membrane disorder in, 1699t, 1701
Dobutamine, for cardiomyopathy, dilated, 884, 911
　　for heart failure, 731–732
　　for hypotension, 184t, 185
Docusate, for constipation, 132t
Dog erythrocyte antigen system, in transfusion, 353, 1798
Döhle bodies, 1845, *1845,* 1848
Dominance aggression, in cats, 160, 160t, 162
　　in dogs, 156, *157,* 158t
Dopamine, for heart failure, 731
　　for hypercalcemia, 344
　　for hypotension, 184t, 185
　　for pancreatitis, 1363t
　　for renal failure, 1627–1628
Doppler echocardiography. See also
　　Echocardiography.
　　color, 835t, *848,* 848–849
　　continuous-wave, 835t, 839–842, *844,* 847t, 847–848
　　in heart failure, 709, 710
　　of cardiomyopathy, hypertrophic, feline, *897, 899, 902,* 904–905
　　of congenital heart disease, 740–741
　　of patent ductus arteriosus, 747–748, *748*
　　of pericardial constrictive disease, 935
　　of pulmonic stenosis, congenital, 765, *766*
　　of ventricular septal defect, 757–758, *758*
　　principles of, 839–842, *841–844*
　　pulsed-wave, 835t, 839–847, *842–844,* 845t, *846*
Doppler ultrasonography, in blood pressure measurement, 179, 184–185
　　of arteriovenous fistula, 971, *971*
　　of renal blood flow, 1612
Double-outlet right ventricle, 783
Doxorubicin, for lymphoma, 510–512, 511
　　for multiple myeloma, 519
　　for sarcoma, of bone, 536, 537
　　　of soft tissue, 534
　　for thyroid tumors, with hyperthyroidism, 1417
　　in cancer treatment, 485t, *486,* 486–488
　　toxicity of, and cardiomyopathy, 878, 914
Doxycycline, dosage of, in renal failure, 1649t
　　for bacterial infection, 391t
　　for bronchopulmonary disease, 1056, 1057, 1059t
　　for ehrlichiosis, 404, 405
　　for lung infection, 1065t
　　for periodontitis, 1132
　　for Rocky Mountain spotted fever, 402

Doxycycline *(Continued)*
　　for thrombocytopenia, 1819
Dramamine, with D-penicillamine, for lead toxicity, 362
Drentse patrijshond, gastritis in, 1165
Drisdol. See *Vitamin D.*
Droncit (praziquantel), for fluke infestation, of pancreas, 1363t, 1364
　　for intestinal parasitosis, 1221t
　　for *Paragonimus* infestation, of lung, 1065t
Drowning, animal rescued from, lung disorders in, 1086–1087
Drugs. See also specific drugs, e.g., *Ampicillin,* and classes, e.g., *Corticosteroids.*
　　absorption of, 295–296
　　adverse reactions to, 320–325, 323t
　　　and diarrhea, 1214
　　　and eruptions, with pruritus, 33t, 34t
　　　drug interactions and, 324
　　　identification of, 322
　　　incidence of, 321–322
　　　type A, 320–324, 323t
　　　type B, 321, 324–325
　　distribution of, 296–297
　　dose-response relationship in, 294
　　dosing regimens for, 298–300, *299*
　　elimination of, 297–298
　　metabolism of, 297
　　movement of, *294,* 294–298, *295*
　　over-the-counter, 318–320
　　toxicity of, and anemia, aplastic, 1813
　　　hemolytic, 1800–1801, 1801t
　　　non-regenerative, 1812, 1812t
　　　with folate deficiency, 1809
　　　and arthritis, 1883
　　　and pancreatitis, 1350
　　　and platelet dysfunction, 1826, 1826t
　　　and stomach ulcers, 1165–1166
　　　and thrombocytopenia, 1822, 1822t
　　　and tremors, 141
　　　renal failure and, 1648–1650, 1649t
　　　to ear, 992, 999t, 999–1000
　　　to liver, 457, 1272–1274, 1326t, 1327–1329
　　　to urinary tract, 1778, 1779t
Duchenne muscular dystrophy, 3t, 688
Duct of Cuvier, atrophy of, and pericardial defects, 925–927
Ductus arteriosus, patent, 745–750, 1976t, 1985t. See also *Patent ductus arteriosus.*
Dulcolax, for constipation, 132
Dumbcane, toxicity of, 364
Duodenum. See also *Small intestine.*
　　anatomy of, 1182, *1184, 1185*
　　juice of, examination of, 1213
　　　in bacterial overgrowth, 1224
　　reflux from, 1174
　　　and gastritis, 1165
　　　and pancreatitis, 1350
Duphalac syrup, for constipation, 132
Dura mater, ossification of, and spinal cord compression, 627
Dwarfism, 1897t, 1897–1898, *1898,* 1899t, *1900,* 1983t, 1987t
Dyes, in food, adverse reactions to, 252
　　in liver function testing, 1290
Dysautonomia, 680
　　and anisocoria, 660t
　　and megaesophagus, 1150t, 1151
　　of bladder, and atony, 93
　　and incontinence, 1742
Dysbetalipoproteinemia, 1986t
Dyschezia, 129, 132–133, 133t
　　causes of, 1258t, 1258–1259
Dyschondroplasia (osteochondrosis), 1869–1870, *1870*

Dyschondroplasia (osteochondrosis) *(Continued)*
　　nutrition in, 245–250, *246,* 249t, *250*
Dyscoria, 1987t
Dysfibrinogenemia, 1839, 1839t
Dyshematopoiesis, familial, 1791t, 1990t
Dyslipoproteinemia, 291
Dysmetria, in brain disorders, 561
Dysmyelinogenesis, 588, 1992t
Dysphagia, 114, 114t, *115*
　　in renal failure, 1636t, 1636–1637
　　pharyngeal disorders and, 1026–1029
　　ptyalism with, 109
Dyspnea, 166–169, 167t, *168*
　　in heart failure, 705
　　pneumothorax and, 1110
Dysraphism, cranial, 1979t, 1991t
　　spinal, 645, *646*
Dystocia, 1530–1536, 1596
　　assessment of, 1530, *1531*
　　diagnosis of, 1530–1531
　　fetal causes of, *1531,* 1532t, *1534,* 1534–1536
　　frequency of, 1530
　　maternal causes of, 1531–1534, 1532t, *1533*
Dystrophin, genetic defect of, and cardiomyopathy, 877
Dysuria, 89–92, *91*
　　idiopathic, 1743–1746
　　in urethral obstruction, 1720
　　liver disease and, 1273t, 1275

Ear, cancer of, radiotherapy for, 497t
　　disorders of, 986–1002
　　　and deafness, 1000t, 1000–1002
　　　congenital, in cats, 1977t
　　　in dogs, 1986t
　　　drug toxicity to, 992, 999t, 999–1000
　　　furosemide and, 715
　　external canal of, anatomy of, 992
　　　inflammation of, 992–994
　　　client information on, 1974
　　　management of, 989t, 990t, 994–997
　　inner, anatomy of, 997
　　　disorders of, and weakness, 12
　　　inflammation of, 999
　　middle, anatomy of, 997
　　　inflammation of, 990t, 997–999
　　otodectic mite infestation of, 34t, 59t, 61, 989t, 990t, 992
　　pinna of, carcinoma of, 988–991
　　　client information on, 1926
　　　dermatoses of, 987t, 988–992, 989t, 990t
　　　disorders of, 986–992
　　　differential diagnosis of, 986, 987t
Easter lily, toxicity of, 364
Ebstein's anomaly, tricuspid valve dysplasia in, 775, *775*
Ecchymoses, diagnosis of, 220, *221*
　　pathophysiology of, 218–220, 219t
　　treatment of, 220–222
Echidnophaga fleas, in skin infestation, 59, 59t, *60*
Echinacea, in cancer management, 378t
Echinococcosis, of small intestine, 1221, 1221t
　　zoonotic, 383t
Echocardiography, 834–871
　　contrast, 835t, 838–839, *841*
　　Doppler, color, 835t, *848,* 848–849
　　　continuous-wave, 835t, 839–842, *844,* 847t, 847–848
　　　principles of, 839–842, *841–844*
　　　pulsed-wave, 835t, 839–847, *842–844,* 845t, *846*

Echocardiography (Continued)
  errors in, 866, 867t
  in hyperthyroidism, 857t, 1403
  M-mode, 834–838, 835t, 839, 840
  of aorta, 852–853, 856t, 858
  of aortic regurgitation, 857t, 871
  of aortic stenosis, 866–869, 868
  of atrial septal defect, 755–756, 756, 854t
  of atrium, left, 850t, 851, 854–857, 856t, 859
    right, 852, 856t, 858–859, 859
  of cardiomyopathy, dilated, 857t, 909–910,
    910
    hypertrophic, 857t
      canine, 888–889, 889
      feline, 897, 899, 901–902
    restrictive, 857t, 904–905
  of congenital heart disease, 740–741
    cyanotic, 780
  of dirofilariasis, 857t, 947, 947, 959
  of endocarditis, bacterial, 857t
  of heart failure, 707, 709–710
  of infective endocarditis, 798
  of mitral insufficiency, 791–792, 792
  of mitral regurgitation, 857t, 869–870
  of mitral stenosis, 847, 847t, 848, 870
  of mitral valve, 856t, 857
    dysplastic, 776, 778, 854t
  of patent ductus arteriosus, 747–750, 748,
    751, 854t
  of pericardial constrictive disease, 935
  of pericardial effusion, 857t, 930, 931–933,
    935, 935–936
  of pulmonary artery, 852–853, 857t, 859
  of pulmonic insufficiency, 871
  of pulmonic stenosis, 847, 847, 868, 869
    congenital, 762–766, 766, 854t
  of subaortic stenosis, 770, 771, 772, 854t
  of tetralogy of Fallot, 839, 841, 854t
  of thromboembolism, 916, 916
  of tricuspid insufficiency, 795, 796
  of tricuspid regurgitation, 857t, 870, 870
  of tricuspid stenosis, 847, 847t, 870, 871
  of tricuspid valve, 857t, 859
    dysplastic, 854t
  of valvular function, 866–871, 867, 870, 871
  of vena cava, 857t, 859
  of ventricle, left, 856t, 857–858
    in diastolic function assessment, 843,
      845t, 845–846, 861–866, 865t
    in size estimation, 849t, 850t, 851–852,
      853
    in systolic function assessment, 859–861,
      862t–864t
    right, 850t, 852, 857t, 859, 859
  of ventricular outflow, 842, 843–845, 845t
  of ventricular septum, 856t, 858
    with congenital defect, 757–758, 758, 759,
      854t
  two-dimensional, 834, 835t, 836–838, 839t
Eclampsia, 1394–1396, 1538
  and hyperthermia, 8
Ectodermal defect, congenital, 1995t
Ectrodactyly, 1895, 1895, 1975t
Ectromelia, 1975t, 1983t
Ectropion, 1987t
Edema, fetal, and dystocia, 1534
  in glomerular disease, 1675, 1675
  in ischemic myelopathy, with fibrocartilagi-
    nous embolism, 635
  mediastinal, 1094–1095
  of brain, after portosystemic shunt ligation,
    1314
    in coma, 147
    in hepatic encephalopathy, 1334
    trauma and, 578–580

Edema (Continued)
  treatment of, 577
    with seizures, 150t
  of cornea, in glaucoma, 69
  of larynx, 1030
  of lymphatic system, congenital, 1979t, 1990t
    peripheral, 977t, 977–980, 978, 979
  of optic nerve, brain tumors and, 585
  of prepuce, 84, 84t
  of vulva, 80, 81t
  pulmonary, 1081–1083, 1083
    in renal failure, 1622–1624, 1623
    with cardiomyopathy, hypertrophic, 906–
      908
    with mitral insufficiency, 790, 793–795
  subcutaneous, 63–66, 64
  with hepatic failure, 1302t
  with intervertebral disk extrusion, 631
  with lymphoma, mediastinal, 508, 508
Edrophonium, for arrhythmia, 832
EDTA, in chelation therapy, for lead toxicity,
    362
  in cancer management, 377
Effusion, pericardial, diagnosis of, 928–931,
    929–933
  management of, 931–933, 933
  pathophysiology of, 924–925, 926
  pleural, 186–189, 1102–1109. See also Pleural
    effusion.
Eggplant, toxicity of, 364
Ehlers-Danlos syndrome, 1981t, 1995t
Ehrlichiosis, 402–406
  and anemia, 199, 203, 1811
  and arthritis, 1878
  and meningitis, spinal, 616–619
  and thrombocytopenia, 1819–1821, 1821
  leukocyte inclusions in, 1846, 1846
  neurologic disorders in, multifocal, 606
  zoonotic, 383t
Eisenmenger's syndrome, auscultation of, 739t
  in cyanotic heart disease, congenital, 780
  with ventricular septal defect, 754–755
Ejection fraction, left ventricular,
    echocardiographic measurement of, 860,
    863t, 864t
Ejection sounds, cardiac, 171
Ejection time, left ventricular, echocardiographic
    measurement of, 861, 862t, 864t
Elavil. See Amitriptyline.
Elbow, dysplasia of, 1870–1872, 1871, 1984t
  luxation of, congenital, 1984t
Electrocardiography, 800–822
  in dirofilariasis, 947, 948, 959
  in hyperkalemia, 227–228
  in hypomagnesemia, 232–233
  in pericardial constrictive disease, 934
  in pericardial effusion, 929–930, 930
  in thromboembolism, 915
  normal findings in, 800–801, 804–806
  of accelerated idioventricular rhythms, 816
  of atrial extrasystoles, 810–811, 811
  of atrial fibrillation, 812–813, 813
  of atrial flutter, 812, 812
  of atrial septal defect, 755, 755
  of atrial standstill, 820, 821
  of atrial tachycardia, 811–812, 812
  of atrioventricular blocks, 817, 817–819
  of bundle branch blocks, 817–818, 820, 821
  of cardiomyopathy, dilated, canine, 879–880,
    880, 880t, 881–883, 882
    feline, 901t, 909
    hypertrophic, canine, 888
      feline, 897, 899, 901t, 904
  of cardiopulmonary arrest, 192
  of conduction disorders, 816–820, 817–821

Electrocardiography (Continued)
  with excitation disorders, 820–822, 822,
    823
  of congenital heart disease, 740
  of endocarditis, infective, 798
  of escape rhythms, 818–820
  of heart failure, 707
  of hypoadrenocorticism, 1494–1495, 1495,
    1498
  of mitral insufficiency, 790–791
  of mitral valve dysplasia, 776
  of patent ductus arteriosus, 747, 747
  of preexcitation syndromes, 821, 822
  of pulmonic stenosis, 761
  of respiratory sinus arrhythmia, 809–810, 810
  of sick sinus syndrome, 821–822, 823
  of sinoatrial blocks, 816
  of sinus bradycardia, 809, 810
  of sinus tachycardia, 809, 809
  of subaortic stenosis, 770, 770
  of torsades de pointes, 815, 816
  of tricuspid insufficiency, 795
  of ventricular extrasystoles, 813–814, 814
  of ventricular fibrillation, 815, 816
  of ventricular flutter, 815
  of ventricular parasystole, 816, 817
  of ventricular septal defect, 756–757
  of ventricular tachycardia, 814–815, 815
  of wandering pacemaker, 810, 811
  principles of, 801, 801–802
  rhythm disturbances in, classification of, 806
    clinical aspects of, 807–808
    identification of, 808, 809t
    indicence of, 806–807, 808t
    of atrial excitability, 810–813, 811–813
    of junctional excitability, 813, 813
    of sinus excitability, 808–810, 809–811
    of ventricular excitability, 813–816, 814–
      817
  techniques of, 802–804, 803
Electrocoagulation, for anal sacculitis, 1266
Electroencephalography, 575
  in coma, 146
  in vision loss, acute, 20
  of tumors, 585
Electrolytes. See also specific elements, e.g.,
    Potassium.
  clearance of, in renal function assessment,
    1604t, 1605
  imbalances of, and weakness, 11–12
    diuretics and, in heart failure, 716
    in renal failure, 1624, 1628t, 1628–1629
    in small intestinal disorders, 1206
    treatment of, 340–346, 341, 343, 345
  transport of, fluid dynamics in, 326, 326–327,
    327
    in large intestine, 1240
Electromechanical dissociation, in
    cardiopulmonary arrest, 192
Electromyography, in spinal cord disorders, 610
Electrophoresis, serum protein, in multiple
    myeloma, 517, 517
Electroretinography, in acute vision loss, 18–19
Elimination trials, in diagnosis of food reactions,
    255–256, 256
Elixophyllin. See Theophylline.
Elliptocytosis, 1990t
  and hemolytic anemia, 1791t, 1792
  genetics in, 3t
Elmiron, for urinary tract disorders, idiopathic,
    1745–1746
Elokomin fluke fever agent, and salmon-
    poisoning disease, 406, 1219
Emaciation, 72–74, 73. See also Cachexia.
Embolism. See also Thromboembolism.

IND

Embolism (Continued)
  fibrocartilaginous, and spinal cord ischemia,
    635–636
  induced, for patent ductus arteriosus, 750
  pulmonary, and weakness, 13
Emesis. See Vomiting.
Emollient laxatives, 131, 132t
Emphysema, in cystitis, 1778, 1779t
  pulmonary, congenital, 1994t
  subcutaneous, 63–66, 65
    chest wall trauma and, 1100
    with pneumomediastinum, 1094
Emulsoil, for constipation, 132
Enalapril (Enacard), for cardiomyopathy, dilated,
    883, 884
  hypertrophic, 905–907
  for glomerulonephritis, 1672t, 1673
  for heart failure, 718–722, 720t
  for hypertension, 182
    in renal failure, chronic, 1653–1654
  for mitral insufficiency, 793
Enamel, fracture of, 1137t, 1137–1140, 1138
  junction of, with cementum, anatomy of,
    1127, 1127
Encephalitis, 591
  cerebrospinal fluid examination in, 574, 574t,
    575
  distemper virus and, 595–596
  feline infectious peritonitis virus and, 596
  fungal infection and, 597
  herpes canis virus and, 596
  in pug, 598, 606, 1992t
  parvovirus and, 596
  protozoal, 596–597
  rabies and, 594–595
  with myelitis, 591, 627
    borna disease virus and, 450–451
    granulomatous, 628
Encephalitozoon cuniculi infection,
    polysystemic, 416
Encephalocele, 1979t
Encephalomyelitis, 591, 627
  borna disease virus and, 450–451
  granulomatous, 628
Encephalopathy, hepatic, 550–551, 1272, 1274t,
    1275
  and ptyalism, 108
  dietary protein in, 260, 1332–1334, 1333t
  hyperammonemia in, 1278t, 1286–1287
  in renal failure, acute, 1624
    chronic, 1638t, 1638–1639
  management of, 1302t
    in acute disorders, 1332t–1334t, 1332–
      1335
    with portosystemic shunt, congenital, 1311–
      1315
  ischemia and, 548–549, 549t
  metabolic, 548, 555–556
  spongiform, 451, 599
    congenital, 1980t
  uremic, 550
Endocardial fibroelastosis, 784, 1976t, 1985t
Endocarditis, and arterial thromboembolism, 966
  infective, 796–799, 797
    echocardiography of, 857t
    murmur with, 172
  Löffler's, 903
Endochondral ossification defect, and growth
    failure, 74
Endocrine disorders, 1369–1508. See also
    specific disorders, e.g., Hypothyroidism.
  and weakness, 12
  paraneoplastic, 501
  skin lesions in, 26
Endodontic treatment, indications for, 1135–1136

Endodontic treatment (Continued)
  of fractured teeth, 1137t, 1137–1140, 1138
  of non-fractured teeth, 1136–1137, 1138
Endometrium, cystic hyperplasia of, and
    mucometra, 1591, 1592
  and prolonged anestrus, 1524, 1524–1525
  in breeding management, 1516, 1518
  with pyometra, 1549–1555, 1550t, 1552,
    1553, 1554t, 1555, 1592
    diagnosis of, 1550t, 1550–1551, 1552,
      1553
    pathophysiology of, 1549–1550
    treatment of, 1551–1555, 1553, 1554t,
      1555
Endomyocardial fibrosis, 903, 904
Endorphins, production of, acupuncture and, 370
Endoscopy, in esophageal disease, 1143
  of gastrointestinal tract, in gastrinoma, 1504
  of large intestine, 1238, 1242–1243, 1243t
    in diarrhea, 125, 126
  of respiratory system, 1037, 1037, 1038t, 1041
  of small intestine, 1212, 1212
    in diarrhea, 125
  of stomach, 1159
    in ulcer diagnosis, 1167, 1167
Endosulfan, toxicity of, 357–359
Endothelin, in heart failure, 701
End-systolic volume index, echocardiographic
    measurement of, 860, 863t, 864t
Endurance, loss of, liver disease and, 1273t,
    1276
Enemas, 131, 132t
  and hyperphosphatemia, 1396
  in management of hepatic failure, 1302t
  over-the-counter, 319–320
Energy, in diet, 237–238
  for kittens, 242
  in enteral nutrition, 279, 279t–281t, 280
  in heart disease, 265–266, 268t
  in orthopedic developmental disorders, 246–
    247, 249t
  in parenteral nutrition, 281, 282t
  in renal failure, 1631
English ivy, toxicity of, 364
Enilconazole, for aspergillosis, 474, 475t
  nasal, 1018
Enophthalmos, 1978t, 1988t
Enostosis, 1899–1901, 1901, 1984t
Enrofloxacin, concentration of, and clinical
    outcome, 304–305
  for bacteremia, with liver disorders, 1335
  for bacterial infection, 391t
  for bronchopulmonary disease, 1056, 1059t
  for enteritis, with Salmonella infection, 1218
  for lung infection, 1065t
  for otitis externa, with Pseudomonas aerugi-
    nosa infection, 990t, 996
  for otitis media, 990t, 999
  for prostatitis, 1693
Entamoeba histolytica infection, of large
    intestine, 1245–1246
  of small intestine, 408–410, 409t, 410t
Enteral nutrition, 275–281, 276, 278, 279,
    279t–281t
  client information on, 1945
Enteritis. See Small intestine.
Enterobacter infection, antibiotics for, 303,
    305–306
Enterochromaffin cells, carcinoid tumors of,
    1508
Enteroclysis, 1208
Enterococcus infection, of skin, antibiotics for,
    305
Enterocolitis, granulomatous, 1249
  in renal failure, 1637

Enterocytes, dysfunction of, 1197
  function of, 1186, 1186–1187
  in immune response, 1194, 1195
  loss of, in villous atrophy, 1197
Enteroglucagon, 1501
Enterostomy, for enteral nutrition, 279
Enthesophytes, in degenerative joint disease,
    1864, 1864
Entropion, 1978t, 1988t
Enzyme-linked immunosorbent assay, for
    antithyroglobulin antibodies, in
    hypothyroidism, 1425
  for dirofilariasis, 943t, 945
  for feline immunodeficiency virus infection,
    436–437
  for feline leukemia virus, 425, 426
  for parvovirus infection, 420, 421
  for progesterone, in breeding management,
    1518
Eosinopenia, 1852
  in hyperthyroidism, 1403, 1403t
Eosinophilia, 1851t, 1851–1852
  in dirofilariasis, 947
  in Löffler's endocarditis, 903
  in splenomegaly, 1858t, 1858–1859
Eosinophilic colitis, 1248
Eosinophilic diseases, of lungs, 1065t,
    1071–1072
Eosinophilic enteritis, 1228–1229
Eosinophilic gastritis, 1163
Eosinophilic granuloma complex, 1118, 1118
Eosinophilic meningitis, cerebrospinal fluid
    examination in, 574t
Eosinophilic plaque, and pruritus, 34t
Eosinophilic pustulosis, sterile, and pruritus, 33t
Eosinophils, in inflammation, steroid effects on,
    311
  in skin lesions, in cytology, 53
  in tracheal inflammation, 1042
  production of, 1842
Ependymoma, 584t, 585t
Ephedrine, for cough, 165t
  for tracheal disease, 1043t
Epidermal dysplasia, congenital, 48, 1995t
Epidermal growth factor, receptors of, in small
    intestine, 1185–1186
Epidermal necrolysis, toxic, 57
Epidermoid cyst, of spinal cord, 643
Epidermoid tumor, of brain, 584t
Epidermolysis bullosa, congenital, 1995t
Epididymis, anatomy of, 1586
Epidural space, injection into, for pain, 23, 24t
Epilepsy. See Seizures.
Epinephrine, for anaphylactic reaction, to
    hyperimmune serum, for tick paralysis, 673
  for bronchopulmonary disease, 1059t
  for hypotension, 184t
  in cardiopulmonary resuscitation, 192, 192t
Epi-Otic, for otitis externa, 989t, 994, 996
Epiphyses, dysplasia of, 1984t
Epiprenum aureum, toxicity of, 364
Episcleritis, 67, 69
Epistaxis, diagnosis of, 213–216, 214t, 216
  pathophysiology of, 213
  treatment of, 216, 216–217
Epithelial cells, in urine, 1607, 1607–1609, 1608
  of small intestinal mucosa, 1183–1186, 1186t
Epithelial neoplasia, of skin, 55, 524t, 524–526
Epitheliogenesis imperfecta, 1981t, 1994t
Epithelioma, cornifying, 525
Epogen. See Erythropoietin.
Epoietin. See Erythropoietin.
Epstein-Barr virus, and Burkitt's lymphoma, 481
Epulides, 1114, 1115, 1117
Equine morbillivirus infection, in cats, 452

Ergocalciferol. See *Vitamin D.*
Erosions, of skin, 39–43, 40t, *41, 42t*
Erythema, necrolytic migratory, 51
   glucagonoma and, *1507, 1507–1508*
Erythema chronicum migrans, in Lyme disease, 28
Erythema multiforme, 29
Erythrocytes, congenital defects of, 1989t–1990t
   in anemia. See *Anemia.*
   in polycythemia, 203–206. See also *Polycythemia.*
   in urine. See *Hematuria.*
   loss of, stroma-free hemoglobin for, 334
   production of, *1784,* 1784–1786, *1786*
   transfusion of, 351
Erythrocytosis, paraneoplastic, 502–503
   primary, 515t, 516
Erythroleukemia, 1853
Erythromycin, concentration of, and bacterial susceptibility, 303t
   for bacterial infection, 391t
   for gastric motility disorders, 1175–1176
   for staphylococcal pyoderma, 46t
Erythropoiesis, *1784,* 1784–1786, *1786*
   failure of, and anemia, 200–202, *201,* 202t
Erythropoietin, for anemia, in renal failure, 1655–1656
   with feline leukemia virus infection, 429
   in polycythemia, 203–204, *205,* 206
Escape rhythms, 818–820
Escherichia coli infection, and colitis, 1244
   and enteritis, 1218, *1218*
   antibiotics for, 303, 305–306
Esmolol, for arrhythmia, 824t, 827, 828t, 830
   supraventricular, with hypotension, 184t
Esophagus, achalasia of, cricopharyngeal, 1145, 1976t, 1985t
   anatomy of, 1142–1143
   compression of, vascular ring anomalies and, 1145
   disorders of, and gagging, 111, 112t
      diagnosis of, 1143–1145, *1144*
      in hiatal hernia, *1152,* 1152–1153
      polyphagia with, 106, 107
      with ptyalism, 108
   diverticula of, 1145–1146
      congenital, 1985t
   enlargement of, 1149–1151, 1150t
      client information on, 1946
      congenital, 1977t, 1986t
      polyphagia with, 106, 107
   fistula of, from lung, 1060, 1147, 1994t
   foreign bodies in, 1146–1147
   gastric intussusception into, 1153, *1153*
   inflammation of, 1147–1149, 1150t
   intubation of, for enteral nutrition, 275–277, *276*
   neoplasia of, 1147
   physiology of, 1143
   reflux into, 1151–1152
   regurgitation from, 114–117, *116,* 117t, 1143
   stricture of, 1148–1149, *1149*
Estradiol, for prostatic hypertrophy, 1691–1692
   in abortion induction, 1545–1546
   in estrous cycle, 1510, 1511, *1511,* 1589
Estrogen, and bone marrow toxicity, with neutrophilia, 1849, *1849*
   excess of, and anemia, 1811
      in prolonged estrus, 1523
   for prostatic hypertrophy, 1691–1692
   in abortion induction, 1545–1546
   in cystic endometrial hyperplasia, with pyometra, 1549
   in estrous cycle, 1520, 1589
      and timing of artificial insemination, *1576*

Estrogen *(Continued)*
   in parturition, 1528
   in persistent proestrus, and infertility, 1564–1565
Estrous cycle, canine, 1510, *1510,* 1520–1522
   abnormalities of, 1520, *1521,* 1522–1526, *1523, 1524*
      in infertility, 1560–1565, *1561–1563, 1565*
      and timing of artificial insemination, 1575–1576, *1576*
   anestrus in, 1510, *1510,* 1514–1516, *1516*
   follicular phase of, 1510–1511, *1510–1513*
   in breeding management, 1516–1518, *1517*
   luteal phase in, *1510,* 1510–1514, *1514, 1515*
   normal variations in, 1522
   ovulation in, 1510, *1510,* 1511, *1514*
   pre-ovulatory luteinization in, 1511
   feline, 1587–1590, *1590*
      estrus induction in, 1595, *1595*
      prolonged estrus in, 1591
   management of, client information on, 1933, 1934
   progestins for, and growth hormone excess, 1370–1371, *1371,* 1373
   pyometra development in, 1550
   vaginal discharge in, 81t–84t, 82
Ethacrynic acid, for heart failure, 714
1,2-Ethanediol. See *Ethylene glycol.*
Ethanol, for ethylene glycol toxicity, 361, 1626t
   injection of, for hyperparathyroidism, 1391
      for hyperthyroidism, 1415
Ethical issues, in cardiopulmonary resuscitation, 193
Ethmoid bone, cribriform plate of, anatomy of, 1003, *1003*
Ethylenediaminetetraacetic acid (EDTA), in chelation therapy, for lead toxicity, 362
   in cancer management, 377
Ethylene glycol, toxicity of, 361
   and hypocalcemia, vs. hypoparathyroidism, 1394
   client information on, 1965
   to kidney, and acute renal failure, 1616
      diagnosis of, 1622, *1622*
      management of, 1625, 1626t
      prognosis of, 1632
      ultrasonography in, 1612
   to liver, management of, 1625, 1626t
Etodolac, for pain, 24t, 25
Etretinate, for lymphoma, cutaneous, 528
   for pinnal dermatosis, 988–991, 989t
   for sebaceous adenitis, 48
Euphorbia pulcherrima, toxicity of, 364
Eurytrema procyonis infestation, of pancreas, 1363t, 1364
Eutocia, 1528–1530. See also *Parturition.*
Evening primrose oil, in cancer management, 378t
Evoked potentials, visual, 575
   in acute vision loss, 19
Evoked responses, brain stem auditory, 575
   in deafness, 1001–1002
Exencephaly, 1979t
Exercise, and hyperthermia, 7–8
   in diabetes mellitus, 1448–1449
   in dirofilariasis, 937–938, 943
   in weight control, 70
Exophthalmos, systemic disease and, 984
Exostoses, cartilaginous, congenital, 1983t
   multiple, 539, 540, 1899, *1901*
      and spinal cord disorders, 642–643
   vitamin A excess and, 1907, *1908*
   with spinal cord compression, 629–630

Extensor carpi radialis reflex, testing of, 568
Extensor reflex, crossed, testing of, 570–571, *571,* 571t
Extracellular matrix, tumor invasion through, *482,* 482–483
Extrasystoles, atrial, 810–811, *811*
   ventricular, 813–814, *814*
Exudates, in pleural effusion, *187,* 188, 1105, 1105t
Eye(s), antibiotic penetration of, 301
   disorders of, as signs of systemic disease, 984–985, 985t, 986t
      blastomycosis and, 459, 462
      coccidioidomycosis and, 465, 466
      congenital, in cats, 1977t–1978t
      in dogs, 1987t–1989t
      cryptococcosis and, 469, 470
      diabetes and, 1458
      drugs for, over-the-counter, 320
      feline immunodeficiency virus infection and, 435
      herpesvirus infection and, 446, 447
      hypertension and, 180, *181,* 182
      in hyperparathyroidism, 1380
      renal failure and, 1639
      with cutaneous hypopigmentation, 55, 57
      with hyperlipoproteinemia, 291
   in coma, 145–146, 146t
   in cranial nerve examination, *563,* 563–566, *564,* 567t
   in granulomatous meningoencephalitis, 598
   in neurologic examination, 657–661, *658, 659t,* 660t, *661*
   plant toxicity to, 364
   radiation injury to, in nasal tumor radiotherapy, 1022–1023
   redness in, differential diagnosis of, 66–69, *67, 68*
   vision loss in, acute, 17t, 17–20, 18t, *19*
Eyelashes, deviation of, 1989t
Eyelids, congenital defects of, 1977t, 1987t, 1988t
   inflammation of, and conjunctivitis, 66
   systemic disease and, 984

Face, defects of, with cranial defects, 1975t
Facial nerve, anatomy of, 664t
   examination of, 563, *563, 565,* 565–566, 567t
   inflammation of, idiopathic, 680–681
   paralysis of, idiopathic, 582–583, 1000
Failure to thrive, 4
   small intestinal disorders and, 1201, *1201*
Fainting, 13t, 13–16, *14*
   in hypertrophic cardiomyopathy, 906
   with mitral insufficiency, 789
Fallot's tetralogy, 780–782, *781, 782,* 1976t, 1985t
   auscultation of, 739t
   echocardiography of, 839, *841,* 854t
   ventricular septal defect in, 751, *754*
Familial Mediterranean fever, and arthritis, 1882–1883
Famotidine, for gastrinoma, 1506, 1506t
   for gastroenteritis, in renal failure, 1648
   for ulcers, gastrointestinal, 1168
      in renal failure, 1629, 1630t
      with coagulopathy, in acute liver disorders, 1335
Fanconi's syndrome, 1708–1709, 1996t
Fasciitis, necrotizing, streptococcosis and, 396
Fat. See *Lipids.*
Fatigue, 10
Fatty acids, for atopic dermatitis, client information on, 1973

Fatty acids (Continued)
  for cachexia, paraneoplastic, 500
  in diet, 239, 240
    in renal disease, 271
  omega-3, in diet, in renal failure, 1646–1647,
    1647t, 1658
Faucitis, and ptyalism, 109
Fear, and aggression, in cats, 160t, 162
  in dogs, 158, 158t
Febantel, for intestinal parasitosis, 1221t
Feces, acholic, liver disease and, 1273t, 1276
  blood in, causes of, 1240, 1240t, 1258, 1259
    with diarrhea, 122t, 123
  elimination of, anorectal physiology in, 1258
    inappropriate, as behavioral problem, 158–
      160, 159
    incontinent, 129, 133–135, 134, 134t,
      1268t, 1268–1269
  examination of, in large intestinal disorders,
    1241, 1242, 1242t
    in small intestinal disorders, 1203t, 1204–
      1207, 1206, 1207, 1207t
  in diarrhea. See Diarrhea.
  in pancreatic exocrine insufficiency, 1360,
    1360–1361, 1361
Feeding. See Diet.
Felbamate, for seizures, 151t
Felicola lice, in skin infestation, 59t, 60
Feline immunodeficiency virus. See
  Immunodeficiency virus infection.
Feline leukemia virus. See Leukemia virus
  infection.
Femoral artery, pulse in, 174, 175
Femoral nerve, injury to, signs of, 663t
Femur, head of, aseptic necrosis of, 1873, 1874,
  1984t
Fenbendazole, for Capillaria feliscati infestation,
    of urinary tract, 1741
  for fluke infestation, of pancreas, 1363t, 1364
  for giardiasis, of small intestine, 1222
    with parvovirus management, 421
  for lungworm infestation, 1065t, 1069–1071
  for parasitosis, intestinal, 1220, 1221t
    of urinary tract, 1779t
  for protozoal infection, 410t
Fentanyl, for pain, 24, 24t
  with adrenal surgery, for hyperadrenocorti-
    cism, 1475–1476
Fenthion, for dirofilariasis, 952
Fenugreek, in cancer management, 378t
Ferrous sulfate, for anemia, iron deficiency, 1788
  paraneoplastic, 504
  with renal disease, 1808
Fertility, disorders of. See Infertility.
α-Fetoprotein, in liver disease, 1285
Fetus. See Pregnancy.
  delivery of, 1528–1536. See also Parturition.
Fever, 6–9, 7t, 8, 9
  and cachexia, 73, 74
  and growth failure, 75
  paraneoplastic, 505–506
  with brain inflammation, management of,
    593–594
  with hepatic amyloidosis, in Shar Pei, 1323
  with infective endocarditis, 797
  with tetany, in hypoparathyroidism, 1397
Fiber, in diet, diarrhea responsive to, 1252
  for inflammatory bowel disease, 1249t,
    1249–1250
  in diabetes mellitus, 261, 1447–1448, 1448t
  in gastrointestinal disorders, 259–260
  in renal failure, 1647
Fibrillation, atrial, electrocardiography of,
    812–813, 813
  with cardiomyopathy, dilated, 879

Fibrillation (Continued)
  ventricular, electrocardiography of, 815, 816
    treatment of, 193
Fibrin, in vasculitis, 972
Fibrinogen, deficiency of, 1838, 1839, 1839t
Fibrinolysis, physiology of, 1830–1832, 1833
  tests of, 1835
Fibroadenoma, of mammary glands, with
    hyperplasia, 1591–1592, 1592, 1593
Fibrocartilaginous embolism, and spinal cord
    ischemia, 635–636
Fibrodysplasia ossificans progressiva, 1980t
Fibroelastosis, endocardial, 784, 1976t, 1985t
Fibrosarcoma, of bone, 538, 1911
  oral, 1115, 1115–1118, 1116, 1117t
Fibrous dysplasia, of bone, 1905, 1905
Filaribits. See Diethylcarbamazine.
Filaroides hirthi infestation, of lung, 1065t, 1070
Filaroides osleri infestation, of trachea, 1038t,
    1044, 1044–1045
Finasteride, for prostatic hypertrophy, 1692
Fipronil, for cheyletiellosis, 49
  in flea control, client information on, 1971
Fish oils, for hyperlipidemia, 289
  for renal failure, 1646–1647, 1647t, 1658
Fish-tank granuloma, 384t
Fissures, of pinna, 991
Fistula, arterioportal, 1979t, 1991t
  arteriovenous, 969–971, 970, 971
    hepatic, 1317–1318
      and portosystemic shunt, 1316
      ultrasonography of, 1292
  bronchoesophageal, 1060, 1994t
  esophageal, 1147
  oronasal, tooth loss and, 1129
  perianal, 1264–1266
  urethrorectal, 1743, 1751
Flagyl. See Metronidazole.
Flail chest, 1100
Flatulence, 135–136, 136
  client information on, 1940
  small intestinal disorders and, 1201
Fleas, and allergic dermatitis, vs. adverse food
    reactions, 254, 255
  as vectors, of bartonellosis, 386, 399
  bites of, sensitivity to, and otitis externa, 992
  in skin infestation, 59t, 59–60, 60
    and pruritus, 32, 33, 33t, 34t, 35–36
    client information on, 1971
Flecainide, for arrhythmia, 824t, 826t, 827
Flexor reflexes, testing of, 568, 570, 571t
Florinef (fludrocortisone), for
    hypoadrenocorticism, 1496–1498
    after adrenalectomy, for hyperadrenocorti-
      cism, 1487
Flosequinan, for cardiomyopathy, 884
Fluconazole, for blastomycosis, 461
  for dermatophytosis, 49
  for fungal infection, 456–457, 475t
    with encephalitis, 597
  for Malassezia infection, in otitis externa, 996
Flucytosine, for central nervous system infection,
    593t
  for cryptococcosis, 471
  for fungal infection, 457, 475t
    of urinary tract, 1741
Fludrocortisone, for hypoadrenocorticism,
    1496–1498
    after adrenalectomy, for hyperadrenocorti-
      cism, 1487
Fluid, balance of, small intestine in, 1191–1193,
    1192, 1193
  deprivation of, diagnostic, in diabetes insip-
    idus, 1375, 1376, 1378
    in polyuria, 86, 87, 87t, 88t, 89, 1604–
      1605

Fluid (Continued)
  drug solubility in, 296, 297
  dynamics of, 325–327, 326, 327
  imbalance of, in dehydration. See Dehydra-
    tion.
    neurologic signs of, 549t, 549–550
    small intestinal, and diarrhea, 1199, 1199t,
      1199–1200
  in edema. See Edema.
  intake of, in calcium oxalate urolithiasis,
    1727–1728, 1765
    in heart disease, sodium in, 266
    in hypernatremia, 228–232, 230t, 231
  metabolism of, in diabetes insipidus, nephro-
    genic, 1706–1707
  osmotic pressure of, 327–328, 328
  retention of, in heart failure, 702t, 703
  transport of, in large intestine, 1240
Fluid therapy, colloids in, 329t, 329–331,
    331t–333t
  crystalloids in, 328–329, 329t, 330t
  in anemia, with blood loss, 1786
  in calcium disorders, 344, 345
  in cardiomyopathy, 911
  in diabetes mellitus, with ketoacidosis, 1444t,
    1444–1445
  in diarrhea, 1214–1215
  in enteritis, with parvovirus infection, 1216
  in gastritis, acute, 1161
  in hepatic failure, 1302t
  in hypoadrenocorticism, 1496
  in liver disorders, acute, 1332, 1334t
  in potassium imbalance, 342–344, 343
  in renal failure, 1652
  in shock, with gastric dilatation and volvulus,
    1172, 1174
  in sodium imbalance, 340–342, 341
  maintenance requirements in, 340
  planning for, 334–340, 336, 338t–339t
  purpose of, 325
Fluke infestation, and salmon-poisoning disease,
    406, 1219
  of pancreas, 1363t, 1364
Flumenazil, for hepatic encephalopathy, 1334
Flumethasone, dosage of, 313t
  potency of, 312t
Flunixin meglumine, for shock, with gastric
    dilatation and volvulus, 1172
Fluocinolone, for otitis externa, 989t, 995, 996
Fluorescent antibody test, for distemper, 418
Fluoroacetate, in rodenticides, toxicity of, 360
Fluoroscopy, in dysphagia, 1027
  of pericardial effusion, 928, 930
  of trachea, 1041
Fluoxetine, for behavioral disorders, in cats, 160t
  in dogs, 156, 158t
Flutamide, for prostatic hypertrophy, 1692
Flutter, atrial, 812, 812
  ventricular, 815
Fly infestation, 59t, 60
Fly strike dermatitis, of pinna, 988
Foamy virus infection, 452
  in polyarthritis, 1881
Folate, absorption of, from small intestine, 1190,
    1191
  blood level of, in small intestinal disorders,
    1208–1210, 1210t
    with bacterial overgrowth, 1224
  deficiency of, and neutrophil hypersegmenta-
    tion, 1846
    in anemia, 1809
    in pancreatic exocrine insufficiency, 1358,
      1363, 1363t
  in diet, 239t
  malabsorption of, in inflammatory bowel dis-
    ease, 1227

Follicles, dysplasia of, congenital, 1994t
hair loss from. See *Alopecia.*
inflammation of, 43, 44, 47
Follicle-stimulating hormone, in estrous cycle, 1589
Follicular cysts, ovarian, and infertility, 1564–1565
and prolonged estrus, *1521, 1523,* 1523–1524, *1524*
Follicular phase, of estrous cycle, 1510–1511, *1510–1513*
Folliculitis, 43, 44, 47
Fomepizole, for ethylene glycol toxicity, 361
Food. See *Allergy, to food* and *Diet.*
Footpad, collagen disorder of, congenital, 1995t
Foramen magnum, cerebellar vermis herniation through, 144, 144t
dysplasia of, 1984t
Foramen ovale, in heart development, 750–751
patent, 751
Foreign bodies, and epistaxis, 213, 215
and granuloma, 37
and otitis externa, 992
and tracheal obstruction, 1050–1053
aspiration of, and pneumonia, 1084–1086, *1085*
in airway, bronchoscopy of, 1038t
in bronchi, 1060
in esophagus, 1146–1147
in osteomyelitis, 1912, *1913*
in pharynx, 1027–1029
in stomach, and outlet obstruction, 1169
Fox terrier, ataxia in, 629, 1991t
Foxes, rabies in, 388
Foxglove. See *Digitalis.*
Foxhound, renal amyloidosis in, 1699t, 1701
Fracture, of ribs, and flail chest, 1100
of tooth, endodontic treatment of, 1137t, 1137–1140, *1138*
with bone cyst, 1904
Francisella tularensis infection, zoonotic, 385t
Franklin-modified Vim-Silverman needle, in renal biopsy, 1613, *1613*
FreAmine, in fluid therapy, 329t
Frenulum, penile, persistent, 1594, 1994t
Frontal sinuses. See *Nasal sinuses.*
Frontline (fipronil), for cheyletiellosis, 49
in flea control, client information on, 1971
Frostbite, of pinna, 991
Fructosamine, in monitoring, with insulin therapy, for diabetes, 1452–1453, 1453t
α-Fucosidosis, 3t, 1992t
and peripheral neuropathy, 670
Fundus, of stomach, anatomy of, 1155, *1155*
Fungal infection, after glucocorticoid therapy, 316
and arthritis, 1878
and cystitis, 1778, 1779t
and encephalitis, 597
and granuloma, 37
and hyperpigmentation, 58
and hypopigmentation, 57
and meningitis, spinal, 616–619, 618t
and meningoencephalitis, cerebrospinal fluid examination in, 574, 574t
and nasal discharge, 196, 197
and pruritus, 32, 33t, 34, 34t
and rhinitis, 1018–1019
computed tomography of, 1009–1012, *1013, 1014*
with epistaxis, 215
and scaling dermatosis, 49
and skin erosions, 40t, 42
and urethritis, in dog, 1778, 1779t
of bone, 1912

Fungal infection *(Continued)*
of intestine, client information on, 1947
large, 1246–1247
small, 1219–1220
of lung, 1066–1068, *1067, 1068*
of nervous system, multifocal, 606
of urinary tract, 1741
systemic, 453–475
Aspergillus in, *473,* 473–475
Blastomyces dermatitidis in, 458–462, *459–461*
Candida species in, 475
Coccidioides immitis in, 465–468, *466–468*
Cryptococcus neoformans in, 468–471, *469, 470*
diagnosis of, 454, 455t
drugs for, 454–457, *457,* 475t
geographic distribution of, 453, *454*
Histoplasma capsulatum in, 462–465, 463t, *464*
hyalohyphomycosis in, 475
phaeohyphomycosis in, 475
skin lesions with, 28
Sporothrix schenckii in, *91,* 471–472, *472*
zygomycosis in, 475
Fungizone. See *Amphotericin B.*
Furazolidone, for giardiasis, of small intestine, 1222
for protozoal infection, 410, 410t
Furosemide, dosage of, in renal failure, 1649t
for ascites, 139
for brain edema, 147
traumatic, 579–580
with inflammation, 593t
for cardiomyopathy, dilated, canine, 883
feline, 911
for cholecalciferol rodenticide toxicity, 360
for congestive heart failure, in dirofilariasis, 949t
for edema, with hepatic failure, 1302t
for heart failure, 714–716
angiotensin-converting enzyme inhibitors contraindicated with, 719–720
with mitral insufficiency, 794
for hypercalcemia, 344
for hypertension, in renal failure, 1654
for intracranial pressure elevation, 577
for lung disorders, 1065t
for pulmonary edema, with hypertrophic cardiomyopathy, 906–908
with mitral insufficiency, 793
for renal failure, 1627
in cardiopulmonary resuscitation, 192t
Furunculosis, 44
anal, 1264–1266
Fusion kidney, 1982t, 1996t
Fusobacterium infection, antibiotics for, 303

Gag reflex, in cranial nerve examination, 566, 567t
Gagging, 111, 112t, *113*
Gait, disorders of, in ataxia, 142
examination of, in brain disorders, 559t, 560–561
Galactocerebrosidase deficiency, in globoid cell leukodystrophy, 1992t
peripheral neuropathy in, 670
spinal cord demyelination in, 627–628
β-Galactosidase deficiency, in gangliosidosis, 589, 590t, 1980t, 1992t
Galactostasis, 1538
Galastop. See *Cabergoline.*
Gallbladder, anatomy of, 1340, *1341*

Gallbladder *(Continued)*
anomalies of, 1979t, 1991t
bifid, 1344
disorders of, cystic, 1344
diagnosis of, *1341,* 1341–1342
inflammation of, 1341–1344, *1342, 1343*
lithiasis of, 1341–1344, *1343*
physiology of, 1340–1341
radiography of, in liver disease, 1291
ultrasonography of, 1292
Gallium, in contrast imaging, of soft tissue sarcoma, 531
Gallop heart sounds, 170
Gallop rhythm, in heart failure, 707
Gammaglobulin, elevated blood level of, in liver disease, 1284
paraneoplastic, 505
Gamma-glutamyl transpeptidase, in liver disease, 1279t, *1282,* 1283
Ganglioneuritis, sensory, 675
Ganglioneuroblastoma, peripheral, 677
Ganglioneuroma, peripheral, 677
Gangliosidosis, 1980t, 1992t
GM$_1$, 589, 590t
genetics in, 3t
leukocyte inclusions in, 1847, *1847*
GM$_2$, and peripheral neuropathy, 670
Gastric acid, drugs reducing, over-the-counter, 319
secretion of, *1156,* 1156–1157
excessive, gastrinoma and, 1503–1506, 1505t, 1506t
in pancreatic enzyme insufficiency, 1362, 1363t
Gastric arteries, anatomy of, 1155
Gastric inhibitory polypeptide, 1501
Gastric veins, anatomy of, 1155
Gastrin, 1500, 1503
in digestion, 1156, *1156*
Gastrinoma, 1503–1506, 1505t, 1506t
Gastritis, acute, 1160–1162
chronic, 1162–1165
in renal failure, acute, 1629, 1630t
chronic, 1636, 1636t
with enteritis. See *Gastroenteritis.*
Gastrocnemius reflex, testing of, 568
Gastroenteritis, and ulcers, 1166
coronavirus and, 422
hemorrhagic, 1162, 1214
and diarrhea, 123
in renal failure, 1648
salmonellosis and, 390, 391
Gastroesophageal intussusception, 1153, *1153*
Gastroesophageal reflux, 1151–1152
Gastrointestinal tract, 1113–1269. See also specific structures, e.g., *Colon.*
bleeding in, and melena, 126–129, 127t, *128*
carcinoid tumors of, 1508
disorders of, and cachexia, 73, 74
and flatulence, 135–136, *136*
and growth failure, 74–77, 75t, *76*
and vomiting, 117–121, 118t, *118–120*
client information on, 1941–1943, 1945–1947
congenital, in cats, 1976t–1977t
in dogs, 1985t–1986t
in adverse food reactions, 254
in hyperthyroidism, 1401t, 1401–1402
in renal failure, 1635–1637, 1636t
nutritional management in, 258–260
pancreatic exocrine insufficiency and, 1359
parvovirus and, 420–421
endocrine system of, 1500–1503
disorders of, 1503–1508, 1505t, 1506t, *1507*
lymphoma of, 508, 508t, 509t

IND

Gastrointestinal tract *(Continued)*
  protozoal infection of, 408–411, 409t, 410t
  toxicity to, chemotherapy and, 486
    plants and, 364–365
Gastrostomy, for enteral nutrition, 277–279, *278, 279,* 1945
Genetic defects, 2–5, 3t
  and cardiomyopathy, dilated, 877
    hypertrophic, 896, 906
  and congenital disorders, in cats, 1975t–1982t
    in dogs, 1983t–1996t
  and deafness, 1000, 1000t
  and heart malformations, 743–744
  and pancreatitis, 1350
  control of, breeding programs in, 5
  diagnostic tests for, 4–5
  frequency of, 2
  in carcinogenesis, 478–481, 479t
  in osteogenesis imperfecta, 1896
  in sexual developmental disorders, 1581–1585, *1582–1584*
  inheritance patterns in, 2–4, 3t
  prognosis of, 5
  signs of, 4
  treatment of, 5
Genitalia. See *Reproductive system.*
Gentamicin, concentration of, and bacterial susceptibility, 303t
  dosage of, in renal failure, 1649t
  for bacteremia, with liver disorders, 1335
  for bacterial infection, 391t
  for central nervous system infection, 593t
German shepherd, peripheral neuropathy in, with aging, 667
  renal cystadenocarcinoma in, 1699t, 1701
  spinal muscular atrophy in, 666, 1992t
  sudden cardiac death in, during sleep, 154
Giant axonal neuropathy, 667
Giant cell granuloma, central, 1905
Giardiasis, and diarrhea, 123, *124,* 126
  enteric, 408–411, 409t, 410t
  fecal examination for, 1206, *1206,* 1207
  of small intestine, 1222
  treatment of, with parvovirus management, 421
Gibbs-Donnan effect, 328, *328*
Ginger, in cancer management, 378t
Gingiva, anatomy of, 1127, *1127*
Gingivitis, 1118, 1127
  signs of, 1129, *1129,* 1129t
Glanzmann's thrombasthenia, 1824t, 1826
Glass ionomers, in dental restoration, 1141
Glaucoma, *68,* 69
  and anisocoria, 659t
  blastomycosis and, 459, 462
  congenital, 1978t, 1988t
Glioblastoma, 584t
Glipizide, for diabetes, 1449, 1449t, *1450*
  toxicity of, to liver, 1329
Globoid cell leukodystrophy, 589, 590t, 1980t, 1992t
  and peripheral neuropathy, 670
  genetics in, 3t
  spinal cord demyelination in, 627–628
Globulins, blood level of, in small intestinal disorders, 1206
  in cerebrospinal fluid, 574t, 575
  in cryoprecipitate, for von Willebrand's disease, 1825
  transfusion of, 351
  in liver disease, 1278t, 1284
Glomerular filtration rate, decreased, angiotensin-converting enzyme inhibitors and, 719
  in renal failure, acute, 1617–1619, *1618*

Glomeruli. See also *Kidney(s).*
  drug filtration in, 297
  function of, 1662–1663, *1663*
    tests of, 1601–1603, *1602,* 1602t
Glomerulonephritis, clinical findings in, 1669t, 1669–1670
  complications of, 1674–1675, *1675, 1676*
  diagnosis of, *1670,* 1670–1671
  familial, 1699t, 1700, 1701
  pathogenesis of, 1663–1667, *1664–1666,* 1666t, 1667t
  prognosis of, 1675–1676
  treatment of, 1672t, 1672–1674
Glomerulosclerosis, diabetes and, 1459
Glossitis, and ptyalism, 109
  plant toxicity and, 364
Glossopharyngeal nerve, anatomy of, 664t
  examination of, 563, 566, 567t
Glossopharyngeal neuralgia, 1029
Glottis, stenosis of, after laryngeal surgery, 1031
Glucagonoma, *1507,* 1507–1508
Glucan synthesis, inhibitors of, for fungal infection, 457
Glucocerebrosidosis, 589, 590t, 1992t
Glucocorticoids, 307–317. See also *Corticosteroids.*
Glucophage, for diabetes, 1449–1451
Glucose, absorption of, from small intestine, 1187–1188, *1189,* 1210
  blood level of, decreased. See *Hypoglycemia.*
  for hyperkalemia, 342
  in cerebrospinal fluid, 575
  in diabetes. See *Diabetes.*
  in urine, 1605–1606, 1704
    renal tubular defects and, 1996t
  intolerance to, in pancreatic exocrine insufficiency, 1357–1358
  toxicity of, to pancreatic islet cells, in diabetes, 1440, *1440*
  with insulin and potassium, for septic shock, 184t
Glucose-6-phosphate dehydrogenase deficiency, 1990t
Glucosidase deficiency, lysosomal, 1290, 1992t
Glucosuria, 1704
  renal tubular defect and, 1996t
Glucotrol (glipizide), for diabetes mellitus, 1449, 1449t, *1450*
  toxicity of, to liver, 1329
β-Glucuronidase deficiency, in mucopolysaccharidosis, skeletal abnormalities with, 1897
Glutamine, in diet, in gastrointestinal disorders, 259
Glutathione, depletion of, in acetaminophen toxicity, to liver, 1327, 1331–1332
Gluteal muscle, superficial, transfer of, in perineal herniorrhaphy, 1260
Gluten-sensitive enteropathy, 254, 1232–1233, 1986t
Glyburide, for diabetes mellitus, 1449
L-Glycericaciduria (hyperoxaluria), and calcium oxalate urolithiasis, 1725t, 1726
  primary, 1996t
  with peripheral neuropathy, in shorthaired cats, 670
Glyceryl guaiacolate (guaifenesin), for cough, 165t
  for tracheal disease, 1043t
Glycogen storage diseases, 1290, 1322–1323, 1986t
  and megaesophagus, 1150t
  and myopathy, 689
  in Norwegian Forest cats, and peripheral neuropathy, 671

Glycogenolysis, genetics in, 3t
Glycogenosis, 1980t, 1992t
Glycolic acid. See *Ethylene glycol.*
Glycoproteins, in platelets, 1817, 1818
Glycopyrrolate, in cardiopulmonary resuscitation, 192t
Glycosaminoglycans, for urinary tract disorders, idiopathic, 1745–1746
  metabolism of, in mucopolysaccharidosis, spinal cord dysfunction with, 638–639
Glycosides, in plant toxicity, 365
Glycosylated hemoglobin, in monitoring, with insulin therapy, for diabetes, 1452–1453, 1453t
Gnathostoma infestation, and gastritis, 1165
Goblet cells, of small intestine, 1185
Golden retriever, hypomyelination in, 668–669, 1992t
  renal dysplasia in, 1699t, 1701
GoLYTELY, before colonoscopy, 1242
Gonadectomy. See *Sterilization.*
Gonadotropin, human chorionic, and testosterone production, 1594
  for cryptorchidism, 1597, 1597t
  for libido stimulation, 1597, 1597t
  for ovulation failure, 1562
  for remnant ovarian tissue, after sterilization, 1596
  in estrus induction, 1595
  pregnant mare serum, in estrus induction, 1595
Gonadotropin-releasing hormone, and testosterone production, 1594
  drugs affecting, in contraception, 1544
  for cryptorchidism, 1597, 1597t
  for libido stimulation, 1597, 1597t
  for prolonged estrus, 1524
  for remnant ovarian tissue, after sterilization, 1596
  in estrous cycle, 1514–1515, 1520
Goodpasture's syndrome, 1072
Granular lymphocytes, leukemia of, 1854–1855, *1855*
Granulation, of neutrophils, anomalous, 1847, 1978t
Granulocyte colony-stimulating factor, 1842
  for aplastic pancytopenia, with estrogen toxicity, 1822
  for feline leukemia virus infection, 429
  for neutropenia, 1848–1849
  for parvovirus infection, 421
Granulocyte-macrophage colony-stimulating factor, 1842
Granulocytopathy syndrome, 1850, 1990t
Granuloma, cutaneous, 36, 37
  eosinophilic, oral, 1118, *1118*
  giant cell, central, 1905
  in blepharitis, systemic disease and, 984
  in urethritis, 1778, 1779t
  Mycobacterium marinum and, 384t
  of brain, 591
  of nervous system, 556
  subcutaneous, 63
  uterine stump, 1567, *1569*
  with meningoencephalitis, cerebrospinal fluid examination in, 574, 574t
Granulomatosis, of lungs, 1072, *1072, 1073*
  eosinophilic, 1071, 1072
  lymphomatoid, 974, 1072, 1077–1078
Granulomatous dermatitis, periadnexal multinodular, 520
Granulomatous enteritis, 1229
Granulomatous enterocolitis, 1249
Granulomatous gastritis, 1163

Granulomatous meningoencephalitis, 597–598
  multifocal, 606
Granulomatous meningoencephalomyelitis, 628
Granulomatous splenitis, 1858t, 1859
Greyhound, polyarthritis in, 1879–1880
Griseofulvin, for dermatophytosis, 49
  toxicity of, and anemia, 1812
Groundhogs, rabies in, 388
Growth, deficiency of, after prepubertal
    gonadectomy, 1540
  failure of, 74–77, 75t, 76
    in dwarfism, 1897t, 1897–1898, 1898,
      1899t, 1900, 1983t, 1987t
    retardation of, in hypothyroidism, 1422, 1422
Growth factors, in carcinogenesis, 478, 479t
Growth hormone, in acromegaly, 1370–1373,
    1370–1373
  in pregnancy, and insulin resistance, 1528
Growth plates, disorders of, 1869, 1901–1903,
    1902
  physiology of, 1887–1888, 1888
Guaifenesin, for cough, 165t
  for tracheal disease, 1043t
Guanine nucleotide binding proteins, in
    carcinogenesis, 478, 479t
Gums, anatomy of, 1127, 1127
  inflammation of, 1118, 1127
    signs of, 1129, 1129, 1129t
Gut-associated lymphoid tissue, 1239
Gyromita species, toxicity of, 364, 1329

Hageman trait, 1839, 1839t
Hair, congenital defects of, 1981t, 1982t, 1995t
  hyperpigmentation of, 55, 56, 57–58
  hypopigmentation of, 55–57, 56
  loss of, 29–31, 30
    chemotherapy and, 487
    congenital, 1981t, 1994t, 1995t
    in hypothyroidism, 1421
    pinnal, nonpruritic, 1421
Hair balls, and gastric outlet obstruction, 1169
Hair follicles, dysplasia of, 1994t
  inflammation of, 43, 44, 47
  tumors of, 525
Half-life, of drugs, 298, 300
Hamartoma, cutaneous, 36
Hammondia infection, enteric, 408, 409t
Hantavirus infection, zoonotic, 384t
Head, fetal, abnormalities of, and dystocia,
    1534–1536
  posture in, in brain disorders, 559t, 559–560
Hearing, loss of, 1000t, 1000–1002
  congenital, 1977t, 1986t
  furosemide and, in heart failure, 715
Heart, 691–936. See also specific structures, e.g.,
    Atrium, and disorders, e.g., Endocarditis.
  arrhythmia of, treatment of, 822–833. See also
    Arrhythmia.
  congenital disorders of, 737–786
    angiography in, 741–742
    breed predilection to, 738, 738t
    cardiac catheterization in, 742, 742–743,
      743
    causes of, 743–744
    classification of, 744–745
    clinical approach to, 892–893
    cyanotic, 779–784, 781–784
    echocardiography of, 740–741, 854, 854t
    electrocardiography in, 740
    history in, 738
    imaging in, 740–741
    in aortic coarctation, 786
    in aorticopulmonary septal defect, 785–786

Heart (Continued)
    in atrioventricular valve dysplasia, 774–778,
      775–779
    in cats, 1976t
    in cor triatriatum, 778–779
    in dogs, 1985t
    in endocardial fibroelastosis, 784
    in patent ductus arteriosus, 745–750, 746–
      752
    in persistent right aortic arch, 784–785, 785
    in pulmonic insufficiency, 773, 773, 774
    in pulmonic stenosis, 759–767, 761–767
    in subaortic stenosis, 768–772, 769–772
    in tetralogy of Fallot, 780–782, 781, 782
    laboratory tests in, 739–740
    multiple anomalies in, 784
    physical examination in, 738–739, 739t
    prevalence of, 744, 744t
    septal defects in, 750–759, 753–760
    venous anomalies in, 785, 786
    vs. peritoneopericardial hernia, 784
  diastolic function of, 896, 897
  dilatation of, with mitral regurgitation, pericar-
    dial restriction of, 924
  disorders of, and chylothorax, 1107
    and cough, 163, 163t, 165, 165t, 166
    and cyanosis, 207, 207t, 209
    and hepatic venous outflow obstruction,
      1318, 1318t
    and hypotension, 185, 185, 186
    and pulse abnormalities, arterial, 174–177,
      175, 176
      venous, 177–179, 178
    and syncope, 13t, 14, 15–16
    and weakness, 11
    client information on, 1949, 1951, 1952
    diet in, 262–268, 264t–268t
    in hyperkalemia, 227–228
      with hypoadrenocorticism, 1494–1495,
        1495, 1498
    in hyperthyroidism, 1401t, 1402–1403
    in hypokalemia, 227
    in hypomagnesemia, 232–233
    in hypothyroidism, 1422, 1426–1427
    in renal failure, acute, 1623
      chronic, 1638, 1638, 1639
    obesity with, 71, 266
    pericardial disorders and, 923–936. See also
      Pericardium.
    sleep-associated, 154
    with pectus excavatum, 1101, 1101
    with pulmonary hypertension, 1080–1081
  electrocardiography of, 800–822. See also
    Electrocardiography.
  function of, pericardium in, 924
  in cardiac arrest, during anesthesia, acupunc-
    ture for, 372, 372
  in cardiopulmonary arrest, 189, 192
    resuscitation from, 190t, 190–193, 191, 192t
  left ventricular hypertrophy in, in hyperten-
    sion, 180
  murmurs of, 171, 171t, 171–174, 173
  myocardial disease of. See also Cardiomyopa-
    thy.
    in cat, 896–918
    in dog, 874–891
  toxicity to, chemotherapy and, 486–487
    plants and, 365
  transient sounds in, abnormal, 170, 170–172,
    173
  valvular disorders of, 787–799. See also spe-
    cific valves, e.g., Mitral valve.
Heart failure, causes of, 692, 692
  diastolic, 695–697, 696t, 698
  systolic, 692–695, 693–697, 694t

Heart failure (Continued)
  compensation in, 697–699, 698, 699
    central, 703–705, 704t
    neurohumeral activation in, 699–701, 700t
    peripheral, 701–703, 702t, 703
  congestive, with arteriosclerosis, 971
    with valvular insufficiency, client informa-
      tion on, 1952
  evaluation of, 707t, 707–710, 708t
  fluid therapy in, 330t
  progression of, 710–711, 711
  right-sided, with pulmonary hypertension, in
    mitral insufficiency, 794
  signs of, 705t, 705–707
  treatment of, 713–734
    abdominocentesis in, 733
    angiotensin-converting enzyme inhibitors in,
      713–714, 718–723, 720t
    anxiolytic, 733–734
    bipyridine compounds in, 732–733
    bronchodilators in, 734
    cough suppressants in, 734
    digitalis glycosides in, 726–731
    diuretics in, 714–717
    oxygen in, 733
    principles of, 713–714
    sympathomimetics in, 731, 731–732
    thoracentesis in, 733
    vasodilators in, 717, 717–718, 723–726
Heartgard, for dirofilariasis, 949–951, 950t, 961
Heartworm. See Dirofilariasis.
Heat stroke, 7
Hedera helix, toxicity of, 364
Heinz bodies, in anemia, 200t, 1785, 1801t,
    1801–1802
  with renal disease, 1808
Helicobacter infection, 391, 391t, 392
  and gastric ulcers, 1168
  and gastritis, 1163–1164
  and hepatitis, 1331
Heller's myotomy, for megaesophagus, 1151
Helminthiasis, of small intestine, 1220–1221,
    1221t
Hemangiosarcoma, 529, 531
  client information on, 1922
  of bone, 538, 1912
  of right atrium, and pericardial effusion, 928,
    932, 932–933
  treatment of, 534
Hematemesis, 120, 120, 121
Hematochezia, 126–129, 127t, 128
  causes of, 1240, 1240t, 1258, 1259
  with diarrhea, 122t, 123
Hematoma, of pinna, 992
  of spleen, 1858
  subcutaneous, 36, 37, 39
Hematopoiesis, cyclic, 1824t, 1826, 1990t
  neutrophils in, 1849–1850
Hematuria, 96, 97t, 98, 99t
  causes of, 1606t, 1607
  detection of, 1606, 1606, 1607, 1607
  idiopathic urinary tract disorders and, 1743–
    1746
  in urethral obstruction, 1720
  localizing signs of, 1748, 1748t
Hemeralopia, 1988t
Hemerocallis species, toxicity of, 364
Hemihopping, in neurologic examination, 561
Hemimelia, 1894, 1894, 1975t
Hemiplegia, spinal cord disorders and, 611
Hemistanding, in neurologic examination, 561,
    561
Hemivertebrae, 621, 622, 1984t
Hemiwalking, in neurologic examination, 561
Hemobartonellosis, 406–407

IND

Hemobartonellosis (Continued)
  and anemia, hemolytic, 1799t, 1799–1800
    non-regenerative, 1811
  and thrombocytopenia, 1821
  screening for, in blood donors, 348, 349
  with feline immunodeficiency virus infection,
    437, 437t
Hemodialysis, for renal failure, acute, 1631t,
    1631–1632
  chronic, 1646, 1658–1659
Hemoglobin, desaturated, in cyanosis, 206–210.
    See also Cyanosis.
  disorders of, in polycythemia, 204
  glycosylated, in monitoring, with insulin ther-
    apy, for diabetes, 1452–1453, 1453t
  in dyspnea, 166, 167t
  stroma-free, in red blood cell replacement,
    334
  synthesis of, defect of, and anemia, 201, 202,
    202t, 1790–1792, 1791t
Hemoglobinuria, 96, 98, 99
Hemolysis, and anemia, 198–200, 1789–1803.
    See also Anemia, hemolytic.
  and jaundice, 211, 212
  congenital nonspherocytic disorders and,
    1989t
Hemophilia, 1839, 1839t, 1979t, 1989t
  and arthropathy, 1873
  genetics in, 3t
Hemoptysis, diagnosis of, 217, 217t, 217–218
  pathophysiology of, 213
  treatment of, 218
  with melena, 127
Hemorrhage, after renal biopsy, 1671
  and anemia, 198, 200, 202t, 1786–1789, 1788
  and spinal cord disorders, 628–629, 629
  coagulation disorders and, in liver disease,
    1284–1285
  from nasal cavity, 213–217, 214t, 216
  in alimentary tract, and melena, 126–129,
    127t, 128, 1200–1201, 1201t
    in hepatic failure, 1302t
  in brain, 580–582
  in gastroenteritis, 1162, 1214
    and diarrhea, 123
  in hemostatic disorders, 1833–1834, 1834,
    1835t
  in myelomalacia, progressive, 643–644, 648
  in renal failure, acute, 1625, 1629–1630
    chronic, 1639–1640
  into superficial tissue, diagnosis of, 220, 221
    pathophysiology of, 218–220, 219t
    treatment of, 220–222
  mediastinal, 1095
  of nervous system, 607
  periodontal disease and, 1129
  postpartum, in cat, 1596
  time testing of, in platelet disorders, 1819
  uterine, postparturient, 1536
  vaginal, in prolonged estrus, 1523
  volume replacement for, 325–346. See also
    Fluid therapy.
  vulvar, 1570
  with intervertebral disk extrusion, 631
  with pleural effusion, 187, 188
Hemostasis, disorders of, and bleeding,
    1833–1834, 1834, 1835t
    and thrombosis, 1834–1836, 1835t, 1836,
      1837, 1839–1840, 1840t
    coagulation defects in, 1836–1839, 1838,
      1839t, 1840t
    in disseminated intravascular coagulation,
      1840–1841, 1841
  physiology of, 1829–1833, 1830–1833, 1833t
Heparin, action of, 1830, 1833t

Heparin (Continued)
  dosage of, in renal failure, 1649t
  for lung disorders, 1065t
  for thromboembolism, arterial, 968
    in cats, 917
    in dirofilariasis, 949t
    in hemolytic anemia, immune-mediated,
      1797
    preventive use of, with surgery, for hypera-
      drenocorticism, 1475
    pulmonary, 1065t, 1080
      with hyperadrenocorticism, 1483
  for thrombosis, venous, 1840
  for vascular neuropathy, 679
  in blood storage, 350, 350t
  in lavage, for pyothorax, 1107
Hepatic veins, acute disorders of, 1330
  obstruction of, 1318t, 1318–1319
Hepatitis, and encephalopathy. See
    Encephalopathy, hepatic.
  breed predisposition to, 1274
  chronic, diagnosis of, 1298t, 1298–1301,
    1299t
    infectious, 1306–1307
    treatment of, 1301–1304, 1302t, 1303t
  client information on, 1939
  dietary management in, 260
  in cats, 1308–1311, 1309
  infectious, 419, 419t, 1330–1331
  lobular dissecting, 1308
    with cholangitis, 1308–1311, 1309, 1342,
      1343
Hepatocutaneous syndrome, 28, 1272, 1337
Hepatoid cell adenoma, 1267–1268
Hepatomegaly, 137, 1276–1277
Hepatozoonosis, leukocyte inclusions in, 1846,
    1846
  polysystemic, 413–414
Herbal medicine, in cancer management, 377,
    378t
Herbicides, toxicity of, 363
Hermaphroditism, 1583, 1593, 1980t, 1993t
Herniation, diaphragmatic, 1098–1099, 1099
  congenital, 1975t, 1983t
  hiatal, 1152, 1152–1153
    and megaesophagus, 1150t
    congenital, 1975t, 1983t
  inguinal, congenital, 1975t, 1983t
  of brain, 144, 144t
  of intervertebral disks, 630, 630–633, 631,
    633
    treatment of, 633–635
  perineal, 1259–1260
  peritoneopericardial, 784, 1099, 1099
    congenital, 925–927, 927, 935, 936, 1975t,
      1983t
  pleuroperitoneal, congenital, 1975t, 1983t
  umbilical, 1975t, 1983t
Herpesvirus infection, 422
  and conjunctivitis, 66
  and encephalitis, 596
  and fetal loss, 1528
  and Kaposi's sarcoma, 481
  and pseudorabies, 595
  and rhinitis, 1018
  and tracheobronchitis, 419
  and vaginitis, 1567
  feline, type 1, 446–448
  of nervous system, 604–605
  of urinary tract, 1711
  transmission of, in mating, 1577–1578
Hetastarch, in fluid therapy, 329t, 329–331,
    331t–333t, 333–334
    for shock, with gastric dilatation and volvu-
      lus, 1172

Heterobilharziasis, of large intestine, 1246
Heterochromia, of iris, 1978t, 1988t
Heterodoxus lice, in skin infestation, 59t, 60, 60
Hexacarbons, toxicity of, to peripheral nerves,
    673t
β-Hexosaminidase deficiency, in gangliosidosis,
    1992t
Hiatal hernia, 1152, 1152–1153
  and megaesophagus, 1150t
  congenital, 1975t, 1983t
Hip, dysplasia of, 1872–1873, 1873, 1975t,
    1984t
  luxation in, 1867
  nutrition in, 245–250, 246, 249t, 250
Hirudin, action of, 1830, 1833t
His bundle, conduction blocks of, 817–818, 820,
    821
  stenosis of, congenital, 1985t
Histamine, in food, adverse reactions to, 253
  in gastric acid secretion, 1156, 1156–1157
  in gastrointestinal endocrine system, 1503
Histidine, in diet, 239t
  in gastrointestinal endocrine system, 1502
Histiocytoma, cutaneous, 527
Histiocytosis, 520–521, 521
  in ulcerative colitis, 1249, 1249
  malignant, 1855
    of lung, 1078
  nodular lesions in, 36
Histocompatibility antigen, in sexual
    differentiation disorders, 1584
Histoplasmosis, 462–465, 463t, 464
  and lymphadenopathy, hilar, with bronchial
    compression, 1059, 1060
  and meningitis, spinal, 616, 617
  geographic distribution of, 453, 454
  in leukocyte inclusions, 1846, 1846
  intestinal, client information on, 1947
  of large intestine, 1246
  of lung, 463, 464, 1066–1067
  of small intestine, 1220
HIV infection, cat scratch disease with, 382, 386
Holly, toxicity of, 364
Homatropine, with hydrocodone, for cough, 165t
    with heart failure, 734
    for tracheal disease, 1043t
Homeopathic medicine, in cancer management,
    376
Hookworm infestation, blood loss in, and
    anemia, 1787
  of large intestine, 1246
  of small intestine, 1220–1221, 1221t
  of spinal cord, 647
  zoonotic, 387
Hopping, in neurologic examination, 562, 562
Horner's syndrome, computed tomography in, of
    mediastinum, 1094
  pupils in, 660t, 660–661, 661
Hornet stings, hepatic reaction to, 1329
Horseshoe kidney, 1982t, 1996t
Human chorionic gonadotropin. See
    Gonadotropin, human chorionic.
Human immunodeficiency virus (HIV) infection,
    cat scratch disease with, 382, 386
Humerus, medial condyle of, osteochondritis
    dissecans of, 1871–1872
Humidification, of airway, for pulmonary
    disorders, 1062–1063
Humidity, and otitis externa, 993
Huskies, atopic dermatitis in, with zinc
    deficiency, 48–49
  laryngeal paralysis in, 669, 1994t
Hyaline casts, in urine, 1608, 1609
Hyalohyphomycosis, 475
Hycodan, for cough, 165t

Hycodan (Continued)
  with heart failure, 734
  for tracheal disease, 1043t
Hydralazine, for cardiomyopathy, dilated, 884
  for heart failure, 723–724
  for hypertension, in renal failure, 1654
  for mitral insufficiency, 793, 794
  for pulmonary hypertension, in dirofilariasis, 949t
Hydration deficit. See Dehydration.
Hydrocephalus, 587, 1980t, 1992t
  fetal, and dystocia, 1534
  with cerebellar degeneration, in bull mastiff, 589
Hydrochlorothiazide, for diabetes insipidus, 1707
  for edema, pulmonary, with hypertrophic cardiomyopathy, 908
    with mitral insufficiency, 793
    with hepatic failure, 1302t
  for heart failure, 716
  for urolithiasis, calcium oxalate, 1728
    preventive use of, 1769–1770
Hydrocodone, for bronchopulmonary disease, 1056, 1059t
  for cough, 165t
    with heart failure, 734
  for tracheal disease, 1043t
Hydrocortisone, before canine hyperimmune serum administration, to cats, for tick paralysis, 673
  for hypoadrenocorticism, 316, 1496
  for otitis externa, 989t, 995
  for steroid withdrawal syndrome, 317
  potency of, 312t
  structure of, 309
  with adrenalectomy, for hyperadrenocorticism, 1486–1487
Hydrometra, 1591, 1592
Hydromyelia, 652, 653
Hydroxycoumarins, in rodenticides, toxicity of, 359–360
Hydroxyethyl starch (hetastarch), for shock, with gastric dilatation and volvulus, 1172
  in fluid therapy, 329t, 329–331, 331t–333t, 333–334
Hydroxyflutamide, for prostatic hypertrophy, 1692
Hydroxylases, in hypoadrenocorticism, 1489
5-Hydroxytryptamine, in gastrointestinal endocrine system, 1502, 1503
  receptors of, antagonists of, for vomiting, in gastritis, 1162
Hydroxyurea, for myeloproliferative disease, 515–516
  for polycythemia, 206, 516
  in cancer therapy, 489
Hydroxyzine, for cough, 165t
Hymen, incomplete perforation of, 1567, 1568
Hymenopteran stings, hepatic reaction to, 1329
Hyperadrenocorticism, 1460–1487
  after gonadectomy, prepubertal, 1540
  and bone loss, 1908
  and hyperpigmentation, 57, 58
  and hypertension, 180, 181, 182
  and myopathy, 687–688
  and neurologic disorders, 551, 607
  and obesity, 71
  and polyuria, 85t, 85–89, 86, 87t, 88t, 1374, 1375
  client information on, 1929
  complications of, 1482–1485, 1484t
  diagnosis of, adrenocorticotropic hormone stimulation test in, 1469, 1469–1471, 1470t, 1485
    computed tomography in, 1473

Hyperadrenocorticism (Continued)
    dexamethasone in, 1470–1472, 1471, 1485–1486
    for pituitary-dependent disease, vs. tumor-induced, 1472, 1472–1473
    history in, 1463, 1463t
    hypertension in, 1465–1466
    imaging in, 1465t, 1466, 1467, 1467t
    liver function tests in, 1464–1465, 1465t
    magnetic resonance imaging in, 1473, 1474, 1475
    physical examination in, 1463t, 1463–1464, 1464
    urinalysis in, 1465, 1465t
    urinary glucocorticoid assay in, 1467–1469, 1468, 1469
  hypothyroidism with, 1424, 1426, 1466
  in cats, 1485t, 1485–1487
  in dogs, 1460–1485
  pathophysiology of, 1461–1462, 1462
  polyphagia with, 105–107
  prognosis of, 1487
  signalment in, 1462–1463
  skin lesions in, 26
  steroid withdrawal and, 317
  treatment of, 1473–1487
    ketoconazole in, 1481–1482, 1486
    L-deprenyl in, 1482
    metyrapone in, 1486
    mifepristone in, 1482
    o,p′-DDD in, 1476–1481, 1477, 1479, 1480, 1486
    surgical, 1473–1476
    trilostane in, 1482
Hyperaldosteronism, and hypokalemia, 225, 226
  renal tubular dysfunction in, 1706
Hyperammonemia, in liver disease, 1278t, 1286, 1286–1287
Hyperammonuria, and ammonium urate urolithiasis, 1724, 1725t
Hyperbilirubinemia, diagnosis of, 211, 211–212
  in hemolytic anemia, 1789, 1790
    immune-mediated, 1794–1795
  in liver disease, 1276, 1278t, 1287, 1287–1288
  pathophysiology of, 210–211
Hypercalcemia, 233–234, 234, 344, 345
  and polyuria, 87t, 87–88
  and weakness, 12
  fluid therapy in, 330t
  in hyperparathyroidism, 1379–1392. See also Hyperparathyroidism.
  in hypoadrenocorticism, 1492t, 1493
  in multiple myeloma, 517, 519
  in renal failure, 1643
  with anal sac tumors, 1267
  with malignancy, 501, 501–502
    bone loss and, 1908
Hypercalcitoninism, in orthopedic developmental disorders, 246
Hypercalciuria, and urinary calculi, calcium oxalate, 1725t, 1726
  calcium phosphate, 1728, 1729, 1729t
  in renal tubular dysfunction, 1706
Hypercarnitinuria, 1705
Hyperchloremia, 234
Hyperchylomicronemia, 291. See also Hyperlipidemia.
  and peripheral neuropathy, 669–670
  congenital, 1977t, 1986t
Hyperemia, conjunctival, with systemic disease, 984
Hypereosinophilic syndrome, 1852
  in Löffler's endocarditis, 903
  splenomegaly in, 1858–1859

Hyperestrogenism, and anemia, non-regenerative, 1811
  in prolonged estrus, 1523
Hypergammaglobulinemia, in liver disease, 1284
  paraneoplastic, 505
Hyperglycemia, and glucosuria, 1704
  in diabetes, 1440, 1440, 1443, 1443t. See also Diabetes mellitus.
Hyperimmune plasma, for parvovirus infection, 421
Hyperimmune serum, canine, for tick paralysis, 673
Hyperinsulinemia, paraneoplastic, in cachexia, 499, 500
Hyperkalemia, 342, 343
  after transfusion, 355
  and myopathy, 688
  causes of, 227, 228t
  diagnosis of, 227–228, 229
  in hemolytic anemia, 1791t, 1792
  in hypoadrenocorticism, 1491–1492, 1492t, 1493, 1498
    electrocardiography in, 1494–1495, 1495, 1498
  in hypoaldosteronism, 1706
  in renal failure, 1624, 1628, 1628t
  in small intestinal disorders, 1206
  renal tubular secretion defect and, 1706
  treatment of, 228, 230t
Hyperkeratosis, digital, congenital, 1995t
Hyperlactatemia, paraneoplastic, in cachexia, 499
Hyperlipidemia, 283–284, 291
  cholestasis and, 290
  diagnosis of, 286–288, 288
  genetics in, 3t
  glomerular disease and, 1675
  hypoadrenocorticism and, 290
  in diabetes mellitus, 289–290
  in hypothyroidism, 290
  in pancreatitis, 289, 1349
  nephrotic syndrome and, 290
  ocular disorders with, 291
  primary, idiopathic, 288–289
    in Briard dogs, 291
Hypermagnesemia, 233, 346
  in renal failure, 1643
Hypernatremia, 340–342, 341
  causes of, 228–230, 230t
  diagnosis of, 230–232, 231
  fluid therapy in, 330t
  in renal failure, 1624
  treatment of, 231, 232
  with hyperosmolality, neurologic signs of, 550
Hyperosmolality, in hyponatremia, 222t, 223, 550
  neurologic signs of, 550
Hyperostosis, calvarial, 1903
  diffuse idiopathic skeletal, and spinal cord dysfunction, 623, 623–624
Hyperoxaluria, and calcium oxalate urolithiasis, 1725t, 1726
  primary, 1996t
  with peripheral neuropathy, in shorthaired cats, 670
Hyperparathyroidism, alcohol injection for, 1391
  in cats, 1392
  medical therapy for, 1388–1389
  nutritional secondary, 1396
    bone loss in, 1906, 1906–1907
  pathology of, 1391–1392
  primary, and bone disorders, 1908, 1909
    diagnosis of, 1380–1387, 1381t, 1382–1387
      differential, 1387t, 1387–1388, 1388t
    etiology of, 1379

IND

Hyperparathyroidism (Continued)
  pathophysiology of, 1379–1380
  signs of, 1380
  prognosis of, 1392
  surgery for, 1389, 1389–1390
    hypocalcemia after, 1390, 1390, 1391, 1391t
  with hyperphosphatemia, in renal failure, 1656–1657
    calcitriol for, 1642–1643
    chronic, 1641–1643, 1642, 1646, 1647t
Hyperphosphatemia, 344
  enemas and, 1396
  in hyperparathyroidism, 1381–1385, 1384
    calcitriol for, 1642–1643, 1656–1657
  in hypoadrenocorticism, 1492, 1492t
  in renal failure, 1641–1643, 1642, 1646, 1647t
    management of, 1650–1651
Hyperphosphaturia, in renal tubular dysfunction, 1706
Hyperpigmentation, 55, 56, 57–58
Hyperproteinemia, in heart disease, 263, 265t
Hyperpyrexic syndrome, 7
Hypersensitivity reactions, and lung disorders, 1065t, 1071–1073, 1072, 1073
  and otitis externa, 992–993
  and vasculitis, 972–973
  small intestinal, 1198
  to drugs, 321, 324–325
    in chemotherapy, 487
Hypersomatotropism (acromegaly), 1370–1373, 1370–1373
  and cardiomyopathy, 914
  and obesity, 71
  polyphagia with, 105
Hypersthenuria, 1604
Hypertension, and cardiomyopathy, 914
  assessment of, 179–182, 181, 182
  in cardiac tamponade, 924–925, 926
  in glomerular disease, 1675
  in renal failure, 1637–1638, 1638
    and retinopathy, 1639
    management of, 1653–1654
  management of, 182
    low-sodium diet in, 262, 264t–268t, 268
  obesity with, 71–72
  pathophysiology of, 179–180, 180t
  pulmonary, 1080–1081
    and heart failure, in mitral insufficiency, 794
    echocardiography of, 844–845, 847t
    in cyanotic heart disease, congenital, 780
    in dirofilariasis, 949t
    in Eisenmenger's syndrome, 739t, 754–755, 780
    with patent ductus arteriosus, 748–749, 750, 751
  venous, in heart failure, 705
  with hyperadrenocorticism, 1465–1466
Hyperthermia, 6–9, 7t, 8, 9
Hyperthyroidism, 586, 1400–1417
  and cardiomyopathy, 913–914, 1403
  and digitalis toxicity, to myocardium, 729
  and hypertension, 180, 181, 182
  and neurologic disorders, 551, 607
  and polyuria, 87t, 88
  causes of, 1400
  client information on, 1931
  clinical features of, 1400–1403, 1401t
  echocardiography in, 857t
  ethanol injection for, 1415
  laboratory tests in, 1403t, 1403–1407, 1404, 1406, 1407
  liver enzymes in, 1284
  medical treatment of, 1408t, 1409–1412, 1410, 1411t

Hyperthyroidism (Continued)
  polyphagia with, 105, 106
  radioactive iodine for, 1408t, 1413–1415, 1414
  radionuclide imaging in, 1407–1409, 1408, 1409
  surgery for, 1408t, 1412–1413
  tumors and, 1415–1417
Hypertrophic osteodystrophy, 1901–1903, 1902
Hypertrophic osteopathy, paraneoplastic, 503, 503
  secondary, 1903, 1903–1904
Hyperuricosuria, and ammonium urate urolithiasis, 1724, 1725t
Hyperventilation, and syncope, 15
  for intracranial pressure elevation, 577
Hyperviscosity, of blood, in multiple myeloma, 516, 519
  in polycythemia, 204
Hypervitaminosis A, and bone disorders, 1907–1908, 1908
  and exostoses, with spinal cord compression, 629–630
Hypervitaminosis D, and bone disorders, 1909
Hypervolemia, fluid therapy and, in renal failure, 1622, 1623, 1623t, 1627
  with hyponatremia, 222t, 223
Hypoadrenocorticism, 1488–1498
  adrenocorticotropic hormone stimulation test in, 1495, 1498
  after adrenalectomy, 1487
  and hyperkalemia, 229
  and hyperlipidemia, 290
  and liver dysfunction, 1336
  and polyuria, 87t, 88
  clinical findings in, 1491, 1491t
  congenital, 1986t
  electrocardiography in, 1494–1495, 1495, 1498
  etiology of, 1489
  fluid therapy in, 330t
  hypotension in, 1494
  hypothyroidism with, 1422, 1424, 1427, 1466
  imaging in, 1494, 1494
  in cats, 1498
  laboratory tests in, 1491–1494, 1492t, 1493
  neurologic signs of, 551
  o,p'-DDD and, in treatment of hyperadrenocorticism, 1481
  pathophysiology of, 1489–1490, 1490
  treatment of, 1496–1498
    steroids in, 316
Hypoalbuminemia, and hypocalcemia, vs. hypoparathyroidism, 1394
  in dirofilariasis, 947
  in glomerular disease, 1671
  in hypoadrenocorticism, 1493
  in liver disease, 1278t, 1284
  in systemic inflammatory response syndrome, 327
  with portosystemic shunt, congenital, 1312
Hypoaldosteronism, renal tubular dysfunction in, 1706
Hypocalcemia, 233, 344, 345
  after surgery, for hyperparathyroidism, 1390, 1390, 1391, 1391t
  after thyroidectomy, 1413
  after transfusion, 355
  and neurologic dysfunction, 586
  and weakness, 11–12
  differential diagnosis of, 1394–1396, 1395, 1396t
  in renal failure, 1643
  in tetany, puerperal, 1538
  neurologic signs of, 550

Hypocalcemia (Continued)
  paraneoplastic, 502
  with hypoparathyroidism, 1392–1399. See also Hypoparathyroidism.
Hypochloremia, 234
  in hypoadrenocorticism, 1491–1492, 1492t
Hypochondroplasia, and dwarfism, 1898
Hypocitraturia, and calcium oxalate urolithiasis, 1725t
Hypoglossal nerve, anatomy of, 664t
  examination of, 563, 566
Hypoglycemia, and neurologic disorders, multifocal, 607
  in dystocia, 1532
  in hypoadrenocorticism, 1492t, 1492–1493
  in liver disease, 1290, 1302t, 1332
  in neonate, 244, 1977t, 1987t
  in pregnancy, 1528
  insulin and, in treatment of diabetes, 1455
  insulinoma and, 502, 1430–1434, 1432t, 1433, 1434t
  neurologic signs of, 549, 549t, 586
  paraneoplastic, 502
  with portosystemic shunt, congenital, 1312
Hypogonadism, and bone growth disorders, 1908
  and obesity, 71
Hypokalemia, 342–344, 343
  and myopathy, 688
  and polyuria, 87t, 88
  causes of, 223–225, 225t
  diagnosis of, 225–227, 226
  diuretics and, in heart failure, 715, 716
  in diabetes mellitus, with ketoacidosis, 1444t, 1445, 1446
  in Fanconi's syndrome, 1708, 1709
  in hyperaldosteronism, 1706
  in liver disorders, 1302t, 1332, 1334t
  in renal failure, acute, 1628–1629
    chronic, 1644, 1651
  neurologic signs of, 550, 550
  treatment of, 226, 227
  with digitalis toxicity, 729, 730
  with hypomagnesemia, 232
Hypoluteodism, and fetal loss, 1525, 1528
Hypomagnesemia, 232–233, 346
  diuretics and, in heart failure, 716
  renal tubular dysfunction and, 1706
Hypomyelination, 588, 1992t
  and tremor, 140–141
  genetics in, 3t
  in golden retriever, 668–669, 1992t
Hyponatremia, 341, 342
  causes of, 222t, 222–223
  diagnosis of, 223, 224
  diuretics and, in heart failure, 715, 716
  in hypoadrenocorticism, 1491–1492, 1492t
  in renal failure, 1624
  in small intestinal disorders, 1206
  treatment of, 223, 224
  with hypo-osmolality, neurologic signs of, 549–550
Hypo-osmolality, in hyponatremia, 222t, 222–223
  neurologic signs of, 549–550
Hypoparathyroidism, 1392–1399
  clinical features of, 1391t, 1393
  congenital, 1977t
  diagnosis of, 1393, 1394t
  histology in, 1399
  pathophysiology of, 1392–1393
  prognosis of, 1399
  treatment of, 1396t, 1396–1399, 1398t
Hypophosphatemia, 344–346
  and hemolytic anemia, 1802
  in diabetes, with ketoacidosis, 1444t, 1445

Hypophosphatemia (Continued)
in hyperparathyroidism, 1381, 1381t, 1384
with anal sac tumors, 1267
Hypophysis. See Pituitary.
Hypopigmentation, 55–57, 56
Hypoproteinemia, in heart disease, 263, 265t
in malabsorption, with diarrhea, 125
Hypoprothrombinemia, 1839, 1839t
Hypospadias, 1584, 1584, 1585, 1981t, 1993t
Hyposthenuria, definition of, 1604
liver disease and, 1291
Hypotension, assessment of, 183–185, 185
in heart failure treatment, hydralazine and, 724
nitroprusside and, 726
vasodilators and, 718
in hypoadrenocorticism, 1494
management of, 184t, 185, 185–186
pathogenesis of, 183, 183t
postural, and syncope, 13–15
Hypothalamus, in polyphagia, 104–105
in temperature regulation, 6, 6
Hypothermia, 9, 9–10
in renal failure, 1625
Hypothyroidism, 1419–1428
and constipation, 1252–1253
and growth failure, 77, 1422, 1422
and hyperpigmentation, 57, 58
and infertility, 1558
and megaesophagus, 1150, 1150t
and myopathy, 687
and neurologic disorders, 551, 607
peripheral, 671–672
and obesity, 70–71
and prolonged anestrus, 1524
client information on, 1932
congenital, 1977t, 1987t
and dwarfism, 1897, 1898
diagnosis of, 1422–1426, 1423
epidemiology of, 1421
hypercholesterolemia in, 290
in cats, 1427–1428
pathogenesis of, 1420–1421
prognosis of, 1427
signs of, 1421t, 1421–1422, 1422
skin lesions in, 26
treatment of, 1426–1428, 1427
with hyperadrenocorticism, 1424, 1426, 1466
Hypotrichosis, 1982t, 1995t
Hypoventilation, blood gas analysis in, 1038–1039, 1039
Hypovitaminosis A, and bone deformity, 1908–1909
Hypovolemia, and shock, fluid therapy in, 330t
gastric ulcers with, 1166
in hypernatremia, 230, 232
in renal failure, 1622, 1623t
management of, 1626–1627
Hypoxemia, in cyanotic heart disease, congenital, 779
oxygen for, 1061–1062, 1062
Hypoxia, and encephalopathy, 548–549, 549t
and neurologic dysfunction, 586
of brain, trauma and, 579
Hysterectomy. See Ovariohysterectomy.
Hytakerol, for hypoparathyroidism, 1397–1398, 1398t

Ibutilide, for arrhythmia, 830
Ichthyosis, 48, 1995t
Icterus. See Hyperbilirubinemia.
liver disease and, 1276
Idioventricular rhythms, accelerated, 816

Iduronate–2–sulfatase deficiency, in mucopolysaccharidosis, skeletal abnormalities with, 1896
α-L-Iduronidase deficiency, in mucopolysaccharidosis, 1979t, 1980t
skeletal abnormalities with, 1896
spinal cord dysfunction with, 638
Ileocolic intussusception, 1251–1252
Ileocolic orifice, 1238, 1238
Ileoscopy, in diarrhea, 125, 126
Ileum, anatomy of, 1183, 1184
electrolyte absorption from, 1192, 1193, 1193
Ileus, adynamic, 1234
and diarrhea, 1200, 1200t
radiography in, 1208, 1208t
Ilex species, toxicity of, 364
Imidacloprid, in flea control, client information on, 1971
Imidocarb, for babesiosis, with hemolytic anemia, 1799t, 1800
for protozoal infection, 410t
for thrombocytopenia, 1819
Imipenem, concentration of, and bacterial susceptibility, 303t
with cilastatin, for lung infection, 1065t
Immiticide. See Melarsomine.
Immune complexes, in glomerulonephritis, 1663–1666, 1664, 1665, 1666t
Immune system, congenital defects of, 1990t
disorders of, skin lesions in, 29, 40t, 43
in anemia, hemolytic, 199, 200t, 1793–1798, 1794t, 1795
client information on, 1960
non-regenerative, 1810
in arthritis, 77–80, 78t, 79, 1879–1883, 1880
client information on, 1961
treatment of, 1883–1885
in hyperthermia, 7, 7t, 8, 8
in hypoadrenocorticism, 1489
in islet cell destruction, in diabetes, 1439
in lung disorders, 1065t, 1071–1073, 1072, 1073
in myositis, 687
in thrombocytopenia, 1821–1822
client information on, 1960
with purpura, 219, 219t, 220
modulators of, for feline leukemia virus infection, 429–430
of colonic mucosa, 1239, 1239t
suppression of, feline leukemia virus and, 427
Immunoaugmentive therapy, in cancer management, 377
Immunodeficiency, severe combined, 3t, 1990t
neutrophils in, 1850
Immunodeficiency virus infection, feline, 433, 433–438, 435, 435t, 436, 437t
and enteritis, 1217
and neurologic disorders, 599, 605–606
and sleep reduction, 155
client information on, 1956
diagnosis of, 436–437
diseases associated with, 434–438, 435, 435t
pathogenesis of, 434
prevention of, 436
screening for, in blood donors, 349
species specificity of, 438
treatment of, 437t, 437–438
human (HIV), cat scratch disease with, 382, 386
Immunofluorescent testing, for feline immunodeficiency virus infection, 436
for feline leukemia virus, 425, 426
in dirofilariasis, 958
Immunoglobulin A, in small intestinal immune response, 1195

Immunoglobulin A (Continued)
selective deficiency of, 1990t
Immunoglobulins, human, transfusion of, 353
in hemolytic anemia, 1793, 1796, 1797
in hypergammaglobulinemia, paraneoplastic, 505
Immunoreactivity, trypsin-like, in pancreatic exocrine insufficiency, 1359–1360, 1360
ImmunoRegulin, for feline immunodeficiency virus infection, 437, 437t, 438
for feline leukemia virus infection, 430
Immunosuppression, for aplastic anemia, 1813
for glomerulonephritis, 1672, 1672t
Imodium A-D (loperamide), for diarrhea, 319, 1215
with histoplasmosis, 464
Impedance audiometry, in deafness, 1001
Impetigo, pustules in, 43–44
Imuran. See Azathioprine.
Incontinence, fecal, 129, 133–135, 134, 134t, 1268t, 1268–1269
urinary. See Urinary incontinence.
Indanediones, action of, 1830, 1833t
toxicity of, 359–360
Indarubin, in cancer management, 378t
Inderal. See Propranolol.
Infarction, and nervous system injury, 556, 607
myocardial, hypertrophic cardiomyopathy and, 905
of bone, medullary, 1904, 1904
renal, 964, 965
Infertility, canine, female, assessment of, 1555–1558, 1556, 1557
management of, 1558–1565, 1559–1563, 1560t, 1565
male, 1578–1580
semen evaluation in, 1571–1574, 1572t
feline, female, 1591–1592, 1592, 1593, 1595, 1595
male, 1594–1595
Inflammation, chronic, and anemia, 202
and weakness, 11
neutrophils in, 1844–1845, 1845
of nervous system, 556
systemic response syndrome in, 327
fluid therapy in, 335, 337
Inflammatory bowel disease, 1225t, 1225–1228, 1226, 1227t
client information on, 1947
food reactions in, 254
idiopathic, 1247–1251, 1248, 1248t, 1249, 1249t
liver disorders with, 1336
Inguinal hernia, congenital, 1975t, 1983t
Inhalation injury, 1083, 1087–1088
Inositol–1,4,5–triphosphate, in platelet activation, 1817, 1817–1818
Insecticides, toxicity of, 357–359
and megaesophagus, 1150t
to peripheral nerves, 673t
Insects. See also specific types, e.g., Fleas.
in skin infestation, 58–60, 59t, 60
Insemination, artificial, 1574–1577, 1576
client information on, 1934
semen collection for, 1571–1572
Insulin, elevated blood level of, paraneoplastic, 499, 500
for hyperkalemia, 342
in diabetes, 1438–1459. See also Diabetes mellitus.
resistance to, in pregnancy, 1528
with glucose and potassium, for septic shock, 184t
Insulin-like growth factor, 1370
Insulinoma, 1429–1438

IND

Insulinoma *(Continued)*
  and hypoglycemia, 502
  and obesity, 71, 72
  diagnosis of, 1430–1434, *1432,* 1432t, *1433,*
    1434t
  etiology of, 1429
  in cats, 1437–1438
  pathophysiology of, 1429–1430, 1430t
  polyphagia with, 105
  prognosis of, 1437
  signalment of, 1429, *1429,* 1430t
  treatment of, 1434t, 1434–1437, *1435,* 1435t,
    1437
Integrins, in platelet activation, *1817,* 1818
Interceptor. See *Milbemycin.*
Intercostal arteries, aberrant, and esophageal
    compression, 1145
Interferon, for feline immunodeficiency virus
    infection, 437, 437t
  for feline leukemia virus infection, 430–431
    with anemia, 1811
  for peritonitis, feline infectious, 441
  in hyperthermia, 7, 7t
  in periodontal disease, 1128
Interleukins, in hyperthermia, 7, 7t, *8*
  in metastatic tumor growth, 483
  in periodontal disease, 1128
Intervertebral disks. See *Disks.*
Intestines. See *Colon* and *Small intestine.*
Intra-arachnoid cysts, and spinal cord
    dysfunction, 645–647, *646*
Intracranial pressure, increased, cerebral edema
    and, in hepatic encephalopathy, 1334
  trauma and, 579, 580
  treatment of, 577
Intravascular coagulation, disseminated. See
    Coagulation, disseminated intravascular.
Intron A. See *Interferon.*
Intussusception, gastroesophageal, 1153, *1153*
  of large intestine, 1251–1252, *1252*
Inulin, in glomerular function testing, 1602t,
    1603
Iodine, for fungal infection, 475t
  in diet, 239t
    in orthopedic developmental disorders, 247–
      248
    in radionuclide imaging, in hyperthyroidism,
      1407–1409, *1408, 1409*
  radioactive, for hyperthyroidism, 1408t, 1413–
    1415, *1414,* 1417
    client information on, 1931
  stable, for hyperthyroidism, 1412
  with povidone, for anal sacculitis, 1266
    for otitis externa, 989t, 995
Ipecac syrup, in induction of vomiting, 319
Ipodate, for hyperthyroidism, 1412
Ipomoea violace, toxicity of, 365
Ipronidazole, for protozoal infection, 410, 410t
Iris, absence of, 1987t
  cyst of, congenital, 1978t, 1988t
  disorders of, and anisocoria, 659t
  heterochromia of, 1978t, 1988t
  muscles of, in pupillary function, 657
Iron, deficiency of, in anemia, 199, 202–203,
    1787–1789, *1788,* 1809
    of chronic disease, 1807, *1807*
  in diet, 239t
  toxicity of, 362
Iron sulfate, for anemia, in renal failure, 1654
Irritable bowel syndrome, 1200, 1200t, 1252
  food reactions in, 254
Iscador, in cancer management, 377
Ischemia, and pancreatitis, 1350, 1363t
  in cardiomyopathy, hypertrophic, 897
  of brain, 548–549, 549t, 556, 580–582

Ischemia *(Continued)*
  of peripheral nerves, 678–679
  of spinal cord, fibrocartilaginous embolism
    and, 635–636
    trauma and, 647–648
  volvulus and, with gastric dilatation, 1173
Islet cells, pancreatic, in diabetes. See *Diabetes
    mellitus.*
    tumors of, and gastrin hypersecretion,
      1503–1506, 1505t, 1506t
    and insulin secretion, 1429–1438. See
      also *Insulinoma.*
Isoerythrolysis, in neonate, 1797–1798
Isoleucine, in diet, 239t
  in gastrointestinal endocrine system, 1502
Isoniazid, for tuberculosis, 394
Isoproterenol, cardiac stimulation with,
    echocardiography of, *840*
  for arrhythmia, 828t
Isoptin (verapamil), for arrhythmia, 824t–826t,
    829t, 830–831
    supraventricular, with hypotension, 184t
  for cardiomyopathy, hypertrophic, 890
Isosorbide dinitrate, for heart failure, 725
Isospora infection, of small intestine, 1221–1222
Isosthenuria, definition of, 1604
  in hyperparathyroidism, 1385
  liver disease and, 1291
Isotretinoin, for ichthyosis, 48
  for lymphoma, cutaneous, 528
  for sebaceous adenitis, 48
Isuprel (isoproterenol), cardiac stimulation with,
    echocardiography of, *840*
  for arrhythmia, 828t
Itching, 31–36. See also *Pruritus.*
Itraconazole, for blastomycosis, 460
  for coccidioidomycosis, 467
  for cryptococcosis, 471
    with feline immunodeficiency virus infec-
      tion, 437t
  for dermatophytosis, 49
  for fungal infection, 456–457, *457,* 475t
  for histoplasmosis, 464
  for *Malassezia* infection, in otitis externa,
    990t, 996
  for pythiosis, of small intestine, 1220
Ivermectin (Ivomec), for cheyletiellosis, 49, 62
  for demodicosis, 62
    client information on, 1970
  for dirofilariasis, 949–952, 950t, 954, 961
  for lungworm infestation, of trachea, 1045
  for mite infestation, of external ear canal,
    989t, 995–996
    of nasal cavity, 1018
    of pinna, 988, 989t
  for notoedric mange, 61
  for parasitosis, intestinal, preventive use of,
    1220, 1221, 1221t
    of lung, 1070
    of urinary tract, in dogs, 1779t
  for scabies, 50–51
Ivy, toxicity of, 364
Ixodes ticks, as vectors, of borreliosis, 28, 396
  bites of, and paralysis, 672–673
  in skin infestation, 59t, 61

Jack Russell terrier, ataxia in, 629, 1991t
Jamshidi needle, in bone biopsy, 1891–1893,
    1892
Japanese yew, toxicity of, 365
Jaundice. See *Hyperbilirubinemia.*
Jaw, articulation of, with temporal bone,
    instability of, 1868

Jaw *(Continued)*
  development of, deciduous teeth in, 1123
  dropped, in trigeminal neuropathy, 582
  giant cell granuloma of, 1905
  osteopathy of, with cranial osteopathy, 1898,
    1900, 1901, 1983t
Jejunostomy, for enteral nutrition, 279
  client information on, 1945
Jejunum, anatomy of, 1182–1183, *1184*
  electrolyte absorption from, 1191, *1192*
Jequirity bean, toxicity of, 364–365
Jerusalem cherry, toxicity of, 364
Jimsonweed, toxicity of, 365
Joints, bacterial infection of, antibiotics for, 306
  disorders of, classification of, 1862, 1862t
    congenital, in cats, 1975t
      in dogs, 1983t, 1984t
    degenerative, 1862–1866, *1863,* 1863t, *1864*
      noninflammatory, classification of, 77–
        79, 78t
      diagnosis of, *79,* 79–80
    developmental, 1869–1873, *1870, 1871,
      1873, 1874*
    in Scottish fold cat, 1874
    sarcoma and, 1874, *1875*
    with hemophilia, 1873
  inflammation of, 77–80, 1875–1885. See also
    Arthritis.
  luxation of, *1867,* 1867–1868, *1868*
  meniscal tears in, with cruciate ligament rup-
    ture, 1868
  neuropathic disorders of, 1868
  trauma to, 1866–1867
  tumors of, 535, 538–539
Jugular vein, distention of, with pericardial
    constrictive disease, 934
  incision of, for heartworm removal, 951, *951,
    961*
  pulse in, 177–179, *178*
Junctional atrioventricular node, in rhythm
    disturbances, 813, *813*

Kanamycin, dosage of, in renal failure, 1649t
Kaposi's sarcoma, 481
Kartagener's syndrome, 1059
Keflex. See *Cephalexin.*
Keflin (cephalothin), concentration of, and
    bacterial susceptibility, 303t
  dosage of, in renal failure, 1649t
  for lung infection, 1065t
Kennel cough, 419t, 419–420, 1043t, 1043–1044
Keratinization, and otitis externa, 989t, 993
Keratitis, *67,* 69
  herpesvirus infection and, 446
  systemic disease and, 984–985
Keratoacanthoma, 525
Keratoconjunctivitis, radiation injury and, in
    nasal tumor therapy, 1022
Keratoconjunctivitis sicca, 66
  systemic disease and, 984–985
Keratopathy, band, in hyperparathyroidism, 1380
Keratosis, 36
  actinic, and nasal carcinoma, 1019, *1020*
Kernicterus, 211
Ketamine, in anesthesia, before catheterization,
    for urethral obstruction, 1734
  for gonadectomy, prepubertal, 1541
  for liver biopsy, 1296t
  in sedation, for blood donation, 349
Ketoacidosis, in diabetes mellitus, in diagnosis,
    1442–1444
  pathophysiology of, 1441–1442
  treatment of, 1444t, 1444–1447

Ketoconazole, for blastomycosis, 460–461
  for coccidioidomycosis, 467
  for cryptococcosis, 471
  for dermatophytosis, 49
  for epidermal dysplasia, in West Highland
    white terrier, 48
  for fungal infection, 456–457, 475t
  for histoplasmosis, 464
  for hyperadrenocorticism, 1481–1482, 1486
  for *Malassezia* infection, in dermatitis, 50
    in otitis, 990t, 996
Ketones, in urinalysis, 1605–1606
Ketoprofen, for fever, 9
  for pain, 24t
Key-Gaskell syndrome, and megaesophagus,
  1150t, 1151
Kidney(s). See also *Renal.*
  amyloidosis of, 1667–1674. See also *Amy-
    loidosis.*
  disorders of, and adverse drug reactions, 323t,
    324
    and anemia, 1808
    and cachexia, 74
    and diabetes insipidus. See *Diabetes insip-
      idus.*
    and hyperchloremia, 234
    and hyperlipidemia, 290
    and hypokalemia, 225, *226,* 227
    and hyponatremia, 222t, 222–223, *224,*
      1644, 1651
    and polyuria, 85t, 85–89, *86,* 87t, 88t
    and proteinuria, 100–102, *101*
    congenital, in cats, 1982t
      in dogs, 1996t
    dextran and, 333
    diabetes mellitus and, 1458–1459
    diet in, 269–271, 271t, 272t, 273–274
    evaluation of, biopsy in, 1612–1613, *1613*
      clinical, 1600–1601, *1601*
      glomerular function tests in, 1601–1603,
        1602, 1602t
      microbiologic, 1610–1611
      radiography in, 1611–1612
      tubular function tests in, 1603–1605,
        1604t
      ultrasonography in, 1612
      urinalysis in, 1605–1610, 1606t, *1606–
        1611,* 1607t
    familial, 1698–1703, 1699t
    hypertension and, with hyperadrenocorti-
      cism, 1466
    in heart failure, 702t, 703
    in hyperkalemia, 228, *229*
    in hyperthyroidism, 1402, 1403t, 1404
    in multiple myeloma, 516–517, 519
    skin lesions with, 28
    with dirofilariasis, 947
  erythropoietin production in, in polycythemia,
    203, 204
  glomerular function in, 1662–1663, *1663*
  glomerular inflammation in, 1663–1676. See
    also *Glomerulonephritis.*
  in bilirubin metabolism, 211
  in drug elimination, 297
  infarction of, 964, *965*
  inflammation of, hyperadrenocorticism and,
    1482
  lymphoma of, 508, 508t
  steroid effects on, 311
  toxicity to, amphotericin B and, 455–456,
    1616
    chemotherapy and, 487, 487t
    ethylene glycol and, client information on,
      1965
    furosemide and, in heart failure, 715–716

Kidney(s) (*Continued*)
  transplantation of, 1632, 1659t, 1659–1660
  tubular disorders in, 1704–1709, 1709t. See
    also *Renal tubules.*
  tumors of, 542
  vascular disorders in, and hypertension, 180–
    182, *181*
Kitten. See *Neonate.*
Klebsiella infection, antibiotics for, 303,
  305–306
Knee, synovitis of, 1883–1885
Krabbe type globoid cell leukodystrophy, 589,
  590t, 1980t, 1992t
  and peripheral neuropathy, 670
  genetics in, 3t
  spinal cord demyelination in, 627–628
Krebs-Henseleit cycle, 1286, *1286*

Labetalol, for arrhythmia, 827
Labor. See *Parturition.*
Labrador retriever, myopathy in, 688–689, 1993t
Lacrimal punctum, imperforate, 1988t
Lactase, deficiency of, 1197
Lactate, elevated blood level of, paraneoplastic,
  499
Lactate dehydrogenase, in liver disease, 1283
  in pleural effusion, 1105
Lactation, disorders of, 1538
  in neonatal nutrition, 241–244, 243t
  in pseudopregnancy, 1526
  management of, 1596
Lactitol, for hepatic encephalopathy, 1333
Lactose, intolerance to, 253
Lactulose, for constipation, 132
  for hepatic encephalopathy, 1333, 1334t
  for portosystemic shunt, congenital, 1314,
    1315
Laminectomy, for intervertebral disk disease,
  1919
Lanoxin. See *Digoxin.*
Lansoprazole, for gastric ulcers, 1168
Laparoscopy, for liver biopsy, 1296t, 1297
Large intestine. See *Colon.*
Larva migrans, zoonotic infection and, 386–387
Larvae, in chigger infestation, and pruritus, 33t
  in heartworm disease, 937, *937, 938,* 958–
    959. See also *Dirofilariasis.*
Laryngitis, 1030
Larynx, disorders of, 1029–1031
  hypoplasia of, 1981t, 1994t
  paralysis of, congenital, 1994t
    in Dalmatian, with polyneuropathy, 668
    nerve degeneration and, 669
  physiology of, 1025, 1026
Lasalocid, toxicity of, to peripheral nerves, 673t
Lasix. See *Furosemide.*
Lassitude, 10
Latissimus dorsi muscle, in surgery, for
  cardiomyopathy, 885
Lavage, bronchoalveolar, 1038
  in tracheal disorders, 1042
  for pyothorax, 1106–1107
Laxatives, 131, 132t
  over-the-counter, 319–320
Lead, accumulation of, in bone, 1909, *1910*
  toxicity of, 361–362
    and megaesophagus, 1150t
    to central nervous system, 586
    to peripheral nerves, 673t
Leflunomide, for arthritis, 1884–1885
Legg-Calvé-Perthes disease, 1873, *1874,* 1984t
Leiomyoma, of stomach, 1176, 1177
Leiomyosarcoma, colorectal, 1253–1254

Leishmaniasis, and arthritis, 1878–1879
  and hypopigmentation, 57
  polysystemic, 410t, 415
  skin lesions in, 28
Lenses, cataracts of, and vision loss, 17, 17t
    congenital, 1977t, 1987t
    diabetes and, 985, 1458
    systemic disease and, 985
  congenital defects of, 1977t, 1978t, 1987t,
    1988t
Lente insulin, for diabetes mellitus, 1451–1452
Lenticonus, 1988t
Leprosy, 393, 394
Leptospirosis, 391t, 397–398
  and anemia, 199
  and renal failure, 1617, 1622, 1631
  of liver, 1307, 1337
  zoonotic, 384t
Lethargy, 10
Leucine, in diet, 239t
Leukemia, and anemia, 1814–1815
  and thrombopoietic disorders, 1823
  lymphoblastic, acute, 514, *514, 1854, 1854*
    chronic, 1855, *1855*
  lymphocytic, *514,* 514–515
  myeloid, *1853,* 1853–1854, *1854*
  nonlymphoid, 515t, 515–516
  of granular lymphocytes, 1854–1855, *1855*
  undifferentiated, acute, 1854
Leukemia virus infection, feline, 424–432
  and anemia, aplastic, 1813
    non-regenerative, 1810t, 1810–1811
  and enteritis, 1217
  and lymphoma, 508t, 509
  and lymphopenia, 1851
  and rectal cancer, 1261
  and urinary incontinence, 1742
  client information on, 1957
  diagnosis of, 425–426
  epidemiology of, 424–425
  management of, 428–432
  pathogenesis of, 426–427
  prevention of, 427–428, *429*
  screening for, in blood donors, 349
Leukocyte adhesion protein deficiency, in
  granulocytopathy syndrome, 1850, 1990t
Leukocyte esterase reaction, in urinalysis, 1606
Leukocytes, 1842–1855. See also specific types,
  e.g., *Neutrophils.*
  changes in, in disease prognosis, 1852
  in brain inflammation, 591–592
  in cerebrospinal fluid, 574, 574t
  in urinary tract infection, *98,* 99, 1607, *1607,*
    1607t, 1678, 1680
  inclusions in, 1846–1848, *1846–1848*
  production of, 1842
Leukocytosis, in hemolytic anemia, 1794
  in hyperthyroidism, 1403, 1403t
  of brain, 591–592
  paraneoplastic, 504–505
Leukoderma, 55–57, *56*
Leukodystrophy, globoid cell, 589, 590t, 1980t,
  1992t
  and peripheral neuropathy, 670
  genetics in, 3t
  spinal cord demyelination in, 627–628
  metachromatic, 589, 590t, 1980t
Leukoencephalomyelopathy, in rottweilers, 589,
  636
Leukogram, stress, 1844
Leukotrichia, 55–57, *56*
Leukotrienes, in inflammation, steroid effects on,
  310
Levamisole (Levasol), for dirofilariasis, 949, 952
  for lungworm infestation, 1070, 1071

IND

Level bite, 1125, *1126*
Levothyroxine, for hypothyroidism, 551,
    1426–1428, *1427*
    after thyroidectomy, 1413
    with megaesophagus, 1150, 1150t
L-form bacterial infection, 391t, 392–393
    and arthritis, 1877–1878
Lhasa apso, renal dysplasia in, 1699t,
    1701–1702
Lice, skin infestation by, 59t, 60, *60*
    and pruritus, 33t
Lichenoid dermatitis, 37
Lichenoid-psoriasiform dermatosis, congenital,
    1995t
Lick dermatitis, 36, 37
Lidocaine, for arrhythmia, 824t–826t, 826, 828t
    for pain, 23, 24t
    for ventricular arrhythmia, with hypotension,
        184t
    for ventricular tachyarrhythmia, in digitalis
        toxicity, 730
    for ventricular tachycardia, in cardiomyopathy,
        dilated, 911
        right ventricular, 913
    in anesthesia, for liver biopsy, 1296t
    in cardiopulmonary resuscitation, 192t
Lieberkühn's crypts, 1238–1239
Light, and pupillary reflex, in cranial nerve
        examination, 563–564, *564*, 567t
    in neurologic examination, 659, 660, 660t
    in vision loss, acute, 18–19, *19*
    neuroanatomy of, 657–658, *658*
Lilies, toxicity of, 364, 365
Limbs, anomalies of, 1894, 1975t, 1983t, 1984t
    rear, weakness of, in diabetes, 1442, *1442*
    segmental hemiatrophy of, 1895–1896
    shortening of, and joint disorders, 1869
Lime sulfur, for mange, notoedric, 61
    pinnal, 988, 989t
Limping kitten syndrome, calicivirus and, 448
Linognathus lice, in skin infestation, 59t, 60, *60*
Linoleic acid, in diet, 240
Lip, cleft, 1976t, 1985t
    small, congenital, 1977t, 1986t
    tightness of, with malocclusion, 1126
Lipidosis, hepatic, 1329–1331, 1330t
    client information on, 1944
    obesity with, 72
    sphingomyelin, 589, 590t, 1980t, 1992t
Lipids, absorption of, from small intestine, 1189
    blood level of, elevated, 283–284, 286–291.
        See also *Hyperlipidemia.*
    digestion of, in small intestine, 1187, *1189*
    drug solubility in, 296, 297
    function of, 284
    in diet, in enteral nutrition, 280, 281t
        in gastrointestinal disorders, 259
        in heart disease, 265t
        in hepatic disease, 261
        in orthopedic developmental disorders, 247,
            249t
        in parenteral nutrition, 281, 282, 282t
    in feces, in pancreatic exocrine insufficiency,
        1361, *1361*
        malabsorption and, 1205
    metabolism of, 284–286, 285t, *285–287*
        disorders of, and megaesophagus, 1150t
        and peripheral neuropathy, 669–670
        in liver disease, 261, 1290
Lipiduria, 99
Lipofuscinosis, ceroid, 589, 590t, 1980t, 1992t
Lipopolysaccharide, in periodontal disease, 1128
Lisinopril, for heart failure, 720t, 722–723
    for myocardial infarction, 905
Lissencephaly, 588, 1992t

Listeriosis, 594
Lithiasis, of gallbladder, 1341–1344, *1343*
    of urinary tract. See *Urinary tract, lithiasis of.*
Lithotripsy, in dogs, 1759
Liver, abscess of, 1292, 1337
    amyloidosis of, 1323, 1337
    arteriovenous fistula in, 970, 1292, 1316–
        1318, 1979t, 1991t
    biopsy of, in hyperadrenocorticism, 1471
    blood vessels of, anomalies of, 1979t
        urate urolithiasis with, 1772, 1774, 1774t
    cirrhosis of, 1299–1301, *1300,* 1304–1306,
        1305
    cysts of, 1322, *1322,* 1979t
    disorders of, acute, and bacteremia, 1335–
        1336
        and coagulopathy, 1335
        classification of, 1326t, 1326–1327, 1327t
        decompensation in, 1336
        diagnosis of, 1331
        infectious, 1330–1331
        treatment of, 1331–1336, 1332t–1334t
    and adverse drug reactions, 323t, 323–324
    and coagulation factor deficiencies, 1836
    and encephalopathy. See *Encephalopathy,*
        hepatic.
    and gastric ulcers, 1166
    and growth failure, 75t, 77
    and jaundice, diagnosis of, *211,* 211–212
        pathophysiology of, 210–211
    and necrolytic dermatitis, 28, 1272, 1337
    and osteodystrophy, 1908
    and platelet dysfunction, 1826
    congenital, 1979t, 1991t
    dietary management in, 260–261
    laboratory tests in, 1277–1278, 1278t, *1280,*
        1281
        biopsy for, 1294–1298, *1295,* 1296t,
            1939
        for ammonia, 1278t, *1286,* 1286–1287
        for bile acids, 1278t, *1288,* 1288–1290
        for bilirubin, 1278t, *1287,* 1287–1288
        for carbohydrate metabolism, 1290
        for enzymes, 1278–1282, 1279t, *1282*
        for hematologic abnormalities, 1291
        for lipid metabolism, 1290
        for plasma proteins, 1278t, 1284–1286
        organic dye excretion in, 1290
        urinalysis in, 1290–1291
        radiography in, 1291–1292
        signs of, 1272–1277, 1273t, *1274,* 1274t
        skin lesions with, 26–28
        ultrasonography in, 1292
        vascular, 1330
        with intestinal disease, 1336
    enlargement of, 137, 1276–1277
    failure of, and polyuria, 87t, 88
        fluid therapy in, 330t
    fibrosis of, 1299, 1304, 1308
    hemangiosarcoma of, 531
    in drug elimination, 297
    in glycogen storage disorders, 1322–1323
    in lipid metabolism, 284–286, *285–287*
    inflammation of. See *Hepatitis.*
    leptospirosis of, 1337
    lipidosis of, 1329–1331, 1330t
        client information on, 1944
        obesity with, 72
    microvascular dysplasia in, 1315–1316, 1991t
    nodular hyperplasia of, 1319–1320
    portosystemic shunts in. See *Portosystemic*
        shunts.
    toxicity to, anticonvulsants and, 1307
        bee stings and, 1329
        carprofen and, 1307–1308, 1327–1328

Liver *(Continued)*
    diethylcarbamazine and, 1307–1308
    drugs and, 1326t, 1327–1329
    fluconazole and, 457
    itraconazole and, 457
    ketoconazole and, 457
    methimazole and, 1328, 1411
    oxibendazole and, 1307–1308
    plants and, 1326t, 1329, 1332
    thiacetarsamide and, 948
    tumors of, 1320t, 1320–1322
    urea cycle in, disorders of, 1286, *1286,* 1287,
        1323, 1987t, 1991t
    venous outflow from, obstruction of, 1318t,
        1318–1319
Lobar consolidation, pulmonary, 1088, *1089*
Lobster-claw deformity, 1895, *1895,* 1975t
Löffler's endocarditis, 903
Lomustine, toxicity of, and anemia, 1812
Loperamide, for diarrhea, 319, 1215
    with histoplasmosis, 464
Lopressor (metoprolol), for arrhythmia, 824t,
    827, 828t, 830
    for tachyarrhythmia, with mitral insufficiency,
        794–795
Lotensin. See *Benazepril.*
Lotrimin (clotrimazole), for aspergillosis, 474,
    475t, 1018–1019
Louse infestation, of skin, 59t, 60, *60*
    and pruritus, 33t
Lufenuron, for coccidioidomycosis, 457, 475t
    in flea control, client information on, 1971
Lugol's solution, for hyperthyroidism, 1412
Lung(s). See also *Respiratory tract.*
    agenesis of, unilateral, 1981t
    auscultation of, in mitral insufficiency, 790
    biopsy of, 1038, 1074–1075
    cystic-bullous disease of, 1083–1084
    disorders of, and dyspnea, 166–169, 167t, *168*
        and hemoptysis, 217t, 217–218
        bronchial, 1055–1061, *1056, 1057,* 1058t,
            1059t, *1060*
        bronchoscopy in, 1037, *1037,* 1038t
        humidification for, 1062–1063
        immune-mediated, 1065t, 1071–1073, *1072,*
            1073
        in renal failure, 1623–1624, 1630
        near drowning and, 1086–1087
        obesity and, 1088
        oxygen supplementation for, 1061–1062,
            1062
        vascular, and hypertension. See *Hyperten-*
         sion, pulmonary.
        ventilatory support for, 1063
    edema of, 1081–1083, *1083*
        in renal failure, 1622–1624, *1623*
        with cardiomyopathy, hypertrophic, 906–
          908
        with mitral insufficiency, 790, 793–795
    esophageal fistula to, 1060, 1147, 1994t
    in heartworm disease. See *Dirofilariasis.*
    infection of, bacterial, 1063–1066, 1065t
        blastomycosis in, 459, *459–461*
        coccidioidomycosis in, 465, 466, *466*
        fungal, 1066–1068, *1067, 1068*
        histoplasmosis in, 463, *464*
        morbillivirus and, 452
        protozoal, 1066
        viral, 1063
    inflammation of, aspiration and, 1084–1086,
        1085
        with dysphagia, 114, *115*
        client information on, 1955
    lobar consolidation in, 1088, *1089*
    lymphomatoid granulomatosis in, 974, 1072,
        1077–1078

Lung(s) (*Continued*)
mineralization of, 1088
parasitosis of, 1065t, 1068–1071, *1069,* 1083–1084
thromboembolism in, 1078–1080, *1079, 1080*
hyperadrenocorticism and, 1483
trauma to, *1083,* 1084–1088, *1085*
tumors of, bronchoscopy of, 1038t
in malignant histiocytosis, 1078
lymphomatous, *1077,* 1077–1078
metastatic, 1075–1077, *1076, 1077*
from oral cancer, 1114–1115
primary, 1073–1075, *1074, 1075*
Lungworm infestation, 1068–1071, *1069*
of trachea, *1044,* 1044–1045
Lupus, discoid, 55, 57
Lupus erythematosus, systemic, and megaesophagus, 1150t
arthritis in, 78, 80, 1882
treatment of, 1883–1885
hypopigmentation in, 57
lungs in, 1072
skin lesions in, 29
Lutalyse. See *Prostaglandins.*
Luteal phase, in estrous cycle, *1510,* 1510–1514, *1514, 1515*
Luteinization, pre-ovulatory, 1511
Luteinizing hormone, in estrous cycle, 1510–1516, *1511, 1514, 1515,* 1520, 1522, 1589
and timing of artificial insemination, 1575–1576, *1576*
Lym Dyp (lime sulfur), for mange, notoedric, 61
Lyme disease. See *Borreliosis.*
Lymph nodes, evaluation of, in hypercalcemia, 1388
Lymphadenitis, 977, 977t
Lymphadenopathy, hilar, fungal infection and, 1067–1068
lymphoma and, 1077, *1077*
with bronchial compression, 1059–1060, *1060*
mediastinal, 1095t, 1096, *1096*
Lymphangiectasia, of small intestine, *1229,* 1229–1230, *1230*
and nutrient delivery blockade, 1198
congenital, 1976t, 1985t
with chylothorax, 1107, *1107*
Lymphangioma, 980
Lymphangiosarcoma, 980
Lymphangitis, 977, 977t
Lymphatic system, congenital disorders of, 1989t, 1990t
fluid dynamics in, 326
in tumor metastasis, 481, 483
peripheral, anatomy of, 975–976
disorders of, 976–977, 977t
Lymphedema, congenital, 1979t, 1990t
peripheral, 977t, 977–980, *978, 979*
Lymphoblastic leukemia, acute, 514, *514,* 1854, *1854*
chronic, 1855, *1855*
Lymphocytes, granular, leukemia of, 1854–1855, *1855*
in colonic mucosal immunity, 1239
in feline immunodeficiency virus infection, 434
in glomerulonephritis, 1663–1664
in inflammation, steroid effects on, 310–311
in lymphoma, cutaneous, 49
in mycosis fungoides, 508, *508*
in skin lesions, in cytology, 53
in small intestinal immune response, 1195–1196, *1196*
with plasma cells, in gastritis, chronic, 1162, 1163

Lymphocytic choriomeningitis, zoonotic, 384t
Lymphocytic leukemia, *514,* 514–515
Lymphocytic portal hepatitis, 1309
Lymphocytic-plasmacytic colitis, 1247–1248, *1248,* 1248t, 1249t
Lymphocytic-plasmacytic enteritis, 1227–1228
Lymphocytic-plasmacytic infiltrates, in gastritis, 1162–1163
Lymphocytic-plasmacytic splenitis, 1858t, 1859
Lymphocytic-plasmacytic synovitis, 78–80
of knee, 1883–1885
Lymphocytosis, 1850–1851, 1851t
Lymphography, 979
Lymphoma, 507–514
and cachexia, 499
Burkitt's, 481
classification of, 507, 507t, 508t
client information on, 1923
cutaneous, 528
T-cell, 49, 508, *508*
diagnosis of, 508–510, *509,* 510t
epitheliotrophic, 42
etiology of, 507
feline immunodeficiency virus infection and, 436, *436*
hepatic, ultrasonography of, 1292
mediastinal, 508, *508,* 508t, 509t, 1095–1096, *1096*
of brain, primary, 584t
of kidney, 542
of lung, *1077,* 1077–1078
of pharynx, 1029
prognosis of, 512–514, *513,* 513t
signs of, 507–508, *508*
treatment of, 510–512, 511t, *512*
Lymphomatoid granulomatosis, 974, 1072, 1077–1078
Lymphopenia, 1851, 1851t
in hyperthyroidism, 1403, 1403t
in stress leukogram, 1844
Lymphosarcoma, of colon, 1253–1254
of rectum, 1253–1254, 1260–1262
of small intestine, 1234, *1235*
of stomach, 1176, 1177
Lynxacarus radovskyi mite infestation, 59t, 61
Lysine, in diet, 239t
Lysodren. See *o,p'-DDD.*
Lysosomal glucosidase deficiency, 1290, 1992t
Lysosomal storage diseases, 589, 590t, 1980t, 1992t
leukocyte inclusions in, 1847, *1847*

Machinery murmurs, 172–174
Macrocytosis, familial, 1990t
in hemolytic anemia, 1791t
Macroglobulinemia, Waldenström's, 516, 517
Macrophages, in feline immunodeficiency virus infection, 434
in hyperthermia, 7, 7t, *8*
in inflammation, steroid effects on, 311
in lung, in dirofilariasis, 942, *942*
in skin lesions, 53
Magnesium, blood level of, decreased, 232–233, 346
diuretics and, in heart failure, 716
renal tubular dysfunction and, 1706
elevated, 233, 346
in renal failure, 1643
functions of, 232
in diet, 239t
in calcium oxalate urolithiasis, 1727
in heart disease, 265t
Magnesium ammonium phosphate urolithiasis, in cats, 1711–1712, *1712, 1713,* 1723t, 1730t, 1730–1732, 1731t

Magnesium ammonium phosphate urolithiasis (*Continued*)
in dogs, 1758t, 1760–1763
with calcium oxalate lithiasis, 1765–1766, *1766,* 1770, *1771*
Magnesium chloride, in cardiopulmonary resuscitation, 192t, 193
Magnesium sulfate, for torsades de pointes, 815
for ventricular arrhythmia, with hypotension, 184t
Magnetic resonance imaging, in congenital heart disease, 741
in hyperadrenocorticism, 1473, *1474, 1475*
of bone disorders, 1891
of brain, 576
of nasal cavity, 1012–1013, *1016*
of pericardial effusion, 931
Malabsorption, and diarrhea, 125–126
in pancreatic exocrine insufficiency, 1208, 1358
of fat, medium-chain triglycerides for, 259
signs of, 1203, 1205
small intestinal disorders and, 1200, 1200t, 1201
Malamute, atopic dermatitis in, with zinc deficiency, 48–49
polyneuropathy in, 667–668
renal dysplasia in, 1699t, 1700
Malassezia infection, and dermatitis, with crusting, 49–50
with pruritus, 32, 33t, 34, 34t
and hyperpigmentation, 58
and otitis externa, 990t, 993, 994, 996
and skin erosion, 40, 42
in epidermal dysplasia, in West Highland white terrier, 48
Malassimilation. See *Malabsorption.*
Malnutrition, anorexia and, 102–103
in neonate, 244
in pancreatic exocrine insufficiency, 1358
in renal failure, 1648, *1648*
with cachexia, 73
Malocclusion, *1123,* 1124–1126, *1125, 1126*
Maltese dog, bile acids in, postprandial, 1289
encephalitis in, 598
Mammary glands, absence of, 1980t
disorders of, postparturient, 1538
examination of, in infertility, 1558
hyperplasia of, fibroadenomatous, 1591–1592, *1592, 1593*
in lactation, disorders of, 1538
in neonatal nutrition, 241–244, 243t
in pseudopregnancy, 1526
management of, 1596
tumors of, 544–545
after sterilization, 1542, *1542*
client information on, 1928
Mandible, articulation of, with temporal bone, instability of, 1868
development of, deciduous teeth in, 1123
dropped, in trigeminal neuropathy, 582
giant cell granuloma of, central, 1905
osteopathy of, with cranial osteopathy, 1898, *1900, 1901,* 1983t
Manganese, in diet, 239t
in orthopedic developmental disorders, 248
Mange, 59t, 61. See also *Mite infestation.*
of pinna, 988, 989t
Mannitol, for cerebral edema, 147
after portosystemic shunt ligation, 1314
in hepatic failure, 1302t
traumatic, 579–580
with inflammation, 593t
for intracranial pressure elevation, 577
for renal failure, 1627

Mannitol (Continued)
for renal injury, in prevention of acute failure, 1625
in cardiopulmonary resuscitation, 192t
Mannosidosis, 1980t
Manx cats, sacrocaudal dysgenesis in, 645, 1975t
Marax, for cough, 165t
Mare, pregnant, serum gonadotropin from, in estrus induction, 1595
Marijuana, toxicity of, 365
Marrow. See Bone marrow.
Mass lesions. See also Tumors.
cutaneous, 36–39, 38
Massage, in cancer management, 375–376
Mast cell tumors, and gastric ulcers, 1166
client information on, 1924
of skin, 526–527
radiation therapy for, 116, 117t
Mast cells, 1852–1853
in tracheal inflammation, 1042
Mastectomy, client information on, 1928
Mastication, muscles of, inflammation of, 687
Mastiff, bull, cerebellar degeneration in, with hydrocephalus, 589
Tibetan, hypertrophic neuropathy in, 669, 1992t
Mastitis, postparturient, 1538
Maxilla, development of, deciduous teeth in, 1123
giant cell granuloma of, central, 1905
Mebendazole, for intestinal parasitosis, 1221t
Meckel's diverticulum, 1976t, 1985t
Medetomidine, for pain, 24t
Median nerve, injury to, signs of, 663t
Mediastinum, air in, 1092, 1092, 1094
tracheal trauma and, 1053, 1053
anatomy of, 1091, 1092t
disorders of, diagnosis of, 1091–1094, 1092–1094
edema in, 1094–1095
hemorrhage in, 1095
inflammation of, 1094
lymphoma of, 508, 508, 508t, 509t, 1095–1096, 1096
mass lesions in, 1093, 1095t, 1095–1096, 1096
Mediterranean fever, familial, and arthritis, 1882–1883
Medium-chain triglycerides, for cachexia, paraneoplastic, 500
for malabsorption, 259
for small intestinal disorders, 1223
Medroxyprogesterone, for behavioral disorders, 160, 160t
reproductive, 1597, 1597t
for eosinophilic granuloma complex, 1118
for prostatic hypertrophy, 1692
in contraception, 1543–1544
Medullary bone infarction, 1904, 1904
Medulloblastoma, 584t
Megace. See Megestrol acetate.
Megacolon, and abdominal distention, 137
and constipation, 129–132, 1253
congenital, 1976t
perineal herniorrhaphy with, 1260
Megaesophagus, 1149–1151, 1150t
client information on, 1946
congenital, 1977t, 1986t
polyphagia with, 106, 107
Megakaryoblastic leukemia, 515t, 515–516, 1853–1854
Megakaryocytes, disorders of, 1823
Megestrol acetate, and diabetes, with hyperlipidemia, 290

Megestrol acetate (Continued)
for behavioral disorders, 160, 160t
reproductive, 1597, 1597t
for prostatic hypertrophy, 1692
in pregnancy maintenance, 1596
Meglumine, for leishmaniasis, 410t, 415
Melanoderma, 55, 56, 57–58
Melanoma, of skin, 526
oral, 1114–1118, 1115, 1116, 1117t
oropharyngeal, 1029
perianal, 1268
Melanotrichia, 55, 56, 57–58
Melarsomine, for dirofilariasis, 948–949, 949t, 951t
client information on, 1953
complications with, 952, 952–954, 953
evaluation of, 954
Melatonin, in estrous cycle, 1590
Melena, 126–129, 127t, 128, 1200–1201, 1201t
Melphalan, for multiple myeloma, 505, 518
Menace reaction, in cranial nerve examination, 563, 563, 567t
in vision evaluation, 18
Mendelian disorders, 2, 3, 3t. See also Genetic defects.
Meningioma, 584, 584t, 585t
pleocytosis with, cerebrospinal fluid examination in, 574t
radiotherapy for, 497t
Meningitis, 591, 597
arthritis with, 1882
bacterial, 597, 603–604, 605, 606
cerebrospinal fluid examination in, 574, 574t, 575
noninfectious, multifocal, 606
pilonidal sinus and, 643
spinal, 616–619, 618t
feline infectious peritonitis and, 627
with arteritis, steroid-responsive, 621–622
Meningocele, 1979t
Meningoencephalitis, 627
borna disease virus and, 450–451
cerebrospinal fluid examination in, 574, 574t, 575
granulomatous, 597–598, 628
multifocal, 606
Meniscus, medial, injury of, with cruciate ligament rupture, 1868
Mental status, examination for, in brain disorders, 559, 559t
Meperidine, for pancreatitis, 1353, 1363t
N-2-Mercaptopropionylglycine, for cystine urinary calculi, 1730, 1776, 1776t
6-Mercaptopurine, for arthritis, 1884–1885
Mercury, toxicity of, 362
to peripheral nerves, 673t
Meridians, in acupuncture, 367–369, 368
Mesalamine, for inflammatory bowel disease, 1250
Mesenchymal neoplasia, of skin, cytology of, 55
Mesenteric arteries, occlusion of, 966
Mesostigmata mite infestation, 59t, 61
Mesothelioma, pleural, and effusion, 1108, 1109
Messenger RNA, in steroid receptors, 310
Mestinon (pyridostigmine), for megaesophagus, 1150, 1150t
for myasthenia gravis, 676
Metabolic acidosis, in renal failure, acute, 1624, 1629
chronic, 1640, 1647t, 1652
Metabolic alkalosis, in renal failure, acute, 1624, 1629
Metabolic disorders. See also specific disorders, e.g., Lipidosis.
and anemia, 1810

Metabolic disorders (Continued)
and cachexia, 72–74, 73
and coma, 146t
and growth failure, 75
and obesity, 70, 71, 72
and scaling dermatosis, 48
and skin ulcers, 40t, 42
and syncope, 16
and tremors, 141
and vomiting, 118t, 119, 121
and weakness, 12
congenital, 3t, 4–5
in cats, 1977t
in dogs, 1986t–1987t
of bone, 1905–1909, 1906–1910
of nervous system, 548–550, 549t, 550, 555–556, 607
Metachromatic leukodystrophy, 589, 590t, 1980t
Metaldehyde, toxicity of, 357
Metalloproteinases, in periodontal disease, 1128
in tumor invasion, 482
Metals, toxicity of, 361–363
Metaphyses, disorders of, 1869, 1901–1903, 1902
in bone growth, 1887–1888, 1888
Metastasis, 481–483, 482. See also Cancer.
Metestrus, 1510, 1510–1514, 1514, 1515, 1520–1522
Metformin, for diabetes, 1449–1451
Methanol, toxicity of, 361
Methemalbumin, in pancreatitis, 1352–1353
Methemoglobinemia, 1790–1792, 1791t, 1801t, 1801–1802, 1990t
in cyanosis, 207, 209–210
in naphthalene toxicity, 357
Methimazole, for hyperthyroidism, 1408t, 1409–1411, 1410, 1411t
before surgery, 1412–1413
client information on, 1931
toxicity of, to liver, 1328, 1411
Methionine, in diet, 239t, 240
Methotrexate, for cholangiohepatitis, 1310
for lymphoma, 511t
Methoxamine, in cardiopulmonary resuscitation, 192, 192t
Methylene blue, for hemolytic anemia, 1802
Methylmalonic aciduria, with vitamin B$_{12}$ deficiency, 1706
Methylprednisolone, dosage of, 313t, 314, 314t
for bronchial asthma, 1058
for central nervous system inflammation, 593t
for cerebral edema, 147
traumatic, 579
with seizures, 150t
for eosinophilic granuloma complex, 1118
for inflammatory bowel disease, 1227
for shock, 316
for spinal cord trauma, 315–316, 648–649
maintenance therapy with, 315
potency of, 312, 312t
structure of, 309
4-Methylpyrazole, for ethylene glycol toxicity, 1626t
Methyltestosterone, for libido stimulation, 1597, 1597t
Methysergide challenge test, for Scotty cramp, 588
Metoclopramide, for gastric motility disorders, 1175
for gastroesophageal reflux, 1152
for megaesophagus, 1150–1151
for urine retention, 95t, 96
for vomiting, in gastritis, 1161
in renal failure, acute, 1629, 1630t
chronic, 1648

Metoclopramide (Continued)
in induction of lactation, 1596
with enteral nutrition, 280
Metoprolol, for arrhythmia, 824t, 827, 828t, 830
for tachyarrhythmia, with mitral insufficiency, 794–795
Metritis, 1536–1537, 1596
Metronidazole, for bacterial infection, 391t
with feline immunodeficiency virus infection, 437, 437t
for central nervous system infection, 593t
for gastritis, with lymphocytic-plasmacytic infiltrates, 1163
for giardiasis, of small intestine, 1222
for Helicobacter infection, with gastritis, 1164
for hemobartonellosis, 407
for hepatic encephalopathy, 1333, 1334t
for inflammatory bowel disease, 1250
for intestinal bacterial overgrowth, 1225
with histoplasmosis, 464
with pancreatic exocrine insufficiency, 1363t, 1363–1364
for meningitis, spinal, 618
for protozoal infection, 409–410, 410t
in intestinal bacterial alteration, for portosystemic shunt, 1314, 1315
toxicity of, to central nervous system, 586
Metyrapone, for hyperadrenocorticism, 1486
Mexiletine (Mexitil), for arrhythmia, 824t–826t, 826, 827, 828t
Mibolerone, for pseudopregnancy, 1526
for shortened estrous cycle, 1525, 1560–1562
in contraception, 1544
Miconazole, for Malassezia infection, in otitis externa, 990t, 996
Microcheilia, 1977t, 1986t
Microcornea, 1978t, 1988t
Microcytosis, familial, 1990t
in hemolytic anemia, 1791t, 1792
Microfilariae, in heartworm disease, 937, 937, 938, 938t, 939, 939t. See also Dirofilariasis.
Micronase, for diabetes, 1449
Microphthalmos, 1978t, 1988t
Microsporum infection, and scaling dermatosis, 49
zoonotic, 383t
Microvascular dysplasia, hepatic, 1315–1316, 1991t
Microvillar membrane, damage to, 1197, 1198
Midazolam, in anesthesia, for prepubertal gonadectomy, 1541
Mifepristone, for hyperadrenocorticism, 1482
in abortion induction, 1545
Migrating myoelectric complex, in gastric emptying, 1159
in small intestinal motility, 1190
Milbemycin, for demodicosis, 62, 1970
for dirofilariasis, 950t, 951, 952, 954, 961
for scabies, 51
in prevention of intestinal parasitosis, 1220, 1221, 1221t
Milk, in neonatal nutrition, 241–244, 243t
production of, disorders of, 1538
in pseudopregnancy, 1526
management of, 1596
Milrinone, for cardiomyopathy, 884
for heart failure, 733
Mineralization, pulmonary, 1088
Mineralocorticoids, deficiency of, 1490, 1490, 1496, 1497. See also Hypoadrenocorticism.
Minerals, in diet, 238–239, 239t
Minimum inhibitory concentration, of antibiotics, 303t, 303–305, 304
Minocycline, for bacterial infection, 391t
Miosis. See Pupils.

Misoprostol, for gastrinoma, 1506, 1506t
for stomach ulcers, 1168
in renal failure, 1629, 1630t
with steroid therapy, for hemolytic anemia, 1797
Mistletoe, toxicity of, 364
Mitaban. See Amitraz.
Mite infestation, 59t, 61–62, 62
and crusting, 50–51
and hyperpigmentation, 57, 58
and otitis externa, 989t, 990t, 992–993, 995–996
and pruritus, 32, 33t, 34, 34t, 35, 35
and rhinitis, 1018
and scaling dermatosis, 49
demodectic, client information on, 1970
of pinna, 988, 989t
Mitochondrial inheritance, 3
Mitotane. See o,p′-DDD.
Mitotic inhibitors, in cancer therapy, 488–489
Mitral insufficiency, 787–795
client information on, 1952
complications of, 794–795
differential diagnosis of, 792
echocardiography in, 791–792, 792
electrocardiography in, 790–791
etiology of, 788
management of, 792–794
murmur with, 172, 789–790, 792
pathology of, 787–788, 788–789, 789
physical examination in, 789–790
prevalence of, 787
progression of, 787, 788
radiography in, 790, 791
signs of, 789
Mitral regurgitation, cardiac dilatation in, pericardial restriction of, 924
echocardiography of, 857t, 869–870
in cardiomyopathy, hypertrophic, 902
in heart failure, 706
Mitral stenosis, echocardiography of, 847, 847t, 848, 870
Mitral valve, dysplasia of, auscultation of, 739t
congenital, 774–778, 775–779
echocardiography of, 856t, 857
in blood flow measurement, 843, 845t, 845–846, 861–865, 865t
malformations of, 1976t, 1985t
Mobitz types, of atrioventricular block, 817, 817, 818
Moderator bands, left ventricular, in cardiomyopathy, 913, 913
Monocytic leukemia, 1853, 1854
Monocytosis, 1852, 1852t
Monoethylene glycol. See Ethylene glycol.
Morbillivirus infection, and canine distemper, 418–419, 419t
in cats, 452
Morning glory, toxicity of, 365
Morphine, for anxiety, in heart failure, 733
for pain, 23, 24t, 25
in lung disorders, 1065t
in pulmonary edema, 1065t, 1082
Mosaicism, sexual developmental disorders in, 1582–1583
Mosquitoes, as vectors, of dirofilariasis, 937–939, 937–939
Motilin, 1501
Motility, of large intestine, 1239–1240, 1240t
of small intestine, 1190–1191
disorders of, and diarrhea, 1200, 1200t
of stomach, disorders of, 1174–1176
physiology of, 1158–1159
Motion, detection of, in evaluation of vision, 18
Motor neurons, congenital disorders of, 1992t

Motor neurons (Continued)
in ocular sympathetic tract, 658
in spinal cord disorders, in lesion localization, 612, 614
in spinal segmental reflex testing, in brain disorders, 566–571, 571t
loss of, in developmental disorders, 666–667
Mouth, cancer of, radiotherapy for, 497t, 1117
disorders of, and dysphagia, 114, 114t, 115
dental. See Periodontium and Teeth.
with ptyalism, 108, 109, 110
examination of, in renal disorders, 1601, 1601
in small intestinal disorders, 1205
inflammation of, 1118–1119
plant toxicity and, 364
uremia toxins and, in renal failure, 1629
lesions of, in eosinophilic granuloma complex, 1118, 1118
in renal failure, 1636–1637
pain in, and anorexia, 103
regurgitation into, 114–117, 116, 117t
tumors of, 1114–1116, 1114–1118, 1117t
ulcers in, uremia toxins and, renal disorders and, 42, 1601, 1601, 1629
Moxidectin, in prevention of dirofilariasis, 955
MTH-68, in cancer management, 377
Mucinosis, cutaneous, 1995t
Mucinous hypertrophy, cystic, of gallbladder, 1344
Mucocele, pharyngeal, 1028
salivary, 1119, 1119–1120, 1120
Mucometra, 1591, 1592
Mucomyst (N-acetylcysteine), for acetaminophen toxicity, to liver, 1332
for hemolytic anemia, 1802
Mucopolysaccharidosis, 1979t, 1980t, 1984t
and spinal cord dysfunction, 638–639
genetics in, 3t
leukocyte inclusions in, 1847, 1847
skeletal abnormalities in, 1896–1897
Mucosa, buccal, inflammation of, periodontal disease and, 1129
in gastric physiology, 1157–1158
of large intestine, immune system in, 1239, 1239t
of small intestine, anatomy of, 1183, 1184
disruption of, 1198, 1198t
inflammation of, 1198
pale, in liver disease, 1276
vaginal, in estrous cycle, 1510–1513, 1512–1515
Mucosa-associated lymphoid tissue, function of, 1193–1196, 1194t, 1194–1196
Müllerian ducts, 1581
Multifactorial inheritance, 3–4
Multiple cartilaginous exostoses, 539, 540, 1899, 1901
and spinal cord disorders, 642–643
Multiple myeloma, 505, 516–519, 517, 518
Murmurs, cardiac, 171, 171t, 171–174, 173
in atrial septal defect, 755
in atrioventricular valve dysplasia, 776, 776
in congenital heart disease, 738–739, 739t
in infective endocarditis, 797
in mitral insufficiency, 172, 789–790, 792
in patent ductus arteriosus, 746–747, 747, 749
in pulmonic stenosis, 761
in subaortic stenosis, 769–770
in ventricular septal defect, 756
with hypertension, in renal failure, 1638
with pectus excavatum, 1101
Muscle(s), atrophy of, in spinal cord disorders, 611
disorders of, congenital, 1980t

IND

Muscle(s) (Continued)
   paraneoplastic, 506, 506t
   renal failure and, 1639
   skeletal, atrophy of, in heart failure, 701–703
      disorders of, 685–689, 686t
      physiology of, 684–685, 685t
   tone of, in spinal cord disorders, 611, 613, 614
   weakness of, 10–13, 11t
      in brain disorders, 560–561
      in diabetes, 1442, *1442*
      in hyperthyroidism, 1401
Muscular dystrophy, 688–689
   X-linked, 3t, 688, 1980t
Musculocutaneous nerve, injury to, signs of, 663t
Mushrooms, toxicity of, 364, 365
   to liver, 1329, 1332
Mutations. See *Genetic defects.*
Mutilation, acral, 669, 1994t
Myasthenia gravis, 675–676, 1980t
   and megaesophagus, 1149, 1150, 1150t
   with hypothyroidism, 1421–1422
Mycobacterial infection, 391t, 393–394
   and enteritis, 1219
   of lung, 1065–1066
Mycobacterium lepraemurium infection, 393, 394
Mycobacterium marinum infection, zoonotic, 384t
Mycoplasma infection, and arthritis, 1878
Mycosis, 453–475. See also *Fungal infection.*
Mycosis fungoides, 508, *508*
Mycotoxins, and tremor, 598–599
Mydriasis. See *Pupils.*
Myectomy, for cardiomyopathy, hypertrophic, 890
Myelin, disorders of, and tremor, 140–141
   congenital, 588, 1991t, 1992t
   in peripheral nerves, 662, *662,* 665–666
      loss of, 674
   in spinal cord, loss of, in globoid cell leuko-dystrophy, 627–628
      in leukoencephalomyelopathy, 636
Myelitis, distemper and, 626–627
   feline infectious peritonitis and, 627
   in feline polioencephalomyelitis, 598, 627
   pilonidal sinus and, 643
   with infectious meningitis, 616
Myeloblastic leukemia, 1853
Myelodysplasia, 639, 1854
   and anemia, 1814, *1815*
   congenital, 1992t
Myelofibrosis, and anemia, 1813–1814, *1814*
Myelogenous leukemia, 515t, 515–516
Myelography, 610
   in atlantoaxial subluxation, 615, *616*
   in calcinosis circumscripta, 619, *619*
   in intervertebral disk herniation, 632–633
   in spinal neoplasia, 641
   in spondylomyelopathy, cervical, 620
Myeloid leukemia, *1853,* 1853–1854, *1854*
Myeloma, and bone infiltration, 1912
   multiple, 505, 516–519, *517, 518*
Myelomalacia, hemorrhagic, progressive, 643–644, 648
Myelomonocytic leukemia, 1853, *1853*
Myelopathy, degenerative, 622–623
   in Afghan hound, 1991t
Myeloproliferative disorders, 515–516
   and platelet disorders, 1823
Myelosuppression, chemotherapy and, 485t, 485–487, *486*
Myocarditis, 914
   parvovirus and, 420

Myocarditis (Continued)
   viral, cardiomyopathy after, 877
Myocardium. See also *Heart.*
   contractility of, in heart failure, 708
   digitalis toxicity to, 729–730
   failure of, 694, *694*
   hypertrophy of, in heart failure, 703–705, 704t
      pressure overload and, 694, *696*
   myopathy of. See also *Cardiomyopathy.*
      in cat, 896–918
      in dog, 874–891
Myoclonus, distemper and, 626
Myoelectric complex, migrating, in gastric emptying, 1159
   in small intestinal motility, 1190
Myofibers, in skeletal muscle, 684, 685t
Myoglobinuria, 96, *98, 99*
Myosin, slow, in heart failure, 704t, 705
Myositis, 686t, 686–687
Myotomy, Heller's, for megaesophagus, 1151
Myotonia, non-dystrophic, 689
Myristica fragrans, toxicity of, 365
Myxedema, 1421, 1422, 1426
Myxomatous degeneration, of mitral valve, and chronic valvular insufficiency, 787–788, *789*

Naloxone, for septic shock, 184t
   in cardiopulmonary resuscitation, 192, 192t
Nanophyetus salmonicola infestation, of small intestine, and diarrhea, 406, 1219
Naphthalene, toxicity of, 357
   and hemolytic anemia, 1802
Narcolepsy, 155
   congenital, 1980t, 1992t
Narcotics, for pain, 23, 24, 24t
Nares, agenesis of, 1981t
   congenital stenosis of, 1994t
Nasal cavity, anatomy of, 1003, *1003, 1004*
   aspergillosis of, *473,* 473–474
   bleeding from, diagnosis of, 213–216, 214t, *216*
      pathophysiology of, 213
      treatment of, *216,* 216–217
   computed tomography of, 1009–1012, *1011–1015,* 1022, 1023, *1023*
   cryptococcosis of, *469,* 469–470
   diagnostic sampling from, 1038
   discharge from, 194t, 194–197, *195, 196,* 197t
   disorders of, and dyspnea, 167t, 169
      diagnostic approach to, 1003–1004
   examination of, access for, caudal, 1016
      dorsal, 1016–1017
      rostral, 1013–1016
      ventral, 1017–1018
   fistula to, tooth loss and, 1129
   hypopigmentation of, acquired idiopathic, 55, 57
   inflammation of, 1018–1019
   intubation of, for enteral nutrition, 275–276, *276*
   magnetic resonance imaging of, 1012–1013, *1016*
   radiography of, 1005–1009, *1006–1008, 1010*
   regurgitation into, 114–117, *116,* 117t
   tumors of, 1019–1023, *1021, 1023*
      radiotherapy for, 497t, 1021–1023, *1023*
Nasal sinuses, anatomy of, 1003, *1003, 1004*
   disorders of, and gagging, 111, 112t, *113*
   dorsal access to, 1016–1017
   tumors of, 1021–1023, *1023*
      radiotherapy for, 497t
Nasopharynx, intubation of, client information on, 1945

Natriuretic peptides, in heart failure, 701
Naturopathic medicine, in cancer management, 376–377
Nausea, 117. See also *Vomiting.*
Near drowning, and lung disorders, 1086–1087
Necrolysis, toxic epidermal, 29
Necrolytic dermatitis, superficial, and pruritus, 33t
   liver disease and, 28, 1272, 1337
Necrolytic migratory erythema, 51
   glucagonoma and, *1507,* 1507–1508
Necrotizing fasciitis, streptococcus and, 396
Necrotizing vasculitis, microscopic, 973
Nemaline myopathy, 689, 1980t
Neomycin, dosage of, in renal failure, 1649t
   for hepatic encephalopathy, 1333, 1334t
   for otitis externa, 990t, 995
   in intestinal bacterial alteration, for portosys-temic shunt, 1314, 1315
Neonate, adverse drug reactions in, 322–323
   congenital disorders in, in cats, 1975t–1982t
      in dogs, 1983t–1996t
   diet for, 241–244, 243t
   hemolytic anemia in, alloimmune, 1797–1798
   kernicterus in, 211
   streptococcosis in, 395–396
   temperature measurement in, 242–244
Neoplasia. See *Tumors* and specific types, e.g., *Sarcoma.*
Neorickettsia infection, and salmon-poisoning disease, 406, 1219
Neosporosis, and encephalitis, 596–597
   and fetal loss, 1527–1528
   and myositis, 687, 688
   of nervous system, multifocal, 606
   of spinal cord, 644–645
   polysystemic, 413
Neostigmine, for myasthenia gravis, 676
Nephritis. See also *Glomerulonephritis.*
   and polyuria, 87, 87t
   hyperadrenocorticism and, 1482
Nephrotic syndrome, and hyperlipidemia, 290
Nerium oleander, toxicity of, 365
Nerve sheath tumors, malignant, spinal, 640
   peripheral, 677–678
Nervous system, 547–689. See also specific structures, e.g., *Facial nerve.*
   central. See also *Brain* and *Spinal cord.*
      antibiotic penetration of, 301
      disorders of, and fecal incontinence, 1268t, 1268–1269
         and vomiting, *118,* 118–119
         in blastomycosis, 459, *459*
         in cryptococcosis, 469
         in hypernatremia, 230, 232
         in spongiform encephalopathy, 451, 599, 1980t
         morbillivirus and, in cats, 452
         pituitary tumors and, with hyperadreno-corticism, 1484t, 1484–1485
      feline immunodeficiency virus in, 434–436, *436*
      glucose consumption in, 1430
      hypomyelination of, genetics in, 3t
      in coma, 144–147, *145,* 145t, 146t
      in polyphagia, 104–105, 107
      in seizures, 148–152. See also *Seizures.*
      in sleep disorders, 152–155, *153*
      in stupor, 144–147, *145,* 146t
      lymphoma of, 512, 584t
   disorders of, and arthropathy, 1868
      and ataxia, 142–143
      and fecal incontinence, 133, 134t
      and megaesophagus, 1150t
      and regurgitation, 115, 117t

Nervous system *(Continued)*
    and tremors, 139–141, *140,* 606–607
    and weakness, 12
    anoxia and, 586
    as signs of systemic disease, 548–551, 549t, *550*
    congenital, in cats, 1979t–1980t
      in dogs, 1991t–1993t
    degenerative, 607
    diabetes and, 1458
    in constipation, 129, 130, 130t, *131*
    in hypothyroidism, 1421–1422
    in renal failure, 1624
    lead toxicity and, 361–362, 586
    paraneoplastic, 506, 506t
    pupillary examination in, 657–661, *658, 659t,* 660t, *661*
    rabies and, 419t, 422–423, 449–450, 594–595
    in heart failure, compensatory mechanisms in, 699–701, 700t
    in pain perception, 20–21
    in pruritus, 31–32
    inflammation of. See also *Meningitis* and *Meningoencephalitis.*
      borna disease virus and, 450–451
      multifocal, 603–606, 604t, *605, 606*
    metabolic disease of, 607
    peripheral, disorders of, 662–681
      and fecal incontinence, 1268, 1268t, 1269
      developmental, 666–671
      evaluation of, 662–665, 663t, 664t
      hypothyroidism and, 671–672
      in acquired demyelinating neuropathy, 674
      in botulism, 672
      in brachial plexus neuritis, 674–675
      in chronic relapsing neuropathy, 674
      in dancing Doberman disease, 679–680
      in diabetes mellitus, 671
      in distal denervating disease, 679
      in distal symmetric polyneuropathy, 679
      in dysautonomia, 680
      in myasthenia gravis, 675–676
      in paraneoplastic syndromes, 677–678
      in polyradiculoneuritis, 673–674
      in renal failure, 1638t, 1638–1639
      in sensory ganglioneuritis, 675
      in tick paralysis, 672–673
      mechanisms of, 665–666
      toxic, 673, 673t
      vascular disorders and, 678–679
    inflammation of, idiopathic, facial, 680–681
      trigeminal, 680
    structure of, 662, *662*
    trauma to, 678
    tumors of, 676–677
    vestibular dysfunction in, idiopathic, 681
    toxicity to, 607
      plants and, 365
    tumors of, 556, 607
    vascular disease of, 607
Nettles, toxicity of, 365
Neupogen. See *Granulocyte colony-stimulating factor.*
Neural tube, closure of, defects of, 1979t, 1980t, 1991t
Neuralgia, glossopharyngeal, 1029
Neurilemoma, 677
Neurinoma, 677
Neuritis, facial, idiopathic, 680–681
    of brachial plexus, 674–675
    optic, and anisocoria, 660t
    trigeminal, idiopathic, 680
Neuroaxonal dystrophy, 589, 642, 1980t, 1992t

Neuroblastoma, peripheral, 677
Neurofibroma, 677
Neurofibrosarcoma, 677
Neuroma, after tail docking, and pruritus, 33t
Neuromuscular junction, disorders of, and regurgitation, 115, 117t
    paraneoplastic, 506, 506t
Neuronopathy, progressive, in cairn terrier, 666, 1992t
Neurons, congenital disorders of, 1992t
Neurotensin, 1501–1502
Neurotoxins, endogenous, 549t, 550–551
Neutering. See *Sterilization.*
Neutropenia, 1848t, 1848–1849
    chemotherapy and, 485–486, *486*
Neutrophilia, 1842–1844, *1844,* 1844t, *1845*
    estrogen-induced myelotoxicity and, 1849, *1849*
    in pyometra, with cystic endometrial hyperplasia, 1550
Neutrophils, granulation of, anomalous, 1847t, 1978t
    hypersegmentation of, 1845–1846
    in gastritis, 1160
    in inflammation, 1844–1845, *1845*
    in inflammatory bowel disease, 1249
    in skin lesions, in cytology, 53
    in stress leukogram, 1844
    in synovial fluid, in joint inflammation, 79, 80
    inclusions in, 1846–1848, *1846–1848*
    inherited defects of, *1849,* 1849–1850
    morphologic abnormalities of, 1845, *1845*
    pools of, 1842, *1843*
    production of, 1842
    transfusion of, 351
Nevi, 36, 1982t, 1995t
Newborn. See *Neonate.*
Niacin, in diet, 239t, 239–240
Niclosamide, for intestinal parasitosis, 1221t
Nicotine, toxicity of, 357, 365
Nictitating membrane, protrusion of, systemic disease and, 984
Niemann-Pick disease, and peripheral neuropathy, 670–671
Nifedipine, for arrhythmia, 830, 831
Nifurtimox, for trypanosomiasis, 410t, 416
Nightshade, toxicity of, 364
Nitrates, for heart failure, 724–726
Nitric oxide, in heart failure, 701
Nitrofurantoin, dosage of, in renal failure, 1649t
Nitrogen, in dietary protein, 237
    metabolism of, disorders of, and aminoaciduria, 1704–1705
      and uricaciduria, 1705–1706
      and xanthinuria, 1706
    urea. See *Urea nitrogen.*
Nitroglycerin, for heart failure, 724–725
Nitroprusside, for cardiomyopathy, dilated, 884
    for heart failure, 725–726
      with mitral insufficiency, 794
Nitroscanate, for intestinal parasitosis, 1221t
Nizatidine, for gastric motility disorders, 1176
    for gastric ulcers, 1168
    for gastrinoma, 1506, 1506t
Nizoral. See *Ketoconazole.*
Nocardiosis, 391t, 395
    and meningitis, spinal, 616
Nociception, 20–21. See also *Pain.*
Nocturia, 89, 90
    in renal failure, 1637
Nodular dermatofibrosis syndrome, 28
Nodular hyperplasia, adrenocortical, and hyperadrenocorticism, 1461–1462
    of liver, 1319–1320
Nodular panniculitis, sterile, 36, 37

Nodules, in histiocytosis, 36
    of pinna, 987t, 991–992
Nolvasan (chlorhexidine), for anal sacculitis, 1266
    for oral disorders, with renal failure, 1629, 1630t
    for otitis externa, 989t, 994
Nonsteroidal anti-inflammatory drugs, and stomach ulcers, 1165–1166
    for degenerative joint disease, 1865–1866
    for fever, 9
    for pain, 24, 24t, 25
Norepinephrine, for hypotension, 184t
Normosol-R, in fluid therapy, 328, 329t, 330t
Norpace, for arrhythmia, 825, 825t, 826t, 828t
Norvasc (amlodipine), for arrhythmia, 824t, 830, 831
    for hypertension, 182
    in renal failure, 1653–1654
Norwegian Forest cat, glycogen storage disease in, 671
Nose, 1003–1023. See also *Nasal cavity.*
Nostrils, agenesis of, 1981t
    congenital stenosis of, 1994t
Notoedres cati infestation, 59t, 61
    of pinna, 988, 989t
Novartis (desoxycorticosterone), for hypoadrenocorticism, 1496–1498
    after adrenalectomy, 1487
NPH insulin, for diabetes mellitus, 1451–1452
Nuclear transcription factors, genetic defects of, and cardiomyopathy, 877
    in carcinogenesis, 478, 479t
Nucleus pulposus. See *Disks, intervertebral.*
Nutmeg, toxicity of, 365
Nutrition. See *Diet.*
Nymphomania, 1595
Nyquist limit, in echocardiography, 841, *842*
Nystagmus, congenital, 1978t
    in cranial nerve examination, 565, 567t
Nystatin, for otitis externa, 990t, 995

Obesity, 70–72, *71*
    after prepubertal gonadectomy, 70, 1540
    and pulmonary disorders, 1088
    in heart disease, 71, 266
Obturator muscle, transfer of, in perineal herniorrhaphy, 1260
Obturator nerve, injury to, signs of, 663t
Occlusion, dental, *1123–1126,* 1124–1126
Octreotide, for gastrinoma, 1506, 1506t
    for pancreatic islet cell tumors, 1434t, 1435t, 1437, *1437*
Oculomotor nerve, anatomy of, 664t
    examination of, 562–565, *564,* 567t
    palsy of, and anisocoria, 660t
Odontoid process, in atlantoaxial subluxation, *615,* 615–616, *616,* 1984t
Odontoma, 1114
Oleander, toxicity of, 365
Olfactory function, 562
    impaired, and anorexia, 103
Olfactory nerve, anatomy of, 664t
Oligodendroglioma, 584t, 585t
Oligodontia, 1122
Oligozoospermia, 1579
Oliguria, in renal failure, 1623
Ollulanus tricuspis infestation, and gastritis, 1164–1165
Omega-3 fatty acids, in fish oil, for hyperlipidemia, 289
    for renal failure, 1646–1647, 1647t, 1658
Omeprazole, for esophagitis, 1148, 1149

Omeprazole (Continued)
with megaesophagus, 1150t
for gastric ulcers, 1168
in renal failure, 1629, 1630t
for gastrinoma, 1506, 1506t
for gastroesophageal reflux, 1152
for Helicobacter infection, with gastritis, 1164
Oncogenes, in carcinogenesis, 478, 479t
Oncovin. See Vincristine.
Onions, toxicity of, and Heinz body anemia, 1801
o,p'-DDD, for hyperadrenocorticism, client information on, 1929
in cats, 1486
in long-term therapy, 1481
monitoring of, 1470
overdose of, 1481
pituitary-dependent, 1476–1479, 1477, 1479, 1480
with adrenal tumors, 1479–1480
Ophthalmoplegia, and anisocoria, 661
Opioids, in gastrointestinal endocrine system, 1502
Opisthorchis felineus infestation, of pancreas, 1363t, 1364
Optic nerve, anatomy of, 664t
congenital defects of, 1978t, 1988t
disorders of, and vision loss, 17, 18t
edema of, brain tumors and, 585
examination of, 562–564, 563, 564, 567t
in pupillary light reflex, 658, 658
inflammation of, and anisocoria, 660t
systemic disease and, 985, 986t
Oral tolerance, in small intestinal immune response, 1196
Orbifloxacin, concentration of, and clinical outcome, 304–305
Orbit, forward eye displacement in, systemic disease and, 984
Orchiectomy. See Sterilization.
Orchitis, 1594
Organochlorine insecticides, toxicity of, 357–359
Organophosphates, toxicity of, 359
and megaesophagus, 1150t
to peripheral nerves, 673t
Ormetroprim/sulfadimethoxine, for staphylococcal pyoderma, 46t
Oronasal fistula, tooth loss and, 1129
Orthopnea, 166
Os penis, congenital deformity of, 1981t, 1994t
Oscillometry, in blood pressure measurement, 184–185
Oslerus osleri infestation, of trachea, 1038t, 1044, 1044–1045
Osmotic pressure, 327–328, 328
Ossification, of dura mater, and spinal cord compression, 627
Osteoarthritis, 1862–1866, 1863, 1863t, 1864
Osteochondritis dissecans, 1869
of medial condyle of humerus, 1871–1872
Osteochondrodysplasia, and dwarfism, 1897–1898, 1899t, 1900
Osteochondroma, congenital, 1983t
Osteochondromatosis, 539, 540, 1899, 1901
and spinal cord disorders, 642–643
Osteochondrosarcoma, 1912
multilobular, 538
Osteochondrosis, 1869–1870, 1870
nutrition in, 245–250, 246, 249t, 250
Osteodystrophy, anticonvulsants and, 1908
hepatic, 1908
hypertrophic, 1901–1903, 1902
in hyperparathyroidism, with hyperphosphatemia, in renal failure, 1642, 1642–1643
renal, 1907

Osteogenesis imperfecta, 1896
Osteoma, 539
Osteomyelitis, 1912–1914, 1913, 1914
aspergillosis and, 474
blastomycosis and, 459
periodontal disease and, 1129
vertebral, and spinal cord dysfunction, 624–626, 625, 626
Osteopathy, craniomandibular, 1898, 1900, 1901, 1983t
hypertrophic, metaphyseal, 1901–1903, 1902
paraneoplastic, 503, 503
secondary, 1903, 1903–1904
with pulmonary neoplasia, 1073–1074
Osteopetrosis, 1896
Osteophytes, in spondylosis deformans, 650–652, 651
Osteoporosis, congenital, 1975t, 1984t
Osteosarcoma, client information on, 1925
in cats, 539–540, 1912
in dogs, 536–537, 1910, 1910–1911
Osteosclerosis, and anemia, 1813
Oti-Cleans, for otitis externa, 989t, 994, 996
Otitis externa, 992–994
client information on, 1974
management of, 989t, 990t, 994–997
Otitis interna, 999
Otitis media, 990t, 997–999
Otodectes mite infestation, 59t, 61
and otitis externa, 989t, 990t, 992
and pruritus, 34t
Otomax, for otitis externa, 990t, 995, 996
Ovaban. See Megestrol acetate.
Ovaries, agenesis of, 1981t
anatomy of, 1586
cysts of, and anestrus, 1525
and infertility, 1562, 1562, 1564–1565
follicular, and prolonged estrus, 1521, 1523, 1523–1524, 1524
hypoplasia of, 1981t
in estrous cycle, 1510, 1511
premature failure of, 1525
remnant tissue from, after sterilization, 1596
tumors of, 544–545
and infertility, 1562
and prolonged estrus, 1523, 1523, 1524
Ovariohysterectomy, and obesity, 70
for pyometra, with cystic endometrial hyperplasia, 1551–1553
in pregnancy prevention, 1542, 1542–1543
prepubertal, 1539–1541
stump granuloma after, 1567, 1569
stump pyometra after, 1551, 1553
Overactivity, and weakness, 12–13
Overweight, 70–72, 71
after prepubertal gonadectomy, 70, 1540
and pulmonary disorders, 1088
in heart disease, 71, 266
Oviducts, anatomy of, 1586
obstruction of, and infertility, 1559
Ovulation, 1510, 1510, 1511, 1514, 1587–1588
failure of, management of, 1562
induction of, 1595
Oxacillin, concentration of, and bacterial susceptibility, 303t
for central nervous system infection, 593t
for staphylococcal pyoderma, 46t
Oxalate, in plants, toxicity of, 364
in urolithiasis, in cats, 1723t, 1725t, 1725–1728, 1732
in dogs, 1758t, 1763–1764
urine level of, increased, primary, 1996t
with peripheral neuropathy, 670
Oxfendazole, for intestinal parasitosis, 1221t
Oxibendazole, in prevention of intestinal parasitosis, 1221t

Oxibendazole (Continued)
toxicity of, to liver, 1307–1308
Oxtriphylline, for cough, 165t
Oxybutinin, for bladder dysfunction, 1739t
Oxygen, blood level of, assessment of, 1038–1039, 1039
in congenital heart disease, measurement of, catheterization for, 743
in cyanosis, 206–210. See also Cyanosis.
in polycythemia, 203–205
deprivation of, in brain, trauma and, 579
neurologic signs of, 548–549, 549t, 586
in cardiopulmonary resuscitation, 190
in therapy, for heart failure, 733
for lung disorders, 1061–1062, 1062
for smoke inhalation, 1087
Oxymorphone, in anesthesia, for liver biopsy, 1296t
for prepubertal gonadectomy, 1541
in sedation, for gastric decompression, for dilatation, with volvulus, 1173
Oxypolygelatin, in fluid therapy, 329t, 329–332, 331t, 332t
Oxytetracycline, for bacterial infection, with feline immunodeficiency virus infection, 437t
for ehrlichiosis, 404
for intestinal bacterial overgrowth, 1225
with pancreatic exocrine insufficiency, 1363t, 1363–1364
Oxytocin, for dystocia, client information on, 1936
for placental retention, 1596
for uterine inertia, in dystocia, 1532, 1596

P wave, 804. See also Electrocardiography.
Pacemaker, for arrhythmia, 832t, 832–833
wandering, electrocardiography of, 810, 811
Paclitaxel, in cancer management, 378t
Pain, assessment of, 21, 21–23
management of, 23–25, 24t, 25t
over-the-counter drugs in, 318
oral, and anorexia, 103
pathophysiology of, 20–21
perception of, in neurologic examination, 568–571, 570–572, 571t
in spinal cord disorders, 612
Palate, cleft, 1976t, 1985t
soft, elongated, 1027, 1985t
Palm, cycad, toxicity of, to liver, 1329
Palpebral reflex, in cranial nerve examination, 565, 565–566, 567t
Panacur. See Fenbendazole.
Panalog, for otitis externa, 990t, 995
Pancreas, anatomy of, 1345, 1345
disorders of, skin lesions with, 28
exocrine insufficiency of, and diarrhea, 122–123, 125, 1359
and malabsorption, 1208, 1358
diagnosis of, 1358–1361, 1360, 1361
etiology of, 1355, 1355–1356
pathophysiology of, 1356, 1356–1358, 1357
prognosis of, 1364
treatment of, 1361–1364, 1363t
with polyphagia, 105–107
fluke infestation of, 1363t, 1364
hypoplasia of, 1991t
inflammation of, 1347–1355. See also Pancreatitis.
islet cells of, in diabetes, 1438–1441, 1439, 1440. See also Diabetes mellitus.
tumors of, and gastrin hypersecretion, 1503–1506, 1505t, 1506t

Pancreas *(Continued)*
    and insulin secretion, 1429–1438. See also *Insulinoma.*
    and pancreatic peptide hypersecretion, 1506–1507
    physiology of, 1345t, 1345–1347, *1346, 1346t, 1347*
    tumors of, 1364
       and glucagon hypersecretion, *1507*, 1507–1508
Pancreatic polypeptide, 1502, 1503
    hypersecretion of, islet cell tumor and, 1506–1507
Pancreatin, for pancreatic exocrine insufficiency, 1361–1362, 1363t
Pancreatitis, 1347–1355
    and diarrhea, 1254
    and exocrine insufficiency, 1355
    and hypocalcemia, vs. hypoparathyroidism, 1394
    client information on, 1948
    diagnosis of, 1350–1353, *1351, 1352,* 1353t
    etiology of, 1349–1350
    hyperlipidemia in, 289, 1349
    liver enzymes in, 1284
    pathophysiology of, 1347–1349, *1348,* 1348t, *1349,* 1349t
    prognosis of, 1354–1355
    treatment of, 1353–1354, 1363t
    with hyperadrenocorticism, 1465, 1483
Pancreazyme, for pancreatic exocrine insufficiency, 1361–1362, 1363t
Pancytopenia, in aplastic anemia, 1812–1813
    estrogen therapy and, 1822
Panleukopenia, parvovirus infection and, 444–446
    with aplastic anemia, 1813
Panniculitis, nodular, sterile, 36, 37
Panniculus reflex, testing of, 568–570
Panosteitis, congenital, 1984t
Pansteatitis, 28–29
Pantothenic acid, in diet, 239t
Papilloma, of skin, 525
    oral, 1114, *1114*
Papillomavirus infection, and cervical cancer, 481
Papules, 44, 46
    of pinna, 987t, 991–992
Paracentesis, of salivary mucocele, 1119, *1120*
Paragonimus kellicotti infestation, of lung, 1065t, 1068–1070, *1069*
    cysts in, 1083–1084
Parainfluenza virus infection, and tracheobronchitis, 419t, 419–420
    of nervous system, 604–605
Paralysis, in spinal cord disorders, 611
    in lesion localization, 613–615
    of diaphragm, 1100
    partial, with ataxia, 142, 143
    periodic, with hypokalemia, 225
    tick bites and, 672–673
Paramyxovirus infection, and thrombocytopenia, 1821
Paranasal sinuses. See *Nasal sinuses.*
Paraneoplastic syndromes, 498–506. See also *Cancer.*
Paraphimosis, 1594
Paraplegia, spinal cord disorders and, 611
Parapoxvirus ovis, PIND-ORF derivative of, for feline leukemia virus infection, 431
Paraprostatic cysts, 1693–1694
Paraquat, toxicity of, 363
Parasitosis. See also specific infestations, e.g., *Leishmaniasis.*
    and anemia, 199, 200t, 1787

Parasitosis *(Continued)*
    and aortic aneurysm, 968, *969*
    and arthritis, 1878–1879
    and cough, 163t
    and diarrhea, 123, *124,* 126
    and gastritis, 1164–1165
    and myositis, 687
    and rhinitis, 1018
       with epistaxis, 215
    client information on, 1970, 1971
    leukocyte inclusions in, 1846, *1846*
    of biliary tract, 1343
    of central nervous system, 582
    of large intestine, 1241, *1245,* 1245–1246, *1246*
    of lung, 1068–1071, *1069*
       cysts in, 1083–1084
    of pancreas, 1363t, 1364
    of skin, 42, 58–62, 59t, *60, 62*
    of small intestine, 1219–1221, 1221t
       and diarrhea, acute, 1214
       fecal examination for, 1206, *1206,* 1207, *1207*
    of spinal cord, 647
    of urinary tract, 1741, 1779t
    systemic, skin lesions with, 28
    urinalysis in, 1606t, 1610
    zoonotic, 383t, 386–389
Parasystole, ventricular, 816, *817*
Parathyroid glands, hyperfunction of, 1379–1392. See also *Hyperparathyroidism.*
    hyperplasia of, primary, 1987t
    hypofunction of, 1392–1399. See also *Hypoparathyroidism.*
Parenteral nutrition, 281–282, 282t
    in cancer cachexia, 500–501
    in hepatic lipidosis, client information on, 1944
    patient selection for, 275
Paresis, with ataxia, 142, 143
Parlodel. See *Bromocriptine.*
Paromomycin, for cryptosporidiosis, 410, 410t, 1222
Paroplatin. See *Carboplatin.*
Parotid glands, congenital enlargement of, 1986t
    disorders of, 1119–1120
Paroxetine, for behavioral disorders, in cats, 160, 160t
    in dogs, 156, 158t
Parturition, behavioral disorders after, 1538–1539
    client information on, 1935, 1936
    completion of, 1530
    disorders of, 1530–1536, 1596. See also *Dystocia.*
    in cat, 1588, 1596
    interval between births in, 1530
    litter size in, 1528
    physiology of, 1528–1529
    puppy loss after, 1536
    signs of, 1529
    stages of, 1529–1530
    tetany after, 1394–1396, 1538
    uterine disorders after, 1536–1538, *1537*
Parvaquone, for protozoal infection, 410t
Parvovirus infection, and anemia, aplastic, 1813
    and encephalitis, 596
    and enteritis, 1215–1216
    canine, 419t, 420–422
    client information on, 1958
    feline, 444–446
    of nervous system, 604–605
Parvus et tardus pulse, 174, *175,* 177
Pasteurella infection, and meningitis, spinal, 616
    of skin, antibiotics for, 305

Pasteurella infection *(Continued)*
    zoonotic, 384t
Pasteurella multocida infection, and skin abscess, 399
Patella, luxation of, 1873
    congenital, 1975t, 1984t
Patellar reflex, testing of, 568, *570,* 571t
Patent ductus arteriosus, 745–750, *746–752,* 1976t, 1985t
    blood pressure in, echocardiographic measurement of, 847, 847t
    client information on, 1951
    clinical findings in, 746–749, *747–751*
    echocardiography of, pulsed-wave, *844*
    management of, 749–750, *752*
    murmur with, 172
    pathogenesis of, 745, *746*
    pathophysiology of, 745–746, *746*
Patent foramen ovale, 751
Pau d'Arco, in cancer management, 378t
Paxil (paroxetine), for behavioral disorders, in cats, 160, 160t
    in dogs, 156, 158t
Peace lily, toxicity of, 364
Pectus carinatum, 1100, 1101
Pectus excavatum, *1100,* 1100–1101, *1101,* 1975t
Pediculosis, of skin, 59t, 60, *60*
    and pruritus, 33t
Pelger-Huët anomaly, 1849, *1849,* 1979t, 1990t
Pellicle, 1127
Pelvic canal, narrow, and dystocia, 1534
Pelvic diaphragm, perineal hernia through, 1259–1260
Pelvic limb, reflexes of, testing of, 568, *569, 570,* 571t
Pelvic plexus, injury to, signs of, 663t
Pemphigus foliaceus, 51
    and pruritus, 34t
Penicillamine, for cystine urinary calculi, 1776–1777
    for hepatic copper accumulation, 1301, 1303t, 1306
    for lead toxicity, 362
Penicillin, concentration of, and clinical outcome, 304
    dosage of, in renal failure, 1649t
    for bacterial infection, 391t
    for central nervous system infection, 593t
    for meningitis, spinal, 618
    for mushroom toxicity, to liver, 1332
    hypersensitivity to, 324
    in artificial insemination, 1574
Penis, anatomy of, 1586
    disorders of, 1594
       congenital, 1981t, 1994t
       with preputial discharge, 83, 84, 84t
    frenulum of, persistent, 1594, 1994t
Pentamidine isethionate, for *Pneumocystis carinii* infection, of lung, 1066
Pentastarch, in fluid therapy, 329, 329t, 330, 331t, 333–334
Pentatrichomonas hominis infection, of large intestine, 1245
    of small intestine, 408–411, 409t, 410t
Pentobarbital, for seizures, 151t
    for strychnine toxicity, 360
    overdose of, acupuncture for, 372, *372*
Pentosan polysulfate sodium, for urinary tract disorders, idiopathic, 1745–1746
Pentosuria, 1704
Pentoxifylline, for dermatomyositis, 26
Pepcid. See *Famotidine.*
Pepsin, in gastric physiology, 1158
Pepsinogens, in gastric physiology, 1158

IND

Peptide histidine-isoleucine, 1502
Peptide YY, 1502
Pepto-Bismol (bismuth subsalicylate), for diarrhea, 318–319
    for *Helicobacter* infection, with gastritis, 1164
Percorten-V (desoxycorticosterone), for hypoadrenocorticism, 1496–1498
    after adrenalectomy, 1487
Perfusion, deficit of, fluid therapy for, 335–337, *336,* 338t–339t
    mismatch of, with ventilation, pulmonary thromboembolism and, 1078, 1079
Perianal fistula, 1264–1266
Perianal gland, cancer of, radiotherapy for, 497t
Perianal tumors, 1267–1268
Pericardiectomy, for effusion, 932–933
Pericardiocentesis, for effusion, 931–932, *933*
Pericardium, anatomy of, 923–924
    congenital defects of, 925–927, *927*
    constrictive disease of, diagnosis of, 933–935
        pathophysiology of, 925, *926*
        treatment of, *934,* 935
    cysts of, congenital, 927–928
    disorders of, 923, 924t
        in cats, *934, 935,* 935–936
    effusion in, diagnosis of, 928–931, *929–933*
        echocardiography of, 857t, *935,* 935–936
        management of, 931–933, *933*
        pathophysiology of, 924–925, *926*
    function of, 924
    mass lesions in, 925
    peritoneal communication with, through diaphragmatic hernia, 784, 1099, *1099*
        congenital, 925–927, *927, 935,* 936, 1975t, 1983t
Perineal hernia, 1259–1260
Perineal reflexes, testing of, 568, *570,* 571t
Periodontal ligament, anatomy of, 1127, *1127*
Periodontium, anatomy of, 1127, *1127*
    care of, terminology in, 1127
    disease of, antimicrobial therapy for, 1132–1133
        client information on, 1940
        complications of, 1128–1129
        pathobiology of, 1128
        prevention of, 1130–1134, *1134*
        signs of, 1129t, 1129–1130, *1129–1131,* 1130t
        systemic diseases with, 1128
Periosteal proliferative arthritis, 1880–1881
Periostitis, polyostotic, 1903
Peripheral nerve disorders, 662–681. See also *Nervous system, peripheral.*
Peritoneal dialysis, for renal failure, acute, 1631t, 1631–1632
    chronic, 1646
    in pancreatitis, 1354
Peritoneopericardial hernia, 784, 1099, *1099*
    congenital, 925–927, *927, 935,* 936, 1975t, 1983t
Peritonitis, 137–139, *138*
    feline infectious, 438–443, 440t, *442*
        and encephalitis, 596
        and enteritis, 1217
        and neurologic disorders, 605
        and pericardial disease, *934,* 935
        and pleural effusion, 440t, 440–441, 1102, 1103, 1105t, 1107
        and pulmonary disease, 1063
        and spinal cord inflammation, 627
        cerebrospinal fluid examination in, 574t, 575
        diagnosis of, 440t, 440–441
        epidemiology of, 441–442, *442*
        pathogenesis of, 439

Peritonitis *(Continued)*
        prevention of, 442–443
        signs of, 439–440
        treatment of, 441
Periuria, 1716–1718, 1717t
Permethrin, in flea control, client information on, 1971
Peromelus ascelus, 1975t
Peroneal nerve, injury to, 663t
Persian cat, polycystic kidneys in, 1699t, 1702
Pertussin (dextromethorphan), for cough, 165t, 319
    in heart failure, 734
    in tracheal disease, 1043t
Petechiae, diagnosis of, 220, *221*
    pathophysiology of, 218–220, 219t
    treatment of, 220–222
Peyer's patches, 1186
    in small intestinal immune response, 1194, *1194,* 1195, *1195*
Peyote, toxicity of, 365
Phaeohyphomycosis, 475
Pharyngitis, 1028
Pharynx, disorders of, 1026–1029
    and dysphagia, 114, 114t, *115*
    and gagging, 111, 112t, *113*
    in swallowing, 1025, *1026*
    intubation through, for enteral nutrition, 276
        client information on, 1945
    salivary mucocele in, 1119, 1120, *1120*
Phenazopyridine, for urinary tract disorders, idiopathic, 1744–1745
Phenobarbital, and osteodystrophy, 1908
    and thyroid hormone deficiency, 1424
    for seizures, 150t, 151, 151t
    toxicity of, to liver, 1307
    with aminophylline, for cough, 165t
        for tracheal disease, 1043t
Phenol, with electrocoagulation, for anal sacculitis, 1266
Phenothiazines, for anxiety, in heart failure, 733–734
    for fever, 9
Phenoxybenzamine, for bladder dysfunction, 1739t
    for tick paralysis, 673
    for urine retention, 95t
Phenylalanine, in diet, 239t
Phenylbutazone, for degenerative joint disease, 1866
    toxicity of, and anemia, 1812
Phenylephrine, for arrhythmia, 832
Phenylpropanolamine, for urinary tract dysfunction, 320, 1739t
Phenytoin, and osteodystrophy, 1908
    for arrhythmia, 829t
    for digitalis toxicity, 730, 829t
Pheochromocytoma, neurologic signs of, 551
    skin lesions with, 26
Philodendron species, toxicity of, 364
Phimosis, 1594
Phlebectasia, cutaneous, 974
    parenteral nutrition and, 281
Phlebitis, 975, *975*
Phlebotomy, for patent ductus arteriosus, 750
    in polycythemia, 204–206, 516
Phocomelia, 1894
Phonocardiography, in mitral valve dysplasia, *776*
    of atrial septal defect, 755, *755*
Phoradendron flavescens, toxicity of, 364
Phosphofructokinase deficiency, 1990t
    and hemolytic anemia, 1791t, 1792
    and myopathy, 689
    genetics in, 3t, 4–5

Phospholipases, in platelet activation, 1817, *1817,* 1818
Phosphorus, blood level of, decreased. See *Hypophosphatemia.*
    elevated. See *Hyperphosphatemia.*
    clearance of, in renal function assessment, 1604t, 1605
    in diet, 239t
        in calcium oxalate urolithiasis, 1726, 1727, 1765
        in heart disease, 265t
        in hyperparathyroidism, 1906
        in orthopedic developmental disorders, 247
        in renal disease, 270–271, 273t, 274, 274t
        in renal failure, 1646, 1647t
    in enemas, 131, 132t
    in urine, elevated level of, in renal tubular dysfunction, 1706
Photodynamic therapy, for squamous cell carcinoma, of skin, 525
Phrenic nerves, in diaphragmatic paralysis, 1100
Phthiraptera infestation, of skin, 59t, 60, *60*
    and pruritus, 33t
Phycomycosis. See *Pythiosis.*
Physaloptera infestation, and gastritis, 1164
Physes, in bone growth, 1887–1888, *1888*
Pickwickian syndrome, 1088
Pigmentation, deficiency of, 55–57, *56*
    excess of, 55, *56, 57*–58
    in urine, 96–99, 97t, *98,* 99t
Pilocarpine, for dysautonomia, 680
Pilonidal sinus, and spinal cord disorders, 643
Pindolol, for arrhythmia, 829t
PIND-ORF, for feline leukemia virus infection, 431
Pinna, carcinoma of, 988–991
    client information on, 1926
    dermatoses of, 987t, 988–992, 989t, 990t
    disorders of, 986–992
    differential diagnosis of, 986, 987t
Piroxicam, for bladder cancer, 542
    for pain, 24t, 25
    for urinary tract disorders, idiopathic, 1745
Pitressin. See *Antidiuretic hormone.*
Pituitary, adenoma of, 584t
    cancer of, radiotherapy for, 497t
    disorders of, and diabetes insipidus, 1374–1379, *1375, 1378*
        and dwarfism, 1897, 1987t
        and hyperadrenocorticism, 1461, 1462. See also *Hyperadrenocorticism.*
        medical treatment of, 1476–1479, *1477, 1479, 1480*
        surgery for, 1476
    tumors of, and acromegaly, 1371, 1373
        signs of, 1484t, 1484–1485
Placenta, retained, 1536
    in cat, 1596
    sites of, subinvolution of, 1537, *1537*
Plague, zoonotic, 384t
Plants, products of, in cancer management, 377, 378t
    toxicity of, 363–365
        to liver, 1326t, 1329, 1332
Plaque, eosinophilic, and pruritus, 34t
    periodontal, 1127–1130, 1129t, *1129–1131,* 1130t
    removal of, 1130–1133
Plasma, drug concentration in, changes in, over time, 294–298, *295*
    dosing regimen and, 298–300, *299*
    fresh frozen, transfusion of, 351, *352,* 354
    hyperimmune, for parvovirus infection, 421
    in semen analysis, 1573
    in volume replacement, 329, 331, 332t, 333t

Plasma cells, in neoplasia, 516–520, *517, 518*
  in skin lesions, 53
Plasmacytoma, cutaneous, 527
  solitary, 519–520
Plasmacytosis, with lymphocytosis. See *Lymphocytic-plasmacytic* entries.
Plasma-Lyte A, in fluid therapy, 328, 329t, 330t
Plasminogen activator, tissue, for thromboembolism, 917, 1840
Platelet-activating factor, in glomerulonephritis, 1664
Platelets, disorders of, and epistaxis, 214t, 214–215, *216*
  and purpura, 218–220, 219t, *221*
  congenital, 1979t
  diagnosis of, 1818t, 1818–1819, 1819t, *1820, 1821*
  functional, 1823–1827, 1824t–1826t
  in thrombocytopenia, 1819–1823. See also *Thrombocytopenia.*
  in thrombocytosis, 1823
  physiology of, *1817,* 1817–1818, *1818,* 1818t
  production of, disorders of, 1823
  transfusion of, 351
Platinum compounds, and gastritis, 1162
  for cancer, 485t, 486, 487, 487t, 489
    of bladder, 542
    with radiotherapy, 495, 496
  for osteosarcoma, 536–537
    after amputation, 1911
  for squamous cell carcinoma, nasal, 1020, *1021*
  toxicity of, and renal failure, 1616–1617
Platynosomum fastosum infestation, of biliary tract, 1343
Play, aggression in, 162
Pleocytosis, and leukocytosis, of brain, 591–592
  with meningioma, 574t
Pleural effusion, 186–189, *187,* 1102–1106, *1103–1106*
  chyle in, *187,* 188–189, 1102, 1103, *1103, 1104,* 1105t, *1107,* 1107–1108
  hyperkalemia with, 229
  in peritonitis, feline infectious, 440t, 440–441, 1102, 1103, 1105t, 1107
  in pneumothorax, 1109, *1109,* 1110
  in renal failure, 1623–1624
  pus in, 1103, 1104, 1105t, *1106,* 1106–1107
  with cardiomyopathy, dilated, 911
  with heart failure, thoracentesis for, 733
  with neoplasia, 1108–1109
Pleuroperitoneal hernia, congenital, 1975t, 1983t
Plugs, urethral, 1732–1739. See also *Urethra, plugs in.*
Pneumocystosis, 410t, 416
  congenital, 1990t
  of lung, 1066
Pneumomediastinum, 1092, *1092,* 1094
  tracheal trauma and, 1053, *1053*
Pneumonia. See *Lung(s).*
Pneumonyssoides caninum infestation, and rhinitis, 1018
Pneumothorax, *1109,* 1109–1110
  lung cysts and, 1083–1084
  subcutaneous emphysema with, 63, 65
Poikilocytes, in hemolytic anemia, 1791t
  in liver disease, 1291
Poinsettia, toxicity of, 364
Pointer, acral mutilation in, 669, 1994t
  spinal muscular atrophy in, 666, 1993t
Polioencephalomyelitis, 598, 627
Pollakiuria, 89, 90
Polyarteritis, juvenile, 973
  with meningitis, and arthritis, 1882
Polyarteritis nodosa, 973–974

Polyarthritis. See also *Arthritis.*
  classification of, 77–79, 78t
  diagnosis of, *79,* 79–80
  idiopathic, treatment of, 1883
  in greyhound, 1879–1880
  progressive, 1880–1881
Polychondritis, relapsing, of pinna, 991
Polychromasia, in anemia, 200t
Polycoria, 1988t
Polycystic disease, of kidneys, 1698, 1699t, 1700–1702, 1982t, 1996t
  with hepatic cysts, 1322
Polycythemia, and epistaxis, 214t, 215
  cyanosis with, 207
  diagnosis of, 204–206, *205*
  pathophysiology of, 203–204, *204*
  treatment of, 206
Polycythemia vera, 515t, 516
Polydactyly, 1894–1895, *1895,* 1975t, 1984t
Polydipsia, evaluation of, 85t, 85–89, *86,* 87t, 88t
  history of, 1600
  in diabetes insipidus, *1376,* 1377–1378
    nephrogenic, 1707
  in hyperparathyroidism, 1380 ,
  in renal failure, 1637
  with polyuria, liver disease and, 1273t, 1275, 1290–1291
Polyhydroxidine iodine, for otitis externa, 989t, 994
Polymerase chain reaction test, for feline leukemia virus, 425–426
Polymyositis, and megaesophagus, 1150, 1150t
  immune-mediated, 687
Polyneuropathy, distal symmetric, 679
  in Dalmatian, with laryngeal paralysis, 668
  in malamute, 667–668
  in rottweiler, 668
Polyostotic periostitis, 1903
Polyphagia, 104–107, 105t, *106*
  in pancreatic exocrine insufficiency, 1358–1359
  with cachexia, 73
Polyps, in cystitis, 1778–1780, 1779t
  nasopharyngeal, 1028
  of middle ear, inflammatory, 999
  of rectum, 1254, *1254,* 1260–1262
  of stomach, 1176
Polyradiculoneuritis, acute, 673–674
Polystyrene resin, with sorbitol, for hyperkalemia, in renal failure, 1628
Polyuria, and incontinence, 89, 90, *91*
  evaluation of, 85t, 85–89, *86,* 87t, 88t
    water deprivation test in, *86,* 87, 87t, 88t, 89, 1604–1605
  with polydipsia, liver disease and, 1273t, 1275, 1290–1291
  with portosystemic shunt, congenital, 1311–1312
  in acromegaly, 1371
  in diabetes insipidus, 1374–1379. See also *Diabetes insipidus.*
  in hyperparathyroidism, 1380
  in renal failure, 1637
  urine color in, 96–99
Pompe's disease, 1322, 1323
  and myopathy, 689
Poodle, demyelination in, 1991t
  renal dysplasia in, 1699t, 1702–1703
Porphyria, and hemolytic anemia, 1791t, 1792
  congenital, 1977t
Portal hepatitis, lymphocytic, 1309
Portal vein, acute disorders of, 1330
  arterial fistula to, intrahepatic, 1979t, 1991t
  thrombosis of, 1336

Portosystemic shunts, and bile acid elevation, 1289
  congenital, 1311–1315, 1979t, 1991t
    breed predisposition to, 1274
  dietary management of, 260
  hepatic venous outflow obstruction and, 1319
  multiple acquired, *1316,* 1316–1317, *1317*
  radiography of, 1291
  ultrasonography of, 1292
  urate urolithiasis with, 1772, 1774, 1774t
Post-caval syndrome, in dirofilariasis, 941, 943, *945*
Postural hypotension, and syncope, 13–15
Posture, examination of, in brain disorders, 559t, 559–562, *561, 562*
  in diabetes, 1442, *1442*
  visual placing reaction in, 18
Potassium, absorption of, from intestine, *1192, 1193*
  blood level of, decreased. See *Hypokalemia.*
    elevated. See *Hyperkalemia.*
  clearance of, in renal function assessment, 1604t, 1605
  diuretics sparing, for heart failure, 716
  in diet, 239t
    and calcium oxalate urolithiasis, 1726, 1765
    in heart disease, 263, 265t
    in parenteral nutrition, 282t
    in renal disease, 270, 273t, 274, 274t
    in renal failure, chronic, 1647t, 1647–1648
  in erythrocytes, congenital elevation of, 1990t
  with glucose and insulin, for septic shock, 184t
Potassium bromide, for seizures, 150t, 151, 151t
  with liver disease, 1307
Potassium citrate, for calcium oxalate urolithiasis, 1728
  preventive use of, 1769
  for metabolic acidosis, in renal failure, 1652
Potassium iodide, for hyperthyroidism, 1412
Povidone-iodine, for anal sacculitis, 1266
  for otitis externa, 989t, 995
Poxvirus infection, 450
PR segment, 804. See also *Electrocardiography.*
Pralidoxime chloride, for insecticide toxicity, 359
  with megaesophagus, 1150t
Praziquantel, for fluke infestation, of pancreas, 1363t, 1364
  for intestinal parasitosis, 1221t
  for *Paragonimus* infestation, 1065t, 1069–1070
Prazosin, for bladder dysfunction, 1739t
  for urine retention, 95t
Precose, for diabetes, 1448
Prednisone/prednisolone, and thyroid hormone deficiency, 1424
  client information on, 1960
  dosage of, 313t, 313–314, 314t
  effect of, on liver enzyme concentrations, *1282,* 1282–1283
  for anaphylaxis, 184t
  for anemia, hemolytic, immune-mediated, 1796
    infection-associated, 1800
    paraneoplastic, 504
  for arthritis, 1884
  for bronchial asthma, 1058
  for bronchopulmonary disease, 1059t
  for central nervous system inflammation, 593t
  for cholangiohepatitis, 1310
  for cough, 165t
  for degenerative joint disease, 1866
  for demyelinating neuropathy, acquired, 674
  for dirofilariasis, 943, 949t, 951, 960, 961

IND

Prednisone/prednisolone *(Continued)*
for edema, in brain trauma, 579
for eosinophilic disease, of lungs, 1065t, 1072
for eosinophilic granuloma complex, 1118
for esophageal stricture, 1149
for gastritis, with lymphocytic-plasmacytic infiltrates, 1163
for hepatitis, chronic, 1301
with copper accumulation, 1306
for hypoadrenocorticism, 1496, 1498
for hypothyroidism, with neurologic signs, 551
for inflammatory bowel disease, 1227, 1250
for intracranial pressure elevation, 577
for lung disorders, 1065t
for lymphangiectasia, small intestinal, 1230
for lymphocytic leukemia, 514–515
for lymphoma, 510, 511, 511t
for mast cell tumors, of skin, 527
for megaesophagus, 1150, 1150t
for meningitis, spinal, with arteritis, 621–622
for multiple myeloma, 518, 519
with hypergammaglobulinemia, 505
for otitis externa, 989t, 995
for pancreatic exocrine insufficiency, 1363t, 1364
for pancreatic islet cell tumors, 1434t, 1437
for pansteatitis, 29
for perianal fistula, 1265
for pulmonary thromboembolism, 1079–1080
for shock, with gastric dilatation and volvulus, 1172
for thrombocytopenia, immune-mediated, 1822
paraneoplastic, 505
potency of, 312, 312t
structure of, *309*
with trimeprazine, for cough, 165t
for tracheal disease, 1043t
Preexcitation, ventricular, 821, *822,* 1976t, 1985t
Pregnancy, adverse drug reactions in, 323
and parturition. See *Parturition.*
and vaginal discharge, 81t–84t
diagnosis of, 1519
diet in, 237
duration of, 1527
failure to achieve. See *Infertility.*
fetal death in, 1527–1528, 1592
hypoluteodism and, 1525, 1528
hypoglycemia in, 1528
immunodeficiency virus transmission in, 433–434
insulin resistance in, 1528
maintenance of, 1596
physiology of, 1527, 1588–1590
prevention of, *1542,* 1542–1544
client information on, 1933
prepubertal gonadectomy in, 1539–1541
streptococcosis in, 395–396
termination of, 1544–1548, *1547*
toxoplasmosis in, zoonotic, 388, 389
Pregnant mare serum gonadotropin, in estrus induction, 1595
Preload, in cardiac output, 693
in heart failure, assessment of, 708
Prepuce, anomalies of, 1981t, 1994t
discharge from, 83–84, 84t
Preservatives, in blood storage, 350t, 350–351
Pressure point diagnosis, in acupuncture, 366, *367*
Prilosec. See *Omeprazole.*
Primaxin, for lung infection, 1065t
Primidone, and osteodystrophy, 1908
Primrose oil, in cancer management, 378t
Prions, and spongiform encephalopathy, 451
Procainamide, for arrhythmia, 824t–826t, 825–826, 829t

Procainamide *(Continued)*
ventricular, with hypotension, 184t
ProcalAmine, in fluid therapy, 329t
Procan SR (procainamide), for arrhythmia, 824t–826t, 825–826, 829t
ventricular, with hypotension, 184t
Prochlorperazine, for vomiting, in gastritis, 1161
in renal failure, 1629, 1630t
Proestrus, 1510–1511, *1510–1513,* 1520
in cat, 1587
persistent, and infertility, *1561,* 1564–1565
prolonged, *1521,* 1523
Progesterone, deficiency of, and fetal loss, 1528
for eosinophilic granuloma complex, 1118
for prolonged estrus, 1524
in contraception, 1543–1544
in cystic endometrial hyperplasia, with pyometra, 1549
in estrous cycle, *1511,* 1511–1513, *1514, 1515,* 1520–1522
and timing of artificial insemination, 1576, *1576*
in breeding management, 1516, *1517,* 1518
in cat, 1589
in parturition, 1528
inhibition of, in abortion induction, 1544–1547, *1547*
Progestins, and diabetes mellitus, with hyperlipidemia, 290
and growth hormone excess, 1370–1371, *1371,* 1373
for behavioral disorders, 160, 160t
reproductive, 1597, 1597t
for prostatic hypertrophy, 1692
in contraception, 1543–1544
in pregnancy maintenance, 1596
Prognathism, 1986t
Program, for coccidioidomycosis, 457, 475t
in flea control, client information on, 1971
Prolactin, in estrous cycle, 1513–1514, *1514–1516,* 1516
in pregnancy, 1589–1590
inhibition of, in abortion induction, 1546–1547, *1547*
Promodulin, for peritonitis, feline infectious, 441
Promyelocytic leukemia, 1853
Pronestyl (procainamide), for arrhythmia, 824t–826t, 825–826, 829t
ventricular, with hypotension, 184t
Propafenone, for arrhythmia, 824t, 826t, 827, 829t
Propantheline, for bladder dysfunction, 1739t
for urinary tract disorders, idiopathic, 1745
Propionibacterium acnes, for feline immunodeficiency virus infection, 437, 437t, 438
for feline infectious peritonitis, 441
for feline leukemia virus infection, 430
Propofol, in anesthesia, for gonadectomy, prepubertal, 1541
for liver biopsy, 1296t
Propranolol, dosage of, in renal failure, 1649t
for arrhythmia, 824t–826t, 827–830, 829t
for cardiomyopathy, dilated, 911
hypertrophic, in cats, 905–907
in dogs, 890
for hyperthyroidism, 1412
Proprioception, disorders of, and ataxia, 142
with spinal cord disorders, 611–612
in lesion localization, 614
segmental reflex testing of, 566–568, *567–570,* 571t
in neurologic examination, 561, *561*
Propulsid. See *Cisapride.*
Propylene glycol, for otitis externa, 989t, 994

Propylene glycol *(Continued)*
toxicity of, 361
Proscar, for prostatic hypertrophy, 1692
Prostaglandin E, analogs of, for gastrinoma, 1506, 1506t
for stomach ulcers, in renal failure, 1629, 1630t
with steroid therapy, for hemolytic anemia, 1797
Prostaglandins, analogs of, for stomach ulcers, 1168
for metritis, in cat, 1596
postparturient, 1537
for placental retention, in cat, 1596
for pyometra, 1596, 1937
with cystic endometrial hyperplasia, *1553,* 1553–1555, 1554t, *1555*
in abortion induction, 1544–1547, *1547*
in gastric physiology, 1158
in gastrointestinal endocrine system, 1503
in glomerulonephritis, 1664
in inflammation, steroid effects on, 310
in parturition, 1528
in periodontal disease, 1128
Prostate, anatomy of, 1586, 1687, *1687*
antibiotic penetration of, 302
calculi of, 1696
cysts of, 1689t, 1693–1694
disorders of, diagnosis of, 1687–1691, 1688t, 1689t, *1689–1691*
in cat, 1594
hypertrophy of, and preputial discharge, 83, 84, 84t
benign, 1688, 1689t, 1691–1692
inflammation of, 1689t, 1692–1693, *1693*
physiology of, 1687
squamous metaplasia of, 1692
tumors of, 542–543, 1689t, 1694–1696, *1695, 1696*
Prostigmata mites, 59t, 61–62, *62.* See also *Cheyletiellosis* and *Demodicosis.*
Prostigmin, for myasthenia gravis, 676
Prostin. See *Prostaglandins.*
Protamine zinc insulin, for diabetes, 1451–1452
Protein, absorption of, from small intestine, 1189, *1190*
digestion of, in adverse food reactions, 255
in small intestine, 1187, *1188*
drug binding to, 296
in cerebrospinal fluid, 572, 574t, 575
in degenerative myelopathy, 623
in diet, 237, 239t
in enteral nutrition, 280, 280t, 281t
in gastrointestinal disorders, 259
in glomerulonephritis, 1673–1674
in heart disease, 263, 265t
in hepatic encephalopathy, 260, 1332–1334, 1333t
in orthopedic developmental disorders, 248, 249t
in parenteral nutrition, 281, 282, 282t
in portosystemic shunt, 1313–1314
in renal disease, 270, 272–273, 273t, 274t
in renal failure, acute, 1631
chronic, 1646, 1647t, 1650
in urolithiasis, calcium oxalate, 1726, 1727, 1764
in plasma, in liver disease, 1278t, 1284–1286
in serum, electrophoresis of, in multiple myeloma, 517, *517*
loss of, enteropathy and, 1201–1202, 1202t, 1211
malabsorption of, in pancreatic exocrine insufficiency, 1358
with diarrhea, 125

Protein (Continued)
  metabolism of, in metabolic acidosis, in renal failure, 1640
Protein C, in coagulation inhibition, 1829–1830, 1833t
Protein S, in coagulation inhibition, 1829–1830, 1833t
Proteinuria, 98, 100–102, 101
  in dirofilariasis, 947
  in glomerular disease, 1670, 1670–1671
  in glomerular function testing, 1602t, 1603
  in renal failure, 1644, 1658
  measurement of, 1605
Proteolysis, fecal, in pancreatic exocrine insufficiency, 1360, 1360–1361
Proteus infection, antibiotics for, 303, 305–306
Prothrombin, deficiency of, 1839, 1839t
Prothrombin time, in liver disease, 1278t, 1285–1286
Proto-oncogenes, in carcinogenesis, 478, 479t
Protopam Chloride (pralidoxime chloride), for insecticide toxicity, 359
  with megaesophagus, 1150t
Prototheosis, 416
  and meningitis, spinal, 616–619, 618t
  client information on, 1947
  of large intestine, 1247
Protozoal infection, and arthritis, 1878–1879
  and encephalitis, 596–597
  and fetal loss, 1527–1528
  and meningoencephalitis, cerebrospinal fluid examination in, 574, 574t
  of lung, 1066
  of nervous system, multifocal, 606
  of small intestine, 408–411, 409t, 410t, 1221–1222
  of spinal cord, 644–645
  polysystemic, 410t, 411–416
Prozac, for behavioral disorders, in cats, 160t
  in dogs, 156, 158t
Pruritus, 31–36, 33t, 34t, 35
  and alopecia, 29, 30
  diagnosis of, 32–35, 33t, 34t, 35
  in adverse food reactions, 254, 254, 257
  in pyoderma, 44, 46, 46–47
  pathophysiology of, 31–32
  treatment of, 35, 35–36
Pseudoallergic drug reactions, 325
Pseudoaneurysm, arterial, 968–969
Pseudocyesis, 1525–1526, 1591
Pseudohermaphroditism, 1584, 1593, 1981t, 1994t
Pseudohyperkalemia, 227, 228t, 229
Pseudohypokalemia, 225
Pseudohyponatremia, 222t, 223
Pseudomonas infection, and otitis externa, 989t, 990t, 993, 995, 996
  and pneumonia, 1064
  antibiotics for, 303, 305–306
Pseudo-neoplasms, cutaneous, 36
Pseudopregnancy, 1525–1526, 1591
Pseudorabies, 423, 451–452, 595
  ptyalism in, 108
Psilocybin, toxicity of, 365
Psittacosis, and abortion, 1592
  and conjunctivitis, 66
  zoonotic, 384t
Psoriasiform dermatosis, lichenoid, congenital, 1995t
Psychogenic dermatitis, and pruritus, 33t
Psychological disorders. See also Behavior.
  and anorexia, 102–104, 103
  and polydipsia, 88, 88t
Ptyalism, 107–109, 110
Puberty, in cat, female, 1587

Puberty (Continued)
  delayed, 1595
  male, 1590
  in dog, delayed, 1522
Pug, encephalitis in, 598, 606, 1992t
Pulex fleas, in skin infestation, 59, 59t, 60
Pulmonary. See also Lung(s).
Pulmonary artery, echocardiography of, 852–853, 857t, 859
  thromboembolism of, glomerular disease and, 1675, 1676
  transposition of, with aorta, 783–784
Pulmonary atresia, 782–783, 783
Pulmonary capillary wedge pressure, in heart failure, 707–708
Pulmonary edema, 1081–1083, 1083
  in renal failure, 1622–1624, 1623
  with cardiomyopathy, hypertrophic, 906–908
  with mitral insufficiency, 790, 793–795
Pulmonary embolism, 1078–1080, 1079, 1080
  and weakness, 13
  hyperadrenocorticism and, 1483
Pulmonary emphysema, congenital, 1994t
Pulmonary function testing, 1039
Pulmonary hypertension. See Hypertension, pulmonary.
Pulmonary veins, blood flow in, echocardiography of, 846, 846–847, 865, 865t
Pulmonic insufficiency, 796
  client information on, 1952
  congenital, 773, 773, 774
  echocardiography of, 871
Pulmonic stenosis, 759–767, 1976t, 1985t
  auscultation of, 739t
  blood pressure in, echocardiographic measurement of, 847, 847t
  cardiac catheterization in, 742, 743, 762
  clinical findings in, 761–766, 763–766
  echocardiography of, 868, 869
  in tetralogy of Fallot, 780–782, 782
  management of, 766–767, 767
  murmur with, 172
  natural history of, 766
  pathology of, 759–760, 761–763
  pathophysiology of, 760–761
Pulp, endodontic treatment of, 1135–1140, 1137t, 1138
Pulseless disease, and syncope, 16
Pulses, arterial, 174–177, 175, 176
  venous, 177–179, 178
Pulsus alternans, 174, 177
Pulsus paradoxus, 174, 177
  in cardiac tamponade, with pericardial effusion, 928, 929
Pupils, anomalies of, 1988t
  congenital defects of, 1978t
  dilation of, in glaucoma, 68, 69
  in cranial nerve examination, 563–564, 564, 567t
  in neurologic examination, 657–661, 658, 659t, 660t, 661
  light reflex of, in vision loss, acute, 18–19, 19
  neuroanatomy in, 657–658, 658
  persistent membranes on, 1988t
  size of, in coma, 145, 146t
Puppy. See Neonate.
Purpura, diagnosis of, 220, 221
  pathophysiology of, 218–220, 219t
  thrombocytopenic, idiopathic, and epistaxis, 214–215
  treatment of, 220–222
Pustular dermatosis, subcorneal, and pruritus, 33t
Pustules, 43–47, 45, 46, 46t
  cytologic sampling from, 52

Pustules (Continued)
  of pinna, 987t, 991
Pustulosis, eosinophilic, sterile, and pruritus, 33t
Pyelonephritis, and polyuria, 87, 87t
  hyperadrenocorticism and, 1482
Pylorus, anatomy of, 1155, 1155
  hypertrophy of, and gastric outlet obstruction, 1169, 1169–1170
  in motility, 1158
  stenosis of, congenital, 1977t, 1986t
Pyoderma, 43–47, 45, 46, 46t
  and hyperpigmentation, 57, 58
  and pruritus, 32–35, 33t, 34t
  and skin erosion, 40–42
  and skin ulcers, 40–42
  crusting in, 49
Pyogranuloma, cutaneous, 36, 37
  in actinomycosis, 395
  in nocardiosis, 395
Pyometra, and polyuria, 87, 87t
  and vaginal discharge, 81t–84t
  client information on, 1937
  in cat, 1596
  with cystic endometrial hyperplasia, 1549–1555, 1550t, 1552, 1553, 1554t, 1555, 1592
    diagnosis of, 1550t, 1550–1551, 1552, 1553
    pathophysiology of, 1549–1550
    treatment of, 1551–1555, 1553, 1554t, 1555
Pyothorax, 1103, 1104, 1105t, 1106, 1106–1107
Pyrantel, for intestinal parasitosis, 1220, 1221, 1221t
  with ivermectin, for dirofilariasis, 949–951, 950t
Pyrethrin insecticides, toxicity of, 359
Pyrethroid insecticides, toxicity of, 359
Pyridostigmine, for megaesophagus, 1150, 1150t
  for myasthenia gravis, 676
Pyridoxine. See Vitamin B_6.
Pyrimethamine, for protozoal infection, 410, 410t
Pyriproxifen, in flea control, 1971
Pyrogens, endogenous, 7, 7t
  exogenous, 6–7, 7t
Pyruvate kinase deficiency, 3t, 1989t
  and hemolytic anemia, 1791t, 1792–1793
Pythiosis, 453–454
  and gastric outlet obstruction, 1170
  itraconazole for, 456, 1220
  of intestine, client information on, 1947
    large, 1246–1247
    small, 1219–1220
Pyuria, 98, 99, 1607, 1607, 1607t, 1678, 1680

Q fever, 385t, 407
QRS complex, 804–805. See also Electrocardiography.
Quadriplegia, spinal cord disorders and, 611
Quibron, for cough, 165t
  for tracheal disease, 1043t
Quinacrine, for giardiasis, of small intestine, 1222
Quinidine, digoxin displacement by, 728
  for arrhythmia, 824t–826t, 824–825, 829t

Rabies, 419t, 422–423
  and encephalitis, 594–595
  and ptyalism, 108, 109
  in cats, 449–450
  zoonotic, 387–388
Raccoons, rabies in, 388

IND

Radial artery, arteriovenous fistula of, ultrasonography of, 971, *971*
Radial nerve, injury to, signs of, 663t
Radiation, and carcinogenesis, 481
Radiation therapy, for brain tumors, 494, 497t, 586
　for cancer, 489–496
　　as primary treatment, 493
　　biology of, 489–492, *491, 492*
　　goals of, 492–493
　　squamous cell, of skin, 525
　　tumor types treated with, 496, 497t
　　with chemotherapy, 495–496
　　with surgery, 493–496, *494, 496*
　for hyperadrenocorticism, 1486
　for intranasal tumors, 1021–1023, *1023*
　for lymphoma, 512, *512*
　for mast cell tumors, *116*, 117t, 527
　for oral tumors, 497t, 1117
　for osteosarcoma, 1911
　for rectal tumors, 1262
　for sarcoma, of soft tissue, 497t, *532, 533*, 534
　for spinal cord tumors, 642
　for squamous cell carcinoma, nasal, 1020
　for thyroid tumors, with hyperthyroidism, 491, 497t, 1417
Radiator fluid. See *Ethylene glycol.*
Radioactive iodine, for hyperthyroidism, 1408t, 1413–1415, *1414*
　client information on, 1931
　with thyroid tumors, 1417
Radiofrequency ablation, for arrhythmia, 832
Radiography. See also specific techniques, e.g., *Angiocardiography.*
　contrast, of arterial occlusion, 967, *967*
　　of esophagus, 1143, *1144*
　　　fistula in, 1147
　　　stricture in, 1148, *1149*
　　of gastric ulcers, 1167
　in hyperadrenocorticism, 1465t, 1466
　in hyperparathyroidism, 1387, 1388
　in hypoadrenocorticism, 1494, *1494*
　of arthritis, bacterial, 1876, *1877*
　of bone cyst, 1904, *1904*
　of bone disorders, 1889–1890, 1891t
　　in rickets, 1907, *1907*
　of bone infarction, medullary, 1904, *1904*
　of bone loss, in hyperparathyroidism, nutritional secondary, 1906, *1906*
　of cartilage cores, retained, 1898, *1900*
　of craniomandibular osteopathy, 1898, *1900, 1901*
　of digital anomalies, 1894, 1895, *1895*
　of dirofilariasis, in cats, *957, 958,* 959
　　in dogs, 944t, *945,* 945–947, *946*
　of elbow dysplasia, 1871, *1871*
　of enostosis, 1900, *1901*
　of femoral head necrosis, aseptic, 1873, *1874*
　of gastroesophageal intussusception, 1153, *1153*
　of heart, in atrial septal defect, 755, *755*
　　in cardiomyopathy, dilated, canine, 880, *881*
　　　feline, 909, *909*
　　　hypertrophic, canine, 888, *889*
　　　feline, 899, *901*
　　in congenital disease, 740
　　in mitral insufficiency, 790, *791*
　　in mitral valve dysplasia, 776, *777*
　　in patent ductus arteriosus, 747, *747,* 750, *752*
　　in pulmonic insufficiency, 773, *773*
　　in pulmonic stenosis, 761–762, *763*
　　in subaortic stenosis, 770, *770*
　　in tetralogy of Fallot, *781,* 781–782

Radiography (Continued)
　in thromboembolism, 915
　in ventricular septal defect, 757, *757*
　of hiatal hernia, 1152, *1152*
　of hip dysplasia, 1872, *1873*
　of joint disease, degenerative, *1863, 1864,* 1864–1865
　of joint luxation, 1867, *1867, 1868*
　of joint swelling, 80
　of kidney, 1611–1612
　of large intestine, 1241–1242, *1243*
　of metaphyseal osteopathy, 1901–1902, *1902*
　of multiple cartilaginous exostoses, 1899, *1901*
　of nasal cavity, 1005–1009, *1006–1008, 1010*
　of ossification disorders, in congenital hypothyroidism, 1897, *1898*
　of osteochondrodysplasia, 1897, *1900*
　of osteochondrosis, 1870, *1870*
　of osteomyelitis, *1913,* 1913–1914, *1914*
　of osteopathy, hypertrophic, 1903, *1903*
　of osteosarcoma, 1910, *1910*
　of pancreatitis, 1351
　of pericardial effusion, 928, *929, 930*
　of peritoneopericardial hernia, 927, *927*
　of portosystemic shunt, 1291
　　congenital, 1313, *1313*
　　multiple acquired, 1317, *1317*
　of prostate, 1688–1689, *1689,* 1689t
　　neoplasia in, 1695, *1695*
　of pyometra, with cystic endometrial hyperplasia, 1551, *1552*
　of radial agenesis, 1894, *1894*
　of rheumatoid arthritis, in dogs, 1879, *1880*
　of small intestine, 1207–1208, 1208t, *1209*
　of tracheal disorders, 1040–1041, *1041*
　of tricuspid insufficiency, 795
　of urinary calculi, *1718, 1722,* 1722t, 1722–1724, 1723t, *1724,* 1756
　of urinary tract disease, 1749, 1751t
　of volvulus, with gastric dilatation, 1172, *1172*
Radioimmunoassay, for progesterone, in breeding management, 1518
Radionuclide imaging. See *Scintigraphy.*
Radius, agenesis of, 1894, *1894,* 1984t
　dysplasia of, 1984t
　hemimelia of, 1975t
Rales, 1035t
Ranitidine, for esophagitis, 1148, 1149
　for gastric motility disorders, 1176
　for gastric ulcers, 1168
　　in renal failure, 1629, 1630t
　　with coagulopathy, in liver disorders, 1335
　for gastrinoma, 1506, 1506t
　for gastroenteritis, in renal failure, chronic, 1648
　for gastroesophageal reflux, 1152
Rapid eye movement sleep, behavioral disorders related to, 154–155
Rat-bite fever, zoonotic, 385t
Rectum, anatomy of, 1257–1258
　disorders of, and fecal incontinence, 1268, 1268t, 1269
　　congenital, 1976t, 1985t
　　diagnosis of, 1258t, 1258–1259
　　with perineal hernia, 1259–1260
　examination of, in small intestinal disorders, 1205
　fistula of, from urethra, 1751
　function of, 1258
　prolapse of, 1262–1263
　scintigraphy of, in liver disease, 1291–1292
　stricture of, 1263t, 1263–1264
　tumors of, *1253,* 1253–1254, *1254,* 1260–1262

Red blood cells. See *Erythrocytes.*
Red clover, in cancer management, 378t
Red eye, 66–69, *67, 68*
　radiation injury and, in nasal tumor therapy, 1022
Reflex(es), Babinski, testing of, 570
　biceps, testing of, 568, *568*
　pupillary light, in cranial nerve examination, 563–564, *564,* 567t
　　in neurologic examination, 659, 660, 660t
　　in vision loss, acute, 18–19, *19*
　　neuroanatomy in, 657–658, *658*
　retractor oculi, in cranial nerve examination, 566, 567t
　spinal, abnormalities of, 611
　　segmental, examination of, 566–571, *567–572,* 571t
Reflux, from duodenum, 1174
　and gastritis, 1165
　and pancreatitis, 1350
　gastroesophageal, 1151–1152
Reglan. See *Metoclopramide.*
Regurgitation, 114–117, *116,* 117t
　in esophageal disease, 1143
　in megaesophagus, 1149
Relaxin, in pregnancy, 1589
Relefact, in thyrotropin-releasing hormone stimulation test, in hyperthyroidism, 1406
Renal failure, acute, 1615–1632
　clinical consequences of, 1622–1625, *1623,* 1623t
　diagnosis of, 1620–1622, *1621, 1622*
　etiology of, 1615–1617, 1616t
　management of, dialysis in, 1631t, 1631–1632
　　medical, 1625–1631, 1628t, 1630t
　　transplantation in, 1632
　pathophysiology of, 1617–1620, *1618, 1619*
　prevention of, 1625, 1626t
　prognosis of, 1632
　and hypocalcemia, vs. hypoparathyroidism, 1394
　chronic, 1634–1660
　　and osteodystrophy, 1907
　　causes of, 1634–1635
　　client information on, 1963
　　diagnosis of, 1644, *1645*
　　gastrointestinal effects of, 1635–1637, 1636t
　　hypercalcemia in, hyperparathyroidism with, *1384–1386,* 1385–1386, 1388
　　incidence of, 1634
　　laboratory tests in, 1640–1644, *1642*
　　management of, 1645–1646, 1646t
　　　dialysis in, 1646, 1658–1659
　　　diet in, 1646–1648, 1647t, *1648*
　　　drug dosage changes in, 1648–1650, 1649t
　　　in anemia, 1654–1656
　　　in dehydration, 1652
　　　in hyperphosphatemia, 1650–1651
　　　in hypertension, 1653–1654
　　　in hypokalemia, 1651
　　　in metabolic acidosis, 1652
　　　transplantation in, 1659t, 1659–1660
　　prognosis of, 1645
　　progression of, *1657,* 1657–1658, 1658t
　　uremia in, 1625, 1629–1630, 1630t, 1635, 1636t. See also *Uremia.*
　definition of, 1600
　diet in, 271t, 271–273, 273t, 274t
　drugs for, over-the-counter, 319
　fluid therapy in, 330t
Renal tubules, dysfunction of, and acidosis, with hyperchloremia, 234
　familial, 1699t, 1700–1702

Renal tubules (Continued)
function testing of, 1603–1605, 1604t
in diabetes insipidus, 1706–1707
in Fanconi's syndrome, 1708–1709
in metabolic disorders, and acidosis, 1707–1708, 1709t
of carbohydrates, 1704
of electrolytes, 1706
of nitrogen, 1704–1706
of vitamin B₁₂, 1706
ischemia of, in renal failure, 1619, 1619–1620
obstruction of, in renal failure, 1619
physiology of, 1704
Renin-angiotensin-aldosterone system, in heart failure, 700–701, 702t, 703
Renovascular hypertension, 180–182, 181
Reovirus infection, 451
and tracheobronchitis, 419
Reperfusion injury, after surgery, for gastric dilatation and volvulus, 1173
Reproductive system, 1509–1598. See also specific structures, e.g., Ovaries.
anatomy of, in cats, 1586–1587
breeding management of, artificial insemination in, 1574–1577, 1576
canine, 1516–1519, 1517
client information on, 1933, 1934
contraception in, 1542, 1542–1544
in control of genetic defects, 5
pregnancy termination in, 1544–1548, 1547
semen evaluation in, 1571–1574, 1572t
developmental disorders of, 1581–1585, 1582–1584
in cats, 1980t–1981t
in dogs, 1993t–1994t
estrous cycle in. See also Estrous cycle.
canine, 1510–1516
feline, 1587–1590
in cats, 1585–1598
in infertility, canine, female, assessment of, 1555–1558, 1556, 1557
management of, 1558–1565, 1559–1563, 1560t
male, 1578–1580
feline, female, 1591–1592, 1592, 1593, 1595, 1595
male, 1594–1595
in parturition, 1528–1530
in dystocia, 1352t, 1530–1536, 1531, 1533, 1534
in postpartum period, 1536–1539, 1537
in pregnancy, 1527–1528
in sterilization, prepubertal, 1539–1541
tumors of, 542–543
Respiration, difficulty in, 166–169, 167t, 168
in pneumothorax, 1110
disorders of, and cyanosis, 207, 207t, 209, 209, 210
in metabolic encephalopathy, 548
pleural effusion and, 186
in heart failure, 705
interruption of, during sleep, 154
larynx in, 1026
Respiratory acidosis, blood gas analysis in, 1039
Respiratory arrest, in anesthesia, acupuncture for, 372, 372
with cardiac arrest, 189, 192
resuscitation from, 190t, 190–193, 191, 192t
Respiratory distress syndrome, acute, 1082, 1083
tracheal collapse and, 1047
Respiratory sinus arrhythmia, 809–810, 810
Respiratory tract, 1033–1110. See also specific structures, e.g., Trachea.
antibiotic penetration of, 301–302
disorders of, and cough, 162–166, 163t, 164, 165t

Respiratory tract (Continued)
and dyspnea, 166–169, 167t, 168
and gagging, 111, 112t, 113
and tachypnea, 166–169, 168
and weakness, 13
congenital, in cats, 1981t
in dogs, 1994t
diagnosis of, 1035–1039, 1037, 1038t, 1039
feline immunodeficiency virus infection and, 435
herpesvirus infection and, 446, 447
history in, 1034–1035
in hyperthyroidism, 1401t, 1402
morbillivirus and, 452
obesity with, 71
physical examination in, 1035, 1035t
endoscopy of, 1037, 1037, 1038t, 1041
radiography of, 1036
scintigraphy of, 1037
ultrasonography of, 1036–1037
Retching, with gagging, 111
with vomiting, 117
Reticulocytes, in anemia, 198, 198t
of chronic disease, 1807, 1808
in erythropoiesis, 1784, 1784–1786, 1786
Reticulosis, inflammatory, 597–598, 606
Retina, degeneration of, hyperadrenocorticism and, 1463–1464
sudden acquired, weight gain with, 105–107
disorders of, and anisocoria, 660t
and vision loss, 17, 17t
congenital, 1978t, 1988t, 1989t
diabetes and, 1458
hypertension and, in renal failure, 1639
Retinitis, distemper and, 418
systemic disease and, 985, 986t
Retinoids. See Vitamin A.
Retractor oculi reflex, in cranial nerve examination, 566, 567t
Retriever, golden, hypomyelination in, 668–669, 1992t
renal dysplasia in, 1699t, 1701
Labrador, myopathy in, 688–689, 1993t
Retrovir (AZT), for feline immunodeficiency virus infection, 437, 437t
PIND-ORF derivative of, for feline leukemia virus infection, 431
Retroviral infection, and anemia, 1810t, 1810–1811
and immunodeficiency, 433–438. See also Immunodeficiency virus infection.
and leukemia, 424–432. See also Leukemia virus infection.
in carcinogenesis, 480–481
syncytium-forming virus in, 452, 1881
Reverse sneezing, 194, 195, 1029
Rex mutant, 1982t
Rhabditic dermatitis, and pruritus, 33t
Rheum species, toxicity of, 364
Rheumatic disorders, calicivirus and, feline, 448–449
Rheumatoid arthritis, 78, 1879, 1880, 1885
Rhinitis, 1018–1019
computed tomography of, 1009–1012, 1013–1015
radiography of, 1005–1009, 1007, 1008
with epistaxis, 215
Rhinoscopy, 1013–1015
in nasal discharge, 196–197, 197t
of respiratory system, 1037
Rhinosporidium seeberi infection, and rhinitis, 1018
Rhodococcus equi infection, 391t, 396
Rhonchus, 1035, 1035t
Rhubarb, toxicity of, 364

Rhythmol, for arrhythmia, 824t, 826t, 827, 829t
Ribavirin, for peritonitis, feline infectious, 441
Riboflavin, absorption of, from small intestine, 1190
in diet, 239t
Ribonucleic acid (RNA), messenger, in steroid receptors, 310
Ribs, fracture of, and flail chest, 1100
Ricinus communis, castor oil from, for constipation, 132
toxicity of, 365
Rickets, 1907, 1907
Rickettsial infection, 400–407
and anemia, non-regenerative, 1811
and arthritis, 1878
and ehrlichiosis. See Ehrlichiosis.
and hemobartonellosis. See Hemobartonellosis.
and meningitis, spinal, 616–619, 618t
and Q fever, 385t, 407
and Rocky Mountain spotted fever. See Rocky Mountain spotted fever.
and salmon-poisoning disease, 406, 1219
and thrombocytopenia, 1819–1821, 1821
and typhus, 385t, 402
leukocyte inclusions in, 1846, 1846
of brain, and vasculitis, 591, 598
of nervous system, multifocal, 606
Rifampin, concentration of, and bacterial susceptibility, 303t
for bacterial infection, 391t
for central nervous system infection, 593t
Rimadyl. See Carprofen.
Ringer's solution, in fluid therapy, 328, 329, 329t, 330t
in lavage, for pyothorax, 1106–1107
RNA, messenger, in steroid receptors, 310
Robitussin-DM, for cough, 165t
for tracheal disease, 1043t
Rocaltrol. See Vitamin D.
Rocky Mountain spotted fever, 400–402
and meningitis, spinal, 616–619
and thrombocytopenia, 1819
cerebrospinal fluid examination in, 574t
neurologic disorders in, multifocal, 606
zoonotic, 385t
Rodenticides, toxicity of, 359–361, 1837
Roferon. See Interferon.
Root canal therapy, in fractured teeth, 1137t, 1137–1140, 1138
in non-fractured teeth, 1136–1137, 1138
indications for, 1135–1136
Rotavirus infection, 451
Rotenone, toxicity of, 359
Rottweiler, glomerular disease in, 1699t, 1702
leukoencephalomyelopathy in, 589, 636
neuroaxonal dystrophy in, 642
polyneuropathy in, 668
spinal muscular atrophy in, 666, 1993t
Round cell tumors, of skin, 526–528
cytology of, 55
Roundworm infestation, and gastritis, 1165
of small intestine, 1220, 1221t
RU 486, for hyperadrenocorticism, 1482
in abortion induction, 1545
Rutin, for chylothorax, 1108

Sacculitis, anal, 1266–1267
Sacrocaudal dysgenesis, 645, 1975t
Saline, for shock, with gastric dilatation and volvulus, 1172
in fluid therapy, 328, 329, 329t, 330t
in lavage, for pyothorax, 1106–1107

Salivary glands, disorders of, *1119*, 1119–1120, *1120*
  excessive secretion from, 107–109, *110*
  parotid, congenital enlargement of, 1986t
Salmon calcitonin, for rodenticide toxicity, 360
Salmonellosis, 390–391, 391t
  and colitis, 1244
  and enteritis, 1217–1218
  zoonotic, 385t
Salmon-poisoning disease, 406, 1219
Samoyed, renal basement membrane disorders in, 1699t, 1702
San Joaquin Valley fever. See *Coccidioidomycosis.*
Sandostatin, for gastrinoma, 1506, 1506t
  for pancreatic islet cell tumors, 1434t, 1435t, 1437, *1437*
Sarcocystis infection, enteric, 408, 409, 409t
Sarcoma, after vaccination, against feline leukemia virus, 428
  and aortic thrombosis, *967*
  and arthropathy, 1874, *1875*
  client information on, 1922, 1925, 1927
  Kaposi's, 481
  of bone, 536–540, *1910*, 1910–1912
  of colon, 1253–1254
  of esophagus, 1147
  of lymphatic system, peripheral, 980
  of mouth, *1115*, 1115–1118, *1116*, 1117t
  of rectum, 1253–1254, 1260–1262
  of small intestine, 1234, *1235*
  of soft tissue, assessment of, *530*, 530–531
    classification of, 529, 529t
    pathogenesis of, 529
    treatment of, 531–534, *532*, 533t
      radiotherapy in, 497t, *532*, 533, 534
  of stomach, 1176, 1177
Scabies, 59t, 61
  and crusting, 50–51
  and pruritus, 32, 33t, 34, 34t, 35
  of pinna, 988, 989t
Scaling, 47–49, *50*
Scapula, sarcoma of, surgery for, 537
Schiff-Sherrington sign, 613
Schistocytes, in anemia, 200t, 1803
Schnauzer, giant, vitamin B₁₂ malabsorption in, 1850, 1986tt
  miniature, renal dysplasia in, 1699t, 1702
Schwann cells, 662, *662*, 665–666
  dysfunction of, in developmental disorders, 668–669
Schwannoma, 677
Sciatic nerve, injury to, signs of, 663t
Scintigraphy, colorectal, in liver disease, 1291–1292
  in glomerular function testing, 1602t, 1603
  in hyperparathyroidism, 1387, 1388
  in hyperthyroidism, 1407–1409, *1408*, *1409*
    with thyroid tumors, 1416
  in hypothyroidism, 1426
  of biliary tract, 1341–1342
  of bone disorders, 1890
  of kidneys, in amyloidosis, 1668–1669
  of lymphatic system, 979
  of portosystemic shunt, congenital, 1313, 1315
  of respiratory system, 1037
  of small intestine, 1208
  of somatostatin receptors, in gastrinoma, 1505
Scleritis, *67*, 69
Scoliosis, with hydromyelia, 652, *653*
Scottish fold cat, arthropathy in, 1874, 1975t
  ear abnormality in, 1874, 1977t
Scottish terrier, cramping in, 588
Scratching, 31–36. See also *Pruritus.*
Sebaceous glands, disorders of, and otitis externa, 989t, 993

Sebaceous glands *(Continued)*
  inflammation of, 48
  tumors of, 525
Seborrhea, and otitis externa, 989t, 993
  congenital, 1982t, 1995t
  of pinna, 988, 989t
  primary, 47–48
Secretin, 1501
  in diagnosis of gastrinoma, 1504–1505
Sedation, cardiac effects of, echocardiography of, 842–843, 845t
  for blood donation, 349
Seizures, 148–152, *149*, 150t, 151t
  after portosystemic shunt ligation, 1314
  and weakness, 12
  brain trauma and, 579, 580
  brain tumors and, 585
  client information on, 1920
  diagnosis of, *149*, 150–151
  dobutamine and, in cardiomyopathy treatment, 911
  genetic predisposition to, 1991t
  hypernatremia and, 230, 232
  in hepatic failure, 1302t
  in hyperthermia, 8
  in hypoparathyroidism, 1393
  management of, 150t, 151t, 151–152
  pathophysiology of, 148–150
  ptyalism with, 108
  with coma, 147
Selectins, in inflammation, 1844–1845
Selenium, in diet, 239t
Semen, artificial instillation of, 1574–1577, *1576*
  client information on, 1934
  collection of, 1571–1572
  evaluation of, 1571–1574, 1572t
    in cats, 1586–1587
    in prostatic disease, 1688
  in infertility, 1578–1580
  pathogen transmission in, 1577–1578
Sensory nerves, disorders of, developmental, 669, 1992t
  and acral mutilation, 669, 1994t
  in ganglioneuritis, 675
  with spinal cord disorders, 611–612
Separation anxiety, 158
Sepsis, after periodontal treatment, prevention of, 1133
  and cholestasis, 1336–1337
  neutrophil response in, 1843, 1844
  with hypotension, *185*, 186
  with liver disorders, 1335–1336
  with shock, management of, 184t
Serine-threonine kinases, in carcinogenesis, 478, 479t
Serotonin, in gastrointestinal endocrine system, 1502, 1503
Sertoli cell tumor, skin signs of, 26
714-X, in cancer management, 377
Severe combined immunodeficiency, 3t, 1990t
  neutrophils in, 1850
Shaker syndrome, 598–599
Shar Pei, amyloidosis in, renal, 1699t, 1702, 1996t
  with fever, 1323
  tight lip syndrome in, 1126
Shih Tzu, renal dysplasia in, 1699t, 1701–1702
Shivers, 139–141, *140*
  brain disorders and, 598–599
  cerebellar hypoplasia and, 588
  generalized, 606–607
Shock, fluid therapy in, 330t, 335, 337, 338t
  glucocorticoids for, 315, 316, 1172
  hypovolemic, fluid therapy in, 330t
    gastric ulcers with, 1166

Shock *(Continued)*
  toxic, streptococcosis and, 396
  with gastric dilatation and volvulus, 1172
  with sepsis, management of, 184t
Short-bowel syndrome, 1235–1236
Shortening fraction, left ventricular, echocardiographic estimation of, 860, 862t, 864t
Shoulder, luxation of, congenital, 1984t
Shunts, cardiac, and cyanosis, 207, 207t, 209, 779
  in fetus, 750–751
  in patent ductus arteriosus, 745–747
  in tetralogy of Fallot, 781, 782
  septal defects and, 751–759. See also *Atrial septal defect* and *Ventricular septal defect.*
  with pulmonic stenosis, 760
  portosystemic. See *Portosystemic shunts.*
Siamese cat, Niemann-Pick disease in, and peripheral neuropathy, 670–671
Siberian husky, atopic dermatitis in, with zinc deficiency, 48–49
  laryngeal paralysis in, 669, 1994t
Sideroleukocytes, 1848
Signal aliasing, in echocardiography, 841, *842*
Signal averaging, in electrocardiography, 803
Silibinin, for mushroom toxicity, to liver, 1332
Silica, in urolithiasis, 1758t, 1777
Silver sulfadiazine (Silvadene), for *Pseudomonas aeruginosa* infection, in otitis externa, 990t, 996
Simethicone, for borborygmus, 136
Sinoatrial blocks, 816
Sinoventricular rhythm, 820, *821*
Sinus(es), nasal. See *Nasal sinuses.*
  pilonidal, and spinal cord disorders, 643
Sinus rhythm, disturbances of, 808–810, *809–811*
Siphonaptera infestation, 59t, 59–60, *60*. See also *Fleas.*
Skeletal disorders, 1887–1914. See also *Bone(s).*
Skin, bacterial infection of, and abscesses, 391t, 398–399
  antibiotics for, 305
  crusting on, 47, 49–51, *50*
  disorders of, as signs of internal disorders, 26–29, *27*
    congenital, in cats, 1981t–1982t
      in dogs, 1994t–1995t
    cytology of, 51–55, *52*, 53t, *54*
    drugs for, over-the-counter, 319
    feline immunodeficiency virus infection and, 435
    in adverse food reactions, 253–254, *254*, 1231, 1231t
    in blastomycosis, 459
    in hypothyroidism, 1421, 1421t
    in necrotizing vasculitis, 973
    in sporotrichosis, *471*, 472, *472*
    liver disorders and, 1272
  erosions of, 39–43, 40t, *41*, 42t
  examination of, in small intestinal disorders, 1205
  histiocytosis of, 520
  hyperpigmentation of, 55, *56*, 57–58
  hypopigmentation of, 55–57, *56*
  inflammation of. See *Dermatitis.*
  lymphoma of, 49, 508, *508*, 509t, 512, *512*, 528
  mass lesions in, 36–39, *38*
  papules on, 44, 46
  parasitosis of, 42, 58–62, 59t, *60*, *62*
  pustules on, 43–47, *45*, *46*, 46t
  scaling on, 47–49, *50*

Skin (Continued)
  tumors of, 36–39, 38, 523, 523t
    diagnosis of, 523–524
      cytology in, 53t, 54, 55
    digital, 525
    epithelial, 55, 524t, 524–526
    mast cell, 526–527
    melanomatous, 526
    radiotherapy for, 491, 492, 492, 497t
    round cell, 526–528
    squamous cell, 42, 524–525
  ulcers of, 39–43, 40t, 41, 42t, 52
    with liver disease, 1272
Skull, congenital defects of, 1975t, 1983t
  osteopathy of, with mandibular osteopathy,
    1898, 1900, 1901, 1983t
  radiography of, in brain disorders, 575–576
    in hydrocephalus, 587
Skunks, rabies in, 388
Skye terrier, hepatic copper accumulation in,
  1306
Sleep, disorders of, 152–155, 153
Slo-Bid. See Theophylline.
Small intestine, 1182–1236. See also
    Gastrointestinal tract.
  algal infection of, 1219, 1947
  anatomy of, 1182–1187, 1184–1186, 1186t
  bacterial flora of, 1193
    overgrowth of, 1223t, 1223–1225, 1224t
      tests for, 1211–1212
      with histoplasmosis, 464
  bacterial infection of, 1207, 1217–1219, 1218
  congenital defects of, 1976t, 1985t, 1986t
  disorders of, acute, 1213t, 1213–1215
    and borborygmus, 1201
    and diarrhea, 122t, 122–126, 1182, 1183t,
      1198–1200, 1199, 1199t, 1200t
    and flatulence, 1201
    and malabsorption, 1200, 1200t, 1201
    and melena, 127t, 127–129, 1200–1201,
      1201t
    and pancreatic exocrine insufficiency, 1356–
      1357, 1357, 1363t, 1363–1364
    and protein loss, 1201–1202, 1202t
    and vomiting, 118t, 119–121, 120
    chronic idiopathic, 1222–1223
    diagnosis of, 1202, 1203, 1204
      biopsy in, 1212t, 1212–1213, 1213, 1213t
      clinical findings in, 1203t, 1203–1205,
        1205t
      endoscopy in, 1212, 1212
      history in, 1202–1203, 1203t, 1205t
      laboratory tests in, 1205–1212, 1206,
        1207, 1207t, 1210t, 1211
      scintigraphy in, 1208
      ultrasonography in, 1208, 1210
    in basenji, 1228
    in food allergy, 1230–1232, 1231t
    in food intolerance, 1233
    in gluten sensitivity, 254, 1232–1233, 1986t
    pathophysiology of, 1197t, 1197–1198,
      1198, 1198t
    radiography of, 1207–1208, 1208t, 1209
    signs of, 1182, 1183t
  fungal infection of, 1219–1220
  ileus in, adynamic, 1234
  in digestion, 1187, 1187t, 1188, 1189
  in fluid balance, 1191–1193, 1192, 1193
  in lipid metabolism, 284, 285, 286
  inflammation of, 1225t, 1225–1227, 1226,
    1227t
    and arthritis, 1883, 1885
    eosinophilic, 1228–1229
    granulomatous, 1229
    liver disorders with, 1336

Small intestine (Continued)
    lymphocytic-plasmacytic, 1227–1228
  lymphangiectasia in, 1229, 1229–1230, 1230,
    1976t, 1985t
  motility of, 1190–1191
  mucosa-associated lymphoid tissue in, func-
    tion of, 1193–1196, 1194t, 1194–1196
  nutrient absorption from, 1187–1190, 1189–
    1191
  obstruction of, 1233–1234
  parasitosis of, 1219–1221, 1221t
    migration of, to lung, 1071
  permeability of, testing of, 1210, 1211
  protozoal infection of, 408–411, 409t, 410t,
    1221–1222
  shortness of, 1235–1236
  sprue in, 1228
  tumors of, 1198, 1234–1235, 1235
  viral infection of, 1207, 1215–1217
Smell, impaired sense of, 562
  and anorexia, 103
Smoke inhalation, and lung injury, 1083,
  1087–1088
Sneezing, 194–197, 195, 197t
  reverse, 194, 195, 1029
Sodium, absorption of, from intestine,
    1187–1188, 1189, 1191–1193, 1192, 1193
  blood level of, decreased. See Hyponatremia.
    elevated. See Hypernatremia.
  clearance of, in renal function assessment,
    1604t, 1605
  excretion of, furosemide and, in heart failure,
    714, 715
  in diet, 239t
    and calcium oxalate urolithiasis, 1764–1765
    in glomerulonephritis, 1673
    in heart disease, 262–263, 264t, 266t–268t,
      266–268
    in mitral insufficiency, 794
    in renal disease, 271, 273t, 274t, 1647t
  in osmolality, 328
  renal tubular reabsorption of, 1706
  retention of, in glomerular disease, 1675, 1675
    in heart failure, 702t, 703
Sodium bicarbonate. See Bicarbonate.
Sodium chloride, and hypertension, 179–180
  for shock, with gastric dilatation and volvulus,
    1172
  in fluid therapy, 328, 329, 329t, 330t
  in lavage, for pyothorax, 1106–1107
Sodium fluoroacetate, in rodenticides, toxicity
  of, 360
Sodium iodide, for fungal infection, 475t
Sodium nitroprusside, for cardiomyopathy,
    dilated, 884
  for heart failure, 725–726
    with mitral insufficiency, 794
Sodium phosphate, in enemas, 131, 132t
Sodium polystyrene resin, with sorbitol, for
  hyperkalemia, in renal failure, 1628
Sodium stibogluconate, for leishmaniasis, 410t
Sodium sulfate, for acetaminophen toxicity, to
  liver, 1332
Soft palate, elongated, 1027, 1985t
Solanum species, toxicity of, 364
Solu-Delta-Cortef. See Prednisone/prednisolone.
Solu-Medrol. See Methylprednisolone.
Somatostatin, for pancreatic islet cell tumors,
    1434t, 1435t, 1437, 1437
  function of, 1370, 1370
  in gastrointestinal endocrine system, 1501–
    1503
  receptors of, scintigraphy of, in gastrinoma,
    1505
Sonography. See Ultrasonography and
    Echocardiography.

Sorbitol, with sodium polystyrene resin, for
    hyperkalemia, in renal failure, 1628
Sotalol, for arrhythmia, 824t–826t, 829t, 830
  for tachycardia, with right ventricular cardio-
    myopathy, 913
SPA, for feline immunodeficiency virus
    infection, 437, 438
  for feline leukemia virus infection, 430
Spaniel, cocker, hepatitis in, 1306
  renal basement membrane disorder in,
    1699t, 1701
  springer, alpha-fucosidosis in, 3t, 1992t
    and peripheral neuropathy, 670
Spastic pupil syndrome, 660t
Spasticity, in brain disorders, 561
Spathiphyllum species, toxicity of, 364
Spavin, 1866–1867
Spaying. See Sterilization.
Spermatozoa. See Semen.
Sphenoidal sinus. See Nasal sinuses.
Spherocytes, in anemia, 199, 200, 200t
  hemolytic, 1795, 1795
Sphingomyelinosis, 589, 590t, 1980t, 1992t
Spina bifida, 645, 646, 1980t, 1984t
Spinal accessory nerve, anatomy of, 664t
  examination of, 563, 567t
Spinal column, disorders of, disk disorders and,
    acupuncture for, 371, 373, 634
Spinal cord. See also Nervous system, central.
  demyelination of, in globoid cell leukodystro-
    phy, 627–628
  in leukoencephalomyelopathy, in rottwei-
    lers, 636
  disorders of, 608–653
    and colonic dysfunction, 1254
    and fecal incontinence, 1268t, 1268–1269
    and urinary incontinence, 1742, 1743
    calcinosis circumscripta and, 619, 619
    degenerative, 622–623
    dermoid cyst and, 643
    diagnosis of, 609–610
    disk disorders and, 630, 630–633, 631, 633
      client information on, 1919
      treatment of, 633–635
    dural ossification and, 627
    epidermoid cyst and, 643
    exostoses and, in hypervitaminosis A, 629–
      630
    hydromyelia and, 652, 653
    in ataxia, 142–143, 611, 613–615, 629
    in diffuse idiopathic skeletal hyperostosis,
      623, 623–624
    in discospondylitis, 624–626, 625, 626
    in myelodysplasia, 639
    in neuroaxonal dystrophy, 642
    in osteochondromatosis, 642–643
    in progressive hemorrhagic myelomalacia,
      643–644, 648
    in spina bifida, 645, 646, 1980t, 1984t
    intra-arachnoid cysts and, 645–647, 646
    localization of, 612t–614t, 612–615
    mechanisms of, 608–609
    mucopolysaccharidosis and, 638–639
    paraneoplastic, 506, 506t
    pilonidal sinus and, 643
    signs of, 557, 557t, 610–612
    spondylosis and, cervical, 619–621
    spondylosis deformans and, 650–652, 651
    synovial cysts and, 652
    syringomyelia and, 652
    vascular malformations and, 652–653
    vascular tumors and, benign, 652–653
    vertebral anomalies and, 621, 622, 1976t
    vertebral stenosis and, 650
      lumbosacral, 636t, 636–638, 638, 639

IND

Spinal cord (Continued)
  with atlantoaxial subluxation, 615, 615–616, 616
  with hemorrhage, 628–629, 629
  in sacrocaudal dysgenesis, 645
  inflammation of, 616–619, 618t
    feline infectious peritonitis and, 627
    in distemper, 626–627
    in feline polioencephalomyelitis, 627
    in granulomatous meningoencephalomyelitis, 628
    with arteritis, steroid-responsive, 621–622
  ischemia of, fibrocartilaginous embolism and, 635–636
  nematode infestation of, 647
  protozoal infection of, 644–645
  segmental reflexes of, examination of, 566–571, 567–572, 571t
  trauma to, 647–650
    glucocorticoids for, 315–316, 648–649
  tumors of, 639–642, 641
    radiotherapy for, 494, 497t
Spinal fluid. See Cerebrospinal fluid.
Spinal muscles, atrophy of, in developmental disorders, 666, 667
Spine. See also Spinal cord.
  anomalies of, 621, 622, 1975t, 1976t, 1983t, 1984t
  intervertebral disk disorders in. See Disks, intervertebral.
Spirillosis, zoonotic, 385t
Spirocerca infestation, and aortic aneurysm, 968, 969
  and cancer, 480
  and gastritis, 1165
  of spinal cord, 647
Spironolactone, for ascites, 139
  with protein-losing enteropathy, 1202
  for edema, with hepatic failure, 1302t
  for heart failure, 716
  for pulmonary edema, with hypertrophic cardiomyopathy, 908
  with mitral insufficiency, 793
Spleen, enlargement of, 1858t, 1858–1859
  liver disease and, 1277
  hemangiosarcoma of, 531, 534
  mass lesions of, benign, 1858
  physiology of, 1857
Splenectomy, anemia after, 199
  for hemolytic anemia, 1797
Splenic artery, anatomy of, 1155
Splenomegaly, 1858t, 1858–1859
  liver disease and, 1277
Spondylitis, and spinal cord dysfunction, 624–626, 625, 626
  ankylosing, 651
Spondylomyelopathy, cervical, 619–621
Spondylosis deformans, 650–652, 651
Spongiform encephalopathy, 451, 599
  congenital, 1980t
Sporanox. See Itraconazole.
Sporotrichosis, 91, 471–472, 472
  zoonotic, 385t, 472
Spotted fever. See Rocky Mountain spotted fever.
Spotton, for dirofilariasis, 952
Sprains, 1867
Spraying, of urine, 160, 160t
Springer spaniel, alpha-fucosidosis in, 3t, 1992t
  and peripheral neuropathy, 670, 1992t
Sprue, 1228
Squamous cell carcinoma, nasal, 1019–1021, 1021
  of salivary glands, 1119
  of skin, 42, 524–525

Squamous cell carcinoma (Continued)
  crusting in, 51
  of tonsils, 1029
  oral, 1115, 1115–1118, 1116, 1117t
Squamous metaplasia, of prostate, 1692
Squirrels, rabies in, 388
ST segment, 804, 805. See also Electrocardiography.
Staining, in cytology, of skin lesions, 52–53
  of muscle fibers, 685t, 686
Stance, examination of, in brain disorders, 559t, 560
Staphylococcal infection, and discospondylitis, 624, 625, 626
  and meningitis, spinal, 616, 618
  and otitis externa, 990t, 993, 995
  and pyoderma, 43, 44, 46t, 49
  and struvite urolithiasis, 1730, 1731
  antibiotics for, 302–303, 305–306
Staphylococcal protein A, for feline immunodeficiency virus infection, 437, 438
  for feline leukemia virus infection, 430
  in anemia, 1811
Starling's law, in fluid dynamics, 326, 327
Status epilepticus. See Seizures.
Steatorrhea, 1361, 1361
  malabsorption and, 1205
Sterilization, 1542, 1542–1543
  and obesity, 70, 1540
  client information on, 1933
  in prostatic hypertrophy, 1691
  prepubertal, 1539–1541
    and bone growth disorders, 1908
  remnant ovarian tissue after, 1596
Steroids, 307–317. See also Corticosteroids.
  anabolic, for anemia, in renal failure, 1655
Stertor, 195, 1035, 1035t
Stibogluconate sodium, for leishmaniasis, 410t
Stomach. See also Gastrointestinal tract.
  anatomy of, 1154–1156, 1155
  bleeding in, and melena, 127, 127t
  dilatation of, with volvulus, 1170–1174, 1171, 1172
    and megaesophagus, 1150t
    client information on, 1943
  disorders of, and vomiting, 118t, 119–121, 120
  evaluation of, 1159–1160
  enlargement of, 137
  erosions of, 1165–1167
  inflammation of, acute, 1160–1162
    chronic, 1162–1165
    in renal failure, 1636, 1636t
    with enteritis, coronavirus and, 422
    hemorrhagic, 123, 1162, 1214
    in renal failure, 1648
    salmonellosis and, 390, 391
  intubation of, for enteral nutrition, 277–279, 278, 279, 1945
  intussusception of, into esophagus, 1153, 1153
  motility disorders of, 1174–1176
  outlet of, obstruction of, 1168–1170, 1169
  physiology of, 1156, 1156–1159
  reflux from, 1151–1152
  tumors of, 1176–1177
  ulcers of, 1165–1168, 1167
    bleeding from, coagulopathy and, with liver disorders, 1335
    steroids and, 1797
    uremia toxins and, in renal failure, 1629, 1630t
Stomatitis, 1118–1119
  and ptyalism, 109
  plant toxicity and, 364
  uremia toxins and, in renal failure, 1629

Stomatocytosis, 1989t
  in hemolytic anemia, 1791t, 1792
Strabismus, congenital, 1978t, 1987t
Stranguria, 89, 90
Stratum corneum, scaling diseases of, 47–48
Streptobacillosis, zoonotic, 385t
Streptococcosis, 391t, 395–396
  and enteritis, 1218
Streptokinase, for thromboembolism, 917, 1840
Streptomycin, dosage of, in renal failure, 1649t
  in artificial insemination, 1574
Stress, and urinary tract disorders, 1746
  and weakness, 12–13
Stridor, 195, 1035, 1035t
Stroke, 966
Stroke volume, in arterial pulse pressure, 175–177
  in heart failure, 693, 693–694
Strongyloides infestation, of small intestine, 1221, 1221t
Struvite urolithiasis, in cats, 1711–1712, 1712, 1713, 1723t, 1730t, 1730–1732, 1731t
  in dogs, 1758t, 1760–1763, 1761t, 1762t
    with calcium oxalate lithiasis, 1765–1766, 1766, 1770, 1771
Strychnine, in rodenticides, toxicity of, 360
Stupor, 144–147, 145, 146t
Subaortic stenosis, 768–772, 769–772. See also Aortic stenosis, subvalvular.
Subchondral bone cyst, 1905
Subclavian arteries, malformation of, and esophageal compression, 1145
Subcutaneous space, accumulations in, 62–66, 64, 65
Sublingual gland, mucocele of, 1119, 1119–1120, 1120
Succimer, for lead toxicity, 362
Sucralfate, for esophagitis, 1148, 1149
  after foreign body ingestion, 1146
  with megaesophagus, 1150t
  for gastric ulcers, 1168
    in renal failure, 1629, 1630t
  for gastrinoma, 1506, 1506t
  for gastritis, with Helicobacter infection, 1164
  for gastroesophageal reflux, 1152
Sulbactam, with ampicillin, for lung infection, 1065t
Sulfadiazine, for lung infection, 1065t
  for neosporosis, with myositis, 687
Sulfadimethoxine, for Isospora infection, of small intestine, 1222
  for protozoal infection, 410, 410t
  for staphylococcal pyoderma, 46t
Sulfamethoxazole, with trimethoprim. See Trimethoprim.
Sulfamidase deficiency, in mucopolysaccharidosis, skeletal abnormalities with, 1896–1897
Sulfasalazine, for diarrhea, with histoplasmosis, 464
  for inflammatory bowel disease, 1250
  for vasculitis, microscopic necrotizing, 973
  of pinna, 989t, 991
Sulfisoxazole, dosage of, in renal failure, 1649t
Sulfonamides, for Pneumocystis carinii infection, of lung, 1066
  for protozoal infection, 410, 410t
  toxicity of, and anemia, 1812
  trimethoprim with. See Trimethoprim.
Sulfonylurea drugs, for diabetes mellitus, 1449, 1449t, 1450
Sunlight, and carcinoma, 481
  client information on, 1926
  with nasal keratosis, 1019, 1020
  and pinnal dermatitis, 988–991, 989t

Suppressor genes, in carcinogenesis, 478–479
Suprascapular nerve, injury to, signs of, 663t
Surfak, for constipation, 132t
Swallowing, disorders of, 114, 114t, *115,*
    1026–1029
    physiology of, 1025, *1026*
Sweat glands, tumors of, 525–526
Swimmer's ear, 989t, 990t, 996
Syncope, 13t, 13–16, *14*
    in hypertrophic cardiomyopathy, 906
    with mitral insufficiency, 789
Syncytium-forming virus infection, 452
    in polyarthritis, 1881
Syndactyly, 1894, *1895,* 1975t, 1984t
Synechiae, posterior, and anisocoria, 659t
Synovial cell sarcoma, 538–539
Synovial cysts, spinal, 652
Synovial fluid, examination of, in arthritis, 79,
    79, 1879
    in degenerative joint disease, 1865
Synovitis, lymphocytic-plasmacytic, 78–80
    of knee, 1883–1885
Syringomyelia, 652
Syrup of ipecac, in induction of vomiting, 319
Systemic inflammatory response syndrome, 327
    fluid therapy in, 335, 337
Systemic lupus erythematosus. See *Lupus
    erythematosus.*
Systolic clicks, 171

T lymphocytes, in colonic mucosal immunity,
    1239
    in feline immunodeficiency virus infection,
        434
    in glomerulonephritis, 1663–1664
    in inflammation, steroid effects on, 310
    in lymphoma, cutaneous, 49
        in mycosis fungoides, 508, *508*
    in small intestinal immune response, 1195–
        1196, *1196*
T wave, 804, 805. See also *Electrocardiography.*
T₃, deficiency of, 1419–1428. See also
    Hypothyroidism.
    excess of, 1400–1417. See also *Hyperthyroid-
    ism.*
T₄, deficiency of, 1419–1428. See also
    Hypothyroidism.
    excess of, 1400–1417. See also *Hyperthyroid-
    ism.*
Tachyarrhythmia, in cardiomyopathy,
    hypertrophic, 898, 905
    in digitalis toxicity, 730
    in mitral insufficiency, and pulmonary conges-
        tion, 794–795
    supraventricular, in hypotension, 184t
Tachycardia, atrial, electrocardiography of,
    811–812, *812*
    in cardiomyopathy, canine, 878
    in heart failure, 703, 704t
    reflex sympathetic, hydralazine and, in heart
        failure, 724
    sinus, electrocardiography of, 809, *809*
    ventricular, electrocardiography of, 814–815,
        815
        in cardiomyopathy, feline, 905, 911, 913
Tachykinins, 1502
Tachypnea, 166–169, *168*
Taenia infestation, of small intestine, 1221,
    1221t
Tagamet. See *Cimetidine.*
Tail, absence of, in Manx cats, 645, 1975t
    congenital defects of, 1975t, 1983t
    docking of, neuroma after, and pruritus, 33t

Tamponade, cardiac, mitral insufficiency and,
    795
    pericardial disorders and, 924–925, *926*
        treatment of, 931–933, *933*
Tapetal hypoplasia, 1978t, 1989t
Tapeworm infestation, of small intestine, 1221,
    1221t
Tartar, periodontal, 1127
Taurine, deficiency of, and cardiomyopathy,
        263–264
    dilated, canine, 878
        feline, 908–912, *909, 910*
    for cardiomyopathy, hypertrophic, 906
    for hepatic encephalopathy, 1335
    in diet, 240
Taxus cuspidata, toxicity of, 365
Tea, in cancer management, 378t
Tears, artificial, over-the-counter, 320
Technetium scans. See *Scintigraphy.*
Teeth, care of, client information on, 1940
    congenital defects of, 1976t
    deciduous, retention of, 1122–1123
    development of, 1123–1124
    endodontic treatment of, in fractured teeth,
        1137t, 1137–1140, *1138*
        in non-fractured teeth, 1136–1137, *1138*
        indications for, 1135–1136
    loss of, giant cell granuloma and, 1905
    number of, variations in, 1122
    occlusion of, *1123–1126,* 1124–1126
    periodontal disorders of, 1127–1134. See also
        Periodontium.
    restorative treatment of, 1140–1141
    types of, 1122
Tegison (etretinate), for lymphoma, cutaneous,
        528
    for pinnal dermatosis, 988–991, 989t
    for sebaceous adenitis, 48
Telangiectasia, renal, in corgi, 1698, 1699t, 1703
Telomeres, in carcinogenesis, 479
Temaril-P, for cough, 165t
    for tracheal disease, 1043t
Temperature, and otitis externa, 993
    changes in, before parturition, 1529
    decreased, in renal failure, 1625
    maintenance of, in neonates, 242–244
    regulation of, 6, *6*
        in hyperthermia, 6–9, 7t, *8, 9*
        in hypothermia, *9,* 9–10
Temporomandibular joint, instability of, 1868
Tendons, contracture of, trauma and, 1867
Tenesmus, 129, 132–133, 133t
    causes of, 1258t, 1258–1259
    perineal hernia and, 1259
Tenormin. See *Atenolol.*
Tenosynovitis, 1867
Teratozoospermia, in dog, 1579
Terbinafine, for fungal infection, 457, 475t
Terbutaline, for bronchopulmonary disease,
        1059t
    for tracheal disease, 1043t
Terramycin. See *Oxytetracycline.*
Terrier, ataxia in, hereditary, 629, 1991t
    bull, acrodermatitis in, 48, 1994t, 1995t
        renal basement membrane disorder in,
            1699t, 1701
    cairn, neuronopathy in, progressive, 666
    hepatic copper accumulation in, 1304–1306,
        1305, 1991t
    West Highland white, epidermal dysplasia in,
        48, 1995t
    Wheaten, glomerular disease in, 1699t, 1702
    Yorkshire, encephalitis in, 598
Territorial aggression, in cats, 160, 160t
    in dogs, 156, *157*

Testicles, anatomy of, 1586
    cancer of, 543–544
    hypoplasia of, 3, 1594, 1981t, 1994t
    inflammation of, 1594
    removal of. See *Sterilization.*
    Sertoli cell tumor of, skin signs of, 26
    torsion of, 1594
    undescended, in cat, 1593, 1597t, 1597–1598,
        1981t
        in dog, 1584–1585, 1993t
Testosterone, for bladder dysfunction, 1739t
    for libido stimulation, 1597, 1597t
    in contraception, 1543
    production of, 1590–1591, 1594
Tetanus, 391t, 398, 604
Tetany, hypocalcemia and, 233
    in hypoparathyroidism, 1392
        management of, 1396t, 1396–1397
    puerperal, 1394–1396, 1538
        and hyperthermia, 8
Tetracycline, concentration of, and bacterial
        susceptibility, 303t
    dosage of, in renal failure, 1649t
    for bacterial infection, 391t
    for ehrlichiosis, 404, 405
    for hemobartonellosis, with hemolytic anemia,
        1799–1800
    for intestinal bacterial overgrowth, with histo-
        plasmosis, 464
    for lung infection, 1065t
    for periodontitis, 1132
    for protozoal infection, 410t
    for rickettsial infection, with arthritis, 1878
        with spinal meningitis, 619
    for Rocky Mountain spotted fever, 402
    for thrombocytopenia, 1819
    toxicity of, to liver, 1328
Tetralogy of Fallot, 780–782, *781, 782,* 1976t,
        1985t
    auscultation of, 739t
    echocardiography of, 839, *841,* 854t
    ventricular septal defect in, 751, *754*
2,3,2-Tetramine, for hepatic copper
        accumulation, 1303t
Tetraplegia, spinal cord disorders and, 611
Thallium, toxicity of, 362
    to peripheral nerves, 673t
Theophylline, for bronchial asthma, 1058, 1059t
    for bronchitis, 1056
    for bronchopulmonary disease, 1059t
    for cough, 165t
    for pneumonia, bacterial, 1064
    for pulmonary hypertension, 1081
    for respiratory disorders, with heart failure,
        734
    for tracheal disease, 1043t
Thevetia peruviana, toxicity of, 365
Thiabendazole, for intestinal parasitosis, 1221,
        1221t
    for lungworm infestation, of trachea, 1045
    for mite infestation, of external ear canal,
        990t, 995
Thiacetarsamide (Caparsolate), for dirofilariasis,
        948, 949t, 951t
    client information on, 1953
    complications with, *952,* 952–954, *953*
    evaluation of, 954
    in cats, 949t, 960
Thiamine, absorption of, from small intestine,
        1190
    deficiency of, neurologic dysfunction with,
        549, 586, 593t
    for lead toxicity, 362
    in diet, 239, 239t
Thioproline, for peritonitis, feline infectious, 441

IND

Thirst, excessive. See *Polydipsia.*
Thistle, in cancer management, 378t
Thoracentesis, for pleural effusion, *187,* 187–188, 1103–1104
in heart failure, 733
with cardiomyopathy, dilated, 911
for pneumothorax, 1110
Thoracic limb, reflexes of, testing of, 566–568, *568,* 571t
Thorax, air in, *1109,* 1109–1110
lung cysts and, 1083–1084
subcutaneous emphysema with, 63, 65
compression of, in cardiopulmonary resuscitation, 190–192
pus accumulation in, 1103, 1104, 1105t, *1106,* 1106–1107
wall of, deformity of, in pectus carinatum, 1100, 1101
in pectus excavatum, *1100,* 1100–1101, *1101,* 1975t
trauma to, 1100
tumors of, 1101–1102
Thorazine (chlorpromazine), for hemobartonellosis, 407
for vomiting, in gastritis, 1161
in renal failure, 1629, 1630t
Thorn apple, toxicity of, 365
Threonine, in carcinogenesis, 478, 479t
in diet, 239t
Thrombasthenia, Glanzmann's, 1824t, 1826
Thrombasthenic thrombopathia, 1824t, 1826, 1990t
Thrombin, in hemostasis, 1829, *1832*
Thrombocytopenia, 1819t, 1819–1823, *1821, 1822t*
and epistaxis, 214–215
and purpura, 218–220, 219t, *221*
chemotherapy and, 486
client information on, 1960
cyclic, *Ehrlichia platys* and, 405
essential, 515t, 515–516
in transfusion reactions, 355
paraneoplastic, 505, 505t
Thrombocytosis, 1823
Thromboembolism, 1840
and absent arterial pulse, 177
and peripheral nerve injury, 678–679
arterial, peripheral, 964–968, *965,* 965t, *967*
cardiomyopathy and, 914–918, *915–917*
during adrenal surgery, for hyperadrenocorticism, prevention of, 1475
glomerular disease and, 1675, *1676*
in dirofilariasis, after adulticidal therapy, 947, 949t, 952–953, *953*
in hemolytic anemia, 1797
pulmonary, 1078–1080, *1079, 1080*
hyperadrenocorticism and, 1483
Thrombopathia, 1823–1827, 1824t–1826t
congenital, 1979t
thrombasthenic, 1824t, 1826, 1990t
Thrombophlebitis, parenteral nutrition and, 281
Thromboplastin time, activated partial, in liver disease, 1278t, 1285–1286
Thrombopoiesis, 1818, 1818t
Thrombosis, arterial, peripheral, 964–968, *965,* 965t, *967*
in hemostatic disorders, 1834–1836, 1835t, *1836, 1837,* 1839–1840, 1840t
of nervous system, 607
of portal vein, 1336
venous, *974,* 974–975, *975*
Thrombovascular necrosis, proliferative, of pinna, 991
Thromboxane A₂, in platelet activation, 1817, *1817*

Thromboxanes, in glomerulonephritis, 1664
Thymus, disorders of, 1096–1097
congenital, 1979t, 1990t
tumors of, *1093,* 1097
and megaesophagus, 1150t
exfoliative dermatitis with, 28
Thypinone, in thyrotropin-releasing hormone stimulation test, in hyperthyroidism, 1406
Thyroid, function of, in orthopedic developmental disorders, iodine and, 247–248
testing of, in hyperadrenocorticism, 1466
hyperfunction of, 1400–1417. See also *Hyperthyroidism.*
hypofunction of, 1419–1428. See also *Hypothyroidism.*
physiology of, 1419–1420, *1420*
tumors of, radiotherapy for, 491, 497t, 1417
Thyroid-stimulating hormone response test, in hyperthyroidism, 1407
in hypothyroidism, 1425
Thyrotoxicosis, 1400–1417. See also *Hyperthyroidism.*
Thyrotropin-releasing hormone stimulation test, in hyperthyroidism, 1406–1407, *1407*
in hypothyroidism, 1425
Thyroxine, deficiency of, 1419–1428. See also *Hypothyroidism.*
excess of, 1400–1417. See also *Hyperthyroidism.*
Tibetan mastiff, hypertrophic neuropathy in, 669, 1992t
Tibial nerve, injury to, signs of, 663t
Tibialis reflex, anterior, testing of, 568, *570*
Tibiotarsal joint, swelling of, with glomerular disease, 1670
Ticarcillin, concentration of, and bacterial susceptibility, 303t
for *Pseudomonas aeruginosa* infection, in otitis externa, 996
Ticks, as vectors, of borreliosis, 28, 396
of ehrlichiosis, 403
of Rocky Mountain spotted fever, 400–402, 616
bites of, and paralysis, 672–673
in skin infestation, 59t, 61
Tiletamine, in anesthesia, for prepubertal gonadectomy, 1541
Tinidazole, for protozoal infection, 410
Tirilizad mesylate, for spinal cord trauma, 649
Tissue factors, in hemostasis, 1829, *1831, 1832,* 1833t
Tissue plasminogen activator, for thromboembolism, 917, 1840
Tobacco, toxicity of, 365
Tobramycin, dosage of, in renal failure, 1649t
Tocainide, for arrhythmia, 824t–826t, 826–827, 829t
Tocopherol. See *Vitamin E.*
Tomato, toxicity of, 364
Tongue, disorders of, and ptyalism, 109
inflammation of, plant toxicity and, 364
Tonocard (sotalol), for arrhythmia, 824t–826t, 829t, 830
for tachycardia, with right ventricular cardiomyopathy, 913
Tonsils, inflammation of, 1028
tumors of, 1029
Tooth. See *Teeth.*
Toprol XL (metoprolol), for arrhythmia, 824t, 827, 828t, 830
for tachyarrhythmia, with mitral insufficiency, 794–795
Torbugesic. See *Butorphanol.*
Torovirus infection, and enteritis, 1217

Torsades de pointes, 815, *816*
Tortoiseshell cat, testicular hypoplasia in, 3, 1981t
Toxic epidermal necrolysis, 29
Toxic milk syndrome, 1538
Toxic shock, streptococcosis and, 396
Toxicity, 357–365. See also *Drugs* and specific agents, e.g., *Ethylene glycol* and affected organs, e.g., *Liver.*
Toxocariasis, intestinal, migration from, to lung, 1071
of small intestine, 1220, 1221t
of spinal cord, 647
zoonotic, 386, 387
Toxoplasmosis, and encephalitis, 596–597
and fetal loss, 1527–1528
and myositis, 687
enteric, 408, 409t, 410t, 410–411
of nervous system, multifocal, 606
of spinal cord, 644–645
polysystemic, 410t, 411–413
with feline immunodeficiency virus infection, 437, *437*
zoonotic, 388–389
Trachea, anatomy of, 1040
anomalies of, 1981t, 1994t
collapse of, 1043t, 1046–1050, *1048, 1049*
bronchoscopy of, 1038t
client information on, 1950
cytologic specimen from, in dirofilariasis, 956–957
disorders of, 1040–1054
and dyspnea, 166–169, 167t, *168*
bacterial cultures in, 1041–1042
cytology in, 1041, 1042
endoscopy in, 1041
history in, 1040
pathophysiology of, 1040
physical examination in, 1040
radiography of, 1040–1041, *1041*
hypoplasia of, 1045, *1046*
inflammation of, infectious, 1043t, 1043–1044
noninfectious, 1042–1043, 1043t
with bronchitis, 419t, 419–420, 1043t, 1043–1044
with laryngitis, 1030
lungworm infestation of, *1044,* 1044–1045
mass lesions of, obstructive, 1050–1053, *1051, 1052*
stenosis of, segmental, 1045–1046
trauma to, *1053,* 1053–1054, *1054*
Tracheobronchitis, infectious, 419t, 419–420, 1043t, 1043–1044
Tracheoscopy, 1041
Transforming growth factors, in metastatic tumor growth, 483
in small intestine, 1186
Transfusion. See *Blood transfusion.*
Transmissible venereal tumors, 545
Transplantation, of bone marrow, for anemia, 1815–1816
for genetic disorders, 5
of kidney, for renal failure, acute, 1632
chronic, 1659t, 1659–1660
Transposition, of great arteries, 783–784
Transudates, in pleural effusion, *187,* 188, 1105, 1105t
Tranxene, for behavioral disorders, 156, 158t
Trauma, and arteriovenous fistula, 969–971, *970, 971*
and hyperpigmentation, 57–58
and nervous system injury, 556, 678
and pancreatitis, 1350
and pneumothorax, 1109, 1110
to brain, 578–580, *579, 580,* 581t

Trauma (Continued)
  to genitalia, 1593
  to joints, 1866–1867
  to larynx, 1030–1031
  to lung, 1083, 1084–1088, 1085
  to pharynx, 1028–1029
  to spinal cord, 647–650
    and urinary incontinence, 1742
    glucocorticoids for, 315–316, 648–649
  to trachea, 1053, 1053–1054, 1054
  to urinary tract, 1752–1753, 1778, 1779t
  to veins, 974
Tremors, 139–141, 140
  brain disorders and, 598–599
  cerebellar hypoplasia and, 588
  generalized, 606–607
Trephination, of nasal sinuses, 1017
Tresaderm, for otitis externa, 990t, 995
Triamcinolone, dosage of, 313t, 314, 314t
  for eosinophilic granuloma complex, 1118
  for otitis externa, 990t, 995
  potency of, 312t, 313
  structure of, 309
Triamterene, for heart failure, 716
  for pulmonary edema, with mitral insuffi-
    ciency, 793
Tribrissen. See Trimethoprim.
Tricalcium phosphate, in urolithiasis, 1777
Triceps reflex, testing of, 566–568, 568, 571t
Trichiasis, 1978t, 1989t
Trichodectes lice, in skin infestation, 59t, 60, 60
Trichomoniasis, of large intestine, 1245
  of small intestine, 408–411, 409t, 410t
Trichophyton mentagrophytes infection, and
    scaling dermatosis, 49
Trichuris infestation, of large intestine, 1245,
    1245
Tricolor cat, testicular hypoplasia in, 3, 1981t
Tricuspid insufficiency, 795–796
  client information on, 1952
  murmur with, 172
  with pulmonic stenosis, 765–766
Tricuspid regurgitation, echocardiography of,
    857t, 870, 870
Tricuspid stenosis, echocardiography of, 847,
    847t, 870, 871
Tricuspid valve, atresia of, 783, 784
  dysplasia of, 1985t
    auscultation of, 739t
    congenital, 774–778, 775, 777–779, 1976t
    echocardiography of, 854t
  echocardiography of, 843, 845t, 846–847,
    857t, 859
Tricyclic antidepressants, for behavioral
    disorders, in cats, 160, 160t
    in dogs, 156, 158t
  for pain, 24t, 25
Trientine hydrochloride, for hepatic copper
    accumulation, 1301–1302, 1303t
Trigeminal nerve, anatomy of, 664t
  examination of, 562, 565, 565–566, 567t
  inflammation of, 680
  motor dysfunction of, 582
Trigger points, in acupuncture, 370, 372–373
Triglycerides, blood level of, elevated, 286–291.
    See also Hyperlipidemia.
  digestion of, in small intestine, 1187, 1189
  medium-chain, for cachexia, paraneoplastic,
    500
    for malabsorption, 259
    for small intestinal disorders, chronic idio-
      pathic, 1223
  metabolism of, 284, 285t, 285–287
Triiodothyronine, deficiency of, 1419–1428. See
    also Hypothyroidism.

Triiodothyronine (Continued)
  excess of, 1400–1417. See also Hyperthyroid-
    ism.
Trilostane, for hyperadrenocorticism, 1482
Trimeprazine, for cough, 165t
  for tracheal disease, 1043t
Trimethoprim, with sulfonamides, and thyroid
    hormone deficiency, 1424
  concentration of, and bacterial susceptibil-
    ity, 303t
  dosage of, in renal failure, 1649t
  for bacterial infection, 391t
  for lung infection, 1065t
  for prostatitis, 1693
  for protozoal infection, 410, 410t
  for staphylococcal pyoderma, 46t
  toxicity of, to liver, 1328
Trochlear nerve, anatomy of, 664t
  examination of, 562, 564, 564, 565, 567t
Truncus arteriosus, defect of, in
    aorticopulmonary septal defect, 785–786
Trypanosomiasis, polysystemic, 410t, 415–416
Trypsin, in defense against pancreatic
    autodigestion, 1346, 1346t, 1346–1347,
    1347
Trypsin-like immunoreactivity, in pancreatic
    exocrine insufficiency, 1359–1360, 1360
Trypsinogen, in pancreatitis, 1353, 1353t
Tryptophan, in diet, 239t, 239–240
Tuberculosis, 391t, 393–394, 1065–1066
  and enteritis, 1219
Tularemia, zoonotic, 385t
Tumor necrosis factors, in cachexia, in heart
    disease, 265
  in hyperthermia, 7, 7t
Tumors. See also Cancer and specific types,
    e.g., Sarcoma.
  adrenal, and hyperadrenocorticism, 1461,
    1462, 1462. See also Hyperadrenocorti-
    cism.
  and arthritis, 1883
  and bone loss, with hypercalcemia, 1908
  and cardiomyopathy, 914
  and cough, 163t
  and epistaxis, 215
  and gastric outlet obstruction, 1170
  and gastric ulcers, 1166
  and hypercalcemia, 233
  and pleural effusion, 186, 189
  and thrombocytopenia, 505, 505t, 1822–1823
  and tracheal obstruction, 1050–1053, 1051,
    1052
  and venous obstruction, 975, 975, 976
  carcinoid, intestinal, 1508
  client information on, 1921–1928
  genital, in male cat, 1594
  in birth canal, and dystocia, 1532–1534
  intracranial, and polyuria, 1375
  metastasis of, biology of, 481–483, 482
  obesity with, 71, 72
  of anal sacs, 1267
  of biliary tract, 1320, 1320–1322, 1343
  of bone, 535–540, 1910, 1910–1912
  of brain, 494, 497t, 577, 583–586, 584t, 585t
  of colon, 1253, 1253–1254
  of ear, otitis externa and, 996–997
  of esophagus, 1147
  of genitalia, 542–545
  of joints, 535, 538–539, 1874, 1875
  of larynx, 1031
  of liver, 1320t, 1320–1322
  of lung, bronchoscopy of, 1038t
    in malignant histiocytosis, 1078
    lymphomatous, 1077, 1077–1078
    metastatic, 1075–1077, 1076, 1077

Tumors (Continued)
  primary, 1073–1075, 1074, 1075
  of mammary glands, 544–545, 1928
    after sterilization, 1542, 1542
  of mediastinum, 1095t, 1095–1096, 1096
  of mouth, 1114–1116, 1114–1118, 1117t
  of nasal cavity, 1019–1023, 1021, 1023
    computed tomography of, 1009, 1012, 1014
    magnetic resonance imaging of, 1012, 1016
    radiography of, 1009, 1010
  of nervous system, 556, 607
  of ovaries, 544–545
    and infertility, 1562
    and prolonged estrus, 1523, 1523, 1524
  of pancreas, 1364
    and glucagon hypersecretion, 1507, 1507–
      1508
  of pancreatic islet cells, and gastrin hypersecre-
      tion, 1503–1506, 1505t, 1506t
    and insulin secretion, 1429–1438. See also
      Insulinoma.
    and pancreatic peptide hypersecretion,
      1506–1507
  of pericardium, 925
  of peripheral nerves, 676–677
  of pharynx, 1029
  of pituitary gland, 1484t, 1484–1485
    and acromegaly, 1371, 1373
  of prostate, 542–543, 1689t, 1694–1696, 1695,
    1696
  of rectum, 1253, 1253–1254, 1254, 1260–
    1262
    and stricture, 1263, 1264
  of salivary glands, 1119
  of skin. See Skin, tumors of.
  of small intestine, 1198, 1234–1235, 1235
  of spinal cord, 494, 497t, 639–642, 641
  of stomach, 1176–1177
  of thoracic wall, 1101–1102
  of thymus, 1093, 1097
    and exfoliative dermatitis, 28
    and megaesophagus, 1150t
  of thyroid, and hyperthyroidism, 1415–1417
  of urinary tract, 541–542, 1717t, 1739–1740
  of vagina, 1570, 1570
  perianal, 1267–1268
  subcutaneous, 63, 64, 65
  thoracic, and pleural effusion, 1108–1109
    hypertrophic osteopathy with, 1903–1904
  vascular, benign, and spinal cord compression,
    652–653
Tussigon (hydrocodone/homatropine), for cough,
    165t
  with heart failure, 734
  for tracheal disease, 1043t
Tussionex, for cough, 165t
Twins, conjoined, 1975t, 1983t
Tylosin, for intestinal bacterial overgrowth, 1225
  with histoplasmosis, 464
  with pancreatic exocrine insufficiency,
    1363–1364
  for protozoal infection, 410t
Tympanic membrane, anatomy of, 997
  perforated, in otitis media, 997–999
Tympanometry, in deafness, 1001
Typhus, 402
  zoonotic, 385t
Tyrosinase deficiency, 1995t
Tyrosine, in diet, 239t
Tyrosine kinases, in carcinogenesis, 478, 479t
Tyrosinemia, 1995t
Tyzzer's disease, 392, 1218–1219
Tzanck's method, in cytology of pustules, 52

Ulcerative colitis, and arthritis, 1883, 1885
  histiocytic, 1249, 1249

IND

Ulcers, gastrointestinal, 1165–1168, *1167*
   and melena, 127
   bleeding from, coagulopathy and, with
      acute liver disorders, 1335
   gastrinoma and, 1503–1506, 1505t, 1506t
   steroids and, 1797
   uremia toxins and, in renal failure, 1629,
      1630t
   with hepatic failure, 1302t
   in esophagitis, 1148
   of mouth, renal disorders and, 1601, *1601,*
      1629
   of pinna, vasculitis and, 991
   of skin, 39–43, 40t, *41,* 42t
      cytologic sampling from, 52
   with liver disease, 1272
Ulna, dysplasia of, 1984t
   retained cartilage cores in, 1898, *1900*
Ulnar nerve, injury to, signs of, 663t
Ultralente insulin, for diabetes mellitus,
   1451–1452
Ultrasonography, in blood pressure measurement,
   179, 184–185
   in hyperadrenocorticism, 1465t, 1466, *1467,*
      1467t, 1486
   in hyperparathyroidism, 1387, *1387,* 1388
   in hypoadrenocorticism, 1494, *1494*
   of arteriovenous fistula, 971, *971*
   of biliary tract, 1292, 1321, 1341, *1341*
   of brain, 576
   of cystic endometrial hyperplasia, 1524, *1524*
   of heart, 834–871. See also *Echocardiography.*
   of hepatobiliary tumors, 1321
   of intestine, in diarrhea, 125
      small, 1208, *1210*
   of kidney, 1612
      in renal failure, 1621, *1621*
   of liver, 1292, 1321
      in biopsy guidance, 1297
      in cirrhosis, 1300, *1300*
      in portosystemic shunt, congenital, 1312–
         1313
   of mediastinum, 1093, *1093*
   of ovarian follicular cyst, 1523, *1523*
   of pancreatic islet cell tumors, 1431, *1432*
   of pancreatitis, *1351,* 1351–1352
   of pleural effusion, 1104–1105
   of prostate, 1689, *1689,* 1689t
      inflamed, 1692, *1693*
      neoplasia in, 1696, *1696*
   of pyometra, with cystic endometrial hyperpla-
      sia, 1551, *1553*
   of respiratory system, 1036–1037
   of sarcoma, of soft tissue, 531
   of urinary tract, calculi in, 1722t, 1722–1724,
      1756, *1760*
      in incontinence, 92
Ultraviolet light, and carcinogenesis, 481
   client information on, 1926
   with nasal keratosis, 1019, 1020
   and pinnal dermatitis, 988–991, 989t
   sensitivity to, in xeroderma pigmentosa, ge-
      netic mutation and, 479
Umbilical cord, aplasia of, 1981t
Umbilical hernia, 1975t, 1983t
Uncinaria stenocephala infestation, of small
   intestine, 1220–1221, 1221t
Unconsciousness, in coma, 144–147, *145,* 145t,
   146t
   hypernatremia and, 230, 232
   myxedema and, 1422, 1426
Unisyn, for lung infection, 1065t
Urachus, anomalies of, 1982t, 1996t
   diverticula of, 1712, *1718,* 1718–1719, 1752
   persistent, 1752

Urate, in urolithiasis, in cats, 1723t, 1724–1725,
   1725t
   in dogs, 1758t, 1770–1775, 1773t, 1774t
Urea cycle, disorders of, 1286, *1286,* 1287,
   1323, 1987t, 1991t
Urea nitrogen, blood level of, in glomerular
   function testing, 1601–1602, *1602,* 1602t
   in hyperparathyroidism, 1381t, 1385
   in hypoadrenocorticism, 1492, 1492t
   in hypoparathyroidism, 1393, 1394t
   in renal failure, 1641
   increased, angiotensin-converting enzyme in-
      hibitors and, 719
Uremia. See also *Renal failure.*
   and encephalopathy, 550
   and neurologic dysfunction, 586
   and oral ulceration, 42, 1601, *1601,* 1629
   and pancreatitis, 1350
   definition of, 1600
   dietary management of, 271t, 272, 272t, 274
   in renal failure, acute, 1625, 1629–1630,
      1630t
      chronic, 1635, 1636t
Ureterocele, 1752, 1982t, 1996t
Ureters, ectopic, 1982t, 1996t
   and incontinence, 92, 1743
Urethra, anomalies of, 1982t, 1996t
   bacterial infection in, 1593–1594
   discharge from, in prostatic disease, 1688
   fistula to, from rectum, 1743, 1751
   in hypospadias, 1584, *1584,* 1585, 1981t,
      1993t
   inflammation of, 1778, 1779t, 1780
   obstruction of, and urine retention, 93t, 93–96,
      94
   plugs in, in cats, complications of, 1737–
      1739, 1739t
      composition of, 1719, 1719t
      diagnosis of, 1733, 1733t
      epidemiology of, 1719
      pathogenesis of, *1732,* 1732–1733, *1733,*
         1733t
      pathophysiology of, *1720,* 1721
      prevention of, 1739
      treatment of, 1733–1737, *1735,* 1735t–
         1737t
   prolapse of, 1751–1752
   sphincter of, incompetence of, and inconti-
      nence, 1742, 1743
      diethylstilbestrol for, and vaginal bleed-
         ing, vs. prolonged estrus, 1523
   stricture of, 1752
   trauma to, 1752
   tumors of, 542
Urethrocystography, in prostatic disease, 1689,
   1689
   of vesicourachal diverticula, 1718, *1718*
Uric acid, in urine, 1705–1706
   in urolithiasis, in cats, 1723t, 1724–1725,
      1725t
   in dogs, 1758t, 1770–1775, 1773t, 1774t
Urinalysis, 1605–1610, 1606t, *1606–1611,* 1607t
   in hyperadrenocorticism, 1465, 1465t
   in hyperparathyroidism, 1385
   in incontinence, 92
   in liver disease, 1290–1291
   in pyometra, with cystic endometrial hyperpla-
      sia, 1550–1551
   in renal failure, 1621
   in urinary tract disease, 1748–1749
   in urinary tract infection, 1680–1681
Urinary bladder. See *Bladder.*
Urinary incontinence, after sterilization, 1540,
   1543
   diagnosis of, 90–92, *91*

Urinary incontinence *(Continued)*
   in cats, 1741–1743
   incidence of, 1748
   pathophysiology of, 89–90
   treatment of, 92
      over-the-counter drugs in, 320
Urinary tract, 1599–1780. See also specific
   structures, e.g., *Kidney(s).*
   disorders of, and tenesmus, 132, 133, 133t
      congenital, in cats, 1982t
         in dogs, 1996t
      glucocorticoids and, 316
      in cats, 1710–1746
         and incontinence, 1741–1743
         classification of, 1713, 1714t
         client information on, 1967
         etiopathology of, 1710–1713, *1711–1713*
         idiopathic, 1743–1746
         incidence of, 1713–1714
         morbidity rates in, 1714–1716, *1715,*
            1715t, *1716*
         pathophysiology of, 1716, 1717t
      in dogs, 1747–1780
         epidemiology of, 1748, *1748*
         localizing signs of, 1748, 1748t
      with spinal cord disorders, 610–611
   diverticula in, vesicourachal, 1712, *1718,*
      1718–1719, 1752
   infection of, 1678–1686, 1710–1711, 1740–
      1741
      antibiotics for, 305–306
      client information on, 1964
      diagnosis of, 1679–1682, *1684*
      discospondylitis with, 624
      in cats, 1717t, 1740–1741
      pathogenesis of, 1679
      treatment of, 1682–1686, *1684,* 1685t, 1780
      with bladder catheterization, for urethral ob-
         struction, 1737, 1737t
      with lithiasis, 1755, 1761–1763
   lithiasis of, client information on, 1966
      diet in, 271t, 272t, 274
      hyperadrenocorticism and, 1482–1483
      in cats, 1719–1732
         calcium oxalate, 1723t, 1725t, 1725–
            1728, 1732
         calcium phosphate, 1723t, 1728–1729,
            1729t
         cystine, 1723t, 1729–1730
         diagnosis of, 1721–1724, *1722,* 1722t,
            1723t, *1724*
         epidemiology of, 1719t, 1719–1720
         morbidity rate in, 1714–1716, *1715,*
            1715t
         pathogenesis of, 1711–1712, *1712, 1713*
         pathophysiology of, *1720,* 1720–1721,
            1721t
         struvite, 1711–1712, *1712, 1713,* 1723t,
            1730t, 1730–1732, 1731t
         treatment of, monitoring of, 1732
         urate, 1723t, 1724–1725, 1725t
      in cystinuria, 1705
      in dogs, 1753–1778
         calcium oxalate, 1758t, 1763–1764
            etiology of, *1764,* 1764–1766, *1766*
            management of, 1766, *1767*
            prevention of, 1766t, 1766–1770, *1767,
               1768,* 1769t, 1770t, *1771*
         calcium phosphate, 1758t, 1777
         composition of, 1753–1754, 1754t, 1757,
            1758t
         compound, 1777–1778
         cystine, 1758t, 1775t, 1775–1777, 1776t

Urinary tract *(Continued)*
  diagnosis of, 1748–1750, 1751t, 1755–1757, 1756t, 1758t
  incidence of, 1748, 1753
  management of, 1757–1759, *1759–1761,* 1778
  pathophysiology of, 1754–1755
  rare materials in, 1778
  silica, 1758t, 1777
  struvite, 1758t, 1760–1763, 1761t, 1762t
    with calcium oxalate lithiasis, 1765–1766, *1766,* 1770, *1771*
  urate, 1758t, 1770–1775, 1773t, 1774t
  in hyperparathyroidism, 1380
  in uricaciduria, 1705–1706
  in xanthinuria, 1706
  with portosystemic shunt, congenital, 1311–1312, *1312*
  obstruction of, in hyperkalemia, 228, *229*
  toxicity to, chemotherapy and, 487, 487t
  trauma to, 1752–1753, 1778, 1779t
  tumors of, 541–542, 1717t, 1739–1740
Urination, excessive. See *Polyuria.*
  in inappropriate location, 1716–1718, 1717t
Urine, blood in. See *Hematuria.*
  discoloration of, 96–99, 97t, *98,* 99t
  laboratory tests of. See *Urinalysis.*
  protein in, *98,* 100–102, *101.* See also *Proteinuria.*
  retention of, urethral obstruction and, 93t, 93–96, *94*
  specific gravity of, 1603–1605, 1604t
  spraying of, 160, 160t, 1596–1597, 1597t
Urobilinogen, in bilirubin metabolism, in liver disease, 1287, *1287,* 1288
Urogenital sinus, abnormal development of, 1569
Urohydropropulsion, in urolith removal, 1759, *1760, 1761*
Ursodeoxycholic acid, for cholangiohepatitis, 1310
  for liver disease, 1304
Urticaceae, toxicity of, 365
Urticaria, 37, 39
  in transfusion reactions, 355
Uterus, anatomy of, in cats, 1586
  artificial insemination of, 1577
  disorders of, and vaginal discharge, 81t–84t, 83
    postparturient, 1536–1538, *1537*
  endometrium of. See *Endometrium.*
  in dystocia, 1530–1534, 1532t, *1533,* 1596
  obstruction of, and infertility, canine, 1559
  pus in. See *Pyometra.*
  removal of. See *Ovariohysterectomy.*
  tumors of, 545
Uvea, cysts of, anterior, 1987t
Uveitis, 68, 69
  and anisocoria, 659t
  blastomycosis and, 459, 462
  systemic disease and, 985, 985t
Uveo-dermatologic syndrome, 55, 57

Vaccination, against atopic dermatitis, 1973
  against calicivirus infection, 448, 449
  against distemper, 1959
  against feline herpesvirus infection, 447–448
  against feline infectious peritonitis, 442
  against feline leukemia virus, 428, *429,* 1957
  against parvovirus infection, 1958
  against rabies, 450, 595
  and sarcoma, 1927
  anemia after, 199

Vaccination *(Continued)*
  client information on, 1927, 1957–1959, 1973
  in contraception, 1544
  protocol for, canine, 419t
Vacuolation, cytoplasmic, 1845, *1845*
Vagina, anatomy of, 1566, *1566*
  abnormalities of, 1567–1569, *1569*
    in cats, 1586
  artificial insemination of, 1576
  atresia of, 1981t
  bacterial flora of, 1518–1519, 1559, 1560t, 1567
  discharge from, 80–83, 81t–84t
  examination of, 1566–1567
    in infertility, 1556–1558, *1557*
  in dystocia, 1530–1536, *1531,* 1532t, *1533*
  in estrous cycle, 1510–1513, *1511–1515,* 1520, 1590. See also *Estrous cycle.*
  inflammation of, 1567, *1568, 1569*
  laceration of, 1570
  prolapse of, 1570
    congenital, 1994t
  septate bands in, 1522, *1522*
  tumors of, 545, 1570, *1570*
Vaginal fold, prolapse of, *1569,* 1569–1570
Vagus nerve, anatomy of, 664t
  examination of, 563, 566, 567t
  in electrocardiography, inhibition of, 806, *807*
  stimulation of, 806, *807*
Valine, in diet, 239t
Valium. See *Diazepam.*
Valley fever. See *Coccidioidomycosis.*
Valvular heart disease, 787–799. See also specific valves, e.g., *Mitral valve.*
Valvuloplasty, balloon, for pulmonic stenosis, 766, 767, *767*
  for subaortic stenosis, 772
van den Bergh bilirubin fractionation, 1288
Vanadium, for diabetes, 1451
Vancomycin, concentration of, and bacterial susceptibility, 303t
Varicose veins, 974
Vascular ring anomalies, and esophageal compression, 1145
Vasculitis, arterial, 972–974
  in brain, infection and, 591
  of lungs, immune-mediated, 1065t, *1072,* 1072–1073, *1073*
  pinnal, 989t, 991
Vasculopathy, cutaneous, congenital, 1995t
Vasoactive amines, in food, adverse reactions to, 253
Vasoactive intestinal polypeptide, 1502
Vasodilators, endogenous, in heart failure, 701
  for cardiomyopathy, dilated, 884
  for heart failure, *717,* 717–718
  for pulmonary hypertension, 1081
Vasopressin. See *Antidiuretic hormone.*
Vasospasm, arterial, 974
Vasotec. See *Enalapril.*
Veins. See also specific vessels, e.g., *Portal vein.*
  arterial fistula to, 969–971, *970, 971*
  inflammation of, 974–975, *975*
  occlusion of, 975, *975, 976*
  pulses in, 177–179, *178*
  thrombosis of, *974,* 974–975, *975*
  trauma to, 974
  varicose, 974
Vena cava, cannulation of, for parenteral nutrition, 281, 282
  disorders of, and hepatic venous outflow obstruction, 1318, 1318t
  echocardiography of, 857t, 859
  left cranial, persistent, *785,* 786
  obstruction of, *974–976, 975*

Venereal tumors, transmissible, 545
Venography, of brain, 576
Ventilation, support of, in pulmonary disease, 1063
Ventilation-perfusion disorders, pulmonary thromboembolism and, 1078, 1079
Ventricle(s), left, contraction of, and pulse pressure, arterial, 175–177
    venous, 177
  echocardiography of, 856t, 857–858
    in diastolic function assessment, *843,* 845t, 845–847, *846,* 861–866, 865t
    in size estimation, 849t, 850t, 851–852, *853*
    in systolic function assessment, 859–861, 862t–864t
  function of, in heart failure, 709
  moderator band increase in, in cardiomyopathy, 913, *913*
  outflow from, echocardiography of, *842,* 843–845, 845t
    obstruction of, in hypertrophic cardiomyopathy, 898, *899*
    in subaortic stenosis, congenital, 768–772, *769–772*
  right, double-outlet, 783
  echocardiography of, 850t, 852, 857t, 859, *859*
  hypertrophy of, in tetralogy of Fallot, 780–782, *781*
  myopathy of, and arrhythmia, *912,* 912–913
  outflow from, obstruction of, in pulmonic stenosis, 759–767. See also *Pulmonic stenosis.*
Ventricular asystole, in cardiopulmonary arrest, 192
Ventricular extrasystoles, 813–814, *814*
Ventricular fibrillation, electrocardiography of, 815, *816*
  treatment of, 193
Ventricular flutter, 815
Ventricular gallop, 170
Ventricular parasystole, 816, *817*
Ventricular preexcitation syndrome, 821, *822,* 1976t, 1985t
Ventricular septal defect, 750–759, 1976t, 1985t
  auscultation of, 739t
  blood pressure in, echocardiographic measurement of, 847, 847t
  client information on, 1951
  clinical findings in, 756–758, *757–759*
  echocardiography of, 757–758, *758, 759, 844,* 854t
  in tetralogy of Fallot, 751, *754,* 780–782, *782*
  management of, 758–759, *760*
  natural history of, 758
  pathogenesis of, 751, *754*
  pathophysiology of, 751–755
  with pulmonary atresia, 782–783, *783*
Ventricular septum, echocardiography of, 856t, 858
Ventricular tachyarrhythmia, in digitalis toxicity, 730
Ventricular tachycardia, electrocardiography of, 814–815, *815*
  in cardiomyopathy, 905, 911, 913
Verapamil, for arrhythmia, 824t–826t, 829t, 830–831
  supraventricular, with hypotension, 184t
  for cardiomyopathy, hypertrophic, 890
Vermis, cerebellar, hypoplasia of, 1991t
Vertebrae, anomalies of, 621, *622,* 1975t, 1976t, 1983t, 1984t
  disorders of, and spinal cord dysfunction. See *Spinal cord.*

Vesicles, of pinna, 987t, 991
Vesicourachal diverticula, 1712, *1718, 1718–1719,* 1752
Vestibular system, anatomy of, 997
  disorders of, and ataxia, 142
    congenital, 1980t, 1992t
    idiopathic, 582, 681, 1000
    signs of, 557t, 559, *559*
  peripheral, idiopathic dysfunction of, 681
Vestibule, of vagina, anatomy of, 1566, *1566,* 1586
  examination of, 1566–1567
  in infertility, 1557
Vestibulitis, and weakness, 12
Vestibulocochlear nerve, anatomy of, 664t
  examination of, 563–565, *564,* 567t
Videofluorography, in dysphagia, 1027
Villi, atrophy of, 1197
  and pancreatic exocrine insufficiency, 1357, *1357*
  crypt cells of, 1183, *1184,* 1193
Vim-Silverman needle, Franklin-modified, in renal biopsy, 1613, *1613*
Vinblastine, in cancer management, 378t
Vinca alkaloids, and thrombocytosis, 1823
Vincristine, for lymphoma, 510–512, 511
  for mast cell tumors, of skin, 527
  for multiple myeloma, 519
  for thrombocytopenia, paraneoplastic, 505
  in cancer therapy, 378t, 485t, 487–489
  toxicity of, to peripheral nerves, 673t
Vinegar, in ear cleansing, for otitis externa, 989t, 994, 996
Viokase-V, for pancreatic exocrine insufficiency, 1361–1362, 1363t
Viral inclusions, in leukocytes, 1847, *1847*
Viral infection. See also specific diseases, e.g., *Rabies.*
  and anemia, 1810t, 1810–1811
  and arthritis, 1878
  and cachexia, 74
  and hepatitis, 419, 419t
  and myocarditis, cardiomyopathy after, 877
  and rhinitis, 1018
    with epistaxis, 215
  and skin ulcers, 40, 40t
  and thrombocytopenia, 1821
  and tracheobronchitis, 419t, 419–420
  in carcinogenesis, 480–481
  of lung, 1063
  of small intestine, 1215–1217
    fecal examination for, 1207
  of urinary tract, 1711, *1711,* 1740, 1743
Virchow's triad, 915
Viscerocutaneous reflexes, in acupuncture, 366
Vision, loss of, acute, 17t, 17–20, 18t, *19*
  hypertension and, 180, *181,* 182
Visken, for arrhythmia, 829t
Visual evoked potentials, 575
  in vision loss, acute, 19
Vitadee. See *Vitamin D.*
Vitamin A, absorption of, from small intestine, 1190
  deficiency of, and bone deformity, 1908–1909
  excess of, and bone disorders, 1907–1908, *1908*
    and exostoses, with spinal cord compression, 629–630
  for lymphoma, cutaneous, 528
  for sebaceous adenitis, 48
  for seborrhea, 48
  in diet, 239, 239t
    in orthopedic developmental disorders, 248
Vitamin B complex. See also *Folate.*
  in diet, 239t, 239–240

Vitamin B complex *(Continued)*
  in renal failure, 1647t
Vitamin B$_1$ (thiamine), absorption of, from small intestine, 1190
  deficiency of, neurologic dysfunction with, 549, 586, 593t
  for lead toxicity, 362
  in diet, 239, 239t
Vitamin B$_2$ (riboflavin), absorption of, from small intestine, 1190
  in diet, 239t
Vitamin B$_6$ (pyridoxine), absorption of, from small intestine, 1190
  for calcium oxalate urolithiasis, 1728
  in diet, 239t
  in renal failure, 1647t
  toxicity of, to peripheral nerves, 673t
Vitamin B$_{12}$ (cobalamin), absorption of, from small intestine, 1190, *1191*
  congenital defect of, 1850, 1986t
  deficiency of, and neutrophil hypersegmentation, 1846
    in anemia, 1809
    in inflammatory bowel disease, 1227
    in pancreatic exocrine insufficiency, 1358, 1363, 1363t
    in small intestinal disorders, 1208–1210, 1210t
      with bacterial overgrowth, 1224
    methylmalonic aciduria with, 1706
    treatment of, 5
  excess of, in small intestinal disorders, 1208–1210, 1210t
  in diet, 239t
Vitamin C (ascorbic acid), for acetaminophen toxicity, to liver, 1332
  for methemoglobinemia, in naphthalene toxicity, 357
  in diet, 240
  in orthopedic developmental disorders, 248
Vitamin D, absorption of, from small intestine, 1190
  blood level of, in hyperparathyroidism, 1386
  deficiency of, in renal osteodystrophy, 1907
    in rickets, 1907, *1907*
  excess of, and bone disorders, 1909
  for hyperparathyroidism, in renal failure, 1656–1657
  for hypoparathyroidism, 1397–1398, 1398t
  in diet, 239, 239t
    in orthopedic developmental disorders, 248
  in rodenticides, toxicity of, 360
  resistance to, with hypocalcemia, after surgery, for hyperparathyroidism, 1390
Vitamin E, absorption of, from small intestine, 1190
  deficiency of, and pansteatitis, 28–29
    in pancreatic exocrine insufficiency, 1358, 1362–1363, 1363t
  for hepatic copper accumulation, 1303t
  for liver disease, 1304
  in diet, 239t, 240
Vitamin K, absorption of, from small intestine, 1190
  deficiency of, and coagulation disorders, 1836–1837, 1839
    in liver disease, 1278t, 1285, 1335
    in pancreatic exocrine insufficiency, 1358, 1363t
  for anticoagulant rodenticide toxicity, 360
  in diet, 239, 239t
Vitiligo, 55–57, 1995t
Vitreous, hyperplastic, primary, 1988t
Vitreous humor, disorders of, and vision loss, 17, 17t

Volvulus, and megaesophagus, 1150t
  with gastric dilatation, 1170–1174, *1171, 1172*
  client information on, 1943
Vomiting, and hypokalemia, 225
  diagnosis of, *119,* 119–121, *120*
  drugs for, over-the-counter, 319
  drugs inducing, over-the-counter, 319
  hydralazine and, in heart failure, 724
  in adverse food reactions, 254
  in gastric outlet obstruction, 1169, 1170
  in gastritis, 1160
  in renal failure, acute, 1629
    chronic, 1636, 1636t, 1648
  liver disease and, 1273t, 1274–1275
  parvovirus infection and, 445
  pathophysiology of, 117–119, *118,* 118t
  vs. regurgitation, 115
    in esophageal disease, 1143
  with diarrhea, 122t
von Gierke's disease, 1322–1323
von Willebrand factor antigen, decreased, with hypothyroidism, 1422
von Willebrand's disease, 1824t, 1824–1825, 1825t, 1979t, 1989t
  and purpura, 219, 219t
  client information on, 1962
  genetics in, 3t, 5
  testing for, in blood donors, 348
Vulva, anatomy of, 1586
  abnormalities of, 1569
  atresia of, 1981t
  edema of, 80, 81t
  examination of, in infertility, 1556
  hemorrhage from, 1570
  in estrous cycle, 1510, *1511*
  tumors of, 545, 1570

Waldenström's macroglobulinemia, 516, 517
Wallerian degeneration, of peripheral nerves, 665
Wandering pacemaker, electrocardiography of, 810, *811*
Warfarin (coumarin), action of, 1830, 1833t
  for glomerulonephritis, 1672t, 1674
  for lung disorders, 1065t
  for thromboembolism, 917
    arterial, 968
    pulmonary, 1065t, 1080
      with hyperadrenocorticism, 1483
  for thrombosis, venous, 1840
  in rodenticides, toxicity of, 359–360
Wasp stings, hepatic reaction to, 1329
Wasting, chronic, 11
Water. See *Fluid.*
Waxy casts, in urine, 1609, *1609*
Weakness, 10–13, 11t
  in brain disorders, 560–561
  in diabetes, 1442, *1442*
  in hyperthyroidism, 1401
Wegener's granulomatosis, of lungs, 1072
Weight, and adverse drug reactions, 322
  assessment of, in orthopedic developmental disorders, 249, 249t
  excessive, 70–72, *71*
    after gonadectomy, prepubertal, 70, 1540
    and pulmonary disorders, 1088
    in heart disease, 71, 266
  gain of, glucocorticoids and, 316
    in heart disease, 266
    in kittens, 242, 243
    in puppies, 241, 243
    with polyphagia, 105–107, *106*
  loss of, dysphagia and, 114
    in cachexia, 72–74, *73*

Weight *(Continued)*
in heart disease, 265–266
paraneoplastic, 499–501
regurgitation and, 115
small intestinal disorders and, 1201, *1201*
with diarrhea, 122, 122t
with heart failure, 706
with polyphagia, 105, *106,* 107
Weimaraner, neutrophil defect in, 1850, 1990t
Welsh corgi, renal telangiectasia in, 1698, 1699t, 1703
Wenckebach atrioventricular block, electrocardiography of, 817, *818*
West Highland white terrier, epidermal dysplasia in, 48, 1995t
hepatic copper accumulation in, 1305, 1991t
Wheat, gluten in, sensitivity to, and enteropathy, 254, 1232–1233, 1986t
Wheaten terrier, glomerular disease in, 1699t, 1702
Wheelbarrowing, in neurologic examination, 561–562, *562*
Wheezing, 195, 1035, 1035t
Whelping. See *Parturition.*
Whipworm infestation, blood loss in, and anemia, 1787
of large intestine, 1245, *1245*
White blood cells. See *Leukocytes.*
White dog shaker syndrome, 598–599
Willebrand's disease. See *von Willebrand's disease.*
Wobbler syndrome, 1983t
cervical spondylomyelopathy and, 619–621
Wolffian duct, 1581
aplasia of, 1980t, 1993t
Woodchucks, rabies in, 388
Wry mouth, 1125, *1126*

Xanax, for behavioral disorders, 156, 158t
Xanthine oxidase inhibitors, for urate urolithiasis, 1773, 1775
Xanthinuria, 1706
Xanthochromia, of cerebrospinal fluid, 573
Xanthoma, 37
Xenodyne, for otitis externa, 989t, 994, 995
Xeroderma pigmentosum, genetic mutation in, 479
X-linked recessive inheritance, 3, 3t
in muscular dystrophy, 3t, 688, 1980t
XO syndrome, 1582, 1993t
XX hermaphroditism, 1583
XX male syndrome, 1583–1585
XX pseudohermaphroditism, 1994t
XX sex reversal, 1583, 1994t
XXX syndrome, 1582, 1981t, 1993t
XX/XXY chimeras, 1583, *1583*
XX/XY chimeras, 1583, *1583,* 1981t, 1993t
XXY syndrome, 1582, *1582, 1583,* 1981t
XY pseudohermaphroditism, 1994t
Xylocaine. See *Lidocaine.*
ᴅ-Xylose, absorption of, from small intestine, 1188, 1210
XY/XY chimeras, 1583

Yellow oleander, toxicity of, 365
Yersinia enterocolitica infection, and colitis, 1244–1245
Yersinia infection, and enteritis, 1218
Yersinia pestis infection, zoonotic, 384t
Yew, toxicity of, 365
Yorkshire terrier, encephalitis in, 598

Zantac. See *Ranitidine.*
Zidovudine (AZT), for feline immunodeficiency virus infection, 437, 437t
PIND-ORF derivative of, for feline leukemia virus infection, 431
Zinc, chondrodysplasia responsive to, 1909
deficiency of, and scaling dermatosis, 48–49
for hepatic copper accumulation, 261, 1302–1303, 1303t
in diet, 239t
in orthopedic developmental disorders, 247
toxicity of, 362
and hemolytic anemia, 1802
Zinc oxide, for skin disorders, 319
Zinc phosphide, in rodenticides, toxicity of, 360–361
Zinc sulfate, in diagnosis of intestinal parasitosis, 123
Zolazepam, in anesthesia, for prepubertal gonadectomy, 1541
Zoonotic infection, 382–389, 383t–386t
and cat scratch disease, 382–386, 399
and coccidioidomycosis, 468
and larva migrans, 386–387
and pruritus, 32
and rabies, 387–388
and sporotrichosis, 385t, 472
and toxoplasmosis, 388–389
protozoal, 410–411
Zygomatic salivary gland, mucocele of, 1119, 1120
Zygomycosis, 475
of small intestine, 1220
Zymogens, in defense against pancreatic autodigestion, *1346,* 1346–1347, *1347*
in pancreatitis, 1348, *1348,* 1349, 1349t

ISBN 0-7216-7258-2

ABNORMAL LABORATORY FINDINGS (continued from front endsheet)

Potassium (*Continued*)
Acidosis
  Diabetic ketoacidosis
Diffuse tissue damage
  Massive muscle trauma
  Post-ischemic reperfusion
Dehydration
Hypoaldosterone
Drugs
  Propranolol
  Potassium-sparing diuretics
  ACE inhibitors

Decreased
Alkalosis
Dietary deficiency (feline)
Potassium-free fluids
Bicarbonate administration
Drugs
  Penicillins
  Amphotericin B
  Loop diuretics
GI fluid loss (K$^+$-rich)
Hyperadrenocorticism
Hyperaldosterone
Insulin therapy
Renal
  Postobstructive diuresis
  Renal tubular acidosis
  Dialysis

Hypokalemic periodic
  paralysis
  Burmese
  Pit Bull
Renal failure
  Chronic polyuric

Protein, total
  Increased
Dehydration (albumin and
  globulin)
Hyperglobulinemia
Spurious
  Hemolysis
  Lipemia

  Decreased
Hemorrhage
  External plasma loss
  GI loss
Overhydration
Liver failure
Glomerular loss

Sodium
  Increased
Hyperaldosterone
GI fluid loss (Na$^+$-poor)
  Vomiting
  Diarrhea
Diabetes insipidus
Renal failure
Dehydration

Insensible fluid loss
  Fever
  Panting
  High ambient
    temperature
Decreased water intake
  Limited water access
  Primary adipsia
Increased salt intake
  Intravenous
  Oral
Spurious
  Serum evaporation

  Decreased
Hypoadrenocorticism
Diabetes mellitus
GI fluid loss (Na$^+$-rich)
  Vomiting
  Diarrhea
  Hookworms
  Burns
Chronic effusions
Excess ADH
Diuretics
Hypotonic fluids
Diet (severe sodium
  restriction)
Psychogenic polydipsia
Renal failure (polyuric)

Spurious
  Hyperlipidemia

Thyroxine (T$_4$)
  Increased
Hyperthyroidism
Anti-T$_4$ autoantibodies

  Decreased
Hypothyroidism
Nonthyroid illness
Drugs
  Corticosteroids
  Phenobarbital

Triiodothyronine (T$_3$)
  Increased
Hyperthyroidism
Anti-T$_3$ autoantibodies

  Decreased
Hypothyroidism

**Trypsinogen-like
immunoreactivity (TLI)**
  Increased
Pancreatitis
Postprandial

  Decreased
Pancreatic exocrine insufficiency

CONDITIONS ASSOCIATED WITH HEMATOLOGIC CHANGE

White blood cells (WBC)
  Increased
Infection
  Bacterial
  Systemic mycosis
Inflammation
  Immune-mediated disease
  Tissue trauma
  Neoplasia
  Tissue necrosis
Physiologic leukocytosis
Metabolic
  Stress
  Glucocorticoids
Associated with responsive anemia
  Hemolytic anemia
  Hemorrhagic anemia
Leukemia

  Decreased
Decreased production
Increased consumption

Red blood cells (RBC)
  Increased
Dehydration
Polycythemia
Splenic contraction

  Decreased
RESPONSIVE ANEMIAS
Blood loss: acute or chronic
  Hemorrhage (internal or external)
    Trauma
    Gastrointestinal hemorrhage
      Ulcers
      Neoplasia
    Coagulopathies
      Congenital
      Acquired
    Ectoparasites
      Fleas
      Ticks
    Endoparasites

Hookworms
Coccidia
Hematuria
Hemolytic anemias
  Microangiopathic
    Dirofilariasis
    Vascular neoplasia
    Vasculitis
    Disseminated intravascular
      coagulation
  Parasitic
    Babesia
    Hemobartonella felis
  Infectious
    Leptospirosis
    E. coli
  Oxidant injury
    Onions
    Kale
    Phenothiazines
    Methylene blue
NON-RESPONSIVE ANEMIAS
Renal failure
Chronic disease
  Infectious disease
  Inflammatory disease
  Neoplasia
Endocrine disease
  Hypothyroidism
  Hypoadrenocorticism
  Hyperestrogenism
    Diethylstilbestrol (high multiple
      doses)
    Estradiol cyclopentylpropionate
    Sertoli cell tumor
Idiopathic aplastic anemia
Red cell aplasia
Myeloproliferative disease
Myelophthisis
Hypersplenism
Drugs
  Chloramphenicol
  Chemotherapeutics
Iron deficiency

Nutritional
  Chronic blood loss
Lead poisoning
Infectious
  Retrovirus
    Feline immunodeficiency
      virus
    Feline leukemia virus
  Ehrlichia

Hemoglobin (Hb)
  Increased
Dehydration
Polycythemia
Splenic contraction

  Decreased
Hemorrhage
  Acute
  Chronic
Decreased production

Hematocrit
  Increased
Dehydration
Polycythemia
Splenic contraction

  Decreased
Hemorrhage
  Acute
  Chronic
Decreased production

Neutrophils
  Increased
Increased production
  Infection
    Bacterial
    Systemic mycosis
      Coccidioidomycosis
      Histoplasmosis
      Blastomycosis
      Aspergillosis

Protozoal
  Hepatozoon
  Toxoplasmosis
  Neosporidiosis
Inflammation
  Immune-mediated diseases
  Tissue trauma
  Neoplasia
  Tissue necrosis
Associated with responsive anemia
  Hemolytic anemia
  Hemorrhagic anemia
Demargination
  Stress
  Glucocorticoids
Chronic granulocytic leukemia

  Decreased
Decreased production
  Myelophthisis
    Myeloproliferative disease
    Lymphoproliferative disease
    Metastatic neoplasia
  Myelofibrosis
  Drug induced
    Chloramphenicol
    Trimethoprim-sulfa
    Cyclophosphamide
    Azathioprin
    Griseofulvin
  Idiopathic hypoplasia/aplasia
    Cyclic neutropenia
    Immune-mediated (steroid-
      responsive)
  Hypersplenism
  Infectious
    Ehrlichia
    Parvovirus
    Retroviruses
      Feline immunodeficiency virus
      Feline leukemia virus
        Aplastic anemia
        Myelodysplasia
        Panleukopenia-like syndrome